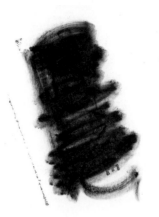

Microbiology

Microbiology

Fourth Edition

Bernard D. Davis, MD

Adele Lehman Professor of Bacterial Physiology, Harvard Medical School, Boston, Massachusetts

Renato Dulbecco, MD

Distinguished Research Professor, The Salk Institute, San Diego; Senior Clayton Foundation Investigator Professor Emeritus, Departments of Pathology and Medicine, University of California, San Diego, School of Medicine, La Jolla, California

Herman N. Eisen, MD

Whitehead Institute Professor of Immunology, Department of Biology and Center for Cancer Research, Massachusetts Institute of Technology, Cambridge, Massachusetts

Harold S. Ginsberg, MD

Higgins Professor of Microbiology and Medicine, Columbia University College of Physicians and Surgeons, New York, New York

With 29 Additional Contributors

J. B. LIPPINCOTT COMPANY

Philadelphia

Grand Rapids *London*
New York *Sydney*
St. Louis *Tokyo*
San Francisco

Acquisitions Editor: Lisa McAllister
Developmental Editor: Richard Winters
Project Editor: Marian A. Bellus
Manuscript Editor: Judith Bronson
Indexer: Barbara Littlewood
Design Coordinator: Caren Erlichman
Book Designer: Arlene Putterman
Cover Designer: Anita Curry
Production Manager: Carol Florence
Production Coordinator: Pamela Milcos
Compositor: Bi-Comp, Inc.
Printer/Binder: The Murray Printing Company

Fourth Edition

6   5   4   3

Library of Congress Cataloging in Publication Data
Microbiology / Bernard D. Davis . . . [et al.]. — 4th ed.
        p.   cm.
    Rev. ed. of: Microbiology, including immunology and molecular genetics. 3rd ed. c1980.
    Includes bibliographies and index.
    ISBN 0-397-50689-9
    1. Medical microbiology.   2. Immunology.   3. Molecular genetics.
I. Davis, Bernard D., 1916–   . II. Microbiology, including immunology and molecular genetics.
    [DNLM: 1. Microbiology.   QW 4 M626]
QR46.M5393 1990
616′.01—dc19
DNLM/DLC
for Library of Congress   89-2338
                                                                     CIP

The authors and publisher have exerted every effort to ensure that drug selection and dosage set forth in this text are in accord with current recommendations and practice at the time of publication. However, in view of ongoing research, changes in government regulations, and the constant flow of information relating to drug therapy and drug reactions, the reader is urged to check the package insert for each drug for any change in indications and dosage and for added warnings and precautions. This is particularly important when the recommended agent is a new or infrequently employed drug.

Dedication

To our wives,
who have remained remarkably patient through four editions.

List of Contributors

Porter W. Anderson, Jr., PhD
Chapter 31
Professor of Pediatrics and Microbiology
University of Rochester
Rochester, New York

John P. Atkinson, MD
Chapter 17
Professor of Medicine
Professor of Microbiology and Immunology
Washington University School of Medicine
Investigator
Howard Hughes Medical Institute
St. Louis, Missouri

Robert Austrian, MD
Chapter 23
John Herr Musser Professor and Chairman (Emeritus)
Department of Research Medicine
University of Pennsylvania School of Medicine
Philadelphia, Pennsylvania

Joel B. Baseman, PhD
Chapter 37
Professor and Chairman
Department of Microbiology
Graduate School of Biomedical Sciences
University of Texas Health Science Center at San Antonio
San Antonio, Texas

Robert M. Chanock, MD
Chapter 40
Chief, Laboratory of Infectious Diseases
National Institute of Allergy and Infectious Diseases
Bethesda, Maryland

Wallace A. Clyde, Jr, MD
Chapter 40
Professor of Pediatrics and Microbiology
University of North Carolina School of Medicine
Attending Physician
North Carolina Memorial Hospital
Chapel Hill, North Carolina

R. John Collier, PhD
Chapter 22
Professor of Microbiology and Molecular Genetics
Harvard Medical School
Boston, Massachusetts

Bernard D. Davis, MD
Chapters 1–10
Adele Lehman Professor of Bacterial Physiology
Harvard Medical School
Boston, Massachusetts

Renato Dulbecco, MD
Chapters 44–50, 64, 65
Distinguished Research Professor
The Salk Institute
San Diego
Senior Clayton Foundation Investigator and Professor Emeritus
Departments of Pathology and Medicine
University of California, San Diego, School of Medicine
La Jolla, California

Herman N. Eisen, MD
Chapters 12–20
Whitehead Institute Professor of Immunology, Department of Biology and Center for Cancer Research, Massachusetts Institute of Technology, Cambridge, Massachusetts

Stanley Falkow, PhD
Chapters 27, 28
Professor of Microbiology and Medicine
Department of Microbiology and Immunology
Stanford University Medical School
Palo Alto, California

Malcolm L. Gefter, PhD
Chapter 16
Chairman
ImmunLogic Pharmaceutical Corporation
Cambridge, Massachusetts

Ronald J. Gibbons, PhD
Chapter 42
Forsyth Dental Center
Harvard School of Dental Medicine
Boston, Massachusetts

Harold S. Ginsberg, MD
Chapters 51–63
Eugene Higgins Professor of Medicine and Microbiology
Columbia University College of Physicians & Surgeons
New York, New York

Emil C. Gotschlich, MD
Chapter 26
Professor and Senior Physician
Rockefeller University
New York, New York

George S. Kobayashi, PhD
Chapters 36, 43
Professor
Washington University School of Medicine
Associate Director, Clinical Microbiology Laboratory
Barnes Hospital
St. Louis, Missouri

Stephen Lory, PhD
Chapter 29
Assistant Professor
Department of Microbiology
University of Washington
Seattle, Washington

Maclyn McCarty, MD
Chapter 24
Professor Emeritus
Rockefeller University
Physician-in-Chief Emeritus
Rockefeller University Hospital
New York, New York

John J. Mekalanos, PhD
Chapter 27
Professor
Department of Microbiology and Molecular Genetics
Harvard Medical School
Boston, Massachusetts

Stephen I. Morse, MD, PhD (Deceased)
Chapter 31
Assistant Professor
Rockefeller University
New York, New York

Richard P. Novick, MD
Chapter 25
Director
Public Health Research Institute
Research Professor
Department of Microbiology
New York University School of Medicine
New York, New York

Margaret Pittman, PhD, Hon FAAP, LLD
Chapter 32
Guest Worker
Center for Biophysics Evaluation and Resource Division
Food and Drug Administration
Bethesda, MD

David H. Raulet, PhD
Chapter 15
Associate Professor of Biology
Department of Biology and Center for Cancer Research
Massachusetts Institute of Technology
Cambridge, Massachusetts

John B. Robbins, MD
Chapter 32
Chief
Laboratory of Developmental and Molecular Immunity
National Institute of Child Health and Human Development
National Institutes of Health
Bethesda, Maryland

Julius Schachter, PhD
Chapter 39
Professor of Epidemiology
Department of Laboratory Medicine
University of California, San Francisco
San Francisco, California

Samuel C. Silverstein, MD
Chapter 21
John C. Dalton Professor of Physiology
Chairman
Department of Physiology and Cellular Biophysics
Columbia University College of Physicians & Surgeons
New York, New York

Sigmund Socransky, DDS
Chapter 42
Forsyth Dental Center
Harvard School of Dental Medicine
Boston, Massachusetts

Thomas H. Steinberg, MD
Chapter 21
Assistant Professor of Medicine and of Cell Biology and
Physiology
Washington University School of Medicine
Assistant Attending Physician
Barnes Hospital
Jewish Hospital
St. Louis, Missouri

Morton N. Swartz, MD
Chapters 30, 33, 34, 41, 42
Professor of Medicine
Harvard Medical School
Chief, Infectious Disease Unit
Massachusetts General Hospital
Boston, Massachusetts

Joseph G. Tully, PhD
Chapter 40
Chief, Mycoplasma Section
Laboratory of Molecular Microbiology
National Institute of Allergy and Infectious Diseases
Frederick Cancer Research Facility
Frederick, Maryland

Fred Winston, PhD
Chapter 11
Associate Professor of Genetics
Department of Genetics
Harvard Medical School
Boston, Massachusetts

Charles L. Wisseman, Jr, MD
Chapter 38
Professor Emeritus
Department of Microbiology and Immunology
University of Maryland at Baltimore School of Medicine
Baltimore, Maryland

Emanuel Wolinsky, MD
Chapter 35
Professor Emeritus of Medicine and Pathology
Case Western Reserve University School of Medicine
Head of Microbiology
Member of Infectious Diseases Division
Cleveland Metropolitan General Hospital
Cleveland, Ohio

Preface

When the first edition of this text appeared, bacterial genetics and molecular genetics were rapidly growing fields, and *Escherichia coli* had become the favored model organism for exploring universal properties of cells. The late William Barry Wood, Jr., who initiated the book and was responsible for the section on pathogenic bacteria, frequently discussed the hope that genetic and molecular approaches would soon become equally pertinent to studies closer to disease. By the third edition this process was well advanced in virology, and it was increasingly influencing studies of bacterial pathogenesis and of the immune responses. In the present edition our earlier hope has been realized: current advances in all aspects of the field rely heavily on molecular and genetic studies.

To make room for the new material we no longer attempt to review all the relevant principles and procedures that have emerged in the now immense discipline of molecular genetics, and we have condensed the coverage of intermediary metabolism. Accordingly, the section on bacterial physiology and genetics has been extensively reorganized, and nearly every paragraph has been rewritten. Our understanding of gene regulation continues to grow in depth and in importance; our emphasis is on its physiological aspects, and not on the wealth of information now available on DNA and protein sequences and on molecular interactions at the atomic level. We have added a short chapter on yeasts, because these eukaryotic microbes are proving increasingly useful as models for many features of animal cells.

The sections on immunology, bacterial pathogens, and virology continue to integrate biological and medical aspects; the book is designed for medical students with a strong interest in science, as well as for graduate students and investigators. The section on immunology has been largely rewritten, and the former chapter on transplantation immunity has been broadened to include major sections on autoimmune and immunodeficiency diseases, particularly AIDS. The section on virology has been extensively revised to reflect the increased knowledge of the viral genomes and their encoded gene functions as well as new insights into the mechanisms of pathogenesis of each viral disease. The DNA and the RNA oncogenic viruses now each require a chapter, and coverage of the retroviruses has been greatly increased, including a major section on the virus of AIDS.

Despite pressure for space, it still seems important to present science as a growing enterprise and not simply a body of knowledge. We therefore have tried, so far as possible, to continue to present the material in a historical perspective, and to indicate briefly the nature of the evidence underlying each major conclusion.

The sections on Immunology and on Virology are published separately as paperback books: General Immunology by Eisen, and Virology by Dulbecco and Ginsberg.

B. D. Davis
R. Dulbecco
H. N. Eisen
H. S. Ginsberg

Preface to the First Edition

"What is new and significant must always be connected with old roots, the truly vital roots that are chosen with great care from the ones that merely survive."

This principle, professed by the composer Bela Bartok, is as applicable to science as it is to music. Indeed, it highlights the most difficult aspect of writing a modern textbook of microbiology, for few branches of natural science have been so rapidly altered by recent advances. Only a few years ago microbiology was largely an applied field, concerned with controlling those microbes that affect man's health or his economic welfare, but with the recent development of molecular genetics, stemming largely from the study of microbial mutants, microbiology has rapidly been drawn to the center of the biological stage.

As a result, infectious disease no longer constitutes the sole bridge between microbiology and medicine. An additional, rapidly broadening span is provided by the use of microbes as model cells in the study of molecular genetics and cell physiology, for the principles and the successful approaches developed in such studies will surely prove widely applicable to human cells, which can now be cultured much like bacteria. In addition, studies at a molecular level are also rapidly providing a deeper insight into problems directly related to infectious disease, including the action of chemotherapeutic drugs, the structure of antibodies and cellular antigens, and the nature of viruses. Hence to prepare the student for the scientific medicine of his future it has seemed to us desirable to increase emphasis on the molecular and genetic aspects of microbiology. At the same time, the authors, having all had clinical experience, are vividly aware of the importance of providing a thorough understanding of host-parasite relationships and mechanisms of pathogenicity, even though many aspects cannot yet be explained in molecular terms.

In short, we have tried to identify the "truly vital roots" of classical bacteriology, immunology, and virology, and to engraft upon them the recent molecular advances. To keep the volume to a reasonable size we have eliminated much traditional information that did not seem to have either theoretical or practical importance for the student of medicine. Moreover, the clinical and epidemiological aspects of infectious diseases have been largely left for later courses in the medical curriculum, and we have provided only a small number of selected references, primarily for access to the original literature and not for documentation. In the hope of making the book more useful and versatile, we have included in smaller type a good deal of material that seemed not essential for an introduction to the subject, but still likely to interest many readers.

The demands of the medical curriculum frequently lead to a condensed memorizing of conclusions; yet courses in the basic medical sciences should surely illustrate the scientific method as well as transmit a body of information. We have therefore briefly reviewed the history of many major discoveries in order to show how scientific advances may depend on new concepts or technics, or on ingenious experiments, or an alertness to the significance of unexpected observations. Moreover, we have endeavored throughout to indicate the nature of the evidence underlying the conclusions presented—for otherwise the student sees only the shadow and not the substance of science.

This book is designed primarily as a text for students and investigators of medicine and the allied professions: hence the exposition proceeds from general principles to specific pathogenic microorganisms. However, we hope that the discussion of general principles will also prove useful to graduate students and investigators in the biological sciences.

The preparation of this volume has been a truly cooperative effort: the chapters drafted by each author have been critically reviewed by most or all of the others. We are deeply grateful for the education and for the warm friendships that have resulted.

A new book of this size will inevitably contain errors and weaknesses. We shall welcome corrections and suggestions for future editions.

B. D. Davis
R. Dulbecco
H. N. Eisen
H. S. Ginsberg
W. B. Wood, Jr.

Acknowledgments

We are grateful to the contributors who revised various chapters. It is also a pleasure to acknowledge the skillful help and the patience of the publisher's staff and our several secretaries.

We are especially indebted to the following colleagues for their generosity in reviewing various chapters:

BARRY R. BLOOM, PHD
JULIAN B. FLEISCHMAN, PHD
DAN G. FRAENKEL, PHD
EDWARD J. GOETZL, MD
DONALD GOLDMAN, MD
FRED KARUSH, PHD
ROBERTO KOLTER, PHD
LISA A. STEINER, MD
PHANG C. TAI, PHD
THEODORE TSOMIDES, BSC
REED WICKNER, MD

Contents

* Deceased

Microbiology

Part One

Bacterial Physiology and Bacterial Genetics

Bernard D. Davis

1

Evolution of Microbiology and of Microbes

There are similarities between the diseases of animals or man and the diseases of beer and wine. . . . If fermentations were diseases one could speak of epidemics of fermentation.
—L. Pasteur

Evolution of Microbiology

THE FIRST MICROSCOPIC OBSERVATIONS

Although the epidemic spread of some diseases long suggested that some kind of agent was being transmitted, it was remarkably difficult for people to imagine the existence of living organisms too small to be seen, or to believe that they could harm large hosts. Their existence was not generally accepted until 1677, when they were seen by Antony van Leeuwenhoek, a cloth merchant in Delft, Holland, who had little education but great patience and curiosity. He achieved great magnification with a simple (one-lens) microscope by grinding lenses of extremely small size and hence high curvature; and in letters published by the Royal Society in London he described a wholly new, previously invisible world, including "animalcules" (now recognized as bacteria and protozoa) whose motility showed that they were alive. But although Leeuwenhoek is regarded as the father of microbiology, he did not really found it as a science—that is, a cumulative, public body of knowledge—because he kept his methods secret. Microorganisms (microbes) did not become accessible to others until the development of an effective compound (multi-lens) microscope 150 years later.

The advance of microbiology to an experimental science, and even the natural history of describing what microorganisms exist, required the development of an appropriate methodology. In particular, the identification and study of particular organisms uncontaminated by others required reliable methods for sterilization and aseptic transfer. Development of such methods was stimulated by a long controversy over a scientific issue with religious overtones: the spontaneous generation of life.

SPONTANEOUS GENERATION

Because organic matter generally decomposes quickly outside the living body, it was natural to assume that the responsible agents, from maggots to microbes, were constantly arising by spontaneous generation. Spallanzani (1729–1799) really solved the problem by showing that an infusion of meat would remain clear indefinitely if boiled and properly sealed.* However, it could still be argued that the absence of decomposition might be attributable to the limited supply of air.

This argument was rebutted when Schroeder and von Dusch replaced sealed glass with the cotton plug, which is still used today to exclude airborne contaminants. Nevertheless, the controversy continued, for some investigators were unable to reproduce the alleged stability of dust-free sterilized organic infusions. Louis Pasteur (1822–1895) then showed that boiled medium could remain clear in a "swan-neck" flask, open to the air through a sinuous horizontal tube in which dust particles would settle as air reentered the cooling vessel (Fig. 1–1). He also demonstrated that in the relatively dust-free atmosphere of a quiet cellar or of a mountain top, sealed flasks could be opened and then resealed with a good chance of escaping contamination.

Pasteur's experiments were a public sensation. Although his contributions were in principle no more decisive than those of his predecessors, his zeal and skill as a polemicist were largely responsible for laying the ghost of spontaneous generation. Because of his crusading spirit, as well as his experimental skill and intuitive genius, Pasteur was, for the nineteenth century, in Dubos' words, "not only the arm but also the voice, and finally the symbol, of triumphant science." For example, from a lecture delivered at the Sorbonne in 1864:

I have taken my drop of water from the immensity of creation, and I have taken it full of the elements appropriate to the development of microscopic organisms. And I wait, I watch, I question it!—begging it to recommence for me the beautiful spectacle of the first creation. But it is dumb, dumb since these experiments were begun several years ago; it is dumb because I have kept it sheltered from the only thing man does

not know how to produce, from the germs which float in the air, from Life, for Life is a germ and a germ is Life. Never will the doctrine of spontaneous generation recover from the mortal blow of this simple experiment!

THE PROBLEM OF SPORES. Despite Pasteur's dramatic success, it turned out that his accusations of technical incompetence did not really explain why his opponents' boiled infusions stubbornly refused to remain clear. The key difference was their use of infusions of hay, whereas Pasteur used yeast extract. The decisive experiments were performed by the British physicist John Tyndall, whose interest in atmospheric dust led him into this biological problem. After bringing a bale of hay into his laboratory, Tyndall could no longer achieve sterility in the same room by boiling, and he showed that the hay had contaminated his laboratory with an incredible kind of living organism: one that could survive boiling. In the same year (1877), Ferdinand Cohn demonstrated the resistant forms as small, refractile **spores** (see Ch. 2), a special stage in the life cycle of the hay bacillus (*Bacillus subtilis*). Because even the most resistant spores are readily sterilized in the presence of moisture at 120°C, the autoclave, which uses steam under pressure, became the hallmark of the bacteriology laboratory.

THE ROLE OF MICROBES IN FERMENTATIONS

We have seen that practical men proceeded to preserve foods while the savants continued to dispute spontaneous generation. Useful fermentations† have an even longer history of achievement without a theoretical foundation: lost in antiquity are the origins of leavened bread, wine, or the fermentations that preserve food through the accumulation of lactic acid (soured milk, cheese, sauerkraut, ensilage).

In the 1830s, with the development of adequate microscopes, several investigators concluded that the microscopic globules found in the sediment of wine were alive and that their metabolic activities caused the alcoholic fermentation. However, because these yeasts were not motile, it was not certain that they were alive; and Liebig, the father of biochemistry, insisted that they were a byproduct of the fermentation, which he considered a purely chemical process attributable to a self-perpetuating instability of the grape juice when exposed to air. Liebig's authority was eventually overturned by Pasteur.

---

* Indeed, the soundness of this discovery was confirmed in the early nineteenth century, when a Parisian confectioner, Appert, competing for a prize offered by Napoleon, developed the art of preserving food by canning.

† In general usage, the term **fermentation** refers to the microbial decomposition of vegetable matter, which contains mostly carbohydrates, whereas **putrefaction** refers to the formation of more unpleasant products by the decomposition of high-protein materials such as meat or eggs. (For a more rigorous definition of fermentation see Ch. 4.) The etymology of the word ferment (L. *fervere*, to boil) and its figurative use today reflect the heating and bubbling that are generated in a vat of fermenting grape juice.

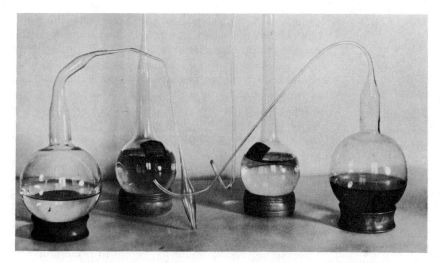

Figure 1–1. Pasteur's swan-neck flasks. After their use in his studies on spontaneous generation, these flasks were sealed, and they have since been preserved, with their original contents, in the Pasteur Museum. (Courtesy of Institut Pasteur, Paris)

Educated as a chemist, Pasteur became interested in fermentations through discovering optical isomerism as a property of certain fermentation products (e.g., tartaric acid). In 1857, he showed that different kinds of microbes are associated with different kinds of fermentation: spheres (now known as yeast cells) in the alcoholic fermentation, and smaller rods (lactobacilli) in the lactic fermentation.*

In the course of establishing the nature of fermentation, Pasteur founded the study of **microbial metabolism** and developed profound insight into many of its problems. In particular, he showed that **life is possible without air,** that indeed some organisms (obligatory anaerobes) are even inhibited by air, and that fermentation is much less efficient than respiration in terms of the growth yield per unit of substrate consumed.

SELECTIVE CULTIVATION. Because the nature of a specific fermentation depends on the organism responsible, how can a given kind of substrate, when not deliberately inoculated with a particular microbe, regularly undergo a given kind of fermentation? Pasteur recognized that the explanation lay in the principle of selective cultivation: various organisms are ubiquitous, and the one best adapted to a given environment eventually predominates. For example, in grape juice the high sugar concentration and the low protein content (i.e., low buffering power) lead to a low pH, which favors the outgrowth of acid-resistant yeasts. In milk, in contrast, the much higher protein and lower sugar content favor the outgrowth of fast-growing but more acid-sensitive bacteria.

An excess of the wrong organism in the starting inoculum, however, can grow out sufficiently to cause formation of a product with a poor flavor; hence, specific microbes play a role in "diseases" of beer and wine, as well as in different normal fermentations. This finding led Pasteur to a most fruitful suggestion: **that specific microbes might also be causes of specific diseases in man.** With an eye always to practical as well as to theoretical problems, Pasteur developed the procedure of gentle heating (**pasteurization**) to prevent the spoilage of beer and wine by contaminating microbes. This process was later used to prevent milkborne diseases of man. Even more impressive and valuable was Pasteur's development of an attenuated bacterial vaccine, against anthrax, by growing the organism at elevated temperature. This procedure is now known to "cure" this bacterium of a plasmid that carries a gene essential for virulence.

Pasteur's demonstration of microbial specificity was a victory in another controversy. Investigators did not then know that they were dealing with mixed cultures, and so when transfer of the same culture to different media yielded organisms of quite different appearance it is understandable that many opted for **pleomorphism:** the doctrine that the same organism adopted very different forms in different environments. The victory of **monomorphism,** which emphasizes the fixed properties of each organism, contributed greatly to the development of microbiology. However, it was an oversimplification that also delayed the development of bacterial genetics, for it discouraged the recognition of genotypic changes arising within a strain and of phenotypic changes within a genotype.

* As in many scientific disputes, the losing argument possessed at least a grain of truth. The view of fermentation as a chemical rather than a vital process was ultimately vindicated in 1897, although in a profoundly modified form, when Edouard Buchner accidentally discovered that a cell-free extract made by grinding yeast cells with sand fermented a concentrated sugar solution added to preserve the extract.

SOIL MICROBIOLOGY; GEOCHEMICAL CYCLES

For most of the century after Pasteur, microbiology remained largely an applied and descriptive field dominated by medical bacteriology. But it is important to recognize also the beneficent and essential roles of most microbes in the geochemical cycles that sustain life—especially because the popular image of a hostile microbial world has no doubt contributed to the recent public anxiety over novel engineered bacteria. In fact, human pathogens constitute only a small fraction of all bacterial species: most microbes (present in many kinds of soil at densities of 10^6 to 10^7 per gram) attack organic matter only after it is dead and buried, each kind of organism hydrolyzing and metabolizing only a particular set of compounds.

The principal role of microbes in nature is thus geochemical: mineralization of organic carbon, nitrogen, and sulfur (i.e., conversion to CO_2, NH_3 or NO_3^-, SO_4^{2-} or S^{2-}) so that these elements can be used cyclically for growth of higher plants and animals. In specialized niches, various bacteria have evolved the ability to use an astonishing variety of energy sources, such as H_2, CO, Fe^{2+}, or S. Unlike natural compounds, many synthetic organic compounds, such as polystyrene, are not biodegradable because no microbes have yet evolved that can attack them.

Microbes also participate in the synthesizing half of the cycle, not only in increasing their own mass, but also in ways that are essential for higher organisms. Algae and some bacteria, as well as higher plants, reduce CO_2 to organic compounds by photosynthesis, **nitrogen-fixing** bacteria reduce atmospheric N_2 to NH_3, and the **nitrifying** bacteria enhance soil fertility by converting the volatile NH_3 into the nonvolatile nitrate.

THE DEVELOPMENT OF MICROBIAL AND MOLECULAR GENETICS

For many years, bacteria remained completely outside the growing field of genetics. The small size of the organisms prevented recognition of their chromosome, the lack of sexual reproduction prevented identification of separate units of inheritance (genes), and the extremely rapid multiplication made it difficult to determine whether the adaptation of a culture to a new medium was genotypic (i.e., involving selection of rare mutants) or physiological (involving reversible alterations in all the cells). With the development of bacterial genetics in the 1940s bacteria were found to have real advantages in the study of universal features of cell physiology, including a somewhat simpler structure than eukaryotic cells (although one surprisingly similar in its fundamental molecular features), the possibility of introducing small blocks of genetic material, and extremely rapid multipli-

cation. But by far the greatest advantage lies in the possibility of selecting rare mutants and rare genetic recombinants from populations of billions of individuals. These mutants have proved to be sharp tools for dissecting complex intracellular processes. Moreover, the selection of rare recombinants extended the resolving power of genetic mapping from the dimensions of individual genes to those of individual nucleotides.

Avery's work on transformation in the pneumococcus first revealed gene transfer in bacteria—an essential step in developing bacterial genetics. Even more important, it showed that DNA is the genetic material. This discovery, and the elucidation of the structure of DNA by Watson and Crick, founded **molecular genetics.** In the rapid advance of this field, the development of a methodology for recombining DNA molecules *in vitro,* and for cloning the resulting recombinant molecules in bacteria and in yeast cells (Chs. 8 and 11), has provided tools of remarkable power, both for studying the genes of any organisms and for the industrial production of proteins of medical importance.

Microbiology and Medicine

THE GERM THEORY OF DISEASE

Among the major classes of disease, infections have undoubtedly presented the greatest burden to mankind: not only were they a leading cause of death, but these deaths were often especially tragic because they were so frequent among the young. Moreover, by their epidemic nature, infections have disabled and terrorized communities and have determined the fate of armies and nations: thus smallpox permitted a few dozen Spaniards to take over a flourishing Mexican civilization. Clearly, the control over infectious diseases and over microbial pollution of the environment has been the greatest achievement of medical science. Today, it is easy to take these advances for granted while focusing on problems created by technology, but an earlier public enshrined Pasteur and Robert Koch (1843–1910) as national heroes.

EPIDEMIOLOGIC EVIDENCE. The discovery of infectious agents was long preceded by the concept of **contagious** disease; i.e., one initiated by **contact** with a diseased person or with objects contaminated by that person. But despite the logical arguments for invisible, transmissible agents, such leading physicians as William Harvey continued, like Hippocrates and Galen, to ascribe epidemics to miasmas: poisonous vapors created by the influence of planetary conjunctions or by disturbances arising within the earth. The difficulty arose in part because many **communicable** diseases are not **contagious** (i.e., spread by contact) but rather are transmitted indirectly by air, water, food, or insects. Indeed, until the agents were shown to be particulate it was quite logical to invoke poisoned air to explain the mysterious spread of such diseases.

The evidence supporting the germ theory accumulated slowly and from several directions. **Experimental transmission** was undertaken in the eighteenth century by the renowned surgeon John Hunter, who boldly inoculated himself with pus from a patient with gonorrhea, unfortunately acquiring syphilis in the bargain; and in an early use of experimental animals, Villemin transmitted tuberculosis from humans to guinea pigs in 1865, 20 years before identification of the agent. **Indirect transmission** was recognized in the 1840s, when Semmelweis in Vienna and Oliver Wendell Holmes in Boston blamed obstetricians moving with unwashed hands from one patient to the next for the prevalence of puerperal sepsis in hospitals; but those pioneers encountered enormous resistance from the insulted physicians. John Snow demonstrated the waterborne transmission of an enteric infection more directly, and with less resistance, when he terminated a localized epidemic of cholera in London in 1854 by closing the contaminated source of water for the neighborhood, the now famous Broad Street pump. The efficacy of other **preventive measures** also lent support to the germ theory: in 1796, Jenner introduced vaccination (*L. vacca*, cow) against smallpox with material from lesions of a similar, milder disease of cattle. Moreover, in the 1860s, Joseph Lister, building on Pasteur's evidence for the ubiquity of airborne microbes, introduced antiseptic surgery by demonstrating the value of a disinfectant, phenol, as well as of cleanliness in preventing serious wound infections.

Nevertheless, such epidemiologic evidence, although logically convincing, did not carry the weight of a direct demonstration of the etiologic agents.

RECOGNITION OF AGENTS OF INFECTION

Fungi, being larger than bacteria, were the first agents to be recognized—in 1836 by Bassi, for a disease of silkworms, and 3 years later by Schönlein, for a human skin disease (favus).

The etiologic role of bacteria was first established with anthrax, a disease which offered several advantages for these studies: the organism is unusually large; the disease, found primarily in cattle and sheep, can be conveniently transmitted to small animals; and dense bacterial populations may appear terminally in the blood. Indeed, in 1850, Davaine saw rod-shaped bodies in the blood of sheep with anthrax, and he later transmitted the disease by inoculating as little as 10^{-6} ml of blood. But however suggestive this evidence, to a skeptical world these microscopic bodies might have been a result rather than the cause of the disease. Koch provided unequivocal proof that they were indeed the cause by infecting animals with organisms isolated in pure culture. This approach became the key to establishing various bacteria as pathogens.

PURE CULTURES. Lister used the awkward method of limiting dilutions, in which the source material is diluted until the individual inocula each contain either one infectious particle or none. Koch meticulously perfected the techniques of identification that are used today, including the use of **solid media,** on which individual cells give rise to separate colonies, and the use of **stains.** Koch's genius is perhaps best reflected in his patient modifications of his own earlier methods, which finally led to the identification of the tubercle bacillus in 1882: because this organism grows very slowly, the usual 1 to 2 days of cultivation had to be extended to several weeks, and because it is so impervious, the usual few minutes of staining had to be extended to 12 hours.

After identifying the tubercle bacillus, Koch formalized the criteria, introduced by Henle in 1840 but known as **Koch's postulates,** for distinguishing a pathogenic from an adventitious microbe: (1) the organism is regularly found in the lesions of the disease, (2) it can be isolated in pure culture on artificial media, (3) inoculation of this culture produces a similar disease in experimental animals, and (4) the organism can be recovered from the lesions in these animals. These criteria have proved invaluable in identifying pathogens, but they cannot always be met: some organisms (including all viruses) cannot be grown on artificial media, and some are pathogenic only for man.

The powerful methodology developed by Koch introduced the "Golden Era" of medical bacteriology. Between 1879 and 1889, various members of the German school isolated (in addition to the tubercle bacillus) the cholera vibrio, typhoid bacillus, diphtheria bacillus, pneumococcus, staphylococcus, streptococcus, meningococcus, gonococcus, and tetanus bacillus.

VIRUSES

The term virus (L., poison) was long used as a synonym for "infectious agent," but it became restricted some decades ago to agents smaller than bacteria (hence separable by filtration) and unable to multiply outside a living host. These characteristics, however, overlap with those of some especially small bacteria (*Rickettsiae, Chlamydiae*). Viruses are now sharply defined in terms of their characteristic structure and their **mode of replication;** i.e., dissociation into components after entering a host cell, use of host machinery to synthesize the components coded for by the viral genes, and formation of new units by reassembly rather than by cellular enlargement and division.

The first virus to be recognized as filterable was a

plant pathogen, tobacco mosaic virus, discovered independently by Ivanovski in Russia in 1892 and Beijerinck in Holland in 1899. Filterable animal viruses were first demonstrated for foot-and-mouth disease of cattle by Löffler and Frosch in 1898 and for a human disease, yellow fever, by the U.S. Army Commission under Walter Reed in 1900. Viruses that infect bacteria (**bacteriophages**) were discovered by Twort in England and by d'Herelle in France in 1916 to 1917.

For the first third of this century, viruses could be detected only by their pathogenic effects on living hosts. Progress was slow until methods were developed, first with bacteriophages and then with animal viruses, for growing viruses as **plaques** on a layer of host cells, analogous to the growth of individual bacteria as colonies on solid media. This technique permitted precise assays and quantitative genetic studies. In addition, electron microscopy and molecular studies made it possible to analyze the mechanism of viral reproduction.

With the resulting dramatic expansion of virology, it has been recognized that the agents of acute viral diseases are only the most conspicuous members, but not the bulk, of the viral kingdom: more and more viruses are being identified that have delayed effects or no apparent effect at all. In addition, the genetic discontinuity between virus and cell has become blurred, with the finding that viruses can become integrated into host chromosomes and can also capture host genes. These developments suggest that viruses have evolved from cellular chromosomes and that they have evolved not primarily as parasites but as agents for transmitting blocks of genetic material from one organism to another.

THE HOST RESPONSE; IMMUNOLOGY

Vertebrates infected by a microbial parasite exhibit a specific immune response, which contributes to recovery and also protects against reinfection. Analysis of this response has given rise to the field of immunology. This field has now grown, in several ways, far beyond its origins in the study of infectious disease. Thus, the same responses are elicited when foreign substances of nonmicrobial origin gain access to the tissues (e.g., pollens, insect venoms, drugs, foreign serum or other proteins, transplanted tissues) and sometimes when cancer cells arise in the host. Moreover, studies of the molecular mechanisms of the immune response are often most conveniently carried out by using small molecules, rather than microbes or their components, as the stimuli. In other directions, immunologic methods are widely used for quantitative detection of various compounds and for probing the structures of proteins. Nevertheless, immunologic concepts and techniques are very important in identifying various microbes, understanding their

pathogenicity, preventing infection, and identifying individuals who have been infected.

Whereas the term **immunity** is usually reserved for the presence of highly specific antibodies and immune cells induced in the host in response to foreign materials, the broader concept of **resistance** to various infectious diseases encompasses in addition many other, much less specific factors. These include **phagocytic cells** that engulf the parasites, **enzymes** that attack them, **nutritional variables** that may promote or limit microbial multiplication, and specific **surface receptors** on host cells that interact with surface components on the parasite and thus affect its adherence and penetration. The presence or absence of these receptors on different cells influences the distribution of the agents in the body, whereas variations between individuals influence their susceptibility to the agent.

CONTROL OF INFECTIOUS DISEASES

Identification of the agents of various infectious diseases soon led to several remarkably effective methods of control. First, in technologically advanced countries environmental **sanitation*** and improved personal **hygiene** have strikingly reduced the incidence of certain diseases and sometimes even eliminated them, particularly those spread by water or food (e.g., typhoid, cholera) or by insects (e.g., typhus, yellow fever). However, a knowledge of these diseases is still essential for the physician, because they are still important in some regions, and they may be spread by travelers. Second, **vaccination** has eliminated smallpox throughout the world and has drastically reduced the incidence of several other serious epidemic diseases (e.g., diphtheria, whooping cough, poliomyelitis). It has been especially valuable for diseases transmitted by respiratory droplets, whose distribution is difficult to control. However, for many organisms, vaccination is not effective or feasible. Third, in the most striking advance in medical bacteriology since the 1880s, the development of **antibacterial chemotherapy** has dramatically reduced the severity and the incidence of many infectious diseases. Table 1–1 illustrates the impact of these several approaches.

In principle, it should ultimately be possible to eradicate all those organisms that are obligatory human pathogens. However, most pathogens are also widely carried by man without causing disease or have reservoirs in lower animals or in the soil; hence, we cannot expect to achieve eradication.

---

* Sanitary measures began to be developed, largely on aesthetic grounds, long before the germ theory of disease. A major advance was the popularization of indoor toilets through the invention, by Thomas Crapper in Victorian England, of the trap and air vent that block the return of sewage gas.

–3. Classification of Kingdoms of elled Organisms

es (bacteria)	Rigid wall (except mycoplasmas)*
	Diameter 1–2 μm
	Photosynthesis:
	Non-oxygenic (sulfur bacteria)
	Oxygenic (cyanobacteria)
	None (most bacteria)
	Movement by simple rotating flagella
eukaryotes)	
molds and yeasts)	Rigid wall
	Diameter greater than prokaryotes
	No photosynthesis
	Rigid wall
	Cell size greater than prokaryotes
	Oxygenic photosynthesis
	Many form large multicellular plantlike
	organisms (seaweeds) but with
	limited cell differentiation
	Some forms motile by cilia-like undulat-
	ing flagella
a	Flexible cell membrane
	No photosynthesis
	Movement ameboid or by cilia or cilia-
	like flagella

bacteria ordinarily have rigid walls, the group that lacks them plasmas) are now sometimes classified as prokaryotes but not as

of these divisions contains a wide variety of mor-cal forms. The algae, being photosynthetic, do ct humans, but they are occasional sources of d toxins. With the fungi and the protozoa, as with otes, only a tiny fraction of species are patho-his text will consider pathogenic fungi, but not a, which are traditionally presented in the medi-iculum along with the metazoan parasites. sification within the prokaryote kingdom pre-ecial problems, which we will now consider.

RIA

eny Versus Determinative Key

ssification of organisms (**taxonomy**) has two pur-One is purely descriptive: to group organisms of ne kind and to describe the basis for that group-that the information collected about a given kind pooled and compared. The ordering of the enti-such a scheme could then be simply a matter of ience, providing a **determinative key** for apply-uccession of criteria to an unknown specimen e correct description is reached. The second pur-to provide a "natural," phylogenetic classification ns at depicting the lines of evolutionary descent necting the specific units (**taxons**) in the succes-

sive categories (species, genus, family, tribe, order, class, and kingdom) in a **hierarchical family tree.**

The fundamental unit of taxonomy is the **species:** the group of organisms of a particular "kind." With most animals and plants, which reproduce sexually, this grouping is not based on morphological and physiologi-cal similarities alone: a species can be sharply defined as a group whose members can mate in nature and form fertile offspring only with members of the same group. The evolution of sexual reproduction clearly required such fertility boundaries, for whereas sex greatly ad-vanced the rate of evolution by increasing the genetic variety that natural selection can act on, crosses between individuals with excessive genetic differences would result in wasteful formation of progeny with unworkable combinations of genes. Accordingly, when two popula-tions in a species are reproductively separated (usually by a geographic barrier), they accumulate differences in their total gene pool, and the resulting races (sub-species), which are still interfertile, eventually evolve into separate species. The transitional forms disappear rap-idly, as they evolve into stable new species with a more harmonious (coadapted) set of genes.

With bacteria, in contrast, there are no such sharp natural species boundaries. Multiplication is asexual (clonal), each individual giving rise by successive **binary fissions** to a **clone:** a set of individuals who are geneti-cally identical except for rare mutations. Moreover, the rare transfers of genes between organisms involve only small blocks of DNA rather than zygote formation. Ac-cordingly, bacterial species have to be defined in a differ-ent way.

THE MEANING OF BACTERIAL SPECIES. Because of this mode of inheritance, one might expect to find a truly continuous genetic spectrum in bacteria in nature. In fact, this has not occurred, because a mutation that im-proves one genome may decrease the fitness of another. Accordingly, as noted above, evolution selects for a **bal-anced genome,** well adapted to a particular range of environments. Because of the resulting discontinuities between groups, a bacterial species can be defined as a **cluster of strains** (individual isolates) with a high de-gree of phenotypic similarity and with significant dif-ferences from related groups. The persistence of stable species despite the extremely rapid multiplication of bacteria reflects the action of natural selection in two directions: not only **divergent selection,** which gives rise to new species, but also **stabilizing selection,** which eliminates excessive deviations from a well-adapted norm.

Because this method of defining species is somewhat arbitrary, taxonomists can themselves be classified into "lumpers" and "splitters." The art of the systematic bacteriologist lies in identifying the discontinuities be-

Disease	1900	1983
Pneumonia	175	23
Influenza	27	0.6
Tuberculosis	175	0.8
Intestinal diseases	143	0.2
Typhoid	31	0
Diphtheria	40	0

Microbiology and Evolution

Although Darwinian evolution is the principle that unites all biology, the growing science of evolutionary biology, initially built on the comparative morphology and physiology of animals and plants and on morpho-logical sequences in a stratified fossil record, was not readily applicable to the microbial world. Indeed, there is no evidence that Pasteur and Darwin had any interest in each other's work (although we can now interpret Pasteur's selective cultivation as an elegant and rapid example of natural selection). The barriers began to be removed when comparative biochemistry revealed the same amino acids and metabolic cofactors and the same glycolytic pathway in the microbial and the visible world.

Today, as we shall see later in this chapter, DNA se-quences provide reliable measures of phylogenetic rela-tions, including those between different bacteria and be-tween bacteria and higher organisms. Indeed, for the latter, these studies now provide much more direct evi-dence for evolutionary continuity than the fragmentary fossil record; and without this continuity, studies on bac-terial cells could not have the relevance that they do for our understanding of human cells.

TELEONOMY. Molecular genetics has also united the two main streams of biology: one concerned with origins and the other with structure and function. This union has legitimized teleologic considerations in biology. **Teleol-ogy** (Gr. *tele*, goal), as originally formulated by Aristotle, proposed that structures or mechanisms are found in a living organism because they have value or purpose for that organism, and because some agency—a "final cause"—had foreseen this value. After Darwin, biologists could profitably employ the same concept in a modified form, substituting the hindsignt of natural selection for divine foresight. Because the term teleology continued to have supernaturalistic connotations, the term **teleon-omy** has been introduced: it implies simply that an or-ganism's genetic characteristics reflect evolutionary ad-aptation to its environment.

Although teleonomic reasoning was long suspect in biochemistry, we can now unequivocally define the

"purpose" or "goal" of an enzyme (i.e., its function in the overall economy of a cell) in two ways: by observing the effects of mutations that alter the enzyme and by identi-fying regulatory responses to various metabolites that have been programed into it (or into its gene) by evolu-tion. indeed, such regulatory mechanisms would have little meaning without the concept of a purpose, that is, the increased metabolic efficiency for which natural se-lection inexorably presses.

POPULATION GENETICS OF BACTERIA

The epidemiology of infectious diseases—the study of the factors that influence their distribution—can be seen as an applied branch of evolutionary biology. It thus deals with the principal components of Darwinian evolu-tion: genetic variation and natural selection.

The complex ecological interactions with their hosts influence the evolution of pathogenic bacteria. Many species include a wide variety of strains with different surface antigens, and some species even have mecha-nisms for producing successive antigenic variants within a strain during the course of an infection. The advantage for the bacteria is obvious: a host that has developed an immune response to a particular surface antigen will remain susceptible to organisms with a different antigen.

For example, the virus of myxoma, a highly lethal dis-ease of rabbits, was introduced into Australia to reduce crop destruction by a plague of these animals; and at first, this biological warfare was dramatically effective. Within a few years, however, the rabbit population recov-ered its initial density through the outgrowth of mutant strains with increased resistance to myxoma. In addi-tion, a less virulent mutant strain of the virus outgrew the original form, evidently because it did not kill off its hosts so rapidly and hence had more opportunity to spread.

Another relevant evolutionary principle is that suc-cessful competition depends not on a single, powerful gene, but on having a **balanced (coadapted) set of genes,** whose mutual interactions produce an effective organism. Pathogenicity, in particular, is multifactorial: to cause disease, an infecting bacterium not only must yield products that harm the host but also must have many other attributes, including the ability to adhere to specific surfaces, to grow under the conditions there, to resist various host defenses, and to survive during trans-mission between hosts. Moreover, as the myxoma story illustrates, a moderately virulent organism may be more successful in maximizing its progeny than an extremely virulent organism, which kills off its host rapidly.

The complexity of pathogenicity also makes it ex-tremely unlikely that the introduction of foreign DNA into a nonpathogenic bacterium by genetic engineering will inadvertently convert it into a pathogen. It is equally unlikely that such altered organisms would spread, because they would almost certainly be less competitive in a natural environment than the parental strain, which has been adapted by a long process of evolutionary selection. Accordingly, there is little basis for the widespread fear that the use of molecular recombination in the domestication of nonpathogenic microbes for industrial or agricultural purposes, supplementing the classic genetic techniques, will lead to the accidental spread of harmful organisms.

Other aspects of bacterial population genetics will be considered below (The Meaning of Bacterial Species).

ROLE OF MICROBES IN HUMAN EVOLUTION

Infectious diseases also affect the evolution of the host. Although the three million years of hominid evolution have been associated with an extraordinarily rapid increase in intelligence and manual dexterity—the features most responsible for man's dominating position—the selection pressures changed markedly 10,000 years ago, when the development of agriculture and then urbanization permitted the formation of larger, more freely communicating groups. As J. B. S. Haldane pointed out, under these changed conditions epidemic diseases must have become an increasingly prominent cause of death; and the resulting selection for increased resistance to these diseases would blunt the selection for more interesting traits.*

The gene for sickle-cell hemoglobin provides a particularly clear example of selection by infectious disease. This gene is prevalent in malarial regions of Africa, where it protects heterozygotes against falciparum malaria, although at the cost of serious disease in the homozygotes. Infections have probably also influenced the distribution of the broader group of genes for host cell-surface antigens (blood group substances, histocompatibility antigens) because these cell constituents influence the attachment and penetration of various parasites.

Selection pressure from infections was strong: a century ago in the United States (and still today in some parts of the world), 25% to 50% of children died of these diseases before reaching puberty. Today this figure is below 2%.

PROKARYOTES AND EUKARYOTES

The world of microbes was initially divided between the two existing kingdoms: bacteria and fungi, with rigid cell walls, were assigned to the plants, and protozoa, with

* It is a well-established principle that selection for one trait will interfere with the efficiency of selection for another. For example, a school may select its student body on the basis of both ability to pay tuition and personal qualities; but if scholarships are used to eliminate the first selection, the second will become more effective because of the enlarged pool of applicants.

flexible cells, to the animals. When the electron microscope revealed fundamental differences in cell organization, the bacteria were reclassified as the kingdom of **prokaryotes†** (Gr., primitive nucleus), whereas all other organisms became the superkingdom of **eukaryotes** (Gr., true nucleus). Eukaryotic cells contain a nucleus with a nuclear membrane enclosing multiple chromosomes and a mitotic apparatus to ensure their equipartition, after replication, to the two daughter cells. The single prokaryotic chromosome does not require a mitotic apparatus and is not enclosed in a nuclear membrane.

Another striking difference is that **introns** (nontranslated regions) are abundant in the genes of eukaryotes but are virtually absent in those of prokaryotes. Although this feature suggested that prokaryotic genes are more primitive, it is striking that introns are also rare in the eukaryotic yeast cells. It has therefore been suggested that introns arose early in evolution to accelerate recombination of protein domains and expansion of the genome, but in organisms that devote most of their energy to cell replication the costs of maintaining introns outweigh their advantages.

Prokaryotes have many additional distinctive features, listed in Table 1–2.

The **mitochondria** of eukaryotic cells and the **chloroplasts** that carry out photosynthesis in plants resemble bacteria in the simple circular structure of their chromosome and in the size, RNA sequences, and antibiotic sensitivity of their ribosomes. These organelles therefore appear to have evolved from prokaryotes that entered and became symbiotic in eukaryotic cells. This inference is supported by the widespread presence of such **endosymbiosis** today: typical bacteria, capable of living free, are found within cells of many protozoa, plants, and animals, where they carry out processes that are valuable for the host. Examples include cellulose digestion in insects and nitrogen fixation in the roots of plants.

A wide evolutionary gap (the real "missing link" in evolution) separates the prokaryotes from the eukaryotes, whose further evolution depended on aggregation, differentiation, and specialization of cells, rather than on any radical change in cell design. Hence, yeasts, which offer the experimental advantages of single-celled organisms, are widely used as model cells for studying the molecular genetics of eukaryotes (Ch. 11).

PRECELLULAR EVOLUTION AND THE ORIGIN OF LIFE

Although the work of Pasteur and of Tyndall dispelled earlier claims of spontaneous generation of life from

† The British spelling originally introduced was procaryote and eucaryote, but for consistency with such terms as karyotype, many prefer to transliterate the Greek kappa as *k*.

TABLE 1–2. Features Distinguishing Prokaryotes from Eukaryotes

A single, circular chromosome (nucleoid) instead of a nucleus with multiple chromosomes

No nuclear membrane or mitotic apparatus

No true histones, nucleosomes

No introns in genes for proteins and rare in genes for tRNAs

Transcription is coupled with translation. No terminal polyadenylation of mRNA (except in archaebacterial)

mRNA usually polygenic

Initiator tRNA is formylmethionyl instead of methionyl (except in archaebacteria)

Ribosome is 70S instead of 80S; moderate differences in shape, length of rRNA molecules, and number of protein molecules

Cell wall with unique residues (in eubacteria: muramic acid, D-amino acids, often diaminopimelic acid)

No steroids or phosphatidyl choline in membrane

No endocytotic vesicles or cytoskeleton

No endoplasmic reticulum (but autotrophic bacteria have extensive invaginations of the cytoplasmic membrane)

No mitochondria or other membrane-bounded organelles (rare exceptions)

No triglyceride fats; carbon storage as poly-β-hydroxybutyric acid in some groups

Movement by flagellar rotation

Unique metabolic capacities: N_2 fixation; anaerobic respiration (with inorganic electron acceptor other than O_2); non-oxygenic photosynthesis

---

nonliving matter **under experimental conditions,** Darwin's theory of evolution (published within 2 years of Pasteur's first paper on spontaneous generation) logically required such an initial origin of life preceding the evolution of the contemporary living world. In the 1920s, Oparin in the Soviet Union and Haldane in England suggested that the appearance of the first cell was preceded by a period of **chemical, prebiotic evolution,** during which various organic compounds were formed with the aid of UV light, lightning, volcanic heat, inorganic surface catalysis, and concentration by freezing or cycles of drying. Because the primitive earth lacked the agents that now make organic substances unstable (microbes and atmospheric oxygen), these substances could accumulate. Polymerization in these thin "soups" of organic compounds would eventually yield protein catalysts, followed by the enclosure of an autocatalytic system in a membrane-bounded cell; and as the cells exhausted the building blocks in the "soup," they would evolve biosynthetic pathways. In support of this hypothesis, Miller and Urey showed that various amino acids could be formed by the action of an electric spark on a gas mixture (H_2O, NH_3, CH_4, and H_2) that simulated the atmosphere of the primitive earth.

However, with the advent of molecular genetics, the problem of the origin of life became better formulated as the **origin of genetic information,** because the unique feature of living systems is the **storage and translation of information in macromolecules.** Since the early

system for replicating and expanding inf have to provide catalysts as well as templ molecule, RNA was probably the first inf romolecule, combining these functions came dependent on DNA and proteins retaining several other functions in infor Indeed, some RNAs have recently been pable of serving as a catalyst (althou slowly cleaving their own chain at speci expanding chain lengths by ligating the the cleavage.

Woese and Eigen have offered mode **biotic evolution was Darwinian.** In t polymerization of activated ribonucleo presence of short polyribonucleotides tion toward production of their own early evolution, competitive selectior that were most effective in promoting tion in this way could make the pro more accurate, thereby increasing the be replicated without too many erron tually, the storage of information wo reverse transcription, to the more st DNA, whereas catalysis would be sh flexible and efficient protein enzymes shift from RNA to DNA replication is n we have no evidence on what kind c chinery for translation might have pr 100-component version.

This model for prebiotic evolution ical evolution is built into the natur under appropriate chemical and phy continuity from a precellular to a c be inevitable, depending on natural of successive steps rather than on a probability (the aggregation of a wide formed molecules into the first cell) of this conclusion, bacterial fossils strated, by morphological and chem earliest sedimentary rocks, laid dov lion years after the formation of the lion years ago.

Classification

PROTISTS

In the nineteenth century, Haeckel single-celled organisms as a new k With the subsequent separation of the eukaryotes, as described abov became restricted to unicellular briefly describes the principal divis organisms. In addition, a few org ate, sharing properties of two divi

tween species on the basis of stable and fundamental properties while ignoring those properties that fluctuate readily.

Molecular taxonomy based on DNA or protein sequences has been used primarily to measure evolutionary relatedness between species (see below), but it also can shed light on the population structure of a species—in particular, on the widespread assumption that the mechanisms for occasional transfer of chromosomal genes between bacteria would eventually randomize the distribution of these genes within a species. This conclusion was not borne out by the study of the distribution of electrophoretic variants of several dozen obligatory enzymes in *E. coli.* Among several thousand isolates these forms were clustered in only a few hundred patterns. In contrast, within each of these groups there was considerable variation in non-obligatory traits, often carried by plasmids: surface antigens, and enzymes for using alternative nutrients. These findings suggest that although movement of DNA between bacteria in nature may be substantial, effective lateral flow of chromosomal genes, resulting in integration and survival in progeny, is actually very slow: despite the enormous crop of *E. coli,* the number of clones, each with a specific set of chromosomal genes, is quite small, perhaps because the genes within each set are especially well coadapted. This demonstration of the clonal structure of a species makes the concept of a bacterial species more meaningful and less arbitrary.

DIAGNOSTIC IDENTIFICATION OF A SPECIES. Medical bacteriologists learned to rely on properties that are relatively easy to recognize. The useful traits include shape, size, color, staining, motility, capsule, colonial morphology, formation of characteristic fermentation products, ability to metabolize various substrates, antibiotic sensitivity, and habitat (including the host range and pattern of disease for pathogens). Specific surface macromolecules, usually detected with antibodies, are useful not only in identifying species but also in identifying **groups,** and even narrower **types,** within a species. The terms "serovar" (serotype), "morphovar," or "biovar" are sometimes used for variants within a species: they are defined, respectively, by characteristic serologic reactions, morphological features, and special biochemical or physiological properties.

The deeper layers of the bacterial wall and the membrane differ much less among related organisms than the surface macromolecules, for their interactions impose structural constraints, and they are subject to less selection pressure from such agents as antibodies, enzymes, and bacteriophages. Hence, immunologic or chemical characterization of these deeper components is a frequent basis for grouping species into a genus. Other fundamental properties include the pattern of the flagella responsible for motility, the energy-yielding pathways, and chemical composition (especially of the wall and the membrane); gas–liquid chromatography of membrane lipids is a valuable tool. Nucleic acid sequences will be discussed below.

By consulting published descriptions, comparing **"type cultures"** (standard strains) that are maintained in several countries, and exchanging strains, bacteriologists can communicate with each other. Following the Linnean tradition of zoology and botany, each "species" (plural spp.) of bacterium is assigned an official Latin **binomial** (in italics), with a capitalized genus (plural genera) followed by an uncapitalized species designation. Unitalicized vernacular names may be derived from, or may be identical with, the official name (e.g., pneumococcus = *Diplococcus pneumoniae,* now *Streptococcus pneumoniae;* salmonella = *Salmonella* spp.)

In virology, which developed more recently, a proposed binomial system has been controversial.

The principal guide to bacterial classification is a large cooperative effort: *Bergey's Manual of Determinative Bacteriology.* Its **descriptions** of species are relatively stable, but the **nomenclature** undergoes occasional changes that now require the approval of an official international body. For example, the same organism has been called *Bacillus typhosus, Bacterium typhosum, Eberthella typhosa,* and *Salmonella typhi.*

The ordering of the higher taxons is more arbitrary than the definition of species. For example, general microbiologists have grouped more than 80 species, with a wide range of properties, in the single genus *Pseudomonas,* whereas the extensive study of the family *Enterobacteriaceae* by medical bacteriologists has resulted in dividing a small set of species, much more similar to each other, into several genera. The still higher groupings provide primarily a determinative key with shaky phylogenetic implications.

Table 1–4 lists some of the major "families" of bacteria, including selected nonpathogens. The major distinction between gram-positive and gram-negative is based on a fundamental difference in the structure of the cell envelope (Ch. 2).

NUMERAL TAXONOMY. To avoid arbitrary judgments, some investigators, with the aid of computers, have revived an old approach to taxonomy in which a large number of characters are determined and given equal weight in grouping strains. The **similarity coefficient** for two strains is the number of positive phenotypic characters that they share divided by the total number positive in either (or in both).

Molecular Taxonomy

Molecular genetics has now provided a much more reliable basis than phenotypic similarity for measuring relat-

TABLE 1–4. Main Groups of Eubacteria

Gram-Positive

Cell Shape	Motility	Other Characteristics		Genera	Families
Cocci	Nearly all permanently immotile	Cells in cubical packets Cells irregularly arranged		*Sarcina* *Micrococcus* *Staphylococcus*	Micrococcaceae
		Cells in chains Lactic fermentation of sugars }		*Streptococcus* *Leuconostoc*	Streptococcaceae
Straight rods	Nearly all permanently immotile	Lactic fermentation of sugars Propionic fermentation of sugars Oxidative, weakly fermentative		*Lactobacillus* *Propionibacterium* *Corynebacterium* *Listeria* *Erysipelothrix*	Lactobacillaceae Propionibacteriaceae
	Motile with peritrichous flagella or immotile	Endospores produced	Aerobic Anaerobic	*Bacillus* *Clostridium*	Bacillaceae

Gram-Negative, Excluding Photosynthetic Forms

Cell Shape	Motility	Other Distinguishing Characteristics		Genera	Families
Cocci	Permanently immotile	Aerobic Anaerobic		*Neisseria* *Veillonella*	Neisseriaceae
				Brucella *Bordetella* *Pasteurella* *Haemophilus*	Brucellaceae
Straight rods	Motile with peritrichous flagella and related immotile forms	Facultative anaerobic	Mixed acid fermentation of sugars	*Escherichia* *Erwinia* *Shigella* *Salmonella* *Proteus* *Yersinia*	Enterobacteriaceae
			Butylene glycol fermentation	*Enterobacter* *Serratia*	
		Aerobic	Free-living nitrogen fixers	*Azotobacter*	Azotobacteraceae
			Symbiotic nitrogen fixers	*Rhizobium*	Rhizobiaceae
	Motile with polar flagella	Aerobic	Oxidize inorganic compounds	*Nitrosomonas* *Nitrobacter* *Thiobacillus*	Nitrobacteraceae
			Oxidize organic compounds	*Pseudomonas* *Acetobacter* *Legionella*	Pseudomonadaceae
		Facultative anaerobic		*Campylobacter* *Zymomonas* *Aeromonas*	
Curved rods	Motile with polar flagella	Comma-shaped Spiral	Aerobic Anaerobic	*Vibrio* *Desulfovibrio* *Spirillum*	Spirillaceae

(Continued)

TABLE 1–1. Deaths per 100,000 in the U.S. From Selected Infectious Diseases

Disease	1900	1983
Pneumonia	175	23
Influenza	27	0.6
Tuberculosis	175	0.8
Intestinal diseases	143	0.2
Typhoid	31	0
Diphtheria	40	0

Microbiology and Evolution

Although Darwinian evolution is the principle that unites all biology, the growing science of evolutionary biology, initially built on the comparative morphology and physiology of animals and plants and on morphological sequences in a stratified fossil record, was not readily applicable to the microbial world. Indeed, there is no evidence that Pasteur and Darwin had any interest in each other's work (although we can now interpret Pasteur's selective cultivation as an elegant and rapid example of natural selection). The barriers began to be removed when comparative biochemistry revealed the same amino acids and metabolic cofactors and the same glycolytic pathway in the microbial and the visible world.

Today, as we shall see later in this chapter, DNA sequences provide reliable measures of phylogenetic relations, including those between different bacteria and between bacteria and higher organisms. Indeed, for the latter, these studies now provide much more direct evidence for evolutionary continuity than the fragmentary fossil record; and without this continuity, studies on bacterial cells could not have the relevance that they do for our understanding of human cells.

TELEONOMY. Molecular genetics has also united the two main streams of biology: one concerned with origins and the other with structure and function. This union has legitimized teleologic considerations in biology. **Teleology** (Gr. *tele*, goal), as originally formulated by Aristotle, proposed that structures or mechanisms are found in a living organism because they have value or purpose for that organism, and because some agency—a "final cause"—had foreseen this value. After Darwin, biologists could profitably employ the same concept in a modified form, substituting the hindsight of natural selection for divine foresight. Because the term teleology continued to have supernaturalistic connotations, the term **teleonomy** has been introduced: it implies simply that an organism's genetic characteristics reflect evolutionary adaptation to its environment.

Although teleonomic reasoning was long suspect in biochemistry, we can now unequivocally define the "purpose" or "goal" of an enzyme (i.e., its function in the overall economy of a cell) in two ways: by observing the effects of mutations that alter the enzyme and by identifying regulatory responses to various metabolites that have been programed into it (or into its gene) by evolution. Indeed, such regulatory mechanisms would have little meaning without the concept of a purpose, that is, the increased metabolic efficiency for which natural selection inexorably presses.

POPULATION GENETICS OF BACTERIA

The epidemiology of infectious diseases—the study of the factors that influence their distribution—can be seen as an applied branch of evolutionary biology. It thus deals with the principal components of Darwinian evolution: genetic variation and natural selection.

The complex ecological interactions with their hosts influence the evolution of pathogenic bacteria. Many species include a wide variety of strains with different surface antigens, and some species even have mechanisms for producing successive antigenic variants within a strain during the course of an infection. The advantage for the bacteria is obvious: a host that has developed an immune response to a particular surface antigen will remain susceptible to organisms with a different antigen.

For example, the virus of myxoma, a highly lethal disease of rabbits, was introduced into Australia to reduce crop destruction by a plague of these animals; and at first, this biological warfare was dramatically effective. Within a few years, however, the rabbit population recovered its initial density through the outgrowth of mutant strains with increased resistance to myxoma. In addition, a less virulent mutant strain of the virus outgrew the original form, evidently because it did not kill off its hosts so rapidly and hence had more opportunity to spread.

Another relevant evolutionary principle is that successful competition depends not on a single, powerful gene, but on having a **balanced (coadapted) set of genes,** whose mutual interactions produce an effective organism. Pathogenicity, in particular, is multifactorial: to cause disease, an infecting bacterium not only must yield products that harm the host but also must have many other attributes, including the ability to adhere to specific surfaces, to grow under the conditions there, to resist various host defenses, and to survive during transmission between hosts. Moreover, as the myxoma story illustrates, a moderately virulent organism may be more successful in maximizing its progeny than an extremely virulent organism, which kills off its host rapidly.

The complexity of pathogenicity also makes it extremely unlikely that the introduction of foreign DNA into a nonpathogenic bacterium by genetic engineering will inadvertently convert it into a pathogen. It is equally unlikely that such altered organisms would spread, because they would almost certainly be less competitive in a natural environment than the parental strain, which has been adapted by a long process of evolutionary selection. Accordingly, there is little basis for the widespread fear that the use of molecular recombination in the domestication of nonpathogenic microbes for industrial or agricultural purposes, supplementing the classic genetic techniques, will lead to the accidental spread of harmful organisms.

Other aspects of bacterial population genetics will be considered below (The Meaning of Bacterial Species).

ROLE OF MICROBES IN HUMAN EVOLUTION

Infectious diseases also affect the evolution of the host. Although the three million years of hominid evolution have been associated with an extraordinarily rapid increase in intelligence and manual dexterity—the features most responsible for man's dominating position— the selection pressures changed markedly 10,000 years ago, when the development of agriculture and then urbanization permitted the formation of larger, more freely communicating groups. As J. B. S. Haldane pointed out, under these changed conditions epidemic diseases must have become an increasingly prominent cause of death; and the resulting selection for increased resistance to these diseases would blunt the selection for more interesting traits.*

The gene for sickle-cell hemoglobin provides a particularly clear example of selection by infectious disease. This gene is prevalent in malarial regions of Africa, where it protects heterozygotes against falciparum malaria, although at the cost of serious disease in the homozygotes. Infections have probably also influenced the distribution of the broader group of genes for host cell-surface antigens (blood group substances, histocompatibility antigens) because these cell constituents influence the attachment and penetration of various parasites.

Selection pressure from infections was strong: a century ago in the United States (and still today in some parts of the world), 25% to 50% of children died of these diseases before reaching puberty. Today this figure is below 2%.

PROKARYOTES AND EUKARYOTES

The world of microbes was initially divided between the two existing kingdoms: bacteria and fungi, with rigid cell walls, were assigned to the plants, and protozoa, with

---

* It is a well-established principle that selection for one trait will interfere with the efficiency of selection for another. For example, a school may select its student body on the basis of both ability to pay tuition and personal qualities; but if scholarships are used to eliminate the first selection, the second will become more effective because of the enlarged pool of applicants.

flexible cells, to the animals. When the electron microscope revealed fundamental differences in cell organization, the bacteria were reclassified as the kingdom of **prokaryotes†** (Gr., primitive nucleus), whereas all other organisms became the superkingdom of **eukaryotes** (Gr., true nucleus). Eukaryotic cells contain a nucleus with a nuclear membrane enclosing multiple chromosomes and a mitotic apparatus to ensure their equipartition, after replication, to the two daughter cells. The single prokaryotic chromosome does not require a mitotic apparatus and is not enclosed in a nuclear membrane.

Another striking difference is that **introns** (nontranslated regions) are abundant in the genes of eukaryotes but are virtually absent in those of prokaryotes. Although this feature suggested that prokaryotic genes are more primitive, it is striking that introns are also rare in the eukaryotic yeast cells. It has therefore been suggested that introns arose early in evolution to accelerate recombination of protein domains and expansion of the genome, but in organisms that devote most of their energy to cell replication the costs of maintaining introns outweigh their advantages.

Prokaryotes have many additional distinctive features, listed in Table 1–2.

The **mitochondria** of eukaryotic cells and the **chloroplasts** that carry out photosynthesis in plants resemble bacteria in the simple circular structure of their chromosome and in the size, RNA sequences, and antibiotic sensitivity of their ribosomes. These organelles therefore appear to have evolved from prokaryotes that entered and became symbiotic in eukaryotic cells. This inference is supported by the widespread presence of such **endosymbiosis** today: typical bacteria, capable of living free, are found within cells of many protozoa, plants, and animals, where they carry out processes that are valuable for the host. Examples include cellulose digestion in insects and nitrogen fixation in the roots of plants.

A wide evolutionary gap (the real "missing link" in evolution) separates the prokaryotes from the eukaryotes, whose further evolution depended on aggregation, differentiation, and specialization of cells, rather than on any radical change in cell design. Hence, yeasts, which offer the experimental advantages of single-celled organisms, are widely used as model cells for studying the molecular genetics of eukaryotes (Ch. 11).

PRECELLULAR EVOLUTION AND THE ORIGIN OF LIFE

Although the work of Pasteur and of Tyndall dispelled earlier claims of spontaneous generation of life from

---

† The British spelling originally introduced was procaryote and eucaryote, but for consistency with such terms as karyotype, many prefer to transliterate the Greek kappa as *k*.

TABLE 1–2. Features Distinguishing Prokaryotes from Eukaryotes

A single, circular chromosome (nucleoid) instead of a nucleus with multiple chromosomes

No nuclear membrane or mitotic apparatus

No true histones, nucleosomes

No introns in genes for proteins and rare in genes for tRNAs

Transcription is coupled with translation. No terminal polyadenylation of mRNA (except in archaebacterial)

mRNA usually polygenic

Initiator tRNA is formylmethionyl instead of methionyl (except in archaebacteria)

Ribosome is 70S instead of 80S; moderate differences in shape, length of rRNA molecules, and number of protein molecules

Cell wall with unique residues (in eubacteria: muramic acid, D-amino acids, often diaminopimelic acid)

No steroids or phosphatidyl choline in membrane

No endocytotic vesicles or cytoskeleton

No endoplasmic reticulum (but autotrophic bacteria have extensive invaginations of the cytoplasmic membrane)

No mitochondria or other membrane-bounded organelles (rare exceptions)

No triglyceride fats; carbon storage as poly-β-hydroxybutyric acid in some groups

Movement by flagellar rotation

Unique metabolic capacities: N_2 fixation; anaerobic respiration (with inorganic electron acceptor other than O_2); non-oxygenic photosynthesis

nonliving matter **under experimental conditions,** Darwin's theory of evolution (published within 2 years of Pasteur's first paper on spontaneous generation) logically required such an initial origin of life preceding the evolution of the contemporary living world. In the 1920s, Oparin in the Soviet Union and Haldane in England suggested that the appearance of the first cell was preceded by a period of **chemical, prebiotic evolution,** during which various organic compounds were formed with the aid of UV light, lightning, volcanic heat, inorganic surface catalysis, and concentration by freezing or cycles of drying. Because the primitive earth lacked the agents that now make organic substances unstable (microbes and atmospheric oxygen), these substances could accumulate. Polymerization in these thin "soups" of organic compounds would eventually yield protein catalysts, followed by the enclosure of an autocatalytic system in a membrane-bounded cell; and as the cells exhausted the building blocks in the "soup," they would evolve biosynthetic pathways. In support of this hypothesis, Miller and Urey showed that various amino acids could be formed by the action of an electric spark on a gas mixture (H_2O, NH_3, CH_4, and H_2) that simulated the atmosphere of the primitive earth.

However, with the advent of molecular genetics, the problem of the origin of life became better formulated as the **origin of genetic information,** because the unique feature of living systems is the **storage and translation of information in macromolecules.** Since the early

system for replicating and expanding information might have to provide catalysts as well as templates in the same molecule, RNA was probably the first informational macromolecule, combining these functions before they became dependent on DNA and proteins (with RNA then retaining several other functions in information transfer). Indeed, some RNAs have recently been shown to be capable of serving as a catalyst (although inefficiently), slowly cleaving their own chain at specific sites, and also expanding chain lengths by ligating the ends created by the cleavage.

Woese and Eigen have offered models in which **prebiotic evolution was Darwinian.** In the nonenzymatic polymerization of activated ribonucleosides *in vitro*, the presence of short polyribonucleotides can bias the reaction toward production of their own complements. In early evolution, competitive selection of those chains that were most effective in promoting their own replication in this way could make the process progressively more accurate, thereby increasing the length that could be replicated without too many erroneous copies. Eventually, the storage of information would be shifted, by reverse transcription, to the more stable, less versatile DNA, whereas catalysis would be shifted to the more flexible and efficient protein enzymes. But although the shift from RNA to DNA replication is not hard to envision, we have no evidence on what kind of rudimentary machinery for translation might have preceded the present 100-component version.

This model for prebiotic evolution implies that biological evolution is built into the nature of matter, and so under appropriate chemical and physical conditions, its continuity from a precellular to a cellular phase would be inevitable, depending on natural selection in a series of successive steps rather than on a single event of low probability (the aggregation of a wide variety of randomly formed molecules into the first cell). In indirect support of this conclusion, bacterial fossils have been demonstrated, by morphological and chemical evidence, in the earliest sedimentary rocks, laid down within only a billion years after the formation of the earth's crust 4.5 billion years ago.

Classification

PROTISTS

In the nineteenth century, Haeckel proposed to group all single-celled organisms as a new kingdom, the **protists.** With the subsequent separation of the prokaryotes from the eukaryotes, as described above, the term "protist" became restricted to unicellular eukaryotes. Table 1–3 briefly describes the principal divisions of the unicellular organisms. In addition, a few organisms are intermediate, sharing properties of two divisions.

TABLE 1–3. *Classification of Kingdoms of Single-Celled Organisms*

Prokaryotes (bacteria)	Rigid wall (except mycoplasmas)*
	Diameter 1–2 μm
	Photosynthesis:
	Non-oxygenic (sulfur bacteria)
	Oxygenic (cyanobacteria)
	None (most bacteria)
	Movement by simple rotating flagella
Protists (eukaryotes)	
Fungi (molds and yeasts)	Rigid wall
	Diameter greater than prokaryotes
	No photosynthesis
Algae	Rigid wall
	Cell size greater than prokaryotes
	Oxygenic photosynthesis
	Many form large multicellular plantlike organisms (seaweeds) but with limited cell differentiation
	Some forms motile by cilia-like undulating flagella
Protozoa	Flexible cell membrane
	No photosynthesis
	Movement ameboid or by cilia or cilia-like flagella

* Because bacteria ordinarily have rigid walls, the group that lacks them (the mycoplasmas) are now sometimes classified as prokaryotes but not as bacteria.

Each of these divisions contains a wide variety of morphological forms. The algae, being photosynthetic, do not infect humans, but they are occasional sources of ingested toxins. With the fungi and the protozoa, as with prokaryotes, only a tiny fraction of species are pathogens. This text will consider pathogenic fungi, but not protozoa, which are traditionally presented in the medical curriculum along with the metazoan parasites.

Classification within the prokaryote kingdom presents special problems, which we will now consider.

BACTERIA
Phylogeny Versus Determinative Key

The classification of organisms (**taxonomy**) has two purposes. One is purely descriptive: to group organisms of the same kind and to describe the basis for that grouping, so that the information collected about a given kind can be pooled and compared. The ordering of the entities in such a scheme could then be simply a matter of convenience, providing a **determinative key** for applying a succession of criteria to an unknown specimen until the correct description is reached. The second purpose is to provide a "natural," phylogenetic classification that aims at depicting the lines of evolutionary descent by connecting the specific units (**taxons**) in the succes-

sive categories (species, genus, family, tribe, order, class, and kingdom) in a **hierarchical family tree.**

The fundamental unit of taxonomy is the **species:** the group of organisms of a particular "kind." With most animals and plants, which reproduce sexually, this grouping is not based on morphological and physiological similarities alone: a species can be sharply defined as a group whose members can mate in nature and form fertile offspring only with members of the same group. The evolution of sexual reproduction clearly required such fertility boundaries, for whereas sex greatly advanced the rate of evolution by increasing the genetic variety that natural selection can act on, crosses between individuals with excessive genetic differences would result in wasteful formation of progeny with unworkable combinations of genes. Accordingly, when two populations in a species are reproductively separated (usually by a geographic barrier), they accumulate differences in their total gene pool, and the resulting races (subspecies), which are still interfertile, eventually evolve into separate species. The transitional forms disappear rapidly, as they evolve into stable new species with a more harmonious (coadapted) set of genes.

With bacteria, in contrast, there are no such sharp natural species boundaries. Multiplication is asexual (clonal), each individual giving rise by successive **binary fissions** to a **clone:** a set of individuals who are genetically identical except for rare mutations. Moreover, the rare transfers of genes between organisms involve only small blocks of DNA rather than zygote formation. Accordingly, bacterial species have to be defined in a different way.

THE MEANING OF BACTERIAL SPECIES. Because of this mode of inheritance, one might expect to find a truly continuous genetic spectrum in bacteria in nature. In fact, this has not occurred, because a mutation that improves one genome may decrease the fitness of another. Accordingly, as noted above, evolution selects for a **balanced genome,** well adapted to a particular range of environments. Because of the resulting discontinuities between groups, a bacterial species can be defined as a **cluster of strains** (individual isolates) with a high degree of phenotypic similarity and with significant differences from related groups. The persistence of stable species despite the extremely rapid multiplication of bacteria reflects the action of natural selection in two directions: not only **divergent selection,** which gives rise to new species, but also **stabilizing selection,** which eliminates excessive deviations from a well-adapted norm.

Because this method of defining species is somewhat arbitrary, taxonomists can themselves be classified into "lumpers" and "splitters." The art of the systematic bacteriologist lies in identifying the discontinuities between species on the basis of stable and fundamental properties while ignoring those properties that fluctuate readily.

Molecular taxonomy based on DNA or protein sequences has been used primarily to measure evolutionary relatedness between species (see below), but it also can shed light on the population structure of a species—in particular, on the widespread assumption that the mechanisms for occasional transfer of chromosomal genes between bacteria would eventually randomize the distribution of these genes within a species. This conclusion was not borne out by the study of the distribution of electrophoretic variants of several dozen obligatory enzymes in *E. coli*. Among several thousand isolates these forms were clustered in only a few hundred patterns. In contrast, within each of these groups there was considerable variation in non-obligatory traits, often carried by plasmids: surface antigens, and enzymes for using alternative nutrients. These findings suggest that although movement of DNA between bacteria in nature may be substantial, effective lateral flow of chromosomal genes, resulting in integration and survival in progeny, is actually very slow: despite the enormous crop of *E. coli*, the number of clones, each with a specific set of chromosomal genes, is quite small, perhaps because the genes within each set are especially well coadapted. This demonstration of the clonal structure of a species makes the concept of a bacterial species more meaningful and less arbitrary.

DIAGNOSTIC IDENTIFICATION OF A SPECIES. Medical bacteriologists learned to rely on properties that are relatively easy to recognize. The useful traits include shape, size, color, staining, motility, capsule, colonial morphology, formation of characteristic fermentation products, ability to metabolize various substrates, antibiotic sensitivity, and habitat (including the host range and pattern of disease for pathogens). Specific surface macromolecules, usually detected with antibodies, are useful not only in identifying species but also in identifying **groups,** and even narrower **types,** within a species. The terms "serovar" (serotype), "morphovar," or "biovar" are sometimes used for variants within a species: they are defined, respectively, by characteristic serologic reactions, morphological features, and special biochemical or physiological properties.

The deeper layers of the bacterial wall and the membrane differ much less among related organisms than the surface macromolecules, for their interactions impose structural constraints, and they are subject to less selection pressure from such agents as antibodies, enzymes, and bacteriophages. Hence, immunologic or chemical characterization of these deeper components is a frequent basis for grouping species into a genus. Other fundamental properties include the pattern of the flagella responsible for motility, the energy-yielding pathways, and chemical composition (especially of the wall and the membrane); gas–liquid chromatography of membrane lipids is a valuable tool. Nucleic acid sequences will be discussed below.

By consulting published descriptions, comparing **"type cultures"** (standard strains) that are maintained in several countries, and exchanging strains, bacteriologists can communicate with each other. Following the Linnean tradition of zoology and botany, each "species" (plural spp.) of bacterium is assigned an official Latin **binomial** (in italics), with a capitalized genus (plural genera) followed by an uncapitalized species designation. Unitalicized vernacular names may be derived from, or may be identical with, the official name (e.g., pneumococcus = *Diplococcus pneumoniae*, now *Streptococcus pneumoniae*; salmonella = *Salmonella* spp.)

In virology, which developed more recently, a proposed binomial system has been controversial.

The principal guide to bacterial classification is a large cooperative effort: *Bergey's Manual of Determinative Bacteriology*. Its **descriptions** of species are relatively stable, but the **nomenclature** undergoes occasional changes that now require the approval of an official international body. For example, the same organism has been called *Bacillus typhosus*, *Bacterium typhosum*, *Eberthella typhosa*, and *Salmonella typhi*.

The ordering of the higher taxons is more arbitrary than the definition of species. For example, general microbiologists have grouped more than 80 species, with a wide range of properties, in the single genus *Pseudomonas*, whereas the extensive study of the family *Enterobacteriaceae* by medical bacteriologists has resulted in dividing a small set of species, much more similar to each other, into several genera. The still higher groupings provide primarily a determinative key with shaky phylogenetic implications.

Table 1–4 lists some of the major "families" of bacteria, including selected nonpathogens. The major distinction between gram-positive and gram-negative is based on a fundamental difference in the structure of the cell envelope (Ch. 2).

NUMERAL TAXONOMY. To avoid arbitrary judgments, some investigators, with the aid of computers, have revived an old approach to taxonomy in which a large number of characters are determined and given equal weight in grouping strains. The **similarity coefficient** for two strains is the number of positive phenotypic characters that they share divided by the total number positive in either (or in both).

Molecular Taxonomy

Molecular genetics has now provided a much more reliable basis than phenotypic similarity for measuring relat-

TABLE 1—4. *Main Groups of Eubacteria*

		Gram-Positive			
Cell Shape	*Motility*	*Other Characteristics*		*Genera*	*Families*
Cocci	Nearly all permanently immotile	Cells in cubical packets Cells irregularly arranged		*Sarcina Micrococcus Staphylococcus*	Micrococcaceae
		Cells in chains Lactic fermentation of sugars		*Streptococcus Leuconostoc*	Streptococcaceae
Straight rods	Nearly all permanently immotile	Lactic fermentation of sugars Propionic fermentation of sugars Oxidative, weakly fermentative		*Lactobacillus Propionibacterium Corynebacterium Listeria Erysipelothrix*	Lactobacillaceae Propionibacteriaceae
	Motile with peritrichous flagella or immotile	Endospores produced	Aerobic Anaerobic	*Bacillus Clostridium*	Bacillaceae

		Gram-Negative, Excluding Photosynthetic Forms			
Cell Shape	*Motility*	*Other Distinguishing Characteristics*		*Genera*	*Families*
Cocci	Permanently immotile	Aerobic Anaerobic		*Neisseria Veillonella*	Neisseriaceae
				Brucella Bordetella Pasteurella Haemophilus	Brucellaceae
Straight rods	Motile with peritrichous flagella and related immotile forms	Facultative anaerobic	Mixed acid fermentation of sugars	*Escherichia Erwinia Shigella Salmonella Proteus Yersinia*	Enterobacteriaceae
			Butylene glycol fermentation	*Enterobacter Serratia*	
		Aerobic	Free-living nitrogen fixers	*Azotobacter*	Azotobacteraceae
			Symbiotic nitrogen fixers	*Rhizobium*	Rhizobiaceae
	Motile with polar flagella	Aerobic	Oxidize inorganic compounds	*Nitrosomonas Nitrobacter Thiobacillus*	Nitrobacteraceae
			Oxidize organic compounds	*Pseudomonas Acetobacter Legionella*	Pseudomonadaceae
		Facultative anaerobic		*Campylobacter Zymomonas Aeromonas*	
Curved rods	Motile with polar flagella	Comma-shaped Spiral	Aerobic Anaerobic	*Vibrio Desulfovibrio Spirillum*	Spirillaceae

(Continued)

TABLE 1—4. Main Groups of Eubacteria (Continued)

	Other Major Groups	
Characteristics	Genera	Orders or Families
Acid-fast rods Ray-forming rods (actinomycetes)	*Mycobacterium* *Actinomyces* *Nocardia* *Streptomyces*	Actinomycetales
Spiral organisms, motile	*Treponema* *Borrellia* *Leptospira* *Spirocheta*	Spirochetales
Small, pleomorphic; lack rigid wall Small intracellular parasites	*Mycoplasma* *Rickettsia* *Coxiella* *Chlamydia*	Mollicutes Rickettsiaceae Chlamydiaceae
Intracellular parasites; borderline with protozoa	*Bartonella*	Bartonellaceae

(Modified from Stanier RY et al: The Microbial World. Englewood Cliffs, NJ, Prentice-Hall, 1963)

edness in bacteria and in higher organisms as well. The underlying principle is that the progressive divergence of organisms in evolution is directly reflected in the DNA. The differences are measured in terms of DNA composition, sequence homology as assessed by hybridization of DNA (or of RNA with DNA), and DNA, RNA, and protein sequences. The results have verified many previously inferred phylogenetic groupings but have contraindicated others.

Closely related bacterial species also exhibit similarities in more classic genetic parameters: the efficiency of transfer of genes and the arrangement of homologous genes on their chromosomes.

BASE RATIOS. The G + C content of DNA can be inferred from its buoyant density or its melting temperature, both of which increase with G + C content because GC pairs are held together by three hydrogen bonds and AT pairs by two. The melting temperature (T_m = 50% melting) is easily measured because the melting of a stretch of DNA into single strands increases its UV absorption. In addition, the range of spread in density or in melting shows how widely the pieces of DNA in the test mixture differ in composition. The results of such studies have shown that the small accessory replicating units present in many strains (plasmids, Ch. 8) often differ markedly in density from the chromosome, whereas the chromosomal fragments (of a few thousand base pairs) show remarkable homogeneity. It thus appears that the machinery for translating the genetic information in each organism is adapted to a particular DNA composition.

The range of DNA composition in bacteria is remarkably wide: whereas the whole phylum of vertebrates ranges only from 36% to 44% G + C, bacteria range from 25% to 75%, yet there is no corresponding difference in amino acid composition of the proteins. This is possible because for most amino acids, the genetic code provides alternative codons (especially in the 3' base; Ch. 6).

Studies of DNA composition have yielded some surprises. For example, the important pathogen *Staphylococcus* and the nonpathogen *Micrococcus*, long placed in the same family on the grounds of their very similar morphology, are at opposite ends of the scale: 30% to 40% and 65% to 75% G + C, respectively. Also, various streptococci and lactobacilli, traditionally grouped together as lactic acid bacteria because of their characteristic fermentation, have a G + C content of 38% to 40%, but *Lactobacillus bifidus* has 56% and so has been assigned to a new genus, *Bifidobacterium*. On the other hand, other groups with considerable spread are still each considered a single genus, including some of medical interest: *Bacillus*, *Corynebacterium*, *Proteus*, and *Pseudomonas*.

NUCLEIC ACID HYBRIDIZATION. DNA—DNA **hybridization** is conveniently measured, after making the samples single-stranded, by adsorbing the DNA from one organism to nitrocellulose filter, which is then annealed with the labeled DNA from a second organism. Occasional mismatches within a sequence weaken but do not prevent hybridization. Accordingly, altering the **stringency** of the conditions (by changing the annealing temperature or the salt concentration) yields information not only on the extent of the homologous regions but also on the degree of their homology.

Whereas significant hybridization occurs between

TABLE 1–5. *Hybridization of Radioactive* E. coli *DNA or* rRNA *with DNA of Various Enterobacteria**

Immobilized DNA	E. coli DNA (%)	E. coli *Ribosomal* RNA (%)
E. coli	100	100
Shigella	86	92
Salmonella	43	79
Proteus	9	76

* The total DNA of the test organisms was made single-stranded and was immobilized on nitrocellulose filters, which were than incubated at annealing temperature with radioactively labeled DNA or rRNA from *E. coli*. The values for the tightly bound radioactivity are expressed as the fraction of that obtained with *E. coli* hybridized with itself, normalized at 100 percent.

even the most distant vertebrates (and reveals 99% homology between man and the chimpanzee), the long evolutionary divergence of bacteria has yielded a very different picture: only very closely related organisms exhibit any DNA hybridization (Table 1–5). However, **rRNA–DNA hybridization** has proved valuable over a broader range (Table 1–5), because the components of the ribosome must fit each other closely on most of their surfaces, and so they conserve their sequences much more than soluble proteins do. Moreover, ribosomal RNA (rRNA) is relatively easy to isolate. But this interaction still has a restricted range: the single genus *Pseudomonas* contains several independent rRNA–DNA groups, which do not hybridize with each other.

NUCLEIC ACID SEQUENCING. The earlier studies on rRNA used two-dimensional chromatography ("fingerprinting") to compare the frequency of identical short oligonucleotides produced by endonuclease T_1, which cleaves on the 3' side of each guanosine residue. Complete rRNA sequences, obtained by reverse transcription to DNA, have provided a more powerful tool, and the conservation of "signature nucleotides" in certain positions has proved to be a better index of relatedness. Such comparisons of rRNAs permit organisms to be arranged in a **dendrogram:** a branching family tree plotting the connections between various taxons against a quantitative estimate of similarity, such as the similarity coefficient S_{AB} (the proportion of oligonucleotides that are shared; see Ch. 25, Fig. 25–3).

With the development of methods for cloning genes and for rapidly sequencing DNA, it became possible to measure precisely the degree of relatedness of an unlimited number of homologous genes and also to relate these genotypic changes to phenotypic differences; protein sequences can be inferred or can be determined directly. The results show that certain parts of a protein or RNA are more conserved than others. Because DNA sequences diverge so widely among bacteria, rapid diag-

nostic methods are being developed commercially that use short DNA sequences, characteristic of a particular organism, as **hybridization probes** to test suitably treated colonies on a plate for the presence of complementary DNA.

Measurements of evolutionary distances by comparison of homologous molecules are complicated by the fact that different molecular lineages and different parts of a sequence evolve at different rates; accordingly, the changes subject to selection and the neutral mutations (which do not affect function and hence are free of selection) must be averaged. In addition, attempts to measure great distances face two further limitations. First, a particular sequence may not have evolved along with the rest of the genome but rather may have been introduced by lateral transfer (especially in prokaryotes) from another organism (**polyphyletic** origin). Accordingly, the evolutionary branches inferred from sequences will be more reliable if a monophyletic origin can be demonstrated by showing that several different highly conserved sequences, (e.g., cytochromes, proton-translocating ATPase, DNA and RNA polymerases, ferredoxins) yield parallel results. Second, the assumption of a molecular clock, based on genes accumulating mutations at a relatively constant rate for each protein, appears to be valid for many proteins over long periods of evolution, but over even longer periods, structure–function relations set a limit to the divergence of amino acid sequences.

Evolutionary conservation has also been studied by comparing the secondary structure of rRNAs (deduced from cross-linking and from calculation of maximal base pairing). Figure 1–2 shows the striking similarity in shape of the rRNAs of an archaebacterium (see below) and a eubacterium, which are separated by a great evolutionary distance. On the other hand, the shapes of RNAs or of proteins, like those of the organs observed by morphologists, are subject to **convergent evolution,** in which distant lineages may end up, through selection pressures, with similar structures in order to perform the same function.

The molecular genetic approach to bacterial taxonomy has revolutionized the study of the early phases of evolution, and the results have also confirmed most of the earlier inferences about bacterial classification within narrow groups; but they also have shown that the higher taxons in the phenotype-based bacterial family tree have little phylogenetic significance. Nevertheless, it is doubtful that a phylogenetic taxonomy will quickly replace the traditional determinative schemes, whose higher level taxons can be useful as mnemonic devices without any pretense of phylogenetic validity. In an additional contribution to evolution, the short generation time of bacteria makes possible refined study of the mechanisms of evolution at a molecular level.

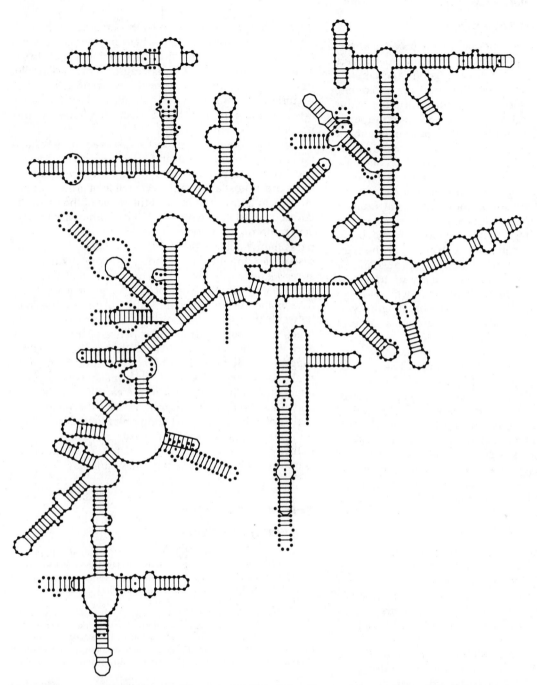

Figure 1–2. Secondary structure of bacterial 16S rRNA. A line diagram of the sequence of the archaebacterium *Halobacterium volcanii* is superimposed on the sequence (*solid dots*) of the eubacterium *Escherichia coli.* Cross-bars indicate hydrogen bonding that orders the secondary structure; the actual sequences of the two molecules differ much more than the secondary structures. (Courtesy of R Gutell and CR Woese)

Archaebacteria and Eubacteria

Differences in rRNA sequences reveal a broad gap between two groups of prokaryotes: a small, specialized group, now designated as the subkingdom **Archaebacteria,** and all the others, called **Eubacteria**. Subsequent studies have revealed additional unique properties of the archaebacteria: a modified cell wall without muramic acid (Ch. 2), membrane lipids containing glyceryl ethers (rather than esters) and polyisoprenoid (rather than alkyl) chains, introns, and some unique enzyme cofactors.

The archaebacteria include the methane bacteria (which derive energy from the conversion of CO_2 and H_2 to CH_4 and H_2O and are important in industrial systems for converting garbage to useful fuel), extreme halophiles (which require the high salt concentrations of brine lakes), and thermoacidophiles (which thrive at the high temperatures and acidity of geothermal springs and of coal deposits exposed to air). Moreover, in the thermoacidophiles the membrane is not a bilayer, as in all other organisms: instead, lipids of double length (with eight isoprenoid units), with a polar group (a glycerol diether) at each end, traverse the whole membrane, forming a monolayer that evidently prevents their melting at the high temperatures of the normal habitat.

The metabolism of the methanogens originally suggested that they might be ancient ("archae-") relics of bacteria adapted to the atmosphere of the primitive earth and preceding the eubacteria. However, in their rRNAs and in some other respects (introns; sensitivity to diphtheria toxin), they are closer to the eukaryotes than to the eubacteria, suggesting that the path from an earlier, extinct urbacterium to eukaryotes may have passed through relatives of archaebacteria.

The Range of Bacteria

The bacteria found in soil, in decomposing organic matter, and in bodies of water are a substantial fraction of the total terrestrial biomass. It is estimated that each person carries some 10^{14} bacteria (more than the number of his or her own cells!) and that the total human population excretes from its collective gut 10^{22} to 10^{23} bacteria per day.

Bacteria have evolved to fill an enormous variety of ecological niches. Their physical environments range from hot springs at 90°C to refrigerated foods, and from distilled water with trace contaminants to the Dead Sea; and their energy-yielding mechanisms range from the oxidation of Fe^{2+} to Fe^{3+} or of H_2S to H_2SO_4 to a special form of photosynthesis that cannot yield O_2. At hydrothermal vents at the rifts between tectonic plates, deep in the ocean floor, some large worms and clams derive their food from organs filled with autotrophic, CO_2-fixing bacteria, which acquire energy by oxidizing the H_2S welling up into the superheated water—a unique exception to the rule that animal life ultimately depends on the products of photosynthesis. Elsewhere in the ocean depths are "baryophiles" that require the ambient high hydrostatic pressure and low temperature. This variety illustrates the capacity of nature to evolve proteins whose requirements for stability and for effective conformations are quite different from those encountered in an anthropocentric biochemistry.

Although the era of explosive discovery of new bacteria is over, the few thousand species described in *Bergey's Manual* undoubtedly represent an incomplete set: these are almost all organisms capable of growth in pure culture on known media, and the range of the yet-undiscovered population with symbiotic or otherwise unfamiliar requirements is unknown. For example, a bacterial parasite on bacteria, *Bdellovibrio* (Lt. *Bdellus*, leech), was discovered only in 1962, although the organism is widespread and easily isolated. This very small bacterium bores a hole in the wall of a specific host bacterium (enzymatically and mechanically), occupies the space between the protoplast and the wall, grows to several times its initial length at the expense of the protoplast, and then divides into cells of the original length. A **magnetotactic** bacterium, recently isolated from muddy shallows, contains crystals of a magnetic iron oxide (magnetite), which orient it in the earth's magnetic field and thus direct its swimming toward the nearer magnetic pole: the downward component of that movement brings the organism to the low oxygen tension on which it thrives. Clearly, the natural historian's approach of Leeuwenhoek is still revealing new "animalcules."

Selected Reading

HISTORY; GENERAL

Brock TD (ed and trans): Milestones in Microbiology. Englewood Cliffs, NJ, Prentice-Hall, 1961. Reprinted by the American Society for Microbiology, 1975. An excellent selection of classic papers with helpful annotations; probably the best introduction to the history of the field.

Bulloch W: The History of Bacteriology. Cambridge, Oxford University Press, 1960; Paperback edition, New York, Dover, 1979. A detailed account, with emphasis on medical bacteriology.

Cairns J, Stent GS, Watson JD (eds): Phage and the Origins of Molecular Biology. Cold Spring Harbor, Cold Spring Harbor Laboratory, 1966

Collard P: The Development of Microbiology. Cambridge, Cambridge University Press, 1976. An excellent short history.

Dobell C: Antony van Leeuwenhoek and His "Little Animals." Originally published 1932; reprinted in paperback by New York, Dover, 1960

Dubos RJ: Louis Pasteur: Free Lance of Science. Boston, Little, Brown, 1950

Dubos RJ: The Professor, the Institute and DNA. New York, Rockefeller University Press, 1976. On the life and scientific achievements of OT Avery.

Jacob F: The Logic of Life: A History of Heredity. Pantheon, 1974

Lechevalier HA, Solotorovsky M: Three Centuries of Microbiology.

New York, McGraw-Hill, 1965; paperback edition, New York, Dover, 1974

Porter JR: Antony van Leeuwenhoek: Tercentenary of his discovery of bacteria. Bacteriol Rev 40:260, 1976

Stanier RY, Ingraham JL, Wheelis ML, Painter PR: The Microbial World, 5th Ed. Englewood Cliffs, NJ, Prentice-Hall, 1986. An excellent survey of general microbiology.

Starr MP, Stolp H, Truper HG, Ballows A, Schlegel HG: The Prokaryotes. New York, Springer, 1981. A useful source of information on the diversity of bacteria.

Valley–Radot R: The Life of Pasteur. Originally published 1901; reprinted in paperback by New York, Dover, 1960. This biography is detailed and chronological; that of Dubos (see above) is more interpretive.

EVOLUTION AND CLASSIFICATION

Barghoorn ES: The oldest fossils. Sci Am May 1971, p 30

Brenner DJ: Impact of modern taxonomy on clinical microbiology. Am Soc Microbiol News 49:58, 1983

Bergey's Manual of Systematic Bacteriology, 18th Ed. Vol 1: Krieg NR, Holt JG (eds), 1984; Vol 2: Sneath PHA, Holt JG (eds), 1985. Baltimore, Williams & Wilkins. Publication of the remaining two volumes is scheduled soon. This is the definitive work on bacterial taxonomy.

Carlile MJ, Collins JF, Moseley BEB (eds): Molecular and Cellular Aspects of Microbial Evolution: 32nd Symposium of the Society of General Microbiology. Cambridge, Cambridge University Press, 1981

Cech TR: Self-splicing RNA: Implications for evolution. Int Rev Cytol 93:3, 1985

Cowan ST: Manual for the Identification of Medical Bacteria. Cambridge, Cambridge University Press, 1974

Darnell, JE, Doolittle, WF: Speculations on the early course of evolution. Proc Natl Acad Sci USA 83:1271, 1986

Deley J, Kersters K: Biochemical evolution in bacteria. In Florkin M, Stotz EH (eds): Comprehensive Biochemistry, Vol 29B, p 1. Amsterdam, Elsevier, 1975

Eigen M, Gardiner W, Schuster P, Winkler–Oswatitsch R: The origin of genetic information. Sci Am April 1981, p 88

Fox GE et al: The phylogeny of prokaryotes. Science 200:457, 1980

Jannasch HW, Taylor CD: Deep-sea microbiology. Annu Rev Microbiol 38:487, 1984

Kandler O, Schleifer NH: Systematics of bacteria. Progr Bot 42:234, 1980

Lake JA: Evolving ribosome structure: Domains in archaebacteria, eubacteria, eocytes and eukaryotes. Annu Rev Biochem 54:507, 1985

Margulis L: Symbiosis in Cell Evolution. San Francisco, WH Freeman, 1981

Mayr E: Populations, Species, and Evolution. Cambridge, MA, Harvard University Press, 1970

Meyer TE, Cusanovich MA, Kamen MD: Evidence against use of bacterial amino acid sequence data for construction of all-inclusive phylogenetic trees. Proc Natl Acad Sci USA 83:217, 1986

Muto A, Osawa S: The guanine and cytosine content of genomic DNA and bacterial evolution. Proc Natl Acad Sci USA 84:166, 1987

Olsen GF, Lane DJ, Giovannoni SJ, Pace NR: Microbial ecology and evolution: A ribosomal RNA approach. Annu Rev Microbiol 40:337, 1986

Oparin AI: The Origin of Life on Earth, 3d Ed. New York, Academic Press, 1957

Schleifer KH, Stackebrandt E: Molecular systematics of prokaryotes. Annu Rev Microbiol 37:143, 1983

Selander RK, Caugant DA, Whittam TS: Genetic structure and variation in natural populations of *Escherichia coli*. In Neidhardt FC et al (eds): *Escherichia coli* and *Salmonella typhimurium*: Cellular and Molecular Biology. Washington, DC, American Society for Microbiology, 1987

Selander RK: Protein polymorphism and the genetic structure of natural populations of bacteria. In Ohta T, Aoki K (eds): Population Genetics and Molecular Evolution. New York, Springer, 1985

Van Niel CB: Natural selection in the microbial world. J Gen Microbiol 13:201, 1955

Woese CR: Bacterial evolution. Microbiol Rev 51:221, 1987

Woese CR, Wolfe RS (eds): The Bacteria: A Treatise on Structure and Function, Vol 8: The Archaebacteria. New York, Academic Press, 1985

Bacterial Architecture

Overview

Most bacteria have a diameter of about 1 μm (10^{-3} mm), so the light microscope, with a resolving power of 0.2 μm, can distinguish only their gross forms: spherical cocci (L., berry), rod-shaped **bacilli** (L., stick), and the curved **vibrios, spirilla,** and **spirochetes** (Fig. 2–1). (The term "bacillus" is also used, capitalized and italicized, as the name of a specific genus.) The electron microscope reveals a distinctive architecture (Fig. 2–2), with a simpler internal structure than eukaryotic cells (Ch. 1, Table 1–2). The only visible structures in the **cytoplasm** are the nuclear body, ribosomes, mesosomes (see below), and sometimes irregular granules of **reserve materials:** glycogen, **poly-β-hydroxybutyric acid** (a source of energy in many *Bacilli*), or polymetaphosphate (which stains metachromatically with certain dyes). Not present are endoplasmic reticulum, a nuclear membrane, and, except in photosynthetic species, organelles.

In contrast to the interior, the **cell envelope** surrounding the cytoplasm is more complex in prokaryotes than in eukaryotes, with a **cytoplasmic membrane** (also termed cell membrane or plasma membrane) and a rigid **cell wall.** The gram-negative organisms have an additional **outer membrane** and a **periplasmic space** (including the wall) between the two membranes. One specialized group, the mycoplasmas, lack the rigid wall. External to the envelope, bacteria may or may not carry flagella and a loose capsule or slime layer.

Gram-negative organisms have a thinner wall than gram-positive organisms, and usually have protruding protein rods (fimbriae). Gram-positives have a thick wall, which may be covered by a sheet of protein or of polysaccharide. The gram-positives also have protruding chains of teichoic acids, and a few gram-positives can form spores, which have even thicker walls.

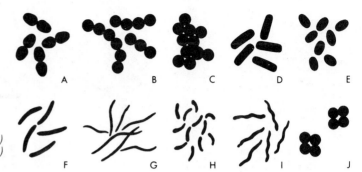

Figure 2–1. Bacterial forms. *(A)* Diplococci. *(B)* Streptococci. *(C)* Staphylococci. *(D)* Bacilli. *(E)* Coccobacilli. *(F)* Fusiform bacilli. *(G)* Filamentous bacillary forms. *(H)* Vibrios. *(I)* Spirilla. *(J)* Sarcinae.

The composition of a typical bacterium, in terms of its principal classes of components and their origins, is presented in Figure 2–3.

This chapter will consider the structures characteristic of most bacteria, and also the composition and formation of the rigid wall that determines the cell shape, the composition of the cell membranes, and the special features of spores. Later chapters will deal with special structures of less typical bacteria (actinomycetes, spirochetes, mycoplasmas, rickettsias, and chlamydias).

PROTOPLASTS AND SPHEROPLASTS

The cytoplasmic membrane is ordinarily pressed against the wall by an internal osmotic pressure that exceeds that of the external medium. When the wall is digested by lysozyme (see below), or when its synthesis is blocked in growing cells, the cell lyses. The wall thus protects bacteria against lysis and allows them to grow over a wide range of osmotic pressures. It is also rigid enough to give bacterial cells their characteristic shape.

In sufficiently hypertonic media cell contraction separates the membrane from the wall (**plasmolysis;** Fig. 2–4). (This observation demonstrates the existence of a distinct wall, with the membrane normally held against it by turgor.) Also, in such media (e.g., containing 20% sucrose or 0.5M KCl), digestion of the wall leads, not to lysis, but to formation of an **osmotically sensitive sphere.** These bodies are called **protoplasts** (consisting of the cytoplasmic membrane and its contents) when derived from gram-positive organisms and **spheroplasts** (with a fragmented outer membrane in addition) when derived from gram-negative organisms. Both these bodies maintain appropriate intracellular concentrations of small molecules through the function of the cytoplasmic membrane, and they can grow briefly (without cell division) and can regenerate the wall. They are useful for performing experimental genetic transfers that would be impeded by the wall.

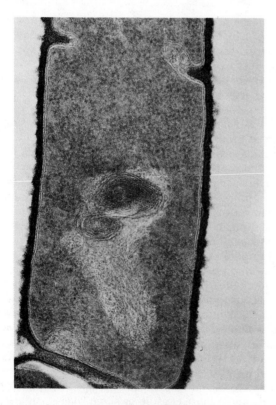

Figure 2–2. Section of portion of gram-positive *Bacillus subtilis,* including a completed but not yet cleaved **septum** at one end of the cell and a beginning septum forming an equatorial ring in the midzone of the cell. Note the well-defined **plasma membrane** ("double track" lining the inner surface of the dense wall) continuous with the small **vesicular mesosome** at one portion of the growing septum. Also note the two large concentric **lamellar mesosomes** in the nuclear region; their connection to the plasma membrane is not seen in this section. (Courtesy of A Ryter)

PROCEDURES

GRAM STAIN. In the identification of most medically important bacteria the gram stain, developed by Christian Gram in Denmark in 1884, is fundamental. In this procedure the cells are stained with a basic dye (crystal violet), treated with an iodine–KI mixture to fix the stain, washed with acetone or alcohol, and counterstained

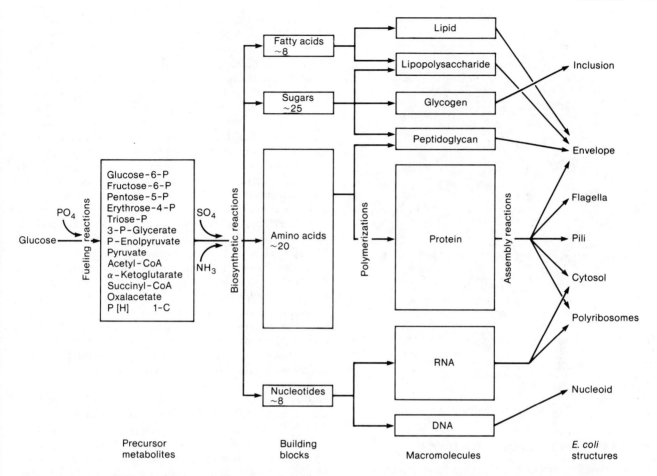

Figure 2–3. Overall view of metabolism leading to production of an *E. coli* cell from glucose. The size of each box is proportional to need. (After Ingraham JL et al: Growth of the Bacterial Cell, Sunderland, MA, Sinauer Associates, 1983)

with a paler dye of a different color (e.g., safranin). Whereas most bacteria take up the initial violet stain, only gram-positive ones retain it during the subsequent steps; gram-negative ones are thus decolorized by the organic solvent and hence show the counterstain. This empiric procedure was used for classifying bacteria for nearly 75 years before its mechanism was traced to the cell wall: the gram-positive organisms have a much thicker wall, which prevents elution of the dye–I_2 complex. As cultures age, gram-positive cells often become gram-negative because the wall deteriorates.

Special stains used for certain organisms (mycobacteria, corynebacteria, legionella, rickettsias) will be described in the corresponding chapters.

OTHER PROCEDURES. Objects that are too thin for resolution in the light microscope (e.g., certain spirochetes) can be seen by **darkfield microscopy,** in which they refract or reflect light entering from the side of the field of vision. In **electron microscopy,** shadowcasting with metal vapor reveals the shapes of appendages; negative staining (by drying in the presence of an electron-dense material) reveals finer surface structure; thin sections stained with a heavy metal resolve intracellular structures; freeze-fracturing creates new surfaces at natural lines of cleavage between the wall and membrane or between the two leaflets of a membrane; and antibodies tagged with ferritin or gold particles can be used to localize an antigen.

To obtain **cell extracts** by **lysis,** for biochemical studies, special methods are required to disrupt the tough walls of bacteria: grinding a wet paste with an abrasive; sonication (application of high-intensity sonic or supersonic vibrations); or explosive release of high pressure (usually past a needle valve in a French press). In a particularly gentle method that preserves long chains of DNA or RNA, protoplasts or spheroplasts are lysed osmotically or by treatment with a detergent.

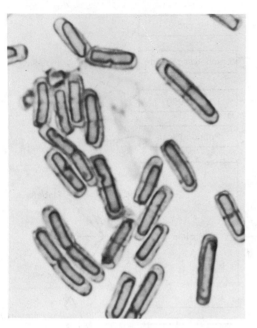

Figure 2—4. Plasmolysis of *Bacillus megaterium*. The cells on a slide were successively treated with ether vapor (which loosens the attachment of membrane to wall), air dried, postfixed with Bouin's fluid (which cause contraction of the protoplast), and stained with Victoria blue (which enhances the visibility of the membrane enclosing the protoplast). (Courtesy of C Robinow)

OPTIONAL APPENDAGES AND LAYERS

The outer surfaces of various bacteria carry a wide variety of materials and structures that are not essential for growth but that strongly influence the interactions with the environment.

FLAGELLA **(L.,** *FLAGELLUM:* **WHIP).** Engines of motility called flagella are found on many rod-shaped or curved bacteria. **Motility** can be seen under the microscope in a liquid medium (in a hanging drop or under a cover slip); it can also be recognized by tests for the spread of visible growth in cultures in semisolid medium (such as 0.3% agar.

In flagella a long (3- to 12-μm) filament with a loose spiral shape protrudes from the cell surface; it consists of molecules of a globular protein (**flagellin**) aggregated in a tight helical chain. Flagella exhibit marked serologic specificity in various bacterial strains. They are too thin (12–25 nm) to be seen by light microscopy unless heavily coated or aggregated by a precipitating agent such as tannic acid. Their structure, formation, and function will be further discussed in Chapter 4 (Motility).

Some species exhibit **polar** flagellation, with one or a few flagella at one or at both poles of the cell. In others, flagellation is **peritrichous** (Gr. *trichos* [pronounced trĭ-

kus], hair), with flagella attached along the cylinder as well (Fig. 2–5). This characteristic separates most bacteria into two orders, *Eubacteriales* (peritrichous) and *Pseudomonadales* (polar). (On the basis of other shared characteristics, many organisms lacking flagella are also assigned to these two groups.)

The number of flagella, and hence the vigor of bacterial movement, differs widely among species. Organisms such as *Proteus* that have a huge number (Fig. 2–5C) form a thin, spreading film ("swarm") when grown on the surface of the usual agar media. Among pathogens, motility is found predominantly in organisms that are adapted to growth in liquid (e.g., the gut, urine) but not in those that are adapted to tissues.

Other types of locomotion are also seen in bacteria. In spirochetes, a long, helical cell surrounds an axial filament from each end, resembling linear flagella; the cell spiral moves by rotating around the linear filament rather than vice versa. This form of motion is evidently better adapted than flagellar rotation for swimming through viscous fluids. Certain organisms (mycoplasmas, myxobacteria, cyanobacteria, and some oral bacteria) exhibit a slow gliding movement on solid surfaces. The mechanisms of contraction giving rise to these two kinds of movement are not well understood.

FIMBRIAE (PILI); ADHESINS. Most gram-negative bacteria have a set of additional filamentous appendages, called fimbriae (L., fringes) or pili (L., hairs). These are straight rigid rods, shorter and thinner than flagella (Fig. 2–6), composed of a single, highly hydrophobic protein, **pilin** (mol. wt. 17,000–25,000), tightly aggregated in a helical chain. Both flagella and fimbriae can be removed from cells by mechanical agitation, and they are rapidly regenerated during further cell growth.

Autoradiography shows that fimbriae grow by addition at the base, whereas flagella grow by flow of flagellin molecules through the hollow filament to the tip. Moreover, like other proteins that are exported into or across the membrane (Ch. 6), pilin is synthesized as a precursor with a leader segment that is cleaved when it enters the membrane, and the pilus is assembled from the processed molecules in the membrane. Flagella, in contrast, have a complex base, and the pilin evidently enters the flagellar lumen directly rather than via the membrane, as it is synthesized without the leader segment needed to enter the membrane (Ch. 6).

Most fimbriae, present in several hundred per cell, function as **adhesins,** mediating adhesion to specific surfaces (including coaggregation of different bacterial species in dental plaque). They therefore play an important role in pathogenesis, as has been established especially for the gonococcus (Ch. 26) and for pathogenic strains of *E. coli;* efforts are being made to develop vaccines based on these antigens. Through a reversible ge-

Figure 2–5. Flagella. *(A)* Flagellated bacillus stained with tannic acid–basic fuchsin, a flagellar stain. *(B)* Electron micrograph of palladium-shadowed bacillus, showing peritrichous flagellation. (>13,000) *(C)* Highly motile form of *Proteus mirabilis* ("swarmer") with innumerable peritrichous flagella. *(A,* Leifson E et al: J Bacteriol 69:73, 1955; *B,* Labaw LW, Mosley VM: Biochim Biophys Acta 17:322, 1955; *C,* Hoeniger JFM: J Gen Microbiol 40:29, 1965)

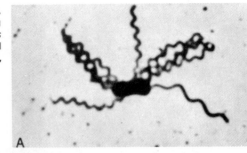

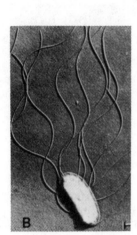

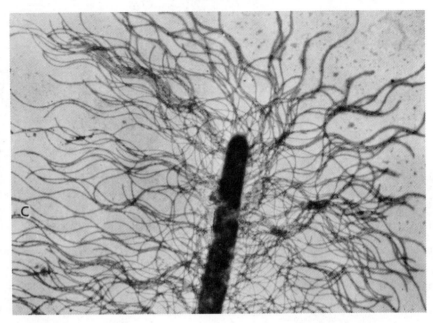

netic regulatory mechanism (Phase Variation; Ch. 7) bacteria shift rapidly between being fimbriated (Fim⁺) or not (Fim⁻). The former state promotes initial colonization but also increases susceptibility to phagocytosis; hence, its loss after colonization appears to promote tissue invasion.

A bacterium may possess several types of fimbriae, which differ in thickness and length, antigenic specificity, protein sequence, and specificity of the host glycoprotein receptor to which they attach. Most enterobacteria have type 1 fimbriae, 7 nm in diameter and 0.5 to 2 μm long, which attach to a variety of host cells, including erythrocytes (hemagglutination). They are classed, like some other fimbriae, as **mannose sensitive,** because mannose inhibits their hemagglutination by competing with the host cell receptor. It appears that the adhesin may not be the pilin but a special protein at the tip, because type 2 fimbriae have the same major antigen but not the same capacity for attachment. Most adhesins are **lectins;** i.e., proteins with high affinity for binding to specific carbohydrates.

Pathogenic strains of *E. coli* usually have additional, thinner fimbriae that are highly specific in their affinity for various epithelial cells: for example, in the human urinary tract or in the intestinal tract of particular species. Their hemagglutination is **mannose resistant.**

In addition to the fimbriae that function in adhesion, conjugating gram-negative bacteria have a special **sex pilus** (conjugal pilus) on the male (donor) cell, which initiates contact with the recipient cell (Ch. 7). Although the terminology has been controversial, the term "fimbriae" is now generally used for most of these structures, reserving "pilus" for the sexual appendage.

OTHER ADHESINS. In gram-positive bacteria a protein or a polysaccharide **surface layer,** rather than fimbriae, serves as specific adhesin. Streptococci form a fuzzy **fibrillar layer** of such protein, whose fibrils are shorter and more closely packed than fimbriae. Many bacteria have a two-dimensional crystalline array of protein on their surface (Fig. 2–7), sometimes in more than one layer.

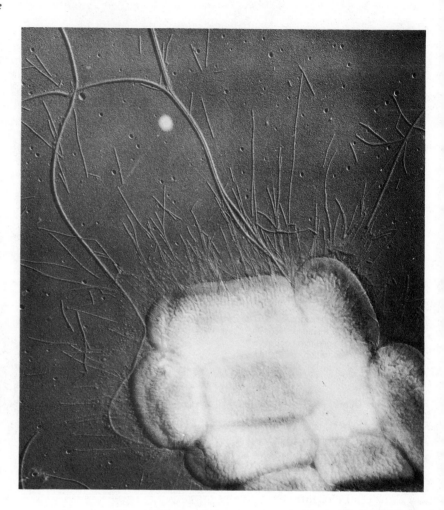

Figure 2–6. Pili. Piliated strain of *Escherichia coli* grown in liquid medium without aeration. Each cell possesses hundreds of pili (diameter 7 nm), and their presence promotes aggregation. Many isolated, broken pili are also seen. A few flagella, much longer and of larger diameter (14 nm), extend from the cells to the edge of the photograph. (Platinum shadowed: >45,000, reduced; courtesy of Charles C Brinton, Jr)

Flagella may serve not only for locomotion but also for specific adhesion. In *Vibrio cholerae*, the flagella are coated by the same lipopolysaccharide as the cell surface.

CAPSULES. The loose gels called capsules are easily seen by **negative staining** (e.g., suspension in India ink), appearing as a clear zone between the opaque medium and the refractile (or stained) cell body. Some capsules have a well-defined border, whereas others form a **slime layer** that trails off into the medium. Electron micrographs do not reveal any detail, and the fixation procedure produces artificial condensates unless the gel is stabilized by antibody.

Capsules are of particular importance in pathogenic bacteria because they protect from phagocytosis; however, slime layers may also function as adhesins. With most pathogens, capsule production is a stable property, and its loss in laboratory cultures usually eliminates pathogenicity. Conversely, the normally noncapsulated, nonpathogenic *Pseudomonas aeruginosa* frequently infects the lungs of cystic fibrosis patients, where the accumulated mucous fluid rapidly selects for encapsulated mutants that are somehow better adapted to that environment.

Soluble capsular substance may be released by partial hydrolysis or by diffusion from a loosely attached layer, and by competing with antibody it can interfere with tests that depend on the interaction of antibody with the bacteria. The thickness of the capsule can vary with nutrition and with temperature, as well as with mutations.

Immunologically distinct capsules are found in different strains (**types**) of many bacterial species. These are conveniently typed by the "**Quellung**" (Ger., swelling) reaction (Ch. 23, Fig. 23–1), in which binding of antibody increases the refractility and apparent thickness of the capsule. Most capsules consist of relatively simple polysaccharides, with repeating units of two or three sugars; representative pneumococcal structures are presented in Chapter 23. The variety of possible hexose stereoisomers

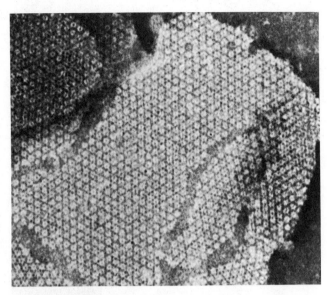

Figure 2–7. Regular hexagonal array of granules on the outer surface of isolated cell wall of a spirillum. Similarly regular rectangular arrays are found on many gram-positive bacteria, but the layer bearing the pattern is easily lost in preparation. (Negatively stained; ×204,000, reduced; courtesy of RGE Murray)

and of linkages, and the occasional incorporation of unusual sugars (C5, deoxy, uronic acids, etc.) can yield thousands of different trisaccharides. The chains are often attached to a membrane phospholipid, and they are built up, before this final attachment, on a membrane carrier lipid, as described for other surface polymers (see Peptidoglycan Biosynthesis, below).

Not all capsules are polysaccharides. Some *Bacilli* have simple polypeptide capsules. Bacteria that utilize hydrocarbons in the environment have emulsifying molecules, containing both hydrophilic polysaccharide and hydrophobic fatty acid residues.

NONSPECIFIC BACTERIAL ADHESION; BIOFILMS. Although bacteria can be best studied quantitatively as suspensions in aqueous media, in nature and in animal hosts they are often attached to surfaces. This process involves not only initial colonization of specific loci through the action of adhesins, as described above, but also nonspecific adhesion. The scanning electron microscope has revealed that moist surfaces in nature are almost universally covered with a biofilm: bacteria embedded in a tough film of adhesive polymer that they secrete. Because it often contains a polysaccharide, it has been called a **glycocalyx.**

Bacterial adhesion has long been of interest to investigators of soil, of corrosion, and of oral microbiology; only recently has its general importance in infectious disease been recognized. For example, in skin, even after vigorous scrubbing, *Staphylococcus epidermidis* cells can still be seen, surrounded by amorphous material, in crypts in the keratin created by bacterial proteolysis. Moreover, intravascular or other catheters passing through the skin invariably develop a biofilm of these relatively avirulent organisms (Fig. 2–8), which are not harmful as long as the numbers released to the circulation do not overwhelm the host defense mechanisms. Similarly, after different streptococci have specifically colonized different mucous surfaces (e.g., teeth, gums, tongue), the sticky polysaccharides they excrete strengthen the adhesion. Chronic systemic lesions (e.g., endocarditis, osteomyelitis, urinary tract infection) involve much thicker deposits. The glycocalyx slows bacterial growth, protects against phagocytes, and inhibits the penetration of antibodies and antimicrobial drugs.

NUCLEAR BODY (NUCLEOID)

In bacteria the high concentration of ribosomes makes the cytoplasm as basophilic as the nuclear region. The usual basic dyes therefore fail to reveal a discrete nuclear body, although one can be shown by special stains for DNA. In electron microscopy, after fixation by the usual methods, thin sections show a centrally located mass, much less heavily stained than the cytoplasm and free of ribosomes. Because this structure lacks a nuclear membrane it is called a **nucleoid** rather than a nucleus.

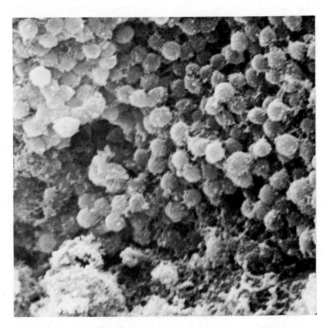

Figure 2–8. Scanning electron micrograph of cocci embedded in a polysaccharide matrix (which contracts into fibers on drying) forming a layer on the surface of an intraperitoneal catheter. (Courtesy of JW Costerton)

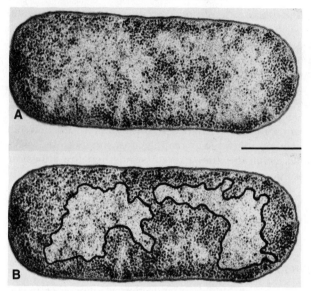

Figure 2–9. Section of a freeze-substituted growing cell of *E. coli*. The lobulated nucleoid is free of the densely staining ribosomes that pack the rest of the cytoplasm. *(A)* is identical to *(B)* except that an outline has been drawn around the borders of the nucleoid. (Hobot JA et al: J Bacteriol 162:960, 1985)

Defined as the region that excludes ribosomes, the nucleoid represents about 10% of the cell volume, although DNA is only 2% to 3% of the cell's dry weight. Genetic studies (Ch. 7) and electron microscopy after gentle lysis show that bacteria contain a **single, covalently closed, circular chromosome.** However, because growing bacteria replicate their DNA through most or all of a cycle of cell division, the nucleoid usually contains a partly replicated chromosome (see Ch. 9; DNA Replication.) In *E. coli* the chromosome contains 3×10^6 base pairs, and its length is about 1000 times the diameter of the cell.

The existence of a localized nucleoid can also be demonstrated in living cells by phase contrast examination of organisms growing in media of appropriate refractive index. However, its structural details have been uncertain in electron micrographs. Earlier methods, which allowed cells to cease growth before fixation, produced bodies with a compact, markedly fibrillar structure (see Fig. 2–2), but this now appears to be the structure of an inactive chromosome. The structure present in growing cells is retained better by rapid freezing of such cells, followed by freeze-substitution (dehydration at low temperature). This technique has revealed a highly lobulated ribosome-free central body distributed through much of the cytoplasm, with a granular fine structure containing short fibrils (Fig. 2–9).

If cells are gently lysed in ordinary media the structure of the nucleoid is lost, and the chromosome is widely dispersed (Fig. 2–10A). However, with a sufficiently high concentration of divalent cations to neutralize the electrostatic repulsion of the nucleic acid chains, the intact nucleoid can be isolated. Such preparations

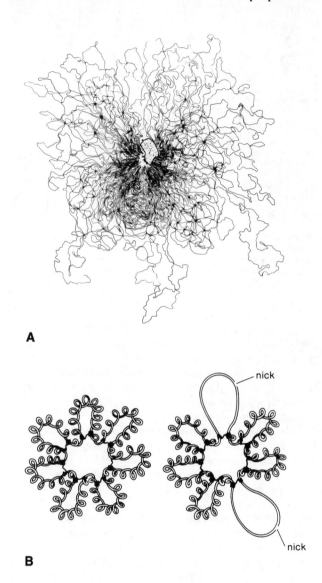

A

B

Figure 2–10. Different states of the chromosome. *(A)* Looping out of DNA from an exploded bacterial cell, spread on a surface layer of a basic protein. (Courtesy of L MacHattie). *(B)* Diagram of supercoiled DNA. Part **A** represents seven domains (actual number is about 50 in a bacterial chromosome), each supercoiled and prevented from uncoiling by a set of proteins (linked pair of small solid circles at the base of each domain) that hold the ends of a domain together. The small loops depicted in each domain may each be wound around a nucleosomal set of proteins, thus decreasing the unwinding tension in the double helix created by the supercoil. In part **B**, two domains have been nicked by a break in one strand, allowing free rotation of the helix and hence relaxation of the supercoiling. (Pettijohn DE, Sinden RR: In Nanninga N [ed]: Molecular Cytology of Escherichia coli. New York, Academic Press, 1985)

contain about 60% DNA, 30% RNA, and 10% protein. They have made possible biochemical studies of the organization of the bacterial chromosome.

SUPERCOILING. The chromosome in the isolated nucleoid is folded in much the same manner as eukaryotic chromosomes, with considerable negative supercoiling; i.e., a partial untwisting of the double helix, which increases the number of nucleotides per Watson–Crick turn from 10 (as in relaxed, noncircular DNA) to 10.5. The resulting tension within the helix provides energy for separating the two strands, as required for replication and for transcription. The extent of supercoiling can be measured from its effect on various physical properties of the DNA; it is carefully maintained by a balance between its formation by DNA gyrase and its relaxation by topoisomerase I. The tension from negative supercoiling is also regulated by formation of loops of DNA, each wound around a protein body. Each loop removes a turn of the helix and thus relieves tension, just as does the coiling of a twisted garden hose into loops.

In eukaryotes the multi-protein bodies around which DNA loops, the **nucleosomes,** have been well defined. In lysates of prokaryotes they are less stable and less well understood. They appear to contain two **DNA-binding proteins, HU** and **protein 1,** which are present in the nucleoid in a ratio of 1 per 150 to 200 base pairs (similar to the histones in eukaryotic nuclei). Moreover, like the histones, protein HU is small (9700 daltons), basic, and highly conserved (in this case, over the whole prokaryotic kingdom). The granular chromosomal structures revealed by electron microscopy (Fig. 2-9) have about the same frequency as protein HU and probably correspond to the bacterial nucleosomes.

LONG-RANGE FOLDING. To maintain tension in a supercoiled double helix, the ends must be held together in some way. With the relatively short chains of viruses and plasmids, as we will see later, this resistance to uncoiling is provided by the closed circular structure of the DNA. The bacterial chromosome is also a closed circle, but in addition, it is folded into about 100 separately coiled **domains,** which are seen to protrude when the cell is lysed under gentle conditions (Fig. 2–10*A*). Because denaturants eliminate these loops and release the chromosome as a single circle, it appears that proteins attached at the base of each domain restrain it from relaxing. Nascent RNA also contributes to folding of the chromosome: treatment of isolated nucleoids with RNase makes them less compact without destroying the domains.

The chromosomal domains are topographically independent, as shown by nicking of double-stranded DNA by DNase to create a single-stranded swivel, which allows free rotation and hence relaxes a supercoil: limited nicking of the nucleoid *in vitro* relaxes domains sepa-

rately (Fig. 2–10*B*), as shown by quantitation of the decrease in supercoiling. This organization of the chromosome into domains permits one region to be relaxed in the cell (e.g., for replication or repair) without affecting the function of the others, and it probably participates in the coordinate regulation of expression of genes within the same domain.

Unlike animals, bacteria have relatively little noncoding DNA in their chromosomes. However, many bacteria have several hundred copies of a 20- to 40-base palindrome outside their genes; and although the function of these structures is not certain, they may well be involved in chromosomal organization. They differ in sequence among species, suggesting that they also serve to maintain species barriers.

ACCESS TO GENES. As will be discussed in Chapter 6, messenger RNA (mRNA) in bacteria, while attached to DNA and being transcribed, is simultaneously translated by ribosomes. Because no ribosomes penetrate the nucleoid, transcription presumably occurs on invisible loops of DNA projecting from its surface. Supporting this inference, in thin sections, gold-labeled antibodies to single-stranded DNA stain only the edge of the nucleoid, whereas antibodies to double-stranded DNA stain the central region. Moreover, when protein synthesis is halted by chloramphenicol freeze-substituted preparations reveal a much more compact nucleoid.

The nucleoid thus does not have a sharp boundary. It cannot be a static structure, since a large fraction of the genes in a bacterium are being transcribed and translated at a given time; moreover, the kinetics of response of an inducible gene to its inducer indicates that any gene has access to ribosomes within a few seconds. It thus appears that the exposure of loops to the surface is a highly dynamic process. RNA polymerase can penetrate the nucleoid, but it is not clear how its attachment, or the subsequent transcription, rapidly exteriorizes the corresponding region of DNA.

REPLICATION. Because bacteria contain only one kind of chromosome, they do not require a mitotic apparatus to segregate the products of replication coordinately to the daughter cells. Instead, the chromosome is attached to the membrane, often via an invagination called a **mesosome** (see Mesosomes, below), in the region where a septum will be formed. Replication originates at a specific DNA sequence in the chromosome (*oriC*), proceeds in both directions around the chromosome, and terminates at a specific sequence. The membrane attachments of the daughter chromosomes are then separated by the growing septum.

The completed daughter chromosomes appear to be initially interlocked (catenated). Mutations in **DNA gyrase** show that this enzyme is required for daughter separation. This remarkable enzyme creates supercoiling by cleaving a strand of DNA, rotating the ends around the second strand, and rejoining them; and it evidently can also allow another DNA chain to pass through a temporary opening first in one strand and then in the other, thus separating a catenated pair of circles.

Molecular aspects of chromosome replication are further described in Chapter 8 (Chromosome Replication).

Cell Wall

Among the several layers constituting the bacterial **cell envelope,** the wall is responsible for the shape of the cell and for protection against osmotic lysis. In sections fixed by OsO_4 the wall of gram-positive bacteria appears as an electron-dense layer 20 to 50 nm thick surrounding a cytoplasmic membrane of about 8 nm (see Fig. 2–2). Gram-negative bacteria have a much thinner wall and an additional, closely apposed outer membrane; the wall is not easily seen, but its digestion by lysozyme shows that it lies between the two membranes (Fig. 2–11).

The wall presents a unique problem in cellular architecture. Other complex cell components (e.g., membrane, ribosomes) assemble spontaneously, but the wall must insert new blocks into a sheet that is already held together by covalent bonds. Its growth and its develop-

ment of a specific shape therefore entail a finely regulated pattern of enzymatic opening as well as closure of bonds.

PEPTIDOGLYCAN STRUCTURE

Purified cell walls can be prepared, for chemical analysis, by mechanically disrupting the cells (e.g., by ultrasound, by an abrupt release of high pressure, or by shaking with glass beads) and then separating the insoluble envelope from the soluble contents; attached proteins and membrane can be removed by proteases or detergents. In such preparations, the wall retains its basic outline (Fig. 2–12). Although peptidoglycan is the main component, responsible for rigidity, the wall also contains covalently attached chains of other materials.

The peptidoglycan has a very similar structure in all bacteria (except arachaebacteria: Ch. 1). As in the example in Figure 2–13, the **backbone** is a glycan chain: a repeating disaccharide of N-acetylglucosamine (GlcNAc) and its lactyl ether, N-acetylmuramate (MurNAc). **Muramic acid** (L., *murus*, wall) is unique to bacterial peptidoglycan. Each disaccharide carries a **tetrapeptide** substituent of alternating L and D amino acids, and **peptide bridges** link the terminal COOH of one tetrapeptide to an NH_2 group of a tetrapeptide on a neighboring glycan chain. The linked NH_2 group is on **diaminopimelate** (ly-

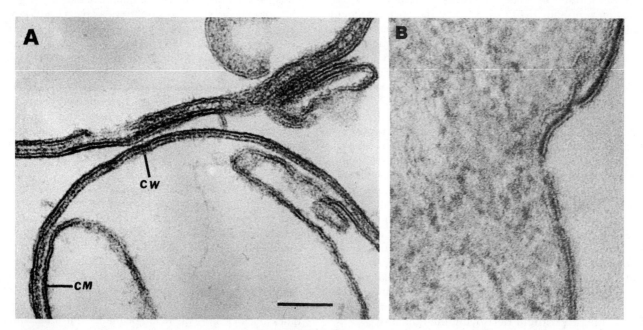

Figure 2–11. Cell wall of gram-negative bacteria. *(A)* Separation of the cytoplasmic membrane *(CM)* from the cell wall *(CW)* in purified envelope of *E. coli.* *(B)* Partial dissolution of peptidoglycan layer of the cell wall of *E. coli* on brief treatment with lysozyme. The upper half of the section of wall has a thick, dense band outside the plasma membrane and separated by a clear layer of constant thickness from an outer, thin, dense band; untreated cells have the same structure. In the lower half, lysozyme has removed much of the thick layer, but a thinner residue remains. Thus, in this gram-negative wall, the peptidoglycan is fused with the outer layer, which is left after peptidoglycan removal. (*A,* Schnaitman CA: J Bacteriol 108:545, 1971; *B,* courtesy of RGE Murray; see Can J Microbiol 11:547, 1965)

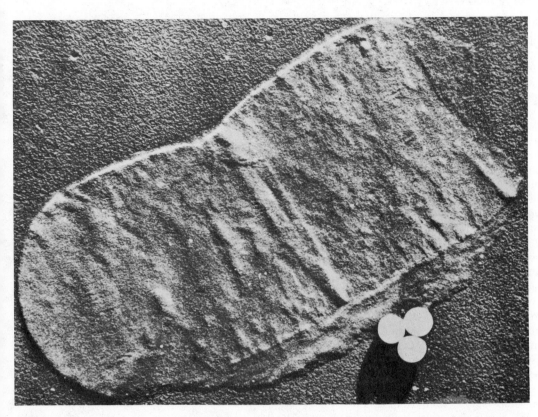

Figure 2–12. Shadow-cast electron micrograph of purified wall preparation from *Bacillus megaterium.* Note flattened structure compared with intact cell. Latex balls are 0.25 μm. (Salton MRJ, Williams RC: Biochim Biophys Acta 14:455, 1954)

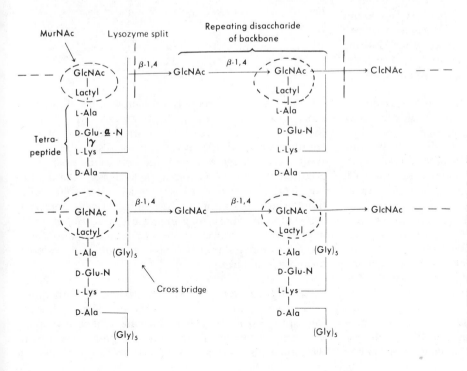

Figure 2–13. Structure of peptidoglycan of *Staphylococcus aureus.* The polysaccharide chains (backbone) are β-1,4-linked polymers of alternating residues of *N*-acetylglucosamine (GlcNAc) and its 3-D-lactic ether (MurNAc, *N*-acetylmuramic acid; structure in Fig. 2–14). (The chain can also be considered a substituted homopolymer of GlcNAc, but because the lactic ether bond is very stable, the muramic acid is ordinarily recovered as such in hydrolysates.) The COOH of the lactic group is attached to a tetrapeptide, which is in turn linked by a peptide cross-bridge to a tetrapeptide on a neighboring polysaccharide chain (which may be above, below, or in the depicted plane). Teichoic acid chains are attached to occasional MurNAc residues.

sine with an additional, terminal COOH) in most bacteria but on lysine in gram-positive cocci.

The peptidoglycan structure was dissected largely through the use of enzymes. **Lysozyme** (ordinarily obtained from egg white but also present in body fluids) hydrolyzes a specific glycoside bond in the glycan chain, yielding the disaccharide GlcNAc–MurNAc carrying various substituents. Bacteriolytic enzymes specific for other linkages were obtained from various sources (especially snails, which digest bacteria), and their use yielded a variety of other fragments. Identification of these compounds and of accumulated biosynthetic intermediates (see Biosynthesis, below) revealed the structure.

The entire peptidoglycan of a cell is thus **one giant, bag-shaped, covalently linked molecule,** called the **murein sacculus.** In *E. coli*, it is one layer thick, whereas in some gram-positive bacteria the amount of peptidoglycan corresponds to 20 layers or more. Because the layers do not peel apart in isolated walls the glycan chains are evidently cross-linked between the concentric sheets as well as within them. The strength of the murein sacculus depends on its extensive cross-linking, for the average chain length in *E. coli* is only about 30 disaccharides, as determined by quantitation of the terminal residues. (The growing end of a chain, attached to a carrier, is a reducing group, but when it is released the cell converts this group to the more stable, nonreducing, 1,6-anhydro-N-AcMur.)

Several features contribute to the toughness of the peptidoglycan. Its glycan chain has a particularly compact link (β-1,4), like the chitin (a poly-N-acetylglucosamine) of fungal cell walls and arthropod exoskeletons. Alternating L and D amino acids, as in the tetrapeptide, also form more compact polymers than either kind of monomer alone. In addition, the glycan structure predicts extensive hydrogen bonding between parallel chains.

Although these features make the murein sacculus firm enough to retain its shape, its rigidity is only relative: it undergoes extensive bending in spirochetal motility, and the flexible cross-links, as in a stretch fabric, permit osmotic changes to expand and contract the volume of bacterial cells substantially. The thin gram-negative wall is highly permeable, and the cell relies on the porosity of the outer membrane to limit the access of molecules to the cytoplasmic membrane (see below). In gram-positive bacteria the thicker wall provides that function, with a porosity of about 1.1 nm (mol. wt. 1200).

Peptidoglycans of various organisms differ in various features: amino acids 2 and 3 of the tetrapeptide, the structure of the cross-linking bridge, and the frequency of cross-links (Table 2–1). In the single layer in gram-negative organisms the glycan chains are often brought close together by a direct bond between tetrapeptides, without an additional bridging sequence. Pathogens of-

---

TABLE 2–1. Peptidoglycan Variations in Gram-Positive Bacteria

Type structure

Variations in tetrapeptide

α
Position 2: D-Glu-COOH
α
D-Glu-CONH$_2$
α
D-Glu-Gly
Position 3: L-Lys
meso-DAP
L,L-DAP
L-Ornithine
L-α,γ-Diaminobutyric acid
L-Homoserine
L-Glu
L-Ala

Variations in cross-bridge from D-Ala (position 4) of one tetrapeptide to NH$_2$ or COOH in another tetrapeptide:
  To NH$_2$ at position 3 via
    Direct peptide bond (i.e., COOH of D-Ala to NH$_2$ of Lys)
    (Gly)$_5$
    (L-Ala)$_4$–L-Thr
    (Gly)$_3$–(L-Ser)$_2$
    L-Ser–L-Ala
    L-Ala–L-Ala
    D-Asp-NH$_2$
    D-Asp–L-Ala
    Standard tetrapeptide
To COOH at position 2 (requiring a diamino acid in the cross-bridge):
    D-Ornithine
    D-Diaminobutyric acid
    Gly–L-Lys

---

ten have a higher frequency of cross-links than most other species (e.g., 75% in *Staph. aureus*), which makes them more resistant to lysis by the lysozyme they encounter in body fluids. In various organisms the initially synthesized structure may undergo various post-incorporation modifications, including loss of N-Ac and addition of O-Ac on glycoside residues, as well as shifts in the number and positions of cross-links. As cells approach the stationary phase they increase the degree of cross-linking and the concentration of covalently bound lipoprotein—changes that increase strength and evidently promote long-term survival.

WALL-LESS PROKARYOTES. Many bacteria, both gram-positive and gram-negative, give rise occasionally to wall-less, spherical forms called **L-forms.** Unlike mycoplasmas (Ch. 40), which have evolved a pattern of growth without walls, L-forms can revert to normal cells. Although some L-forms may result from mutations, in most, the change is only phenotypic; i.e., formation of the wall has become uncoordinated and evidently ceases for lack of acceptor molecules. L-forms will be further discussed in Chapter 41.

ADDITIONAL COMPONENTS OF GRAM-POSITIVE WALLS; TEICHOIC ACIDS

The wall of gram-positive bacteria also contains long-chain polymers, called teichoic acids (Gr., *teichos*, wall), which protrude at the surface and provide much of the wall's antigenic specificity. They also play a role in wall morphogenesis (see Autolysins, below). Teichoic acids consist of chains of as many as 30 **glycerol** or **ribitol** (a 5-C polyhydric alcohol) residues with phosphodiester links and with various substituents (sugars, choline, D-alanine) that provide the specificity:

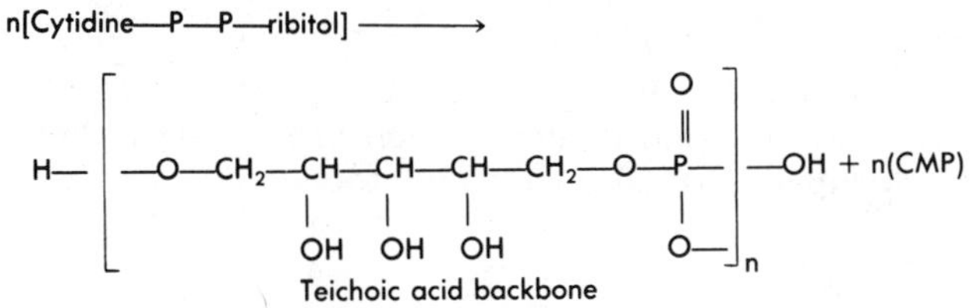

n[Cytidine—P—P—ribitol] ⟶

Teichoic acid backbone
(polyribitol phosphate)

There are two classes of cell-bound teichoic acid. All gram-positive bacteria have a **lipoteichoic acid** traversing the peptidoglycan: one end of the chain is linked to a glycoplipid in the membrane, while the other end is exposed on the exterior. Some organisms also have a **wall teichoic acid,** which is attached to MurNAc residues. In addition, large amounts of free soluble teichoic acid may be excreted.

Under phosphate limitation, which prevents teichoic acid production, *B. subtilis* makes instead **teichuronic acid:** chains of glycosidically linked uronic acid residues with free COOH groups and various substituents. The wall thus appears to require highly acidic polymers, with either phosphate or COOH groups.

Gram-positive organisms may also have a covalently bound true polysaccharide (e.g., *Streptococcus* C carbohydrate) or an external protein layer (e.g., *Streptococcus* M protein). The protein layers sometimes form a beautifully regular array (see Fig. 2–6). Gram-negative organisms, whose peptidoglycan is covered by the outer membrane, evidently do not provide a proper base for such surface structures.

PEPTIDOGLYCAN BIOSYNTHESIS

Synthesis of peptidoglycans has four main stages: (1) synthesis of a water-soluble, nucleotide-linked precursor in the cytoplasm; (2) its transfer from the nucleotide to a membrane lipid, followed by addition of substituents; (3) addition of this prefabricated block to a linear glycan chain on the far side of the membrane; and (4) cross-linking to an adjacent chain.

SOLUBLE INTERMEDIATES. Park discovered that penicillin-treated staphylococci accumulate a novel kind of compound, a short peptide attached to a nucleotide; but its significance remained obscure until the wall was purified several years later and found to contain the same few amino acids. Thus began a long mutual interaction of studies on wall synthesis and on penicillin action.

The principal accumulated compound is the uridine nucleotide of MurNAc, whose lactic carboxyl is attached to a **pentapeptide** (Fig. 2–14). The accumulation also of

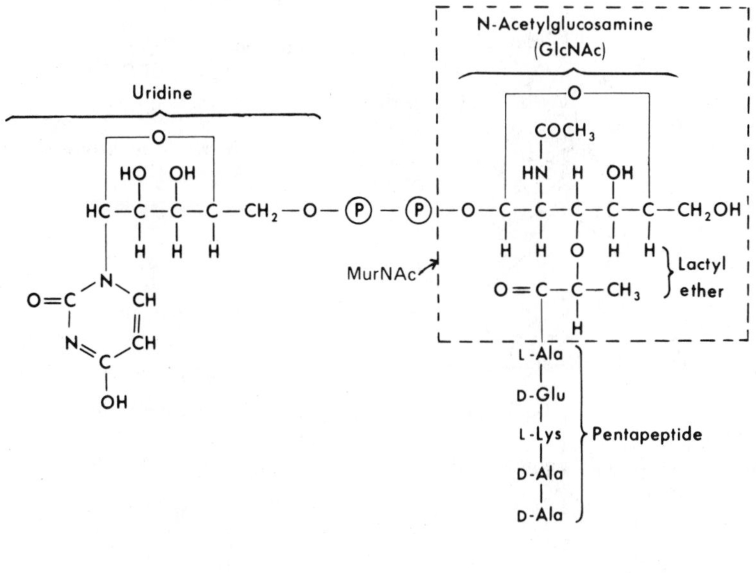

Figure 2–14. Structure of UDP-MurNAc-pentapeptide, a uridine nucleotide from penicillin-treated *Staph. aureus*.

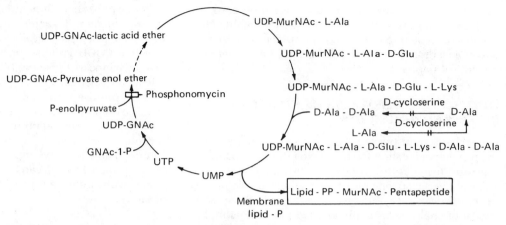

Figure 2–15. Pathway of biosynthesis of the UDP-muramic-pentapeptide wall precursor in *Staph. aureus.* The individual amino acids are added with the use of energy from ATP. The sites of action of various inhibitors, which have been useful in working out this pathway, are indicated. (After Strominger JL, Tipper DJ, Am J Med 39:708, 1965)

smaller precursors, and Strominger's separation of the enzymes, then established the biosynthetic sequence (Fig. 2–15). This process utilizes 15 different enzymes for the successive additions of the monomers and of the terminal D-Ala–D-Ala as a dipeptide.

LIPID-ATTACHED INTERMEDIATES. The next two stages (Fig. 2–16), which will incorporate radioactively labeled precursor into acid-insoluble peptidoglycan chains, can also be carried out *in vitro* with a particulate (i.e., membrane-derived) enzyme preparation. The first part of this process transfers P-MurNAc–pentapeptide from the nucleotide to the phosphate of a **membrane carrier lipid, undecaprenol-P** (also called **bactoprenol-P**):

$$H - (CH_2 - \overset{\overset{\textstyle CH_3}{\textstyle |}}{C} = CH - CH_2)_{11} - OP$$

Still facing the cytoplasm, the lipid-attached intermediate adds GlcNAc and any bridging sequence. (The five Gly residues of this sequence in staphylococci are enzymatically transferred from aminoacyl-tRNAs.)

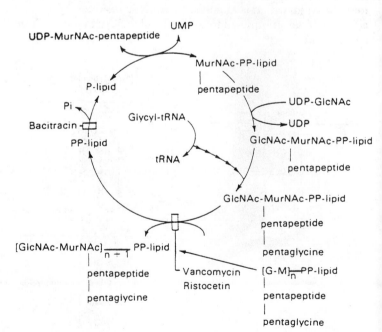

Figure 2–16. Lipid carrier cycle in peptidoglycan synthesis in *Staph. aureus.* The carrier lipid is undecaprenol, which enters the cycle as a monophosphate and builds up a substituted disaccharide unit attached as a pyrophosphate. That unit, on the carrier, serves as recipient for transfer of a growing chain of n units from an identical carrier. The latter is then recycled. (Modified from Matsuhashi M et al: Proc Natl Acad Sci USA 54:587, 1965; Ghuysen JM: Bacteriol Rev 32:425, 1968)

GLYCAN POLYMERIZATION. The **transglycosylation** reaction of glycan polymerization is carried out, like protein synthesis (Ch. 6), by "head synthesis": the reducing end of an existing glycan chain (acceptor), attached to one molecule of lipid carrier, is transferred from it to the disaccharide of the incoming subunit (donor) on an identical carrier. The released carrier (**undecaprenol-PP**) then loses a P, thus regenerating the form that can accept a precursor. The energy released by this P–P hydrolysis is presumably used to promote the reaction and perhaps also to promote reorientation of the undecaprenol-P toward the inner face of the membrane.

How a carrier lipid transfers the donor subunit from the cytoplasmic face of the membrane to a site of chain elongation, and how the lipid moves back, is obscure. It would not be thermodynamically possible for the undecaprenol to flip-flop in a way that dragged the attached highly polar precursor through the lipid of the membrane from one face to the other. Alternatively, whereas most of the cytoplasmic membrane surface is not attached to the peptidoglycan, the contacts between the growing end of the peptidoglycan chain (attached to undecaprenol in the membrane), the adjacent **transglycosylase,** and the donor subunit on another undecaprenol may require a discontinuity in the membrane leaflets, blurring the distinction between the inner and outer faces. The precursor might reach the enzyme at such an edge without passing through the membrane lipid. The electron microscope demonstrates such adhesion zones but cannot provide any detail (Fig. 2–17).

CROSS-LINKING. Because the **transpeptidation** reaction (Fig. 2–18), like transglycosylation, takes place outside the cytoplasm, it does not have access to ATP. The source of the energy is the terminal D-Ala on the pentapeptide, which is displaced by a free NH_2 from a neighboring glycan chain. The pentapeptide of the precursor thus is converted to the tetrapeptide of the murein.

STEPS INHIBITED BY VARIOUS ANTIBIOTICS

The interference by **penicillin** with wall formation was traced to inhibition of the **transpeptidation** reaction. Moreover, electron microscopy shows that penicillin-treated cells accumulate amorphous material between the membrane and the wall. There is a close structural analogy between D-Ala–D-Ala and the β-lactam ring of penicillin (and other β-lactam antibiotics), and that high-

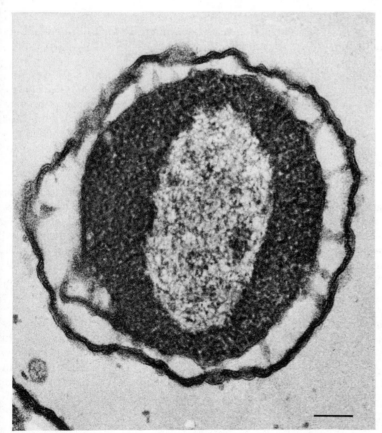

Figure 2–17. Areas of adhesion between the wall and inner membrane of *E. coli.* After plasmolysis (shrinkage in 20% sucrose for 2 minutes), the cells were fixed in formaldehyde and OsO_4, embedded, and sectioned. Numerous duct-like extensions from membrane to wall are seen; these are the sites of attachment of various phages to the outer surface of the wall and the probable sites of synthesis of outer membrane. (Bayer ME: J Gen Microbiol 53:395, 1968)

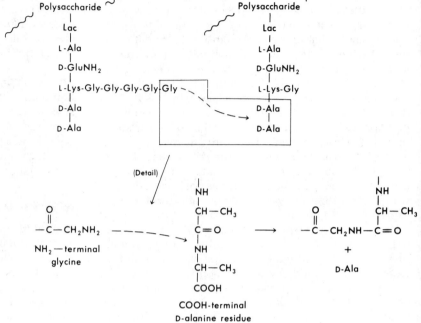

Figure 2–18. The penicillin-sensitive transpeptidation reaction in *Staph. aureus,* which completes the cross-link between different peptide side chains: the D-Ala → D-Ala peptide bond (CO → NH) is replaced by a similar D-Ala → Gly bond. Other species use other cross-links than the pentaglycine bridge (Table 2–1).

energy ring (Ch. 10) reacts with the transpeptidase to form a stable covalent bond, thus inactivating both the enzyme and the β-lactam (suicide inhibition). The normal substrate, D-Ala–D-Ala, reacts with the same group on the enzyme, but it then undergoes transpeptidation.

Other antibiotics act on other steps in peptidoglycan synthesis. **Cycloserine,** a structural analogue of D-Ala, competitively inhibits both the racemization of L-Ala to D-Ala and the conversion of the latter to the dipeptide D-Ala–D-Ala. **Fosfomycin (phosphonomycin),** an antibiotic analogue of P-enolpyruvate, irreversibly inhibits its conversion to the ether-linked lactyl group of UDP-MurNAc (see Fig. 2–15). **Moenomycin** blocks transfer of muramyl peptide to the growing chain. **Vancomycin** blocks transpeptidation through the unusual mechanism of binding, not to the enzyme, but to D-Ala–D-Ala in several intermediates and also in peptidoglycan. **Bacitracin** also binds to a substrate, undecaprenol-PP, blocking the dephosphorylation required to recycle it to its active form, undecaprenol-P.

These antibiotics will be further considered in Chapter 10.

PEPTIDOGLYCAN MORPHOGENESIS

Wall morphogenesis involves complex modifications of peptidoglycan synthesis, with hydrolytic as well as polymerizing reactions regulated in space as well as in time. The β-lactams have played a key role in the limited

advances that have been made so far in understanding these reactions.

PENICILLIN-BINDING PROTEINS. Because the reaction of transpeptidase with β-lactams yields stable products, the enzyme could be easily identified after reaction with a radioactively labeled β-lactam, and also easily purified by affinity chromatography with a β-lactam attached to a gel. Such labeling, combined with gel electrophoresis, revealed that there are not one but about six penicillin-binding proteins (PBPs) in a bacterium, numbered in order of decreasing molecular weight. Differences in their function have been elucidated by several approaches, including differential inhibition by various β-lactams, alteration in mutants, and characterization of the purified enzymes.

These studies have shown that *E. coli* PBP-la and PBP-lb are involved in **elongation of the cylinder** and that their inactivation by an antibiotic causes rapid lysis; either, but not both, can be eliminated by mutation without loss of viability. PBP-2 is involved in **cell shape,** as its specific inactivation by mecillinam causes the cells to round up for a generation or two before death. PBP-3 is involved in **septum formation,** as its specific inhibition by azthreonam causes formation of long filaments before cell death. These are all sites of lethal action. Incidentally, an old observation that sublethal concentrations of penicillin cause bacilli to grow as long filaments can now be explained by partial inactivation of the PBP-3.

Enzymatic studies further showed that these three PBPs are **double-headed** enzymes, carrying out both **transglycosylation** and **transpeptidation.** The β-lactams inactivate only the latter reaction. (This explains why cells accumulate amorphous peptidoglycan in their presence; and the accumulation of a nucleotide-attached precursor may be attributable to an indirect impairment of transglycosylation by the wall disorganization.) Since antibiotics that block transglycosylation also prevent transpeptidation it appears that the incoming subunit must be transglycosylated before it can be cross-linked.

The smaller PBPs 4, 5, and 6 are **D,D-carboxypeptidases,** which release the terminal D-Ala from a pentapeptide and thus form tetrapeptide with a free terminus (which cannot enter a cross-link). These enzymes also can act as an **endopeptidase** on existing cross-links, again releasing the tetrapeptide terminus. They evidently function only in guiding morphogenesis and not in polymerization, and they can all be eliminated without lethal effect.

AUTOLYSINS. PBPs are not the only enzymes involved in wall morphogenesis. Lysis by penicillin was long assumed to be secondary simply to mechanical bursting of the peptidoglycan by expansion of the growing protoplast, but further study in the pneumococcus has shown that it depends on autolytic enzymes: primarily an **amidase** that splits the bond between tetrapeptides and the glycan, and a **glycosidase** that cleaves the glycan. When these enzymes are rendered inactive (by growth at low pH or by certain mutations) penicillin becomes **bacteriostatic** rather than lytic. However, these "autolysins," and additional murein hydrolases that attack other bonds, have presumably evolved for a role in morphogenesis rather than to permit bacteria to self-destruct.

This function of the several murein hydrolases probably depends on their specific distribution in various regions of the membrane and on the effects of physical tensions in the peptidoglycan on their access to various bonds. Teichoic acid evidently plays a regulatory role: when the choline in the teichoic acid in pneumococci is replaced by ethanolamine the growing cells fail to split into diplococci and penicillin is only bacteriostatic.

TOPOLOGY OF THE PEPTIDOGLYCAN CHAINS. When the wall of rod-shaped bacteria has been loosened by partial hydrolysis, electron micrographs suggest that the glycan chains are oriented perpendicular to the cell axis, probably in a tight spiral. Similarly, the growing septum at sites of cell division normally exhibits concentric rings. The mechanism of insertion of new chains into an already cross-linked peptidoglycan is obscure. The 100 or more adhesion zones of the cytoplasmic membrane (see Fig. 2–17) are presumably each sites of insertion, moving around the axis of the cell.

Structural models suggest that each glycan chain forms a helix with four disaccharide subunits per turn. In a single-layered peptidoglycan with this structure only alternate side chains could be linked to adjacent chains, whereas the others would face above or below the plane of the sheet. The observed cross-linking of 50% in *E. coli* fits this model. Multi-layered gram-positive walls may have more extensive cross-linking.

Cytoplasmic Membrane

The cytoplasmic membrane in bacteria (also called the **inner membrane** in gram-negatives), like other membranes, consists primarily of a mosaic of proteins embedded in a bilayer of phospholipids whose polar groups are exposed at the two surfaces (Fig. 2–19). It also contains a small amount of the carrier lipid undecaprenol-P, as described above, and in some organisms it is traversed by chains of poly-β-hydroxybutyrate and polyphosphate, which together may form a pore for ion transport. It differs from eukaryotic membranes in lacking sterols. This thin **osmotic barrier** retains metabolites and ions, and it excludes external compounds larger than glycerol unless they can enter via specific transport systems or can dissolve in the lipid.

The bacterial cytoplasmic membrane carries out many additional functions that are distributed among several membranes in higher organisms, including active concentration of nutrients and ions (Ch. 4), lipid synthesis, protein secretion (Ch. 6), and electron transport (Ch. 4). It is also responsible for assembling the several more external layers of the cell envelope, and for flagellar motility and chemotaxis (Ch. 4). Gel electrophoresis after membrane solubilization by detergents reveals more than 100 different proteins.

The insolubility of membrane proteins blocked their study until the discovery that they can be solubilized by detergent without losing their enzymatic or their serologic reactivity. Some membrane enzymes are active only when associated with a specific phospholipid. When bacteria are disrupted mechanically the membrane fragments form closed **vesicles,** some right side out and some inverted, with which certain functions (such as electron transport and protein secretion) can be studied. Membrane function can be further analyzed by incorporating specific proteins into artificial vesicles (**proteoliposomes**) made by dialyzing away detergent from solubilized phospholipid–protein mixtures.

Whether a particular membrane protein is exposed on one surface of the membrane in the cell, the other, or both can be determined by radioactive labeling or enzymatic digestion of the outer surface (in cells) and the inner surface (accessible in inverted vesicles). How the proteins reach these positions will be discussed in Chapter 6.

LAYERS   COMPONENTS

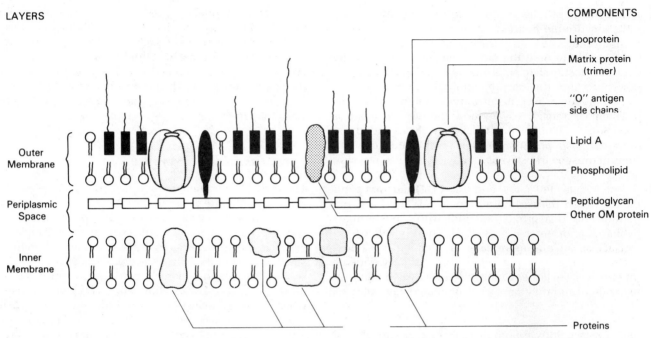

Figure 2–19. Diagram of a gram-negative cell envelope. Components are listed on the right. The trimers of matrix protein of the outer membrane are associated with lipoprotein and with LPS of variable polysaccharide length, and lipoprotein is covalently bound to peptidoglycan. The diagram also illustrates some general properties of membranes (see Cytoplasmic Membrane). Phospholipid molecules are illustrated with a *circle* for the polar groups, and a *line* for each fatty acid acyl moiety.

Lipid molecules are much less specific in their mutual attractions than are proteins and nucleic acid chains, and so they readily exchange their contacts within either leaflet of a membrane bilayer (but not between leaflets). Membranes can therefore be viewed as two-dimensional fluids.

MESOSOMES

Electron micrographs of gram-positive bacteria show large, irregular, convoluted invaginations of the cytoplasmic membrane, called mesosomes. **Septal mesosomes** project into the cytoplasm in advance of the growing peptidoglycan in cell division (see Fig. 2–2), and they provide the site of attachment of the enzymes of DNA replication to the membrane. **Lateral mesosomes,** attached to nonseptal regions, evidently function in **protein secretion,** as they increase in number during induced formation of a major secretion product, penicillinase, in a *Bacillus*. Photosynthetic bacteria have a more elaborate internal membranous structure, with parallel lamellae that contain many copies of the apparatus of photosynthesis—a process in which energy transfer, just as in electron transport, involves embedded proteins creating a potential across a membrane.

CELL DIVISION

Division of bacteria starts with ingrowth of the cytoplasmic membrane, which may or may not be extensive enough to be called a mesosome. The accompanying ingrowth of wall eventually creates a complete transverse **septum** (cross-wall), which is thicker than the peripheral wall. Septal cleavage progresses inward from the periphery and leads to cell separation. In gram-negative organisms the enzymes responsible for the cleavage are presumably attached to the outer membrane, but how gram-positives localize an enzyme within a thick peptidoglycan septum is unknown.

Differences in the details of septum formation and cleavage create characteristic differences in bacterial shape and arrangement. For example, linked cocci are formed by **incomplete cleavage** of the septum. Streptococci form long chains in this way by synthesizing successive septa in parallel orientation, whereas staphylococci form three-dimensional clumps by beginning each new septum perpendicular to the preceding one.

The **equatorial zone** around a growing septum is a major region of growth and shaping of the peripheral wall, as can be demonstrated in gram-positive bacteria by staining with fluorescent antibody to a surface constituent, followed by growth without labeling (Fig. 2–20).

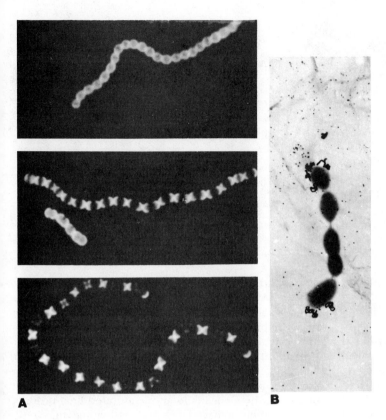

Figure 2–20. Equatorial growth of gram-positive cell wall. (*A, Top*) Streptococci, with surface Ag stained with fluorescent Ab. The two samples below were taken after 15 and 30 minutes of growth without Ab: fresh, unstained wall has been deposited in each cell in an equatorial ring, which separates the older, stained parts of the cell. Each stained portion remains attached to the similar portion of the adjacent cell, forming an "X." (*B*) Pneumococcus with wall of original cell labeled in its teichoic acid with ³H-choline and then grown for several generations with ethanolamine, which promotes formation of chains of cells rather than separation into diplococci. Electron microscope radioautographs reveal localization of silver grains (from disintegration of ³H) only at ends of chain, indicating formation of new wall between conserved halves of original, labeled wall. (*A,* Cole RM: Bacteriol Rev 29:326, 1965; *B,* Briles EB, Tomasz A: J Cell Biol 47:786, 1970)

In gram-negatives the fluidity of the outer membrane prevents such fixed staining, but an equatorial zone of rapid peptidoglycan assembly can be demonstrated by incorporation of labeled diaminopimelate, or by the initial bulging in this region in cells whose wall assembly has been disorganized by penicillin.

In *E. coli* serial sections have shown a **periseptal annulus:** a pair of continuous circumferential contacts between the membranes and the peptidoglycan enclosing the region of septum formation. One might expect such a structure to be weak because of an abundance of "loose ends" of the growing peptidoglycan chain; and, indeed, on limited autolysis staphylococci release their wall as hemispheres.

Many genes contribute to the orderly process of cell division. Mutants with impaired peptidoglycan synthesis may form fragile cells; those that cannot form septa yield long filaments; and still others develop various aberrant shapes. One interesting mutation frequently initiates septum formation near the end rather than at the middle of a cell, yielding **minicells** (Fig. 2–21) that lack a chromosome. Because they often include plasmids (small units of DNA; see Ch. 7) minicells are useful in genetic studies, for they allow specific labeling of the products coded for by the plasmids. Cells without a wall (myco-

plasmas) divide slowly and grow best in the depths of agar, whose fibers may help to pinch off daughter cells.

Bacterial Lipids

Fatty Acids

The apolar components of bacterial membrane lipids are predominantly 14-C to 18-C fatty acid chains, either saturated or monounsaturated; unlike eukaryotes, **prokaryotes do not have polyunsaturated chains.** Unusual fatty acids are frequent, containing methyl branches, a cyclopropane ring, a β-hydroxy group, or extremely long chains (e.g., mycolic acids, with two branches totalling 83-C, in mycobacteria; see Ch. 35).

The biosynthesis of fatty acids proceeds, as in higher organisms, by successive addition of acetyl residues to the chain at its carboxyl end. In this process, briefly reviewed in Figure 2–22, CO_2 is added to acetyl coenzyme A to form the more reactive malonyl-CoA, a step that explains the absolute requirement of bacteria for CO_2 (Ch. 4). Initiation by acetyl-CoA leads to the common, even-numbered straight-chain fatty acids, whereas those with an odd-numbered chain or with a subterminal methyl branch are formed by initiation with propionyl-

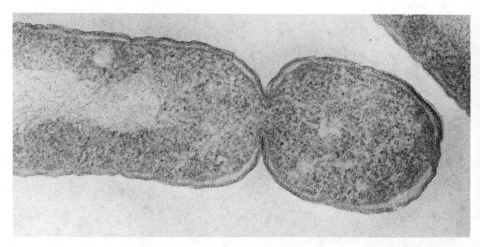

Figure 2–21. *E. coli* mutant producing a minicell without chromosome. (Adler HI et al: Proc Natl Acad Sci USA 57:321, 1967)

CoA or with an acyl-CoA derived from a branched-chain amino acid.

Unsaturation

Bacteria growing aerobically make their unsaturated fatty acids, just as do plants and animals, by O_2-linked removal of hydrogen from a saturated fatty acid. Bacteria growing in the absence of O_2 cannot use this route, and they solve the problem by retaining a double bond present in an intermediate. Ordinarily, the double bond formed in the course of incorporating each acetate residue is *trans*, and it is reduced in the next step; but at a certain chain length, anaerobes form a *cis* double bond instead. That bond is not a substrate for the reduction, and so it is retained during further chain growth.

At low temperatures, membrane lipids become effectively solid rather than fluid, impairing membrane function. Unsaturated fatty acids, which lower the temperature of solidification, are required: mutants unable to make them die unless supplied with these compounds. Moreover, bacteria shifted to growth at a lower temperature adapt by increasing the proportion of unsaturated fatty acids. The mechanism is remarkably direct and simple: the enzyme that forms a *cis* instead of a *trans* double bond, and hence leads to an unsaturated final product, is increasingly active relative to the other enzymes in the pathway at lower temperatures.

In another interesting modification, when growth ceases the cells convert their unsaturated fatty acid residues to the more stable **cyclopropane fatty acids** by adding a methylene group from S-adenosyl-methionine across the double bond. This change presumably helps to preserve the viability of nongrowing cells.

Complex Lipids

In most of the lipids of bacteria other than the lipopolysaccharide of the outer membrane, two of the hydroxyls of glycerol are attached to hydrocarbon chains through ester linkages in eubacteria and ether linkages in archaebacteria; the third hydroxyl is attached to a substituted phosphate in phosphatides or to a polysaccharide in glycolipids. In *E. coli* most of the phosphatide in the outer membrane is the neutral phosphatidylethanolamine, whereas the cytoplasmic membrane contains in addition the acidic phosphatidylglycerol and diphosphatidylglycerol (cardiolipin). Phosphatidyl serine, phosphatidyl choline (lecithin), and phosphatidyl inositol are uncommon in bacteria.

Although most bacteria do not contain sterols, **mevalonic acid** (3,5-dihydroxy-3-methylvaleric acid), an intermediate in their synthesis in yeasts and higher organisms, was initially discovered as a bacterial growth factor. It was later found to be a precursor of several minor but

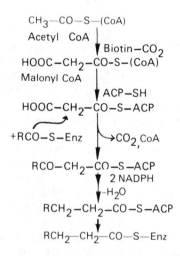

Figure 2–22. Chain elongation in fatty acid biosynthesis. *ACP-SH*, acyl carrier protein; *RCO-*, growing chain. The elongated acyl group is transferred from -S-ACP to -S-Enz, recycling the ACP-SH.

essential products in bacteria. These include the polyiso-prenoid membrane carrier lipid, undecaprenol; carot-enoids; and side chains on quinone cofactors of electron transport. Moreover, the membranes of many bacteria contain **hopanoids:** pentacyclic saturated derivatives of mevalonic acid.

Outer Membrane

ORGANIZATION AND FUNCTIONS

The outer membrane (**OM**) of bacteria differs in impor-tant ways from the inner membrane (**IM**).

1. Whereas the IM is held in place against the wall by the turgor pressure of the protoplast except at excessive external osmotic pressure, retention of the OM requires attachments to the underlying wall. When the wall is fragmented mechanically these adhesions persist and the OM behaves as part of the wall, but when the pepti-doglycan is digested the released OM fragments form vesicles, like typical membrane fragments. In some or-ganisms (e.g., neisserias) the OM is loosely held and is easily fragmented.

2. In the inner leaflet of the OM, as in both leaflets of the IM, phosphatides are the principal lipids, but in the outer leaflet of the OM the lipid is lipopolysaccharide (**LPS).**

3. Because polysaccharides are denser than protein or lipid, the vesicles derived from OM are denser than those from IM; hence, they can be separated by equilibrium density centrifugation.

4. A major function of the OM is to provide a **molecu-lar sieve,** which allows diffusion only of relatively small molecules; it excludes enzymes (e.g., lysozyme) that might attack the peptidoglycan, which would otherwise be very susceptible because it is so thin in gram-nega-tives.

5. The LPS units, each with six long fatty acid chains (see below), cohere more closely than phosphatides, each with two chains; moreover, all the chains in LPS are saturated. Accordingly, the OM is less fluid than the IM. It is also less soluble in mild detergents, a property that can be used to separate the two fractions in the prepara-tion of membrane fragments.

6. The more coherent OM is also less easily distorted or dissolved by detergents or organic solvents and less permeable to hydrophobic molecules, including many antibiotics. The resulting protection against attack by bile salts can explain why the bacteria in the upper gut are all gram-negative.

7. On the other hand, proteins of the immune system (antibody plus complement) can attack the OM, but they cannot reach the IM in gram-positive organisms. Hence this mechanism can kill only gram-negative bacteria.

8. Electrophoretic gels of solubilized membrane reveal a large variety of proteins in the IM, corresponding to its many functions; but the variety is more limited in the OM.

ACCESSIBILITY TO LYSOZYME. Because of the barrier presented by the OM, lysozyme cannot convert gram-negative cells into spheroplasts unless the peptidoglycan is first made accessible e. g., by freezing and thawing, which damages the OM without regularly killing the cell. Lowering of the concentration of Mg^{2+} by chelation by EDTA, or its replacement by Ca^{2+} in the medium, are also effective, because the strength of the OM depends in part on ionic cross-linking of anionic charges at its surface by Mg^{2+}. Treatment with Ca^{2+} also permeabilizes cells to DNA (see Genetic Transformation; Ch. 7).

LIPOPROTEIN. The firm binding of OM to the underlying peptidoglycan depends primarily on a small **lipoprotein** (mol. wt. 7200) that is present in about 250,000 copies per *E. coli* cell. It is covalently linked to about one-tenth of the tetrapeptides in the peptidoglycan. The reaction that links the terminal D-Ala of the tetrapeptide to the car-boxy-terminal lysine of the protein is similar to the trans-peptidation described above. The other end of the pro-tein chain is attached to the OM by an embedded hydrophobic substituent on its amino-terminal cysteine (Fig. 2–23). The formation of this special lipid terminus will be described in Chapter 6 (Signal Peptides).

PORINS. Electron microscopy with negative staining re-veals frequent protein trimers, each subunit containing a pore with a diameter of about 1 nm. These proteins (porins), with molecular weights in the range of 35,000, can also be extracted from the cell envelope as trimers. The porins bind noncovalently to the peptidoglycan: they remain attached when the OM lipid is dissolved by mild detergents but are released by stronger solvents.

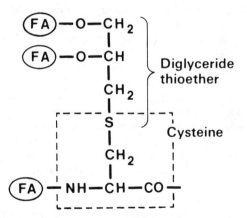

Figure 2–23. Lipid-substituted N-terminal cysteine of lipoprotein (mol. wt. 7200) of outer membrane. *FA,* long-chain fatty acid.

This attachment may ensure continuation of the porin channel into the peptidoglycan.

Genetic studies have shown that *E. coli* has two major porins, called **OmpC** and **OmpF** (for *o*uter *m*embrane *p*rotein), with permeability cutoffs of about mol. wt. 500 and 600, respectively. Growth in media of low osmolarity (as ordinarily encountered in nature) induces formation of the more permeable porin, whereas media of high osmolarity (as encountered in the animal host) repress that gene and induce the one for the less permeable porin. Phosphate limitation induces formation of a third porin, **PhoE**, which particularly admits negatively charged molecules. Another major protein band, OmpA, is important for the structural integrity and shape of the cell rather than for permeability. Mutations eliminating one or even two of these proteins are not lethal, and in compensation, the amounts of the remaining porins increase.

The function of porins was established by observing the effects of their mutations on OM permeability and by incorporating them into artificial vesicles containing LPS as well as phosphatides: the presence of a porin allowed escape of radioactive sugars initially enclosed in the vesicles. The exclusion limit (the largest oligosaccharide that could cross) provided a rough measure of pore size. More refined, kinetic measurements have been made on the basis of liposome swelling or of conductivity across a flat membrane. Most informative have been measurements of the rate of hydrolysis of a substrate by an enzyme present in excess in the periplasm of intact cells. (Kinetic studies of entry without hydrolysis have limited use because small molecules reach equilibrium within less than 1 second.)

It is now clear that all OM pores transfer sufficiently small molecules but that specific features of the porin surface influence the rate for larger molecules. Thus, study of the hydrolysis of various β-lactams by a β-lactamase in the periplasm has shown that positive charge increases, and hydrophobicity or negative charge decreases, entry through OmpC or OmpF. This property may protect gram-negative organisms against damage to the IM by the bile salts in the intestinal environment. Conversely, PhoE, with a smaller pore originally thought to be specific for phosphates, strongly favors anions. In these responses, charges on the protein surface lining the pore evidently aid the entry of permeants with opposite charges and repel those with like charges.

SPECIFIC CHANNELS. A small number of porins, inducible in small amounts, show much greater specificity. Their permeants, which are likely to be encountered in low concentration or are too large to pass through the usual porins, include maltodextrin, nucleosides, various Fe chelates, and vitamin B_{12}. Although these systems originally seemed to resemble passive carrier proteins (Ch. 4, Facilitated Diffusion), they now appear to be porins also. Thus, although the system for maltose is specific for maltodextrins the size of trisaccharides and larger and is very efficient in transferring maltose, it also passes smaller molecules (hexoses, amino acids) nonspecifically.

PHAGE RECEPTORS. In addition to their roles in growing cells, some of the OM proteins also serve as receptors for specific phages and for bacteriocins (Ch. 7), whose evolution has evidently taken advantage of their presence. Organisms with mutations that eliminate or alter these proteins are therefore easily isolated because the mutation confers resistance to the lethal agent. Indeed, the attachment site of phage lambda was discovered, and hence named **LamB**, before its more important function as the maltose receptor was recognized.

LIPOPOLYSACCHARIDE STRUCTURE

LPS, also known as **endotoxin**, is responsible for the toxicity of the gram-negative cell envelope. It can be extracted from cells by 45% phenol at 65°C, but on dilution in aqueous media it forms aggregates, whose variation in size (up to more than 10^6 daltons) influences its biological effects. However, solubilization in hot detergent solutions shows that the units each have one polysaccharide chain. Mild acid hydrolysis yields two moieties: the lipid-soluble **lipid A** and the water-soluble **polysaccharide O antigen** (O Ag).

LIPID A. Among *Enterobacteriaceae* the structure of lipid A (actually a glycolipid) is virtually constant. It consists of a β-1,6-D-glucosamine disaccharide with all but one of the hydroxyl and amino groups substituted (Fig. 2–24). The substituents include the O polysaccharide, six long alkyl chains on four fatty acid residues, and groups that give the outer surface of the cell a strongly negative charge: phosphate and a characteristic sugar acid, **2-keto-3-deoxyoctulonic acid (KDO)**. In various other gram-negative bacteria lipid A differs in detailed structure and in toxicity.

THE CORE. The O Ags of various wild-type, "smooth" (S) *Salmonella* strains each consist of a long specific chain linked to lipid A by a uniform core of five different kinds of sugar. (Other groups of *Enterobacteriaceae* have similar but not identical cores.) Many "rough" (R) mutants lack only the specific chain, because of a block in the formation or incorporation of a particular sugar. Other R strains are blocked at various steps in the formation of the core, and the composition of their LPS revealed the sequence of the *Salmonella* core, depicted in Figure 2–25. Because the most extreme R mutations that have been isolated all retain the three KDO residues adjacent

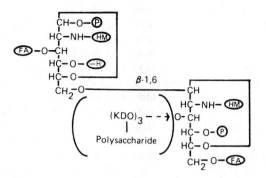

Figure 2–24. Structure of unit of lipid A from *Salmonella* lipopolysaccharide. Some of the 1-phosphate groups are replaced by a pyrophosphate group. Brackets enclose the three units of ketose-linked ketodeoxyoctonate (*KDO*, 3-deoxy-D-mannooctulosonic acid), which link the lipid to a variable polysaccharide and may be considered part of lipid A. *HM*, β-hydroxymyristic acid (a C_{14}-saturated fatty acid characteristic of lipid A); *FA*, other long-chain fatty acids. One of the HM residues has its hydroxyl group esterified with a myristic acid. The fatty acids are very similar in all enterobacteria studied but are quite different in some other gram-negative organisms (e.g., *Pseudomonas, Brucella*). (After Rietschel T et al: Eur J Biochem 28:166, 1972)

to the lipid A in LPS, these are evidently essential for viability and hence are functionally part of lipid A.

SPECIFIC O ANTIGENS. The specific chains attached to the core consist of a repeating sequence of a linear trisaccharide or a branched tetrasaccharide or pentasaccharide. The lengths differ even in the same organism,

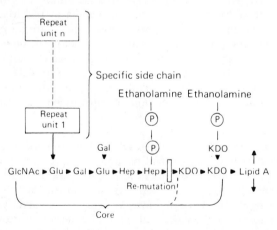

Figure 2–25. Structure of the core of *Salmonella* lipopolysaccharide (*Hep*, L-glycero-D-mannoheptose). The sugars are attached with their reducing group toward the lipid A (1 → 4, etc.); hence, there are no free reducing groups.

In the core biosynthesis, from right to left, a specific enzyme adds each residue. The genes for the core transferases map in a cluster (the *Rfa* locus), whereas those for the synthesis or transfer of a component of a specific, repeating chain (Fig. 2–26) map in another cluster (*Rfb* locus; see Chap 8 for definition of locus). Re ("extreme rough") mutants have the least LPS compatible with viability.

ranging up to 40 repeat units. The O Ag layer is thus a mat of "whiskers" attached to lipid A embedded in the membrane.

Antibodies are useful in identifying specific O Ag chains, and they were also helpful in determining their structures. An antibody to an O Ag recognizes at least a pair of sugars and the specific link between them, and so these structures can be inferred from the oligosaccharide or glycoside that is most effective in competitively inhibiting the reaction.

Loss of the specific O Ag does not affect the permeability of the OM. However, "deep rough" mutations eliminating most of the core perturb the morphogenesis of the OM, and some phosphatide is then incorporated into its outer leaflet. These strains are also more sensitive to lysozyme and more permeable to hydrophobic antibiotics. Conversely, selection for mutants with increased resistance to multiple antibiotics yields strains with various other changes in the structure of the LPS.

LIPOPOLYSACCHARIDE SYNTHESIS

LPS is synthesized on the IM by three different processes, whose products are assembled there and then transferred to the OM.

Lipid A is synthesized by the addition of the fatty acids and KDO to the glucosamine disaccharide. Lipid A, with its hydrophobic chains embedded in the membrane, then serves as the primer and the carrier for building up the **core polysaccharide.** Each successive sugar is added from a nucleoside diphosphate sugar (Ch. 5) by a specific enzyme.

The **repeat units** of the **specific chains** are built up on another lipid carrier, **undecaprenol-P** (Fig. 2–26), adding each specific residue by "tail addition" to a free end in the cytoplasm. We have already encountered undecaprenol-P as the carrier for the assembly of peptidoglycan, teichoic acids, and capsular polysaccharides. It probably carries the precursors of these different products to the same opening in the peptidoglycan, where they interact with appropriate enzymes.

When an O Ag subunit is completed, it is incorporated, by "head addition," into the longer chain; i.e., the growing chain, attached to undecaprenol-P, is transferred to the incoming subunit on another undecaprenol-P (Fig. 2–26). This process, like the synthesis of a protein or fatty acid, permits synthesis of a long chain whose free end may wander far from the site of growth.

When the chain reaches the proper length (or happens to encounter the transferase), it is transferred to the free end of a core already built up on lipid A, thus completing the LPS.

TRANSFER TO THE OUTER MEMBRANE. After formation on the cytoplasmic surface of the IM, the LPS is trans-

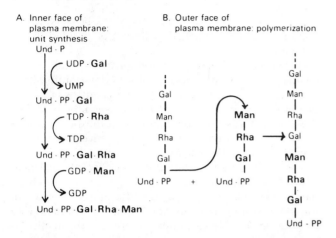

A. Inner face of
plasma membrane:
unit synthesis

B. Outer face of
plasma membrane: polymerization

Figure 2–26. Biosynthesis of repeating chain of LPS of *Salmonella newington.* *(A)* Inner face of plasma membrane: unit synthesis. *(B)* Outer face of plasma membrane: polymerization. *Und,* undecaprenol (a C_{55} polyisoprenol) carrier lipid. The nucleoside diP sugars (UDP-galactose, TDP-rhamnose, GDP-mannose) are synthesized as described in Chapter 5. The chemically reactive reducing group (C-1) of a sugar, by which it is linked to the nucleoside diP, is involved in its transfer to a growing repeat unit *(A),* in transfer of the "head" end of the growing chain to each additional repeat unit *(B),* and in final transfer (not shown) of the chain to the free end of a core chain. (After Robbins PW et al: Science 158:1536, 1967. Copyright © 1967 by the American Association for the Advancement of Science)

ferred to the OM through regions where the two membranes are connected across holes in the peptidoglycan. The existence of such holes can be demonstrated in osmotically shocked cells, which exhibit regular, small protrusions of the IM. These are probably also the site of the **adhesion zones** (also known as **Bayer junctions**) of stretched IM attached to peptidoglycan, seen in plasmolyzed cells (see Fig. 2–17). Thus, when a Gal⁻ mutant is grown without galactose and then briefly with galactose, so that it briefly forms a "smooth" LPS (containing galactose) on a background of "rough" LPS, staining with labeled antibody to the newly formed O Ag shows that it first appears directly above the adhesion zones and then slowly disperses. Proteins can move from the IM to the OM by a similar route (see Ch. 6, Fig. 6–11).

We do not know the detailed structure of these adhesion zones, or whether precursors of peptidoglycan and of the OM flow through the same zones or through separate ones. The mechanisms that direct the flows to the OM are also unknown. The adhesion zones evidently contain specific proteins that are exposed to the exterior, as they also serve as sites for attachment of certain bacteriophages.

THE PERIPLASM; OSMOREGULATION

Gram-negative bacteria maintain a significant aqueous volume in the periplasmic space (periplasm) between the IM and the OM (and hence including the peptidoglycan). It contains a specific set of proteins, including enzymes such as RNases or phosphatases that digest impermeable molecules, enzymes such as penicillinase that inactivate harmful substances, and binding proteins specific for various permeants, which function in membrane transport and in chemotaxis (see Ch. 4).

Periplasmic proteins can be released in several ways: by converting the cell to a spheroplast; by treatment with chloroform; or by **osmotic shock,** in which the cells in a chilled hypertonic medium are exposed to EDTA and then rapidly poured into a chilled solution of low tonicity. Presumably the EDTA loosens and partly releases the LPS layer, the cold makes it more brittle, and the hypertonicity of the periplasm places stress on the membranes.

PERIPLASMIC OSMOREGULATION. The periplasm also contains variable concentrations of a **membrane-derived oligosaccharide (MDO),** which regulate its osmolarity. MDO consists of (1,2)-β-D-glucans of six to ten glucose units (just large enough to be retained within the OM) substituted with multiple acidic groups; their counterions increase the contribution to osmolarity. In enterobacteria the concentration is very low after growth in a medium of high osmolarity (e.g., 300 osM, the range within the bacterium and in animal body fluids), whereas after growth at low osmolarity (such as in the sewage to which enteric bacteria also must be adapted), it can reach 7% of the dry weight of the cell. Although the bacteria can survive abrupt shifts of osmolarity, optimal growth evidently requires that they maintain an optimal volume of the periplasm, and the osmolarity provided by the MDO molecules does so by opposing the turgor pressure of the protoplast (the difference between the internal and external osmotic pressures) against the peptidoglycan. The high concentration of macromolecules in the periplasm makes it highly viscous, as shown by the low rate of lateral diffusion of introduced fluorescent proteins.

CYTOPLASMIC OSMOREGULATION. Variations in the external osmotic pressure also lead to compensatory shifts in the intracellular concentration of various ions and metabolites, especially K⁺. The mechanism of this **osmoregulation** is not known. Moreover, the maximal external osmotic pressure at which bacteria can grow is increased by adding compounds that serve as **osmoprotectants,** because the cell can concentrate them to especially high levels and thus prevent separation of the cytoplasmic membrane from the wall. (Although this separation is not lethal, it apparently interferes with wall synthesis.) In *E. coli,* proline and betaine (N,N,N-triMe-glycine) are particularly effective osmoprotectants, but why is not clear. Osmoprotection may be important for pathogens where tissue disintegration releases a high concentration of small molecules.

Gram-positive organisms, with their thick walls, can maintain a higher turgor pressure than gram-negatives, and they tend to be more resistant to inhibition of growth by hypertonic media. They predominate in regions such as the skin that are subject to dehydration.

Spores

When the supply of C, N, or P is limited, certain bacteria develop highly resistant, dormant forms called **spores** (Gr., seed) or **endospores;** the surrounding mother cell is called the **sporangium.** Spore-formers are limited to the aerobic *Bacilli*, the anaerobic clostridia, and a few sarcinae and actinomycetes. These organisms are all gram-positive, and sporulation clearly depends on the ability to form a thick wall.

Like the exospores of fungi and of certain actinomycetes and the seeds of higher plants, endospores are **cryptobiotic:** that is, they have no metabolic activity but can recover from this dormancy. Unlike the spores and seeds of the immotile and relatively large fungi and plants, which serve primarily for dissemination, the spores of bacteria serve to promote survival under adverse conditions: heat, drying, freezing, toxic chemicals, and radiation. Although resistance to heat has received the most attention, the principal ecological role of spores is probably **survival in the dry state.** Viable *Bacilli* have been isolated from soil specimens stored for more than 300 years.

Spores are important in medical bacteriology as the causes of a few diseases and also as the most refractory cells in the preparation of sterile materials. In addition, their formation (**sporulation**) and the restoration of the vegetative state (**germination**) have aroused wide interest as a simple unicellular model for cell differentiation. The regulatory processes involved will be briefly described here, although some of the relevant principles of molecular genetics will not be presented until later chapters.

FORMATION AND STRUCTURE

Spores are impervious to stains. They are also unusually dehydrated and hence refractile; in the light microscope the first visible stage in sporulation is the formation of a region of increased refractility at one end of a cell. The refractility gradually increases and the spore is completed in 6 to 8 hours. It is released thereafter by autolysis of the sporangial wall. In a well-sporulating culture most cells form a spore.

Spores of most species are smooth-walled and ovoid, but in some they are spherical or have characteristic ridges. In *Bacilli*, they fit within the cell diameter, whereas in the slender *Clostridia*, they cause a bulge, which may be either terminal ("drumstick") or more central (Fig. 2–27).

In electron micrographs, the first detectable step in sporulation is the condensation of a newly replicated chromosome into an **axial filament** (Fig. 2–28), which moves to a pole of the cell. There it triggers a specialized **asymmetric** cell division, in which a **double layer** of cytoplasmic membrane invaginates, without peptidoglycan, to form a **spore septum.** The periphery of this septum migrates as a double membrane toward the forespore pole and finally engulfs the chromosome and surrounding cytoplasm to form the **forespore** (Fig. 2–29).

SPORE INTEGUMENT. The two membrane layers of the forespore, derived as extensions of the mother cell membrane, become differentiated and give rise to the special-

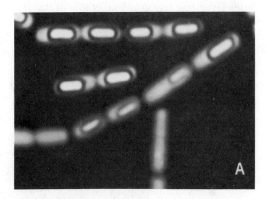

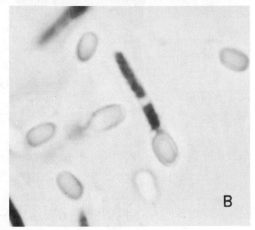

Figure 2–27. Spores seen by the light microscope. *(A) Bacillus cereus:* elongated subterminal spores, nigrosin stain. *(B) Clostridium pectinovorum:* large terminal spores and spores freed from parent cell (sporangium); cells stained with I_2 (which stains granulose). (×3600; courtesy of C Robinow)

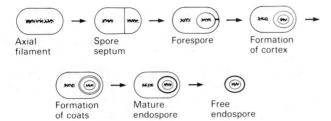

Axial filament → Spore septum → Forespore → Formation of cortex →

Formation of coats → Mature endospore → Free endospore

Figure 2–28. Stages in sporulation.

ized spore integument (envelope), which occupies more than half the spore volume. Several layers can be distinguished (Fig. 2–30).

1. The innermost layer, enclosing the **protoplast (core),** is the **germ cell membrane.**

2. **The cortex** is a thick, concentric, laminated structure laid down between the two forespore membranes. The facing surfaces of the membranes correspond to the wall-synthesizing surface of the parental cell membrane, and each forms a characteristic kind of peptidoglycan. The outer layer has few cross-links (6% of the muramate residues in *B. subtilis*), which promotes its rapid autolysis during later germination. The thin inner layer (spore wall) is more tightly cross-linked, and it persists longer

during germination, providing osmotic stability for the protoplast and also a primer for restoration of the vegetative cell wall. In the loose outer peptidoglycan most of the muramate residues are blocked from cross-linking, often by condensing their lactyl COOH with their NH_2 group to form the following lactam:

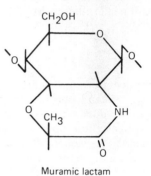

Muramic lactam

3. **The coat,** a keratin-like protein layer rich in S–S groups, constitutes as much as 80% of the total protein; it is presumably formed by the sporangium and is deposited outside the outer spore membrane after the cortex has been completed and the maturing spore has become refractile. The dozen or more coat proteins cannot be

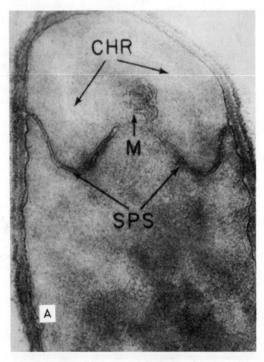

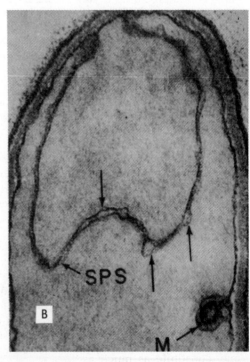

Figure 2–29. Early stage in sporulation. *(A)* The protoplasm at one end of the cell containing a chromosome *(CHR)* is cut off from the rest of the cell by a transverse spore septum *(SPS)* formed by ingrowth of a double membrane and mesosome *(M)* from the protoplasmic membrane of the other cell. *(B)* The periphery of this double membrane moves toward the tip of the cell, ultimately enclosing the whole forespore. (Ohye DF, Murrell WG: J Cell Biol 14:111, 1962)

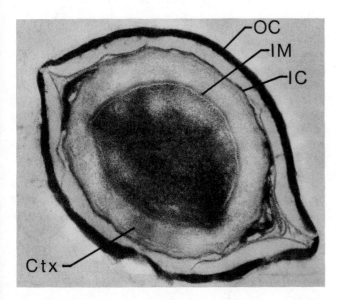

Figure 2–30. Electron micrograph of sectioned spore of *B. megaterium*. The core is surrounded successively by the inner membrane *(IM)*, cortex *(Ctx)*, inner coat *(IC)*, and outer coat *(OC)*. With other methods of fixation, the cortex is much denser and is seen to be laminated. (×11,200; courtesy of P Fitz–James)

solubilized unless the S–S groups are reduced, and this impervious, highly cross-linked layer is responsible for the resistance of spores to toxic chemicals. (In *Clostridium perfringens* [Ch. 34] an enterotoxin is formed only during sporulation and is serologically related to coat proteins.)

4. **The exosporium,** present on some spores, is a loose protein–lipid membrane of unknown function.

SMALL MOLECULES. Although Ca^{2+} is absent from most bacteria, active transport systems for this ion appear in the mother cell early in sporulation, and the completed spore contains a high concentration. The Ca^{2+} is chelated by a roughly equivalent amount of **dipicolinic acid,** which is formed in the sporangium from diaminopimelate (a precursor also of the peptidoglycan):

$$HOOC-\text{(pyridine ring)}-COOH$$

Dipicolinic acid

(Pyridine-2,6-dicarboxylic acid; for biosynthesis,
see bacterial pathway to lysine, Ch. 5)

Dipicolinate is almost unique to bacterial spores, and it may constitute as much as 15% of their weight. It is located primarily in the core, as shown by the attenuation of the β-emission of the ^{3}H-labeled compound by the surrounding envelope and by immuno-electron mi-

croscopy; electron probe X-ray microanalysis has demonstrated the same location for the Ca^{2+}.

SPORE DEHYDRATION. The expulsion of essentially all the water from the maturing spore requires a good deal of energy; the mechanism is not firmly established. The cortex appears to play a key role, as its impairment by mutation or by penicillin prevents effective dehydration.

COMPOSITION OF THE CORE

The core contains everything necessary for resuming growth, and in stable form; it lacks the components of the vegetative cell that are particularly unstable or can be replaced readily early in germination. It includes a chromosome and small amounts of each component of the protein-synthesizing machinery: ribosomes, tRNAs, and accessory protein factors and enzymes. Two unstable cell components, mRNA and nucleoside triphosphates, are absent, but there is a supply of their more stable precursors, the nucleoside monophosphates and diphosphates (Table 2–2). Amino acids and their biosynthetic enzymes are virtually absent, but on germination, they are supplied by hydrolysis of small soluble **storage proteins** constituting about 20% of the total protein. (These proteins have the additional function of binding to the DNA, where they reverse UV-induced damage.) Energy for initiating replenishment of missing constituents is stored as the stable 3-P-glycerate, which is readily converted to the P donor P-enolpyruvate.

PROTEINS AND HEAT RESISTANCE. The extent of thermal resistance of spores is probably set by their proteins. A few enzymes in spores are derived from corresponding vegetative cell enzymes by cleavage and are more resistant, and the specific new enzymes induced by sporulation are also stable. However, many enzymes are iden-

TABLE 2–2. Levels of Metabolites in Dormant Spores and in Growing Cells of B. megaterium

	Amount (µmol/g)	
Compound	*Spores*	*Growing Cells*
ATP	3	725
ADP + AMP	544	195
GTP + CTP + UTP	<10	680
G + C + U nucleotides	530	860
Deoxyribonucleotides	<1.5	181
Phosphoglyceric acid	6,800	—
Amino acids*	150	1,400

(After Setlow P: In *Spores VI*, p 443. Washington, DC, American Society for Microbiology, 1975.)

* Setlow P, Primus G, ibid., p 451; germinating instead of growing cells.

tical in the two kinds of cells and are not especially thermostable in solution. Their striking stability in spores must therefore depend on the intracellular environment. A significant factor is **dehydration,** which increases the stability of proteins in the test tube, especially in the presence of appropriate protective materials. Ca dipicolinate also appears to play a large role, for mutations that reduce its concentration cause a parallel reduction in resistance to killing by heat.

REGULATORY CHANGES IN SPORULATION

TRIGGERS. How nutritional deprivation initiates sporulation is not well understood, but there is evidence for correlation with a decrease in the level of energized guanine nucleotides (GTP and GDP), and also for the accumulation of a novel purine metabolite, $3',5'$-p_3Ap_3. Another early event in sporulation is the appearance of one or more intracellular **proteases.** These enzymes increase protein turnover, providing the starving mother cell and the developing spore with the amino acids needed for synthesis of new proteins; but they may also be involved in specific cleavages that contribute to regulation. Starving cells of *B. subtilis* excrete a **peptide that promotes sporulation;** hence, the process is more efficient in dense cultures.

GENE REGULATION. Sporulation involves a shift in the activity of several hundred genes, some in the sporangium and others in the core. Studies of mRNA and of enzymes show that many vegetative enzymes continue to be made, others are turned off, and genes unique to sporulation are turned on. The mRNAs from sporulating cells are in general more stable than those from vegetative cells, and they often have long **polyA tails** (like eukaryotic messengers), which may protect them from exonucleases.

The ordered temporal sequence of seven morphological stages in sporulation (Fig. 2–28) is accompanied by an equally complex set of successive stages in gene expression, as shown by shifts in the patterns of pulse-labeled proteins detected by gel electrophoresis.

An important regulatory mechanism is a shift in the **sigma factors** in the cell: the elements that select the set of transcription initiation sites (promoters) recognized by each **RNA polymerase** (Ch. 9). In sporulating *B. subtilis* the chief sigma factor, designated σ^{55} on the basis of size (in Kd), is replaced by σ^{29}, which selects a different, although overlapping, set of promoters. There is then an intricate cascade of regulatory mechanisms, including further shifts in sigma factors.

The main approach to analyzing this sequence of regulatory stages has been the isolation of a large number of **sporulation-negative (spo⁻)** mutants. These are grouped in terms of the stage at which they are arrested,

and their different loci on the chromosome are designated by letters: *spoOA* (for those blocked at the earliest stage) to *spoOK*. Mutants defective in germination are more difficult to isolate. Other approaches to understanding regulation include isolation of the proteins being formed at each stage; isolation of the mRNAs; cloning *spo* genes and identification of their products; and study of the regulatory responses of these genes by fusion of their regulatory region to a gene that yields an easily identified product (Chap. 8, Gene Manipulation).

Molecular genetic analysis has shown that one new sigma factor, σ^{27}, is a composite, formed in the mother cell by recombining portions of two genes (see Chap. 9, Promoter and Sigma Variation). The loss of the intervening DNA is acceptable because the mother cell is discarded.

GERMINATION

The process of converting a spore into a vegetative cell can be divided into three stages: **activation, germination (initiation),** and **outgrowth.** The overall process, often also called germination, is much faster than sporulation: it requires about 90 minutes in a rich medium from onset to cell division.

ACTIVATION. Although some bacterial spores will germinate spontaneously in a favorable medium, others remain **dormant** unless they are activated by some traumatic agent, such as heat, low pH, or an SH compound. **Aging,** with its multiple, undefined consequences, is probably the most important natural cause. Activation presumably damages the impermeable coat, because grinding with glass powder is also effective. Similarly, the seeds of many higher plants will not germinate until an outer coat has been damaged. The requirement for activation spreads out germination in time and space, thus promoting survival of the strain by preventing uniform germination in response to conditions that are only temporarily favorable.

GERMINATION. Unlike activation, germination requires water and a **germination agent,** which differs in different species (e.g., alanine, dipicolinate, Mn^{2+}). The agent penetrates the damaged coat and triggers conversion of a membrane-bound spore-lytic enzyme into an active, soluble form, which hydrolyzes the cortical peptidoglycan. This digestion is no doubt promoted by the **loose crosslinking** of the outer layer of peptidoglycan and possibly also by loss of bound Ca^{2+} ions.

OUTGROWTH. In a nutrient medium germination leads to immediate outgrowth, whereas starvation or inhibition of protein synthesis allows rehydration but not formation of a vegetative cell. In outgrowth the vegetative σ

factor is restored early, and vegetative growth is gradually resumed. Protein synthesis increases progressively as the initially scanty machinery is expanded by protein and RNA synthesis; the vegetative cell wall builds up on the cell membrane; and, after about an hour, DNA synthesis begins. The cell, twice its initial volume, then begins to burst out of the spore coat.

SUMMARY

We have seen that bacterial endospores are differentiated cells formed within a vegetative cell; they encase a genome in an insulating, dehydrated vehicle that makes the cell ametabolic and resistant to various lethal agents but permits subsequent germination in an appropriate medium. Spores are formed by the invagination of a double layer of cell membrane, which closes off to surround a chromosome and a small amount of cytoplasm. A thin spore wall, and a thicker cortex with a much looser peptidoglycan, are synthesized between the two layers; outside the cortex is a protein coat, rich in disulfide cross-links. Selective synthesis, hydrolysis, and uptake of metabolites yield a core containing the minimal complement of the stable constituents necessary for the resumption of growth. The stages of sporulation are presented diagrammatically in Figure 2–28.

The keratinlike properties of the coat account for the resistance to staining and to attack by deleterious chemicals, whereas the dehydration and the accumulation of Ca dipicolinate contribute to the heat resistance. We do not know the mechanism by which these cells become essentially completely dehydrated, but the cortex appears to play a major role. In germination, following activation by mechanical or chemical damage to the surface coat, the attack of a lytic enzyme on the peptidoglycan of the cortex permits uptake of water and loss of Ca dipicolinate by the core.

Sporulation involves the action of specific proteases and an extensive shift in the pattern of gene transcription, brought about in part by shifts in the sigma factors of RNA polymerase. The sequential regulatory processes in this microbial differentiation are being analyzed through the use of mutants blocked at various stages in sporulation.

Selected Readings

BOOKS AND REVIEW ARTICLES

Aronson AI, Fitz–James P: Structure and morphogenesis of the bacterial spore coat. Bacteriol Rev 40:360, 1976

Beachey EH (ed): Bacterial Adherence. London, Chapman and Hall, 1980

Benz R: Porin from bacterial and mitochondrial outer membranes. CRC Crit Rev Biochem 19:145, 1985

Bitton G, Marshall KC (eds): Adsorption of Microorganisms to Surfaces. New York, John Wiley, 1980

Doetsch RN, Sjoblad RD: Flagellar structure and function in eubacteria. Annu Rev Microbiol 34:69, 1980

Donachie WD, Begg KJ, Sullivan NF: Morphogenes of *Escherichia coli*. In Losick R, Shapiro L (eds): Microbial Development, p 27. Cold Spring Harbor, Cold Spring Harbor Laboratory, 1984

Drlica K: Biology of bacterial deoxyribonucleic acid topoisomerases. Microbiol Rev 48:273, 1984

Drlicka K, Rouviere–Yaniv J: Histonelike proteins of bacteria. Microbiol Rev 51:301, 1987

Dworkin M: Developmental Biology of the Bacteria. Menlo Park, Benjamin/Cummings, 1985

Frere JM, Joris B: Penicillin-sensitive enzymes in peptidoglycan biosynthesis. CRC Crit Rev Microbiol 11:299, 1985

Gaastra W, De Graaf FK: Host-specific fimbrial adhesins of noninvasive enterotoxigenic *Escherichia coli* strains. Microbiol Rev 46:129, 1982

Inouye M (ed): Bacterial Outer Membranes as Model Systems. New York, Wiley-Interscience, 1987

Keilin D: The problem of anabiosis or latent life: History and current concepts. Proc R Soc Lond [Biol] 150:149, 1959

Levinson H et al (eds): Sporulation and Germination. Washington, DC, American Society for Microbiology, 1981

Losick R, Youngman P: Endospore formation in *Bacillus*. In Losick R, Shapiro L (eds): Microbial Development. Cold Spring Harbor, Cold Spring Harbor Laboratory, 1984

Losick R, Youngman P, Piggot PJ: Genetics of endospore formation in *Bacillus subtilis*. Annu Rev Genet 20:625, 1986

Lugtenberg B, Van Alphen L: Molecular architecture and functioning of the outer membrane of *Escherichia coli* and other gram-negative bacteria. Biochim Biophys Acta 737:51, 1983

Nanninga N (ed): Molecular Cytology of *Escherichia coli*. New York, Academic Press, 1985

Neidhardt FC (ed): *Escherichia coli* and *Salmonella typhimurium*: Cellular and Molecular Biology. Washington, DC, American Society for Microbiology, 1987. Includes several pertinent chapters.

Nikaido H, Vaara M: Molecular basis of bacterial outer membrane permeability. Microbiol Rev 49:1, 1985

Ogden GB, Schaechter M: Chromosomes, plasmids, and the bacterial cell envelopes. In Leive L (ed): Microbiology—1985, p 282. Washington, DC, American Society for Microbiology, 1985

Osborn MJ, Wu HCP: Proteins of the outer membrane of gram-negative bacteria. Annu Rev Microbiol 34:369, 1980

Ottow JCG: Ecology, physiology, and genetics of fimbriae and pili. Annu Rev Biochem 29:79, 1975

Pettijohn DE, Sinden RR: Structure of the nucleoid. In Nanninga N (ed): Molecular Cytology of *Escherichia coli*. New York, Academic Press, 1985

Savage DC, Fletcher MM (ed): Bacterial Adhesion: Mechanisms and Physiological Significance. New York, Plenum Press, 1985

Sleytr UB, Meissner P: Crystalline surface layers on bacteria. Annu Rev Microbiol 37:311, 1983

Sutherland IW: Biosynthesis and composition of gram-negative bacterial extracellular and wall polysaccharides. Annu Rev Microbiol 39:243, 1985

Symposium: Molecular concepts of lipid A. Rev Infect Dis 6:427, 1984

Tomasz A: The mechanism of the irreversible effects of penicillins. Annu Rev Microbiol 33:113, 1979

Ward JB: Teichoic and teichuronic acids: Biosynthesis, assembly, and location. Microbiol Rev 45:211, 1981

Waxman DJ, Strominger JL: Penicillin-binding proteins and the mechanism of action of B-lactam antibiotics. Annu Rev Biochem 52:825, 1983

SPECIFIC ARTICLES

Broyles SS, Pettijohn DE: Interaction of the *Escherichia coli* HU protein with DNA. J Mol Biol 187:47, 1986

Burman LG, Park JT: Molecular model for elongation of the murein sacculus of *Escherichia coli*. Proc Natl Acad Sci USA 81:1844, 1984

Gotschlich EC, Frazer BA, Nishimura O, Robbins JB, Liu TY: Lipid on capsular polysaccharide of gram-negative bacteria. J Biol Chem 256:8915, 1981

Hobot JA, Villiger W, Escaig J, Maeder M, Ryter A, Kellenberger E: Shape and fine structure of nucleoids observed on sections of ultrarapidly frozen and cryosubstituted bacteria. J Bacteriol 162:960, 1985

Kennedy EP: Osmotic regulation and the biosynthesis of membrane-derived oligosaccharides in *Escherichia coli*. Proc Natl Acad Sci USA 79:1092, 1982

Macalister TJ, MacDonald B, Rothfield LI: The periseptal annulus: An organelle associated with cell division in gram-negative bacteria. Proc Natl Acad Sci USA 80:1372, 1983

Nikaido H, Rosenberg EY, Foulds J: Porin channels in *Escherichia coli:* Studies with β-lactams in intact cells. J Bacteriol 153:232, 1983

3

Growth and Death of Bacteria

This chapter will deal with the predominant mode of growth of bacteria, in which the individual cells in a clone interact autonomously with the environment. However, we should note that under some circumstances bacteria communicate with each other by means of specific excreted products, resulting in density-dependent **social interactions.** For example, at late stages in the culture cycle, pneumococci excrete a protein that promotes the uptake of DNA, some streptococci excrete a pheromone (mating hormone), and the differentiation of some Bacilli into spores is promoted by a peptide that they excrete under conditions of starvation.

Nutrient transfers between **different** types of organisms are more common and probably are partly responsible for the frequent presence of mixed infections in natural environments (including the indigenous flora of the human body).

Bacterial Growth

Bacteria are generally encountered in nature as mixtures but are studied as pure cultures. These are most conveniently isolated on solid media, because each colony can be derived from a single cell (or from an aggregate of identical cells with those species whose cells do not separate regularly after division). Growth in liquid medium is used for many kinds of physiological studies and for large-scale cultivation. We should note that the concept of purity in microbiology—freedom from any contaminating organisms—is quite different from that in chemistry, where contaminating compounds are tolerated within specified limits.

Bacteria are quantitated in terms either of **mass,** for biochemical studies, or of **cell number,** for studies of genetics or of infectivity. The ratio of mass to number is constant under conditions of steady-state growth, but it varies with the growth rate.

Cell mass can be measured in terms of dry weight or of some chemical component (nitrogen, DNA). The most practical index is **turbidity,** which can be conveniently followed in a growing culture, even without sampling, by photoelectric measurement of the decrease in transmission (**optical density; OD**). This decrease is attributable mostly to light scattering by the highly refractile bacteria (solid content about 25% compared with 1% to 2% in the medium). The OD is greater the lower the wavelength, but it is generally measured above 490 nm in order to avoid light absorption by the yellow products of autoclaving of the medium. The OD is proportional to bacterial density between 0.01 mg dry weight (about 10^7 cells) and 0.5 mg per ml, but as cultures approach full growth (1–2 mg per ml), the ratio falls.

Viable cell number is determined by inoculating a fixed volume of a series of 10-fold or 100-fold dilutions on a solid medium ("plating"), incubating, and counting the colonies in those Petri plates that are not too crowded (fewer than 400 colonies). Precision is limited by the statistical sampling error: the **standard deviation** (SD) is the square root of the number counted.

The **total cell number** can be counted either under the microscope (in special chambers) or in an electronic particle analyzer that detects the effect of a particle on electrical impedance (e.g., the Coulter counter). Total cell number is ordinarily identical with the viable count except under conditions that cause cell death. With bacteria that aggregate, or those that fail to separate regularly at division (e.g., streptococci), plate counts yield the number of **colony-forming units** (CFU) rather than the number of cells.

GROWTH IN LIQUID MEDIUM
Growth Cycle

When bacteria are inoculated into fresh medium, the growth curve usually exhibits three phases: **lag, exponential** (also called **logarithmic** or **log**), and **stationary** (Fig. 3–1). The cessation of growth may be secondary to exhaustion of a required nutrient or of oxygen or to accumulation of an inhibitory product, usually organic acids or alcohol. When a specific metabolite such as an amino acid is growth-limiting the level of the resulting plateau provides a measure of its initial concentration and thus can be used for **bioassays.**

In the slowing of growth as cells approach the stationary phase, and during starvation in that phase, the cells become smaller by as much as a factor of 4 and undergo striking changes in composition. In particular, the ribosomes (see Ch. 9; Cell Composition and Growth Rate) cease being made and begin to break down, and the

resulting supply of amino acids and nucleotides permits continued synthesis of the macromolecules required for further cell division without an increase in total mass.

When stationary cells are inoculated into fresh medium, they reverse these changes. Accordingly, the turbidity increases only gradually, as ribosomes and other depleted components are restored, until growth becomes exponential. The increase in cell number lags even more, because the cells have to become larger before they begin to divide. Both these transitions are shown diagrammatically in Figure 3–1.

With a large inoculum from an exponentially growing culture transferred to the same kind of medium, the lag may be negligible. However, with small inocula growth may be slowed by trace inhibitors contaminating the medium (e.g., soap, heavy metal ions), or it may be delayed until the metabolic activity of the cells causes accumulation of the CO_2 required for growth (Ch. 4).

After sufficient time in the stationary phase, cells of some species (e.g., the pneumococcus) begin to lyse, but many other species (e.g., *E. coli*) undergo progressive loss of viable number without loss of turbidity (sometimes called the **death phase**). There is evidence that in this phase the adaptive process of ribosome degradation becomes suicidal; i.e., it eliminates the last ribosome, thus preventing the protein synthesis required for regeneration of ribosomes.

During long-term storage of a culture, nutrients released by lysis of some cells may permit outgrowth of mutants that are more resistant to the limiting conditions.

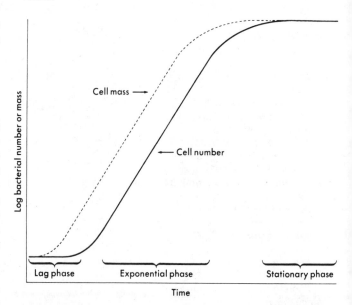

Figure 3–1. Phases of bacterial growth starting with an inoculum of stationary-phase cells. Note that the classic phases, defined in terms of cell number, do not precisely coincide with the phases of changing growth in terms of protoplasmic mass.

Exponential Kinetics

In the exponential phase of growth the rate of increase of bacterial mass at any time is proportional to the mass present:

$$dB/dt = \alpha B \qquad (1)$$

where B is bacterial mass, t is time, and α is the **instantaneous growth rate constant** for that culture (i.e., the relative increase per unit time). Hence:

$$dB/B = \alpha dt (\text{or } d \ln B = \alpha dt) \qquad (2)$$

$$B_t = B_0 e^{\alpha t}; \text{ and integrating:} \qquad (3)$$

$$\ln B_t/B_0 = \alpha t, \text{ or } \ln B_t = \ln B_0 + \alpha t \qquad (4)$$

Hence, in this phase, a plot of the logarithm of B against time gives a straight line (Fig. 3–1). This semilogarithmic plot is generally used for bacterial growth curves. It is often convenient to express growth rate in terms of **doubling time** (t_D), also called the **mean generation time** (**MGT**). It is obtained by setting B_t at $2B_0$ (i.e., one doubling) in equation 4:

$$\ln B_t/B_0 = \ln 2 = \alpha t_D$$

$$t_D = (1/\alpha) \ln 2 = 0.69(1/\alpha)$$

$$1/t_D = \mu = 1.45\alpha$$

The reciprocal of the MGT, μ $(= 1/t_D)$, is the **exponential growth rate constant,** expressed as generations per hour. It is 1.45 times the instantaneous growth rate constant α, because the value of B, and hence of αB, is constantly increasing during exponential growth; and at the end of doubling, the rate of cell synthesis is twice what it was at the beginning.

Figure 3–2 demonstrates the curvature of exponential growth when plotted linearly, rather than logarithmically, against time. Precisely the same curve would be obtained if cell number were measured instead of cell mass, because ordinary bacterial cultures are **asynchronous:** because the cells at any moment are randomly distributed in the division cycle, the rate of division rises continuously rather than discontinuously. The growth of a hypothetical perfectly synchronized culture is compared in Figure 3–3.

The linear relation between logarithm of number (or mass) and time is obtained regardless of the base of the logarithm. Logarithms to the base 10 are conventional, but the base 2 is more pertinent because the unit of growth then represents a doubling (one generation). The conversion is made through the relation:

$$\log_2 x = \log_{10} x / \log_{10} 2 = 3.3 \log_{10} x$$

It is convenient to remember that $2^{10} = 1024$; i.e., 10 generations equal a 1000-fold increase and 20 generations a million-fold. In exponential growth plotted in terms of the conventional $\log_{10}$, an increase of 0.3 units equals one generation.

From these considerations, it is evident that exponential growth must be more the exception than the rule in the life of bacteria. A bacterium that doubles in 20 minutes will yield 10 generations (10^3 cells)

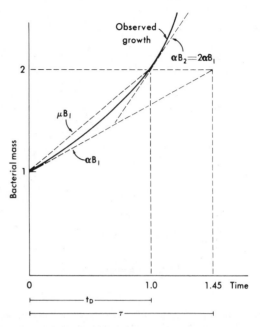

Figure 3–2. Kinetics of exponential growth. B_1, initial bacterial mass, B_2, doubled mass, t_D, doubling time, τ, instantaneous generation time, α, instantaneous growth rate constant, μ, exponential growth rate constant.

in 3.3 hours and 10^9 cells in 10 hours, whereas a bacterium doubling every 60 minutes would require three times as long. (These rates are approximately the values for many species on a rich and on a minimal medium, respectively.) Hence, single cells yield visible colonies (about 10^6–10^7 cells) in overnight cultures. Furthermore, because the volume of an average bacterium is 1 μm^3, or 10^{-12} cm^3, the volume of the earth (about 4×10^{27} cm^3) is equivalent to 4×10^{39} bacteria; and the progeny of our rapidly growing cell would reach this volume in only 45 hours if growth remained exponential. Fortunately, something becomes limiting earlier.

The Chemostat

Though cells harvested in exponential growth are adequate for many physiological studies, they have been growing in an ever-changing environment. Continuous-flow cultures, in a device called the chemostat (Fig. 3–4), yield cells in truly steady-state growth in a medium of constant composition. In this instrument, fresh medium flows into a stirred growth chamber at a constant rate; each drop causes a drop of culture to overflow, and so the volume of growing culture is constant. A **growth-limiting concentration** of a specific required nutrient in the medium determines the **cell density** in the steady-state culture, and the **rate of flow of the medium** determines the **rate of growth.** The chemostat thus permits the indefinite growth of bacteria in a constant medium with independent control of the growth rate and population density. It has made possible very precise analysis of mutation rates and of regulation of enzyme formation.

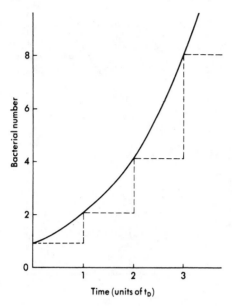

Figure 3–3. Arithmetical plot of the increase in cell number in asynchronous *(solid line)* and hypothetic synchronous *(broken line)* exponential growth. In either type of growth, mass would follow the solid line.

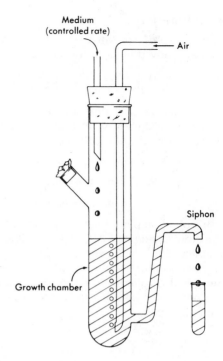

Figure 3–4. Simplified diagram of the chemostat. (For a detailed description, see Novick A, Szilard L: Proc Natl Acad Sci USA 36:708, 1950)

Because the mass of growing bacteria remains constant, growth is **linear** rather than exponential. The observed doubling time is therefore the instantaneous generation time (τ), as shown in Figure 3–2.

Synchronized Growth

In a growing bacterial culture, the cells are distributed among all stages in the division cycle;* hence chemical analyses yield only average values. However, variations in a cell during its division cycle are pertinent to the study of DNA replication and cell wall morphogenesis, and they may also affect mutability, susceptibility to damage to DNA, and uptake of DNA or other molecules. Techniques have therefore been sought for synchronizing the growth of bacteria; i.e., for producing cultures in which all the cells would be in approximately the same part of the division cycle. Synchronization can be achieved by mechanically separating small cells, produced by a recent division, from the larger cells in later stages of the division cycle. In one procedure, cells are wedged in the **pores of a membrane filter;** subsequent reverse flow of fresh, warm medium through the filter provides a continuous supply of "newborn" cells derived by fission from the permanently trapped cells. The released cells are accumulated in a chilled tube, and when incubated in

fresh medium their divisions are synchronous for several generations. Thereafter, the times of division become scattered—a loss of synchronization also seen in the division times of single cells on solid media, observed under the microscope. Causes may be lack of precise equipartition of cytoplasm in cell division and stochastic variation in the timing of replication and of division.

During a synchronized doubling of cell size, the synthesis of the principal constituents proceeds exponentially (Fig. 3–5) except that DNA synthesis proceeds linearly until the chromosome is replicated (Ch. 7). Accordingly, **exponential growth, $dB/dt = \alpha B$, is a property of the growing cell** and not simply a statistical property of the culture: a cell on the verge of dividing has twice as many enzyme molecules and ribosomes as a cell just formed, and it grows twice as fast.

GROWTH ON SOLID MEDIUM
Solidifying Agents

The earliest method available for enumerating bacteria or for isolating pure cultures (clones)† was **extinction**

---

* Although a culture may reasonably be referred to as "old" if harvested after a long stationary incubation or long-term storage, it is ambiguous to speak of bacterial cells themselves as old, because they do not have a life cycle that includes generation of progeny, senescence, and death.

† A **clone** is defined as a group of organisms derived by vegetative reproduction from a single parental organism. Thus, any pure culture of bacteria is a clone, and the progeny of a mutant arising in it are a subclone.

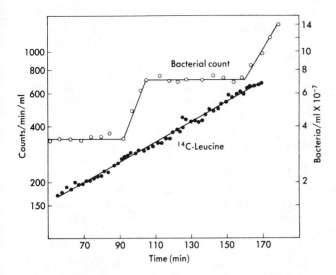

Figure 3–5. Exponential synthesis of protein in an *E. coli* culture synchronized by filtration. Protein synthesis was measured as incorporation of radioactive leucine from the medium into cell components precipitated with trichloroacetic acid. (Adapted from Abbo FD, Pardee AB: Biochim Biophys Acta 39:478, 1960)

dilution; i.e., dilution up to loss of infectivity. An important advance was the introduction of **solid media** by Koch. **Agar,** a polysaccharide derived from certain seaweeds, proved to be an ideal substance. It is nontoxic to bacteria, and very few attack it. At 1.5% to 2% agar, the surface is wet enough to support growth but dry enough to keep colonies separate. (Exceptionally motile organisms, such as *Proteus*, require about 5% agar to prevent swarming). After melting at 80° to 100°C, agar solutions remain fluid at temperatures down to 45° to 50°, which most bacteria can withstand briefly; and after solidifying at room temperature, the solutions remain solid far above 37°. The fibrous structure of the gel is fine enough to prevent motility of bacteria within it but coarse enough to permit diffusion of even macromolecular nutrients.

Agar is primarily a polymer of galactose, with one sulfate per 10 to 50 residues, and these bind polyvalent cations preferentially. A sulfate-free fraction, **agarose,** is available for special purposes.

Uses of Solid Media

We have already noted the utility of plating as a means of **enumerating viable cells** and **isolating pure cultures.** Another important use is to **identify organisms.** A practiced eye can recognize a variety of species in a throat or stool culture on the basis of the appearance of the colonies; the presumptive diagnosis can then be confirmed by further tests.

In using a **selective** solid medium (see below) to **isolate pure cultures** from a naturally occurring mixture,

the colonies may overlap, and even feed, viable cells of other species that cannot grow on the medium used. Accordingly, a colony from the first plate should be streaked again to yield single colonies on **a second plate of the same medium;** one of these colonies can then be used to furnish the stock culture.

Agar plates lend themselves to a variety of **special applications.** For example, on a heavily seeded plate, the **antimicrobial sensitivity** of a strain is specified by the zones of inhibition around paper disks each containing a known amount of a particular agent. Similarly, with an auxotroph, the response to a growth factor on a disk can be recognized from the zone of surrounding growth. **Syntrophism** (cross-feeding) between adjacent streaks of two auxotrophic mutants has been very useful in identifying strains that accumulate and others that respond to a biosynthetic intermediate. The same phenomenon is sometimes seen as **satellite growth** of some organisms around colonies of others on diagnostic plates.

Colonial Morphology

SURFACE TEXTURE. One of the most important diagnostic features of a colony is the texture of its surface, ranging from rough (R) to smooth (S) to mucoid (M) (Fig. 3–6). **Smooth** colonies reflect the presence of a capsule or other surface component that promotes a compact cellular orientation. **Rough** colonies have a dry and sometimes wrinkled surface; they are formed by cells that lack such a component or that grow as filaments. Different degrees of roughness within a species are often correlated with differences in virulence.

Thus with the tubercle bacillus, **virulence** is associated with a lipophilic surface component that causes the cells to adhere to each other in serpentine **cords** that form rough colonies, whereas mutations to decreased virulence are often associated with a smoother colony. With many organisms, in contrast, **virulent strains** form a surface component associated with a **smooth** colony: polysaccharide side chains on the outer membrane in gram-negative organisms (e.g., *Enterobacteriaceae*), and a capsule in gram-positive organisms (e.g., pneumococci; Fig. 3–6). In the former, a capsule may also be formed, yielding a **mucoid** or **glossy** colony.

Capsule formation, and therefore colonial morphology, sometimes depends on environmental as well as on genetic factors. Some nonmucoid *Enterobacteriaceae* become mucoid if grown at a low temperature or in a medium with an excess of carbon and limited nitrogen or phosphorus. Mucoid colonies may be huge and even liquid because of the volume of capsular material produced.

SIZE. Colony size provides a more sensitive comparison of growth rate than does the most careful direct measurement of growth rate in liquid medium. Thus, the latter cannot detect directly a 1% difference in the growth rate of two organisms. However, growth from one cell to the 10^7 cells of a colony involves about 23 generations; and if the differential of 1% is maintained through this period, the faster grower multiplies through $(1.01/1)^{23} = 1.3$ times as many generations and hence yields a proportionately larger colony.

Differential media may reveal specific characteristics without being selective and are very useful in bacterial identification. **Blood agar,** containing 5% sheep or horse blood, can reveal production of a hemolysin.

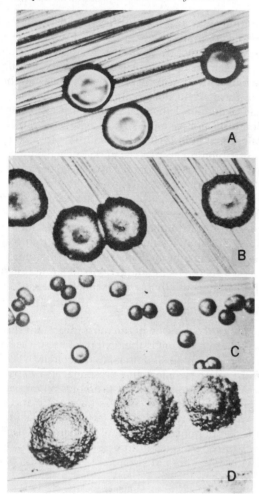

small to reveal characteristic morphology, and their extensive production of acid can obscure the staining of fermenting colonies and can cause diffuse nonspecific hemolysis.

In diagnostic work, the bacteria in a colony are often further identified by overnight growth in tubes of various media (**fermentation tubes**), which test for the ability to carry out various biochemical reactions. Some tests can be carried out directly, and hence rapidly, on the initial colonies; for example, catalase or oxidase production.

Selective Media

The predominant cell types in a mixed population can be readily cloned on a plate by simple dilution. Minor components, however, require selective media. Selective

Figure 3–6. Variations in colonial morphology of pneumococcus strains. *(A)* Smooth colonies of capsulated, nonfilamentous cells. *(B)* Rougher colonies of capsulated but filamentous variant. *(C)* Nonfilamentous noncapsulated variant. *(D)* Roughest variant, filamentous and noncapsulated. All photographs ×18 after 24 hours of incubation at 36°C on blood agar. (Austrian R: J Exp Med 98:21, 1953)

In **fermentation plates,** utilization of the particular sugar provided is revealed by indicator dyes, such as an eosin–methylene blue (EMB) mixture, which not only changes color but precipitates in the presence of acid; hence, the colony itself is stained, and precipitation is sufficiently localized to demarcate stained **sectors** in a colony that contains a mutant subclone (Fig. 3–7). Fermentation plates are used largely for facultative organisms; they are effective even when incubated in air, because such organisms convert sugars to organic acids faster than they can burn the latter to CO_2.

A fermentation plate must contain other nutrients besides the test sugar, to permit the growth of fermentation-negative organisms. When such negative colonies are fully grown, they may give rise, on long-term incubation, to positive **papillae** (Fig. 3–7) derived from mutant cells arising late in the growth of the colony. Through similar selection, colonies on old plates are frequently warty and irregular.

In **diagnostic bacteriology,** it is important to deal with well-separated colonies; **crowded colonies** are too

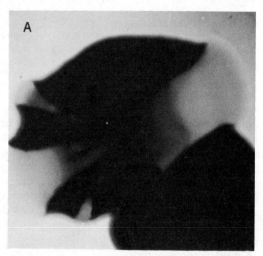

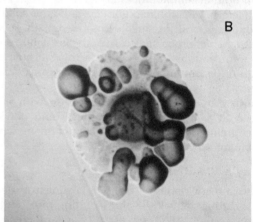

Figure 3–7. *(A)* Lac⁻ (unstained) sectors in colony derived from an ultraviolet-irradiated Lac⁺ *E. coli* cell, plated on EMB-lactose medium, which stains only Lac⁺ cells. Note sharp demarcation of sectors and adjacent Lac⁺ colony without Lac⁻ mutants. *(B)* Lac⁺ papillae, arising late in Lac⁻ colony incubated for several days on EMB-lactose medium. *(A,* courtesy of HB Newcombe; *B,* courtesy of V Bryson)

liquid media **enrich** the population with respect to the desired organisms, whereas solid media permit direct **isolation.**

Organisms that can utilize a given sugar are easily screened for by making that compound the only carbon source. Similarly, the use of a minimal medium will exclude fastidious organisms. Selection in the opposite direction (nonutilizers; requirement for specific factors) is not always possible and is indirect; i.e., it is based on **selective inhibition** of the unwanted organisms (e.g., by unfavorable pH, salts, specific inhibitors).

Surface antigens (Ags) are the basis for two newer methods for isolating rare bacteria: adsorption by antibodies (Abs) fixed on a column and separation by a cell sorter that recognizes immunofluorescent staining.

Sterilization and Disinfection

The early arts of civilization included practical means of preventing putrefaction and decay long before the role of microorganisms in these processes was appreciated. Perishable foods were preserved by drying, by salting, and by acid-producing fermentations. Embalming was practiced in ancient Egypt, but the essential oils used were probably less important than the dry climate. As was noted in Chapter 1, the canning of food was introduced 50 years before Pasteur's research gave it a rational basis. Similarly, calcium hypochlorite and phenol were introduced in the early nineteenth century to deodorize sewage, garbage, and wounds even before their germicidal action was recognized.

The subsequent need for pure cultures in bacteriology required the development of reliable methods for not merely reducing but eliminating viable microorganisms; i.e., sterilization. These techniques were then rapidly adapted to prevent the spread of infectious disease.

Definitions

Sterilization denotes the use of physical or chemical agents to eliminate **all** viable microbes from a material, whereas **disinfection** generally refers to the use of germicidal chemical agents to destroy the potential **infectivity** of a material and need not imply elimination of all viable microbes. **Sanitizing** refers to procedures used to lower the bacterial content of utensils used for food without necessarily sterilizing them. **Antisepsis** usually refers to the topical application of chemicals to a body surface to kill or inhibit pathogenic microbes.

A **bacteriostatic** agent prevents further multiplication but allows the inhibited cell to remain viable; i.e. to resume multiplication in an adequate medium when the agent is removed or diluted. **Bactericidal** action damages the cell irreversibly, so it cannot resume multiplication. **Chemotherapeutic** agents (Ch. 10) may be either bacteriostatic or bactericidal, but disinfectants must be bactericidal.

In further contrast to the highly selective chemotherapeutic agents, disinfectants must be effective against all kinds of microbes, must be relatively insensitive to their metabolic state, and need not be harmless to host cells. They are widely used for skin antisepsis in preparation for surgery. For prophylactic application to open wounds or for topical application to superficial infections, they have been largely replaced by various antibiotics, which are painless and less damaging to the tissues.

CRITERIA OF VIABILITY

With killing by heat or by other methods that disrupt the cell membrane, a useful indirect criterion of cell death is staining by dyes that do not penetrate the normal membrane. This test is not useful, however, for methods of killing that act by damaging DNA or other internal constituents.

Tests for damaged cells' viability may give quite different cell counts in different media. For example, spores "sterilized" by Hg^{2+} can be **"resurrected"** by a wash in H_2S solution, which displaces Hg^{2+} from its inhibitory complexes with -SH groups in cell constituents.

The problem of defining viability assumes practical importance in the preparation of vaccines, which are often sterilized as gently as possible in order to retain maximal immunogenicity. Killing is ordinarily tested in culture media, but it is necessary to be sure that the organisms have also lost the ability to initiate infection in the animal body.

Sterilization is not identical with **destruction** of bacteria or their products. Accordingly, in preparing solutions for intravenous administration, it is necessary to minimize prior bacterial contamination, because **pyrogenic** bacterial products (which can survive autoclaving or filtration) may subsequently produce a febrile response.

CLASSES OF LETHAL ACTION

On theoretical grounds, there appear to be only three general ways to kill a cell: irreparable damage to its genome, to its envelope, or to certain classes of proteins. With most proteins, denaturation of all the molecules should not be lethal, for if the corresponding gene is intact and the required energy and building blocks are supplied, the cell should be able to regenerate that protein. The same should be true of RNAs. However, **complete elimination of any protein that is required for protein synthesis** (RNA polymerase, ribosomal proteins, or the enzymes and protein factors of protein synthesis) would prevent the protein synthesis required for regeneration of the missing species.

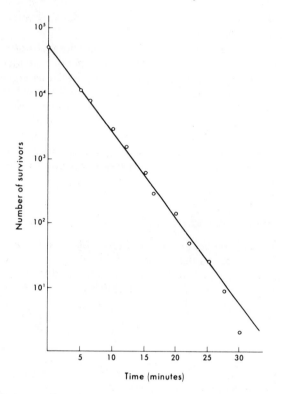

Figure 3–8. Exponential killing by heat of spores of a thermophilic bacillus. Number of survivors is plotted on a logarithmic scale against time of exposure to 120°C. (After Williams CC et al: Food Res 2:369, 1937)

Many bactericidal agents exhibit **first-order kinetics,** in which the viable number declines exponentially:

$$\ln n = \ln n_0 - kt$$

Surprisingly, similar kinetics have been observed for the action of heat (Fig. 3–8) or of chemical disinfectants such as phenol. Hence, even though these agents must damage many different proteins in a cumulative manner, the lethal event cannot be the denaturation of the last of many molecules of a given species, for this process would give a multi-hit curve with a long lag and then a steep decline. The one-hit (exponential) curve suggests, instead, a single irreparable damage to the DNA or a sudden opening of a hole in the membrane.

PHYSICAL AGENTS
Heat

Heat is generally preferred for sterilizing materials except those that it would damage. The agent penetrates clumps and reaches sites that might be protected from a chemical disinfectant. Fungi, most viruses, and the vegetative cells of various pathogenic bacteria are sterilized

within a few minutes at 50° to 70°C and the spores of various pathogens at 100°. The spores of some saprophytes, however, can survive boiling for hours. Because absolute sterility is essential for culture media and for the instruments used in major surgical procedures, it has become standard practice to sterilize such materials by steam in an **autoclave** at a temperature of 121°C (250°F) for 15 to 20 minutes.

At altitudes near sea level, this temperature is attained by steam at a pressure of 15 lb per square inch (psi) in excess of atmospheric pressure. In Denver, at an altitude of 5000 ft, a pressure 3 psi higher is required. The rapid action of steam depends in part on the large latent heat of water (540 cal/g): cold objects are thus rapidly heated by condensation on their surface. The steam pressure may be maintained in an outer jacket while the central chamber is decompressed, so that condensation water is evaporated rapidly.

In using an autoclave, it is important that flowing steam be allowed to displace the air before building up pressure, for in steam mixed with air, the temperature is determined by the partial pressure of the water vapor. Thus, if air at 1 atm (15 psi) remains in the chamber and steam is added to provide an additional gauge pressure at 1 atm, the average temperature will be only 100° (that of steam at 1 atm). Moreover, heating will be uneven because the air will tend to remain at the bottom of the chamber.

Pasteurization is now used primarily for milk. It consists of heating at 62°C for 30 minutes or, in "flash" pasteurization, at a higher temperature for a fraction of a minute. The total bacterial count is generally reduced by 97% to 99%. Pasteurization is effective because the common milkborne pathogens (tubercle bacillus, *Salmonella*, *Streptococcus*, and *Brucella*) do not form spores.

KINETICS. The sensitivity of an organism to heat is often expressed in practical work as the **thermal death point:** the lowest temperature at which a 10-minute exposure of a given volume of a broth culture results in sterilization. The value is about 55°C for *E. coli*, 60° for the tubercle bacillus, and 120° for the most resistant spores.

For precise studies, this qualitative endpoint has been replaced by quantitative determination of the numbers of survivors at different times. Because killing by heat turns out to have simple exponential kinetics, the rate of killing can be expressed in terms of the **rate constant** k in the exponential decay curve. Another convenient index, the **decimal reduction time,** D (the time required for a ten-fold reduction of viability), is inversely proportional to the rate of killing. Its logarithm varies linearly with temperature (Fig. 3–9), and from the slope of the curve, it can be seen that the rate of killing (of the spores studied in this figure) increased about ten-fold with a rise of 10°.

MOIST HEAT AND DRY HEAT. Sterilization by heat involves **protein denaturation** and the **melting of membrane lipids** as a consequence of the disruption of multiple weak bonds. Among these, hydrogen bonds between a $>C=O$ and an $HN<$ group are more readily

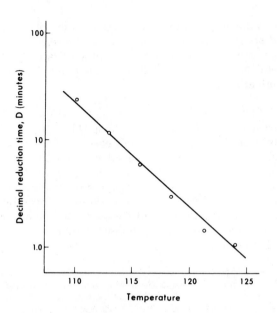

Figure 3–9. Rate of killing of spores of a thermophilic bacillus at various temperatures, in terms of the time required for a ten-fold reduction in viability. (Schmidt CF: In Reddish CF [ed]: Antiseptics, Disinfectants, Fungicides, and Sterilization. Philadelphia, Lea & Febiger, 1957)

broken if they can be replaced with hydrogen bonds to water molecules (Fig. 3–10). Accordingly, sterilization requires a **higher temperature for dry than for wet material.** Reliable sterilization of glassware and instruments in a dry oven requires 160°C for 1 to 2 hours. In addition, bacteria and viruses, like isolated enzymes, are more stable in an aqueous medium when the water concentration is reduced by the presence of a high concentration of glycerol or glucose.

The role of water in heat denaturation of proteins is illustrated by the usefulness of steam in pressing woolen fabrics (i.e., in shifting the multiple weak bonds between fibrous molecules of keratin).

Freezing

When a suspension of bacteria is frozen, the crystallization of the water results in the formation of tiny pockets of concentrated solutions of salts, which do not themselves crystallize unless the temperature is lowered below the eutectic point (about −20°C for NaCl); at this temperature, the solution becomes saturated, and the salt also crystallizes. The localized high concentrations of salt, and possibly the ice crystals, damage the bacteria, as shown by their increased sensitivity to lysozyme. Only some of the cells are killed, but repeated cycles of freezing and thawing result in a progressive decrease in the viable count.

PRESERVATION. Once frozen, the surviving cells retain their viability indefinitely if the temperature is kept below the eutectic points of the various salts present: a satisfactory temperature is provided by solid CO_2 (−78°) or liquid N_2 (−180°), but not by a household freezing unit (about −10°C).

In preserving bacteria, viruses, or animal cells by freezing, it is helpful to add a relatively high concentration of glycerol, DMSO, or protein. These agents promote amorphous, vitreous solidification instead of crystallization on cooling, thus avoiding local high concentrations of salt. Similarly, protein-rich materials (milk, serum) are added in the preservation of bacteria by **lyophilization** (desiccation from the frozen state).

Ultraviolet Radiation

With radiation of decreasing wavelength, the killing of bacteria first becomes appreciable at 330 nm and then increases rapidly. The sterilizing effect of sunlight is attributable mainly to its content of UV light (300–400 nm). Most of the UV light approaching the earth from the sun, and all of that shorter than 290 nm, is screened out by the ozone in the outer regions of the atmosphere; otherwise, organisms could not survive on the earth's surface.

UV absorption by bacteria is attributable chiefly to the purines and pyrimidines of nucleic acids, with an average maximum at 260 nm. In addition, the aromatic rings of tryptophan, tyrosine, and phenylalanine in proteins absorb more moderately, with an average maximum at 280 nm. The sterilization action spectrum (i.e., the efficiency of sterilization by radiation of various wavelengths) parallels the absorption spectrum of the bacteria, suggesting that absorption by either nucleic acid or protein can have a lethal effect.

MECHANISM. Lethal mutations make only a small contribution to UV killing: the principal mechanism is alterations in the DNA that block its replication or transcription. Because most of these alterations can be repaired (Ch. 8), the quantum efficiency of UV sterilization is ordi-

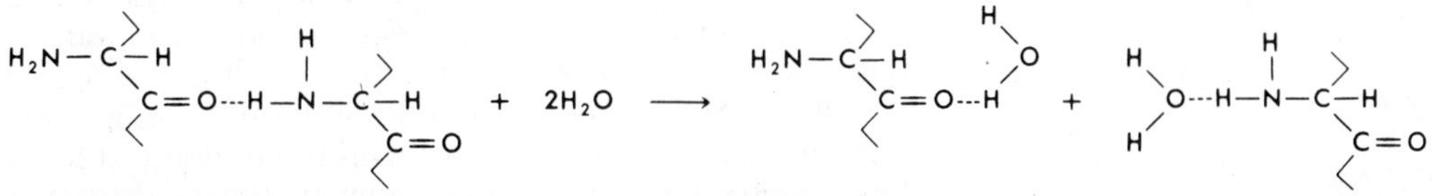

$$H_2N-C{\overset{\diagup}{\underset{\diagdown}{}}}H \quad {\overset{H}{\underset{\diagdown}{}}}{\underset{\diagdown}{}}C{=}O{\cdots}H{-}N{-}C{\overset{\diagup}{\underset{\diagdown}{}}}H \quad + \ 2H_2O \longrightarrow \quad H_2N-C{\overset{\diagup}{\underset{\diagdown}{}}}H \quad C{=}O{\cdots}H \quad + \quad O{\cdots}H{-}N{-}C{\overset{\diagup}{\underset{\diagdown}{}}}H$$

Figure 3–10. Role of water in promoting the denaturation of protein by heat by facilitating disruption of intramolecular hydrogen bonds between peptide groups.

narily very low. The rest of the cellular machinery is still functional; hence heavy irradiation of host cells followed by infection with a phage restricts subsequent synthesis of mRNA and proteins to those coded for by the phage.

PRACTICAL USES. Inexpensive low-pressure mercury vapor lamps, emitting 90% of their radiation at 254 nm, are widely used to decrease airborne infection. Its effectiveness in public places seems uncertain, but it has been convincingly demonstrated in hospital wards and in animal houses, where the infected individuals cannot make close contact with other individuals. In laboratory areas used for culture transfers, UV lamps are similarly useful to decrease contamination and the infection of workers. It is important to protect the eyes (glass is opaque to UV), as excessive exposure of the cornea to UV causes severe irritation, with a latent period of about 12 hours.

IONIZING RADIATIONS. The lethal and mutagenic actions of X-ray and other ionizing radiations will be discussed in Chapter 8. This mechanism is not convenient for routine laboratory use, but intense sources of radioactivity are now being used to sterilize food. Public fear of danger from the irradiation is unwarranted, as the activated mutagenic molecules produced by the irradiation are extremely short-lived.

Photodynamic Sensitization

In the presence of certain fluorescent dyes (e.g., methylene blue, rose bengal), strong **visible light** denatures proteins and sterilizes bacteria and viruses. These dyes retain an absorbed quantum for a comparatively long time (10^{-6}–10^{-8} seconds), during which the energy sometimes is transferred to another molecule instead of being emitted as fluorescence. This transfer leads to oxidation of certain residues in proteins (especially histidine and tryptophan) and in nucleic acids.

Even in the absence of added dyes, intense visible light is capable of killing bacteria, presumably via physiologically occurring photosensitizing substances such as **riboflavin** and **porphyrins.** It is therefore inadvisable to expose bacterial cultures to direct sunlight even when protected by UV-absorbing glass. For example, BCG vaccine in glass ampules can lose all viability and effectiveness on exposure to bright sunlight in outdoor field stations.

Psoralen markedly increases sensitivity to killing by near-UV, which causes it to form cross-links between the two strands of DNA.

MECHANICAL AGENTS
Ultrasonic and Sonic Waves

In the supersonic (ultrasonic) range, with a frequency of 15,000 to several hundred thousand per second, sound waves denature proteins, disperse a variety of materials, and sterilize and fragment bacteria. The effect has not been of practical value as a means of sterilization, but it is useful for disrupting cells for experimental purposes (**sonication**).

Filtration

Bacteria-free filtrates may be obtained by the use of filters with a maximum pore size not exceeding 400 nm. This procedure is used for solutions that cannot tolerate sterilization by heat (e.g., sera and media containing proteins or labile metabolites). The early, rather adsorptive filters of asbestos or diatomaceous earth were replaced by unglazed porcelain or sintered glass, and these in turn have been replaced by nitrocellulose membrane filters of graded porosity.

Membrane filters can also be used to recover bacteria quantitatively for chemical or microbiological analysis. Moreover, when incubated on a solid nutrient medium, cells on the filter can give rise to colonies, and these can conveniently be exposed to a succession of different media by transfer of the filter.

CHEMICAL AGENTS

Among the many chemicals (including nutrients such as O_2 and fatty acids) that are bacteriostatic and even bactericidal at sufficiently high concentrations, the term **disinfectant** is restricted to those that are rapidly bactericidal at low concentrations. Unlike most chemotherapeutic agents, which interact with active metabolic systems, most disinfectants act either by dissolving lipids from the cell membrane (detergents, lipid solvents) or by damaging proteins or nucleic acids (denaturants, oxidants, alkylating agents, sulfhydryl reagents).

The rate of killing by disinfectants increases with concentration and with temperature. Anionic compounds are more active at low pH and cationic compounds at high pH, which promote penetration and increase opposite charges in cell constituents.

Determination of Disinfectant Potency

Ever since Lister began spraying surgical operating rooms with phenol, this compound has been considered the standard disinfectant, although it is required in a relatively high concentration—0.9%—to sterilize a suspension of *Salmonella typhosa* under standard conditions in 10 minutes. The **phenol coefficient** of a compound is the ratio of the minimal sterilizing concentration of phenol to that of the compound. In the official test of the U.S. government, a broth culture is diluted 1/10 with various concentrations of the test compound; the endpoint is the lowest concentration that yields, after incubation for 10 minutes at 20°C, sterile loopful samples. The germicide is generally recommended for use at five times this concentration.

The phenol coefficient provides a reasonable index for comparing various phenol derivatives, but it is less satisfactory for other agents, which may differ in their concentration–action curves and in their susceptibility to neutralization by the environment. Thus, the concentrations of a disinfectant, c, required to sterilize a bacterial population in time t generally correspond to a curve that may be fitted by the equation $(c^n t = k)$. Whereas phenol has the remarkably high concentration coefficient (n) of 5 to 6, oxidants such as hypochlorite have a value of about 1.

The effectiveness of a disinfecting procedure often depends strongly on the "cleanness" of the material. The presence of a large amount of organic matter (e.g., in excreta or discarded cultures) rapidly neutralizes the action of many agents, either by chemical reaction (e.g., with oxidants) or by adsorption. Moreover, drying may encase bacteria in crystals and thus protect them from bactericidal gases. Different kinds of disinfectants are therefore used for different purposes, such as skin antisepsis, sanitizing food containers, or rendering discarded cultures harmless.

As with killing by heat (see Fig. 3–8), the sensitivity of an organism to a disinfectant can be expressed more precisely as the slope of the semilogarithmic curve for killing as a function of time. However, the curves for chemical disinfection are often imperfectly exponential. Hence, the endpoint remains of practical value.

Specific Chemical Agents

ACIDS AND ALKALIS. Strongly acid and alkaline solutions are actively bactericidal. However, mycobacteria are relatively resistant, it being common practice to liquefy sputum before plating by exposure for 30 min to 1N NaOH or H_2SO_4. Boric acid has been used as a mild antiseptic.

With weak organic acids the presence of undissociated molecules promotes penetration into the cells, and the increasing activity with chain length suggests a direct action of the organic compound itself. (Long-chain fatty acids will be considered under Surface-Active Agents.) Lactic acid is the natural preservative of many fermentation products, and salts of propionic acid (CH_3CH_2COOH) are frequently added to foods to retard mold growth.

SALTS. Pickling in brine or treatment with solid NaCl has been used for many centuries as a means of preserving perishable meats and fish. Bacteria differ widely in susceptibility.

HEAVY METALS. The various metallic ions can be arranged in a series of decreasing antibacterial activity. With small inocula, Hg^{2+} and Ag^+, at the head of the list, are effective at less than 1 part per million (ppm) because of their high affinity for -SH groups. The antibacterial action of Hg^{2+} can be reversed readily by sulfhydryl compounds.

Various organic mercury compounds (e.g., Merthiolate, Mercurochrome), in which one of the valences of Hg is covalently combined, have been used as relatively nonirritating antiseptics. Silver has long been used in various forms as a mild antiseptic. Copper salts have great importance as fungicides in agriculture but not in medicine.

HALOGENS. Iodine combines irreversibly with proteins (e.g., by iodinating tyrosine residues), and it is an oxidant. **Tincture of iodine** (a 2%–7% solution of I_2 in aqueous alcohol containing KI) is a reliable antiseptic for skin and for minor wounds, but it has a painful and destructive effect on exposed tissue. I_2 complexes spontaneously with detergents to form **iodophors,** which provide a readily available reservoir of bound I_2 in equilibrium with free I_2 at an effective but nonirritating concentration.

Chlorine was the antiseptic introduced (as chlorinated lime) by O. W. Holmes in Boston in 1835 and by Semmelweis in Vienna in 1847 to prevent transmission of puerperal sepsis by the physician's hands. Chlorine combines with water to form hypochlorous acid (HOCl), a strong oxidizing agent:

$$Cl_2 + H_2O \rightleftharpoons HCl + HOCl$$

or

$$Cl_2 + 2NaOH \rightleftharpoons NaCl + NaOCl + H_2O$$

Hypochlorite solutions (200 ppm Cl_2) are used to sanitize clean surfaces in the food and the dairy industries and in restaurants; and Cl_2 gas, added at 1 to 3 ppm, is widely used to disinfect water supplies and swimming pools. Chlorine is a reliable, rapidly acting disinfectant for such "clean" materials.

The "chlorine demand" of a water supply increases with its content of organic matter, and chlorination must be titrated to a definite level of free Cl_2. This reactivity of Cl_2 is a virtue in the sanitizing of food utensils: residual traces of chlorine will be destroyed rapidly on subsequent contact with food, leaving no flavor or odor.

OTHER OXIDANTS. Hydrogen peroxide (H_2O_2) in a 3% solution was once widely used as an antiseptic, but bacteria differ greatly in their susceptibility, as some species possess catalase. **Peracetic acid** ($CH_3CO-O-OH$), a strong oxidizing agent, is used as a vapor for the sterilization of chambers for germ-free animals.

ALKYLATING AGENTS. Formaldehyde and ethylene oxide replace the labile H atoms on $-NH_2$, -OH, -COOH, and -SH groups (Fig. 3–11). The reactions of formaldehyde are in part reversible, but the high-energy epoxide bridge of ethylene oxide leads to irreversible reactions. These alkylating agents, in contrast to other disinfectants, are nearly as active against spores as against vegetative bacterial cells, presumably because they can penetrate eas-

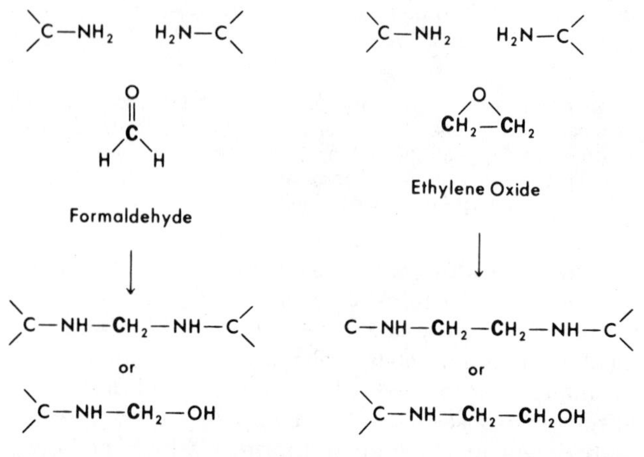

Figure 3–11. Reactions of formaldehyde and ethylene oxide with amino groups. Similar condensations may take place with other nucleophilic groups. Bridges may be formed between groups on the same molecule or on different molecules.

ily, being small and uncharged, and do not require H_2O for their action.

Formaldehyde is usually marketed as a 37% aqueous solution (Formalin). It also may be used as a gas for sterilizing dry surfaces.

Ethylene oxide, a highly water-soluble gas, has proved to be reliable for gaseous disinfection of heat-sensitive objects: plasticware; surgical equipment; hospital bedding; and books, leather, etc. handled by patients. Its action is slower than that of steam, and it is more expensive and presents some hazard of residual toxicity (vesicant action). Indeed, the potential hazards of mutagenicity and carcinogenicity for humans deserve careful investigation, as formaldehyde and ethylene oxide, like other alkylating agents, have been shown to be mutagenic.

SURFACE-ACTIVE AGENTS (SURFACTANTS). Synthetic detergents, like fatty acids (soaps), contain both a hydrophobic and a hydrophilic portion: They therefore form micelles (large aggregates) in aqueous solution in which only the hydrophilic portion is in contact with water, and they can similarly form a layer that coats and solubilizes hydrophobic molecules. Anionic detergents are only weakly bactericidal, perhaps because they are repelled by the net negative charge of the bacterial surface; they are more effective against gram-negative than gram-positive organisms. Nonionic detergents are not bactericidal and may even serve as nutrients.

Cationic detergents, however, are active against all kinds of bacteria. The most effective types are the **quaternary** compounds, containing three short-chain alkyl groups as well as a long-chain alkyl group (e.g., benzalkonium chloride; Fig. 3–12). These compounds are widely

used for skin antisepsis and for sanitizing food utensils. They act by disrupting the cell membrane. In addition, their detergent action provides the advantage of dissolving lipid films that may protect bacteria. In the absence of adsorbing molecules, they may be rapidly bactericidal at concentrations as low as 1 ppm, and unlike many other disinfectants, they are not poisonous to man. Their activity is neutralized by soaps and phospholipids, because oppositely charged surfactants precipitate each other.

PHENOLS. Phenol (C_6H_5OH) is both an effective denaturant of proteins and a detergent, and it causes cell lysis. Its antibacterial activity is increased by halogen or alkyl substituents on the ring, which increase the polarity of the phenolic–OH group and make the molecule more surface active. With increasing chain length, the potency of phenols at first increases, but then it decreases, presumably because of low solubility. Phenols are more active when mixed with soaps, which increase their solubility and promote penetration.

A mixture of **tricresol** (mixed ortho-, meta-, and para-methylphenol) and soap is a widely used disinfectant for discarded bacteriologic materials. Its action is not impaired by the presence of organic matter because it must be used in a relatively high concentration.

Halogenated bis-phenols, such as **hexachlorophene** (below) are bacteriostatic in very high dilutions.

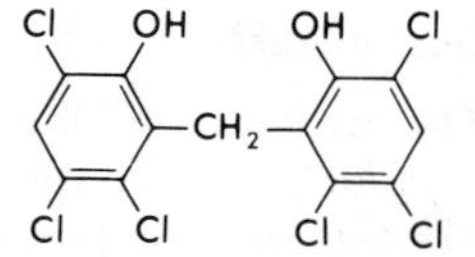

Hexachlorophene is widely used as a skin antiseptic (especially mixed with a detergent, as pHisoHex). However, its absorption through inflamed skin may cause serious systemic toxicity.

Alkyl esters of *p*-hydroxybenzoic acid are used as a preservative in foods and pharmaceuticals: they act on bacteria much like an alkyl-substituted phenol, but when taken by mouth, they are nontoxic because they are rapidly hydrolyzed, yielding the harmless free *p*-hydroxybenzoate.

The **essential oils** of plants, which have been used since antiquity as preservatives and antiseptics, contain

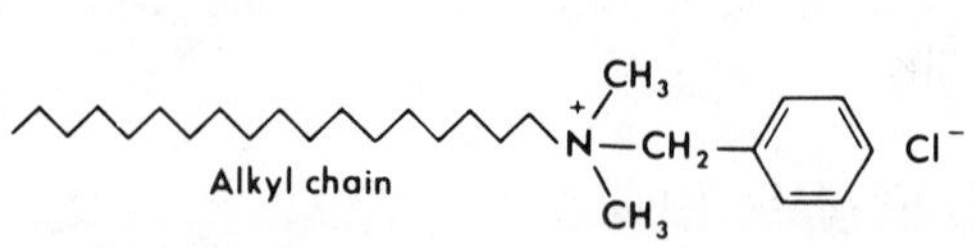

Figure 3–12. Benzalkonium chloride (benzyldimethyl alkonium chloride; Zephiran), a typical quaternary ammonium detergent; the long-chain alkyl group is a mixture obtained by the reduction and amination of the fatty acids of vegetable or animal fat.

a variety of phenolic compounds, including thymol (5-methyl-2-isopropylphenol) and eugenol (4-allyl-2-methoxyphenol); the latter is used in dentistry as an antiseptic in cavities.

ALCOHOLS. The disinfectant action of the aliphatic alcohols increases with chain length up to 8 to 10 carbon atoms, above which the water solubility becomes too low. Although **ethanol** (CH_3CH_2OH) has received widest use, **isopropyl alcohol** ($CH_3CHOHCH_3$) is less volatile and slightly more potent and is not subject to legal restrictions.

The disinfectant action of alcohols, like their denaturating effect on proteins, involves the participation of water. Ethanol is most effective in 50% to 70% aqueous solution: at 100%, it is a poor disinfectant.

Other organic solvents, such as ether, benzene, acetone, or chloroform, also kill bacteria but are not reliable disinfectants. However, the addition of a few drops of toluene or chloroform, which dissolve slightly in aqueous solutions, will prevent the growth of fungi or bacteria. **Glycerol** is bacteriostatic at concentrations exceeding 50% and is used as a preservative for vaccines and other biologicals because it is not irritating to tissues.

Selected Reading

GROWTH

Campbell AM: Synchronization of cell division. Bacteriol Rev 21:263, 1957

Gray TRG, Postgate JR (eds): The Survival of Vegetative Microbes. 26th Symposium, Society for General Microbiology. Cambridge University Press, 1976

Hitchens AP, Leikind MC: The introduction of agar-agar into bacteriology. J Bacteriol 37:485, 1939

Ingraham JL, Maaloe O, Neidhardt FC: Growth of the Bacterial Cell. Sunderland, MA, Sinauer Associates, 1983. Especially Chapters 5 (Growth of Cells and Cultures) and 6 (Growth Rate as a Variable)

Monod J: La technique de culture continue: Théorie et applications. Ann Inst Pasteur Lille 79:390, 1950

Schaechter M: Going after the growth curve. In Schaechter M, Neidhardt FC, Ingraham JL, Kjeldgaard NO (eds): The Molecular Biology of Bacterial Growth, p 370. Boston, MA, Jones and Bartlett, 1985

Spudich JL, Koshland DE Jr: Nongenetic individuality: Chance in the single cell. Nature 262:467, 1976

Symposium: Continuous culture methods and their application. In Recent Progress in Microbiology, 7th International Congress of Microbiology, Stockholm, 1958. Springfield, IL Charles C Thomas, 1959

Tempest DW: The place of continuous culture in microbiological research. Adv Microbiol Physiol 4:223, 1970

DEATH

Albert A: Selective Toxicity, 5th Ed. London, Methuen, 1978

Beuchat LR: Injury and repair of gram-negative bacteria, with special consideration of the involvement of the cytoplasmic membrane. Adv Appl Microbiol 23:219, 1978

Block SS (ed): Disinfection, Sterilization, and Preservation. Philadelphia, Lea & Febiger, 1968

Bruch CW: Gaseous sterilization. Annu Rev Microbiol 15:245, 1961

Chick H, Browning CH: The theory of disinfection. Med Res Coun Syst Bacteriol [Lond] 1:179, 1930

Hugo WB (ed): Inhibition and Destruction of the Bacterial Cell. New York, Academic Press, 1971

Phillips CB, Warshowsky B: Chemical disinfectants. Annu Rev Microbiol 12:525, 1958

Wells WF: Air-borne Contagion and Air Hygiene. Cambridge, MA, Harvard University Press, 1955

4

Nutrition; Energy; Membrane Transport; Chemotaxis

> When it is possible to catalogue the substances required by pathogenic bacteria for growth, it will probably be found that most of them are . . . important in animal metabolism, and . . . it is equally probable that some will be new.
> —J. H. Mueller, *J Bacteriol* 7:309 (1922)

Nutrition

ORGANIC GROWTH FACTORS

From the days of Pasteur, the culture media used for bacteria were "broths," obtained by cooking animal or vegetable tissues. Mueller initiated the study of bacterial nutrition by fractionating such complex mixtures in an effort to identify the specific required compounds, an approach that soon revealed the previously unknown amino acid methionine.

Subsequent studies showed that the nutritional requirements of various bacteria range widely, from single sources for C and for N to requirements even more complex than those of mammalian cells. The more complex requirements, however, do not reflect greater metabolic complexity: on the contrary, all bacteria make their nucleic acids and proteins from the same building blocks, and their specific organic requirements reflect the absence of the corresponding biosynthetic pathways. With this recognition of the underlying **metabolic unity,** the field of bacterial nutrition has become chiefly of practical interest. However, it still presents challenges: for example, the leprosy bacillus, the treponeme of syphilis, and the rickettsias still cannot be cultivated in artificial media.

The specific growth requirements of bacteria and yeasts could be used for **quantitative microbial assays** for amino acids and vitamins. These assays, much simpler than those in mammals, were used in the isolation of most of the vitamins essential for mammals—for example, a growth factor for a *Lactobacillus* proved to be identical with a hematopoietic factor in patients with pernicious anemia, vitamin B_{12}.

Not surprisingly, those bacteria that have been adapted in evolution to growth in the soil or in natural waters often have simple organic growth requirements. Those adapted to growth in animal tissues or milk or on mucous surfaces may have very complex requirements. These include not only various amino acids and vitamins but also nucleic acid bases, inositol and choline (as components of phospholipids or cell walls), hemin (or porphyrin), unsaturated fatty acids, mevalonic acid (a precursor of isoprenoid compounds), and polyamines.

INORGANIC REQUIREMENTS

CARBON DIOXIDE. The flow of carbon from the glycolytic pathway to the tricarboxylic acid (TCA) cycle requires incorporation of CO_2 into pyruvate or P-enolpyruvate. Accordingly, without added CO_2, the initiation of growth by a small inoculum in minimal medium may have a long lag until the culture has built up its own CO_2. Added TCA cycle intermediates, or the biosynthetic products of the cycle that are present in a rich medium, markedly decrease this dependence. However, even in a rich medium measures that lower the normal pCO_2 (such as use of freshly autoclaved medium) may prevent growth, for the lipids of the cell cannot all be supplied from without, and in their biosynthesis, the acetyl donor, acetyl-CoA, must be activated by attachment of CO_2 to form malonyl-CoA (see Fig. 2-22). Hence all growing cells have an absolute requirement for an adequate pCO_2.

Many pathogens, genetically adapted to the relatively high pCO_2 in the mammalian body, initiate growth better at a pCO_2 higher than that found in air (about 0.03% outdoors); they presumably have some enzyme with a low affinity for CO_2. Elevated pCO_2 is conveniently provided in a **candle jar,** in which a candle is allowed to burn until it extinguishes itself.

INORGANIC IONS. The inorganic ions required in substantial quantity are PO_4^{3-}, K^+, and Mg^{2+}. In the absence of organic sources of N and S, NH_3 and SO_4^{2-} (or a reduced product) are also required. Unlike mammalian cells, most bacteria can thrive in a broad range of concentrations of the required ions, including the very dilute solutions found in natural waters, but they maintain constant internal concentrations by means of active transport systems in their membranes (discussed later in this chapter).

TRACE ELEMENTS. Iron is required, not only for cytochromes in aerobes, but also for ferredoxins (protein factors of low redox potential) in anaerobes and for reduction of ribonucleotides to deoxyribonucleotides in almost all organisms. Its uptake will be described below (Membrane Transport). Other trace metal ion requirements include Zn^{2+}, Mn^{2+}, and Cu^{2+}; Mo^{2+} is required for N_2 fixation and nitrate reduction. Co^{2+} is required for vitamin B_{12}, and because plants do not contain this vitamin, bacteria may be its ultimate source for man. Ca^{2+} does not appear to be required by vegetative bacteria, but it is a significant constituent of bacterial spores (Chap. 2).

AEROBIOSIS AND ANAEROBIOSIS

Bacteria differ markedly in the effect of O_2 or its absence on their growth, in ways that are important for pathogenesis and also for the isolation and identification of the organism.

   1. **Obligate aerobes** (e.g., the tubercle bacillus and some spore-forming bacilli) require O_2 and lack the capacity for substantial fermentation.

   2. **Obligate anaerobes** (e.g., clostridia, propionibacter) can grow only in the absence of O_2. A subgroup, called **microaerophiles,** prefer or even require O_2 at low tension.

   3. **Facultative organisms** (e.g., many yeasts, enterobacteria) can grow without air but also can perform respiration. A facultative organism makes either a fermentative or a respiratory set of enzymes, depending on the conditions. In the shift from aerobic to anaerobic growth, about 50 new enzymes are induced, as shown by acrylamide gel electrophoresis.

   4. **Aerotolerant anaerobes** (e.g., most lactic acid bacteria) resemble facultative organisms in growing either with or without O_2, but their metabolism remains fermentative.

SUPEROXIDE. Obligate anaerobes are not only inhibited but rapidly killed by air. The poison is superoxide (O_2^-), a highly reactive free radical that is formed from O_2 as an intermediate in flavoprotein-linked oxidations. In aerobic organisms **superoxide dismutase** destroys this compound by the reaction:

$$2\,O_2^- + 2H^+ \rightarrow H_2O_2 + O_2$$

The absence of this enzyme in obligate anaerobes accounts for their sensitivity to oxygen poisoning, for mutations that inactivate it in facultative anaerobes also make them sensitive.

Superoxide dismutase occurs in several forms. A permanent (constitutive) form in *E. coli* is Fe^{2+} dependent;

O_2 induces the synthesis of an additional Mn^{2+}-dependent form; and a Cu^{2+}-dependent form is characteristic of eukaryotes and a few prokaryotes.

METHODS. Aerobic growth on solid media is straightforward (although the center of a colony, and even the layers below a thin dental plaque, may be anaerobic). However, aerobic growth in liquid medium ordinarily requires agitation. Moreover, the solubility of O_2 in water is low (about 5 μg/ml in equilibrium with air at 34°C); and because this amount would be consumed in less than 10 seconds by a fully grown culture of an aerobe, the diffusion of O_2 across the air–water interface may limit growth to 1 to 2 mg dry weight per ml in a culture aerated by swirling in a flask. Increasing the area of the air–water interface, as by bubbling through a porous sparger, will support heavier growth.

In the cultivation of **obligate anaerobes,** O_2 tensions as low as 10^{-5} atmospheres can be inhibitory. A sulfhydryl compound such as **sodium thioglycollate** ($HSCH_2COONa$) added to the medium permits some strict anaerobes to be grown in tubes exposed to air. Anaerobic growth in large volumes is discussed below (Fermentations), and practical methods for incubating plates anaerobically are described in Chapter 27.

In nature, mixed cultures are the rule, and the strict anaerobes may depend on facultative neighbors to scavenge oxygen.

PHYSICAL AND IONIC REQUIREMENTS

Most bacteria can withstand a considerable range of temperature, osmotic pressure, and pH. Moreover, in filling all possible ecological niches the bacterial world has evolved members that can grow under conditions too extreme for any other organisms: temperatures exceeding 100°C, pH below 1.0, salinity up to 30% NaCl. The properties of the macromolecules in these experiments of nature can shed light on the relation between macromolecule structure and stability.

TEMPERATURE. Most bacteria can grow over a **temperature range** of 30° or more but have a narrow range for optimal growth. Below the optimum, the decline in growth rate with decreasing temperature at first has a slope typical of enzyme reactions, but then it becomes very steep, giving rise to a fairly well-defined **minimal growth temperature** (Fig. 4–1). Above the optimum, the growth rate decreases steeply with increasing temperature, giving rise to a sharply defined **maximum growth temperature.** It is not certain whether the upper and the lower limits are set by properties of the membrane lipids or by effects on protein conformation; the initiation process in protein synthesis is particularly sensitive to low temperature.

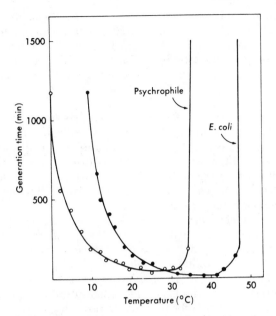

Figure 4–1. Effect of temperature on the generation time of a typical mesophile *(Escherichia coli)* and a psychrophilic pseudomonad. (After Ingraham JL: J Bacteriol 76:75, 1958; modified according to data of Ron EZ, Davis BD: J Bacteriol 107:391, 1971)

The **temperature range** for growth of an organism is a characteristic of considerable taxonomic value. Most bacteria are **mesophiles.** Those found in the mammalian body have a temperature optimum of 37° to 44°C, but many others found in nature grow better at 30°. The protein composition of an organism differs little over the lower part of this range, but in the upper part there is a dramatic shift to "heat shock proteins," discussed in Chapter 9.

Psychrophiles (predominantly pseudomonads) can grow at low temperatures, many down to 0°C. These organisms are important in spoilage of refrigerated foods and are also found in naturally cold waters and soils. **Thermophiles** (predominantly bacilli), in contrast, may have temperature optima as high as 50° to 55°, with tolerance to 100°. They are found especially in hot springs and compost heaps. Thermophiles (e.g., *Bacillus stearothermophilus*) are useful as sources of exceptionally stable forms of enzymes.

The existence of thermophiles shows that nature can evolve proteins with stability far beyond the usual range. Conversely, many temperature-sensitive mutants isolated in the laboratory form an altered enzyme that denatures at ordinary incubation temperatures.

COLD SHOCK. Although bacteria are often preserved in the refrigerator, the sudden chilling of exponentially growing cells of some species (*E. coli, Pseudomonas*) results in substantial killing (>90%). This phenomenon is not observed with gradual cooling or with stationary-phase cells, and hypertonic media offer protection. The mechanism evidently involves damage to the cell membrane.

pH. In bacteria adapted to growth in different pH ranges, the pumps in the membrane are so adjusted that the internal pH is relatively close to neutrality. The pH range tolerated by most microorganisms extends over 3 to 4 units, but rapid growth may be confined to 1 unit or less. *E. coli* cannot withstand a pH much above 8 or below 4.5, whereas pathogens adapted to tissues have a narrower range. Vinegar-forming *Acetobacter* and sulfur-oxidizing bacteria can tolerate the acid that they produce up to 1N (pH ~ 0 for sulfuric acid). In contrast, a few bacterial species (urea splitters, *Alcaligenes faecalis*, the cholera vibrio) thrive at pH 9.0 or more. Most yeasts and molds are relatively acid-tolerant, and this feature is exploited in selective media for their cultivation.

The lower pH cutoff point depends in part on the concentrations of organic acids in the medium; a lower pH increases the proportion of an acid in the undissociated (and hence more permeable) form, thus making it more inhibitory. Hence, a lactate-producing fermenter inhibits itself when it reaches a certain concentration of free lactic acid rather than a given pH.

In a culture growing aerobically on a limiting amount of sugar, the pH often falls and then rises as acid accumulates and then is utilized. To restrict pH changes during growth, media are often heavily buffered, and for fine control, automatic continual titration is sometimes employed.

OSMOTIC PRESSURE. Because of their rigid wall, most bacteria can grow over a rather wide range of osmotic pressure. Changes in osmotic pressure induce changes in composition, discussed in Chapter 2 (Periplasm).

HALOPHILES. Na^+ and Cl^- are not widely required by bacteria, although moderate concentrations are generally tolerated. Most bacteria isolated from the ocean, however, are slightly halophilic, requiring NaCl in a concentration approaching that of their natural habitat (3.5%). In addition, moderate and extreme halophiles, with NaCl requirements up to 20% and with optima approaching saturation (slightly above 30%), are found in flats and lakes where salt water is evaporated and in pickling fluids.

Like other cells, halophilic bacteria do not have a significant intracellular concentration of NaCl. Instead, the high Na^+ concentration of the medium functions osmotically to permit the intracellular accumulation of a high concentration of K^+, required by the ribosomes and

many enzymes of these organisms. However, in some halophiles, the integrity of the cell wall specifically requires a high Na^+ concentration.

PRACTICAL BACTERIAL NUTRITION

Although media of chemically defined composition are valuable for special purposes, the traditional rich "soups" are still generally employed in diagnostic bacteriology: they are less expensive, and initiation of growth by small inocula is often more reliable. These media are based primarily on **meat digest** (tryptic digest, peptone, nutrient broth), the soluble product of enzymatic hydrolysis of meat or fish. Many types are marketed, differing in the source material or in the method of preparation and often in suitability for cultivating specific organisms.

To provide vitamins and coenzymes, media are often further enriched with **meat extract (meat infusion)** or **yeast extract,** which contain the stable small molecules released from the cells and concentrated by boiling. Yeast extract is rich in nucleotides. **Casein hydrolysate** is often used as an inexpensive source of amino acids in chemically defined, relatively rich media. In the usual acid hydrolysate (e.g., Casamino acids), tryptophan and glutamine have been destroyed. Enzymatic hydrolysates contain all the amino acids, but mostly as small peptides.

Blood, in **blood agar,** provides not only nutrients but also a diagnostically useful index of hemolysis. Some organisms thrive best in media containing **serum** (e.g., 20%), which provides not only nutrients but also a **protective, nonnutrient growth factor, albumin:** a protein whose versatile affinity protects cells from such toxic compounds as fatty acids (soaps) and heavy metal ions. Starch also binds fatty acids. Protective growth factors are especially valuable in promoting the initiation of growth by small inocula, for with inhibitors that bind tightly, the ratio of inhibitor to cell number is more important than the concentration of inhibitor.

ATTACK ON NONPENETRATING NUTRIENTS: EXOENZYMES

Microbes can take up nutrients of low molecular weight, including not only sugars and amino acids but also oligopeptides, nucleosides, and small organic phosphates such as glycerol phosphate. However, the macromolecules in the organic matter returned to the soil must be digested, and for this purpose various bacteria, protozoa, and fungi produce a variety of **extracellular** or **surface enzymes** (exoenzymes). With pathogens, these enzymes often play a role in disease by attacking tissue constituents. Gram-negative organisms also have **periplasmic** enzymes retained between the two membranes. The mechanism of enzyme secretion will be discussed in Chapter 6.

Extracellular enzymes include polysaccharidases (amylase, cellulase, pectinase); mucopolysaccharidases (hyaluronidase, chitinase, lysozyme, neuraminidase); nucleases; lipases; and phospholipases. Some proteases are released from the cells as inactive zymogens, which catalyze their own activation. Protease formation can be repressed by a high concentration of amino acids in the medium.

Recognition of various hydrolases is useful in diagnostic work. Extracellular protease is generally detected by the liquefaction of gelatin (denatured collagen) around a colony, and lecithinase by the formation of an opaque product from egg yolk.

ALTERNATIVE CARBON SOURCES

The microbial world has evolved extraordinary diversity in its energy-yielding patterns and its ability to use different foods. Indeed, as a result of its genetic creativity and the evolutionary pressure to maximize microbial growth, it appears that all naturally occurring organic compounds are attacked by some microbe, thus maintaining the geochemical cycle of carbon between the atmosphere and organic matter (Chap. 1). Efforts are being made to domesticate and extend this capacity in the elimination of toxic wastes.

In each sample of soil, many different kinds of organisms play different roles in this process of mineralizing organic matter, and different nutritional conditions select for very different populations. Many organisms have only a narrow range of foodstuffs, but some pseudomonads (a major group of soil scavengers) can use more than 100 carbon sources.

Because the microbes in the world are the product of a long evolutionary adaptation to the available substrates, it is not surprising that many synthetic compounds are not attacked. However, their accumulation is likely to be transient, because the genetic adaptation of the huge microbial population is rapid: strains that attack novel compounds by the evolution of new enzyme specificities have been isolated in the laboratory, and they are no doubt also being selected in nature. Meanwhile, **biodegradable** substitutes are being sought for those persistent toxic compounds that are concentrated by plants and animals.

The genetic capacity to metabolize a given substrate may or may not be expressed, depending on the immediate history of the cells. This **adaptive enzyme formation,** which led to the study of gene regulation (Ch. 9), was first recognized by Karström in Finland in 1931 during a study of the lactic acid bacteria important in the formation of cheese: nongrowing cells (e.g., in buffer) could ferment most sugars only if grown on them. However, the enzymes of glucose metabolism were **constitutive;** i.e., glucose could be fermented regardless of the C source used during growth. This pattern evidently evolved because glucose is by far the most common sugar encountered (in polymers) in nature. In the following description of metabolic patterns, glucose therefore will be used as the prototype.

The immediate principles of living bodies would be, to a degree, indestructible if, of all the organisms created by God, the smallest and apparently most useless were to be suppressed. And because the return to the atmosphere and to the mineral kingdom of everything which had ceased to live would be suddenly suspended, life would become impossible.
—Louis Pasteur

Energy Metabolism

FERMENTATIONS

Long before the development of microbiology, humans discovered the fermentation of stored grape juice into wine, accompanied by the evolution of gas (L., *fervere*, to boil). Pasteur's demonstration of the role of microbes, described in Chapter 1, led to his definition of fermentation as "life without air"—at that time a bold suggestion.

Pasteur recognized that in a fermentation, the organism derives metabolic energy by its "property of performing its respiratory function, somehow or other, with the oxygen existing combined in sugar." Because the principal products of fermentations accumulate in large amounts, their identification initiated the study of microbial metabolism, and later studies on the "somehow or other" led to a redefinition of fermentation as **metabolism in which organic compounds serve as both the electron donors and the electron acceptors.**

A fermentation must balance: the average level of oxidation; i.e., the number of moles of C, H, and O, must be the same in the products as in the substrates. For example,

$$C_6H_{12}O_6 \rightarrow 2\ C_3H_6O_3\ (CH_3CHOHCOOH)$$
Glucose   Lactic acid
$$C_6H_{12}O_6 \rightarrow 2\ CH_3CH_2OH\ +\ 2\ CO_2$$
Ethanol

In liquid of significant depth, O_2 from the air is consumed by the organisms near the surface, and so the depths are anaerobic; in addition, in fermentations that evolve CO_2, this heavier gas displaces O_2 at the surface. For these reasons, most bacteria have retained a fermentative metabolism (although it is much less energy-efficient than respiration), and the alcohol fermentation in vats of grape juice could be recognized long before the concept of anaerobiosis arose.

The anaerobic metabolism of carbohydrates yields various pleasant-smelling products. **Putrefaction** refers to a fermentation, primarily of proteins (as in infected tissues), that yields ill-smelling products.

Source of Energy in Fermentation

The energetics of fermentation may be considered from several points of view. In **thermodynamic** terms, fermentations proceed because the products have a lower energy content than the substrates. Thus, the molar free energy difference (ΔF) between one mole of glucose and two moles of lactate* (at neutral pH) is 58 Kcal. This difference arises essentially from the much lower energy level of the carboxyl group and H_2O compared with the same atoms in carbonyl or hydroxyl groups. Fermentation may thus be viewed, in terms of **bond energy**, as a regrouping of atoms in organic molecules to yield low-energy products. Similar considerations explain the much higher energy yield (688 Kcal) of oxidizing all the C and H of glucose to CO_2 and H_2O.

In terms of **intermediate metabolism**, the generation of ATP† from ADP + P_i involves a free energy gain (ΔF) of 8 Kcal, and to carry out that reaction in a fermentation, a sequence of spontaneous, energy-losing reactions must lead up to an organic phosphate that can transfer its P to ADP because its energy of hydrolysis ($-\Delta F$) exceeds that amount. Fermentations involve the formation of a few such high-energy intermediates: 1,3-di-P-glycerate, P-enolpyruvate, and acetyl-P are the main ones. Their transfer of a P to ADP is called substrate-level phosphorylation; ATP formation in respiration (see below) does not employ such intermediates.

Coenzymes

A variety of coenzymes (cofactors), of relatively low molecular weight and high thermostability, were initially distinguished from enzymes because they could be removed from extracts by dialysis, with a consequent loss of enzymatic activity; and activity could be restored by supplying the supernatant fluid from an extract in which the enzymes had been denatured by boiling. Such cofactors include (1) CoA for acyl transfer; (2) thiamine pyrophosphate (TPP) for transferring groups derived from a ketone (e.g., decarboxylation of α-keto acids); and (3) biotin for CO_2 transfer. Various biosynthetic reactions employ pyridoxal phosphate for amino acid transamina-

---

* For organic acids, terms such as "lactic acid" and "lactate" will generally be used interchangeably in this volume; the formula will generally be written as the free acid, although at the usual pHs, organic acids are largely ionized.

† Abbreviations: The phosphate group (-PO_3H_2) is symbolized by the letter P in the names of compounds and by a circled P in structural formulas; P_i = inorganic phosphate; ~P = high-energy phosphate. ADP and ATP = adenosine 5'-di- and triphosphate; NAD^+ and NADH = the oxidized and the reduced forms of nicotinamide adenine dinucleotide (NAD = DPN [diphosphopyridine nucleotide]); $NADP^+$ and NADPH = the comparable forms of nicotinamide adenine dinucleotide phosphate (NADP = TPN); CoA = Coenzyme A.

tion, decarboxylation, and racemization; tetrahydrofolate for 1-C group transfer and reduction; and cobamide (from vitamin B_{12} [cobalamin]) in methyl group transfers and certain reductions.

Redox cofactors play an important role in directing metabolic flow: in order to ensure a smooth flow of energy and to promote economy, the cell contains cofactors of different redox potential: ferredoxin, lipoic acid, NAD and NADP, flavins, and hemes. For example, the fermentative formation of lactate from pyruvate by lactic dehydrogenase employs the cofactor NAD, whose redox potential favors lactate; whereas the reverse reaction in respiration, by lactic oxidase, employs a flavin cofactor, whose higher redox potential favors the oxidation.

Similar considerations explain why the same cytoplasmic pool contains two different pyridine nucleotides, NAD and NADP, that are very similar in structure and in redox potential. In an aerobic culture, NAD is present predominantly in the oxidized form, because it is directly linked to the powerful oxidizing system of electron transport, whereas NADP, reduced by the pentose phosphate pathway and by isocitric dehydrogenase, is predominantly kept in the reduced form (NADPH) because it lacks that link. Hence, the cell can carry out its reductive biosynthetic reactions (e.g., α-ketoglutarate $\rightarrow$ glutamate; acetate $\rightarrow$ fatty acids) by linkage with NADPH, while it uses the more highly oxidized NAD in dehydrogenations.

In order of generally increasing potential, the redox cofactors common to bacterial, plant, and animal cells are lipoic acid, NAD and NADP, flavins, and hemes. Flavins and hemes are tightly (sometimes covalently) bound to proteins, and the different proteins endow them with a wide range of redox potentials. Some anaerobic bacteria, and plants, also have **ferredoxins:** small proteins of mol. wt. 6000 to 10,000 containing eight atoms of Fe complexed with acid-labile S that readily yields H_2S. This form of S gives them an exceptionally low standard redox potential, similar to that of the H_2 electrode (-417 mv):

$$2\,H^+ + 2\,e^- \rightleftharpoons H_2.$$

Ferredoxin is used in the release of H_2 gas by certain anaerobes, photosynthesis, N_2 fixation, and the utilization of H_2 as a fuel for respiration.

Flavodoxins, containing flavin mononucleotide rather than Fe, have a similar low potential and can replace ferredoxins in certain reactions. They are synthesized by many bacteria, especially in low-Fe media.

Thioredoxin is a widely distributed small protein that functions in several reductions: of ribose to deoxyribose, of disulfides in proteins, and of sulfate.

Glycolysis; Alternative Fates of Pyruvate

A number of fermentations are based on the **glycolytic (Embden–Meyerhof) pathway** (Fig. 4–2). This pathway

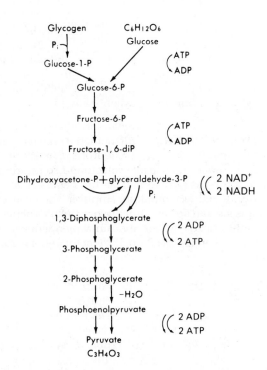

Figure 4–2. The glycolytic formation of pyruvate (Embden–Meyerhof pathway). Sum: glucose + 2 ADP + 2P$_i$ + 2NAD$^+$ → 2 pyruvate + 2ATP + 2 NADH + 2 H$^+$. *Double arrows* signify two moles reacting per mole of glucose.

generates ATP twice: first through the oxidation of glyceraldehyde-3-P (triose-P) by NAD$^+$ and again through the conversion of P-enolpyruvate to pyruvate. To balance the fermentation and allow the NAD to recycle, the NADH produced in the net oxidation to pyruvate must be reoxidized at the expense of the reduction of some substrate. For this purpose, microbes have evolved a variety of pathways (Fig. 4–3) adapted to different nutritional conditions. Because each fermentation converts most of the glucose to a single product (e.g., lactic acid in the homolactic fermentation) or to very few, this process is quantitatively the principal overall biochemical activity of the fermenting organism and hence the easiest to study biochemically. Accordingly, fermentations dominated the early study of intermediary metabolism.

LACTIC FERMENTATION. This is the simplest fermentation: a one-step reaction, catalyzed by NAD-linked lactic dehydrogenase (really a pyruvate reductase), reduces pyruvate to lactate. No gas is formed. Because two ATP molecules are consumed in the formation of hexose diphosphate from glucose, and because four ATP molecules are subsequently produced, the net yield is two ATPs per hexose. This fermentation is the first stage in cheese manufacture; it is also identical with the glycolysis in mammalian cells.

The **homolactic fermentation,** which forms only lac-

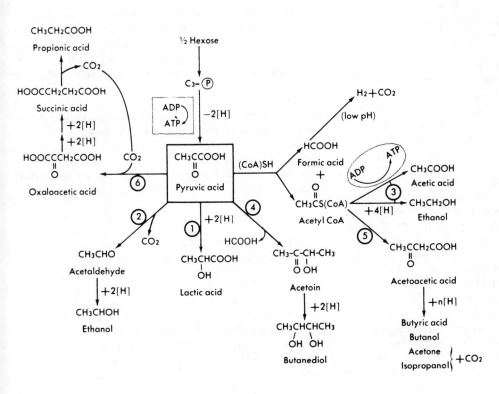

Figure 4–3. Key role of pyruvate in principal fermentations. (1) Lactic *(Streptococcus, Lactobacillus)*. (2) Alcoholic (many yeasts, few bacteria). (3) Mixed acid (most *Enterobacteriaceae*). (4) Butanediol *(Enterobacter)*. (5) Butyric *(Clostridium)*. (6) Propionic *(Propionibacterium)*. (For abbreviations, see text footnote.)

tate, is characteristic of many of the lactic bacteria such as *Lactobacillus casei, Streptococcus cremoris,* and pathogenic streptococci. Others carry out a rather different, **heterolactic, fermentation** (see Phosphogluconate Pathways, below), which converts only half of each glucose molecule to lactate. Both these fermentations are responsible for the souring (acidification) of milk and certain other foods (sauerkraut, pickles), which preserves them as long as they are kept anaerobic; these processes also provide interesting flavors (especially highly developed in the secondary fermentations of lactic acid and amino acids in cheeses).

ALCOHOL FERMENTATION. Pyruvate is converted to CO_2 plus acetaldehyde, which is then reduced to ethanol in an NAD-linked reaction. This fermentation is characteristic of yeasts; as a major product, ethanol is uncommon in bacteria.

THE MIXED ACID (FORMIC) FERMENTATION. Most *Enterobacteriaceae* dispose of their substrate partly through a lactic fermentation but mostly by splitting pyruvate (without net oxidation or reduction) to formate and acetyl-CoA; the latter in turn generates an ATP via acetyl-*P* (Fig. 4–3). Because this reaction does not absorb the two [H] released in forming pyruvate, fermentation balance requires that an equal amount of pyruvate be reduced by pathways absorbing more [H]: (1) formation of ethanol from acetyl-CoA, and (2) reduction (after carboxylation) to succinate. The formic fermentation thus yields three ATPs per glucose fermented (compared with two in the lactic fermentation).

GAS FORMATION. In the mixed acid fermentation, as the pH drops below 6, "gas-formers" (e.g., *E. coli*) reduce the accumulation of acid by forming an enzyme, formic hydrogenlyase, that converts formic acid (HCOOH) to CO_2 and H_2. *Enterobacteriaceae* that do not form this enzyme (e.g., *Shigella*) produce acid but no gas (like homolactic fermenters). Gas formation is an important diagnostic test.

Intestinal gas accumulates when bacteria in the colon produce H_2 and CO_2, and in some people CH_4, faster than these compounds can be absorbed. The substrates increase in the colon when disorders of peristalsis or of pancreatic or biliary secretion impair their absorption in the small intestine; in addition, some foods contain carbohydrates that cannot be absorbed in the small intestine but can be metabolized by the much more numerous bacteria in the colon. Impaired colonic peristalsis also promotes the formation of free gas, because it hinders the convection of fluid to the mucosal surface, where dissolved gases are transferred to the blood.

In the **methane fermentation,** a major process in ruminants, various methane bacteria use H_2 formed by other organisms to reduce CO_2 to CH_4, yielding a small amount of energy. Curiously, among humans the presence of CH_4 in intestinal gas appears to be an unusual familial trait, which may reflect variations in establishing the intestinal flora early in life: it is highly correlated among siblings but not between spouses.

BUTANEDIOL (ACETOIN) FERMENTATION. This pattern, observed in *Enterobacter* (formerly *Aerobacter*), and also in certain other *Enterobacteriaceae* and some species of *Bacillus,* involves formation of acetyl-P and formate, as in the mixed acid fermentation. However, the electron acceptor is acetoin, formed from two molecules of pyruvate (by head-to-head condensation) and then reduced to butylene glycol (in the reactions, TPP = thiamine pyrophosphate):

$$CH_3\text{—}CO\text{—}COOH + TPP \rightarrow [CH_3\text{—}CHO]\text{—}TPP + CO_2$$

"Active acetaldehyde"

$$[CH_3\text{—}CHO]\text{—}TPP + CH_3\text{—}CO\text{—}COOH \rightarrow CH_3\text{—}CO\text{—}\underset{OH}{\overset{COOH}{\underset{|}{\overset{|}{C}}}}\text{—}CH_3$$

Acetolactate

$$\xrightarrow{-CO_2} CH_3\text{—}CO\text{—}CHOH\text{—}CH_3 \xrightarrow{[2H]} CH_3\text{—}CHOH\text{—}CHOH\text{—}CH_3$$

Acetoin (acetylmethyl carbinol)   2,3-Butylene glycol

This fermentation, like the alcohol fermentation, yields only neutral products and produces two ATPs per glucose. Exposure to air oxidizes some of the butylene glycol to acetoin, which is readily recognized by a specific color test (**Voges—Proskauer**). In sanitary engineering, this test is of considerable diagnostic value in discriminating between *E. coli*, which reaches bodies of water primarily from the mammalian gut, and *Enterobacter*, originating primarily from vegetation.

The formation of neutral rather than acidic products permits the fermentation of larger amounts of carbohydrate without self-inhibition and therefore the production of more gas; hence the old name *Aerobacter aerogenes.*

PROPIONIC FERMENTATION. In the propionic fermentation of lactate (which is ordinarily an endproduct), one mole of lactate provides ATP via its conversion to acetyl-P, and to balance the oxidation, two moles of lactate are reduced, via oxalacetate and succinate, to propionate. In the formation of Swiss cheese this late fermentation occurs after the completion of the lactic fermentation and the coagulation of the casein: the propionic acid contributes to the flavor and the CO_2 creates the characteristic holes.

BUTYRIC–BUTYLIC FERMENTATION. The butyric–butylic pattern of pyruvate reduction is seen in certain strict anaerobes. The initial scission yields acetyl-CoA plus two [H] and CO_2. Two acetyl residues are then condensed, not head to head as in acetoin, but head to tail as in fatty acid synthesis. The resulting acetoacetyl-CoA undergoes several reactions, in varying proportions: decarboxylation and reduction by the H_2 (activated by ferredoxin) to yield acetone, isopropanol, butyric acid, and *n*-butanol.* These patterns are useful for classification (e.g., *Bacteroides;* Ch. 28).

MIXED AMINO ACID FERMENTATIONS. Fermentations of amino acid mixtures occur where there is considerable proteolysis; they are prominent in putrefactive processes, including the gangrene associated with anaerobic wound infections. Certain amino acids or their deamination products serve as electron donors and others as acceptors. In addition, decarboxylation of various amino acids, and further reactions, yield products that are pharmacologically active (e.g., histamine) or malodorous (e.g., indole from the breakdown of tryptophan, and the even more mephitic -SH compounds derived from cysteine and methionine). More pleasant, empirically selected fermentations of minor constituents are responsible for the characteristic flavors of various wines and cheeses, whereas the toxic effect of poorly fermented wines is largely attributable to longer-chain aldehydes derived from amino acids.

Phosphogluconate Pathways

Whereas the Embden–Meyerhof pathway is the most widely used way of metabolizing glucose, two other pathways begin by oxidizing glucose-6-P to P-gluconate. The **ketodeoxygluconate (Entner–Doudoroff) pathway** (*C* in Fig. 4–4) cleaves the P-gluconate into two 3-C fragments; it is the primary route in pseudomonads, and *E. coli* also uses this pathway to metabolize gluconate (which cannot enter glycolysis). A **heterolactic fermentation,** in contrast, decarboxylates the P-gluconate to pentose-P and finally yields approximately equal quantities of lactate, ethanol, and CO_2 (*B* in Fig. 4–4).

E. coli also decarboxylates P-gluconate to pentose-P in initiating the **hexose monophosphate shunt,** through which a minor part of its supply of hexoses flows. The pentose-P (and that derived from dietary pentoses) can then be fermented by a complex series of 2-C and 3-C transfers that convert it to triose-P, or it can be oxidized.

---

* The use of this fermentation for the industrial production of acetone was developed by Chaim Weizmann in England in 1915. This scientific contribution, which solved an urgent problem in explosives manufacture in World War I, promoted the Balfour Declaration and thus contributed eventually to the founding of the state of Israel, with Weizmann as its first president.

This alternative to glycolysis does not serve simply as an option or reserve: glycolysis generates NADH, whereas the shunt generates NADPH, and so the two pathways distribute reducing power as needed between the two factors.

Adaptive Value of Different Fermentations

With the glycolytic pathway having evidently evolved as a particularly effective central mechanism, the diversity of final products reflects the selection of variants that best fit different ecological opportunities. Thus, as we have already noted in Chapter 1, grape juice is much richer in sugar than is milk but poorer in protein (i.e., buffering power). Hence, in the fermentation of grape juice, lactic acid bacteria soon produce a self-inhibitory pH, whereas the yeasts, although slower growing, produce a neutral product and outgrow the bacteria. (In addition, grape juice fails to meet the requirement of these bacteria for various amino acids.) Milk, in contrast, supports the growth of either organism, and the faster-growing bacteria soon predominate.

Similarly, the vertebrate colon, with a meager supply of unabsorbed carbohydrates and growth factors, selects for enteric bacteria (e.g., *E. coli*), which have no specific growth requirements and extract as much energy as possible from their fermentation. In contrast, *Enterobacter*, which grows primarily on vegetation, can ferment larger concentrations of carbohydrate (to butanediol) but with a less efficient energy yield.

It is evident that nature selects for a variety of fermentative talents, which might be compared to sprinters and long-distance runners.

SUBSTRATE-SPECIFIC PATHWAYS. The first steps in the metabolism of most substrates convert them to some intermediate in a central pathway (glycolysis or the TCA cycle). The specific connecting pathway is often quite short. For example, a single step will convert fructose to fructose-6-P or will yield glucose from sucrose or from lactose; three steps are necessary to convert galactose to glucose-1-P; and two convert glycerol to dihydroxyacetone-P.

RESPIRATION
Respiratory Metabolism

TRICARBOXYLIC ACID CYCLE. Complete oxidation converts organic compounds to CO_2 and H_2O. In the commonest pattern (Table 4–1), pyruvate, from the glycolytic pathway, is oxidized to acetyl-CoA and CO_2, and the acetyl-CoA is oxidized via the **TCA cycle** (Fig. 4–5) in the process called **terminal respiration.** Respiration of glucose yields about ten times as much free energy and 18 times as much ATP as does fermentation (Table 4–1). It

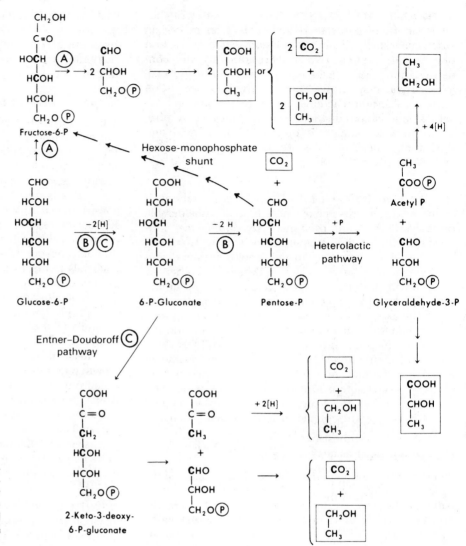

Figure 4–4. Alternative ways of metabolizing glucose to lactate and/or ethanol. Glucose-3,4-^{14}C yields alcohol labeled *(heavy letter)* either *(A)* in neither C atom (Embden–Meyerhof pathway), *(B)* in the CH_2OH (heterolactic pathway), or *(C)* in the CH_3 (ketodeoxygluconate pathway).

also permits the use of fuels such as fatty acids that are too reduced to be fermented.

In each of the oxidative steps in the TCA cycle, a pair of hydrogens from substrates is used to reduce FAD or NAD^+, but no ATP is formed directly. These reduced cofactors are then ultimately oxidized by O_2 (or alternative electron acceptors such as nitrate in some bacteria), in the process of electron transport (see below), which provides the energy from respiration in useful form. The energy that is not ultimately used in biosynthesis or in minor additional outlets appears as heat.

THE GLYOXYLATE CYCLE. In each turn of the TCA cycle, the oxalacetate that combines with acetate is regenerated. However, when this compound (and α-ketoglu-

tarate) are siphoned off into biosynthesis (Fig. 4–5), the cycle will soon run down unless a 4-C acid is replenished. In growth on a sugar, this replenishment occurs by carboxylation of pyruvate. However, growth on acetate or a fatty acid alone presents a problem, because aerobic cells are incapable of reducing acetate to pyruvate. Bacteria evolved a solution, which has been lost by mammals (with consequent acidosis when they metabolize too much fat relative to carbohydrate). In this pathway (Fig. 4-5), the presence of acetate without sugar induces the formation of two enzymes that bypass the two reactions of the TCA cycle, between isocitrate and succinate, that release two CO_2. Instead isocitrate is split to yield glyoxylate and succinate, and then the glyoxylate is combined with another acetate to rejoin the cycle at malate.

TABLE 4-1. Energetics of Metabolism

Reaction	No. of ATP generated	$-\Delta F$ (Kcal)	Efficiency* (%)
Glucose → 2 Lactic acid	2	58	28
Glucose → 2 Ethanol + 2 CO_2	2	57	28
Glucose + 6 O_2 → 6 CO_2 + H_2O			
Stages:			
Glucose $\xrightarrow{-4[H]}$ 2 Pyruvate (substrate)	2		
(2 NAD)	6		
$\xrightarrow{-4[H]}$ 2 AcCoA + 2 CO_2 (2 NAD)	6		
$\xrightarrow{-16[H]}$ 4 CO_2 + 4 H_2O (6 NAD, 2 FAD)	22		
Total	36	688	44

ΔF = free energy difference; $-\Delta F$ = energy of hydrolysis.

* Assuming ΔF of ATP formation = 8 Kcal.

The result is the net formation of malate from two acetates.

INCOMPLETE OXIDATIONS. Respiratory metabolism does not always proceed all the way to CO_2 and H_2O. *Acetobacter* oxidizes ethanol to acetic acid much faster than it can utilize the latter, thus converting wine to vinegar. In a parallel pattern, *E. coli* growing aerobically on glucose initially forms only those TCA cycle enzymes that are required for biosynthesis, and it carries the oxidation of glucose only as far as acetate, extracting about one-third the energy available from complete respiration. After a critical concentration of acetic acid has accumulated, it induces formation of the missing TCA enzymes, and the cell can then oxidize the accumulated acetic acid.

Respiring organisms are used in the commercial production of many metabolic products (e.g., antibiotics, amino acids, citric acid), and in the search for palatable **single-cell protein** from inexpensive feedstocks such as petroleum or wood.

Dioxygenases add molecular oxygen across a double bond. These reactions do not yield energy, but they convert a refractory compound (e.g., one with a benzenoid ring) into one that is useful as a fuel or for other purposes.

Electron Transport

In aerobic bacteria, as in the mitochondria of eukaryotic cells, the electrons from various donors, transferred to NADH or a flavoprotein, are funneled into the electron transport (ET) system, from which most of the energy goes into ATP synthesis (oxidative phosphorylation). After years of fruitless efforts by biochemists to discover phosphorylated intermediates like those observed in fermentation, Peter Mitchell recognized the role of a radically different, *chemiosmotic* process, which depends on the asymmetric (vectorial) orientation of the involved proteins in the ion-impermeable membrane of a closed vesicle or a cell. The transport of electrons in this system, ultimately to O_2, is accompanied by the extrusion of pro-

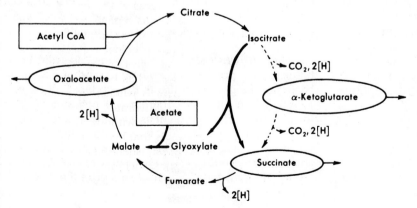

Figure 4-5. Krebs TCA cycle and within it the "glyoxylate bypass" *(heavy arrows)*. The glyoxylate cycle substitutes these reactions, which conserve carbon, for the two decarboxylative reactions of the TCA cycle *(dashed arrows)*, which release carbon as CO_2. In an organism growing on acetate alone, the glyoxylate cycle provides net 4-C (and thus 3-C) synthesis to replenish the biosynthetic drain *(circled compounds)*. Because the glyoxylate cycle involves two oxidative steps linked to electron transport, it also provides some energy, but most of the cell's energy is derived from the simultaneous oxidation of other acetate molecules via the TCA cycle.

tons to the exterior. The resulting **electrochemical proton gradient (protonmotive force; pmf** or **Δp)** across the membrane provides a source of energy that is tapped by various kinds of transmembrane machinery, through which the protons flow downhill: for **phosphorylating ADP to ATP,** for **active transfer** of various permeants, and for **motility.**

Using protons instead of electrons, this biological system is comparable to the wired electric supply into which we can plug alternative appliances. Moreover, just as some motors can serve reversibly as generators, transducing electrical and mechanical energy in either direction, so the ATP-generating and the active transport systems across biological membranes are reversible under appropriate circumstances.

The Δp resulting from the pumping out of protons has two components: a gradient of H^+ concentration (ΔpH, more acidic outside), and a gradient of electrical charge (the membrane potential, $\Delta\psi$), more negative inside and hence increasing the force attracting the protons back across the membrane. In volts, the relation is:

$$\Delta p = \Delta\psi - 0.06\,\Delta pH.$$

The mechanism of proton extrusion is not well understood.

The ΔpH can be eliminated by ionizable lipid-soluble reagents, such as dinitrophenol, which shuttle back and forth in the membrane in both ionized and un-ionized form until they have equilibrated the H^+ concentration on the two sides. The $\Delta\psi$ can be short-circuited by a system such as the K^+-specific ionophore valinomycin (in the presence of K^+) that allows a cation to flow freely across the membrane and thus to establish electrical neutrality.

COMPONENTS. All the components of the ET chain are fixed in the membrane in a specific orientation. Each carrier reversibly transfers electrons, some with and others without protons, between the two carriers with the next lower and the next higher redox potential. Although there are a dozen or more electron carriers in the total system, they are grouped in three physically separate multi-protein respiratory complexes, each of which harvests a fraction of the large redox potential difference between H_2 and O_2 and uses this energy to extrude two H^+ against a considerable electrochemical gradient. Electron transfer from each respiratory complex to the next is carried out by a diffusible single molecule shuttling between them.

The ET systems of bacteria differ in their details but in general accord with the following sequence:

1. The complex of lowest potential, the **NADH dehydrogenase,** contains many proteins, including flavoproteins and **iron-sulfur proteins;** in the latter, linkage

with H_2S imposes a low redox potential on the Fe. This complex accepts two H, as a pair of protons and a pair of electrons, from the redox cofactor NADH:

$$NADH + H^+ \rightarrow NAD^+ + 2\,H^+ + 2\,e^-.$$

The two H^+ are extruded, and the two e^- are passed along the ET chain.

Other flavoprotein dehydrogenases (e.g., succinic, lactic, fatty acyl-CoA) each accept two H directly from the corresponding substrate; without a soluble redox cofactor, this transfer is at a higher redox potential and does not result in proton extrusion.

2. A small, reversibly reducible quinone anchored by a long alkyl chain transports two H by shuttling in the membrane between a dehydrogenase and a cytochrome. In most gram-negative bacteria, just as in mitochondria, this quinone is a benzoquinone, **ubiquinone;** in most gram-positives, it is a naphthoquinone, **menaquinone.**

3. In *E. coli*, ubiquinol is oxidized by both the **cytochrome d** and the **cytochrome o** complex; the former predominates when the oxygen tension is low and the latter when it is high. Each complex contains multiple cytochromes and functions as an **oxidase,** collecting electrons from four hemes and transferring them to molecular O_2. The cytochrome d, but not the cytochrome o, complex also contains Cu^{2+}, like the oxidase of mitochondria.

Cytochrome c is a small cytochrome that differs from most others in being loosely attached to the cytoplasmic membrane surface and water soluble. Its sequence is highly conserved in evolution. It is present, along with **cytochrome c oxidase,** in mitochondria and in many aerobic bacteria but not in facultative organisms such as *E. coli*. In the **oxidase test,** widely used in diagnostic bacteriology, cells containing these components rapidly oxidize N,N-dimethyl-*p*-phenylenediamine into a colored product, which stains the colonies.

Cytochromes differ not only in their proteins, but also in some details of their hemes. Whereas the cytochromes in mitochondria of diverse origin are relatively uniform, those from various bacteria have greater diversity and are designated with numerical subscripts (e.g., cytochromes b_{558} and b_{595} in the d complex) based on the wavelength of their absorption peak in the reduced state.

BACTERIORHODOPSIN. A large, pigmented transmembrane protein present in purple photosynthetic bacteria, bacteriorhodopsin, is similar to the rhodopsin of the vertebrate eye. It illustrates the fundamental simplicity of the electrochemical gradient as a mechanism for storing energy. Under illumination, its covalently bound chromophore loses a proton on one side of the membrane and converts from *trans* to *cis* form, whereas regeneration of the *trans* form, which can occur in the dark, employs a proton from the other side. The overall process thus causes proton translocation. Strikingly, this single protein alone, embedded in an artificial vesicle, can create such a light-driven proton gradient; and when coupled with other required proteins, described in the next section, this gradient can drive ATP formation.

Oxidative Phosphorylation

ATPase (ATP synthetase), a large complex of many proteins, is responsible for using the energy of Δp to convert ADP + P_i into ATP. it consists of a transmembrane complex, F_0, together with another complex, F_1, bound on its cytoplasmic surface by a stalk and projecting into the cytoplasm. The flow of protons down the thermodynamic gradient through F_0 transmits energy to F_1, which can use it to create a high-energy phosphate bond. In mitochondria the P/O ratio (ATP formed per O reduced) is three, reflecting a remarkably efficient conversion of energy from ET into ATP energy—about 50%, which is far better than the efficiency of electric motors made by man. Whether the efficiency is equally high in bacteria cannot be demonstrated, because part of the Δp energy is used directly for transport and for motility and because the ATP is not stored but is made in the cytosol and hence is rapidly used.

Artificial vesicles provide the strongest evidence that the ET system and the ATPase are linked only through the proton gradient: incorporation of the complete ATPase into such vesicles, together with **any one** of the respiratory complexes (or with bacteriorhodopsin plus illumination), results in ATP generation. This interaction is equally effective regardless of the evolutionary distance between the sources of the two components, which supports the model of linkage by protons but not linkage by specific contacts between macromolecules.

A striking feature of the membrane ATPase reaction is its reversibility: anaerobic organisms, generating ATP but not ET, use ATP hydrolysis by the membrane ATPase to generate Δp. In facultative organisms, *unc* mutants, **uncoupled** in this reaction (in both directions), can grow aerobically on glucose, deriving ATP from glycolysis and Δp from ET; but they cannot grow either on succinate (for lack of ATP) or anaerobically on glucose (for lack of Δp). This finding emphasizes that Δp is a major form of currency in energy metabolism.

Because bacteria function under a much wider range of environmental conditions than mitochondria, they differ more widely in the proportions of the two components of Δp. Thus under anaerobic conditions, where the ATPase reaction pumps protons but there is no pumping of electrons by the ET system, $\Delta \psi$ is low, and the cells develop a higher ΔpH. Similarly, a low external pH causes bacteria to develop a higher ΔpH and hence a compensatory lower $\Delta \psi$. The low $\Delta \psi$ impairs the entry of cationic antimicrobials, such as the aminoglycosides, and so their activity is sensitive to acidity and to anaerobiosis (see Chap. 10, Aminoglycosides).

AUTOTROPHIC METABOLISM
Chemoautotrophy and Anaerobic Respiration

In contrast to the **heterotrophic** metabolism of animals and most bacteria, based on use of organic compounds as fuels, **autotrophic** metabolism uses various other sources of energy and reducing power to synthesize organic compounds from CO_2. The main form is photosynthesis, by plants, algae, and bacteria. However, the bacterial world also has evolved another form, chemoautotrophy, which derives energy from the oxidation of various **inorganic electron donors,** such as H_2, H_2S, Fe^{2+}, NH_3, and NO_2^-.

In a related use of inorganic fuels, called **anaerobic respiration** (or more precisely **anaerobic ET**), the **electron acceptor** is NO_3^-, SO_4^{2-}, or CO_2, instead of O_2; the metabolism may be autotrophic, with H_2 as electron donor, or heterotrophic, with various organic compounds. Indeed, while autotrophic metabolism is not found in pathogens, anaerobic ET, with **nitrate** as terminal electron acceptor, in a short, flavoprotein-dependent ET system, is common among heterotrophs (including *E. coli*), probably because nitrate is universally present as the principal form of storage of N in soil.

Chemoautotrophy and anaerobic respiration are unique to bacteria.

Photosynthesis

In photosynthesis, energy from light is used to provide both energy and reducing power for a succession of reactions that convert CO_2 to triose-P and hence to other cell constituents. In this process, a photon of absorbed visible light is converted to chemical energy by causing a charge separation at the photocenter of a chlorophyll molecule (a protein-bound Mg^{++}-tetrapyrrole pigment) embedded in a membrane. The energized chlorophyll ejects an electron, which is accepted by an adjacent ferredoxin molecule; and the positive charge on the resulting chlorophyll free radical is then neutralized by donation of an electron from a cytochrome on the other side of the insulating membrane. These reactions occur very rapidly, and the large potential difference between the oxidized cytochrome and the reduced ferredoxin is then used in either of two ways, whose proportions vary with the needs of the cell, to convert ADP to ATP via ET or to transfer electrons from reduced ferredoxin to NADPH, which is then used in biosynthetic reductions.

In the familiar photosynthesis of higher plants (which permits them to grow simply on CO_2, H_2O, and some inorganic ions), the oxidized chlorophyll is reduced at the expense of oxidizing water:

$$H_2O \rightarrow \tfrac{1}{2} O_2 + 2\,H^+ + 2\,e^-$$

But a very high redox potential, exceeding that of O_2, is necessary for this reaction; and a single quantum of light does not provide enough energy to create the difference between this potential $(+0.82\text{ v})$ and the very low potential of reduced ferredoxin (-0.42 v). Accordingly, plants evolved their remarkable capacity to metabolize water, and thus to eliminate their dependence on other fuels, by coupling two photoactivated chlorophyll reaction centers in series, much like a pair of electrical batteries. Some bacteria, however, retain a more primitive type of photosynthesis, employing only one reaction center, and therefore requiring a more easily oxidized electron donor than water such as H_2 or H_2S.

Non-oxygenic photosynthetic bacteria are obligate anaerobes. The process is very restricted in location today, but in the primitive earth, with H_2 and no O_2 in the atmosphere, it no doubt contributed to the initial accumulation of organic compounds. The next stage was the evolution of **oxygenic photosynthesis** in the **cyanobacteria** (blue-green bacteria), and evolution then transferred this process to plants by evidently incorporating cyanobacteria into their cells as chloroplasts.

Autotrophic Assimilation of CO₂

Autotrophic cells use the ATP and the reducing power supplied by photosynthesis (or by chemoautotrophy) to reduce CO_2 to triose-P. These "dark reactions" of photosynthesis can be shown to take place after a pulse of light has activated chlorophyll. Only the initial steps in the fixation of CO_2 involve novel enzymes, in the following reaction:

CH₂O (P)   [CH₂O (P)]   CH₂O (P)
| | CHOH
C=O   C—OH   CO₂ |
| || COOH
CHOH → C—OH →   +
| | Carboxy-   COOH
CHOH   CHOH dismutase |
| | CHOH
CH₂O (P)   CH₂O (P) |
                                     CH₂O (P)

Ribulose di-P   3-P-glycerate

At this stage the assimilated C is still at the fully oxidized carboxy level. To serve as a general source of C 3-P-glycerate is reduced to triose-P, by NADPH plus energy provided by ATP (Fig. 4–6). The ribulose-P that initiated the fixation is regenerated by the normal pathway of pentose metabolism, the Calvin cycle (not shown), which transfers fragments between carbohydrates of 3, 4, 5, 6, and 7 C atoms. By this circuitous route 3 pentose plus 3 CO_2 regenerate 3 pentose and yield 1 triose as the net gain.

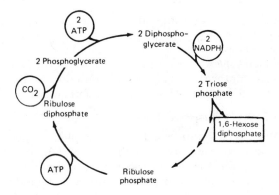

Figure 4–6. The ribulose-diP cycle requires three moles of ATP and two moles of NADPH per mole of CO_2 converted to carbohydrate.

Nitrogen Cycle; Nitrogen Fixation

A discussion of the autotrophic reduction of CO_2 would be incomplete without noting a parallel property that is unique to certain bacteria and algae: the ability to reduce atmospheric nitrogen to a form useful for biosynthesis. In the geochemical nitrogen cycle, the N in decomposing organic matter is at first largely converted to NH_3. This volatile compound is then stabilized in the soil by oxidation, through the action of **nitrifying** bacteria, to nonvolatile nitrate, which can be reduced by plants to organic amino compounds. However, some NH_3 is lost to the atmosphere, especially in anaerobic regions of the soil, where **denitrifying** bacteria reduce nitrate to N_2. Maintenance of the biosphere therefore requires constant fixation of atmospheric nitrogen by soil bacteria. Efforts are under way to transfer the *nif* (nitrogen fixation) genes from *Klebsiella* into crop plants in order to eliminate the need for nitrogen fertilizer.

The most important group of nitrogen fixers are the members of the genus *Rhizobium* (Gr. *rhizo*, root), which form symbiotic N_2-fixing nodules in the roots of the plants that they infect. However, various free-living bacteria (including *Azotobacter*) fix N_2 for their own metabolic needs. Some bacteria (e.g., *Rhodospirillum rubrum*) can fix both CO_2 and N_2.

Membrane Transport
ALTERNATIVE MECHANISMS

The cytoplasmic membrane of bacteria, like that of higher cells, provides an osmotic barrier that is permeable to very few substances. It is porous to H_2O and to uncharged organic molecules up to the size of glycerol; and O_2, CO_2, and nonpolar organic molecules such as tetracycline penetrate by solution in the lipid of the membrane. Both processes have the kinetics of **simple**

diffusion: the **flux** in either direction is proportional to the concentration on the entering side, so the rate of **net transfer** is proportional to the concentration difference between the two sides. These kinetics also apply to the transfer of most molecules across the outer membrane by diffusion through large pores (Ch. 2).

Molecules larger than glycerol and all ionized molecules (including H^+) require **specific transport systems.** Some of these are capable only of **passive carrier transport,** whereas others are linked to an energy source and can mediate **active transport.** This usually means transfer against a concentration gradient; but for charged molecules, taking into account membrane potential, active transport is defined as movement from a lower **electrochemical potential** on one side of a membrane to a higher potential on the other side.

Active Transport

Bacteria were long regarded as semipermeable bags of enzymes, because they seemed too small to possess a variety of specific transport systems and because they attack a variety of small molecules with the same kinetics as enzymes in solution. Even after bacteria were shown to concentrate mineral ions and amino acids, it was not certain how much was bound to intracellular molecules and how much was free. Yet it is now clear that bacteria required early evolution of a membrane with specific and active transport systems, in order to retain intermediary metabolites, maintain specific intracellular concentrations of mineral ions and H^+, and scavenge nutrients efficiently from the dilute solutions encountered in nature.

The decisive evidence for specific transport systems was the demonstration that the ability of a bacterial cell to take up and to concentrate specific nutrients can be turned on and off either by induction or by mutation. In particular, G. Cohen and J. Monod showed that the inducible *lac* operon contains not only a gene for β-galactosidase (*lac-z*) but also a gene for a corresponding transport system in the membrane (*lac-y*). Moreover, this system not only mediates downhill transport of β-galactosides that are rapidly hydrolyzed (and hence not concentrated), but it can also concentrate non-metabolizable analogues such as methyl-β-thiogalactoside more than 100-fold. (Specific inducible transport systems in bacteria were called **permeases,** but the systems are fundamentally the same as those found earlier in mammalian cells, and most of them are not enzymes, as implied by the suffix -ase, that convert a substrate into another compound.)

KINETICS. Active transport is usually studied by incubating cells with a radioactively labeled permeant, rapidly filtering the culture, and measuring the radioactivity accumulated by the cells. This accumulation must be shown to be still in the form of the compound supplied and not in a metabolic derivative. With amino acids, whose entry is much faster than their incorporation into protein, this is not a problem. However, sugars are usually metabolized as fast as they can enter, and so to analyze the kinetics of their transport systems it is necessary to block metabolism (e.g., by a mutation) or to use a non-metabolized analogue.

The kinetics of the active transport systems of bacteria are the same as those in other cells, and they will not be described in detail here. Briefly, these carrier systems are saturable, with a K_m and a V_{max}, like the activity of an enzyme. What makes active transport possible is that the apparent K_m for efflux from the interior is higher than that for influx in the opposite direction.

The K_m and V_{max} of influx are calculated from the rate of initial entry, before efflux has become significant. The value of the K_m of efflux can be calculated from a comparison of the internal and external concentrations after equilibrium is reached, as efflux then equals influx, and so the degree of saturation of the carrier, dependent on concentration and affinity, must be the same on the two sides. Because an increase in the concentration of an extracellular permeant above the saturating level cannot further raise the intracellular concentration, hypertonic concentrations of sugars and salts can provide osmotic protection of protoplasts and spheroplasts even though these substances can enter the cell.

Passive Carrier-Mediated Systems (Facilitated Diffusion)

Passive systems also have saturable, Michaelis kinetics, but they are not linked to an energy source; hence, they are incapable of active transport, and the K_m is the same on both sides of the membrane. This process is frequently designated as facilitated diffusion, because the flow is only downhill; but it is more fundamentally related to active transport than to diffusion. Indeed, systems capable of active transport systems also function as passive carriers when energy is not needed (i.e., downhill transport of a rapidly metabolized permeant) or when the energy supply is removed.

Cells adapted to a high ambient sugar concentration, such as yeasts and erythrocytes, often possess passive carriers. However, in bacteria, which have to be able to acquire nutrients from dilute solution, no such systems have been identified in the inner membrane. (Glycerol induces a change in the membrane that increases its uptake, but it is not saturable and hence appears to be a small pore rather than a carrier). The outer membrane of bacteria, which lacks a source of energy, has a few kinds of pores that exhibit specificity, but perhaps less than that of carrier systems (Chap. 2).

Specific Transport Systems

Many **sugar transport systems** have been described, with properties similar to that for β-galactosides. They have a moderately high affinity for a specific sugar (or a group of related sugars), with K_m about 10^{-4}M. There are also systems for taking up disaccharides and even short oligosaccharides: for example, the maltose system can also take up maltodextrins. Additional mechanisms of sugar uptake, the phosphotransferase system, will be discussed below.

Amino acids are actively concentrated by a set of transport systems with higher affinities (K_m between 10^{-6} and 2×10^{-8}) than the transport systems for sugars. This difference correlates with the concentrations of these compounds generally found in the microbial environment and also with the rate at which the cells can metabolize them. Other factors being equal, an increased affinity of a carrier should be associated with a lower rate of release of its permeant from the binding site and hence a lower turnover (V_{max}); and in fact, mutants selected for increased affinity do pay the price of a lower rate of uptake.

The set of specificities for amino acid uptake in *E. coli* is complex: single carriers (generally constitutive) each transport a group of similar compounds (aromatic; aliphatic; basic; Gly–Ser–Ala; Cys–DAP). In addition, a low concentration of some of these amino acids induces the formation of "scavenger" high-affinity individual carriers. This array permits the uptake of many different amino acids, over a wide range of concentrations, efficiently and without mutual interference. But interference can occur: an excess of phenylalanine may be innocuous to an organism that can make its own tyrosine but inhibitory to an auxotroph requiring tyrosine—a possible model for the damaging effect of phenylalanine in phenylketonuric humans, who cannot convert this compound to tyrosine.

Oligopeptide transport systems, which may encounter an enormous variety of peptides, exhibit much less specificity than the systems for amino acids. *E. coli* has three systems: one for any dipeptide, one for aliphatic tripeptides, and one for any oligopeptide up to a length of six residues. Peptides that enter the cell are rapidly hydrolyzed, yielding amino acids. This property, and the nonspecificity of the systems, makes it possible to introduce nonpermeating compounds by coupling them to peptides (**portage** or **"piggyback" transport**). Originally demonstrated for amino acid analogues, this system also offers promise for other antimicrobial agents, linked to peptides by bonds that become labile on peptide hydrolysis.

Inorganic ions (K^+, Mg^{2+}, PO_4^{3-}) are maintained by membrane transport systems at a relatively constant intracellular level of the free ions (in addition to that bound in ribosomes and elsewhere). Mutations that impair the transport of a specific ion markedly increase the concentration required for growth. *E. coli* uses two systems for P_i: a constitutive low-affinity one for ordinary uptake, and a high-affinity "scavenger" system that is repressed by P_i until its concentration becomes low.

E. coli also has systems for **extruding Na$^+$ and Ca^{2+}.** In bacteria these systems presumably function only to eliminate unwanted ions that leak into the cell, but in higher organisms they have evolved into elaborate signalling mechanisms. In addition, the adaptation to altered osmotic pressure involves **pressure-sensitive gated ion channels.**

REGULATION OF FORMATION OF TRANSPORT SYSTEMS. Many transport systems for optional nutrients are formed only when induced by the presence of their substrate. Two paths of induction are known: internal and external. The classical *lac* system exemplifies the **internal** path: the slow initial entry of the inducer (which cannot yet be metabolized) leads to its interaction with the cytoplasmic repressor of the *lac* operon (Ch. 9), which then induces formation of the transport system. The ability of that system to concentrate a nonmetabolized inducer creates an interesting **positive feedback:** the concentration required for maintaining the induction is lower than that required for its initiation. The other, **external** path is characteristic of substances that would be very rapidly metabolized after entry (e.g., citrate, glycerol phosphate, glucose-6-P) and so cannot raise their intracellular concentration by slow nonspecific entry. These inducers must therefore act by transmitting information across the membrane, thus preceding in evolution the extensive use of this process in eukaryotic cell regulation.

Nonspecific Entry

"Cryptic" mutant cells, which do not have the *lac* transport system but make cytoplasmic β-galactosidase, hydrolyze lactose at a very low rate (less than 1% of that with a transport system). Such nonspecific slow entry is probably important for the action of many antimicrobial agents. The mechanism is not certain. The rates are linearly proportional to concentration, which suggests diffusion through an imperfection in the osmotic barrier. However, attachment with low affinity to a system specific for another, similar compound might give the same result, since the early part of a Michaelis-Menten curve is linear.

Limited membrane damage can greatly increase nonspecific entry or exit of small molecules and ions by diffusion while retaining the enzymes within the cell. Thus, in the commercial production of amino acids by auxotrophic mutants, the yield may be increased by controlled membrane damage (e.g., by penicillin). In transfer in the other direction, membrane damage by toluene facilitates measurement of the concentration of intracellular enzymes by making them freely accessible to substrates.

Mechanism of Active Transport

CARRIER PROTEINS. The first carrier protein to be identified in the solubilized total membrane proteins was that of the *lac* system of *E. coli*. It was recognized by radioactively labeling proteins on the cell surface: the labeling of one electrophoretic peak was decreased by the presence of the permeant (masking the binding site for transport), and it was eliminated by mutations that eliminated the transport system. In a fully induced cell, this protein is about 4% of the membrane protein (about 8000 molecules); hence, the total class of transport proteins must constitute a large fraction of the cytoplasmic membrane. However, the classic biochemical approach to analyzing molecular mechanisms (by isolating and recombining the individual components) was unsuccessful when applied to active transport: removal of the carrier from the membrane not only destroys the characteristic asymmetric (vectorial) orientation of the process and its linkage to an energy supply but it often also destroys the capacity of the carrier to bind the permeant.

VESICLES. Kaback showed that closed membrane vesicles, which form spontaneously when bacterial membranes are fragmented, provide a simplified system that remains active. Using energy derived from the protonmotive force (see Electron Transport, above), "right-side out" vesicles (i.e., with the cytoplasmic surface inside) can concentrate the substrates of those transport systems that have fixed binding proteins in the membrane. In a further simplification, carrier proteins can be purified and then incorporated into such vesicles with the aid of detergents and sonication. Even better, they are also active, like the ATPases described above under Oxidative Phosphorylation, when incorporated into artificial vesicles (proteoliposomes) reconstituted from phospholipids and proteins.

In these vesicles, a single protein, such as the purified *lac* carrier protein (Fig. 4–7), can carry out active transport if an electrochemical proton gradient is provided— for example, by incorporating the cytochrome oxidase complex into the same vesicles. Moreover, the behavior of this reconstituted system fulfills a significant prediction from the general model for active transport described above: the carrier changes its K_m when a membrane potential is imposed.

SYMPORT, ANTIPORT, AND CONFORMATION. The *lac* system acts by symport: the proton flow downhill from the higher external electrochemical potential to the lower internal one carries with it the β-galactoside. In other, *antiport*, systems, the proton flow inward is associated with permeant flow outward (e.g., Ca^{2+} extrusion). The interactions of permeant and protons are symmetrical, like the interaction of the membrane ATPase: in the absence of a proton gradient, downhill flow of lactose can cause uphill flow of protons.

To say that flow of protons through the *lac* carrier brings the permeant with it by symport does not answer the question of how; even less does it explain passive transport by active transport systems deprived of energy. Although there is little direct evidence, certain features can be logically inferred. Because the same site on the carrier evidently binds the permeant on either side of the membrane, and because proteins as a whole do not flip-flop in the membrane, a conformational change within the transmembrane protein, rather than between it and its surround, must permit the binding site to face either way. Moreover, this shift in the distance moved by the binding site could be short, as suggested in Figure 4–8. To account for passive transport, the shift between the two orientations would have to be spontaneous and reversible; while in active transport, the movement of a proton must be responsible for a further conformational change, which alters the K_m in one of the two orientations. In symport, the affinity would be higher when the carrier is facing the outside, and in antiport, it would be higher when facing the inside.

In mammalian cells the ET system resides in the mitochondria, the ATP that it produces then transfers energy to the plasma membrane, and an ATP-driven Na^+–K^+ pump there establishes a Na^+ gradient that drives most symport and antiport. Bacteria, however, have the energy of a proton gradient directly available at the cell surface (under aerobic conditions), rather than transduced by ATP from mitochondria at a distance, and they rarely employ cations other than H^+ for symport and antiport.

Periplasmic Binding Proteins

In gram-negative bacteria, specific periplasmic binding proteins (PBP) bind certain permeants and then transfer them to a cognate **acceptor complex of proteins** in the membrane, which actively transports them to the cytoplasm. Different PBPs (or a group of related ones) interact with different membrane acceptors. This interaction is obligatory for transport by these membrane systems and also for providing a signal for chemotaxis (see below): if a specific PBP is eliminated by mutation, or if all the periplasmic proteins are released by osmotic shock, these responses disappear. The mechanism for supplying energy to these active transport systems is not certain, but it appears to depend on ATP or acetyl-P rather than on a proton gradient.

The system is more efficient than one-protein active transport systems for scavenging dilute permeants, because binding to the PBPs (which greatly outnumber the

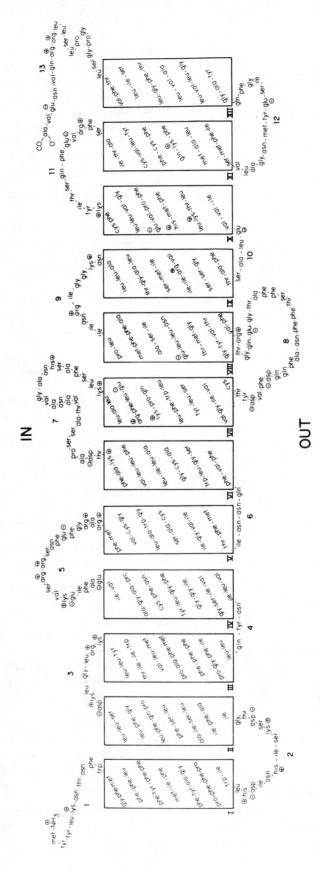

Figure 4–7. Sequence of the *lac* transport protein. The formation of 12 hydrophobic α-helices and their embedding in the membrane are inferred from the amino acid sequence of the protein. (Courtesy of Ronald Kaback)

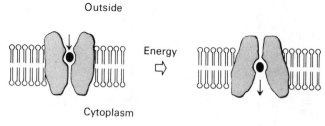

Outside

Energy

Cytoplasm

Figure 4–8. Model for conformational change in membrane binding protein, accepting permeant on one side of membrane and discharging it on the other side. In active transport (not shown), application of energy changes the affinity for the permeant on one side. (After Singer SJ: Annu Rev Biochem 43:805, 1974)

cognate membrane units) hinders diffusion of a dilute permeant from the periplasmic space back into the medium. *E. coli* has such systems for only certain amino acids and certain sugars (e.g., galactose and ribose but not glucose or lactose), perhaps because these permeants are more likely to be encountered in dilute solution.

Phosphotransferase Systems

Obligate and facultative anaerobes, which derive much less energy than aerobes from their fuels, and a very few aerobes utilize an especially economical **group translocation** system for transporting certainly commonly encountered sugars: instead of expending a high-energy phosphate on the transport alone, they utilize it both for transport and for the first step in metabolism of the sugar, its conversion to the 6-phosphate. The result is not active transport, in a strict sense, but it is metabolically equivalent. This **group translocation** system was discovered by Roseman through the observation that mutations in certain proteins eliminate the uptake of several sugars. The substrates in *E. coli* include glucose, fructose, mannose, and the corresponding hexitols and hexosamines.

The system includes both generic proteins and sugar-specific proteins. As outlined in Figure 4–9, in the generic reactions, in the cytoplasm, Enzyme I transfers P from P-enolpyruvate to a histidine (thus retaining a high-

energy bond) on a protein of 9000 daltons named HPr. In the membrane, each substrate is passively transferred by a specific protein (Enzyme II) to the cytoplasmic surface, where it is phosphorylated by P-HPr and then released; the transfer is direct for some sugars and involves an additional sugar-specific cytoplasmic Enzyme III for others. The two generic proteins are constitutive; the specific ones are induced by their substrates.

This system may have evolved such complexity because it also participates in a network of regulation, acting on both the formation and the activity of various transport systems and enzymes involved in peripheral catabolic pathways. For example, the extent of phosphorylation of HPr influences the formation of cyclic AMP (which represses the genes for utilization of non-preferred fuels; Ch. 9); and in further modulation of this control, a high level of ATP causes a kinase to inactivate HPr by a second phosphorylation, on a serine. Moreover, glucose Enz III, when not phosphorylated (i.e., after reaction with glucose), inhibits many transport systems by binding to their cytoplasmic surface. The Enz IIs also participate in chemotaxis (see below).

The various kinds of transport systems found in *E. coli* are depicted in Figure 4–10. The use of different systems for different sugars in the same organism may reflect adaptation to the likelihood of encountering them at high or low concentration and under anaerobic or aerobic conditions.

Ionophore Antibiotics

Some small antibiotics make the membrane specifically permeable to certain cations, in one of two ways.

1. **Valinomycin** (a cyclic molecule containing three repeats of the sequence L-lactate, L-valine, D-hydroxyisovalerate, and D-valine) can fold around a K^+ ion in a way that creates a cavity of just the right size, with six O atoms surrounding and coordinating with the cation, while the hydrophobic portions of the molecule lie on its exterior. The molecule dissolves in the membrane lipid and diffuses back and forth, as a **carrier,** between the two faces; and because the competition between the K^+ and H_2O for the coordinating O atoms is so balanced, this shuttle rapidly equilibrates the internal and the external

Enzyme I
(Cytoplasm)

P-enolpyruvate + HPr $\rightleftharpoons$ Pyruvate + P-HPr (Reaction 1)

Enzyme II, III
(Membrane)

P-HPr + Sugar $\longrightarrow$ Sugar-P + HPr (Reaction 2)

―――――――――――――――――――――――――――――

P-enolpyruvate + Sugar $\longrightarrow$ Sugar-P + Pyruvate (Over-all reaction)
(outside)   (inside)

Figure 4–9. The phosphotransferase transport system. Each sugar uses a specific enzyme II (which accepts the sugar) and some also use a specific enzyme III (to accept -P from P-HPr).

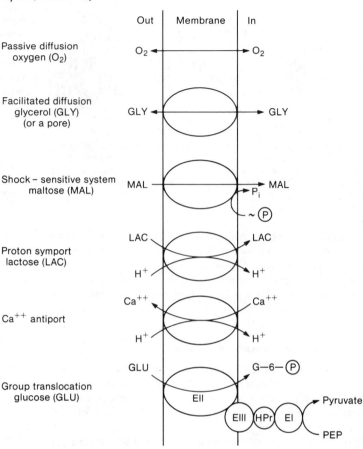

Figure 4–10. Classes of membrane transport observed in *E. coli.*

K^+. The resulting short-circuiting of the membrane potential has been very useful in studying the protonmotive force.

2. **Gramicidin A,** an open-chain hydrophobic polypeptide of 15 residues (with modified termini) enters the membrane and forms a **channel** through which specific cations can pass.

Lowering the temperature, which converts the membrane lipid from a fluid to an essentially frozen state, distinguishes the two mechanisms. Cold inactivates the diffusible carrier antibiotic but not the channel former, which does not need to move in the lipid.

Iron Uptake: Siderophores

Fe(II) (the form present under anaerobic conditions) is highly soluble, and so anaerobes can take up iron as easily as other metal ions. Under aerobic conditions, however, iron is present as Fe(III), which is not readily accessible to cells because it forms a hydroxide with very low solubility $(10^{-18}M)$ at neutral pH. To facilitate its uptake, aerobic bacteria (both obligate and facultative) excrete small compounds, called siderophores (Gr., iron-bearers), that solubilize Fe(III) and transport it into cells via specific membrane receptors. Mycobacteria have siderophores (mycobactins) that are attached to their hydrophobic surface.

Siderophores solubilize Fe(III) by **chelation** (gr. *chelos;* claw)—a process in which a metal ion is coordinated with two electronegative O or N atoms. The siderophores formed by microbes are much more powerful chelators than any synthesized by chemists, because they combine three chelating ligands, properly spaced, in a single molecule (Fig. 4–11). More than 100 different siderophores are known. They fall into three groups: **ortho-diphenols** (catechols), **α-hydroxy acids** (especially citrate), and **hydroxamic acids** (RCONHOH).

In *E. coli* a single operon repressible by a high Fe concentration codes for the enzymes that synthesize a siderophore (**enterochelin**). It also codes for a membrane protein, which is presumably the receptor for the siderophore; it is found in the outer membrane, and the mechanism of transport across the inner membrane is not clear.

In the cell the release of the Fe from its tight binding to the siderophore is accomplished in two ways. With ferrichrome (a fungal siderophore), reduction of the

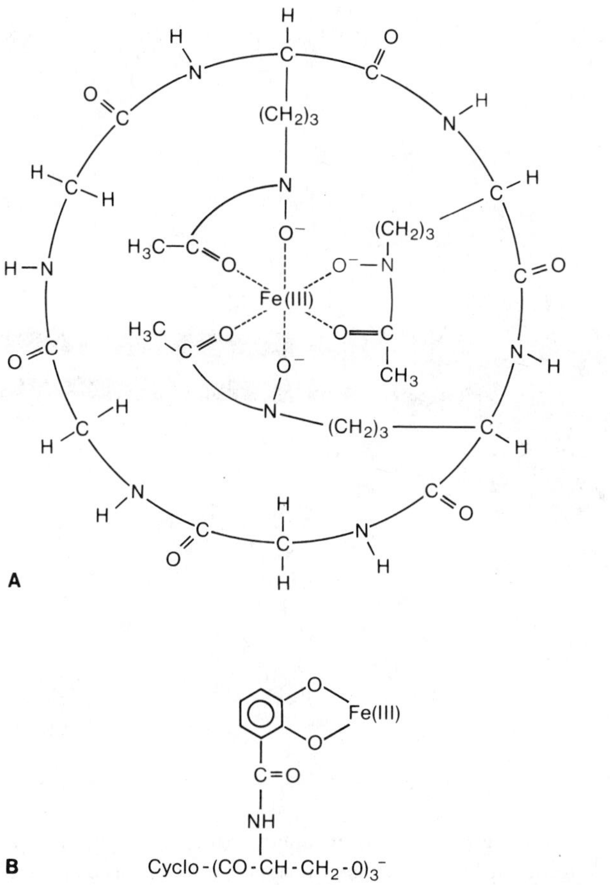

A

B   Cyclo-(CO-CH-CH$_2$-O)$_3^-$

Figure 4–11. Two siderophores. *(A)* Ferrichrome, from the fungus *Ustilago*, is a cyclic hexapeptide containing three glycines and three acetylhydroxamates of ornithine. *(B)* Enterobactin, from *E. coli*, is a cyclic trimer of 2,3-dihydroxybenzoyl serine (a catechol). The hydroxamate and the catechol groups are chelators, and in each of these molecules, they are appropriately spaced so that all three can coordinate especially well with an Fe(III), thus satisfying all six of its coordination valences.

Fe(III) to Fe(II) releases it and allows the siderophore to recycle. Enterochelin, in contrast, is hydrolyzed within the cell, so each molecule functions only once.

The importance of ensuring adequate uptake of Fe is illustrated by the multiple mechanisms in *E. coli*. It (1) can assimilate Fe slowly via a low-affinity pathway without siderophores; (2) synthesizes enterochelin; (3) may harbor plasmids that code for a siderophore **(aerobactin)** ordinarily made by another organism, *Enterobacter*; (4) can be induced to form a system for transport of ferric citrate; and (5) even has receptors for some siderophores that it does not itself make. Indeed, because of the specificity of their receptors, siderophores may play an important role in nature in the competition between different bacteria for a limiting supply of Fe.

Fe uptake is increasingly recognized as an important

factor in pathogenesis. Variables include the limited supply of Fe in host fluids and cells, the effect of pH and anaerobiosis on its solubility, the effect of fever on siderophore formation, and the competition between siderophores and Fe-binding proteins of the host (transferrin, lactoferrin). In fact, transferrin, a protein that transports Fe in the blood in mammals, was discovered through its antibacterial action.

Motility and Chemotaxis

Motility, which revealed bacteria to Leeuwenhoek as living organisms, is useful to these organisms because it is associated with chemotaxis: movement toward a more concentrated supply of a nutrient (Fig. 4–12). This property was discovered in 1881 by Engelmann, who observed that bacteria under a coverslip on a microscope slide swam toward air but not toward N_2 at the periphery. In addition to such **positive chemotaxis** toward an **attractant,** bacteria exhibit **negative chemotaxis** away from various **repellants** (e.g., phenol, acid). The basic mechanisms of motility and chemotaxis, elucidated quite recently, have aroused wide interest, not only because of their novel features, but also as possible simple models for some aspects of the nervous system. Moreover, the similar process of **phototaxis** in photosynthetic bacteria—movement toward light, mediated by pigment proteins in the membrane—may be regarded as a precursor of the visual system. We will consider first the motor and then the sensory components of chemotaxis.

FLAGELLA
Structure

Bacterial flagella are thin helical **filaments** several times the length of the cell (see Fig. 2–5), connected by a short **hook** to a **basal body** embedded in the cell envelope (Fig. 4–13). The flexibility of the hook permits the helical filament to have an attachment perpendicular to the wall, and it also allows parallel filaments to rotate as an aggregated group (see below).

Filaments can be isolated from cells by mechanical agitation followed by differential centrifugation. Cross-sections show that they are tubes with a narrow empty core. They are made of molecules of a single globular protein, **flagellin** (mol. wt. 40,000), which are disaggregated by heat and can spontaneously reassemble to form filaments. The hook, which can be isolated from mutants that overproduce it, also has a simple composition. The basal body is more complex (Fig. 4–13). In gram-positive bacteria two rings embedded in the inner membrane surround a central rod, whereas gram-negative bacteria have an additional pair of rings embedded in the outer

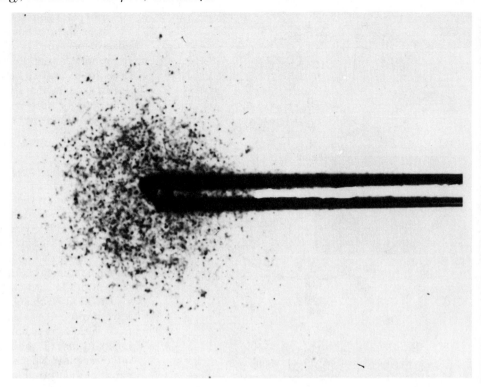

Figure 4–12. Positive chemotaxis of *E. coli* cells toward the tip of a capillary containing a concentrated solution of glucose. (Courtesy of J. Adler)

membrane. In *E. coli* about 30 genes (*fla*) influence the structure and assembly of flagella.

Incorporation of a radioactively labeled amino acid has shown that the filament grows by **addition of flagellin molecules at the tip.** The hook molecules, and then the flagellin molecules, move outward through the hollow core. It appears that the flagellin molecules move more slowly the longer the path, thus self-regulating the length of the filament.

Flagellar Rotation

Bacterial flagella were long assumed to create their curvature by a whiplike motion, like the cilia of higher organisms. However, in 1973 Howard Berg showed, by attaching polystyrene beads, that the filament has an essentially rigid helical structure and rotates like a propeller. The energy is supplied by the protonmotive force: the downhill flow of protons across the cytoplasmic membrane applies an electrostatic force to an inner ring of the flagellar basal body, just as the flow of electrons in an electric motor induces a magnetic force. Other rings presumably serve as bushings, tight enough to prevent substantial leakage of even very small molecules.

In addition to the basal body, coded for by *fla* genes, the flagellar motor involves two membrane proteins, coded for by *mot* genes, whose mutations paralyze the flagella. Graded restoration of the missing product by

attaching its gene to an easily controlled regulatory element leads to stepwise increases in rotational speed. The number of steps suggests that the motor contains about 16 independent force-generating units.

Bacterial flagella are the only known example of rotary motion in biology, perhaps because it becomes too difficult to maintain a tight, perfectly circular seal at larger dimensions.

CHEMOTAXIS

The positive chemotactic response to nutrients (see Fig. 4–12) and the negative response to repellants were naturally assumed to be related to the effects of these substances on the energy supply. However, in 1969, Julius Adler showed that chemotaxis involves specific sensory responses (i.e. to information rather than to energy). Thus many foodstuffs are not attractants (i.e., bacteria "taste" only a small sample of their environment); some nonmetabolizable analogues are active; and many different chemotaxis (*che*) mutations can eliminate the response without affecting any other aspect of metabolism. The development of methods for quantitating chemotaxis has aided analysis of the mechanism. Most conveniently, isolated bacteria deposited in soft agar (i.e., dilute enough to permit swimming) containing a dilute nutrient form a spreading ring as the multiplying organisms

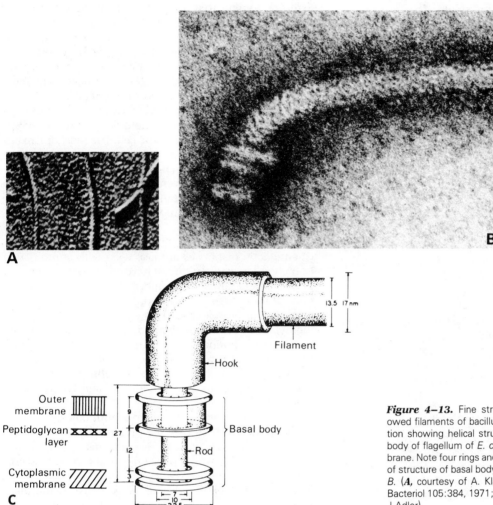

Figure 4–13. Fine structure of flagella. (***A***). Metal-shadowed filaments of bacillus in Fig. 2–7*B,* at higher magnification showing helical structure. (***B***) Negatively stained basal body of flagellum of *E. coli* freed of attached wall and membrane. Note four rings and thick, hooklike sheath. (***C***) Diagram of structure of basal body, inferred from preparations such as *B.* (***A,*** courtesy of A. Klug; ***B,*** DePamphilis ML, Adler J: J Bacteriol 105:384, 1971; ***C,*** courtesy of ML DePamphilis and J Adler)

exhaust the food within the ring and move toward fresh nutrient at the periphery.

Biased Random Walk

The recognition that gradients are sensed in terms of information, rather than of energy supply, raised the problem of how a cell could sense the tiny difference in concentration over its length of 2 μm. By developing an automatic tracking microscope, Howard Berg revealed the answer: not directed movement along the gradient but a biased random walk, with changes too rapid to be recognized visually. Without a gradient, *E. coli* cells swim in a straight line for 1 to 2 seconds, then "twiddle" or "tumble" aimlessly for 0.1 to 0.2 seconds, which randomizes the direction of their next run. In a chemotactic gradient the linear runs are lengthened in the direction of an attractant (or shortened in the direction of a repellant). This modulation of a random walk thus recognizes concentration differences over a distance about 20 times the length of the cell, and it yields **net movement** along a gradient. The frequent reorientations are more effective than a long stretch of continuous movement would be, because Brownian movement rapidly causes an object with so little inertia to deviate from a straight line.

Direction of Rotation

The two phases of cell motion depend on the direction of rotation of the flagella. When it is counterclockwise, the flagella form parallel intertwined bundles in which the rotating filaments slide past each other, as is possible for left-handed helices rotating counterclockwise. This coordinated rotation drives the cell steadily forward. When it is reversed, the bundles fly apart; moreover, the reversed torque alters the interactions of the flagellin units and hence the shape of the filament. The consequence is erratic "tumbling."

Sensory Adaptation; Methylation

The remarkable feature of this system is its response to a **change** in concentration of the stimulant rather than to the absolute concentration. Adler found that chemotactic stimulation is associated with increased methylation of a membrane protein, and various *che* mutations that blocked this reaction eliminate chemotaxis. Using a temporal rather than a spatial gradient (i.e., exposing cells to an abrupt large change in concentration), which caused the continuous run to last several minutes before restoration of tumbling (Fig. 4–15), Koshland could show that carboxyl groups on several glutamic residues on the cytoplasmic domain of the stimulated transducing protein are cumulatively methylated (by S-adenosylmethionine) at a constant rate, until the new level of methylation (which inhibits the response) balances the new concentration of the attractant. The methylase and a demethylase, as well as their genes, have been isolated.

Although the regulation of the methylation and demethylation reactions is not completely understood, it appears that the activation of signal synthesis on the cytoplasmic domain also makes the transducer protein a substrate for methylation, which resets the responsiveness of the system as it adapts to each new concentration of stimulant. The "memory" in this system derives from the lag of the slow methylation behind the rapid release of signal.

Excitation and Signal Transmission

The excitation of chemotaxis is mediated by transmembrane proteins that function as transducers, much like the receptors for various hormones in animal cells. In *E. coli* three of these proteins, named for their strongest stimulators, are responsible for most of the responses: Tsr (for serine), Tar (for aspartic acid), and Tgr (for glucose and ribose). Tsr, for example, has a receptor on its external domain that interacts with serine or with certain sugars complexed with their periplasmic binding protein. This external interaction leads to an interaction of the cytoplasmic domain with the *che* products.

Mutations have shown that four *che* genes are involved in a part of signal transmission based on phosphorylation by ATP and dephosphorylation (Fig. 4–14). Because all the flagella shift gears in synchrony, the stimulus from the sensory to the motor system must be rapidly transmitted throughout the cell. The mechanism appears to be diffusion of a labile substance generated at the transducers: with *E. coli* grown as long filamentous cells and stimulated externally in a localized region by iontophoretic ejection from a micropipette, the flagellar response extended for only a few micrometers.

Alternative Mechanisms

Chemotactic responses are also seen with stimuli such as high or low pH that do not have cognate receptors but may act by altering the conformation of some component of the systems described. Moreover, whereas chemotaxis can be inactivated by elimination of either the methylase or the demethylase, it is restored to some degree by the elimination of both; and methylation does not seem to be involved in the chemotactic response to O_2 and to sugars that enter via the phosphotransferase system. The presumed alternative system has not been identified.

Another mechanism is seen in **osmotaxis** (i.e., a negative response to high osmotic pressure). This response, and the accompanying adaptive changes in internal ion concentrations, involve **pressure-sensitive ion channels,** which have been demonstrated by electrical studies with patch clamps (as in nerve cells), using giant spheroplasts of *E. coli*, derived from the long filaments, without septa, that form during growth in the presence of cephalexin.

Adaptive Value

Both flagella and the chemotactic apparatus are subject to regulation: for example, catabolite repression by glucose (Ch. 9). Moreover, the pathogen *Vibrio parahaemolyticus* forms a single polar flagellum when growing in liquid but hundreds of lateral flagella, permitting a swarming type of movement, when growing on a surface. The evolutionary value of chemotaxis and motility is further suggested by the observation that the pathogen *Salmonella*, which grows in the lumen of the intestine, is motile, whereas the closely related *Shigella*, which invades the epithelium, is nonmotile (as are many pathogens whose habitat is restricted to tissues and mucous surfaces). Moreover, in the colon of experimental animals nonmotile mutants of *E. coli* survived less well than the motile parent. The role of chemotaxis in pathogenesis has not been extensively explored.

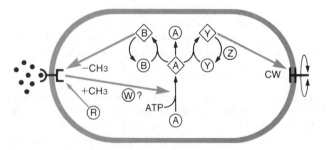

Figure 4–14. Proposed cycle of phosphorylation in the transmission of a signal to the flagella. In response to a stimulus from the membrane transducer, the product of gene *cheA* undergoes autophosphorylation and then transfers its phosphate to the products of *cheB* and *cheY;* CheZ completes the cycle by dephosphorylating CheY. Phosphorylation is designated by a shift from a circle to a box. (Parkinson JS: Cell 53:1, 1988)

A.

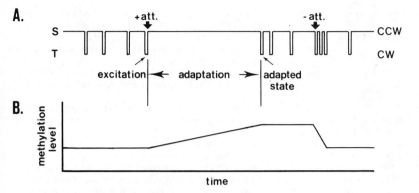

B.

Figure 4–15. Relation of level of methylation of a chemotaxis-transducing protein to sensitivity of bacteria subjected to an abrupt rise and then an abrupt fall in the concentration of an attractant (designated att.). *S,* periods of swimming, 2 to 3 seconds without excitation and longer after excitation; swimming is caused by counterclockwise (CCW) rotation of the flagella. *T,* brief periods of twiddling (ca. 0.2 seconds) caused by clockwise (CW) rotation. The increased methylation of the protein in response to an attractant lags behind its other biochemical response, which results in a signal that prolongs swimming. (Hazelbauer GL, Harayama S: Int Rev Cytol 81:33, 1983)

Bacterial chemotaxis is an interesting model for studying receptor function, sensory transduction, and chemomechanical energy conversion at a molecular level. Moreover, it has led to the discovery that chemotaxis in leukocytes also is associated with changes in the extent of protein methylation. However, although progress in our understanding of bacterial chemotaxis has been dramatic, we still do not know the nature of the transmitted signal, the motor, or its reversible switch.

Selected Reading

BOOKS AND REVIEW ARTICLES

Adler J: Chemotaxis in bacteria. Annu Rev Biochem 44:341, 1975

Ames, GF-L: Bacterial periplasmic transport systems: Structure, mechanism, and evolution. Annu Rev Biochem 55:397, 1986

Antonucci TK, Oxender DL: The molecular biology of amino-acid transport in bacteria. Adv Microb Physiol 28:146, 1986

Boyd A, Simon MI: Bacterial chemotaxis. Annu Rev Physiol 44:501, 1982

Bullen JJ, Griffiths E (eds): Iron and Infection. New York, John Wiley, 1987

Bullen JJ, Rogers HJ, Griffiths E: Role of iron in bacterial infection. Curr Topics Microbiol Immunol 80:1, 1978

Crosa JH: The relationship of plasmid-mediated iron transport and bacterial virulence. Annu Rev Microbiol 38:69, 1984

Dickerson RE: Cytochrome c and the evolution of energy metabolism. Sci Am 242(3):137, 1980

Downie JA, Gibson F, Cox GB: Membrane adenosine triphosphatases of prokaryotic cells. Annu Rev Biochem 48:103, 1979

Fridovich I: Oxygen: Boon or bane. Am Sci 63(1):54, 1975

Gottschalk G: Bacterial Metabolism, 2nd Ed. New York, Springer, 1986

Haddock BA, Hamilton WA (eds): Microbial Energetics. Society General Microbiology Symposium No. 27, Cambridge, Cambridge University Press, 1977

Harold FM: The Vital Force: A Study of Bioenergetics. New York, WH Freeman, 1986

Hazelbauer GL, Harayama S: Sensory transduction in bacterial chemotaxis. Int Rev Cytol 81:33, 1983

Ingledew WJ, Poole RK: The respiratory chains of *Escherichia coli.* Microbiol Rev 48:222, 1984

Kaback RM: Active transport in *Escherichia coli:* Passage to permease. Annu Rev Biophys Biophys Chem 15:279, 1986

Knowles CJ (ed): Diversity of Bacterial Respiratory Systems. Boca Raton, FL, CRC Press, 1980

Koshland DE Jr: Biochemistry of sensing and adaptation in a simple bacterial system. Annu Rev Biochem 50:765, 1981

Landick RC, Oxender, DL: Bacterial periplasmic binding proteins. In Martinosi A (ed): Membranes and Transport: a Critical Review, p 81. New York, Plenum Press, 1982

Martonosi AN (ed): Bioenergetics of Electron and Proton Transport. New York, Plenum Press, 1985

Macnab RM, Aizawa SI: Bacterial motility and the bacterial flagellar motor. Annu Rev Biophys Bioeng 13:51, 1984

Morris JG: The physiology of obligate anaerobiosis. Adv Microb Physiol 12:169, 1975

Mitchell P: Keilin's respiratory chain concept and its chemiosmotic consequences (Nobel lecture). Science 206:1148, 1979

Neilands JB: Microbial envelope proteins related to iron. Annu Rev Microbiol 36:285, 1982

Neilands JB: Significance of aerobactin and enterobactin in siderophore-mediated iron assimilation in enteric bacteria. In Schlessinger D (ed): Microbiology 1983, p 284. Washington, DC, American Society for Microbiology, 1983

Nunn WD: A molecular view of fatty acid catabolism in *Escherichia coli.* Microbiol Rev 50:179, 1986

Ornston LN, Sokatch JR (eds): The Bacteria, Vol VI: Bacterial Diversity. New York, Academic Press, 1978. Includes comprehensive articles on pathways for utilizing organic foods, energy-yielding pathways, and bacterial photosynthesis.

Parkinson JS: Genetics of bacterial chemotaxis. Symp Soc Gen Microbiol 31:265, 1981

Postma PW, Lengeler JW: Phosphenolpyruvate : carbohydrate phosphotransferase systems of bacteria. Microbiol Rev 49:232, 1985

Racker E: From Pasteur to Mitchell: A hundred years of bioenergetics. Fed Proc 39:210, 1980

Rosen BP: Recent advances in bacterial ion transport. Annu Rev Microbiol 40:263, 1986

Saier MH: Mechanisms and Regulation of Carbohydrate Transport in Bacteria. New York, Academic Press, 1985

Scarborough GA: Binding energy, conformational differences, and the mechanism of trans-membrane solute movements. Microbiol Rev 49:214, 1985

Silverman M: Building bacterial flagella. Quart Rev Biol 55:395, 1980

Springer MS, Goy MR, Adler J: Protein methylation in behavioural control mechanisms and in signal transduction. Nature 280:279, 1979

Stoeckenius W: The purple membrane of salt-loving bacteria. Sci Am 226(4):58, 1976

Weinberg ED: Iron withholding: A defense against infection and neoplasia. Physiol Rev 64:65, 1984

Wikstrom M, Krab K, Saraste M: Proton-translocating cytochrome complexes. Annu Rev Biochem 50:623, 1981

Yoch DC, Caruthers RP: Bacterial iron-sulfur proteins. Microbiol Rev 43:384, 1979

SPECIFIC ARTICLES

Belas R, Simon M, Silverman M: Regulation of lateral flagella gene transcription in *Vibrio parahaemolyticus*. J Bacteriol 167:210, 1986

Block SM, Berg HC: Successive incorporation of force-generating units in the bacterial rotary motor. Nature 309:470, 1984

Hess JF, Bourret RB, Simon MI: Histidine phosphorylation and phosphoryl group transfer in bacterial chemotaxis. Nature 336:139, 1988

Kingsbury WD, Boehm JC, Perry D, Gilvarg P: Portage of various compounds into bacteria by attachment to glycine residues in peptides. Proc Natl Acad Sci USA 81:4573, 1984

Levitt MD, Ingelfinger FJ: Hydrogen and methane production in man. Ann NY Acad Sci 150:75, 1968

Martinac B, Buechner M, Delcour AH, Adler J, Kung C: Pressure-sensitive ion channel in *Escherichia coli*. Proc Natl Acad Sci USA 84:2297, 1987

Rudd KE, Menzel R: *his* operons of *Escherichia coli* and *Salmonella typhimurium* are regulated by DNA supercoiling. Proc Natl Acad Sci USA 84:517, 1987

Segall JE, Ishihara A, Berg HC: Chemotactic signalling in filamentous cells of *Escherichia coli*. J Bacteriol 161:51, 1985

Stock J, Borczuk A, Chiou F, Burchenal JEB: Compensatory mutations in receptor function: A reevaluation of the role of methylation in bacterial chemotaxis. Proc Natl Acad Sci USA 82:8364, 1985

5

Biosynthesis and Its Regulation; Allostery

Biosynthesis

Although glycolysis, pyruvate oxidation, and the TCA cycle were originally discovered as energy-yielding (catabolic) pathways, various of their intermediates initiate the biosynthetic (anabolic) pathways to the building blocks and other essential metabolites of the cell, as Figure 5–1 outlines. Hence, the former pathways are now called central or **amphibolic** (Gr. *amphi*, either).

Long after the central pathways had been dissected, by selective inhibition and fractionation of their enzymes, the biosynthetic branches remained recalcitrant, because each involves a much smaller flow of material. Beadle and Tatum, seeking markers for genetic studies in a simple unicellular eukaryote, the bread mold *Neurospora crassa*, provided a new approach by isolating a variety of auxotrophic mutants, each blocked in a biosynthetic reaction and hence requiring the product of that pathway for growth. Study of these organisms contributed to the later development of molecular genetics by revealing a one-to-one relation between genes and enzymes, but an unexpected dividend was the further finding that each mutant accumulates the precursor of the blocked reaction. Subsequently, similar mutants in bacteria proved more convenient than those of the mold. Moreover, analysis of the kinetics of their accumulation of intermediates later revealed the basic mechanism of regulation of metabolic pathways: modulation of the activity of special regulatory enzymes by interaction with specific metabolites.

The biosynthetic pathways found in microbes proved to be nearly uniform throughout the living world. They

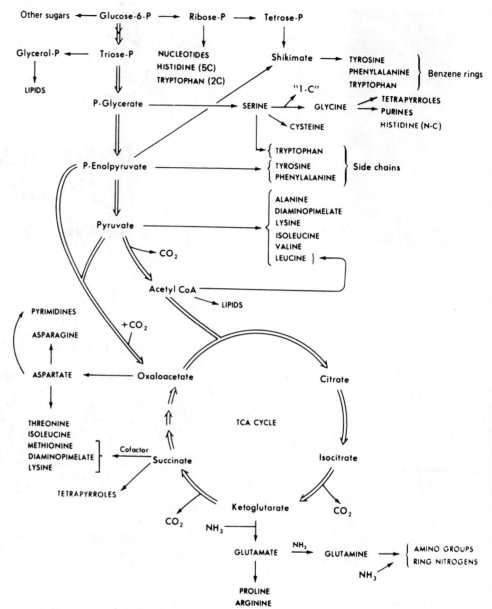

Figure 5–1. Relation of amphibolic pathways *(heavy arrows)* to main anabolic pathways. End products are in capitals. "1-C" is a 1-carbon fragment.

are described in biochemistry texts, and this chapter will deal with only selected aspects of the subject. The synthesis of lipids and of cell-wall constituents has been described briefly in Chapter 2, and the formation of informational macromolecules (nucleic acids, proteins) will be considered in later chapters.

METHODS FOR ANALYZING BIOSYNTHETIC PATHWAYS

Microbes have offered several advantages in the study of biosynthesis. In particular, while growing cells nor-

mally contain biosynthetic intermediates in only trace amounts, auxotrophic mutants excrete a precursor in large amounts, often exceeding the weight of the cells. In addition, **cross-feeding (syntrophism)** of one mutant by a precursor accumulated by another has often revealed that accumulation (Fig. 5–2), and it provides a convenient bioassay. Most of the steps in the biosynthesis of the amino acids have been identified through study of accumulated intermediates.

Some compounds that satisfy the growth requirement of an auxotroph are not true intermediates—for example, free purines and pyrimidines, which many organ-

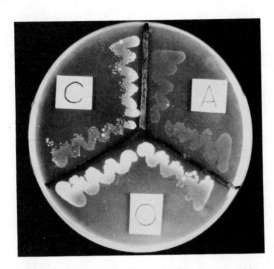

Figure 5–2. Cross-feeding between different bacterial mutants blocked in the same pathway. Note that a streak of mutant A, growing slightly on medium containing a trace of arginine, stimulates the growth of adjacent streaks of mutants C and O, whereas C similarly stimulates O but not A. These interactions establish the biosynthetic sequence ornithine (O) → citrulline (C) → arginine (A).

isms can utilize as a source of nucleotides, via "salvage" pathways.

Another valuable approach has been the incorporation of radioactively labeled C or H, either from specific precursors competing with glucose, or from specific positions in glucose into specific positions in the product. Some steps have been revealed only by separation of the enzymes in vitro.

These several methods have yielded a nearly complete map of biosynthesis in *E. coli*. Most sequences include a virtually irreversible reaction, usually ATP-linked, that ensures unidirectional flow.

BIOSYNTHESIS FROM ALTERNATIVE FUELS

The amphibolic pathways presented in Figure 5–1 are characteristic of aerobic growth on sugars. However, other nutritional conditions, which are no less "normal," shift the directions of flow in these pathways in bacteria, just like the gluconeogenesis observed in mammals. The following are some examples.

TCA CYCLE FUELS. With a fuel that enters metabolism via the TCA cycle, C flows into the glycolytic pathway via two intermediates, P-enolpyruvate and pyruvate. The P-enolpyruvate, formed from oxaloacetate and ATP, initiates biosynthesis of many compounds via reversed glycolysis, which utilizes the usual glycolytic enzymes for its reversible reactions but requires three new enzymes for the others. The pyruvate, derived from the TCA cycle either by oxidative decarboxylation of malate or by direct

decarboxylation of oxaloacetate, is used for terminal respiration and for certain biosynthetic reactions (Fig. 5–1).

ANAEROBIOSIS. When a facultative organism shifts from aerobic to anaerobic metabolism, it can no longer carry out the entire TCA cycle, which requires terminal respiration. To meet its biosynthetic needs, it converts the cycle into a pair of linear pathways branching from oxaloacetate, as shown in Figure 5–3. An oxidative branch, retained from the original cycle, continues to form α-ketoglutarate. However, α-ketoglutarate oxidase, which forms succinate, is no longer made, and instead, a new, reductive branch makes succinate by reversing its usual oxidation to oxaloacetate. For this purpose, the NAD-linked succinate dehydrogenase is replaced by a flavin-linked fumarate reductase, which favors the reductive reaction.

ACETATE; THE GLYOXYLATE PATHWAY. Like mammals, aerobic and facultative bacteria cannot assimilate acetate (or higher fatty acids) by reversing the oxidative decarboxylation of pyruvate, but many of them can assimilate it by another route, converting two acetates to malate by employing a "glyoxylate bypass" of part of the TCA cycle, described in Chapter 4 (see Fig. 4–5). An organism growing on acetate will funnel part of it through this pathway, to meet its biosynthetic needs, and part through the regular TCA cycle, to supply energy and α-ketoglutarate.

In contrast to facultative organisms, many obligatory anaerobes have a redox cofactor (a ferredoxin) whose potential is low enough for formation of pyruvate from acetyl-CoA by reductive carboxylation. These organisms can therefore incorporate acetate into carbohydrates without the glyoxylate pathway.

AMINO ACIDS

The L-amino acids found in proteins are grouped into a small number of biosynthetic families, each arising from a specific amphibolic intermediate (see Fig. 5–1). The nine amino acids synthesized by man arise by pathways of one to three enzymes each, totalling only 13 enzymes, whereas the pathways to the 11 required amino acids range from 6 to 13 enzymes each. Dispensing with the latter pathways has thus obviated genes for about 60 enzymes.

In addition to the 20 L-amino acids that are recognized in the genetic code, some amino acids in bacteria, just as in higher organisms, are modified after incorporation into structural proteins (e.g., ε,ε-N-dimethyl lysine in pili, like the hydroxyproline in collagen). In addition, various D-amino acids are found in cell-wall polypeptides and antibiotics. They are made in two steps: a racemase interconverts L- and D-alanine, and a special trans-

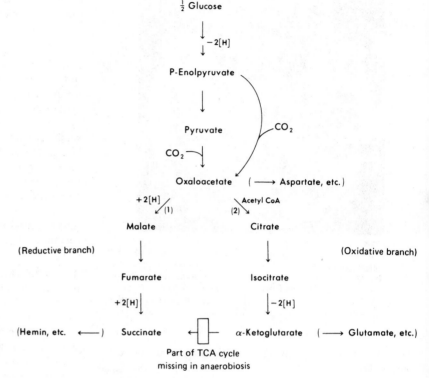

Figure 5–3. Biosynthesis of TCA intermediates in anaerobic growth on glucose in *E. coli*. The TCA cycle becomes split into a reversed reductive branch *(1)* and a normal oxidative branch *(2)*.

aminase transfers the D-amino group from D-alanine to various keto acids.

The reader is referred to biochemistry texts for the specific pathways to the amino acids and for the structures of many of the compounds mentioned below. We will comment on features that are unusual or that illustrate significant principles.

The Glutamate Family

Glutamate and **glutamine** are formed by reductive amination of α-ketoglutarate by two different pathways, as depicted below under Regulation of Nitrogen Assimilation. Glutamate serves as the source, by transamination via pyridoxal-P, of the α-amino group of all other amino acids, whereas the amide group of glutamine provides N at a higher energy level in the biosynthesis of many other compounds. Glutamate also provides the C skeleton of **proline, arginine,** and the **polyamines.**

Arginine is built up via ornithine by the same reactions found in the urea cycle in mammalian liver, except that the arginine is an endproduct instead of being cleaved by arginase to release urea. Arginine and ornithine are also precursors of polyamines (see below).

The Aspartate Family

Aspartate is synthesized by transamination of oxaloacetate. It gives rise to **asparagine, methionine, threonine,** and parts of **diaminopimelate (DAP), lysine,** and **isoleucine.** The branches of this biosynthetic tree (along with the feedback reactions that regulate their activity) are depicted in Figure 5–8, below. Aspartate is also a direct precursor of the pyrimidine ring, and it supplies N atoms to purines and to the guanidino group of arginine.

Methionine can derive its methyl group in *E. coli*, surprisingly, in two ways: with 5-methyltetrahydrofolate or with cobamide (from vitamin B_{12}) as a coenzyme. It plays a central role in metabolism, serving as donor, via **S-adenosylmethionine,** for methylations of RNA and DNA and for the cyclopropane ring in some fatty acids.

Diaminopimelate ($HOOC - CHNH_2 - (CH_2)_3 - CHNH_2 - COOH$) is a component of the peptidoglycan of most bacteria, and it also gives rise, by decarboxylation, to **lysine.** Its synthesis is initiated by the formation of aspartic semialdehyde and its condensation with pyruvate.

Lysine is the only amino acid that is synthesized by quite different routes in different organisms. In fungi and in plants, which do not contain DAP, its synthesis starts with the condensation of acetyl-CoA with α-ketoglutarate.

The Pyruvate Family: Aliphatic Amino Acids

Alanine is derived in most bacteria by transamination of pyruvate but in some bacilli by direct reductive amination. It provides 3-C fragments for the synthesis of **valine,**

isoleucine, and **leucine.** These pathways are unusual in having a single set of enzymes that catalyze two parallel sequences whose substrates differ by a -CH_2- group.

The Serine Family: 1-C Fragments

Serine is formed by the reactions:

3-P-Glycerate → 3-P-Hydroxypyruvate → 3-P-Serine → Serine

Serine in turn can transfer CH_2OH to **tetrahydrofolate (THF),** giving rise to glycine plus a 1-C fragment (hydroxymethyl-THF). In addition, the glycine can react with THF to yield a second molecule of HOCH_2-THF, plus CO_2 and NH_3.

All these reactions are readily reversible; hence, the cell can make serine from glycine, as well as the reverse; and it can make the two compounds (and 1-C fragments) in whatever proportions are needed.

1-C TRANSFER. The hydroxymethyl-THF derived from serine or glycine is used in a variety of biosynthetic reactions: it can be isomerized to 5,10-methylene-THF, reduced to 5-Me-THF, or oxidized to 5,10-methenyl-THF and its isomer 1-formyl-THF. At these various levels of oxidation, it provides the methyl group of methionine or of thymine, the formyl group of formyl-Met-tRNA (see Initiation, Chap. 6), or closure of the two rings in purines. Inhibition of THF synthesis (by sulfonamides) or of its function (by trimethoprim) are important chemotherapeutic mechanisms.

Cysteine is formed from serine by the incorporation of H_2S. Sulfate, a common source of S, is activated by ATP to yield 3'phosphoadenosine-5'phosphosulfate, which is then reduced to H_2S. The SH group of cysteine provides the S in methionine via an intermediate, cystathionine, in which the S links (as a thioether) the two C skeletons.

Histidine

This amino acid is formed by a complicated route in which the source of its 5-C backbone, 5-phosphoribosyl-1-pyrophosphate, adds an N–C fragment from ATP and then an NH_2 group from glutamine. Subsequent reactions lead to the amino alcohol histidinol, whose terminal CH_2OH is oxidized to yield histidine.

This pathway is unique among amino acid syntheses in having no COOH in its intermediates until the last step. Because these intermediates contain other ionizable groups (phosphate and then the imidazole ring), this pathway does not violate an interesting general principle in intermediary metabolism: **all intracellular intermediates contain ionizable groups** (such as the "extra" phosphates that participate in glycolysis without affecting its energetics). These groups presumably improve the retention of the metabolite in the cell and the efficiency of its interactions with enzymes.

Aromatic Compounds

The key to this pathway was the discovery of mutants of *E. coli* that each require five aromatic compounds (tyrosine, phenylalanine, tryptophan, *p*-aminobenzoate, and *p*-hydroxybenzoate). Certain of these mutants were found to accumulate, and others to grow on, **shikimic acid** (see below), a hydroaromatic compound that is found in certain plants. The pathway starts by condensation of erythrose-4-P with P-enolpyruvate, followed by cyclization, further transformations, and then addition of another enolpyruvyl group to form the main branch compound, **chorismic acid** (Gr., fork):

Shikimic Acid   Chorismic Acid

In further steps the pyruvyl group of chorismic acid shifts its attachment to the ring and becomes the 3-C side chain, and aromatization is achieved by removing either two [H] or H_2O, yielding the ketoacids of **tyrosine** and **phenylalanine,** respectively. In forming **tryptophan,** chorismic acid releases the pyruvyl group to yield anthranilate (*o*-aminobenzoate), which is converted to the indole ring and then adds a 3-C side chain from serine. Tryptophan, the least common amino acid in most proteins, has the longest biosynthetic pathway, comprising 15 enzymes (including the common aromatic pathway).

Chorismic acid is also the source of several additional aromatic compounds, which enter into various cofactors: *p*-aminobenzoate (→ folic acid), *p*-hydroxybenzoate (→ benzoquinones), and 3,4-dihydroxybenzoate (→ naphthoquinones and various siderophores). The folic acid pathway is the site of action of the sulfonamides and some other chemotherapeutic agents (Chap. 10).

OTHER PATHWAYS
Polyamines

The simplest polyamine, the diamine **putrescine** (1,4-diaminobutane), is made by two pathways: the decarboxylation of ornithine, or the decarboxylation of arginine followed by conversion of the guanidino to an amino group. The triamine **spermidine** is made by addition to putrescine of a -(CH_2)_3NH_2 group from S-adenosylmethionine. (The tetramine spermine, present in eukaryotic cells, has not been found in bacteria).

Polyamines bind readily to nucleic acids, forming ionic cross-links between phosphates on the two strands of a double helix and thus increasing resistance to strand separation. In bacterial cells they appear to be located mainly in ribosomes, because their total concentration roughly parallels that of the ribosomes under different growth conditions.

It has been difficult to determine the role of polyamines in the cell because they are partially interchangeable with the inorganic polycation Mg^{2+} in many functions, although they are less effective. Accordingly, mutants blocked in their synthesis still grow, although more slowly; and in extracts, the rate or the accuracy of several important processes is improved when some of the Mg^{2+} is replaced by a polyamine. These reactions include protein synthesis, the secretion of proteins into membrane vesicles, and the methylation of tRNA. It thus seems likely that polyamines serve to optimize and regulate a number of functions of nucleic acids by providing fine control, through reversible ionic cross-links, over the opening and closing of double-stranded regions.

In some viral particles polyamines are present in amounts sufficient to neutralize a large fraction of the negative charges on the DNA or RNA. Their cross-linking of the nucleic acid (presumably between, as well as within, double strands) evidently promotes its tight packing within the viral coat.

Nucleotides

Purine and pyrimidine nucleotides serve several functions. Besides being building blocks for (1) nucleic acids and (2) many coenzymes, they are (3) carriers for the transfer and the transformations of many cell constituents (sugars, wall peptides, complex lipids); (4) covalent modifiers of the activity of many enzymes; and (5)constituents of some antibiotics. The pathways to the nucleotides were elucidated largely in animal tissues by isotopic and enzymatic methods.

These pathways further exemplify a feature of intermediary metabolism that was noted above under Histidine Biosynthesis: the importance of being ionized. Purine nucleotides are built up from a ribose-P chain, and all the intermediates have a phosphate group (and no COOH). Pyrimidine nucleotides, in contrast, start with aspartate and retain a COOH group until ribose-P is incorporated.

PENTOSES. Ribose-5-P can be formed from glucose-6-P in *E. coli* either oxidatively, via decarboxylation of 6-P-gluconic acid, or non-oxidatively, by a series of transfers of 2-C and 3-C fragments. Only the first of these pathways generates the biosynthetic reductant NADPH from NADP, so the choice contributes to the cell's adjustment of the production of NADH, used for energy production, and NADPH, used for biosynthesis.

Deoxyribose residues are formed by NADPH-linked reduction of the ribose of the nucleoside diphosphates (or the triphosphates in some organisms) of A, G, and C. In that reduction *Lactobacillus* employs vitamin B_{12}, which is present in its normal habitat (milk). *E. coli*, which usually grows in a less rich environment, uses instead a small protein cofactor, **thioredoxin**, in which a pair of SH groups on adjacent cysteines have a sufficiently low redox potential.

If the thymine (5-Me-uracil) of DNA were similarly made by reduction of UDP or UTP, followed by methylation of the product, the DNA would inevitably incorporate U as well as T, and U is less accurately read in DNA replication. This source of error is eliminated by forming dTTP from dCMP, with deamination and methylation of the ring, by a sequence that avoids dUDP:

$$dCDP \rightarrow dCMP \rightarrow dUMP \rightarrow dTMP \rightarrow dTDP \rightarrow dTTP$$

As further protection against error, *E. coli* has a specific dephosphorylase for dUTP, and also an N-glycosidase that cleaves any dU that may be inserted in DNA.

Sugars

Polysaccharides, which provide much of the surface specificity of bacteria, differ widely in their components. Most of the novel sugars are formed from glucose by reactions at the level of **sugar nucleotides (nucleoside diphosphate sugars).** These are formed by specific pyrophosphorylases (named after the reverse of the biosynthetic reaction):

$$\text{Nucleoside-P-P-P + Hexose-1-P} \rightleftharpoons$$

$$\text{Nucleoside-P-P-hexose + P-P}$$

The sugar nucleotides may undergo conversion to isomers (Fig. 5–4A), amino sugars, deoxy sugars, sugars with a terminal methyl group, or uronic acids. They are also the donors in the transglycosylation reactions that incorporate the sugars into specific polysaccharides. In addition, sugar nucleotides are involved in the conversion of some sugars, utilized as fuels, to glucose phosphate, as shown in Figure 5–4B.

Intermediates in these pathways are often accumulated, as in amino acid biosynthesis, by mutants blocked in the synthesis (or in the transfer) of a particular sugar. Figure 5–5 outlines some pathways that have been worked out in this way. It should be noted that synthesis of the different monomers of a particular polysaccharide from glucose starts by attaching that residue to different nucleotides—a feature that may improve the specificity or the regulation of the enzymes of these pathways.

Polysaccharides

CAPSULES. The specific heteropolymeric polysaccharides of capsules are formed much like those of lipopolysaccharides, as has been described in Chapter 2. Each repeating subunit is formed on a nucleotide carrier, then transferred to a lipid carrier in the membrane, and finally polymerized on the outer surface of the membrane.

In a very different process, important in the bacterial adhesion that contributes to dental caries, certain lactic

A Biosynthetic formation of galactose from glucose

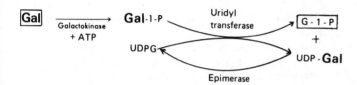

D-Glucose-1-P (G-1-P)   Uridine diphosphate glucose (UDPG)   Uridine diphosphate galactose (UDP Gal)

B Utilization of galactose (Gal) as carbon source

Figure 5–4. Epimerization of galactose and glucose. The anabolic sequence from glucose to galactose *(A)* evidently employs the same isomerase as the pathway for the amphibolic utilization of galactose *(B)*, for a *gal⁻* mutant of *E. coli* that lacks this enzyme has lost the ability both to use galactose as a carbon source and to make a galactose-containing wall polysaccharide from glucose. These two sequences are also found in mammalian cells.

bacteria form a sticky homopolymer from exogenous sucrose (glucose-1,2-fructoside) by a simple reaction in which the energy of the glycoside bond is used to polymerize one of the two residues. Some species release and absorb the fructose moiety and polymerize the glucose (= dextrose) to a high-molecular-weight **dextran;** others free the glucose and polymerize the fructose (levulose) to

a **levan:**

$$n \text{ Sucrose} \longrightarrow (\text{Glucose})_n + n \text{ Fructose}$$
$$\text{or}$$
$$n \text{ Glucose} + (\text{Fructose})_n$$

In these polymers, the predominant linkage is α-1,6, in contrast to the α-1,4 of starch or glycogen.

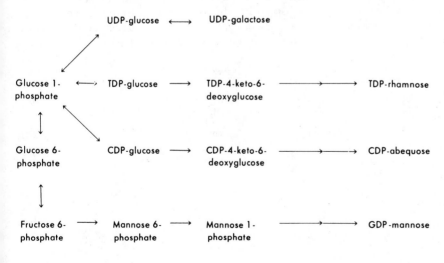

Figure 5–5. Biosynthesis of the precursors of a specific wall polysaccharide (O ag) of group B *Salmonella.* (Nikaido H et al: J Bacteriol 91:1126, 1966)

Cellulose (poly-β-1,4-glucose), the principal structural material of higher plants, is also formed by some acetobacters: obligate aerobes that oxidize ethanol to acetic acid, forming vinegar. The cellulose forms an extracellular mat that traps cells and is floated by bubbles of CO_2 to the surface.

Glycogen (poly-α-1,4-glucose) is an intracellular storage material in many bacteria. Just as in mammals, it is formed from UDPG (Fig. 5–4) and is utilized via phosphorolysis [glycogen + $nP_i \rightarrow$ n(glucose-1-P)].

Nonprotein Polypeptides

HOMOMERIC POLYPEPTIDES. The anthrax bacillus forms a capsule of polyglutamic acid, which is essential for virulence. In contrast to proteins, whose synthesis costs more than four ~P per residue, these noninformational polypeptides are synthesized by a simple enzymatic mechanism that uses only one ~P per residue. Some short peptides (glutathione; the peptides of peptidoglycan) are also made by a simple enzymatic mechanism with a separate enzyme to recognize each successively added residue.

Peptide antibiotics (10–20 residues) are synthesized by a mechanism intermediate in complexity between protein synthesis and homopolymer synthesis. The sequence is determined by a sequence of sites on a complex, **multiheaded enzyme.** An example is the synthesis by *Bacillus brevis* of **gramicidin S,** a head-to-tail ring of two pentapeptides:

L-Leu-D-Phe-L-Pro-L-Val-L-Orn
| |
L- Orn-L-Val--L-Pro-D-Phe-L- Leu

In this process the amino acids are activated as aminoacyladenylates (as in protein synthesis), and each is then transferred to a high-energy thioester link with an -SH on an enzyme. Enzyme I racemizes phenylalanine and then transfers the D-Phe to Enzyme II, a large multienzyme complex that also attaches the other four residues in specific sites. Pantetheine-P, a long prosthetic group located in the middle of these sites on the enzyme, accepts on its terminal SH the growing peptide from each site and transfers it to the next residue, as shown in Figure 5–6. Enzyme II is thus analogous to a primitive ribosome with a template for a fixed sequence built in.

Heterotrophic CO_2 Fixation

In heterotrophic organisms, the large production of CO_2 from organic fuels long masked the fact that these organisms also assimilate a small amount of CO_2. However, in contrast to autotrophic CO_2 fixation, this C is not reduced sufficiently to be incorporated into derivatives of the glycolytic pathway. Instead, it enters into the following limited number of reactions:

1. Carboxylation of pyruvate or of P-enolpyruvate, the largest route of heterotrophic CO_2 fixation. In these reactions, CO_2 yields one of the carbons of oxaloacetate (or malate) and thus of aspartate, glutamate, and their numerous derivatives.

2. Formation of carbamyl-P, which contributes both the guanidino C or arginine and C-2 of the pyrimidine ring.

3. Contribution of C-6 of the purine ring.

4. CO_2 participates cyclically, without being assimilated, in fatty acid biosynthesis (Fig. 2–22).

Regulation of Biosynthesis; Allostery
INTRACELLULAR REGULATION

While neural and hormonal mechanisms were long known to regulate the interactions of organs and cells in higher organisms, the presence of sophisticated regulatory mechanisms within the simple bacterial cell, coordinating the metabolic pathways outlined in Figure 5–1, was at first surprising. Their early evolution evidently reflects the strong selection pressure for maximizing growth rate and efficiency in the utilization of foodstuffs.

Intracellular metabolic regulation depends on **feedback loops,** in which the concentration of certain metabolites affects the activity of key, regulatory enzymes. The molecular basis is **allostery** (Gr. *allos*, other; *stereos*,

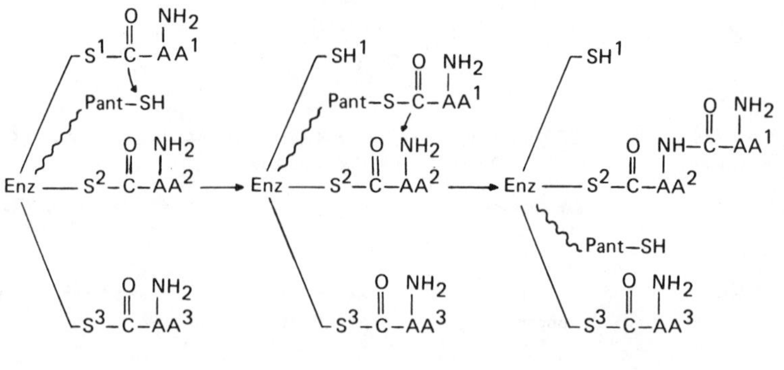

Figure 5–6. Peptidyl transfer by transthiolation in the synthesis of a peptide antibiotic on a multienzyme complex. The pantetheine *(Pant-SH)* is attached at one end to some central position in the protein. Its free, reactive-SH end can accept an amino acid *(A)* or peptide from a thioester and transfer it to the amino group of the next amino acid in the sequence.

shape), a process in which the binding of a small **effector** molecule at a specific regulatory site on a protein influences its conformation and hence its activity.

Initially elucidated in bacteria as the inhibition of a biosynthetic enzyme by the endproduct of the pathway, allosteric responses were later found to have a much broader significance. They regulate energy-yielding as well as biosynthetic pathways, and also membrane transport systems; and they permit transmembrane proteins to convey information from the outside to the inside of the cell. They provide the molecular basis for the responses to most hormonal, sensory, and pharmacologic stimuli and for nerve conduction and transmission. Complementing information storage in macromolecular sequences, they provide information about concentrations, and its translation into conformational responses is now recognized as a key aspect of life processes.

We should further note that the discovery of allostery has had a profound effect on the goals of biochemistry. In contrast to physiologists, biochemists were long reluctant to engage in teleonomic speculations or inferences—asking not only what activity or structure is present in an organism, but why. But the question is no longer speculative: the function of a reaction can be inferred reliably from its regulatory responses (because these clearly evolved in relation to its role in the overall economy of the cell), as well as from the phenotypic consequences of eliminating it by mutation.

The structural and the mechanistic features of allostery are now major topics in protein chemistry; we will restrict our discussion to the discovery of the phenomenon and to its physiologic functions. The regulation of RNA and protein synthesis (i.e., of gene expression), which also depend on allostery, will be considered in Chapter 9.

FEEDBACK LOOPS

Two observations first suggested that the endproduct of a biosynthetic pathway exerts **feedback inhibition** of the activity of enzymes already present. First, in a bacterial culture growing on radioactive glucose the labeling of an amino acid by endogenous synthesis ceases immediately when the same amino acid, unlabeled, is provided exogenously. Second, the accumulation of precursors by auxotrophic mutants, described earlier in this chapter, begins only as the endproduct is exhausted; and if the endproduct is added again, the accumulation ceases within a few seconds (Fig. 5–7). In 1957, Umbarger, studying the biosynthesis of isoleucine and valine, and Pardee, studying pyrimidine nucleotides, discovered the mechanism: the endproduct, acting directly on the first enzyme of its pathway, instantly inhibits its activity. This basic mechanism thus turned out to be much simpler than the already known feedback regulation of enzyme

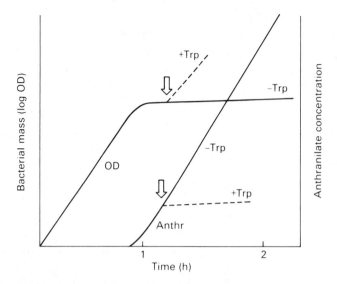

Figure 5–7. Feedback inhibition by an endproduct. A trytophan auxotroph growing on limiting Trp begins to accumulate a precursor (anthranilate) in the medium at the time when growth ceases, as determined by optical density (OD). Addition of Trp to part of the culture stops the accumulation, with simultaneous resumption of growth. In extracts the inhibition of accumulation occurs in seconds.

formation by endproducts acting on a repressor or activator of the gene (Chap. 9).

The regulation of biosynthesis also sometimes involves **positive effectors.** For example, aspartate transcarbamylase, the first enzyme in the pathway to pyrimidines, not only is inhibited by the endproduct cytidine triphosphate but is stimulated by ATP, the endproduct of a parallel pathway (see Fig. 5–11, below). Similarly, in mammals as well as in bacteria, when ATP utilization is increased, the resulting increase in the level of AMP stimulates regulatory enzymes in various catabolic pathways and thus increases the supply of energy.

In addition to the noncovalent interactions with effector molecules just described, enzyme activity can also be regulated by **chemical modification,** as will be described below.

BRANCHED PATHWAYS

Branched pathways present a special problem in regulation, for if feedback from one branch blocked the common pathway, its other branches would be starved. Several solutions have evolved. One is the formation of **isoenzymes** (isozymes: different enzymes for the same reaction). For example, in the aspartate family of biosynthesis, whose initial common pathway has three branches, *E. coli* makes three species of the first enzyme, aspartokinase (Fig. 5–8), all of which contribute to a common pool of the same product (aspartyl phosphate) but

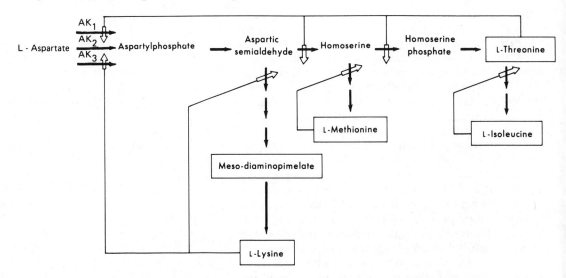

Figure 5–8. Sites of endproduct inhibition in *E. coli* in the family of amino acids derived from aspartate. *Thick lines,* biosynthetic pathway; *thin lines,* inhibition; AK_1, AK_2, AK_3, isozymic aspartokinases. AK_1 and AK_3 are subject to endproduct repression of enzyme formation (see below), as well as to inhibition of enzyme actions; AK_2 is not inhibitable, but it is repressed by methionine.

are subject to feedback inhibition by different endproducts. In addition, at each **fork** in the pathway, the **initial enzyme of each branch** is inhibited by the appropriate endproduct. A "valve" thus regulates the flow at each branch, just as in a proper hydraulic system.

Three additional mechanisms for regulating branched pathways have been discovered (Fig. 5–9). First, **cumulative inhibition** is seen with glutamine synthetase, which plays a key role in nitrogen assimilation (see below): many endproducts each cause only partial inhibition, even at high concentrations, and their effects are additive. Second, in **concerted feedback,** a single enzyme responds to a mixture of two or more endproducts but not to individual ones (at physiologic concentrations). Third, in **sequential feedback,** the endproduct inhibits only the initial enzyme of its branch, and the resulting accumulation of the preceding intermediate inhibits the first enzyme in the common pathway. Different organisms may employ different mechanisms for the same pathway, but the reasons are not clear.

PSEUDOFEEDBACK INHIBITION BY ANALOGUES

Regulatory mechanisms have evolved that can discriminate accurately even between metabolites with a very similar structure (e.g., isoleucine and leucine). However, synthetic analogues have not had the evolutionary opportunity to select for similar specificity, so they often can deceive regulatory mechanisms, just as they can deceive enzymes. For example, 5-methyltryptophan mimics the feedback effect of tryptophan on the first enzyme

of the tryptophan pathway (pseudofeedback inhibition), thus preventing growth unless tryptophan is added.

Growth in the presence of the analogue selects readily for mutants with an altered enzyme that is resistant to pseudofeedback inhibition, and these enzymes are often

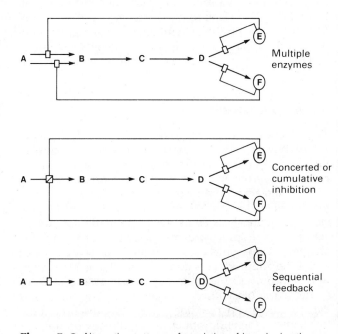

Figure 5–9. Alternative patterns of regulation of branched pathways. Concerted and cumulative inhibition are similar in their response to the mixture of endproducts, but only the latter shows a partial response to the individual products.

also resistant to inhibition by the normal endproduct. Such cells therefore synthesize in excess, and excrete, that product—a commercially useful property.

THE FUNCTIONS OF FEEDBACK INHIBITION

Feedback inhibition was discovered through its sparing of endogenous synthesis in response to **exogenously supplied metabolites.** This response releases material and energy for other syntheses, which explains why bacteria grow faster in a rich than in a minimal medium. But feedback inhibition has a broader physiological function: it also governs the amounts of **endogenously synthesized endproducts,** so that they are formed in the required proportions without wasteful overproduction. The proof, just noted, is that loss of feedback inhibition of a pathway by mutation results in excretion of the endproduct.

It has often been suggested that endproduct repression of the formation of biosynthetic enzymes (Chap. 9) provides coarse regulation, and endproduct inhibition of enzyme activity fine regulation, of biosynthesis. However, mutations that markedly increase the level of the enzymes of a pathway do not cause excretion of the endproduct if feedback inhibition is normal. It therefore seems clear that feedback repression of enzyme production provides economy only in macromolecule synthesis, whereas feedback inhibition of enzyme activity provides economy in small molecule biosynthesis.

The direct regulation of key enzymes also indirectly affects the activity of others, by influencing the amount of the metabolites in the **intracellular metabolite pool.** This pool can be obtained for analysis by rapidly lysing the cells and inactivating their enzymes (e.g., by pouring a culture into boiling water or into trichloroacetic acid solution). In steady-state growth each intermediate is at a concentration below saturation of the next enzyme, so the enzymes normally are working at less than capacity. This **reserve capacity** makes possible a rapid response to an increased demand for a particular metabolite.

ALLOSTERIC TRANSITIONS AND THEIR COOPERATIVE KINETICS

The **effector** and the **substrate** of an allosteric enzyme have quite different shapes, and they bind to different sites on the protein. Nevertheless, with most allosteric enzymes the conformational interaction between the two sites causes the two ligands to exhibit **competitive antagonism.** The reason is that these enzymes have the special property of possessing two stable conformations: the active one has high affinity for the substrate and low affinity for the inhibitory effector, whereas the opposite is true of the inactive conformation. The effector, complexing reversibly with its site, stabilizes or induces the inac-

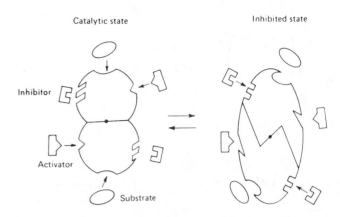

Oligomeric enzyme

Figure 5–10. Regulatory changes in an allosteric enzyme. This model assumes spontaneous transitions in tertiary structure, which can be stabilized by binding various ligands (indicated by *arrow*). The inhibitory effector stabilizes the inactive state of the enzyme; the substrate (and, for some enzymes, the stimulatory effector) stabilizes the active state. (After Changeux JP: Sci Am April 1965, p 36. Copyright © 1965 by Scientific American, Inc. All rights reserved.)

tive conformation, while the substrate, complexing with the catalytic site, stabilizes or induces the active conformation (Fig. 5–10). Positive effectors may act either by helping to stabilize the active site or by blocking the binding of a negative effector. In most allosteric enzymes the catalytic site and the effector site are on different subunits.

With some allosteric enzymes binding of the negative effector does not decrease affinity for the substrate but instead decreases the turnover number (V_{max}). With these enzymes, the interaction with the two ligands is not competitive: an excess of substrate cannot overcome the inhibition.

COOPERATIVE KINETICS. Although in principle an enzyme with a single active site could exhibit allosteric behavior, in fact, allosteric enzymes possess multiple, symmetrically arranged subunits whose contacting surfaces are complementary when the subunits are all in the active or all in the inactive conformation. This feature has profound physiological significance, because it permits the subunits to influence each other's conformation. Accordingly, the binding of substrate to a subunit, stabilizing the active conformation, favors the same conformation for the symmetrical subunit, thus increasing its affinity for the second molecule of bound ligand. As a result, the enzyme exhibits **cooperative kinetics** rather than the usual first-order mass-law kinetics, as shown in Figure 5–11: the variation of activity with substrate concentration is **sigmoidal,** reflecting a steeper rise in activ-

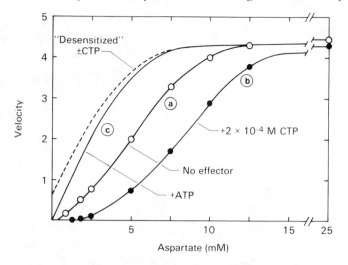

Figure 5–11. Kinetics of an allosteric enzyme, aspartate transcarbamylase from *E. coli*. This initial enzyme of the pathway to pyrimidine nucleotides converts aspartate plus carbamyl phosphate to carbamyl aspartate. In these experiments enzyme activity in an extract is measured at various concentrations of aspartate, with the other substrate constant.

Solid lines, native enzyme. The sigmoid middle curve *(A)*, obtained without effectors, indicates cooperative interaction of multiple substrate molecules with an enzyme molecule. *(B)* The endproduct of the reaction, cytidine triphosphate (CTP), causes feedback inhibition, which is overcome competitively by increased concentrations of aspartate. *(C)* Conversely, ATP is stimulatory, and because it was added at a high enough concentration to stabilize all the enzyme molecules in a fully active conformation, the kinetics are of the Michaelis–Menten type, with a hyperbolic curve (i.e., binding of the first molecule of substrate by such a stabilized enzyme does not influence the binding of additional molecules). ATP and CTP can antagonize each other's effects.

Dashed line, enzyme "desensitized" by heating at 60°C or by treatment with $10^{-6}M$ Hg^{2+}, which separates the catalytic from the regulatory subunits. The sigmoidal shape is lost, as is inhibitability by CTP. (After Gerhart JC, Pardee AB: J Biol Chem 237:891, 1962)

ity over a given percentage increase in concentration. The response to effector concentration is similarly sigmoidal (not shown).

When the subunits are separated or the connection between them is weakened by mild denaturation ("desensitization"), the allosteric response is destroyed, and the catalytic subunit carries out the reaction with first-order kinetics (Fig. 5–11). (Before the concept of allostery arose, the special kinetic properties of allosteric enzymes were seen occasionally but were considered an anomaly caused by impurities, and these enzymes therefore were "purified" until they gave, because of unrecognized separation of subunits, the expected first-order kinetics.)

Allosteric enzymes are ordinarily stable in either of two symmetrical states in which all the identical subunits have the same conformation (tight = inactive, relaxed = active). Monod, Wyman, and Changeux have

been able to interpret many of the kinetics of these enzymes in terms of a model in which the switches between these two states are entirely spontaneous and ligands influence the proportions only by stabilizing the state to which they can bind. However, Koshland has shown that the intermediate forms can sometimes be detected, and so the ligands may use their binding energy not only to stabilize, but also to induce the conformation that they fit. The rather large differences between the T (tight) and R (relaxed) conformations have now been identified for some allosteric enzymes by X-ray crystallography, and the responsible interactions between residues are being defined.

PHYSIOLOGICAL AND EVOLUTIONARY SIGNIFICANCE. The sigmoid curves of Figure 5–11 resemble the oxygen dissociation curve of hemoglobin, which permits a large fraction of the bound O_2 in blood to be transferred between the lungs and tissues with only a moderate pO_2 difference. In allosteric enzymes, similarly, the higher-order kinetics cause a large change in enzyme activity in response to small changes in the concentration of a substrate or of a regulatory effector. The physiological consequence, in both cases, is efficient **homeostasis,** maintaining the concentration of a compound (O_2 or a biosynthetic product) in the organism within a narrower range. The marvelous homeostatic property of hemoglobin thus derives from a property of proteins that had already evolved in bacteria.

COVALENT MODIFICATION OF ENZYMES; CASCADE REGULATION OF NITROGEN ASSIMILATION

Some enzymes are regulated not by noncovalently binding an effector but by the enzymatic, covalent attachment (and detachment) of a modifying group. For example, when *E. coli*, having exhausted a supply of glucose, shifts to growth on the accumulated acetate, it not only forms the enzymes of the glyoxylate cycle (see Fig. 4–5), but it rapidly shifts part of the flow of isocitrate from the TCA to that cycle by **phosphorylating,** and thus inactivating, some of the competing isocitrate dehydrogenase molecules. Other reversible covalent modifications of enzymes, found more extensively in eukaryotes, include methylation, acetylation, and ADP-ribosylation; and another, adenylylation, seems to be unique to prokaryotes. Some covalent modifications are involved in an elaborate **cascade** of regulatory enzymes, which amplifies both the range of the response and its sensitivity to changes in the intensity of the signal.

The best known example in bacteria, worked out by Magasanik and by Stadtman, is the assimilation of inorganic nitrogen (NH_3); mostly via glutamate (which provides the amino groups of most amino acids) and one-fifth via its derivative glutamine (whose amide group provides nitrogen atoms for many other biosyntheses). This pathway is central to virtually all biosynthesis, and because the cell cannot concentrate NH_3 (which is permeable in its unionized form) it has developed another mechanism for using low concentrations. At high concentrations NH_3 enters glutamate by reaction (1) and glutamine by reaction (2):

$$NH_3 + \alpha\text{-ketoglutarate} \xleftrightarrow[\text{dehydrogenase}]{\text{Glutamic}} \text{glutamate} + NADP^+ \quad (1)$$
$$+ H_2O + NADPH + H^+$$

$$\text{Glutamate} + NH_3 \xrightarrow[\text{synthetase}]{\text{Glutamine}} \text{glutamine} + ADP + P \quad (2)$$
$$+ ATP$$

However, when NH_3 is supplied at a low concentration, directly (<0.1 mM NH_4^+) or by derivation from a slowly degraded source, the equilibrium of reaction (1) is unfavorable. The NH_3 is then all taken up, at the expense of ATP hydrolysis, via glutamine in reaction (2), and the glutamine in turn yields glutamate by reaction (3):

$$\text{Glutamine} + \alpha\text{-ketoglutarate} \xrightarrow[\text{synthetase}]{\text{Glutamate}} 2 \text{ glutamate} \quad (3)$$
$$+ NADP^+ + NADPH + H^+$$

The sum of reactions (2) and (3) is thus the same as reaction (1), plus the hydrolysis of ATP.

The shifts between the two modes of assimilation involve a cycle of changes in the structure (as well as in the concentration) of glutamine synthetase (GS). A high NH_3 level increases the ratio of glutamine to α-ketoglutarate, which triggers a sequence that causes the specific activity of GS (i.e., the activity per molecule present) to be decreased by covalent addition of adenylyl (= AMP) groups (reaction 4); and when the NH_3 level drops, the enzyme is reactivated by reaction (5):

$$\text{GS (active)} + ATP \rightarrow \text{GS-AMP (inactive)} + PP \quad (4)$$

$$\text{GS-AMP} + P_i \rightarrow \text{GS} + ADP \quad (5)$$

The enzyme has 12 identical subunits, which can each attach one AMP group; and the activity of a GS molecule is proportional to the number of its unmodified subunits.

The adenylylation is controlled by two levels of regulation (Fig. 5–12). First, an unmodified enzyme complex carries out reaction (4), and its uridylylated derivative carries out reaction (5). Second, two additional enzymes add or remove, respectively, this UMP group; and it is these enzymes that are responsive to the ultimate effector in this cascade: the ratio of α-ketoglutarate to glutamine. Thus, low NH_3 results in accumulation of α-ketoglutarate and a short supply of glutamine, which leads to high uridylylation and low adenylylation, and therefore to high activity of GS. High NH_3 has the opposite effects.

This **indirect feedback inhibition** of GS by glutamine, through regulation of its adenylylation, is sup-

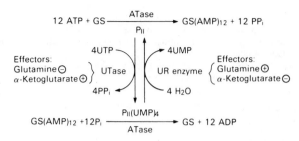

Figure 5–12. Covalent modifications of glutamine synthetase (GS) and its regulatory protein. GS can reversibly add 1 to 12 AMP groups, which are transferred by adenylyl transferase (ATase) complexed with a regulatory protein, P_{II}. Whether ATase carries out the addition (from ATP) or the removal (yielding ADP) depends on whether or not the P_{II} is uridylylated. The extent of this uridylylation is determined by still other enzymes (uridylyl transferase; uridylyl release enzyme), and glutamine and α-ketoglutarate govern the cascade of reactions by their promotion (+) or inhibition (−) of the activity of these opposing enzymes.

plemented by **direct feedback inhibition** by endproducts of pathways to which glutamine contributes nitrogen; for example, tryptophan, histidine, glycine, glucosamine-6-P, and several nucleotides. The subunits of GS thus possess remarkably polyvalent allosteric sensitivity, in addition to their regulation by covalent modification.

Cascades of regulatory enzymes, and regulation by covalent modification, are much more prominent in eukaryotic than in prokaryotic cells.

Selected Reading

Cozzone AJ: Protein phosphorylation in bacteria. Trends Biochem Sci, Sept 1984, p 400

Cunin R, Glansdorff N, Pierard A, Stalon V: Biosynthesis and metabolism of arginine in bacteria. Microbiol Rev 50:314, 1986

Herrmann KM, Somerville RD (eds): Amino Acid Biosynthesis and Genetic Regulation. Menlo Park, CA, Benjamin/Cummings, 1985

Holmgren A: Thioredoxin. Annu Rev Biochem 54:237, 1985

Kornberg HL: Anaplerotic sequences in microbial metabolism. Angew Chem [Eng] 4:558, 1965

Lipmann F: Bacterial production of antibiotic polypeptides by thiol-linked synthesis on protein templates. Adv Microb Physiol 21:228, 1980

Mandelstam J, McQuillen K: Biochemistry of Bacterial Growth, 2nd Ed. New York, Wiley-Interscience, 1973

Monod J, Changeux J-P, Jacob F: Allosteric proteins and cellular control systems. J Mol Biol 6:306, 1963

Neidhardt FC, Ingraham JL, Low KB, Magasanik B, Schaechter M, Umbarger HE (eds): *Escherichia coli* and *Salmonella typhimurium*: Cell and Molecular Biology. Washington, DC, American Society for Microbiology, 1987. Many pertinent chapters.

Pittard J, Gibson F: The regulation of biosynthesis of aromatic amino acids and vitamins. Curr Top Cell Regul 2:29, 1970

Stadtman ER, Chock PB: Interconvertible enzyme cascades in metabolic regulation. Curr Top Cell Regul 13:53, 1978

Stadtman ER, Ginsburg A: The glutamine synthetase of *E. coli*: Structure and control. In Boyer P (ed): The Enzymes, 3rd Ed, Vol 10, p 755. New York, Academic Press, 1974

Tabor CW, Tabor H: Polyamines in microorganisms. Microbiol Rev 49:81, 1985

Tonn SJ, Gander JE: Biosynthesis of polysaccharides by prokaryotes. Annu Rev Microbiol 33:169, 1979

Troy FA II: The chemistry and biosynthesis of selected bacterial capsular polymers. Annu Rev Microbiol 33:519, 1979

Umbarger HE: Amino acid biosynthesis and its regulation. Annu Rev Biochem 47:533, 1978

Yamada K, Kinoshita G, Tsunoda T, Aiota K (eds): The Microbial Production of Amino Acids. New York, Wiley (Halsted), 1972

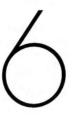

6

Protein Synthesis and Localization

Protein Synthesis

The translation of genetic information into proteins with unlimited variations in sequence, and with great accuracy, requires an extraordinarily complex mechanism, quite different from the sequences of individual enzymatic reactions that constitute the rest of metabolism. In the elucidation of this process, biochemists, asking how proteins are synthesized, and molecular geneticists, asking how genes are expressed, found themselves working on the same problem.

Effective analysis began in the 1950s, when Zamecnik and Hoagland incorporated radioactively labeled amino acids into protein in extracts of liver cells and then demonstrated a requirement for particulate components (ribosomes), transfer RNAs (tRNAs), and enzymes that charge the tRNAs with amino acids. Meanwhile, genetic studies in bacteria led to the discovery of a labile messenger RNA (mRNA) (see Chap. 9; Messenger RNA). Synthetic polyribonucleotides used as artificial messengers led to elucidation of the genetic code and also of many features of ribosome action, but their translation bypassed normal initiation; the introduction of phage RNA as a uniform natural messenger later revealed the initiation process. The simultaneous transcription and translation of phage or plasmid DNA finally extended synthesis *in vitro* from polypeptides to defined proteins, because this DNA contains relatively few genes, and so the product of each is a significant fraction of the total.

Although the mechanism of protein synthesis was largely worked out in bacteria, very similar systems have now been elucidated in mammalian cells. In this brief review we will emphasize the features characteristic of prokaryotes. We will also consider a more recently developed topic, the export of proteins into or across membranes. The effects of various antibiotics on protein synthesis, which have contributed to our understanding of this process, will be reviewed in Chapter 10.

THE MICROCYCLES OF CHAIN ELONGATION
Transfer RNA

Translation from a language of four nucleotides to one of 20 amino acids is carried out by the tRNA molecules and their charging enzymes (**aminoacyl-tRNA synthetases**). Each enzyme attaches a specific amino acid to a corresponding tRNA by an ester bond between the carboxyl of the amino acid and a hydroxyl of the 3'-terminal nucleotide. On the ribosome, the tRNA in turn recognizes a particular trinucleotide **codon** in mRNA, thus serving as an "adapter" between the codon and the corresponding (cognate) amino acid.

In a planar representation all tRNAs have a similar cloverleaf shape, with four double-stranded stems (arms) and three loops; but further folding creates an L shape that fits more compactly on the ribosome (Fig. 6–1). The anticodon (which recognizes the complementary codon in mRNA) is located in a loop at the opposite end from the amino acid attachment. The other two loops have fairly constant sequences whose pairing with complementary sequences on the ribosome contributes to its ability to recognize all aminoacyl-tRNAs (aa-tRNA) interchangeably. The stems of various tRNAs are similar in length but have different sequences, which contribute, along with the anticodon, to specific recognition by an aminoacyl-tRNA synthetase. In all tRNAs, the 3'-terminal sequence, which attaches the amino acid, is CCA, and this uniform sequence is evidently recognized by the region of the ribosome that forms the peptide bond with any incoming amino acid.

The requirements for accuracy are very stringent (less than one error in 10,000), because with an average chain length of several hundred residues even an error rate of one in 1000 in either the charging of tRNA or the codon–anticodon pairing, would result in a high proportion of faulty proteins. High fidelity in the charging is achieved by a two-step process: formation of aminoacyl-AMP on the enzyme, and covalent transfer of the amino acid to the tRNA. Errors that slip past the first step can be corrected in the second step ("editing"). A similar editing process ensures fidelity in codon–anticodon pairing, as will be described below.

The Bacterial Ribosome

The ribosome, with a sedimentation constant of 70S and a molecular weight of about three million, dissociates reversibly at low Mg^{2+} into two subunits (30S and 50S); its limited dissociation under physiologic conditions is important in its function. This function involves **microcycles** of amino acid addition and also a **macrocycle** of

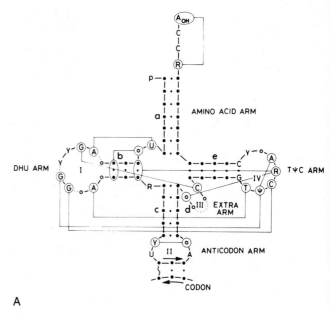

A

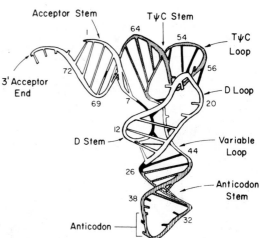

B

Figure 6–1. tRNA. (**A**) Generalized cloverleaf model. I through IV, unpaired regions (loops); a through e, base-paired regions; solid small circles with centered dots, base pairs; P, purine; Y, pyrimidine; T, ribothymidine; ψ, pseudouridine. Arrow shows 5' → 3' direction. Letters indicate nucleotides common to all sequences (which often have substituents; not indicated). Circled nucleotides joined by light lines are known to be paired or adjacent in the tertiary structure. (**B**) Folded structure. (**A**, Levitt M: Nature 224:759, 1969; **B**, courtesy of Alexander Rich)

chain initiation and termination. In each microcycle the growing polypeptide shuttles back and forth between a tRNA bound noncovalently in the **A (aminoacyl)** site and one in the **P (peptidyl)** site. The microcycle has three main steps (Fig. 6–2): recognition, peptidyl transfer, and translocation.

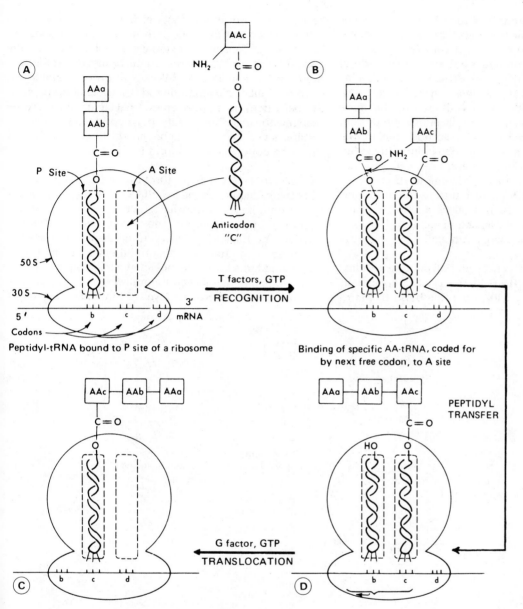

Figure 6–2. Steps in microcycle. *(A)* Peptidyl–tRNA bound to peptidyl (P) site of a ribosome. *(B)* Binding of specific aa–tRNA, coded for by next free codon, to aminoacyl (A) site. *(C)* Peptide chain transfer to A site by formation of peptide bond with aa–tRNA bound to that site. *(D)* Movement of peptidyl–tRNA, along with corresponding region of mRNA, from A to P site, ejecting free tRNA.

RECOGNITION. A **trinucleotide codon** in the mRNA, positioned in the recognition region of the ribosome, specifies the binding in the A site of an **aminoacyl-tRNA** that has a complementary anticodon. The 20 amino acids are present as cytosolic **ternary complexes** containing aminoacyl-tRNA, GTP, and the protein **elongation factor EFTu.** EFTu comprises a large fraction (ca. 5%) of the total bacterial protein, because virtually every aminoacyl-

tRNA molecule awaiting recognition is complexed with it, and rapid protein synthesis requires a relatively high concentration. After recognition, the EFTu is released as a complex with GDP, and dissociation of this complex by another elongation factor, **EFTs,** frees EFTu for another cycle.

Recognition has two steps: the initial binding of the ternary complex in the neighborhood of the A site, which is **reversible,** and hydrolysis of the GP, which provides energy from **irreversible** binding of the aa-tRNA in the A site, where it can accept peptidyl transfer. These two steps provide an opportunity for **editing (proofreading)** in the following way (Fig. 6–3). The initial, reversible binding step effectively rejects most incorrect aa-tRNAs. However, nearly cognate ones, with two of the three bases correct, are not rejected rapidly enough to prevent a few from moving forward into the second step. In that step, the GTP hydrolysis, altering the conformational interaction between the ribosome and the EFTu, provides a second opportunity for the ribosome to discriminate between a correct aa-tRNA, which it locks into the A site, and an incorrect one, which it releases along with the EFTu·GDP. (The fidelity of translation will be further discussed below under Ribosomal Ambiguity.)

PEPTIDYL TRANSFER. The nascent polypeptide, residing as **peptidyl-tRNA (pp-tRNA)** in the P site, replaces its ester bond to the tRNA with a peptide bond to the α-amino group of the aa-tRNA in the A site. The chain is thus transferred from the P to the A site and becomes one residue longer. This step can be carried out by the 50S subunit, and it depends on the **peptidyl transferase center** on that particle rather than on a separable enzyme. Unlike recognition and translocation, peptidyl transfer does not require an external factor or a source of energy: the ester bond of the polypeptide to tRNA, in the P site, is at a somewhat higher energy level than the new peptide bond that it will form in the A site.

TRANSLOCATION. The pp-tRNA moves back from the A to the P site, displacing the free tRNA left in the P site by the preceding peptidyl transfer. The mRNA moves with the pp-tRNA by the length of one codon, bringing the next codon into the A site. However, the displaced free tRNA does not leave the ribosome until the next microcycle: it is retained in a third site (not shown in the figure), where it presumably helps keep the mRNA properly aligned.

The translocation step involves binding of a cytosolic

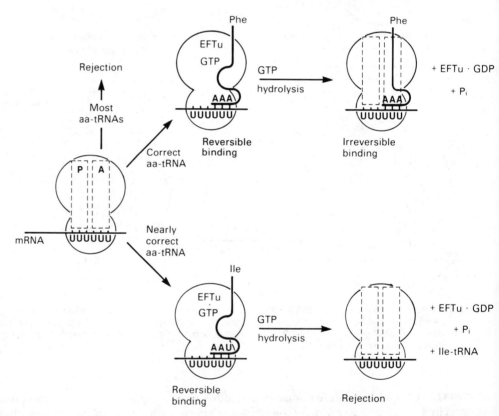

Figure 6–3. Proofreading in the two-step recognition of aa–tRNA. The initial reversible binding of a ternary complex (aa–tRNA·EFTu·GTP) probably involves a site that overlaps with the A site, as the aa–tRNA recognizes a codon that must already be in position in the A site. However, the aa–tRNA is not fully in the A site (i.e., is not able to receive peptidyl transfer) until after GTP hydrolysis and ejection of EFTu·GDP. This second step not only makes the binding of a correct aa–tRNA irreversible but somehow also allows recognition and ejection of an incorrect aa–tRNA (i.e., one whose anticodon pairs with only two nucleotides instead of three in the codon). Grossly incorrect aa–tRNAs are rejected in the first step.

elongation factor, EFG, complexed with GTP. Hydrolysis of the GTP on the ribosome provides the energy for a major conformational change, which shifts the pp-tRNA and the mRNA; the EFG●GDP complex is released and spontaneously dissociates. This movement of the pp-tRNA from one site to another, while retaining a firm attachment, is the least understood aspect of ribosome function.

Energy Cost

We have seen that in the synthesis of certain oligopeptides by a sequence of specific enzymes (see Chap. 5, Fig. 5–6), the peptide bond (a low-energy bond) can be formed at the cost of only one ~P. Protein synthesis, however, utilizes more than four ~P per peptide bond: release of a pyrophosphate (and hence two ~P) from ATP in the charging of tRNA, hydrolysis of a phosphate from GTP in the EFTu and in the EFG cycle, and a further energy drain in the turnover of mRNA. Protein synthesis therefore consumes a large fraction of the energy in a growing bacterial cell.

This price is evidently needed to optimize several features of protein synthesis: an unlimited choice of sequences, high speed (ca. 15 residues per second), high accuracy (whose cost increases with speed), and reliable retention of the expensive growing chain. The mechanistic principles include precise alignment of numerous ligands on the ribosome and an orderly succession of their attachment, alteration of state, and detachment; each of these actions imposes a different conformation on the ribosome. In addition, energy from GTP hydrolysis allows firm binding to be combined with mobility, ensures the unidirectional flow of the cycle, and makes editing possible.

THE MACROCYCLE

The macrocycle in the translation of each gene consists of chain initiation, elongation, termination, and reinitiation (Fig. 6–4). Successive initiations follow each other rapidly, creating a **polysome** (mRNA carrying multiple ribosomes: see Fig. 6–7A, below).

The early elucidation of the ribosomal microcycle and also of the genetic code depended on a fortunate and unrecognized artefact: synthetic polynucleotides were translated by using artificially high concentrations of Mg^{2+} (which increases their strength of binding) and thus permitting them to bypass proper initiation. When a natural messenger (phage RNA) became available, its physiological initiation was found to require dissociation of the ribosome and hence to have a lower Mg^{2+} optimum.

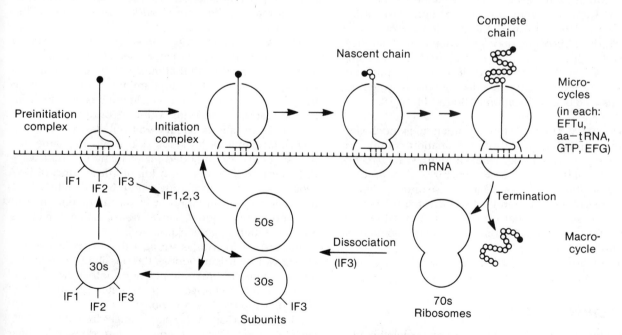

Figure 6–4. Overall scheme of protein synthesis portrayed as successive microcycles of chain elongation within a macrocycle of initiation, termination, dissociation, and reassociation during initiation.

INITIATION. For initiation, a special sequence in the mRNA codes for the binding of a ribosome (see Interactions with mRNA, below), and slightly downstream, at the beginning of a gene, AUG (or, rarely, GUG) codes for binding a special **initiating tRNA, N-formyl-Met-tRNA$_F$,** to the P site in the initiating ribosome. When the growing polypeptide chain extends into the cytosol, it encounters an enzyme that removes its formyl group, and in many proteins the initial Met is also removed (occasionally along with a few additional residues).

Internal AUGs in a gene also code for Met, but they lack the preceding ribosome-binding sequence, and they bind a different tRNA, Met-tRNA$_M$. The aminoacyl stems in these two tRNAs differ slightly in length; in addition, just as in peptidyl-tRNA (which also binds to the P site), f-Met-tRNA lacks the charged NH$_2$ group found on other aa-tRNAs.

The cycle of **ribosome dissociation and reassociation** in initiation (Fig. 6–4) involves three **initiation factors, IF1, 2,** and **3** (which were not needed for translating synthetic polynucleotides). In the **macrocycle** the free 70S ribosome is released at termination, and IF3 serves as a **dissociation factor** by binding to the 30S subunit and thus shifting the equilibrium strongly toward dissociation. The separated small subunits then bind IF1 and IF2, forming a reservoir of **initiating small subunits** (which contain virtually all of the IF molecules in the cell). These subunits, along with GTP, form a preinitiation complex with mRNA and f-Met-tRNA, and release of the dissociating IF3 permits the large subunit to be added. Much as in recognition, formation of the final, stable 70S initiation complex requires hydrolysis of the GTP followed by release of the remaining factors and GDP. The binding of one ribosomal subunit to the mRNA, followed by the other, may be required for attaching mRNA in a way that is highly stable and yet permits it to move across the ribosome in a deep groove between the subunits (see below, Location of Bound Ligands).

TERMINATION. The final step (termination) is much simpler than initiation. The three termination codons are recognized by two protein **release factors: RF1** recognizes UAG or UAA, and **RF2** recognizes UAA or UGA. Binding of either factor results in release of the polypeptide by hydrolysis of its bond to tRNA (i.e., peptidyl transfer to H$_2$O). An additional cytosolic protein, **ribosome release factor,** speeds the release of the ribosome from the mRNA after polypeptide release.

Termination will be further discussed below under Suppression.

THE GENETIC CODE

A frameshift mutation involving insertion or deletion of a single base results in garbled translation of the subsequent sequence. However, the studies by Crick and associates with phage showed that three frameshift mutations in the same direction (in a region whose sequence was not important) restore the reading frame, so that distal translation continues in the original sequence. The genetic code was thus shown to be read in a continuous sequence of triplets (codons) without intervening punctuation.

The specific codons began to be identified in 1961, when Nirenberg found that **poly(U),** a synthetic homopolymer of uridylic acid, codes for **polyphenylalanine.** Moreover, the trinucleotide UpUpU alone can bind PhetRNA to ribosomes under ionic conditions that amplify its weak binding strength. Studies of the translation of various random synthetic polymers revealed the composition of most codons, and binding studies with trinucleotides revealed their sequences. However, there were several uncertainties, and these were removed by Khorana's studies on the translation of polynucleotides with known repeating sequences. For example, ACACAC . . . is read as alternating triplets, yielding His–Thr–His–Thr . . . . Finally, studies in intact cells confirmed the code by showing that various mutations in a gene led to the predicted changes in a protein sequence.

Among the 64 triplets of the four-letter genetic code (Fig. 6–5), three code for termination (UAG = amber, UAA = ochre, and UGA = opal), and the remaining 61 for 20 amino acids. The code is thus redundant, with two or more codons for almost every amino acid. However, there are fewer tRNAs than codons, because some recognize more than one codon as a result of ambiguity ("wobble") in reading the 3' nucleotide, which is less tightly paired with the anticodon.

The redundancy of the code is not simply a matter of filling space. Instead, as Figure 6–5 shows, the assignment of codons is such that most one-base substitutions will code either for the same amino acid or for a functionally similar one. This arrangement has obvious value for the gradual process of evolution, because it ensures that such mutations usually will not destroy function. The redundancy of the code also allows the same protein sequence to be coded for in many different ways, thus permitting flexibility in important features of DNA sequence other than coding. These include sites affecting frequency of mutation or of recombination, restriction and modification (Chap. 8), transposable sequences, and regulation of gene expression.

Because GC pairing is stronger than AT pairing (three versus two hydrogen bonds), the possibility of selecting for variations in DNA composition (both localized and total) without a change in the proteins produced is of particular interest. As was noted in Chapter 1, the proportion of G + C among bacteria ranges from 30% to 70%, yet the overall protein composition does not differ widely. Most of the variation in DNA composition is at-

First letter of triplet (5' end)	Second letter of triplet				Third letter of triplet (3' end)
	U	**C**	**A**	**G**	
U	Phe Phe Leu Leu	Ser Ser Ser Ser	Tyr Tyr Ochre Amber	Cys Cys Opal Try	U C A G
C	Leu Leu Leu Leu	Pro Pro Pro Pro	His His Gln Gln	Arg Arg Arg Arg	U C A G
A	Ileu Ileu Ileu Met	Thr Thr Thr Thr	Asn Asn Lys Lys	Ser Ser Arg Arg	U C A G
G	Val Val Val Val or Met	Ala Ala Ala Ala	Asp Asp Glu Glu	Gly Gly Gly Gly	U C A G

Figure 6–5. The genetic code. *Glu, Asp,* glutamic and aspartic acid; *Gln, Asn,* glutamine and asparagine; *ochre, amber, opal,* terminator codons. *Shaded triplets* code for polar amino acids. This diagram also summarizes the pattern of degeneracy. *Brackets* at the right of amino acids indicate codons that are recognized by the same tRNA, in which wobbling of the 5'-end base of the anticodon leads to ambiguous reading of the 3' end of the codon. Some codons are recognized by more than one anticodon, as indicated by overlapping brackets.

tributable to differences in the 3' position of the codons, where substitutions usually do not affect codon specificity (Fig. 6–5).

NEAR-UNIVERSALITY OF THE CODE. Because an evolutionary shift in the code would simultaneously alter many proteins and hence might be lethal, it was not surprising that the genetic code appeared initially to be universal. However, some exceptions have been encountered, particularly in mitochondria. For example, in human mitochondria, UGA codes for tryptophan instead of for stop, and there are two additional initiation codons and two new stop codons. The evolution of these differences might ensure that these organelles persist autonomously within the cell instead of having their genes absorbed into the nuclear genome. More surprisingly, a shift in the reading of a single codon also has been found in mycoplasma and in the cytoplasm of the protozoon *Tetrahymena.*

UNUSUAL AMINO ACIDS. In addition to the standard 20 amino acids, modified amino acids are found in some proteins in prokaryotes as well as in eukaryotes: for example, hydroxyproline or acetyllysine in structural proteins, and reversibly phosphorylated serine or tyrosine in some regulatory proteins. These modifications all occur **posttranslationally.** In addition, in *E. coli* a few enzymes contain a novel amino acid, **selenocysteine** (cysteine with the sulfur replaced by selenium), in which the SeH group creates a lower redox potential than SH. Surprisingly, this modification is made on the serine on a special minor seryl-tRNA, and the resulting twenty-first standard amino acid is then coded for by UGA, which is

evidently spared as a stop codon in some contexts in mRNA.

RIBOSOMES

We will now consider the properties of the ribosome in greater detail.

Structure

Although the basic features of ribosomes are the same in all cells, differences in structural components, overall architecture, and evolutionary origins can distinguish five categories: (1) the 80S ribosomes occur in the cytoplasm of all eukaryotes; (2) the mitochondrial ribosomes form a highly diverse group, ranging from 55S for mammals to 75S for higher plants; (3) the plastid ribosomes, in the chloroplast, are unique to the plant kingdom; (4) the ribosomes of archaebacteria resemble the 80S ribosomes of eukaryotes in several characteristics (e.g., antibiotic sensitivity); and (5) the ribosomes of eubacteria, discussed in this chapter, are 70S in size.

A rapidly growing *E. coli* cell contains about 15,000 ribosomes per genome. Almost all are engaged in protein synthesis, as Figure 6–6 shows: 80% are **polysomes.** About 10% of the particles are 30S and 50S subunits stabilized by complexing of the 30S with initiation factors, as described above. When initiation is blocked but chain elongation continues, the "runoff" ribosomes accumulate as free 70S particles (Fig. 6–6*B*). These can be distinguished from complexed 70S ribosomes (i.e., the shortest polysomes), because the attached ligands make the latter more resistant to dissociation at low Mg^{2+} concentrations.

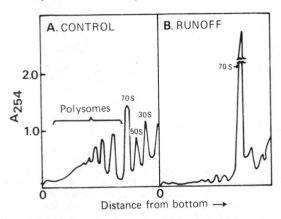

Figure 6–6. Production of 70S ribosomes by runoff in *E. coli.* Control growing cells *(A)* were rapidly chilled by pouring the culture onto ice. Runoff cells *(B)* were slowly cooled, which allowed the ribosomes to complete their chains but not to reinitiate. (A smaller sample was analyzed because of the high 70S peak.) The cells were gently disrupted by treatment with lysozyme (to lyse the wall) and deoxycholate (to lyse the membrane). The lysates were analyzed in a sucrose gradient (see Fig. 10–4, Chap. 10). Similar results were obtained when net runoff was promoted (1) by starvation for a required amino acid or a required nucleic acid base, (2) by treatment with puromycin to release ribosomes prematurely, or (3) by treatment with actinomycin to cause depletion of mRNA. (After Subramanian AR et al: Cold Spring Harbor Symp Quant Biol 34:233, 1969)

Each subunit is composed of about two-thirds rRNA and one-third r-proteins. The small subunit contains one 16S RNA molecule and 21 different r-proteins, named S1 to S21 according to their decreasing size. The large subunit contains 23S RNA (mol. wt. 1.1×10^6), 5S RNA (mol. wt. 40,000), and proteins L1 to L34 (one shared with the small subunit). Drastic conditions are required to dissociate and solubilize the tightly associated components of the ribosome, but after separation, the individual proteins are soluble and renature readily.

RECONSTITUTION (ASSEMBLY). Nomura's achievement in reconstituting active subunits from their solubilized components has greatly advanced the study of ribosomal structure and function. For example, genetic resistance to streptomycin could be localized in protein S12, because the incorporation of this protein (but not of others) from a streptomycin-resistant ribosome yielded resistant hybrid ribosomes. Moreover, "assembly mapping" has suggested that in the cell, r-proteins assemble on RNA while it is growing: the region of rRNA that is synthesized early binds certain proteins directly, whereas other proteins bind only after various members of the first group have been assembled into an intermediate particle. The assembly of the very complex ribosome without a template or enzymatic modification emphasizes the importance of spontaneous, specific aggregation of macromolecules in the general process of morphogenesis.

TOPOGRAPHY. Electron microscopy shows that each ribosomal subunit has a highly irregular shape (Fig. 6–7B), presenting different images in different orientations. Long study of these images and other information on the **topographic relations** of various proteins to each other and to specific regions of RNA have led to models such as that presented in Figure 6–8. The techniques used have included covalent cross-linking between proteins, identification of regions of RNA that can be cross-linked to different proteins, analysis of nucleoprotein fragments released by partial digestion of the RNA, identification of RNA sequences that are protected by binding various r-proteins, energy transfer (as a measure of distance) between fluorescent dyes attached to various pairs of proteins and then fitted into reconstituted ribosomes, and neutron scattering by reconstituted ribosomes containing specific deuterated proteins. Perhaps the most powerful tool for studying the surface has been **immuno-electron microscopy,** in which the two identical binding sites on an antibody to a specific r-protein (or to a ligand of the ribosome) link two ribosomes (or subunits) symmetrically, and the attachment site can be localized by the orientation of the particles.

The RNAs and the proteins are extensively interdigitated, with various regions of both exposed at the surface. Figure 6–8 indicates the exposed protein locations. Among these, L7 and L12 (which are identical except that L7 has an amino-terminal acetyl group) have four copies rather than the usual one per ribosome. The function of this acetylation, whose extent differs under different conditions, is not known. The exceptionally elongated and large protein S1 (mol. wt. 61,000) is attached at one end to the ribosome while the rest, which has a high general affinity for RNA, floats free, suggesting that it may serve to "catch" mRNA and steer it to initiation.

Each rRNA has extensive secondary structure (see Chap. 1, Fig. 1–2), with pairing between distant as well as adjacent regions in the sequence. rRNAs are extraordinarily conserved in evolution, in sequence as well as in shape. As was discussed in Chapter 1, the ability of RNA to serve both in information storage and in catalysis supports the view that it preceded proteins in evolution. However, its role as a major component of the ribosome may depend on another property: alternative patterns of base pairing permit the rRNAs to be folded in a number of alternative specific ways, which suggests that they may be better equipped than an aggregate of proteins to provide the wide variety of conformations required in the cycles of protein synthesis.

Because the components are so intricately interwoven, a mutational change at one site on the ribosome may alter the conformation at another. Thus, certain mutations in protein S12 impair binding of streptomycin although that protein does not appear to be part of the binding site. Similarly, binding of any ligand decreases

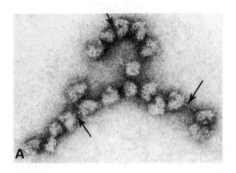

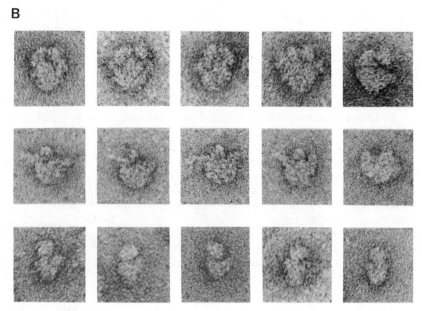

Figure 6–7. Electron micrograph of negatively stained polysomes and ribosomes. *(A)* Polysomes; arrows show mRNA strand connecting the ribosomes. *(B)* Various views of *E. coli* 70S ribosomes (top row), 50S subunits (middle row), and 30S subunits (bottom row). *(A,* Nonomura Y, Blobel G, Sabatini D: J Mol Biol 60:303, 1971. Copyright © by Academic Press Inc. [London] Ltd.; *B,* courtesy of M Boublik)

the conformational mobility of the ribosome, as shown by the decreased number of groups accessible on the surface. This restriction is important in the action of antiribosomal antibiotics, for some of these can bind only to free, initiating ribosomes and not to ribosomes engaged in chain elongation (Chap. 10).

LOCATION OF BOUND LIGANDS. Cross-linking and immuno-electron microscopy indicate that the mRNA, with

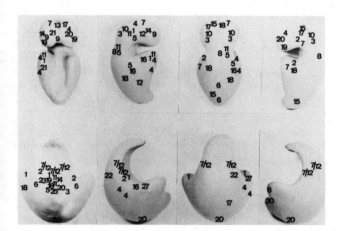

Figure 6–8. Three-dimensional model of *E. coli* ribosomal subunits with approximate locations of antibody-binding sites for individual proteins. *Above:* model for 30S subunit in successive 90° rotations. *Below:* same for 50S subunit. The orientation of the two subunits in the 70S ribosome forms a channel between them. (Courtesy of M Stoffler-Meilicke)

about 80 residues protected by the ribosome, runs through a deep cleft between protuberances in the small subunit and then in a deep groove between the subunits. The tRNAs in the A and the P sites are also located largely in that cleft, and an exposed loop of the 16S RNA has been identified that can be cross-linked to a base of the tRNA anticodon. Another region of the tRNA can be cross-linked to the large subunit, but the topography of the A and the P sites has not yet been resolved sufficiently to reveal the mechanism of translocation. The binding of the tRNAs depends on two sets of forces: nonspecific interaction of any tRNA with the ribosome and specific interaction of codon with anticodon. Part of the nonspecific binding depends on the complementarity of the TΨC and the DHU loops (see Fig. 6–1) to accessible regions of rRNAs.

In the growing polypeptide about 25 residues are protected from enzymatic digestion, and the orientation of secreting ribosomes bound to the membrane suggests that the nascent chain emerges from a region distant from the 30S subunit. Ribosomes have now been crystallized, and x-ray studies have demonstrated a **tunnel** through the 50S subunit.

Interactions with mRNA

RIBOSOME-BINDING SITES IN mRNA. Bacterial ribosomes initiate at the correct AUG, and not at those later in the gene, by recognizing a preceding sequence in the mRNA. Thus, in various *E. coli* mRNAs, the segment that is protected by initiating ribosomes was found to share, at about 10 nucleotides before the initiating AUG, a sequence with greater or lesser resemblance to a purine-rich "consensus sequence," AGGAGGU. Moreover, this **Shine–Dalgarno sequence** is complementary to a sequence in the 3′-terminal region of all 16S RNAs, and it was shown to be paired with that region in ribosomes blocked at initiation. Confirming its role in initiation, mutations in the Shine–Dalgarno sequence decrease the efficiency of translation.

In an important regulatory mechanism, differences in the closeness of the initiation sequence of various natural messengers to the consensus influence the frequency of initiation of translation. Bacterial groups that have diverged in evolution differ somewhat in their optimal sequence, and so ribosomes may read messengers from distant species (e.g., gram-positive versus negative) inefficiently.

In a remarkable further variation, in a gene transcript of phage T4 an untranslated 60-nucleotide internal sequence is not spliced out, like the introns of eukaryotic messengers, but is apparently bypassed by the ribosome by an unknown mechanism.

POLYGENIC MESSENGERS. Most bacterial messengers correspond to several genes. Usually, there is an untranslated spacer region containing a Shine–Dalgarno sequence between successive genes, suggesting that the ribosomes are released and then reattached at these junctions. Some adjacent genes, however, have no spacer; and, indeed, the A of a terminal UAA may also serve in the initiating AUG of the next gene. Whether and how ribosomes "read through" such overlaps is not certain.

OVERLAPPING GENES. Whereas most genetic sequences are translated into unique products, some overlap; i.e., the same DNA sequence is translated into different polypeptides. In bacteria these alternative translations remain in phase but use alternative initiation or termination sites or both. Some viruses use the information in the DNA even more economically by translating a sequence in more than one of its three possible coding phases, and by transcribing both strands in the same region.

Eukaryotic Ribosomes

Eukaryotic cytoplasmic ribosomes (80S) are about 50% larger than those of bacteria. The major RNA molecules are greater in molecular weight (18S and 28S), whereas the proteins are greater in number rather than in size. The elongation factors of eukaryotes, named EF-1 and EF-2, correspond to EFTu and EFG, respectively, and these factors of either group do not cross-react with ribosomes of the other group.

Initiation shows even greater differences. In eukaryotes the initiating Met-tRNA is not formylated, and the initiating AUG is simply the one nearest the 5′ end, without a Shine–Dalgarno sequence. Eukaryotes also employ a more extensive set of initiation factors, perhaps because they regulate gene expression at the level of initiation of translation much more than do prokaryotes. Other features of eukaryotic mRNA are described in Chapter 9 (Messenger RNA).

The formylation of the initiating Met in prokaryotes, but not in eukaryotes, has had a curious evolutionary consequence, of importance for medicine. Some pathogenic bacteria excrete small amounts of short peptides that start with f-Met (presumably breakdown products), and these are powerful chemoattractants and activators for mammalian leukocytes.

MODIFICATIONS OF ACCURACY

Various genetic and environmental factors can influence the accuracy of translation. These have been recognized primarily through their ability to **suppress** the effect of various mutational defects (i.e., to restore function). Suppressors have been of interest primarily as experimental tools. One major group alters the specificity of a tRNA, while another group of mutations, and also environmental factors, decrease the ability of the ribosome to enforce fidelity in translation. Other mechanisms of suppression will be described in Chapter 8.

Suppression by Altered tRNAs

NONSENSE SUPPRESSORS. Nonsense-suppressing mutants allow translation to continue beyond a nonsense (terminator) mutation in another gene because they insert an amino acid at the nonsense codon. Although mutant, they are designated as su^+ because they support growth, just as trp^+ designates the ability to grow without tryptophan. Amber suppressor mutations were discovered as mutations that not only reversed a mutational defect in a cell but also permitted the growth of certain phage mutants, which have an amber (UAG) mutation in an essential gene, and hence cannot grow in wild-type cells. Each su^+ mutation replaces a single base in an anticodon in a tRNA, so that it reads a particular nonsense codon instead of its original codon.

Because each base has three possible replacements, eight different tRNAs, coding for different amino acids, can yield the amber su^+ anticodon in one step; the ninth codon adjacent to amber is a terminator, UAA.

Any su^+ tRNA competes with the release factor for translation of the amber codon, and so an amber mutant gene in su^+ cells or extracts will yield both the amber fragment and a protein of normal length (Fig. 6–9). **The efficiency of nonsense suppression,** defined as the proportion of completed chains to total chains of the mutant protein, depends on the concentration of the su^+ tRNA in the cell and on the effectiveness of its competition with release factors. Moreover, the misreading that

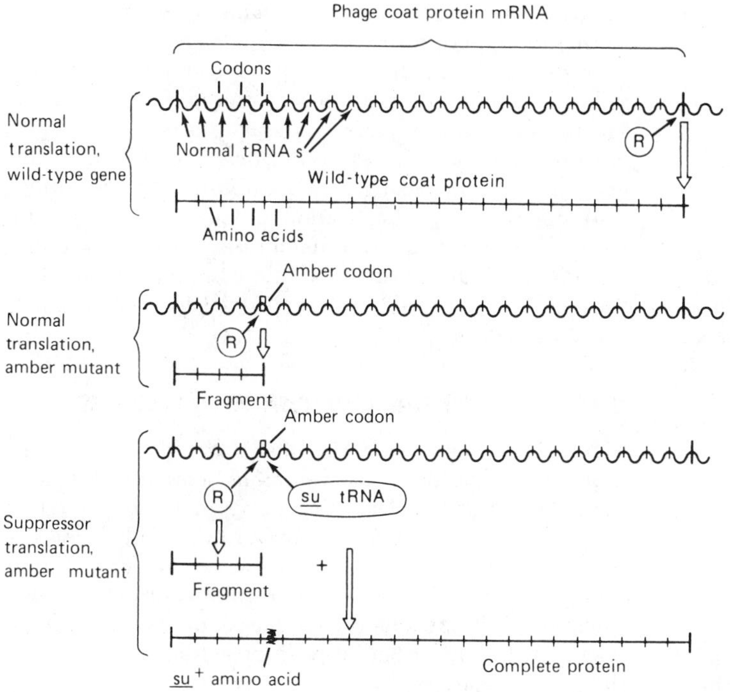

Phage coat protein mRNA

Codons

Normal translation, wild-type gene

Normal tRNA s

Wild-type coat protein

Amino acids

Amber codon

Normal translation, amber mutant

Fragment

Amber codon

Suppressor translation, amber mutant

Fragment

+

Complete protein

su⁺ amino acid

Figure 6–9. Genetic suppression of nonsense mutation. In the translation of an amber mutant gene (in a cell or in extracts), an *su*⁺ tRNA reads the amber codon (UAG) in competition with an *R* (release) protein. A particular suppression causes incorporation of a particular amino acid at the amber site, corresponding to the *su* tRNA present; the various amber *su* tRNAs are derived from those tRNAs in which a replacement of one nucleotide can yield the required anticodon ($\overline{\text{CUA}}$), which reads $\overline{\text{UAG}}$ in antipolar fashion. The **efficiency** of suppression is the fraction of the readings yielding complete protein. The rate of cell growth restored by an *su*⁺ mutation depends not only on its efficiency but also on the frequency of harmful interference of the *su* tRNA with normal termination elsewhere in the genome.

corrects the mutational error at one site will create errors elsewhere in the genome: hence, suppressors lower the growth rate. Because amber suppressors often have high efficiency (30% to 75%) and little effect on growth rate, while ochre suppressors are all weak (4% to 12% efficiency) and slow growth, it appears that cells use the amber (UAG) codon for termination less frequently than ochre (UAA) and hence can tolerate its misreading better.

Because an *su*⁺ tRNA has lost the ability to read its normal codon, its formation is not compatible with viability unless the cell possesses an additional tRNA for that codon or unless it has been made diploid for that tRNA.

Missense suppressors, which also have a tRNA with an altered anticodon, will be discussed in Chapter 8 (Suppression of Mutations).

Ribosomal Ambiguity

Ribosomal ambiguity (ram) mutations, located at certain sites in ribosomal protein S4 or S5, also increase misreading, presumably by distorting the alignment of codon and anticodon. Unlike tRNA mutations, they are not specific for a codon or for an amino acid replacement.

Ribosomal ambiguity can also be induced **phenotypically** by the distorting effect of aminoglycoside antibiotics on the ribosome; its importance for their action will be discussed in Chapter 10. In addition, ribosomal ambiguity can be increased by agents with a less specific ef-

fect, including elevated Mg^{2+}, elevated temperature, and alcohol (observable in "drunk" cells as well as *in vitro*). These effects are perhaps less remarkable than their background: the ability of the conformationally flexible ribosomal particle to maintain the codon–anticodon alignment with such precision under widely differing conditions.

NORMAL AMBIGUITY. We have seen that cells have evolved elaborate editing mechanisms in the charging of tRNA and in ribosomal function to decrease the errors in translation. Nevertheless, within these mechanisms, they have not selected for the greatest possible accuracy: streptomycin-resistant mutations in protein S12 of the ribosome **decrease** the background error rate (as well as opposing the increased ambiguity induced by *ram* mutations). However, this increased accuracy is achieved at the expense of a decreased rate of translation per ribosome. Evidently, there is **selection for an optimal balance between accuracy and rate** rather than for maximal accuracy, for the longer the delay between the reversible and the irreversible steps in recognition on the ribosome, the greater the opportunity for the editing process to discriminate between correct and nearly correct codon–anticodon pairing.

Coding Ambiguity

Various mutations can also be suppressed by introducing base analogues into mRNA, much like the ambiguous replication (mutagenesis) caused by incorporated base analogues in DNA (Chap. 8). Thus, **5-fluorouracil,** which can be incorporated extensively into RNA in place of U, is occasionally misread in translation as C rather than U.

Protein Localization

In the early 1960s Palade discovered that animal cells contain not only free ribosomes, which release their proteins to the cytoplasm but also membrane-bound ribosomes (the rough endoplasmic reticulum), which are involved in protein secretion. The difference resides not in the ribosomes but in their product, as was discovered serendipitously during early studies on immunoglobulin synthesis in extracts, in which Milstein and coworkers found that the product was not the expected chain but rather a larger precursor; moreover, the additional segment, of about 3000 daltons, was amino terminal and was cleaved by a membrane enzyme. Those workers therefore suggested that in protein secretion a hydrophobic amino-terminal **signal peptide** (later also known as **leader peptide**) initiates binding of the ribosome to the cell membrane and then is removed. Blobel subsequently showed that similar signal peptides are also present in the precursors of integral membrane proteins and that the mechanism of protein translocation can be studied with membrane vesicles in cell extracts.

Membrane-bound ribosomes are also present in prokaryotes, but their recognition was long delayed because they could not be distinguished from free ribosomes in the dense prokaryotic cytoplasm. Prokaryotes offer certain experimental advantages, particularly the use of mutants that are altered in protein translocation. In addition, because the outside of the membrane is accessible to manipulation (unlike the lumen of the endoplasmic reticulum), cotranslational secretion (i.e., secretion during chain growth) could be established unequivocally by radioactively labeling proteins on the cell surface with a nonpenetrating reagent, disrupting the cells, and showing that some labeled peptide chains were still attached to membrane-bound ribosomes.

Study of the mechanism of protein translocation has rapidly become one of the liveliest areas of cell biology. The term **secretion** refers to passage across a membrane (into the periplasm in gram-negative bacteria or to the exterior in gram-positives) while **export** or **translocation** refers to any localization outside the cytoplasm, whether into or beyond a membrane. Although the discovery of cotranslational secretion initiated interest in the field, we will see that much translocation is post-translational.

SIGNAL PEPTIDES AND THE EARLY STEPS

Signal peptides in bacteria differ widely in length (generally 16–32 residues) as well as in sequence, but they have three common features, shown in Table 6–1: (1) an initial cationic sequence of two to five residues with a terminal NH_2 and one to three Lys or Arg residues or both; (2) a central "core" of hydrophobic or neutral residues; and (3) a consensus cleavage sequence with a small residue (Ala, Gly, or Ser) at positions -1 and -3 relative to the site of cleavage.

The positive charges provide ionic bonds to surface phosphates on the membrane, whereas the hydrophobic core evidently initiates entry, as mutations that introduce a polar residue within it prevent attachment to the membrane. Cleavage requires that its site reach the outer surface of the cytoplasmic membrane, because the active site of the leader peptidase faces that surface. After the signal peptide has been cleaved, it is rapidly digested. The signal peptides in bacteria are very similar to those of proteins that enter the endoplasmic reticulum in eukaryotes, and members of either group often can function in the other.

Bacterial **lipoproteins** have a special amino terminus embedded in the membrane, with Cys substituted with a diglyceride on its SH and a fatty acyl group on its free NH_2 (see Chap. 2; Fig. 2–23). Their precursors therefore

TABLE 6–1. *Some Signal Sequences of* E. coli

Protein	Charged Segment	Hydrophobic Segment*
Periplasmic protein Alkaline phosphatase	Met Lys	Gln Ser Thr Ile Ala Leu Ala Leu Leu Pro Leu Leu Phe Thr Lys Ala ↓ Arg Thr Pro
Outer membrane protein Lipoprotein	Met Lys Ala Thr Lys	Leu Val Leu Gly Ala Val Ile Leu Gly Ser Thr Leu Leu Ala Gly ↓ Cys Ser Ser
Excreted toxin Heat-labile toxin, β-subunit	Met Asn Lys Val Lys	Cys Tyr Val Leu Phe Thr Ala Leu Leu Ser Ser Leu Tyr Ala His Gly ↓ Ala Pro Gln

* Arrow denotes site of proteolytic cleavage.

have a different consensus sequence whose cleavage yields an amino-terminal Cys. In their processing the diglyceride is first attached to the Cys and a special lipoprotein peptidase in the membrane then removes the leader peptide. In a few bacterial proteins, such as the β-lactamase of *B. licheniformis*, the precursor is initially cleaved in this way to yield a membrane-bound lipoprotein, and a second cleavage of some of the molecules then releases a water-soluble form of the enzyme to the medium. This process resembles the synthesis of some hormones (e.g., parathormone) in animals as pre-proproteins, which undergo two successive cleavages in the course of their secretion.

Cleavable leader peptides are not universal in protein export. They are generally involved in initiating secretion, and also in transfer of an amino-terminal hydrophilic sequence that will protrude from the external surface of the membrane. In contrast, with membrane proteins whose amino terminus is embedded or protrudes on the cytoplasmic side, a hydrophobic chain of about 20 residues enters the membrane but is not cleaved, and the subsequent sequences either remain in the cytoplasm or lead to multiple hydrophobic transmembrane segments (see Chap. 4, Fig. 4–7), which similarly enter without cleavage.

In general, cell-surface antigens cross the membrane once, whereas transport proteins cross multiple times to create a channel. The loops accessible on the exterior can be identified by proteolysis or by binding of monoclonal Ab. The OM maltose porin, LamB, crosses the membrane 17 times.

PROTEIN FACTORS. Initiation of protein translocation involves protein factors as well as a signal sequence. In animal cells Walter and Blobel have demonstrated a **signal recognition particle (SRP)**, containing six polypeptides and a 7S RNA molecule, that attaches to free ribosomes and binds the signal peptide as it emerges. In some *in vitro* systems it arrests further chain elongation, and on interacting with an SRP receptor ("docking" protein) on the membrane, it is released, allowing elongation to be resumed. Such translational arrest might be useful in preventing growing chains from becoming tightly folded as they protrude in the cytoplasm, before the ribosome reaches the membrane. Bacteria also appear to have cytoplasmic translocation factors, reversibly bound to ribosomes and membrane, but there is no evidence for translational arrest.

SORTING MECHANISMS IN TRANSLOCATION

Because the same signal can initiate entry of secreted proteins and of membrane proteins, the choice between the two fates must be determined by later sequences in the chain. Cogent evidence for this assumption, and for a special secretory channel, has been provided by experiments of Beckwith and coworkers in which a large, easily measured cytoplasmic protein, β-galactosidase, was fused genetically to an amino-terminal segment (including the signal sequence) of either a periplasmic or an inner membrane (IM) protein. When the amino-terminal moiety came from a periplasmic protein the fusion protein, whose galactosidase sequence is evidently incompatible with secretion, became stuck in the membrane; moreover, it apparently blocked a secretory channel, as precursors of several exportable proteins accumulated in the cytoplasm. When the amino-terminal moiety was a segment of an IM protein the fused protein was again fixed in the IM. However, a sufficiently long IM segment (but not a short one) evidently contained a "**stop-transfer**" signal that moved the protein out of a secretory channel into the lipid, because there was no interference with export of other proteins.

The stop-transfer signal appears to be simply a sufficiently long hydrophobic segment in the proper context. Thus, in certain membrane proteins (phage f1 coat protein; cell-bound immunoglobulins in animal cells), a single hydrophobic carboxy-terminal sequence provides an anchor in the membrane, whereas if it is eliminated by mutation the residual protein is secreted. The stop-transfer signals of other membrane proteins are probably similar, although not necessarily carboxy-terminal; and as we have noted, many membrane proteins have multiple hydrophobic transmembrane sequences.

After a protein has been moved out of the secretory pathway it may be destined for one or another membrane. In eukaryotic cells the numerous differentiated membranes derived from the endoplasmic reticulum appear to have similar signal peptides and therefore must be directed to their different destinations by internal sequences, while the mitochondria are autonomous and require special signal sequences on their imported proteins. In bacteria the main differentiation is between IM and OM, but there are also specialized locations, such as the septum, the invaginations that initiate spore formation, and pili. The route from the IM to the OM appears to be essentially the same for proteins as that established earlier for the OM lipids: flow through the intermembrane junctions (Chap. 2, Fig. 2-17; see also Fig. 6-11 below). Both components can be shown by labeling to appear first in relatively few sites in the OM, similar in number to those junctions.

The sequences that "ticket" proteins for the OM, and the mechanism of the selective flow of these proteins to that destination, are not known. However, various distinct OM proteins have regions with substantial sequence homology, and some have shown affinity *in vitro* for lipopolysaccharide. In eukaryotic cells, glycosylation, occurring after proteins have crossed the endoplasmic membrane, contributes to sorting them into various membranes, but this process does not appear to occur in bacteria.

POSTTRANSLATIONAL TRANSLOCATION

As noted above, in prokaryotes much translocation is cotranslational in the sense that part of a chain protrudes outside the membrane before the rest has been completed. However, the process turned out not to be cotranslational in a stricter sense, that of being obligatorily and closely coupled to synthesis. Kinetic studies indicate that nascent secretory chains accumulate a substantial length between the ribosome and the membrane before they begin to appear on the *trans* side, and when further synthesis is blocked by chloramphenicol transfer to the *trans* side continues for a few minutes. Evidently, synthesis is faster than transfer, and folding of the accumulating chain on the *cis* side does not prevent subsequent chain transfer.

Indeed, a radical dissociation of secretion from synthesis has been observed *in vitro*—that is, completely posttranslational translocation into vesicles added to the system only after chains have been completed and synthesis has been stopped. Moreover, this effect has even been found with proteins that are made on membrane-bound ribosomes and hence are evidently secreted cotranslationally in cells. Binding of ribosomes to the membrane thus does not appear to be essential for translocation, at least for some proteins, although it probably increases the efficiency of the process.

The mechanism of transfer of already folded proteins is not certain, but passage of highly polar, water-soluble proteins through the lipid of the membrane as a folded particle seems excluded on thermodynamic grounds. The alternative of an energy-utilizing process of translocation through some kind of machinery, pulling the chain through the membrane linearly or in small domains (and reversing any accumulated folding when necessary), would provide a unitary mechanism for cotranslational and posttranslational translocation. In support of this model, Schatz has shown that in the posttranslational uptake of an enzyme by mitochondria, stabilization of the folded conformation by complexing with an analogue of the substrate prevents entry. Proteins evidently differ in their ease of unfolding: in *E. coli* the **SecB protein antagonizes protein folding,** and mutations in that gene affect the secretion of some proteins, whereas others, which fold less tightly (as shown by sensitivity to protease), do not require the assistance of this unfolding factor. The leader peptide also delays folding, a second mechanism by which it promotes export.

ENERGY SOURCES. Mutants and inhibitors that eliminate the protonmotive force impair protein translocation by bacteria and by mitochondria. However, with the development of posttranslational translocation, *in vitro* ATP was no longer required for simultaneous protein synthesis, and it could then be shown that translocation also requires ATP. This finding increases the resemblance of the process in these systems to that in the endoplasmic reticulum, which has no protonmotive force. How ATP is used in protein translocation is not known.

THE MOLECULAR MECHANISM OF PROTEIN SECRETION

The nature of the channel through which proteins are transferred across a membrane has remained elusive. Genetic studies have revealed mutations in several *sec* genes (A, B, Y), which block the secretion of many proteins, as well as *prl* mutants that suppress the effect of an impaired signal sequence, perhaps by altering the channel with which it interacts. The *sec* proteins have been isolated (through their genetic fusion with a known protein), but their function in a membrane machinery has not been established.

Nevertheless, the accumulated biochemical information has suggested a model that can account in general terms for the thermodynamic and topographic problems of protein translocation (Fig. 6–10). Like some known membrane transport systems (e.g., the sodium channel), the protein translocator would be composed of several transmembrane polypeptide subunits bound to each other by complementary interfaces and with hydrophobic groups facing the surrounding lipid and polar groups facing a central aqueous pore. A hydrophobic signal sequence (cleavable or not) could be intercalated in a loose interface between two subunits in a hydrophobic region peripheral to the central pore. Subsequent to this entry, the polypeptide chain would not be threaded continuously; instead, a contractile mechanism (reminiscent of translocation on the ribosome) would cause the translocator to intercalate successive segments (subdomains) of a roughly fixed length, sufficient to traverse the membrane. If a subdomain is polar, it would slip into the polar, central region of the interface, whereas hydrophobic subdomains would be located in the peripheral, more hydrophobic, region, from which they could be displaced into the membrane lipid. While speculative, this model can account in general terms not only for secretion but also for the insertion of successive internal hydrophobic sequences of membrane proteins, oriented in either direction and connected by short or long hydrophilic sequences on either side of the membrane.

SECRETION TO THE EXTERIOR BY GRAM-NEGATIVE BACTERIA

In gram-positive bacteria, with a single membrane, secretion across that membrane is synonymous with release

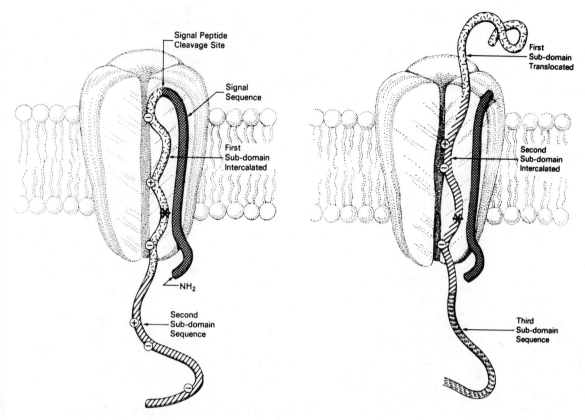

Figure 6–10. Schematic representation of two stages in a proposed model for the secretion of a hydrophilic protein via the interface between two component polypeptides of a translocator channel; the polypeptide on the *cis* side is removed from the diagram to expose the interface. In the stage shown at the left, the hydrophobic signal sequence is intercalated into the interface, with its cleavage site at the external surface of the membrane, whereas the immediately following sequence of approximately 20 hydrophilic residues forms the first subdomain bound within the interface, with its charged residues facing into the aqueous channel of the translocator. In the stage at the right, the signal peptide has been cleaved but not yet released, the first subdomain has been translocated, and the second subdomain is intercalated in the interface. (Singer SJ, Maher PA, Yaffe MP: Proc Natl Acad Sci USA 84:1015, 1987)

from the cell. With gram-negative bacteria, however, release requires transfer past a double membrane. Because the OM has no source of energy, a protein that has been secreted into the periplasm by an energy-dependent process cannot be further secreted by a similar process across the OM. However, some oligomeric proteins, such as cholera toxin, are secreted rapidly into the periplasm, where the accumulated subunits aggregate to form the final protein, and it is then slowly released to the exterior. The mechanism appears to involve specific translocator proteins in the OM, since other periplasmic proteins are not released, and mutations in specific OM proteins can interfere with toxin release.

Some monomeric proteins, such as exotoxin A of *Pseudomonas aeruginosa*, appear to use a different mechanism of release, which bypasses the periplasm and does not involve true secretion across any membrane. This toxin is normally processed and secreted so fast that neither it nor a precursor can be detected in the cells. However, perturbation of the membrane by 10% ethanol blocks these processes and causes a larger precursor to accumulate; moreover, it is located on the outer surface of the cells, as shown by its accessibility to protease. Evidently, in the normal process, the precursor is initially anchored by its hydrophobic signal sequence to the IM, flows to the OM through the intermembrane junctions (as is known for OM proteins), and is cleaved in the course of that transit, releasing the free toxin on the far side. The structure of the intermembrane junctions is not known, but one possibility, involving continuity of the two leaflets, is depicted in Figure 6–11.

Protein secretion is important for the pathogenicity of many bacteria. In addition, in biotechnology, the yield of a protein from a cloned gene in bacteria can often be

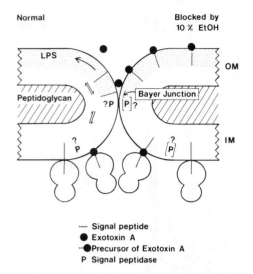

Normal   **Blocked by 10 % EtOH**

---- Signal peptide
● Exotoxin A
•●Precursor of Exotoxin A
P Signal peptidase

Figure 6–11. Model of protein excretion via the Bayer junction in gram-negative bacteria. The growing precursor of exotoxin A is held to the inner face of the IM by its signal peptide, together with a subsequent region. After chain completion, the product is transported laterally via a Bayer junction to the outer surface of the outer membrane, and in transit, it is cleaved by a signal peptidase, P, resulting in release to the medium. In the presence of EtOH (right half of diagram), the peptidase *(P)* fails to cleave the precursor, which then ends up in the OM surrounded by lipopolysaccharide *(LPS)*. Removal of EtOH restores normal processing and excretion of newly synthesized exotoxin but not of the accumulated precursor. (Lory S, Tai PC, Davis BD: J Bacteriol 156:695, 1983)

increased by fusion to a leader sequence that causes it to be secreted rather than to accumulate in the cell.

Selected Reading

PROTEIN SYNTHESIS: BOOKS AND REVIEW ARTICLES

Fournier MJ, Ozeki H: Structure and organization of the transfer ribonucleic acid genes of *Eschericia coli* K12. Microbiol Rev 49:379, 1985

Giri L, Wittmann HG, Witmann–Liebold B: Ribosomal proteins: Their structure and spatial arrangement in prokaryotic ribosomes. Adv Protein Chem 36:11, 1984

Gold L, Pribnow D, Schneider T, Shineding S, Singer BS, Stormo G: Translational initiation in prokaryotes. Annu Rev Microbiol 35:365, 1981

Gorini L: Informational suppression. Annu Rev Genet 4:107, 1970

Hardesty B, Kramer G (eds): Structure, Function, and Genetics of Ribosomes. New York, Springer, 1986

Kozak M: Comparison of initiation of protein synthesis in procaryotes, eucaryotes, and organelles. Microbiol Rev 47:1, 1983

Kurland CG, Gallant JA: The secret life of the ribosome. In Kirkwood TBL, Rosenberger RF, Gaslas DJ (eds): Accuracy in Molecular Processes, p 127. London, Chapman & Hall, 1986

Noller HR, Lake JA: Ribosome structure and function: Localization of rRNA. In Bittar E (ed): Membrane Structure and Function, Vol 6, p 217. New York, John Wiley, 1984

Nomura M, Tissieres A, Lengyel P (eds): Ribosomes. Cold Spring Harbor, NY, Cold Spring Harbor Laboratory, 1974

Subramanian AR: Structure and functions of ribosomal protein S1. Prog Nucleic Acids Res Mol Biol 28:101, 1983

Weissbach H, Pestka S: Molecular Mechanisms of Protein Synthesis. New York, Academic Press, 1977

Wittmann HG: Architecture of prokaryotic ribosomes. Annu Rev Biochem 52:35, 1983

Woese CR, Gutell R, Gupta R, Noller HF: Detailed analysis of the higher-order structure of 16S-like ribosomal ribonucleic acids. Microbiol Rev 47:621, 1983

PROTEIN LOCALIZATION: BOOKS AND REVIEW ARTICLES

Bankaitis VA, Ryan JP, Rasmussen BA, Bassford PJ Jr: The use of genetic techniques to analyze protein export in *Escherichia coli.* Curr Top Membrane Transport 24:105, 1985

Gething M-J (ed): Protein Transport and Secretion. Cold Spring Harbor, NY, Cold Spring Harbor Laboratory, 1985

Michaelis S, Beckwith J: Mechanism of incorporation of cell envelope proteins in *Escherichia coli.* Annu Rev Microbiol 36:435, 1982

Pugsley AP, Schwartz M: Export and secretion of proteins by bacteria. FEMS Microbiol Rev 32:3, 1985

Randall LL, Hardy SJS: Export of protein in bacteria. Microbiol Rev 48:290, 1984

Silhavy TJ, Benson SA, Emr SD: Mechanisms of protein localization. Microbiol Rev 47:313, 1983

Watson MEE: Compilation of published signal sequences. Nucleic Acids Res 12:5145, 1984

Wu HC, Tai PC (eds): Protein Secretion and Export in Bacteria. Curr Top Microbiol Immunol, vol 125, 1986

PROTEIN LOCALIZATION: SPECIFIC ARTICLES

Baty D, Mercereau–Puijalon D, Perrin D, Kourilsky P, Lazdunski C: Secretion into the bacterial periplasmic space of chicken ovalbumin synthesized in *Escherichia coli.* Gene 16:79, 1981

Boeke JD, Model P: A prokaryotic anchor sequence: Carboxy terminus of bacteriophage f1 gene III protein retains it in the membrane. Proc Natl Acad Sci USA 79:5200, 1982

Chen L, Rhoads D, Tai PC: Alkaline phosphatase and OmpA protein can be translocated posttranslationally into membrane vesicles of *Escherichia coli.* J Bacteriol 161:973, 1985

Chen L, Tai PC: ATP is essential for protein translocation into *Escherichia coli* membrane vesicles. Proc Natl Acad Sci USA 82:4384, 1985

Dodd DC, Bassford PJ Jr, Eisenstein BI: Dependence of secretion and assembly of type 1 fimbrial subunits of *Escherichia coli* on normal protein export. J Bacteriol 159:1077, 1984

Koshland D, Botstein D: Evidence for posttranslational translocation of β-lactamase across the bacterial inner membrane. Cell 30:893, 1982

Mackman N, Holland IB: Secretion of a 107 kDalton polypeptide into the medium from a haemolytic *E. coli* K12 strain. Mol Gen Genet 193:312, 1984

Maher PA, Singer SJ: Disulfide bonds and the translocation of proteins across membranes. Proc Natl Acad Sci USA 83:9001, 1986

Michaelis S, Guarente L, Beckwith J: In vitro construction and characterization of *phoA–lacZ* gene fusions in *Escherichia coli.* J Bacteriol 154:356, 1983

Nielsen JBK, Caulfield MP, Lampen JO: Lipoprotein nature of *Bacillus licheniformis* membrane penicillinase. Proc Natl Acad Sci USA 78:3511, 1981

Nikaido H, Wu HC: Amino acid sequence homology among the major outer membrane proteins of *Escherichia coli.* Proc Natl Acad Sci USA 81:1048, 1984

Oliver DB, Beckwith J: Identification of a new gene (*secA*) and gene product involved in secretion of envelope proteins in *Escherichia coli*. J Bacteriol 150:686, 1982

Smit J, Nikaido H: Outer membrane of gram-negative bacteria XVIII: Electron microscopic studies on porin insertion sites and growth of cell surface in *Salmonella typhimurium*. J Bacteriol 135:687, 1978

Smith WP, Tai PC, Thompson RC, Davis BD: Extracellular labeling of nascent polypeptides traversing the membrane of *Escherichia coli*. Proc Natl Acad Sci USA 74:2830, 1977

Talmadge K, Stahl S, Gilbert W: Eukaryotic signal sequence transports insulin in *Escherichia coli*. Proc Natl Acad Sci USA 77:3369, 1980

Von Heijne G: How signal sequences maintain cleavage specificity. J Mol Biol 173:243, 1984

Walter P, Gilmore R, Blobel G: Protein translocation across the endoplasmic reticulum. Cell 38:5, 1984

Wolfe PB, Silver P, Wickner W: The isolation of homogeneous leader peptidase from a strain of *Escherichia coli* which overproduces the enzyme. J Biol Chem 257:7898, 1982

7

Gene Variation and Transfer

Classical genetics, beginning in 1900, recognized units of inheritance by recombining alternative forms (alleles) in the progeny by recombination, and by correlating their frequency of segregation or linkage in recombination with their positions on chromosomes. However, neither recombination nor chromosomes could be demonstrated in bacteria. Moreover, because drastic genetic changes in bacterial populations often occurred far too rapidly (e.g., overnight) to seem to fit the evolutionary process of mutation and selection, genotypic changes (arising in a single cell) were misinterpreted as phenotypic adaptations (reversible changes in all the cells of a population). Not until the 1940s was it realized that the speed of genotypic change in bacterial cultures in a new environment can be very rapid because of extremely rapid multiplication, together with the exceptionally strong selection pressure for new variants. The discovery of gene transfer in bacteria then showed that these organisms possess transferable units of inheritance (genes), linked on a chromosome, and bacterial genetics soon provided essential tools for the rapidly emerging field of molecular genetics.

Auxotrophic mutations, creating requirements for various growth factors, have been particularly useful in the development of microbial genetics. The **one-gene–one-enzyme** hypothesis (later refined as one-gene–one-polypeptide) emerged from the studies of Beadle and Tatum on auxotrophs of the mold *Neurospora*, and it began to reveal the molecular connections between genes and the traits of formal genetics. Moreover, recombinations between auxotrophs to yield easily selected prototrophs were the basis for the discovery of gene transfer by conjugation and by transduction.

Particularly important was the development of "**fine-structure genetics**" by Benzer in phage and Yanofsky in bacteria. Because the mapping of mutations in higher organisms, by measurements of recombination frequencies, does not have a high enough resolution to distinguish sites within most genes, recombinations were believed to occur at special positions between genes. However, in bacteria and their viruses the resolving power of genetic mapping is greater by many orders of magnitude because of the possibility of quantitatively selecting very rare recombinants (i.e., those between very close sites on the DNA). The results revealed several novel, fundamental principles: (1) mutations and recombinations can occur at any nucleotide in the continuous DNA of the chromosome; (2) the gene is a segment and not a separate molecule in that sequence; and (3) changes at various sites within a gene are colinear with changes in the corresponding polypeptide.

With these findings, **a gene can be defined as a sequence that codes for a functional product;** moreover, the sequence can define a gene in positive terms, without having to rely on the allelic differences of classical genetics.

Complementation

Because some enzymes contain several different polypeptides, whose inactivation by mutation can have the same phenotypic effect, a practical way to distinguish genes is the **complementation test:** if a cell is made heterozygous for two different mutations with the same phenotype, and if they are in the same gene, the cell will not produce the normal product; but if they are in different genes the two normal alleles will complement each other and allow normal enzyme production and growth. Complementation can also be observed in vitro, by mixing extracts of two phenotypically similar mutants altered in different genes.

Though mutants altered in the same polypeptide generally do not complement each other, they can exhibit such **intragenic complementation** when the polypeptides are part of an oligomeric protein. The explanation is that some pairs of defective polypeptides interact conformationally in a way that restores some enzymatic activity. Though this effect makes complementation a less sharp criterion for defining a gene, it does not restore the full activity, observed with intergenic complementation.

This chapter will discuss primarily the physiological aspects of bacterial variation and gene transfer; the more detailed molecular mechanisms will be covered in the next chapter. Phage genetics will be postponed until Chapter 45.

RANDOM VERSUS DIRECTED CHANGE

The development of bacterial genetics was delayed by a long-standing popular preference for an anthropomorphic, guided process in evolution, instead of the stark role of chance and selection. Application of this prejudice to the microbial world suggested that drug-resistant bacteria emerged through some unknown process by which the drug "trained" the bacteria. Luria and Delbruck settled the issue, in 1943, in a classical experiment called **fluctuation analysis,** as described in Figure 7–1. If the mutations to resistance arose spontaneously, before exposure to the agent, parallel cultures in liquid medium should have their first mutation at different times, and the resulting differences in the number of subsequent cell divisions before completion of growth would yield wide variation in the number of resistant colonies recovered. If, however, the resistant variants did not arise until they were directed (with a low probability) by the agent in the test plate, the samples from various tubes should all be equivalent, just as in aliquots from a single flask, and the fluctuation in the number of colonies should reflect the simple statistics of that random probability of induction by the agent on each plate. The

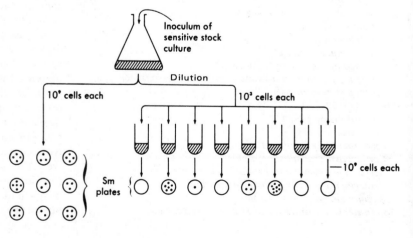

Figure 7–1. Fluctuation analysis of mutation to streptomycin *(Sm)* resistance. A small number of sensitive cells were inoculated in a flask containing 100 ml of broth, and also in 100 tubes each containing 1 ml of the same medium. After full growth was reached, 1-ml samples were inoculated in plates of medium containing the drug, and the number of Sm-resistant colonies appearing after overnight incubation was determined. The fluctuation in their number was much greater among the samples that had grown out in separate tubes than among those from the same flask. (Based on similar experiment with phage by Luria SE, Delbruck M: Genetics 28:491, 1943)

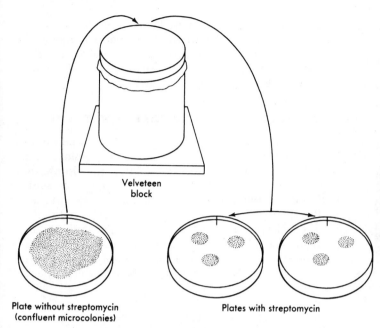

Velveteen
block

Plate without streptomycin
(confluent microcolonies)

Plates with streptomycin

Figure 7–2. Use of replica plating to demonstrate undirected, spontaneous appearance of streptomycin-resistant mutants. About 10^5 sensitive cells were spread on a plate of drug-free solid medium and allowed to reach full growth (10^{10}–10^{11} cells). Sterile velveteen, covering the flat end of a cylindrical block, was pressed lightly on this continuous heavy lawn ("master plate") and then successively on two plates of medium containing streptomycin at a concentration that killed sensitive cells. A few colonies of resistant cells appeared on each plate, usually in coincident positions, and cells harvested from the corresponding positions on the master plate yielded a much larger proportion of resistant colonies than cells harvested from other parts of the plate. Evidently, resistant clones, arising in the absence of drug on the master plate, were the source of most of the resistant colonies on the replica plates.

results showed conclusively that the resistant mutants had appeared spontaneously before exposure; i.e., they were only selected, not directed, by the inhibitor.

Lederberg subsequently demonstrated the same conclusion more directly by growing a continuous lawn of bacteria from a heavy inoculum of sensitive cells on drug-free medium and **replica plating,** after outgrowth, onto several plates of drug-containing medium. The lawn contained a few clusters of resistant cells, each derived from a single mutated cell that appeared before exposure to the drug (Fig. 7–2).

With these findings, and with the observation that UV irradiation increases the frequency of such mutants (just as in higher organisms), it became clear that inheritance in bacteria is governed by mutable unit factors; i.e., genes.

Mutations

PHENOTYPIC CLASSES

A **mutation** can be defined as **any change in the base sequence of the DNA.** Some mutations are **silent;** i.e., without demonstrable phenotypic effect (although important for evolution as a basis for further change). Initial studies focused on mutations that inactivate a function, but others may reduce its expression ("leaky" mutants) or may cause overexpression, by altering either the **structure** of a gene product or its **amount** (through alterations in regulatory sequences). "Wild type" refers to the functional form of a gene commonly found in nature,

but that classical term has now lost much of its meaning: at the level of DNA sequence the wild-type gene in a species may have different alleles (polymorphism). With enzymes the alternative forms are more or less identical in function, but with surface proteins they may provide alternative antigenic specificity rather than a single wild-type function.

Mutations are designated in capitalized Roman letters (Lac⁻, His⁻, etc.) for the phenotype that has lost a function, and in italics (*lacZ* or *lacY*) for the corresponding genotypes. The minus sign to indicate the defect is usually omitted from the genotype; Z and Y designate different genes that lead to the same phenotype; and numbers are often added to designate a particular isolate. Where necessary, the wild-type strain is designated as plus (e.g., *lac*⁺); and the wild-type gene product, when not identified biochemically, is designated like the gene but capitalized and not in italics (e.g., SecB).

The following phenotypic classes of mutations have been useful in genetic studies:

1. Inability to use a carbon source (Lac⁻, Ara⁻).

2. Inability to synthesize a required small molecule (His⁻, Thi⁻). Such mutants are called **auxotrophs,** whereas the wild type is a **prototroph** with respect to that essential metabolite.

3. Resistance to antibiotics and other inhibitors (Str^R, Azi^R, phage^R).

4. Alteration of cell-surface components (flagellin, pili, LPS, capsule), which may affect **colonial morphology** (Fig. 7–3) or may be recognized as **antigenic variants.** These classes are especially important for pathogenicity,

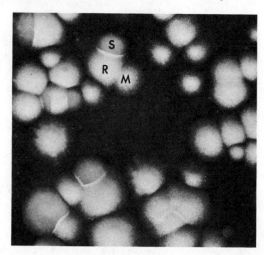

Figure 7–3. Rough *(R)* and smooth *(S)* colonies of *Brucella abortus*. Because of the difference in the reflection of light in the photograph, the R colonies appear considerably lighter than the S colonies, as well as more stippled. (Courtesy of W Braun)

for such changes may be selected rapidly when pathogens isolated from a host are cultured in an artificial medium in the laboratory, and they affect virulence. Reversible shifts between alternative antigens, especially in flagella or pili, are called **phase variation** (see Chap. 8).

5. Loss of excretion of a detectable product (enzymes, hemolysins, toxins).

6. Alteration of cell shape, motility.

The various kinds of molecular change in DNA that can give rise to mutations will be described in Chapter 8.

CONDITIONAL MUTATIONS

While auxotrophic mutations can be recovered because the missing product can be provided exogenously, that is not possible for many mutations. However, **conditional mutants** (also called **conditional lethals**) for these functions can be recovered and maintained under **permissive conditions,** while their expression can be studied under **nonpermissive conditions.** Two classes of conditional mutants are used. First, **temperature-sensitive (*ts*) mutations** prevent expression of a gene at normal growth temperature but not at a low temperature. Usually the product protein denatures at the customary temperature of growth but not at a lower temperature, but sometimes the *ts* element is regulatory. Some mutations are **cold-sensitive,** usually impairing assembly of multicomponent systems. Second, **suppressible mutations** can be maintained in a cell carrying an extragenic suppressor mutation, described in Chapter 6, and their effect can be expressed by transfer to a cell lacking the suppressor. Conditional mutations have been indispensable in identifying the many genes whose inactivating

mutations would otherwise be lethal. Thermosensitivity is also useful in determining whether a mutation that decreases activity is located in a structural or in a regulatory gene: if the product is more thermolabile, the mutation must be in its structural gene.

DETECTION AND SELECTION OF MUTANTS

Bacteria are **haploid;** i.e., they lack the paired homologous chromosomes present in higher, **diploid** organisms. Accordingly, **heterozygosity** and **dominance,** so prominent in classic genetics, are not present to influence the expression of mutations except under the special circumstances that produce partial diploids (see below). Because bacteria normally multiply asexually, the progeny of a single organism constitute a **clone:** a genetically identical group of individuals. If a mutation arises within a clone, the progeny of that cell constitute a subclone.

SCREENING AND SCORING. Quantitative screening of rare mutants or recombinants (e.g., one colony from 10^9 cells plated) is possible for certain phenotypes: fermentation-positive, prototrophic, and drug- or phage-resistant. Mutations in the opposite direction, or to alterations in appearance or in the excretion of various products, cannot be quantitatively screened, but they can be readily **scored** on appropriate plates (e.g., ones that will stain only fermentation-positive colonies). **Replica plating** (Fig. 7–2) is useful in scoring large numbers of colonies on a variety of media.

The **penicillin method** for enriching for **auxotrophic mutants** (Fig. 7–4), is based on the fact that this antibacterial agent kills only growing cells. Hence in a minimal medium auxotrophs, which cannot grow, largely survive in its presence, while the predominant parental cells, which can grow, are selectively killed. An intermediate cultivation is required between mutagenesis and exposure to penicillin, because the expression of an auxotrophic mutation has a **phenotypic lag.** One cause is **nuclear segregation:** because most growing bacterial cells have more than one copy of their chromosome, a recessive mutation (e.g., an inactive biosynthetic gene) cannot be expressed until separated from the parental allele present in a companion chromosome. A second cause is **phenomic lag:** a change in the genome is not reflected in the **phenome** (i.e., the total set of products of the genome) until the enzyme molecules previously formed by the gene have been diluted out.

MUTATION RATES

With bacterial mutations that are easy to select quantitatively from large populations (e.g., mutations to resistance or to prototrophy), it is possible to detect small

E. coli culture

↓ Mutagen

Mixture of killed parental,
live parental, and a few live
mutant genotypes

↓ Intermediate cultivation
in enriched medium

Phenotypic expression
of mutant genotype (Fig. 8-8)

↓ Penicillin in minimal
medium

Selective killing
of parental cells

↓ Plate on enriched
medium

Colonies from surviving
cells, with parental type
much decreased in frequency

↓ Parallel inoculation of
each colony on minimal
and enriched medium

Growth of parental clones
on both media, auxotrophic
mutants only on enriched medium

↓ Inoculation of mutant
colony in minimal pour
plate

Identification of growth
requirement(s) of mutant by
"spot tests" with growth factors

Figure 7–4. Penicillin method for selecting auxotrophic mutants of bacteria. Similar results may be obtained with other agents that also kill only growing cells; for example, metabolite analogues such as 8-aza-guanine; or radioactive metabolites that release lethal irradiation during long-term storage after their incorporation.

increments to the background "spontaneous" mutation rate. Many weakly mutagenic substances have thus been detected, expanding enormously the class of recognized mutagens (see Ames test, Chap. 8). The spontaneous rate in bacteria is often approximately 10^{-6} for the mutations, in a large number of sites in a gene, that can cause loss of function. It is as low as 10^{-9} for a mutation, such as streptomycin resistance, that depends on a limited variety of changes in a small region of the gene (change of function).

DEFINITION OF MUTATION RATE. In growth at different rates the **spontaneous mutation rate** (i.e., the probability of appearance of a given type of mutant) remains relatively constant **per cell division** rather than per cell per unit of time. Accordingly, it is customary to define mutation rate, α, as

$$\alpha = m/d,$$

where m is the number of **mutations** and d the number of cell **divisions.**

In a population grown from a small inoculum, the value of d essentially equals the final number of cells, as each division produces one additional cell. However, the value of m is not simply the **mutant frequency** (the total number of mutants present in a population), because that frequency includes the accumulated progeny of mutations that arose before the most recent generation, and so it becomes higher the later a culture is harvested. Special methods are therefore necessary to determine the mutation rate (see Appendix to this Chap.).

MUTATIONS IN THE STATIONARY PHASE. Mutations appear not only in growing cells, where they can be expressed in terms of frequency per generation, but also in the stationary phase, despite the lack of substantial growth and cell division. In colonies on plates that have been incubated for many days such mutants are often seen as papillae, i.e. regions of renewed growth. Their frequency fluctuates widely with time and with conditions, and so the focus on quantifiable mutation rates led to neglect of this class. Nevertheless, their existence is not surprising, since damage is known to occur to non-replicating as well as to replicating DNA (Chap. 8).

These stationary-phase mutations have unexpected properties. Their appearance can be enormously accelerated by the presence of a substrate that makes them adaptive (e.g., lactose causing reversion from Lac$^-$ to Lac$^+$); they are generally delayed until after several days in the stationary phase; they can then appear in numbers far beyond what would be expected from the rates observed in the growth phase; and they may even require two distinct mutations (each infrequent in growing cells) to produce the adaptive phenotype. It thus appears that in starving cells potential substrates can selectively influence mutation rates in a manner that is useful for the cell. The mechanisms that accelerate mutations in late stationary phase, and that respond to substrates, are obscure. However, the phenomenon is important since bacteria in nature often alternate between feast and famine. Moreover, the phenomenon has interesting evolutionary implications: for while a Lamarckian specification of mutations by the environment is incompatible with basic principles of molecular genetics, a biassing of mutation frequencies by the environment could similarly result in adaptive evolution, instead of pure random mutation and selection.

SUPPRESSION OF MUTATIONS

Mutations that reverse the phenotypic effect of an earlier mutation usually do not restore the original allele of the gene (true reversions) but rather are **pseudorevertants;** most are located at a different site from the first mutation, as shown by genetic crosses that segregate the two and restore the original mutant phenotype. In classic genetics this compensatory interaction occurring between two genes was named **genetic suppression.**

Studies in bacteria have demonstrated several mechanisms. **Extragenic** suppressor mutations (i.e., in another gene, usually for a tRNA) create errors in translation that occasionally correct the effect of the first mutation, whereas in **intragenic** suppressor mutations, a second alteration in the mutated gene restores its function. Because extragenic suppressors impair the fidelity of translation they are likely to be selected against in nature, but as tools in research they have revealed innumerable genes whose mutations would otherwise be lethal (and hence not recoverable; see Conditional Mutations, above). Some suppressors are codon-specific, some are gene-specific, and others cause generalized errors. They will be described in Chapter 8.

In addition to genetic suppression, **phenotypic suppression** of the effects of mutations can be induced by factors that decrease the fidelity of translation. These include antibiotics acting on the ribosome, and incorporation of ambiguously translated base analogues into mRNA (see Chap. 6, Ribosomal Ambiguity; Coding Ambiguity).

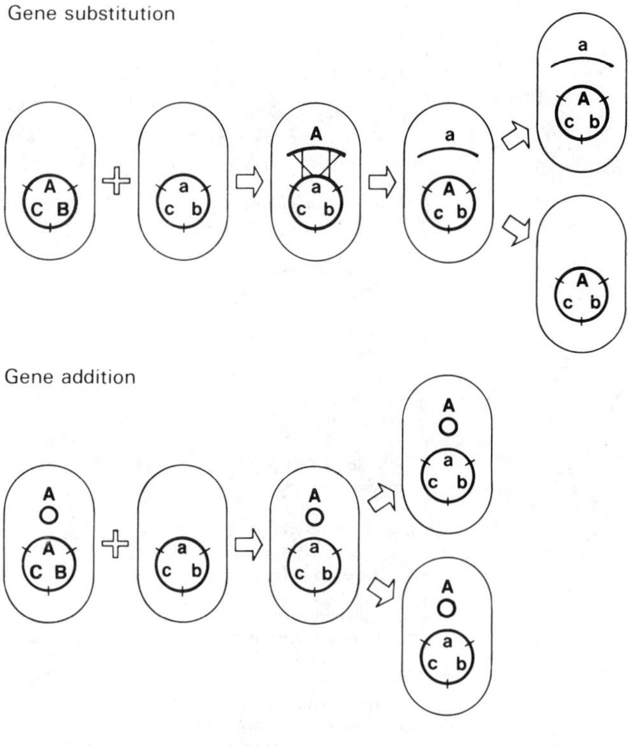

Figure 7–5. Two types of gene transfer in bacteria: substitution and addition.

Gene Transfer

EVOLUTIONARY SIGNIFICANCE

Genetic diversity, on which evolution depends, arises not only from mutations (as the ultimate source of novelty) but also from a powerful additional mechanism, **recombination of genes from different individuals.** In eukaryotes the evolution of sex made this process a regular feature of reproduction. However, more primitive forms of recombination evolved much earlier, in prokaryotes, as an occasional exception to clonal reproduction. Three mechanisms are known: **transformation** (uptake of naked DNA); **conjugation** (plasmid-mediated mating between cells in contact); and **transduction** (infection by a nonlethal virus carrying bacterial genes). Unlike zygote formation, these processes transfer only a part of a genome (**exogenote**) from a donor into a recipient cell, creating a **merozygote** (Gr. *meros*, part).

After entering the cell some exogenotes **substitute,** while others **add,** novel genes in the recombinant (Fig. 7–5). Thus, with a **chromosomal fragment,** which cannot multiply, the stable association of any of its genes with the cell depends on a double crossover that incorporates part of the fragment into the chromosome, usually by substitution for a homologous region. However, when the introduced DNA is a **replicon**—a viral genome

or a plasmid (see below), which can replicate autonomously—it creates a stable merodiploid.

We should note that the term "**recombination**" is used in two senses: the assembly of new combinations of genes from two sources, or the molecular process of crossing over between two DNA chains. The latter may include rearrangements within a genome (see Chap. 8, Recombination, for molecular mechanisms).

Conjugation and transduction, which protect the DNA during its transit, may have evolved later than transformation. It seems likely that viruses evolved from plasmids. Their freer movement between cells then permitted them to function not only as agents of gene transfer but also as parasites, undergoing evolutionary selection for maximizing their reproduction.

SPREAD OF GENES. Genes can be transferred not only between members of the same bacterial species but also, less efficiently, between species. With substitutive transfers, dependent on DNA homology, efficiency falls off rapidly with evolutionary distance. Plasmids, in contrast, do not depend on sequence homology for persistence in a new host, and some (but not all) have a broad host range. Transfers by plasmids of overlapping host range can connect even very different organisms (Fig. 7–6), suggesting that genes flow slowly throughout the microbial

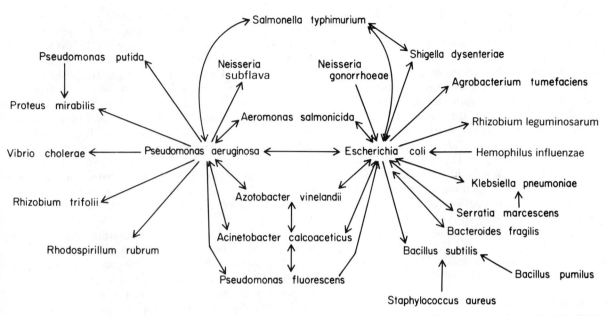

Figure 7–6. Flow of plasmids, either by transformation or by conjugation, known in 1979. (Young FE, Mayer L: Rev Infect Dis 1:55, 1979)

world and that transformation can take up DNA from any source.

TRANSFORMATION

Transformation in bacteria was discovered adventitiously in the course of a study of virulence in pneumococci. Virulent strains form smooth (S) colonies, owing to the presence of a type-specific polysaccharide capsule, whereas avirulent variants, often emerging on repeated transfer in culture, have lost the capacity to make the capsule and hence form rough (R) colonies. When a large number of R cells are inoculated in a mouse, S cells emerge again and kill the animal. In 1928, Griffith in England discovered that injection of heat-killed S pneumococci into mice along with the live R pneumococci not only accelerated the latter's reversion to the S form but also could transform their type; i.e., killed cells of one S type could impose that type on R cells derived from another type (Fig. 7–7). Working before bacterial variation was linked to genetics, Griffith failed to recognize the profound implication of the phenomenon: that a substance conferring a new heritable property must itself be replicated.

Identification of the Transforming Substance

Avery, who had discovered the role of the pneumococcal capsule in virulence, then extended the study of transformation to the test tube, using anti-R serum to agglutinate R cells and thus allow S cells to be recognized by their diffuse growth. In 1944, after years of work with this difficult assay, Avery, MacLeod, and McCarty, all medical investigators without extensive biochemical training,

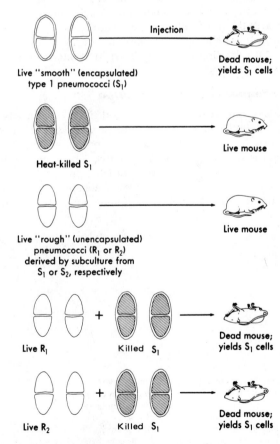

Figure 7–7. The Griffith experiment. Rough (R) cells not only apparently reverted to smooth (S) cells of the parental type during association with heat-killed S cells of the same type but also were transformed to a different S type by heat-killed cells of that type.

succeeded in isolating the "transforming principle" and identifying it as DNA (Fig. 7–8).

This revolutionary discovery not only identified the material of heredity but also showed that bacteria can transfer genes. It thus laid the foundation for two fields, molecular genetics and bacterial genetics. Nevertheless, it was slow to be appreciated and was never given the recognition of a Nobel Prize. In retrospect, we can see several reasons: virulence was not readily seen as a genetic trait in an organism with no known genetics; DNA seemed too simple to be the genetic material; and phage workers, who had been pursuing the nature of the gene in this simplest of all organisms, were reluctant to believe that studies on pathogenicity had inadvertently solved the problem. The role of DNA was not rapidly accepted until it was confirmed in phage: in 1952, Hershey and Chase showed that the DNA from infecting phage labeled with radioactive P enters the cell, whereas most of the protein, labeled with radioactive S, remains outside.

It is remarkable that bacterial gene transfer was first discovered as transformation, because free DNA is highly susceptible to mechanical and enzymatic damage: In addition, the nutritionally fastidious, fragile pneumococcus is one of the most difficult bacteria to work with. The key was Avery's lifelong concentration on the pneumococcus—the leading cause of death in Western countries when he started.

Mechanisms of Transformation

Transformation has been observed in a wide variety of genera, both gram-positive and gram-negative. By extending it to genes that could be sharply selected (e.g., drug resistance, fermentative ability), it became possible to quantitate the effectiveness of DNA preparations and also the **competence** of cells to accept DNA. In the pneumococcus the DNA fragment must be double-stranded, without nicks, and with mol. wt. 3×10^5 to 10^7 or more. In synchronized cultures, the proportion of competent cells varies regularly during the cycle of cell division, suggesting that entry occurs through zones of wall synthesis. Moreover, in an unsynchronized culture competence goes through a peak during the culture cycle, and at that stage the supernatant fluid contains a protein **competence factor** whose addition to other cultures increases their competence. With improved techniques, it has become possible to transform 5% of the cells for a given marker (compared with Avery's 10^{-4}), and to achieve nearly one transformant for a given marker per gene-equivalent of DNA taken up.

Three distinct mechanisms of transformation have been recognized.

1. The pneumococcus and some other gram-positive bacteria bind double-stranded DNA nonspecifically (i.e., any DNA competes), and the molecules are cut, by an endonuclease in the membrane, to a length of 7 to 10 Kb, of which **only one strand enters.** The membrane evidently provides an unwinding mechanism. In consequence, there is an **eclipse** period of about 5 minutes during which the transforming DNA is protected within the cell from external DNase but cannot be recovered in active form. The single-stranded DNA forms a **heteroduplex** by hybridizing with one strand of homologous recipient DNA and displacing the other strand (see Chap. 8, Recombination). After becoming covalently integrated, the introduced genes have recovered transforming activity.

2. In the gram-negative *Haemophilus*, uptake depends on a specific sequence of about ten nucleotides that is much more numerous in this organism than in other species. A membrane protein binds this sequence, and **the DNA enters as a double strand**. In the gram-negative *Neisseria*, transformation occurs only in piliated strains.

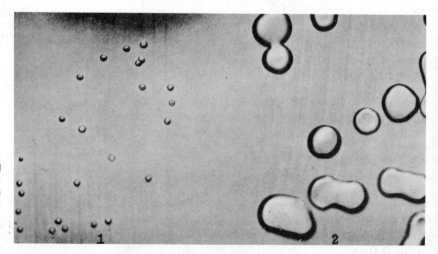

Figure 7–8. Transformation of R to S pneumococci by DNA from S cells. *(1)* Colonies on blood agar of an R variant derived from type 2 pneumococci. *(2)* Colonies from cells of the same strain that had grown in the presence of DNA from type 3 pneumococcus plus antiserum to R cells (see text). (Type 3 forms especially glistening mucoid colonies.) (Avery OT et al: J Exp Med 79:137, 1944)

3. With enteric bacteria transformation has been observed only after **artificial modification** of the cell envelope: conversion to **spheroplasts** or permeabilizing the envelope to DNA by heating in the presence of $CaCl_2$. This modified surface permits the cell to take up **double-stranded fragments. Electroporation**—the application of high-voltage pulses permeabilizes the cell envelope and permits efficient uptake of DNA in a wide variety of gram-positive as well as gram-negative bacteria.

TRANSFECTION. Such permeabilized cells can also take up the **intact double-stranded DNA of viruses or plasmids.** The mechanics are those of transformation but the DNA is more stable, and it yields a stable merodiploid, with gene addition rather than replacement. When the introduced replicon is a viral genome, the process has been called transfection because it results in infection, but it seems more logical to apply the term also to plasmids, reserving "transformation" for chromosomal fragments that cannot replicate autonomously.

Significance of Tranformation and Transfection

Transformation can be used for genetic mapping over short distances by linkage measurements, as described below under Transduction. It can also be used to quantitate the relative number of copies of various genes, and hence to identify the origin of replication and the sequence of genes in the chromosome. Though transformation is less convenient than transduction and conjugation for mapping, in recent years transfection has become indispensable for cloning recombinant DNA in plasmid or viral vectors (Chap. 8). Transformation has been extended to yeasts and to animal cells.

Since the uptake of random pieces of DNA in transformation involves special enzymes it is evidently an evolved mechanism, occurring in nature, rather than an artefact. Moreover, it may have epidemiological significance, for in the peritoneal cavity of a mouse injected with pairs of pneumococcal strains of low virulence, recombinants with increased virulence can be selected.

TRANSDUCTION

Transduction of bacterial genes by a bacteriophage, like transformation, introduces only a small fraction of a bacterial chromosome. Because the surrounding phage coat protects the DNA from damage, transduction is much easier to perform and more reproducible than transformation. Originally discovered by Lederberg and Zinder in *Salmonella*, it has been observed in a wide range of bacteria.

Two mechanisms are known. In **generalized transduction** the phage picks up fragments of host DNA at random; hence it may transfer any genes. In **specialized transduction** phage DNA that has been integrated into the host chromosome is excised along with a few adjacent genes, which the phage can then transfer. Detailed consideration of these processes will be deferred to Chapter 46. We shall consider here only the use of generalized transduction for obtaining desired recombinants and for mapping the bacterial chromosome.

In generalized transduction, the phage coat occasionally encloses a fragment (ca. 1%) of the disintegrating host chromosome, instead of the phage genome (Fig. 7–9). Such a **transducing particle,** released from the cell along with normal phage, can then inject its DNA into a recipient cell, just as in phage infection. After the DNA penetrates the cell it frequently recombines with a homologous region of the chromosome.

Mapping by Transduction

The population of transducing phage particles includes an assortment of segments of relatively uniform length derived at random from the donor chromosome (Fig. 7–10). Each bacterial gene should therefore be represented with more or less equal frequency. The distance between two mutational sites that can **cotransduce** in the same particle can be estimated in two ways: from the

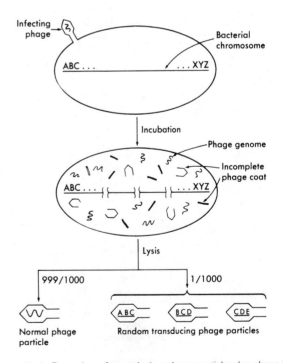

Figure 7–9. Formation of transducing phage particles by phage-infected bacterium. The entry of the phage genome leads to its replication and also to formation of all the other components that are finally assembled into the mature phage (Chap. 45). In this assembly, the coat occasionally encloses a fragment of bacterial DNA instead of the usual phage DNA, thus forming a transducing particle.

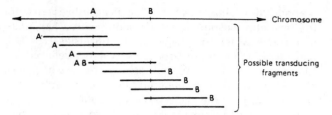

Figure 7–10. Relation of the distance between two markers to the frequency of their joint transduction. The various segments indicate possible fragments of cellular DNA of the proper length for transfer in phage particles. The probability of including any marker in a fragment is proportional to its length, but the probability of including two markers is proportional to the difference between that length and the intermarker distance. Therefore, the frequency of cotransduction falls sharply with increasing distance between A and B. As a first approximation, the breaks that form transducing fragments are randomly located, and the lengths of the fragments are uniform. Refined studies, however, have revealed some preference in sites and some variation in length.

frequency of **joint transduction** of distinct genes, or from the frequency of **recombination** between sites within a gene.

TRANSDUCTIONAL RECOMBINATION. Studies of transduction and recombination have been extremely valuable in fine-structure mapping. One mutant strain is transduced with phage from various strains carrying other mutations in the same gene, and the wild-type recombinants are selected on an appropriate medium. Their frequency **increases** with the distance between the sites of mutation in donor and recipient (Fig. 7–11). This procedure can detect even the lowest possible frequencies: those of recombinations between mutations in adjacent nucleotides.

JOINT TRANSDUCTION. With **cotransduction** of two markers from the same donor incorporation into the recipient requires a pair of crossovers within the ends of the transducing fragment but outside the pair of markers (Fig. 7–10). Hence unlike transductional recombination, where frequency is roughly proportional to the distance between the markers, with cotransduction the frequency falls off rapidly with increasing distance, and it ceases with linkage distances that exceed the total length of the fragments—about 1% that of the chromosome.

The use of transduction in mapping is further discussed below (The Genetic Map). The use of two-factor and three-factor crosses for mapping will be discussed in Chapter 8, Appendix.

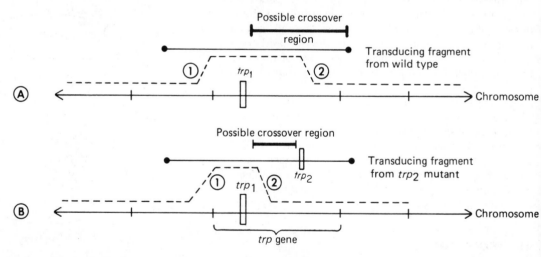

Figure 7–11. Recombination between a transducing and a recipient marker in same gene. (**A**) A *trp*⁻ recipient is transduced with phage from a wild-type donor. Of the set of transducing fragments (Fig. 7–10) carrying a normal replacement for the defective *trp₁* site, one typical member is shown. Given a crossover (1) to the left of the *trp₁* site, the second crossover (2) required for recombination may occur anywhere to the right of that site, up to the end of the fragment. (**B**) The same experiment is performed with transducing phage from another *trp*⁻ mutant (*trp₂*). To produce a prototrophic recombinant, the second crossover must now occur between *trp₁* and *trp₂*; otherwise, the correction of one defect in the cell will be accompanied by the introduction of another.

With various donors, the shorter the distance between their *trp*⁻ site and *trp₁*, the lower the frequency of prototrophic recombinants. In "self-transduction" of *trp₁* × *trp₁*, none are obtained.

The sequence of *trp₁* and *trp₂* relative to an outside marker (in another gene) can be determined unequivocally by a three-factor cross with two different alleles of the marker in the two parents. In a reciprocal transduction, with either strain serving as donor in the *trp₁* × *trp₂* cross, one donor will bring in a nearby unselected marker to the right of the cross and the other will bring in one to the left.

CONJUGATION

Because living organisms share so many properties, microbiologists had occasionally looked for sexual reproduction in bacteria under the microscope, but without success. The discovery of transformation and of mutable genes in bacteria renewed interest in the subject, and in 1946, Lederberg, leaving medical school to take up the problem, demonstrated the formation of prototrophic recombinants in a mixed culture of two double auxotrophs (Fig. 7–12). The use of double auxotrophs was essential, because the rate of recombination (about 10^{-6} per cell) was similar to the rate of formation of prototrophs by reversion of single auxotrophs.

Conjugation requires cell contact, and it can simultaneously transfer a large number of markers. These features suggested zygote formation. However, despite the hope for unifying the new genetics of bacteria as much as possible with that of higher organisms, crosses between various sets of mutations failed to yield the consistent linear map of classic genetics.

Mechanism of Gene Transfer

POLARITY. A serendipitous observation of Hayes in London, introducing streptomycin (Str) during a cross rather than in the screening of the products, provided proof that conjugating bacteria do not form zygotes. The presence of the antibiotic blocked recombination between a particular sensitive strain and resistant strain, but not between the same pair with the alleles for sensitivity and for resistance reversed. There are thus two mating types, functioning asymmetrically; since Str kills cells by blocking protein synthesis (Chap. 10), while allowing DNA synthesis and energy production, cells can serve as **genetic donors (males)**, contributing DNA to the cross, even af-

ter being killed; but the **recipients (females)** must remain viable. Another difference between donor and recipient is that the former contributes unselected markers much less frequently, suggesting that it transfers only part of a chromosome.

THE F PLASMID. The donor property of male cells is created by the presence of the **F agent (fertility factor)**, a plasmid that codes for a conjugation apparatus and can transfer chromosomal genes. Moreover, **transfer of the plasmid itself occurs with high frequency:** when genetically labeled F^+ and F^- cells are grown together at sufficient densities, most of the F^- cells become F^+ within an hour. The low frequency of transfer of bacterial genes thus turns out to be due to infrequent joining of the chromosome to the plasmid, rather than to infrequent conjugation. The plasmid was subsequently demonstrated directly by ultracentrifugation and by electron microscopy.

Balancing its rapid spread, the plasmid is easily lost, especially during long-term incubation in the stationary phase (which is frequent in nature); otherwise all strains would soon be F^+. Hence in the early studies the various mutant stocks were all interfertile (thus concealing the polarity of mating), because each contained a mixture of the two mating types. The F agent turned out to be the first of a large group of **conjugative plasmids,** which will be discussed below.

The F plasmid causes transfer of the chromosome by integrating into it, so that in conjugation, in which DNA transfer is initiated at a specific plasmid sequence (*oriT*; origin of transfer), the attached chromosome follows. The **mechanism of integration** of plasmid into chromosome is a single crossover between the two rings of DNA at certain sites on the chromosome, yielding an enlarged single ring (see Fig. 7–14 below). This process can equally be viewed as an integration of the chromosome into F, which interrupts the transfer of F; and because part of the sequence of F then enters at the start and part at the end of transfer, the recipient cell remains F^- except when the entire chromosome is rarely transferred (see Chap. 8, Plasmids). The integration is stable, so strains that have integrated the plasmid can be isolated as **Hfr (high frequency of recombination)** cultures.

Kinetics of Mating

Going beyond the classic studies of recombinant frequencies, Wollmann and Jacob in Paris used high-frequency transfers to study the process of gene transfer directly. A Str^S prototrophic donor was mated with a Str^R polyauxotrophic recipient, and at intervals, samples were plated on media containing Str and various growth factors, thus identifying Str^R recombinants carrying various prototrophic genes derived from the donor. More-

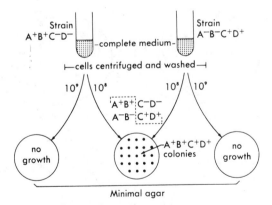

Figure 7–12. Diagrammatic representation of the initial experiment of Lederberg (1946). The mutants were cultivated in a medium that included growth factors A, B, C, and D; the test for recombination and the control tests for reversion were carried out in a minimal medium lacking these factors.

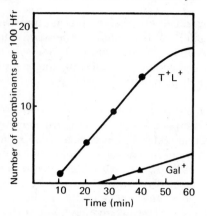

Figure 7–13. Kinetics of conjugation studied by interrupting further chromosomal transfer, as well as further pair formation, at various times. Cross: HfrH *str^s thr^+ leu^+ gal^+* × F^− *str^R thr^− leu^− gal^−*. Exponential broth cultures were mixed at time 0 (10^7 Hfr + excess of F^− cells/ml) and aerated in broth. At intervals, samples were diluted, agitated briefly in a Waring blender, and plated (1) on glucose minimal medium plus streptomycin to select *thr^+ leu^+ str^R* recombinants; and (2) on galactose minimal medium plus threonine, leucine, and streptomycin to select *gal^+ str^R* recombinants. (After Wollman EL, Jacob F, Hayes W: Cold Spring Harbor Symp Quant Biol 21:141, 1956)

over, mating could be **artificially interrupted** at various times after mixing by mechanical agitation (by means of a Waring blender, rapid pipetting back and forth, or vibration). This experiment revealed the **time of initial entry of each gene:** that required to form the earliest mating pairs and transfer the required length of chromosome. The results (Fig. 7–13) led to the following conclusions.

1. The genes are transferred in a **fixed order.**

2. There is a **gradient of decreasing transmission** with increasing distance from the origin; i.e., the transfer is spontaneously interrupted at more or less random times, so it rarely includes the entire chromosome. (Spontaneous interruption can be hindered by mechanical support of the mating pair on agar or wedged in membrane filters.)

3. Different Hfr strains have different origins, depending on the site of integration of the plasmid; and different strains inject in opposite directions, depending on the polarity of the integration. The number of sites of integration is limited, indicating some specificity in the process of recombination.

4. The overlaps between the sequences introduced by different Hfr strains provided the first evidence for a **circular chromosome** (Fig. 7–14)—a characteristic of all

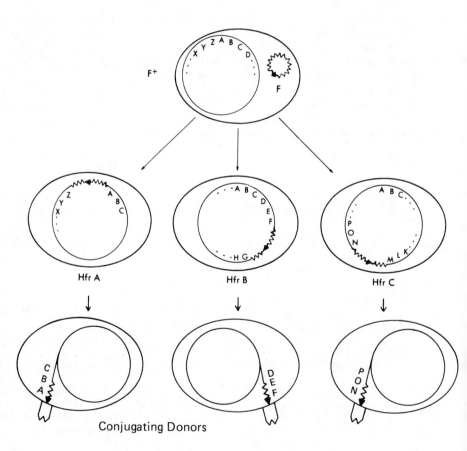

Figure 7–14. Formation of different Hfr strains by integration of F agent at different locations on the bacterial chromosome. Site of initial entry of the Hfr chromosome in conjugation (origin) is depicted as an *arrowhead* in the middle of F.

Conjugating Donors

replicating DNA in bacteria—as was subsequently demonstrated directly by electron microscopy after gentle lysis with detergent to remove organizing proteins (Chap. 2, Fig. 2–10).

With this development, **distances on a chromosome,** previously measured only in terms of recombination frequencies, **could be measured directly** in units of time. At 37°C transfer of the entire chromosome requires about 100 minutes; i.e., 1% (45 Kb or 15 μm), corresponding to 20 recombination units (i.e., 20% crossing over), is transferred per minute.

F' Plasmids

The integration in an Hfr strain is reversible at low frequency, usually restoring the original F⁺. However, excision may be imprecise and carry a segment (of variable length) from either adjacent region of the host chromosome; the resulting **hybrid plasmid** is called **F'**. Because these hybrids are transmitted to F⁻ cells with high effi-

ciency and they are easily separated from the chromosome in lysates, they are very useful for the transfer and the isolation of selected genes.

The transferred F' plasmid can have several fates: (1) it can replicate autonomously; (2) its segment from the donor chromosome can recombine by a double crossover with the homologous recipient segment (as in transformation); or (3) a single crossover can integrate the plasmid, resulting in duplication of its chromosomal segment. This last integration is unstable, because homologous recombination between the two copies can excise one, together with any sequence between them.

The Genetic Map

With the several unique features of bacterial conjugation thus elucidated, a consistent chromosome map of *E. coli* could be constructed. Figure 7–15 presents some of the known markers, expressing the distances in terms of time of entry: total about 100 minutes. Mapping by inter-

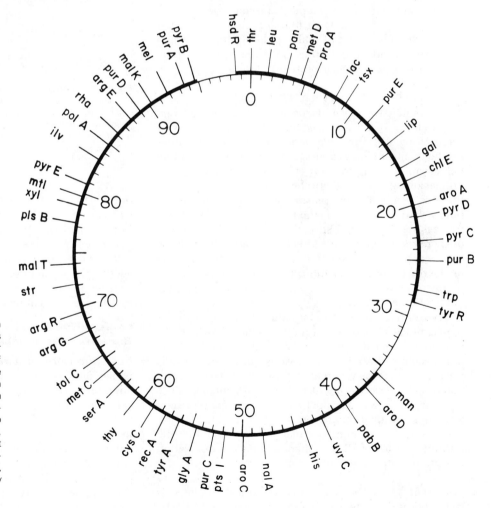

Figure 7–15. Map of a few genes in the chromosome of *E. coli*. Numbers represent minutes required for transfer (broth, 37°C) from the origin (zero) of the first Hfr strain isolated, HfrH. The parts of the circle in *heavy lines* contain markers whose distances have been confirmed by cotransduction. In the earlier literature, the map was calibrated to a total of 90 rather than 100 minutes, and so the positions of genes distant from the origin were given lower numbers. (Modified from Bachmann BJ, Low KB, Taylor AL: Bacteriol Rev 40:116, 1976)

rupted mating is ideal for long distances in the chromosome (>5 minutes on the map), complementing the use of cotransduction and recombination frequencies for short distances.

A genetic map is important not only for understanding the organization of the genome and for making evolutionary comparisons, but also for the creation of specific genotypes. In particular, one can obtain recombinants with desired nonselectable genes by taking advantage of their linkage to selectable markers. Additional ways of mapping bacterial genes are noted in Chapter 8, Appendix.

Physiology of Conjugation

F PILI. The F plasmid codes for the formation of a special **sex pilus,** and mating is initiated by attachment of its tip to a **receptor** (the product of the *ompA* gene) on an F⁻ cell. That major OM protein is also present in F⁺ cells, but their F plasmid codes for a product that covers it, which explains the low F⁺ × F⁺ fertility; otherwise, identical F⁺ cells would uselessly exchange plasmids. *E. coli* K12 has one to three sex pili per male cell, and these are readily distinguishable from the large number of other pili by their adsorption of **male-specific phages,** which infect cells by adsorbing either to the main protein, pilin (Fig. 7–16), or to a special protein at the tip.

REPRESSION OF PILUS FORMATION. Unlike the F agent, most conjugative plasmids ordinarily cause only rare cells to form sex pili, because the plasmid codes also for a repressor of the *tra* **(transfer) operon,** which codes for the conjugation apparatus. However, when a cell that has escaped the repression encounters a new population lacking the plasmid and hence lacking its repressor, the first recipient of the plasmid immediately forms sex pili and transfers the plasmid, and repetitions of this process result in rapid spread of the plasmid to previously plasmid-free cells. Within a generation or so, however, each recipient cell accumulates repressor and hence ceases pilus formation. The mixing of donor and recipient populations thus results in a transient wave of conjugational activity.

The repression of pilus formation between episodes of plasmidial spread to a virgin population provides two evident advantages: economy of synthesis and protection against infection by the widespread male-specific phages—a sort of venereal disease of bacteria. Fortunately for the development of bacterial genetics, the F agent of strain K12 had lost the capacity for repressor formation during its long protected growth in the laboratory, and the resulting permanent formation of pili permitted it to reveal the phenomenon of conjugation despite the low frequency of integration.

TRANSFER. After the pilus attaches to a recipient it is retracted and the two cells form a stable contort. The

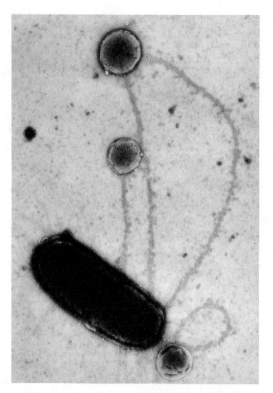

Figure 7–16. Attachment of an F⁺ *E. coli* cell by means of F pili to three F⁻ minicells (products of mutants that occasionally separate a small cell without a nucleus). The few long F pili are covered with F-specific MS2 phage particles. These phages are icosahedral (Chap. 46); other filamentous male-specific phages have been found to adsorb only to the tips of F pili. (After Curtiss R III et al: J Bacteriol 100:1091, 1969)

donor DNA is then replicated in a special way and is transferred as a single strand, which is promptly copied in the recipient. The mechanisms and the regulation of plasmid DNA transfer will be described in Chapter 8. Conjugative and normal DNA replication apparently proceed at the same rate, because it requires 90 minutes to transfer the length of the chromosome linearly and 45 minutes to replicate it bidirectionally.

Conjugation in Gram-Positive Bacteria; Pheromones

In gram-positive bacteria, conjugation does not depend on sex pili; instead, the donor cells form a protein **adhesin** on the surface that causes aggregation with recipient cells. In addition, in *Streptococcus faecalis*, recipient cells excrete small (mol. wt. ca. 1000) peptide **sex pheromones** that each elicit a mating response, including adhesin formation, in donor cells carrying the corresponding conjugative plasmid. The acquisition of the plasmid by a recipient causes its production of that pheromone to cease (although pheromones for other plasmids are still made).

PROTOPLAST FUSION

Zygote formation with bacterial protoplasts has recently been achieved experimentally with a procedure developed earlier with plant cell protoplasts: brief exposure to 40% polyethylene glycol. Under these conditions protoplasts undergo occasional fusion, and on resynthesis of the cell wall they segregate stable haploid recombinants, with a total frequency of about 10^{-4}. Much rarer fusion of protoplasts also occurs without the fusing agent, which suggests that this form of gene transfer may occur in nature.

Plasmids

GENERAL PROPERTIES

Plasmids are a highly diverse group of **extrachromosomal genetic elements:** circular, double-stranded DNA molecules with the capacity for autonomous replication in cells. The first one to be discovered, the F factor, was revealed by its ability to transfer chromosomal genes. Many more kinds of plasmids lack that property but can be recognized because they carry genes that affect host metabolism. More recently, physical methods (centrifugation, electron microscopy, or gel electrophoresis) applied to cell lysates have revealed that plasmids are extremely widespread, being present in virtually all bacterial genera tested and including small **cryptic forms** (i.e., with no detectable phenotypic effect). Moreover, similar extrachromosomal elements are found in yeasts and cells of higher eukaryotes.

Most plasmids are cyclic and supercoiled, whereas the chromosomal DNA is ordinarily recovered in a lysate as fragments, which cannot be supercoiled. Because supercoiling markedly affects the intercalation of ethidium bromide in double-stranded DNA and thus electrophoretic mobility (determined in gels) and density (determined by ultracentrifugation in CsCl), its use permits easy recognition and isolation of plasmids. However, rare kinds of plasmids are found in cells in linear form (although some circularize for replication), and these kinds are harder to detect.

Those plasmids and viruses that can integrate into the chromosome were originally called **episomes,** but the term has fallen into disuse because membership depends on the sensitivity of the test.

PHENOTYPIC EFFECTS. Plasmids may be regarded as symbionts of bacteria. In general, the chromosome carries all the genes essential for growth, whereas plasmids carry **optional genes** that confer additional properties (Table 7–1); hence, cells that have lost their plasmids are still viable. Among the optional properties, plasmids broaden the range of organic compounds that can be degraded, detoxify Hg^{2+} and other harmful materials,

TABLE 7–1. *Observed Phenotypic Effects of Plasmids on Bacteria*

Trait	Bacterial species
Fertility	Most gram-negative organisms; *Streptococcus faecalis; Streptomyces*
Resistance to:	
Various antibiotics	Widespread
Various metal ions	Widespread
Ultraviolet irradiation	*E. coli*
Phages	*E. coli*
Serum bactericidal activity	*E. coli*
Ethidium bromide	*Staphylococcus aureus*
Production of:	
Bacteriocins	Widespread
Proteases (cheese)	*Strep. lactis*
Exotoxin	*Clostridium botulinum*
Enterotoxin	*E. coli, Staph. aureus*
Exfoliatin	*Staph. aureus*
Surface antigens	*E. coli*
Hemolysins	*E. coli, Strep. faecalis*
H_2S	*E. coli*
Chloramphenicol	*Streptomyces*
Siderophores	Widespread
Metabolism of:	
Various sugars	Widespread
Hydrocarbons (toluene, xylene, camphor, salicylate, etc.)	*Pseudomonas*
Tumorigenesis in plants	*Agrobacterium tumefaciens*

and produce bacteriocins (proteins that kill other strains of the same bacterial species). They also code for the enzymes that produce some antibiotics, and in pathogens their most important effects are coding for virulence factors or for resistance to various antibiotics.

Bacterial properties that depend on plasmids may fluctuate easily. In addition to the gain or loss of a plasmid, the genetic composition of the plasmids fluctuates, in part because the genes that affect the host phenotype are present in highly mobile segments of DNA, called **transposons,** and these also code for an enzyme that mediates their loss or their transfers between plasmids or between a plasmid and the chromosome (see Chap. 8). Finally, since accessory genes on plasmids code for optional functions, their natural selection depends entirely on their value for the host cell under specific circumstances.

SIZE AND CONJUGATION. Plasmid sizes range from 1.5 to 400 Kb, compared with 1 Kb for an average gene and 4500 for the *E. coli* chromosome. The sizes are also expressed in other terms: 1 μm length = 2 megadaltons [1 Mdal = 10^6 daltons] = 3 Kb.

The large plasmids (e.g., F), 60 to 120 Kb long, are mostly **conjugative** (also called **self-transmissible**); i.e., they code for an apparatus that mediates their transfer to another cell. The small plasmids, 1.5 to 15 Kb long, are **nonconjugative.** However, they often have sequences that can recognize the apparatus supplied by certain conjugative plasmids, and so they can be **mobilized** by the presence of the latter in the same cell. They also may be transferred occasionally by **integration** into the conjugative plasmid. Plasmids (especially small ones) may also be transferred by **transduction** and by **transfection** of their DNA (see Transformation, above); the latter process is seen in the test tube but may not be important in nature.

COPY NUMBER REGULATION. In growing cultures, each plasmid maintains a characteristic number of copies per chromosome. These are generally correlated inversely with size, ranging from one for large plasmids to 50 for some small ones. Regulation depends in part on host genes but primarily on a **replication repressor** coded for by the plasmid. Copy number may be increased by a mutation in the repressor gene, or, with some strains ("relaxed"), by blocking the formation of repressor protein by chloramphenicol.

The mechanisms of plasmid replication, copy number regulation, and equipartition in cell division will be discussed in Chapter 8. Here, we may simply note that all plasmids must have an origin of replication and genetic elements that regulate their copy number; together, these constitute the **basic replicon.** This pair of elements in large plasmids may be separated from the remainder, forming **miniplasmids.** Conjugative plasmids also code for a set of special enzymes and membrane proteins (including pili) involved in transfer to other cells.

Small, multicopy plasmids can be segregated into minicells (Chap. 2), which lack a chromosome. These cells can be separated easily from the larger, complete cells, and their synthesis of labeled new mRNA and proteins can then be conveniently used to identify the products of plasmid genes.

CLASSIFICATION

Because plasmids exhibit extraordinary variety, often can infect a wide range of host bacteria, and are promiscuous in exchanging genes, classification has been a problem. For a physician, the **phenotypic pattern** of antibiotic resistance of the organism is usually of most interest. However, for epidemiologic analysis of the spread of pathogenic bacteria and of plasmids (including such challenges as hospital epidemics and transfer from agricultural animals to humans), this classification is not adequate, because unrelated plasmids can produce the same phenotype, and the same plasmid may alter its phenotype by gain or loss of a gene. Several more stable properties are therefore used to detect identity or genetic continuity of different isolates.

Because cells are often infected with multiple plasmids, it is useful to identify a bacterial strain by agarose **gel electrophoresis** of its lysate, conveniently performed with a colony lysed with detergent in a well in the gel before electrophoresis. Each **plasmid-size** yields a single band, but some also form multiples: either molecules consisting of two or more copies of the plasmid in tandem sequence, or **concatenates** (two linked circles). A band of novel size may be a very different plasmid, or it may be a known one that has gained or lost a transposon: In the latter case electrophoretic comparison of **restriction endonuclease fragments** of two isolated plasmids will reveal many fragments of identical size as well as some differences (see Chap. 10, Fig. 10–24).

Conjugative plasmids offer another basis for classification: the **specificity of the transfer apparatus.** One aspect of this specificity is the sex pilus, which has been found in 15 serologically distinct types in enterobacteria, the most common being F and I (named for colicinogen I; see below). The repression of pilus formation (see Physiology of Conjugation, above) also exhibits specificity: among conjugative plasmids some inhibit formation of pili when added to the original, derepressed F plasmid in *E. coli* K12, but others have a different, non cross-reactive repressor of pilus formation.

INCOMPATIBILITY GROUPS

The most fundamental basis for classifying plasmids has been the incompatibility, in the same cell, of different plasmids that share the same specific system (*ori, rep*) for regulating replication and hence copy number. The reason for the incompatibility is **chance segregation:** when two plasmids of the same group start with the same numbers in a cell, statistical fluctuations in the occupancy of the shared initiator proteins, replication repressor, and partitioning system will cause differences in the partition at cell division. One or the other then becomes slightly predominant, and any numerical advantage will be amplified at subsequent generations until each cell contains only one kind. In contrast, if plasmids recognize different regulators there is no competition at division, and so they are compatible. Accordingly, plasmids with the same partition specificity form an incompatibility group: its members cannot coexist for many cell generations unless each carries a gene for which there is strong selection.

Incompatibility groups are usually tested for in **mixedly infected cells,** using a selective marker to ensure initial acceptance of the second plasmid and then cultivating without selection. A more refined test for homology is **replicon typing by DNA hybridization** with probes specific for sequences in a particular replication system. This procedure is simpler than the direct incompatibility test; it is effective even with the rare plasmids that have two replication systems (which confuse the direct test); and it distinguishes minor from major differences. In particular, with those plasmids that are regulated by countertranscribed ("antisense") RNA (Chap. 8), small changes in the regulatory sequence readily evolve; and hybridization with a probe can identify them as close relatives, whereas incompatibility tests may classify them as independent types.

More than 20 incompatibility groups have been found in enterobacteria, and the F-like plasmids in *E. coli*, which mobilize the chromosome, form six major incompatibility groups (I to VI). They can be collected into overgroups, each with the same type of pilus. The many incompatibility groups found among plasmids permit multiple infections of a cell. Some plasmids can shuttle between genera, but rarely between gram-positive and gram-negative organisms. Although the genetic components theoretically can be combined randomly, most members of an incompatibility group are similar in size, copy number, host range, and pilus morphology and serology.

CONJUGATIVE TRANSPOSONS

We have noted above that the streptococci (gram-positive) have a rather different mechanism of conjugation than the enterobacteria (gram-negative), lacking sex pili and involving pheromones. Another difference in streptococci, and also in some gram-positive anaerobes, is that their conjugative apparatus is sometimes coded for by a sequence that appears to reside exclusively in the chromosome, where it can be activated to generate the apparatus of conjugation and to form a copy that enters it; free plasmids are not found in lysates. These conjugative transposons appear to have all the elements of a conjugative plasmid except for those required for autonomous replication.

RESISTANCE PLASMIDS (R FACTORS)

The group of conjugative plasmids known as R factors are of special medical interest and are much more widely distributed than are F plasmids. They were discovered in 1959 in Japan as the cause of a rapid increase in multiple drug resistance in *Shigella*, and they were also found to move freely between this pathogen and ordinary *E. coli* strains. Since then they have increased greatly in prevalence as a result of the worldwide extensive use of antibiotics; but they also have been found at low frequency in strains stored before the use of antibiotics in therapy—possibly because of the existence of antibiotics in nature. R plasmids occasionally carry genes for other traits as well (see Table 7–1), including the ability to detoxify Hg^{2+} by reduction to the volatile elemental Hg. The surprising prevalence of this trait suggests that toxic levels of Hg^{2+} have long been present in natural waters.

Resistance plasmids are the most common cause of acquired antibiotic resistance, and their spread creates a threat to chemotherapy, as will be discussed in Chapter 10. They have been encountered not only in *Enterobacteriaceae* but also in the most prevalent enteric organism, the anaerobic *Bacteroides*. Nonconjugative plasmids coding for penicillinase are also common, and are not closely related to the enteric R factors.

STRUCTURE AND DISSOCIATION. R factors are large plasmids with two functionally distinct parts. One is the **resistance transfer factor (RTF),** about 80 Kb long, containing the basic replicon plus the extensive set of genes required for conjugation. The other part is the smaller **resistance determinant,** which varies widely in size and in its content of **transposons** (see Chap. 8) carrying genes for various kinds of drug resistance. For example, the widely distributed transposon Tn1 carries ampicillin resistance, and Tn10 carries tetracycline resistance.

R plasmids may dissociate, forming a replicon that carries the genes for conjugation but not the R determinant (i.e., an RTF) and a replicon with the converse loss (Fig. 7–17). These products may be segregated into daughter cells, in nature as well as in the laboratory. Cells carrying an autonomous R determinant are re-

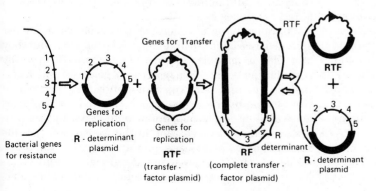

Figure 7–17. Diagram of hypothetical formation of resistance factors and their observed occasional segregation of an RTF and a resistance-determinant plasmid. These two forms may be found in the same cell or in different cells; when in the same cell, they can reversibly associate and dissociate.

vealed by infection with an RTF, which can cause spread of the resistance genes; the mechanism is usually reversal of the dissociation to form a **cointegrate.**

GENE AMPLIFICATION. In cells containing a plasmid with a gene for resistance to a given drug, growth with subinhibitory concentrations of the drug often causes the emergence of cells with high resistance. Such cells contain plasmids in which multiple tandem copies of the resistance determinant have been formed by recombination between daughter strands during replication. The role of the drug is thus selective, as in other forms of resistance. In human cells, similar mechanisms are important in the development of resistance to cancer chemotherapy.

BACTERIOCINOGENS AND BACTERIOCINS

In 1925, Gratia in Belgium discovered that a protein released by a strain of *E. coli* inhibited the growth of a limited number of other strains. Subsequently, some 20 such **colicins,** of different specificity and action, were recognized and designated by letters. They are widespread: 20% of tested enteric bacteria yielded colicins against a single test strain of *E. coli.* Similar substances have been isolated from many genera. The group as a whole are now called **bacteriocins.**

The formation of a given bacteriocin is due to a corresponding plasmid, called a **bacteriocinogen** (and identified by the same letter). Most bacteriocinogens repress their bacteriocin formation, and the escape of an occasional cell from repression, followed by lysis, appears to be responsible for the small amount of bacteriocin normally present in culture filtrates. Moreover, UV irradiation can induce some bacteriocinogenic strains to form and release bacteriocin, just as it induces certain strains carrying a temperate phage to form infectious phage (Chap. 46). Both effects are attributable to activation of the SOS bacterial system (see Chap. 8, Repair of DNA Damage), leading to destruction of the *lexA* repressor of the colicin gene (and of many others).

Some large bacteriocinogens are conjugative, but small ones are not. Among the former, colicinogen V (ColV) forms F pili, and ColI forms I pili.

Bacteriocinogens have a simple genetic organization. For instance, ColE1 has three main genes: *cea* specifies the colicin (which initially accumulates in the periplasmic space); *imm* for a membrane protein that makes the cells **immune** to the colicin that they produce; and *lys* for a small lipoprotein that makes the cell membrane permeable to exit of the colicin. Copy number is controlled by a small antisense RNA, which prevents initiation of DNA replication (Chap. 8).

MECHANISMS OF ACTION OF BACTERIOCINS. Bacteriocins are generally proteins of mol. wt. 50,000 to 80,000

(some much smaller ones are called **microcins**). They have a narrow antimicrobial spectrum, limited to strains closely related to the one forming the bacteriocin, and are very potent: one molecule is often sufficient to kill a bacterium. They attach to specific **OM receptors** and select for **resistant** bacterial mutants, which lack effective receptors. Some bacteriocins also select for bacterial mutations to **tolerance,** in which the receptors still bind the bacteriocin, but alterations in the cytoplasmic membrane prevents its penetration.

Some colicins (El, I, K) kill by creating **ion channels** in the cytoplasmic membrane, which inhibit energy transduction. Others are **nucleases,** which act after entering the cell: ColE2 attacks DNA, and E3 stops protein synthesis by cleaving a specific fragment from the 16S RNA in a ribosome (Chap. 6).

The small immunity protein acts in the producing cell by reversibly binding the bacteriocin. ColE3 is found in the medium mostly as such a complex; after it adsorbs to the receptors on the target cell it dissociates, and enzymatically active colicin enters the cell.

SIGNIFICANCE OF PLASMIDS

While classical genetic recombination depends on DNA homology, as observed in meiotic recombination in higher species and in bacterial transformation, plasmids have played a key role in the recognition of additional mechanisms that do not require extensive homology. These bring about such recombinational events as gene transposition, gene amplification, and integration of plasmids or temperate viruses into the chromosome, and it is now clear that these events also occur in higher organisms. The evolutionary value of plasmids and viruses in producing novel genotypes by "horizontal" gene transfer depends on their ability to recombine with unrelated DNA sequences in this way.

Plasmids and viruses were probably both derived ancestrally from cell chromosomes by cyclization of a small excised segment of DNA, which presumably contained the site for initiating replication. They have evolved different mechanisms of transmission but are closely related in other ways. Some entities, called **phasmids,** can replicate as autonomous plasmids and also can be transferred as viruses in a coat.

Plasmids have a variety of practical effects. Their spread of resistance to antibiotics is best known, but they also play a valuable role in the geochemical cycle by providing an economical reservoir of genes for the degradation of complex organic compounds. In experimental work **transposons** in conjugative plasmids or in phages are widely used as **insertional mutagens.** In this process, a drug resistance gene in the transposon permits selection of recipients, and among these, insertion of the transposon will have interrupted genes at random, creating a variety of defects. The resulting mutants are stable, because after transposons have had time to express their genes in a new recipient they repress their further transposition (much like activation and then repression of pilus formation by conjugative plasmids).

More recently, plasmids have become invaluable as vectors in the molecular recombination and cloning of DNA (Chap. 8). They have the advantage over viruses in that the size of the inserted DNA is not limited.

Appendix: Determination of Mutation Rate

One reliable method for determining the true mutation **rate** is to measure the slope of the increase in mutant **frequency** with continued growth. Especially smooth curves are obtained in the chemostat (see Fig. 3–4, Chap. 3), an apparatus that provides prolonged steady-state growth with a constant population size. This method is applicable only when the mutant multiplies at the same rate as the wild type.

Another method utilizes mutation on solid medium, in which the progeny of an early mutant can be held together in a colony. For example, 10^5 streptomycin-sensitive cells may be spread on a porous membrane on nonselective medium and allowed to grow to 10^9 cells (determined by enumerating the cells washed off a plate grown in parallel). When the membrane is then transferred to a drug-containing plate, the progeny of each mutation to resistance, whether a single cell or a clone, will give rise to one colony.

A widely used statistical method is based on the Poisson distribution of random, chance mutations in a series of identically inoculated and incubated tubes of culture medium. The probability that X mutations occur in a tube $(P_{(x)})$ depends on m, the average number of mutations per tube, averaged over all the tubes, and is

$$P_{(x)} = (m^x/x!)e^{-m}$$

where e is 2.718, the base of natural logarithms. The value of m cannot be measured directly, because, as we have seen, the number of mutants in any tube does not measure the number of mutational events in that tube. However, the number of tubes containing **no** mutants corresponds to the Poisson prediction, which reduces in this case to:

$$P_{(0)} = e^{-m}$$
$$\text{or} \quad \ln P_{(0)} = -m$$

Hence, from a determination of the proportion of mutant-free tubes, $P_{(0)}$, one can calculate the average mutation frequency per tube, m. For example, an average of one mutation per tube yields $P_{(0)} = e^{-1} = 1/e = 0.37.$[*]

[*] For a more extensive discussion of the use of the Poisson distribution see Appendix, Chapter 44.

Selected Reading

BOOKS AND REVIEWS

Bachmann B: Linkage map of *Escherichia coli* K-12, edition 7. Microbiol Rev 47:182, 1983

Bradley DE: Morphological and biological relationships of conjugative pili. Plasmid 4:155, 1980

Campbell A: Evolutionary significance of accessory DNA elements in bacteria. Annu Rev Microbiol 35:55, 1981

Clewell DB: Plasmids, drug resistance, and gene transfer in the genus *Streptococcus*. Microbiol Rev 45:409, 1981

Clewell DB, Gawron–Burke C: Conjugative transposons and the dissemination of antibiotic resistance in streptococci. Annu Rev Microbiol 40:635, 1986

Crosa JH: The relationship of plasmid-mediated iron transport and bacterial virulence. Annu Rev Microbiol 36:69, 1984

Elwell LP, Shipley PL: Plasmid-mediated factors associated with virulence of bacteria to animals. Annu Rev Microbiol 34:465, 1982

Foster TJ: Plasmid-determined resistance to antimicrobial drugs and toxic metal ions in bacteria. Microbiol Rev 47:361, 1983

Goodgal S: DNA Uptake in *Haemophilus* transformation. Annu Rev Genet 16:168, 1982

Hartl DL, Dykhuisen DE: The population genetics of *Escherichia coli*. Annu Rev Genet 18:31, 1984

Hopwood DA: Genetic studies with bacterial protoplasts. Annu Rev Microbiol 35:237, 1981

Hotchkiss RD: Gene, transforming principle, and DNA. In Cairns J, Stent GS, Watson JD (eds): Phage and the Origins of Molecular Biology, p 180. Cold Spring Harbor, NY, Cold Spring Harbor Laboratory, 1966

Ippen–Ihler K, Minkley EG Jr: The conjugation system of F, the fertility factor of *Escherichia coli*. Annu Rev Genet 20:593, 1986

Koniski J: The bacteriocins. In Ornston LN, Sokatch JR (eds): The Bacteria, Vol VI. New York, Academic Press, 1978

Koniski J: Colicins and other bacteriocins with established modes of action. Annu Rev Microbiol 36:125, 1982

Levy S, Clowes RC, Koenig EL (eds): Molecular Biology, Pathogenicity, and Ecology of Bacterial Plamids. New York, Plenum Press, 1981

Manning PA, Achtman M: Cell-to-cell interactions in conjugating *Escherichia coli*: The involvement of the cell envelope. In Inouye M (ed): Bacterial Outer Membranes: Biogenesis and Functions, p 409. New York, John Wiley, 1986

Neidhardt FC, Ingraham JL, Low KB et al: *Escherichia coli* and *Salmonella typhimurium*: Cellular and Molecular Biology. Washington, DC, American Society for Microbiology, 1987. Several relevant papers.

Novick RP: Plasmid incompatibility. Microbiol Rev 51:381, 1987

Piggot PJ, Hoch JA: Revised genetic linkage map of *Bacillus subtilis*. Microbiol Rev 49:158, 1985

Sanderson KE, Roth JR: Linkage map of *Salmonella typhimurium*, edition VI. Microbiol Rev 47:410, 1983

Scaife J, Leach D, Galizzi A (eds): Genetics of Bacteria. New York, Academic Press, 1985

Scott JR: Regulation of plasmid replication. Microbiol Rev 48:2, 1984

Seifert HS, So M: Genetic mechanisms of bacterial antigenic variation. Microbiol Rev 52:327, 1988

Shapiro JA (ed): Mobile Genetic Elements. New York, Academic Press, 1983

Stewart GJ, Carlson CA: The biology of natural transformation. Annu Rev Microbiol 40:211, 1986

Willetts N, Skurray R: The conjugative system of F-like plasmids. Annu Rev Genet 14:41, 1980

Willetts N, Wilkins B: Processing of plasmid DNA during bacterial conjugation. Microbiol Rev 48:24, 1984

SPECIFIC ARTICLES

Avery OT, MacLeod C, McCarty M: Studies on the chemical nature of the substance inducing transformation of pneumococcal types. J Exp Med 79:137, 1944

Couturier M, Bex F, Bergquist PL, Maas WK: Identification and classification of bacterial plasmids. Microbiol Rev 52:375, 1988

Cairns J, Overbaugh J, Miller S: The origin of mutants. Nature 334:142, 1988

Ehrenfeld EE, Kessler RE, Clewell DB: Identification of pheromone-induced surface proteins in *Steptococcus faecalis* and evidence of a role for lipoteichoic acid in formation of mating aggregates. J Bacteriol 168:6, 1986

Hall BG: Adaptive evolution that requires multiple spontaneous mutations. Genetics 120:887, 1988

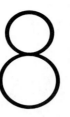

Molecular Aspects of DNA Replication and Variation

This chapter will review a number of features of DNA metabolism, some of which have been discussed from a more physiological perspective in Chapter 7.

Chromosome Replication

As noted in Chapter 2, a bacterial cell contains at least one chromosome in the form of a cyclic DNA molecule associated with proteins and folded into 50 to 100 domains with independent supercoiling. Replication is strictly regulated and occurs at a defined phase of the cell cycle; through its association with the plasma membrane, the chromosome also controls the division of the cell. We will consider here the molecular mechanisms and the regulation of chromosome replication.

BIDIRECTIONAL REPLICATION. In all bacterial genomes, replication of DNA occurs at a **growing point (fork)** that moves linearly from an **origin** to a **terminus. Radioautographic imaging** of the replication by Cairns clearly showed, as was suggested earlier by the variation of Hfr strains in conjugation (Chap. 7, Fig. 7–14), that the **E. coli chromosome is cyclic throughout replication** (Fig. 8–1). **Genetic evidence** for **bidirectional** replication was obtained in synchronized cultures by observing either peaks of mutagenesis at the growing fork (Fig. 8–2) or regions of autoradiographic labeling (Fig. 8–3), or by electron microscopy in bacteriophages (see Fig. 45–8). **Unidirectional replication** occurs more rarely; for example, in the cyclic DNAs of some plasmids, and in conjugation.

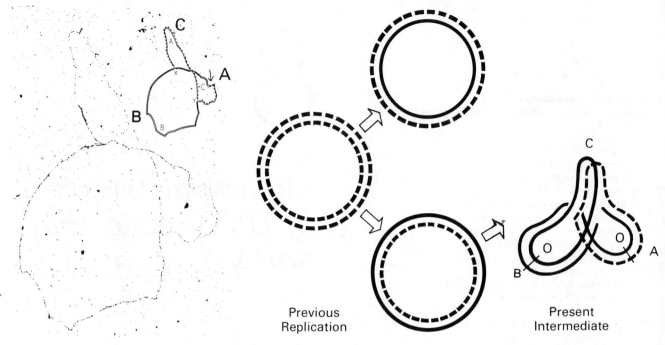

Figure 8–1. Radioautograph of *E. coli* DNA after labeling for about 1.8 generations showing a replicating chromosome with three branches (*A, B,* and *C*). Of these, *B* is probably newly replicated, because it has the highest grain density. A possible interpretation is given. *Dashed lines,* unlabeled strands; *continuous lines,* labeled strands; *O,* possible origin of replication. This type of replicative intermediate is referred to as a **theta** (θ) or **Cairns intermediate.** (Cairns J: Cold Spring Harbor Symp Quant Biol 28:43, 1964)

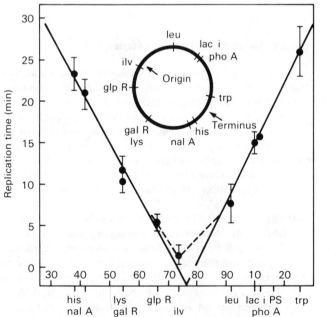

Figure 8–2. Replication of various *E. coli* mutant markers, determined as the moment of highest frequency of induction of mutations by nitrosoguanidine, which acts mostly on sites undergoing replication. For synchronization cells were exposed to nalidixic acid, which halts DNA replication, and then it was removed, which initiates a new wave of replication at the origin. Brief exposure at intervals to nitrosoguanidine then yielded equidistant points of mutagenesis on either side from the origin, which is located at about 80 min on the standard genetic map (see Fig. 7-15). (Modified from Hohlfeld R, Vielmetter W: Nature New Biol 242:130, 1973)

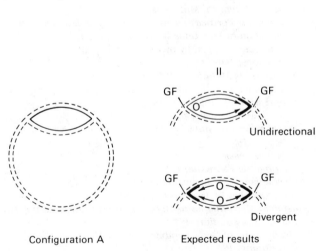

Figure 8–3. Radioautographic evidence for divergent replication of the bacterial chromosome. Synchronous cultures of germinating *Bacillus subtilis* spores at the start of the second round of replication were exposed first to a low concentration of ^{3}H-thymidine and then briefly, before extraction of the DNA, to a high concentration. *(I)* When extracted, the chromosome was in configuration A, where the *continuous lines* indicate radioactive atoms (irrespective of grain density). *(II)* The different positions of the parts with high grain density under the two models of unidirectional or divergent replication are shown; *heavy lines* represent the heavily labeled DNA. Experimental results clearly conformed to the expectations of the divergent replication model. O, origin; GF, growing fork. (Modified from Gyurasitis EB, Wake RG: J Mol Biol 73:55, 1973)

***UNITS OF REPLICATION (REPLICONS).* Chain initiation** and **elongation** require different proteins (as well as shared ones), because at the nonpermissive temperature some *ts E. coli* mutants are blocked in one process and others in the other. Moreover, mutations that block chromosome synthesis do not prevent synthesis of bacteriophage DNA in the same cell, while some *ts* mutations of the F plasmid (Chap. 7) do not affect replication of cellular DNA. These and related findings define units of DNA replication (**replicons**) characterized by specific **origins, initiating proteins,** and **termination mechanisms,** and by separate **elongating proteins.**

ROLE OF MEMBRANE IN REPLICATION. Electron microscopy shows that the bacterial DNA is always attached to the cell membrane, sometimes via a **mesosome** (Chap. 2). The attachment probably occurs at the growing point, because after a short exposure to a radioactive precursor, the DNA just synthesized is found preferentially associated with the membrane fraction when the cell is lysed.

The end of replication occurs at a well-defined **terminus.** Electron microscopy has revealed that the mesosome is then split by localized growth of the membrane, segregating the daughter DNA molecules to the daughter cells. Some large plasmids (Chap. 7) segregate together with the chromosome, suggesting that they are attached to the same mesosome. The cell membrane therefore appears to have a role like that of the mitotic spindle that segregates the multiple chromosomes of higher cells.

MECHANISMS OF REPLICATION OF THE BACTERIAL CHROMOSOME
Initiation

Though DNA sequences can be replicated *in vitro* by a single repair enzyme, DNA polymerase I, replication of the chromosome is a complex process that requires a large number of proteins. Their identification depended on preceding genetic studies in *E. coli:* isolation of various ts mutants for DNA replication (*dna*) defined the set of proteins; extracts of these mutants facilitated *in vitro* **assays;** and **cloning of the replication origin (oriC)** permitted study of initiation *in vitro.*

The **initiation complex** includes the replication origin (*oriC*) and several proteins. The *oriC* is made up of 245 nucleotides, most of which are conserved in related strains, and it contains characteristic sites for binding several proteins, including one that attaches to the membrane.

Twelve proteins are required for *in vitro* initiation. The work of A. Kornberg and others has elucidated the roles of several of them (Fig. 8–4). First, **DnaA protein–ATP complexes** bind to five nine-base pair-long sites in *oriC* (**dnaA boxes**) (see Fig. 8–5) with almost identical sequences, forming a tight complex. **DnaA protein** also evidently binds to membrane, and the latter plays a spe-

cific role, as the recycling of the active protein by release by ADP after ATP hydrolysis requires the presence of membrane containing unsaturated fatty acid residues. Then **DnaB helicase,** binding to three 13-base-pair repeats, becomes associated with the structure to form a longer **prepriming complex,** which includes approximately 50 base pairs of DNA. The role of the helicase is to unwind the duplex DNA using energy from hydrolysis of nucleoside triphosphates; this unwinding allows the attachment of **single-strand binding (SSB) protein,** which keeps the strands separate. Extensive unwinding by the helicase also requires the swivel activity of **DNA gyrase.** The next step is the formation of a **primosome** with the attachment of the **DnaG primase,** which synthesizes the RNA primer while the helicase unwinds the DNA helix ahead of synthesis.

Chain Elongation

While the **leading strand,** which grows in $5' \rightarrow 3'$ direction, has a single primer, the **lagging strand** grows in an **overall** $3' \rightarrow 5'$ direction by initiating separate **Okazaki fragments,** each elongating in $5' \rightarrow 3'$ direction (Fig. 8–6). All RNA primers are extended as DNA by **DNA polymerase III** holoenzyme. After DNA is synthesized the primers are removed (probably by RNase H), the resulting gaps are filled by DNA polymerase I, and the various fragments are joined by polynucleotide ligase.

Initiation causes the formation of **two replication forks,** which proceed in opposite directions under the action of helicase, primase, SSB, and DNA polymerase III. The error rate of *in vivo* replication is very low owing to the **editing function** of DNA polymerase III through its $3' \rightarrow 5'$ exonuclease action on incorrectly paired regions. On the template of the lagging strand, the primosome probably moves ahead of synthesis, periodically building a primer. Finally, the two forks meet at the **terminus** *terC,* which is at about 180° in respect to *oriC* on the circular chromosome. This region also mediates attachment of the chromosome to the cell membrane and determines the partitioning of the daughter genomes to the two daughter cells; its deletion causes segregation of some genome-free cells. The dissociation of the replication machinery at the terminus requires the participation of the **DnaT protein.**

In vivo replication also requires **RNA polymerase** (as well as primase), as shown by its sensitivity to rifampin (Chap. 7). This enzyme apparently destabilizes the helix during local transcription beginning at DnaA-repressed promoters; this allows the productive interaction of DnaA and DnaB proteins (see Fig. 8–4).

Regulation of DNA Replication

In vivo, a new initiation is not linked to termination but occurs after a specific ratio of origins to cell mass is reached; it is thus linked to the growth rate. This regulation depends on the concentration of several proteins,

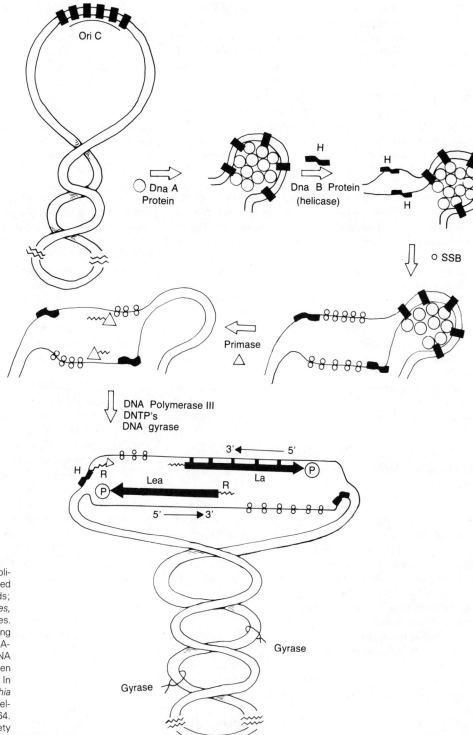

Figure 8–4. Initiation of DNA replication at *oriC* as part of a supercoiled chromosome. *Thin lines,* old strands; *thick lines,* new strands; *wavy lines,* RNA; *black squares,* DnaA boxes. *Lea,* leading strand; *La,* lagging strand; *SSB,* single-stranded DNA-binding protein; Δ, primase; *P,* DNA polymerase III. (Data from McMacken R, Silver L, Georgopoulos C. In Neidhardt FC et al [eds]: *Escherichia coli* and *Salmonella typhimurium:* Cellular and Molecular Biology, p 564. Washington, DC, American Society for Microbiology, 1987)

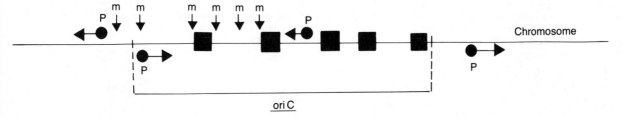

Figure 8–5. Organization of the *E. coli* origin of replication. *Black squares,* DnaA boxes; *P,* promoters; *m,* GATC methylation sites. (Data from McMacken R, Silver L, Georgopoulos C: In Neidhardt FC et al [eds]: *Escherichia coli* and *Salmonella typhimurium:* Cellular and Molecular Biology, p 564. Washington, DC, American Society for Microbiology, 1987)

including DnaA and DnaB, RNA polymerase, and possibly proteins for attachment to the envelope. A requirement for GATC methylation of adenine in **both** strands (see Fig. 8–5) prevents a new initiation until the strand formed in the previous round of replication is methylated, by Dam protein. The need for these constituents explains why initiation is prevented by inhibitors of protein and RNA synthesis; the relation of the limiting factor(s) to cell mass is not clear.

Modifications of DNA; Restriction Endonucleases

Studies of bacteriophage multiplication (see Host Induced Modification and Restriction; Chap. 45) showed that many bacteria contain various **restriction endonucleases,** which cleave DNA at specific short **target sequences.** To prevent autodigestion the cells must also carry a **modifying enzyme,** cognate to their restriction enzyme, that specifically methylates the target sequence and thus protects it against cleavage. The endonucleases have important evolutionary implications, and also important practical applications in DNA cloning (see Gene Manipulation, below).

The **target sequences** for **class II** endonucleases are **palindromes** of between four and ten bases; the enzyme, which is a dimer, cuts the two strands symmetrically within the target (Table 8–1). The two cuts are often staggered, leaving short single-stranded complementary tails (**cohesive ends**); but some enzymes cut both strands at the same place, producing **blunt ends.** The targets for **class I** and **class III** enzymes are not palindromes, and the cuts occur far from the target at a **cleavage** site, which, for class I enzymes, can be as far as 7000 base pairs away.

The type II modifying enzymes generate either N^6-methyladenine or 5-methylcytosine, whereas those of

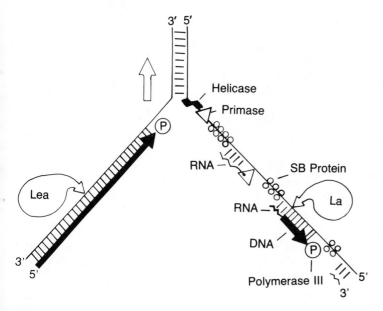

Figure 8–6. Chain elongation. The growing fork moves as shown by the arrow. Synthesis is continuous on the leading strand *(Lea)* and discontinuous on the lagging strand *(La)*. *Heavy line,* newly synthesized chains; *thin lines,* parental strands. (Data from McMacken R, Silver L, Georgopoulos C: In Neidhardt FC et al [eds]: *Escherichia coli* and *Salmonella typhimurium:* Cellular and Molecular Biology, p 564. Washington, DC, American Society for Microbiology, 1987)

TABLE 8–1. *Examples of Some Target Sites and of Various Cutting Modes of Restriction Endonucleases*

Name and Bacterial Species	Target Site*	Type of Ends Produced		
Eco R1	5'-G↓A A T T C-3'	-G-3'	5'-A A T T C-	5'-ended tails
Escherichia coli†	3'-C T T A A G-5'↑	-C T T A A-5'	3'-G-	
Hae 1	5'-Pu G C G C↓Py-3'	-PuG C G C-3'	5'-Py-	3'-ended tails
Haemophilus aegyptius 1	3'-Py↑C G C G Pu-5'	-Py-5'	3'-C G C G Pu-	
Hpa 1	5'-G T T↓A A C-3'	-G T T-5'	3'-A A C-	Blunt ends
Haemophilus parainfluenzae	3'-C A A↑T T G-5'	-C A A-3'	5'-T T G-	

* Arrow are sites of cuts.
† Carrying an *fi⁺* R factor.
P = purine; Py = pyrimidine.

types I and III methylate only adenines. With type I, three subunits of the same enzyme are responsible for recognition, modification, and cleavage.

The genes for Type II and III restriction modification systems are all in plasmids; with some type I systems (such as *Eco B* in *E. coli* B and *Eco K* in *E. coli* K), they are chromosomal.

EVOLUTIONARY CONSIDERATIONS

One biological consequence of restriction is obvious: the destruction of DNA of bacteriophages or plasmids attempting to infect a new host. Hence, restriction may have evolved as a **defense of bacteria** against these parasites, and also as mechanisms of competition among plasmids or phages specifying different restriction endonucleases. In addition, the endonucleases may contribute to genetic variability by promoting insertions within the targets, just as in recombination *in vitro*.

Modification must have evolved as a **defense against autorestriction.** Thus with modified (MM) and unmodified (00) phage f1 DNA, and with artificial heteroduplexes modified in one strand only (0M), a purified enzyme cleaves 00 DNA rapidly but leaves 0M and MM uncleaved. In addition, 0M is rapidly modified to MM, whereas 00 is modified only slowly. Thus, the enzyme respects its own DNA (MM), rapidly destroys foreign DNA (00), and rapidly modifies its own replicating DNA (0M, because the newly made strand is at first unmodified).

Mechanisms of Recombination

Genetic recombination is recognized by analysis of the distribution of markers (identifiable alleles) among the progeny derived from a cross between two parental genomes. We shall examine here the molecular events.

Genetic studies with eukaryotes indicated that classical recombination involves the extremely precise pairing of homologous chromosomes (**synapsis**), for a cross between two different mutants regularly yields the wild-type and the reciprocal recombinant (double mutant) with no other genetic changes in either. Studies in fine-structure genetics in phage or bacteria (Chap. 7) localized the site of recombination between **two adjacent nucleotides.** Thus, if one of the glycines in tryptophan synthetase is replaced by glutamic acid, arginine, or valine, crosses between pairs of these mutants yield a very low frequency of recombinants in which the glycine has been restored (Fig. 8–7). These results would have appeared extraordinary before the genetic code was dis-

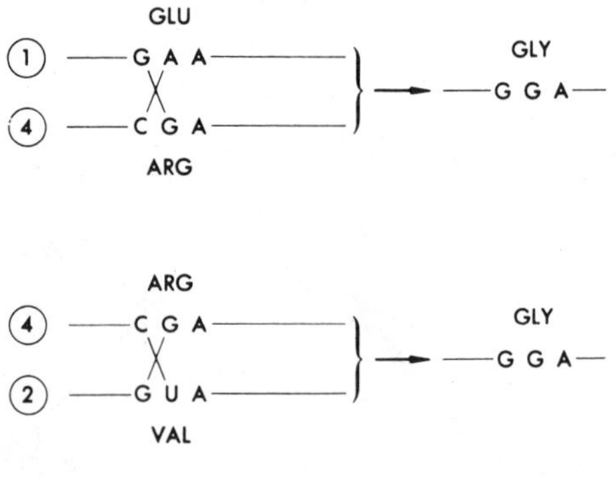

Figure 8–7. Recombination within a codon. The crosses involved three mutants of the A protein of tryptophan synthetase (*numbers on the left*) with different amino acids replacing the glycine. The nucleotide composition of the codons is inferred from the amino acid changes in the mutants and the restoration of glycine in the recombinants. As would be expected from the known codon, the cross of mutants 1 and 2 fails to restore glycine. Recombination is indicated as a reciprocal crossover but may have occurred by gene conversion. (Data from Yanofsky C: Cold Spring Harbor Symp Quant Biol 28:581, 1963)

covered, but they are now easily understood as the consequence of rare recombination **within a codon.**

The **molecular aspects of recombination** have been revealed primarily by a combination of formal genetic analysis in fungi and molecular studies with phages.

CROSSING OVER. The process of crossing over, which is studied by the recombination of **distant markers,** occurs by **breakage and reunion of DNA molecules.** The evidence derives from a classic experiment of Meselson and Weigle with bacteriophage lambda (Fig. 8–8), which also showed the participation of **limited DNA synthesis of the repair type** in recombination. Similarly, in eukaryotes, recombination occurs during meiosis, **after** the DNA has replicated, and it is also accompanied by a small amount of repair synthesis.

DIFFERENT TYPES OF RECOMBINATION

The double strand of DNA allows the original base sequence to be perfectly conserved in crossover because ordinarily only one strand of each parental molecule is broken at any time. In addition, the broken DNA ends are kept together by a complex of proteins. The characteristics of the cuts, and of the mechanism of sequence conservation, distinguish different types of recombination.

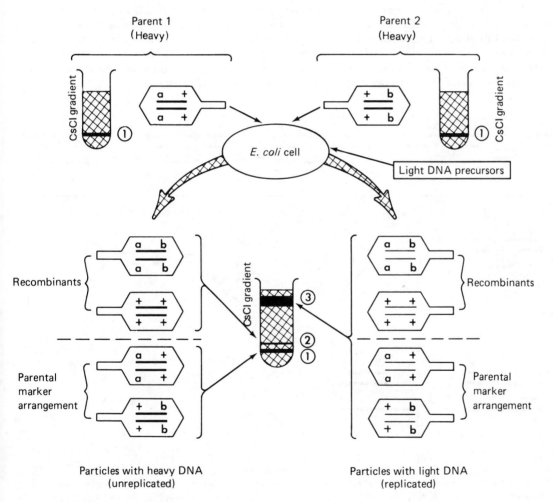

Figure 8–8. Scheme of the Meselson and Weigle experiment showing recombinant formation by breakage and reunion of molecules of phage λ DNA. The experiment involves mixed infection of bacteria with two genetically marked phages *(above)*. These DNAs contain heavy atoms and have a high buoyant density, as determined in CsCl gradients. The bacteria they infect do not contain heavy atoms, so the newly made DNA is of lower buoyant densities. The progeny DNA *(below)* is mostly of light densities *(3)*, but a small proportion *(1)*, retaining the high density of the parental phage, is unreplicated, as shown by the marker arrangement. The most significant fraction is in *(2)*, with intermediate density and recombinant genotype. This DNA derives from parental DNA that underwent recombination by breakage and reunion with progeny DNA.

Generalized Recombination

The generalized type of recombination is initiated by a single strand cut, which in some cases is the consequence of DNA damage or repair (e.g., breaks produced by ionizing radiation, strand incision during excision repair; see below). A specific mechanism is nicking by **exonuclease V,** the product of the *recB, recC,* and *recD* genes. *In vitro* experiments show that nicking preferentially occurs near instigator *Chi* sites, (crossover hotspots, 5'-GCTGGTGG-3'), which occur about every 5000 base pairs in *E. coli* DNA. The enzyme binds to the DNA helix where it is interrupted, such as a natural end or a double-strand cut, even at a considerable distance away, and then travels to the *Chi* site at a great speed (300 base pairs/second), unwinding the DNA ahead and rewinding behind it. The exchanges may occur as much as 10 Kb away from the nick at the *Chi* site, but the frequency decreases with the distance.

After nicking, the **RecBCD** enzyme unwinds the helix, releasing the nicked from the continuous strand (Fig. 8–9,*1*). This separation allows the central step in recombination, **strand invasion,** to take place, catalyzed by the **RecA** protein, which also plays an important role in SOS repair (see Repair of DNA Damage, below). The end of the nicked strand, coated with RecA protein, associates with a duplex DNA (**synapsis**). The association is nonhomologous at first but becomes homologous as the two DNAs slide past each other and come into register. The invading strand forms a helix with the complementary strand of the duplex, displacing the other strand. The helical segment slowly grows in 5' → 3' direction on the invading strand while ATP is hydrolyzed, giving rise to a stretch of **heteroduplex DNA** with one strand from each parental molecule. The process is not blocked by even extensive mismatches such as deletions or insertions of 100 or so bases on one of the DNAs: they will be corrected later (see Repair of DNA Damages, below). (If the invading single-stranded DNA is cyclic it makes a homologous association with a strand of the duplex, but no true helix is formed. This joint is labile and dissolves on removal of the RecA protein.)

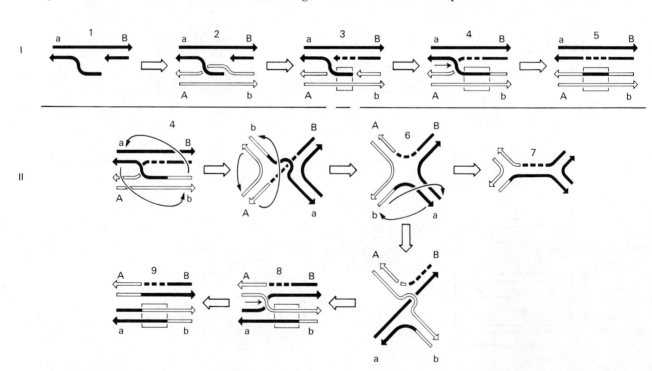

Figure 8–9. Model of reciprocal recombination. *(Panel I) (1)* A DNA duplex carrying markers **a** and **B** is nicked and partially unwound by the *RecBCD* protein. *(2)* The free strand pairs with a complementary sequence of another intact duplex that carries complementary markers **A** and **b.** Such **strand invasion** is facilitated by gyrase, which unwinds the duplex. After assimilation, the recipient duplex is nicked by an endonuclease. *(3)* Elongation of the assimilated strand by a polymerase causes a **strand displacement** in the upper duplex and creates a **heteroduplex segment** *(boxed)* in the lower duplex. *(4)* Covalent attachment of the ends generates an **integrated molecule.** *(5)* Cutting the bridge by an endonuclease *(arrow)* and resealing releases two recombinants with a **heteroduplex patch** and the flanking markers still in parental arrangement (**aB** and **Ab**). *(Panel II)* Intermediate 4 undergoes a series of isomerizations, generating a figure X *(6)*. This generates a different intermediate *(8)*, which, after bridge cutting, produces two molecules *(9)* that are **recombinants for the flanking markers** (**AB** and **ab**) and again contain heteroduplex tracts *(boxed)*. Figures H *(7)* can be generated from 6. (Modified from Meselson MS, Radding CM: Proc Natl Acad Sci USA 72:358, 1975)

The synapsis formed by the invading strand then evolves by a series of events according to the model of Figure 8–9, steps 1 and 2, which is based on the electron microscopic observation of **recombination intermediates** with an X or H shape (Fig. 8–10). Finally, **resolution** of the intermediates, probably carried out by the RecBCD enzyme, yields separate recombinant molecules.

Site-Specific Recombination

The site-specific type of recombination is *recA* independent; the two parental DNAs break and rejoin at sites of very limited homology that are recognized by specific **recombinases.** This process is used especially for inversion of DNA segments (see Phase Variation, below) and for integration of transposons or phage genomes into the bacterial chromosome.

Finally, an **illegitimate recombination,** of obscure mechanism, occurs at a low frequency in the bacterial chromosome using neither extensive homology nor specific sites; it is important as a source of gene duplication and deletion.

CONSEQUENCES OF RECOMBINATION

The model of Figure 8–9 predicts that a segment of **heteroduplex DNA**—with strands from each parent— will be produced by strand invasion at the site of crossing over and that the recombination intermediate can segregate into molecules either with or without recombination of markers at the two sides. The validity of these predictions can be demonstrated in bacteriophage recombination. In cells mixedly infected by wild-type and mutant phage, 1% of the progeny phage are heterozygous for the mutation: on subsequent replication, half of the progeny of such a particle are mutant and half wild type.

With phage DNAs differing at three not closely linked markers (e.g., *ABC, abc*), molecules heterozygous at the middle marker (*Bb*) are frequently recombinant for the outside markers (*Ac* or *aC*), showing the association of heterozygosity with crossing over. The heteroduplex segment is estimated to extend to about 2000 base pairs; hence molecules can be heterozygous for several markers only when these are closely linked. In eukaryotes formation of the heteroduplex DNA in crossing over is indicated by the phenomenon of gene conversion (see below).

The formation of heteroduplex DNA without crossover of flanking markers (**patch recombination**) is frequently observed in fungi and is revealed by gene conversion.

GENE CONVERSION

In recombination between phage genomes distinguished by several markers, more than one crossover may be observed in the same DNA molecule. If these occur independently the frequency of multiple crossovers should equal, as a first approximation, the product of the frequencies of each crossover by itself. With distant markers, this is indeed observed. However, multiple crossovers are considerably more frequent between closely linked markers for which phage DNA molecules are heterozygous. Distant markers flanking this group often do not show enhanced recombination.

The mechanism was revealed by studies in fungi, in which the spores in each ascus (Chap. 11) define the four products resulting from recombination among four

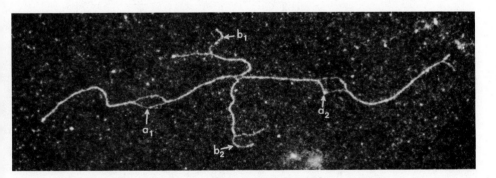

Figure 8–10. Electron micrograph of a recombination intermediate of colicin E1 DNA. After the two partners were linearized by cutting with restriction endonuclease Eco R1, the DNA was spread in the presence of a high concentration of formamide, which denatures AT-rich regions. The local denaturations *(arrows)* allow the identification of homologous regions in the two molecules taking part in recombination. In this intermediate, the homologous arms are characterized, one by an internal *(a),* the other by a terminal *(b)* denaturation; clearly, the homologous arms are in *trans* configuration. This intermediate corresponds to the X figure predicted by the model of Figure 8–9, configuration 6. (Potter H, Dressler D: Proc Natl Acad Sci USA 73:3000, 1976)

chromatids (each a duplex DNA molecule) in one meiosis (Fig. 8–11). In a cross of mutant (m) and wild type (wt), the ratio of mutant to wild type in each ascus is normally 2:2, but occasionally, it is 3:1 or 1:3. This exceptional result, called gene conversion, implies that a part of one chromatid, instead of being exchanged, becomes **changed** to match a chromatid deriving from the other parent, because it replaces one allele by another without recombination of flanking markers. Gene conversion is responsible for almost all recombinations between very closely linked markers in fungi, and possibly in phage and higher organisms as well.

Gene conversion is caused by formation of **heteroduplex DNA** (Fig. 8–12), followed by **correction of its mismatch** (see Repair of DNA Damages, below). Once initiated, a correction may extend to other mismatched sites in nearby hybrid DNA, causing the simultaneous conversion of two or more markers. In support of the proposed mechanism, gene conversion is absent in mutants defective for the endonuclease that initiates correction. Moreover, heteroduplex DNA made *in vitro* by annealing the DNAs of two phage strains differing at several alleles; after transfection into cells the heterozygosity often disappears (i.e. only one allele is recovered in the progeny).

MECHANISMS OF ANTIGENIC VARIATION

Antigenic variation is an important mechanism used by pathogenic microorganisms for escaping the neutralizing activity of antibodies produced by the animal host. The two main mechanisms are site-specific inversion and gene conversion.

Site-Specific Inversion

Regulation of gene expression by inversion of an adjacent sequence is fairly common: it accounts for the re-

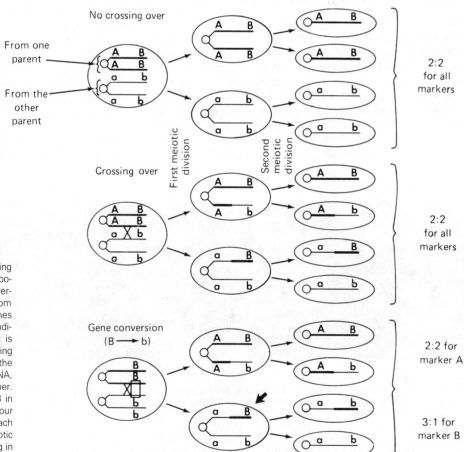

Figure 8–11. Chromatid segregation during meiosis in ascomycetes showing the composition of asci and the effect of gene conversion. The double-stranded chromatids from the two parents are identified by single lines of different thickness. The *boxed area* indicates where gene conversion occurs. It is represented as associated with crossing over, but the association is not required; the *heavy arrow* points to the heteroduplex DNA, with marker B on one strand, b on the other. Mismatch correction then converts the B in one strand to b. Asci are shown with four spores, but often they contain eight, each spore being doubled by a subsequent mitotic division. The events presumably occurring in the boxed area are shown in Figure 8–12.

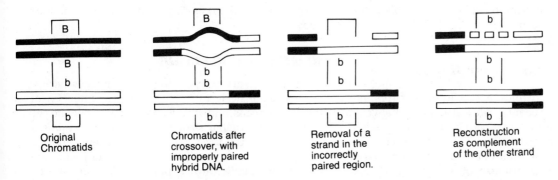

| Original Chromatids | Chromatids after crossover, with improperly paired hybrid DNA. | Removal of a strand in the incorrectly paired region. | Reconstruction as complement of the other strand |

Figure 8–12. Hypothetical molecular events in gene conversion, representing the two chromatids (each a double-stranded helix) of Figure 8–11 *(boxed area).* Incorrect pairing in hybrid DNA *(boxed)* may activate a mismatch-correction mechanism to form a correctly paired DNA, thus eliminating the information of one of the strands.

versible variation of flagellar antigens (**phase variation;** Chap. 7) in *Salmonella* and for change of host range in several bacteriophages (see Mu, Chap. 46). In *Salmonella* flagellin (the protein H antigen) is made in either of two distinct forms, H1 and H2, and a site-specific inversion of a 900-base-pair DNA segment contains the promoter for gene *H2* and also for gene *rh1*, which specifies a repressor of the distant *H1* gene. Figure 8–13 shows how the inversion of that DNA segment (by a mechanism described in Fig. 8–26, below) determines whether H1 or H2 is made. Inversion is specified by gene *hin* (for H inversion) within the inverting segment.

A similar switching system, employing highly homologous recombinases, is responsible for changes in the host range in several bacteriophages (see Mu, Chap. 46).

The exchanges leading to inversion start by pairing at short inverted repeats flanking the inverting segment, to form a stem-loop. The recombinase breaks the DNA chains at the repeats and rejoins them by exchanging partners. This **site-specific recombination** is similar to that of transposon resolvases (see Transposons, below). Inversions are controlled by a protein **factor for inversion stimulation, Fis,** whose binding to **enhancer sequences** (see Chap. 9, Enhancers) increases the frequency of inversion as much as 200-fold.

Flagellar phase variation has a much higher frequency than most mutational changes (ca. 10^{-4}). Moreover, inversions are not simply a source of occasional variation but can be a form of regulation of gene expression at a populational level. Thus in a culture of a cyanobacterium deprived of nitrogen recombinational switching turns on the apparatus of nitrogen fixation in as much as 10% of the cells. The capacity of bacteria for high-frequency recombination in specific regions may also be viewed as a forerunner of the similar, more highly developed, process in the genes for immunoglobulins in vertebrates.

Gene Conversion

Certain human pathogens (*Neisseria gonorrhoeae, Borrelia hermsii*) display dramatic sequential antigenic changes. *N. gonorrhoeae* clones shift the specificity of their pilin (the protein of pili, which mediate adhesion to the urethral mucosa) with a frequency of 10^{-4} to 10^{-3} per cell generation. The organism has one expressed gene for pilin and several silent, defective ones. The transcribed gene readily changes sequence by gene conversion with the silent genes, and sometimes by recombination; the recombination occurs more frequently with DNA fragments transformed from lysed cells than by rearrangement within the chromosome. In trypanosomes

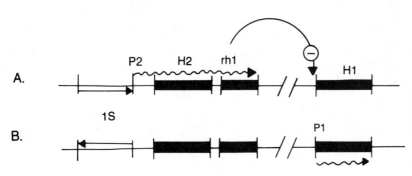

Figure 8–13. Schematic representation of the variation of flagellar antigen in *Salmonella.* The invertible segment *(IS)* contains the promoter *(P).* In orientation *A* it promotes transcription of *H2* and *rh1,* and the latter in turn represses *H1.* In the opposite orientation, *B, H2* and *rh1* are not transcribed, and *H1* is therefore expressed. *Heavy lines,* genes; *wavy lines,* mRNA.

a similar genetic organization leads to even more extensive variation in a coat protein.

DNA Damages and Their Repair

Various physical or chemical agents in the environment, including mutagenic agents, cause structural changes in DNA. Many of these changes are completely repaired, whereas those that are not may result in mutations or in lethal damage. The alterations are of several types: (1) **spontaneous deamination** of 5-methylcytosine to thymidine; (2) **chemical alterations of bases** by deaminating or monofunctional alkylating agents; (3) **dimerization of two adjacent pyrimidines** on the same strand under the action of UV light (here, the connected pyrimidines form either a cyclobutane ring or a pyrimidine–pyrimidone (6–4) dimer [Fig. 8–14]; UV light also causes other, less frequent pyrimidine changes. Dimers block replication, and, by blocking transcription, cause the **functional inactivation of genes** situated beyond the dimer in the same transcription unit); (4) **cross-links** between the two strands, caused mainly by UV and by bifunctional alkylating agents such as mechlorethamine (nitrogen mustard), psoralen in the presence of light, and mitomycin; (5) **breaks** of one or both strands, mostly by ionizing radiations, through the formation of highly reactive radicals in the water surrounding the DNA or by the decay of radioactive atoms (e.g., ^{32}P, ^{3}H) incorporated in the DNA; and (6) **gaps** in the growing strand caused by inhibition of DNA synthesis, which are then widened by exonuclease V, the *recBCD* product (see Recombination, above).

MECHANISMS OF REPAIR

The mechanisms for repairing DNA damages have been studied extensively in *E. coli*; they are similar in other microorganisms and in eukaryotic cells. **Direct repair** restores the original structure; in **indirect repair** a lesion in one strand is bypassed during replication; or is excised and then rebuilt by copying the intact strand; and in **postreplication repair** the damages are eliminated by recombination between the sister strands after replication. The latter two mechanisms repair lesions of many kinds.

Direct Repair

PHOTOREACTIVATION. Photoreactivation was discovered through the observation that parallel platings of a bacterial suspension exposed to UV light yield highly variable numbers of colonies, depending on how long the inoculated plates remain on the laboratory bench before being placed in a dark incubator. The cause is an enzyme that combines specifically with pyrimidine dimers: on irradiation with light of the long-UV or short-visible region, the enzyme cleaves the dimers, restoring the original pyrimidine residues. Photoreactivation occurs with UV-damaged RNA as well as DNA. UV-irradiated virus particles do not contain the photoreactivating enzyme, but in infected cells the cellular enzyme can act on the viral nucleic acid.

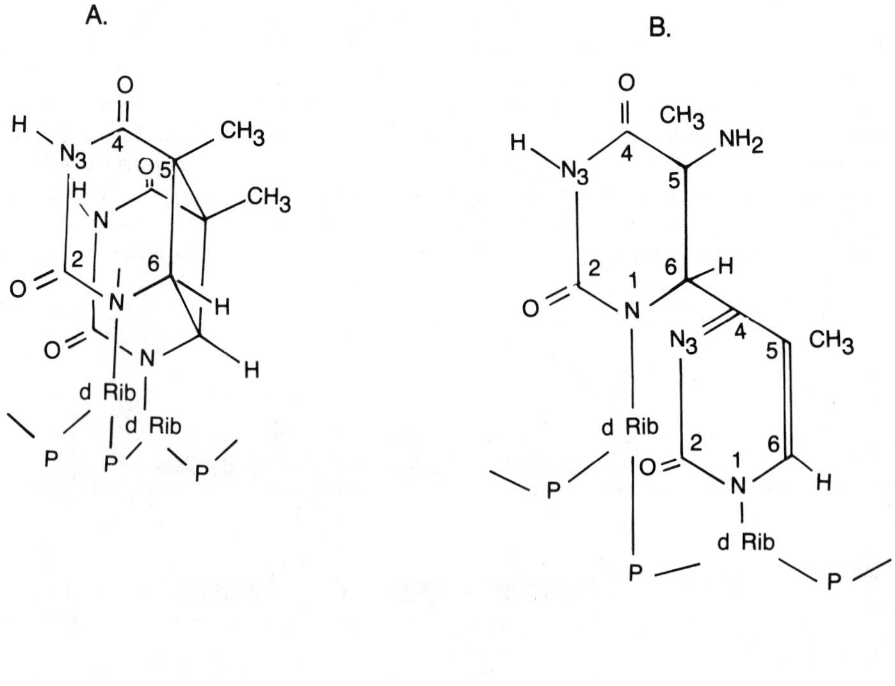

Figure 8–14. Pyrimidine photoproducts produced by UV light. (**A**) Thymine dimer. (**B**) Pyrimidine–pyrimidone (6–4) photoproducts. (**B**, from Franklin WA, Doetsch PW, Haseltine WA: Nucleic Acids Res 13:5317, 1985)

Photoreactivation increases, sometimes enormously, the viable fraction of UV-treated bacteria or viruses. After maximal photoreactivation other, less frequent, damages remain.

ADAPTIVE RESPONSE TO ALKYLATING AGENTS. N-methyl-N'-nitro-N-nitrosoguanidine (MNNG) and similar agents generate strongly mutagenic O-methylated purines and pyrimidines, such as O^6-methylguanine, and also methyl phosphotriesters, in DNA. In their repair a **transferase** irreversibly transfers the methyl group of either lesion to cysteine residues of the enzyme itself; hence one enzyme molecule removes only one methyl group. However, after this **suicidal** action the protein becomes an activator of its own gene (and of several others). This type of direct repair is thus **inducible** becoming more active during exposure to the mutagen.

REMOVAL OF METHYLATED BASES (AP SITES). The protein induced in the adaptive response to alkylating agents also induces gene *alkA*, which specifies DNA glycosylase II. This enzyme and a noninducible glycosylase I release 3-methyl purines and O^2- and O^4-methylpyrimidines from alkylated DNA, thus generating **AP (apurinic and apyrimidinic) sites;** They also remove purines with bulky adducts. The repair is then completed by an **AP endonuclease,** which cleaves the strand at the AP site, allowing resynthesis from the complementary strand by polymerase I.

Indirect Repair: SOS System

Damages that are not directly repaired block chain elongation during replication. The major mechanisms for overcoming this block are provided by the **SOS system,** a set of about 20 **din (damage-inducible)** genes that are normally repressed. Their derepression affects a number of cell functions related to DNA metabolism and to the restoration of DNA synthesis after damage.

All the *din* genes are under negative control of the ***lex A* repressor,** which binds to very similar sequences of about 20 genes (the **SOS box**). Under normal conditions, the repressor is abundant, and the genes are inactive. However, the single-stranded regions or distorted helical segments of damaged DNA, in the presence of the single-strand binding protein (SSB), bind the product of *recA* in a way that changes its conformation: instead of its usual major function in homologous recombination, it now becomes **activated** as a very specific **protease,** cleaving LexA (and also some repressors of prophage induction: Chap. 46). In support of this mechanism, a constitutively activated *recA* mutant (*recA441*) expresses SOS functions in the absence of DNA damage: its RecA protein is activated by single-stranded DNA segments present physio-logically, as in the replicating fork, which do not activate the normal RecA protein.

The major mechanism of repair by the SOS system is **bypass repair.** The oligomeric enzyme specified by genes *umu C,D* adapts DNA polymerase III to the irregular template opposite a lesion such as a pyrimidine dimer, and the result is that the undamaged strand provides the information for both double strands being formed. This synthesis is **error-prone,** for while it depends on polymerase III, the editing function of that enzyme is inhibited.

The SOS System also activates **excision repair.** The **UV endonuclease** specified oligomeric by *din* genes *uvr A,B,C* cuts the altered strand at both sides of lesions produced by UV and other agents, several bases away. The nucleotides between the cuts are removed and then replaced by the action of polymerase I, copying the intact strand. This repair is **not error prone.**

The genes that are derepressed by the elimination of LexA include *recA* and *lexA* themselves. Accordingly, after the damage is repaired normal levels and functions of these proteins are rapidly restored.

The following forms of indirect repair do not involve the SOS system.

MISMATCH REPAIR. Mismatches (noncomplementary bases) arise occasionally either during DNA replication despite the editing function of the polymerase, or during strand completion in recombination (see above). They are repaired by excising a segment of the new strand that includes the mismatch, and then rebuilding the strand. The new strand is not methylated until after a delay, and the enzyme identifies and attacks this strand (rather than its correct partner) because it lacks adenine methylation in GATC sequences (see above, DNA Replication). This type of correction requires the products of the genes *mutH*, *mutL*, *mutS*, and *mutU*: the *mutH* protein probably cleaves the unmethylated GATC sequence, the *mutS* and *mutL* proteins bind to the mismatch, and the *mutU* protein (a helicase) together with SSB protein unwinds the DNA helix between the mismatch and the cleaved GATC sequence. This segment, which can be as much as 1000 bases long, is removed and replaced by new synthesis. In this way, the original sequence is restored. In many organisms GATC sequences are not methylated, and the new strand is identified by transient nicks left during synthesis; this repair is independent of GATC sequences and the *mutH* protein. Mismatch correction increases the fidelity of replication 100- to 1000-fold.

POSTREPLICATION REPAIR. In bacteria in which mutations have eliminated other forms of repair, the presence of even hundreds of pyrimidine dimers per cell may still

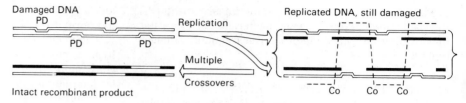

Damaged DNA
PD   PD   Replication   Replicated DNA, still damaged
PD   PD
Multiple
Intact recombinant product   Crossovers   Co   Co   Co

Figure 8–15. Repair of pyrimidine dimers by recombination. When DNA containing dimers *(PD)* replicates the new strands *(heavy lines)* have corresponding gaps. Multiple crossovers *(Co)* between the two daughter helices restore an intact molecule. Evidence for this mechanism was obtained by growing *E. coli* cells in heavy isotopes (^{13}C, ^{15}N). The cells were then irradiated and transferred to light isotopes (^{12}C, ^{14}N) in the presence of ^3H-thymidine. Shortly after irradiation, the label was in short strands of light density; after repair, it was in long strands of density intermediate between light and heavy. Sonication to break the strands produced short pieces, some light, some heavy. (Rupp WD et al: J Mol Biol 61:25, 1971)

not abolish viability, because undamaged regions in either DNA strand may be replicated. Recombination between the newly replicated segments, whose gaps do not usually coincide (Fig. 8–15), results in repair.

FACTORS DETERMINING SENSITIVITY TO DNA-DAMAGING AGENTS

Sensitivity to the lethal effects of UV light is measured by the slope of the survival curve (see Appendix, this chap-

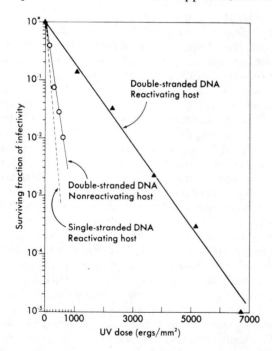

Figure 8–16. UV inactivation of the single-stranded and double-stranded DNA of bacteriophage φX174 (Chap. 45). Each DNA in solution was exposed to increasing doses of UV light and then assayed for infectivity in the dark on spheroplasts of two *E. coli* strains, one capable and the other incapable of carrying out repair. The proportion of the residual titer is plotted against the dose of irradiation. (Data from Yarus M, Sinsheimer RL: J Mol Biol 8:614, 1964. Copyright © by Academic Press Inc. [London] Ltd.)

ter). Repair is very efficient owing to the duplication of the genetic information in the complementary strands: with double-stranded DNA as many as 2500 dimers may be needed for a single lethal hit. In contrast, single-stranded DNA is very sensitive in the dark: it cannot be repaired by dimer excision or by recombination but only by error-prone SOS synthesis during replication (Fig. 8–16). Organisms with double-stranded DNA may become much more sensitive as a result of mutations affecting repair: among these are the *phr*⁻ mutants lacking photoreactivation, which normally can eliminate up to 90% of UV damages; *recA*⁻ mutants; *mut*⁻ mutants defective in mismatch repair; mutations in gene *uvrA,B,C,* which together specify the UV endonuclease; and ligase-deficient mutants, which cannot carry out reconstruction.

Mutations

CLASSES OF CHANGE IN DNA SEQUENCE

The changes in various kinds of mutations can be precisely identified in terms of base sequences in DNA and amino acid sequences in the protein. The DNA changes include **nucleotide replacements, deletions, insertions,** and **rearrangements** (Table 8–2). Among replacements, in **transitions,** a purine is replaced by a purine and a pyrimidine by a pyrimidine (e.g., AT → GC), whereas in **transversions,** a purine is replaced by a pyrimidine and vice versa (e.g., AT → TA or CG) (Fig. 8–17). **Shifts of the reading frame** are secondary to the insertion or deletion of, usually, a single nucleotide.

Nucleotide replacements, **single-nucleotide** deletions, and even large insertions, are **point mutations;** i.e., they all give wild-type recombinants with each other, and they undergo true reversion through appropriate replacements, insertions, or deletions. However, **larger deletions** give wild-type recombinants only with other strains that can replace the entire deleted region, and they do not revert. Because of this genetic stability, they

TABLE 8–2. *Main Properties of Different Kinds of Mutations*

Nature of Nucleic Acid Change	*Effect on Coding Properties*	*Recombinational Behavior*	*Production of Reversions*	*Consequences for Protein*		*Other Properties*
				Structure	*Function*	
Nucleotide replacement	Missense	Point mutation	Yes	Amino acid substitution	1. None 2. Temperature-sensitive 3. Lost	CRM may be present
	Nonsense	Point mutation	Yes	Premature termination of polypeptide chain	Usually lost	Extragenic suppression
Microdeletion: microinsertion		Point mutation	Yes	Frameshift	Usually lost	Intragenic suppression
Insertion		Point mutation	Yes	Altered	Usually lost	May introduce terminator codons
Deletion		Segment	No	Altered	Usually lost	
Silent				1. No amino substitution 2. Amino acid substitution with little effect on overall structure	Conserved	

CRM = Cross-reacting material.

are especially useful for metabolic and genetic studies where reversions would interfere.

These properties afford criteria for the recognition of various kinds of mutations. Most difficult to recognize are insertions, which behave formally like point mutations (i.e., they can revert). They can be distinguished readily only if the inserted DNA has special properties (e.g., contains recognizable genes). In addition, with small DNAs, electron microscopy shows unpaired areas

in **heteroduplexes** formed by a deletion or an insertion mutant and a wild-type DNA strand.

CONSEQUENCES OF MUTATIONS FOR PROTEIN STRUCTURE

Mutational consequences are outlined in Table 8–2. Among the replacements, **missense mutations** cause the substitution of one amino acid for another; the protein may remain functional (although often with quantitative alterations) if the substitution does not markedly affect its tertiary structure or its active site. Altered enzymes often exhibit increased sensitivity to heat denaturation even at normal temperature, causing *ts* mutations. Other altered enzymes lose function while remaining recognizable immunologically as a **cross-reacting material** (CRM). **Nonsense (terminator) mutations** prematurely terminate the growing peptide chain, almost always destroying its function.

A **shift of the reading frame** causes the production of a **jumbled distal sequence;** the resulting loss of function can be corrected by another shift in the opposite direction if the jumbled region is small and not in a critical position (Fig. 8–18). **Larger deletions** destroy function except in rare cases when they remove small unessential parts of proteins. Deletions at the boundary between two genes, if in frame, cause the two polypeptide chains to be synthesized as a single chain (**gene fusion),** often with partial retention of one or both functions. **Insertions,** usually caused by transposons (see

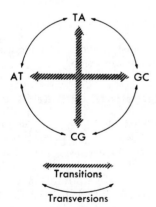

Figure 8–17. Classes of nucleotide replacement. When a mutation substitutes one nucleotide for another in a strand, at the next replication, the new nucleotide is paired with its regular partner. The resulting pair is represented. Example: if, in the upper TA pair, T is replaced by C, the result is the lower CG pair. Note that each base pair can undergo one kind of transition and two kinds of transversions.

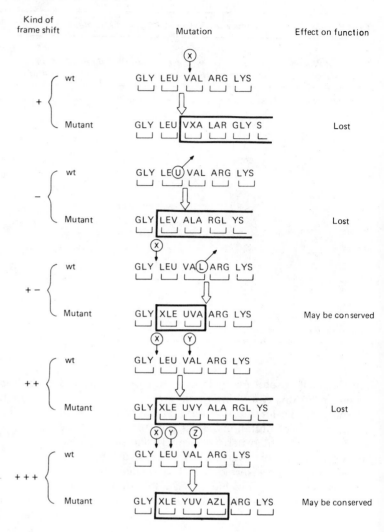

Figure 8–18. Effect of frameshifts on a sequence of bases that are read three at a time from the left. The sequences are arbitrary, but in order to emphasize the consequences of frameshifts, the three letters in each codon *(underlined)* are the first letters of amino acids (glycine, leucine, valine, arginine, lysine). **Plus frameshift** means the insertion, and **minus** the deletion, of a nucleotide. The scheme shows that two mutations of opposite signs can correct each other except for the region between them, two of the same sign cannot, but three of the same sign can. The *heavy lines* indicate the abnormal region. If these stretches are short, the function of the gene may be conserved.

below) or prophages (Chap. 46), frequently destroy the function of the protein; moreover, when they introduce terminator codons, they affect the expression of distal genes (**polarity,** Chap. 9).

INDUCTION OF MUTATIONS

The induction of mutations by a **mutagenic agent** was first shown in 1927 by Muller applying x-rays to the fruit fly *Drosophila*. With bacteria, which do not require the penetrating power of x-rays, the more convenient UV irradiation is equally effective. Powerful chemical mutagens were subsequently discovered. In addition, through the selection of rare mutants from large populations of bacteria, a slight mutagenic action was later demonstrated for many chemicals (e.g., formaldehyde, caffeine, Mn^{2+}) and even for elevated temperature. Bacteria thus provide sensitive test systems for detecting potential environmental human mutagens.

ACTION OF CHEMICAL MUTAGENS

Chemical mutagens fall into several main groups in relation to the DNA change they cause: (1) base analogue; (2) deaminating agents; (3) alkylating agents; and (4) acridine derivatives. The alkylating agents may be monofunctional (attacking one DNA strand) or bifunctional (and hence able to cross-link two strands). Additional agents, of less significance, include Mn^{2+} and formaldehyde. Some agents (base analogues, acridines, Mn^{2+}) **require replication for their action** because they affect only the product of replication, whereas the chemically reactive agents and radiation cause mutations **even in a nonreplicating template,** including transforming DNA or phage DNA *in vitro*. However, a very reactive, strongly mutagenic alkylating agent, **nitrosoguanidine, acts only on cells;** it interacts with single-stranded regions at the growing fork of replicating DNA and thus produces mutations in closely linked clusters.

We shall now consider the mechanisms by which these agents cause mutations.

Mutations Formed During Repair of DNA Damage

Errors arising from the inducible SOS system are responsible for most mutations induced by UV light, x-rays, or ³²P decay, as well as by some carcinogens and cross-linking agents. The importance of this system is shown by the requirement for active *recA*, *lexA*, and *umuC/D* genes (see SOS System, above) for the production of mutations, and by the phenomenon of **Weigle mutagenesis:** a high frequency of mutations in the progeny of phage lambda (Chap. 46) grown in cells irradiated with UV light (hence activating the SOS system) before being infected. Some plasmids, such as pKM101, express genes that enhance SOS repair even without DNA damage. Their presence increases the sensitivity of the Ames test for mutagens (see below). In contrast, excision repair mediated by the *uvrABC* genes or by the AP endonuclease has high fidelity and rarely causes mutations.

Studies with genes of known sequence show that most mutations induced by UV and other agents through the SOS system occur at the sites of lesions and are concentrated at some sites (**hot spots**), which depend on the mutagen used.

Induction of Mutations by Mispairing

Certain base analogues, such as **5-bromouracil** (5-BU) or its deoxynucleoside 5-bromodeoxyuridine (5-BUdR), cause **transitions.** In growing cells these analogues are converted to the corresponding nucleoside triphosphates and can be incorporated into DNA in place of thymine (T). Indeed, 5-BU so closely resembles T that its substitution for as much as 90% of the T in bacteriophages is compatible with subsequent normal replication. However, it tends to undergo a transient internal rearrangement (**tautomerization**) from the keto to the enol state, in which it mispairs with G instead of with A (Fig. 8–19). (In addition, exposure to blue or UV light causes strand breaks at the sites of incorporation.) **2-Aminopurine** also causes transitions, its tautomerization causing it to be read as either A or G.

The tautomerization of 5-BU within the DNA causes **replication errors,** which are expressed as mutations at the next generation when the two strands separate. In addition, its tautomerization in the triphosphate precursor can cause it to be recognized as though it were dCTP, leading to an **incorporation error,** which is expressed immediately. Because of this double action, 5-BU can

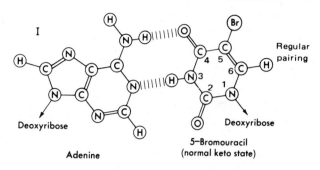

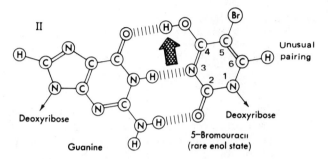

Figure 8–19. Regular and unusual base pairing of 5-BU. *(I)* Regular base pairing (in the common keto form) with adenine. *(II)* Base pairing (in rare enol form) with guanine; the *heavy arrow* indicates the displacement of the proton in the tautomerization of 5-BU.

induce **reversion** of the mutations that it has produced (Fig. 8–20). Hence, mutations of unknown origin can be defined operationally as transitions if 5-BU induces them to undergo true reversion.

Several **reactive mutagens** (which do not require growth) induce more selective transitions. **Nitrous acid** (Fig. 8–21) deaminates A to hypoxanthine (which resembles G) and C to U. **Hydroxylamine** specifically converts C to a derivative that pairs with A, producing a GC → AT transition, which is not reversed by hydroxylamine. **Monofunctional alkylating agents,** such as ethyl ethanesulfonate (EES), produce a similar transition, primarily through formation of O⁶-methylguanine, which mispairs with T instead of C. **Heat** produces GC → AT transitions by deaminating C to U.

Mutations Induced by Intercalation

Acridine derivatives cause **reading frameshifts** by intercalating between DNA bases. Usually only one base is skipped or inserted in the new strand. Unknown mutations can be identified as frameshifts if they can be reversed by acridine or by a second frameshift (Fig. 8–18) but not by mutagens of the preceding groups.

These mutations preferentially affect replicating DNA, which has single-strand gaps, and their frequency is increased when the closing of gaps is slowed by

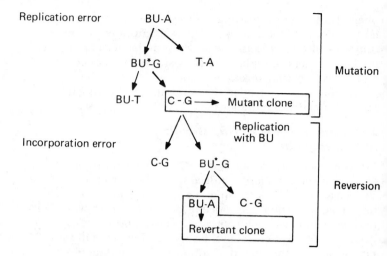

Figure 8–20. Induction of mutations and their reversions by 5-BU: an incorporation error corrects a previous replication error. The sequence can be inverted, a replication error correcting a previous incorporation error. *BU**, transient enol form.

mutational impairment of DNA ligase. They also seem to require the presence of **short runs of the same base pair,** which promote **illegitimate** (i.e., shifted) **pairing** of a free end and the uninterrupted strand (Fig. 8–22). As is suggested in the model of this figure, the intercalated acridine may act by stabilizing the temporary illegitimate pairing until the gap is closed.

Deletions

The ends of many deletions coincide with the end of repeated sequences, either with the same orientation or in opposite orientations, suggesting that they are produced by recombination between regions of homology at different sites in a chromosome. Deletions may also result from **cross-links** between the complementary strands, under the action of nitrous acid, bifunctional alkylating agents, or irradiation. Apparently, a segment of DNA around the cross-link is not replicated, while the segments on either side replicate and join with each other. Excision of transposable elements, along with adjacent segments (see below), is also an important cause of deletions.

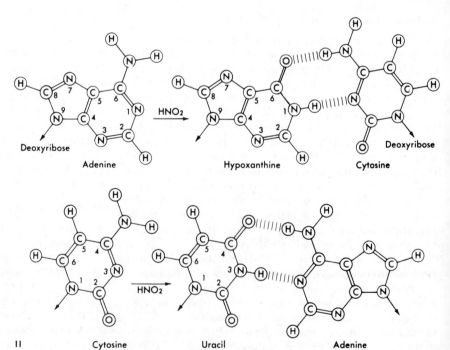

Figure 8–21. Oxidative deamination of DNA by nitrous acid and its effects on subsequent base pairing. *(I)* Adenine is deaminated to hypoxanthine, which pairs with cytosine instead of with thymine. *(II)* Cytosine is deaminated to uracil, which pairs with adenine instead of with guanine.

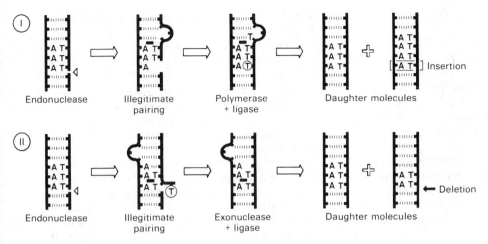

Figure 8–22. Possible mechanism of frameshift by acridines at sites of single-base reiterations near a single-strand break. The intercalated acridine molecules (*thick lines* between base pairs) would stabilize the illegitimate pairing long enough to allow repair, leading to base insertion (*I*) or deletion (*II*).

INFLUENCE OF SITE ON THE FREQUENCY OF MUTATIONS. The presence of mutational hot spots shows that the sequence surrounding a certain base has a determining effect by controlling the probability either of damage or of its repair. It seems that the former effect plays the predominant role, for *uvr B⁻* mutants, which do not carry out excision repair, have the same hot spot distribution as wild-type cells.

SPONTANEOUS MUTATIONS

Studies of sequences show that spontaneous mutations are mostly frameshifts, deletions, and transversions. They are produced by various mechanisms, including the imperfect fidelity of replication, and also limited background activation of the SOS system; the constitutively activated SOS product in a *recA* mutant increases their rate. Background mutagens (radiation, chemicals) appear to play only a small role.

Mutations Affecting Mutability

Certain mutations increase or decrease the spontaneous mutation rate in bacteria and in phage. These **mutator** mutations alter proteins that participate in DNA repair or in replication—for example, the editing function of the DNA polymerase. In *E. coli* these mutations favor TA → GC transversions.

These findings help explain the large variations in the proportion of G + C observed among different organisms, for after the introduction of a mutator gene with TA → GC bias in an *E. coli* strain the proportion of G + C increased about 0.5% in 1500 generations. The viable substitutions must occur where they have acceptable consequences for the proteins; i.e., mostly in the third bases of codons.

The ease of isolation of mutants with an increased or a decreased mutation rate suggests that **natural selection favors some intermediate value** of the rate. This value is correlated, in various organisms, with the size of the genome (Table 8–3), so that the **rate per genome, rather than per nucleotide,** is relatively constant. An advantage of higher mutation rates under some circumstances has been demonstrated by chemostat experiments (Chap. 3, Fig. 3–4), in which an *E. coli* mutator strain outgrew the wild type.

TABLE 8–3. Spontaneous Mutation Rates in Different Organisms

Organism	AT Base Pairs per Genome	Mutation Rate per AT Base Pair Replication	Total Mutation Rate per Genome
Bacteriophage λ	4.8×10^4	2.0×10^{-8}	1.2×10^{-3}
Bacteriophage T4	1.8×10^5	1.7×10^{-8}	3.0×10^{-3}
Salmonella typhimurium	4.5×10^6	2.0×10^{-10}	0.9×10^{-3}
E. coli	4.5×10^6	2.0×10^{-10}	0.9×10^{-3}
Neurospora crassa	4.5×10^7	0.7×10^{-11}	2.9×10^{-4}
Drosophila melanogaster	2.0×10^8	7.0×10^{-11}	1.4×10^{-2}
E. coli with a mutator mutation	2.0×10^6	3.5×10^{-6}	

(Data from Drake JW: Nature 221:1132, 1969)

SUPPRESSION OF MUTATIONS

Reversion of mutations by suppression has been briefly discussed in Chapter 7. A number of mechanisms have been identified.

1. **Nonsense suppressors.** As was discussed in Chapter 6 (Fig. 6–9), altered tRNAs, which insert various amino acids at a specific nonsense (terminator) codon, allow translation to continue beyond a nonsense mutation.

2. **Missense suppressors** also alter the anticodon of a tRNA so that it reads an incorrect codon. When this error in translation inserts an effective amino acid at a site where a mutation has made a protein defective, it restores function. Members of this class are theoretically possible in great variety, but they are encountered only infrequently. Most of them replace a larger amino acid by glycine, whose unobtrusive presence is apparently more easily tolerated than other substitutions.

3. **Frameshift suppressors.** Frameshift mutations cause garbled downstream translation (see Fig. 8–18), but when an extra base has been added to a codon, a mutant tRNA that reads that sequence of four bases (as a result of an extra base in its anticodon) restores translation.

4. **Generalized translational suppressors** are not codon-specific, like the above mechanisms: they increase misreading randomly by altering the ribosome (see Chap. 6, Ribosomal Ambiguity).

5. **Metabolic suppressors** may supply or bypass the function of an inactivated enzyme by altering the specificity or increasing the concentration of another enzyme. Alternatively, when an enzyme has reduced affinity for its substrate or cofactor, a second mutation that increases the concentration of that ligand may restore function. Metabolic suppressors are infrequent and are **gene-specific** rather than codon-specific.

6. **Polarity suppressors** alter transcription termination factor Rho, thus reversing the effect of some mutations that cause premature termination. They will be discussed in Chapter 9.

7. **Subunit complementation** is an important class of **gene-specific** suppressions involving conformational interactions between proteins that form stable complexes (many enzymes; ribosomes). We have already noted that mutations in two different subunits in a complex enzyme can yield normal function in a heterozygote (complementation), whereas mutations in two different sites in the same subunit do not. However, in the homodimers formed in the latter, the conformational effects of the two mutant polypeptides on each other sometimes restore partial function. A similar compensation may arise between functionally interacting proteins. For example, altered leader sequences (see Chap. 6) can be compensated for by alterations in a protein involved in their translocation.

8. **Intracodon suppressors,** one type of intragenic suppressor, may restore the original amino acid (but not the original DNA sequence) by yielding a synonym of the original codon, thus creating a **silent mutation;** or they may yield a codon for another amino acid, similar enough to the original to restore function to the protein.

9. Another intragenic suppressor, **amino acid replacement at a distant site** in the same polypeptide as the primary mutation, can sometimes restore an attraction or a repulsion required for proper folding.

10. A second **frameshift mutation** in the same gene can suppress the effect of a first if it is opposite in direction and if the changes in the segment between the two mutations do not destroy function (see Fig. 8–18).

IN VITRO MUTAGENESIS

After many decades in which geneticists could enrich their supply of mutants only by random mutagenesis, in which only a tiny fraction of the mutants would be in any desired region, the dream of directed mutagenesis has been fulfilled. **Mutations within a restricted target** (but at random bases) are often obtained by first **generating a single-stranded region** and then introducing mutations, either by sodium bisulfite (which deaminates C to U in single-stranded but not double-stranded DNA) or by using a mutagenic polymerase, such as reverse transcriptase, to fill the gap. The required single-stranded target can be created around a known restriction endonuclease site by exposing the DNA to the enzyme in the presence of ethidium bromide, which intercalates between successive bases and limits the action of the endonuclease to cutting a single strand ("nicking") rather than both. The gap is then widened by exonuclease treatment. After exposure to bisulfite and then repair of the gap, the DNA contains mutations at random sites within the target.

In another approach, not requiring recognition by a restriction enzyme, the DNA is exposed in the presence of RecA protein to a **single-stranded oligodeoxynucleotide** with the same sequence as the site. As in strand invasion (see Recombination, above), the oligonucleotide anneals to its complementary strand, exposing the other, unpaired strand to mutagenesis.

A third approach is to **mutagenize a synthetic double-stranded oligonucleotide** with a reactive mutagen such as nitrous acid or hydroxylamine and then introduce it into the homologous gene by *in vitro* recombination (see below).

In a related method, a generalized transducing lysate is heavily mutagenized or is prepared from heavily mutagenized cells, and transductants that have incorporated a selectable marker (which may be a transposon; see below) in a desired region are obtained. In these transductants, any gene closely linked to the selected marker has a high probability of having acquired a mutation.

Even more localized mutations are obtained by **synthesizing a single-stranded sequence** from a gene of interest but with one base difference. A vector carrying the gene is separated into single strands, the oligonucleotide is annealed to the complementary strand, and the remaining single-stranded part is copied with polymerase. The double-stranded vector is introduced into a host cell, where its replication segregates a mutant and a wild-type molecule.

DNA REPAIR AND MUTAGENESIS IN HIGHER ORGANISMS

Repair

Repair mechanisms capable of removing damages produced by UV light or by certain carcinogenic agents (such as N-acetyl-2-acetylaminofluorene) have been recognized in higher organisms. Exposure of cells to carcinogens or UV light probably induces error-prone repair, as it increases the infectivity of UV-irradiated viruses.

The significance of DNA repair in humans is dramatically demonstrated in patients with the rare fatal autosomal recessive disease **xeroderma pigmentosum.** Homozygotes for this gene have defects of various types in the repair of UV damage. Complementation tests, carried out by measuring repair in heterokaryons (obtained by fusing cells of two individuals), identify at least nine complementation groups, affecting incision, recognition of AP sites, photoreactivation, or postreplication repair. Repair defects have also been recognized in homozygotes of other recessive hereditary diseases: ataxia telangiectasica, Fanconi's anemia, and Bloom's disease. Individuals affected by all these diseases frequently develop cancers, probably as a result of somatic mutations during error-prone repair.

Mutagenesis

Most work in higher organisms has been carried out with ionizing radiation because of its ability to penetrate. Some mutagenic chemicals, such as alkylating agents, are also active, but others may not reach the DNA in germ cells. Some mutagens require **metabolic activation.** In the **Ames test,** the mutagenic activity of such compounds is measured by using bacterial strains with auxotrophic mutations of different classes, plus mutations that decrease repair and a plasmid with a mutation that enhances SOS response. The bacteria are incubated with the test substance in the presence of a liver extract to carry out the metabolic activation; in this way even labile mutagenic intermediates can be recognized. With this system many carcinogens score as mutagens, suggesting that **somatic mutations** cause cancer.

Exposure to chemicals with potential mutagenic action, and the relation between mutagenesis and carcinogenesis, are serious problems for human health, but are easily exaggerated. Low-level exposure to mutagens is inevitable: the Ames test reveals their presence in many food plants, and in the pyrolysis products of browning in cooking.

Transposable Elements

Cells contain a variety of transposable elements that can become inserted at many places in the bacterial chromosome, and can be excised, by **site-specific recombination.** An important feature is that after transposing with high frequency under some conditions they become quite stable under others.

Transposable elements are not replicons, for they lack an origin of replication. Nevertheless, during transposition, they are usually **duplicated,** leaving the original element intact and inserting a copy elsewhere and thus increasing the total number in the cell. In this transfer, an enzyme (**transposase**) specified by a gene of the element itself interacts with its ends and with target sequences in the recipient DNA. The enzymes of different transposable elements recognize different targets, which differ in abundance.

Transposable elements are important in several ways. They provide valuable tools for genetic studies in microorganisms; they contribute rather large steps in evolution; and they mobilize drug resistance genes for transfer to other bacteria (Chap. 7).

Insertion sequences (ISs), the simplest transposable elements, were discovered as mutagens, whose transposition into a gene usually inactivates it. They are rather short (150–1500 base pairs), with inverted repeats of 15 to 40 base pairs at the ends; hence on denaturation and self-annealing, they generate "lollipop" figures (Fig. 8–23). Large ISs contain the gene for the transposase. **Transposons** are larger and contain additional genes, often for antibiotic resistance.

Prokaryotic transposons belong to three classes. **Class I** are bounded by two ISs (which can also be transposed separately). The ISs contain the transposition genes, while the intervening DNA contains selectable genes (e.g., for resistance to toxic substances or for prototrophy). For example, Tn10 carries a gene for tetracycline resistance and Tn5 one for kanamycin resistance. **Class II transposons** are bounded by two short repeats, 30 to 40 base pairs long, instead of terminal ISs. Tn3, with a gene for ampicillin resistance, is an example. **Class III**

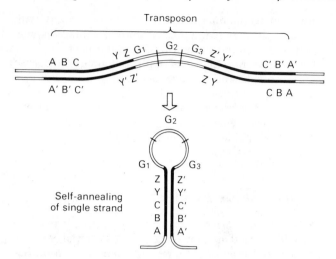

Figure 8–23. Complex transposon. Self-annealing of the inverted ISs *(heavy lines)* on one strand produces the "lollipop" figure visible in electron micrographs, with the bacterial genes (G1–G3) in the single-stranded loop. *AB . . . Z,* nucleotide sequence; *A'B' . . Z',* its complement.

transposons are phages and are discussed in Chapter 65.

MECHANISM OF TRANSPOSITION

Some transposons (e.g., Tn7) can integrate essentially at a single site, like the lambda bacteriophage genome (see Chap. 46), causing the appearance of **hot spots** for transposition. Others (e.g., Tn10) integrate at many sites, which are related in sequence. Finally, others (such as IS1) integrate almost anywhere, although they prefer certain sequences.

Transposition can give rise to **simple insertions** or to **cointegrates** (Fig. 8–24). In simple insertion a conservative transposition displaces the transposon from its location to a new location without replication (Fig. 8–24A). In cointegrate formation (Fig. 8–24B), each strand of the transposon is copied, resulting in two complete copies separated by a host chromosome segment and integrated in **direct orientation** (i.e., reading in the same direction). When a transposon on a plasmid (a cyclic replicon) transposes in this way onto another plasmid it causes fusion of the two plasmids, to form a longer plasmid with a copy of the transposon at each junction.

Transposons integrated at the new location are usually flanked by a duplication of a short segment of host DNA (Fig. 8–24B). They can be precisely excised by the transposase, as shown by the reactivation of a gene inactivated by the insertion. The duplication occurs because transposition initiates with two staggered nicks in the target replicon, five to ten base pairs apart, and a nick at each end of the transposon in the donor replicon; after joining, the segment originally between the nicks in the target is duplicated (Fig. 8–25). The nicking–joining event is caused by the replicon's transposase.

Transposons of class II can **resolve** the cointegrate, regenerating the two original replicons but each now containing the transposon (see Fig. 8–24). In this way, the transposon spreads and increases in number. Resolution can occur by homologous recombination catalyzed by RecA protein, or by a **resolvase** specified by a transposon gene. The resolvase produces a reciprocal recombination only between specific *res* sites of the two transposons present on the same DNA chain. It acts like a transposase: the enzyme uses the energy from a cleaved phosphodiester bond to make a new bond. Two transposons on a **cyclic plasmid** can be resolved when they are in the same orientation, but if the plasmid is linearized by a double-strand cut they can be in either orientation. The difference derives from the complex interwrapping of the two transposons in the synaptic intermediate and the topological constraints of cyclic molecules: resolution of a cyclic plasmid generates two interlinked plasmids, each carrying a copy of the transposon.

The transposing activity is self-regulated. In class II transposons the start of the resolvase gene overlaps the *res* site, whose binding of the resolvase inhibits **transcription.** With class I transposons, if many copies are present their products inhibit **translation** of the transposase messenger (**multicopy inhibition**). Transpositions are therefore frequent when a transposon penetrates a naive host, and it then becomes **self-repressed,** much like the transfer of many conjugative plasmids (Chap. 7).

CONSEQUENCES OF TRANSPOSITION

Transposons may have **positive functional consequences** for the host cells by introducing new genes. They also may **inactivate a host gene,** by interrupting a coding sequence, or by terminating transcription or translation upstream. (The gene can be reactivated by precise excision of the transposon.) Finally, transposons can **activate** neighboring genes by initiating transcription. In this function some transposons act as **switches** for adjacent genes by **reversible recombination between inverted repeats:** in one direction, they initiate transcription; in the other, they either fail to initiate it or terminate it (Fig. 8–26).

Transposons also have broader effects on gene arrangements, which derive from the mechanism of transposition (see Fig. 8–24).

1. A transposon introduced into a plasmid will allow its subsequent **integration** into the cellular chromosome (as in the fusion of two plasmids) flanked by two copies of the transposon.

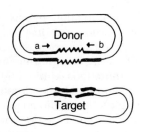

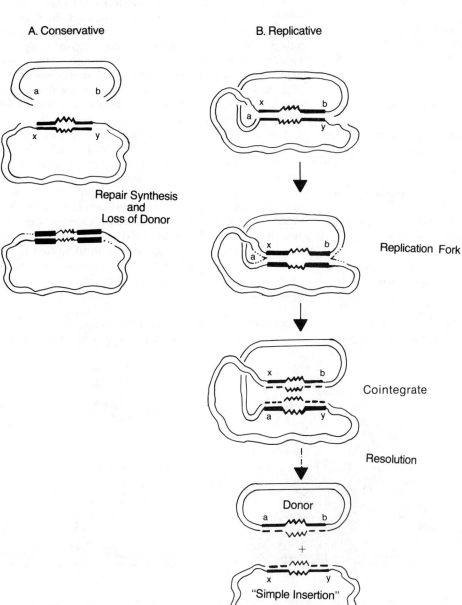

A. Conservative

B. Replicative

Repair Synthesis
and
Loss of Donor

Replication Fork

Cointegrate

Resolution

Donor

+

"Simple Insertion"

Figure 8–24. Model of transposition. *(A)* Simple integration (conservative transposition). *(B)* Cointegrate formation (replicative transposition). Some transposons can resolve the cointegrate. *Heavy lines* between a and b, transposon in donor; *arrows,* terminal repeats; *x, y,* cuts in the target. (Modified from Berg CM, Berg DE. In Neidhardt FC et al [eds]: *Escherichia coli* and *Salmonella typhimurium:* Cellular and Molecular Biology, p 1071. Washington, DC, American Society for Microbiology, 1987)

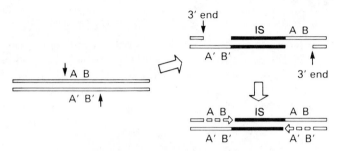

Figure 8–25. Simplified mechanism of insertion of a transposon *(heavy lines)* causing a direct repeat of the host sequences AB/A'B' by formation of two staggered nicks, followed by insertion and filling of the gaps.

2. A transposon inserted into the chromosome may transpose itself to a neighboring target in the chromosome, giving rise to a **duplicative inversion.** This is probably the mechanism by which simple transposons of class I become complex transposons, containing additional genes.

3. A transposon may also **generate a deletion** by being excised along with adjacent DNA.

4. Such excisions may also **mobilize an adjacent plasmid,** along with chromosomal genes (see F' agents, Chap. 7).

5. Homologous recombinations between copies of a transposon may cause **deletion** or **duplication** of intervening chromosomal sequences.

GENETIC APPLICATIONS. Several properties of transposons have made them invaluable tools for genetic studies and genetic manipulation. In particular, transposons are stable after insertion, can inactivate or activate a gene, are easily selected as carriers of drug resistance, and can be used to produce a high frequency of mutation without multiple mutations within a cell. (With chemical mutagens or radiation multiple mutations are not rare, and so the multiple phenotypic changes observed in a mutant may or may not all be due to the same mutation.)

Transposition can be used to link a selectable marker (drug resistance) to any genes of interest. Such strains can then be used for efficiently transferring nonselectable genes, and for obtaining specific regions of DNA for localized mutagenesis (see *In Vitro* Mutagenesis, above). Even more, in a **genomic library** of such a strain (see Molecular Cloning, below), clones carrying the desired gene can be isolated by a probe for the transposon (**transposon tagging**).

For example, in an amber suppressor host strain (Chap. 6) Tn10 can be maintained in a "suicide" phage, with amber mutations in essential genes; and when this phage infects a nonsuppressor strain only these cells that have integrated the transposon into the chromosome will display tetracycline resistance. Among these, strains in which the insertion has inactivated a desired gene are readily identified. Alternatively, those in which Tn10 is adjacent to that gene can be identified by cotransduction, in which the desired gene complements a defective recipient, while the transposon introduces drug resistance.

EUKARYOTIC TRANSPOSONS. Transposons are present in organisms of every kind. The first were in fact discov-

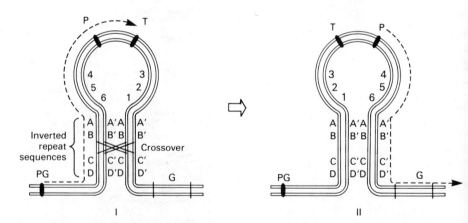

Figure 8–26. Inversion of IS2 acting as a switch controlling an adjacent gene. A crossover between the inverted repeat sequences causes an inversion of the loop between the sequences. The original direction can be similarly restored by a second crossover. The loop contains a transcription terminator *(T)* and a promoter *(P)*. In orientation *I,* transcription from the promoter *PG,* which normally initiates transcription of gene *G,* is terminated at *T,* inactivating the function of gene *G.* In the opposite orientation *(II),* promoter *P* initiates transcription, and *G* is transcribed even if there is no initiation at *PG. Dashed lines,* transcription; *A,B,1,2,* etc., base sequences; *primed letters,* sequences complementary to unprimed ones.

ered in plants, not bacteria, by Barbara McClintock. The **Ty** transposons of yeast (Chap. 11) are related to retroviruses (Chap. 65) and, like them, transpose by **reverse transcription.** They also cause chromosomal rearrangement. *Drosophila* contain several types of transposons. The **P-elements** are similar to bacterial class II transposons, and **copia-like elements** are similar to yeast's Ty; they cause mutations by insertion into cellular genes. Flies contain many defective P-elements that are incapable of autonomous transposition, but they can be mobilized by a competent element carried by a sperm into an egg cell, causing mutations and chromosomal rearrangements (**hybrid dysgenesis**).

In vertebrates transposons related to retroviruses are present as repeated sequences and are transcribed only at certain developmental stages. Among plants, maize contains transposons similar to those of class II in bacteria. As in *Drosophila*, the cells contain inactive transposons, whose mobilization by the introduction of an active transposon causes genetic instability.

Plasmids: Mechanisms of Replication and Conjugation

The important roles of plasmids in bacterial physiology and genetics have been discussed in Chapter 7. The underlying molecular mechanisms will be examined here.

GENETIC CONSTITUTION

The genomes of plasmids are made up of two main regions: one specifies **functions for autonomous existence** and replication within the host; the other specifies the **functions that give an advantage** to the plasmid—and therefore to the host—such as conjugation or antibiotic resistance. The latter genes are not essential, and their deletion leaves a **miniplasmid** containing a cluster of **autonomy genes** (also called **replication drive unit**); they may be as little as one-tenth or less of the original genome. Many plasmids also express **recombinases** similar in function to those specified by transposons (see above), which carry out integration.

The replication drive units contain four elements: the origin of vegetative replication, genes specifying proteins for replication, genes controlling the number of copies of a plasmid in a cell, and genes for the regular partition of the progeny plasmids to the daughter bacteria at division. All other functions needed for replication (such as precursors or enzymes) are supplied by the cell. **Replication** is initiated by proteins that bind to several tandem repeats at the **origin for vegetative replication** (*ori*V) and then proceeds unidirectionally or bidirectionally, depending on the plasmid.

MECHANISMS OF COPY NUMBER CONTROL

Copy number control is carried out by a **repressor of multiplication,** the concentration of which increases with the number of copies. Some are proteins, and when they are depleted by blocking protein synthesis the copy number increases markedly.

Many plasmids utilize an **RNA repressor,** rather than a protein. It is formed by **countertranscription,** from a sequence overlapping that specifying a larger RNA, but in the opposite direction (i.e., on the opposite strand). In ColE1 the larger RNA generates the primer for DNA replication, and in R1 it specifies a protein needed for initiating DNA replication. Base pairing between the repressor and DNA abolishes the formation of the larger RNA (see Antisense RNA, Chap. 9).

PARTITIONING

It is clear that partitioning does not occur at random, for if plasmid replication is blocked while the bacteria multiply, the number of copies per cell progressively and evenly decreases until all cells have a single copy. Only after that stage do plasmid-free cells appear. This regular distribution is caused by several genes of the plasmids. One acts in *cis*; i.e., controls partitioning of only the plasmids that carry it; others act in *trans*, on other plasmids in the same cell. The *cis*-acting gene is comparable to a chromosome centromere; the proteins specified by the *trans*-acting genes probably bind to the cell membrane, generating specific sites for the attachment of the centromere. Another gene slows bacterial division when the copy number decreases.

The origin of replication is also involved in partitioning, because if it is replaced by the bacterial origin partitioning becomes random. With large plasmids, but probably not with high-copy-number plasmids, partitioning may involve the bacterial membrane in the same way as the regular distribution of the cellular chromosomes to the daughter cells (see DNA Replication, above).

MECHANISM OF CONJUGATION

Conjugation requires the expression of many plasmid genes. In the F plasmid these occupy 33 Kb, about one-third of the genome; they form a cluster whose products are mostly found in the bacterial membranes (Fig. 8–27). Twenty of the genes constitute the **transfer (*tra*) operon** under positive control of the *J* gene, which is in turn repressed by the products of two **fertility-inhibition genes** outside the transfer operon: *fin* P and *fin* O. Most of the *tra* genes are needed for transfer; two (*S* and *T*) make the cell a poor target for a transfer of F from another cell (**surface exclusion**).

Transfer is initiated by **nicking one of the strands at**

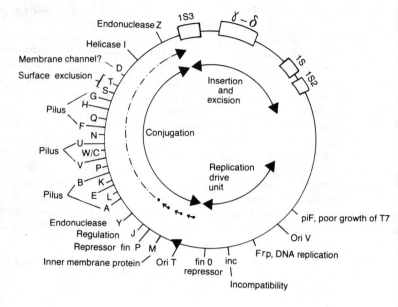

Figure 8–27. Map of the F plasmid. Letters A to Z indicate genes of the transfer *(tra)* operon. *Dashed line,* transcription. Gene *fin0* is inactive in the derepressed F used in experimental work. Insertion elements IS2, IS3, γ–δ provide the sites of integration in various Hfr strains. During conjugation, the order of penetration is *oriT–inc–frp,* etc. The *tra* operon is thus last, and so in transfers from Hfr donors, it enters only after the whole inserted bacterial chromosome. The separation of the *tra* operon and the *inc* gene accounts for the finding of different *inc* groups among plasmids of the same pilus type. *Col V,* colicinogen V.

*ori*T (distinct from *ori*V, the origin of vegetative replication) by the YZ endonuclease, probably located at the inner surface of the cytoplasmic membrane. The enzyme seems to remain connected to the 5′ end of the cut strand, which it moves to the recipient cell through a plasmid-encoded channel. Initiation of transfer requires a signal from cell pair formation, probably via a membrane protein.

Transfer occurs as a single strand, during DNA synthesis by a **rolling-circle model** (Fig. 8–28): the 5′ end of the nicked strand enters the recipient cell, while synthesis by DNA polymerase III elongates the 3′ end in the donor cell using the intact strand as template. The transferred strand is cut when it reaches *ori*T, and sealing

reconstitutes the donor plasmid. The DNA must have precise recognition signals for the various enzymes.

In the recipient cell DNA synthesis by the host polymerase III at the cell membrane builds a new strand complementary to the transferred strand; the linear duplex is then circularized to complete the plasmid, with supercoiling by the host's gyrase.

In the **mobilization** of **nonconjugative plasmids** a conjugative plasmid present in the same cell provides the transfer function; the nonconjugative plasmid must have a functional *mob* gene, an *ori*T-like sequence, and a *nic* function to nick *ori*T. A given nonconjugative plasmid can usually be mobilized by various conjugative plasmids.

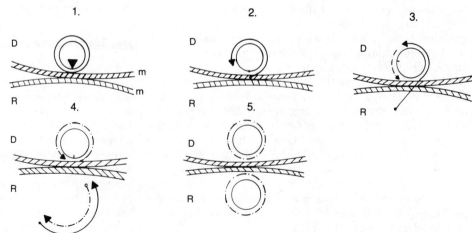

Figure 8–28. Penetration of a plasmid strand in conjugation at a site of apposition of the donor *(D)* and recipient *(R)* cell membrane. *Dots,* 5′ ends; *arrow,* 3′ ends. *Dashed lines,* new synthesis. *(1)* The donor plasmid is nicked *(arrowhead).* *(2)* The nicked 5′ end penetrates the membranes. *(3)* As the donor strand penetrates, it is replaced by new synthesis; the penetrating strand is replicated as it enters the recipient cell. *(4)* Penetration is completed; the donor plasmid is reconstituted. *(5)* The newly acquired DNA is circularized.

Gene Manipulation

For several decades the techniques of gene transfer in bacteria have been used to produce recombinants between different mutations, the classic foundation of genetic studies. The manipulations were then extended to **gene rearrangements,** by the use of **deletions** that cause the **fusion of genes or of operons,** and by the use of **transposons** to move a gene to a new position in the chromosome. When fused genes are in phase they yield fused proteins, and these are very useful. For example, a fusion protein can be isolated by precipitation by antibodies to its known component, and that protein can then be used to raise antibodies that will precipitate the intact unknown protein from wild-type cells. In a widely used procedure for identifying the responses of a regulatory region it is fused to the gene for a protein whose activity is easily assayed—usually the *lacZ* gene. Fusion can also be used to define the region of a protein responsible for a particular activity, and to attach a protein to a sequence that will cause it to be secreted.

In a more recent development, the recombination of DNA into plasmids and phages *in vitro* has made it possible to transfer genes of any origin into bacteria. This technology has been of immense value in studying the sequence, expression, and regulation of genes, and it has had an extraordinary range of uses, both fundamental and practical. This development, accomplished by the integration of a number of earlier esoteric techniques, illustrates vividly the unforeseeable consequences of basic scientific knowledge.

MOLECULAR CLONING (RECOMBINANT DNA)

The basic principle of molecular cloning is to insert a DNA segment into a small replicon (**a vector**), generating a **recombinant (chimeric) vector** capable of replicating in cells. The vector must have an origin of replication responding to factors produced in the host cells—which can be bacteria, yeast, animal, or plant cells—and must have all the genes essential for its replication. For studying the product of the foreign DNA segment, the vector must also provide transcription and translation control signals recognized within the cells. With many proteins production, or conversion to the mature form, requires further steps, such as excision of intervening sequences in RNA or post-translational modifications of the protein (e.g., glycosylation). Since bacteria lack these powers the extension of cloning to yeast and to animal cells has been valuable.

The *in vitro* splicing of DNA into a bacterial replicon followed by multiplication in cells was first accomplished by Berg and Kaiser in 1972 with defined segments of prokaryotic DNA. Originally, the vector and the foreign segment were spliced by building short runs of a base at the 3′ ends of the linearized vector, and of the complementary base at the 3′ ends of the foreign DNA (Fig. 8–29). Annealing and ligation yielded the recombinant molecule. Subsequently, the procedure was greatly simplified by the use of **restriction endonucleases** (see above) that make staggered cuts, leaving overlapping ends. After separation, these complementary (**cohesive**) ends can be made to pair by annealing, and they can then be covalently linked by **polynucleotide ligase.** A given restriction enzyme produces the same self-complementary ends in all its products; hence, in a mixture of a purified vector and some other DNA, both cut with the same enzyme, this treatment will yield both the reconstituted original vector and **recombinants.**

Hybrid vectors prepared by either method can **transfect** *E. coli* cells rendered competent by warming with $CaCl_2$ solution, and the vector is then perpetuated in the cell's progeny (**cloned**). High-copy-number plasmids or phages then yield many copies per cell. Because the efficiency of transfection is low the vectors are made in such a way that cells carrying recombinants can be readily identified. For instance, some vectors contain two antibiotic resistance genes, one of which is inactivated when foreign DNA is inserted into its restriction site. Cells without vector are then sensitive to both antibiotics; those with recombinant vectors are sensitive to one; those with original vectors are sensitive to neither.

After lysis the recombinant vectors can be isolated from the cellular DNA. Cyclic vectors can be separated from bacterial DNA fragments by **equilibrium sedimentation in the presence of ethidium bromide,** owing to their higher buoyant density under these conditions, while viral vectors can be isolated as viral particles. The recombinant DNA can be cleaved at the specific sequences joining its components, using the same enzyme that created the cohesive ends, and the components can be separated on the basis of size by gel electrophoresis.

In this way, **large amounts of a specific segment of DNA of any origin can readily be obtained in pure form.** Available methods then permit easy determination of its sequence. When a sequence appropriate for initiation of translation is encountered the region between that and the next translation termination codon is called an **open reading frame (ORF),** and it often leads to identification of a novel protein.

Vectors

Bacterial vectors are derived from plasmids or from phage genomes. Both have been severely reduced in size so that they can accommodate large foreign segments while retaining the genes required for autonomous replication. By suitable selection procedures, all target sites for certain restriction enzymes except one or two have been eliminated, avoiding excessive fragmentation on exposure to the enzymes. New items affecting function or

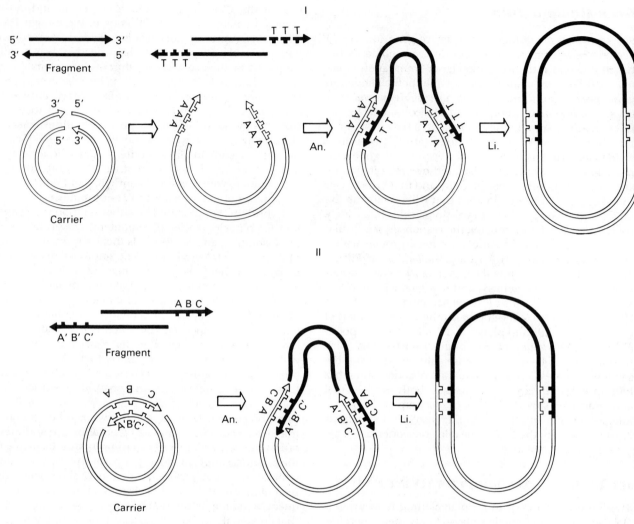

Figure 8–29. Incorporation of a DNA fragment into a vector represented as a cyclic DNA. *(I)* Incorporation mediated by the addition of poly(A) and poly(T) by a terminal transferase. *(II)* Incorporation through cohesive ends formed by restriction endonucleases. *A, B, C,* bases complementary to *A', B', C',* respectively; *An.,* annealing; *Li.,* ligase.

manipulation of the DNA or the protein are often introduced at suitable positions.

The cyclic replicons of nonconjugative plasmids are excellent vectors because they can accommodate variable amounts of foreign DNA, are easy to purify, have selectable genes, and can be made to reproduce to large numbers in a cell. Col EI has the selectable colicin gene, possesses a single site for restriction endonuclease EcoRl within that gene, and in the presence of chloramphenicol can multiply to 1000 to 3000 copies per cell, corresponding to about one-half of the cell's DNA. The most widely used plasmid vector is pBR322, which was obtained by fusing parts of several plasmids. It has a genome of minimum size, plus genes for resistance to tetracycline and to ampicillin, which are used for the selection of recombinants (Fig. 8–30).

The host range has been extended to **eukaryotic vectors,** using yeast plasmids or DNA from viruses. Vectors capable of replicating in both bacteria and eukaryotic cells **(shuttle vectors)** are created by fusing two replicons, one bacterial, the other eukaryotic. Shuttle vectors are useful for many applications, especially those in which they are studied in animal cells but amplified in bacteria or yeasts. Yeast vectors will be discussed in Chapter 11, phage and **cosmid** vectors in Chapter 46, and animal virus vectors in Chapters 48 and 65.

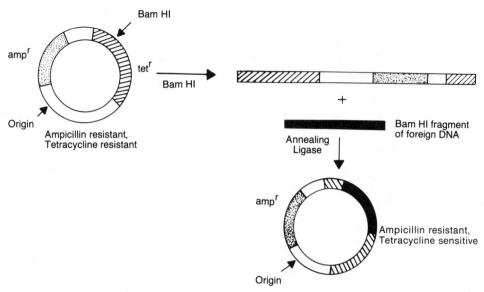

Figure 8–30. Use of plasmid pBR322 in DNA cloning. *Amp*^{r}, ampicillin-resistance gene; *tet*^{r}, tetracycline-resistance gene; *black,* foreign DNA; *Bam HI,* restriction endonuclease for which pBR322 has a single target.

Identification of Specific Cloned Genes

Using the described methods for fragmenting and cloning DNA, the entire genome of a prokaryote or a yeast can be transferred into a set of several thousand clones (**a genomic library),** which can be contained in a single test tube. Bacteria carrying a recombinant vector with a given insert are identified by **colony hybridization,** using radioactive complementary RNA or DNA called **probes.** A transfected culture containing random fragments from a genomic library is seeded on nutrient agar plates; when colonies or plaques (Chap. 44), depending on the vector, are formed, they are transferred in part onto a filter disc briefly applied to the agar. After exposure to strong alkali, to lyse the cells or phages and denature the DNA without displacing it, the filter is hybridized with the radioactive probe.

Several thousand colonies or plaques can be tested per Petri dish; only those containing an insert complementary to the probe will show radioactivity. The intact recombinant vector is then recovered from the original plate, using the radioactive spots on the filter as reference. With these techniques a desired mammalian gene, constituting only about 10^{-6} of the genome, can be isolated readily if a probe is available.

Cloned genes can also be identified by their functional **complementation** of a mutational defect in cells.

cDNA Cloning

Recombinant DNA technology can also be used to obtain the genes that form the mRNA found in a particular class of cells. For this purpose **complementary DNA** copies of the mRNA, called **cDNA,** are generated by **reverse transcription** (see Chap. 65) followed by synthesis of the complementary strand. The ds copy can then be cloned in appropriate vectors.

Expression Vectors

While many vectors are designed merely to clone and amplify the foreign DNA, some are made to obtain large amounts of the protein specified by the inserted gene. In these vectors the inserted gene is under the control of a **promoter** and a **ribosome-binding site** suitable for expression in the host cells. For *E. coli* vectors, the *lac* operator-promoter is frequently used because its inducers can control expression of the fused gene; another especially strong promoter, *tac,* has been artificially constructed as a composite of two other promoters. Suitable for mammalian vectors are the promoter-enhancer sequences of viral genes, especially of tumor viruses, which are active in many cell types. Useful for special purposes are promoters inducible in animal cells: that of the metallothionine gene—a detoxification gene—is activated by zinc, and that of the mouse mammary tumor virus is activated by dexamethasone.

The production of an active eukaryotic protein in bacteria has additional requirements: bacteria do not splice out intervening sequences, do not cleave protein precursors into mature proteins, and do not glycosylate. Some eukaryotic proteins are produced in bacteria in active form: for instance, interferons, whose genes have no intervening sequences, are not cleaved, and either are not glycosylated or retain activity in the absence of glycosylation. The need for splicing intervening sequences can be eliminated by using the **cDNA of the gene,** which lacks them.

In general, proteins that can be secreted are produced

in larger amounts than those that accumulate in the bacterial cell, where foreign proteins tend to undergo denaturation and digestion (in part because the reducing conditions in the cell prevent formation of the disulfide bonds that stabilize most extracellular proteins). Accordingly, expression vectors for foreign protein manufacture often include a leader sequence that initiates secretion and then is cleaved (Chap. 6).

APPLICATIONS OF MOLECULAR CLONING

The introduction of DNA cloning has revolutionized the study of many fields of biology. We will summarize some of its contributions that are most relevant for the study of microbiology.

1. Determination of the **organization of small genomes.** DNA cloning, in conjunction with methods for determining the base sequences, has allowed the complete sequencing of many genomes of viruses and plasmids, often revealing **open reading frames** (see above, Molecular Cloning). The promoter-operator sequences controlling the expression of genes have been identified and the role of their parts determined by directed mutagenesis (see above). In bacterial genomes, the gene rearrangements important for antigenic variation (see above) have been defined. Probes for specific genes or control sequences can be prepared and used to measure precisely the expression of genes and its regulation.

2. Understanding of **eukaryotic cell genetics.** Through DNA cloning, the organization of eukaryotic genes and their control sequences have been determined. Examples of important results are the discoveries of the changes in gene organization that take place during the maturation of antibody-producing cells, those that determine the changes of antigenicity in trypanosomes, and those responsible for mating-type shift in yeast. Comparison of sequences of cloned genes has established the relatedness between many oncogene products and normal growth factors or their receptors. The homology of genes in organisms of different species provides a quantitative molecular basis for measuring evolutionary distances between organisms (Chap. 1). The use of specific probes has determined the precise positions of many genes in chromosomes, including detailed study of the translocations involved in oncogene activation. DNA cloning has allowed the analysis of the complex patterns of changing expression of genes in *Drosophila* development, through recognition of specific mRNAs and proteins. The analysis of the distribution of overlapping fragments generated by different restriction endonucleases allows the determination of maps of chromosome segments. In some cases, these maps permit the identification of genes responsible for hereditary defects, making it possible to identify disease-free heterozygotes and to diagnose the disease during early pregnancy.

3. **Production of valuable substances.** Cells containing a cloned gene in an expression vector can produce large amounts of the product of that gene provided the vector and the host cell are compatible, as discussed above, for both the gene and the protein. For example, recombinant human growth hormone is now produced in bacteria. In the past, this hormone, extracted from pituitary glands taken from cadavers, has been not only in extremely scarce supply, but sometimes also a source of incurable infection, such as that leading to the slow Creutzfeldt–Jakob disease (see Chap. 51). Cloning in yeast has produced the hepatitis B s antigen (see Chap. 63), which is used as a vaccine and was formerly obtained from human blood. Cultures of animal cells now yield factors used for treating hemophilia, formerly also produced from human blood with considerable risk of transmitting hepatitis B or HIV.

4. Studies of **gene replacement** and **gene regulation** in animals. **Transgenic mice** are an interesting example: a nucleus of a fertilized egg is injected with cloned DNA including a suitable control region. The gene becomes integrated at random locations into the DNA of some cells. In the animal developing from the egg it is then possible to study the influence of **cell differentiation** on expression of the gene. A possible future application in humans is **gene therapy,** introducing a cloned gene into cells to compensate for a gene defect. Moreover, molecular genetic techniques are making it possible to advance our understanding of cell differentiation by identifying **transcription factors** in various tissues that turn specific genes on or off. A future possibility in humans is **gene therapy:** introducing a cloned gene into somatic cells (especially of the bone marrow), or into germline cells, to compensate for a defective gene.

Appendix: Genetic Mapping

Genetic mapping aims at determining the order of markers in DNA and the distances between them. It can be achieved by recombinational, topologic, and physical methods.

Determining recombination frequencies is the classic method, intermarker distances being calculated from the proportion of recombinants between markers. The standard procedure uses a **three-factor cross,** involving parents differing in three markers as shown in Figure 8–31. By crossing various overlapping sets of three markers in this way, all the available markers in a chromosome can be ordered in a unique sequence: **the genetic map.** Phenotypically similar markers that map in the same region are assigned to the same or to different genes by means of **complementation tests** (Chap. 7).

Order of markers: A   B   C

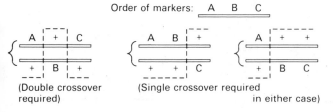

(Double crossover   (Single crossover required
required)   in either case)

Figure 8–31. Three-factor cross. *A, B, C,* the mutant alleles; +, the corresponding wild-type *(wt)* alleles. The test consists of measuring the proportion of wt genomes in the progeny of double-mutant × single-mutant crosses. When the single mutant is the central marker, the cross yields many fewer wt recombinants because two crossovers are required.

Distances are evaluated from the proportion of recombinants between fairly close markers, for with more distant markers multiple crossovers tend to decrease the recombination values, instead of remaining additive; the values asymptotically approach a maximum, with increasing distance, of 50%.

Recombination mapping is generally valid down to fairly short distances. However, it is less accurate for very close markers (e.g., within a gene) because of the role of gene conversion, whose frequency does not depend simply on distance.

Insertion mapping uses a selectable marker inserted near a mutation whose alleles are not readily selected. For example, when a transposon carrying tetracycline resistance (Tn10) is added to a culture of the wild type it will localize in many different sites in different cells before becoming stabilized. Generalized transduction from this heterogeneous population to a culture of the mutant recipient of interest then yields selectable drug-resistant transductants. Among these an occasional clone has replaced the mutant allele, thus recovering the wild-type phenotype; and that gene can then be approximately localized by mapping the closely linked drug resistance gene.

Deletion mapping is based on the inability of a deletion, in a pairwise cross, to produce wild-type recombinants with an overlapping deletion or with any point mutation within the deleted region. **Because the crosses give a simple yes or no answer, the deletion ends and their relation to point mutations can be ordered unambiguously.** This approach gives marker order over any distance, whether minute or large; it is not affected by gene conversions, and it is applicable to many biological systems. Deletion mapping, however, does not provide distances. These can sometimes be obtained by physical mapping of the DNA.

Transduction mapping (Chap. 7) uses **generalized transducing phages.** As will be described in Chapter 46, these transfer DNA segments of **nearly constant length** taken at random from the DNA of the donor cell. In abortive transduction (which does not involve integration) the probability of cotransduction of two genes depends only on the ratio of their physical distances to the known length of the transduced DNA fragments; hence the results afforded an unambiguous way to determine both order and distances. In **stable transduction** the distances are less reliable because the factors that complicate recombination similarly influence integration of the transduced segment.

Physical mapping is the most direct technique. **Protein mapping** is useful for sites within a gene; it can be carried out by measuring the length of the polypeptide chains resulting from the introduction of terminator (nonsense) mutations. **Nucleic acid mapping** is best performed by hybridizing DNA from strains differing by two or more deletions or insertions, to form **heteroduplexes.** Where the two strands lack homology the unpaired DNA forms a "bush," and the length of the paired region between bushes can be determined unambiguously. Time of initial entry in conjugation (Ch. 7, Fig. 7–13) is an indirect form of physical mapping.

Restriction enzyme mapping uses specific fragments produced by restriction endonucleases. The order of cleavage sites for a variety of endonucleases is determined from the overlaps of fragments produced by incomplete digestion (or by different endonucleases). The location of a gene on this restriction site map is then established by various procedures such as marker rescue, or hybridization of fragments to known mRNA or to DNA with deletions (see Chap. 45, Genetic reactivation).

A **comparison of genetic maps** obtained by physical means or by generalized recombination shows a general agreement over long distances or in selected DNA segments. However, there are marked discrepancies over short distances, and "hot spots" where recombination frequencies are abnormally high. These discrepancies show that the local frequency of recombination depends on the DNA sequences.

Appendix: Quantitative Aspects of Killing by Irradiation

We shall consider here certain mathematical relations between the dose of radiation and its lethal effect that are useful for understanding problems involving the uses of radiation in research and for sterilization.

The **inactivation** or **death** of a microorganism is defined as the loss of its ability to initiate a clone: this effect is the consequence of a certain number of **chemical events,** each consisting, for instance, in the unrepaired change of a chemical group or the breaking of a chemical bond. The relation between the dose of radiation and the proportion of surviving organisms can be calculated as follows.

It is assumed that the events occur randomly and independently in the susceptible chemical groups in various individual organisms, with a probability P per group, proportional to the dose, and n groups per organism. If a single such event is sufficient for inactivation, the proportion of surviving organisms (S) that have experienced no such event is, from the Poisson distribution (see Appendix, Chap. 44), $S = e^{-Pn}$. In turn, $P = kD = krt$, where k is a constant that measures the probability of unrepaired damage of the chemical group, D is the dose of radiation, r is the dose rate (i.e., the dose of radiation per unit time), and t is the time. Thus, the basic equation of inactivation is $S = e^{-krtn}$. The equation is used in its logarithmic form: $\log S = -krtn \log e = -Krtn$, where $K = k \log e$.

When the inactivation of bacteria or viruses by UV light, x-rays, or ^{32}P decay is followed by plotting the logarithm of the surviving fraction (S) versus time, the **survival curve** is often seen to be a **straight line**: curve A in Figure 8–32. Such a curve is called a **single-hit** curve because it is generated by a process in which a **single event** in an organism destroys its viability.

The slope of one-hit survival curve, $-Krn$, is the basis for radiation analysis of **target size**; as a first approximation, this slope is proportional to the size of the genome (e.g., n) if the proportion of repaired damages is constant. If K is the same for two different organisms, the ratio of the values of Kn, or **relative target size,** can be determined directly from the slopes of their survival curves. However, differences in efficiency of repair influence the value of K and hence the observed target size.

Other important types of survival curves, called **multiple-hit curves,** are represented by curves B, C, and D in Figure 8–32. They have a shoulder near the origin before becoming linear because several events (hits) must accumulate in a viable unit before it is inactivated. To determine the number of events required for inactivation, the straight part of the survival curve is extrapolated back to intersect the ordinate axis. The position of the intersection measures the number of hits in logarithmic units. Curve B corresponds to 10 hits and curve C to 100 hits; curve D also corresponds to 10 hits but has a different slope. The slope of the straight part of a multiple-hit curve has the same meaning as for a single-hit curve; i.e., it is proportional to the target size of the organism. Thus, curves A, B, and C reflect the inactivation of organisms with the same target size.

Multiple-hit curves are obtained whenever one susceptible component can replace another in the reproduction of the unit whose survival is being measured. For instance, when bacteria are infected by several UV-irradiated virus particles, curves of this type describe the survival of the ability to yield active virus (see Multiplicity Reactivation, Chap. 47). Similarly, in clumps of bacteria the survival of a single organism is sufficient to maintain

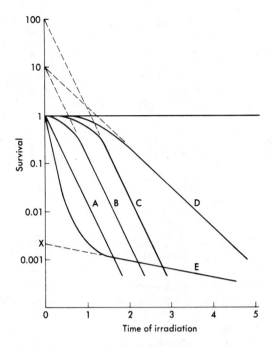

Figure 8–32. Survival curves of microorganisms irradiated by UV light (*A*) Single-hit curve. (*B*) 10-hit curve. (*C*) 100-hit curve. (A, B, and C are for the same target size.) (*D*) 10-hit curve for organisms with a smaller target size than that of B. (*E*) Multi-component curve produced by a population containing organisms with different target sizes. X, proportion of organisms with the smallest target size. The dose rate is assumed to be constant.

the colony-forming ability of a clump. Because the straight part of the curve is reached when the surviving clumps have only one surviving organism, its slope measures the inactivation (and the target size) of the last surviving individual in the clump. Curve A would then describe the inactivation of single organisms, curve B clumps of 10 organisms, and curve C clumps of 100 organisms.

Another mechanism generating multiple-hit curves is a decrease of repair efficiency at high radiation doses. Thus, postreplication repair becomes inefficient when the distances between radiation-induced dimers are short and so recombination is infrequent.

A third type of survival curve is **multicomponent** (E in Fig. 8–32), generated by a population composed of organisms with different target sizes. Those with the large target—more sensitive—are inactivated first with a steep slope, whereas at the end, only the most resistant ones survive, with a shallower slope for their survival curve. The proportion of this group can be estimated by extrapolating back the final straight part of the curve to the ordinate axis (about 2×10^{-3} in Fig. 8–32). Curves of this type are commonly obtained when viruses are exposed to chemical inactivating agents, where the differences in sensitivity depend primarily on differences in penetration. Recognition of these curves is important in the preparation of safe vaccines.

Selected Reading

Berg DE, Howe MM (eds): Mobile DNA. Washington, DC, American Society of Microbiology, 1989

Bingham PM, Kidwell MG, Rubin GM: The molecular basis of P–M hybrid dysgenesis: The role of the P element, a P-strain-specific transposon family. Cell 29:995, 1982

Boeke JD, Garfinkel DJ, Styles CA, Fink GR: Ty elements transpose through an RNA intermediate. Cell 40:491, 1985

Botstein D, Shortle D: Strategies and applications of *in vitro* mutagenesis. Science 229:1193, 1985

Claverys IP, Lacks SA: Heteroduplex deoxyribonucleic acid base mismatch repair in bacteria. Microbiol Rev 50:133, 1986

Demple B, Sedgwick B, Robins P, Totty N, Waterfield MD, Lindahl T: Active site and complete sequence of the suicidal methyltransferase that counters alkylation mutagenesis. Proc Natl Acad Sci USA 82:2688, 1985

Derbyshire KM, Grindley NDF: Replicative and conservative transposition in bacteria. Cell 47:325, 1986

Dohet C, Wagner R, Radman M: Methyl-directed repair of frameshift mutations in heteroduplex DNA. Proc Natl Acad Sci USA 83:3395, 1986

Gellert M, Nash H: Communication between segments of DNA during site-specific recombination. Nature 325:401, 1987

Grindley NDF, Reed RR: Transpositional recombination in prokaryotes. Annu Rev Biochem 54:863, 1985

Gunge N: Yeast DNA plasmids. Annu Rev Microbiol 37:253, 1983

Hanawalt PC, Cooper PK, Ganesan AK, Smith CA: DNA repair in bacteria and mammalian cells. Annu Rev Biochem 48:783, 1979

Howard–Flanders P, West SC, Stasiak A: Role of RecA protein spiral filaments in genetic recombination. Nature 309:215, 1984

Ippen–Ihler K: F-pilin, the membrane, and conjugation. In Leive L (ed): Microbiology, p 265. American Society for Microbiology, Washington, DC, 1985

Johnson RC, Simon MI: Enhancers of site-specific recombination in bacteria. Trends Genet 3:262, 1987

Jones M, Wagner R, Radman M: Mismatch repair and recombination in *E. coli*. Cell 50:621, 1987

Kleckner N: Transposable elements in prokaryotes. Annu Rev Genet 15:341, 1981

Lahue RS, Su S-S, Modrich P: Requirement for d(GATC) sequences in *Escherichia coli* mutHLS mismatch correction. Proc Natl Acad Sci USA 84:1482, 1987

Little JW, Mount DW: The SOS regulatory system of *Escherichia coli*. Cell 29:11, 1982

Loeb LA: Apurinic sites as mutagenic intermediates. Cell 40:483, 1985

Messer W: Initiation of DNA replication in *Escherichia coli*. J Bacteriol 69:3395, 1987

Myers RM, Lerman LS, Maniatis T: A general method for saturation mutagenesis of cloned DNA fragments. Science 229:242, 1985

Radding C: Strand transfer in homologous genetic recombination. Annu Rev Genet 16:405, 1982

Scott JR: Regulation of plasmic replication. Microbiol Rev 48:1, 1984

Shiba T, Saigo K: Retrovirus-like particles containing RNA homologous to the transposable element *copia* in *Drosophila melanogaster*. Nature 302:119, 1983

Smith GR: Chi hotspots of generalized recombination. Cell 34:709, 1983

Stahl FW: Roles of double-strand breaks in generalized genetic recombination. Nucleic Acids Res Mol Biol 33:169, 1986

Stahl FW: Genetic recombination. Sci Am 256(2):91, 1987

Teo I, Sedgwick B, Kilpatrick MW, McCarthy TV, Lindahl T: The intracellular signal for induction of resistance to alkylating agents in *E. coli*. Cell 45:315, 1986

Walker GC: Mutagenesis and inducible responses to deoxyribonucleic acid damage in *Escherichia coli*. Microbiol Rev 48:60, 1984

Willetts N, Wilkins B: Processing of plasmid DNA during bacterial conjugation. Microbiol Rev 48:24, 1984

Wu AM, Kahn R, DasGupta C, Radding CM: Formation of nascent heteroduplex structures by RecA protein and DNA. Cell 30:37, 1982

Zell R, Fritz HJ: DNA-mismatch repair in *Escherichia coli* counteracting the hydrolytic deamination of 5-methyl-cytosine residues. EMBO J 6:1809, 1987

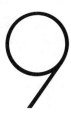

Regulation of Gene Expression

The genetic information is expressed by transcription of segments of DNA into two classes of RNA: labile messenger RNA (mRNA), which is translated into protein (Chap. 6), and stable RNA (ribosomal, transfer, and small RNAs), which is not translated. Genetic and molecular studies have revealed a number of mechanisms for regulating gene expression in bacteria, and these findings have provided a foundation for studying the more intricate regulation of genes in higher organisms.

This chapter will concentrate on the physiological aspects of these responses in the cell; the reader is referred to molecular biology texts for the molecular aspects. We will take up (1) the discovery of the classic mechanism of regulation of the genes for various enzymes by repressors and activators of initiation of their transcription; (2) the relation of this work to the discovery and the metabolism of mRNA; (3) the molecular basis for this regulatory mechanism; and (4) alternative regulatory mechanisms involving transcription termination or translation. We will then discuss processes that involve regulation of large groups of genes, including (5) the protein-synthesizing system; (6) protein breakdown and other responses to various stresses; and (7) DNA replication and cell division.

Before discussing these aspects of regulation we will review the mechanism of DNA transcription.

Transcription of DNA

Physiologic transcription generally reads only one strand in a particular sequence of DNA, but different segments may be transcribed on opposite strands (and consequently in the opposite direction). Transcription is slower than replication and is usually in the same direction; when it is slowed, the replication behind it is also slowed. What happens when the two processes occur in opposite directions and collide is not known.

RNA is synthesized by a **DNA-dependent RNA polymerase,** also called **transcriptase,** which catalyzes the reactions:

$$n(\text{ATP, GTP, UTP, CTP}) \xrightarrow[\text{Enzyme}]{\text{DNA template}}$$

Nucleoside triphosphates

$$\cdot (\text{AMP, GMP, UMP, CMP})n + n(\text{P}\cdot\text{P})$$

Polynucleotide · · · · · · · · · · Pyrophosphate

As in DNA synthesis, the chains grow at the 3' end. In bacteria the initiating 5'-terminal nucleotide retains its triphosphate; in eukaryotes it is capped by a special methylated base.

Purification of RNA polymerase of *E. coli* yields both a **core enzyme** and a **holoenzyme.** The core polymerase is composed of two α chains (mol. wt. 41,000), one β chain (mol. wt. 155,000), and one chain whose similar

size (mol. wt. 165,000) led it to be designated β'. The holoenzyme contains an additional **initiating protein,** called a **sigma (σ) factor.** The factor used in exponential growth in *E. coli* is σ^{70} (mol. wt. 70,000). The interaction of transcriptase with DNA involves three main steps: initiation, chain elongation, and termination (Fig. 9–1). Despite the complexity of the process, it can also be carried out by simpler RNA polymerases (e.g., a single polypeptide of mol. wt. 100,000 coded for by phage T7).

INITIATION

Physiologic initiation requires the holoenzyme, the proper nucleoside triphosphate (always a purine), and a special **promoter** DNA sequence, (see below).

In the initial, reversible step the holoenzyme encloses about five turns (50 base pairs) of the double helix of the promoter in a groove. It then causes the melting of a segment (usually 12 bases long), the **transcription bubble,** by unwinding the DNA one and one-half turns; alterations in chemical reactivity have established the points

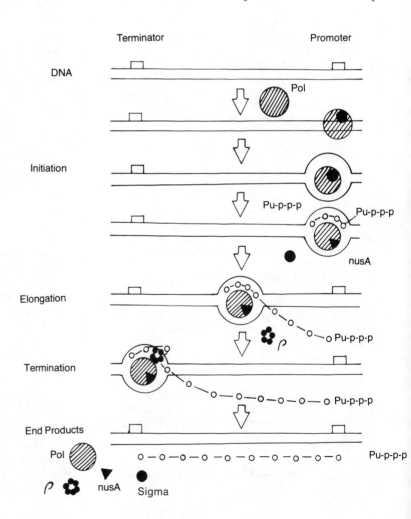

Figure 9–1. Model of transcription.

of contact with the enzyme, and the location and size of the bubble.

The enzyme complex, now bound tightly, intercalates between the separated strands and polymerizes an RNA strand of about ten nucleotides complementary to the template DNA strand. The sigma factor is then replaced by the **nusA protein,** marking the transition from the initiation to the elongation phase. The released σ factor can engage in another initiation cycle.

Promoters differ in their sequences and their strength of binding of polymerase; with some its binding requires the binding of an activator protein immediately upstream (see Cyclic AMP, below). Promoters have similar but not identical sequences in two regions, -35 and -10 with respect to initiation of transcription at $+1$. The "**consensus**" sequence (i.e., the most frequent one) at -35 is TTGACA, while that at -10 is TATAAT, whose AT pairs (weaker than GC) promote the required melting. Thus the weak *lac* promoter, which requires the cooperation of CRP, has a GC pair in its -10 region, and replacement by AT eliminates that requirement. Melting also depends on **negative supercoiling** produced by DNA gyrase, and mutations in that enzyme have pleiotropic regulatory effects.

Under various circumstances cells use different σ factors, which select different promoters, as noted below.

ELONGATION

In the elongation phase the core enzyme assumes a new conformation by interacting with several factors, one of which is the *nusA* protein (Fig. 9–10). The transcription bubble, now about 18 bases long, moves from one to the other end of the transcription unit, which can be several thousand bases long. The growing end of the nascent RNA remains held to the template DNA strand within the bubble by a 12-base hybrid segment. Each cycle of elongation somewhat resembles that on a ribosome (Chap. 6). The polymerase first binds IMP to its **substrate site,** a nucleoside triphosphate that matches the next base of the template; it then cleaves the nucleotide and joins it to the growing chain; then it advances on the DNA helix, opening it ahead and closing it behind by one base, so that the total number of turns remains constant.

PAUSING. Nucleotides are added to the RNA at a rate of 30 to 50 per second. At certain sites, however, the polymerase makes pauses that can last many seconds and are important for function. For instance, in the transcription of phage lambda DNA (see Chap. 46) from the P_R promoter the enzyme pauses at the sixteenth base, and it proceeds further only after binding the phage-specific Q protein. Pausing can be induced either by sequences that form a hairpin in the nascent RNA and thus jam the polymerization mechanism, or by sequences rich in GC.

TERMINATION AND ANTITERMINATION

At termination, the polymerase drops off and the nascent RNA chains leave the DNA template. This process is subject to extensive modulation, which is important in regulating gene function but is not as well understood as initiation of transcription.

There are two classes of terminators. **Strong (Type I) terminators,** at the end of most operons, cause regular termination. **Weak (Type II) terminators** of various strengths, which are found frequently within operons, cause a **pause** in the movement of the polymerase. Interaction with various regulatory proteins then governs the frequency either of termination within an operon (decreasing the transcription of subsequent genes) or of antitermination at the end of an operon (allowing readthrough of subsequent genes).

Strong terminators have a dyadic symmetry in their base sequence, which can form a hairpin; this sequence is immediately followed by a string of 6 to 8 U's. The hairpin in the mRNA evidently binds to the polymerase immediately ahead of it and causes a conformational change that halts further progress, while the following U's, forming weaker bonds than C or G, promote dissociation of the mRNA from the template DNA. The sequence as well as the length of the hairpin influence its interaction with the polymerase.

Weak terminators may form a smaller hairpin than strong ones, or may have none; and no consensus sequence has been recognized. They also do not have a string of U's, and the site of termination at a given terminator is somewhat variable (unlike the precise nucleotide in strong termination).

Termination protein Rho is required by weak terminators, and it accelerates release at strong terminators. This large, hexameric protein binds to a long stretch of mRNA (of about 80 bases) and then moves downstream to a paused polymerase, where its binding, accompanied by ATP hydrolysis, results in termination. The interaction is evidently direct, since defective Rho mutations may be suppressed by polymerase mutations. However, the binding of Rho can be prevented by various **antiterminator** proteins, which also bind to the polymerase-NusA complex. These include certain bacterial Nus proteins (and the N protein of phage lambda: Chap. 46).

Rho cannot reach the polymerase if any ribosomes intervene between its binding site and the polymerase. Its role is therefore especially prominent in **polarity** of operon transcription: premature termination when translation is impaired (see below). A different form of premature termination, involving access to a strong terminator, is responsible for another major regulatory mechanism, attenuation (see below).

PROCESSING

Posttranscriptional changes, which are extensive in the transcripts of eukaryotic genes, also occur in some bacterial transcripts. The rRNA operons contain the three rRNA genes in the order 16S–23S–5S, separated by spacers (which often contain tRNA genes and sometimes protein-coding genes). These products must all be separated from the transcript by processing. All three rRNAs are flanked by long terminal repeats, and the resulting hairpins are the sites of cleavage by RNase III; mature ends are generated by further trimming. The tRNAs are cleaved and trimmed by special endonucleases and exonucleases.

Introns, which are common in eukaryotic genes, are absent in eubacterial genes, but one is curiously present in a gene of bacteriophage T4, where it is excised by self-splicing.

ANTIBIOTICS AFFECTING TRANSCRIPTION

Completion of initiation is blocked by a group of antibiotics with an aromatic chromophore spanned by a long aliphatic bridge (Fig. 9–2): the naturally occurring **rifamycins,** the more effective semisynthetic derivative **rifampin,** and the **streptovaricins.** These antibiotics inhibit bacterial RNA polymerase but not the cytoplasmic enzyme of eukaryotes, and this selectivity has made rifa-

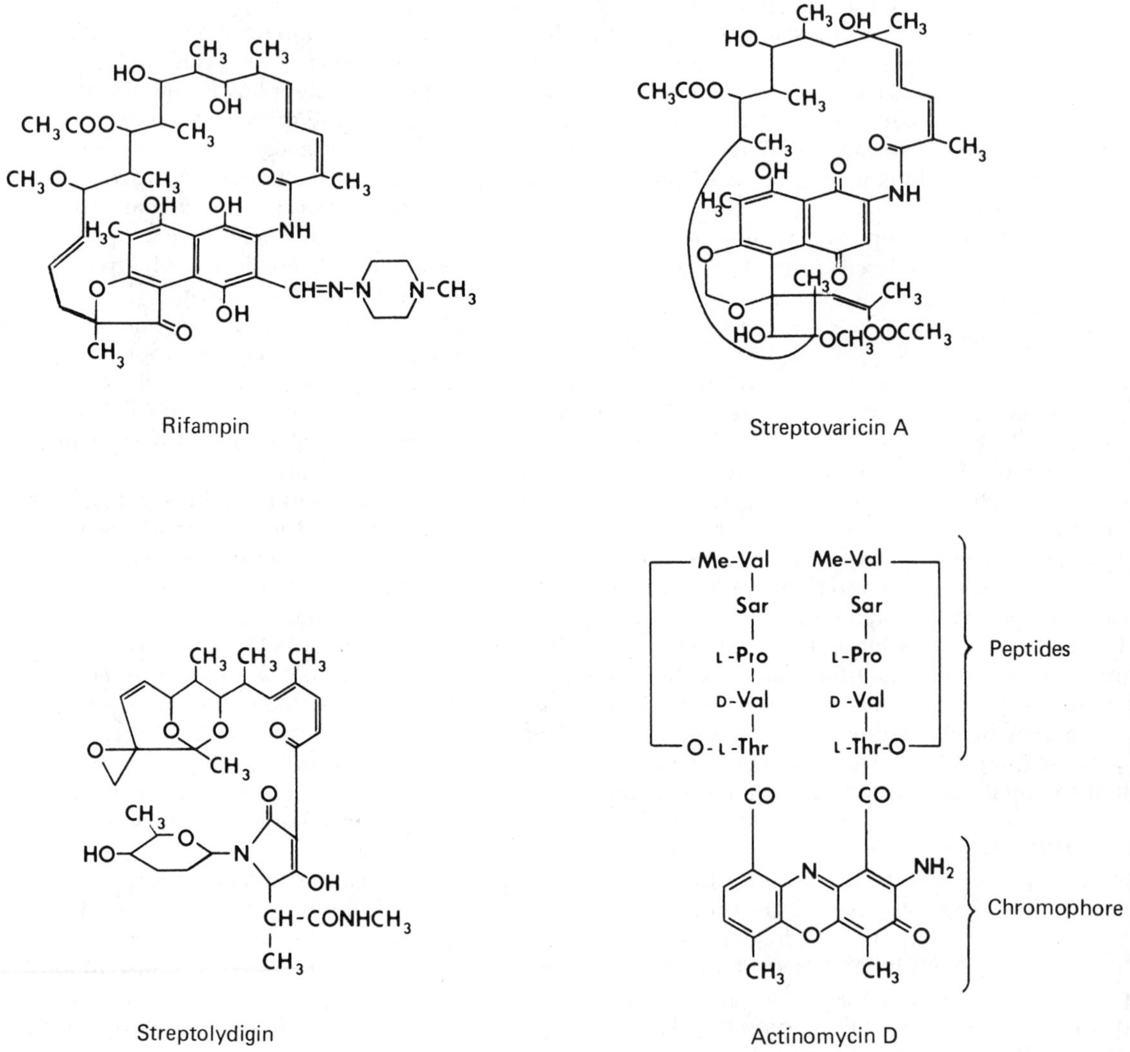

Rifampin

Streptovaricin A

Streptolydigin

Actinomycin D

Figure 9–2. Antibiotics that interfere with initiation of transcription (rifampin, streptovaricin) or chain extension (streptolydigin, actinomycin D.) *Sar,* sarcosine (N-Me-glycine); *Me-Val,* N-Me-L-valine.

mycins useful in antibacterial chemotherapy, especially against tuberculosis. Mutations to resistance have been useful tools for altering the polymerase.

Chain extension can be blocked in two ways. **Streptolydigin** (Fig. 9–2) binds to the polymerase. In contrast, actinomycin D (**dactinomycin**) binds to helical DNA at GC pairs; the chromophore (Fig. 9–2) intercalates into the helix, as demonstrated earlier for acridines, and the attached cyclic peptides appear to bind to the external surface. Like all antibiotics that bind to DNA, dactinomycin inhibits both transcription and replication, but the former process is much more sensitive. Evidently, the unwinding of the helix in replication behind a swivel point can dislodge dactinomycin, whereas the local, transient unwinding in transcription is less forceful.

Many other antibiotics that bind to DNA inhibit both transcription and replication, to different degrees. Some of them have intercalating polycyclic chromophores with attached sugars.

Enzyme Induction and Repression

As was noted in Chapter 4 (Alternative Carbon Sources), many enzymes for utilizing particular foodstuffs are formed only during growth in the presence of that substrate. In the 1940s Monod, at the Pasteur Institute, showed that the formation of **β-galactosidase** can be elicited not only by lactose and other substrates but also by analogues that cannot be utilized (e.g., methyl-β-D-thiogalactoside); hence, the mechanism involves a specific process of **enzyme induction** rather than direct adaptation to the improved nutrition of the cell. The response is rapid: within a minute or two, at a saturating concentration of inducer, the new enzyme becomes a constant fraction (ca. 5%) of the new protein; and on removal of the inducer, its formation ceases equally rapidly.

Induction of β-galactoside is accompanied by formation of an **active transport system** (Chap. 4) for uptake of the inducer. This response leads to an interesting positive feedback: in order to enter the cell initially (by an inefficient mechanism), the inducer must be present at a high concentration; but once the cell has been induced it can concentrate the inducer, and hence lower concentrations can maintain the induced state. However, some inducers are already present as intracellular metabolites (e.g., citrate, glucose-6-phosphate); they must act (in unknown ways) on the cell surface rather than in the cytoplasm.

Most catabolic enzymes are likewise inducible. In contrast, formation of most biosynthetic enzymes is subject to regulation in the opposite direction, **repression,** by an exogenously supplied endproduct (e.g., an amino acid). Nevertheless, these superficially opposite processes—induction and repression—involve fundamentally the same mechanism.

Endproduct repression of enzyme formation parallels the feedback inhibition of enzyme activity (Chap. 5) in the same pathway and is elicited by the same endproduct. However, their effects on the cellular economy and their mechanisms are quite different. Repression is a mechanism for sparing wasteful protein synthesis, and it affects all the enzymes of the pathway; feedback inhibition spares wasteful synthesis of metabolites, and it acts only on the first enzyme. Moreover, in inhibiting an enzyme, the endproduct acts directly on it, whereas in regulating enzyme synthesis the mechanisms are more elaborate.

Some enzymes are subject to both induction and repression: for example, glucose represses the formation of many enzymes inducible by other C sources (see Catabolite Repression, below). Probably all enzymes are normally subject to regulation of their formation, so the term **constitutive,** originally used to designate enzymes that are always present, is now used primarily for mutations that eliminate regulatory responses.

RESERVE CAPACITY FOR ENZYME FORMATION. Although feedback repression was discovered as an economy-promoting response to the exogenous supply of an endproduct, it is at least equally important as a response to the level of endogenously formed endproducts, adjusting the concentration of their enzymes as needed. In normal growth cells use only a fraction of the capacity of most genes, but they tap the full capacity when recovering from repression. For example, long-term growth in the presence of arginine severely represses the enzymes of arginine biosynthesis, and so when the exogenous supply is exhausted growth temporarily ceases. Restoration of protein synthesis is limited by arginine, derived initially as a trickle from protein turnover; but as Figure 9–3 shows, the enzymes that make arginine are preferentially synthesized until they reach their normal level, and growth gradually returns to normal within 10 minutes. This reserve capacity obviously accelerates the adaptation of bacteria to the fluctuating nutrition often encountered in nature.

GENE DOSAGE EFFECTS. When enzymes are regulated by endogenous feedback, their levels are not significantly affected by increasing the number of copies of the corresponding gene per genome, because a slight increase in the level of the signal will decrease the activity of all the copies. However, when a gene is fully induced, or is derepressed by mutation, product synthesis is proportional to the number of gene copies present. This response is of great practical value in the use of recombinant bacteria to make desired proteins.

Branched pathways have special regulatory arrange-

Figure 9–3. Preferential synthesis of a derepressed enzyme of arginine biosynthesis, ornithine transcarbamylase. *(A)* An *arg⁻his⁻* mutant, grown with **excess Arg** and His and transferred to a chemostat with limiting His and excess Arg. **Complete repression** of the enzyme continues. *(B)* The same cells in a chemostat with **limiting Arg** and excess His, show **completely derepressed** synthesis of the Arg enzyme (i.e., because of continued Arg limitation, this enzyme continues indefinitely to be synthesized up to the capacity of the gene). Only the early part of the curve of exponential increase, which finally levels off at 45 arbitrary units per cell, is shown. Thus, 50% of the final level is reached after one generation, 75% after two, etc., just as with a fully induced enzyme. *(C)* An *arg⁺his⁻* mutant, grown with **excess Arg** and His and transferred to a chemostat with limiting His and **no Arg.** The enzyme is initially synthesized at the fully derepressed rate relative to total protein synthesis, as in *B*. However, within about 0.05 generations, the restoration of Arg synthesis in this *arg⁺* strain causes formation of the enzyme to level off at the steady-state, **partly repressed** rate (maintaining 2.5 units per cell) characteristic of the wild type in minimal medium. We thus see that normal synthesis uses only about $\frac{1}{20}$ of the capacity of the gene, while the excess capacity is used for rapid adjustment to deprivation of exogenous arginine. (Gorini L, Maas WK: Biochim Biophys Acta 25:208, 1957)

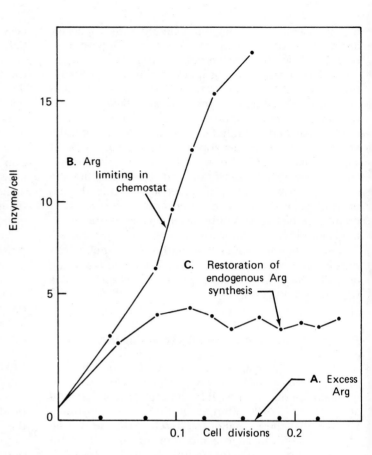

ments to avoid interference by one endproduct with the formation of another. One such arrangement involves **parallel enzymes** subject to different feedback repression (as well as to different feedback inhibition of enzyme activity; see Chap. 5, Fig. 5–8). Another response (e.g., in the synthesis of isoleucine, leucine, and valine) involves **multivalent control,** in which each of the endproducts contributes to regulating formation of the same enzymes; one mechanism, attenuation, will be described below.

Regulation of Initiation of Transcription

REPRESSOR, OPERATOR, AND OPERON

Jacob and Monod recognized that the synthesis of β-galactosidase can be altered by mutations in either of two genes: the structural gene, *lac-z*, or a regulatory gene, *lac-R* (often still called *lac-I* for inducible). Mutations in either gene can prevent formation of the enzyme, but mutations in the z gene also can cause formation of an altered product: a thermosensitive enzyme or an **immunologically cross-reacting material** (CRM). The R gene forms a diffusible cytoplasmic **repressor,** which

can act in *trans* and is dominant in a merozygote (Fig. 9–4); and mutations in this gene can make the cell constitutive for the enzyme.

Induction depends on reversible inactivation of the repressor by complexing with the inducer. In this kind of **negative control** the regulatory proteins are active repressors **until** they bind the **effector** (inducer). In endproduct repression, the relations are reversed: the regulatory proteins are active repressors only **after** binding the effector (**corepressor).** Inducers and corepressors exert an allosteric effect on the conformation of the repressor protein, just as in the feedback regulation of enzyme activity (see Fig. 5–10).

The evidence for a cytoplasmic repressor led to the prediction that it must act on a specific receptor, called the **operator;** if the operator governs only adjacent genes, its mutational inactivation should be dominant and should affect the *lac-z* gene on the same chromosome only (i.e., should act in *cis*). This prediction was confirmed by the isolation of *cis*-**dominant constitutive** (Oᶜ) mutants (Fig. 9–5).

The *lac* system was found to code also for genes for two additional proteins of β-galactoside metabolism, synthesized in coordination with β-galactosidase (Fig.

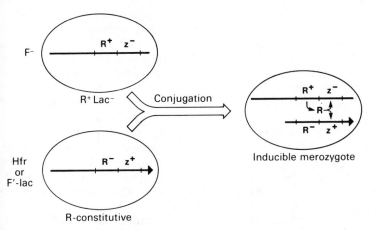

Figure 9–4. Dominance of R⁺*lac* (inducible) over R⁻*lac* (constitutive) allele. *Arrows* in merozygote indicate that the product of the *R* gene influences the activity of a *z* gene in a separate chromosome (*trans* effect) as well as in its own chromosome (*cis* effect). The donor may be either an Hfr or an F'-*lac* cell.

9–6): *lac-y*, for an active transport system, and *lac-a*, for a specific transacetylase, whose acetylation of non-metabolizable β-galactosides promotes their extrusion from the cell. This **unit of transcription** was called an **operon.** It starts with a **promoter (P)** sequence, which binds RNA polymerase and initiates transcription. That binding is blocked by binding of the R protein to the operator sequence, which overlaps the promoter (see below for more detail).

Each *R* gene has its own promoter. In the *lac* system the *R* gene is next to the operon, and occasional read-through from its promoter into the operon results in a very low "basal" level of expression of the uninduced operon. However, in many systems the *R* gene is separated by intervening genes from the operon that it regulates. Moreover, some pathways (e.g., to arginine) involve a **regulon:** a group of several operons that are scattered on the chromosome but nevertheless respond to the same cytoplasmic regulator and hence constitute a functionally coordinated unit.

Operons differ widely in size; one of the largest contains ten genes for enzymes of histidine biosynthesis, which are coordinately regulated (i.e., formed in fixed proportion at various levels of repression). However, the amounts are not necessarily equal: sites of premature termination of transcription between genes may decrease the rate of expression of distal ones, while secondary promoters within an operon can have the opposite effect. Some operons (e.g., *mal*) are **divergent;** i.e., a single operator controls promoters on both sides.

In eukaryotes, each gene resides in a separate operon. Prokaryotes may derive an evolutionary advantage from the clustering of functionally related genes in operons, an evolutionary advantage because they recombine genes by transfer of small blocks of DNA rather than by fusion of gametes.

POSITIVE REGULATION

While most inducible systems exhibit negative regulation by the product of an *R* gene, as just described, others—

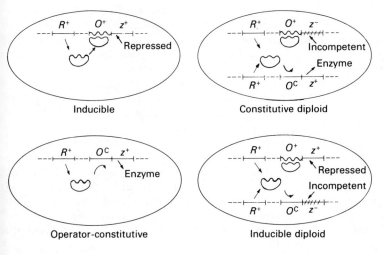

Figure 9–5. Dominance of operator constitutivity (O^C). Repressor *(R)* attaches to the wild-type operator *(O⁺)* (blocking expression of the *cis z⁺* gene) but not to the O^C operator. In isolating O^C mutants, merodiploid cells were used in order to avoid the more frequent (R⁻) constitutive mutants. Thus in an R⁺O⁺z⁺/R⁺O⁺z⁺ cell, mutation of either R⁺ gene to R⁻ would usually be recessive and hence not expressed, whereas mutation of O⁺ to O^C would be dominant and hence would be expressed.

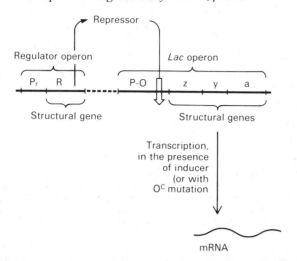

Figure 9–6. Map of the *lac* operon and its regulator operon. Structural genes, *z, y,* and *a* code respectively for β-galactosidase, the β-galactoside transport protein (Chap. 6), and β-galactoside transacetylase. Transcription is initiated at the promoter *(P)*, and its frequency is regulated by the overlapping operator *(O)* locus. The regulator operon is a primitive operon: it has a single structural gene R (for a repressor protein) and a weak promoter (P_r), but no operator.

for example, those for arabinose *(ara)* or maltose *(mal)* utilization and for regulation of phage lambda—involve **positive regulation,** in which the product of the *R* gene complexed with the inducer is required for activation of the genes. The "R" in *R* gene therefore now stands for "regulator" rather than "repressor." In positive regulation the binding of the activator protein adjacent to the promoter strengthens, rather than inhibits, the binding of the RNA polymerase. In general, while repressors bind downstream from, and overlap with, the promoter, activating regulatory proteins bind immediately upstream, providing an adjacent surface that increases binding of the RNA polymerase to an otherwise too weak promoter. Some R proteins can repress one operon and activate others.

The *ara* operon has a particularly elaborate mechanism: its R protein represses in one conformation and activates in the other. Moreover, it acts as a repressor of its own synthesis **(autoregulation),** and so it responds to induction by an initial burst of rapid, unrepressed synthesis, followed by maintenance synthesis at a lower rate. These multiple functions make the operon particularly well fitted to the intermittent exposure of *E. coli* to arabinose in the intestine, allowing rapid adaptive enzyme formation while avoiding overproduction.

MESSENGER RNA

Before considering further how regulatory proteins act, we shall review some features of mRNA. Its translation by ribosomes has been reviewed in Chapter 6.

DISCOVERY OF mRNA. The existence of mRNA as an intermediary in the transfer of information from DNA into protein was discovered by Jacob and Monod in 1961 through genetic studies. The introduction of a z^+ gene into R^-z^- cells led to enzyme synthesis at full rate within a few minutes, just like induction in R^+z^+ cells. Moreover, both these responses evidently involved synthesis of new template RNA, because they were prevented if the cells incorporated base analogues into the new RNA. However, ribosomes were unlikely templates, because studies with isotopes showed that they do not turn over. Accordingly, the DNA of the gene must be transcribed into a complementary RNA, named messenger, that turns over very rapidly.

Biochemical confirmation came within a year, in two ways. 1) After phage infection, which blocks synthesis of host RNA and protein, the newly formed, radioactively labeled RNA has the composition of phage DNA. 2) **Pulse labeling** of uninfected cells with radioactive phosphate (for less than 1 minute) heavily labels a rapidly turning over fraction (Fig. 9–7). In both cases the new RNA is partly complexed with ribosomes; moreover, this fraction ranges widely in molecular weight, thus explaining its failure to be detected in earlier biochemical analyses. Additional proof came later from hybridization of the rapidly labeled RNA to phage DNA in infected cells, and to the cellular DNA in uninfected cells, and from the translation of specific messengers *in vitro* (Chap. 6).

SIMULTANEOUS SYNTHESIS AND TRANSLATION OF mRNA. Transcription and translation take place in the same direction on the RNA ($5' \rightarrow 3'$); hence, in bacteria, where no nuclear membrane separates the two processes, multiple ribosomes can join and move along the mRNA while it is still growing, thus greatly increasing the efficiency of its use (which is essential if it is to turn over rapidly). Electron microscopic examination of gently prepared bacterial lysates reveals "trees" (Fig. 9–8) that confirm this model: a trunk of DNA carries parallel branches bearing ribosomes (i.e. polysomes) connected to the DNA by an RNA polymerase molecule and increasing in length as the polymerase moves from the site of initiation of transcription to that of termination. Each tree corresponds to an operon. The operons for rRNA (which is not translated) carry similar branches but without ribosomes.

Translation keeps pace with transcription, as is seen from the close approach of the ribosomes on polysomes to the attachment of the growing mRNA to DNA (Fig. 9–6). The rate of transcription and translation in *E. coli* at 37°C is about 45 nucleotides, and hence 15 amino acids, per second. *In vitro*, with much more dilute solutions, protein synthesis reaches only about one-tenth this rate.

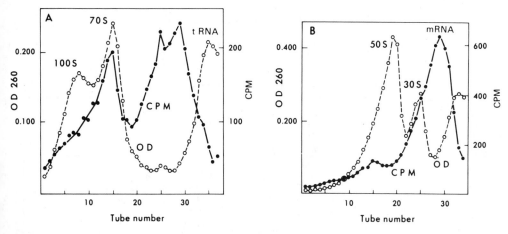

Figure 9–7. Zonal sedimentation of **pulse-labeled** RNA. RNA was labeled in *E. coli* by growth for 20 seconds with ^{14}C-uracil, and further metabolism was stopped rapidly by pouring on ice and adding azide. The cells were lysed by grinding with alumina, the lysates were sedimented in a sucrose gradient with Mg^{2+}-Tris buffer, and fractions were collected through the bottom of the tube and analyzed for RNA (optical density at 260 nm; open circles) and for radioactivity *(CPM)*. *(A)* Extracted and sedimented in 10 mM Mg^{2+}, which preserves the integrity of the ribosomes and their association with mRNA. The pulse-labeled RNA *(closed circles)* sediments partly with the 70S (ribosome) and 100S (disome) peaks and partly as a broad slower peak of free mRNA and nascent rRNA. *(B)* Sedimented in 0.1 mM Mg^{2+}, which dissociates the ribosomes into their 50S and 30S subunits and releases the labeled RNA, now all seen as a broad, slower peak. The lysis by grinding in this early work produced much fragmentation; gentler methods later yielded much longer polysomes, binding a larger fraction of the pulse-labeled RNA. (Gros F et al: Nature 190:581, 1961)

BREAKDOWN OF mRNA. The concentration of an RNA depends on the rates of its breakdown as well as its formation. Hybridization with the DNA of selected parts of the tryptophan operon (Fig. 9–9) after a brief pulse of transcription shows that the mRNA from the first gene begins to disappear before any mRNA from the last gene is made. Hence, overall mRNA breakdown proceeds in the same direction as synthesis and simultaneously with it. The mRNA of this operon is translated about 30 times before destruction.

Complexing with ribosomes stabilizes mRNA, and breakdown appears to be initiated in regions that are at least transiently freed of ribosomes. Thus, when the polysomes in the cell are blocked by chloramphenicol, the mRNA is much more stable; conversely, releasing the ribosomes has the opposite effect (see Polarity, below).

Non-messenger RNAs are evidently stabilized by extensive secondary structure, methylation, and, possibly, absence of sequences suitable for nucleolytic attack. With nascent rRNA the long chains are further protected by the rapid binding of ribosomal proteins.

mRNA breakdown is initiated by cleavage by an **en-**

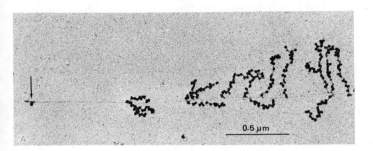

Figure 9–8. Electron micrograph of active operon recovered in gentle lysate of *E. coli*. The rectilinear thin fibers can be destroyed by treatment with DNase, while the attached chains can be destroyed by RNase. (They are also released by protease, because RNA polymerase is essential for their attachment.) Picture illustrates formation of messenger. The growing mRNA chains are essentially fully loaded with ribosomes, and they exhibit an irregular gradient of increasing length along the gene. Most regions of DNA are free of such appended polysomes, which is consistent with other evidence that only a small fraction of the genome is being transcribed at any time. An RNA polymerase molecule (mol. wt. 4×10^5) is visible at the presumptive site of initiation *(arrow)* and at the site of attachment of most chains. (Miller OL Jr et al: Science 169:392, 1970. Copyright © 1970 by the American Association for the Advancement of Science.)

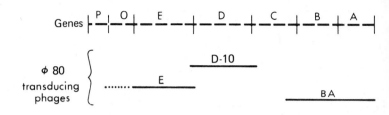

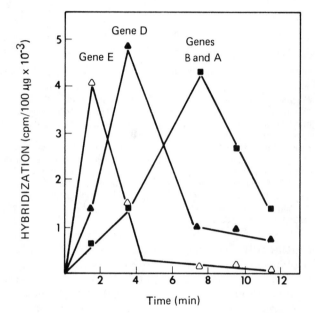

Figure 9–9. Sequential synthesis and degradation of the mRNA of the tryptophan operon in *E. coli*. Cells were derepressed at 0 time to initiate transcription with ³H-uridine present to label the RNA formed. After 1.5 minutes tryptophan was added to restore repression (i.e., to prevent new initiations). At various times, RNA was extracted, and portions were hybridized to the DNA of different transducing φ80 phages carrying selected parts of the operon, as indicated in the upper part of the figure. The curves show that such a pulse of derepression causes a wave of transcription that moves from one end of the operon to the other in about 6 minutes. (After Morse DS et al: Cold Spring Harbor Symp Quant Biol 34:725, 1969)

donuclease at certain preferred sites, and because the remainder of the transcript of that gene is not protected by a continuing entry of ribosomes, its additional sites suitable for cleavage become more accessible to the endonuclease. Although overall breakdown proceeds 5′ → 3′, each cleavage provides a substrate for **exonucleolytic digestion in the opposite direction.** This digestion involves both RNase II (which yields 5′ nucleotides) and polynucleotide phosphorylase (which cleaves by addition of P_i to yield 5′-nucleoside diphosphates); mutants lacking either still grow well, while the double mutants are not viable. The phosphorylase confers the advantage of preserving a high-energy bond; the value of using the less economical hydrolase is not clear, except perhaps when phosphate is limiting.

The kinetics of mRNA breakdown has been studied by labeling the RNA in growing bacteria and then abruptly stopping its synthesis with actinomycin. Breakdown proceeds exponentially, with an average half-life of about 2 minutes at 37°C. The results with briefly labeled

cells show that mRNA constitutes more than half the **total** synthesis of RNA, the rest being the stable RNA. However, mRNA constitutes only a small fraction of the **net** RNA synthesis (i.e., the fraction of the RNA composition of the cell): after steady-state labeling, only 5% of the label is lost after addition of actinomycin.

VARIATION IN mRNA BREAKDOWN. Different mRNAs have different half-lives ranging from 0.5 to 10 minutes, an important mechanism in the regulation of gene expression. The decay of individual messengers, as of total mRNA, is exponential, reflecting random timing of the initiating cleavage. *E. coli* has 500 to 1000 copies of a repetitive, highly conserved sequence, called *rep*, in which an inverted repeat of 35 bases forms a stable stem-loop; some operons have multiple copies. While the functions of these sequences are not certain, deletions show that they protect the upstream RNA from digestion from the 3′-end. In addition, near the 5′-end highly labile mRNAs have a specific site for endonuclease attack. This action initiates rapid decay, involving multiple cleavage of the untranslated distal segment, followed by exonucleolytic digestion of the fragments.

EUKARYOTIC MESSENGERS. Because the DNA and the ribosomes are in separate compartments in eukaryotic cells, eukaryotic mRNA differs from that in prokaryotes in several ways. Most obviously, the transcript, formed in the nucleus, cannot be complexed with ribosomes until it has been transferred to the cytoplasm. In addition, most gene transcripts in mammals, and some coded by phages (but not by the bacteria), have **introns,** which must be spliced out in the processing of messenger. Introns are not present in prokaryotes, where they would prevent the translation of growing mRNA. The eukaryotic messenger is further processed by the formation of a specialized 5' cap and the addition of a long 3'-terminal poly(A) tail, and it is much more stable than prokaryotic mRNA.

It thus appears that bacteria, which can multiply on a much shorter time scale, have lost the benefits of introns (accelerated evolution of novel proteins, and possibly more refined regulation) while gaining a faster adjustment of cell composition to environmental fluctuations through a more immediate use and more rapid turnover of mRNA. Another significant difference is that each mammalian gene has its own operator, evidently providing greater flexibility in cell composition.

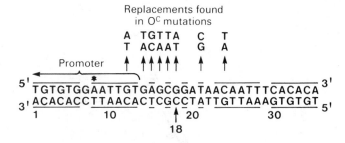

Figure 9–10. The *lac* operator sequence of *E. coli* (i.e., the region protected by *lac* repressor from digestion by DNase). The sequence has extensive dyadic symmetry (see text) with its axis at base pair 18; the bases involved are indicated by lines above and below. The identified point mutations that have yielded an O^c phenotype are indicated; their locations show that the central region of the operator plays an especially large role in binding repressor.

Bases in close contact with the repressor have been identified by several additional approaches. These include (1) influence of repressor binding on methylation of A or G by Me$_2$SO$_4$; (2) UV-induced cross-linking of the protein to DNA containing 5-bromouracil (5-BU, a photoreactive analogue) in place of T; and (3) altered binding of repressor to synthetic sequences in which various analogues have replaced specific single bases. The results indicate that the repressor binds to one side of the operator, alternately contacting bases from one strand and then from the other, in the next half-turn of the helix.

Transcription starts and proceeds, to the right, from base pair 8 (denoted by *asterisk*). The promoter (i.e., the region protected by RNA polymerase from digestion) extends 38 base pairs "upstream" from this point (not shown) and 6 "downstream"; hence roughly half of the promoter (P) and of the operator (O) overlap. (After Ogata R, Gilbert W: Proc Natl Acad Sci USA 74:4973, 1977)

MOLECULAR MECHANISM OF OPERON REPRESSION AND ACTIVATION

We will now consider in somewhat greater detail the interactions of regulatory proteins with operons, including several additional mechanisms that were discovered later.

KINETICS OF BINDING TO DNA. The *lac* repressor, a 150,000-dalton molecule of four identical subunits, binds to double-stranded DNA of the operator, which can be isolated by virtue of its protection by bound repressor from enzymatic digestion or chemical modification ("**footprinting**"). It also can be greatly increased in amount by genetic techniques). The binding can be shown *in vitro* to have extremely high affinity (dissociation constant about 10^{-12}M); hence a very few molecules of repressor suffice. The inducer, whose binding to the repressor greatly decreases affinity for operator DNA (as predicted), actively induces an allosteric change, for it markedly accelerates the otherwise-slow release of already bound repressor. The multivalent binding of the tetrameric repressor and the allosteric cooperativity of the subunits (as noted for allosteric enzymes in Chap. 5, Figs. 5–10 and 5–11) account for the very tight binding

and the striking speed of its reversal in the cell by induction.

Some regulatory proteins repress or activate an operon indirectly, by modifying another protein; hence binding studies are necessary to identify a direct regulator.

The number of repressor molecules in a cell can be titrated in an effect called **transduction escape synthesis:** when the number of copies of the operon introduced by transduction exceeds the number of repressor molecules synthesis is activated.

PROMOTER-OPERATOR SEQUENCES. In the *lac* operon the promoter sequence (P), defined by its protection by RNA polymerase from DNase action in vitro, is about 44 base pairs long, while the operator sequence (O), similarly defined by its protection by the repressor, is about 35 base pairs long. The two sequences overlap extensively, as suggested by binding competition and established by their sequences. As Figure 9–10 shows, the *lac* O region has extensive dyadic symmetry, which fits the binding of a symmetric repressor molecule.

The interactions of repressor and operator are now known in refined detail, including the contact points,

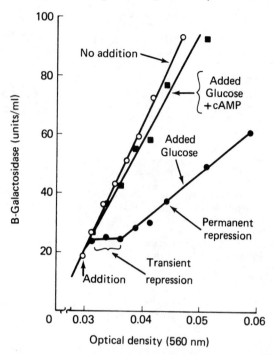

Figure 9–11. Catabolite repression of β-galactosidase synthesis and its reversal by cAMP. Glucose, with or without cAMP, was added to a culture of *E. coli* growing on succinate in the presence of an inducer of the enzyme, isopropyl-β-D-thiogalactoside (IPTG). The cAMP is seen to overcome both the transient (complete) and the permanent (partial) repression by glucose. The brief lag before repression reflects the completion and the translation of already initiated messenger. (After Pastan I, Perlman R: Science 169:339, 1970. Copyright © 1970 by the American Association for the Advancement of Science.)

their relation to the three-dimensional structure of the protein, and the slight conformational changes in both that are induced by the binding.

PROMOTER AND SIGMA VARIATION

The affinity of various promoters for a specific RNA polymerase depends on the degree of their deviations from a promoter **consensus sequence.** This affinity determines the maximal rate of transcription of an operon; the resulting protein production ranges from ten molecules per cell doubling, for some regulatory proteins, to 10^4 to 10^5 for some proteins involved in protein synthesis or in membrane structure. R genes, which require only low-level activity, may be regulated in an inflexible way, by low-level promoters; hence when the *lac-R*$^+$ gene is introduced into growing R$^-$ cells, the conversion from constitutive to inducible requires 60 minutes. Alternatively, as noted above, the *ara* R protein has an autoregulated

reserve capacity and therefore responds more rapidly. Curiously, other low-activity genes, concerned with the synthesis of trace metabolites such as biotin, have repressors, although the economic benefit cannot be large.

Secondary promoters are found within genes in some operons, and they may be created by mutation. They permit weak expression of distal genes despite repression of the proximal genes. **Tandem promoters,** differing in sequence, are found at the beginning of some operons, where their responses to different regulators broaden the range of response.

SIGMA VARIATION. Another important mechanism of operon regulation is the use of various sigma factors, which differ in their affinity for different groups of promoters. Additional sigma factors are induced to activate major groups of genes required for N uptake (the glutamine regulon), or in the responses to various kinds of stress such as heat shock (as discussed at the end of this chapter). Even more dramatic shifts, eliminating the normal sigma factor, are seen in sporulation (Chap. 2) and in phage production (Chap. 45).

The gene for one sigma factor in the sporulating mother cell is a composite, formed from portions of two genes by site-specific recombination within a 5-base-pair repeat. The loss of the intervening DNA affects only the mother cell, a terminally differentiated cell that is later discarded; the spore is in effect a germline cell. Bacteria thus evolved a mechanism for irreversibly rearranging the genome of a differentiated cell—a process that became greatly expanded in eukaryotic cells, especially in immunoglobulin formation.

CYCLIC AMP AND CATABOLITE REPRESSION

Monod's interest in the mechanism of enzyme regulation began with his discovery of a biphasic growth pattern, which he named **diauxie:** *E. coli* growing in a mixture of glucose with either lactose or various other C sources first consumes all the glucose and then adapts, after a few minutes, to utilization of the second, less rapidly used, compound. This "**glucose effect**" obviates the synthesis of many enzymes that would be superfluous, because glucose alone evidently supplies C and energy as rapidly as they can be used.

On the assumption that the system was responding to the level of some catabolic intermediate, the glucose effect was renamed **catabolite repression.** However, the key turned out to be **activation** by a special signal molecule, adenosine-3′,5′-monophosphate (**cyclic AMP, cAMP;** see below), whose level varies **inversely** with the rate of catabolism of the C source.

This information transmitter, discovered by Sutherland in mammalian cells and later in bacteria, is made

Cyclic AMP

from ATP, by the loss of PP, by a membrane-bound **adenyl cyclase.** The complex of cAMP with a 45,000-dalton **cAMP acceptor protein, CAP** (also called CRP), forms an **activator** that is required by many operons concerned with supplying C. The addition of cAMP to cells overcomes the catabolite repression of many C sources (Fig. 9–11); and mutants defective in either adenyl cyclase or CAP have lost the ability to be induced to utilize these fuels. In addition to functioning as an activator, the cAMP-CRP complex **represses** some operons that would increase the demand for C (e.g., glutamine metabolism, central to N uptake).

Because cAMP is formed from ATP, the inhibition of the reaction by the higher energy supply from glucose is paradoxical. However, a nonmetabolizable analogue of glucose can have the same effect. The control appears to be elaborate, depending not directly on the energy supply but rather on the phosphorylation of a protein (III^{Glc}) involved in a phosphotransferase membrane transport system (see Chap. 4). Moreover, its rapid transfer of phosphate to glucose elevates the unphosphorylated form of this protein, which further contributes to the glucose effect by **inducer exclusion:** repression of the formation of transport systems for many other sugars.

Compounds below glucose in the rate of energy supply can repress the response to C sources that are still lower in the hierarchy. Bacilli employ cGMP instead of cAMP.

ENHANCEMENT AND DNA LOOPING

Studies of gene regulation in mammalian cells revealed the frequent presence of **enhancer sequences:** regulatory regions several hundred nucleotides away, on either side, from the promoter of the operon being regulated. Similar regions were discovered later in bacteria (e.g., the *lac* or *ara* operons; lambda phage). The mechanism of transmission of information from such a distance turned out to be formation of a loop of the DNA by interaction between two proteins, each binding tightly to the regulatory sequence at one end of the loop. This mechanism was suggested by *in vivo* experiments with bacterial mutants in which the distance between the regulator and the promoter was varied: effectiveness of regulation alternately increased and decreased with each added half-turn of the DNA helix, as would be expected of a loop, as the proteins would reach each other most easily if they were bound on the same side of the helix. Loops were subsequently formed *in vitro* and demonstrated directly by electron microscopy.

DNA looping evidently broadens the range of proteins that can be used to regulate one operon; one system (*ara*) has been seen to form loops with various enhancer sequences.

REGULATION OF NITROGEN AND PHOSPHATE ASSIMILATION

In the discussion of the largest biosynthetic pathway, that for the assimilation of N from NH_3 or other nitrogenous compounds, Chapter 5 described a **cascade mechanism** for finely adjusting the **activity** of a key enzyme, **glutamine synthetase (GS),** in response to the levels of many metabolites. Magasanik has worked out the similarly elaborate mechanism for regulating the **formation** of the products of a number of genes (*gln*) of nitrogen metabolism, including GS. In this mechanism the same protein PII that regulates GS activity and is itself regulated by a uridylylation cycle also regulates the phosphorylation of another regulatory protein, which controls transcription by a special RNA polymerase initiation factor for the glutamine regulon, sigma-60. In addition, there is a second promoter for GS, controlled by cAMP. Finally, the level of GS is also regulated by its turnover, in which the state of its adenylation affects its inactivation by mixed function oxidases.

The uptake and the metabolism of **phosphate** also involve elaborate regulatory processes. Not only does the **Pho regulon,** responsive to a single R-protein and to the level of P, govern 20 genes, but the level of P also influences at least 40 additional, unidentified genes, as shown by changes in the intensity of the corresponding protein spots (among a thousand others) in two-dimensional chromatograms.

Histidine can provide both C and N, and its utilization is regulated in response to either need. When C becomes limiting induction of the genes for histidine utilization (*hut*) involves cAMP (as in other systems responsive to C starvation); while when N is limiting another mechanism, involving adenylylation of GS, is invoked.

Regulation of Transcription Termination and of Translation

Translation can influence transcription in several ways. One mechanism is passive and global: when protein synthesis is inhibited many products of biosynthesis and of energy metabolism accumulate for lack of an outlet, and they repress their operons. In addition, two more specific, direct mechanisms have been observed: polarity and attenuation.

OPERON POLARITY; ANTITERMINATION

While many operons are transcribed without interruption into a complete messenger, thus yielding equimolar quantities of their several products, others have termination signals of various strengths between their genes. For example, in the *lac* operon, the molar ratio of the successive z, y, and a products is about 5/2/1.

This important regulatory mechanism was discovered through a laboratory artefact: nonsense (termination) mutations not only block translation of the remainder of a gene but also can decrease the transcription of the distal (downstream) genes of the operon, without affecting proximal ones. The degree of inhibition increases with the length of the "dead space" between the termination site and the beginning of the next gene: for the absence of translation in this region exposes weak termination signals, whose formation of a hairpin would be prevented by a stream of ribosomes; and the probability of encountering such a signal naturally increases with the length of the exposed mRNA. Termination factor Rho, which is required by weak signals (see above, Termination), then binds to naked mRNA and moves downstream to interact with the pausing RNA polymerase.

Polarity can be **suppressed** by **mutations in Rho** and also in certain **antitermination proteins** that antagonize the action of Rho. These proteins were discovered because of their key role in regulating the cycles of temperate phages (Chap. 46), but they are also important for bacterial function. Thus, because the long chains of rRNA are not translated, and they inevitably contain weak termination signals, their completion depends on antitermination proteins: mutations in one such, NusB, cause cells to make some incomplete rRNA molecules.

ATTENUATION

A mechanism of operon regulation very different from promotor repression or activation attenuation, was discovered in Yanofsky's studies of the *trp* operon. The derepressed levels of the Trp enzymes, elevated by the genetic inactivation of the repressor, were unexpectedly further elevated by limiting the supply of Trp in an auxotroph, and determination of the sequence of the early part of this operon revealed the basis: variable **premature termination** (**attenuation**) of transcription in a special **leader region** following the promoter.

In this region, of about 200 nucleotides, the early part codes for a **leader peptide** of 14 residues, which overlaps the subsequent **attenuator segment.** This segment can form either of two stem-loop structures (Fig. 9–12) by pairing a short sequence with either of two adjacent sequences, one proximal and the other distal. The distal stem, together with the immediately following string of U's, serves as a **transcription terminator** that releases the polymerase, while the alternative formation of the first stem does not have this effect. Because the preceding leader peptide contains two successive Trp residues, the supply of Trp governs the choice of stems. When Trp is freely available, the flow of ribosomes completing and releasing successive molecules of leader peptide continually covers a sequence that would be required for the proximal stem. The attenuator can then form only the distal stem, resulting in frequent release of the RNA polymerase and thus inhibiting further transcription of the operon. On the other hand, with a limiting supply of Trp the arrest of the ribosomes at the Trp codons in the leader message frees the remainder of that message to form the alternative proximal stem (which is energetically favored), thus preventing attenuation. To prevent the RNA polymerase from escaping before the attenuator mechanism has chosen its stem, the leader region in the mRNA contains a sequence that causes the enzyme to pause.

Most operons for amino acid synthesis have an attenuator. In the Phe and the His operons the leader peptide contains seven copies of the endproduct. In the operon for the branched pathway to Ileu, Leu, and Val (*ilv*), it contains multiple copies of all three, in harmony with the **multivalent regulation** described above.

THE ROLE OF ATTENUATION. Because in cells in steady-state growth the aa-tRNAs are all nearly fully charged, it appears that the attenuators are normally closed. The function of attenuation is thus to provide an emergency response, that is, the highly selective burst of synthesis seen when a cell is starved for a particular endproduct (see Fig. 9–1). In various operons, release of attenuation increases maximal expression by 8 to 20 fold.

Full attenuation thus evidently still allows expression up to the level required for the highest steady-state growth rate, and so the regulation at lower rates must depend on other mechanisms. With the *trp* operon the operator-repressor mechanism can serve this role. However, **most amino acid operons have only an attenuator and no operator,** and so they must use some other

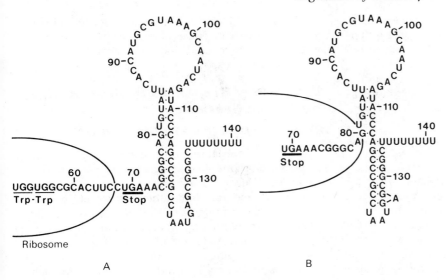

Figure 9–12. Possible secondary structures of mRNA involved in attenuation in the *trp* operon of *E. coli*. The leader sequence starts being transcribed at nucleotide 1 (not shown), and it codes for a 14-residue leader peptide from nucleotide 27 through 68, followed by termination codon UGA *(underlined)*. That peptide contains two Trp residues (codons UGG; *underlined*). If Trp is available the leader peptide is completed, and the leader mRNA sequence is terminated at the attenuator site (141); if Trp is not available the ribosome is held up, and the leader sequence continues to be transcribed, reaching the first structural gene of the operon at nucleotide 163 (not shown).

The connection between leader peptide synthesis and attenuation depends on an effect of the ribosome on the alternative secondary structures of this mRNA. Ribosomes mask a dozen nucleotides on either side of the codon being recognized: hence, a ribosome held up at UGG should not interfere with the formation of **form I** *(A)* of the leader sequence. However, if Trp–tRNA is present, the ribosomes proceed to the end of the peptide, where they interfere with the first stem. The second stem, in **form II** *(B)*, can then form. This secondary structure, extending close to the site of potential premature termination of transcription, promotes this termination, thus linking it to the supply of Trp. (After Lee F, Yanofsky C: Proc Natl Acad Sci USA 74:4365, 1977)

mechanism of response to growth rate, just as in the regulation of ribosomal RNA synthesis (see below). This mechanism is not well understood. One participant appears to be the **host integration factor (HIF),** a protein discovered to be required for integration of temperate phages (Chap. 46) but also later seen to influence expression of host operons.

Other forms of transcriptional attenuation, not involving a leader sequence, have also been found. Induction of the degradative protein tryptophanase is regulated by an **allosteric antiterminator protein,** whose interaction with Trp governs its ability to antagonize the activity of the transcription termination protein Rho at a weak terminator sequence early in the operon. Pyrimidine biosynthesis exhibits another mechanism: the distance between the polymerase and the first ribosome behind it normally allows occasional formation of a termination hairpin at an early site in the operon; but a decreased level of pyrimidine nucleotides, slowing transcription relative to translation, decreases the distance and thus prevents hairpin formation.

TRANSLATIONAL ATTENUATION

Attenuation acting on initiation of translation, rather than on termination of transcription, has also been observed, but in these cases leader peptide synthesis is impaired by an inhibitor rather than by deprivation of aa-tRNA. The best known case involves a gene for an enzyme that methylates a particular base in ribosomal RNA, making the ribosome resistant to erythromycin (Chap. 10). Preceding that gene is an attenuator sequence whose transcript can form two alternative loops, overlapping either the messenger for a leader peptide or the ribosome-binding site of the gene for the enzyme. Because the messengers for the peptide and for the enzyme are out of frame, the latter must initiate by binding a ribosome rather than by readthrough. Normally, continual synthesis of the leader peptide forces formation of the distal loop, thus preventing synthesis of the enzyme. However, erythromycin halts ribosomes after incorporation of a few amino acids, thus allowing the remainder of the leader peptide message, no longer covered by ribosomes, to form the proximal, energetically favored loop. The ribosome-binding site on the message for the enzyme is thus released and the enzyme can be synthesized.

Chloramphenicol uses a similar mechanism in inducing formation of an inactivating enzyme, chloramphenicol transacetylase.

OTHER TRANSLATIONAL REGULATION: ANTISENSE RNA

Regulation at the level of translation appears in general to be less important in prokaryotes than in eukaryotes, except for the attenuation just described, and the regulation of ribosomal protein synthesis discussed below. However, as noted above, factors that influence the stability of mRNA, and variations in the frequency of reinitiation of translation in the middle of a message, also influence gene expression. In addition, RNA that is complementary to an mRNA can form a strong RNA–RNA duplex that blocks translation both *in vitro* and in the cell.

A few such **antisense transcripts,** complementary to a region of mRNA but formed on the chromosome at a separate location (rather than on the opposite DNA strand), occur naturally, as revealed by analysis of the finding that extra copies of a distant region of cellular DNA inhibit the formation of a specific protein (e.g., the outer membrane protein **ompF**). In a more complex example, the cAMP activator protein (CAP) regulates its own production (and that of adenyl cyclase) by **divergent transcription:** its complex with cAMP initiates transcription of the early part of its own operon in the reverse direction, thus forming an RNA that inhibits the normal transcription.

The importance of antisense RNA as a natural regulatory mechanism is not certain. **Artificial antisense sequences** are a useful experimental tool for modifying gene expression in eukaryotes as well as prokaryotes, and they may be candidates for antiviral drugs.

Regulatory Responses to Growth Rate; Ribosome Synthesis

CELL COMPOSITION AND GROWTH RATE

Although the obligatory constituents of the cell, unlike inducible or repressible enzymes, are "constitutive" in the sense of always being present, they are not synthesized at a fixed rate but rather are closely regulated. Indeed, because the size of bacteria varies four-fold in different parts of the growth curve (Chap. 3), there must be some mechanism for broadly adjusting cell composition to the changing conditions.

Maaloe in Denmark introduced a new approach to this problem by replacing the notion of phases in a cell cycle in the classic growth curve with the notion of adaptation to growth at different rates. Moreover, he recognized that growth at a strictly constant rate is **balanced;** i.e., it maintains a constant composition; and in balanced growth at various rates, whether controlled by the composition of the medium or by the chemostat, **the ratio of RNA to DNA is proportional to the growth rate,** whereas the ratio of protein to DNA remains essentially constant. Except at very low growth rates, the variation in RNA concentration is due largely to its major component, rRNA (Table 9–1), and hence it roughly reflects the concentration of ribosomes.

It is thus clear that over a broad range of growth rates the expensive ribosomes are formed only in the amount needed, so they work to capacity; i.e., are equally fully engaged and move along the mRNA at the same rate. This constant output per ribosome is possible, even though ribosomes are more dilute in slower growing

TABLE 9–1. RNA Distribution and Protein Synthesis in S. typhimurium at Various Growth Rates

| Carbon source | Growth rate (generations/h) | DNA (μg/mg bact. dry wt) | rRNA/ DNA | tRNA/ DNA | Protein/ DNA | Protein Synthesis per Hour | |
						Per unit RNA	Per unit rRNA
Broth	2.4	30	8.3	2.0	22	3.7	4.5
Glucose	1.2	35	3.9	2.4	21	2.8	4.6
Glycerol	0.6	37	2.4	2.4	21	1.8	3.6
Glutamate	0.2	40	0.9	2.1	21	1.0	3.3

The growth rate was controlled by providing C sources that differ in their maximum rate of utilization. The cells were harvested at low densities, below 0.15 mg dry weight/m. Above this value, alterations of the medium by the metabolizing cells began to cause unbalanced growth, resulting in progressive changes in cell composition. Conventionally plotted growth is much less sensitive to such changes and appears to remain exponential until about half-way to the saturation level of 1 to 2 mg/ml.

cells, because the rate of translation is ordinarily determined by the rate of initiation, and the concentration of initiating subunits is maintained. (In very slow growth, the ratio of rRNA to growth rate rises for two reasons: the initiating ribosomal subunits become a substantial fraction of the total ribosomes; and with the decreased supply of energy, and possibly of amino acids, the rate of chain elongation becomes somewhat slower.)

The **maximal growth rate** of a bacterium in a rich medium is probably set by two factors: the rate of protein synthesis per ribosome, and the maximal concentration of ribosomes that a cell can support in proportion to its other components. In rapidly growing *E. coli* (doubling time 22 minutes at 37°C), containing about 25,000 ribosomes per genome, the average distance between ribosomes (outside the nuclear region) is about the diameter of a ribosome, and the machinery of protein synthesis contains more than half the total cell protein. It is evidently not possible to sustain a higher concentration of ribosomes without sacrificing the supply of building blocks and energy that their activity requires.

The total **tRNA concentration** does not vary much with growth rate (Table 9–1). This pattern is not surprising, because the concentration required for rapid recognition of each successive codon on a ribosome would be the same whether the ribosomes are concentrated or dilute. Nevertheless, the regulation of the tRNAs is not well understood, for many of their genes are present in operons that produce, in more widely fluctuating quantities, rRNA or ribosomal proteins (see below).

RESPONSE OF SYNTHESIS TO SHIFTS IN GROWTH RATE.
Global regulation of cell composition was further analyzed by studying the **dynamics of the transition** from one steady-state composition to another, and these processes were also found to be very efficient. In an abrupt **upshift** to a richer medium, the ribosome concentration is immediately growth-limiting, and in response the **rate of net RNA synthesis** (largely rRNA) increases **abruptly** (Fig. 9–13), thus rapidly increasing the concentration of the ribosomes. The **rate of protein synthesis,** however, can increase only **gradually,** as the number of ribosomes increases. When the cells reach the ribosome concentration appropriate for the new medium, the rate of rRNA synthesis is reduced, and the total protein rate has risen, to the values that maintain the proper composition. The rapidly increased synthesis of rRNA in an upshift is accompanied by a parallel shift in the synthesis of r-proteins, evidently at the expense of a passive decrease in the synthesis of other proteins, because the total protein synthesis cannot leap forward.

Conversely, in a **downshift** to a poorer medium protein synthesis shifts immediately to the new, lower, rate because of the diminished supply of building blocks and energy; hence, the cells contain idle ribosomes. In response, **rRNA synthesis ceases abruptly,** and there is also breakdown of idle ribosomes. rRNA synthesis resumes only when cell growth and ribosome breakdown have diluted the ribosomes to the level appropriate for the new growth rate.

The rapid increase of rRNA synthesis in an upshift requires the presence of a reservoir of free **RNA polymerase** in addition to that already complexed with DNA. Hence, this enzyme, unlike ribosomes, is not ordinarily adjusted to full use except at the highest growth rate.

GLOBAL REGULATION.
The study of the regulation of the overall composition of the growing cell revealed that

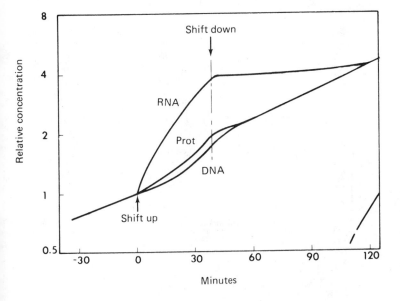

Figure 9–13. Responses of DNA, net RNA, and protein synthesis to shift up and shift down of the medium. The curves are idealized, and the amount of each component per milliliter of culture is normalized to 1.0 at the time of the initial shift. The shift down depicted does not involve a diauxic lag. When there is such a lag, as in adapting to a new C source, the absence of an energy supply temporarily halts net synthesis of all three classes until turnover of mRNA and protein (see text, Protein Breakdown) has built up the required new enzymes.

there are no master controls. Instead, global regulation results from an intricate network of mechanisms. The replication of DNA is regulated at a single origin (see below), while several thousand RNA and protein species are governed individually and in functionally related groups, linked by a network of regulatory effectors and also by the rate of supply of energy and material (i.e., some systems are regulated passively by competition for a limited supply of substrates). In attacking the problem of metabolic regulation, microbiologists, following the lead of physicists, initially sought the simplest possible solutions; but they found that the very different aim of evolution—maximal flexibility and efficiency in adjusting to environmental variations—had led to an elaborate system.

The study of the regulation of cell composition led to study of the regulation of a major component, ribosome synthesis. In addition to the 52 proteins and three RNAs of the ribosome, this synthesis is linked to the formation of about 50 additional proteins and 40 additional RNAs of the **protein-synthesizing system.**

REGULATION OF RIBOSOMAL RNA SYNTHESIS BY ppGpp AND BY FREE RIBOSOMES

In the regulation of ribosome formation, there are two feedback loops, one for rRNA and the other for the r-proteins. Because the rRNA is not released as a free product but rather forms complexes with the proteins while it is still growing, it cannot regulate itself; instead, it is sensitive to the level of inactive ribosomes. Its rate of supply, and hence its rate of complexing with the r-proteins, in turn affects their levels (which are very low), and these then feed back to govern their own formation. The two loops are thus linked.

The genes for the 52 r-proteins are distributed in single copies of about 20 operons, each containing from one to eleven of these genes, and their mRNAs can form enough protein copies to meet the high demands of accelerated growth (see Cell Composition and Growth Rate, below). In contrast, rRNA is not amplified by translation, and so other features are required to provide an adequate supply. Most important is the presence of seven operons (*rrn*) that yield essentially identical rRNAs. (How they fail to diverge genetically is not clear.) Moreover, these operons are clustered in the chromosome around the origin of DNA replication (Fig. 9–14), thus increasing the average number of copies because these regions are duplicated earliest in each round of replication. Finally, the *rrn* operons have two promoters, one able to initiate transcription with exceptional speed; and this speed is continued into chain elongation because it is not limited by coupling to translation. As a further example of economy in evolution, the very slowly growing mycobacteria and mycoplasmas have only one rRNA operon per genome.

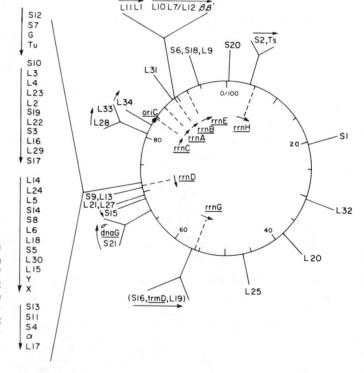

Figure 9–14. Locations of operons for r-proteins *(outside circle)* and for rRNA *(inside circle)* in *E. coli.* Cotranscribed genes include those for elongation factors G and Tu, for subunits α, β, β', and σ of RNA polymerase and for protein translocation protein secY. Note that the directions of transcription are almost all the same as those of the divergent replication of the DNA from its origin at *oriC*, thus minimizing displacement of RNA polymerase by DNA replicase, and that most of these ribosomal operons are located in the half of the chromosome flanking the origin. (Modified from Nomura M, Gourse R, Baughman G: Annu Rev Biochem 53:75, 1984)

The organization and the processing of the individual rRNA segments within the *rrn* transcripts are described above (Transcription of DNA: Processing). The operons for r-proteins often also containing genes for tRNAs and for various other proteins related to protein metabolism (Fig. 9–14). The consequences of these linkages are not clear: not all tRNA genes are linked to r-protein genes, and as was noted in Table 9–1, total tRNA synthesis does not parallel ribosome synthesis closely.

Two methods for regulating rRNA synthesis have been discovered, which respond to two kinds of **idle ribosomes:** those that are blocked in polysomes for lack of an aminoacyl-tRNA, and those that accumulate as free ribosomes when the supply of energy or amino acids is decreased.

ppGpp IN THE RESPONSE TO AMINO ACID DEPRIVAL.
When ribosomes are blocked in polysomes by lack of the next required aminoacyl-tRNA (e.g., by depriving an auxotroph of its required amino acid, or by inactivation of a thermosensitive aminoacyl-tRNA synthetase), rRNA synthesis stops immediately; yet chloramphenicol, which blocks ribosomes **after** they have bound aminoacyl-tRNA, even stimulates this synthesis. The explanation came from studies on mutants with **relaxed control** (*rel⁻*) of rRNA synthesis; i.e., loss of response to deprival of any amino acid. Under such deprival, the wild type, with the normal **stringent control** (*rel⁺*), accumulates a novel nucleotide, **guanosine 3′-diphosphate-5′diphosphate (guanosine tetraphosphate; ppGpp),** as well as ppGppp, but the *rel⁻* cells lack this capacity.

Studies *in vitro* then showed that the wild type, but not certain **relaxed mutants** (*relA⁻*), possess a ribosomal enzyme called **stringent factor.** When the ribosome encounters a codon on mRNA for which the cognate aminoacyl-tRNA is missing it binds the uncharged tRNA instead, which stimulates the stringent factor to synthesize ppGpp(p). In this reaction PP is transferred from ATP to the 3′-OH of GDP (or GTP). The rapid turnover of ppGpp (half-life 30 seconds) in the cell ensures the rapid response of this system.

REGULATION BY FREE RIBOSOMES.
Variations in ppGpp levels correlate well with the response of rRNA synthesis to a decreased supply of an amino acid, but not with the response to slowing of growth by energy limitation. Here, the mechanism appears to be a response to the level of another kind of idle ribosome, the free ribosomes, which increase at the expense of polysomes when the supply of energy (or of an amino acid) is reduced.

Both mechanisms can explain why chloramphenicol stimulates rRNA synthesis: it keeps the level of free ribosomes low (Chap. 10), and by keeping the A site filled in polysomal ribosomes it prevents ppGpp formation.

The mechanisms by which ppGpp and free ribosomes each control rRNA operons are obscure. Not surprisingly, the regulation of such an important process appears to involve additional factors, including an activator upstream from the promoters and a downstream antiterminator.

REGULATION OF RIBOSOMAL PROTEIN FORMATION

Regulation of r-protein synthesis is partly transcriptional but more posttranscriptional (feedback inhibition of translation). Thus, when extra copies of operons for r-proteins are introduced the cells overproduce their messengers but not the proteins.

The mechanism of this translational regulation, worked out by Nomura, depends on the ability of certain r-proteins to bind to a specific sequence in rRNA (Chap. 6) and also to a similar sequence in their mRNA. In each r-protein operon one of the proteins that it produces feeds back to bind to its own messenger, thus regulating the translation of the whole transcript. As long as the process of ribosome assembly removes r-proteins rapidly the corresponding mRNAs (which bind them less strnogly) escape this repression. Conversely, slowing of the synthesis of rRNA increases the level of these proteins and hence their binding to the mRNAs. In an elegant demonstration of this mechanism, genetic manipulations resulting in overproduction of a regulatory r-protein repress formation of the other r-proteins of that operon and impair ribosome synthesis, but overproduction of nonregulatory r-proteins has no such effect.

AUTOREGULATION OF OTHER NONENZYMATIC PROTEINS

The regulatory mechanism demonstrated for r-proteins has been found to apply to several other proteins whose function also involves binding to specific RNA sequences. More broadly, although most studies of gene regulation have involved response to small-molecule effectors, the r-protein autoregulation has shown that the operon mechanism can also respond to variations in the concentration of structural proteins that do not have enzymatic products for the cells to sense. In some cases, direct repression has been observed and in others the formation of antisense RNA (see next section).

Protein Breakdown; Adaptation to Stress

The concentration of each protein in a cell depends on its rate of breakdown, as well as its rate of synthesis. Unlike many kinds of animal cells, whose function requires maintenance rather than growth, bacteria are geared for growth and do not normally turn over most proteins. Indeed, labeling with radioactive amino acids, followed by an excess of unlabeled amino acids, shows that in growing *E. coli* cells, only about 1% of the protein is degraded to amino acids per hour at 37°C. However, a few regulatory proteins, such as a sigma factor that turns on heat shock proteins (see below), and some proteins in phage development, have half-lives as short as 4 minutes, thus permitting rapid reversal of their response.

Breakdown increases greatly under two sets of circumstances: proteins with structural defects are rapidly scavenged, and starvation induces selective attack on certain normal proteins, which then serve as reserve fuels.

DEGRADATION OF DEFECTIVE PROTEINS

The rapid degradation of abnormal proteins in bacteria was revealed by introducing abnormal sequences in various ways: incorporation of an amino acid analogue (Fig. 9–15), misreading induced by an aminoglycoside or by a *ram* mutation (Chap. 6), or premature termination caused by a nonsense mutation or by puromycin. In addition, the commercial production of mammalian proteins cloned in bacteria is frequently hampered by instability when they are accumulated in the cell rather than secreted. How these proteins are recognized as foreign is not clear, but at least some of them are less stable because reducing conditions in the cell prevent disulfide bond formation.

The proteases that eliminate proteins with artificial defects are presumably also used to eliminate the occasional defective products of normal protein synthesis. In support of this assumption, conditions that damage proteins (see Heat Shock, below) also increase the formation of these proteases.

E. coli contains a number of cytoplasmic proteases. A. Goldberg has shown that the elimination of abnormal proteins is initiated by an ATP-dependent endoprotease, originally called **protease La** but now recognized as the **Lon protease,** produced by the *lon* gene (see below); a second ATP-dependent protease also has been discovered. Mutants that lack these proteases are defective in the scavenging process. The Lon protease chops the protein into fairly short polypeptides, which are then digested to amino acids by several peptidases. These endoproteases are larger molecules than those excreted by bacteria, the additional material in the molecule presumably providing specificity and regulation that prevent wanton attack on normal intracellular proteins.

The molecular basis for selective attack on defective proteins was suggested by the finding that when they accumulate in bacteria they form insoluble aggregates (Fig. 9–16), and so they have evidently undergone some degree of denaturation. (Similar aggregates are seen in bacteria overproducing a cloned protein and also in human cells in disease states that result in the accumulation of an abnormal protein.) Because denaturation exposes loops that normally are tightly folded in the molecule, these may be what the endoprotease initially

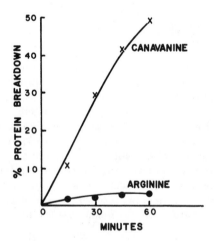

BREAKDOWN of PROTEINS CONTAINING CANAVANINE in E. COLI

Figure 9–15. Accelerated degradation of abnormal proteins. An arginine auxotroph of *E. coli* was incubated for 10 minutes with ^{3}H-leucine to label newly formed protein, plus either arginine or the analogue canavanine, which is well incorporated in place of arginine but does not allow the proteins to fold into their normal conformations. The cells were then incubated with arginine plus excess nonradioactive leucine to chase any leucine released by protein breakdown. Breakdown was measured as loss of acid-precipitable radioactivity. (Courtesy of AL Goldberg)

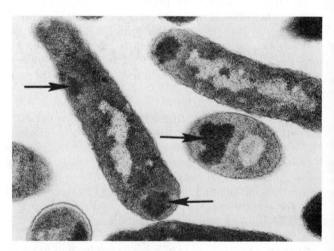

Figure 9–16. Precipitation of abnormal protein in *E. coli* cells. The cells of an arginine auxotroph had been grown for 1 hour with the analogue canavanine instead of arginine. *Arrows,* precipitated aggregates of protein. (×33,000; courtesy of MJ Karnovsky and AL Goldberg)

recognizes. In eukaryotes, but not in bacteria, an additional step is used to identify proteins scheduled for destruction: covalent attachment of a special small protein, ubiquitin.

With each hydrolysis of a peptide, the Lon protease hydrolyzes ATP. Because protein hydrolysis is exergonic and its products are often needed to provide cells with an endogenous source of energy, this expenditure of energy was surprising. A possible explanation is that the endonuclease, after finding an initial site of attack, may use energy from ATP for processive movement to successive sites of cleavage, thus protecting the cell from being clogged with incompletely digested proteins. The ATP requirement may also protect starving cells from excessive autodigestion.

STARVATION-INDUCED BREAKDOWN

In nature bacteria often starve, and their adaptive responses include the breakdown of macromolecules, yielding building blocks for new enzymes that permit the cell to use new substrates. An important substrate for this recycling is the ribosomes, whose breakdown provides amino acids, nucleotides, and probably energy (since polynucleotide phosphorylase yields nucleoside diphosphates). Moreover, in the rapid adjustment of ribosome content to decreasing growth rate, discussed above, cells approaching the stationary phase begin "starvation-induced" breakdown even before growth ceases, thus allowing some continued multiplication that maximizes the number of cells produced from the limited amount of nutrient.

Protein breakdown, in starvation, is regulated by mechanisms closely linked to those that regulate ribosome synthesis (see above). First, in starvation the polysomal ribosomes are converted into free ribosomes, which, as we have seen, provide feedback in regulating ribosome synthesis. Indeed, because they are conformationally more flexible than polysomal ribosomes (which are restricted by their ligands), their greater susceptibility to enzymatic attack may play a direct role in initiating their breakdown. In addition, starvation-induced breakdown is much slower in a *rel* mutant, which cannot make ppGpp; but how this compound regulates rRNA breakdown (as well as synthesis) is unknown. Whether ribosome breakdown is initiated by a protease or an RNase is likewise not known.

Once the degradation of a ribosome has been initiated, the release of its proteins and rRNAs and their subsequent hydrolysis proceed rapidly: intermediates are not seen. Free r-proteins that are overproduced in mutants are also labile. The mechanism is a general one, observed also with other proteins when they are prevented from finding their normal places in a multimeric complex. Evidently, such proteins are more susceptible to proteolysis when in the naked state, which exposes ordinarily hidden surfaces and also may alter conformation.

Because the starvation-induced digestion of normal proteins may thus depend on abnormally exposed loops, and because it also requires ATP, the enzymes involved seem likely to be the same as (or extensively overlapping with) those that remove abnormal proteins. It is not certain what other normally stable proteins besides those of ribosomes are degraded in response to starvation. Unlike rRNAs, the tRNAs are maintained during starvation.

Starvation for C or P induces additional, specific responses: formation of the enzymes that break down corresponding nonprotein storage reserves (glycogen, polymetaphosphate), and changes in surface structure that promote survival. Two-dimensional chromatography shows that starvation induces about 20 proteins, some increased in amount and some novel, in a sequence of several phases; most are of unknown function.

RESPONSES TO STRESS; HEAT SHOCK

E. coli possesses several regulons, each a coordinately regulated set of genes, that are activated by different stresses. First, exhaustion of a C source leading to formation of cAMP (see Catabolite Repression, above) can be viewed as a form of **energy stress.** The second, damage to DNA, induces the **SOS response** (see DNA repair, Chap. 8). Third, in amino acid starvation the **"stringent" response** (involving ppGpp), discussed above, not only influences rRNA synthesis and ribosome breakdown but also stimulates some operons of amino acid biosynthesis. We will now discuss responses to two other kinds of stress: heat and oxidizing chemicals. The signaling nucleotides involved in some of these responses (cAMP, ppGpp, adenylylated nucleotides described below) are called **alarmones.**

HEAT SHOCK. The most extensively studied stress system is called the heat shock response (though it can also be elicited by various chemicals), in which elevated temperature increases formation of a set of 10 to 20 **HSP** (heat-shock proteins); they are also called **HTP proteins,** for high-temperature production. They have aroused great interest because they are universally distributed and have been carefully conserved in evolution: their sequences exhibit similarity in organisms ranging from archaebacteria to higher plants and animals. Some HSP, but not all, are present in smaller amounts at ordinary temperatures. In *E. coli* the group becomes an increasing fraction of the protein synthesized as the temperature is raised above 40°C, and the exclusive products at 50°.

The functions of most HSP are not known. The *lon* gene endoprotease, described above, has been best characterized. Because it initiates the degradation not only of abnormal proteins (including those denatured by heat) but also of labile regulatory proteins, *lon* mutants are highly pleiotropic. For example, by stabilizing the labile SulA protein, which prevents septation, they cause production of long, filamentous cells, hence the name *lon*.

HSP production is regulated by a gene initially called *htpR* but renamed *rpoH* after it was discovered to produce an RNA polymerase sigma factor of 32 Kd (σ^{32}) that competes with the principal factor, σ^{82}. Although the mechanism of its activation is not completely understood, the key may be that the various physical and chemical stimuli of this regulon all cause **denaturation of proteins;** this process exposes loops that can bind the proteases and thus decrease their free level, and through a feedback response, this decrease might then activate *rpoH*. Supporting this model, overproduction of a single abnormal protein resulting from an amber mutation increases the production of HTP proteins.

The increased formation of HTP proteins during brief growth at a moderately elevated temperature increases survival on subsequent exposure to 55°C. Conversely, *rpoH* mutants cannot grow above 34°C. The relation of the many HTP proteins to this protection is obscure; one possibility is protection of DNA from denaturation. In addition, one HSP (GroEL) binds to, and prevents the amorphous aggregation of, proteins destined for assembly and it may also play a role in inhibiting folding that would prevent secretion. It has therefore been called a **chaperonin.**

OXIDATION STRESS. Exposure of bacteria to various oxidants stimulates another regulon, controlled by the *oxyR* gene and comprising about 35 proteins. The activity of this regulon parallels, and may well be controlled by, the level of certain **adenylylated nucleotides:** mostly **diadenosine tetraphosphate (AppppA)** and adenylylated ppGpp (AppppGpp). These compounds had been encountered much earlier, with no evident function, as side products of the action of aminoacyl-tRNA synthetase: when the enzyme, having formed aminoacyl-AMP as an intermediate, finds no supply of tRNA to which to transfer the amino acid, it instead transfers the AMP to various nucleotides by a bond between the 5' phosphates. How oxidants stimulate this reaction, and how the products act, are not known.

The patterns of response to various stresses are complicated and overlapping. Thus, some promoters participate in more than one regulon; some proteins induced by stress also have a basal level essential to normal growth; and some stresses can activate multiple regulons. EtOH stimulates only the HTP system; H_2O_2, quinones, and N-ethylmaleimide (an SH reagent) cause pure oxidation stress; and nalidixic acid and puromycin cause an SOS and some HTP response. Interest in these is increased by the possibility that aging in higher organisms involves the kinds of damage that they prevent.

Regulation of DNA Replication and Cell Division

The rate of synthesis of DNA in growing cells, like that of other informational macromolecules, depends on the frequency of initiation: the subsequent rate of movement of the **growing point** along the chain (or, more precisely, the rate of passage of the chain through the membrane-bound replication machinery) is independent of the growth rate of the cell. Study of the time of doubling of specific genes in **synchronized cultures** (Chap. 3), and also radioautographic detection of newly synthesized DNA in the intact chromosome (recovered by gentle lysis), further showed that replication begins at a fixed **origin** (*oriC*) (located in *E. coli* at 80 minutes on the 100-minute genetic map; see Fig. 9–14) and then proceeds **bidirectionally** in the circular bacterial chromosome.

When the two **replication forks** meet at the **terminus,** about 180° around the circle, the two sister chromosomes are completed and separate. The terminus provides information for the **partition** of the daughter chromosomes to the two progeny cells. The DNA sequences of the origin and the terminus of the *E. coli* chromosome, and some proteins that bind to them, have been identified. Moreover, DNA replication in vitro requires interaction with a phospholipid.

E. coli at 37°C requires about 45 minutes from initiation to completion of a cycle of replication. Hence, in growth with a doubling time of 50 minutes about 90% of the cells are engaged in DNA synthesis and incorporate ^{3}H-thymidine, and in slower growth the gap between rounds of replication is greater. A replication time of 45 minutes for each half of a chromosome of 3×10^6 base pairs corresponds to processive synthesis at the rate of about 500 base pairs per second at each growing point: about ten times the rate of transcription. The difference may be attributable in part to the limitation of transcription by coupling with translation.

THE REPLICON. Studies with *ts* mutants blocked in various aspects of replication led to the concept of a functional unit of regulation of DNA replication, the **replicon,** in which a specific cytoplasmic **initiator** interacts with a corresponding origin. The cell's chromosome and different groups of plasmids and phages each respond to a specific initiator.

Maaloe showed that blockade of protein synthesis allows completion of any current round of replication but prevents initiation of a new round. Because the replication machinery of a chromosome must be doubled at each new initiation, at least some of the newly synthesized protein is probably required for that purpose.

MULTIPLE GROWING POINTS. If the chromosomal replication time is fixed at 45 minutes, how can a cell have a doubling time, in a rich medium, of 25 minutes? The

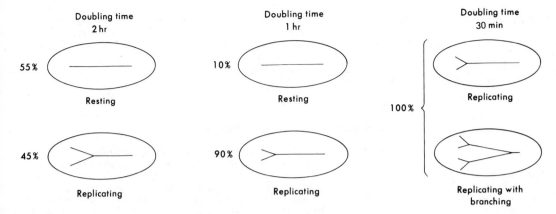

Figure 9–17. States of chromosomal replication in *E. coli* cultures growing at different rates. Numbers denote percentage of the population in each state. For convenience, the cyclic structure of the chromosome is ignored.

solution is the formation of **additional growing points** before completion of the first round of replication (Fig. 9–17); i.e., the already replicated origin on each branch of the fork, which has passed through the membrane-attached site of replication, reattaches to the membrane and forms a new fork. The presence of multiple branches can be demonstrated by quantitating the transforming DNA for different genes in cell lysates: with a doubling time of 50 minutes the ratio of the genes near the origin to that near the terminus is about 2/1, whereas in fast growth it approaches 4/1.

At each growth rate the number of origins has a characteristic ratio to cell mass (and to cell protein); i.e., an initiation occurs after a fixed increment in cell mass. Although the complex, multi-component molecular mechanism of DNA synthesis, including its initiation, has been studied in great detail, the mechanism that relates initiation to cell mass is still not clear.

CELL DIVISION

Cell division normally is triggered by completion of a round of replication of the chromosome. Thus, blockade of DNA synthesis prevents initiation of septum formation while allowing some further growth. Conversely, when starvation for an amino acid has resulted in completion of replication without cell growth, septum formation is evidently initiated, for restoration of the amino acid leads immediately to septum formation and cell division even though the cells have not reached the proper size.

The interval between completion of DNA replication and completion of cell division (i.e., physical cell separation), in *E. coli* at 37°C, is about 20 minutes, creating a **constant phase difference** between the rhythms of replication and of division. Because of this gap, cells in rapid growth, with a branched chromosome, can contain beginning septa while their advanced septa are still incompletely separated. The mechanism linking duplication of the terminus of the chromosome to septum formation is not known. As we have seen, septum formation is inhibited by the labile SulA protein, whose turnover is impaired by mutations in the *lon* gene. Some β-lactam antibiotics, which preferentially inhibit certain morphogenetic enzymes (Chap. 2), also prevent septation.

Selected Reading

BOOKS AND REVIEW ARTICLES

Beckwith J, Davies J, Gallant J (eds): Gene Function in Prokaryotes. Cold Spring Harbor, NY, Cold Spring Harbor Laboratory, 1983

Botsford JL: Cyclic nucleotides in procaryotes. Microbiol Rev 45:620, 1981

deCrombrugghe, Busby S, Buc H: Cyclic AMP receptor protein: Role in transcription activation. Science 224:831, 1984

Doi RH, Wang LF: Multiple procaryotic ribonucleic acid polymerase sigma factors. Microbiol Rev 50:227, 1986

Drlica K: Biology of bacterial deoxyribonucleic acid topoisomerases. Microbiol Rev 48:273, 1984

Dubnau D: Translational attenuation: The regulation of bacterial resistance to the macrolide–lincosamide–streptogramin B antibiotics. CRC Crit Rev Biochem 16:103, 1984

Forst S, Inouye M: Environmentally regulated gene expression for membrane proteins in *Escherichia coli*. Annu Rev Cell Biol 4:21, 1988

Gegenheimer P, Apirion D: Processing of procaryotic ribonucleic acid. Microbiol Rev 45:502, 1981

Goldberg AL, Goff SA: The selective degradation of abnormal proteins in bacteria. In Reznikoff W, Gold L (eds): Maximizing Gene Expression. London, Butterworths, 1986, p 287

Gottesman S, Trisler P, Torres–Cabasa A, Maurizi MR: Regulation via proteolysis: The *Escherichia coli lon* system. In Leive L (ed): Microbiology—1985, Washington, DC, American Society for Microbiology, 1986 p 350.

Helman JD, Chamberlin MJ: Structure and function of bacterial sigma factors. Annu Rev Biochem 57:839, 1988

Helmstetter CE, Pierucci O, Weinberger M, Holmes MR, Tang MS: Control of cell division in *Escherichia coli*. In Ornston LN, Sokatch JR (eds): The Bacteria, Vol VII. New York, Academic Press, 1978

Ingraham JL, Maaloe O, Neidhart FC (eds): Growth of the Bacterial Cell. Sunderland, Mass, Sinauer Associates, 1983

King TC, Sirdeskmukh R, Schlessinger D: Nucleolytic processing of ribonucleic acid transcripts in procaryotes. Microbiol Rev 50:428, 1986

Kolter R, Yanofsky C: Attenuation in amino acid biosynthetic operons. Annu Rev Genet 16:113, 1982

Kornberg A: DNA Replication. San Francisco, WH Freeman, 1980; Supplement 1982

Lamond AI, Travers AA: Stringent control of bacterial transcription. Cell 41:6, 1985

Lindahl L, Zengel JM: Ribosomal genes in *Escherichia coli.* Annu Rev Genet 20:297, 1986

Losick R, Chamberlin M (eds): RNA Polymerase. Cold Spring Harbor, NY, Cold Spring Harbor Laboratory, 1976

Miller JH, Reznikoff WS (eds): The Operon. Cold Spring Harbor, NY, Cold Spring Harbor Laboratory, 1978

McClure WR: Mechanism and control of transcription initiation in procaryotes. Annu Rev Biochem 54:171, 1985

Neidhardt FC, Van Bogelen RA, Vaughn V: Heat shock. Annu Rev Genet 18:295, 1984

Neidhardt FC, Ingraham JL, Low KB, Magasanik B, Schaechter M, Umbarger HE (eds): *Escherichia coli* and *Salmonella typhimurium:* Cellular and Molecular Biology. Washington, DC, American Society for Microbiology, 1987 (Many relevant chapters.)

Nomura M: Regulation of the synthesis of ribosomes and ribosomal components in *Escherichia coli:* Translational regulation and feedback loops. In Booth I, Higgins C (eds): Regulation of Gene Expression. Symposium of the Society for General Microbiology. Cambridge, Cambridge University Press, 1986

Nomura M, Gourse R, Baughman G: Regulation of the synthesis of ribosomes and ribosomal components. Annu Rev Biochem 53:75, 1984

Ptashne M: Gene expression by proteins acting nearby and at a distance. Nature 322:697, 1986

Ptashne M: A Genetic Switch. Cambridge, Mass, Cell Press, 1986

Reznikoff WS, Siegele DA, Cowing DW, Gross C: The regulation of transcription initiation in bacteria. Annu Rev Genet 19:355, 1985

Schleif R: Regulation of the arabinose operon. In Schaechter M, Neidhardt FC, Ingraham JL, Kjeldgaard NO (eds): The Molecular Biology of Bacterial Growth, p 194. Boston, Jones and Bartlett, 1985

Schlesinger MJ, Ashburner M, Tissieres A (eds): Heat Shock: From Bacteria to Man. Cold Spring Harbor, NY, Cold Spring Harbor Laboratory, 1982

Torriani A, Ludtke DN: The Pho regulon of *Escherichia coli.* In Schaechter M, Neidhardt FC, Ingraham JL, Kjeldgaard NO (eds): The Molecular Biology of Bacterial Growth, p 224. Boston, Jones and Bartlett, 1985

Walker R: The Molecular Biology of Enzyme Synthesis: Regulatory Mechanisms of Enzyme Adaptation. New York, John Wiley, 1983

Weisblum B: Inducible resistance to macrolides, lincosamides and streptogramin type B antibiotics: The resistance phenotype, its biological diversity, and structural elements that regulate expression. J Antimicrob Chemother 16 (Suppl A):63, 1985

Yanofsky C: Attenuation in the control of expression of bacterial operons. Nature 289:751, 1981

Yanofsky C: Attenuation and mutations that alter it. Annu Rev Genet 10:1982

SPECIFIC ARTICLES

Bochner BR, Lee PC, Wilson SW, Cutler CW, Ames BN: ApppppA and related adenylated nucleotides are synthesized as a consequence of oxidation stress. Cell 37:225, 1984

Davis BD, Luger LM, Tai PC: Role of ribosome degradation in the death of starved *Escherichia coli* cells. J Bacteriol 166:439, 1986

Duvall EJ, Lovett PS: Chloramphenicol induces translation of the mRNA for a chloramphenicol resistance gene in *Bacillus subtilis.* Proc Natl Acad Sci USA 83:3939, 1986

Goff SA, Goldberg AL: Production of abnormal proteins in *E. coli* stimulates transcription of *lon* and other heat shock genes. Cell 41:587, 1985

Grossman AD, Erickson JW, Gross C: The *htpR* gene product of *E. coli* is a sigma factor for heat shock promoters. Cell 38:383, 1984

Horinouchi S, Weisblum B: Posttranscriptional modification of RNA conformation: Mechanism that regulates erythromycin-induced resistance. Proc Natl Acad Sci USA 77:7079, 1980

Hunt TP, Magasanik B: Transcription of *glnA* by purified *Escherichia coli* components: Core RNA polymerase and the products of *glnF, glnG,* and *glnL.* Proc Natl Acad Sci USA 82:8453, 1985

Mizuno T, Chou M, Inouye M: A unique mechanism regulating gene expression: Translational inhibition by a complementary RNA transcript (micRNA). Proc Natl Acad Sci USA 81:1966, 1984

Ninfa AJ, Magasanik B: Covalent modification of the *glnG* product, NR_I, by the *glnL* product, NR_{II}, regulates the transcription of the *glnALG* operon in *Escherichia coli.* Proc Natl Acad Sci USA 83:5909, 1986

Okamoto K, Freundlich M: Mechanism for the autogenous control of the *crp* operon: transpositional inhibition by a divergent RNA transcript. Proc Natl Acad Sci USA 83:5000, 1986

Sharrock RA, Gourse RL, Nomura M: Defective antitermination of rRNA transcription and derepression of rRNA and tRNA synthesis in the *nusB5* mutant of *Escherichia coli.* Proc Natl Acad Sci USA 82:5275, 1985

Simons RW, Kleckner N: Translational control of IS10 transposition. Cell 34:683, 1983

Stewart V, Yanofsky C: Evidence for transcription antitermination control of tryptophanase operon expression in *Escherichia coli* K-12. J Bacteriol 164:731, 1985

Stragier P, Kunkel B, Kroos L, Losick R: Chromosomal rearrangement generating a composite gene for a developmental transcription factor. Science 243:507, 1989

Vanbogelen RA, Kelley PM, Neidhardt FC: Differential induction of heat shock, SOS, and oxidation stress regulons and accumulation of nucleotides in *Escherichia coli.* J Bacteriol 169:26, 1986

10

Chemotherapy

Origins

More than most fields, chemotherapy was founded by one person, Paul Ehrlich. Fascinated with the concept of selective affinity, he introduced (as a medical student) dyes that are still used for staining basophilic or acidophilic components of tissues. He later formulated the side chain theory to account for the specificity of antigen–antibody reactions, and in 1904, he proposed that there must be chemicals ("magic bullets") with the ability to attach to specific microbes but not to host cells. This **selectivity,** and not antimicrobial potency, is the essential feature of chemotherapy. Today, we would define the selectivity in quantitative terms: the ability to inhibit microbes (and, by extension, cancer cells) at concentrations that can be tolerated by the host.

Ehrlich's successful products—dyes for use against trypanosomes and arsenicals against spirochetes—were not active *in vitro*, and so skeptics claimed that they were only bolstering host defenses (although we now know that they are metabolized by the host to yield an active inhibitor). Hence after Ehrlich's death in 1915 his dream of selective inhibition was largely abandoned until the dramatic success of the sulfonamides in 1935. Medical microbiology then entered a second golden age, comparable to the rapid recognition of specific pathogens half a century earlier.

The history of the sulfonamides illustrates how progress in chemotherapy has depended largely on empiricism and serendipity rather than on logical design. Pursuing Ehrlich's concept, and expecting dyes to bind best to specific tissues, Domagk at the IG Farbenindustrie in Germany showed that the dye Prontosil dramatically cured streptococcus infections. It is fortunate that he tested the chemical in mice, for it would not have shown any activity in cultures. Trefouel in France soon isolated a simple inhibitory breakdown product, **sulfanilamide**

201

(*p*-aminobenzene sulfonamide), from patients' urine, and many more active derivatives, called **sulfonamide drugs,** were then synthesized.

ANTIBIOTICS. The success of sulfonamides revived interest in a phenomenon that has been observed by Pasteur and Joubert in 1877 and subsequently by many others: inhibition of a culture by products of a contaminating microorganism. In one example, Fleming in London in 1929 observed that a colony of the mold *Penicillium notatum* lysed adjacent colonies of staphylococci (Fig. 10–1). The product, called **penicillin,** seemed too unstable to be useful, and it aroused little interest. However, it proved to be stable when purified by Chain at Oxford 10 years later, and Florey showed that it was remarkably effective in patients.

Waksman, a soil microbiologist, then undertook a search for additional inhibitors of microbial origin, now called **antibiotics.** Although the next one proved to be too toxic, his discovery of streptomycin in 1944 proved that a persistent search could be rewarding.

Massive screening, mostly in the pharmaceutical industry, has since yielded several thousand antibiotics, of which roughly 100 have been useful. These have become the largest class of prescription drugs: the production of the β-lactams (the group related to penicillin) exceeds 10^8 pounds per year.

The term "antibiotic" is generally reserved for relatively small molecules. Some bacteria produce antibacterial proteins called bacteriocins (Chap. 7), but these are not of chemotherapeutic use. The term "chemotherapeutic" is sometimes applied only to synthetic antimicrobials and not to antibiotics. However, the two groups overlap, and some compounds discovered as antibiotics (e.g., chloramphenicol) are now produced by chemical synthesis. Antibiotics have proved to be useful not only in therapy but as tools for the study of cell biology.

General Aspects of Chemotherapeutic Action

SENSITIVITY. The sensitivity of an isolate to various antimicrobial agents is of great importance as a guide to therapy. The **minimal inhibitory concentration (MIC),** which prevents outgrowth of a standard inoculum, is usually determined with tubes, microwells, or plates containing two-fold serial dilutions of the drug. Automated methods are available for measuring, within a few hours, whether that concentration inhibits an increase in turbidity in liquid cultures. In general, an organism is considered susceptible if its MIC is at most one-fourth the easily obtainable peak serum level of the drug.

For routine testing, diagnostic laboratories often use an **agar diffusion** method, which is simple and measures the actual level of sensitivity rather than a threshold. In the **Kirby–Bauer test,** small circles of filter paper

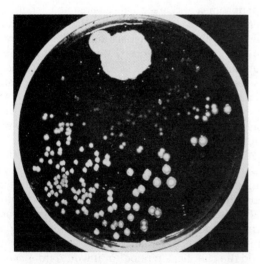

Figure 10–1. The discovery of penicillin. Note lysis of colonies of *Staphylococcus aureus* surrounding a large contaminating colony of *Penicillium notatum*. (Fleming A: Br J Exp Pathol 10:226, 1929)

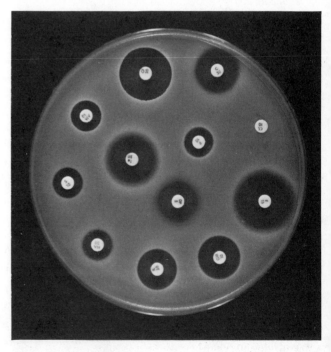

Figure 10–2. Disk assay for antimicrobial sensitivity. Filter paper disks containing appropriate amounts of various antimicrobial agents were placed on a heavily seeded lawn of a culture and incubated overnight. The zones of inhibition show that this organism was sensitive to all but one of the tested agents. (Courtesy Inge Taftegaard.)

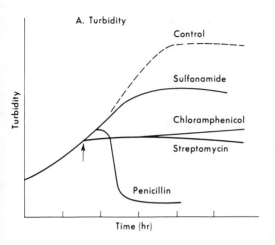

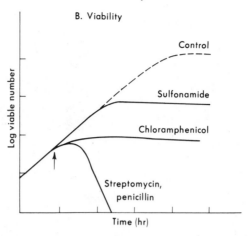

Figure 10–3. Kinetics of antimicrobial action of representative drugs. *(A)* Turbidity. *(B)* Viability. Drug added *(arrow)* to exponentially growing culture.

containing standard quantities of various agents are placed on a heavily seeded lawn of bacteria, and the zones of inhibition are observed after overnight incubation (Fig. 10–2). In this test, which has been calibrated by the MIC, an adequate zone indicates merely that the MIC of that drug for the organism is within the accessible range: the agent with largest zone is not necessarily the best for that particular infection. Sensitivity can also be determined, more rapidly, by automated methods for measuring the increase in the turbidity of liquid cultures.

In evaluating new agents, the **antimicrobial spectrum** (i.e., the set of susceptible organisms) is of particular interest.

BACTERIOSTATIC VERSUS BACTERICIDAL ACTION. Some chemotherapeutic agents are merely bacteriostatic, inhibiting growth reversibly, whereas others are bactericidal, exerting an irreversible and hence lethal action. Although bacteriostatic cultures, like starved ones, eventually die out, the kinetics of bactericidal action is measured in minutes or hours. With most bactericidal agents the **minimal bactericidal concentration (MBC)** is only slightly higher than the MIC.

With agents that cause **lysis** the kinetics of bactericidal action may be observed turbidimetrically. Other bactericidal agents, however, destroy only viability, and the kinetics is observed by sampling at intervals for viability counts (Fig. 10–3).

Bactericidal action results from **irreparable damage at only a limited class of sites.** The effective sites are: (1) the **wall** or the **membrane** (resulting in partial or complete lysis); (2) the **DNA;** or (3) all the copies of a protein-containing component of the **protein-synthesizing apparatus** (including the ribosome), because the complete apparatus is necessary to regenerate a protein. Inactiva-

tion of most enzymes, even if irreversible, is not lethal, because the cell retains the genetic information required for their regeneration, and turnover can supply the required building blocks and energy (See Protein Breakdown, Chap. 9).

APPROACHES TO MECHANISM. An early step is to measure the incorporation of labeled precursors into DNA, RNA, protein, lipid, or wall. The process that is inhibited first is then studied more closely in extracts. Most antibiotics that are selective for microbes interfere with either peptidoglycan synthesis or protein synthesis, but some act on nucleic acid synthesis or on the membrane. The literature on antimicrobial actions is far from straightforward, because inhibition of any component of growth inevitably affects many additional processes.

Synthetic Chemotherapeutic Agents
SULFONAMIDES AND THEIR ANTAGONISTS

Sulfonamides not only launched antibacterial chemotherapy but also aroused great interest in analogues that compete with metabolites, which proved to be a widespread mechanism of drug action.

COMPETITIVE ANTAGONISM. Pursuing the observation that the inhibition of bacterial growth by sulfanilamide was antagonized by something in yeast extract, Woods identified the agent as the previously unknown metabolite **p-aminobenzoate (PAB),** and he further showed that the antagonism is competitive—that is, with a doubling of the concentration of the inhibitor, restoration of growth requires a doubling of the concentration of the antagonist. This finding, and the structural similarity of

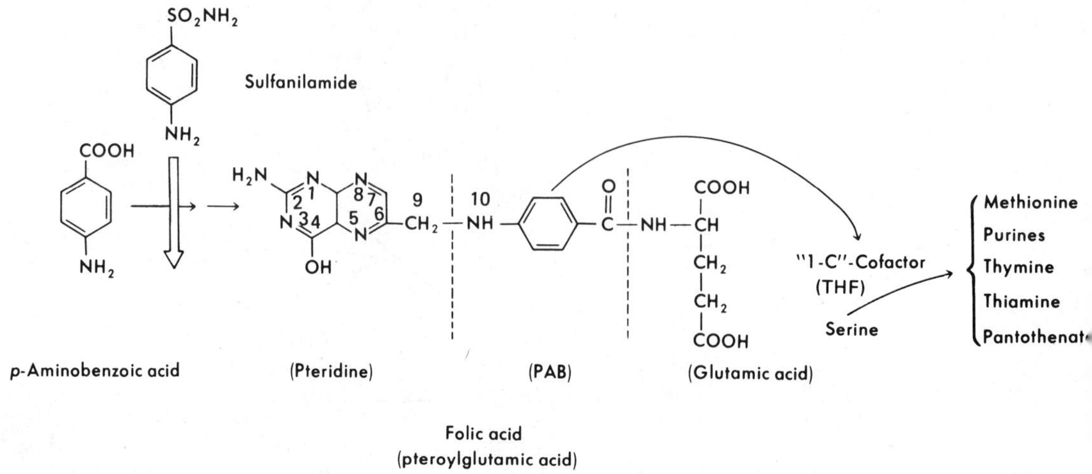

Figure 10–4. Metabolism blocked by sulfonamides. These analogues of *p*-aminobenzoate (PAB) block (and also replace) its condensation with a pteridine to form dihydropteroate (not shown), which condenses with glutamate to form folic acid. This compound and its reduced forms, dihydrofolic acid (DHF) and tetrahydrofolic acid (THF), go through a cycle of reductions and oxidations in the reduction and transfer of 1-C fragments derived from serine; only the products are shown. Trimethoprim, an analogue of DHF, blocks its reduction to THF; hence, trimethoprim and sulfonamides interfere with different steps in the same pathway.

the two compounds (Fig. 10–4), established the principle of growth inhibition by a structural analogue competing with an essential metabolite.

NONCOMPETITIVE ANTAGONISM. PAB was subsequently found to be a precursor of **folic acid,** a cofactor of one-C metabolism in all cells. Mammals obtain this compound in their diet and hence transport it into cells from their body fluids, whereas most bacteria make their folate, via PAB. For this reason it is fortunate for the development of chemotherapy that most bacteria cannot utilize exogenous folate; the few that do (and require it) are insensitive to sulfonamides.

Sulfonamides are also antagonized by a mixture of the products of folate-dependent pathways (Fig. 10–4). This antagonism is noncompetitive; that is, it cannot be overcome by an increase in drug concentration. While some of these antagonists (methionine, serine, and vitamins) are normally present in body fluids, sulfonamides can be effective because purines and thymine do not circulate (they are made as nucleotides and retained within each cell). In support of this conclusion, the virulence of *Salmonella* for mice is lost by mutants auxotrophic for PAB or for purines but not by those auxotrophic for various amino acids. However, **tissue destruction (trauma, burns, pus) releases nucleic acid bases,** and the ineffectiveness of sulfonamides under these conditions is a serious limitation to their use.

Although virtually all bacteria can be inhibited *in vitro* by sulfonamides at an adequate concentration, only a limited spectrum of organisms can be inhibited by the

concentrations attainable in the host. Another limitation is that bacteriostasis is delayed until the folic acid already present has been diluted by cell growth (Fig. 10–3).

SYNERGISTIC SULFONAMIDE THERAPY. **Trimethoprim,** a folate analogue, blocks another enzyme in the folate pathway, dihydrofolate reductase, and it has much lower affinity for the mammalian than for the bacterial enzyme. The combination of inhibitors of two steps in the same pathway results in marked **synergism,** because the incomplete first block impairs accumulation of an antagonistic metabolite behind the second block.

Various sulfonamides differ very little in antimicrobial spectrum, which includes both gram-positive and gram-negative bacteria. Improvements have therefore involved mostly pharmacologic properties. In current use, sulfonamides (e.g., sulfamethoxazole, sulfisoxazole; Fig. 10–5) are generally mixed with trimethoprim. Although they have been extensively replaced by various antibiotics, they are still widely used, especially for infections of the urinary tract.

OTHER PAB ANALOGUES. **Dapsone (diaminodiphenyl sulfone)** (Fig. 10–5) was synthesized as a congener in which the sulfonamide group is replaced by a sulfone group, but it does not appear to compete with PAB. It is effective, by some unknown mechanism, in the treatment only of one infection, leprosy (Chap. 35).

p-Aminosalicylic Acid (PAS) is an analogue of PAB created by a substitution on the ring (Fig. 10–5). It is useful only in the treatment of infection with *Mycobacte-*

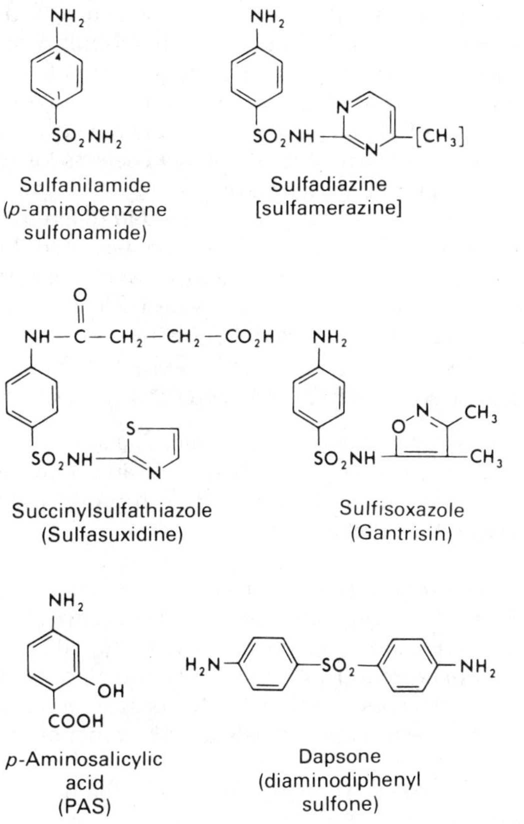

Figure 10–5. Sulfonamides and other PAB analogues.

rium tuberculosis (Chap. 35), whose receptor for PAB evidently differs markedly from that in most bacteria. PAS has an advantage over streptomycin in that it readily reaches intracellular organisms, but it is only bacteriostatic.

FURTHER STUDIES OF COMPETITIVE INHIBITION

Although early studies with enzymes had already established the principle of competitive antagonism by an analogue, the competitive, selective inhibition of intact cells by sulfonamides aroused great interest in the possibility of rationally developing additional chemotherapeutic agents by synthesizing analogues of other essential metabolites. Indeed, thousands of analogues of amino acids, bases, and vitamins were found to be inhibitory. However, they failed to exhibit the required selectivity, for they were modeled on metabolites that, unlike PAB, are essential for the host as well as for the bacteria. Nevertheless, antimetabolites with only slight selectivity have proved useful in the chemotherapy of cancer and of viral infections. Moreover, the concept of structural analogy has explained the action of many other drugs.

OTHER SITES OF COMPETITION. Competitive inhibition, originally ascribed to blockade of the active site of an enzyme, also involves two additional mechanisms. In **competition for transport** into the cell, the essential metabolite can interfere with entry of the analogue and vice versa. In **biosynthetic incorporation** the analogue does not simply block but deceives the enzyme. Both these mechanisms apply to sulfonamides as well as to many other analogues. Indeed, in previous chapters we have noted experiments in which analogues were heavily incorporated into DNA, RNA, or proteins, some with relatively little disturbance of function and others resulting in **lethal synthesis.**

Another mechanism is **pseudofeedback inhibition** (Chap. 9), in which an analogue of the endproduct of a biosynthetic pathway inhibits growth by mimicking the allosteric action of that endproduct on the first enzyme of the pathway.

ISONIAZID

Isoniazid (isonicotinic acid hydrazide; INH) (Fig. 10–6) was synthesized as an intermediate in the search for analogues of PAB, but it turned out to be a remarkably effective agent against tuberculosis, with an action unrelated to PAB. Among its advantages over streptomycin (the only agent then available), it is less toxic, can be given orally, is bactericidal even at very low concentrations (less than 1 μg/ml), and acts on intracellular as well as extracellular organisms; and mutations to resistance arise only in small steps (and often decrease virulence). **Ethionamide** (α-ethylisonicotinylthioamide) resembles INH in structure and in action. Other agents used in treating tuberculosis will be discussed in Chapter 35.

INH has an exceptionally limited antimicrobial spectrum—certain mycobacteria and the related nocardiae and corynebacteria—presumably because it inhibits synthesis of the **mycolic acids:** very long-chain fatty acids that are unique to these organisms (see Chap. 35). Because these compounds, in the waxy outer layer, are linked covalently to the underlying peptidoglycan, the bactericidal action of INH is evidently secondary to interference with wall synthesis.

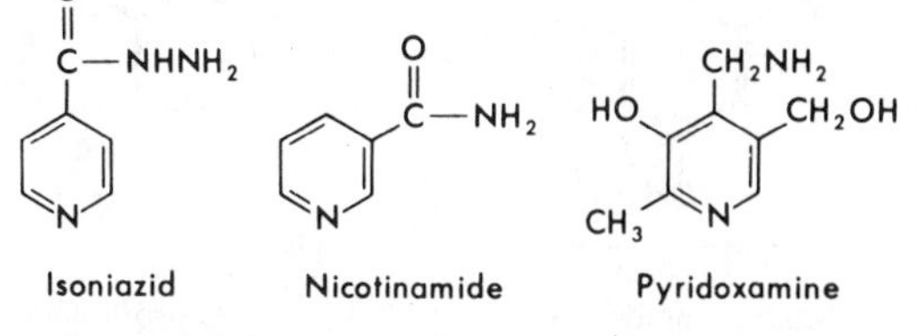

Figure 10–6. Isoniazid (isonicotinic acid hydrazide; pyridine-4-hydrazoic acid) and two metabolites that it resembles.

INH is also an analogue of nicotinamide and of pyridoxine (Fig. 10–6). It can be incorporated enzymatically in place of nicotinamide to form an analogue of NAD, it can inhibit various enzymes that require pyridoxal phosphate (Fig. 10–6) as cofactor, and its toxicity is reported to be antagonized by large doses of pyridoxine. When an antimicrobial has such a multiplicity of biochemical actions it is often difficult to determine which are related to its inhibition of growth. With INH, mycolic acid seems the key because it explains the narrow antimicrobial spectrum.

QUINOLONES

Nalidixic acid (Fig. 10–7), a quinolone (4-oxo-8-azaquinoline), was synthesized in 1962. Its narrow antimicrobial spectrum and rapid selection of resistant mutants virtually restricted its use to infections of the urinary tract, where it is concentrated. However, many years later **fluoroquinolones,** with F substituted at position 6 (Fig. 10–7), were found to have much greater potency and hence a broader spectrum. **Ciprofloxacin** has 600 times the potency of nalidixic acid, which gives it a very broad spectrum, including several types of intracellular bacteria. In addition, the fluoroquinolones have not selected for plasmid-mediated resistance, and chromosomal resistance arises only in small steps. These advantages have revived interest in synthetic antimicrobial compounds, after decades of being eclipsed by antibiotics.

The mechanism of action of quinolones has been studied in detail. These compounds block the action of bacterial, but not mammalian, **DNA gyrase.** This enzyme uses energy from ATP to catalyze the negative supercoiling of closed circles of duplex DNA (Chap. 2), a reaction that is important in chromosome replication, regulation of transcription, and DNA repair. At concentrations well above the MIC quinolones are bactericidal. The reaction requires protein synthesis, perhaps because nicks in the DNA, accumulating when the gyrase is blocked, induce formation of an exonuclease.

Novobiocin, an antibiotic, also inhibits DNA gyrase. Unlike the quinolones, it is **bacteriostatic.**

Bacterial DNA gyrase consists of two A and two B subunits, and certain mutations in subunit A make the cell highly resistant to nalidixic acid (but not to ciprofloxacin). These mutations appear readily *in vitro* but have not been of great clinical importance, suggesting that they decrease virulence. Novobiocin selects for resistant mutants altered in subunit B.

These two sets of mutants altered in different parts of this unusual enzyme have been very useful in the study of its action. In particular, nalidixic acid traps an intermediate in which the DNA has been cleaved and covalently linked to the gyrase-A protein.

OTHER SYNTHETIC ANTIMICROBIALS

We will note briefly two antimicrobials that are useful only for treating chronic urinary tract infections. Because they cannot act systemically, they are not truly chemotherapeutic agents.

NITROFURANS. The nitrofurans are bacteriostatic to a variety of gram-positive and gram-negative organisms; the mechanism is not clear. They cannot attain an effective concentration in body fluids, but they do become sufficiently concentrated in the urine. **Nitrofurantoin** (Fig. 10–8) is the most widely used member of the group.

METHENAMINE. Methenamine, the cyclic product of the condensation of formaldehyde and ammonia (Fig. 10–8), is more a disinfectant than a chemotherapeutic agent: it is not active *in vitro*, but when excreted into an acidic urine, it is hydrolyzed, and the formaldehyde that it releases is bactericidal (see Chap. 3, Disinfectants). A mixture with mandelic acid (methenamine mandelate) is often used to promote acidity of the urine. *Proteus* is resistant because the urease that it forms splits urea to CO_2 and NH_3, thus making the urine alkaline.

Antibiotics

The majority of antibiotics act either on enzymes of peptidoglycan synthesis or on the ribosome. We have described in Chapter 2 actions on peptidoglycan synthesis,

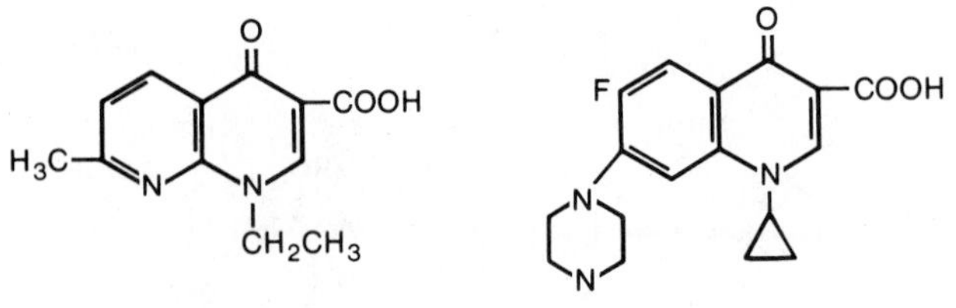

Nalidixic acid   Ciprofloxacin

Figure 10–7. Quinolones.

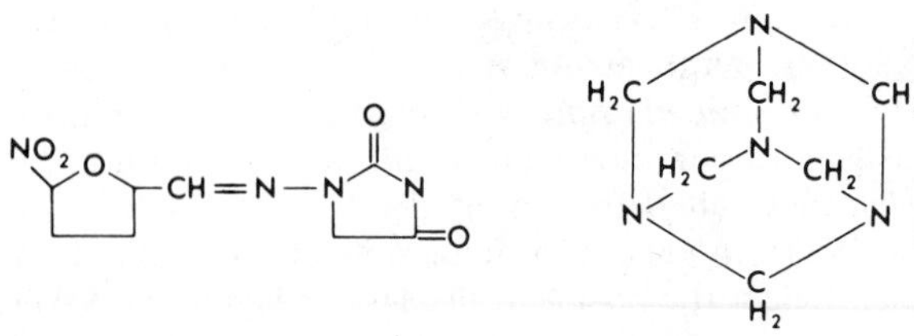

Nitrofurantoin   Methenamine

Figure 10–8. Synthetic compounds used to treat urinary tract infections.

which have been intimately linked with the elucidation of that synthesis; we will discuss here additional aspects of the major group, the β-lactams. We will then consider the antiribosomal group in some detail and will briefly summarize other kinds of antibiotic action.

Antibiotics vary enormously in structure, but most are large, complex molecules, with hydrophobic regions that facilitate diffusion into cells. Their large size may also reflect the value of a broad area of interaction with macromolecular targets. Multiple ring structures are common, some optimizing the conformation of the groups that interact with the target.

PENICILLINS: PRODUCTION AND CHEMISTRY

The first antibiotic, penicillin, proved to be truly a miracle drug. It is rapidly bactericidal, it interferes specifically with a reaction that is unique to the bacteria, and even in high concentrations, it does not have side effects on the host except in allergic patients. Accordingly, unlike most antimicrobials, which have a relatively narrow **therapeutic index** (ratio of toxic to therapeutic dose), penicillin can be given in huge doses without toxic effects. Its action on peptidoglycan synthesis, via penicillin-binding proteins (PBPs), has been described in Chapter 2.

STRUCTURE. The initially isolated penicillin was found to be a mixture of closely related compounds. They share a binucleate structure, **6-aminopenicillanic acid** (6-APA; Fig. 10–9): a **cyclized dipeptide,** formed by condensation of L-cysteine and D-valine, with a β-lactam and a thiazoline ring. Attached is a variable acyl side chain derived from the culture medium. **Benzylpenicillin (penicillin G),** one of the original members, It is as effective as later β-lactams against group A streptococci and certain other organisms. It is also less expensive, in part because it was developed at a time when academic administrators opposed the patenting of any discoveries related to health.

The four-membered β-lactam ring is responsible for key features of the molecule. It holds the amide group in a configuration that makes it a good analogue of the D-Ala–D-Ala bond in the transpeptidation reaction in peptidoglycan synthesis (Chap. 2); it has a strained configuration, so cleavage of its amide bond provides enough energy to form a covalent bond with the enzymes that are inactivated; and this strain also makes the bond unstable, especially when exposed to acid.

Semisynthetic Penicillins

The value of penicillin G is limited by its relatively narrow antimicrobial spectrum: gram-positive cocci and spirochetes and a small number of gram-negative organisms (especially neisserias). Other limitations are its destruction by acid in the stomach (roughly one-fifth of the orally administered drug is usually absorbed), destruction by bacterial β-lactamases, elicitation of allergic responses, and rapid excretion in the urine.

Semisynthetic modifications that overcame various of these limitations were later developed by isolating the precursor 6-APA, either by treatment of penicillin with an amidase or by cultivation of the mold in a medium lacking an acyl donor. This compound can easily be con-

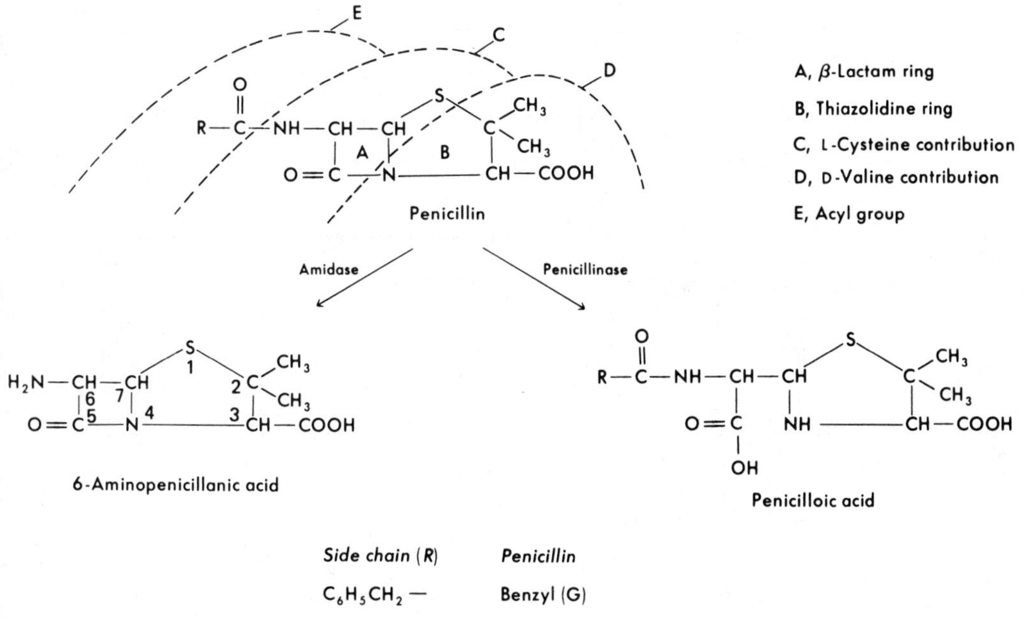

A, β-Lactam ring

B, Thiazolidine ring

C, L-Cysteine contribution

D, D-Valine contribution

E, Acyl group

Side chain (R)	Penicillin
$C_6H_5CH_2$ —	Benzyl (G)

Figure 10–9. Structure and reactions of penicillin.

densed with any carboxylic acid, yielding a virtually un-limited number of possible penicillins. Several are illustrated in Figure 10–10.

One group of these products (e.g., **oxacillin** and the closely related **cloxacillin** and **dicloxacillin; methicillin**), with a bulky substituent near the β-lactam ring, are **resistant to the plasmid-coded staphylococcal β-lactamase,** which has become very prevalent. However, with staphylococci lacking that enzyme, these derivatives are only about one-tenth as potent as benzylpenicillin.

Another semisynthetic group has a broader gram-negative spectrum. In **ampicillin** (Fig. 10–10), the amino group on the side chain evidently improves penetration through the negatively charged outer membrane, but this antibiotic is only half as active as benzylpenicillin against gram-positive organisms, and it also is sensitive to β-lactamases.

As these β-lactams became widely used, resistance to them emerged with various mechanisms (see Resistance to β-Lactams, below). To overcome this problem, and to broaden the antimicrobial spectrum, a wide variety of

additional derivatives were developed. Among these, **amoxycillin** is better absorbed than ampicillin; **azlocillin, mezlocillin,** and **piperacillin** have a broader gram-negative spectrum; and **ticarcillin** has superior activity against a particularly difficult organism, *Pseudomonas aeruginosa.* Unfortunately, all of the penicillins are still susceptible to a plasmid-coded β-lactamase called TEM-1, which is encountered in some enterics and other gram-negative organisms.

Broader changes began with **mecillinam,** which has the same bicyclic nucleus as penicillins but with an amidino (-NH-CH-N-) link to the ring at C-6. Wider structural variations have been achieved by building on nuclei with the same A ring as penicillins but a different B ring, or even with none. The most important group are the cephalosporins.

Cephalosporins

The cephalosporin nucleus is derived from the same amino acids as 6-APA, but one of the methyl groups of valine is incorporated in the ring, yielding a six-membered B ring instead of the five-membered ring of the

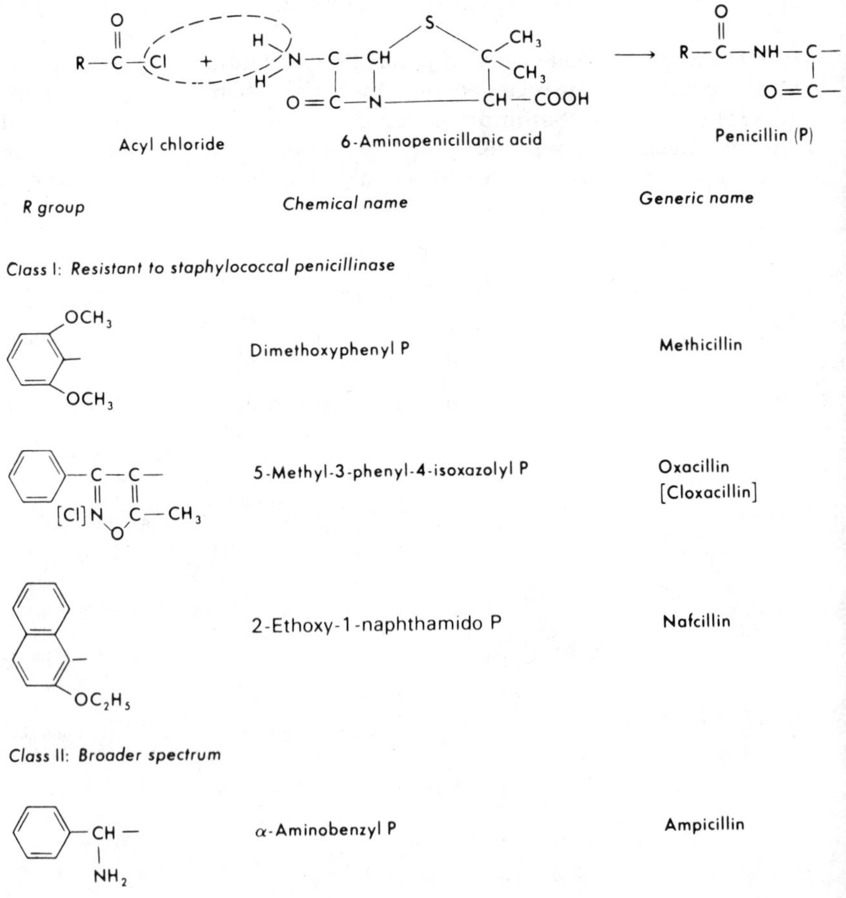

R group	Chemical name	Generic name
Class I: Resistant to staphylococcal penicillinase		
	Dimethoxyphenyl P	Methicillin
	5-Methyl-3-phenyl-4-isoxazolyl P	Oxacillin [Cloxacillin]
	2-Ethoxy-1-naphthamido P	Nafcillin
Class II: Broader spectrum		
	α-Aminobenzyl P	Ampicillin

Figure 10–10. Some semisynthetic penicillins.

penicillins. A cephalosporin was first isolated from a mold of the genus *Cephalosporium,* and the same nucleus is found in the **cephamycins,** produced by streptomycetes rather than by molds. The original cephalosporin was long ignored because of its low potency, but isolation of the precursor **7-aminocephalosporanic acid,** analogous to 6-APA, led to a series of valuable semisynthetic antibiotics.

Cephalosporins were originally introduced for use in patients with allergy to penicillins. This response is evoked by opening of the A ring and attachment of the resulting penicilloic acid (Fig. 10–9) to a protein carrier. Since the allergy is thus directed to the B ring, cephalosporins, with a different B ring, do not cross-react, although they can elicit allergy to themselves in the same way. The first useful cephalosporin, **cephalothin** (Fig. 10–11), has an antimicrobial spectrum somewhat broader than that of penicillin. This antibiotic and the related **cephazolin** are widely used for surgical prophylaxis.

Subsequent derivatives combine a broad spectrum (including *Haemophilus influenzae*) with resistance to β-lactamases of gram-negative organisms; hence they are widely used when the sensitivity of the organism is not known and in mixed infections. They are, however, more expensive than penicillins. Examples include **cephuroxime** and **cefoxitin.** Further derivatives, with greater effectiveness against the anaerobic *Bacteroides* and against the generally resistant *Pseudomonas aeruginosa,* include **cefotaxime** and **cephtriaxone.** In general, increase in activity against gram-negative organisms is accompanied by a decrease in activity against gram-positives.

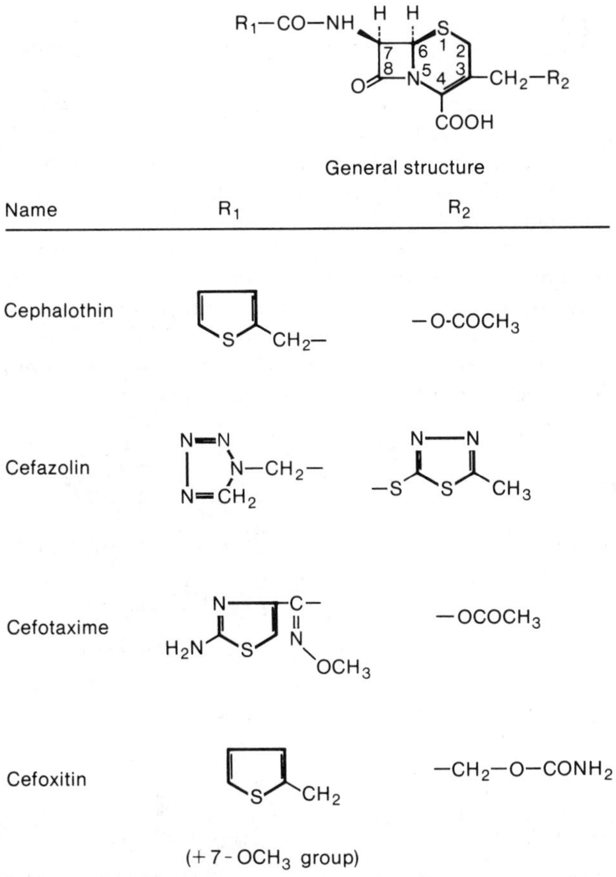

Other β-Lactams

RING SUBSTITUTIONS. **Moxalactam,** with an O instead of S in position 1 of the B ring (an oxacephem nucleus), is produced by a mold and was introduced for clinical use but proved too toxic. **Thienamycin,** a **carbapenem** (with a C replacing the S in ring B of 6-APA), was also discovered as a mold product. The first derivative to be used, **imipenem** (Fig. 10–12), has an exceptionally broad antibacterial spectrum, its relatively small substituents apparently improving its effectiveness against organisms whose outer membrane impedes entry of most β-lactams. Imipenem also binds exceptionally well to PBP2 (see Chap. 2), which may be an advantage because there are relatively few copies of this enzyme per cell. It is administered in combination with cilastatin, a dipeptidase inhibitor that prevents its destruction by a renal enzyme. Additional carba-β-lactams and oxa-β-lactams, with replacements for the S in the ring B, are under development.

Although the β-lactams now available cover the bulk of the spectrum of pathogenic bacteria, there are still problems with listeria, group D streptococci, pseudomonads, and *Bacteroides fragilis.*

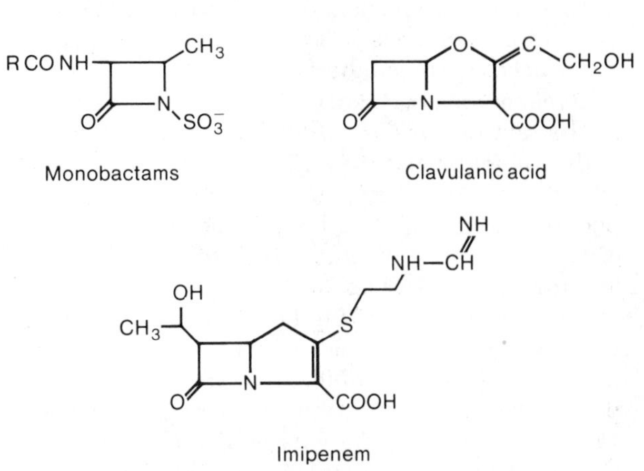

General structure

Name	R₁	R₂
Cephalothin		$-O-COCH_3$
Cefazolin		$-S$ ... CH_3
Cefotaxime		$-OCOCH_3$
Cefoxitin		$-CH_2-O-CONH_2$

(+ 7 - OCH₃ group)

Figure 10–11. Some semisynthetic cephalomycins.

Figure 10–12. Some unusual β-lactams.

MONOBACTAMS. The monobactam group, produced by bacteria rather than by a mold, have a monocyclic β-lactam nucleus without a B ring (Fig. 10–12). Among the products that have been improved by chemical modification, **azthreonam** is relatively specific for the PBPs of various aerobic gram-negative organisms, including *Pseudomonas aeruginosa.* This narrow spectrum has some advantage, in that preservation of the normal throat and gastrointestinal flora prevents colonization by undesirable organisms.

BETA-LACTAMASE INHIBITORS. In addition to efforts to eliminate sensitivity to various β-lactamases, an alternative approach irreversibly inactivates the enzyme by using a substrate with little bactericidal action but with high affinity, such as **clavulanic acid** (an oxa-β-lactam; Fig. 10–12) or **sulbactam** (a penicillanic acid sulfone). When administered together with another, bactericidal, β-lactam (most often amoxicillin), these compounds can increase the antimicrobial effectiveness against β-lactamase-producing organisms.

Other Inhibitors of Peptidoglycan Synthesis

Among other antibiotics that interfere with peptidoglycan synthesis, as noted in Chapter 2, two have clinical use.

Vancomycin, from an actinomycete (*Nocardia*), is a complex heptapeptide of modified aromatic acids condensed into a tricyclic structure and with a disaccharide substituent. It blocks chain extension by **forming a complex with D-Ala–D-Ala,** both on the lipid-borne muramyl peptide and on the growing peptidoglycan chain, and so it does not select for resistant mutants. Impurities in early preparations were largely responsible for a toxicity that discouraged its use, but the drug is now under further investigation. Vancomycin is effective against many gram-positive bacteria, including anaerobes. It is used especially in the presence of allergy or resistance to both penicillins and cephalosporins and in the treatment of the clostridial pseudomembranous colitis induced by some other antibiotics.

Bacitracin, a cyclic peptide (Fig. 10–13), is produced by a strain of *Bacillus subtilis.* It forms a 1/1 **complex with undecaprenyl-PP** and prevents its dephosphorylation, an essential step in the elongation of both the peptidoglycan and the lipopolysaccharide O antigen (Chap. 2). Because of its toxicity, bacitracin is used only for antisepsis (see Chap. 3).

Two unusually small antibiotics are analogues of peptidoglycan precursors that act in the cytoplasm. Because they are highly hydrophilic, they must enter via transport systems for related metabolites. **Cycloserine** (Fig. 10–14) competitively inhibits both the formation of D-alanine from L-alanine and its conversion to the dipeptide D-Ala–D-Ala. The conformation fixed by the ring gives

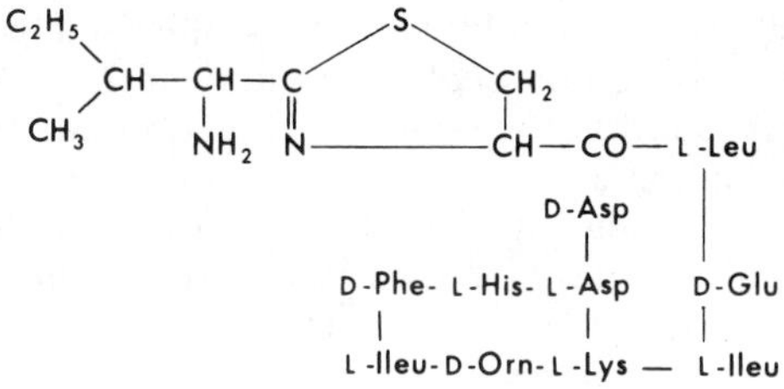

Figure 10–13. Bacitracin A. The portion presented in detail consists of an isoleucine and a cysteine residue condensed to form a thiazoline ring rather than the usual peptide linkage of a polypeptide.

it an affinity for the enzyme 20 times that of the natural substrate. **Fosfomycin (phosphonomycin;** Fig. 10–14), an analogue of P-enolpyruvate, has an epoxide group, which permits irreversible inhibition of the enzyme that converts enolpyruvate to the ether-linked lactyl group of UDP-MurNAc. Fosfomycin enters via a transport system for glycerol-P.

ANTIRIBOSOMAL ANTIBIOTICS

Antibiotics acting on the ribosome can be classified in several ways.

1. The aminoglycosides are **bactericidal,** whereas most others are **bacteriostatic.**

2. Some antibiotics act selectively on **prokaryotic** ribosomes, some (e.g., cycloheximide) only on ribosomes of **eukaryotic cytoplasm,** and others on both. Mitochondrial ribosomes respond like prokaryotic ribosomes to many antibiotics.

3. Some antibiotics (e.g., puromycin, chloramphenicol) act on **polysomal ribosomes;** others (e.g., erythromycin) block only **free, initiating ribosomes,** because their binding sites are not accessible on the more conformationally restricted polysomal ribosomes. The aminoglycosides act on both types, with different effects.

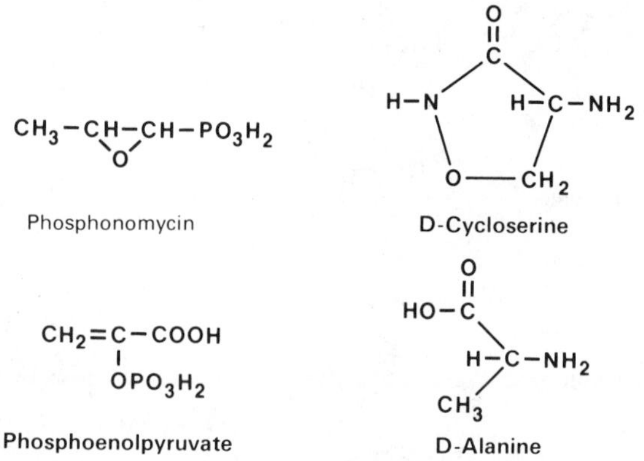

Figure 10–14. Antibiotic metabolite analogues that inhibit peptidoglycan synthesis, with the corresponding metabolites.

4. Some antibiotics bind to the small and others to the large ribosomal subunit, as can be established either by direct binding studies or by identifying the subunit that is altered in resistant mutants. The binding sites can be localized by cross-linking to ribosomal RNA or proteins.

As Chapter 6 emphasized, the ribosome is a conformationally interacting body and not a set of independent enzymes; hence, binding of any ligand (normal or an antibiotic) decreases conformational flexibility and can also affect the conformation at distant sites. Accordingly, although the events on the ribosome can be neatly divided into a sequence of steps, it has often not been possible to define precisely "the" key action of an antibiotic.

STRUCTURE AND UPTAKE. The antiribosomal antibiotics are virtually all large, complex molecules, differing widely in structure but often possessing cationic groups and rings, promoting ionic and stacking interactions with rRNA. Unlike the agents that block peptidoglycan synthesis (at the outer surface of the cytoplasmic membrane), they must enter the cytoplasm. The aminoglycosides are polycationic and highly polar; hence they must induce membrane damage before they can enter the cell extensively. Most of the others, however, have a large hydrophobic region, which promotes entry by diffusion through the membrane lipid.

Table 10–1 summarizes the key actions of selected antiribosomal antibiotics.

Puromycin

Puromycin interferes with protein synthesis by causing premature release of the nascent polypeptide from the ribosome. It serves as an analogue of the terminal aminoacyl-adenosine of aminoacyl-tRNA (Fig. 10–15), binding to part of the A site (on both prokaryotic and eukaryotic ribosomes) and accepting nascent polypeptide (or f-Met) from the P site (see Chap. 6). The resulting peptidyl-puromycin is bound more loosely than aminoacyl-tRNA, and it cannot continue chain elongation, so it is released. The phenyl group in puromycin evidently contributes to the binding energy (suggesting base stacking), as similar analogues of nonaromatic amino acids are much less effective.

Puromycin is not a chemotherapeutic agent, but it has been a very useful reagent for blocking protein synthesis formation (especially in eukaryotic cells), and for study of the peptidyl transfer reaction (see Chap. 6). Moreover, covalent linkage of puromycin to the ribosome has localized its binding site (and hence the peptidyl transferase center) at the interface between the two subunits.

Cells of *E. coli* require a high concentration (ca. 500 μg/ml) of puromycin for the immediate release of nascent chains. Moderate concentrations release longer truncated chains; and, as will be discussed at the end of

TABLE 10–1. *Antibiotics Inhibiting Protein Synthesis*

	Site of Action				
Antibiotic	*Cell Type*	*Subunit*	*Step*	*Altered in Resistant Mutants*	*Specific Effects*
Puromycin	Eu, Pro*	L	R,P	—	Releases peptidyl-puromycin
Tetracyclines	Pro	S	R	—	Block stable binding in A site
Streptomycin	Pro	S	I,R	Protein S12	1. Irreversible: blocks movement of initiation complex 2. Causes misreading by elongating ribosome
Kasugamycin	Pro	S	I	Protein S2; 16S RNA	Blocks formation of initiation complex
Spectinomycin	Pro	S	I	Protein S5	Blocks movement after initiation
Chloramphenicol, lincomycin	Pro	L	P	—	Blocks peptidyl transfer
Sparsomycin	Eu, Pro	L	P	—	Blocks puromycin reaction and stable binding in A site
Erythromycin	Pro	L	P	23S RNA, Proteins L4, L26	Blocks chain extension soon after initiation
Siomycin, thiostrepton	Pro	L	T,R	23S RNA	Irreversible; blocks binding of EFG · GTP, and of EFTu · aa-tRNA · GTP
Kirromycin	Pro	S	R	EFTu	Blocks release of EFTu · GDP
Pulvomycin	Pro	S	R	—	Blocks formation of aa-tRNA · EFTu · GTP
Fusidic acid	Eu, Pro	L	T	EFG	Blocks release of EFG and GDP
Viomycin	Pro	S,L	T	S,L	Blocks P site
Rifamycins	Pro	Transcription		β-Subunit	Block initiation
Streptolydigin	Pro	Transcription		Polymerase	Inhibits extension
Dactinomycin	Eu, Pro	Transcription		—	Binds to DNA

* Eu, pro = eukaryotic, prokaryotic cells; L, S = large, small ribosomal subunit; R = recognition; P = peptidyl transfer; T = translocation, I = initiation.

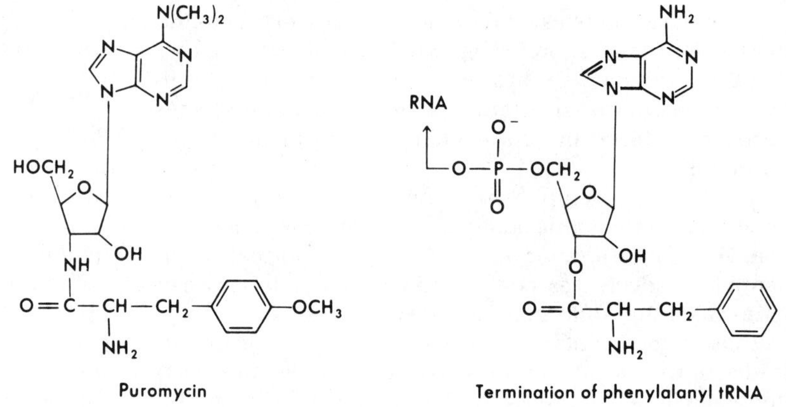

Figure 10–15. Puromycin and its metabolic analogue, the aminoacyl end of tRNA. (After Yarmolinsky MB, de la Haba GL: Proc Natl Acad Sci USA 45:1721, 1959)

the section on aminoglycosides, these cause the membrane to become leaky to small molecules.

Aminoglycosides: General

The aminoglycosides, formed by actinomycetes of the genus *Streptomyces*, are highly polar, polycationic compounds containing an **aminocyclitol** (a cyclohexitol with basic substituents) plus two or more sugars (including at least one amino sugar). In **streptomycin** (Str) and a few other aminoglycosides, the aminocyclitol is a diguanidinoinositol (**streptidine**), while in most it is diamino-2-deoxyinositol (**deoxystreptamine**; Fig. 10–16).

Although the aminoglycosides all share several unique features, Str differs from the deoxystreptamine group in several respects. It binds only one molecule per ribosome; it binds to a different site, as shown by the RNA sequence that it protects from digestion; and one-step mutations can yield highly resistant ribosomes with greatly decreased affinity for the drug. The various members can all be inactivated by various enzymes that attach substituents to specific groups (see Drug Resistance, below). To circumvent this kind of resistance, and also to decrease toxicity, many aminoglycosides have been isolated. However, unlike the diverse β-lactams, the aminoglycosides differ little in antimicrobial spectrum.

The aminoglycosides are active against many gram-positive and gram-negative organisms and also against the tubercle bacillus. The drugs in clinical use include **streptomycin, kanamycin, tobramycin, gentamicin, metilmycin,** and several others. (Gentamicin is formed by a *Nocardia*, and its peculiar spelling results from a bureaucratic ruling restricting the suffix "-mycin" to products of streptomycetes.) **Amikacin** is a semisynthetic derivative of kanamycin, with an NH_2 group derivatized to prevent inactivation by a resistance enzyme. **Neomycin** is potent but also toxic, and it is used only topically. Dihydrostreptomycin, made by reducing the aldehyde group of Str, is virtually identical in action to Str.

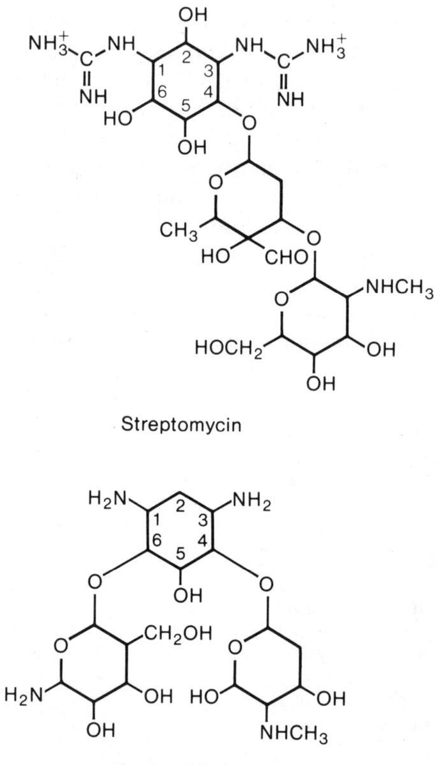

Streptomycin

Gentamicin A

Figure 10–16. Aminoglycosides. All these drugs contain an aminocyclitol ring and one or more amino sugars. In streptomycin, the ring is streptidine: 1,3-diguanidino inositol. In the gentamicins and in many other aminoglycosides, the ring is deoxystreptamine, with two amino instead of guanidino groups. Other gentamicins differ in their substituents on the sugars, some with an additional amino group; and the kanamycins similarly have sugars substituted on positions 4 and 6 of the aminocyclitol ring. Neomycin has two diamino sugars, on positions 4 and 5.

The highly polar polycationic aminoglycosides do not readily cross cell membranes. This impermeability limits their therapeutic use in the following ways:

1. They cannot be absorbed from the intestine, so treatment of systemic infections requires injection. However, oral administration can be used to alter the intestinal flora.

2. They are ineffective against intracellular bacteria.

3. Their uptake by bacteria is antagonized by acid and by salts, especially divalent cations. This property decreases their value for urinary tract infections.

4. Anaerobiosis also antagonizes entry (for reasons discussed below), increasing the MIC for *E. coli* about ten-fold.

5. The rate of entry (and of killing) increases with antibiotic concentration over a wide range (in contrast to the rate of killing by β-lactams, which is limited by the rate of cell growth). Unfortunately, the attainable concentrations are severely limited because aminoglycosides are quite toxic, often causing irreversible damage to the inner ear on long-term administration and also causing nephrotoxicity.

For these reasons the aminoglycosides are not the drugs of choice except in severe infections. They are used in treating tuberculosis, brucellosis, tularemia, and plague, for though the first three of these organisms can multiply within host cells the rapid bactericidal action of the antibiotic interferes with their spread. A particularly important use involves **synergism with β-lactams** in certain life-threatening diseases, especially bacterial endocarditis, and gram-negative sepsis. The basis of this synergism is that even nonlethal degrees of disorganization of the cell wall by β-lactams damage the membrane and facilitate the uptake of aminoglycosides.

Aminoglycosides require concomitant protein synthesis for their bactericidal action (Fig. 10-17), and so they are not active against starving bacteria. However, their mechanism of killing (see below) requires less growth than does killing by B-lactams, and this property may contribute to their value against the slowly growing organisms of bacterial endocarditis.

STREPTOMYCIN RESISTANCE AND DEPENDENCE. Str can select for one-step mutants (*strA*) with a large increase (more than 100-fold) in resistance. These mutants are altered in ribosomal protein S12, as was shown by reassembling sensitive ribosomes with various single proteins obtained from resistant ribosomes. Because the resistance requires a functional protein altered within a small region, the mutation rate is low (10^{-9}) compared with mutations that inactivate various enzymes. Str does not bind to the isolated protein S12, but it binds to specific sequences of the 16S RNA in intact ribosomes.

Selection for resistance also yields **dependent** (*str*^d) mutants, which require Str for growth; the mechanism

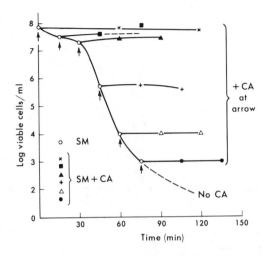

Figure 10–17. Rapid protection by chloramphenicol *(CA)* against killing by streptomycin *(SM)* added to exponentially growing *E. coli* at 0 time. At intervals, samples were transferred *(arrows)* to flasks containing chloramphenicol. These flasks were similarly incubated. Samples were removed for viable counts as noted. (Plotz P, Davis BD: J Bacteriol 83:802, 1962)

will be discussed below. Such mutants have occasionally been encountered in patients. Drug dependence has since also been observed with antibiotics that act on smaller targets than the ribosome (e.g., rifampin, which acts on RNA polymerase).

Mechanism of Aminoglycoside Action

Aminoglycosides have an exceptionally pleiotropic set of effects. The key effect responsible for killing was sought for decades, but it has turned out that the several following effects are all equally important. Because this problem has revealed novel aspects of both ribosome and membrane function we will describe the key findings in some detail.

MEMBRANE DAMAGE AND STR UPTAKE. Uptake of radioactive Str by bacteria is **triphasic** (Fig. 10–18): an immediate adsorption to the exterior; a lag during which there is very little entry; and then rapidly increasing entry to the cell (finally reaching about 100 times the molar concentration of ribosomes). The rapid entry depends on damage to the membrane, for at its onset the cells become leaky to many small molecules. The damage, like killing, requires protein synthesis in sensitive cells. The uptake is irreversible, presumably because of extensive binding to anionic surfaces within the cell.

MEMBRANE POTENTIAL. Str uptake appears to be facilitated by electrophoresis (as well as diffusion) through the channels created by membrane damage, for it is slowed by conditions that lower the membrane potential

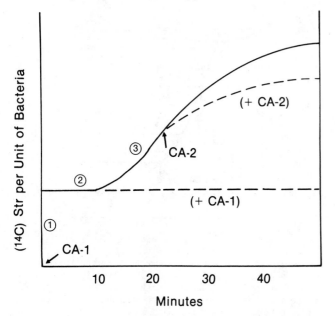

Figure 10–18. Triphasic uptake of streptomycin. ^{14}C-Str was added to a growing culture of *E. coli,* and at intervals, samples were collected on membrane filters, washed with water, and counted. An immediate adsorption (phase 1), which can be washed off by concentrated salt solution, was followed by a lag (phase 2) with little or no detectable uptake and then by a rapid transition to extensive, irreversible uptake (phase 3). Chloramphenicol added with the Str *(arrow CA-1)* prevented the uptake *(dashed line),* indicating that protein synthesis is required during phase 2 to initiate phase 3; but CA added after phase 3 had begun *(arrow CA-2)* allowed already damaged cells to continue to take up the antibiotic. (After Anand N, Davis BD, Armitage AK: Nature 185:23, 1960; Andry K, Bockrath RC: Nature 251:534, 1974)

(negative interior). Anaerobiosis severely reduces the membrane potential, which explains why it delays entry.

ALTERNATIVE EFFECTS. Although bactericidal concentrations of Str **inhibit protein synthesis** starting at about the time when leakiness begins to become detectable, in contrast, sublethal concentrations cause **misreading in protein synthesis:** the antibiotic distorts the ribosome in a way that increases errors, in which codons pair with near-cognate anticodons containing only two of the three complementary bases.

This finding had several important implications. It (1) showed that drugs can affect the accuracy as well as the rate of a reaction; (2) localized the site of aminoglycoside action to the recognition region; (3) led to the isolation of ribosomal ambiguity (*ram*) mutants (Chap. 6), with a similar effect; and (4) explained **Str-dependent mutations:** they evidently distort the recognition region in a way that **restricts** codon–anticodon interaction, and this effect can be compensated for (Fig. 10–19) by the opposite, loosening effect of the antibiotic (or of *ram* mutants). But whether inhibition or misreading was responsible for killing was not clear.

The state of the ribosome determines whether binding of Str will cause blockade or misreading. With chain-elongating polysomes in vitro it causes misreading (over a wide range of concentrations of the antibiotic), while with free, initiating ribosomes it causes the formation of **blocked initiation complexes.** As with other antibiotics described above, these blocks are unstable, allowing the ribosomes to recycle onto, and block, fresh mRNA.

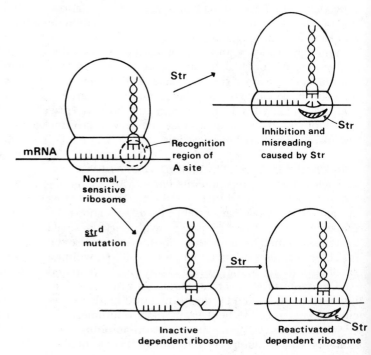

Figure 10–19. Diagram showing how the same distorting effect of streptomycin *(Str)* is believed to impair the activity of sensitive ribosomes but reactivate dependent ribosomes.

StrA mutations eliminate both blockade and misreading. Since the ribosome has only one site for binding a molecule of Str tightly, it appears that the same binding site is exposed in the two states of the ribosome, but its fuller exposure in the more flexible free ribosome results in binding with a more drastic effect.

THE MULTI-STEP MECHANISM. Various experiments have shown that the bactericidal action of aminoglycosides requires protein synthesis during the period of invisible uptake, but not during the later, rapid uptake. This feature has led to the following multi-step model. A few molecules of antibiotic enter the cell, perhaps through transient imperfections in the growing membrane. These molecules bind to polysomal ribosomes (which predominate in growing cells), yielding misread proteins. Some of these proteins enter the membrane, where their misfolding creates aqueous channels. Further entry of the antibiotic then increases autocatalytically, as more misreading leads to more membrane damage. Finally, when enough antibiotic has entered to block all the ribosomes, it irreversibly halts protein synthesis.

PUROMYCIN AND MEMBRANE CHANNELS. This model can also explain the paradoxical finding that high concentrations of puromycin prevent Str uptake (and killing), while moderate concentrations accelerate it. At high concentrations puromycin evidently releases chains that are too short to enter the membrane, while at moderate concentrations they are long enough to enter and cause damage. In addition, the accelerating effect of a moderate concentration of puromycin can be explained by the further observation that it leads to entry of Str even in Str-resistant cells (in which Str does not cause misreading), unexpectedly revealing that truncated chains cause damage to the membrane even without generalized misreading.

Other Antiribosomal Antibiotics

We have seen that aminoglycosides block only initiating ribosomes, and that their action is irreversible because of their irreversible uptake. Among other antiribosomal antibiotics, which are reversible in their uptake and their action, some (erythromycin, spectinomycin, kasugamycin) act only on initiating ribosomes. (The resulting blockade is unstable, as with aminoglycosides.) Others (including chloramphenicol and tetracycline) can block chain-elongating ribosomes.

CHLORAMPHENICOL. Chloramphenicol (Fig. 10–20) is unusual among natural products in containing a nitro and a dichloracetyl group. It binds to the large ribosomal subunit and blocks peptidyl transfer on chain-elongating ribosomes. The effect is direct, as the antibiotic inhibits

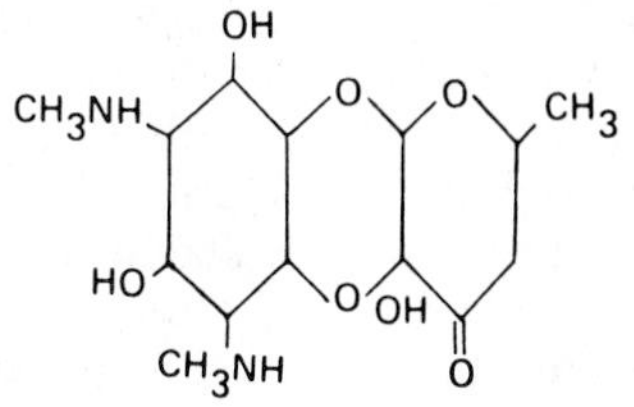

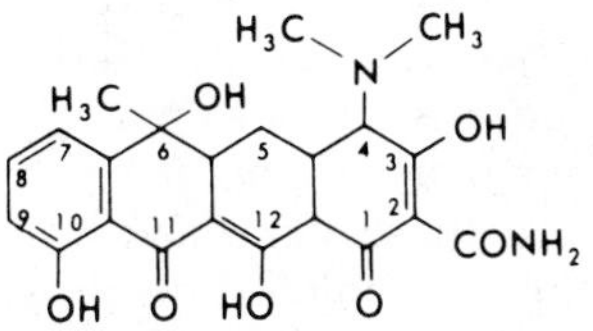

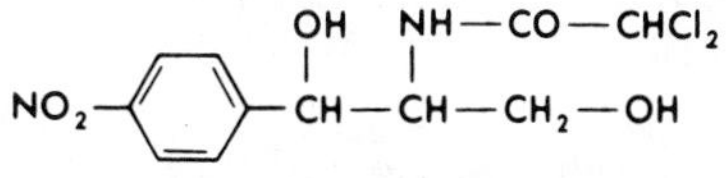

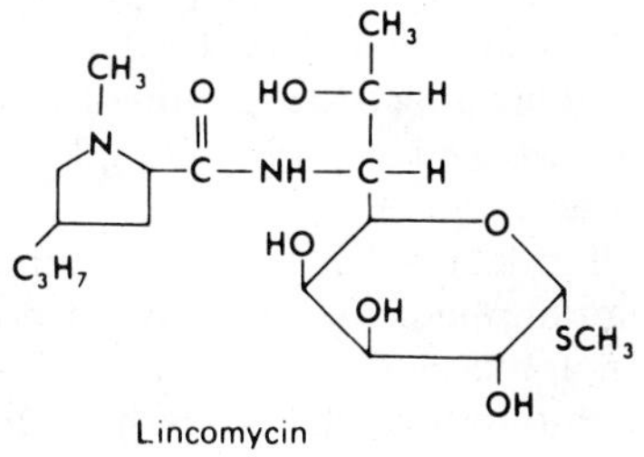

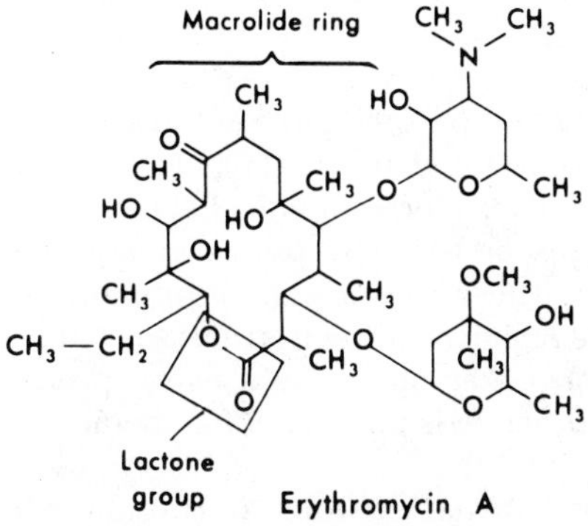

Figure 10–20. Antibiotics that act reversibly on the ribosome. Chlortetracycline is 7-chlorotetracycline; oxytetracycline is 5-hydroxytetracycline; demethylchlortetracycline is chlortetracycline without the 6-methyl group. Erythromycin is one of several macrolides with similar structure and action. Lincomycin has been largely replaced by clindamycin (7-chloro-7-deoxylincomycin). Chloramphenicol has no congeners in clinical use.

the release of f-Met as well as of polypeptides by puromycin. (A block of translocation would stop the reaction with polypeptide, but not that with fMet.) Chloramphenicol has been a very useful reagent in studies of the ribosome cycle because it rapidly stabilizes polysomal ribosomes.

Chloramphenicol and tetracycline were the first "broad-spectrum" antibiotics (effective against a variety of gram-positive and negative bacteria), but that term now also describes many of the newer β-lactams. Chloramphenicol occasionally causes severe blood dyscrasias. This reaction suggests that the drug may reach the mitochondria in bone marrow cells, for the ribosomes of mitochondria, unlike those of the eukaryotic cytoplasm, are sensitive to chloramphenicol. This drug should be used only in serious infections, with periodic checking of blood cell counts, but because it is inexpensive and has a broad spectrum it is used excessively in some underdeveloped countries.

TETRACYCLINE. Tetracycline and its several congeners, containing four fused rings (Fig. 10–20), bind to either subunit. These drugs interfere with binding of aminoacyl-tRNA in the A site. However, GTP hydrolysis is not prevented, and so the block evidently involves **an unstable, distorted binding of aminoacyl-tRNA,** analogous to the unstable blocked initiation complexes noted above for some other antibiotics.

Tetracycline has much the same antibacterial spectrum as chloramphenicol, although the mode of action is quite different. It is especially useful against intracellular bacteria (including rickettsias), perhaps because its hydrophobicity facilitates its diffusion through the membrane. It is also useful against mycoplasmas, which do not form cell walls and hence are insensitive to β-lactams.

SPARSOMYCIN. Sparsomycin blocks two steps: like tetracycline, it prevents stable binding of aminoacyl-tRNA; but in addition, like chloramphenicol, it blocks the release of polypeptides or f-Met by puromycin, and it stabilizes polysomes. These effects suggest binding to the 50S region of the A site, near the transferase center. Sparsomycin acts on eukaryotic as well as on prokaryotic ribosomes and hence is not useful for therapy.

ERYTHROMYCIN; MACROLIDES. The macrolides have a large lactone ring with no N and with one or more amino-sugar and sugar substituents. The group includes **erythromycin** (Fig. 10–20), **oleandomycin, carbomycin, spiramycin,** and **tylosin.** The best-studied member, erythromycin, binds one molecule to free ribosomes (or to their 50S subunits) but not to polysomal ribosomes. Whereas other antibiotics that interact only with free initiating ribosomes cause an immediate block of the initiation complex, erythromycin blocks synthesis only after a short polypeptide has been formed. The blocked peptide is not released by puromycin, implying a block either in peptidyl transfer or in translocation.

Macrolides are effective against a wide variety of gram-positive bacteria and some gram-negatives (including *Legionella* and *Bordetella*). Mutants of *E. coli* resistant to macrolides are altered in proteins L4 or L22. In addition, many species exhibit **inducible resistance,** in which subinhibitory concentrations cause the formation of an enzyme that dimethylates two specific adenine residues in 23S RNA. The ribosome is then resistant to macrolides, and also to lincomycin and streptogramin (**MLS resistance;** see Translational Attenuation, Chap. 9).

LINCOSAMIDES. Lincomycin (see Fig. 10–18) binds to free ribosomes or the 50S subunit but not to polysomal ribosomes. Since MLS resistance applies to lincomycin as well as to erythromycin, the two may bind in the same region of the ribosome. The more potent 7-chloro derivative **clindamycin** is useful clinically, especially against gram-negative anaerobes, but its suppression of this group in the intestine tends to cause **pseudomembranous enterocolitis** by allowing overgrowth of the enterotoxin-producing, gram-positive *Clostridium difficile.*

Streptogramin A resembles lincomycin in its binding, effects on the ribosome, and response to MLS resistance, although it has a very different structure (a large substituted lactone with N atoms). It is used in animal feed but not clinically.

SPECTINOMYCIN. Spectinomycin (Fig. 10–20), like the aminoglycosides, has an aminocyclitol ring, but the rest of the structure is hydrophobic rather than hydrophilic and cationic; hence, spectinomycin can enter without membrane damage, and its action is bacteriostatic. Like aminoglycosides, spectinomycin causes the formation of unstable initiation complexes and selects for resistant mutants with altered ribosomes; but unlike them, it does not cause misreading and does not inhibit polysomal ribosomes. Spectinomycin is particularly useful in the treatment of gonorrhea.

Viomycin and **capreomycin,** highly basic cyclic polypeptides, appear to block the ribosomal P site and hence to **prevent translocation,** as they block the reaction of acetyl-Phe (a substitute for f-Met). Moreover, they interfere with the formation of the 30S initiation complex (in which f-Met-tRNA binds to the P site). They have been used clinically against mycobacteria.

INTERFERENCE WITH ELONGATION FACTORS. Thiostrepton (see Fig. 10–19) and the structurally related **siomycin** are very large polycyclic antibiotics that bind to the large subunit, where they **block the binding of both elongation factors EFTu and EFG.** The site of the binding has been narrowly localized to a complex of protein L11 and a short region of the 23S RNA. Moreover, in the streptomycete that produces the antibiotic, that region in the RNA is methylated, making the ribosome resistant. The site differs from that of the methylation in MLS resistance.

Fusidic acid (Fig. 10–21), a product of the eukaryotic mold *Fusarium*, is a steroid. It **binds to EFG** and inhibits release of the EFG·GDP complex, thus allowing one round of translocation and then fixing the pp-tRNA in the P site because the ribosome cannot bind the EFTu ternary complex until EFG is released (Chap. 6). This antibiotic is useful clinically against gram-positive cocci, especially β-lactam-resistant staphylococci.

Pulvomycin and **kirromycin** are not clinically useful but they are interesting because they **bind to EFTu.** The former blocks the addition of aminoacyl-tRNA to form a ternary complex, whereas the latter blocks release of EFTu·GDP, just as fusidic acid blocks EFG·GDP.

In conclusion, various antibiotics interfere with virtually every aspect of ribosome function, and they have been useful probes for the reaction centers that are involved.

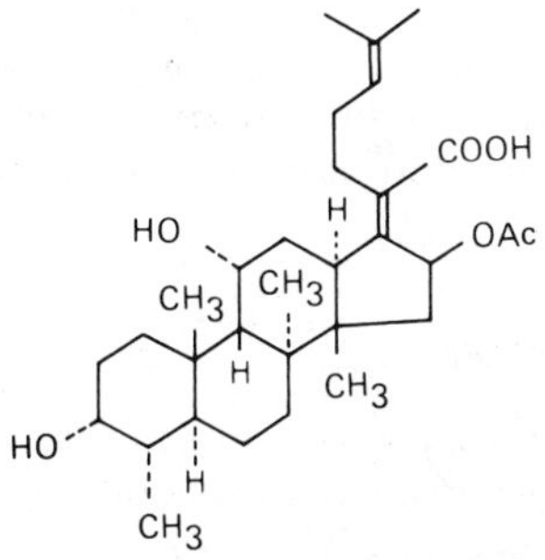

OTHER ANTIBIOTIC ACTIONS

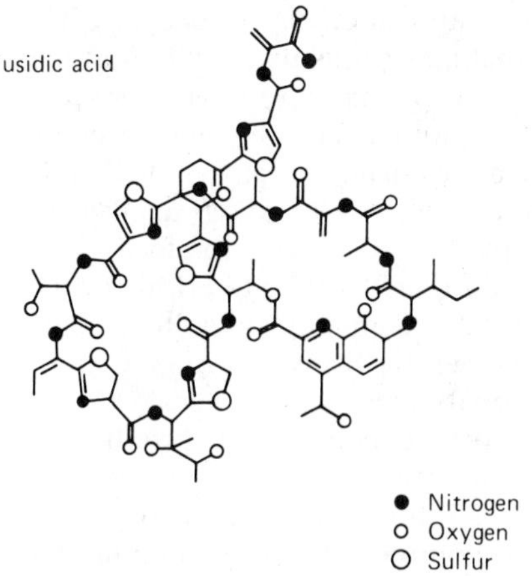

Actions on the Membrane

POLYMYXINS. The polymyxin group of cyclic polypeptides, produced by *Bacillus polymyxa* and related *Bacilli*, resemble cationic detergents in having multiple basic groups (in diaminobutyric acid) and a long alkyl residue (Fig. 10–22). They bind to membranes and are the only antibiotics that are **bactericidal to nongrowing cells.** The damage to the outer membrane (which forms blebs and fragments) can account for the bactericidal action and for its selectivity for gram-negative organisms, because polymyxin remains effective when attached to agarose beads, which cannot penetrate the peptidoglycan. The cytoplasmic membrane is also attacked, the intact wall remaining as a ghost.

Polymyxin is effective at concentrations far below those required for the cationic detergents used as disinfectants. Its selectivity may involve its ability to form complexes with both phosphatidyl ethanolamine and lipopolysaccharide; it has much lower affinity for phosphatidyl choline, an important constituent of animal cell membranes that is not present in bacteria.

Because of its nephrotoxicity, polymyxin B is rarely used systemically except against *Pseudomonas aeruginosa*.

Tyrocidin and the very similar **gramicidin S** are cyclic polypeptides that cause disorganization of the membrane, resulting in leakage of small molecules and in lysis of protoplasts. They were among the earliest antibiotics but proved to be too toxic for systemic use.

Polyene antibiotics complex with **sterols,** as can be shown *in vitro*, and so they are useful against fungi (see Chap. 43) but not against bacteria except for those mycoplasmas that have incorporated sterols. The resulting aqueous pores in the membrane release small molecules from the cytoplasm.

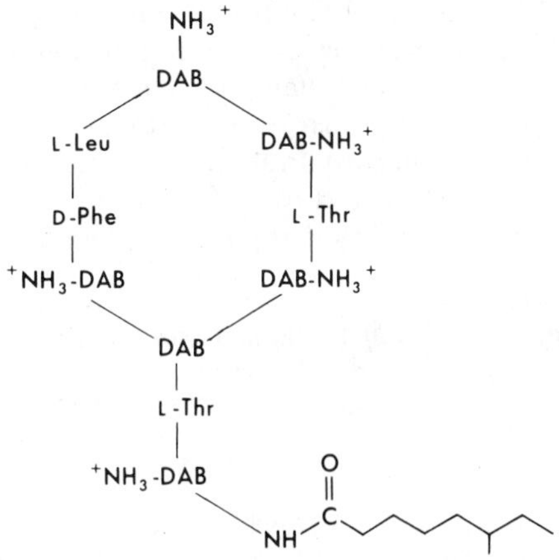

Fusidic acid

Thiostrepton

● Nitrogen
○ Oxygen
○ Sulfur

Figure 10–21. Antibiotics that interfere with translocation.

Figure 10–22. Polymyxin B. *DAB*, α,γ-diaminobutyrate [NH_2CH_2-$CH_2CH(NH_2)$ COOH]. Aliphatic residue is 6-methyloctanoic acid.

IONOPHORES. The ionophore molecules greatly increase the permeability of membranes to specific ions: they form rings that have a nonpolar periphery and therefore spontaneously insert themselves ("dissolve") in membranes, while the interior of the ring closely fits a particular inorganic cation and also provides carbonyl groups that coordinate with it, replacing its normal hydration shell. (Such caged ions are called **clathrates.**) These antibiotics are bactericidal but are not selective enough to be useful in therapy; they are useful as tools for studying membrane physiology.

Several chemical classes of antibiotics have been found to act as ionophores. Some have a covalently closed ring, whereas others are linear but fold into a ring; some are neutral, and others have a carboxyl group (Table 10-2). For example, **valinomycin,** which is highly specific for transporting K, is a cyclic **depsipeptide** (i.e., a chain of alternating α-amino and α-hydroxy acids connected by peptide and ester bonds):

$$[D - \text{hydroxyvalerate} \longrightarrow D - \text{valine} \longrightarrow L - \text{lactate} \longrightarrow L - \text{valine}]_3$$
$$\text{Valinomycin}$$

As atomic models show, the aliphatic side chains readily face outward from the ring and the carboxyl groups face inward, which explains how these compounds form selective pores across membranes.

The carrier function depends either on diffusion or on conformational change of the ionophore within its lipid matrix. Neutral ionophores permit the charged ion to move across the membrane in the direction of the electrical potential, thus eliminating that potential. Acidic ionophores, in contrast, can exchange their metal ion for H^+, thus eliminating the pH difference rather than the potential difference across the membrane.

Other Classes of Antibiotics

INHIBITION OF TRANSCRIPTION. The RNA polymerases of bacteria, phages, and mammalian cells differ markedly, and so their inhibitors may be highly selective.

Rifampin, a semisynthetic derivative of the natural antibiotic **rifamycin,** has an aromatic chromophore spanned by a long aliphatic bridge (Fig. 10–23). It interferes with **initiation** of transcription in bacteria, but not with chain extension. Rifampin binds to RNA polymerase, and probably also to the DNA in the initiation complex. It is an effective inhibitor of many bacteria, but resistant mutants, altered in the B subunit of the polymerase, appear rapidly. Rifampin is used mostly in combined therapy in tuberculosis and bacterial endocarditis and in eradication of carrier states. **Streptolydigin** (Fig. 10–23) binds to RNA polymerase in a different way, which results in blockade of **chain extension.**

Actinomycin D (dactinomycin) (Fig. 10–23) also blocks chain extension in transcription but by interacting with DNA: its aromatic chromophore is intercalated into the helix at GC pairs in DNA, while its cyclic peptide binds to the surface. Like all antibiotics that bind to DNA, it inhibits both replication and transcription, although the latter is more sensitive. Antibiotics that bind to DNA cannot discriminate usefully between bacteria and host cells, but several have proved valuable in studying viruses and in treating viral infections and cancer.

DNA GYRASE. **Novobiocin** acts on bacterial DNA gyrase as we have discussed above in connection with the quinolones. It was used earlier against penicillinase-producing organisms, but it has been displaced by later β-lactams.

OTHER TARGETS. Several antibiotics (e.g., **antimycin, oligomycin**) inhibit mitochondrial ATPase and hence were considered initially to be inhibitors of energy production, but it is not clear whether they act on specific components of the energy-transfer chain or have a more general effect on the organization of the membrane. Among additional effects, **cerulenin** inhibits fatty acid chain growth, **tunicamycin** blocks glycosylation of proteins in eukaryotic cells, **cyclosporin** inhibits immune reactions that contribute to graft rejection, and **ivermectin** can cure filariasis.

ANTIBIOTIC PRODUCTION

The β-lactams are derived from molds, most other antibiotics from actinomycetes (largely of the genus *Streptomyces*), and some from Bacilli. These are all aerobic sporulating organisms, and their formation of antibiotics is intimately related to sporulation.

In the initial screening for novel antibiotics, the yield from a promising strain is ordinarily low, but it can be improved—by as much as 5000 times—by two empiric procedures: screening for higher-yielding mutants (which are evidently altered in regulatory mechanisms) and modifications of the culture medium. Moreover, although aerobic growth is more convenient than anaerobic growth on a laboratory scale, providing adequate aeration for the commercial production of antibiotics in tanks as large as 50,000 gallons required the development of novel fermentation technology.

The complex structures of antibiotics often combine derivatives of two or more groups of metabolites: amino acids, sugars, nucleic acid bases, and intermediates in lipid synthesis. In particular, acetyl-CoA and propionyl-

TABLE 10–2. Classes of Antibiotic Ionophores

Enniatins	Cyclic depsipeptides with ring of 18 atoms
Gramicidins	Cyclic (gramicidin S) and open-chain (A,B,C) peptides
Actins (e.g., Nonactin)	Tetralactone, ring of 32 atoms, 4 methyl or ethyl substituents
Nigericin, monensin	Open-chain: form ring by hydrogen-bonding the terminal COOH to 2 OH groups at other end

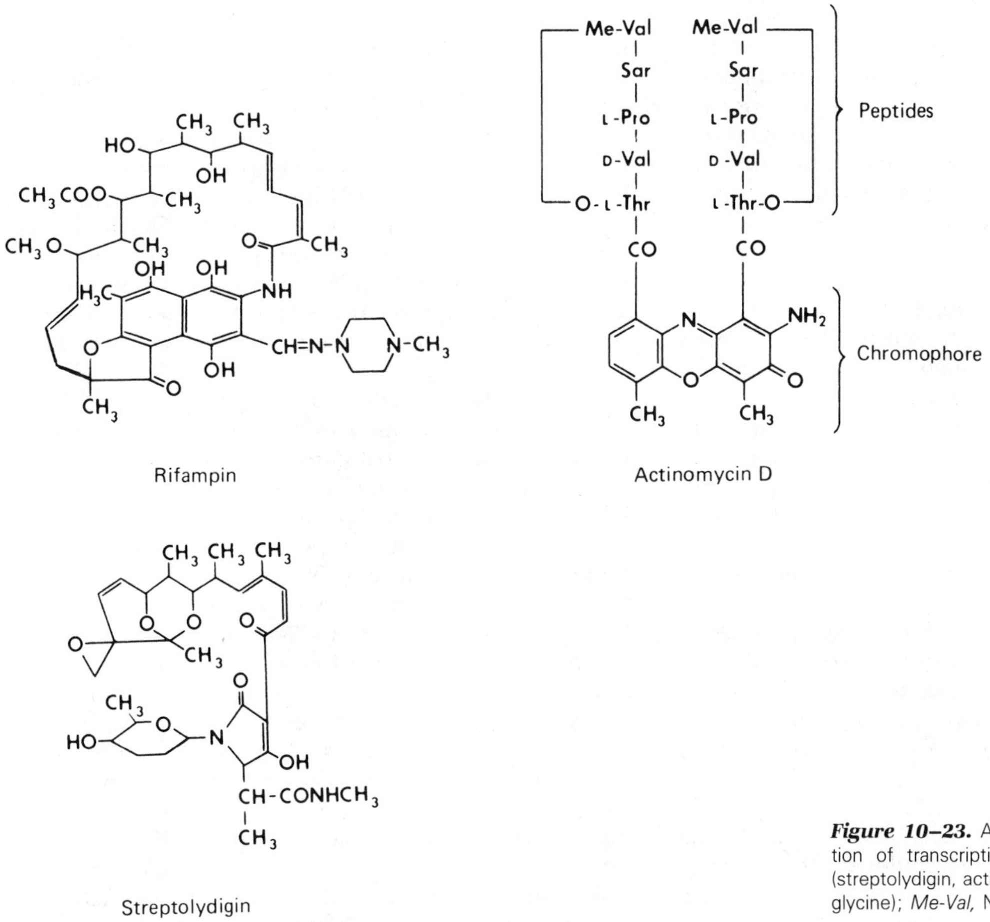

Rifampin

Actinomycin D

Streptolydigin

Figure 10–23. Antibiotics that interfere with initiation of transcription (rifampin) or chain extension (streptolydigin, actinomycin D.) *Sar,* sarcosine (N-Me-glycine); *Me-Val,* N-Me-L-valine.

CoA form long chains, as in fatty acid biosynthesis, but without the reductive steps that yield alkyl chains, and the resulting poly-β-ketones (**polyketides:** $RCO\text{-}CH_2\text{-}CO\text{-}CH_2\text{-}$) can condense internally to form the rings of macrolides, polyenes, tetracyclines, and portions of other antibiotics. Aromatic rings are derived from the shikimate pathway (Chap. 5).

Empiric screening of soil samples for sources of novel antibiotics is continuing, although the yield is dwindling. Semisynthetic antibiotics made by chemical modification of natural products are increasingly important. In addition, the pathways of biosynthesis of many antibiotics have been dissected, and the genes (usually found on plasmids) have been isolated, with the expectation of developing new products by genetic engineering.

ABSENCE OF SELF-INHIBITION. To account for the failure of antibiotics to prevent growth of the organisms that produce them, several mechanisms can be identified. Fungi lack peptidoglycan, and so their production of antibiotics that inhibit its formation presents no problem.

In the few streptomycetes that make β-lactams, the target PBPs are resistant, just as are the ribosomes in the streptomycetes that make macrolides. In contrast, streptomycetes that produce other antibiotics generally have sensitive targets, and the organisms often achieve self-protection by rapid excretion; i.e., failed to accumulate the antibiotic in the cytoplasm in active form. (Thus, whereas commercial production of amino acids is improved by sublethal treatment with penicillin, which makes the cell envelope leaky to the accumulated compound, that treatment has not been useful in antibiotic production.) The aminoglycosides are made in the cell as an inactive phosphorylated derivative, which is dephosphorylated as it is released. Finally, because antibiotics are produced only during sporulation, the organisms may be indifferent to inhibition or to killing that requires growth at this stage.

Secondary Metabolites; Ecological Role

Among microbial products antibiotics are particularly easy to detect, but chromatographic techniques have shown that they are only part of a broader class called secondary metabolites: compounds that are formed only after growth ceases, unlike the **primary metabolites** that contribute to energy production or biosynthesis. They exist in great variety, and some have exhibited useful pharmacologic properties other than antibiotic activity (e.g., cyclosporin, protease inhibitors), like the products of higher plants that became our earlier drugs.

Antibiotics exhibit less biosynthetic specificity than primary metabolites: many organisms excrete a group of closely related variants (e.g., multiple penicillins or multiple kanamycins). Because mutations that block an early step in sporulation block antibiotic synthesis, the two processes are clearly connected, but the mechanisms that relate them are uncertain and may be multiple. There is evidence that some antibiotics play a regulatory role in sporulation. Others, however, may be byproducts of the extensive degradation of the cell envelope that occurs during sporulation, for that structure contains D-amino acids and novel sugars, like many antibiotics. One polypeptide antibiotic, bacitracin, is derived from a vegetative protein that is degraded during sporulation. On the other hand, gramicidin is synthesized from amino acids by an elaborate nonribosomal mechanism of polypeptide formation (Chap. 5, Nonprotein Polypeptides), which could hardly have evolved unless it served the organism.

It is tempting to assume that antibiotic production has evolved as an ecological mechanism for inhibiting competing microorganisms; i.e., **antibiosis,** the opposite of symbiosis. Indeed, it would appear that antibiotics are released in the soil, as plasmids coding for resistance to various antibiotics are found in some soil organisms (in addition to those in which these genes may be related to antibiotic production). On the other hand, several considerations cast doubt on this ecological role: antibiotic producers are only a tiny fraction of all soil microbes and hence do not have a striking advantage; antibiotics generally are formed after growth has ceased rather than during competition for growth; and this ecological mechanism would not account for the nonantibiotic secondary metabolites.

Drug Resistance

Soon after introducing chemotherapy for protozoa, Ehrlich discovered that microorganisms can become resistant in the course of treatment. After the advent of antibacterial chemotherapy, the same phenomenon was encountered on a large scale. It led to an extraordinarily large experiment in interventive population genetics, as the use of a variety of agents selected for changes in the planet's most populous cells, bacteria.

Within 6 years after the introduction of benzylpenicil-lin, the frequency of resistance in staphylococci in British hospitals increased from less than 10% to 60%, and the value now approaches 90% throughout the world. As additional antibiotics were introduced, resistance to most of them emerged, although at lower frequencies. It has not been as troubling with most other pathogens, but it has been particularly important with enterobacteria, and more recently it has appeared even with organisms that long remained sensitive to penicillin: the pneumococcus and the gonococcus. For reasons that are not apparent, some organisms have never developed resistance: for example, group A streptococci to penicillin.

Fortunately, new antibiotics and the fluoroquinolones have maintained or increased the effectiveness of chemotherapy against most pathogens. Some authors have suggested that we will be required, like the Red Queen, to keep running faster and faster merely to stand still. On the other hand, if a bacterial species has been selected in evolution for a sensitive phenotype, the genetic changes responsible for resistance are likely to decrease its fitness to some degree, which should lead to a steady state with a balance between sensitive and resistant variants. In fact, although resistance to newer agents continues to emerge and spread, the frequency of the widespread resistance to the older agents has generally leveled off.

It would be desirable to reserve the term "resistant" for specific strains within a usually sensitive species, using the term **"insensitive"** or **"naturally resistant"** for those species that are excluded from the antimicrobial spectrum of each agent. Insensitivity is usually secondary to a barrier to penetration, especially in gram-negative bacteria.

A strain may become resistant by two very different genetic mechanisms: **mutation in a chromosomal gene** or **infection by a plasmid.** The latter mechanism presents a much more serious problem, because it is more prevalent, it usually involves resistance to multiple agents (including some that do not select for resistance mutations), and it does not substantially decrease the growth rate or the virulence of organisms (as many mutations to resistance do). These two genetic mechanisms are associated with quite different physiologic (phenotypic) mechanisms.

Drug Resistance

PHYSIOLOGIC MECHANISMS OF MUTATIONAL RESISTANCE

The resistant phenotype may be attributable to mutations in various components of the bacterial cell.

1. **Formation of an altered target** is the principal mechanism. For example, in a sulfonamide-resistant pneumococcus, the enzyme for incorporating PAB has a

two-fold decrease in affinity for that substrate and a 100-fold decrease in affinity for the analogue. As was noted above, mutations in various target enzymes can lead to resistance to rifampin, nalidixic acid, novobiocin, or β-lactams, and mutations in a ribosomal protein can cause high-level resistance to streptomycin. Many antibiotics, especially those acting on the ribosome, do not select for a resistant target, presumably because the change would destroy viability; and some mutants that are viable evidently have decreased virulence, as they appear readily in cultures but not in treated patients.

We have noted that ribosomes become resistant to some antibiotics through specific methylation of the RNA, which is often inducible. This mechanism is effective in changing all the ribosomes, whereas a mutation in rRNA sequence would occur in only one of the several copies of this gene.

2. **Decreased access** to the target usually affects multiple agents and is due to decreased permeability of the outer or inner membrane (including loss of a porin). In addition, uptake of aminoglycosides is impaired by mutations that decrease the membrane potential.

Those inhibitors (e.g., amino acid analogues) that enter via a specific transport system can select for mutations that decrease its affinity for the analogue or that even delete it.

3. **Increased level of an enzyme** can be brought about by mutations in its regulation (e.g., in β-lactamase formation) and also by amplification of the number of copies of its gene (which is more important for plasmid-coded enzymes). Gene amplification is particularly important in resistance in cancer chemotherapy in mammals.

4. **Decreased activation of the drug** is seen with purine or pyrimidine analogues, which must be converted to nucleotides before they can interfere with essential reactions. Because these **scavenging enzymes** are not essential for normal biosynthesis, they may be deleted to yield resistant mutants. Compounds requiring activation are important in cancer chemotherapy.

Enzymatic inactivation of the antibiotic is not important in mutational resistance, but it is the usual mechanism, as will be discussed below, in plasmid-borne resistance.

INDUCED PHENOTYPIC RESISTANCE. As was noted above, subinhibitory concentrations of erythromycin induce an enzyme that methylates ribosomal RNA and thus increases resistance. Chloramphenicol similarly induces an enzyme for its own acetylation, and some β-lactamases are inducible by low levels of a β-lactam. When such mechanisms are present, the observed level of resistance depends on the recent history of the tested cells, while with most strains the level of resistance in a given medium is a constitutive property.

PLASMID-MEDIATED RESISTANCE (R FACTORS)

In Japan, the introduction of various chemotherapeutic agents was soon followed by an increasing frequency of strains of the dysentery bacillus with multiple resistance to sulfonamides, streptomycin, chloramphenicol, and tetracyclines, or to two or three of these and later to additional antibiotics. Their frequency increased in one hospital from 0.2% in 1954 to 52% in 1964. The multiple resistance was found to be due not to a mutation, but to a plasmid (**R factor**) that could be transferred by conjugation; moreover, this plasmid was also found in the normal gut flora. But investigators in the West ignored the universality of the microbial world and dismissed R factors as something peculiar to the use of night soil (human excrement) as fertilizer in Japan. They failed to look for these agents for over 5 years.

The R factors are large, self-transmissible plasmids, widely distributed among enterobacteria and also other gram-negative organisms. They include several incompatibility groups (Chap. 7), and they differ widely in their content of **resistance genes (R determinants),** which each code for a particular resistance. These genes are mostly located in **transposons** (Chap. 8) and hence move freely between plasmids, allowing rapid evolutionary change. They occasionally also move into chromosomes: after years of use of an antibiotic resistance genes with strong similarity to plasmid genes have been found in the chromosomes of some bacterial strains. Stored enterobacteria from before the antibiotic era have been found to have plasmids of the same incompatibility groups but with few or no genes for resistance.

NONENTERIC PLASMIDS. Plasmids are also responsible for the common resistance of staphylococci to penicillin, due to a penicillinase. These plasmids are smaller and not self-transmissible, but they can be transferred by transduction or can be mobilized by other plasmids for conjugative transfer. More recently similar plasmids have appeared increasingly in strains of *Haemophilus influenzae* and the gonococcus.

ADVANTAGES. In protecting bacteria against inhibitors mutations have the advantage of being able to create resistance to a chemically novel inhibitor, while resistance plasmids have presumably been selected in evolution only by inhibitors that have long been present in the environment. However, plasmids have many other advantages. These include: (1) multiple resistance; (2) the ability to spread, not only vertically in progeny, but also horizontally, either between pathogenic strains or from a reservoir of other flora; (3) the ability to vary their patterns of resistance in response to selection pressures and to acquire novel resistance genes from distant members of the microbial world; (4) the economy of being eliminated from many cells in a population but then spreading when occasion arises; (5) little effect on the virulence of the bacterium, because they do not alter its essential components; and (6) ready amplification of the number of copies.

As an example of this process of evolutionary spread, with the growing use of cationic detergents as disinfectants in hospitals in recent years the plasmids of staphylococci increasingly carry resistance to these agents.

EPIDEMIOLOGY OF PLASMIDS. As plasmids spread they can fluctuate rapidly in their content of resistance genes. Moreover, the same resistance genes can be found in plasmids that differ in incompatibility groups and in other bases of classification (Chap. 7). In studies of the epidemiology of plasmids, analysis of restriction fragments (Fig. 10–24) has proved more valuable than incompatibility group or phenotype, and it is relatively simple, as plasmid DNA is easily separated from chromosomal DNA. Plasmids that share large regions of DNA evidently have a common recent origin despite significant differences in resistance pattern.

This technique is widely used to monitor the spread of resistance plasmids between organisms and between communities or countries, and to demonstrate the presence of the same plasmids in salmonella strains in cattle and in humans. Unfortunately, resistance to older antimicrobials appears to be especially prevalent in underdeveloped countries, which cannot afford widespread testing or the use of the newer, more expensive antibiotics.

PHYSIOLOGIC ACTIONS OF RESISTANCE FACTORS

Most of the resistance genes on R factors code for an **enzyme that inactivates an antibiotic,** as listed in Table 10–3. Many require a source of an adenylyl or phosphate

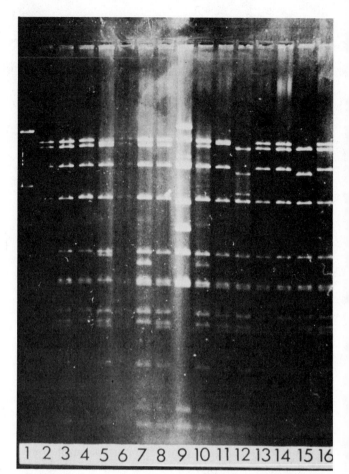

Figure 10–24. Comparison of restriction endonuclease fragments of related resistance plasmids. Gentamicin was used in one hospital for 5 years before resistance began to appear in *Klebsiella* and then in other genera. From resistant strains of several genera, isolated over several years from patients in different parts of the hospital, the resistance plasmid was transferred to *E. coli* K12 (in order to provide a uniform background), extracted, partly purified (on the basis of size), and digested with a restriction endonuclease; and the digests were electrophoresed in an agarose gel. The patterns of fragments are sufficiently similar in the various isolates to show that the resistance was due to the spread of one plasmid but varied enough to show evolution during the spread. Other resistance plasmids yielded very different patterns. (Courtesy of Thomas O'Brien)

group (from ATP) or an acetyl group (from acetyl-CoA), and so they must act in the cytoplasm. Hydrolysis by the β-lactamases, however, can occur on the outer surface of a membrane, in the periplasm, or outside the cell.

Aminoglycosides can be derivatized on various hydroxyl or amino groups: with kanamycin, for example, six different enzymes have been identified, acting on different acceptor groups. Because each enzyme requires a particular configuration, each is specific for very few aminoglycosides. These enzymes are attached to the cy-

TABLE 10–3. Mechanisms of Plasmid-Mediated Resistance

Agent	Reaction
β-Lactams	Hydrolysis of β-lactam ring
Aminoglycosides	O-phosphorylation
	O-adenylylation
	N-acetylation
Spectinomycin	O-adenylylation
Chloramphenicol	O-acetylation
	Reduction of nitro group (? plasmid)
Erythromycin, lincomycin	Methylation of ribosomal RNA
Tetracycline	Extrusion by membrane protein
Sulfonamides	Resistant dihydropteroate synthetase
Trimethoprim	Resistant dihydrofolate reductase
Hg^{2+}	Reduction to Hg (volatile)

toplasmic membrane (presumably on the cytoplasmic surface). Because aminoglycosides enter the cytoplasm at a very low rate, before membrane channels have been formed (see above), they can easily be inactivated as they enter, thus providing a high level of resistance.

A few inactivating proteins act by other mechanisms. Tetracycline, which enters bacteria by diffusion, is **actively extruded** by a plasmid-coded protein in the membrane. The same is true of resistance to Cd^{2+}. Resistance to mercury, however, depends on hydrolysis of organic mercurials and on reduction of Hg^{2+} to the nontoxic, volatile free Hg. Plasmid-coded erythromycin resistance is due to an inducible enzyme that modifies the ribosomal RNA.

RESISTANCE TO ENDOGENOUS ANTIBIOTICS. The plasmid gene that codes for phosphorylation of kanamycin has considerable similarity to the gene (also on a plasmid) in the antibiotic-producing streptomycete, where the same reaction is part of the biosynthetic sequence. Resistance genes may thus have evolved to meet a need in antibiotic producers and then spread to other bacteria. But this mechanism cannot be the only one, for resistance to Cd^{2+} and to Hg^{2+} evidently evolved to protect the bacteria against an exogenous rather than an endogenous inhibitor. Because antibiotics may also be encountered in the environment, resistance to them could have a similar origin.

RESISTANCE TO β-LACTAMS

Study of the action of β-lactamases, using a wide variety of β-lactams, has shown that these enzymes differ in their location as well as in specificity and level of activity. For example, the plasmid-coded β-lactamase encountered in many staphylococci is secreted to the exterior, while that coded by R factors in some enterobacteria is secreted to the periplasm. Many enterobacteria and other bacteria secrete a chromosomally coded β-lactamase, in small amounts, the commonest being called the **TEM enzyme.** In some Bacilli, the chromosome-coded enzyme is exported to the outer surface of the cell membrane (after cleavage of the leader peptide), and part is released to the medium after further cleavage.

Some β-lactamases are constitutive and others are induced by exposure to the antibiotic. In enterobacteria β-lactams insensitive to plasmid-coded resistance (especially methicillin) may select for another kind of resistance, in which a chromosomal β-lactamase has become constitutive and has acquired a more active promoter.

The endogenous, low-level, chromosomally coded β-lactamases are widespread in bacteria without evident selection for resistance. A possible explanation is suggested by their considerable sequence similarity to penicillin-binding proteins (PBPs), which play an essential role in wall morphogenesis (see Chap. 2); moreover, some PBPs eventually hydrolyze the covalently attached β-lactam, thus acting as inefficient penicillinases. Hence, penicillinases may well be modified PBPs that have developed a higher turnover rate for the hydrolysis.

POPULATION DENSITY. β-lactamase in the medium (as with staphylococci) acts by destroying the extracellular supply of antibiotic before many cells have been killed. Accordingly, the observed level of the resistance depends on the population density of the bacteria. This resistance can be recognized in the usual disc assay because a heavy inoculum is used, and it is important in patients because staphylococci form dense populations in localized lesions. Moreover, in mixed infections resistant staphylococci may protect other, sensitive organisms.

In contrast, with resistance due to a periplasmic β-lactamase, just as with that due to cytoplasmic enzymes acting on other antibiotics, the level is a property of the individual cell, because it depends on the competition between the rates of entry and of inactivation.

PENICILLIN-BINDING PROTEINS. PBPs also play a significant role in resistance. Thus, after staphylococcal resistance due to penicillinase production was largely overcome by the introduction of methicillin, strains appeared that had become resistant by altering their PBPs. Such alterations have also been observed in gonococci and pneumococci. Whereas most β-lactams act on (and thus define) several PBPs, in staphylococci mecillinam is nearly specific for PBP2, and mutants altered in this enzyme are highly resistant.

In yet another mechanism, in enterobacteria, resistance can be increased by mutations that eliminate the outer membrane protein OmpF, which forms a more permeable porin than OmpC and hence permits faster entry of β-lactams to the periplasm. Alterations in LPS also affect access.

TOLERANCE; PERSISTERS

We have seen in Chapter 2 that cell lysis by penicillin involves not only blockade of the peptidoglycan cross-linking reaction but also activation of lytic enzymes. In a few bacteria found in nature, and in some pneumococcus mutants, penicillin is bacteriostatic rather than bactericidal over a broad concentration range. This phenomenon is called tolerance rather than resistance, for it does not lower the MIC, and it does not prevent (although it may moderate) the chemotherapeutic response. The failure of penicillin inhibition to lead to lysis in these strains may be due to perturbation of the factors that regulate the hydrolytic steps in wall morphogenesis.

Another kind of bacteriostatic response to penicillin, called "persisters," may have broader significance. In a growing culture killing by the antibiotic is more or less exponential after a lag. However, after extensive killing a few viable cells persist for days and generate colonies when transferred to fresh medium. This is **phenotypic resistance** rather than genotypic, for the progeny of the surviving cells grown out in the absence of the drug show no increase in resistance when the experiment is repeated. The mechanism is not clear, but it appears that in the surviving persisters, penicillin inhibits, perhaps indirectly, a reaction needed for completion of the lytic process that it initiates.

PREVENTION OF RESISTANCE

Mutation to resistance cannot be prevented, but the selection of the products may be preventable. When successive mutations each contribute small increments of resistance the early steps might be prevented by maintaining the drug at a high enough level. A more general approach, applicable even to one-step mutations to high-level resistance, is **combination therapy,** originally suggested by Ehrlich. It has a simple rationale: if one cell in 10^6 mutates to resistance to drug A, and one in 10^7 to drug B (which lacks cross-resistance), only one in 10^{13} will develop both mutations. This approach has been successful in the treatment of tuberculosis.

Plasmids present a more refractory problem than mutations. Their multiple resistance can be selected by a single antibiotic; they can acquire additional resistance genes; and antibiotic treatment promotes their spread in the normal flora (as well as in the pathogen at which it is aimed), providing an additional reservoir for transfer to pathogens. Reagents that cure bacteria of their plasmids have had some success in cultures but they do not seem promising for clinical practice.

Possible responses therefore seem to be restricted to the continued development of new antimicrobial agents by industry, and to avoiding unwarranted use of antibiotics, such as for minor infections or for those in which antibiotics are ineffective. Such abuse by physicians is common (although the definition of what is unwarranted is sometimes controversial). Moreover, in much of the world, over-the-counter sales make the problem much worse. But even if avoiding indiscriminate use would help to ameliorate the problem, it would not eliminate it, for legitimate therapy also selects for resistance plasmids.

ANTIBIOTICS IN ANIMAL FEED

Most feed for cattle and for pigs in many countries now contains subtherapeutic levels of antibiotics, which increase the rate of weight gain, the efficiency of feed conversion to meat, and freedom from bacterial disease (especially in farms with crowding or poor sanitation). Agriculture now accounts for about half the utilization of antimicrobials. The mechanism of the growth promotion is not clear: it may include preventing subclinical disease, altering the removal of nutrients by the intestinal flora, or altering its production of vitamins or mild toxins.

Because food is a major source of *Salmonella* infection in humans, and because many isolates from epidemics (20% to 30% in the United States) carry plasmids with resistance to one or more antimicrobials, the possible contribution of subtherapeutic antibiotics to this distribution has aroused much concern. Indeed, there is no doubt that the use of antibiotics in animals, whether therapeutic or in routine feed, has increased their carriage of bacteria with resistance plasmids. Moreover, one human epidemic of resistant organisms has been traced to meat from cattle carrying the same strain. However, the implications for policy are not automatic, for we are also dealing with large economic and health benefits from improved meat production (and possibly also less overall transmission of pathogens, from healthier livestock); hence, the real issues are (1) the magnitude of the harm balanced against the benefits, and (2) the gain to be expected from now banning subtherapeutic antibiotics.

Unfortunately, there is no scientific basis for estimating the overall balance. However, there is information on the effectiveness of a ban. Certain European countries have prohibited subtherapeutic use of penicillin and tetracycline since the early 1970s, requiring them to be replaced by antibiotics that are not used in humans. After 14 years, the expected decrease in frequency of resistance to the banned antibiotics had not occurred.

In addition, because continued therapeutic use of these antibiotics was still permitted, it is impossible to tell how much of the resistance now observed is attributable to this use and how much persists from selection by the earlier subtherapeutic use. Because both uses in animals have the same economic purpose and similar effects on plasmid distribution, to single out one while allowing the other (because it is less novel and resembles use in humans) seems less logical than to ban all use of certain antimicrobials in animals. However, the costs would be large, the impact on the distribution of resistance plasmids is uncertain, and a "non-human" antibiotic could still select for a plasmid that also carries resistance to other antibiotics. Such legislation therefore seems unlikely.

Clinical Applications

Without attempting to discuss in detail the clinical use of various chemotherapeutic agents, we will briefly review some of the major guiding principles.

BACTERICIDAL VERSUS BACTERIOSTATIC DRUGS

With organisms that grow only outside cells, the bactericidal β-lactams and aminoglycosides are in general more rapidly curative than bacteriostatic agents, although the latter are also often effective. Moreover, bactericidal agents are essential—usually as a synergistic mixture of an aminoglycoside and a β-lactam—in certain circumstances: against the densely packed, sluggish organisms in bacterial endocarditis; in the treatment of meningitis (where the organisms are relatively inaccessible to the immune system, and one tries to achieve a cerebrospinal fluid concentration ten times the minimal bactericidal concentration); and in the treatment of persons with an impaired immune system—an increasing fraction of the hospital population. On the other hand, with intracellular bacteria, bacteriostatic agents have proved to be more effective, as noted below.

Because bactericidal action of antibiotics (except polymyxin) requires bacterial growth, it is repressed in lesions where impaired circulation prevents growth through inadequate nutrition and accumulation of acid. Thus, in the lesions of experimental pneumococcal pneumonia penicillin can be shown to cause lysis of the bacteria in the outer edema zone, while in the more central portions destruction by phagocytes is more prominent. In another limitation, with β-lactams, the "persisters" described above, which are inhibited but not killed, may interfere with rapid eradication.

On the other hand, even early, nonlethal damage to the wall by penicillin in growing bacteria slows the resumption of growth after elimination of the inhibitor, the cells also are more susceptible to destruction by phagocytes, and they may be impaired in their adhesiveness. These effects may be important in therapy, because with periodic administration of the drugs the blood levels are often only intermittently adequate for bacteriostatic or bactericidal action.

With agents that cause bacteriostasis but not killing, eradication of the organisms depends on the immune and the phagocytic mechanisms of the host. The same is often true with bactericidal agents, because nutrient limitations prevent their growth or because some cells are persisters (see above). Fortunately, the **host mechanisms complement those of antimicrobial agents,** for they are effective with quiescent as well as with growing bacteria because they attack the surface rather than the internal metabolism.

In most infections some of the bacteria are relatively inaccessible to host defenses, and so the last stages in the process of eradication are slow; accordingly, chemotherapy, even with bactericidal agents, must be continued for a number of days, even though the bulk of the organisms (and the symptoms) may be eliminated rapidly. There are exceptions, such as the effective treatment of acute gonorrhea in the male with a single large dose of penicillin.

While the rapid lysis by β-lactams helps to eradicate bacteria, it also may cause a transient exacerbation of symptoms through the release of toxic or allergenic constituents. This effect (the **Herxheimer reaction**) is prominent in the treatment of secondary syphilis, in which allergy plays an important role in pathogenesis.

INTRACELLULAR BACTERIA. With obligatory intracellular parasites (rickettsias, chlamydias), the aminoglycosides, which cannot penetrate host cells, are ineffective, and most β-lactams do not penetrate well enough to be useful; hence various bacteriostatic agents are used. With bacteria that can survive and even multiply in phagocytic cells (such as *Brucella, Listerella, Legionella,* and the typhoid bacillus), the bactericidal aminoglycosides, and to a large extent the β-lactams, can act only during extracellular exposure; hence agents that can penetrate (erythromycin, tetracycline, chloramphenicol, rifampin, and ciprofloxacin) are widely used. Similarly, with tubercle bacilli aminoglycosides act only on extracellular cells, while isoniazid (which also is bactericidal) and rifampin have the advantage of acting inside host cells also.

Organisms that can thrive in host cells tend to give rise to chronic diseases and to a persistent carrier state, because they are not rapidly destroyed by the phagocytes and can even become dormant. Similarly bacteriostatic agents acting on sensitive organisms within host cells do not effect a cure as rapidly or reliably as is seen with extracellular parasites.

CHOICE OF CHEMOTHERAPEUTIC AGENT

Ideally, the choice of an antimicrobial agent should be dictated by identification of the infecting organism and knowledge of its sensitivity pattern. However, in acute infections it is often better not to delay therapy while awaiting a laboratory report but to proceed on the basis of a presumptive diagnosis, supported when possible by the simple gram stain. Moreover, in practice, many physicians believe that the presumptive diagnosis often has a high enough probability, and the toxicity of the available agents is low enough, to justify therapy without isolation of the organism unless the expected therapeutic response fails. But because group A streptococcal infection may lead to rheumatic fever, and because elimination of that possibility requires therapy well beyond the asymptomatic period, it is important to test for that diagnosis.

In general, it is not justified to use a broad-spectrum antibiotic on a shotgun basis rather than to choose a less expensive drug with a narrower spectrum and a high probability of being effective. Immune-impaired hospital patients are an exception, because they are exposed to such a range of nosocomial pathogens.

COMBINED THERAPY. Mixtures of antimicrobial agents are appropriate under several circumstances. As was noted above, they are used to prevent emergence of drug resistance (especially in long-term treatment of tuberculosis) and to inhibit the β-lactamase that would destroy an accompanying β-lactam. Especially important is **synergism** between β-lactams and aminoglycosides. Other indications are sepsis caused by a mixed infection (especially abdominal and pelvic abscesses) and grave illness where the organism has not yet been identified.

On the other hand, bacteriostatic inhibition of growth **antagonizes** the **bactericidal** action of either β-lactams or aminoglycosides (see Fig. 10–17), and this effect generally contraindicates such mixtures. However, because agents differ in the kinetics of absorption, distribution, and excretion, the antagonism by bacteriostatic agents, although readily demonstrated *in vitro*, may not be a good model for the effects of such mixtures in the patient, and clinical studies suggest that mixtures may be beneficial in septic mixed infections. In one special kind of antagonism, cefoxitin induces formation of a β-lactamase that can then act on other β-lactams.

HOST FACTORS AFFECTING CHEMOTHERAPY

LOCAL TISSUE FACTORS. When bacteria cause tissue cells to die in a localized area, an **abscess** forms: the lesion is walled off by fibrin and dead cells, circulation is blocked off, the leukocytes cease to function and eventually disintegrate (suppuration), and the bacteria fail to multiply (except at the periphery), although they may survive. Antimicrobial therapy becomes relatively ineffective under these circumstances. The reason does not appear to be failure of the drugs to penetrate, for even if their diffusion through the barrier is slow, it should reach equilibrium (unless they are metabolized). Moreover, experimental subcutaneous pneumococcal abscesses failed to respond to penicillin even when it was injected directly at frequent intervals; similarly, streptomycin has been shown to penetrate caseous tuberculous lesions that it cannot sterilize.

A sounder explanation is the multiple effects of impairment of circulation in the lesion. These include a reduced supply of antibodies, complement, leukocytes, oxygen, and nutrients; impeded removal of waste products (including acids produced by both host cells and bacteria) and bacterial toxins; and the destruction of complement and impaired leukocyte function associated with the latter changes. There are also more specific effects with some agents: as was noted above, acid and

anaerobiosis antagonize the action of aminoglycosides; these antibiotics also are bound by DNA in purulent lesions; and metabolites released from damaged cells antagonize the action of sulfonamides.

Cure of abscesses requires drainage, either spontaneous or surgical. Serous exudate can then replace the bacteriostatic pus, providing nutrients as well as a fresh wave of leukocytes and antibodies.

Foreign bodies, such as splinters of wood, spicules of dead bone (in osteomyelitis), or sutures, decrease the effectiveness of chemotherapy by providing pockets in the surface where bacteria are poorly nourished, accumulate metabolic products, and are sequestered from leukocytes. Even on the smooth surface of a prosthetic joint or heart valve, a layer of sessile bacteria may be protected from leukocytes (and even from antibodies and antibiotics) by a glycocalyx (see Chap. 2). Similarly, with **obstruction** of the urinary, biliary, or respiratory tracts (bronchi or paranasal sinuses), bacterial infections tend to persist despite chemotherapy, because the increased fluid pressure impairs circulation and lymphatic drainage in the tissues lining the obstructed cavity. Lesions associated with a foreign body or obstruction are rarely cured by chemotherapy unless the impediment is removed.

TOPICAL THERAPY. Chemotherapeutic agents are often effective when applied directly to superficial infections, including those of skin, wounds, and eyes; they are also valuable prophylactically in extensive burns. (No benefit can be expected, however, from application of ointments to the superficial drainage of a deep focus.) For such topical application, some of the more toxic antibiotics, including neomycin, polymyxin, and bacitracin, are used, as well as quinolones and such antiseptics (Chap. 3) as cationic detergents and iodophors. β-Lactams and aminoglycosides (other than neomycin) should never be used on the skin, because applications there are particularly prone to induce allergy to the drug and thus to prevent its later use in a life-threatening illness; in addition, this use selects for resistance in the ubiquitous staphylococci, which might then cause a systemic infection. However, to provide high local concentrations at deep sites of infection, these drugs may be injected into the pleural, pericardial, or joint cavities or into the subarachnoid space.

CHEMOPROPHYLAXIS. Antimicrobial prophylaxis is likely to be successful only when directed against an organism that rarely gives rise to mutants resistant to the agent. It has been useful in preventing several diseases: recurrent streptococcal infections in patients with rheumatic fever, bacterial endocarditis in patients with valvular heart disease undergoing dental or other surgical procedures, certain sexually transmitted diseases, and recurrent urinary tract infections. Because the treatment is chronic, and low concentrations are sufficient to eliminate an inoculum that has not yet become established, the doses may be small. Chemoprophylaxis for susceptible hosts has also been useful in terminating epidemics of meningococcal infection and of shigellosis in schools and military installations. Isoniazid appears useful in preventing disease in persons who have recently developed a positive tuberculin test and in individuals undergoing steroid therapy that might reactivate an old tuberculous lesion.

Antibiotic prophylaxis has been invaluable in reducing infection in surgical operations on areas that are likely to be contaminated (abdomen, pelvis, lungs), and in the placement of prostheses. However, it is not a substitute for aseptic technique, and its indiscriminate use may do more harm than good by fostering infection with drug-resistant organisms. Chemoprophylaxis cannot be expected to keep an especially vulnerable organ, such as the urinary bladder with an indwelling catheter, free of bacteria.

SUPERINFECTIONS. One of the most serious and frequent complications of chemotherapy is the outgrowth of minor, insensitive components of the indigenous flora when major components are suppressed. Various antibiotics, especially **clindamycin,** occasionally induce a bacterial enteritis, called **pseudomembranous colitis,** which is caused by outgrowth of *Clostridium difficile.* Long-term treatment with tetracycline can cause a similar enteritis and occasionally **thrush** (oral **moniliasis**) caused by the yeast *Candida.* Although broad-spectrum antibiotics are appropriate where the etiologic agent is not identified or cannot be reasonably inferred, drugs with a narrow spectrum are to be preferred where they are known to be effective, as they have less effect on the normal flora.

The principle underlying superinfections is evolutionary: bacteria populate every available ecological niche, and eliminating any normal flora will lead others to fill the vacuum. The exceptionally rapid spread of staphylococci resistant to penicillin (and more recently to other agents) is a similar process. Thus, staphylococci are a major component of the normal skin flora, and because the skin is so accessible, they are easily transferred between individuals. Accordingly, if the systemic use of penicillin eliminates a sensitive strain from an individual, these features of the organism increase the likelihood that a resistant strain will acquire a foothold. Moreover, such a strain can provide a reservoir, not only for future infection, but also for transfer of its resistance plasmid to more virulent strains (including transfer from *Staph. epidermidis* to *Staph. aureus*).

Selected Reading

BOOKS AND REVIEW ARTICLES

Bartlett JG: Antibiotic-associated pseudomembranous colitis. Rev Infect Dis 1:530, 1979

Baurenfeind A: Classification of β-lactamases. Rev Infect Dis 8:S470, 1986

Broda P: Bacterial Plasmids and their Practical Importance. San Francisco, WH Freeman, 1979

Bryan LE (ed): Antimicrobial Drug Resistance. New York, Academic Press, 1984

Campbell IM: Secondary metabolites and microbial physiology. Adv Microb Physiol 25:1, 1984

Cherubin CE: Antibiotic resistance of *Salmonella* in Europe and the United States. Rev Infect Dis 3:1105, 1981

Chopra I, Ball P: Transport of antibiotics into bacteria. Adv Microb Physiol 23:183, 1982

Cohen ML, Tauxe RV: Drug-resistant *Salmonella* in the United States: An epidemiological perspective. Science 234:964, 1986

Cundliffe E: Self defence in antibiotic-producing organisms. Br Med Bull 40:61, 1984

Davies JE: Resistance to aminoglycosides: Mechanisms and frequency. Rev Infect Dis 5:S261, 1983

Davies JE, Smith DI: Plasmid-determined resistance to antimicrobial agents. Annu Rev Microbiol 32:469, 1978

Davis BD: The mechanism of the bactericidal action of aminoglycosides. Microbiol Rev 51:341, 1987

Foster TJ: Plasmid-determined resistance to antimicrobial drugs and toxic metal ions in bacteria. Microbiol Rev 47:361, 1983

Gale EF, Cundliffe E, Reynolds PE, Richmond MH, Waring MJ: The Molecular Basis of Antibiotic Action. New York, John Wiley, 1981

Gorini L: Streptomycin and misreading of the genetic code. In M Nomura, A Tissieres, P Lengyel (eds): Ribosomes. Cold Spring Harbor, NY, Cold Spring Harbor Laboratory, 1974

Greenwood D, O'Grady F (eds): Scientific Basis of Antimicrobial Therapy. Symposium 38, Society for General Microbiology. Cambridge, Cambridge University Press, 1985. Includes an excellent review on the fluoroquinolones.

Hancock REW: Aminoglycoside uptake and mode of action with special reference to streptomycin and gentamicin. J Antimicrob Chemother 8:249; 429, 1981

Handwerger S, Tomasz A: Antibiotic tolerance among clinical isolates of bacteria. Annu Rev Pharmacol Toxicol 25:349, 1985

Hopwood DA: Extrachromosomally determined antibiotic productions. Annu Rev Microbiol 32:373, 1978

Kerridge D: Mode of action of clinically important antifungal drugs. Adv Microb Physiol 27:1, 1986

Levy SB, Burke JP, Wallace CK (eds): Antibiotic use and antibiotic resistance worldwide. Rev Infect Dis 9:S231, 1987

Lyon BR, Skurray R: Antimicrobial resistance of *Staphylococcus aureus:* Genetic basis. Microbiol Rev 51:88, 1987

Martin JF, Demain AL: Control of antibiotic synthesis. Microbiol Rev 44:230, 1980

Matthew M: Plasmid-mediated β-lactamases of gram-negative bacteria: Properties and distribution. J Antimicrob Chemother 5:349, 1979

Moats WA (ed): Agricultural Uses of Antibiotics. ACS Symposium Series No 320. Washington, DC, American Chemical Society, 1986

Morin RB, Gorman M (eds): Chemistry and Biology of Beta-Lactam Antibiotics. New York, Academic Press, 1982

Neu HC: Beta-lactam antibiotics: Structural relationships affecting *in vitro* activity and pharmacologic properties. Rev Infect Dis 8:S237, 1986

O'Brien TF, Mayer KH, Hopkins JD: Global surveillance of the deployment of antibiotic resistance genes and plasmids. In Antibiotic Resistance Genes: Ecology, Transfer, and Expression. Banbury Report 24. Cold Spring Harbor, NY, Cold Spring Harbor Laboratory, 1986

Rao VSR, Vasudevan TK: Conformation and activity of β-lactam antibiotics. CRC Crit Rev Biochem 14:173, 1983

Salton M, Shockman GD (eds): Beta-Lactam Antibiotics. New York, Academic Press, 1981

Schaeffer P: Sporulation and the production of antibiotics, exoenzymes, and exotoxins. Bacteriol Rev 33:48, 1969

Shaw WV: Chloramphenicol acetyltransferase: Enzymology and molecular biology. CRC Crit Rev Biochem 14:1, 1983

Spratt BG: Penicillin-binding proteins and the future of β-lactam antibiotics. J Gen Microbiol 129:1247, 1983

Takayama K, Davidson LA: Antimycobacterial drugs that inhibit mycolic acid synthesis. Trends Biochem Sci, Dec 1979, p 280

Tomasz A: The mechanism of the irreversible effects of penicillins. Annu Rev Microbiol 323:113, 1979

Turck A: Cephalosporins and related antibiotics: An overview. Rev Infect Dis 4:S281, 1982

Waxman DJ, Strominger JL: Penicillin-binding proteins and the mechanism of action of β-lactam antibiotics. Annu Rev Biochem 52:825, 1983

Weisblum B: Inducible resistance to macrolides, lincosamides, and streptogramin type B antibiotics: The resistance phenotype, its biological diversity, and structural elements that regulate expression. J Antimicrob Chemother 16(Suppl A):63, 1985

Wise R: Antimicrobial potentiating agents. J Antimicrob Chemother 5:121, 1979

SPECIFIC ARTICLES

Cohen SP, McMurry LM, Levy SB: *marA* locus causes decreased expression of OmpF porin in multiple-antibiotic-resistant (Mar) mutants of *Escherichia coli*. J Bacteriol 170:5416, 1988

Mates SM, Eisenberg ES, Mandel LJ, Patel L, Kaback HR, Miller MH: Membrane potential and gentamicin uptake in *Staphylococcus aureus*. Proc Natl Acad Sci USA 79:6693, 1982

Moazed D, Noller HF: Interactions of antibiotics with functional sites in 16S ribosomal RNA. Nature 327:389, 1987

Thompson CJ, Gray GS: Nucleotide sequence of a streptomycete aminoglycoside phosphotransferase gene and its relationship to phosphotransferases encoded by resistance plasmids. Proc Natl Acad Sci USA 80:5190, 1983

11

Fred Winston

Yeast as a Model Eukaryotic Cell

Saccharomyces cerevisiae, one of a large number of species of yeasts found in nature, has been used for millenia for making bread, beer, and wine. Because it is a eukaryote, in many fundamental respects it resembles a mammalian cell more than a prokaryotic cell. At the same time, as a unicellular organism, it is amenable to most of the types of manipulation that one can use with *E. coli*: it can easily be grown in defined medium and can be propagated as colonies on agar plates. The generation time in rich medium is approximately 90 minutes. *S. cerevisiae* has a haploid DNA content about four times that of *E. coli* (approximately 20,000 Kb pairs) but less than one-hundredth that of a mammalian cell.

Many eukaryotic processes can be studied in *S. cerevisiae* by genetic and microbiologic techniques not possible with higher eukaryotes. These processes include cell division, regulation of gene expression, metabolism of mRNA, protein localization, cellular differentiation, and the functions of oncogene homologues. The organism's ability to be propagated mitotically as either haploid or diploid cells provides additional advantages for genetic studies.

The Mitotic Cell Cycle

S. cerevisiae is a **budding yeast.** At the beginning of the cell cycle, a cell has no bud. As the cycle proceeds, a bud emerges from the mother cell, enlarges, and finally separates, initially as a smaller daughter cell (Fig. 11–1). The mother cell retains a ring of chitin, a **bud scar,** where a daughter bud has emerged. In fact, one can determine the age of a cell by the number of bud scars it contains. The ability to monitor the position in the cell cycle by

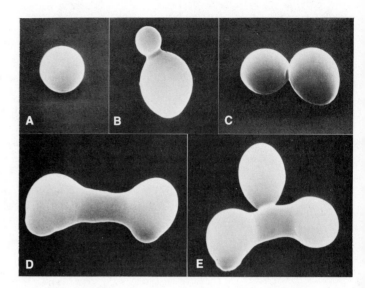

Figure 11–1. Electron micrographs of *Saccharomyces cerevisiae* cells. *(A–C)* Cells that are unbudded, with a small bud, and with a large bud during mitotic growth. *(D)* Cells during conjugation after cellular fusion. *(E)* After growth of the first diploid bud. (Courtesy of Eric Schabtach and Ira Herskowitz)

bud size has aided analysis of both genetic and biochemical aspects of the cell cycle.

The *S. cerevisiae* cell cycle can be divided, as in other eukaryotes, into four phases: G1, which precedes DNA replication; S, during which DNA synthesis occurs; G2; and M, when mitosis and finally cell division occur. Specific landmark events of the cell cycle can be monitored morphologically or biochemically. These events include DNA replication, assembly of the mitotic spindle, nuclear migration to the neck between the mother cell and the daughter bud, and nuclear division.

MITOSIS AND CELL DIVISION-CYCLE MUTANTS. Taking advantage of the landmarks in the *S. cerevisiae* cell cycle, Hartwell and colleagues have isolated mutations in more than 50 different cell division-cycle (*CDC*) genes. Most of these mutants are temperature-sensitive: that is, they are able to grow at 30°C, but at 36°, a given mutant will arrest growth at a particular stage of the cell cycle. Genetic analysis of these mutants has allowed construction of a temporal order for the functions of the *CDC* gene products throughout the cell cycle. Many products of particular *CDC* genes have been identified, including DNA ligase, adenylate cyclase, and thymidylate kinase.

Several genes are involved at a critical stage of the cell cycle, termed **Start.** At this point, the cell must integrate both environmental and intracellular signals to decide whether to continue to the next mitotic cycle or to follow one of the other possible routes: meiosis, conjugation, or entry into stationary phase.

CELL DIVISION IN S. POMBE. Cell cycle studies in another yeast, *Schizosaccharomyces pombe*, have also

helped in understanding certain aspects of cell division, particularly at **Start.** *S. pombe* is very distantly related to *S. cerevisiae*, and its cell division occurs by fission rather than by budding (Fig. 11–2). Nevertheless, certain aspects of cell division are conserved. Most notably, the *cdc2* gene of *S. pombe* and the *CDC28* gene of *S. cerevisiae*

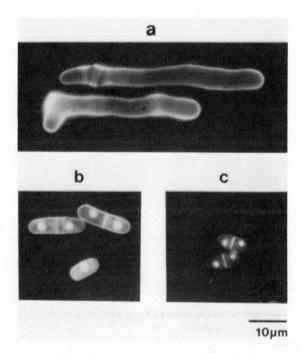

Figure 11–2. *Schizosaccharomyces pombe* cells. Mutations in cell division can inhibit cell division *(a)* or cause premature cell division *(c)*. Wild-type cells are shown in *(b)*. (Courtesy of Paul Nurse)

each encode a protein kinase that is essential for the cell to advance past **Start.** Remarkably, a human gene has been cloned by Lee and Nurse that can complement an *S. pombe cdc2* mutation, and these genes share 63% identity at the amino acid level.

Conjugation and Meiosis

CONJUGATION. Conjugation of haploids to form diploids and regeneration of haploids by meiosis in diploids form the foundation of genetic analysis in *S. cerevisiae.* Haploid *S. cerevisiae* cells can be one of two mating types, **a** or *α,* and conjugation occurs when haploid cells of the opposite mating type are close to each other. The mating type is determined by the state of the *MAT* locus: either *MATa* or *MATα.*

In conjugation, cells of each mating type secrete a peptide **pheromone, *α*-factor** or **a-factor,** that arrests the growth of cells of the opposite mating type at the beginning of the cell cycle. This arrest is followed by cell fusion, forming a **heterokaryon:** a single cell with two haploid nuclei (see Fig. 11–1). Nuclear fusion rapidly follows, resulting in a cell with one diploid nucleus. This cell can now proceed to divide mitotically, as described above.

The ability to work easily with either stable haploid or stable diploid strains greatly facilitates mutational analysis. Propagation in the haploid state allows one to isolate recessive mutations that would not be phenotypically expressed in a diploid. In diploid strains, one can easily analyze the recessiveness or dominance of a mutation and can test for complementation of recessive mutations, as in bacterial merozygotes. In addition, diploids can be used for complementation analysis of recessive mutations.

MEIOSIS. An alternative mode of growth of diploid cells is meiosis. In this process, the homologous chromosomes pair **(synapse)** with each other (i.e., assume parallel, closely adjacent positions), and each chromosome divides without duplicating its centromere (whose attachment to a spindle fiber subsequently guides its migration to one pole or the other during anaphase). Each chromosome thus becomes a pair of identical **chromatids** connected by a centromere. One or more genetic exchanges (crossing over) may then occur at random among the four chromatids, resulting in genetic recombination.

Two meiotic divisions follow. In the first, there are no divided centromeres to separate (as in mitosis); instead, one member of each pair of homologous chromosomes is drawn after its centromere to each pole. In the second meiotic division, the chromosome is already divided into two chromatids, and only the centromere divides; one

product then migrates (as in mitosis) to each pole. Thus the four chromatids are distributed to four different cells, each of which ends up with a haploid set of chromosomes (Fig. 11–3). The individual members of each set are thus derived at random by segregation from either parent and are further reassorted by the genetic recombination occurring at the four-strand stage. (Recombination can also occur during mitotic growth, although at lower frequency. Mitotic recombination is discussed in Chap. 43).

An advantage of yeasts for genetic studies is that all four spores from each meiosis are retained in the same **ascus.** Analysis of their genetic constitution (**tetrad analysis**) allows the most thorough possible description of the genetic events occurring during meiosis. The products of **reciprocal recombination** can be identified, rather than merely deduced from the statistical distribution of genetic markers among the progeny, as with higher organisms.

Diploid cells undergo meiosis when they are starved for N, C, or S. In the laboratory, starvation is usually accomplished by transfer of the organisms into "sporulation medium," which lacks N. A few days later, one can observe microscopically the presence of asci. To analyze the tetrads, incubation with an enzyme, zymolyase, is used to digest away most of the ascus wall; the four spores of each tetrad are separated on an agar surface and allowed to germinate and form colonies, which are then scored for their genetic markers, usually by replica plating. Any mutant phenotype that is caused by a single mutation yields a 2:2 segregation pattern, whereas phenotypes that are caused by more than a single mutation will deviate from this pattern, as shown in Figure 11–3. For example, two mutations segregating independently in a cross will yield asci with segregation patterns for the two phenotypes of 4:0, 3:1, and 2:2 in a ratio of 1:4:1. **Cytoplasmically inherited mutations,** such as those in mitochondrial DNA, will yield segregation patterns of 4:0. Tetrad analysis is the foundation for all yeast genetic analysis, both classic and molecular.

Molecular Genetics

Recent developments in transformation of cells (introduction of DNA) and in recombinant DNA techniques have had a tremendous impact on molecular genetic studies in *S. cerevisiae.* Transformation allows reintroduction of genes altered *in vitro* as well as introduction of genes from heterologous organisms (cloning). This approach is being utilized by biotechnology companies in attempts to produce large quantities of commercially valuable proteins in an easily manipulated eukaryotic microorganism. Yeast cells have some advantages over *E. coli* as a commercial source in that yeast will glycosylate

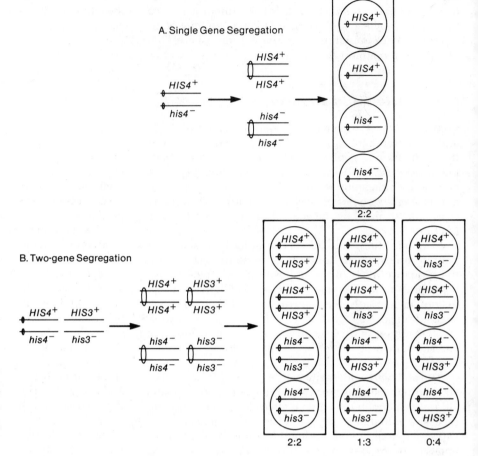

Figure 11–3. Tetrad analysis. (*A*) A single mutation causing a His⁻ phenotype will segregate 2 : 2 in tetrads. (*B*) If two mutations are present, either of which can cause a His⁻ phenotype, then tetrads will exhibit phenotype segregation patterns of 2 : 2, 1 : 3, and 0 : 4 in a ratio of 1 : 4 : 1.

mammalian glycoproteins. In addition, *S. cerevisiae* cells produce no toxins that could contaminate preparations of a foreign protein.

TRANSFORMATION. Exogenous DNA can be taken up in the presence of Ca^{2+} by *S. cerevisiae* spheroplasts, which are produced by digesting the cell wall with zymolyase under hypertonic conditions. In an alternative method, one can transform yeast cells after treatment with lithium acetate.

PLASMID VECTORS. Several types of plasmid vectors are employed in yeast transformations. All contain a selectable marker for transformation into *E. coli* (generally an antibiotic resistance gene, such as ampicillin resistance), a selectable marker for transformation into *S. cerevisiae* (generally to complement an auxotrophy), and an *E. coli* origin of replication, which is important to allow propagation of the plasmid in *E. coli* to prepare large amounts

of plasmid DNA. The three main classes of plasmid vectors are integrating plasmids, high-copy-number autonomous plasmids, and low-copy-number autonomous plasmids.

The **integrating plasmids** have no *S. cerevisiae* origin of replication and can produce a stable transformant only by integration into the host genome. Because this integration occurs by recombination between yeast sequences on the plasmid and homologous sequences in the genome, one can direct a plasmid to integrate in a particular genomic location by including that segment of yeast DNA in the vector. The **high-copy-number autonomous plasmids** contain a segment of a plasmid, called **2 μ circle,** found in most wild-type *S. cerevisiae* cells in around 50 copies. This segment confers autonomous replication and also high copy number. Such vectors are one means of overexpressing certain gene products. The **low-copy-number autonomous plasmids** have a centromere-containing DNA segment that is required to maintain the low copy number and also a second segment that allows for autonomous replication, called an *ars* sequence and believed to be a copy of a chromosomal origin of DNA replication.

Plasmid vectors may also contain useful regulatory elements. For example, if a cloned gene is placed under control of the *S. cerevisiae GAL* promoter, it will be transcribed at very high levels in growth on galactose and will not be expressed in growth on glucose.

CLONING OF S. CEREVISIAE GENES. One can clone yeast genes by isolating a wild-type gene that will complement a recessive mutant defect. First, one constructs a recombinant DNA library from a wild-type yeast strain in a plasmid that can be autonomously propagated in both yeast and *E. coli*. The library contains a large enough population of plasmids to include all *S. cerevisiae* DNA sequences. Second, one transforms this library into a recipient yeast strain that contains a mutation in the gene to be cloned. Third, one screens the transformants for those that have a wild-type phenotype. These transformants presumably contain a plasmid with a wild-type copy of the gene of interest.

This presumption must be verified by two experiments. First, to ensure that the wild-type phenotype is associated with the plasmid, the plasmid is isolated from the yeast transformant and introduced into *E. coli*, recovered from *E. coli*, and retransformed back into the original yeast mutant. Now, every transformant should have a wild-type phenotype.

Even when a clone passes the above tests, the demonstration that it contains the correct gene is not complete. For example, some genes are overexpressed when cloned onto plasmids. This overexpression could compensate for a mutation in a different gene. Therefore, to verify that the clone contains the gene of interest, one must demonstrate genetic linkage of the cloned DNA to the correct genetic locus. To do this, one subclones the cloned DNA segment into an integrating vector that contains another scoreable marker. Transformation by this plasmid results in integration by homologous recombination at the locus corresponding to the cloned fragment. Using this transformant, one can then determine by a genetic cross that the cloned segment had directed integration of the plasmid to the correct locus.

After an *S. cerevisiae* gene has been cloned, one can alter it in any way desired (for example, by deletion of a portion *in vitro*), recombine the mutation into the yeast genome at its proper chromosomal locus (replacing the wild-type allele), and then analyze the mutant phenotype (Fig. 11–4). These molecular approaches rely on the ability of *S. cerevisiae* to perform homologous recombination at a high frequency and an analysis of genetic segregation patterns in tetrads.

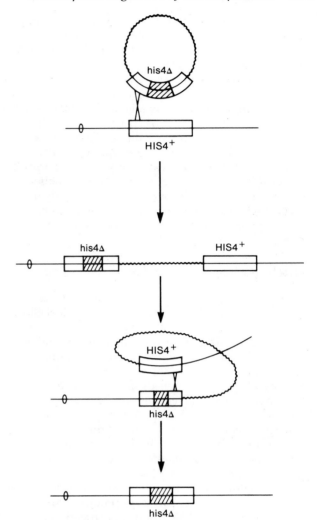

Figure 11–4. Gene disruption by transformation. A deletion mutation is constructed *in vitro* in an integrating plasmid (see text). Transformation results in integration, creating a duplication of the locus, one copy containing the wild-type gene, the other copy containing the deletion mutation. Recombination between the duplications can result in excision of the plasmid, resulting in a strain containing the *in vitro* constructed deletion mutation.

Transcription: Regulation of Gene Expression

Transcription in *S. cerevisiae* involves three RNA polymerase (RNAP) activities analogous to the RNAP I, II, and III of mammalian cells. RNAP A transcribes ribosomal RNA genes, B transcribes messenger RNA, and C transcribes tRNAs and 5S RNA. Yeast mRNA molecules contain polyA additions at the 3' end and a 5' terminal cap composed of either m⁷G(5')pppAp or m⁷G(5')pppGp. Also, some genes contain intervening sequences, but these are relatively rare compared to the frequency in higher eukaryotes.

Regulation of gene expression in *S. cerevisiae* is only beginning to be understood. However, it is already clear that transcriptional regulatory elements are distinctly different from what has been elucidated in *E. coli* and are closely analogous to those of other eukaryotes. In general, one can identify three types of regulatory elements: an **upstream activator sequence** is believed to be equivalent to mammalian **enhancer elements** in governing the frequency of transcription initiation, and a **TATA region** is important for determining initiation of transcription at the third region, the **I site.**

Mating-Type Regulation

Regulation of mating type in *S. cerevisiae* has been studied in particular detail because its novel mechanisms have led to greater understanding of a cell's potential for differentiation. As previously mentioned, the mating type of a haploid cell is determined by whether a single locus, *MAT*, is in one of two states, **a** or **α.** These two alleles, *MATa* and *MATα*, encode distinct gene products. The state of the *MAT* locus regulates a large number of genes, most of which have been identified by isolation of nonmating, or **sterile,** mutants. Some of these genes encode known functions such as the receptors for the mating pheromones and enzymes required for the proteolytic processing of the pheromones.

The mating type is determined by whether the *MATα* locus is expressing its two gene products, *MATα1* and *MATα2*. Genetic analysis has demonstrated that *MATα1* activates α-specific genes such as those that encode the **mating pheromone α-factor,** whereas the *MATα2* gene product represses a-specific genes.

The *MATa* locus products are not necessary for mating type determination: an **a** cell results from the absence of either *MATα1* and *MATα2*. However, gene products from both *MATa* and *MATα* determine the mating behavior of a diploid cell. *MATa1* and *MATα2* together repress *MATα1* and other haploid-specific genes, with the result that the diploids cannot mate but can sporulate.

Mating-Type Interconversion

Whereas most laboratory strains of *S. cerevisiae* are **heterothallic;** that is, exist in one of two stable mating types, some strains are **homothallic** (i.e., do not require two strains for mating) because they can undergo mating-type interconversion at high frequency. The interconversion event occurs by a recombination event between the *MAT* locus and silent copies of mating-type information contained elsewhere in the genome. The two silent copies, *HMLα* and *HMRa*, contain complete α and a information, respectively, that is not expressed. These are referred to as "silent cassettes."

Mating-type interconversion results from a nonreciprocal recombination between a silent copy of mating type (at *HMLα* or *HMRa*) and the *MAT* locus. For example, in a switch from *MATa* to *MATα*, the silent information at *HMLα* is recombined into the *MAT* locus, replacing the *MATa* information that was present there (Fig. 11–5). This recombination event is nonreciprocal because the information at *HMLα* is copied, rather than transferred, to replace the information at *MAT*. Mating-type interconversion requires the *HO* gene, which encodes a site-specific endonuclease; heterothallic strains carry inactive mutant forms.

Chromosome Structure and Segregation

S. cerevisiae strains contain 16 chromosomes, which range in size from 300 to 2000 Kb pairs. Each chromosome is replicated once and is properly transmitted to progeny cells with remarkable fidelity in each cell cycle. Molecular genetic studies have focused on discerning

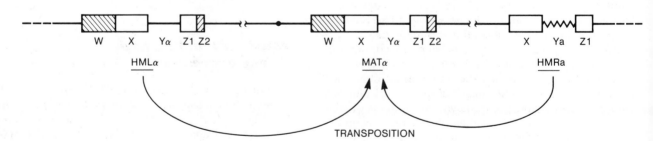

Figure 11–5. Organization of the *S. cerevisiae* mating-type cassettes. Three copies of mating-type information are present on chromosome III. Information at *MAT* is expressed; information at *HMLα* and *HMRa* is silent. During mating-type interconversion, the information at *MAT* is removed and replaced by a nonreciprocal recombination event with information from one of the silent cassettes.

the mechanism of chromosome inheritance and the structure of the DNA at the ends of the chromosomes that is presumably required for proper replication of the ends of a linear molecule. Three components of a chromosome that are required for proper transmission have been cloned.

1. A **centromere** is the region of a chromosome where spindle fibers attach to allow proper segregation during mitosis and meiosis. In *S. cerevisiae*, this region, cloned from at least 10 of the 16 *S. cerevisiae* chromosomes, has two highly conserved sequences that may be the sites of spindle attachment.

2. A **telomere** is the region at the end of a linear chromosome, presumably involved in proper replication of the ends and in the stability of the chromosome. This DNA is a hairpin, with single-stranded nicks and gaps, and specific telomere-binding proteins have been identified; but the functionality of the telomere remains to be determined.

3. *S. cerevisiae* chromosomes each have several **autonomous replication sequences (ars)**, whose cloning into plasmids permits them to replicate autonomously. These sequences are presumed to be the chromosomal origins of DNA replication.

With yeast, it has been possible to construct **artificial chromosomes** by combining centromeres, telomeres, and *ars* sequences. However, small (10–50 Kb) linear artificial chromosomes are at least 100-fold less stable for proper transmission during mitotic or meiotic growth than authentic yeast chromosomes. Artificial chromosomes of 150 Kb are significantly more stable, although still less stable than authentic chromosomes.

Ras Genes

The *RAS* genes, a highly conserved family found in many eukaryotes, were first identified as the oncogenic transforming genes in the Harvey and Kirsten sarcoma viruses. *RAS* proteins bind GTP and contain a GTPase activity. Mutant proteins, differing from the wild type in one of a few amino acid residues and with reduced GTPase activity, have been identified as the transforming agents in a number of human tumors. Little is known about their normal function in vertebrates, and so the presence of similar genes in yeast has aroused much interest. In *S. cerevisiae*, two closely related genes, *RAS1* and *RAS2*, have been identified. Complete loss of both is lethal but not the loss of either alone. They show significant (greater than 60%) amino acid homology to mammalian *RAS* genes, and the human *RAS* gene, under control of a yeast promoter in a plasmid, can substitute functionally for the yeast *RAS* genes.

The powerful genetics available in *S. cerevisiae* has begun to reveal the function of their *RAS* genes. They are required for activation of adenylate cyclase, and the resulting cAMP activates the yeast cAMP-dependent protein kinase. Its targets, and the factors that stimulate the activation, have yet to be identified.

Cell Structure

S. cerevisiae cells possess nearly all of the structures of more complex eukaryotes, including mitochondria, endoplasmic reticulum, Golgi apparatus, vacuoles, and a cytoskeleton. Furthermore, many of the components of these structures such as actin, α-tubulin, and β-tubulin are genetically highly conserved when compared with their other eukaryotic counterparts. The genetics available in *S. cerevisiae* allows several questions in cell biology to be addressed by a molecular genetic approach not possible in other eukaryotes, including studies on protein localization, endocytosis, and the roles of highly conserved cellular proteins such as actin and tubulin.

PROTEIN LOCALIZATION. Localization of proteins in a eukaryotic cell can be considerably more complicated than in a prokaryotic cell because they can be destined for various subcellular compartments, including the mitochondrion, the endoplasmic reticulum, the Golgi complex, the lysosome, the plasma membrane, and the vacuole, an organelle analogous to the mammalian lysosome. Whereas in higher eukaryotes understanding this process has entailed using exclusively biochemical approaches, recent genetic approaches in *S. cerevisiae* have been valuable for understanding protein sorting to different cellular membranes.

A genetic approach to the secretory process in *S. cerevisiae* taken by Schekman and coworkers has resulted in isolation and analysis of a large number of temperature-sensitive **secretory mutants** that are blocked in secretion, bud growth, cell division, and the incorporation of proteins into the plasma membrane. Many mutants accumulate or exaggerate specific secretory organelles such as vesicles, endoplasmic reticulum, and Golgi body.

Molecular analysis has identified segments in the N-terminal region of various proteins that are essential for sorting to the vacuole or to the mitochondrion. In addition, genetic analysis has identified several genes, as in bacteria, that are required for this proper sorting.

Selected Readings

BOOKS AND REVIEW ARTICLES

Mortimer RK, Hawthorne DC: Yeast Genetics. In Rose AH, Harrison JS (eds): The Yeasts, vol. 1, p 368. New York, Academic Press, 1969
Rothstein RJ: One-step gene disruption in yeast. Methods Enzymol 101:202, 1983

Russell P, Nurse P: *Schizosaccharomyces pombe* and *Saccharomyces cerevisiae:* A look at yeasts divided. Cell 45:781, 1986

Sprague GF, Jr, Blair LC, Thorner J: Cell interactions and regulation of cell type in the yeast *Saccharomyces cerevisiae.* Annu Rev Microbiol 37:623, 1983

Strathern JN, Jones EW, Broach JR (eds): The Molecular Biology of the Yeast Saccharomyces: Life Cycle and Inheritance; Metabolism and Gene Expression. Cold Spring Harbor, Cold Spring Harbor Laboratory, 1981

Struhl K: The new yeast genetics. Nature 305:391, 1983

Winston F, Chumley F, Fink GR: Eviction and transplacement of mutant genes in yeast. Methods Enzymol 101:211, 1983

SPECIFIC ARTICLES

Bankaitis VA, Johnson LM, Emr SD: Isolation of yeast mutants defective in protein targeting to the vacuole. Proc Natl Acad Sci USA 83:9075, 1986

Bucking–Throm E, Duntze W, Hartwell LH, Manney TR: Reversible arrest of haploid yeast cells at the initiation of DNA synthesis by a diffusible sex factor. Exp Cell Res 76:99, 1973

Clarke L, Carbon J: Isolation of a yeast centromere and construction of functional small circular chromosomes. Nature 287:504, 1980

Hartwell LH, Culotti J, Reid B: Genetic control of the cell-division cycle in yeast I: Detection of mutants. Proc Natl Acad Sci USA 66:352, 1970

Hartwell LH, Culotti J, Pringle JR, Reid BJ: Genetic control of the cell division cycle in yeast. Science 183:46, 1974

Hartwell LH, Mortimer RK, Culotti J, Culotti M: Genetic control of the cell division cycle in yeast V: Genetic analysis of *cdc* mutants. Genetics 74:267, 1978

Hicks JB, Herskowitz I: Interconversion of yeast mating types I: Direct observations of the action of the homothallism (*HO*) gene. Genetics 83:245, 1976

Hicks JB, Herskowitz I: Interconversion of yeast mating types II: Restoration of mating ability to sterile mutants in homothallic and heterothallic strains. Genetics 85:373, 1977

Hieter P, Mann C, Snyder M, Davis RW: A colony color assay that measures nondisjunction and chromosome loss. Cell 40:381, 1985

Hinnen A, Hicks JA, Fink GR: Transformation of yeast. Proc Natl Acad Sci USA 75:1929, 1978

Holm C, Goto T, Wang JC, Botstein D: DNA topoisomerase II is required at the time of mitosis in yeast. Cell 41:553, 1985

Ito H, Fukuda Y, Murata K, Kimura A: Transformation of intact yeast cells treated with alkali cations. J Bacteriol 153:163, 1983

Johnson LM, Bankaitis VA, Emr SD: Distinct sequence determinants direct intracellular sorting and modification of a yeast vacuolar protease. Cell 48:875, 1987

Kataoka T, Powers S, Cameron S, Fasano O, Goldfarb M, Broach J, Wigler, M: Functional homology of mammalian and yeast *ras* genes. Cell 40:19, 1985

Mackay V, Manney TR: Mutations affecting sexual conjugation and related processes in *Saccharomyces cerevisiae* I: Isolation and phenotypic characterization of nonmating mutants. Genetics 76:255, 1974

Mackay V, Manney TR: Mutations affecting sexual conjugation and related processes in *Saccharomyces cerevisiae* II: Genetic analysis of nonmating mutants. Genetics 76:273, 1974

Murray AW, Szostak JW: Construction of artificial chromosomes in yeast. Nature 305:189, 1983

Novick P, Field C, Schekman, R: Identification of 23 complementation groups required for post-translational events in the yeast secretory pathway. Cell 21:205, 1980

Rothman JH, Stevens TH: Protein sorting in yeast: Mutants defective in vacuolar biogenesis mislocalize vacuolar proteins into the late secretory pathway. Cell 47:1041, 1986

Scherer S, Davis RW: Replacement of chromosome segments with altered DNA sequences constructed *in vitro.* Proc Natl Acad Sci USA 76:4951, 1979

Strathern J, Hicks J, Herskowitz I: Control of cell types in yeast by the mating type locus: The α1–α2 hypothesis. J Mol Biol 147:357, 1981

Struhl K, Stinchcomb DT, Scherer S, Davis RW: High frequency transformation of yeast: Autonomous replication of hybrid DNA molecules. Proc Natl Acad Sci USA 76:1035, 1979

Tatchell K, Chaleff D, Defeo–Jones D, Scolnick E: Requirement of either of a pair of *ras*-related genes of *Saccharomyces cerevisiae* for spore viability. Nature 309:523, 1984

Valls LA, Hunter CP, Rothman JH, Stevens TH: Protein sorting in yeast: The localization determinant of yeast vacuolar carboxypeptidase Y resides in the propeptide. Cell 48:887, 1987

Part Two

Immunology

Herman N. Eisen

12

Introduction to the Immune Responses

The immune system of vertebrates is characterized by a remarkable set of adaptive processes that enable the individual organism to produce, on demand as it were, an immense variety of specifically reactive proteins and cells that can recognize and cause the destruction of an almost limitless variety of foreign substances. These processes, called immune responses, are essential for survival, for they constitute the principal means of natural defense against infection by pathogenic microorganisms; they probably also contribute to defenses against some host cells that undergo transformation into cancer cells.

The Origins of Immunology

It has been known since ancient times that persons who recover from certain epidemic diseases (plague, for example) cannot contract them again. This awareness led to deliberate attempts, beginning in the Middle Ages, to induce immunity against smallpox by inoculating well persons with material scraped from skin lesions of persons suffering from the disease (variolation). The procedure was hazardous, but in the late 18th century, the English physician Jenner used scrapings from skin lesions of people with cowpox (a mild form of smallpox) and thereby established **vaccination** (L. *vacca*, cow) as a simple, safe, and effective procedure. About 100 years later, Pasteur happened to use an old culture of the bacteria of chicken cholera (*Pasteurella aviseptica*) to inoculate some chickens, and instead of becoming ill, the animals proved to be immune when reinoculated with a fresh virulent culture. This observation was subsequently applied to many other infectious diseases, and various procedures were used to diminish the virulence but preserve the immunity-generating activity of microbes.

239

It was found later that immunity to infectious diseases·can also be induced by injecting products or parts of the causative microorganism. Following the demonstration of a powerful toxin in culture filtrates of diphtheria bacilli in 1888, von Behring showed that nonlethal doses of the filtrates could induce immunity to diphtheria. Ehrlich and Calmette similarly established immunity to toxins of nonmicrobial origin, e.g., snake venoms.

A clue to the basis for these immune responses was uncovered in 1890, when von Behring and Kitasato demonstrated that the serum of individuals with induced immunity to tetanus could neutralize the toxin and could confer immunity on normal animals. Moreover, Ehrlich, studying the effects of a plant toxin (ricin) on red blood cells *in vitro*, showed that protection involved combination of the toxin with specifically reactive components of the serum; a similar combination presumably accounted for the effects of immune serum on infectious agents. These observations opened the way to analysis of substances responsible for immunity and also to the effective treatment of several infectious diseases by injecting serum from immune animals.

Within the next 10 years, many specific reactions of immune sera (called **serologic** reactions) were discovered. For example, serum from immunized animals caused **bacteriolysis** (disintegration of cholera vibrios), **precipitation** of soluble components in cell-free culture filtrates of plague bacilli, and **agglutination** or clumping of bacteria. These reactions were all specific: an immune serum reacted only with the substance that had induced the immune response, or, as we shall see later, with substances of similar chemical structure. By about 1900, immune responses were found to extend beyond immunity in a strict sense: similar responses could also be elicited by nontoxic and noninfectious substances, such as proteins of milk or egg white.

Definitions

The inoculated materials and the substances whose appearance in serum they evoke are called **antigens (Ags)** and **antibodies (Abs),** respectively. **An almost limitless number of substances can behave as Ags**—virtually all proteins, many polysaccharides, nucleoproteins, lipoproteins, and synthetic polypeptides, and also an enormous number of small molecules if they are suitably linked to proteins.

An antigen has two properties: (1) **immunogenicity,** i.e., the capacity to stimulate the formation of the corresponding Abs, and (2) the **ability to react specifically** with those Abs. The two properties are not always associated, and the term **immunogen** is often used for the substance that stimulates the formation of the Abs; other substances known as **haptens** (described under Anti-

genic Determinants, below) are not immunogenic by themselves but react specifically with the appropriate Abs. **"Specific" means that the Ag (or hapten) combines, in a highly selective fashion, with the corresponding Ab and not with the multitude of other Abs evoked by other Ags.**

The definition of an Ag is operational: **immunogenicity is not an inherent property of a macromolecule,** as is, for instance, its molecular weight or absorption spectrum. For example, rabbit serum albumin (RSA) isolated from rabbits is not immunogenic in this species, but it can elicit copious amounts of anti-RSA Abs in virtually any other species of vertebrate. Responses to Ags differ markedly with the conditions under which they are administered, e.g., the quantity injected and the route and frequency of injection. **One important condition is that the putative immunogen be somehow recognized as foreign (i.e., not self) by the responding organism.**

The term "**antibody**" refers to the protein or set of proteins that is formed in response to an Ag and that reacts specifically with that Ag (or with related substances). All Abs belong to a family of proteins, the **immunoglobulins (Igs),** whose properties are considered in detail in Chapter 14.

Antigenic Determinants

The reaction between an Ag and the corresponding Ab involves their reversible combination. Often called "**antigen recognition,**" this reaction epitomizes immune specificity and is considered in some detail in Chapter 13. Here, however, it is useful to distinguish between the Ag molecule in its entirety and its **antigenic determinants** or **epitopes:** those restricted portions of the Ag that are recognized by Ab and determine the specificity of Ab–Ag reactions. These areas are much smaller than a macromolecule; they range in size from a small hapten up to a cluster of perhaps 15 to 20 amino acid residues.

The great diversity of antigenic substances was first emphasized by Obermayer and Pick (1903), who attached NO_2 groups to rabbit serum proteins, injected these proteins into rabbits, and found that the resulting serum reacted with nitrated proteins of rabbit, horse, or chicken serum but not with the corresponding unmodified proteins. The Abs formed were evidently capable of specifically recognizing the nitro groups or other uniquely altered structures in the nitrated proteins.

Starting with this observation, Landsteiner explored the chemical basis of antigenic specificity by coupling various aromatic amines to proteins (Fig. 12–1). Rabbits injected with *p*-azobenzenearsenate coupled to rabbit globulin form Abs that react with any proteins that con-

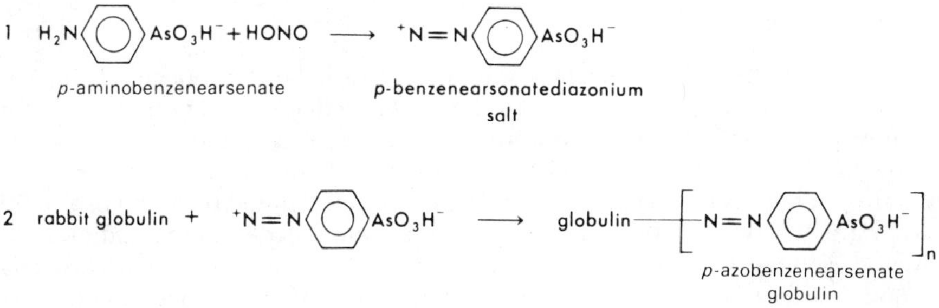

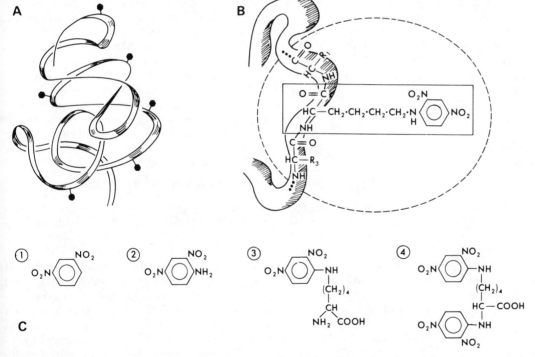

1 $H_2N\langle\bigcirc\rangle AsO_3H^- + HONO \longrightarrow {}^+N=N\langle\bigcirc\rangle AsO_3H^-$

   p-aminobenzenearsenate   *p*-benzenearsonatediazonium
   salt

2 rabbit globulin + ${}^+N=N\langle\bigcirc\rangle AsO_3H^- \longrightarrow$ globulin $\left[-N=N\langle\bigcirc\rangle AsO_3H^- \right]_n$

   p-azobenzenearsenate
   globulin

Figure 12–1. The classic example of attachment of haptens (in this instance, an aromatic amine) to a protein via azo linkage (–N=N–) to form a hapten–protein conjugate.

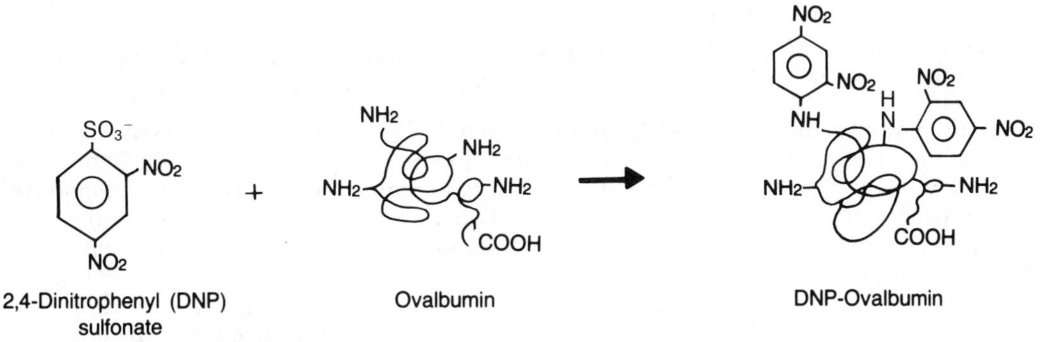

2,4-Dinitrophenyl (DNP)   Ovalbumin   DNP-Ovalbumin
sulfonate

Figure 12–2. A commonly used method for producing a hapten–protein (DNP–ovalbumin) conjugate.

A **B**

C (1) m-dinitrobenzene (2) 2,4-dinitroaniline (3) ε-Dnp-lysine (4) α,ε-bis-Dnp-lysine

Figure 12–3. Distinctions between conjugated proteins, antigenic determinants (or epitopes), haptenic groups, and haptens. *(A)* **Conjugated protein** with substituents represented as solid hexagons. *(B)* A representative **haptenic group:** a 2,4-dinitrophenyl (Dnp) group substituted in the ε-**NH$_2$** group of a lysine residue. The haptenic group is outlined by the solid line, the **antigenic determinant** or **epitope** by the broken line. Amino acid residues contributing to the antigenic determinant need not be the nearest covalently linked neighbors of the ε-Dnp-lysine residue, as shown: they could be parts of distant segments of the polypeptide chain looped back to become close neighbors of the Dnp-lysyl residue. *(C)* Some **haptens** that correspond to the haptenic group in B: (1) m-dinitrobenzene; (2) 2,4-dinitroaniline; (3) ε-Dnp-lysine; (4) α,ε-bis-Dnp-lysine. With respect to Abs specific for the Dnp group, haptens 1, 2, and 3 are univalent (one combining group per molecule), and hapten 4 is bivalent.

241

tain *p*-azobenzenearsenate substituents but not with the proteins in unsubstituted form. Later, it was found that *p*-aminobenzenearsenate itself can combine specifically with these Abs, but it does not evoke their formation. Substances of this type, as noted above, are defined as haptens: they react selectively with appropriate Abs, but they are not immunogenic by themselves. Various aromatic amines (with some important exceptions) do not cross-react with each other's Abs.

Although the formal difference between Ag and hapten is clear, it may be difficult in practice to decide whether a substance is weakly immunogenic or completely nonimmunogenic. Generally, however, small molecules (mol. wt. <1000) are not immunogenic unless covalently linked to proteins *in vitro* (Fig. 12–2) or *in vivo* (see Contact Skin Sensitivity, Chap. 19). The diazo reaction (see Fig. 12–1) introduces azo groups as substituents in tyrosine, tryptophan, histidine, and lysine residues. Other methods (e.g., those shown in Fig. 12–2) for coupling haptens to proteins are now more widely used. An almost unlimited variety of organic molecules can serve as haptens.

Proteins with substituents covalently linked to their side chains are referred to as **conjugated proteins;** and the substituents, sometimes including the amino acid residues to which they are linked, are called **haptenic groups.** Although a haptenic group is thus part of an antigenic determinant, it is not clear just how much of the complete determinant it represents. These distinctions are shown in Figure 12–3.

An Overview of Cellular and Humoral Immunity

Coincident with early studies on the role of serum Abs, Metchnikov discovered that certain phagocytic cells destroy the bacteria they ingest. The resulting controversy between advocates of "humoral" immunity, attributable to Abs, and "cellular" immunity, attributable to cells, was temporarily reconciled by the finding, in 1903, of cooperation between the two components: the coating of particles by Abs (called **opsonization;** Gr., to prepare food) was shown to increase their susceptibility to phagocytosis.

However, a very different kind of cellular immunity was recognized much later as a result of studies of allergy (hypersensitivity)—a state induced by an Ag in which a subsequent response to that Ag causes local inflammation or even, in extreme situations, a generalized reaction with acute shock and death. Although certain allergic states can be transferred by serum Abs, Landsteiner and Chase showed in 1942 that others can be transferred only with living leukocytes, later shown by

the Harrises and by Gowans to be lymphocytes. Lymphocytes were also found to mediate a wide variety of other specific immune responses, e.g., immunity to tubercle bacilli and many other infectious agents, the destruction of virus-infected cells, the accelerated rejection of grafted cells, and resistance to many experimental cancers. As we shall see later, it is these cells that are ultimately responsible for the capacity to discriminate among vast numbers of Ags.

LYMPHOCYTES AND THE CLONAL SELECTION HYPOTHESIS

There are about 10^{12} lymphocytes in an adult human, constituting about 5% to 10% of all cells in the body. They migrate through tissues and circulate in blood and lymph, and about half of them are found in the main lymphatic organs: spleen, thymus, and a multitude of small lymph nodes scattered in all tissues and organs except the central nervous system. These cells are of two major classes, named for the sites where they develop from precursors into immunologically competent cells: **B-lymphocytes** or "**B cells**" in the bone marrow and **T-lymphocytes** or "**T cells**" in the thymus. The essential activity of these cells was predicted in the **clonal selection hypothesis** (due primarily to Burnet). According to this hypothesis, which is now supported by an immense body of experimental evidence and constitutes the central paradigm of immunology, B- and T-cell populations are made up of enormous numbers of diverse clones, each distinguished by the ability to recognize only one or a few similar Ags. It is because there are millions of these clones that an individual can respond specifically to millions of different Ags.

B CELLS AND ANTIBODY STRUCTURE

The recognition of Ags by lymphocytes has been traced to a family of glycoproteins embedded in the cell-surface membrane. These proteins have a similar overall structure in B and T cells. In B cells, they are the same as soluble, circulating Abs except for a modified carboxy-terminal amino acid sequence that anchors them in the cell membrane. Thus a B cell's recognition of an Ag is synonymous with the specific binding of that Ag by the cell's surface Ig. The binding of Ag, together with additional stimuli provided by growth factors secreted by T cells (described below), provides the specific signals that trigger resting B cells (in G_0 of the cell cycle) to proliferate and to differentiate into fully mature B cells. The latter, called **plasma cells,** are adapted to secrete copious amounts of Ig (i.e., Ab).

Although Abs are extraordinarily diverse in their specificity for Ags and fall into several distinct classes in other respects, they have a remarkably similar overall molecular structure (see Chap. 14). Each molecule is made up of an equal number of heavy (H) and light (L) polypeptide chains (approximately 50,000 and 22,000 daltons, respectively), and each H–L pair forms a single Ag-binding site. The number of H–L pairs per antibody molecule varies in different classes of Ig: e.g., two per molecule (H_2L_2) in the commonest class, called IgG, and ten per molecule ($H_{10}L_{10}$) in the IgM class. Amino acid sequences and x-ray crystallographic studies have shown that all Ig chains are made up of repeating domains of about 110 amino acid residues, each folded into a characteristic three-dimensional shape, the "**Ig-fold.**"

The uniqueness of the Igs made by different B-cell clones lies in the amino acid sequences of the amino-terminal domains (the **V** or **variable domain**) of both their H and L chains, which differ from one B-cell clone to another, whereas the other domains (called **C** or **constant domains**) do not necessarily differ among clones. The V domain differences are especially pronounced in three **hypervariable** regions. These regions are not contiguous in the linear sequence, but in the folded Ig molecule, all six regions of each L–H pair (three in VL plus three in VH) are clustered to form the Ag-binding site. Because these sites are essentially complementary in shape to the epitopes that they bind specifically, the hypervariable regions are often called **complementarity-determining regions** (or **CDRs**); the much less variable sequences that separate them within the amino-terminal domain are termed **framework regions** (or **FRs**).

Small characteristic variations in amino acid sequence of C domains distinguish nine different classes or isotypes of H chains (called μ, δ, $\gamma1$, $\gamma2$, etc.) and several different types (also termed isotypes) of L chains (called κ, $\lambda1$, $\lambda2$, and so on). Any given B cell produces an Ig made up of one particular H chain isotype and one L chain isotype (the one cell–one Ab rule). However, in an individual with millions of Ig-producing B cells, the total pool of Igs contain H chains of any class paired with L chains of any type. There will thus be millions of different Ig products in serum, not only because of the 36 possible isotype combinations (9H × 4L), but, more importantly, because of the unique V-domain amino acid sequences of each B-cell clone. The V regions are responsible for Ag specificity, whereas the C regions determine different effector functions once Ag is bound.

In eliciting an Ab response, an Ag usually stimulates many different B-cell clones, yielding a **polyclonal** antiserum. The members of this set of Abs, reacting with the same Ag, differ in the epitopes they recognize or in affinity for a given epitope. This heterogeneity greatly impeded molecular analyses of Abs and their use as diagnostic reagents until Kohler and Milstein found, in 1975, in a discovery with revolutionary consequences, that normal Ab-forming B cells can be fused with "immortal" B cells from tumors of plasma cells (called myeloma tu-mors) to yield cloned hybrid cell lines (**hybridomas**), each of which produces a normal B cell's Ab. Because a hybridoma characteristically results from the fusion of one B cell to one nonsecreting myeloma tumor cell, it secretes large quantities of a uniform **monoclonal Ab (mAb).** Hybridomas can be propagated indefinitely and can be used to produce enormous amounts of pure Abs.

IMMUNOGLOBULIN GENES

If each of the millions of different Igs produced by an individual were encoded by a different gene, a large fraction of the genome would consist of Ig genes. This unlikely possibility was disposed of when the genes that encode Ig H and L chains were identified. Analyses of these genes has also greatly clarified the basis for the one cell (or one clone)–one Ab rule and for the clonal diversity of Abs. Unlike the differentiation during embryonic development of other cell types, which retain a constant (or essentially constant) genome, the B and T cells of the immune system systematically rearrange selected regions of the genome, even in adult life. Several hundred Ig genes are inherited (**germ-line genes**), and they are rearranged and further diversified during B-cell development and even further by additional mechanisms during B-cell responses to antigenic stimulation. These genes fall into three families, for H, κ, and λ chains, each located on a different chromosome and consisting of many gene segments. As first shown by Tonegawa, the V domain of each L chain is encoded by two gene segments, a so-called variable or V gene segment, for amino acids 1–97 or 98, and a joining or J gene segment, encoding positions 98 or 99 to about 112. The V domain of each H chain is encoded by three segments: a V, a J, and one or a few small **diversity** or D segments that differ in length, each typically encoding two to ten amino acids between V and J. Separate C-gene segments encode the C domains of each H and L chain isotype (one for κ, one for each of the three or more types of λ chains, and one for each of the nine H chain classes).

Igs are produced before Ags are encountered. But before an Ig chain can be expressed, the appropriate gene segments have to be recombined or "rearranged." The rearrangements take place as B cells develop from stem cells in bone marrow. In the developing B cell, an H-chain gene is formed by two rearrangements: first a D and a J gene segment are joined, and then a V gene segment joins the linked DJ sequence. Next, an L-chain gene is formed by a single rearrangement linking a V to a J gene segment. Many rearrangements are nonproductive, because many of the V–J and V–D–J joins are out of frame: downstream of such joins, the normal triplet sequence of codons is replaced by a garbled message, usually with frequent nonsense ("stop") codons. Nevertheless, every Ig-producing B cell ends up with one, and only one, productive V–D–J rearrangement for an H chain and only one productive V–J recombination for an L chain (for κ or λ, not both). Hence, each B cell and its progeny (i.e., a B-cell clone) initially produces only a particular H chain and a particular L chain and expresses only a singular pair of VH–VL domains. **These circumstances account for the unique Ag-binding site and specificity for Ag that characterizes the Ig of each B-cell clone.**

IMMUNOGLOBULIN DIVERSITY

The enormous clonal VL–VH diversity that exists before Ags are encountered (the **pre-immune repertoire**) arises from several circumstances.

1. Many V-domain gene segments are inherited (e.g., hundreds of V_K, hundreds of V_H, and multiple Ds and Js).

2. Within each family, recombination apparently can take place between almost any V and any J (or any D) gene segment, giving rise to many alternative combinations (e.g., >200 V_K × 4 J_K = >800 distinctive V–J sequences for κ chains).

3. Variation in the positions of the nucleotide bonds that are cut and joined to make contiguous V–J and V–D–J sequences can generate new codons or **junctional diversity** at each join.

4. Additional nucleotides, not found in germ-line DNA, can be inserted between V–D and D–J during their recombination ("junctional insertions" form what are termed **N regions**).

ANTIGEN-INDUCED CHANGES

Once a productive V–J (for an L chain) and a productive V–D–J (for an H chain) rearrangement occurs in a developing B cell, they persist in that cell's progeny and provide a stable marker of the clone's individuality, even as members of the clone differentiate further through a series of stages into Ig-secreting plasma cells. However, the rearranged genes can still undergo two additional changes as B cells respond to intense antigenic stimulation.

One change is called **heavy (H) chain switching.** The assembled VDJ segment (for an H chain) is initially proximal to the C-gene segment for an H chain of the μ class and is expressed in an IgM molecule. In the switch, the VDJ sequence is translocated downstream on the same chromosome to the C-gene segment for a different H chain class, say a $\gamma1$ chain (see Chap. 14 for the order of gene segments for H chain C domains). In consequence, a VDJ sequence that was expressed in a μ chain becomes expressed in a $\gamma1$. Because the L chain is unaffected by the H chain change, the IgM molecule made before the switch and the IgG1 made afterward have the same V_L

and V_H domains and, therefore, the same specificity for Ag.

In the second change during the immune response, single nucleotide replacements (**somatic mutations**) occur at scattered positions in V-domain sequences, at a rate estimated to be about 1 per 1000 base pairs per cell division in the responding B cells of an intensely immunized (**hyperimmunized**) individual. This extraordinary rate (about 10,000-fold greater than normal mutation rates) can generate thousands of different sequences in a V domain that is encoded by a single V and a single J gene segment. Because many of the amino acid substitutions occur in hypervariable regions, some of them doubtless change the Ab's affinity for its Ag (or even its specificity). It is likely that the resulting intraclonal diversity provides opportunities for Ag at low concentration to bind preferentially to and selectively stimulate those cells whose novel sequences result in higher Ab affinity. This mechanism, reminiscent of mutation selection in the Darwinian evolution of species, accounts for the **progressive increase in affinity (affinity maturation),** and therefore in effectiveness, of Ab that is often observed during prolonged immunization.

PRIMARY VERSUS SECONDARY RESPONSES

The binding of some Ags (principally polysaccharides) to surface Ig on B cells seems, by itself, sufficient to trigger these cells to proliferate and produce the secreted form of their Ig. However, for most Ags, which are proteins, an optimal B-cell response requires additional signals in the form of proteins secreted by neighboring T cells that are specifically stimulated by the same Ag. These proteins (called **lymphokines**), also seem to be required for H chain switching and for the high frequency of somatic mutations in V domains associated with affinity progression. Thus they are also essential for the pronounced differences between the **initial (primary)** and **subsequent (secondary** or **memory)** response to an Ag. The Abs made in the primary response are typically of the IgM class and have low affinity for the Ag. However, as the response progresses, there is a selective expansion of B cells that have switched from production of IgM to IgG Abs and of those whose somatic mutations in V domains increase the Ab's affinity for Ag. These selectively accumulated B cells are poised to produce high-affinity IgG Abs when the organism again encounters the Ag, months and even years later, in what is called the memory (or **anamnestic** or secondary) immune response.

T-CELL SUBSETS

T cells are functionally much more diverse than B cells. The two best characterized types, termed **helper** or T$_H$

cells and **cytotoxic T-lymphocytes** or **CTLs,** can be readily grown in long-term culture as cloned lines. T_H cells characteristically respond to specific antigenic stimulation by secreting *lymphokines*. The lymphokines secreted by some T_H cells (IL-4, IL-5, etc.) stimulate B cells to respond more effectively to Ags. Other lymphokines (interferon-γ), secreted by other T_H cells, stimulate macrophages to release factors that cause slowly evolving inflammation (delayed type hypersensitivity). CTLs, in contrast, act by destroying just those cells (**target** cells) whose Ag they recognize. Some T_H cell lines can also lyse their target cells. Considerable evidence suggests that some T cells, termed **T suppressor** or **Ts,** block the activity of B cells and of other T cells; it is possible that Ts cells are important regulators of immune responses, but they have not yet been routinely cultured successfully, and their properties are not well defined.

THE MAJOR HISTOCOMPATIBILITY COMPLEX

Polyclonal populations of B cells, through their surface Igs, can recognize an enormous variety of Ags. Populations of T cells, through their cell-surface Ag-specific receptors (described below), can also recognize a wide variety of Ags but, in addition, exhibit a striking propensity to recognize at the same time a special set of cell surface glycoproteins encoded by a genetic locus known as the **major histocompatibility complex** or **MHC** (called HLA in man, H-2 in the mouse). Although a B cell, via its surface Ig, can recognize Ag alone, either in solution or on a cell surface, a T cell characteristically recognizes Ag only on the surface of another cell and in conjunction with that cell's MHC-encoded glycoproteins. The recognition of Ag in conjunction with an MHC product is known as **MHC restriction.** There are two principal sets of MHC-encoded glycoproteins, termed I and II, and each restricts Ag recognition by a different T-cell type: **class I MHC glycoproteins restrict CTLs, and class II restrict T_H cells.** A CTL or a T_H cell will thus not respond specifically to a target cell unless that cell has on its surface both the correct ("nominal") Ag and the correct MHC-I or MHC-II glycoprotein (called the "restricting element"). These glycoproteins are also known as **transplantation or histocompatibility (or H) Ags,** because in tissue and organ transplants in which the donor's MHC differs from that of the recipient (**allografts**), the specific T-cell responses they elicit result in vigorous rejection of the grafts. Although the MHC-encoded Ags were discovered in studies of allograft rejection, their natural function is to permit Ag recognition by T cells.

In the MHC complex of man, mouse, and other vertebrates, there are several (typically three) class I and several class II genes, and each is extremely polymorphic, perhaps having more than 50 to 100 allelic variants. Therefore, genetically nonidentical individuals will almost certainly have different sets of class I and class II MHC glycoproteins. Normally, Ag recognition by an individual's T_H cells and CTLs is possible only in conjunction with products of that individual's own class I and II alleles (**self**). However, any particular T cell will usually also have the ability to recognize some nonself (allogeneic) MHC-encoded class I or II molecules, and it is these cross-reactions that cause allografts to be routinely rejected. Analysis of mice whose own thymus has been replaced by a foreign thymus graft has revealed that the ability of a T_H cell or CTL to distinguish between self and nonself MHC products is not fixed in the genome. Instead, this ability is determined by the particular MHC-I and -II molecules that are expressed by certain cells in the thymus, where pre-T-cell precursors develop into immunologically competent T cells (**thymic selection or education**).

The class I and class II MHC glycoproteins are each two-chain molecules (heterodimers) with some domains that have low but distinct amino acid sequence homology to Ig constant regions. Much evidence suggests that these molecules bind peptide fragments of Ags and that it is the MHC–peptide complexes that are recognized by Ag-specific receptors of T cells. Although any particular MHC molecule (class I or class II) must be able to bind many different Ags (perhaps thousands), it binds peptides from only certain Ags and not from others. This selectivity is probably an important source of individual variation in resistance to infection. Thus, an individual whose MHC-I glycoproteins permit that individual's CTLs to recognize a particular viral antigen on virus-infected cells is more likely to destroy those cells and to resist infection by that virus than is an individual whose MHC class I molecules lack this ability. Similarly, only the products of certain class II alleles permit T_H-cell recognition of certain epitopes; hence, only individuals with those class II alleles are able to make optimal B-cell (i.e., Ab) responses to that epitope. Because no individual's MHC alleles are capable of permitting an optimal response to all Ags, the great diversity of these alleles seems to be important for a species' survival, enabling at least some individuals to make effective immune responses against otherwise-lethal infectious agents.

ANTIGEN PROCESSING AND PRESENTATION

Although virtually all nucleated cells express class I molecules (and are thus potential targets for CTLs, when they present a viral or other nonself Ag), class II molecules are expressed only on special **antigen-presenting cells (APCs),** principally macrophages, dendritic cells, and B cells. Optimal production of Abs requires interactions between APCs and T_H cells. The APCs bind, ingest, and cleave protein Ags into peptide fragments that become bound to MHC-II molecules on the cell surface, where they can be recognized by T_H cells. Recognition of the **processed** Ag–MHC-II complex by receptors on T_H cells stimulates these cells to secrete several lymphokines, including **interleukin-2 (IL-2),** and to express receptors for IL-2 on the activated T_H cell's surface. Activated T_H cells also produce **γ-interferon** and a variety of additional factors, including several (IL-4, IL-5, IL-6) that are necessary for optimal responses by various B cells (proliferation, Ig secretion, and H-chain switching and multiple nucleotide substitutions in genes encoding Ig V regions).

Other cells cleave some of the proteins they synthesize (e.g., viral-encoded proteins in virus-infected cells) into peptides that are bound to MHC-I proteins on the cell surface. These cells are lysed if the MHC-I–peptide complex is recognized by CTLs.

ANTIGEN RECEPTORS ON T CELLS

Antigen receptors on T cells (TcR) are responsible for specific Ag-driven responses of T cells. Like Igs on B cells, TcR for Ag is made up on most T cells of two different S–S-linked polypeptide chains (see Chap. 15), termed α and β, each encoded by a set of Ig-like gene segments. Two similar sets of gene segments, termed γ and δ, encode similar heterodimeric Ag-specific T cell receptors (γ/δ) on other T cells. Compared to T_H cells and CTLs, which express α/β receptors, T cells with γ/δ receptors are relatively scarce; they tend to cluster within epithelial layers of skin and intestine where they appear to be cytolytic, as though they lyse cells that are infected by intestinal microbial pathogens.

The strikingly similar structure and organization of the genes for B- and T-cell Ag-recognition molecules indicates that they are all descended from a common ancestral set of rearranging gene segments. Thus, like the Ig gene families, the T-cell α, β, γ, and δ gene families have multiple V-gene segments, a variable number of J segments (ranging from four $J\gamma$ to about 50 $J\alpha$), a few D segments, and a small number of C-gene segments (one for $C\alpha$, two for $C\beta$, and at least four for $C\gamma$). Moreover, the expression of T-cell α, β, γ, and δ gene segments also depends on the joining, within each family, of V to J or D to J and then V to DJ segments. Conserved noncoding signal sequences that flank Ig V and J coding sequences and are probably required for Ig V–J joining are also next to T-cell V and J gene segments and are evidently required for their becoming joined. Finally, the overall amino acid sequence similarities of TcR subunits to Ig H and L chains is unmistakable (about 20% to 35%).

Amino acid sequences deduced from transcripts of rearranged α, β, γ, and δ genes show that their products are integral membrane polypeptide chains (see Chap. 15) with two extracellular domains: an N-terminal variable (V) domain, whose sequence varies from one clone to another, and an adjacent membrane-proximal domain that is not clonally variable and resembles Ig constant (C) domains.

Another T-cell surface glycoprotein, CD3, is closely associated with the Ag-specific α/β and γ/δ receptors. CD3 does not vary from one clone to another and therefore is not itself an Ag-recognizing molecule. However, Abs that bind to CD3 can trigger T cells to proliferate and express effector functions (e.g., T_H cells to secrete IL-2 and γ-interferon and CTLs to lyse cells to which they are adherent). CD3 is made up of five subunits and probably has a transmembrane signalling function in activated T cells.

SOME OTHER IMPORTANT T-CELL SURFACE PROTEINS

Mature T cells express either CD4 or CD8, two cell differentiation (CD) glycoproteins. T_H cells express CD4 (termed T4 on human and L3T4 on mouse cells), whereas cells that express CD8 (termed T8 on human and Lyt-2,3 on mouse T cells) are CTLs, i.e., they have the ability to destroy the cells they recognize (or to develop into such killer cells). In both CD4 and CD8 proteins the N-terminal domain has low but distinct amino acid sequence homology to Ig variable domains, but it does not vary from one clone to another. Abs to CD4 and CD8 can block Ag-triggered T-cell functions, and it is likely that these proteins bind to invariant epitopes on MHC proteins, e.g., **CD8 to class I molecules** (which determine Ag recognition by CTLs) and **CD4 to class II molecules** (which determine Ag recognition by CD4 cells).

In exploring the surface of prospective target cells for the presence of Ag, T cells crawl about and adhere transiently to other cells (**immunologic surveillance**). Adhesion to the other cells seems to depend on several T-cell surface glycoproteins (LFA-1, etc.) that resemble the adhesion molecules on some other cells (granulocytes, etc.) that, like T cells, derive from bone marrow stem cells. Several of the adhesion molecules share a common subunit structure, with one subunit (α) that is unique for each of these proteins and another subunit (β) that is common to all of them.

ID–ANTI-ID NETWORK

Although individuals are tolerant of (i.e., do not react with) antigenic determinants (epitopes) of C domains of their own Igs, they can make Abs to their V domains, which are unique for particular B-cell clones. These unique determinants are called **idiotypes (Ids)**, and Abs to them are anti-idiotypes (anti-Ids). It has been suggested that under some circumstances, immunization with an Ag, call it X, elicits an Ab (anti-X) that, in turn, elicits a second Ab, anti-(anti-X), that is specific for the Id of the first Ab; i.e., the second Ab is an anti-Id. Because the anti-Id and X can each bind to the specific ligand-binding sites of anti-X, it is not surprising that in the absence of X, the appropriate anti-Ids can themselves stimulate (or sometimes suppress) the production of anti-X, presumably by binding, like an Ag, to the corresponding B cells. Anti-Ids that are specific for unique V domains of the Ag-specific receptors of T cells might also affect the responses of these cells. It has been suggested that Id–anti-Id reactions constitute an important regulatory network for B- and T-cell responses under certain circumstances, e.g., shutting off or enhancing immune responses to a particular Ag.

ANTIGEN DESTRUCTION

Ag binding by Abs and T cells triggers reactions that lead to degradation of the Ags and lysis of Ag-bearing cells. Thus, specific Ab–Ag complexes can activate the sequential "cascade" reaction of over 11 serum proteins (collectively called **complement**), with consequences that include enhanced phagocytic destruction of Ags and osmotic lysis of Ag-bearing cells. Abs can also activate macrophages to lyse Ag-bearing cells. In this process, called **antibody-dependent cell-mediated cytotoxicity (ADCC)**, Abs bind specifically both to Ags on target cells and, through particular H-chain C domains, to receptors (termed **Fc receptors**) on macrophages. The result is that the macrophages release highly reactive forms of oxygen (superoxide anion, hydrogen peroxide) that are toxic for target cells. In parallel with Ab-mediated cytotoxicity, CTLs lyse target cells whose surface Ags they recognize (in conjunction with restricting MHC proteins). The lysis results from the release by activated CTLs of toxic granules containing complement-like proteins that create lethal ion channels in membranes of target cells.

All of these degradative reactions are obviously beneficial when the Ags are pathogenic (e.g., bacterial toxins, tumor cells, virus-infected cells that shed virions). However, when the Ags are intrinsically harmless, such as proteins of plant pollens or Ags on cells of a transplanted organ, the same reactions can result in unwanted acute or chronic inflammation (called **allergic or hypersensitivity reactions**). Such reactions are responsible for rejection of kidney and heart allografts and underlie many acute and chronically recurring disorders such as asthma and contact dermatitis.

TOLERANCE OF SELF

Although an individual's B and T cells can collectively respond to a virtually unlimited number of different Ags, they do not normally respond to that individual's own Ags. This selective unresponsiveness or "tolerance of self" has long been recognized as a fundamental feature of immune responses, but the responsible mechanisms are still obscure. When, on certain occasions, self-tolerance fails, the resulting **autoimmune** responses can lead to severe disorders, such as chronic thyroiditis, rheumatoid arthritis, and systemic lupus erythematosus.

Scope of Immunology

Because Ags of pathogenic microorganisms represent only a small fraction of the vast number of substances that induce specific immune responses, there is obviously far more to immunology than immunity in the literal sense. Abs, and particularly mAbs, are now widely used as specific, sensitive reagents to analyze the structure of macromolecules and to measure vast numbers of different substances of physiologic and pathological importance (hormones, toxins, cyclic nucleotides, prostaglandins, etc.). In industry, kilogram amounts of mAbs are being produced to purify interferons and other proteins, and mAbs tagged with radioisotopes or toxins or chemotherapeutic agents are being tested for their ability to find and deliver to tumors therapeutic doses of cytotoxic agents. There is also wide interest in the development of B and T cells, and in their responses to Ags and other stimuli, as models for studying cell differentiation; and genes for Igs and TcRs are being exploited as clonal markers to study human B- and T-cell tumors and as models to study the organization, evolution, and regulation of gene expression in multigene families.

Despite this long (and incomplete) list of widening interest in immunology, the historic role of infectious diseases in the development of the field has left an indelible imprint; this is reflected in the nomenclature. For example, the response to an immunogen is still referred to as "immunization" even when no infectious agent is involved. "Vaccination" is the term reserved for immunization given to establish resistance to an infectious disease.

In the chapters that follow, we shall consider the formation and molecular properties of Abs and their interactions with Ags, and then proceed to the more complex reactions of cellular immunity. Because our understanding of the structure of Abs and TcRs and of the cellular basis for immune responses is extensively based on the use of Ab molecules as analytic reagents, we shall begin with a consideration of specific Ab–Ag reactions.

Selected Reading

Arrhenius S: Immunochemistry. New York, Macmillan, 1907

Burnet FM: The Clonal Selection Theory of Acquired Immunity. Cambridge, The University Press, 1959

Ehrlich P: Studies in Immunity. New York, John Wiley, 1910

Jerne NK: Towards a network theory of the immune responses. Ann Immunol (Paris) 125C:373, 1974

Landsteiner K: The Specificity of Serological Reactions, Rev Ed. Cambridge, Harvard University Press, 1945; reprinted by Dover Publications, New York, 1962 (paperback)

Metchnikoff E: Lectures on the Comparative Pathology of Inflammation. Kegan Paul, Trench, Trubner and Co., 1893; reprinted by Dover Publications, New York, 1968 (paperback)

Topley WWC, Wilson GD: The Principles of Bacteriology and Immunity, 2nd Ed. Baltimore, Williams & Wilkins, 1936

Zinsser H, Enders JF, Fothergill LD: Immunity: Principles and Applications in Medicine and Public Health, 5th Ed. New York, Macmillan, 1939

13

Antibody–Antigen Reactions

Antigen recognition, a cardinal feature of the immune system, is epitomized by the combination of antibody (Ab) with antigen (Ag). Most Ags are proteins, and we rarely know the identity and conformation of their reactive groups (termed antigenic determinants or epitopes), or even their number per Ag molecule or particle. Accordingly, to understand the principles of Ag recognition, we shall first consider the simplest example, the specific reaction of Abs with haptens. Because the distinction between haptens and Ags, based on the difference in immunogenicity (see Definitions, Chap. 12), is largely irrelevant for the present discussion, we shall use the generic term **ligand** to include both.

Reactions with Simple Haptens

Abs to a hapten are usually obtained by immunizing animals with the hapten attached covalently to a protein. The resulting Abs are easily purified (see Affinity Chromatography, Appendix in this chapter), and the formation and properties of specific Ab–hapten complexes can be analyzed by well-defined methods.

VALENCE AND AFFINITY OF ANTIBODIES

In the simplest reaction, a small univalent ligand, with one combining group per molecule, binds **reversibly** to a specific site on the Ab. At low concentrations of ligand, only a small proportion of the Ab's combining sites are occupied by ligand molecules; as the ligand concentration increases, the number of occupied sites rises until all are filled. At saturation, the number of univalent ligand molecules bound per Ab molecule is the **antibody valence.**

If we assume that the binding sites on a population of Ab molecules are equivalent and act independently of each other, the representative binding reaction is

$$S + L \underset{k'}{\overset{k}{\rightleftharpoons}} SL \tag{1}$$

where S is a binding site on Ab, L is ligand, and k and k' are the rate constants for association and dissociation, respectively. The ratio $k:k'$ is the equilibrium (association) constant, K, which is a measure of **affinity**, i.e., the tendency of site and ligand to form a stable complex (SL). Thus:

$$K = \frac{k}{k'} = \frac{[SL]}{[S][L]} \tag{2}$$

where the terms in brackets refer to the concentrations, at equilibrium, of the occupied Ab sites (SL), vacant Ab sites (S), and free (unbound) ligand molecules (L). If the total concentrations of binding sites ($S + SL$) or of ligand molecules ($L + SL$) are known, a measurement at equilibrium of L or S or SL leads to the association constant. It is usually convenient to measure the free ligand concentration, and several methods are available to distinguish free (L) from bound (SL) ligand. The most general one is equilibrium dialysis.

EQUILIBRIUM DIALYSIS. The principles of equilibrium dialysis are shown in Figure 13–1. A solution containing Ab molecules specific for a haptenic group (such as 2,4-dinitrophenyl; Dnp) in one compartment (I for inside), is separated by a membrane (m) from another compartment (O, for outside) that contains a solution of a small univalent ligand (e.g., 2,4-dinitroaniline; see Fig. 12–3, Chap. 12). The membrane is permeable to small molecules (mol. wt. <1000) but not to Abs, and the ligand can diffuse back and forth across the membrane until equilibrium is reached. Thereafter, the concentrations in the two compartments remain unchanged. If compartment I contained only the solvent or a protein that was incapable of binding, the ligand's concentration would ultimately become identical in both compartments; however, if it contains Ab molecules that can bind dinitroaniline, the final (equilibrium) concentration of total ligand in I will exceed its concentration in O. The difference represents ligand molecules bound to Ab molecules. Because the reaction is reversible, the concentrations finally attained are the same, regardless of whether the Ab and ligand are initially placed in the same or in separate compartments (see Fig. 13–1A).

By dividing the numerator (SL) and the denominator (S) of equation 2 by the Ab concentration, the equation may be expressed as

$$K = \frac{r}{(n - r)c} \tag{3}$$

or, more conveniently, as

$$\frac{r}{c} = Kn - Kr \tag{4}$$

where, at equilibrium, **r** represents the number of ligand molecules bound per Ab molecule at **c** free concentration of ligand, and **n** is the maximum number of ligand molecules that can be bound per Ab molecule (i.e., the Ab valence). When a set of values for **r** and **c** is obtained by analyzing a series of dialysis chambers at equilibrium, each with the same amount of Ab but a different amount of ligand, a plot of **r/c** versus **r** (termed the Scatchard plot) should give a straight line of slope—K (negative value of the equilibrium constant), providing all Ab sites are identical (and independent). Hence, linearity or non-linearity of this plot can provide information on the uniformity of equilibrium constants of the binding sites in the sample of Ab molecules. The number of sites per Ab molecule can also be determined by the same plot: when the concentration of unbound ligand (**c**) becomes very large, **r/c** approaches zero and the number of ligand molecules bound per Ab molecule approaches the number of binding sites, or Ab valence.

It is important to recall that the equilibrium constant, K, refers to a "representative" binding site. However, there are multiple binding sites per Ab molecule (see below and Chap. 14), and K reflects the series of individual association constants (κ_i) that describe the binding of ligand to individual sites (i). For a particular site i, κ_i is determined by the total number of binding sites per Ab molecule (n), the number of sites occupied when site i is filled, the number that remain vacant ($n - i$), and the overall or representative association constant K. As shown in the Appendix of this chapter:

$$\kappa_i = \frac{n - i + 1}{i} K \tag{5}$$

Equation 5 means that for a bivalent Ab molecule having (two vacant sites, see IgG, Chap. 14), κ_1, the association constant for binding the first ligand to one of them is $2K$; when the first site is filled, κ_2, the association constant for binding ligand to the second site, is $K/2$. (This fourfold difference ($2K$ versus $K/2$) is a statistical factor; i.e. the ligand is twice as likely to bind to an Ab molecule with two vacant sites than to one with a single vacant site; and it is twice as likely to dissociate from an Ab with two occupied sites than from one with a single occupied site). For an Ab with ten identical binding sites per molecule, the disparity is 100-fold: i.e., κ_1, the association constant for binding the first ligand is $10K$, and κ_{10}, the association constant for binding the tenth ligand, is $K/10$. To emphasize these relations, K, the association constant of the representative site in equations 2 through 5, is termed the **intrinsic association constant** or the **intrinsic affinity.** Equilibrium dialysis and similar meth-

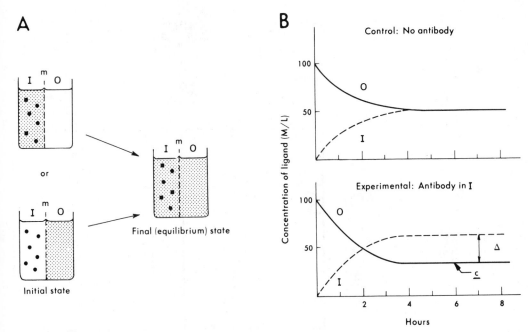

Figure 13–1. Equilibrium dialysis. *(A)* Small univalent haptens (small dots) can diffuse freely between the compartments (I, O), but Ab molecules (large dots) cannot. At equilibrium, the greater concentration of hapten in I is attributable to its binding by Ab. *(B)* Change in hapten concentration with time. Equilibrium is reached in about 4 hours (the time varies with temperature, volumes of the compartments, nature and surface area of the membrane [m], etc.). In *B,* the hapten was initially in compartment O. Its concentration in compartment O is shown by the continuous line (—), and its concentration and in compartment I by the broken line (---). After equilibrium is reached, the concentrations in I and O are equal in the control unit (no Ab) but greater in I than in O in the experimental unit (Ab present in I).

ods measure the total amount of bound ligand rather than the distribution of the bound ligand among different Ab molecules; hence, they provide a direct measure of the intrinsic affinity. When the concentrations of Ab and ligand are expressed in standard terms (moles per liter), intrinsic affinity values can be compared directly with those for any other reversibly interacting pair of molecules, e.g., binding of other ligands to other Abs, or of substrates to enzymes, or of drugs or hormones or lymphokines to cell-surface receptors, etc. (For more on the Scatchard equation and equation 5, see Appendix).

HETEROGENEITY WITH RESPECT TO INTRINSIC AF-FINITY. Figure 13–2 shows representative data for the binding of univalent ligands by Abs of the most prevalent type (mol. wt. 150,000, IgG class, see Chap. 14). Two main points are apparent.

1. As saturation is approached (**c** becomes very large), the limiting value of **r** is 2. Thus, there are two binding sites per Ab molecule. (Less common Abs with five-fold higher molecular weights have ten binding sites per molecule; see IgM, Chap. 14.)

2. For a monoclonal Ab (the uniform Ab molecules secreted by a single clone of Ab-producing cells; see Chap. 14) the relation between r/c and r is linear (e.g.,

Fig. 13–2*D*), showing that the binding sites of such an Ab are identical. However, this relation is characteristically nonlinear for the polyclonal Abs isolated from conventional antisera (see Fig. 13–2*A–C*), because these Abs are produced by many different clones of Ab-producing cells; and even when the Abs are specific for the same epitope, they can differ considerably in intrinsic affinity (>10,000-fold is not unusual). For such a heterogeneous polyclonal population of Abs, an "average" value for intrinsic affinity, K_0, is usually defined, arbitrarily, by the free ligand concentration required for half the Ab binding sites to be occupied (see Table 13–1, footnote).

Some average intrinsic association constants for typical polyclonal Abs are shown in Table 13–1. With different conditions of immunization, differences as great as 100,000-fold in intrinsic affinity are observed among Ab molecules of the same specificity (see Chap. 16).

SPECIFICITY

The specificity of Abs is strikingly evident from differences in their reactivities with sets of closely related simple chemicals, as illustrated in Figures 13–3 and 13–4. Some other examples are seen in the large variations in

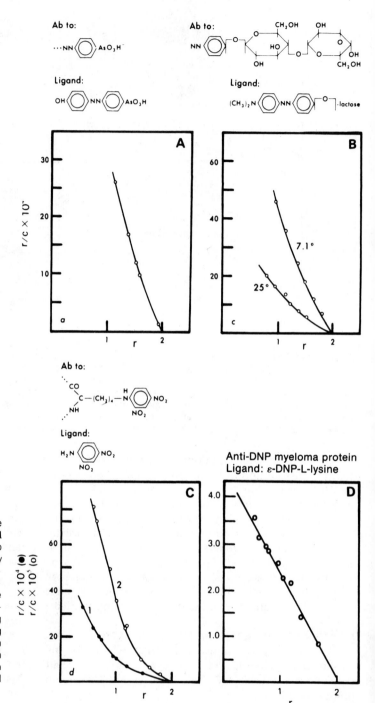

Figure 13–2. Specific binding of ligands plotted according to the Scatchard equation (equation 4). For all Ab–ligand systems (*A* through *C*), the extrapolation shows two combining sites per Ab molecule (mol. wt. 150,000, IgG class; see Chap. 14). In *B*, affinity is higher at 7°C than at 25°C. In *C*, two purified anti-2,4-dinitrophenyl (anti-DNP) Abs differ about 30-fold in affinity for dinitroaniline. In *D*, the anti-DNP protein was produced by a single clone of Ab-producing cells (myeloma tumor; see Chap. 14). Nonlinearity, showing heterogeneity with respect to affinity of binding sites, is pronounced in *B* and *C* but slight in *A*; linearity, showing uniformity of binding sites, is evident in *D*. (*A*, from data in Eisen HN, Karush F: J Am Chem Soc 71:363, 1949; *B*, from Data in Karush F: J Am Chem Soc 79:3380, 1957; *C*, from data in Eisen HN, Siskind G: Biochemistry 3:996, 1964; *D*, from data in Eisen HN et al: Cold Spring Harbor Symp Quant Biol 32:75, 1967)

affinity that result from small differences in ligand structure, shown in Figures 13–5 and 13–6. The following generalizations have been drawn from these and many other examples.

1. The ligands bound most strongly are those that resemble most closely the determinant groups of the im-

munogen. This generalization is part of the broad rule that **Abs react more effectively with the Ag that stimulated their formation than with other Ags;** within this context, the former is designated the **homologous Ag** and the latter heterologous Ags. Similarly, haptens that resemble most closely the haptenic groups of the immu-

TABLE 13–1. Intrinsic Association Constants for Representative Antibody–Ligand Interactions

Antibody Specific for	Ligand	Intrinsic Association Constants (K) (liters/mole)*
p-Azobenzenearsonate	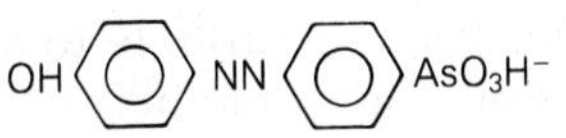 OH ⟨○⟩ NN ⟨○⟩ AsO$_3$H$^-$	3×10^5
p-Azobenzoate	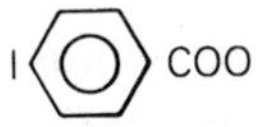 I ⟨○⟩ COO	4×10^4
ε-Dnp-lysyl	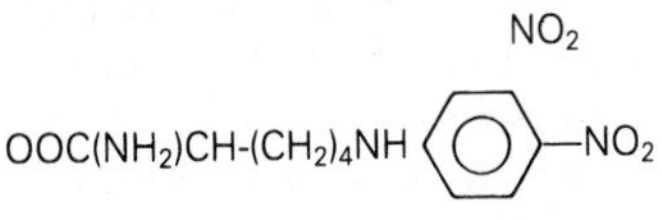 OOC(NH$_2$)CH-(CH$_2$)$_4$NH ⟨○⟩—NO$_2$ (NO$_2$)	1×10^7
p-Azophenyl-β-lactoside	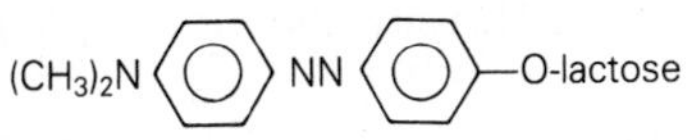 (CH$_3$)$_2$N ⟨○⟩ NN ⟨○⟩—O-lactose	2×10^5
Dnp in mono-Dnp-ribonuclease	Mono-Dnp-ribonuclease	1×10^6

Dnp = 2,4-dinitrophenyl.

* The value listed for each Ab is the reciprocal of free ligand concentration at half-saturation of the Ab. If the dissociation constant, instead of the association, were used, each value would be simply the free ligand concentration (rather than its reciprocal) at half-saturation of Ab. The choice of half-saturation to represent the diverse affinities of a heterogeneous (polyclonal) population of Ab molecules is a convention; it does not reflect a true "average."

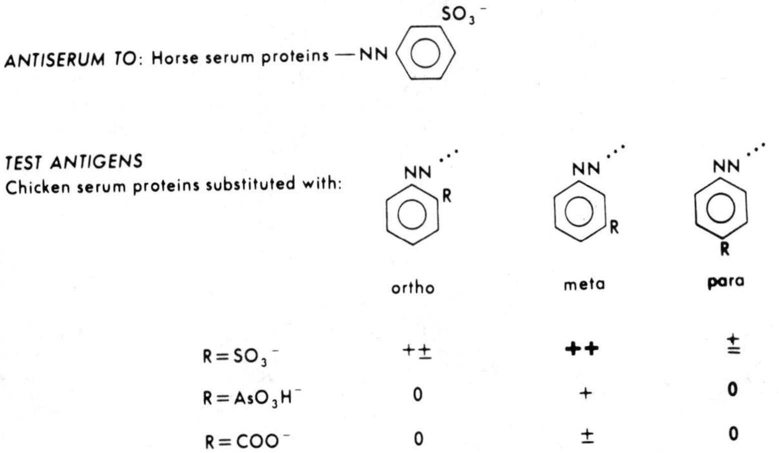

ANTISERUM TO: Horse serum proteins —NN ⟨○⟩ SO$_3^-$

TEST ANTIGENS
Chicken serum proteins substituted with:

	ortho	meta	para
R = SO$_3^-$	+±	++	±
R = AsO$_3$H$^-$	0	+	0
R = COO$^-$	0	±	0

Figure 13–3. Prominent effect of position and nature of acidic substituents of haptenic groups on the reaction between Abs to *m*-azobenzenesulfonate and various test Ags. *R* in the test Ag refers to the acidic substituents SO$_3^-$, AsO$_3$H$^-$, and COO$^-$. The homologous reaction is most intense (largest amount of precipitation) and is shown in heavy type. (Landsteiner K, van der Scheer J: J Exp Med 63:325, 1936)

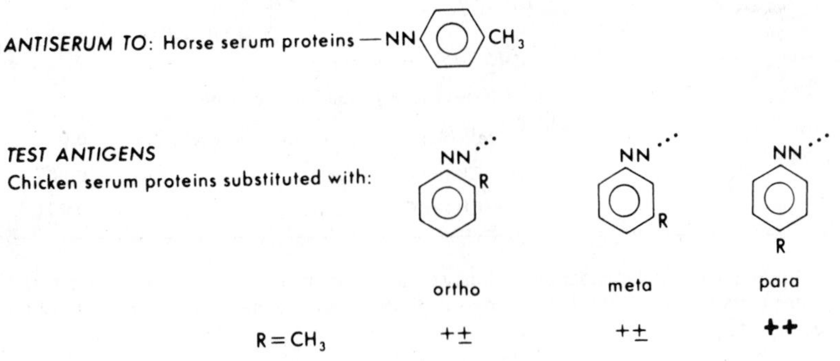

ANTISERUM TO: Horse serum proteins —NN ⟨○⟩ CH$_3$

TEST ANTIGENS
Chicken serum proteins substituted with:

	ortho	meta	para
R = CH$_3$	+±	+±	++

Figure 13–4. Effect of nature and position of uncharged substituents of haptenic groups on the reactions between Abs to the *p*-azotoluidine group and various test Ags. The homologous reaction is shown in heavy type. (Landsteiner K, van der Scheer J: J Exp Med 45:1045, 1927)

nogen are the homologous haptens. However, in view of the random process for generating the amino acid sequences that determine specificity (see Origin of Antibody Diversity, Chap. 14), it is not too surprising that rare Abs (termed **heteroclitic** Abs) are found to have higher affinity for another Ag than for the immunogen.

2. Those structural elements of the determinant group that project distally from the central mass of the immunizing Ag are immunodominant: they are especially influential in determining specificity. Thus, Abs to *p*-azophenyl-β-lactoside and to Dnp bind the terminal residues almost as well as they bind the larger haptenic structures that have these residues as their end groups: for example, compare lactose with a phenyl-β-lactoside (see Fig. 13–5) and dinitroaniline with ε-Dnp-lysine (see Fig. 13–6). A particularly striking example is seen in Abs

to human blood group substances (A, B, etc.) weighing more than a million daltons. Anti-A is specific for the terminal N-acetyl galactosamine residues of A, and anti-B is specific for the terminal galactose residues of B, despite great structural similarity in the rest of these huge mucopolysaccharide molecules. However, nonterminal residues also contribute to specific binding, sometimes decisively: for example, nonterminal mannosyl-rhamnose residues (see Fig. 13–16) in the lipopolysaccharides of various groups of *Salmonella*.

3. Abs are generally as discriminating as enzymes. For instance, some Abs readily distinguish between two molecules that differ only in the configuration about one carbon (e.g., glucose versus galactose, or D- versus L-tartrate; see also Fig. 13–5).

4. The specific binding of a ligand to an Ab molecule

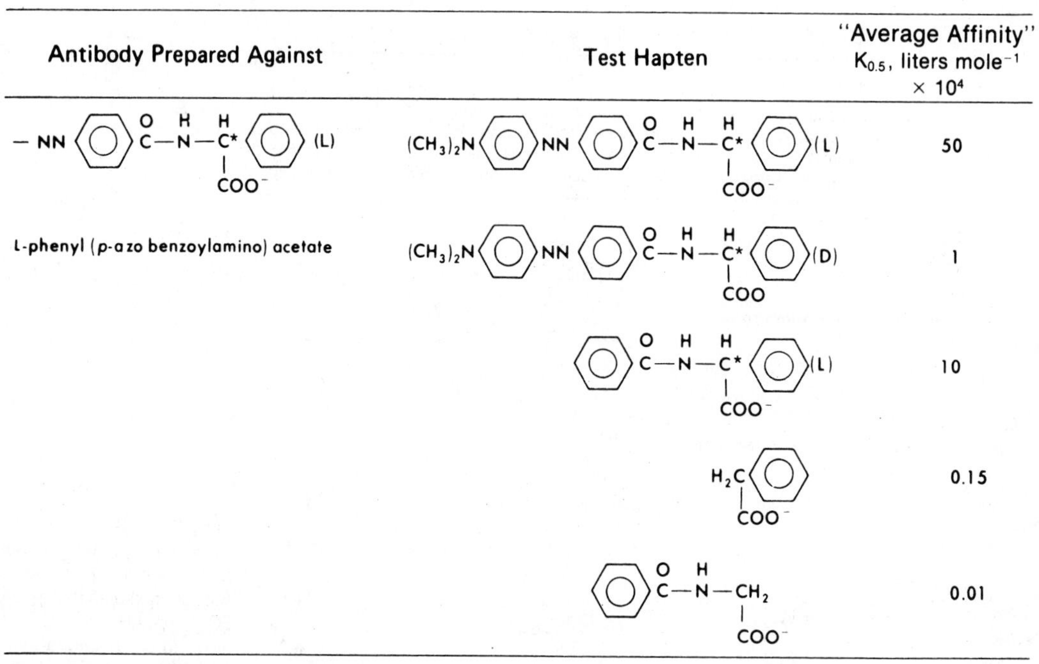

Figure 13–5. Specificity of Ab–hapten reactions; dependence of affinity on the structure of the hapten. In the top panel, the asterisks (*) mark the asymmetric carbon atom (D or L form) in the substituted phenyl acetate. (Karush F: J Am Chem Soc 78:5519, 1956; 79:3380, 1957).

Antibody Prepared Against	Test Hapten	"Average Affinity" $K_{0.5}$, liters mole^{-1} × 10^5
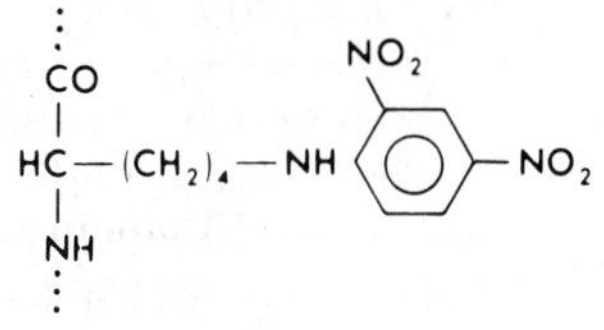 2,4-dinitrophenyl- L -lysyl group of Dnp protein	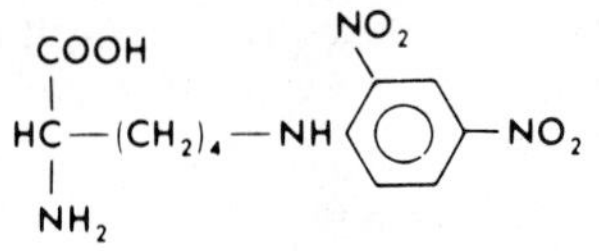 ϵ · Dnp · L -lysine	200
	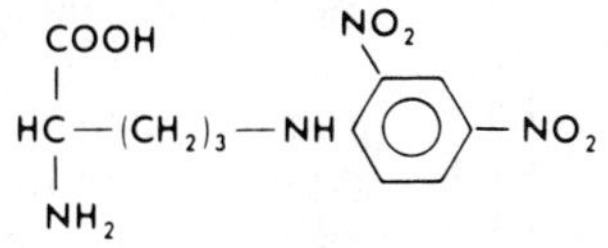 δ · Dnp · L -ornithine	80
	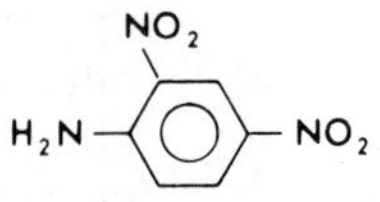 2, 4-dinitroaniline	20
	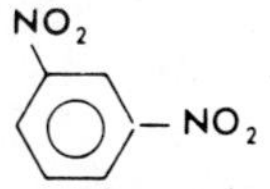 m-dinitrobenzene	8
	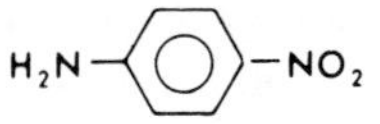 p-mononitroaniline	0.5

Figure 13—6. Specificity of Ab–hapten reactions; dependence of affinity on the structure of the hapten. The haptens that approximate the haptenic group of the immunogen are bound more strongly. (Eisen HN, Siskind GW: Biochemistry 3:996, 1964)

may be regarded as a competitive partition of the ligand between water and Ab-binding sites, which are relatively hydrophobic. Hence, ligands that are sparingly soluble in water, such as dinitrophenyl haptens, tend to form high-affinity complexes with Ab, whereas ligands that are highly soluble in water, such as sugars and organic ions (e.g., benzoate), tend to form more dissociable, lower-affinity complexes.

The strength of the overall bond between an Ab and a ligand reflects the sum of many noncovalent interactions between atomic groups of the ligand and side chains of amino acid residues in the Ab's binding site. The greater the sum, the more stable (i.e., the less dissociable) is the Ab–ligand complex.

Hydrogen bonds and van der Waals interactions account for most of the interactions, and for the latter, bond strength is inversely proportional to distance to the seventh power. Hence the stability of immune complexes is critically dependent on how closely the three-dimensional surface of the ligand fits the three-dimensional

contour of the Ab's combining site. Bulky substituents on ligands can hinder close approach and diminish binding (**steric hindrance**).

Although binding strength depends enormously on **complementarity** between the interacting surfaces, chemical features are also important. For example, binding is greater when the interacting groups attract, such as when an anionic group of the ligand is close to a cationic group of the Ab or a hydrogen-bond acceptor of the ligand is close to a hydrogen-bond donor of the Ab. Trying to understand how Abs and Ags combined, immunologists at the turn of the century imagined that they fit together like a "lock and key." This metaphor is still valid; indeed, it is dramatically reinforced by recent x-ray crystallographic studies of an Ab–Ag complex (see Chap. 14, Fig. 14–25).

SPECIFICITY AND AFFINITY. The specificity of an Ab refers to its capacity to discriminate between ligands of similar structure: **the greater the difference in affinity**

for two closely related structures, the more specific the Ab. However, discrimination depends not only on the magnitude of the difference in affinity for different ligands, but also on how the Ab–ligand reaction is measured. Most assays (e.g., precipitation, below) have an **affinity threshold,** below which reactions are not detected. Consequently, an Ab with only a moderate difference in affinity for its homologous ligand, X, and for a potentially cross-reacting ligand, X', will discriminate sharply between them if the affinity for X is just above and the affinity for X' just below the threshold. In contrast, an Ab with a large difference in affinity for X and for X' will be poorly discriminating if both affinities are well above the threshold. Abs for carbohydrates generally have low affinity for their ligands, and this may account for their extraordinary ability to discriminate between closely related Ags and their resulting great practical value in diagnostic typing of blood-group substances on red blood cells and of bacteria through their cell wall polysaccharides (e.g., salmonellae).

CARRIER SPECIFICITY. In antisera made against a hapten–protein conjugate, some Abs seem to react exclusively with the haptenic group: they combine no better with the immunogen than with other conjugates in which the same hapten is attached to different proteins. However, many other Abs in the same antisera exhibit carrier specificity: for maximal reactivity (highest affinity), they require not only the haptenic group and the amino acid residue to which it is attached but also (in various degrees) neighboring residues of the immunogen. Still other Abs in these antisera react only with epitopes on the protein moiety of the conjugate.

Reactions with Macromolecules

The complexes formed by Abs and small univalent ligands, considered in previous sections, are soluble. With macromolecular Ags, however, the complexes frequently become insoluble and thus precipitate from solution. Although the Abs responsible for this precipitin reaction were once regarded as members of a unique class, called "precipitins," it is now clear that most Abs can precipitate their Ags.

THE QUANTITATIVE PRECIPITIN REACTION

The precipitin reaction was formerly used to measure Abs in serum, but it lacked precision until Heidelberger and Avery found, in 1923, that an important Ag of the pneumococcus was a polysaccharide. With this Ag, it was possible to establish unambiguously that the Abs precipitated from serum are proteins; hence, procedures for measuring proteins in general could be used to ana-

lyze the precipitated Abs because the included Ag did not interfere. The discovery also revealed that some macromolecules besides proteins can be immunogenic.

The precipitin reaction has been replaced as a routine assay by faster and more sensitive methods (see Radioimmunoassays and Enzyme-Linked Assays, below), but it is still important for understanding the general characteristics of Ab reactions with high-molecular-weight Ags. To illustrate the reaction, consider an antiserum prepared by immunizing a rabbit with pneumococci encapsulated by a polysaccharide. When the purified capsular polysaccharide is added to the antiserum (but not to the preimmunization serum), a precipitate appears. Analysis of the washed precipitate reveals only protein and the polysaccharide. Moreover, when the precipitated protein and polysaccharide are separated (see Appendix), the protein recovered is evidently purified Ab because it can be precipitated again, completely and specifically, by a fresh sample of the polysaccharide.

As is shown in Figure 13–7 and in Table 13–2, in a series of tubes with the same volume of antiserum, the amount of protein (i.e., Ab) precipitated from a given volume of antiserum increases with the amount of polysaccharide added up to a maximum, beyond which larger amounts of the Ag lead to progressively less precipitation. The precipitation of a maximum amount of Ab by an optimal amount of Ag may appear inconsistent with the binding reaction discussed earlier, in which the number of Ab sites occupied by ligand increases progressively to saturation without going through a maximum. This apparent discrepancy is attributable to special features of precipitation, which are discussed below under Lattice Theory.

TABLE 13–2. *Precipitin Reaction With a Polysaccharide as Antigen*

Tube no.	Antigen (S3) Added (mg)	Total Protein (or Antibody) Precipitated (mg)	Supernatant Fluid Contains
1	0.02	1.82	Excess Ab
2	0.06	4.79	Excess Ab
3	0.08	5.41	Excess Ab
4	0.10	5.79	Excess Ab
5	0.15	6.13	No Ab, no S3
6	0.20	6.23	Slight excess S3
7	0.50	5.87	Excess S3
8	1.00	3.76	Excess S3
9	2.00	2.10	Excess S3

The Ag (S3) is purified capsular polysaccharide of type 3 pneumococcus. Each tube contained 0.7 ml of antiserum obtained by injecting rabbits repeatedly with formalin-killed encapsulated type 3 pneumococci.

(Based on Heidelberger M, Kendall FE: J Exp Med 65:647, 1937)

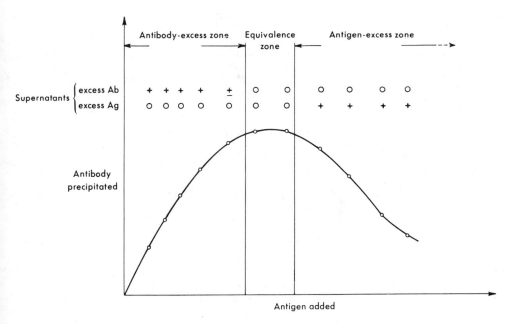

Figure 13–7. Precipitation curve for a monospecific system: one Ag and the corresponding Abs.

When the Ag is a protein instead of a polysaccharide (Table 13–3), the amount of precipitated Ag must be subtracted from the total amount of protein in the precipitate in order to measure the precipitated Ab. The subtraction is simple, because in certain regions of the precipitin curve (Ab-excess and equivalence zones in Fig. 13–7) the total amount of Ag added has been shown (e.g., with radiolabelled Ags) to be precipitated.

ZONES OF THE PRECIPITIN CURVE. Useful information can be obtained from qualitative tests of the supernatant fluids to detect unreacted Ab and unreacted Ag. For this purpose, a portion of each supernatant fluid is mixed with a small amount of fresh Ag (to detect excess Ab), and another portion is mixed with a small amount of fresh antiserum (to detect excess Ag). If the Ag–Ab system is **monospecific,** i.e., consists of only one Ag and the corre-

TABLE 13–3. Precipitin Reaction With a Protein as Antigen

Tube No.	Antigen (EAc) Added (mg)	Total Protein Precipitated (mg)	Antibody Precipitated by Difference (mg)	Supernatant Test	Ab/Ag in Precipitates Weight Ratio	Mole Ratio
1	0.057	0.975	0.918	Excess Ab	16.1	4.0
2	0.250	3.29	3.04	Excess Ab	12.1	3.0
3	0.312	3.95	3.64	Excess Ab	11.7	2.9
4	0.463	4.96	4.50	No Ab, no EAc	9.7	2.4
5	0.513	5.19	4.68	No Ab, trace EAc	9.1	2.3
6	0.562	5.16	(4.60)	Excess EAc	(8.2)	(2.1)
7	0.775	4.56	(3.79)	Excess EAc	(4.9)	(1.2)
8	1.22	2.58	—	Excess EAc	—	—
9	3.06	0.262	—	Excess EAc	—	—

Each tube contained 1.0 ml of antiserum obtained by injecting rabbits repeatedly with alum-precipitated crystallized chicken ovalbumin (EAc).

The Ab content of precipitates in tubes 6–9 could not be determined by difference because too much EAc remained in the supernatants. The latter was measured independently in the supernatants of tubes 6 and 7, allowing an estimate to be made of EAc and Ab in the corresponding precipitates (values in parentheses).

Mole ratio Ab/Ag was estimated by assuming mol wt for EAc and Ab of 40,000 and 160,000, respectively.

(Based on Heidelberger M, Kendall FE: J Exp Med 62:697, 1935)

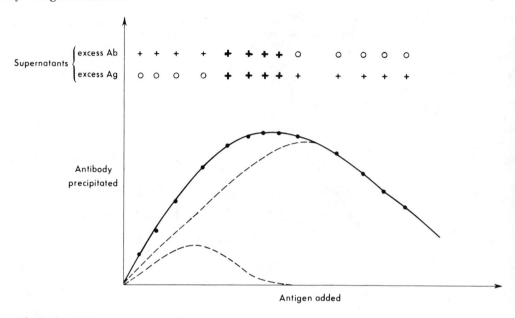

Figure 13–8. Precipitin curve for a multispecific system. The precipitation observed (—•—) is the sum of two or more precipitation reactions (---). The significant difference from the monospecific system shown in Figure 13–7 is that some supernatant fluids have **both** excess Ag and excess Abs (indicated by pluses in heavy type).

sponding Abs, the nonprecipitated reactants are distributed as shown in the precipitin curve of Figure 13–7: on the ascending limb, or **Ab-excess zone,** the fluids contain free Ab; on the descending limb, or **Ag-excess zone,** they contain free Ag. In the **equivalence zone** or equivalence point, the supernatant fluids are usually devoid of both detectable Ab and detectable Ag, and the amount of Ab in the corresponding precipitate represents the total amount of Ab in the volume of serum tested.

However, many Ags considered to be pure by conventional criteria are contaminated by trace amounts of unrelated Ags, which can also provoke immune responses. The precipitin reaction is then the sum of two (or more) independent monospecific reactions. In this situation (Fig. 13–8), supernatant fluids often contain both unreacted Abs and unreacted Ag, because the Ag-excess zone of one system overlaps the Ab-excess zone of another. As we shall see later, the precipitin reaction in agar gel provides a more sensitive test for multiplicity, and it also provides an estimate of the number of different systems.

LATTICE THEORY

One molecule of a typical protein Ag can bind many Ab molecules, and the Ab:Ag ratio in precipitates varies nearly linearly over the Ab-excess zone with the amount of Ag added (Fig. 13–9). With Ab in large excess, the mole ratio greatly exceeds 1. At the other end, the Ag-excess

zone, the mole ratio of Ab:Ag tends toward a limiting value of 1 (see Fig. 13–9).

To account for precipitation, and for varying ratios, Marrack, and Heidelberger and Kendall, suggested that Ab–Ag aggregates could form in such a way that each Ag

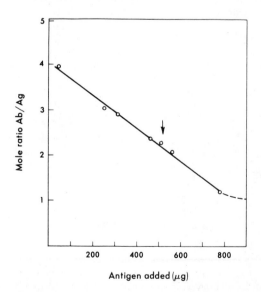

Figure 13–9. Change in the Ab:Ag ratio of precipitates with increasing amount of Ag added to a fixed volume of an antiserum. Chicken ovalbumin (EAc) is the Ag, and the serum is rabbit anti-EAc. The **arrow** marks the equivalence zone. (Data are those of Table 13–3)

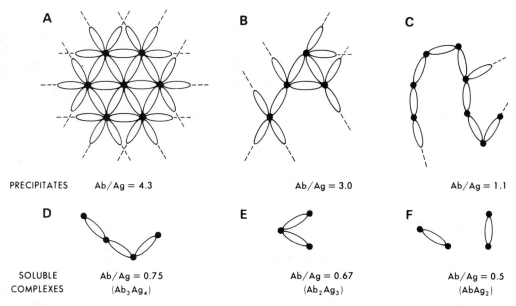

PRECIPITATES   Ab/Ag = 4.3   Ab/Ag = 3.0   Ab/Ag = 1.1

SOLUBLE   Ab/Ag = 0.75   Ab/Ag = 0.67   Ab/Ag = 0.5
COMPLEXES   (Ab_3Ag_4)   (Ab_2Ag_3)   ($AbAg_2$)

Figure 13–10. Schematic diagram of immune precipitates and soluble complexes according to the lattice theory. Numbers refer to mole ratios of Ab to Ag. Dotted lines with precipitates indicate that the complexes continue to extend as shown. The precipitates may be visualized as those found in the Ab-excess zone *(A)*, the equivalence zone *(B)*, and the Ag-excess zone *(C)*. The soluble complexes correspond to those in supernatant fluids in moderate *(D)*, far *(E)*, or extreme *(F)* Ag excess. *Black circles,* Ag molecules; *open ellipses,* Ab molecules (bivalent).

molecule is linked to more than one Ab molecule and each Ab molecule is linked to more than one Ag molecule. When the aggregates exceed some critical mass, they settle out of solution spontaneously. The assumption that Abs are multivalent was validated many years later by equilibrium dialysis with univalent haptens, as noted above (see Fig. 13–2*A*).

As Figure 13–10 shows, alternation of multivalent Ag and Ab molecules (i.e., the lattice theory) accounts for the wide and continuous variations in Ab:Ag ratios in precipitates (Fig. 13–9). When the Ag is labeled and can thus be measured directly, precipitates formed in the presence of excess Ag are found to have Ab:Ag mole ratios that approach 1 as a limiting value, suggesting a large linear aggregate with alternating Ab and Ag molecules (. . . Ab•Ag•Ab•Ag•Ab•Ag . . .). In the region of Ag excess, complexes of even lower Ab:Ag ratios are formed, but they are small and remain in the supernatant fluid as **soluble complexes** (Fig. 13–10*D–F*); they account for the descending limb of the precipitin curve (see Fig. 13–7). The soluble complexes have mole ratios that differ considerably; e.g., 0.75 (Ab_3Ag_4) in slight Ag excess, 0.67 (Ab_2Ag_3) in substantial Ag excess. In extreme excess, the ratio approaches 0.5 ($AbAg_2$), as expected from the bivalence of most Ab molecules.

VALENCE AND COMPLEXITY OF PROTEIN ANTIGENS

The multivalency of many polysaccharides results from their repeating residues (e.g., Fig. 13–14). With proteins, however, the chemical basis for their multivalency is less obvious. Groups of amino acid residues hardly ever recur as repetitive sequences in a single polypeptide chain; hence, each antigenic determinant (epitope), consisting of perhaps 10 to 20 residues, is likely to occur only once per chain. Nevertheless, protein molecules that consist of but a single chain usually behave as though they are multivalent. The reason is that the corresponding antisera are nearly always polyclonal and contain mixtures of Abs to the chain's many different epitopes. Thus, proteolytic cleavage of bovine serum albumin (BSA, one chain of 70,000 daltons) yields several large fragments, each capable of forming a specific precipitate with different sets of Abs in antiserum prepared against the intact BSA molecule. Further evidence is supplied by the model system illustrated in Figure 13–11: the small ligand R–X, in which the functional groups R and X each occur once per molecule, does not precipitate with an anti-R serum or with an anti-X serum but does precipitate with a mixture of the two.

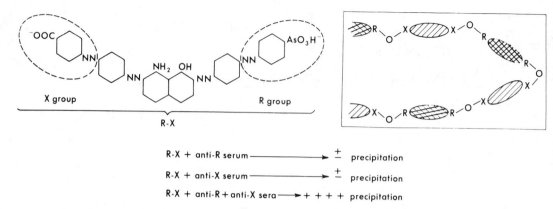

R-X + anti-R serum ⟶ ± precipitation

R-X + anti-X serum ⟶ ± precipitation

R-X + anti-R + anti-X sera ⟶ + + + + precipitation

Figure 13–11. Cooperation between Abs of different specificities (anti-R and anti-X) in the precipitation reaction with a synthetic ligand, R–X. (The small amount of precipitate (±) formed by R–X with anti-R alone or with anti-X alone is probably due to some aggregation of R–X). The inset shows a hypothetical segment of the precipitate with alternation of bivalent anti-R and anti-X antibodies with the R–X antigen (designated R–O–X to indicate the naphthalene spacer). (Based on Pauling L, Pressman D, Campbell DH: J Am Chem Soc 66:330, 1944)

The valence of an Ag depends on the population of Abs with which it reacts. The dependence is illustrated with bovine pancreatic ribonuclease (one chain per molecule), to which one Dnp group has been added (mono-Dnp-RNase). In the antiserum made against this immunogen, some Abs are anti-Dnp and others are specific for various other epitopes. Mono-Dnp-RNase behaves as a multivalent molecule with this antiserum, giving a classic

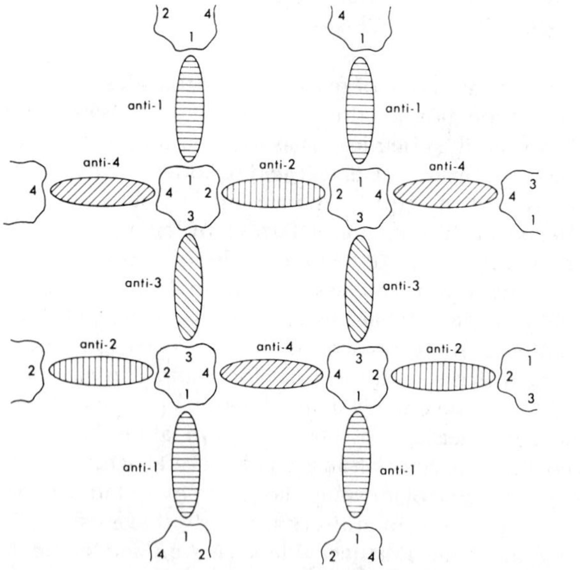

Figure 13–12. Diversity of Abs formed against a single Ag and their cooperation in the precipitation reaction with that Ag. The Ag is assumed to have four epitopes, numbered 1 through 4. Each set of Abs (anti-1, anti-2, etc.) is probably heterogeneous with respect to affinity for the corresponding epitope.

precipitin reaction, whereas if the anti-Dnp molecules are isolated from the antiserum and then mixed with mono-Dnp-RNase, only soluble complexes are formed because the same Ag is univalent with respect to this particular set of Ab molecules. These observations emphasize the operational nature of the definition of Ag valence: **a given molecule of Ag can be univalent with respect to some Ab molecules and multivalent with respect to others.**

Although Ags usually have many different epitopes, it is important to emphasize that **the binding sites of any single Ab molecule are identical.** That they are always specific for the same epitope (**homospecific**) is explained by the symmetrical structure of Ab molecules (see Chap. 14) and by the one cell–one Ab rule (see Chaps. 15 and 16).

All of these considerations lead to the schematic view of the precipitin reaction shown in Figure 13–12: **precipitation of a protein Ag usually depends on a mosaic of epitopes in the Ag and the cooperative effects of Abs against different epitopes.**

NONPRECIPITATING ANTIBODIES. The precipitin reaction involves two distinct stages: rapid formation of soluble Ab–Ag complexes, and slow aggregation of these complexes to form visible precipitates. By measuring free Ag concentrations, it has been found that the specific interactions are completed within a few minutes, whereas precipitate formation usually requires several days to reach completion. However, even with unlimited time, not all Abs precipitate their Ags. One reason is the low affinity of some Abs. To precipitate them, the Ag would have to be added at high concentrations in order

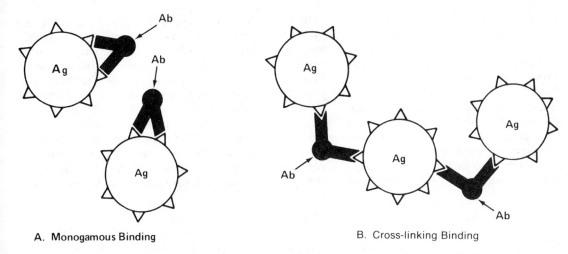

A. Monogamous Binding   B. Cross-linking Binding

Figure 13–13. Monogamous bivalent bonding *(A)* leading to cyclic Ab–Ag complexes, is contrasted with conventional binding *(B)*, which leads to cross-linking of Ag particles (. . . Ag●Ab●Ab . . .). (Based on Hornick CC, Karush F: Immunochem 9:325, 1972)

to occupy a significant proportion of the Ab's combining sites; if this Ag level is in large stoichiometric excess, only small soluble Ab–Ag complexes are formed (see Fig. 13–10*D–F*). Another reason is that some Ab molecules combine preferentially with two (identical) epitopes of a single Ag particle, forming cyclic complexes rather than cross-linked ones (Ag●Ab●Ag; Fig. 13–13). This type of "multivalent" binding (called **monogamous bivalency** by Karush) requires that a given epitope occur repetitively on the Ag surface as in hapten–protein conjugates, polysaccharides, and many multichain proteins; it is commonplace with surface epitopes of viruses and of bacteria and other cells. Abs that combine specifically in this way with cells do not agglutinate (i.e., cross-link) them and are sometimes called **blocking** or **incomplete** Abs (see below).

For Abs that can form monogamous complexes, the equilibrium constant with multivalent ligands can be much higher than with the corresponding univalent ligand. For instance, the reaction between anti-Dnp Abs and Dnp-bacteriophage, with many Dnp groups per phage particle, has an association constant about 100,000-fold greater than the reaction between the same Abs and univalent Dnp-lysine (e.g., 10^{12} versus 10^7 liters/ mole). Evidently the two bonds in the monogamous complex greatly decrease the probability that the Ab–Ag pair will separate: **it is likely that when one bond dissociates, the other will hold the Ab–Ag pair together, allowing the dissociated bond to form again.** Because viral and bacterial surfaces usually have repeating, identical antigenic groups, the formation of such cyclic complexes can explain why exceedingly low concentrations of some Abs (e.g., 10^{-12} moles/liter or about 1.5×10^{-4} μg/ ml) can neutralize pathogenic microbes *in vivo*.

REVERSIBILITY OF PRECIPITATION. After a precipitate has formed, its complexes can dissociate and reequilibrate with the introduction of additional Ag. When the additional Ag is in sufficient excess, small soluble complexes are formed, and the precipitate dissolves. This reversibility provides the basis for many of the procedures used to isolate purified Abs. In practice, however, it may be difficult to observe dissociation. Hence, the formation of Ab–Ag aggregates was formerly believed to be irreversible.

Apparent irreversibility is especially striking with many Ab–virus complexes: some are so stable that they do not perceptibly dissociate even when a mixture of virus and antiserum is diluted many thousandfold, with a corresponding reduction in the concentrations of free virus and free Ab. The extraordinary stability of such complexes probably derives from monogamous multivalent binding (see above), which is made possible especially by the many repeating epitopes characteristically found on the surface of viruses. Even ordinary single-bonded complexes of Ab with small univalent haptens can appear to be irreversible if the intrinsic association constant is sufficiently high ($>10^8$ liters/mole) such an Ab cannot be completely freed of hapten by dialysis. Nevertheless, reversibility can always be demonstrated by "exchange": the addition of free ligand in great excess will replace the ligand molecules that appeared to be irreversibly bound.

AVIDITY VERSUS FUNCTIONAL AFFINITY. As noted before, the stability of Ab–Ag complexes increases with Ab affinity. However, other properties of the heterogenous populations of Ab molecules in antisera are also important for the stability of the complexes formed by antisera and Ags. **One property is diversity itself:** a diverse Ab population that recognizes many epitopes of an Ag will form a more stable lattice with that Ag than a population that recognizes only a few of the epitopes (see Fig. 13–12). Moreover, Abs having more binding sites per molecule will tend to form more stable complexes than Abs with fewer sites per molecule (cf. IgM and IgG Abs, Chap. 14), and nonspecific properties, such as net charge, can have large effects on aggregation and on close packing of macromolecules. Because of these complexities, the term **avidity** is often used as a qualitative (and vague) description of the overall tendency of Abs to combine with a complex Ag. (When measurements of avidity are made, they are typically based on particular assays that are applicable to particular Ab–Ag reactions, e.g., measuring the fraction of total Abs in antisera that are precipitated by particular amounts of Ag; the resulting values cannot be compared from one Ab–Ag system to another.) However, an association constant for the binding of Abs to a multivalent Ag has been measured under some circumstances and found to be greatly enhanced over the association constant for the reaction of the same Abs with the corresponding ligand in univalent form. The enhancement arises because when one Ab–ligand bond

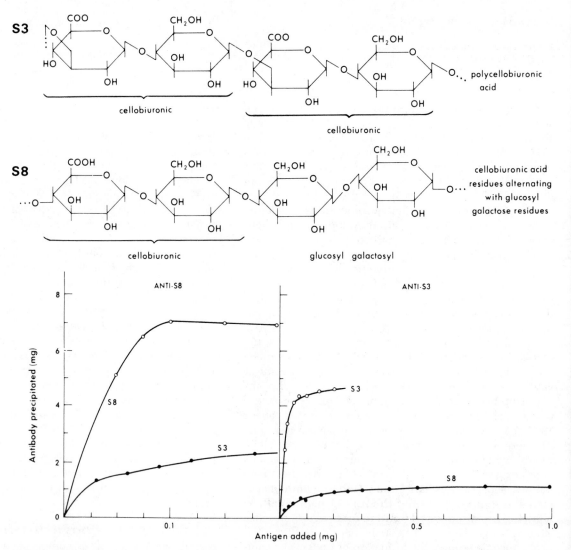

Figure 13–14. Cross-reactions between S3 and S8, capsular polysaccharides of pneumococci of types 3 and 8, respectively. *(Left)* Horse antiserum to type 8 pneumococcus reacted with purified S8 and S3 polysaccharides. *(Right)* Horse antiserum to type 3 pneumococcus, reacted with S3 and S8 polysaccharide. (Based on Heidelberger M: J Exp Med 65:487, 1937; Heidelberger M et al: J Exp Med 75:35, 1942)

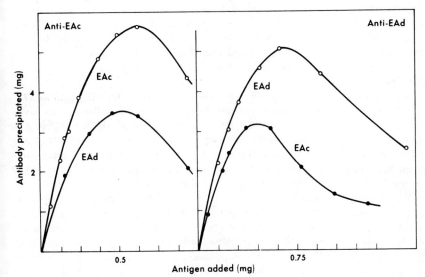

Figure 13–15. Cross-reactions between chicken and duck ovalbumin, EAc and EAd, respectively. *(Left)* Rabbit antiserum to EAc reacted with EAc and EAd. *(Right)* Rabbit antiserum to EAd reacted with EAd and EAc. (Based on Osler AG, Heidelberger M: J Immunol 60:327, 1948)

dissociates, other bonds hold the bivalent (or multivalent) Ab to the multivalent Ag, allowing the dissociated bond to form again (see Monogamous Bivalency, above).

The association constant for the reaction between bivalent (or multivalent) Ab and multivalent ligand has been termed the **functional affinity** to contrast it with intrinsic affinity, which is the association constant for an Ab's representative individual site (see Affinity, above).

CROSS-REACTIONS

Besides reacting with its immunogen, an antiserum almost invariably cross-reacts with certain other Ags (heterologous Ags) that are sufficiently similar to the immunogen; some cross-reactions are illustrated in Figures 13–14, 13–15, and 13–16. Sometimes the apparent cross-reactions are secondary to shared impurities. Most im-

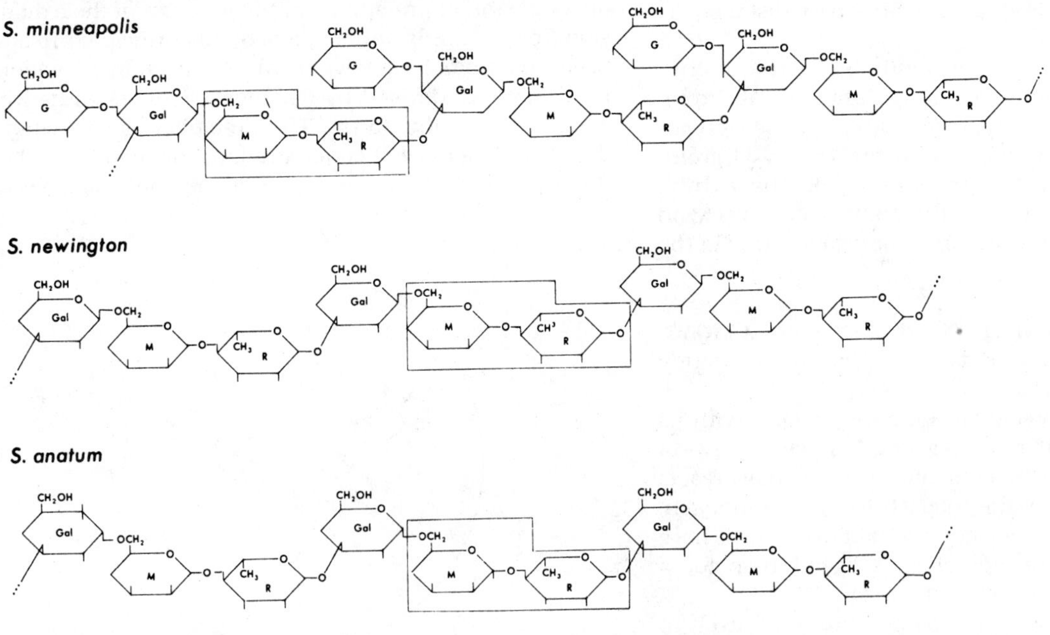

S. minneapolis

S. newington

S. anatum

Figure 13–16. Portion of the cell wall lipopolysaccharide of three strains of salmonellae. The strains are assigned to the same group (O) because of their serologic cross-reaction attributable due to their common mannosyl rhamnose residues (boxed). They are also distinguishable serologically because each has some unique structural feature, e.g., the terminal glucose *(G)* residue in *S. minneapolis,* and the α or β glycosidic bond linking galactose *(Gal)* to mannose *(M)*. (Based on Robbins PW, Uchida T: Fed Proc 21:702, 1962)

munogens are complex mixtures of antigenic molecules. This is obviously true when the immunogen is a cell. It is also usually true, though less obvious, with purified proteins, because these are nearly always contaminated with other proteins. Even at trace levels (e.g., 1%) the contaminants can elicit the formation of Abs. Hence antisera usually consist of several Ab populations, each reactive with a different Ag (e.g., see Fig. 13–24, below).

CROSS-REACTIONS ATTRIBUTABLE TO COMMON OR SIMILAR FUNCTIONAL GROUPS. We have already noted that a single protein contains many different epitopes, each of which can evoke the formation of a corresponding set of Abs. If two different Ag molecules happen to have one or more epitopes in common, they usually cross-react. This type of cross-reaction is frequently observed with polysaccharides, and it provides the basis for classifying many groups of closely related bacteria (see, for instance, Fig. 13–14). For example, the capsular polysaccharide of the type 3 pneumococcus is a linear polymer of cellobiuronic acid residues (β-1,4-glucuronidoglucose), whereas in type 8 pneumococci, these residues alternate with glucosyl-galactose residues. Hence antisera to either Ag cross-react extensively with the other (see Fig. 13–14). Similar cross-reactions with protein Ags are infrequent unless they are closely related in evolution and hence are similar in sequence. Before DNA sequences could be determined, cross-reactions between homologous proteins of closely related species served as a crude indication of evolutionary distance between species.

Cross-reacting groups need not be identical; they need only be sufficiently similar. For example, Abs to *m*-azobenzenesulfonate cross-react with *m*-azobenzenearsonate (see Fig. 13–3) and Abs to the Dnp-lysyl group cross-react with 2,4,6-trinitrobenzene. **All Abs exhibit some cross-reactions:** i.e., they bind some Ags with determinant groups that are not identical to those in the immunogen.

GENERAL CHARACTERISTICS OF CROSS-REACTIONS. The following generalizations are drawn from the study of many cross-reactions.

1. An antiserum precipitates more copiously with its immunogen than with cross-reacting Ags (see Figs. 13–14 and 13–15), because a heterologous ligand usually reacts with only a fraction of the total Ab to the immunogen, and Abs of a given specificity will almost always have greater affinity for the homologous ligand than for a cross-reacting ligand (see Figs 13–5 and 13–6).

2. Different antisera to a given immunogen are likely to differ in the extent of their cross-reactions with heterologous Ags.

3. Fewer cross-reactions are exhibited by low- than by high-affinity Abs (see Specificity and Affinity, above). Be-

cause polysaccharide–antipolysaccharide systems are, in general, characterized by low affinities, this rule accounts for the great specificity of the sera used to type bacteria and red blood cells according to their surface polysaccharide J antigens (see Chap. 23).

REMOVAL OF CROSS-REACTING ANTIBODIES (ADSORPTION AND ABSORPTION). Before an antiserum is sufficiently monospecific for use as an analytic reagent, it is usually necessary to remove certain cross-reacting Abs by binding them to the cross-reacting Ags. Large complexes (e.g., precipitates or Abs bound to cells) are easily removed along with the cross-reacting Abs. However, when the complexes are soluble and difficult to remove, cross-reacting ligand may be added in large excess to saturate the cross-reacting Abs, eliminating them functionally but not physically. In a frequently used method, the antiserum is passed over a column of agarose beads to which the cross-reacting Ag is attached: the cross-reacting Abs stick to the column, and other Abs emerge with the "pass-through." We shall use the terms **adsorption** when Abs are removed by particulate Ags and **absorption** when they are neutralized by reaction with soluble Ags.

PRECIPITIN REACTION IN GELS

When an Ab and its Ag are placed in different regions of an agar gel, they diffuse toward each other and form an opaque band of precipitate at the junction of their diffusion fronts. Simple applications of this principle provide useful methods for analyzing Ab–Ag reactions. A widely used method, devised by Ouchterlony, is illustrated in Figures 13–17 and 13–18. The precipitate forms where the Ab and Ag meet at concentrations that correspond to the equivalence zone in conventional precipitin reac-

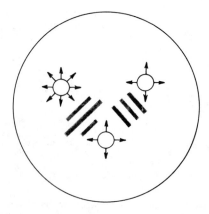

Figure 13–17. Gel diffusion precipitin reaction. The antibodies and antigens diffuse radially from the wells (O) in which they were placed. Darkened areas are opaque bands of precipitate (Ouchterlony method).

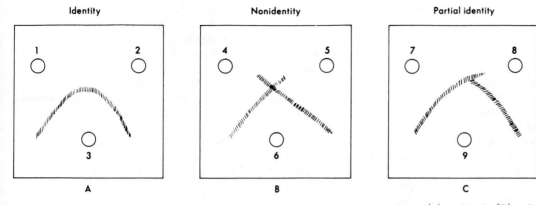

Figure 13–18. Double-diffusion precipitin reactions in agar gel illustrating reactions of identity *(A)*, nonidentity *(B)*, and partial identity *(C)*. In *A*, the same Ag was placed in wells *1* and *2* and the antiserum in well *3*. In *B*, different Ags were placed in wells *4* and *5*, and a mixture of the respective antisera to both were placed in well *6*. In *C*, an Ag and its antiserum were placed in wells *7* and *9*, respectively, and a cross-reacting Ag was placed in well *8*. Because rates of diffusion vary inversely with molecular weight, the curvature of the precipitin band also provides a clue to the molecular weight of the Ag provided Ag and Ab are present in roughly equivalent amounts. If the Ag and Ab have about the same molecular weight, the precipitation band appears as a straight line; if not, the band is concave toward the reactant of higher molecular weight.

tions. If the concentration of either the added Ab or the Ag is raised, the band forms closer to the other well.

The arrangements shown in Figures 13–18 and 13–19 are particularly useful for comparing different Ags for the presence of identical or cross-reacting components. The samples are placed in adjacent wells, and the corresponding Ab is placed in the center well. If the two pre-

cipitin bands fuse completely at their contiguous ends (see Fig. 13–18*A*), the pattern is termed the **reaction of identity:** it is seen whenever indistinguishable Ab–Ag systems react in adjacent fields. If, however, unrelated Ags are placed in adjacent wells and diffuse toward a central well that contains Abs for each of them, the two precipitin bands form independently and cross (**reaction of nonidentity;** see Fig. 13–18*B*). If the Ag in one of the wells and the antiserum in the central well constitute a homologous pair, and if the Ag in an adjoining well is a cross-reacting Ag, the precipitation bands fuse but form a spurlike projection that extends toward the cross-reacting Ag (**reaction of partial identity** or **cross-reaction;** see Fig. 13–18*C*).

From what is known of precipitin reactions in liquid, the spur can be readily interpreted: it represents the reaction between homologous Ag and those Ab molecules that do not combine with the cross-reacting Ag and hence diffuse past its precipitation band. Because these non-cross-reacting Abs represent only a fraction of the total Ab involved in the homologous precipitin reaction (see Figs. 13–14 and 13–15, for example), the spur is usually less dense than the band from which it projects, and it tends to have increased curvature toward the antiserum well.

In the event that neither of the Ags is homologous with respect to the antiserum (i.e., neither is the immunogen), a pattern of partial identity might be observed, with the spur projecting toward the less-reactive Ag, or there might be partial fusion with two crossing spurs, indicating that some Abs react only with one of the cross-reacting Ags and some only with the other.

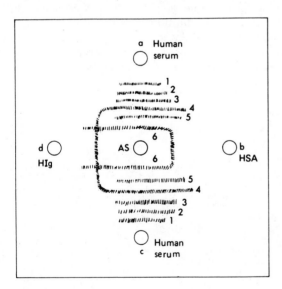

Figure 13–19. Use of purified Ags to identify components of a complex series of precipitin bands. Center well *(AS)* contains rabbit antiserum prepared against unfractionated human serum. Wells *a* and *c* contain human serum; well *b* has purified human serum albumin *(HSA)*, and well *d* has a purified human immunoglobulin *(HIg)*. Thus, band *4* corresponds to HIg and band *6* to HSA.

If one well contains a mixture of different Ags and the facing well contains Abs to several of them, the **number of bands** formed between the wells represents the minimum number of Ab–Ag systems involved. Individual bands may be identified by placing known Ags in adjacent wells, as in Figure 13–19.

Double diffusion in two dimensions provides a simple means for evaluating cross-reactions observed in other assays. Thus cross-reactions that arise from a common impurity can usually be recognized unambiguously. On the other hand, when two purified Ags, such as chicken and duck ovalbumins (see Fig. 13–15), give rise to a cross-reaction, gel diffusion analysis cannot decide whether their common epitopes are identical or only similar: in both cases, partial fusion would be observed, with a spur that extends toward the cross-reacting Ag (see Fig. 13–18C).

AGGLUTINATION REACTIONS

Cells in suspension, such as bacteria or red blood cells, are usually clumped (agglutinated) when mixed with their antisera. The principles are fundamentally the same as those described above for reactions with soluble Ags. Agglutination provides a rapid method for identifying various bacteria, fungi, and types of red blood cells; conversely, with the use of known cells, it can detect and roughly quantitate Abs in sera.

MECHANISMS OF AGGLUTINATION. Agglutination is carried out in physiologic salt solution (0.15M NaCl). The ionic strength is important, for at neutral pH, bacteria ordinarily bear a net negative surface charge, which must be adequately damped by counterions before cells can approach each other closely enough for Ab molecules to form specific bridges between them. Hence, even with Abs bound specifically to bacteria, agglutination may not occur if the salt concentration is too low (e.g., $<10^{-3}$M NaCl). Conversely, the addition of excess salt can lead to agglutination even in the absence of Abs.

When a mixture of readily distinguishable cells, such as nucleated avian red blood cells (RBCs) and nonnucleated mammalian RBCs, is added to a mixture of the respective antisera, each clump that forms consists of cells of one or the other type (Fig. 13–20). Thus, as expected from the lattice theory (above), each cell–Ab system agglutinates independently of the others in the same mixture.

SURFACE VERSUS INTERNAL ANTIGENS OF CELLS. When a bacterial, fungal, or foreign animal cell is introduced as an immunogen, it is broken up in the host animal, and many of its surface and internal components are immunogenic. However, the Abs that cause agglutination are specific for surface determinants. Abs to surface Ags are usually elicited more effectively by using intact cells rather than disrupted ones as the immunogen.

TITRATION OF SERA. When the agglutination reaction is used as a semiquantitative assay, a fixed number of cells is added to a series of tubes, each with the same volume of antiserum at a different dilution, usually increasing in twofold steps. Clumping is detected by direct inspection. The relative strength of an antiserum is expressed as the reciprocal of the highest dilution that causes agglutination. If, for example, a 1:512 dilution causes agglutination but a 1:1024 dilution does not, the titer is 512.

Agglutination titers are not precise ($\pm100\%$), but as indications of the relative Ab concentrations of various antisera with respect to a particular bacterial strain, they

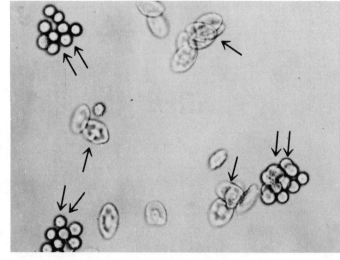

Figure 13–20. Specificity of agglutination, showing that antibodies cross-link only cells having the appropriate surface antigens. Human erythrocytes (small, spherical, non-nucleated) were coated with egg albumin (EA), and duck erythrocytes (large, oval, nucleated) were coated with bovine γ-globulin (BGG). Suspensions of the two erythrocytes were mixed with each other and with a mixture of bivalent F(ab')₂ fragments of anti-EA and anti-BGG antibodies. Note that in the resulting agglutination reaction, there are either clumps of cross-linked human cells *(double arrows)* or of cross-linked duck cells *(single arrows)*, but no clumps having a mixture of both human and duck cells. (Fudenberg H et al: J Exp Med 119:151, 1964)

are useful for following changes in Ab titer during the course of acute bacterial infection (see Diagnostic Applications of Serologic Tests, below). However, titers obtained with different bacteria are not directly comparable: for example, an antiserum to type 1 pneumococcus with 1.5 mg Ab/ml agglutinated the organism at a dilution of 1:800, whereas an antiserum to type 1R pneumococcus with 9.6 mg Ab/ml agglutinated the organism to a titer of only 1:80. Apparently the number, distribution, and chemical properties of the epitopes on the cell surface can markedly influence the titer.

Agglutination reactions are as specific as other serologic reactions, but they can present difficulties because a cell surface has many Ags, and cross-reactions are common. In order to achieve a high level of specificity, it is nearly always necessary to adsorb antisera with cross-reacting cells.

PROZONE. By analogy with the precipitin reaction, it would be expected that agglutinating activity would decline with progressive dilution of an antiserum. Curiously, however, some sera give agglutination reactions only when diluted several hundred- or thousand-fold: when undiluted or slightly diluted, they do not visibly react with the Ag. The latter region of the titration is called the prozone, as in tubes 1–3:

Tube No.	1	2	3	4	5	6	7	8	9
Serum dilution	1:8	1:16	1:32	1:64	1:128	1:256	1:512	1:1024	1:2048
Clumping	0	0	0	+	+	+	+	0	0

Labeled Abs, or the antiglobulin test described below, show that unagglutinated cells in the prozone actually have Abs adsorbed on their surfaces. Indeed, it might be expected that when Ab molecules are in great excess relative to the number of epitopes on the cells, the simultaneous attachment of both sites of a bivalent Ab molecule to different cells would be improbable. Nevertheless, the prozone phenomenon is not attributable simply to Ab excess but often involves special blocking or incomplete Abs.

BLOCKING OR "INCOMPLETE" ANTIBODIES. In certain sera with a pronounced prozone, some of the Abs not only fail to elicit agglutination but inhibit it, as shown by subsequently mixing the Ab-bearing unclumped cells or particles with antiserum at a dilution that would otherwise evoke a clumping reaction. Some sera contain only the inhibitory Abs. These Abs, termed blocking or incomplete Abs, are particularly evident in certain antisera to human erythrocytes (to Rh antigens). They are probably bivalent Abs that engage in monogamous bivalent binding like some nonprecipitating Abs in the precipitation reaction noted above.

A useful test for detecting incomplete or blocking Abs, called the **Coombs** or **antiglobulin test,** is important for recognizing certain hemolytic diseases. It exploits the fact that Ab molecules can be highly immunogenic and elicit Abs to themselves in a foreign species. For example, rabbits injected with human immunoglobulins (HIgs) form anti-HIg that react with most HIg molecules, regardless of their specificities as Abs. Hence erythrocytes with nonagglutinating human Abs bound to their surface can be specifically clumped by rabbit anti-HIg serum.

RADIOIMMUNOASSAYS (RIAs)

Abs, Ags, and many small organic molecules such as drugs are most often measured by sensitive procedures that take advantage of radioactive labels on the Ab or Ag (radioimmunoassay or RIA) or of enzymes linked to Abs (enzyme-linked immunoassays or ELISAs). The RIAs, introduced by Berson and Yalow to measure serum insulin concentrations, are often based on competition for Ab between a radioactive "indicator" ligand (L*) and its unlabeled counterpart (L) in the test sample: the higher the level of L, the less L* is bound (Fig. 13–21). The concentration of L is readily determined by comparison with a calibration curve prepared with purified L at known concentrations (Fig. 13–22).

These assays can be exceedingly discriminating because antisera can be chosen with great specificity for the ligand. The sensitivity is limited primarily by the amount of radioactivity that can be introduced into L*: with carrier-free radioactive iodine (^{125}I) as extrinsic label, as little as 0.01 to 0.1 ng ($0.01–0.1 \times 10^{-9}$g) of ligand can usually be detected.

Because of the extremely low concentrations of Ab and L used in RIAs, Ab–L complexes do not spontaneously form precipitates even if the ligand is multivalent. However, free and bound ligand can still be readily separated and counted. In a widely used method, the Ab–L* complexes are precipitated with antiserum to the Ab moiety of the complex, leaving unbound L* in the supernatant (see Fig. 13–21). The latter approach is feasible because, as noted before, the Abs of one species are usually immunogenic in other species: the resulting antisera (anti-Ig) react with essentially all Igs of the first species, regardless of their specificities as Abs. In the double-Ab

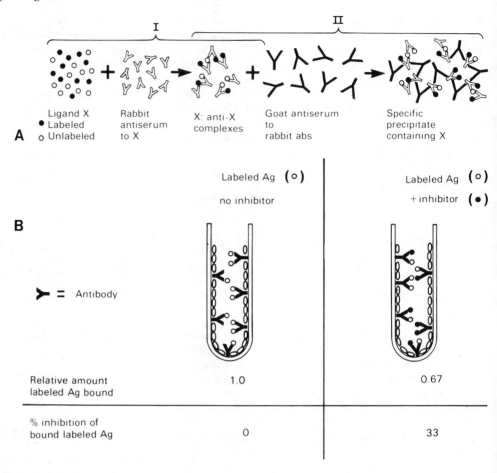

Figure 13–21. *(A)* Radioimmunoassay. The Ab–ligand complexes formed in step I are separated from unbound ligand by specific precipitation in step II with antiserum prepared against the Abs used in step I. The effect of competition between labeled (●) and unlabeled (○) ligand molecules is illustrated in Figure 13–22. *(B)* Solid-phase radioimmunoassay. In contrast to the double-Ab assay illustrated in *A*, in this assay, the Ab is bound noncovalently to a plastic surface, which is then coated with an unrelated protein such as serum albumin to prevent the subsequently added ligands from adhering to plastic. Then the labeled ligand and an unlabeled competitive inhibitor are added. The difference between the amount of labeled ligand added and the amount remaining in solution is the amount bound by the immobilized Ab.

reaction, the first Ab (anti-ligand) is added at a low level to enhance competition between L and L*, i.e., the Ab:L ratio corresponds to the Ag-excess zone in the precipitin reaction (see Fig. 13–7). The second Ab (anti-Ig) is introduced in excess (i.e., Ab-excess zone in Fig. 13–7) to ensure complete precipitation of the first Ab and its bound ligand.

SOLID-PHASE ASSAYS. By taking advantage of the ability of many plastics (polystyrene or polyvinyl, for instance) to adsorb proteins, these assays can eliminate the need for a second Ab (anti-Ig; see Fig. 13-21*B*). The assays are usually carried out in small plastic ("microtiter") trays having many (e.g., 100) depressions or "wells," each for the analysis of a different sample.

To measure a ligand (Ag or hapten, such as insulin or digitalis), the corresponding Ab is first adsorbed to the bottom of a well. An unrelated "filler" protein, such as bovine serum albumin, is then added at high concentration to adsorb to any plastic surface that remains vacant and thereby to prevent nonspecific binding of the subsequently added ligand (L). The L, at unknown concentration in the test sample, and L*, a standard (trace) amount of L in radioactive form (e.g., ^{125}I-labeled), are then added. The more L in the test sample, the less L* binds to the adherent Ab. As in assays based on inhibition of particular Ab–Ag reactions by an added excess of homologous or heterologous Ag, it may be difficult in an RIA to determine whether the inhibitor in the unknown is identical to the indicator L* or just similar enough to cross-react.

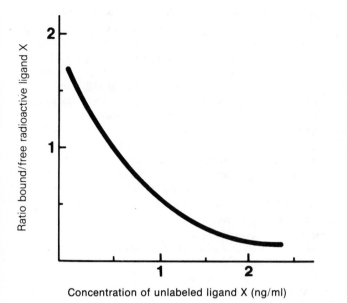

Figure 13–22. Calibration curve for a radioimmunoassay. A fixed amount of radioiodine-labeled ligand X competes with various amounts of unlabeled ligand X for a limiting amount of anti-X Abs.

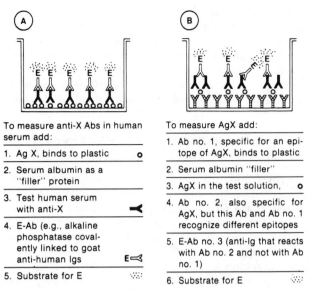

Figure 13–23. Enzyme-linked immunosorbent assay (ELISA test). This technique can measure serum Abs *(A)* or Ag *(B)* and depends on the ability of certain plastics (polystyrene, polyvinyl) to adsorb proteins (Ags, Abs) strongly. Only the component added in step 1 is bound to the plastic, which is then coated with unrelated proteins to make sure that the substances added subsequently stick only specifically to reactants, rather than nonspecifically to the plastic.

To measure Ab, the procedure is reversed: Ag is adsorbed first to the plastic surface, then the unrelated serum albumin "filler" is adsorbed to the remaining vacant space. The test sample containing Ab (Ab no. 1) at an unknown concentration is then added. After several hours, the surface is rinsed. To measure the remaining (bound) Ab no. 1, a second, ^{125}I-labeled, Ab (Ab no. 2, usually an anti-Ig) is added. The amount of ^{125}I-anti-Ig that sticks is proportional to the amount of Ab no. 1 in the test sample.

The second Ab (anti-Ig) can be replaced by **protein A,** a protein from *Staphylococcus aureus* that happens to bind strongly to the constant domain of the most common form of Ab (IgG, see Chap. 14) but does not affect the Ab's ligand-binding activity. Protein A not only reacts specifically with bound (or free) Ab but also can bind to and promote precipitation of Ab–Ag complexes.

ENZYME-LINKED IMMUNOASSAYS (ELISAs)

ELISAs are based on the use of covalently linked enzyme–Ab (E–Ab) complexes in which the catalytic and immunologic activities are preserved. The Ab is bound to its Ag when present, and substrates that yield colored or fluorescent products then measure the linked enzyme. The enzymes used (e.g., alkaline phosphatase, horseradish peroxidase, β-galactosidase) are stable, unlike radioactive labels, and they are simpler and as sensitive to measure. These assays are also useful under conditions such as the physician's office, the home, or underdevel-

oped countries where radioimmunoassays are unavailable or prohibitively costly.

Many variations of ELISA are possible. For instance, to detect Abs (Fig. 13–23), the corresponding Ag, adsorbed to plastic (polystyrene) plates, binds Abs from the test sample (Ab no. 1). The specifically adsorbed Abs are then measured with an E–Ab complex whose Ab (anti-Ig) reacts specifically with Ab no. 1; e.g., E-linked goat antihuman Ig can be used to measure almost any human Ab.

As is suggested by Figure 13–23, the same E–Ab preparation can be used to measure a great variety of Abs and Ags (e.g., human Abs to cytomegalovirus or measles, herpes, rubella, or mumps viruses). Automated devices (ELISA readers) can be used to analyze the products of the enzyme reaction quantitatively and rapidly.

BIOTIN–AVIDIN. The extraordinarily high affinity $(\sim 1 \times 10^{15}$ liters/mole) of avidin, an egg white protein, for biotin (mol. wt. 1000), a vitamin, expands even further the usefulness of ELISA assays. Biotin is readily attached covalently to Abs and many enzymes, such as horseradish peroxidase, without impairing their reactivity with Ags or substrates. To detect a biotinylated Ab, for example when it is bound to an Ag that is immobilized on a plastic surface, a biotinylated enzyme–avidin complex is added. The avidin, having four sites per molecule for biotin, can cross-link several biotinylated enzyme molecules to each other and to each molecule of biotinylated Ab, greatly amplifying the sensitivity of the assay by increasing the number of catalytic sites that become linked to each molecule of ligand-bound Ab. A given biotinylated enzyme–avidin complex is a general reagent and can detect and quantitate any biotinylated Ab, regardless of the species from which it is derived, its isotype, or the Ag with which it reacts.

SYNTHETIC PEPTIDES AS REPRESENTATIVE EPITOPES OF PROTEIN ANTIGENS

In precipitin reactions, Abs to a native protein react poorly, if at all, with that protein in unfolded ("denatured") form. Similarly, Abs to a denatured protein hardly precipitate with the protein in native form. Hence the long-held view that Abs to proteins are **conformation specific:** i.e., that the epitopes they recognize depend on the folded protein's three-dimensional shape rather than on its linear amino acid sequence. Although largely correct, this view has been substantially modified by two developments: (1) the use of sensitive RIAs and ELISAs in place of precipitin reactions and (2) the great number of peptides that have become available as a result of improved methods for their synthesis and purification.

In solution, a native protein normally behaves as though it has a well-ordered and distinctive shape, but small peptides (<20 amino acid residues) generally behave as though they are conformationally disordered. Nevertheless, Abs produced against small synthetic peptides that correspond to segments of a native protein often react in RIAs and ELISAs with the native protein. Conversely, Abs to native proteins react with many of the corresponding synthetic peptides. Although a completely satisfactory explanation for these circumstances is still lacking, these reactions have many practical applications.

MAPPING PROTEIN EPITOPES WITH PEPTIDES. To identify epitopes in a native protein, overlapping short peptides spanning the protein's entire sequence are synthesized and tested individually for their ability to react with Abs raised against the intact protein. This approach can detect epitopes that are made up of contiguous amino acids in a linear sequence (**continuous epitopes**), but it cannot be expected to succeed when an epitope is **discontinuous:** i.e., formed from amino acids that are close neighbors in the folded protein but widely separated in the protein's linear sequence. Most epitopes in native proteins are probably discontinuous (see lysozyme–Ab complexes, Chap. 14, Fig. 14–24).

USE OF PEPTIDES IN CONJUNCTION WITH RECOMBINANT DNA TECHNOLOGY. With recombinant DNA technology, it often happens that a gene is cloned and sequenced before the protein it encodes is identified. It is then possible to use synthetic peptides corresponding to the sequences of amino acids predicted from the sequenced gene to raise anti-peptide antisera (and even mAbs); these antisera can greatly facilitate the identification and isolation of the new protein. Although Abs to the synthetic peptide may react only poorly (and sometimes not detectably) with the corresponding native protein, they often react well with the unfolded protein in the presence of mild detergents, especially in what are termed **"Western blots"** (described below). It is not yet possible to predict accurately which peptides are most likely to elicit Abs that react with the intact protein, but sequences of 10 to 15 amino acids having a balanced mixture of hydrophilic and hydrophobic amino acids are often chosen because they are usually immunogenic and seem likely to be exposed on the surface of proteins in an aqueous environment.

"IMMUNOBLOTS." In immunoblots, Abs, including those to synthetic peptides, detect individual proteins in extremely complex mixtures, as in disrupted cells. The mixture is first subjected to electrophoresis in a polyacrylamide gel in the presence of a high concentration of sodium dodecyl sulfate (SDS), an anionic detergent that binds to virtually all peptide bonds of all proteins. The

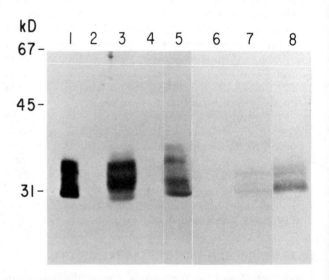

Figure 13–24. Western blots ("immunoblots"). Rabbit Abs were used to detect serine proteases of cytotoxic T lymphocytes (Chap. 19). Lysates of the cells were subjected to electrophoresis and the proteases were detected with anti-protease rabbit Abs, biotinylated goat anti-rabbit immunoglobulins, and avidin-biotinylated horseradish peroxidase complexes. (The latter are revealed as the darkly pigmented products formed by the peroxidase with 4-chloro-1-naphthol and hydrogen peroxidase.) Numbers at left are mol. wt. (Kilodaltons). Cell lysates from cytotoxic T lymphocytes (CTLs) were introduced into lanes 1, 3, and 5, and from non-cytotoxic T lymphocytes into the other lanes. (From Pasternack MS et al: Nature 322:740, 1986)

bound SDS converts the proteins into highly negatively charged rigid rods having approximately the same charge per unit length. Hence, the proteins migrate in an electrical field at rates that are determined primarily by their respective molecular weights. After migration in the electrical field is stopped, the proteins are transferred ("blotted") electrophoretically from the gel to a sheet of nitrocellulose, which binds and immobilizes the transferred macromolecules. To reveal the position of a particular protein (call it X), the nitrocellulose sheet is incubated with an Ab to X (Ab no. 1) and washed, and the position of the adherent Ab no. 1 is revealed by a second Ab (Ab no. 2), which is specific for Ab no. 1 (e.g., if Ab no. 1 is rabbit anti-X, then Ab no. 2 is goat Ab to rabbit Ig). Because Ab no. 2 carries an attached radioactive label, such as ^{125}I, or an attached enzyme, such as horseradish peroxidase, exposure of the nitrocellulose sheet to x-ray film sensitive to ^{125}I or to a chromogenic substrate for the enzyme will reveal the location of Ab no. 2 and thereby of Ab no. 1 and protein X. This simple method provides sensitive, rapid, and highly specific means to identify proteins in crude extracts of tissues and cells and to determine some of their properties, e.g., apparent molecular weight (Fig. 13–24).

Nitrocellulose sheets with transferred DNA are called **Southern blots** after Edward Southern, who invented the process in order to analyze fragments of DNA. **"Northern blotting"** is the term applied (facetiously) when the same procedure is used to analyze transferred RNA. To maintain the geographic motif, nitrocellulose sheets with transferred proteins are commonly termed **"Western" blots** (or immunoblots).

PEPTIDES AS VACCINES. The reactivity of antipeptide Abs with intact proteins has generated much interest in the use of peptides conjugated to carrier proteins as vaccines, particularly when the preparation and administration of conventional vaccines entail a risk of exposure to highly pathogenic microbes. However, several considerations raise questions about the general effectiveness of this approach. One is that whereas Abs to a peptide may have high affinity for the peptide, they are likely to have low affinity for the corresponding protein. Moreover, peptides represent only continuous epitopes, and the discontinuous ones may well be important in the response to complete Ags. Finally, Abs to a single epitope seem unlikely to afford as much protection against infection as the many sets of Abs against the many different epitopes of conventional vaccines. Nevertheless, as we shall see, peptides play a special role in eliciting cellular immune responses: some of these responses are especially critical in defenses against infectious agents (see Chaps. 15 and 19), and some are essential for optimal Ab production (see Chap. 16).

Appendix

AFFINITY CHROMATOGRAPHY
Purification of Antibodies

Methods for purifying Abs are based on the dissociability of Ab–ligand complexes. Two stages are usually involved. First, Abs interact with Ag or hapten that is covalently attached to an insoluble adsorbent. In the most widely used procedure (**affinity chromatography**), antiserum is passed slowly through a column of agarose beads (an **immunoadsorbent**) to which the Ag or hapten has been coupled. Second, after all extraneous serum proteins are washed away, adsorbed Abs are eluted by specific or nonspecific procedures.

SPECIFIC PROCEDURES. With aggregates whose stability depends largely on specific ionic interactions, strong salt solutions (e.g., 1.8M NaCl) elute purified Abs effectively.

When the specific antigenic determinants are simple haptenic groups, such as 2,4-dinitrophenyl, small univalent haptens that encompass the crucial part of the determinant (e.g., 2,4-dinitrophenol) displace the insoluble Ag, yielding soluble Ab–hapten complexes.

It is desirable to use for elution those haptens that are both **weakly bound** by the Ab and **highly soluble.** Highly concentrated solutions of hapten can then elute the Ab in high yield, and the weakly bound hapten is easily removed (e.g., by dialysis), leaving purified Abs.

NONSPECIFIC PROCEDURES. To elute Abs from protein Ags on the immunoadsorbent, it is usually necessary to expose the adsorbed Abs (and the Ag) to conditions that cause reversible denaturation of many proteins, allowing Ab to dissociate from the immobilized Ag. Acids (HCl-glycine or acetic acid) at pH 2–3 are often effective. Because Abs usually regain their native structure on being restored to physiologic conditions, neutralization of the acidified eluate yields purified Ab with most of its activity retained.

YIELD AND PURITY. Abs can be isolated from serum in high yield (usually over 50%) and high purity; i.e., nearly all (>90%) of the recovered protein reacts specifically with the Ag.

USE OF ANTIBODIES TO PURIFY ANTIGENS

Affinity chromatography is also used to isolate Ags from complex mixtures. Purified Abs (preferably monoclonal Abs, see Chap. 14) are attached covalently to agarose beads. When a complex mixture containing Ag is passed slowly through a column of such beads, the Ag is selectively bound. The bound Ag can then be eluted by treating the column with a solvent (e.g., dilute acetic acid) that denatures the Ab, allowing the Ag to dissociate and to be recovered in highly purified form. The denatured Ab is usually readily renatured by washing the column with physiologic buffers (neutral pH, etc.). Many Abs are so stable that a given Ab column can be used repeatedly, with hundreds of denaturing—renaturing cycles, without losing Ag-specific binding activity.

INTRINSIC AFFINITY

The reversible binding of a univalent ligand by Ab is described by the **Scatchard equation** (see Equilibrium Dialysis, equation 4, above), whose derivation follows.

The successive steps in the binding of a univalent ligand (L) by a multivalent antibody (B) with n combining sites can be represented by the reactions on the left and their equilibrium constants on the right.

$$B + L \rightleftarrows BL \qquad k_1 = \frac{[BL]}{[B][L]}$$

$$BL + L \rightleftarrows BL_2 \qquad k_2 = \frac{[BL_2]}{[BL][L]}$$

$$\cdots \qquad \cdots \qquad (10)$$

$$BL_{i-1} + L \rightleftarrows BL_i \qquad k_i = \frac{[BL_i]}{[BL_{i-1}][L]}$$

$$\cdots \qquad \cdots$$

$$BL_{n-1} + L \rightleftarrows BL_n \qquad k_n = \frac{[BL_n]}{[BL_{n-1}][L]}$$

We wish to determine the **average** number of ligand molecules bound per Ab molecule, i.e., the ratio of all bound ligand to all Ab molecules, or L_b/B_t:

$$L_b = BL + 2BL_2 + 3BL_3 \cdots + iBL_i \cdots + nBL_n, \text{ or}$$
$$= B[k_1 L + 2k_1 k_2 (L)^2 \cdots + ik_1 k_2 \cdots k_i(L)^i \cdots \quad (11)$$
$$+ nk_1 k_2 \cdots k_n(L)^n]$$

and

$$B_t = B + BL + BL_2 + BL_3 \cdots + BL_i \cdots + BL_n, \text{ or}$$
$$= B[1 + k_1 L + k_1 k_2(L)^2 \cdots + k_1 k_2 \cdots k_i(L)^i \cdots \quad (12)$$
$$\cdots + k_1 k_2 \cdots k_n(L)^n]$$

Assume that all Ab-combining sites are equivalent and independent. Then for the representative step in which the ith site becomes occupied (third step in equation 10), the concentration of vacant Ab sites (S) is:

$$[S] = [n - (i - 1)][BL_{i-1}] \quad (13)$$

and the concentration of occupied sites (SL) is:

$$[SL] = i[BL_i] \quad (14)$$

When equations 13 and 14 are combined, the equilibrium constant for the ith reaction becomes

$$k_i = \frac{n - i + 1}{i} \cdot \frac{[SL]}{[S][L]} \quad (15)$$

$[SL]/[S][L]$ is defined as K, the **intrinsic association constant,** or the **intrinsic affinity,** for the general reaction in which a representative site binds a ligand molecule (S + L ⇌ SL); i.e.,

$$k_i = \frac{n - i + 1}{i} K \quad (16)$$

The constants for the individual steps in equation 10 can thus be expressed in terms of the intrinsic constant (e.g., $k_1 = nK; k_2 = (n - 1)K/2; k_n = K/n$); this makes it possible to reduce equations 11 and 12, with the aid of the binomial theorem, to*:

$$L_b = nK[B][L](1 + K[L])^{n-1} \quad (17)$$

and

$$B_t = [B](1 + K[L])^n \quad (18)$$

or

$$\frac{L_b}{B_t} = \frac{nK[L]}{1 + K[L]}$$

Since L_b/B_t is r (moles ligand bound per mole Ab) and [L] is c (equilibrium concentration of free ligand), we have

$$r = \frac{nKc}{1 + Kc} \quad (19)$$

which is the same as equation 4 (p 250):

$$\frac{r}{c} = Kn - Kr \quad (20)$$

Intrinsic affinity, K, provides a convenient and rigorous basis for analyzing Ab-combining sites and for comparing sites of different Abs with each other and with those of other proteins. However, the multiplicity of binding sites on Ab molecules and on most Ag particles means that for biologically significant Ab–Ag reactions *in vivo*, the actual equilibrium constants can differ greatly from the intrinsic constants. Because surface Ags on cells and virions occur as repeated copies, they can engage in multivalent binding with Abs, as in monogamous multivalency (see above); the equilibrium constant for formation of multivalent complexes can greatly exceed (up to perhaps 10⁵) the Ab's intrinsic equilibrium constant. The difference is attributable to cooperativity between sites on the same molecule. Such cooperativity is commonplace; for example, the strength of a bond between two polynucleotide strands with many complementary base pairs is enormously greater than the strength of a bond between any single pair of complementary nucleotides.

* This derivation is due to Dr. B. Altschuler, New York University.

TABLE 13–4. Kinetic Properties of Some Antibody–Ligand Interactions

Ab	Ligand	k_1 (liters/mole/second)	k_{-1} (per second)	$t_{1/2}$ (seconds)	K (liters/mole)
Anti-DNP	ε-DNP-L-lysine	8×10^7	1	0.7	10^8
Anti-fluorescein	Fluorescein	4×10^8	5×10^{-3}	140	10^{11}
Anti-bovine serum albumin (BSA)	Dansyl-BSA	3×10^5	2×10^{-3}	350	1.7×10^8

(Data from Mason DW, Williams AF: Kinetics of antibody reaction and the analysis of cell surface antigens. In Weir DM [ed]: Handbook of Experimental Immunology, vol 1: Immunochemistry, 4th ed, chap 3. Oxford, Blackwell Scientific Publications, 1986. Day LA et al: Ann NY Acad Sci 103:611, 1963; Levison et al: Biochem Biophys Res Commun 43:258, 1971)

RATES OF REACTION

The rates at which Abs form complexes with Ags are determined by the forward or association rate constant (k_1 in equation 21) and the backward or dissociation rate constant (k_{-1} in equation 22):

$$\text{association rate} = k_1 (Ab)(L) \tag{21}$$

$$\text{dissociation rate} = k_{-1} (AB \cdot L) \tag{22}$$

where (Ab), (L), and (Ab $\cdot$ L) are concentrations of unbound Ab, unbound ligand, and Ab–ligand complexes. The commonly used units are liters/mole/second for k_1 and 1/second for k_{-1}. The time ($t_{1/2}$) required for half the bound ligand to dissociate from the Ab's combining sites is:

$$t_{1/2} = \frac{0.693}{k_{-1}} \tag{23}$$

Abs and ligands combine at widely different rates. For some small haptens, the forward rates are perhaps the fastest known for biochemical reactions (see Table 13–4), with rate constants of approximately 10^8 liters/mole/second or only about one-tenth the theoretical upper limit of 10^9 liters/mole/second for a diffusion-limited reaction. However, for protein Ags, the forward rate constants are much lower (10^5 liters/mole/second), probably because collisions between an Ab and a protein Ag are nonproductive unless the Ag's epitopes happen to be so oriented that they can be engaged by the Ab's combining site.

Dissociation rate constants vary even more widely than association rate constants. For an Ab that binds a set of related haptens with markedly different affinities, the forward rate constant usually differs only slightly from one ligand to another, but the dissociation rate constants varies enormously. Indeed, differences in affinity of an Ab for various structurally related ligands are deter-

mined largely by the different rates at which the bound ligands leave the Ab's combining sites.

For practical purposes, $t_{1/2}$ provides useful information because it measures the Ab–ligand complex's stability. To illustrate how greatly $t_{1/2}$ can vary, consider the following two fabricated examples:

1. An Ab that binds a protein Ag with high affinity, $K = 1 \times 10^9$ liters/mole, has an association rate constant of 1×10^5 liters/mole/second. Hence the dissociation rate constant is $10^{-4} sec^{-1}$, and $t_{1/2}$ is approximately 10^4 second or 3 hours.

2. Another Ab binds a polysaccharide Ag with low affinity, $K = 1 \times 10^4$ liters/mole, and has an association rate constant of 1×10^7 liters/mole/second. Hence the dissociation rate constant is $10^3 sec^{-1}$, and $t_{1/2}$ is approximately 10^{-3} seconds.

In these examples, which are imaginary but probably not unusual, one Ab–ligand complex is 10 million times more stable than the other (10^4 versus 10^{-3}). For some applications, such as immunofluorescent staining of cell-surface Ags (see Chap. 15), Abs that form very slowly dissociable complexes are required, whereas for other applications, such as affinity chromatography purification of a protein Ag (see above), Abs that form more readily dissociable complexes may be preferred.

THERMODYNAMICS

The formation of the Ab–ligand complex results in a change in Gibbs free energy, ΔG, which is exponentially related to the association constant by

$$\Delta G = \Delta G° + RT \ln K \tag{24}$$

where R is the gas constant (1.987 calories/mole-deg.), T the absolute temperature, and $\ln K$ the natural logarithm of the intrinsic association constant. $\Delta G°$, the standard free energy change, is the gain or loss of free energy in calories, as 1 mole of Ab sites and 1 mole of free ligand combine to form 1 mole of bound ligand. At equilibrium, $\Delta G = 0$ and $\Delta G° = -RT \ln K$.

Values of $\Delta G°$ for various Ab–hapten pairs range from about -5500 to $-12,500$ calories (per mole of hapten bound), corresponding to association constants of 10^4–10^9 liters/mole at 30°.

It is sometimes useful to determine whether the free energy change comes about from a change in the heat content (**enthalpy**) or in the entropy of the system. This determination is based on

$$\Delta G° = \Delta H° - T\Delta S° \qquad (25)$$

where $\Delta H°$ is the change in enthalpy (measured in calories), T is absolute temperature, and $\Delta S°$ is the entropy change. $\Delta H°$ is determined experimentally in sensitive calorimeters or by measuring the intrinsic association

constant (K) at two or more temperatures:

$$\Delta H° = \frac{R \ln \frac{K_2}{K_1}}{\frac{1}{T_1} - \frac{1}{T_2}} \qquad (26)$$

where K_1 and K_2 are intrinsic association constants at temperatures T_1 and T_2. $\Delta H°$ values range from 0, in which case the driving force for complex formation is the $T\Delta S$ term of equation 8, to $-30,000$ calories/mole ligand bound, in which case the decrease in heat content drives the reaction. The formation of apolar or **hydrophobic bonds** is essentially athermal ($\Delta H° \cong 0$), whereas the formation of hydrogen bonds is exothermic ($\Delta H° \cong -1000$ calories/hydrogen bond).

Affinity (intrinsic association constant) decreases with increasing temperature for Ab–ligand reactions where $\Delta H°$ has a negative value, and it is unaffected by increasing temperature when $\Delta H°$ is 0. For most Ab–ligand sys-

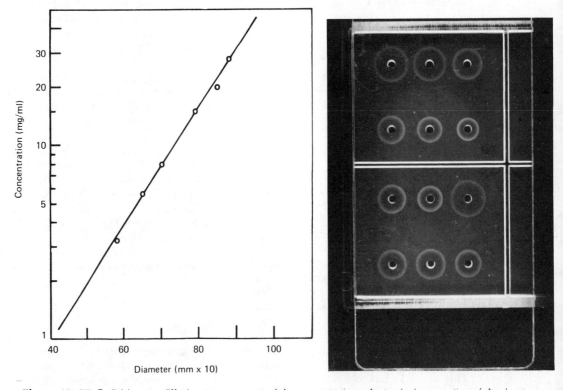

Figure 13–25. Radial immunodiffusion measurement of Ag concentrations. A standard preparation of Ag, human immunoglobulin G (HIgG), was added at six different concentrations to wells in agar containing goat antiserum to HIgG *(upper right panel)*. The diameters of the resulting circular precipitates are plotted on the left. After a longer incubation, when each precipitate has attained its maximum size, linearity is obtained by plotting log Ag concentration versus area or (diameter)². The lower right panel shows six human sera with different concentrations of HIgG. (Courtesy of Dr C Kirk Osterland)

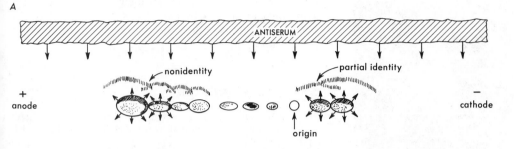

A

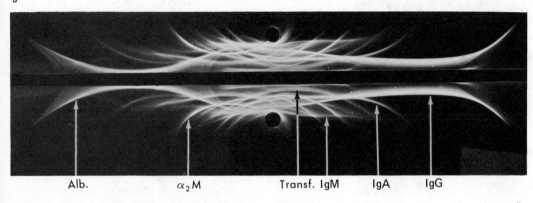

B

Alb. α_2M   Transf. IgM   IgA   IgG

Figure 13–26. Immunoelectrophoresis. *(A)* A thin layer of agar gel (about 1–2 mm) covers a glass slide, and a small well near the center *(origin)* receives a solution containing various Ags. After electrophoresis of the Ags, the current is discontinued, and antiserum is added to the trough. Precipitation bands form as in double diffusion in two dimensions. The apex of each precipitin band corresponds to the center of the corresponding Ag. *(B)* Human serum, placed at the origin, was analyzed with an antiserum prepared against unfractionated human serum. Alb, γ_2M, Transf, etc. refer to various serum proteins. (Courtesy of Dr Curtis Williams)

tems, $\Delta H°$ is unknown: to increase the formation of Ab–ligand complexes, it is therefore a common practice to carry out the Ab–ligand reaction in the cold, i.e., at 4°C rather than at 37°C.

ADDITIONAL METHODS FOR MEASURING ABS AND AGS
Radial Immunodiffusion

Precipitation in agar can be used not only to examine Ab–Ag reactions and cross-reactions but also to measure Ab and Ag concentrations. A procedure that measures Ag concentration is carried out in a layer of agar (e.g., on a glass slide) containing a uniformly dispersed antiserum. Diffusion of the Ag from a well cut in the agar leads to the formation of a ring of precipitation whose area is proportional to the initial Ag concentration (Fig. 13–25).

Immunoelectrophoresis

Immunoelectrophoresis combines electrophoresis with precipitation in agar. The mixture of Ags is introduced into a small well in agar that has been cast on a plate, say an ordinary microscope slide. An electric field applied for 1 to 2 hours causes the proteins to migrate, each with a distinctive electrophoretic mobility. The electric gradient is then discontinued, and antiserum is introduced into a trough whose long axis parallels the axis of electrophoretic migration. The Abs and Ags diffuse toward each other, and precipitation bands form at the intersection of their diffusion fronts. The principles involved in the precipitation stage are those described earlier in this chapter for reactions of identity, nonidentity, and partial identity. Immunoelectrophoresis has revealed as many as 30 different Ags in human serum (Fig. 13–26).

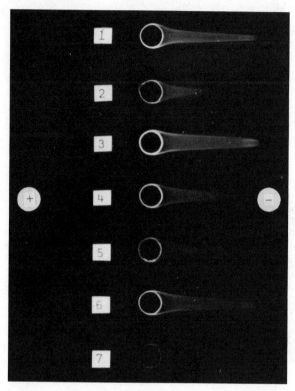

Figure 13–27. Rocket immunoelectrophoresis measurement of Ag concentrations. The rocket-shaped areas of precipitation result from electrophoresing solutions with various concentrations of an Ag into agar that contains the corresponding antiserum. Rocket heights (or areas of precipitates) are linearly proportional to Ag concentration. (Based on Claman HN et al: J Lab Clin Med 69:151, 1967)

Rocket Immunoelectrophoresis

Radial immunodiffusion and electrophoresis have been combined to provide a rapid method for quantitating Ags. By electrophoresing the Ag from solution in a small well into agar that contains the antiserum in excess, the time required to reach maximum precipitation is short-

ened to a few hours (from several days in the radial diffusion method shown in Fig. 13–25). The height of the resulting rocket-shaped zone of precipitation is proportional to Ag concentration (Fig. 13–27).

Selected Readings

Berzofsky JA, Berkower IJ: Antigen–antibody interaction. In Paul WE (ed): Fundamental Immunology, pp 595–644. New York, Raven Press, 1984

Berzofsky JA, Buckenmeyer GK, Hicks G et al: Topographic antigenic determinants detected by monoclonal antibodies to myoglobin. In Celada F, Shumaker V, Sercarz EE (eds): Protein Conformation as Immunological Signal, pp 165–180. New York, Plenum Press, 1983

Crothers DM, Metzger H: The influence of polyvalency on the binding properties of antibodies. Immunochemistry 9:341–357, 1972

Crumpton MJ, Wilkinson JM: The immunological activity of some of the chymotryptic peptides of sperm-whale myoglobin. Biochem J 94:545–556, 1965

DeLisi C, Metzger H: Some physical chemical aspects of receptor–ligand interactions. Immunol Commun 5:417–436, 1976

Hornick CL, Karush F: Antibody affinity III: The role of multivalence. Immunochemistry 9:325–340, 1972

Karush F: The affinity of antibody: Range, variability, and the role of multivalence. In Litman GW, Good RA (eds): Comprehensive Immunology, vol 5: Immunoglobulins, pp 85–116. New York, Plenum Press, 1978

Klotz IM: Protein interactions. In Neurath H, Bailey K (eds): The Proteins, 1st Ed, vol 1, part B, pp 727–806. New York, Academic Press, 1953

Maron E, Shiozawa C, Arnon R, Sela M: Chemical and immunological characterization of a unique antigenic region in lysozyme. Biochemistry 10:763–771, 1971

Nisonoff A, Pressman D: Heterogeneity and average combining site constants of antibodies from individual rabbits. J Immunol 80:417–428, 1958

Richards FE, Konigsberg WH, Rosenstein RW, Varga JM: On the specificity of antibodies. Science 187:130–137, 1975

Scatchard G: The attractions of proteins for small molecules and ions. Ann NY Acad Sci 51:660–672, 1949

Thakur AK, Jaffe ML, Rodbard D: Graphical analysis of ligand-binding systems: Evaluation by Monte Carlo studies. Anal Biochem 107:220–239, 1980

Weir DM, Herzenberg LA, Blackwell C, Herzenberg LA: Handbook of Experimental Immunology.

Yalow R: Radioimmunoassay. Rev Biophys Bioeng 9:327–345, 1980

14

Immunoglobulins and Immunoglobulin Genes

IMMUNOGLOBULINS

For many years, antibodies (Abs) were identified with γ-globulins, the class of plasma proteins with lowest electrophoretic mobility. The level of these proteins was increased by immunization and was lowered when Abs were removed from the serum by specific precipitation with antigen (Ag) (Fig. 14–1). However, some of the electrophoretically faster-moving serum proteins have also been found to exhibit Ab activity; hence **immunoglobulin** (Ig), a more general term, has been introduced. In current usage, Ab and Ig are essentially synonymous, with Ab generally preferred when the ligand is known and relevant; otherwise, Ig is more commonly used.

All Igs are structurally similar, but they are an immensely diversified family that can be arranged into many groups and subgroups on the basis of variations in antigenic properties and amino acid sequences. The first half of this chapter emphasizes the relations between these properties and the two functions that are characteristic of all Ab molecules: (1) specific binding of one or a few ligands, and (2) participation in certain effector reactions, e.g., activating complement proteins (see Chap. 17), stimulating cytotoxic lymphocytes (see Chap. 19), and triggering mast cells to release vasoactive amines (see Chaps. 18 and 19). As we shall see, the ligand-binding and effector functions are carried out by different domains of the Ab molecule. The second half of the chapter describes Ig genes and the mechanisms that permit a

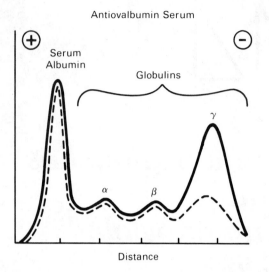

Figure 14–1. Electrophoresis of serum from a rabbit intensively immunized with ovalbumin before (———) and after (– – –) removal of Ab molecules by specific precipitation with ovalbumin. (Tiselius A, Kabat EA: J Exp Med 69:119, 1939)

limited number of these genes to encode an enormous number of different Ig molecules.

IMMUNOGLOBULINS ARE NORMALLY HETEROGENEOUS

The Abs elicited by most Ags are heterogeneous. They differ not only in specificity for different epitopes of the Ag and in affinity but also in electrical charge, reflecting differences in amino acid sequences. During electrophoresis, each of the other serum proteins (such as albumin) migrates as a compact band with a characteristic mobility, because the molecules of each protein have essentially the same net charge at a given pH. Igs, however, migrate as a broad band, because they differ considerably in electrical charge (Fig. 14–2). This heterogeneity, a result of enormous amino acid sequence diversity, greatly hindered efforts to decipher their detailed structure. This difficulty was eventually overcome with two kinds of homogeneous Igs: myeloma proteins and monoclonal Abs (mAbs). Before describing how these Igs helped clarify the structure of Abs, we consider how they are obtained.

HOMOGENEOUS IMMUNOGLOBULINS: MYELOMA PROTEINS AND MONOCLONAL ANTIBODIES

MYELOMA PROTEINS. The most mature cells of the B-cell lineage, called plasma cells (see Chaps. 15 and 16), sometimes become transformed into cancer cells and grow as **plasma cell tumors** (also termed **myeloma tumors**). As with most other tumors, the cells of each myeloma tu-

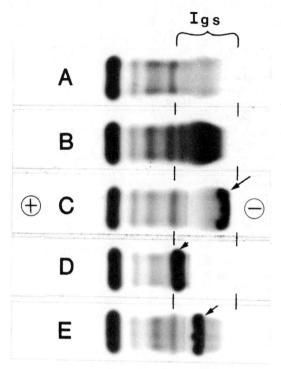

Figure 14–2. Electrophoresis of human sera (at pH 8.4). *(A)* Normal serum; note diffuse Igs, proteins with least mobility to the anode (+). *(B)* Serum with elevated heterogeneous **(polyclonal)** Igs. *(C* through *E)* Sera from three patients with myeloma tumors. Each myeloma protein **(arrow)** is a compact band **(monoclonal** Ig); note their different mobilities. Serum albumin is the compact dark band at left. (Courtesy of Dr C Kirk Osterland)

mor arise from a single progenitor cell—i.e., they constitute a **clone**—and each tumor produces a homogeneous Ig, called a **myeloma protein,** often in huge amounts. In a patient with such a tumor, serum levels of 50 mg of myeloma protein per ml are not unusual.

Myeloma tumors arise spontaneously in many mammals, and they account for about 1% of human cancer. They have been studied particularly intensively in certain inbred strains of mice (BALB/c, NZB), in which they are readily elicited by intraperitoneal injections of substances such as mineral oil or certain plastics that cause chronic peritoneal inflammation. The tumors can be maintained indefinitely by serial passage through mice of the same strain or by growth in culture, providing large amounts of homogeneous Ig for analysis. The tumor cells are also a rich source of DNA and messenger RNA for analyzing Ig genes (see below, this chapter).

Figure 14–2 compares the compact electrophoretic migration of some myeloma (monoclonal) Igs with the diffuse migration of normal (polyclonal) Igs. For most myeloma proteins, the Ags they bind are unknown. But in the few cases where the Ags have been identified, myeloma proteins react like typical Abs, e.g., with similar specificity and affinity and with two binding sites per molecule of approximately 150,000 daltons, located in the proper regions (Fab domains; see Fragmentation, below). These circumstances helped establish that normal, heterogenous Abs consist of many subsets, each as homogeneous as a myeloma protein.

HYBRIDOMAS AND MONOCLONAL ANTIBODIES. Virtually unlimited amounts of a single homogeneous Ab to essentially any Ag can be produced by a remarkable procedure invented by Kohler and Milstein. In this method, a normal B cell is fused with a myeloma cell to yield a hybrid cell (**hybridoma**) having key properties of both parent cells. It produces the B cell's Ig and expresses two important properties of the cancerous myeloma cell: (1) a capacity for limitless growth ("immortality"), and (2) the capacity for synthesizing and secreting prodigous amounts of Ig (about 10,000 molecules/cell/min), perhaps the highest rate of protein production and secretion known for a eukaryotic cell.

Hybridomas are usually produced from special myeloma cell lines that carry two mutational defects. First, they no longer make their own Ig; thus, the hybrid cell's Ig product is exclusively that of the normal B-cell parent. Second, they lack an enzyme required for nucleic acid synthesis, usually hypoxanthine-guanine phosphoribosyl transferase (HGPRT). Hence, a special culture medium, termed HAT, can be used to favor the growth of hybridomas (Fig. 14–3). The medium contains aminopterin (the A in HAT), which forces the cells to depend on HGPRT for synthesis of nucleic acids from hypoxanthine (the H in HAT). Thus, in this medium, the unfused myeloma cells (or myeloma cells fused only to each other) will not grow, and the unfused B cells (or B cells fused only to each other) also will not grow because they normally die out after only a few days in culture in any medium. **The only cells that will grow are hybridomas: their B-cell components provide the required enzyme, and their myeloma cell components provide the capacity for unlimited growth.**

Because the initial fusion is performed between myeloma cells and a population of B cells, often obtained from a mouse spleen, many different hybridomas are obtained. Only rare ones produce Abs of interest, because only a small proportion of spleen B cells make Abs to any particular Ag, even in animals that are repeatedly injected with the Ag ("hyperimmunized"). The useful hybrids are detected through the use of sensitive assays (RIA, ELISA; see Chap. 13) that screen rapidly hundreds of small cultures, each containing thousands of diverse hybridomas. When a positive culture is identified, single clones are grown from its individual cells, and when a clone that secretes the desired Ab (now called an mAb) is identified, it can be expanded to a virtually unlimited extent by growing it in culture or by passing it serially as a peritoneal (ascites fluid–producing) tumor through mice. Hundreds of grams of some monoclonal Abs have been produced for experimental, diagnostic, and industrial purposes.

ANTIGENIC CLASSIFICATION OF IMMUNOGLOBULINS: ISOTYPES, ALLOTYPES, AND IDIOTYPES

Igs from one species elicit immune responses when injected into a different species, and reactions with the resulting antisera divide Igs of the first species into groups that differ in antigenic structure.

Isotypic determinants (Gr. *iso*, same) are shared by all Ig molecules of a given class or **isotype.** Different isotypes have different amino acid sequences and effector functions but they may be specific for the same Ag.

Allotypic determinants (Gr. *allos*, different). The Ig within an isotype can be subdivided into sets, called **allotypes,** that are distinguished by small, heritable antigenic differences. These differences reflect a few amino acid substitutions within otherwise similar amino acid sequences, and they do not affect ligand binding or effector functions. Antiallotypic Abs are generally produced within a species by immunizing an individual who lacks a particular allotype with Igs from those who possess it, yielding **alloantisera.** Because allotypic determinants reflect differences between alternative forms of genes (i.e., alleles), they are valuable probes for exploring Ig genes.

Idiotypic determinants (Gr. *idios*, individual) refer to the distinctive antigenic determinants that are shared by the Igs made by one or a few clones of Ig-producing cells. As we will see later, an Ab's idiotypic determinants are located in or near its ligand-binding sites, and the ability of one Ab to elicit other Abs that react with the first Ab's binding sites has led to the suggestion that the immune responses might be regulated by an idiotype–anti-idiotype network (see Chap. 16).

Classes of Heavy Chains and Types of Light Chains (Isotypes)

Electrophoresis initially identified several classes or isotypes of human Igs (IgG, IgA, and IgM; Fig. 14–4); refined antisera subsequently distinguished four IgG classes (IgG1, IgG2, IgG3, IgG4) and two IgA classes (IgA1, IgA2). Two additional classes, IgD and IgE, present in low concentrations in normal serum, were detected by more sensitive methods, e.g., radioimmunoassays.

HEAVY-CHAIN ISOTYPES. Ig molecules are made up of a heavy (H) and a light (L) polypeptide chain. Each of the nine human Ig classes has an antigenically distinctive heavy chain, named with the corresponding Greek let-

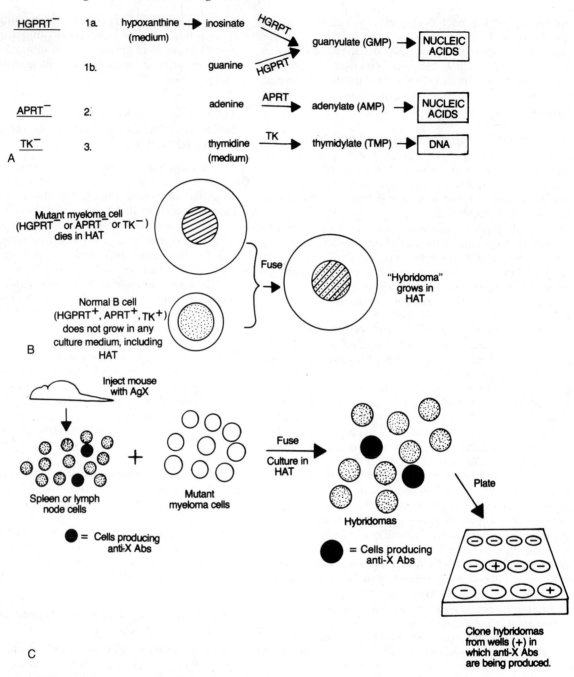

Figure 14–3. Production of mAbs. *(A)* Myeloma cells with a mutation in the enzyme hypoxanthine-guanine phosphoribosyl transferase (HGPRT) or adenine phosphoribosyl transferase (APRT) or thymidine kinase (TK) are chosen as "fusion partners" because they will not grow in the selective HAT medium (*H*, hypoxanthine; *A*, aminopterin; *T*, thymidine) unless fused to normal B cells, which supply the missing enzyme(s). Unfused B cells also do not grow in culture unless fused to the immortal myeloma cells. *(B)* The mutant myeloma cell line is fused to normal B cells from immunized mice, and the fusion mixture is cultured in HAT medium. The only cells that grow are B cell–myeloma cell hybrids. *(C)* Hybrid cells are screened in a series of minicultures (in microtiter wells) to detect those making antibodies to the antigen of interest. Cells in the positively reacting minicultures are then cloned to yield individual hybrids **(hybridomas),** each producing a single mAb.

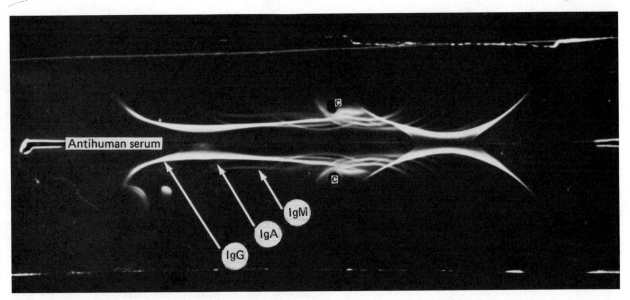

Figure 14–4. Immunoelectrophoresis showing IgG, IgA, and IgM. Human serum in the center well *(c)* was subjected to electrophoresis in agar in 0.1M barbital, pH 8.6; then rabbit antiserum prepared against unfractionated human serum was placed in the long trough, parallel to the axis of migration. Precipitation bands identify three Ig isotypes (IgG, IgA, IgM) and many other serum proteins. (See Fig. 13–25; courtesy of Dr C Kirk Osterland)

ter—e.g., μ chains in IgM, $\alpha 1$ chains in IgG1, $\alpha 2$ chains in IgA2. The L chains are similar in all classes. In a heteroantiserum to a homogeneous human Ig, say a myeloma protein of the IgG3 class, some Abs are specific for the H ($\gamma 3$) chains and others for the L chains.

KAPPA AND LAMBDA LIGHT CHAINS. There are also two main L-chain isotypes. They were distinguished when it was realized that urine from many patients with myeloma tumors contain excreted L chains, unassociated with H chains. The free L chains are named **Bence Jones proteins** after the 19th-century physician who first recognized them. About 10% of myeloma tumors produce only Bence Jones proteins, about 40% produce only complete myeloma proteins, and in the rest, which produce both, the **Bence Jones protein is identical with the myeloma protein's L chain.** Because a patient can excrete huge amounts (3–4 g per day) of Bence Jones protein in the urine, these proteins played an important role historically in working out the detailed structure of Igs.

Antisera to individual Bence Jones proteins distinguish two types of chains, termed **kappa** (κ) and **lambda** (λ). Each normal Ig molecule, regardless of its H-chain class, has one type of L chain or the other, never both. About 60% of human Ig molecules have κ chains; 40% have λ chains. Other vertebrate species also have k and λ chains, as defined by homologous amino acid sequences, but most have predominantly one type (e.g.,

about 95% of all L chains in mice are κ and almost 100% in horses and in birds are λ); a few (e.g., guinea pigs) have, like humans, nearly equal amounts of κ and λ L chains.

To see how H and L chains are arranged in complete Ig molecules, we consider next the structure of the most commonly encountered class of Ig, termed IgG.

THE IgG IMMUNOGLOBULINS
Separation of Heavy and Light Chains

The IgG proteins (mol. wt. 150,000) constitute about 90% of serum Igs. They were known to have many disulfide (S–S) bonds but were thought to have only a single chain per molecule until Edelman discovered that reductive cleavage of all the S–S bonds resulted in a fall in mol. wt. and the appearance of two grossly denatured components. By using milder reducing conditions, Porter selectively cleaved just the interchain S–S bonds, and soluble lower-mol. wt. components could then be separated by exposure to organic acids (acetic, propionic), which disrupt noncovalent hydrophobic bonds and impose many positive charges on polypeptide chains, leading to their mutual repulsion. Gel filtration yielded two components, with essentially 100% yield (Fig. 14–5*A*); the mol. wt. of the heavier (H) was about 50,000 and that of the lighter (L) about 25,000. The original molecule of 150,000 daltons thus consisted of two H chains (2 × 50,000) plus two L chains (2 × 25,000).

Although analysis of antigenic differences and of

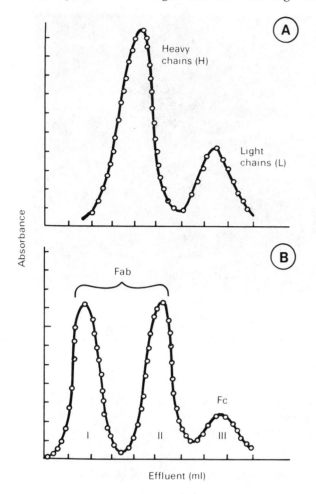

Figure 14–5. *(A)* Separation of H and L chains of IgGs. The protein was reduced and to prevent the liberated -SH groups from again forming S–S bridges, they were alkylated as follows:

$$. . . S\text{-}S\rightarrow . . . SH + I\cdot CH_2\cdot COOH\rightarrow . . . S\cdot CH_2\cdot COOH$$

Gel filtration in an organic acid (1M propionic) yielded H and L chains. *(B)* Separation of Fab and Fc fragments of Igs. The protein was digested with papain; after dialysis (during which some of the Fc crystallized), the digest was chromatographed on carboxymethylcellulose. Two Fab peaks *(I, II)* were seen because of the heterogeneity of the IgG sample; when the fragments are produced from a monoclonal Ig (e.g., a myeloma IgG), the Fab fraction emerges as one large peak, the sum of I + II. *(A,* based on Fleischman JB et al: Arch Biochem Suppl 1:1974, 1962; *B,* based on Porter RR: Biochem J 73:119, 1959)

amino acid sequences have revealed a great variety of H and L chains, we shall see that **any particular Ig molecule has identical H chains and identical L chains.**

Fragmentation with Proteolytic Enzymes: Fab and Fc Fragments

Enzymatic fragmentation of Abs contributed greatly to an understanding of their structure.

PAPAIN DIGESTION. Porter showed that digestion of native rabbit IgG with the enzyme papain split the molecule into fragments with loss of only about 10% of the protein as small dialyzable peptides. Ion-exchange chromatography separated the digest into two kinds of fragments. One had ligand-binding sites and was termed **Fab (antigen-binding fragment).** The other lacked Ag-binding sites but turned out to be surprisingly easy to crystallize; it was termed **Fc (crystallizable fragment)** (Fig. 14–5*B*). There is a single ligand-binding site per Fab fragment, and the total yield of these fragments accounts fully for the ligand-binding activity of the intact molecules.

Of the total digest prepared with papain, about two-thirds is Fab (mol. wt. about 45,000), and one-third is Fc (mol. wt. 50,000). Hence an **intact, bivalent IgG molecule is made up of two univalent Fab fragments joined to one Fc fragment.**

OTHER PROTEASES. Other proteolytic enzymes also split native Igs into large fragments, and pepsin has been especially useful: it cleaves from IgG Abs a bivalent fragment, of mol. wt. about 100,000, which can be split by reduction of one or a few S–S bonds to yield univalent fragments (Fig. 14–6). The latter are indistinguishable from the Fab fragments prepared with papain with respect to ligand-binding activity and antigenicity, but the pepsin fragment has a mol. wt. about 10% higher. To indicate the small difference, the univalent fragment obtained with pepsin is called **Fab′;** the corresponding bivalent fragment is **F(ab′)$_2$.** Fc is broken into many small peptides by pepsin and is not recovered.

Overall Structure

RELATIONS BETWEEN CHAINS AND FRAGMENTS. The immunogenicity of the proteolytic fragments made it possible to match fragments with dissociated chains. Thus, goat antiserum to the isolated Fc fragment of rabbit IgG forms specific precipitates with isolated H chains (as well as with Fc) but not with L chains. In contrast, antiserum to Fab fragments reacts with both L and H chains (Table 14–1). These findings led Porter to propose

TABLE 14–1. Goat Antibodies to Rabbit Fab and Fc Fragments: Precipitation Reaction with Chains Isolated from Rabbit IgG

	Antiserum to	
	Fab	Fc
Heavy chains	+	+
Light chains	+	−

+ = precipitation

− = no precipitation

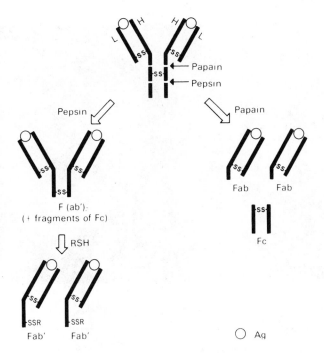

Figure 14–6. Four-chain structure of IgG showing critical interchain S–S bonds and regions susceptible to proteolytic cleavage (papain, pepsin, at arrows). The piece of heavy *(H)* chain within the Fab fragment is the **Fd piece**. The spherical Ag represents an Ag molecule in a ligand-binding site. (Four-chain model from Fleischman JB et al: Biochem J 88:220, 1963; scheme for pepsin digestion based on Nisonoff A et al: Arch Biochem 89:230, 1960)

the structure for IgG shown in Figure 14–6; it fits all the information now available, including x-ray crystallographic studies of Abs. Electron microscopy (Fig. 14–7) and x-ray analysis of single Ab crystals show Ab molecules to be Y shaped, with a "hinge" at the middle of the H chain connecting the Fc to Fab domains; the two ligand-binding sites are at the tips of the Y.

STABILITY. IgG proteins are unusually stable. In serum or as purified Abs, they can remain unaltered for years at 0°C. Moreover, after exposure to denaturing conditions (e.g., 70°C; pH 11 or pH 2; 8M urea), they largely recover their native structure when returned to dilute salt solution at physiologic conditions of pH and temperature; a major factor is the presence of a large number of stabilizing disulfide (S–S) bonds (16–24 per molecule). Four to twelve of these bonds (interchain) link the four chains together; the remainder (intrachain) stabilize their respective conformations (see Figs. 14–10 and 14–11, below).

SYMMETRY. As we shall see later, an Ig-producing cell usually makes only one type of L chain and one type of H chain (see Chap. 16, one cell–one Ig rule). Hence IgG

molecules are symmetric (see Fig. 14–10, below). In any particular molecule, the two light chains are identical, as are the two heavy chains. The two ligand-binding sites (see Chap. 13, Antibody Affinity and Valence) are also identical, for each of these sites is formed by a pair of H–L chains (see below).

IgG Classes

Antigenic analysis with antisera to myeloma proteins distinguishes 4 classes of human IgG (IgG1 through IgG4). Sometimes called subclasses, each class has a distinctive H chain (γ1 through γ4). IgG1, 2, 3, and 4 make up about 70%, 15%, 10%, and 5%, respectively, of human IgG proteins (Figs. 14–8 and 14–11). The distinctive antigenic determinants that characterize each of these classes are located in their Fc segments.

Four classes of IgG have also been identified in the mouse, the only other species in which many myeloma proteins have been intensively studied. Fewer IgG classes have been recognized in other species, probably because their Igs have not yet been analyzed as intensively.

Antigenic differences among the four IgG classes are less pronounced than those between them and the other Ig classes. For example, after Abs to L chains are removed, antiserum prepared against an IgG1 myeloma protein cross-reacts with IgG2, IgG3, and IgG4 but not with IgM, IgA, IgE, or IgD. Amino acid sequence data (below) similarly reveal greater sequence similarities among γ1, γ2, γ3, and γ4 chains than among H chains of other classes (see Table 14–4, Appendix, this Chap.).

Amino Acid Sequences: Variable (V) and Constant (C) Domains

The basis for antigenic differences among Igs has been illuminated by amino acid sequences of chains from monoclonal Igs (myeloma proteins and mAbs). The first extensive sequences were obtained with two human L chains (κ Bence Jones proteins analyzed by Hilschmann and Craig and by Putnam et al). These chains differ from one another in many amino acid residues present at homologous positions in the N-terminal half (now termed the **variable** or **V domain**), whereas the carboxy half (called the **constant** or **C domain**) is the same in all human κ chains (except at two positions; see Allotypes, below). This remarkable distinction between sequence variability in the V domains and constancy in the C domains, illustrated in Figure 14–9, has since been found to be characteristic of all Ig H and L chains.

The IgG γ chains are about twice as long as L chains. The first amino acid sequences revealed linear repeats in both H and L chains, suggestive of repeating domains: each domain has about 110 amino acids with an S–S bond that links two cysteine residues, one about 20 residues from the amino end and the other about 20 residues from the carboxy end. Hence the S–S bond estab-

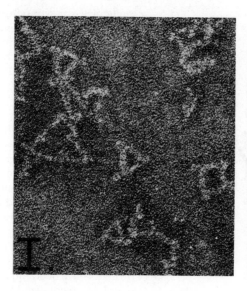

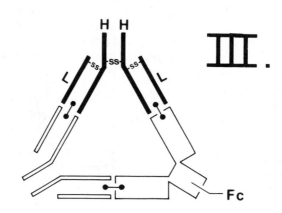

Figure 14—7. Three IgG anti-Dnp Ab molecules joined in a triangular complex by a ligand with two Dnp groups per molecule (Dnp-NH[CH$_2$]$_8$-NH-Dnp). The ligand is too small to be seen. The complex in *I* forms the basis for the diagram in *III*. The picture in *II* was obtained after treatment of the complex in *I* with pepsin, removing the corner projections, which correspond to Fc. (Valentine RC, Green NM: J Mol Biol 27:615, 1967) (*I* and *II*, electron micrographs, ×500,000)

●—● Dnp ligand

lishes a loop of approximately 60 amino acid residues. Similarities in sequence suggested that each of these domains has an approximately similar shape, as was later confirmed by x-ray diffraction of Ig crystals (see Three-Dimensional Structure, below). Comparison of various γ chains showed that, as with κ chains, the variations are localized in the N-terminal (V) domain; the remaining sequence is the same in all chains of a particular class (except for small heritable differences; see Allotypes, below). An IgG molecule has six domains: two in L chains

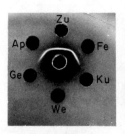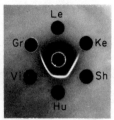

Figure 14–8. IgG classes. Twelve IgG myeloma proteins (each from a human with a myeloma tumor) were tested with monkey antiserum (center well in each panel) to the protein from patient *Zu* after the antiserum had been absorbed with Igs of other classes. Five additional proteins were precipitated *(Ap, Fe, Vi, Hu, Sh)*; hence they belong to the same class as *Zu* (IgG3). The six nonreacting IgGs belong to other classes. (Grey HM, Kunkel HG: J Exp Med 120:253, 1964)

(V_L and C_L) and four in H chains (V_H, C_H1, C_H2, C_H3; Fig. 14–10). Generally, sequence similarity between γ chain isotypes is greater in C_H1 than in C_H2 or C_H3 domains. For instance, human $\gamma1$ and $\gamma2$ are identical at more than 90% of the positions in C_H1 and at only 60% to 70% of the positions in C_H2 and C_H3.

HINGE REGION. A stretch of about 15 amino acid residues between C_H1 and C_H2 corresponds to a flexible junction between Fab and Fc regions in $\gamma1$, $\gamma2$, and $\gamma4$ chains (see Three-Dimensional Structure, below). This "hinge" region has no obvious homology with other domains. It contains the interchain S–S bonds that link together the two H chains of each IgG molecule and the H and L chains of IgG1 molecules (Figs. 14–10 and 14–11).

The few cleavages caused by proteolytic enzymes in native Ig molecules are localized in the hinge region (see Figs. 14–6 and 14–10). The abundance here of residues that confer rigidity on polypeptides (proline and cysteine) evidently exposes this part of the polypeptide backbone to the solvent and to proteolytic enzymes. In contrast to their native form, denatured Igs are extensively degraded into small peptides by many proteases.

Figure 14–9. Variable *(V)* and constant *(C)* segments illustrated by selected amino acid sequences from some human light chains (named *SH*, etc., for the patient from whom the myeloma protein was derived). Sequences are aligned for maximal homology. From positions marked C_L to the COOH terminus (to the right of the vertical dashed line), the κ chains are all alike, as are the λ chains; κ-λ differences are especially easy to discern in C_L (e.g., at positions 118, 119, 120). Amplitude of the jagged line above the sequences represents extent of variability. Note the one-letter code for amino acids. (Based on references in Dayhoff M [ed]: Atlas of Amino Acid Sequence and Structure, vol 5. Silver Spring, National Biomedical Research Foundation, 1972)

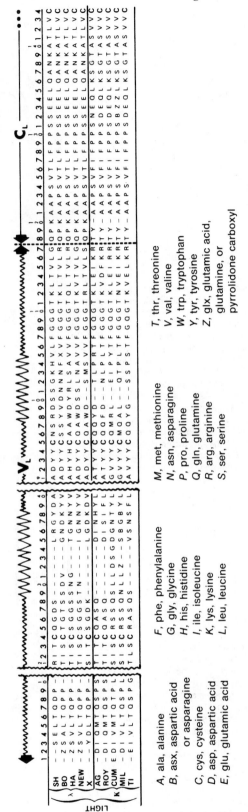

A, ala, alanine
B, asx, aspartic acid or asparagine
C, cys, cysteine
D, asp, aspartic acid
E, glu, glutamic acid
F, phe, phenylalanine
G, gly, glycine
H, his, histidine
I, ile, isoleucine
K, lys, lysine
L, leu, leucine
M, met, methionine
N, asn, asparagine
P, pro, proline
Q, gln, glutamine
R, arg, arginine
S, ser, serine
T, thr, threonine
V, val, valine
W, trp, tryptophan
Y, tyr, tyrosine
Z, glx, glutamic acid, glutamine, or pyrrolidone carboxyl

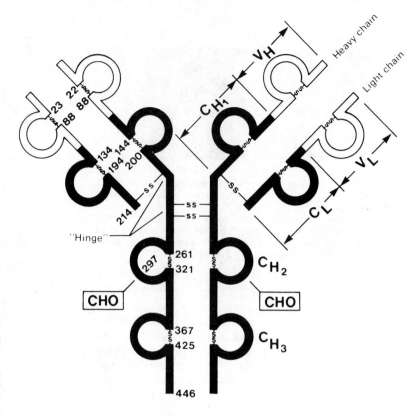

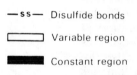

Figure 14–10. Linear periodicity in amino acid sequences of an IgG molecule shows that light *(L)* and heavy *(H)* chains have repeating domains, each with about 110 amino acid residues and an approximately 60-membered S–S bonded loop. Domains with variable sequences are represented by open bars (V_L, V_H); those with constant sequences in a given class of H or type of L are represented by solid lines $(C_L, C_H1, C_H2, C_H3;$ see Fig. 14–9). Numbered positions refer to cysteinyl residues that form S–S bonds, or to the point of attachment of an asparagine-linked oligosaccharide (CHO, see Fig. 14–16). Disulfide (S–S) bonds joining distant parts of the same chain are **intrachain bonds;** those linking L to H or H to H chains are **interchain bonds.** For other arrangements of interchain S–S bonds see Figure 14–11. (Based on Edelman GM: Biochemistry 9:3197, 1970)

—ss— Disulfide bonds

☐ Variable region

■ Constant region

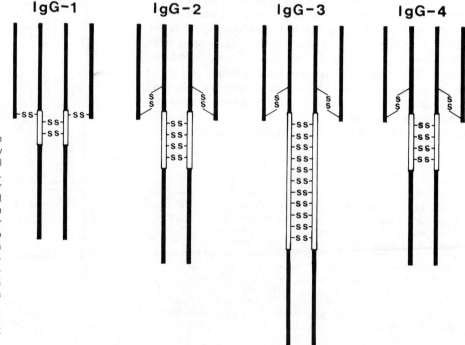

Figure 14–11. Interchain S–S bridges in various human IgG classes. The diversity of these bonds contrasts with the virtual constancy of intrachain S–S bonds (Fig. 14–10). Note that the hinge in γ3 is four times longer than in the other γ chains. All H–H S–S bridges are in the hinge *(open rectangles);* variations in their number and arrangement are probably related to effector and other differences between these classes (e.g., susceptibility to papain digestion). The H chain cysteinyl residue forming the H–L S–S bridge in IgG classes 2, 3, and 4 is about 100 residues closer to the N terminus than in IgG1. (Based on data from Frangione B et al: Nature 211:145, 1969; Michaelson TE et al: J Biol Chem 252:883, 1977)

OTHER IMMUNOGLOBULIN CLASSES

IgM

Because of their abundance in certain antisera (e.g., those prepared in horses to treat many serious bacterial infections in the era before antibiotic therapy) Abs of the IgM class were the first Igs to be isolated as a pure protein. But in the immune response to most Ags, Abs of the IgM class are actually formed only early in the response and at very low levels and are soon overshadowed by larger amounts of IgG Abs to the same Ag (see Chaps. 15 and 16). In humans and other mammals, IgM normally accounts for about 5% to 10% of the serum Igs, and few myeloma proteins are of the IgM class. (The IgMs used to establish the detailed structure outlined in Figure 14–12 below were obtained from humans with a form of lymphatic cancer known as **Waldenstrom's macroglobu-** linemia; in each patient, a clone of neoplastic Ig-producing lymphocytes yields a monoclonal IgM.)

The human IgM molecule (about 900,000 daltons) is a pentamer made up of five four-chain monomers, each with a pair of H (μ) chains and a pair of κ or λ L chains (Fig. 14–12). The μ chains lack a hinge. Instead, they have about 130 more amino acid residues, or one more domain, than γ chains. The extra domain is located (like the hinge in other Ig molecules) between domains that are homologous by amino acid sequence to C_H1 and C_H2 of γ chains. As expected, μ chains from different myeloma tumors differ in the N-terminal (V) domain and not in other (C) domains. The four-chain monomers are linked by two S–S bonds between μ chains (one is in C_H3 and another in C_H4 at the penultimate residue of the μ chain) and also by another chain, called J, described below.

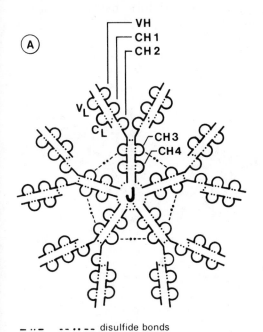

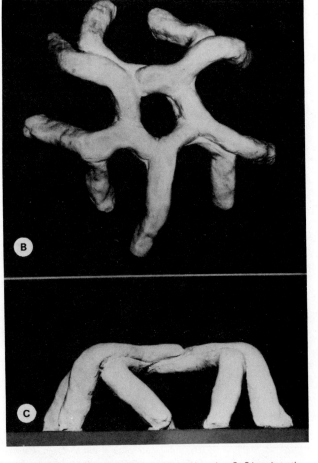

Figure 14–12. Structure of human IgM. (**A**) Five four-chain subunits are joined by S–S bridges and linked by other S–S bonds to the J chain. Hot trypsin (60°C) cleaves between C_H2 and C_H3, yielding ten Fab fragments and one Fc pentamer per molecule. (**B** and **C**) Models of the IgM molecule based on electron microscopy. Top view (**B**) displays flexible subunits. Profile view (**C**) shows the molecule bound at multiple sites to the surface of an Ag. (**A**, based on Putnam FW et al: Science 182:287, 1973; **B** and **C**, based on Feinstein A, Munn EA: Nature 224:1307, 1969; Svehag SE et al: J Exp Med 130:691, 1969)

Under mild reducing conditions, IgM is cleaved into monomers, each with two H (μ) and two L chains. Resembling an IgG molecule, the monomer, sometimes called IgM$_s$, has two ligand-binding sites per molecule but loses its ability to participate in agglutination and many other immune reactions. The dependence of these latter activities on more than two binding sites per molecule is probably attributable to the fact that IgM Abs usually have very low intrinsic affinity for Ag. Accordingly, it is usually necessary for IgM molecules to bind Ags multivalently (see Chap. 13) in order to exhibit biologic activity (see Fig. 14–12C and Appendix, Chap. 13).

(Low-molecular-weight IgM, corresponding to the monomer produced by mild reductive cleavage of the pentameric molecule, also occurs naturally in slightly modified form as the surface Ig of most B-lymphocytes, the precursors of Ab-secreting cells (Chaps. 15 and 16). It also occurs at trace levels in normal human serum and at high levels (about 1 mg/ml) in certain disorders of the immune system such as rheumatoid arthritis and systemic lupus erythematosus.)

J CHAINS. Besides the ten L and ten H chains per molecule, pentameric IgM has one additional chain, called J (see Fig. 14–12). This chain (15,000 daltons) does not share antigenic determinants or amino acid sequences with Igs, but it is probably an essential stabilizing element in the pentameric molecule, where it is S–S bonded to μ chains. J chains also join the H chains of multimeric forms of IgA (Fig. 14–13; also see below). J chains are synthesized in the same cells as the Ig molecules to which they are linked.

IgA

Immunoelectrophoresis of human serum led to the identification of IgA, whose basic structural unit corresponds to the four-chain molecule shown in Figure 14–13 (see also Fig. 14–4). Unlike IgM, which is a pentamer, and IgG, which is uniformly a monomer (i.e., H$_2$L$_2$), **IgA occurs in various polymeric forms: monomers (H$_2$L$_2$), dimers (H$_4$L$_4$), and even higher multimers.** The multimers are S–S linked monomers: mild reduction dissociates them into the basic four-chain Ig molecule (H$_2$L$_2$).

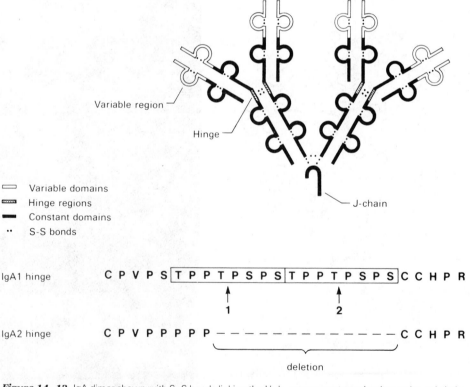

Variable region

Hinge

Variable domains
Hinge regions
Constant domains
S-S bonds

J-chain

IgA1 hinge   C P V P S | T P P T P S P S | T P P T P S P S | C C H P R

                          1   2

IgA2 hinge   C P V P P P P — — — — — — — — — — — C C H P R

deletion

Figure 14–13. IgA dimer shown with S–S bonds linking the H$_2$L$_2$ monomers to each other and to a J chain. The duplicated hinge of the α1 chain is shown in the rectangle; note deletion within the α2 hinge. Arrows point to the threonine–proline bonds cleaved in IgA1 molecules by a streptococcal protease (1) and a gonococcal protease (2), yielding in each case Fabα and Fcα fragments. IgA2 molecules are resistant to these proteases. The secretory piece is shown in Figure 14–14. For amino acid abbreviations, see Figure 14–9. (Based on Plaut AG et al: Science 190:1103, 1975)

IgA normally accounts for less than 10% of the total Ig in human serum but is the principal Ig in external secretions such as colostrum, respiratory and intestinal mucin, saliva, tears, and genitourinary tract mucin. IgA Abs very likely play an important role in protecting mucosal surfaces from invasion by infectious agents. In colostrum, they also help protect the suckling newborn from infection.

The number of IgA classes differs among species, e.g., one in the mouse, three in rabbits. There are two in humans, IgA1 and IgA2, with $\alpha 1$ and $\alpha 2$ H chain isotypes, respectively. In human serum, about 80% of the IgA is monomeric $(\alpha_2 L_2)$ and IgA1; in secretions, about 90% is polymeric (mostly dimers and decreasing amounts of trimers, tetramers, etc.), and IgA1 and IgA2 are about equally represented.

Both $\alpha 1$ and $\alpha 2$ chains have four domains (one V_H, three C_H). A duplicated proline-rich sequence in the hinge region of $\alpha 1$ is largely lacking in $\alpha 2$ chains (see Fig. 14–13). Bacterial proteases from certain streptococci and from gonococci cleave particular bonds in this region of IgA1 molecules, yielding Fabα and Fcα fragments, but IgA2 molecules are entirely resistant. Hence IgA2 Abs might confer greater protection than IgA1 against such bacteria (e.g., gonococci in the genitourinary tract).

The IgA dimer has a single J chain, as in the IgM pentamer (above), and it also has another chain, called **secretory piece (SP),** which is the key to the transport of IgA across the epithelial lining of exocrine glands into external secretions.

SECRETORY PIECE. The transport of IgA into external glandular secretions requires the Ig molecule to traverse glandular epithelial cells. This complex process is made possible by an IgA-specific receptor on the surface of the epithelial cells. After binding IgA, the receptor–IgA complex is taken into these cells by receptor-mediated endocytosis, transported across the cell's entire length, and extruded from the opposite surface into the external secretions (Fig. 14–14). A proteolytic cleavage of the receptor as it is extruded from the epithelial cell leaves a fragment (approximately 70,000 daltons), termed secretory piece, attached by an S–S bond to the secreted IgA molecule.

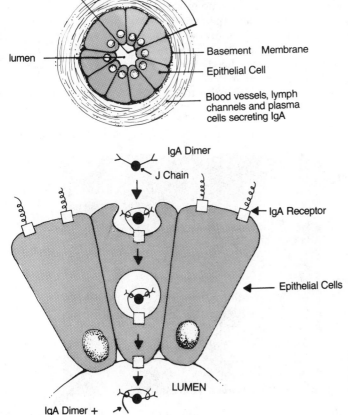

Figure 14–14. Secretion of IgA with attached secretory piece. *(Top)* Cross-section through an exocrine gland. In the expanded view of three epithelial cells *(bottom)*, an IgA dimer is being bound to a receptor and endocytosed by the middle cell, which it traverses to exit on the luminal side bearing an attached piece of the receptor (secretory piece). (From Mostov KE, Simister NE: Cell 43:389, 1985)

Amino acid sequences show that secretory piece of IgA corresponds to the C-terminal half of the receptor, whereas the receptor's N-terminal section, which is responsible for binding IgA, consists of five similar domains, each unmistakably resembling an Ig domain (described below). The striking similarity suggests that this receptor, and also several other cell-surface receptors to be described later, are related to Ig and are members of what has been called the **Ig superfamily.** All members of this family were probably derived in evolution from a common ancestral Ig-like gene that may have encoded a single Ig-like domain (Chap 15, Fig. 15–33).

IgD

These proteins were discovered as myeloma proteins that failed to react with antisera to the other Ig classes known at the time (IgG, IgA, and IgM). Although produced at high levels by rare myeloma tumors, the corresponding normal Igs, termed IgD, are present in normal human sera at extremely low levels, on average about 30 μg/ml or about 0.2% of the total Igs. The overall structure is the same as that of IgG. The mol. wt. of the isolated δ chain is 70,000, suggesting five domains (one V_H, four C_H). A single S–S bond joins L to δ chains and another joins the two δ chains.

Compared with other Igs, IgD molecules are relatively heat labile, and they are also extremely sensitive to proteases: in serum stored in the cold for a few days, IgD is broken down into Fab and Fc fragments, probably through attack by serum enzymes. Although present at only trace levels in serum, IgD is expressed at high levels, along with IgM, on the surface of most mature B lymphocytes. The IgM and IgD on the surface of the same cell line have the same amino acid sequence in the ligand-binding domain and thus must have the same specificity for Ag. However, when the cells are stimulated to make Igs, they produce and secrete IgM, not IgD. The mechanisms responsible for this change are known (see Ig Genes, Fig. 14–39 below), but the role of IgD on the cell surface is not understood.

IgE

IgE proteins were discovered by K. and T. Ishizaka while studying the human Abs (called reagins; see Chap. 18) that mediate certain acute allergic reactions. They found that these Abs were precipitated by rabbit antiserum to reagin-rich fractions of serum Ig but not by antisera to the then-known Ig classes. Thus, these Abs appeared to represent still another Ig class, now called IgE. This suggestion was confirmed by the finding in Sweden of an unusual human myeloma protein that also did not react with antisera to the known Ig classes. Abs to either the Swedish myeloma protein or to reagins reacted specifically with the other (Fig. 14–15).

Only a very few other human IgE myeloma proteins have been identified, but many mAbs of the IgE class have been produced. The IgE molecule (188,000–196,000 daltons) has a pair of ε H chains linked by S–S bonds to a pair of either κ or λ L chains. The carbohydrate content is high (11.5%). The mol. wt. of ε chains (about 75,000, or 61,000–65,000 daltons if carbohydrate is deducted) is slightly higher (by about 3000 daltons) than that of μ chains. As with μ chains, the ε chain has an extra C domain that lies between what correspond to C_H1 and C_H2 of γ chains.

IgE is present in traces in normal human serum, on

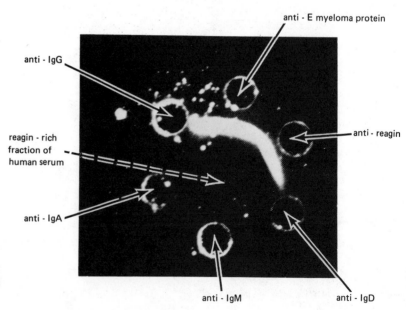

Figure 14–15. Identification of reagins as IgE protein. A reagin-rich fraction of human atopic serum was placed in the center well, and antisera for each of the human Ig classes were placed in peripheral wells. Antisera to reagin and to the myeloma IgE gave reactions of identity. (Ishizaka K. In Merier E [ed]: Immunoglobulins: Biologic Aspects and Clinical Uses. Washington, National Academy Press, 1970)

average, about 0.3 μg/ml, or about 1 in 50,000 serum Ig molecules is IgE. Nevertheless, **Abs of the IgE class are responsible for anaphylactic shock,** an acute allergic reaction that can be explosive and life-threatening (see Chap. 18).

IgE levels are elevated slightly in some people with some reagin-mediated diseases such as severe hay fever and, even more, in those with chronic parasitic infestations of the intestinal tract (e.g., African children with ascariasis, hookworm, or schistosomiasis), where levels as high as 140 μg/ml have been described. Perhaps because of chronic intestinal parasitism, IgE levels are also elevated in laboratory rats, in which a high proportion of myeloma tumors produce IgE myeloma proteins.

As we shall later consider in some detail, the most severe allergic reactions depend on the extremely high affinity of the Fc region of IgE molecules for special cell-surface receptors (Fcε receptors) on tissue mast cells and on basophilic leukocytes. These cells release histamine and other vasoactive amines when multivalent Ag cross-links IgE Abs that are tightly associated with the Fcε receptors (see Chap. 18).

LIGHT-CHAIN ISOTYPES

There is a single class of κ chains. However, there are several classes of λ chains, and the number differs in various species: three in inbred mice (λ1, λ2, λ3) and five or six in humans. Antisera readily distinguish κ from λ chains; some of the λ classes are similarly distinguished from each other, whereas others are so similar in amino acid sequence that they have not been distinguished serologically.

CARBOHYDRATE SIDE CHAINS

Igs are glycoproteins, with carbohydrate making up 3% to 12% of their mol. wt. Oligosaccharide units are attached to one or more positions of all H chains but only rarely to L chains.

Except for some of the carbohydrate on α1 chains, the oligosaccharides are attached via N-glycosidic linkage of an N-acetylglucosamine residue to asparagine in the sequence Asn–X–Ser or Asn–X–Thr of the Ig chains, where Asn is asparagine, X is any amino acid (except proline), and the third position is serine or threonine (Fig. 14–16). During synthesis of Ig chains, the triplet sequence can serve as acceptor for oligosaccharides from transferase enzymes of the Golgi complex (N-acetylglucosamine–asparagine transglycosylase). However, in some chains, some acceptor sites are not glycosylated, perhaps because they are not accessible in the folded chains to the glycosylating enzymes. Some of the oligosaccharides on Ig H chains are shown in Figure 14–15.

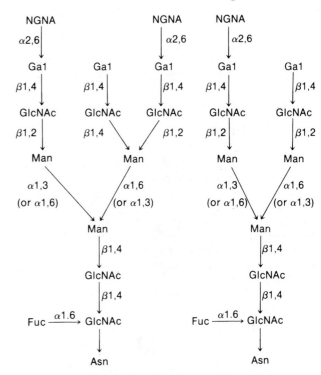

Figure 14–16. Various carbohydrate side chains are found in Igs. The examples shown, in the C_H domain of a mouse IgM, are attached to the amide N of an asparagine (Asn) residue in the triplet sequence Asn–X–Ser/Thr (where X is any amino acid except proline) and the carboxy terminus is serine or threonine. *NGNA*, N-glycolylneuraminic acid; *Gal*, galactose; *GlcNAc*, N-acetylglucosamine; *Man*, mannose; *Fuc*, fucose. (Redrawn from Brenckle and Kornfeld, 1980)

The oligosaccharide branches terminate in galactose, to which sialic acid (N-acetyl neuraminic acid) residues are frequently attached. When circulating Igs have sialic acid removed (by neuraminidase), they become bound to a receptor on hepatocytes with high affinity for terminal galactose of oligosaccharides on glycoproteins. By receptor-mediated endocytosis, the bound Ig is taken into the hepatocytes and degraded. Hence the persistence of Ig in the circulation (usually measured as a half-life) depends on the status of its oligosaccharides. Each Ig class has a characteristic half-life in the circulation, e.g., 23 days for human IgG1. Differences in half-life could mean that the Igs of different classes differ in the structure of their oligosaccharides or their susceptibility to neuraminidase (see Appendix, this Chap., Table 14–5).

ALLOTYPES: GENETIC VARIANTS

The Ags encoded by alternative forms of a gene (termed alleles) are called **alloantigens (alloAgs).** They are characteristically produced by some individuals and not by others of the same species. Many important Ags are alloAgs: for instance, the prominent cell-surface Ags that determine the success or failure of transplanted organs or transfused blood from one individual to another. **Alloantigenic forms of Igs are called allotypes;** they have contributed greatly to our understanding of Ig structure and the organization of Ig genes.

Human Allotypes

A chance observation led to the discovery of human Ig allotypes. Sera from persons with rheumatoid arthritis often contain rheumatoid factors, which are Igs that react with pooled human IgG. For example, they specifically agglutinate human red blood cells (RBC) coated with human anti-RBC Abs of the incomplete type (see Blocking Antibodies, Chap. 13). Rheumatoid factor from some patients was noted to react only with RBC that had been coated with Abs from certain other persons. It was also noted that any particular agglutination reaction could be specifically inhibited only by serum from particular individuals, whose Igs presumably carried the same epitopes as the anti-RBC Abs and therefore competed for the rheumatoid factor (see Appendix, this Chap., Fig. 14–41). By means of such reactions with rheumatoid factors, human Igs can be classified into sets of allotypes, of which the principal sets are called **Gm** on γ chains, **Am** on α chains, and **Km** on κ L chains.

Useful sera for identifying these allotypes also come from other sources. In about 10% of human pregnancies, mothers have Ig allotypes that their babies lack. With transfer of maternal Ig across the placenta, about half of these babies are stimulated to make antiallotype Abs. Antiallotypes are also frequently formed in persons who receive multiple blood transfusions because the donors often have allotypes that the recipients lack. To illustrate the principal features of allotypes we consider the simplest set, **Km** on human κ L chains.

Km ALLOTYPES. As we shall see later, the C domain of human κ chains is encoded by a single gene. This gene has three known allelic forms, and the C domains they encode are distinguished by agglutination reactions (described above) and amino acid substitutions at two positions (153 and 191, Table 14–2). Although separated in the linear sequence by 38 amino acids, x-ray crystallographic studies show that in the folded Ig molecule, the two variant positions are in very close proximity; hence they probably are critical components of the epitope recognized by anti-Km Abs. That the recognition of this epitope depends on Ig conformation, and not only on sequence, is also evident because κ chains lose their reactivity with anti-Km Abs when separated from H chains.

All allotypes, including Km, are inherited as dominant Mendelian traits. Thus, an individual expresses

TABLE 14–2. *Amino Acid Substitutions Corresponding to Km Allotypes in Human κ Chains*

Serologic marker*	Amino Acid At Position	
	153	191
Km(1)	Val	Leu
Km(1,2)	Ala	Leu
Km(3)	Ala	Val

* Km was previously called InV (because Igs with these allotypes inhibited the reactions of a typing serum from patient V). Km(2) is always associated with Km(1), but some individuals are Km(1⁺2⁻). See Fig. 14–17 for the inhibition assay.

one (if homozygous) or two (if heterozygous) but never more than two (because vertebrate cells are diploid).

In a Km-heterozygous individual, the two Km allotypes (for instance, Km1 and Km3) are found at more or less equal levels in total serum Ig, but **the individual Ig molecule has exclusively one allotype or the other,** never both. For instance, if a Km-heterozygous individual has a myeloma tumor that produces a myeloma protein having κ chains, the protein will have only one of the two possible κ allotypes. Observations of this type helped establish the important principle called **allelic exclusion.** As we shall see later, the basis for this principle is that an Ig-producing cell that expresses a particular L-chain gene (κ or one of the λ's) will express only one of that gene's alleles, not both. The same exclusion applies to H chains. It is the basis for **the fundamental rule that each Ig molecule has identical H chains and identical L chains and hence only a single Ag-binding specificity** (the **one cell–one Ig** or **one cell–one Ab** rule).

The geographic and ethnic distribution of allotypes is extremely uneven, and they are of considerable value in studies of population genetics and anthropology; e.g., Km(1,2) is present in 10% to 20% of Europeans and in more than 90% of Venezuelan Indians. Rare individuals lack all of the known Km allotypes, suggesting that there are additional Km alleles.

Gm ALLOTYPES. Each of the four IgG classes has its own set of allotypes (termed Gm) and, in total, more than 20 allotypic γ chain variants have been identified. Like the Km allotypes, the Gm allotypes are expressed at more or less equal levels in Gm-heterozygous individuals. Fragments and isolated chains from myeloma proteins have served to localize the allotypic determinants to particular domains and even to particular amino acid substitutions. Thus, some allotypic determinants of γ1 chains are located in the C_H3 domain (Fc fragment), and others are in the C_H1 domain (Fab fragment). That a single Ig chain has more than one allotypic determinant should not be surprising, because there commonly are a multiplicity of epitopes on a single polypeptide chain (see Appendix, this Chap., Table 14–6). The amino acid substitutions that specify some of the Gm allotypes are known.

Am ALLOTYPES. Genetic variants of IgA have the same overall characteristics as those of κ and γ chains. They were discovered through reactions to blood transfusions: recipients who lack an IgA variant can suffer severe reactions when transfused more than once with blood that contains it. (The first transfusion induces formation of the antiallotype Abs, which then react with that allotype in subsequent transfusions.)

Allotypes in Other Species

RABBIT. These allotypes were recognized by precipitin reactions with antisera from rabbits that had been immunized with Abs from other rabbits. The antisera identify three sets of allotypes, for H, κ, and γ chains. Their inheritance follows the same pattern as in humans (see also below).

MOUSE. Inbred mouse strains simplify the recognition of allotypes. All members of a given strain are virtually identical genetically, and many strains differ in Ig allotypes. Hence antiallotype Abs are readily produced by immunizing mice of one strain with Igs from another strain. Some mouse allotypes are listed in Table 14–7 of the Appendix, this Chapter.

INHERITANCE OF ALLOTYPES. Like κ chain Km allotypes, the allotypic variants of other Ig chains are also inherited as dominant Mendelian traits. H chain allotypes are especially notable, because those of all the H chain classes are inherited together as a single unit, termed a **haplotype,** in which the genes for the various H chain classes are so tightly linked that recombination between them occurs in far less than 1% of progeny. In contrast, allotypes for H chains and κ chains, and also for λ chains in those species (rabbit) where they have been identified, segregate independently. The reason, as we shall see, is that each of the three sets of Ig genes (for H, κ, and λ chains) resides on a different chromosome (Table 14–3).

TABLE 14–3. Chromosome Location of Loci for Human and Mouse Heavy (H) Chains and κ and λ Light Chains

Ig Chain	Chromosome No.	
	Human	Mouse
H	14	12
κ	2	6
λ	22	16

IDIOTYPES: UNIQUE DETERMINANTS OF INDIVIDUAL IMMUNOGLOBULINS

Idiotopes are antigenic determinants (epitopes) that distinguish one monoclonal Ig (e.g., myeloma protein or mAb) from others having the same H and L chain isotypes and allotypes. An Ig's set of idiotopes is called its **idiotype** or **Id.**

Ids were discovered through studies of rabbit Abs and human myeloma proteins. Oudin injected anti-Salmonella Abs from one rabbit into other rabbits with the same allotypes. Some recipients formed Abs (antiidiotypes) that reacted specifically with the Ab used for immunization but not with other Igs from the donor or with anti-Salmonella Abs from other rabbits. In a basically similar observation with human myeloma proteins, Kunkel and colleagues adsorbed a rabbit antiserum to one human myeloma protein with other myeloma proteins having the same H- and L-chain isotypes and allotypes, and they found the residual Abs to be specific for the "individually unique" antigenic determinants (i.e., the Id) of the immunogen.

Although each Ig molecule has a unique or individual Id **(IdI),** shared only by molecules produced by cells of the same clone, some Abs also have cross-reacting Ids **(IdX)** that are present on some other Igs elicited by the same Ag, even in other individuals if their genetic background is the same (e.g., in an inbred mouse strain). One shared IdX, for instance, is present on about 15% of the Abs made against benzenearsonate in all A/J mice; another is present on virtually all Abs made in BALB/c mice to phosphorylcholine. Many Ags, tested in inbred mice, elicit Abs with shared Ids (IdX).

All Ids are located in or near Ag-binding sites. Ids are present in Fab, not Fc, fragments, and their localization in or extremely close to ligand-binding sites is evident because haptens (or Ags) can specifically block the binding of anti-Id Abs: the higher the ligand's affinity, the more effectively it inhibits binding by anti-Id (Fig. 14–17). Because Ag and anti-Id Abs compete for the binding site (Id) of the same Ab, it has been suggested that an epitope of the Ag and the combining site of the anti-Id Abs are structurally similar, as if the anti-Id Ab's combining site is an **internal image** of an epitope of the Ag (Fig. 14–18). We shall later consider several instances in which anti-Id Abs serve as substitutes for Ags (see Chap. 16).

Anti-Id Abs are produced by injecting an Ab (call it Ab-1) isolated from one individual (the donor) into animals of a different species (giving rise to **heteroantisera**) or into genetically different individuals of the same species (giving rise to **alloantisera**). In order to obtain sera containing only anti-Id Abs, the antisera have to be thoroughly adsorbed with the donor's normal Ig (minus Ab-1), removing antiisotypic Abs from the heteroantisera and antiallotypic Abs from heteroantisera and from al-

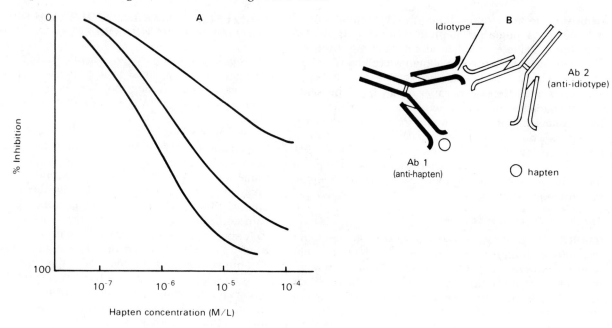

Figure 14–17. *(A)* Specific inhibition of an idiotype/anti-idiotype reaction. The reaction of an anti-idiotypic Ab can be blocked specifically by ligands that bind to the Ab with the idiotype. The inhibition curves *(left)* were obtained with three haptens having different affinity for the Id-bearing Ab: the hapten with highest affinity elicited the lowermost curve at the left, and the hapten with lowest affinity the uppermost curve. *(B)* A hapten competing with an anti-idiotypic Ab *(Ab 2)* for the binding site of the anti-hapten Ab *(Ab 1)*. (Based on Brient BW, Nisonoff A: J Exp Med 132:951, 1970)

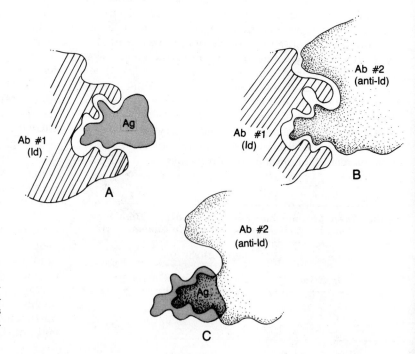

Figure 14–18. Antigen (Ag) and an anti-idiotypic antibody (Ab 2) compete for the binding site of Ab 1, the Id-bearing antibody. Hence the anti-Id's combining site is assumed to mimic the structure of an epitope on the Ag. (See *C* for overlapping structures.)

loantisera. However, anti-Id Abs can often be elicited even when the donor of Ab-1 and the immunized individual are from the same inbred strain of mice and are thus genetically the same. Because the donor and recipients have the same allotypes and isotypes, any Abs produced by the recipient will be specific for the Id of Ab-1. It has even been possible to obtain anti-Id Abs by injecting Ab-1 back into the individual from which it had been previously isolated. These circumstances suggest that anti-Ids Abs might be formed spontaneously against Ids of conventional Abs that arise in response to immunization with an Ag. The possibility that normal immune responses are regulated by such anti-Id/Id interactions will be considered later (see Chap. 16).

COMPARISON OF THE NUMBER OF IDIOTYPES, ALLOTYPES, AND ISOTYPES. There is a great disparity between the total number of idiotypes, isotypes, and allotypes. Thus, in the mouse, there are 12 known isotypes (eight for H chains, three for λ chains, and one for κ chains) and about 30 to 40 known allotypes (i.e., multiple allotypes for almost every isotype), but the number of Ids is essentially equal to the total number of different Igs: more than 10^8 is a guess, but not an exaggerated one. As we shall see, the basis for this vast number lies in the enormous variability of amino acid sequences of the variable (V) segments of Ig chains and in the organization and somatic alterations of the genes that encode them.

VARIABLE DOMAIN: COMPLEMENTARITY-DETERMINING REGIONS (CDRs) AND FRAMEWORK REGIONS (FRs)

Among the Ig chains of any class, the amino acid sequences are the same in their C-terminal constant (C) domains (except for the few substitutions that are responsible for allotypic variants), but sequences differ from one chain to another at many positions in the N-terminal variable (V) domain. In this domain, the variability is especially extreme in **hypervariable regions** (Fig. 14–19). Because these regions form the combining sites that are complementary in shape to ligands (see below), they are also referred to as **complementarity-determining regions (CDRs)**. There are three CDRs in L chains and three in H chains; each consists of about five to ten residues centered at positions 30–35, 50–55, and 95–100. The less-variable sequences on either side of each CDR are called **framework regions** (FRs). Thus each V domain consists of four FRs and three CDRs; in order, from the N-terminus, they are FR1–CDR1–FR2–CDR2–FR3–CDR3–FR4. The conserved amino acids at certain framework positions distinguish three types of V sequences: V_H, associated with H chains; V_κ, associated with κ chains; and V_λ, associated with λ chains.

V GROUPS. Variations within the framework regions further distinguish many groups of V domains or "V groups" (Fig. 14–20). Just how many framework differences between two V sequences justify their assignment to different V groups is arbitrary, but the prevailing view is that V domains with more than three differences in the N-terminal 25 positions belong to different groups. In mice, where about 95% of L chains are κ, there appear to be at least 50 V_κ groups. The recognition of these groups was an early indication that the genome contains many encoding sequences or genes for V regions (see V Gene Segments, below). As we shall see, V region encoding sequences in germ-line DNA also fall into groups, each of which is characterized by similar nucleotide (and amino acid) sequences.

THE ANTIGEN-COMBINING SITE IS FORMED BY HYPERVARIABLE REGIONS OF BOTH HEAVY AND LIGHT CHAINS. Because hypervariable regions differ greatly from one Ab to another, their amino acids were expected to determine the specificity of Ag-binding sites. In accord with this expectation, several Abs with the same ligand-binding specificity were found to have virtually identical residues in the hypervariable regions of their V_L and V_H domains, including residues that are rarely seen in the corresponding positions of chains from randomly selected Igs (Fig. 14–21).

An Ab's binding site is dependent on both its H and its L chains. This requirement is seen in **reconstruction studies** in which an Ab's H and L chains are separated and then mixed and permitted to reassemble spontaneously with each other or with chains from other Abs. H_2L_2 molecules are readily formed, regardless of whether the chains come from the same or different Ab molecules or even from different species (e.g., a human H chain and a rabbit L chain). **However, Ag-binding specificity is reconstituted only when the H and L chains come from the same mAb.** Unlike multichain enzymes, whose binding sites are usually associated with single chains, **the ligand-binding site that characterizes each Ab is formed by a unique pair of H and L chains** (see below).

THREE-DIMENSIONAL STRUCTURE OF ANTIBODIES

X-ray diffraction analysis of single crystals of Fab fragments and of an IgG1 molecule has shown that all domains of H and L chains share the same distinctive three-dimensional shape. Called the **Ig fold**, this distinctive folding pattern is composed of seven to nine β strands labeled A to G from the amino end to the carboxy end of the linear sequence (Fig. 14–22). The strands are arranged in antiparallel orientation into two layers (termed β **sheets**) that are maintained in a closely packed, face-

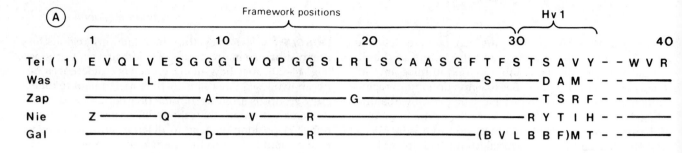

(A)

Framework positions — Hv 1

```
              1              10              20            30                40
Tei ( 1)  E V Q L V E S G G G L V Q P G G S L R L S C A A S G F T F S T S A V Y - - W V R
Was       —————— L —————————————————————————————————— S ————— D A M - - - ——
Zap       ——————————————— A ——————————— G ————————————————— T S R F - - - ——
Nie       Z ————— Q ————— V ———— R ———————————————————— R Y T I H - - - ——
Gal       ——————————— D ————— R ———————————————— (B V L B B F)M T - - - ——
```

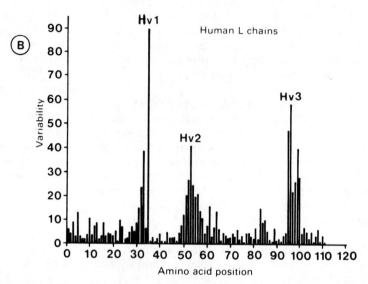

Figure 14–19. Framework and hypervariable (complementarity-determining) regions of V domains of human H chains. Sections with extreme variability are **hypervariable (Hv)** or **complementarity-determining regions (CDRs);** other sections are **framework regions (FRs).** *(A)* Sequences from parts of some human H chains. (Based on Capra D, Kehoe M: Adv Immunol 1975) (See Fig. 14–9 for abbreviations.) *(B)* Variability (ν) at different positions in human L chains demonstrated in a **Kabat-Wu plot,** ν is defined as the number (n) of different amino acids at a given position divided by the frequency (f) of the most common amino acid at that position ($\nu = n/f$). ν can range from 1.0 (no variation) to 400 (20 amino acids, equally frequent). (Based on data compiled by "Prophet Information Handling System," National Institutes of Health, by H Bilofsky, TT Wu, and EA Kabat, 1978)

```
V_KI      1              10              20              30              40
ROY    D I Q M T Q S P S S L S A S V G D R V T I T C Q A S Q D I S - - - - - - I F L N W Y Q Q K P — · · ·
EU     B I Q M T Q S P S T L S A S V G B R V T I T C R A S Z S I B - - - - - T W L A W Y Z Z K P — · · ·
OU     D I Q M T Z S P S S L S A S V G B R V T I T C R A S Z T I S - - - - - S W L B W Y Z (Z K P) — · · ·

V_KII
CUM    E D I V M T Q T P L S L P V T P G E P A S I S C R S S Q S L L A S G D G N T Y L N W Y L Q K A — · · ·
TEW    D I V M T Q S P L S L P V T P G E P A S I S C R S S Q - - H (G B) S - - - - F L N W Y L Q K P — · · ·
MIL    D I V L T Q S P L S L P V T P G E P A S I S C R S S Q N L L Z S - B G B - Y L D W Y L Z K P — · · ·

V_KIII
Ti     E I V L T Q S P G T L S L S P G E R A T L S C R A S Q S V S - - - - - - N S F L A W Y Q Q K P — · · ·
FR4    E (I V L) T Q S P G T L S L S P G E R A T L S C R A S Q S V R - - - - - N N Y L A W Y Q Q R P — · · ·
B6     Z I V L T Z S P G T L S L S P G Z R A A L S C R A S Q S L S - - - - - G N Y L A W Y Q Q K P — · · ·
```

Figure 14–20. Some V region groups (e.g., V_KI, V_KII, V_KIII) illustrated with the N-terminal sequences of nine human κ chains. The framework residues that characterize each group are in boldface. Alignment maximizes homology; dashes (gaps) represent deletions or insertions. Residues in parentheses are known by peptide composition and not actually sequenced. See Figure 14–9 for amino acid abbreviations. (Data are from several laboratories, reviewed by Hood L, Prahl J: Adv Immunol 14:291, 1971)

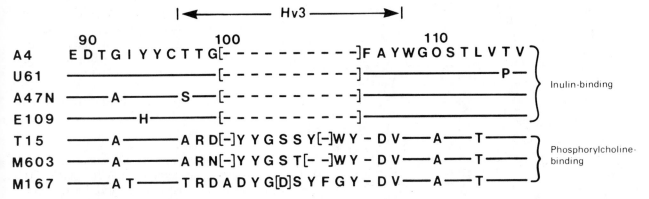

Figure 14–21. Evidence that hypervariable regions determine the specificity of combining sites. Note the similarity of sequences in and around the third hypervariable (Hv) region of H chains from four inulin-binding and three phosphorylcholine-binding myeloma proteins. Bracketed hyphens represent deletions (compared to a prototype sequence). Horizontal lines refer to sequences that are the same as the topmost protein (A4). For amino acid abbreviations, see Figure 14–9. (Vrana M et al: Proc Natl Acad Sci USA 75:1957, 1978)

to-face array by many van der Waals interactions and hydrogen bonds between their respective amino acid side chains and also by an S–S bond that links strand B of one sheet with strand F of the other sheet (see Fig. 14–22). In constant domains, the Ig-fold consists of just the basic seven-stranded structure (A–B–D–E in one sheet and C–F–G in the other sheet), whereas variable domains have one or two additional strands, C′ and C″, between C and D (Figs. 14–22 and 14–23).

An important rule emerging from crystallographic studies of many proteins is that within a large protein family, such as the Igs, **three-dimensional shape is even more highly conserved than is amino acid sequence similarity.** Thus, the alpha carbon backbone of two Ig domains having only about 20% amino acid identity at homologous positions can be superimposed on one another with an almost perfect match.

PAIRED DOMAINS. Many of the conserved amino acids in Igs are necessary for maintaining the Ig-fold (e.g., the cysteine residues that form the intradomain S–S bond). Other amino acids are also conserved in key positions that are essential for the **domain–domain interactions**

that maintain **three pairs of domains** in nearly all Igs: the V_H/V_L pair, which forms the Ag-binding site; the C_H1/C_L pair; and the C_H3/C_H3 pair (Fig. 14–24).

β TURNS, CDRs, AND THE ANTIGEN-COMBINING SITE. The seven to nine strands of the Ig-fold account for only about half of the 110 to 120 amino acid residues of each V or C domain. About half of the remaining residues, or about 25% to 30% of all V-region amino acids, form the loops (termed β turns) that connect the β strands. (The rest of the amino acids are at the N-terminus preceding strand A or at the C-terminus following strand G; see Figs. 14–10 and 14–23). The enormous sequence diversity of V domains, which is responsible for their great diversity in specificity for Ags, is predominantly clustered in CDRs, which are located in certain of the loops that connect certain β strands: B to C (CDR1), C′ or C″ to D (CDR2), and F to G (CDR3). **Although widely separated in the linear sequence, in three-dimensional space, the three CDRs of each V domain are in proximity, and the six CDRs of the paired V_H/V_L domains (three from V_H and three from V_L) form the Ag-combining site.**

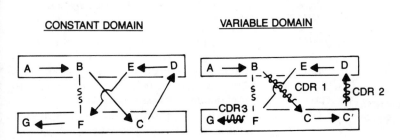

CONSTANT DOMAIN

VARIABLE DOMAIN

Figure 14–22. Diagram of the two β sheets and the β strands that form them in the Ig-fold of constant and variable Ig domains. In each domain seven to nine β strands are arranged in two β sheets (enclosed in rectangular boxes), one with four strands (A, B, D, E) and the other with three strands in constant domains (C, F, G) and four or five in variable domains (C, C′, C″, F, G). Strands B and F are linked by an S–S bond between the two cysteine residues that occupy homologous positions in all Ig domains. Arrows represent the β turns that connect β strands; CDRs are indicated by curves surrounding arrows (in variable domain only). Strand A, N terminus; Strand G, C terminus.

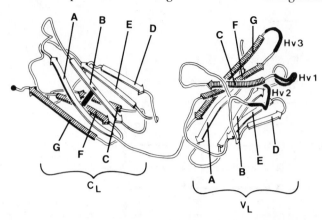

Figure 14–23. Three-dimensional structure of V and C domains of a human light (λ) chain (McG) showing the Ig fold. Thick arrows indicate direction of chain polarity (NH$_2$→COOH). Note that contiguous strands have opposite ("antiparallel") orientation. White arrows represent twisted β strands in one β sheet; hatched arrows in the other β sheet. Each short black bar is the intradomain S–S bond (see Fig. 14–13). Hypervariable (*Hv*) regions are brought together at one end of the molecule. In intact Ig molecules and in Fab fragments, apposition of Hv sections of V$_L$ and V$_H$ forms the ligand-binding site. In V$_L$, strand C is connected to strand D by a greatly elongated loop termed C', or C' and C" (see Fig. 14–22). Based on Schiffer M, et al: Biochemistry 12:4620, 1973.)

Low-resolution x-ray crystallographic analysis (and also electron microscopy; see Fig. 14–7) show that the IgG molecule is Y shaped, with each arm of the Y having a binding site at its tip. **Because the two sites are so far apart, a single Ab molecule can bind simultaneously to identical epitopes on two large Ag-bearing particles, such as virions or bacteria or mammalian cells, causing them to aggregate** (see Agglutination Reaction, Chap. 13).

Small haptens bind to clefts or cavities of complementary shape in the Ab's (or Fab's) combining site. However, in a crystallized immune complex formed by the Fab fragment of a mAb and its protein Ag (hen egg lysozyme),

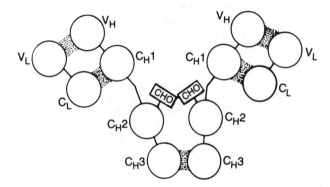

Figure 14–24. Diagram of an IgG molecule showing pairs of interacting domains (indicated by dots between them): V$_H$/V$_L$, C$_H$1/C$_L$, C$_H$3/C$_H$3. The C$_H$2 domains are separated by oligosaccharide (CHO) side chains (see Fig. 14–16) and do not interact with each other.

the Ab's combining site for the protein Ag was seen (Fig. 14–25) as a large, almost flat area (about 20 × 30Å). This site and the Ag's epitope form complementary, interdigitating surfaces, with protruding side chains of one protein molecule accommodated by matching depressions in the other.

In the specific Fab–lysozyme complex, one or more amino acids from each of the six CDRs was seen to make contact with the bound Ag. It is thus apparent why an isolated H or L chain, each with only three CDRs, binds the Ag much less well than does the intact Ig, if at all. With the Fab–lysozyme complex, the H chain's CDR3 made especially numerous contacts, and this CDR probably played a particularly prominent role in the Ab–Ag interaction. A basis for the exaggerated role of this CDR will become apparent in the following section when we consider the genetic mechanisms that are responsible for the great diversity of V domains and, especially, their CDRs.

IMMUNOGLOBULIN GENES

The great diversity of amino acid sequences in myeloma proteins and mAbs makes it clear that an individual's total Ig pool consists of an enormous number, probably millions, of different Ig molecules. What genetic mechanisms are responsible for this diversity? If each Ig were encoded by a conventional gene in germ-line DNA, as was postulated by a **germ-line theory**, the genome would have to contain millions of different Ig genes. However, the uniqueness of each Ig arises in part from its particular H–L pair. Hence, if any H chain can pair with any L chain, far fewer genes would be required. For example, 10^4 L-chain genes and 10^4 H-chain genes could, by random pairing of their products, yield about 10^8 different Igs, each with a distinct V$_H$–V$_L$ pair and a distinct specificity. But even 20,000 Ig genes is an improbable number, because the human genome is estimated to contain a total of only about 50,000 to 200,000 genes. This dilemma was avoided by an alternative **somatic theory**, which postulated that only very few Ig genes are inherited but that they are subjected to enormous diversification in certain differentiating somatic cells.

Ig GENES ARE FORMED BY REARRANGING GENE SEGMENTS

DNA cloning techniques ultimately resolved the debate between germ-line and somatic theories and showed that although there are indeed many germ-line Ig sequences, the great diversity of Igs as proteins arises ultimately from remarkable processes that take place in special somatic cells, the Ig-producing B lymphocytes. In essence, functional Ig genes are generated by rearrang-

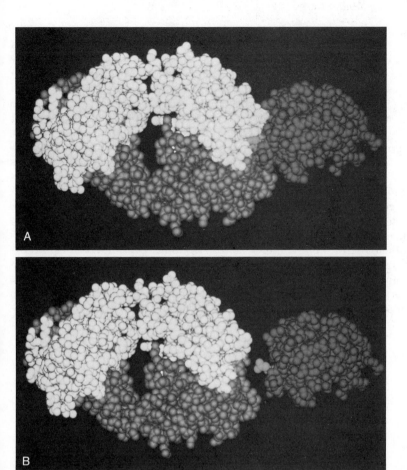

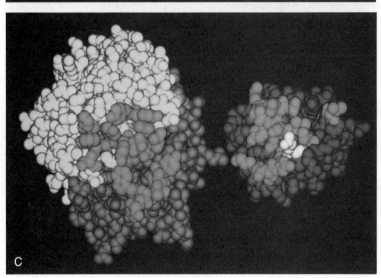

Figure 14–25. Three-dimensional structure of a complex between an antigen (lysozyme) and the Fab fragment of a monoclonal anti-lysozyme antibody. In the Ab's binding site, 17 amino acid residues make close contact with 16 amino acid residues of the Ag; some of the Ag's contact residues are near its N terminus (positions 18–27), and others are close to the C terminus (positions 116–129). The separation of these residues in the linear sequences and their close approximation in the folded Ag molecule are typical of a "discontinuous" epitope. All six of the Ab's CDRs contribute some residues that make contact with the Ag. Lysozyme is the small molecule at the right. In the Fab (left), atoms of the light chain are light and above; those of the heavy chain are darker and below. **(A)** The Fab/lysosyme complex with the Ag (lysosome) occupying the Fab's binding site. **(B)** The Fab and Ag are separated to demonstrate complementarity in shape between the Ag's epitope and the Fab's binding site; note that protuberances of one fit into complementary depressions on the other. **(C)** The Fab and the Ag of part **(B)** have been rotated 90° to face the viewer head-on, in order to highlight those amino acid side chains of the Fab that make contact with amino acid side chains of the Ag. (Amit AG et al: Science 233:747, 1986)

ing small gene segments that are inherited in germ-line DNA. The rearrangements occur in lymphocytes as they develop from immature precursor cells into Ig-producing B cells; **the assembly process itself creates vast sequence diversity.** These processes, which have had a powerful impact on our understanding of how information in genetic material can be amplified, have been found in no other genes so far except those that encode the almost equally diverse antigen-specific receptors of T lymphocytes, described in Chapter 15.

Even before DNA cloning was possible, many observations had pointed to the possibility that an Ig molecule is encoded by more than a single conventional gene. For example, in different κ chains, the same C_κ domain is associated with different V_κ amino acid sequences. Moreover, a rare myeloma tumor was found to produce both an IgM and an IgA myeloma protein in which the identical V_H sequence was associated with C_μ domains in the IgM protein and with C_α domains in the IgA protein. Based on these and other observations, Dreyer and Ben-

nett speculated that an Ig gene is formed by joining any one of many V genes to one C gene to form a complete H or L chain gene.

Striking studies by Tonegawa provided the first direct evidence that two separate genes are actually brought together to make a functional Ig gene. DNA from two sources were compared: from a mouse myeloma tumor that produced a κ chain, and from mouse embryo cells, which do not produce Ig. The DNA from both sources was cleaved with a restriction enzyme into fragments that were separated by electrophoresis. The fragments with encoding sequences for the κ chain were then identified by nucleic acid hybridization using two pieces of κ chain mRNA as probes: one for the complete κ chain (V_κ and C_κ domains), the other (corresponding to the 3' half of the mRNA) for the C_κ domain. As shown in Figure 14–26, in the embryonal cell DNA, the probe for C_κ hybridized to one fragment (containing the C_κ gene), whereas the other probe, for V and C, hybridized to both the fragment with the C_κ gene and to another fragment, pre-

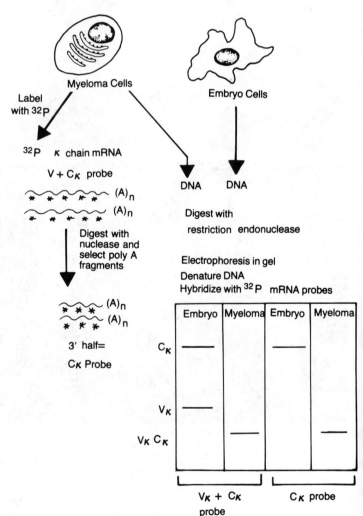

Figure 14–26. Rearrangement of the genome's encoding sequences for a κ chain is shown by comparing DNA from cells that produce no Ig (embryo) with DNA from myeloma cells that produce the κ chain. Asterisks refer to the radioactive label (^{32}P). (Based on Hozumi N, Tonegawa S: Proc Natl Acad Sci USA 73:3628, 1976; adapted from Watson JD, et al: Molecular Biology of the Gene. Vol. 2. The Benjamin/Cummings Publishing Co, Inc, 1987)

sumably containing the V_κ gene segment. In contrast, with DNA from the myeloma tumor, both probes (for V + C and for C alone) hybridized to a **single** fragment. Extension of these results showed that in DNA from cells that do not make Igs (e.g., from embryo, kidney, or liver), the V_κ and C_κ encoding sequences are separated, but in B cells that produce a particular κ chain, the V_κ and C_κ encoding sequences for that chain are on the same fragment (we shall see below that they are actually joined). Similar results have been obtained with probes for the V and C domains of λ chains and of H chains. The encoding sequences that can be brought together to form a functional gene are usually called **gene segments.**

CHROMOSOMAL LOCATION. Are all the gene segments that can be joined to each other located on the same chromosome? The inheritance of allotypes (see above) showed that genes encoding H, κ, and λ allotypes segregated from each other in animal breeding experiments and in human families, as if each of the three sets of genes (for H, κ, and λ) were located on a separate chromosome. To identify these chromosomes, hybrid cell lines made by fusing human to mouse cells have been used. Under selective conditions, the hybrid cells lose many human chromosomes and yield panels of diverse cell lines that contain limited numbers of different human chromosomes. Similarly, many mouse chromosomes are lost from mouse–hamster hybrids. By hybridizing DNA from various hybrid cell lines with probes for V and C regions of various Ig chains, the chromosomes on which the H, κ, and λ gene segments are located have been identified (see Table 14–3). Functional Ig genes are formed by joining gene segments of the same chromosome: $V_\kappa \to C_\kappa$, $V_\lambda \to C_\lambda$, $D \to J_H$, $V_H \to DJ_H$.

Assembly of λ Light Chain Genes

The process by which V and C gene segments are assembled was first established with the gene for a mouse λ chain, the simplest of the Ig genes. Each λ chain gene is formed from four separate segments called, in 5' ("upstream") to 3' ("downstream") order, $L\lambda$, $V\lambda$, $J\lambda$, and $C\lambda$.

$L\lambda$ encodes most of the 15 to 20 amino acids of the "leader" sequence at the N-terminus of the growing polypeptide chain. This hydrophobic sequence is cleaved as it leads the peptide chain through the membrane of the endoplasmic reticulum, and it is absent from the mature Ig molecule.

$V\lambda$ encodes the last four amino acids of the leader and most of the λ chain's variable region, from amino acid positions 1 to 97.

$J\lambda$ encodes the remainder of the variable region, from positions 98 to 110.

$C\lambda$ encodes the entire C domain, from positions 111 to 214.

In a cell that expresses a λ L chain, a V segment (V_λ)

becomes linked covalently to a J segment $(J_\lambda;$ J for "joining") to form an uninterrupted sequence for the entire variable domain. The functional gene thus formed has three exons: $L\lambda$, $V\lambda J\lambda$, and $C\lambda$, separated by two introns (one between $L\lambda$ and $V\lambda J\lambda$ and the other between $V\lambda J\lambda$ and $C\lambda$). Both introns are spliced out of the primary RNA transcript of the rearranged gene to yield a functional λ messenger RNA (Fig. 14–27).

There are three λ chain isotypes (λ1, λ2, and λ3) in inbred mice, and functional genes for all of them are assembled in the same way. Each isotype corresponds to a particular combination of V_λ, J_λ, and C_λ segments. The organization of murine λ gene segments is shown in Figure 14–28. A gene for a fourth λ isotype, λ4, is nonfunctional (termed a "pseudogene") because of a defect in sequence that is incompatible with formation of functional messenger RNA. (Similarities between λ genes suggest that they arose in evolution from the duplication of one set of J_λ–C_λ segments, followed by duplication of the pair.) In humans, where there are more λ chain isotypes (probably about six), λ gene segments resemble those of inbred mice, but their exact number and organization have not yet been fully clarified.)

Assembly of κ Light Chain Genes

The basic strategy for assembling functional genes for κ chains is the same as for λ chains, but the organization of the κ gene locus is quite different. In accord with the much greater abundance of κ than λ chains in mouse Igs (about 20 : 1), there are about 100 times more V_κ than V_λ gene segments (see below).

Each V_κ gene segment, like each of the V_λ gene segments, is separated by about 100 base pairs on its upstream side from a leader sequence (L_κ) (Fig. 14–29). But unlike the λ locus, downstream from the many tandomly arranged L_κ and V_κ segments, there are five closely clustered J_κ segments (one of which is defective), and about 1000 base pairs still further downstream there is a single C_κ gene segment.

In constructing a functional κ gene, one of the 200 to 300 V_κ segments joins one of the four functional J_κ segments (Fig. 14–30). The rearranged V_κ segment brings along all the DNA on its upstream side, including its own L_κ exon and an upstream transcriptional promoter. The intervening DNA between the joined V_κ and J_κ is not always excised and lost from the cell, as occurs with rearranged V_λ gene segments; (the exact process of V_κ–J_κ joining is often complex and sometimes involves a segmental inversion of DNA between the joined segments). When the rearranged V_κ gene is transcribed, RNA splicing removes the intron between L_κ and V_κ, as with λ genes, but splicing out of the second intron extends from the 3' end of the joined J_κ to the 5' end of the C_κ gene segment. The end result is that mRNA for a κ chain has the same overall structure as that for a λ chain: a 5' untranslated

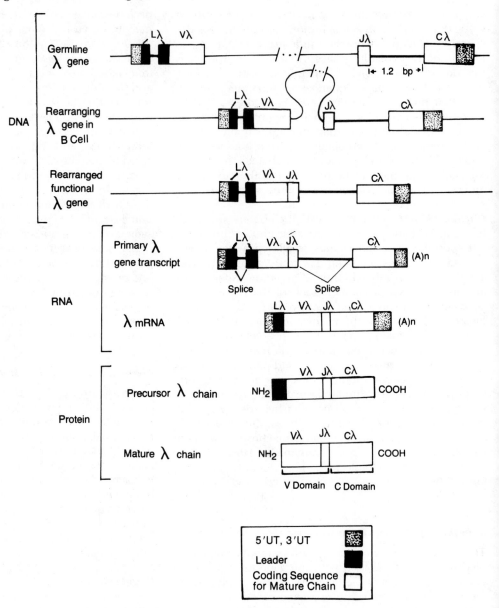

Figure 14–27. Successive stages in the formation and expression of a functional gene for a λ L chain. Thin horizontal lines are double-stranded DNA; thick straight lines are introns; note that they are spliced out when the RNA transcript is converted to messenger RNA (mRNA). Open boxes represent encoding sequences for the λ chain and solid boxes those for the chain's leader *(L)* sequence. Stippled rectangles are sequences of mRNA that are not translated (UT) into protein.

sequence followed by L_κ, V_κ, J_κ, and C_κ encoding sequences and finally by a 3′ untranslated sequence that terminates in polyadenylate (poly [A]) (Fig. 14–29, line 4).

Nucleotide sequence similarities classify V_κ gene segments into groups resembling those suggested by amino acid sequence similarities (see V_κ Groups, above). The V_κ groups are revealed with probes, usually prepared by

synthesizing on a κ-RNA template a complementary DNA **(cDNA)** labeled with [32]P. By digesting mouse DNA with a restriction enzyme, separating the variously sized fragments electrophoretically, and testing them by hybridization in the Southern blotting technique with a probe corresponding to a particular rearranged V_κ gene, a set of several (typically about ten) different fragments will be

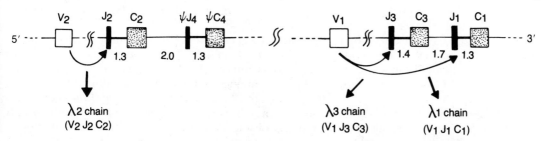

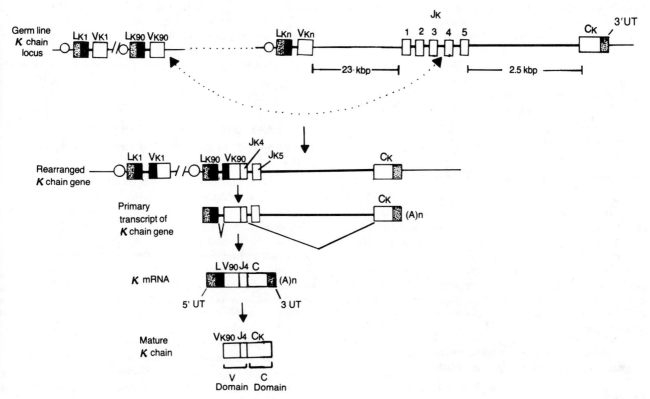

Figure 14–28. Lambda gene locus in the mouse. The arrows indicate the rearrangements that generate genes for the three λ isotypes (λ1, λ2, λ3). J_4 and C_4 are defective ("pseudogenes"). Humans have five or six (perhaps more) λ-chain isotypes. The horizontal line represents double-stranded DNA; breaks in that line indicate unknown lengths between the gene segments shown. L coding sequence not shown. See Figure 14-27 for explanation of the symbols used. Numbers are distances, in kilobases, between the gene segments shown. The V, J, and C segments that form the various λ chain isotypes are given in parentheses. (Based on Blomberg B, et al: Proc Natl Acad Sci 78:3765, 1981 and Miller J, et al: Proc Natl Acad Sci 78:3829, 1981.)

identified, each one homologous to the V_κ probe. Different probes identify different sets. Altogether, it is estimated that there are about 200 to 300 V_κ segments in the mouse genome, but many of them may well be defective. Any of the functional ones appears to be able to join any one of the four functional J_κ segments.

Assembly of H-Chain Genes

The strategy for generating an H or L chain gene is basically the same, but H-chain gene segments are more numerous, and their organization is more complex. As with the κ family, there appear to be several hundred V_H gene

Figure 14–29. Rearrangement and expression of an Ig κ gene. The top line shows a chromosome with V_κ gene segment no. "90" ($V_{\kappa 90}$) rearranging to $J_{\kappa 4}$ (see dotted lines terminating in arrowheads). The splicing of the primary (RNA) transcript to form the mRNA for $V_{\kappa 90}J_{\kappa 4}C_\kappa$ is indicated by the V-shaped lines. The V domain of the mature κ chain is encoded by $V_{\kappa 90}$ and $J_{\kappa 4}$ gene segments. The straight line represents double-stranded DNA; heavy lines are introns (note their elimination when primary RNA transcript is spliced to form mRNA). Open boxes are encoding sequences; stippled boxes are untranslated parts of exons. Solid rectangles encode leader sequences. Circles upstream of the leader (L) segments indicate promoter regions. (Distances not drawn to scale.)

segments, and they are spread out over probably 2 million base pairs. Like V_κ and V_λ, each V_H has about 100 base pairs on its upstream side, an L_H gene segment for a leader, and, upstream of the L_H segment, a transcriptional promoter. At a large but unknown distance downstream of this great array of V_H (and L_H) segments, there are four J_H gene segments.

An important difference between the L and the H gene families is the presence of approximately 12 small additional segments, termed D (for diversity), located between the J_H cluster and the large array of V_H gene segments. Each D segment encodes only about 5 to 15 amino acids. On the downstream side of the J_H cluster, the C domains for each of the H-chain isotypes is represented by a linear array of exons, illustrated for the human isotypes in Figure 14–30. The order (5′–3′) of gene segments for the mouse isotypes is: μ–δ–$\gamma3$–$\gamma1$–$\gamma2b$–$\gamma2a$–ε–α.

In assembling a functional gene for an H chain, two recombinational events are required, not just one as for κ and λ genes. First, one of the D and one of the J_H gene segments are linked (D–J_H joining); then one of the many V_H gene segments joins to form an uninterrupted V_H–D–J_H sequence for the entire V_H domain.

The V_H segments, like the V_κ segments, can be divided into groups, the members of which have very similar sequences and readily cross-hybridize. Some V_H groups have few members (say, 5 to 10), whereas others have many dozens. Altogether, there appear to be at least 300 V_H gene segments. The H-chain locus covers an enormous but still incompletely defined length of DNA: the D–J_H–C_H segments are spread over about 150,000 bp, and it is estimated that the V_H segments span a distance on the order of 2,000,000 bp.

Ig Exons Correspond to Ig Domains

For each of the eight or nine H-chain isotypes, the C gene segment is itself made up of the six distinct exons. These are shown in detail in Figure 14–30 for $C\mu$. Each of the $C\mu$ exons corresponds precisely to a domain of the μ chain; thus, the $C\mu1$ exon specifies the $C\mu1$ domain, the $C\mu2$ exon encodes the $C\mu2$ domain, etc. The exons denoted M_1 and M_2 encode the transmembrane and cytoplasmic amino acid sequences that anchor the H chain in the surface membrane of the cell (B lymphocyte) that synthesized it.

Recognition Sequences for Joining Ig Gene Segments: The 12/23 Spacer Rule

The common strategy used to assemble functional genes for all of the Ig chains (H, κ, and λ) is strikingly revealed further by an underlying shared pattern of noncoding "signal" sequences on the joining side of every V, D, and J segment (i.e., on the downstream side of each V, on the

upstream side of each J, and on both sides of each D segment).

Each signal consists of highly conserved heptamer (7-mer) and nonamer (9-mer) consensus sequences (CACAGTG and ACAAAAACC) separated by a "**spacer**" of variable sequence but fixed length, either 12 (±1) or 23 (±2) nucleotides (nt) (Fig. 14–31). **Only those gene segments that have signal spacers of different length can be joined.** Thus, the signal sequence on the downstream side of each V_κ segment has a 12-nt spacer, whereas the signal on the upstream side of each J_κ segment has a 23-nt spacer. For the λ family, the difference is preserved, but the order is reversed: V_λ spacers have 23 nt, and J_λ spacers have 12 nt. However, the spacers for all V_H and J_H segments are the same (23 nt), and in accord with **the 12/23 spacer rule**, V_H and J_H cannot be joined to each other. But every D segment is flanked on both its upstream and the downstream side by a signal with a 12-nt spacer. Therefore, J_H and D can be joined, and D and V_H can also be joined, and the consistently observed V_H–D–J_H order is thus exactly in accord with the 12/23 spacer rule.

The 12 and 23 spacer lengths correspond to one and two turns in a DNA double helix. Hence, the as-yet-undiscovered "recombinase" enzymes responsible for cutting and joining DNA to link V–J or V–D–J segments may have binding sites that distinguish the heptamer and nonamer signal sequences when they are separated by one or by two turns of the double helix (Fig. 14–32).

SEQUENCE DIVERSITY IN V DOMAINS
Junctional Diversity Due to Imprecise V_L–J_L and V_H–D–J_H Joining

From a myeloma or hybridoma cell line that makes an Ig chain, say a λ chain, the λ mRNA can be copied by the enzyme reverse transcriptase into a **complementary DNA sequence (cDNA),** which can then be replicated or "cloned" to provide enough material to determine its exact nucleotide sequence. When such sequences from cells that express λ chains are compared with the sequences of the corresponding unrearranged V_λ and J_λ segments, there is usually a perfect match over the entire V–J length except at the V–J boundary. At this position, several (usually three or four) alternative codons, for three or four different amino acids, can be found in various λ chains from diverse cell lines. From the nucleotide sequences at the 3′ end of the unrearranged V_λ and at the 5′ end of the rearranged J_λ segments, it is apparent how codons for diverse amino acids can be generated at the V–J junction through variation in the particular nucleotides that are recombined (Fig. 14–33). Similar diversity also occurs at the V_κ–J_κ boundary of κ chains.

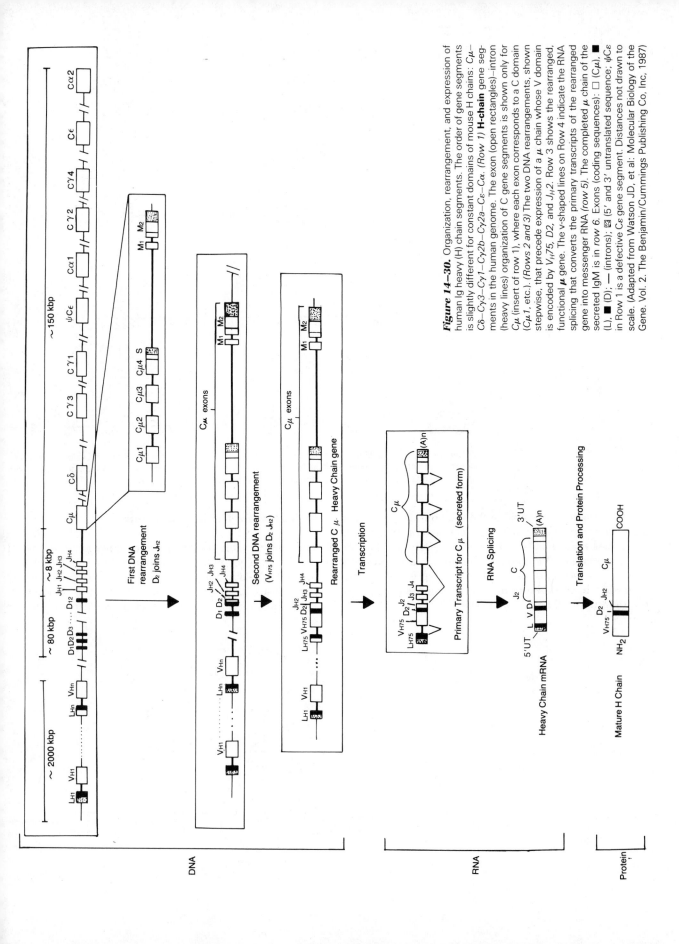

Figure 14–30. Organization, rearrangement, and expression of human Ig heavy (H) chain segments. The order of gene segments is slightly different for constant domains of mouse H chains: $C\mu$–$C\delta$–$C\gamma3$–$C\gamma1$–$C\gamma2b$–$C\gamma2a$–$C\epsilon$–$C\alpha$. (*Row 1*) **H-chain** gene segments in the human genome. The exon (open rectangles)–intron (heavy lines) organization of C gene segments is shown only for $C\mu$ (insert of row 1), where each exon corresponds to a C domain ($C\mu1$, etc.). (*Rows 2 and 3*) The two DNA rearrangements, shown stepwise, that precede expression of a μ chain whose V domain is encoded by V_H75, D_2, and J_H2. Row 3 shows the rearranged, functional μ gene. The v-shaped lines on Row 4 indicate the RNA splicing that converts the primary transcripts of the rearranged gene into messenger RNA (*row 5*). The completed μ chain of the secreted IgM is in *row 6*. Exons (coding sequences): $\square$ (L), $\blacksquare$ (D); — (introns); $\boxtimes$ (5' and 3' untranslated sequence; $\psi C\epsilon$ in Row 1 is a defective $C\epsilon$ gene segment. Distances not drawn to scale. (Adapted from Watson JD, et al: Molecular Biology of the Gene. Vol. 2. The Benjamin/Cummings Publishing Co, Inc, 1987)

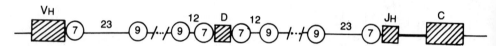

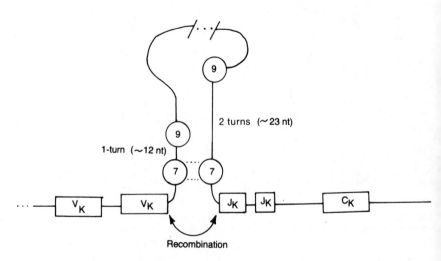

Figure 14–31. The 12/23 bp spacer rule. Each *V, D,* and *J* gene segment is flanked on the side where it joins another segment by the heptamer–spacer–nonamer sequence. Only segments having dissimilar spacer length can be joined (23/12 for *Vλ/Jλ*, 12/23 for *Vκ/Jκ*, and 23/12/12/23 for $V_H/D/J_H$).

The variable amino acid at the V–J boundary can have important consequences for Ig function. For instance, Ig molecules that differ only by a single amino acid at the V–J boundary of the L chain have shown a marked difference (~ 1000-fold) in affinity for a hapten. Thus, **imprecision in the joining of gene segments is another important source of Ig diversity.**

N-Region Nucleotide Additions

The most variable region of Ig molecules is the H chain's third CDR. The amino acids encoded by *D* segments are located in this region, and it is also the site of two joining boundaries, V_H–*D* and *D*–J_H. In addition, this region contains short variable sequences of amino acids, termed **N**

Figure 14–32. Hypothetical substrate for recombination that results in a Vκ → Jκ rearrangement.

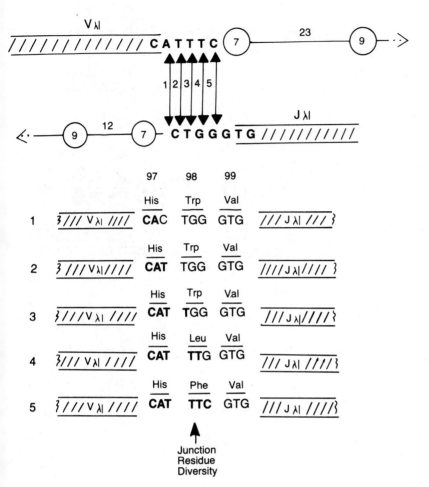

Figure 14–33. Junctional diversity: new codons are generated at the junction of two linked segments (Vλ1 → Jλ1 is shown) by variation in the internucleotide bonds that are cleaved and joined.

regions (Fig. 14–34), that cannot be accounted for by the germ-line V_H, D, and J_H sequences or by junctional diversity at the boundary of these segments. One N region is located at the V_H–D boundary and another at the D–J_H boundary. These sequences might be added by the enzyme called terminal transferase (or one like it), which is present in some immature lymphoid cells and which can add deoxynucleotides more or less at random (in a template-free fashion) to the 3' end of a growing DNA strand.

Gene Conversion

A remarkable additional mechanism for generating diversity has been seen with L chains of chicken Igs. The V regions of all chicken L chains have turned out, surprisingly, to be encoded by just a **single V_λ** gene segment. There are many additional V_λ gene segments, but they all have defects in sequence (i.e., they are pseudogene seg-

ments). However, short stretches of 20 to 30 nt from these defective genes are found in various functional λ genes that encode diverse L chains, as if blocks of sequence from a pseudogene can somehow be exchanged with sequences from the single competent V_λ gene segment. The detailed mechanism for this process, termed **gene conversion,** is not understood, but its consequences are clearly sufficient to result in chicken λ chains with great V-region sequence diversity. It is possible that gene conversion also contributes to sequence diversity of mammalian V_κ domains.

Nonproductive Rearrangements

In forming a functional gene, variable region segments must be joined so that a correct triplet reading frame is preserved. If the joining introduces or deletes one or two nucleotides (or any number not divisible by three), the downstream sequence would be out of frame and hence

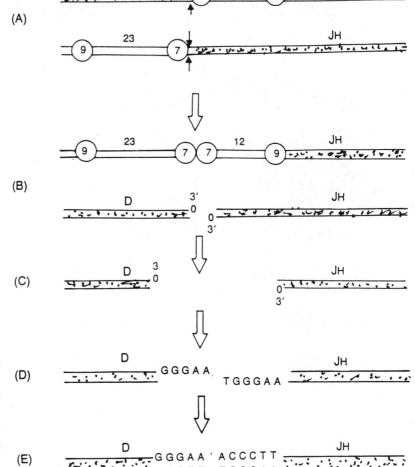

Figure 14–34. A model for N-region diversity attributable to random addition of nucleotides at D–J_H junction. *(A)* D and J_H gene segments are aligned and the four strands of DNA are cut where coding sequences *(stippled)* meet the heptamer signal *(arrows)*. *(B through D)* Before the D and J_H segments are joined, an exonuclease removes deoxynucleotides from all four strands, and new deoxynucleotides are added at random in a template-independent reaction, perhaps by the enzyme termed terminal transferase. *(E)* DNA polymerase replicates the added deoxynucleotides, and ligase finally joins the D and J_H segments. (Based on Alt F, Baltimore D: Proc Natl Acad Sci USA, 79:4118, 1982)

likely to introduce frequent stop codons, preventing translation into a functional chain. Such nonproductive arrangements are common. It appears that as an immature lymphocyte develops into an Ig-producing cell, rearrangements occur first in the H chain locus and then in L chain loci (κ before λ) until a functional Ig is made, and then rearrangements cease. Thus, in many cells that express a κ chain, two V_κ–J_κ rearrangements can be detected by the Southern blotting technique, but only one encodes the κ chain that the cell synthesizes; the other has a nonproductive join.

Because the assembly of the H-chain gene requires two joins, and because there are N-region additions, there are many more opportunities for nonproductive assembly of H-chain than L-chain genes. Indeed, virtually every B-lymphocyte has two V–D–J rearrangements, one defective and the other encoding the H chain made by that cell. It is very likely that many lymphocytes have only nonproductive rearrangements and are thus of no value to the immune system. However, when the benefits

are great enough, nature can apparently afford to waste cells, as in the huge number of sperm that are produced but not used to fertilize ova.

Hypermutation in V Domains

Whereas most of the genetic mechanisms that generate Ig diversity are active in B lymphocytes **before** these cells encounter their Ag, another powerful mechanism is activated **after** the cells respond to Ag, especially under conditions of intensive immunization. Thus, as we have noted above, mouse $\lambda 1$ L chains are encoded by single gene segments for V_λ, J_λ, and C_λ (Fig. 14–28), and so one might expect that in inbred mice, with no known allotypic $\lambda 1$ variants, the amino acid sequence of every $\lambda 1$ chain would be the same except for junctional diversity at the V–J boundary. However, the sequences of many $\lambda 1$ chains differ from each other by many amino acids, and these can be accounted for by single base substitutions in the rearranged gene. The substitutions are found only in V domains. They are also found in V regions of κ and H chains.

The single nucleotide substitutions, termed **somatic mutations,** probably occur at random throughout rearranged V regions, but they are often found clustered in the CDRs. Moreover, most of the substitutions result in codons that encode a different amino acid. (Substitutions that are entirely random are expected one-fourth of the time to be "silent," i.e., not to result in an amino acid substitution.) These circumstances suggest that Igs having the amino acid substitutions provide the cells that express them (as surface receptors for Ag) with a selective advantage during immunization, probably because the mutated Abs have a higher affinity for Ag (Fig. 14–35; see Affinity Changes During Immunization, Chap. 16).

Even a small number of somatic mutations per chain can generate great diversity. For example, with four amino acid substitutions introduced at random in the approximately 30 amino acids of the three CDRs of a single V gene about **10 million different V domain sequences** can be generated. Because amino acid sequences in V regions determine idiotypes, it is clear why **every monoclonal Ig is expected to have unique V region sequences, or a unique combination of V_H and V_L sequences, and a unique idiotype.**

Summary of the Sources of Amino Acid Sequence Diversity in V Domains

1. **Combinatorial Diversity by Random Assembly of Gene Segments.** Because there appear to be about 250 V_κ and four J_κ gene segments, random pairing would generate about 1000 (250 × 4) V_κ–J_κ combinations. Similarly, if there are the same number of V_H segments (250), then, because there are 12 D segments and four J_H segments, random joining of these elements can yield 250 × 12 × 4 or about 12,000 V_H–D–J_H combinations.

2. **Junctional Diversity.** On average, three different amino acids can be found at the junction of each type of joined segments (V–J, V–D, D–J). Hence the number of V_κ

sequences would increase to about 3000 (1000 × 3) and the number of H chains to about 100,000 (12,000 × 3 × 3).

3. **N-Region Additions.** By introducing variations in both the number and the sequences of residues added, the N regions expand the number of H chains far beyond 100,000.

4. **Gene Conversion.** In some Ig gene families (chicken λ chain), and perhaps in some others as well, it appears that stretches of nucleotides are translocated from one V gene segment to another in the same V locus.

5. **Combinatorial Diversity by Random Pairing of H and L Chains.** If any L can be paired with any H chain, there would be well over 10^8 (100,000 H × 3000 L) different Igs (or perhaps about 10^7 if only 10% of the H–L pairs can form stable Ig molecules). These numbers are minimal estimates because they ignore the impact of N regions in greatly expanding the number of H chains.

6. **Somatic Mutations.** An enormous number (probably millions) of different V-region sequences can arise from random single nucleotide substitutions in the V region of a functional Ig gene, especially under conditions of intense immunization.

The known mechanisms for generating sequence diversity in Igs are capable of yielding a number of different Igs (**the Ig repertoire**) that far exceeds 10^8. Since each Ig is produced by a single clone of B lymphocytes (see Chaps. 15 and 16), it appears that what limits the size of the repertoire is the number of clones of Ig-producing cells in the body.

EXPRESSION OF Ig GENES
Transcriptional Enhancers

Each V_H gene segment, whether rearranged or not, has a transcriptional promoter on its upstream side, but only those segments that have been joined to DJ_H segments are vigorously transcribed. The reason is a special transcription-enhancing sequence (about 200 nt long), termed an **enhancer,** that lies in the intron between the J_H cluster and $C\mu$ (Fig. 14–36). Like similar enhancers that

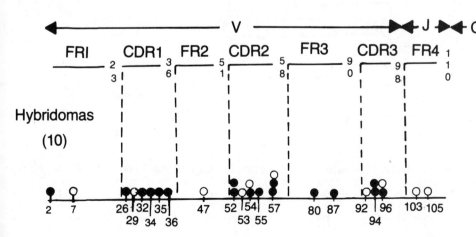

Figure 14–35. Somatic mutations in V regions. The positions of mutations are shown in $\lambda 1$ chains from ten monoclonal Abs (*bottom*) determined by sequencing cDNA from hybridomas making anti-Dnp antibodies in response to hyperimmunization. $\bigcirc$, silent mutations; $\bullet$, replacement mutations, i.e., mutations that result in amino acid substitutions). The V–J junction residues at positions 97 and 98 are not shown. (Based on Tamoto K, Azuma T, Igras V, et al: In Eisen HN, Reilly EB: Adv Immunol 3:337, 1985)

are known for DNA and RNA tumor viruses, the H-chain enhancer augments transcription from promoters located within a few kilobases on either side of it. Hence the promoter of a rearranged V_H gene is close enough to be affected, but promoters of unrearranged **V_H** gene segments are too distant.

The H chain (J_H–C_μ) enhancer exerts its effect only in cells that can make Igs. This remarkable specificity is evident when, by genetic engineering, the enhancer sequence is attached to molecularly cloned genes that are introduced into various cultured cell lines: the introduced (transfected) gene is normally transcribed only in cells of B lineage (such as myeloma cells or hybridomas) and not in nonlymphoid cells, e.g., those of kidney and liver. The power of this enhancer has been exploited in the industrial manufacture of various proteins. For instance, human tissue plasminogen activator (tPA) can be manufactured by mouse myeloma cells that are transfected with the molecularly cloned human tPA gene to which the mouse H-chain enhancer has been attached.

Another sequence, 5′ to each leader (L_H) gene segment, also enhances H-chain transcription and is likewise more effective in B-lymphocytes than in other cells. The κ-chain genes have their own transcriptional en-

hancer, similarly located in the intron between the J_κ cluster and the C_κ gene segment.

Developmental Sequence

The formation of a functional Ig gene in a developing B lymphocyte begins with the joining of a D to a J_H segment. Then a V_H segment joins, forming a V_H–D–J_H exon and a functional H-chain gene. In keeping with the proximity of $C\mu$ exons (see Fig. 14–29) to V_H–D–J_H, the H-gene transcript is translated into a μ chain provided the V_H–D and D–J_H rearrangements maintain the correct triplet reading frame. Once a μ chain is synthesized by a cell, further V_H segment rearrangements in that cell cease, and V_κ–J_κ rearrangements commence. If the first V_κ–J_κ join is nonproductive, rearrangement of a V_κ on the homologous chromosome takes place. It has been suggested that V_λ segment rearrangements take place only if both V_κ rearrangements fail to yield a normal κ chain.

The consequence of this orderly progression is **allelic exclusion,** i.e., the expression by the individual cell, even though it is diploid, of only an H-chain gene of one chromosome and an L-chain gene of one chromosome (Fig. 14–37). For L chains, the exclusion is actually more extensive: mouse cells have eight L-chain alleles (one pair of κ and three pairs of λ), and human cells have about 12

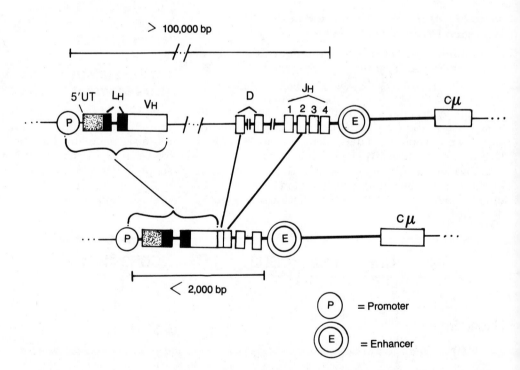

Figure 14–36. The enhancer sequence (*E*) responsible for augmented transcription of rearranged H-chain genes. The distance between the enhancer and the promoter (*P*; upstream of each V_H gene segment) in the unrearranged state (*top line*) is >100 Kb, but after a rearrangement takes place, it is <2 Kb. The horizontal line is double-stranded DNA. Closed rectangles are coding sequences for the leader (*L*) peptide. The stippled rectangle is the 5′ untranslated part of the L_H exon. (Adapted from Gillies SD, et al: Cell 33:1717, 1983.)

to 14 L-chain alleles (one pair of κ, five to six pairs of λ), yet an Ig-producing human or mouse cell expresses only a single L-chain allele. The important consequence of the exclusion is that an Ig-producing cell makes only a single H chain and a single L chain, i.e., a single Ig having specificity for only one (or a few very similar) Ags (the one cell–one Ab rule).

To explain the ordered sequence of gene rearrangements, it has been suggested that the polypeptide chain produced as a result of a productive rearrangement acts as a signal that regulates the ensuing rearrangements. Thus, a μ chain would block further V_H rearrangements and stimulate V_κ rearrangement, and a κ chain, forming a $(\mu\kappa)_2$ molecule, would block additional V_κ or V_λ rearrangements. This model has some support from studies of transgenic κ mice that develop from fertilized ova into

which a rearranged, functional κ gene has been introduced. A large proportion of Ig-producing cells in these mice express the introduced κ "transgene" and lack rearrangements of their indigenous V_κ and V_λ gene segments.

Although vigorous transcription of an H-chain gene occurs only after D–J_H–$C\mu$ segments are joined, some transcripts that correspond to D–J, and the corresponding truncated polypeptide chains, have been found in some lymphocytic tumors, as if there are also active transcriptional promoters near D segments, not just upstream of each V_H segment. If a $DJ_HC\mu$ peptide were to provide a signal for V_H segments to combine with D–J segments, this would explain why D–J_H rearrangements precede V_H–D rearrangements. It is possible that some unrearranged V_H segments and joined D–J_H segments are transcribed (at a low level) because localized unwinding

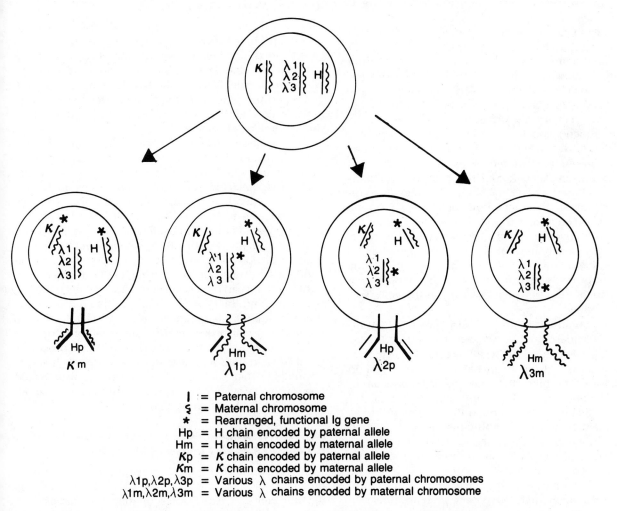

| | = Paternal chromosome
ζ = Maternal chromosome
$*$ = Rearranged, functional Ig gene
Hp = H chain encoded by paternal allele
Hm = H chain encoded by maternal allele
κp = κ chain encoded by paternal allele
κm = κ chain encoded by maternal allele
λ1p,λ2p,λ3p = Various λ chains encoded by paternal chromosomes
λ1m,λ2m,λ3m = Various λ chains encoded by maternal chromosome

Figure 14–37. Allelic and isotypic exclusion. (*A*) B-cell precursor (*top*), not producing Ig, is shown with maternal ($\sim$) and paternal (—) chromosomes containing unrearranged gene segments for κ, λ, and H chains. (*B*) In a B cell that expresses Ig, only one H-chain gene (maternal or paternal) and only one L-chain gene (maternal or paternal for κ or λ1 or λ2 or λ3, etc.) are expressed. For each B cell in inbred mice, there are 32 possibilities, of which four are shown.

of chromatin near them exposes them to "rearrangase" enzyme(s).

Membrane-Bound Versus Secreted Ig: RNA Processing

As cells develop from immature precursors into Ig-synthesizing B lymphocytes, the first Igs produced are IgM molecules that are embedded in the membrane at the cell surface and serve as Ag-specific receptors. After these "virgin" B cells interact with Ag, the newly synthesized IgM molecules are secreted instead of being anchored in the cell membrane. Another difference is that the secreted IgM (termed IgM_s) is a pentamer ($[H_2L_2]_5$) of the basic four-chain molecule (see Fig. 14–12), whereas the membrane-bound IgM (termed IgM_m) is an Ig monomer (H_2L_2). The change from membrane to secreted form results from a change in RNA processing that leads to a different amino acid sequence at the C terminus of the μ chain of IgM_m and IgM_s.

As shown in Figure 14–38, the primary RNA transcript of a rearranged μ chain gene has two potential sites for cleavage and attachment of the polyadenylate residues that mark the downstream end of mRNA. Before Ag stimulation, the B cell uses the downstream poly A site (site no. 2 in Fig. 14–38) and a splicing pattern that results in mRNA for the μ chain of IgM_m. In this chain the carboxy-terminal sequence includes a stretch of 25 hydrophobic amino acids (boxed in Fig. 14–38C), called the membrane domain, followed by a cationic sequence, Lys–Val–Lys, at the C terminus. As is characteristic of all protein chains that are anchored in cell membranes (**integral membrane proteins**), the membrane domain's 25 amino acids can form an α-helix of sufficient length to span the membrane; its hydrophobicity also ensures strong interactions with membrane lipids. The positively charged sequence that follows it is also characteristic of integral membrane proteins; by extending into the cytoplasm, it helps to anchor the polypeptide firmly in the cell's surface membrane.

After Ag stimulation, the H-chain gene's RNA transcript is polyadenylated at site no. 1 (see Fig. 14–38), removing the sequences for the membrane and cytoplasmic domains. As a result, the μ chains of secreted IgM no longer have a C terminus that can anchor the μ chain in the cell membrane. Moreover, the new C-terminal sequence of 19 amino acids, termed the S segment in Fig. 14–34C, includes a cysteine at the penultimate position (circled at the bottom of Fig. 14–38); this cysteine forms the S–S bond between monomeric units in the pentameric, secreted IgM_s molecule. The S segment is spliced out of the RNA transcript when it is processed to form mRNA for the membrane form of the μ chain. However, upstream of these C-region alterations, the μ chains of the secreted and the membrane forms are precisely the same. Because the change from IgM_m to IgM_s does not

affect the molecule's L chain, the two IgM forms made by a B cell have the same V_H and V_L domains, which means that they have the same Ag-binding activity and the same idiotype. A B cell that is stimulated to switch from producing membrane-bound to secreted IgM also begins producing J chains, which are necessary for stabilizing the pentameric secreted IgM.

The other Ig classes also exist as either membrane-bound Ag-specific receptors on the B-cell surface or as soluble Igs that are secreted. In all classes, the two forms arise from the same kind of alternative RNA processing that determines whether the H-chain's C-terminal sequence can anchor it in the cell's membrane. Just how the binding of an Ag to surface Ig causes a B cell to alter its pattern of RNA processing is not understood.

RNA Processing Is Responsible for IgM and IgD Production by The Same Cell

Although the Ag-specific receptors on newly developed (immature) B cells are IgM_m molecules, many mature B cells express a membrane-bound form of IgD in addition to IgM_m. This double expression does not violate the one cell–one Ab rule, because the two Igs have the same L chain and the same V_H domain and hence the same Ag-binding sites (and the same idiotype); they differ only in the C domains of their H chains.

The expression by one cell of a μ chain and a δ chain with identical V domains can be explained by variations in processing of the rearranged H-chain gene's primary RNA transcript. This transcript can be exceedingly long (>15 kb), extending downstream to the Cδ gene segments or even further (Fig. 14–39). If it is cleaved and polyadenylated at the end of all the Cμ exons (site 1 or 2 in Fig. 14–39), the resulting RNA encodes a μ chain, but if the site of polyadenylation is further downstream, beyond the Cδ exons (site 3 or 4 in Fig. 14–39), then conventional splicing can remove all of the RNA between the V_H–D–J_H exon and the Cδ exons. The resulting mRNA would then encode the membrane form of IgD (IgD_m). Why the immature B cell processes H-chain RNA transcripts to yield only IgM_m and why the mature B cell processes them to yield both IgM_m and IgD_m is not clear. It seems improbable that such an elaborate mechanism would have evolved unless it has an important role in the development or the function of B cells.

Repetitive Sequences in H-Chain Genes Permit B Cells to Switch Classes of H Chains

Before encountering its Ag, the virgin B cell expresses only IgM_m or IgM_m and IgD_m, but after reacting with the Ag, the cell can express Igs of different classes. The switch entails a shift in the H-chain constant region but not in the L chain or in V_H region and thus no change in Ag-binding specificity.

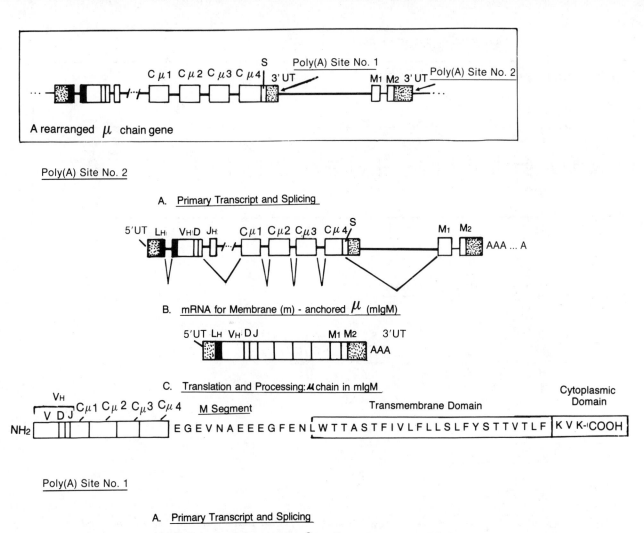

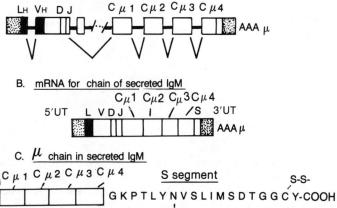

Figure 14–38. RNA processing determines whether IgM is anchored in the cell membrane or secreted. To make membrane-anchored IgM, the primary transcript of the rearranged μ gene (*boxed, at top*) is cleaved at site no. 2, and multiple adenylate residues are added (polyadenylation); the splicing pattern shown then yields mRNA for a membrane-anchored μ chain. To make the secreted IgM, polyadenylation takes place at site no. 1, and a different splicing pattern at the 3' end yields mRNA for the μ chain of secreted IgM. Note that the membrane-anchored μ chain has a lysine-rich sequence at the C terminus preceded by 25 hydrophobic amino acids, as is characteristic of many integral membrane proteins. All these amino acids are missing in the μ chain of secreted IgM, which is shorter and has an entirely different sequence at the C terminus; note that its penultimate cysteine (SH) links the monomers of the secreted IgM pentamer (see Fig. 14–12). For one-letter code for amino acids see Figure 14–9. (Adapted from Hood L, et al: Immunology, 2nd ed. The Benjamin/Cummings Co, 1984.)

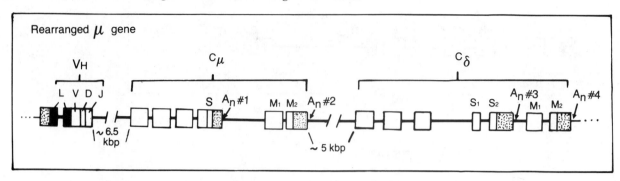

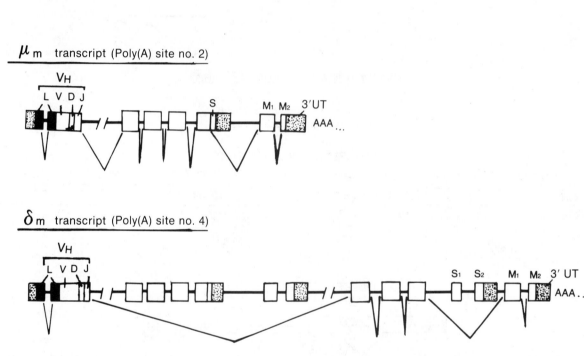

Figure 14–39. Alternative sites of polyadenylation explain how a single B cell can express both IgM and IgD with the same V_H domain. Polyadenylation at site no. 2 and the splicing pattern shown yield RNA for the membrane-anchored μ chain (μm) of an mIgM (see Fig. 14–38). However, polyadenylation at site no. 4 and a different splicing pattern yields mRNA for the membrane-anchored chain (δm) of mIgD. At site no. 1, polyadenylation results in secreted IgM (see Fig. 14–38); only trace amounts of secreted IgD are found in serum, presumably because polyadenylation rarely occurs at site no. 3.

The switch from one class to another is accomplished by recombination between special **switching sequences** in the intron upstream of the C exons for each H-chain class (except for Cδ). These sequences are 2 to 10 kb long, and their many short repeats probably promote recombination. In switching from production of a μ chain to expression of, say, a γ1 chain, recombination takes place between the two corresponding switch sequences; hence, the resulting γ1 chain has the same V_H–D–J_H exon as the previously expressed μ chain (Fig. 14–40). It is significant that the potent transcriptional enhancer in the intron between the J_H cluster and the $C\mu$ exons is upstream of the switching sequence ($C\mu_s$) in this intron. Therefore, **every switch recombination carries the enhancer with it, ensuring active transcription of the H-chain gene regardless of the H-chain class expressed.** Each switch recombination generates a new, chimeric sequence: e.g., in a μ/γ1 switch, the 5′ end is from the μ switch and the 3′ end is from the γ1 switch. B cells can switch successively from μ to γ1 to α, etc. As we shall see in Chapter 15, certain regulatory proteins that are secreted by T cells stimulate B cells to undergo particular switch recombinations (e.g., interleukin-4 promotes switching to the ε gene and production of IgE).

A.

<u>A functional μ heavy chain gene</u>

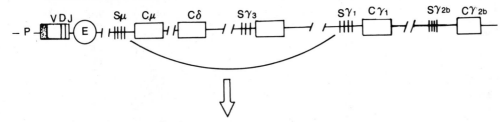

⇩

B.

<u>A functional γ1 heavy chain gene</u>

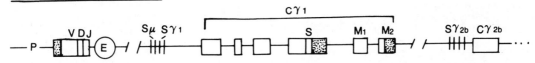

Figure 14–40. DNA recombination between switching *(S)* sequences permits class switching from IgM to other Ig classes (except IgD, to which it takes place by alternative RNA processing [Fig. 14–39]). *S* sequences lie 2 to 3 Kb upstream of *C* genes for each H-chain class (except for the δ chain of IgD) and consist of long (2–10-kb) repeats of many short, conserved sequences (indicated by multiple vertical lines for *Sμ, Sγ3, Sγ1, Sγ2b . . .*). Because the enhancer *(E)* sequence lies upstream of *Sμ*, it is carried along with the rearranged *V$_H$–D–J$_H$* from *Cμ* to other C gene segments (*Cμ→Cγ1* is shown) in *(A)*. Note the resemblance of the exon–intron organization of *Cγ1* in *(B)* to that of *Cμ* in Figure 14–38; like *μ* chains, *γ1* chains can be expressed with a C terminus that anchors IgG1 in the cell membrane or with the different and shorter one of the *γ1* chain in secreted IgG1. The alternative forms exist for all other H-chain C genes as well.

Appendix

TABLE 14–4. Amino Acid Sequence Similarity Among Selected Ig Domains: A Key to the Evolution of Igs*

Domains That Are Compared	% Similarity
V$_\kappa$ domains from the same V$_\kappa$ group	73–87†
V$_\kappa$ domains from different V$_\kappa$ groups	51–68
V$_\kappa$ vs V$_\lambda$ domains	43–50
C$_\kappa$ vs C$_\kappa$ (Hu vs. Mo)	60
C$_\lambda$ vs C$_\lambda$ (Hu vs. Mo)	69
C$_\kappa$ (Hu) vs C$_\lambda$ (Mo)	36
C$_\kappa$ (Mo) vs C$_\lambda$ (Mo)	35
C$_\kappa$ (Mo) vs C$_\lambda$ (Hu)	34
C$_H$1 vs C$_H$2 vs C$_H$3, all within C$_\gamma$1	30–33
C$_\kappa$ or C$_\lambda$ vs C$_\gamma$1 (C$_H$1) or C$_\alpha$1 (C$_H$3)	23–27
V$_\lambda$ vs C$_\lambda$ / V$_{\kappa I}$ vs C$_\lambda$ / V$_{\kappa II}$ vs C$_\kappa$	12–18‡

* Domains from mouse Igs are denoted (Mo); all other domains are from human Igs (Hu). Percent homology means percent of positions in the linear sequence that are occupied by identical amino acids.

† Cross-hybridize in Southern blots under stringent conditions.

‡ Proteins selected at random (e.g., hemoglobulin and Igs) have close to the 5% homology expected (because there are 20 amino acids). Hence there is only 7% corrected homology (12% − 5%) (Between C$_\lambda$ and V$_\lambda$1 [human]); nevertheless, these domains have very similar overall shape in 3 dimensions (the Ig-fold).

(Based on Nisonoff A: Introduction to Molecular Immunology, 2nd ed. Sinauer, Sunderland, MA, 1984, p 77)

TABLE 14–5. Some Properties of Classes of Human Immunoglobulins*

Property	IgG				IgA		IgM	IgD	IgE
	IgG1	IgG2	IgG3	IgG4	IgA1	IgA2			
Sedimentation coefficient (S)	7	7	7	7	7–13	7–13	19	7	8
Molecular weight ($\times 10^{-3}$)	150	150	150	150	150–600	150–600	900	?	190
Heavy chains	γ1	γ2	γ3	γ4	α1	α2	μ	δ	ε
Light chains: κ/λ ratio	2.4	1.1	1.4	8.0	1.4	1.6	3.2	0.3	?
Carbohydrate (%, approx.)	3	3	3	3	7	7	12	13	11
Average conc. in normal serum (mg/ml)	8	4	1	0.4	3.5	0.4	1	0.03	0.0001
Half-life in serum (days, in vivo)	23	23	8	23	6	(6?)	5	3	2.5
Heavy chain allotypes	Gm	Gm	Gm	Gm		Am			
Earliest Ab in primary immune responses†							+		
Most abundant Ab in most late immune responses†	←――――――― + ―――――――→								
Conspicuous in mucinous exocrine secretions					+	+			
Transmitted across placenta†	+	±	+	+	0	0	0	?	−
Effector functions									
Principle surface Ig on B cells†							+	+	
Binds to macrophage Fc receptors	+ +	+	+ +	±					
Complement fixation‡	+ +	+	+ +	0§	0§	0§	+ +	?	0§
Sensitizes human mast cells for anaphylaxis ¶									+

* For hinge region differences see Fig. 14–15 and Table 14–2.

† Chapters 15 and 16.

‡ Chapter 17.

§ Can activate complement via the alternate mechanism (Ch. 17).

¶ Chapter 18; IgE molecules are reagins, responsible for atopic allergy.

TABLE 14–6. Allotypes of C_H Regions of Human IgG and IgA

Ig Class	Allotype		Location of Epitopes
	Alphabetical Designation	Numerical Designation[a]	
IgG1	G1m(a)	G1m(1)	C_H3
	(x)	(2)	C_H3
	(f)	(3)	C_H1
	(z)	(17)	C_H1
IgG2	G2m(n)	G2m(23)	C_H2
IgG3	G3m(b0)	G3m(11)	C_H3
	(b1)	(5)	C_H2
	(b3)	(13)	C_H3
	(b4)	(14)	C_H2
	(b5)	(10)	C_H3
	(c3)	(6)	
	(c5)	(24)	
	(g)	(21)	
	(s)	(15)	
	(t)	(16)	
	(u)	(26)	
	(v)	(27)	
IgA2		A2m(1)	
		A2m(2)	

[a] The alphabetical designations were introduced first and are still occasionally used.

(After WHO Committee Report (1976) and Nisonoff A: Introduction to Molecular Immunology, 2nd ed. Sinauer, Sunderland, MA, 1984)

TABLE 14–7. *Allotypes on C_H Regions of Mouse Igs of Various Classes*

| Ig Haplotype[a] | Prototype Strain | Locus and Chain | | | | | | |
		Igh-1 γ_{2a}	Igh-2 α	Igh-3 γ_{2b}	Igh-4 γ_1	Igh-5 δ	Igh-6 μ	Igh-7 ε
a	BALB/c	a	a	a	a	a	a	a
b	C57BL	b	b	b	b	b	b	b
c	DBA/2	c	c	a	a	a	[c]	
d	AKR	d	d	d	a	a		a
e	A	e	d	e	a	e	e	a
f	CE	f	f	f	a	a		
g	RIII	g	c	g	a	a		
h	SEA	h	a	a	a	a		
j	CBA	j	a	a	a	a	a	a
k	KH-1[b]	k	c	a	a			
l	KH-2[b]	l	c	a	a			
m	Ky[b]	m	b	b	b			
n	NZB	e	d	e	a	a	e	

[a] Haplotype refers to the cluster of linked C gene segments for all H chain classes (see Fig. 14–30).

[b] Wild mice.

[c] Not determined.

(Nisonoff A: Introduction to Molecular Immunology, 2nd ed. Sinauer, Sunderland, MA, 1984)

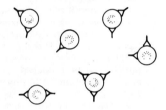

+ test Ig (same allotype as the indicator)
+ human Abs to the indicator's allotype

no agglutination (inhibited by test Ig)

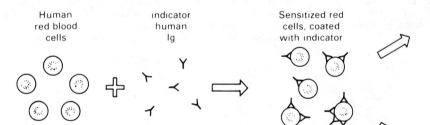

Human red blood cells

indicator human Ig

Sensitized red cells, coated with indicator

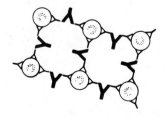

+ test Ig (different allotype than the indicator)
+ human Abs to the indicator's allotype

agglutination

Figure 14–41. Assay to identify human allotypes. In the inhibition assay for Gm and Km allotypes shown here, the indicator Ig is nonagglutinating Ab specifically bound to RBCs. In the assay for some other allotypes, other means are used to adsorb the indicator Ig to RBCs. (Based on Grubb R, Laurell AB: Acta Pathol Microbiol Scand 39:195, 390, 1956)

Selected Readings

BOOKS AND REVIEW ARTICLES

Davies DR, Metzer HA: Structural basis of antibody function. Annu Rev Immunol 1:87–117, 1983

Koshland ME: The coming of age of the immunoglobulin J chain. Annu Rev Immunol 3:425–454, 1985

Nisonoff A, Hopper JE, Spring SB: The Antibody Molecule. New York, Academic Press, 1975

Tonegawa S: Somatic generation of antibody diversity. Nature 302:575–581, 1983

Weill JC, Reynaud C-A: The chicken B cell compartment. Science 238:1094–1098, 1987

Williams A: The year of the Ig superfamily. Immunol Today 8:298–303, 1987

Yancopoulos GD, Alt FW: Regulation of the assembly and expression of variable-region genes. Annu Rev Immunol 4:339–368, 1986

SPECIFIC ARTICLES

Amit AG, Mariuzza RA, Phillips Sev, Poljak RJ: Three-dimensional structure of an antigen-antibody complex at 2.8 Å resolution. Science 233:747–753, 1986

Coleclough C, Perry R, Kanjalainen K, Weigert M: Aberrant rearrangements contribute significantly to the allelic exclusion of immunoglobulin gene expression. Nature 290:372, 1981

Desiderio SV, Yandopoulos GDM, Paskind M, Thomas E, Boss MA, Landau N, Alt FW, Baltimore D: Insertion of N regions into heavy chain genes is correlated with expression of terminal deoxytransferase in B cells. Nature 311:752–755, 1984

Early P, Huang H, Davis M, Calame K, Hood L: An immunoglobulin heavy chain variable region gene is generated from three segments of DNA: V_H, D and J_H. Cell 19:981, 1980

Early P, Rogers J, Davis M, Calame K, Bond M, Wall R, Hood L: Two mRNAs can be produced from a single immunoglobulin mu gene by alternative RNA processing pathways. Cell 20:313–319, 1980

Edelman GM: The covalent structure of an entire γG-immunoglobulin molecule. Proc Natl Acad Sci USA 63:78–85, 1969

Eisen HN, Reilly EB: Lambda chains and genes in inbred mice. Annu Rev Immunol 3:337–365, 1985

Gillies SD, Morrison SL, Oi VT, Tonegawa S: A tissue-specific transcription enhancer element located in the major intron of a rearranged immunoglobulin heavy chain gene. Cell 33:717–728, 1983

Grosschedl R, Baltimore D: Cell-type specificity of immunoglobulin gene expression is regulated by at least three DNA sequence elements. Cell 41:885, 1985

Grosschedl R, Weaver D, Baltimore D, Constantini F: Introduction of a μ immunoglobulin gene into the mouse germ line: Specific expression in lymphoid cells and synthesis of functional antibody. Cell 38:647, 1984

Kabat EA, Wu TT, Bilofsky H, Reid–Miller M, Perry H: Sequences of Proteins of Immunological Interest, vol 1. US Department of Health and Human Services, Washington, DC, 1983

Kohler G, Milstein C: Continuous cultures of fused cells secreting antibody of predefined specificity. Nature 256:495–497, 1975

Levitt D, Cooper MD: Mouse pre-B cells synthesize and secrete μ heavy chains but not light chains. Cell 19:617, 1980

Lewis S, Gifford A, Baltimore D: Joining of Vκ to Jκ gene segments in a retroviral vector introduced into lymphoid cells. Nature 308:425, 1984

Max EE, Seidman JG, Leder P: Sequences of five potential recombination sites encoded close to an immunoglobulin κ constant region gene. Proc Natl Acad Sci USA 76:3450–3454, 1979

Mostov K, Friedlander M, Blobel G: The receptor for transepithelial transport of IgA and IgM contains multiple Ig-like domains. Nature 308:37, 1984

Nelson K, Haimovich J, Perry R: Characterization of productive and sterile transcripts from the Ig H-chain locus: Processing of μm and μs mRNA. Mol Cell Biol 3:1317, 1983

Porter RR: Structural studies of immunoglobulins. Science 180:713–716, 1973

Reynand CA, Anguez V, Dahan A, Weill JC: A single rearrangement event generates most of the chicken Ig light chain diversity. Cell 40:283, 1985

Ritchie KA, Brinster RL, Storb U: Allelic exclusion and control of endogenous immunoglobulin gene rearrangement in κ transgenic mice. Nature 312:517–520, 1984

Seidman JG, Max EE, Leder P: A κ-immunoglobulin gene is formed by site-specific recombination without further somatic mutation. Nature 280:370–375, 1979

Shimuzu A, Honjo T: Ig class switching. Cell 36:801, 1984

15

David H. Raulet
Herman N. Eisen

Cellular Basis for Immune Responses

In stimulating immune responses, antigens (Ags) elicit many molecular and cellular changes. In this chapter, we consider the principal cellular changes, focussing primarily on **lymphocytes,** the cells that recognize Ags, and on cells that process and present Ags for recognition, mainly macrophages and dendritic cells but also some lymphocytes and other cells.

Until the 1960s, about all that was known about lymphocytes was that these unremarkable-looking cells (Fig. 15–1) circulate and tend to accumulate in areas of chronic inflammation. They are among the most abundant cells in vertebrates, constituting about 5% to 10% of all cells in the adult human (about 10^{12} lymphocytes). If collected into a single organ, they would weigh as much as the human brain.

Clonal selection (see Chap. 12) was originally proposed to account for the great diversity of Abs before the identity of antibody (Ab)-producing cells was established. Since then, we have learned (through means described below) that these cells are lymphocytes but that only about half of all lymphocytes, called B cells, have this capacity. The other half, called T cells, do not make immunoglobulins (Igs), but they also recognize Ags (via Ag-specific receptors termed T-cell receptors or TcR). With improved cell culture techniques, it has been possible to grow many lymphocytes as cloned cell lines: their specificity for Ags has established beyond doubt that both B- and T-cell populations are made up of an enormous number of different clones, each specific for one antigenic determinant (epitope) or a few cross-reacting ones.

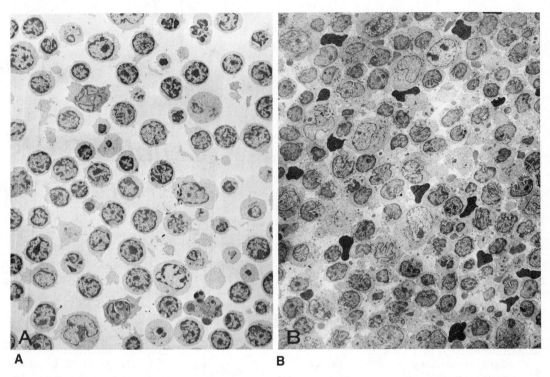

Figure 15–1. Lymphocytes in lymph from the thoracic duct. *(A)* From a rat. (Zucker-Franklin D: Semin Hematol 6:4, 1969) (×2400) *(B)* From a human. (Zucker-Franklin D: J Ultrastruct Res 325, 1963) (×1200)

Primary Lymphatic Organs

BONE MARROW

Self-renewing, multipotential hematopoietic (Gr. *haima*, blood; *poiesis*, forming) **stem cells** give rise to lymphocytes, macrophages, and dendritic cells as well as to all other blood cells. The stem cells appear initially during development in the head end of the mammalian embryo and then in blood islands of the yolk sac and later in the fetal liver. Just before birth, they are found in bone marrow, where they persist during adult life. In adult mice, some stem cells are present in the spleen; in humans, when the bone marrow is destroyed by disease or irradiation, stem cells and active hematopoiesis become evident in the spleen and sometimes even in the liver.

Besides renewing themselves, dividing stem cells yield **progenitor cells** that are programed to differentiate along various developmental lineages, giving rise to erythrocytes, granulocytes (including neutrophils, eosinophils, and basophils), macrophages, platelets, and lymphocytes (Fig. 15–2). Some cells of the lymphocyte lineage develop within the bone marrow into Ig-producing

lymphocytes, called **B cells** because they mature in **b**one marrow.* Others migrate from bone marrow to the thymus, where they develop into Ag-recognizing lymphocytes called **T cells** because they mature in the **t**hymus. Having acquired surface receptors for Ag in the **primary lymphatic organs** (bone marrow and thymus), both kinds of lymphocytes, called **virgin B and T cells** because they have not yet interacted with Ag, circulate around the body, residing temporarily in secondary lymphatic organs such as the spleen, lymph nodes, and Peyer's patches of the intestine (Fig. 15–3).

THYMUS

The thymus, a lymphoepithelial organ, consists essentially of a mass of lymphocytes, a much smaller number

---

* Before it was accepted that Ab-producing lymphocytes (B cells) mature in the mammalian bone marrow, it had been discovered that in chickens these cells mature in a special thymus-like organ termed the **bursa of Fabricius.** The bursa arises as an outpouching at the hind end of the developing gut. Its extirpation about the time of hatching results in chickens that cannot make Abs.

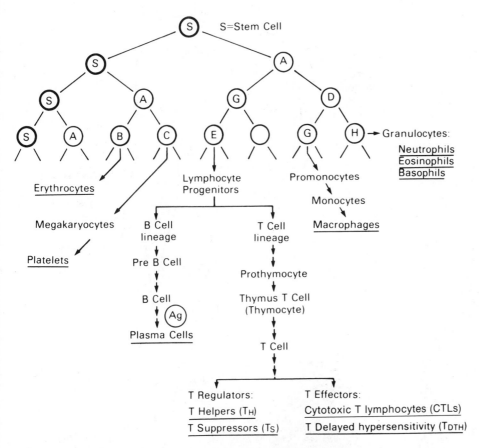

Figure 15–2. Hematopoiesis. Self-renewing pluripotential stem cells give rise to more stem cells (S) and to various progenitors (A, B, C, . . . F) of diverse lineages (erythrocytes, platelets, various granulocytes, macrophages, and diverse lymphocytes). The terminally differentiated "end cells" (underlined) differ in life expectancy; e.g., erythrocytes, 120 days; granulocytes, 12 h; plasma cells (Ab-secreting form of B lymphocytes), 3–4 days.

of epithelial cells, and some macrophages and dendritic cells (Fig. 15–4). It develops in the embryo from branchial pouches of the pharynx: epithelial buds grow out, pinch off, and migrate (in higher vertebrates) to the midline of the upper thorax, where they eventually become populated by thymic lymphocytes (called **thymocytes**). Through experiments on the transfer of cells from various tissues of mice having a distinctive chromosomal marker to mice that lack the marker but are otherwise the same genetically, it has been shown that thymocytes derive from migratory bone marrow cells. Frequent mitotic figures in the thymus and rapid incorporation of radioactive thymidine into DNA show that the immigrant cells divide rapidly, but only a small proportion of their progeny survive and become mature T cells. The sequence of their developmental changes is considered later (T-Cell Development).

The thymus is larger at birth than in the adult. It begins to atrophy around puberty or in occasional rapid bursts after severe stress, probably in response to high levels of adrenocorticosteroids, which cause immature thymocytes to lyse.

Nude mice, which lack a thymus (as well as hair), are valuable for analyzing T-cell function. Their primary defect, in epithelial-cell function, is inherited as a recessive trait. Mature, functional T cells are almost totally missing, and so these mice do not mount cell-mediated immune responses; hence, unlike normal mice, they do not reject skin grafts from other mouse strains or even from other species (e.g., chicken skin grafts grow and even form feathers). For this reason, nude mice are sometimes used to maintain human cancer cells, some of which can be propagated indefinitely by serial transfer from one nude mouse to another. Most lymphocytes in nude mice

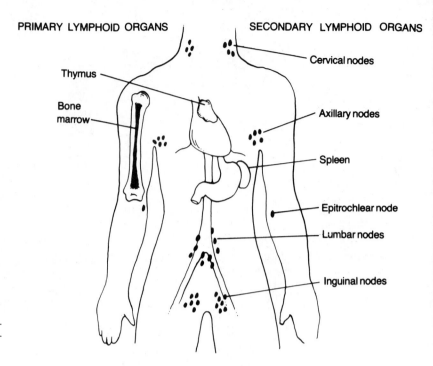

PRIMARY LYMPHOID ORGANS   SECONDARY LYMPHOID ORGANS

Cervical nodes

Thymus

Bone marrow

Axillary nodes

Spleen

Epitrochlear node

Lumbar nodes

Inguinal nodes

Figure 15–3. Distribution of human lymphoid tissue. (Modified from ES Golub, Immunology, A Synthesis. Sinauer Assoc Inc, Sunderland, MA, 1987)

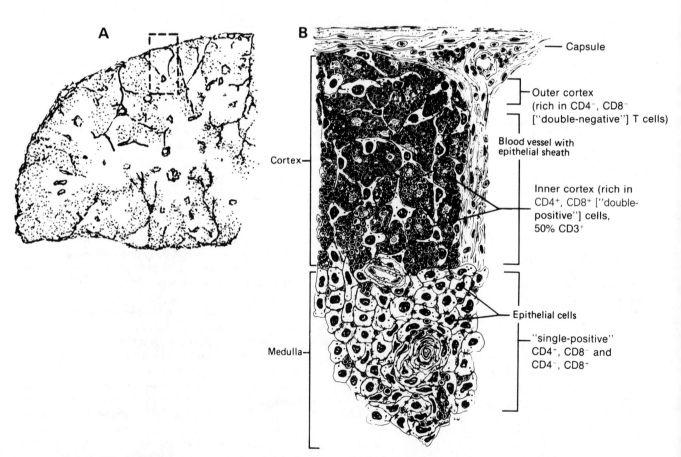

A

B

Capsule

Outer cortex (rich in CD4⁻, CD8⁻ ["double-negative"] T cells)

Blood vessel with epithelial sheath

Cortex

Inner cortex (rich in CD4⁺, CD8⁺ ["double-positive"] cells, 50% CD3⁺)

Epithelial cells

Medulla

"single-positive" CD4⁺, CD8⁻ and CD4⁻, CD8⁺

Figure 15–4. Anatomy of the thymus. **(A)** The darkly stippled cortex consists of a dense mantle of immature T cells (thymocytes) surrounding the lightly stippled medulla, which is made up of epithelial cells plus T cells that are virtually as mature as T cells in peripheral tissues and blood (see T-Cell Differentiation, this Ch.). **(B)** Portion of a thymus lobule (area enclosed in A) in greater detail. (Based on Weiss L: Cells and Tissues of the Immune System. Englewood Cliffs, Prentice-Hall, 1972)

are B cells; they can function normally if the appropriate T cells are provided.

Secondary Lymphatic Organs

LYMPH NODES

These small bean-like structures (normally less than 1 cm in humans) are generally located at the junction of interconnecting lymphatic channels. They contain an extensive reticular fiber network in which lymphocytes and Ag-presenting cells (macrophages and dendritic cells) are enmeshed and in which Ags tend to become trapped (see Ag Entrapment, below). Densely packed small lymphocytes form a **cortex** that surrounds a loosely structured **medulla** (Fig. 15-5). Through the use of distinctive cell surface Ags as markers (see below), T and B cells can be distinguished from each other. Both cell types enter lymph nodes from circulating blood by penetrating through specialized venules. In the cortex B cells are clustered in distinct nodules and T cells fill the intervening areas. Although the distinction between B- and T-cell areas is clear, some B cells are seen in T areas and vice versa.

There are two kinds of nodules. In a **primary nodule,** small nondividing ("resting") B cells form a compact spherical mass. In a **secondary nodule,** a collar of small nondividing B cells surrounds a central mass of large, rapidly dividing B cells called the **germinal center.** Germinal centers differ in size according to the intensity of antigenic stimulation: they are greatly enlarged in secondary responses to Ags, when Ab production is especially vigorous (see Chap. 16), and they are essentially absent in germ-free mice (which are maintained under conditions that greatly limit exposure to environmental Ags).

On leaving the cortex, B and T cells migrate to sinusoidal spaces of the medulla, from which they are carried out of the lymph node in efferent lymphatic vessels.

SPLEEN

Like other secondary lymphatic organs, this large vascular structure (about 200 g in an adult human) has a cortex made up of densely packed B and T cells and a loosely structured medulla (Fig. 15–6). It differs from lymph nodes in that the medulla is external to the cortex rather than the reverse. In addition, its many wide sinusoidal vascular channels are packed with erythrocytes. This "red pulp" is where aged erythrocytes are destroyed. As in lymph nodes, the cortical areas of the spleen (called the **white pulp**) have B cells packed into primary and secondary nodules with T cells dispersed in between.

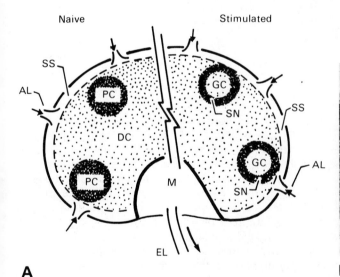

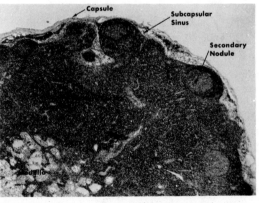

A **B**

Figure 15–5. Mammalian lymph node. *(A)* Schematic view. "Naive" lymph nodes—i.e., before antigenic stimulation—have multiple primary nodules (PC, primary cortex) separated by a tertiary, or diffuse, cortex (DC). After intense antigenic stimulation, primary nodules become secondary nodules (SN) with prominent germinal centers (GC). The lymphocytes of primary and secondary nodules are mainly B cells; those of the diffuse cortex are mainly T cells. AL and EL are afferent and efferent lymphatic channels, respectively (see Fig. 15–7). SS, the subcapsular sinus, has crisscrossing reticulum fibers that extend throughout the node. The central portion (M) is less packed with cells (see Medulla in B). *(B)* Human lymph node. The secondary nodule label points to a germinal center with its surrounding mantle of small B lymphocytes. The tertiary cortex is a mass of T cells. (×45) (B, Weiss L: Cells and Tissues of the Immune System. Englewood Cliffs, Prentice-Hall, 1972)

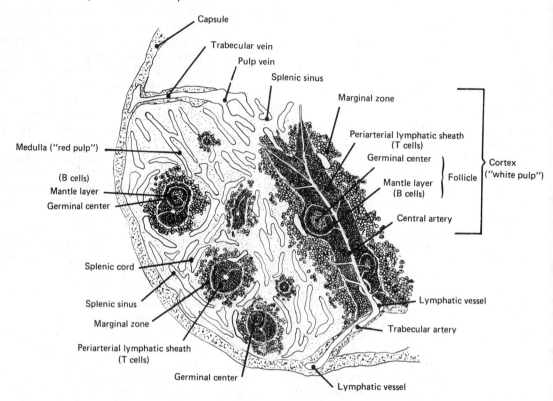

Figure 15—6. Representative area of the spleen showing masses of lymphoid cells (white pulp) distributed around the central arteries. T cells make up the periarterial lymphatic sheath; B cells form the mantle layer around germinal centers. (Weiss L: Cells and Tissues of the Immune System. Englewood Cliffs, Prentice-Hall, 1972)

GUT-ASSOCIATED LYMPHATIC STRUCTURES

Dozens of lymph nodes are found in the peritoneal cavity in membranes attached to the gastrointestinal tract. However, several special gut-associated lymphatic tissues (sometimes referred to as **GALT**) are located directly in the wall of the intestinal tract and in the nasopharynx, with which the intestinal tract is in direct continuity. In humans, the largest and most important of these are tonsils in the pharynx, adenoids in the nasopharynx, the appendix (at the junction of small and large intestine), and many **Peyer's patches,** distributed as ovoid nodules along the small intestine. Like lymph nodes, the gut-associated lymphatic organs contain masses of small lymphocytes, many clustered into distinct nodules, often with prominent germinal centers. Some nodules are intimately interdigitated with the overlying epithelium, forming **lymphoepithelial** structures resembling those seen in the thymus and also in the bursa of Fabricius, a structure found only in birds, where it is an important site of B-cell development (see footnote, p. 320).

LYMPHOCYTE CIRCULATION

Blood normally contains about 5×10^6 leukocytes per milliliter, of which about one-fourth are lymphocytes. Approximately another one-fourth are monocytes (which are precursors of tissue macrophages), and the rest are polymorphonuclear leukocytes (also called granulocytes, mostly neutrophils but also a small proportion—ca 1–2%—of eosinophils and basophils). Lymphocytes migrate from blood vessels to lymphatic channels by crossing endothelial cells of specialized postcapillary venules in the cortex of secondary lymphatic organs. After a period of several hours to several days in the cortex, depending on whether Ag is encountered (see below), the lymphocytes migrate to the medulla, from which they leave via thin-walled efferent lymphatic channels. These fine vessels penetrate through most tissues and organs of the body, linking up lymph nodes and forming a collecting system for lymph fluid (which resembles dilute serum), lymphocytes, and occasionally Ag-bearing particles such as bacteria. Small lymphatics join larger

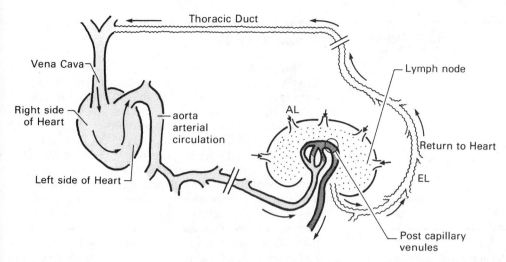

Figure 15–7. Circulation of lymphocytes. Lymphocytes leave the blood stream at postcapillary venules (small veins) in a lymph node, exiting from the node in efferent lymph channels that merge with the lymph channels from hundreds of other lymph nodes to form, eventually, the large collecting thoracic duct. This empties into the great veins (subclavian and vena cava) returning blood from the venous circulation to the right side of the heart. A typical lymph node is normally much less than 1/1000 the size of the heart. AL = afferent lymph channel carrying lymph to the lymph node from nearby tissue spaces. EL = efferent lymph channel, carrying lymph from the lymph node toward the thoracic duct. (Redrawn from Gowans JL: Hosp Pract 3 (3):34, 1968)

ones, like tributaries of a river, culminating finally in a single large vessel in the thorax (the **thoracic duct**) that empties into a major vein (the subclavian, Fig. 15–7), mixing lymph with blood being returned to the heart for another round of circulation. A complete circuit for a lymphocyte is estimated to require about 24 h, or longer if it encounters an Ag (see Ag Entrapment, below).

Lymphocytes make up virtually 100% of cells in the lymph that can be collected from the thoracic duct (see Figs. 15–1 and 15–7).

In a separate circulatory pathway, lymphocytes exit from blood vessels in the spleen and, after several hours in splenic tissue, make their way into the venous and lymphatic channels that leave the spleen for further recirculation.

HOMING PATTERNS

Although the secondary lymphatic organs all have a similar organization (e.g., a cortex with B cells aggregated into primary and secondary nodules and with T cells spread diffusely between the nodules), they exhibit characteristic differences. For instance, B cells that produce IgA or IgE are much more frequent in gut-associated lymphatic structures than in lymph nodes of the extremities. Moreover, the ratio of T:B cells is about 2.5/1 in lymph nodes but 0.5/1 in spleen and in Peyer's patches. These variations probably reflect different patterns of

"homing" of various circulating B and T cells by transfer across venules into different lymphatic tissues.

The ability of circulating lymphocytes (but not most other blood cells) to penetrate across postcapillary venules of lymphatic organs implies that they and endothelial cells of these venules may have complementary receptors. Indeed, Abs that specifically block the binding of B and T cells to endothelial cells distinguish between two "homing receptors" on lymphocytes, one apparently responsible for the adhesion of some lymphocytes to Peyer's patch venules and of others to lymph node venules. The homing receptor to lymph nodes appears to be an unusual branched glycoprotein, covalently linked by its lysine side chains to **ubiquitin,** a small protein found in all eucaryotic cells. Other receptors may account for other variations in the distribution of B and T cells; for example, intravenously injected IgA-bearing B cells localize in the intestinal lining and in other IgA-secreting epithelia (see IgA, Secretory Piece, Chap. 14), such as in the lactating mammary gland.

ANTIGEN ENTRAPMENT

Ags entering the body by different routes are trapped in different lymphatic structures. Small antigenic particles in blood (e.g., bacteria, virions) tend to be trapped in the spleen. The brain, spinal cord, and eye lack lymphatic channels, and Ags carried away from these tissues in

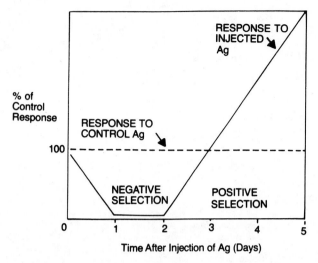

Figure 15–8. Interaction of circulating lymphocytes with a tissue-localized Ag. Within 1 day after Ag is injected into a mouse, Ag-specific T cells disappear from thoracic duct lymph and become sequestered in lymphoid tissues. After extensive proliferation, the activated progeny of these lymphocytes reenter the circulation in expanded numbers. This sequence of events can be used to obtain a population of lymphocytes that is depleted of particular Ag-specific T cells ("negative selection") or enriched for these cells ("positive selection"). The solid line represents responses to the Ag of **thoracic duct lymphocytes** taken from the Ag-injected mouse, as percent of the responses of the corresponding cells from uninjected (control) mice. The responses to an unrelated (control) Ag is shown by the dashed line. (Based on Sprent J: Cell Immunol 2:171, 1971)

blood also tend to be trapped in spleen. However, most Ags enter the body via the respiratory and intestinal tracts and are carried by lymphatic channels to nearby (**regional**) lymph nodes. There, they are taken up by Ag-presenting cells (B cells, macrophages, dendritic cells) and presented (usually as peptide fragments) for recognition by T cells (see below).

If a circulating lymphocyte encounters an Ag that it recognizes in a lymphatic organ, it will temporarily cease to circulate and will proliferate and differentiate locally into lymphoblasts, which leave after about 2 days to resume the circulatory circuit. Because of this detention, the intact animal can be used as a "filter" to separate lymphocytes specific for different Ags by injecting a mouse intravenously with a heterogeneous population of lymphocytes, some of which are specific for a trapped Ag, and then collecting the cells in thoracic duct lymph (Fig. 15–8). For the first 1 to 2 days, the collected cells are depleted of the Ag-specific cells ("negative selection"); in contrast, a few days later, these cells emerge as lymphoblasts and make up an increased proportion of the thoracic duct cells ("positive selection").

Lymphocyte Subpopulations: B and T Cells

Freshly isolated lymphocytes from blood, thoracic duct lymph, or secondary lymphatic organs are relatively uniform in appearance. Nearly all are small ($\sim$6–8 μm diam.) and in the G_0 stage of the cell cycle; that is, they are nondividing cells with relatively little cytoplasm and RNA. The first clear evidence for functionally different subsets emerged from analysis of the effects of removing the thymus. When it was removed from mice within 2 days after birth (neonatal thymectomy), the animals had, at maturity, a dramatically impaired ability to make either humoral or cellular immune responses to Ags, but if thymus lymphocytes were injected into these defective mice their immune responsiveness was restored. Because removal of the thymus from an adult had little effect, it seemed initially that all lymphocytes required for immune responses originated in the thymus and that once sufficient numbers of these cells had left to populate the periphery, the thymus was no longer required.

This simple picture was subsequently modified by **adoptive transfer** experiments in which mice were subjected to high doses of ionizing radiation and then injected with cells that had been manipulated outside the body (Fig. 15–9). Because cells of hematopoietic origin are much more radiosensitive than most other cells, the radiation eliminates the host's own lymphocytes (which would otherwise confound the experiment), making it possible to analyze the function of the injected cells. (The dose of radiation [650–1000 rad] is adjusted to ensure the survival of the host animal for at least the period of the experiment, typically 1 to 2 weeks. If a source of pluripotent hematopoietic stem cells is injected, such as bone marrow cells, fetal liver cells, or spleen cells, the mice survive indefinitely despite doses of up to 1200 rads.)

The irradiated mice do not produce Abs in response to Ag stimulation unless they are injected with the appropriate cells. Spleen cells confer the ability to respond, but thymocytes or bone marrow cells do not. However, a mixture of bone marrow cells and thymocytes are as effective as spleen cells. This striking finding indicated that **two kinds of cells are required for an Ab response:** one thymus derived (T-lymphocytes), the other bone marrow derived (B-lymphocytes), with both being present in the spleen. The experiment did not establish which of the two produced Ab. Subsequently, combinations of bone marrow and thymus cells from mice that express different Ig allotypes (see Chap. 14) established that the allotype of the Ab produced depended on the B cells and not on the T cells. **Hence, B cells produce Ab and T cells serve an auxiliary role.**

T and B cells and subsets of these cells differ not only in function but also in many of their cell surface proteins,

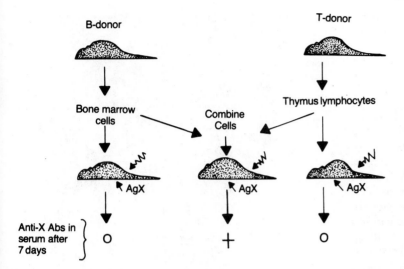

Figure 15—9. Cooperation (synergy) between B (bone marrow-derived) and T (thymus-derived) cells in Ab responses demonstrated by "adoptive transfer." The irradiated adoptive hosts serve as an *in vivo* "test tube" in which the transferred cells can respond to Ags. Abs are produced when a **mixture** of bone marrow cells and thymus cells are transferred but not when either is transferred alone. (Based on Claman HN et al: J Immunol 97:828, 1966)

often termed **markers.** Before considering the lymphocyte subsets and their interactions, we describe here their distinctive markers, some of which have crucial roles in lymphocyte function and specificity. In reviewing the markers, it is useful to be aware that in order to produce Abs in response to most Ags, B cells require "help" from only a subset of T cells, termed T-helper (T$_H$) cells; the other principal T-cell subset, called cytotoxic T lymphocytes or CTLs, kill cells whose Ags they recognize.

Abs to cell-surface markers, especially monoclonal Abs (mAbs), are useful for separating lymphocyte subsets. For instance, Abs (plus complement, see Chap. 17) to the markers on one set of lymphocytes can destroy these cells, leaving a population enriched for another set **(negative selection).** Or, in a process called **panning** (as in panning crude ore for gold nuggets), the Abs are adsorbed to the surface of a plastic dish; when cells are then added, those that express the corresponding marker adhere specifically to the dish, leaving other cells in suspension. The adherent cells can be recovered (by scraping them off gently) as a population enriched for one set **(positive selection),** or the nonadherent population can be collected as another enriched population (negative selection).

Many surface markers of human, mouse, and rat lymphocytes have been identified by the use of Abs, and the corresponding genes or cDNA clones have been isolated. Their nucleotide sequences have revealed homologues between species, and although the markers in different species have been assigned various names, a unifying nomenclature has been proposed and will be adopted here. Some of the most important markers are listed in Table 15–1; a few of them are considered below.

B-CELL MARKERS

IMMUNOGLOBULINS. Surface membrane-bound Ig (mIg) on B cells serves as the Ag-specific receptor for these cells. Because T cells do not express Ig genes, **mIg is an unambiguous marker for B cells.**

C3bi RECEPTOR. This B-cell marker is a receptor for a fragment (C3bi) of complement factor 3 (see Chap. 17). Absent on T cells, it is also a receptor for Epstein–Barr virus, which infects human B cells and can transform them into tumor cells.

T-CELL MARKERS

Thy-1. In mice this Ag is an unambiguous marker on T cells, distinguishing them from B cells. Its discovery illustrates the power of alloimmunization. Abs to Thy-1 were first produced by injecting mice of one strain (AKR) with thymocytes from mice of another strain (C3H; see Mouse

---

TABLE 15–1. Some Common Markers on Human and Mouse T Cells

Name			Tissue Distribution†	
			Thymus %	*Periphery** %
Generic	*Human*	*Mouse*		
CD 1	T6	TL(?)	15	~0
CD 2	T11	?	95	100
CD 3	T3	T3	30–40	100
CD 4	T4	L3T4	80	50–75
CD 5	T1	LYT-1	100	100
CD 8	T8	LYT-2,3	80	25–50

* Spleen, lymph nodes, and so on.

† Values are percent of cells with the indicated marker.

Strains, below). The resulting antiserum reacted with all thymocytes and with about 30% of spleen cells from the donor C3H mice but not with any AKR cells. The C3H Ag thus detected is now called Thy-1.2. Its allelic counterpart in AKR mice, called Thy-1.1, is detected with antiserum produced by the reciprocal immunization (AKR thymocytes into C3H mice).

That Thy-1$^+$ cells are T cells was established by destroying them with antiserum to Thy-1 plus complement, see Chap. 17) in a spleen cell population and showing that the surviving cells could serve in adoptive transfer (see above) to replace the required B cells but not the T cells. Supplementation of the transferred cells with a source of T cells, for example, thymocytes, restored the Ab response. About half of all mouse lymphocytes are Thy-1$^+$ (i.e., T cells); the others are mIg$^+$ (B cells). Thy-1 is also present in membrane vesicles of neuronal cells ("synaptosomes"), but its function there as well as on T cells is unknown. The Thy-1 homologue in human T cells has not been identified.

CD2. Human T cells were first distinguished from B cells by their capacity to bind sheep red blood cells (SRBC), forming distinctive rosettes: lymphocytes surrounded by a necklace-like array of SRBC (Fig. 15–10). The SRBC-binding protein of the T-cell surface is a glycoprotein, called CD2 (previously termed T11 and LFA-2), whose natural ligand (termed LFA-3) is present on a great variety of other cells (see Cell Adhesion Molecules, this chapter). Some Abs to CD2 activate T cells as though in response to antigenic stimulation.

CD3. A set of at least five proteins (γ, δ, ε, zeta, and p21) forms a complex that is present on all mature T cells of humans and mice. This CD3 complex (also called T3) is closely associated with the Ag-specific receptors on T cells, and Abs that bind to CD3 (like Abs to the receptors) activate T cells as though in response to Ag-bearing cells.

CD4. The two major subsets of T cells, T$_H$ cells and CTLs, are distinguished by a pair of structurally related cell-surface glycoproteins called CD4 and CD8. Mature T cells express one or the other. Immature T cells can express both ("double-positive" cells) or neither ("double-negative" cells) (see T-Cell Development, below).

Two subsets of T$_H$ cells, T$_H$1 and T$_H$2, express CD4 (CD4$^+$, CD8$^-$). Both respond to epitopes on Ag-presenting cells by secreting proteins called lymphokines (see below). T$_H$2 cells are the principal helper T cells for B cells; that is, their interaction with B cells promotes B-cell proliferation and secretion of Ig. The helper effect is exerted in part through the lymphokines (such as IL-4, IL-5, and IL-6) they secrete. T$_H$1 cells do not produce these lymphokines but instead secrete other lymphokines, such as γ-interferon, that promote inflammatory

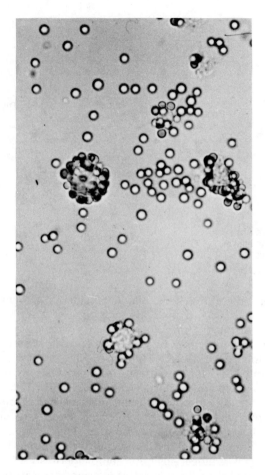

Figure 15–10. Appearance of a rosette: red blood cells bound to receptors on lymphocytes. Essentially all human T cells form rosettes with sheep red blood cells. (For the responsible adhesion molecules, see Cell Adhesion Molecules, this Chap.)

responses (see delayed-type hypersensitivity, DTH, Chap. 19). T$_H$1 cells also secrete the T-cell growth factor IL-2 and therefore may be important regulators of T-cell activity. T$_H$1 and T$_H$2 cells are not routinely distinguished, and we shall refer to them collectively as T$_H$ cells.

On human T cells, CD4 happens to serve as the receptor for human immunodeficiency virus (HIV), the causative agent of acquired immune deficiency syndrome (AIDS); hence this virus's propensity to destroy CD4$^+$ cells and to cripple immune defenses by eliminating T-helper cell activity. Some macrophages also express CD4 and are subject to infection by HIV. The structure of the CD4 protein and its partial resemblance to Igs are described at the end of this chapter.

CD8. Most CD8$^+$ T cells destroy cells whose surface Ags they recognize; hence, **CD8$^+$ cells are cytotoxic T lym-**

TABLE 15–2. Antigens Recognized by CD4⁺ and CD8⁺ T Cells

T Cell Subset	Phenotype	MHC Molecules Recognized
T_H1	CD4⁺CD8⁻	MHC-II
T_H2	CD4⁺CD8⁻	MHC-II
CTL	CD4⁻CD8⁺	MHC-I

phocytes (**CTLs**); they are also referred to as **T$_c$ cells** or **T-killer cells (T$_k$)**. Some CD8⁺ cells, called T suppressor or T$_s$ cells, appear to block immune responses by secreting suppressor factors that act on T$_H$ or on B cells.

ANTIGENS RECOGNIZED BY CD4⁺ AND CD8⁺ T CELLS. As we shall see below, T cells recognize peptide fragments of Ags in conjunction with one of the two main classes of cell-surface glycoprotein of the major histocompatibility complex (MHC): either class I (MHC-I) or class II (MHC-II) proteins. **CD8⁺ cells recognize Ags (or peptide fragments of Ags) in conjunction with MHC-I, whereas CD4⁺ cells recognize them in conjunction with MHC-II** (Table 15–2). Only special Ag-presenting cells (APC) express MHC-II; hence CD4⁺ T cells react only with APC. However, MHC-I is expressed on the surface of all cells except erythrocytes, and so **CD8⁺ cells can react with virtually any cell in the body.**

Because T cells recognize Ags only in conjunction with MHC molecules, all specific T-cell interactions with other cells are critically influenced by the MHC. Accordingly, we next consider general features of the MHC. A more detailed account of MHC genes and proteins is given at the end of this chapter, along with the structural features of other key components of T cells (the T-cell receptor for Ag (TcR), CD3, CD4, CD8, etc.).

The Major Histocompatibility Complex (MHC)

MOUSE STRAINS AND HISTOCOMPATIBILITY ANTIGENS

The roots of modern cellular immunology, with its understanding of the role of the MHC, lie in studies of tissue grafts exchanged between mice. The early immunogeneticists realized that these studies required genetically homogeneous strains, which could be generated by continuous **inbreeding;** that is, through brother–sister matings over many generations. This procedure leads to an increasing proportion of loci that are homozygous; after 20 generations, virtually all loci are homozygous, and all members of the resulting **inbred strain** have essentially the same genome.

Skin grafts exchanged between two members of the same inbred strain are accepted, whereas those between members of two different strains are always rejected. The cause is an immune reaction, primarily involving T cells, and the responsible Ags on the grafted cells are called **transplantation** or **histocompatibility** (or **H) Ags.** The compatibility of skin grafts exchanged between mice of many different strains indicated that in inbred mice, there are more than 30 genetically distinguishable loci for the H Ags (see Chap. 20).

With one exception, these loci (H-1, etc.) encode Ags, called "minors," that elicit weak graft rejection responses (evident weeks or months after grafting). The exceptional locus, **H-2,** encodes Ags that elicit intense reactions leading to rapid graft rejection (in about 10–12 days). Although H-2 gene products can cause dramatic graft rejection, their physiological significance is far more profound, for as we shall see, T cells only recognize foreign antigens when they are associated with H-2 proteins. There are many genes at the H-2 locus, but they are all inherited together in a tightly linked cluster called the **major histocompatibility complex or MHC.** Each linked cluster or **haplotype** of H-2 alleles is designated (in mice) by a letter superscript, H-2ᵃ, H-2ᵇ, etc. (Table 15–3).

CONGENIC STRAINS. To analyze the H loci, breeding programs have been devised to yield pairs of **congenic** strains that differ at only a single locus. Congenic strains that differ at the MHC locus (H-2) are especially valuable. Their production, illustrated in Figure 15–11, starts with a cross between two inbred strains, A and B, that differ in their MHC. The final resulting strain, called A.B, has the entire genome of one parental strain (A) except for a small chromosomal region that includes the MHC of the other strain (B). A comparison of the responses of congenic strain pairs, such as A and A.B, makes it possible to determine rapidly the biologic effects of differences at the MHC locus.

RECOMBINANT CONGENIC STRAINS. These strains differ by only one or a few genes in the MHC locus. About 1% of the progeny of a cross between two MHC-different congenic strains (say A.B and A.C) have novel combinations of the parental MHC genes, a result of rare recombinations. By subjecting these progeny to the same inbreeding program that produces congenic strains, recombinant congenic strains that differ from each other by only one or a few MHC genes are derived (Fig. 15–12).

Table 15–3 lists some of the more than 100 inbred mouse strains that are available and their MHC haplotypes. There are also available about 75 MHC-congenic strains and a large number of recombinant congenic strains that differ by just one or a few MHC genes (Table 15–4).

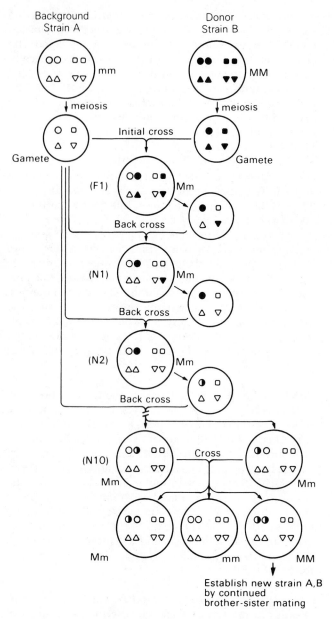

Background Strain A

Donor Strain B

Figure 15—11. Production of congenic strain A.B. Following an initial cross between an inbred A mouse and an inbred B mouse and a back-cross of the F1 generation to strain A, a series of successive back-crosses to strain A is carried out with progeny that possess the strain B marker of interest (M; e.g., a particular alloantigen). Offspring of the tenth back-cross generation (N10) are intercrossed, and progeny that are homozygous for M (e.g., they have the alloantigen of the B strain, not of the A strain) are then inbred by successive brother–sister matings to establish the new congenic A.B strain. This strain is identical genetically with inbred strain A except for the transferred chromosomal segment of strain B that bears the allele of interest. The principle is a general one: a congenic strain can be established for any gene. (If the transferred allele codes for a histocompatibility Ag and leads to graft rejection, the congenic A.B line is sometimes called a congenic resistant (CR) line, because it resists being killed by a tumor graft.) Strain A is the "background" strain, and strain B is the "donor" strain. (Courtesy of Dr RJ Graff; based on Snell GD: J Gen 49:87, 1948)

TABLE 15–3. MHC Haplotypes in Mice

Inbred Strains	MHC Haplotype	Composition of MHC-Haplotype			
		K	A	E	D
C57BL/6, C57BL/10, 129	H-2^b	b	b	b	b
BALB/c, DBA/2	H-2^d	d	d	d	d
Caracul	H-2^f	f	f	f	f
CBA, C3H, AKR	H-2^k	k	k	k	k
DBA/1, SWR	H-2^q	q	q	q	q
SJL	H-2^s	s	s	s	s
A*	H-2^a	k	k	k	d*

* Strain A is a natural MHC recombinant between the H-2^k and H-2^d haplotypes.

Immunization of mice of one strain with cells from an MHC-different congenic strain, say A.B cells (the "donor") injected into A mice (the "recipient"), yields alloantisera and mAbs that can identify MHC Ags of the donor by immunofluorescence or immunoprecipitation or by Ab-dependent cytotoxicity assays in which Abs plus complement (see Chap. 17) kill cells that bear the appropriate surface Ags (see Appendix, this chapter).

CLASSES OF MHC GENES. The MHC contains three classes of genes. Some of their key properties are summarized briefly here. The Class I and II genes and their products are discussed extensively later in this chapter; the Class III genes and their products are considered in Chapters 17 and 18.

Class I genes encode the principal subunits of MHC-I glycoproteins. Called **H-2 K, D,** and **L** in mice and **HLA-A, -B,** and **-C** in humans (see below), the proteins they encode are present on virtually all cells. These proteins elicit the intense responses of CD8$^+$ T cells (CTLs) that play a major role in rejection of allografts. They also form complexes with peptide fragments of viral Ags on virus-infected cells: recognition of the complexes by CD8$^+$ CTLs results in destruction of virus infected cells.

Class II genes encode cell-surface glycoproteins that are expressed by Ag-presenting cells (principally B cells, macrophages, and dendritic cells). Together with peptide fragments of Ags, the class II proteins form the epitopes that are recognized by T helper cells (CD4$^+$ T cells). Hence, the MHC-II proteins are critically involved in responses to nearly all Ags, including the intense reactions leading to allograft rejection. (In humans but not in mice, activated CD4$^+$ [T$_H$] cells also express MHC-II genes and might also serve as Ag-presenting cells.)

Class III genes encode three proteins of the complement cascade (C2, C4, Bf; see Chap. 17) and two cytotoxic proteins (tissue necrosis factor and lymphotoxin, see

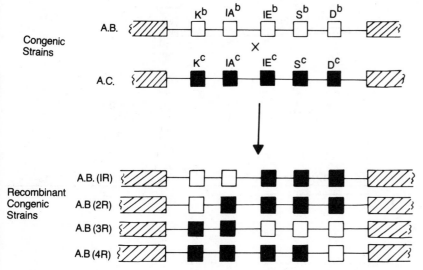

Figure 15–12. Some hypothetical recombinant congenic strains (A.B.(1R), etc.) derived from matings between mice of two congenic inbred strains (A.B × A.C), which have the same genome except for the MHC (B in one strain, C in the other). The various recombinant progeny arose from crossovers at different points in the section of the genome shown.

Chap. 19). These proteins are involved in diverse immune reactions that destroy cells, not necessarily in connection with allografts.

Analysis of recombinant congenic mouse strains, indicates that the order of loci within the mouse MHC (i.e., H-2) is **K–A–E–S–D** (Fig. 15–13), where K and D are class I loci, A and E are class II loci, and S corresponds to the class III locus. At the end of this chapter, we shall consider a more detailed map of MHC genes.

MHC IN OTHER SPECIES. An MHC has been found in bony fish, birds, and some amphibians, and it is probably present in some form in all vertebrates. The order of class I, II, and III genes in the human and the mouse is compared in Figure 15–13.

THE HUMAN HLA COMPLEX

In humans, the proteins encoded by the MHC are termed HLA (**h**uman **l**eukocyte **a**ntigens) because of the circumstances under which they were identified (see below). They are also specified by class I, II, and III loci that are homologous to the mouse MHC loci (Fig. 15–13). However, the human genes have been analyzed by different means because the breeding programs used in analyzing the mouse H-2 complex are obviously inapplicable to humans. HLA alleles were first recognized by the human alloAbs that appear following multiple blood transfusions (in which donors' white blood cells bear Ags that the recipient lacks), and pregnancies (in which the mother is exposed to the father's HLA Ags on fetal leuko-

TABLE 15–4. Some Congenic Inbred Strains of Mice Derived From Inbred Strains C57BL/10 (termed B10) or A as Background Strains and Various Inbred Donor Strains

Background Strain	Congenic Strain Designation	MHC (H-2) Haplotype	Donor Strain	Other Inbred and Congenic Strains With the Same MHC (H-2) Haplotype
B10 MHC type = b	B10.D2	d	DBA/2	DBA/2, BALB/c
	B10.A	a	A	A/J
	B10.BR	k	C57BR	C3H, CBA, AKR, BALB.K
	B10.Q	q	DBA/1	DBA/1, SWR
	B10.S	s	A.SW	A.SW, SJL
A MHC type = a	A.BY	b	B10	B10, C57BL/6, 129, BALB.B
	A.CA	f	Caracul	B10.M
	A.SW	s	Swiss	SJL, B10.S

Modified from Hood LE, Weissman IL, Wood WB, Wilson JH: Immunology, 2nd edition. Benjamin/Cummings Co, Inc, 1984.

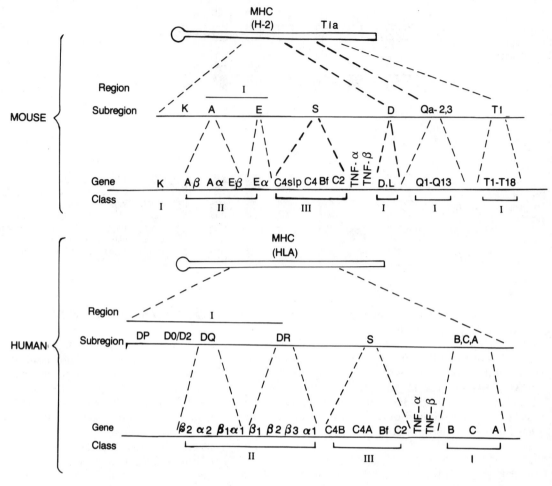

Figure 15–13. MHC locus in mouse (chromosome 17) and human (chromosome 6). Subregions were defined by analyzing cells from genetically related humans and from recombinant congenic strains of mice with antisera. MHC-II genes are interspersed between MHC-I genes (K, D, L) in the mouse, whereas in humans and most other species, the MHC-I genes (B, C, A) are contiguous. The Qa and Tla genes are not considered part of the MHC, although they encode proteins that are very similar to MHC-I molecules; in mice, there are 10 to 13 highly conserved genes in the Qa-2,3 region (Q1–Q13) and 13 to 18 highly conserved genes in the T1 region (T1–T18). By "gene conversion" (described later in this chapter), the Qa genes may be responsible for diversifying sequences of MHC-I genes. Map distances are not drawn to scale.

cytes that cross the placenta). Multiple pregnancies involving the same father lead to especially high-titered antisera. The Abs in these sera were initially recognized by white blood cell agglutination (leukoagglutination), but they are currently measured by cytotoxicity assays: the Abs (plus complement) damage leukocytes having the appropriate surface Ags.

MIXED LYMPHOCYTE REACTION. The genes that encode the HLA Ags have been studied by analyzing white blood cells from human families (especially those with many children) using human anti-HLA alloantisera and the mixed lymphocyte reaction (**MLR**). In this reaction, pe-

ripheral blood mononuclear cells (B and T cells and monocytes) from two individuals are incubated together in the presence of ^{3}H-thymidine (^{3}H-TdR). If the individuals differ in MHC-I or MHC-II, the T cells proliferate and incorporate ^{3}H-thymidine into their DNA. The reaction can be made **one-way** by treating cells from one individual with mitomycin C or ionizing radiation to block DNA replication. The MHC-I or MHC-II Ags that are responsible for a given reaction can sometimes be identified by alloantisera or monoclonal Abs that block the MLR.

All MHC-I and MHC-II genes on one chromosome are inherited together as a tightly linked cluster or haplotype. Hence, each person inherits two MHC haplotypes, one from each parent, and transmits one to each child. Thus, among the children born to two heterozygous parents having no haplotype in common, one in two siblings, on average, will share one haplotype; only in those having two identical haplotypes (a probability of 1 in 4) will the MLR be negative (i.e., no increase above background in ^{3}H-thymidine incorporation into DNA). In contrast, negative MLRs between unrelated individuals are extremely rare (perhaps 1 in 10,000), because there are a great many allelic variants of each of the MHC genes; that is, the MHC-I and MHC-II genes are extremely **polymorphic.** The genetic mechanisms that generate their extreme polymorphism are referred to below (MHC Molecules and Genes).

Although haplotypes are inherited with fidelity, in about 1% of children, the HLA-A and HLA-B alleles represent recombination between A and B loci; recombinations between B and C are rarer (see Fig. 15–13). The recombinations provided key opportunities for mapping the gene order in the HLA locus.

Antigen Recognition by T Cells

T CELLS RECOGNIZE ANTIGENS ON OTHER CELLS: MHC RESTRICTION

B cells react with Ags that are either in solution or on a cell surface, but a T cell characteristically reacts only with Ag on the surface of another cell. The difference became understandable when it was realized that T cells recognize Ags only in association with MHC glycoproteins, which are normally present only on the surface of cells.

A clear demonstration of the role of MHC proteins came from studies of CTL lysis of virus-infected target cells, where Ags encoded by the viral genome are expressed on the cell's surface. If mice are inoculated with such a virus, CTL recovered several days later from the spleen will normally lyse target cells only if they are infected with the same virus and if they express the same MHC haplotype as the CTL (Fig. 15–14). These remark-

able findings suggested that **CTL are specific for both viral Ag and MHC gene products:** the MHC products are said to "restrict" Ag recognition by CTL, and the phenomenon is called **MHC restriction.** By testing virus-infected cells from various recombinant congenic strains of mice, it became clear that CTLs recognized Ag in conjunction with MHC-I proteins. Other studies indicated that T_H cells are also MHC restricted, but by MHC-II proteins. However, only special Ag-presenting cells (B cells, macrophages, dendritic cells) normally express these proteins, and thus it is only these cells that normally activate T_H cells. All cells express MHC-I and are therefore susceptible to being lysed by CTLs.

In inbred mice, each cell expresses two or three MHC-I proteins (K and D in some strains; K, D, and L in others), and each of these proteins can restrict Ag recognition. If we consider just K and D, then in an MHC-heterozygous mouse (with, say, MHC haplotypes H-2^a and H-2^b) infected with virus X, there are potentially four sets of anti-X CTLs, recognizing X + H-2K^a, X + H-2K^b, X + H-2D^a, or X + H-2D^b. Humans have as many as six MHC-II genes per haplotype, and so in an individual who is heterozygous at each of them, there might be as many as 12 sets of T_H cells that are specific for a given epitope, each recognizing it in association with a different MHC-II protein. However, not all MHC-I and MHC-II proteins can restrict recognition of all Ags. Indeed, there is considerable selectivity, and any given Ag is usually recognized only in association with one or a few of the several possible restricting elements. For example, in H-2^d mice, a major influenza virus Ag is restricted by H-2K^d but not by H-2D^d.

A SINGLE TcR RECOGNIZES ANTIGEN IN CONJUNCTION WITH AN MHC-I OR MHC-II PROTEIN.
Although it was initially considered that each T cell might have two receptors, one for an Ag and the other for an MHC protein, **one receptor, called the TcR, has been shown to be specific for both Ag and MHC.** As described in detail below, the TcR has striking similarities to mIg on B cells: it is made up of two different S–S-linked subunits, and

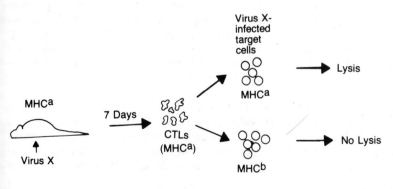

Figure 15–14. MHC restriction of Ag recognition by CTLs. CTLs specific for virus X are elicited by challenging mice (MHC^a) with virus X. The CTLs lyse virus-infected target cells from MHC^a mice, but not those from MHC^b mice. (Based on RM Zinkernagle, PC Doherty: Nature 251:547, 1974)

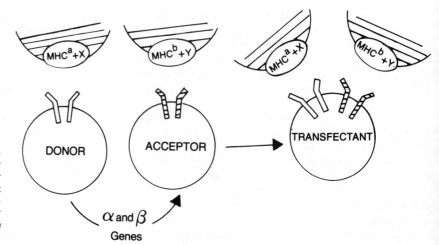

Figure 15–15. T-cell specificity transferred with the TcR α and β genes. The α and β genes were transfected from a donor CTL (specific for MHC^a + X) to an acceptor CTL (specific for MHC^b + Y). The transfected cells lyse targets that express either MHC^a + X **or** MHC^b + Y. Transfection of the α and β gene alone did **not** transfer specificity. (Based on Dembic et al: Nature 320:232, 1986)

the genes that encode them are assembled, as are Ig genes, from V, D, J, and C gene segments (see TcR Genes, below). When the assembled TcR genes of a CTL line specific for a particular Ag and MHC-I protein were transfected into another CTL specific for a different Ag–MHC-I combination, the donor cell's specificity was conferred on the recipient cell (Fig. 15–15), showing that **a single TcR can recognize specifically a distinct Ag–MHC-I** combination. The TcR on T_H cells has likewise been shown to recognize specific Ag–MHC-II combinations. Because a TcR's combining site is probably similar to that of an Ig (see Chap. 14), it follows that **the recognized ligand is probably a binary Ag–MHC complex.** Before considering the nature of this complex, we will briefly consider another feature of T cells: their great propensity to recognize foreign MHC molecules in the apparent absence of other Ags.

ALLOREACTIVITY

Far older than the discovery of MHC restriction was the observation that normal T cells from one mouse strain react vigorously to the different (allogeneic) MHC-I and MHC-II glycoproteins of other mouse strains. This phenomenon, called "alloreactivity," is the basis for rapid rejection of MHC-different tissue allografts. It is not surprising that T cells recognize allogeneic MHC molecules as foreign; what is remarkable is the potency of the response, which is attributable to the extraordinarily **high frequency** of alloreactive T cells. It is estimated by limiting dilution analysis (see Appendix, this chapter) that 1% to 10% of T cells recognize any given allogeneic MHC protein; for comparison, the frequency of T cells reactive to typical viral Ags associated with a self-MHC molecule is probably 0.01% or less. Because there are many MHC alleles, it appears that **most T cells are reactive with one or several allogeneic MHC proteins.** Indeed, T cell clones that recognize Ags associated with self-MHC

molecules normally cross-react with one or more allogeneic MHC molecules. Why this is so is not established, but it is possible that a propensity to react with MHC molecules of the species may be inherent in the germline pool of genes encoding TcRs.

PROCESSING OF EXTRINSIC ANTIGENS INVOLVES PROTEOLYSIS

It has long been known that T_H cells recognize altered or "processed" forms of Ag on special APCs, principally macrophages, B cells, and dendritic cells. Agents (e.g., chloroquine and ammonium chloride) that raise pH in lysosomes and interfere with degradation of ingested proteins, block effective Ag presentation by APC. This finding suggests that proteolysis in lysosomes is essential for protein Ag presentation to T cells. Furthermore, if APCs are first incubated with glutaraldehyde to block metabolic ("processing") activities and then with an intact protein Ag, they cannot present the Ag to T cells, whereas if glutaraldehyde-fixed APC are incubated with the Ag after it has been cleaved with a protease, effective presentation occurs. Moreover, in cultures containing APC, T_H cells that were elicited by immunization with an intact protein Ag can be stimulated to proliferate by small peptides (10 to 20 amino acids in length) derived from the Ag. It thus appears that **APC present protein Ags as peptide fragments for T_H-cell recognition.** These observations explain why unfolding a protein Ag usually does not abolish its recognition by T cells even though it usually greatly decreases its recognition by Abs (see Peptides, Chap. 13).

DEGRADED FORMS OF ANTIGEN INTERACT DIRECTLY WITH MHC GLYCOPROTEINS. Once a protein Ag is taken into an APC and degraded, the peptide fragments must find their way back to the cell surface for T-cell recognition to occur. The route is not known, but it is likely that on the cell surface, the peptides are bound selectively by MHC glycoproteins, as, in the test tube, immunogenic peptides bind to purified MHC-II glycoproteins with affinities (equilibrium constants) that can approach 10^{-6} M. Compared with Ab–hapten interactions having similar affinities, the rate constant for the association step is extremely low ($k_a = \sim 1 M^{-1} s^{-1}$), and the rate constant for the reverse step is extraordinarily low ($k_d = \sim 10^{-6} s^{-1}$, corresponding to a half-time for dissociation of about 10 days). A particular peptide may bind well to some MHC-II proteins and not detectably to others, and the differences usually correlate with the high or low Ab responses of MHC-different mice to the corresponding Ag.

MHC-LINKED IMMUNE RESPONSE GENES

Long before MHC restriction was discovered, it was found that guinea pigs and mice with different MHC haplotypes can differ in their responses to particular protein Ags, particularly those with few epitopes per molecule. The effect is Ag-specific, as animals that are low responders to some Ags are high responders to others, and the ability to produce a high Ab response to a given Ag is genetically dominant: heterozygotes produced by crossing high responders with low responders are high responders. The responsible genes were denoted **immune response** or **Ir genes,** and they were subsequently discovered (see below) to be identical to MHC-II genes. In at least some cases, the low-responder phenotype results from failure of a given Ag to interact with particular MHC-II glycoproteins. Some of the landmark experiments that led to these conclusions are summarized below.

Ir GENES ENCODE MHC-II PROTEINS. To produce Abs against Ir gene products, mice of one strain were immunized with spleen cells from a strain that expressed different Ir gene alleles. Such antisera, and mAbs derived from similar immunizations, react with MHC-II glycoproteins, which are expressed primarily on APC, but not (in mice) on T cells.

That particular Ir gene alleles and particular MHC-II alleles are inherited together could mean either that they are identical or that they are closely linked in the MHC gene complex. Proof of their identity came from studies with **transgenic mice.** As noted below, although most mouse strains express two different MHC-II molecules (A and E), some strains do not express the E molecule owing to a mutation. Such strains also do not respond to immunization with certain Ags. To prove that nonresponsiveness to such an Ag, call it X, is secondary to the failure to express the E MHC-II molecule, an E gene isolated by recombinant DNA technology was injected into fertilized eggs of the E-defective mouse strain. Stable transgenic mouse strains derived from the embryos ex-

pressed the donor E gene and also responded to Ag X. Thus **proteins specified by MHC-II genes control an animal's ability to respond to particular Ags.**

In the experiment cited, the injected E gene is an Ir high-responder allele for the response to Ag X. Another allele might be responsible for a low response to Ag X for various reasons: for example, it might not be expressed at all (like the E mutant noted above). More often, it *is* expressed but is incompatible with a response to Ag X for one of several reasons. Perhaps the most common one is that it fails to bind Ag X. Thus, peptides from an immunogenic protein often fail to bind significantly *in vitro* to MHC proteins from mice of low-responder strains (in contrast to high responders). In other instances, however, immunogenic peptides of an Ag bind strongly to a low-responder MHC-II protein, and yet no T cells reactive to the complex are elicited. In this case, there appears to be a "**hole**" in the repertoire of T cells and their Ag-specific receptors; that is, T cells with receptors reactive with the complex do not exist in the animal. A possible explanation is that the complex of low-responder MHC-II and the immunogenic peptide mimics a complex of the MHC-II and a "self" Ag, to which the animal is tolerant (see T-Cell Self Tolerance, below). According to still another possibility, the immunogenic peptide binds to the low-responder strain's MHC-II proteins, and there are T_H cells that recognize the complex, but they are prevented from responding to it by $CD8^+$ T cells that act as suppressors.

PRESENTATION OF ANTIGENS IN ASSOCIATION WITH CLASS I MHC PROTEINS. Viral infections elicit CTLs that recognize viral Ags in association with MHC-I proteins on infected target cells. These Ags were initially expected to be the viral envelope glycoproteins, which are expressed as integral membrane proteins on virus-infected cells. However, analyses of various target cells infected with different influenza-virus variants suggested that most anti-influenza CTLs react specifically against a viral nucleoprotein (NP) that is not expressed on the infected cell's surface. Moreover, fibroblasts that are not infected with the virus become specific targets for anti-influenza CTLs when a small (15 amino acids) synthetic peptide corresponding to a sequence in the NP is simply adsorbed to the fibroblast surface provided that the fibroblast expresses the appropriate MHC-I protein. Thus, like MHC-II-restricted T_H cells, MHC-I-restricted CTLs can recognize peptide fragments of Ags, presumably bound directly to MHC-I molecules on the target-cell surface.

ANTIGEN-PROCESSING PATHWAYS

The T cells elicited by immunization with an **extrinsic** protein Ag (e.g., bovine serum albumin injected into a mouse) are MHC-II-restricted $CD4^+$ cells, that is, T_H cells.

But viral Ags, which are synthesized within the infected animal's cells and might therefore be termed **intrinsic** Ags, can be restricted by either MHC-I or MHC-II glycoproteins; hence, they can elicit both T_H and CTL cells. It is therefore likely that extrinsic and intrinsic Ags are processed by different pathways.

As noted before, the extrinsic Ags are degraded by lysosomal proteases in APC, and some of the resulting peptides bind to the cell's MHC-II proteins and serve as epitopes for T_H cells. However, the intrinsic Ags are essentially equivalent to other cellular (self) proteins, and they are probably degraded to peptides by the same proteolytic pathway that is responsible for the cleavage and turnover of most cellular proteins. In this pathway, the protein **ubiquitin** becomes covalently linked to some of the cell's protein molecules by means of the enzyme **ubiquitin ligase,** rendering them susceptible to cleavage by proteases within the same cell. How the resulting peptides bind to MHC-I and make their way to the cell surface is not known.

Cell–Cell Interactions in the Humoral (Antibody) Response

There appears to be more than one pathway by which T_H cells enhance the production of Abs by B cells. In the most important pathway, termed **cognate** interaction, T_H cells and B cells recognize different epitopes on the same Ag particle or molecule; hence, contact between the cells appears to be required. A second pathway, which may operate at high Ag concentrations, does not require such contact. In addition, the humoral response also involves **accessory cells,** which have **no clonally distributed specificity for Ag.** Instead, they function both as APC and as activators of specific T_H cells in the initial phases of the immune response. Once activated, these T_H cells can then interact with and help specific B cells.

The principal accessory cells are dendritic cells and macrophages. Both originate from bone marrow stem cells, are relatively adherent (e.g., to glass and plastic surfaces), and express MHC-II glycoproteins. The expression of MHC-II is constitutive in dendritic cells but inducible by a lymphokine—immune interferon (γ-IFN)—in macrophages. Another difference is that macrophages, but not dendritic cells, are phagocytic. B cells normally express MHC-II proteins and can likewise function as APC (see below) but are relatively ineffective as activators of **resting** T cells. Under some pathological conditions (see Chap. 20), other cells (e.g., endothelial cells, pancreatic islet β cells in Type I diabetes, thyroid cells in thyroiditis) are induced to express MHC-II proteins, and it is possible that they then also function as APCs.

COGNATE T_H-CELL–B-CELL COOPERATION

How exactly do T_H cells, B cells, and accessory cells interact in the course of an immune response? A widely accepted model is illustrated in Figure 15–16. As noted before, in the initial step protein Ags are taken into the accessory cells, which fragment them and present the peptides bound to MHC-II glycoproteins on the cell surface. In addition, Ags bind specifically to the corresponding mIg receptors on B cells and are then internalized and similarly processed and presented by these B cells. "Resting" T_H cells that recognize the peptide–MHC-II complex on the accessory cells become **activated:** they leave the G_0 stage of the cell cycle, enlarge, proliferate, and interact with those B cells that present the Ag. Moreover, the activated T cells secrete several proteins (see Lymphokines and Interleukins, below) that act on B cells, causing them to undergo cell division and terminal differentiation into Ab-secreting cells (plasma cells, see Chap. 16).

THE CARRIER EFFECT. An important feature of Ag-recognition in T_H cell–B cell cooperation emerged from studies of the Ab response to multiple spaced injections of animals with a hapten conjugated to a "carrier" protein. As we shall see later (see Chap. 16), when an animal is given one injection ("primed") with a hapten (A) coupled to a carrier (protein X), a second injection of the same Ag (A–protein X) several weeks later elicits a vigorous secondary Ab response (high serum levels of IgG Abs having high affinity for A). However, if the second injection is made with A attached to another carrier protein (Y), the secondary response hardly occurs unless the animal has also been previously primed with protein Y itself.

Analysis of the carrier effect showed that T cells recognize the carrier protein and that the hapten and carrier must be **physically linked** for effective T cell–B cell cooperation to occur (Fig. 15–17). For example, the T and B cells that cooperate in the response can be elicited in separate mice immunized (primed) with protein Y or with the hapten A conjugated to protein X. When a mixture of T cells (anti-Y) from the first donor and B cells (including anti-A) from the second are transferred to irradiated adoptive hosts, they mount a secondary anti-A response to a challenge ("boosting") with a new conjugate, of A to protein Y. In contrast, boosting with a mixture of free protein Y and a conjugate of A with protein Z is ineffective. Hence, cooperating T_H cells and B cells **can recognize different epitopes of an Ag** (e.g., A and peptides of protein Y), but the epitopes that they recognize must be physically linked for optimal effectiveness. For conventional protein Ags, having no attached hapten, the same principal applies: usually one epitope (E1, Fig. 15–16) is recognized by the B cell and another (E2) by the cooperating T_H cell, but E1 and E2 have to be parts of the

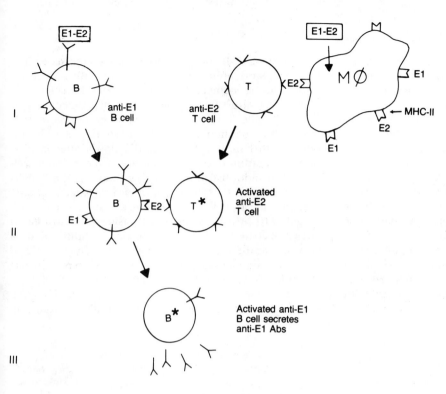

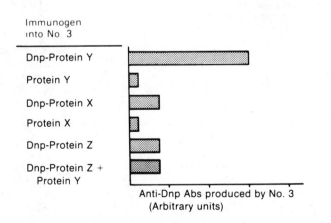

Figure 15–16. A model of T–B–macrophage interactions leading to antibody secretion. For simplicity the Ag is shown with only two epitopes, E1 and E2. In stage I, the Ag binds to the E1-specific mIg receptor on the B cell and is internalized and "processed." Fragments of the Ag, including one corresponding to E2, bind to MHC-II molecules and appear at the cell surface (stage II). Also in stage I, the E1-E2 Ag is processed and presented by Ag-presenting cells (e.g., macrophages) to T cells specific for E2–MHC-II. In stage II, the activated T cell (T*) provides inductive signals ("help") to the B cell by virtue of its recognition of E2–MHC-II on the B cell. In stage III, the activated B cell (B*) begins to secrete E1-specific Abs. Thus the cooperation of an anti-E2 T_H cell with an anti-E1 B cell results in production of anti-E1 Ab in response to Ag (E1-E2).

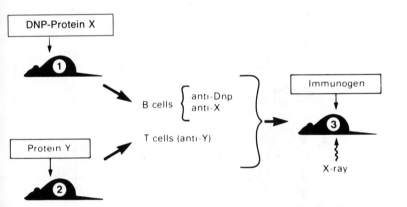

Figure 15–17. Carrier effect analyzed by adoptive transfer. Mouse no. 1, primed against DNP and protein X, provided B cells. Mouse no. 2, primed against protein Y, provided T cells. No. 3 mice were given, in order: (1) sufficient X- or γ-irradiation (e.g., 600 r) to inactivate its own lymphatic system, (2) a mixture of B cells from mouse no. 1 and T cells from mouse no. 2, and (3) various immunogens as noted. One week later, the anti-Dnp Ab responses of no. 3 mice were measured by analyzing either its serum Ab concentration or the number of spleen cells secreting anti-Dnp Abs in a hemolytic plaque assay. The most intense response is elicited with Dnp-protein Y, indicating that the carrier (protein Y) and hapten must be physically linked. (Based on Ovary Z, Benacerraf B: Proc Soc Exp Biol and Med 114:72, 1963, and Mitchison A: Eur J Immunol 1:18, 1971)

337

same Ag molecule, just as in a hapten–protein conjugate. The epitopes recognized by T_H cells and B cells **need not** be different, although in most instances they are. The reason is that T cells recognize "linear epitopes" present on small peptides, whereas B cells usually recognize "conformational epitopes," which depend on the protein antigen's native configuration (see Chap. 13).

COGNATE T–B COOPERATION IS MHC RESTRICTED. The carrier effect suggested that a T_H cell is linked to the B cell that it helps by an **Ag bridge** between the Ag-specific receptors of the two cells. This simple view had to be modified, however, when adoptive transfer experiments showed that T_H cells recognize only Ags that are associated with MHC molecules (not with mIg) on the B-cell surface. For example (Fig. 15–18), in MHC-heterozygous ($MHC^k \times MHC^b$)F_1 mice that have been immunized with SRBC, one set of T cells recognizes Ags (SRBC) in associa-

tion with MHC-II^k (in a complex designated as SRBC–MHC-II^k), and another set recognizes SRBC–MHC-II^b. Those that recognize SRBC–MHC-II^k can be selectively expanded by transferring the total T-cell population, and injecting SRBC, into heavily irradiated homozygous H-2^k mice, which contain MHC-II^k Ag-presenting cells. (Compared with lymphocytes, APCs die slowly after irradiation and continue to function *in vivo* over the short period of an adoptive transfer experiment.) If the T cells recovered from these animals several days later (greatly enriched for T_H cells that recognize SRBC–MHC-II^k) are mixed with MHC^k B cells and transferred to irradiated ($MHC^k \times MHC^b$)F_1 hosts, an injection of SRBC elicits a vigorous anti-SRBC Ab response. However, if MHC^b B cells are used instead of MHC^k B cells, the Ab response is much lower, similar to that obtained with unprimed T_H cells. Because the latter result is obtained even if a large excess of MHC^k APCs is included in the inoculum, the

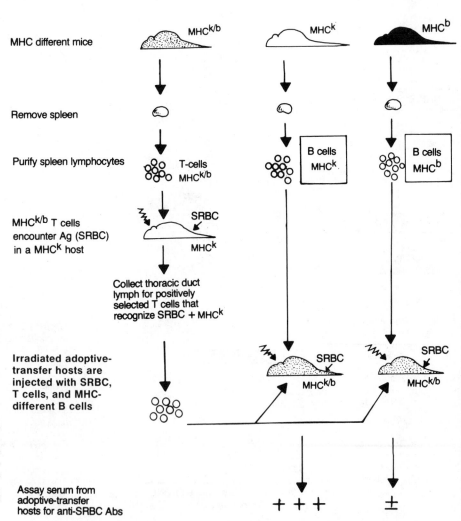

Figure 15–18. A demonstration that T-cell–B cell interactions are MHC restricted. The subset of T cells from MHC$^{k/b}$ mice specific for SRBC/MHC^k is enriched by exposing them to SRBC in MHC^k mice. These T cells support a secondary Ab response to SRBC in irradiated MHC$^{k/b}$ adoptive hosts that are given MHC^k but not MHC^b B cells. (Based on J Sprent et al: J Exp Med 147:1159, 1978)

low response is not attributable to a failure to activate the T_H cells. Instead, it occurs because **effective cooperation between a T_H cell and a B cell requires the T_H cell to recognize Ag–MHC-II complexes on the B cell it helps.**

SPECIFICITY OF T-CELL–B-CELL COOPERATION. Although cooperating T_H cells and B cells can see different epitopes on an Ag, the specificity of the resulting Ab production comes about in part because the B cells efficiently process only those Ags that they bind specifically via their mIg receptors (see Fig. 15–16). Thus, B cells that are exposed to Ag concentrations as low as 1×10^{-9} moles/liter can take up that Ag and present it effectively to T_H cells only if the B cells have mIg with sufficient affinity for the Ag. Otherwise, more than 1000-fold higher Ag concentrations are required, and at these high concentrations, Ags probably enter the B-cell processing pathway via an uncharacterized nonspecific mechanism similar to that of APCs.

B-CELL ACTIVATION SIGNALS IN COGNATE T_H-CELL–B-CELL COOPERATION. The activation signals passed from T_H cells to B cells in cognate cooperation probably consist in part of several of the known **lymphokines** (including IL-4, IL-5, and IL-6, see below). Although critically important, these proteins, which are secreted by activated T_H cells and stimulate B cells, are probably not sufficient, as attempts to substitute them for T_H cells have thus far not succeeded (at the low Ag concentrations at which cognate T_H-cell–B-cell cooperation occurs). Whether the binding of Ag to B-cell mIg receptors is also an activation signal per se or simply operates to pass Ags into the processing pathway is also not clear.

NONCOGNATE T_H-CELL–B-CELL COOPERATION

Under certain conditions, B cells can be activated without direct contact with T_H cells. For instance, a high concentration of intact (bivalent) rabbit Ab to mouse Ig (causing "cross-linking" of mIg on mouse B cells) is sufficient, in the presence of lymphokines (derived from T cells) and in the absence of T cells, to trigger purified B cells to proliferate and secrete Ig. This finding suggests that B cells might also be activated *in vivo* by high concentrations of multivalent Ags (which would likewise cross-link mIg on the corresponding B cells) provided that lymphokines (from activated T cells) are present.

CELLULAR REQUIREMENTS FOR INDUCTION OF CTLs

In nonimmune animals, **precursors of CTLs (pCTLs)** exist as "resting" $CD4^-CD8^+$ T cells, which lack cytolytic activity. Stimulation with Ag results in their activation: the cells enlarge, enter into the mitotic cycle, proliferate, and acquire specific cytolytic activity. Ags must be presented to pCTL in association with MHC-I proteins. Because virtually all cells in the body express MHC-I proteins, it is possible that pCTLs do not require a specialized Ag-presenting cell. Indeed, *in vitro* studies suggest that even fibroblasts can activate pCTL.

$CD4^+$ T_H cells can augment activation of $CD8^+$ CTLs, but they may not be required. Because $CD8^+$ resting pCTL do not express MHC-II proteins, there can be no necessity for them to be recognized by T_H cells (as in B cell responses); hence, it is unlikely that T_H-cell–pCTL interaction occurs by direct cell contact. Rather, Ag-activated T_H cells efficiently secrete several diffusible lymphokines (see below) that can act on pCTLs at some distance, inducing them to proliferate and differentiate into mature killer cells. Although some lymphokines are also produced by activated pCTLs (see below), lymphokine production by T_H cells is probably more efficient and may include factors not produced by CTL. Lymphokines that influence the proliferation and acquisition of cytolytic activity by pCTL include interleukin-2, interleukin-4, and less well characterized differentiation factors.

SUPPRESSOR T CELLS

There is evidence that immune responses to a variety of Ags can be inhibited by cells called **T-suppressor cells** (T_s). T_s-cell activity, when present, is manifested in the $CD4^-CD8^+$ T-cell population. T_s cells are reported to bear a marker called **IJ,** which seems to distinguish them from $CD4^-CD8^+$ CTLs, and they appear to bind free Ags without MHC restrictions. Hence, their Ag-specific receptors probably differ from those on T_H cells and CTLs.

It is thought that the main function of T_s cells is to inhibit or **down-regulate** immune responses, but the mechanisms are obscure. They appear to secrete soluble factors that inhibit specific T_H cells and that can also shut off selectively the transcription of Ig H or L chain genes in some model myeloma cell lines. In addition, they may have a role in sustaining nonresponsiveness to certain self Ags (see Tolerance, below). T_s cells are not well characterized, perhaps because it has been difficult to derive clonal cell lines with reproducible properties.

Cytokines and Their Receptors

A variety of proteins have profound effects on lymphocyte proliferation and terminal differentiation into effector cells. These include **lymphokines,** produced by T lymphocytes, and **monokines,** produced by APCs (Table 15–5). These proteins, collectively termed **cytokines,** are not specific for Ags, but their production, and also the

TABLE 15–5. Cytokines and Their Receptors

Cytokine	M_r	Producing Cell Types	Responding Cell Types	Activities
IL-1α and IL-1β	15–17kDa	Several, including monocytes	Several	Stimulates acute-phase protein synthesis and endogenous pyrogen production. Cofactor in T- and B-cell responses.
IL-2	15kDa	T cells	T cells, CTL, B cells	Growth factor
IL-3	28kDa	T cells	Mast cells, hematopoietic stem cells	Growth factor
IL-4	20kDa	T cells	T cells, B cells	Growth factor. Increases B-cell MHC glycoprotein expression. Promotes IgG1, IgE production by B cells.
IL-5	18kDa	T cells	B cells (T cells?)	Stimulates B-cell growth and Ig secretion.
γ interferon	17kDa	T cells	Several	Anti-viral activity. Induces MHC Class II glycoprotein expression by macrophages. Augments T-cell responses.
IL-6	21kDa	Several, including T cells	B cells, T cells	Stimulates Ig secretion by B cells. Stimulates T-cell activation and IL-2 production. Growth factor for myeloma and hybridoma cells.

responses to them, are dependent on Ag stimulation. Indeed, **the clonal response of lymphocytes depends on these proteins as well as on Ags.**

Cytokines are a subclass of extracellular factors that affect cell proliferation and differentiation. **Endocrine** cells produce hormones that act on other cells located elsewhere in the body (e.g., the pituitary secretes the thyroid-stimulating hormone that acts on thyroid cells). In **paracrine** growth, a factor made by one cell acts on nearby cells of the same or of different type (e.g., a cytokine secreted by macrophages acts on dendritic cells). In **autocrine** systems, a cell secretes factors required for its own growth. In all instances, a cell's responsiveness to a protein factor depends on its expression of a surface receptor for that factor. Some of the cytokines described below act as paracrine and others as autocrine factors; some act as both.

INTERLEUKIN-2 (IL-2)

The best-characterized lymphokine is interleukin 2 (IL-2), a single-chain protein of 15 Kd. It is required for growth by most T cells, and it is a cofactor in activating B cells to secrete Ig (see Noncognate T_H-Cell–B-Cell Cooperation, above). It may also be a B-cell growth factor.

Resting T cells do not secrete IL-2 and have no IL-2 mRNA. In response to Ag–MHC stimulation of T cells, IL-2 mRNA accumulates, reaches peak levels at around 20 hours, and then falls to very low levels over the next 2 days. Reexposure to Ag–MHC several days later elicits

the same cycle. Thus, **Il-2 production is a transient response to Ag–MHC stimulation.** (Many, but not all, cloned T_H cell lines produce IL-2. Some cloned CTL lines also produce IL-2 but generally at a much lower level.)

IL-2 RECEPTORS. Cells responsive to IL-2 express cell-surface IL-2 receptors (IL-2R). There are at least two forms, with very different affinities for IL-2; both usually coexist on the same cell. An activated T cell usually expresses approximately 5000 high-affinity IL-2R (K_d, 10^{-11} M) and approximately 50,000 low-affinity IL-2R (K_d, 3×10^{-8}M). Because IL-2 is active at concentrations (10^{-9}M) that saturate high- but scarcely bind to low-affinity IL-2R, binding to low-affinity IL-2R is apparently not necessary for function. It is probably significant for its function that IL-2 bound to high-affinity IL-2R is rapidly internalized by the cells.

Two subunits of IL-2R have been identified. A 50-Kd glycosylated transmembrane protein was identified with mAbs that bind to T cells and block IL-2 binding. A second subunit (70 Kd) was identified by chemical cross-linking to the 50-Kd subunit. It appears that either subunit alone has low affinity for IL-2 (as shown by transformed cell lines that express one subunit or the other); when the two subunits are associated (noncovalently), they form the high-affinity IL-2R. Regulation of expression of the subunits may control the number of high-affinity IL-2R per cell and hence the responsiveness of cells to IL-2.

Resting T-lymphocytes express no detectable IL-2R as

measured by the binding either of IL-2 or of mAbs to the 50-Kd subunit. Following Ag–MHC stimulation *in vitro*, mRNA for the 50-Kd subunit accumulates in T cells, high- and low-affinity IL-2R appear on the cell surface, and the cells become responsive to IL-2. Peak levels of IL-2R are present a few days later but decline thereafter to very low levels. The decline is paralleled by loss of responsiveness to IL-2. The cycle is repeated on reexposure to Ag–MHC. Therefore, **like IL-2 production, expression of IL-2R and responsiveness to IL-2 are transient and inducible responses to Ag–MHC stimulation.**

IL-2 AND CELLULAR INTERACTIONS. A resting CD4$^+$ T cell makes neither IL-2 nor IL-2R. The expression of both (which is necessary for the cell to enter cell cycle, proliferate, and differentiate into an effector T_H cell) requires multiple signals, including, for example, cross-linking the cell's Ag-specific receptors by Ag–MHC-II complexes on accessory cells and soluble factors produced by the accessory cells (possibly interleukin-1 and interleukin-6; see below). For subsequent rounds of activation of T-cell lines, cross-linking of the T-cell's Ag receptor may be sufficient, at least for T_H cells.

INTERLEUKIN-4

Interleukin-4 (IL-4, also called B-cell stimulating factor-1) is a 20-Kd protein growth factor for B cells and some T cells. It also induces increased expression of MHC-II glycoproteins on B cells and promotes production of IgG1 and IgE. IL-4 is produced by T_H cells (of the T_H2 subset) following Ag–MHC-II stimulation, and it serves as **an autocrine growth factor for these cells.** Like IL-2, **it also acts as a paracrine factor** (because T cells and B cells that do not produce IL-4 can respond to the IL-4 provided by other T_H cells). IL-4 also has some activities outside the immune system; for example, it stimulates fibroblasts to secrete growth factors.

THE SPECIAL ROLE OF ACCESSORY CELLS IN T-CELL ACTIVATION

We have seen (see Fig. 15–16) that dendritic cells and macrophages play an important role in initiating immune responses. Although dendritic cells, macrophages, and B cells all express MHC-II molecules and can present Ags to T cells, the B cells are ineffective at **initiating** the response of resting T cells. The ability of macrophages and dendritic cells to initiate these responses is probably attributable to their capacity to provide special signals to resting T cells. The cytokine IL-1, which is produced by macrophages but not by dendritic cells, may play some role in T-cell activation. Another cytokine, **IL-6,** also has potent activity in activating resting T cells,

and it is produced by a variety of cell types, including macrophages. It is also possible that macrophages and dendritic cells provide nondiffusible signals to T cells via contacts between their membrane proteins.

T-Cell Development

DIFFERENTIATION

As will be discussed in detail below, differentiating T cells are subjected to **selection,** based on their specificity for Ags, in order to ensure that an individual's mature T cells do not react with self Ags (i.e., are self-tolerant) but can recognize foreign Ags in association with self-MHC proteins. To understand the selection mechanisms, it is important to distinguish stages in T-cell differentiation.

That T lymphocytes differentiate within the thymus was first shown by transplantation experiments. If thymus lobes are transplanted to nude mice—which lack a thymus and are T-cell deficient—the grafts are rapidly vascularized and become seeded with immigrant T-cell progenitors from the animal's bone marrow. Within a few weeks, functional T cells appear within the grafted thymus lobe, and they subsequently migrate to the secondary lymphoid organs. Hence, the thymus provides an effective environment for the differentiation of T cells from immature precursors. (It may not be the only site, as a small number of functional T cells can be found in the spleen and lymph nodes of old nude mice. Where these T cells mature is not known.)

A valuable approach to the study of T-cell development is to delineate thymocyte **subpopulations** and the sequence of their appearance during fetal ontogeny. In the mouse, the first hematopoietic cells to colonize the thymus, around day 11 to 14 of gestation, express the Thy-1 antigen but lack CD4 and CD8 (**double-negative thymocytes**). The cellularity of the thymus increases exponentially until birth and more slowly thereafter. During this time, new thymocyte subpopulations appear (Fig. 15–19). For instance, by day 16 of gestation, cells that express both CD4 and CD8 markers (**double-positive thymocytes**) appear and soon become the dominant subpopulation. Later (around day 19), cells that express **either** CD4 or CD8 appear (the mature T-cell phenotypes; here called **single-positive thymocytes**). When analyzed *in vitro*, these cells are fully functional T cells. After birth (on about day 20 of gestation), the proportions of the different thymocyte subpopulations stabilize so that thymocytes with double-negative, double-positive, and single-positive (mature) phenotypes represent about 5%, 80%, and 15% of the total, respectively.

The lineage relations among the major thymocyte subpopulations are only partly resolved. Double-negative thymocytes appear to include progenitors of other thymocytes. In one study, heavily irradiated mice were inoc-

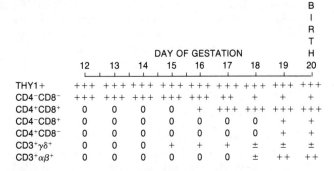

Figure 15–19. Development of T cells in the fetal mouse thymus. The following cell markers were analyzed from day 12 to 20 of gestation: Thy-1, CD4, CD8, CD3, and the Ag-specific heterodimeric receptors (α, β and γ,δ). CD4$^-$ CD8$^-$ are "double negative" cells; CD4$^+$ CD8$^+$ are "double positive" cells; CD4$^+$ CD8$^-$ and CD4$^-$ CD8$^+$ are "single positive" (mature) T cells. CD3 is only expressed together with the α,β receptor or the γ,δ receptor. 0, ±, +, ++, +++ refer to the relative abundance of cells having the indicated markers.

ulated with purified double-negative thymocytes with marker alleles that distinguished them from the host's cells. The inoculated cells migrated to the thymus and differentiated into double-positive thymocytes and mature T cells. In another approach, explanted thymus lobes from early embryos, containing only double-negative cells, were cultured *in vitro* (thus preventing further influx of cells into the thymus), and they differentiated

into double-positive and single-positive thymocytes over the next 2 weeks.

This developmental order is consistent with the derivation of single-positive from double-positive cells. Alternatively, both may be derived directly from double-negative thymocytes, with a delayed appearance of single-positive cells (Fig. 15–20). In either case, it is clear that most double-positive thymocytes die within the thymus, perhaps because they fail to pass several "tests": **only T cells that (1) express functional Ag-specific receptors; (2) are self-tolerant; and (3) can react with Ags in association with the individual's own MHC proteins are allowed to leave the thymus** (see below for T-Cell Tolerance and Thymus Selection).

It is within the thymus, and not before, that the genes encoding Ag-specific T-cell receptor (TcR) subunits undergo rearrangement and are expressed, resulting in the surface expression of functional TcR. As we shall see later, the TcR is made up of two subunits, termed α and β, both encoded by Ig-like genes that are not expressed until they are assembled from gene segments that resemble those of Ig genes (see Chap. 14 and below). Definitive rearrangements of the β genes are detectable in double-negative thymocytes by day 15 of gestation, whereas functional α-gene rearrangement and expression is delayed until day 17. The complete TcR α–β molecule (associated with the CD3 polypeptides) is not expressed on fetal double-negative thymocytes; it is first detected on double-positive thymocytes at day 17 and on single posi-

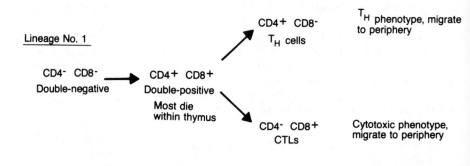

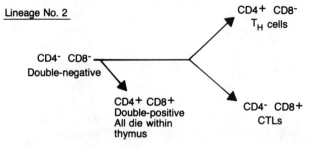

Figure 15–20. Two possible maturation pathways for T cells within the thymus. In both pathways, double-negative thymocytes are the progenitors of both double-positive thymocytes and mature T cells. Although double-positive thymocytes may be intermediates in T-cell differentiation, most die within the thymus.

tive thymocytes at the time of their appearance just before birth. Selection of cells on the basis of the receptor's specificity must therefore occur in the double-positive stage or during a transition phase to single-positive.

(Although embryonic double-negative thymocytes do not detectably express the α–β TcR molecule, a small proportion—5% to 10%—of these cells express a similar receptor composed of subunits called γ and δ (see below), also associated with CD3. In adult mice, cells of the same phenotype (CD4$^-$, CD8$^-$, CD3$^+$, γ–δ cells) are found in small numbers in the thymus and secondary lymphoid organs, but in larger numbers in intestinal epithelium and in epidermis. Their function and the specificity of their receptors are not yet known.)

Thymocyte subpopulations occupy different areas within the thymus. The vast majority of mature, single-positive thymocytes are found in the medulla. In the cortex, most of the cells are double-positive. The small percentage of double-negative thymocytes are distributed diffusely and possibly concentrated just under the capsule, and subcapsular thymocytes labeled by an injected fluorescent tag appear to migrate in toward the medulla as they differentiate. Exposure of the differentiating T cells to cortical epithelial cells, which express both MHC-I and MHC-II proteins, may be involved in the selection processes discussed below. In addition, the inward migration of differentiating T cells may expose them to bone marrow-derived dendritic cells, which are concentrated near the junction of cortex and medulla. Eventually, thymocytes with a mature phenotype reach the medulla, from which they are presumed to be exported directly to the periphery.

SELF–NONSELF DISCRIMINATION

The formation of the T-cell repertoire is influenced by two related but seemingly contradictory requirements. To avoid immune reactions against self Ags (autoimmunity), thus ensuring **self-tolerance,** T cells that can react with **self Ags,** including self-MHC proteins, must be somehow ablated or **selected against.** But T cells must also be self-MHC restricted, and those that can react with Ags associated with self-MHC I and -II proteins must be **selected for** during T-cell development; this phenomenon, termed **thymic selection,** ensures that an individual's pool of functional T cells are useful in the context of his or her own MHC glycoproteins. Our current understanding of thymic selection (sometimes termed **thymic education**) and the induction of T-cell tolerance of self-Ags are considered below.

Selection against Autoreactive T Cells: Self-Tolerance

Allelic variants of a protein are generally immunogenic in those individuals of the species who do not produce

them. Such alloimmune responses to the protein products of allogeneic MHC-I and -II genes are especially intense (see Allograft Rejection, Chap. 20, and Alloreactivity, above). Thus, while the prevention of autoimmunity requires that T-cell clones be deleted, paralyzed, or suppressed if they are potentially reactive with any self-Ag, it is especially critical to eliminate T-cell clones that react with self-MHC proteins.

The fate of skin grafts provides a powerful tool for studying tolerance of MHC glycoproteins (Chap. 20). These grafts are rapidly rejected unless the host is tolerant of these Ags. With this simple assay, it became apparent that tolerance of self-MHC glycoproteins is **acquired** during an individual's development. The first experimental evidence involved the transfer of cells from one inbred mouse strain into advanced embryos of an MHC-different strain. Once mature, the recipient animals were found to accept permanently (i.e., to be tolerant of) skin grafts from mice of the donor strain. A similar transfer of cells into older (postnatal) mice usually fails to induce tolerance. Hence, it appears that **if T cells are confronted with Ags early in their program of differentiation, they are "tolerized" rather than immunized.**

THYMUS CHIMERAS. A more useful way to study the induction of tolerance is with experimental mice in which developing hematopoietic cells encounter foreign MHC proteins in various tissues. Because T cells reach maturity in the thymus, studies of induction of tolerance to allogeneic MHC proteins in transplanted thymus grafts have been of particular interest. To ensure that the full program of T-cell differentiation occurs in the allogeneic thymus, it is transplanted into mice that have normal bone marrow but lack a thymus and are therefore T-cell deficient; for example, nude mice. T-cell deficient mice can also be derived from normal mice by surgical removal of the thymus (thymectomy), followed by heavy irradiation to destroy hematopoietic cells (including T cells), and finally reconstitution with bone-marrow stem cells syngeneic with the recipient; after 6 to 8 weeks, all hematopoietic cell types, except T cells, will differentiate from the injected bone marrow cells. Such mice are called "TxBM" (thymectomized, irradiated, bone-marrow reconstituted) mice.

To test for induction of tolerance to MHC glycoproteins, a TxBM mouse of strain B is given an MHC-different thymus graft from an F_1 hybrid between strains A and B; that is, an $(A \times B)F_1$ animal. About 6 to 8 weeks later, virtually all of the mouse's peripheral T lymphocytes are of strain B genetic origin but have differentiated in the $(A \times B)F_1$ thymus graft. Significantly, these T cells do not make an immune response to strain A cells, although they can respond to cells from a strain having unrelated MHC glycoproteins (strain C). Thus, the strain B T cells in these animals are specifically tolerant to MHC glycoproteins of strain A, which are expressed by cells of the donor thymus graft. Transplantation of fully allogeneic strain A thymus lobes to strain B TxBM mice yields similar results.

During their differentiation, the strain B T cells are confronted with MHC^a glycoproteins expressed by several cell types in the strain A thymus graft, including thymic epithelial cells, and the bone marrow-derived cell types that were resident in the thymus at the time of transplantation: macrophages, dendritic cells, and thymocytes. Which of these cell types must express MHC^a in order to "tolerize" immigrant strain B-thymocytes? One way to answer the question is to treat thymus grafts before transplantation with agents that selectively ablate different cell types. In one such experiment, thymus lobes from strain A were treated briefly *in vitro* with **deoxyguanosine,** which is toxic to thymocytes, dendritic cells, and macrophages but not to epithelial cells. Remarkably, when the treated thymus lobes (strain A) were transplanted into nude mice (strain B), the strain B T cells that developed in them did not become tolerant of strain A MHC glycoproteins (Fig. 15–21). Hence, T cells are not rendered tolerant of MHC glycoproteins that are expressed only by thymic epithelial cells, and it appears that deoxyguanosine-sensitive cells (possibly dendritic cells or the thymocytes themselves) are required. (Although T cells that differentiate in MHC-different, deoxyguanosine-treated thymus grafts do not become tolerant

of the foreign MHC glycoproteins, they also do not reject these specially treated thymus allografts. The reason is that these grafts lack accessory cells of strain A, and induction of alloreactivity and allograft rejection requires T cells to be stimulated by APC that bear allogeneic MHC-II proteins; see p. 341 and Passenger Leukocytes and Graft Rejection, Chap. 20.)

Tolerance is established at least in part by deletion of clones of self-reactive T cells during their differentiation in the thymus. Direct evidence for this view has come from the use of a monoclonal Ab to a particular variable region of an Ag-specific TcR. This Ab happens to react with those TcR that are specific for a particular MHC-II protein (called IE^d). Therefore, the Ab can be used to monitor for the presence or absence of IE^d-reactive T cells. In mice that express the IE^d protein, the frequency of anti-IE^d T cells is severely depressed among T cells in peripheral tissues, but within the thymus, these T cells are found among the immature CD4$^+$,CD8$^+$ (double-positive) T cells, not among those with a mature phenotype (i.e., either CD4$^+$ or CD8$^+$). Hence, it appears that potentially self-reactive T cells (in this case against IE^d, an MHC-II protein) are deleted or aborted before they acquire a mature phenotype.

MECHANISMS OF T-CELL TOLERANCE INDUCTION. How self-reactive T cells are ablated is not known. A widely held belief is that ablation mechanisms act selectively on

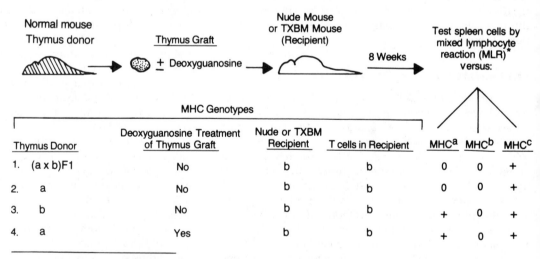

Thymus Donor	Deoxyguanosine Treatment of Thymus Graft	Nude or TXBM Recipient	T cells in Recipient	MHC^a	MHC^b	MHC^c
1. (a x b)F1	No	b	b	0	0	+
2. a	No	b	b	0	0	+
3. b	No	b	b	+	0	+
4. a	Yes	b	b	+	0	+

*In the MLR assay- no reaction (0) means tolerance was induced
proliferation (+) means tolerance was not induced

Figure 15—21. Induction of tolerance to MHC molecules with thymus grafts. In a nude mouse recipient or a TxBM recipient of an allogeneic thymus graft, the recipient's stem cells (MHC^b) can differentiate into T cells within the MHC-different graft (MHC$^{a/b}$ or MHC^a). Such T cells are nonresponsive (tolerant) to MHC^a molecules when tested in the mixed lymphocyte reaction (MLR). However, if the MHC^a thymus graft is depleted of hematopoietic cells by deoxyguanosine treatment before grafting, the MHC^b T cells that differentiate in the graft are responsive (i.e., not tolerant) to cells bearing MHC^a molecules (cf. lines 2 and 4). Therefore, MHC^a-type hematopoietic cells in the thymus graft are necessary for imposing tolerance to MHC^a. (Based on von Boehmer H, Schubiger K: Eur J Immunol 14:1048, 1984)

those T cells that bind with high avidity to self components. Thus, during their differentiation, T cells may go through a stage where Ag recognition is a tolerogenic rather than an immunogenic stimulus. Whatever the mechanism, the end result is that **the developing self-reactive T cell is either killed or paralyzed: it never becomes a mature T cell.** Although genes encoding many self-Ags are not expressed by cells within the thymus, there is some evidence that such Ags find their way to the thymus, perhaps by circulating blood, where they might stick to dendritic cells. Thus, T cells reactive to self-Ags that are not synthesized within the thymus may also be tolerized within the thymus.

(Besides clonal deletion at an early stage in T-cell differentiation, other mechanisms may tolerize self-reactive mature T cells in the periphery. It has

been suggested that exposure to Ags sometimes leads to an active state of **suppression,** in which self-reactive T cells are held in check by Ag-specific suppressor T cells.)

Selection for Recognition of Self-MHC: Thymic Education

MHC-restricted T cells generally distinguish products of different MHC alleles with a high degree of specificity, and each individual of a given species must have the **potential** to produce T cells that are restricted by an enormous number of different MHC glycoproteins (on the order of 100 alleles for each of the MHC-I and -II genes). However, a given individual inherits only two MHC haplotypes, which include only a few (up to about 10) MHC-I and -II genes. Does this mean that most of an individual's T cells are not useful for recognizing Ags in

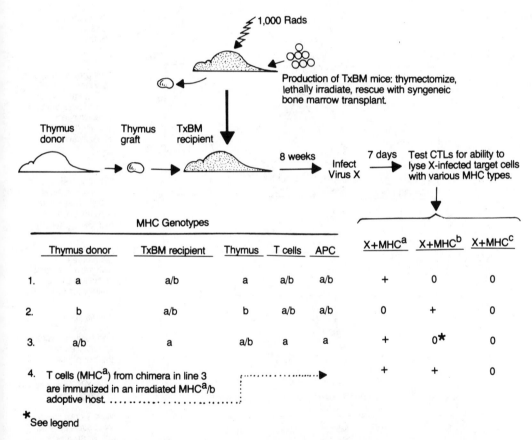

		MHC Genotypes				X+MHC^a	X+MHC^b	X+MHC^c
	Thymus donor	TxBM recipient	Thymus	T cells	APC			
1.	a	a/b	a	a/b	a/b	+	0	0
2.	b	a/b	b	a/b	a/b	0	+	0
3.	a/b	a	a/b	a	a	+	0*	0
4.	T cells (MHC^a) from chimera in line 3 are immunized in an irradiated MHC^a/b adoptive host.					+	+	0

*See legend

Figure 15—22. An experiment to demonstrate thymus selection. TxBM mice are produced by thymectomy followed by irradiation and reconstitution with **syngeneic** bone marrow. Such mice, which are similar to athymic nude mice, are then grafted with thymus lobes of various MHC types. After allowing time for differentiation of T cells in the transplanted thymus, the mice are immunized with virus X, and 1 week is allowed for induction of virus X-specific CTLs. If the MHC$^{a/b}$ TxBM mice received an MHC^a thymus, most of the CTL are MHC^a restricted, showing that the thymus selects T cells that are restricted to its own type of MHC molecules. Conversely, if an MHC^a TxBM mouse receives an MHC$^{a/b}$ thymus, the thymus selects T cells that are either MHC^a- **or** MHC^b-restricted. However, to reveal the MHC^b-restricted CTLs, the T cells must be immunized in a host that includes MHC^b-bearing APC (line 4). (Based on Zinkernagel RM, et al: J Exp Med 147:882, 1978, and Bevan M, Fink P: Immunol Rev 42:3, 1978)

association with his or her own (self) MHC glycoproteins? The answer appears to be that although an individual has the **potential** to produce T cells that can be restricted by virtually all MHC glycoproteins of the species, a **thymic selection mechanism operating during T-cell development favors the maturation of those cells that are restricted by self-MHC glycoproteins.**

At first glance, it would seem that the simplest way to demonstrate thymus selection would be to test the capacity of T cells from strain A mice (MHC^a) to respond to Ags associated with MHC^b glycoproteins on strain B APCs. However, this approach is precluded, because T cells of strain A mice respond extremely vigorously to strain B MHC glycoproteins, obscuring other immune responses (see Alloreactivity, above).

To avoid such alloreactivity, systems have been developed in which the T cells are **tolerant** of both MHC^a and MHC^b glycoproteins. Thus, thymus selection was first noted in chimeric mice (see above), and the critical studies involved thymus grafts (Fig. 15–22). First, MHC-heterozygous mice of the cross (A × B)F$_1$ were thymectomized then heavily irradiated and reconstituted with syngeneic [(A × B)F$_1$] bone-marrow stem cells. Over the next several weeks, most hematopoietic cell types regenerated; however, T cells were missing because these TxBM mice lacked a thymus. They were then grafted with thymus lobes from strain A **or** strain B mice, and after several weeks, the (A × B)F$_1$ bone-marrow-derived T cells, which had differentiated in the transplanted thymus, were tested for their capacity to respond to Ags associated

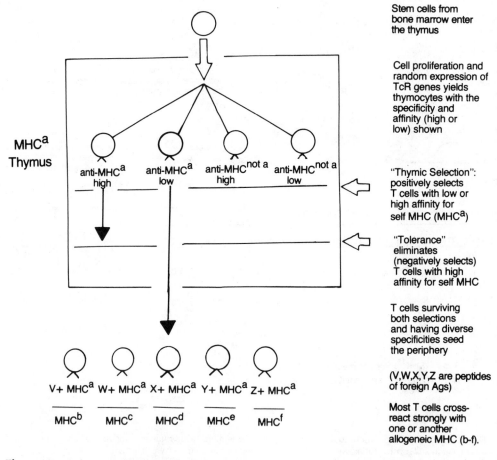

Figure 15–23. A speculative model of selections imposed on developing T lymphocytes in the thymus. T cells first express the TcR within the thymus. In the first selection, those thymocytes that express TcR with significant (low or high) affinity for thymic MHC molecules (expressed by thymic epithelial cells) are positively selected, either by selective proliferation or by selective survival. In the second stage, those cells that express TcR with high affinity for thymic MHC molecules (expressed by thymic dendritic cells) are negatively selected (eliminated). The cells that survive both selections have TcR with low affinity for self-MHC molecules but may have high affinity for (a) self-MHC molecules that are modified by association with peptides of a foreign Ag or (b) foreign (allogeneic) MHC molecules (MHC^b, MHC^c, etc.).

with various MHC^a or MHC^b glycoproteins. Strikingly, those T cells that had differentiated in thymus grafts of strain A origin responded well to Ags associated with MHC^a glycoproteins but poorly to Ags associated with MHC^b glycoproteins. T cells that had differentiated in a strain B thymus had the opposite behavior.

The reverse procedure yields concordant results. Strain A thymectomized irradiated mice, reconstituted with strain A bone marrow and transplanted with thymus lobes of (A × B)F$_1$ mice, generate T cells that recognize Ags that are associated with either type MHC^a or MHC^b. **Thus, developing cells are selected in the thymus for ability to recognize Ags associated with the MHC type of the thymus.** Both T$_H$ cells (MHC-II-restricted) and CTLs (MHC-I-restricted) are selected by thymus MHC glycoproteins. Experiments with deoxyguanosine-treated thymus lobes (see Tolerance Induction, above) suggested that a deoxyguanosine-**resistant** cell is responsible for selecting T cells with the appropriate specificity for MHC. The best candidates are cortical thymic epithelial cells, which express both MHC-I and MHC-II glycoproteins and survive deoxyguanosine treatment. Thus, **clonal deletion of self-reactive cells and selection of self-MHC-restricted T cells appear to be imposed by different cell types within the thymus: marrow-derived cells in tolerance and epithelial cells in thymus selection.** These processes may therefore occur at separate sites and stages within the thymus.

The mechanism of thymus selection is unknown. It is difficult to propose a simple model as to how T cells reactive to, for example, MHC^a plus an Ag "X" can be selected during differentiation **when X is not present.** A reasonable suggestion (Fig. 15–23) is that although such T cells do not react strongly enough with MHC^a alone to trigger T-cell effector functions, they may react with sufficient avidity for selection within the thymus. Perhaps those T-cell clones with low but significant avidity for self-MHC glycoproteins often have high avidity for MHC^a glycoproteins modified by bound peptides of a foreign Ag. Thus **thymus selection may be a kind of clonal selection that operates during T-cell development to shape the repertoire of Ag-specific T cells. The further deletion of those cells with high avidity for self-Ags, imposing self-tolerance, completes the formation of the repertoire.** These views, while somewhat speculative, fit the existing data.

The Major T-Cell Surface Proteins and Their Genes

The preceding sections of this chapter have referred to many of the cell-surface proteins that distinguish between lymphocyte subpopulations and described the role that some of them play in immune functions of B and T cells. In this section, we focus on the proteins themselves and their genes, relying heavily on the wealth of information provided by molecular gene cloning.

MHC CLASS I AND CLASS II PROTEINS AND GENES

MHC-I PROTEINS. These molecules are made up of two noncovalently associated subunits. An α chain, 45 Kd, encoded by an MHC-I gene, is anchored as an integral protein in the cell membrane. A small β chain, 12 Kd, encoded by a gene on another chromosome, is firmly associated noncovalently on the cell surface with the α chain (Fig. 15–24).

The α chain has five domains (Fig. 15–24). Three, termed $\alpha1$, $\alpha2$, and $\alpha3$ in order from the N terminus, are external to the cell membrane. The fourth is a sequence of about 22 predominantly hydrophobic amino acid residues that spans the cell membrane. The fifth, on the cytoplasmic side of the membrane, is a short C-terminal sequence containing several lysine and arginine residues, as is characteristic of cytoplasmic domains of integral membrane proteins.

The β chain is also known as **β_2-microglobulin** because of its small size and amino acid sequence homology with Igs (see Ig Superfamily, below, and Fig. 15–34). Many years before it was identified as a subunit of MHC-I protein, β_2-microglobulin was discovered as a free protein at high concentration in the urine of persons with severely impaired kidney function, such as immediately after receipt of a renal allograft.

MHC-II PROTEINS. Like MHC-I, the MHC-II proteins are also heterodimers but both of their subunits, also called α and β, are anchored in the cell-surface membrane (see Fig. 15–24). The two chains have similar domain structure and molecular mass (α is 30–33 Kd and β is 27–29 Kd). In each chain, two extracellular domains, termed (in order from the N terminus) $\alpha1$ and $\alpha2$ for the α chain and $\beta1$ and $\beta2$ for the β chain, are followed by (1) a transmembrane sequence of 20 to 22 predominantly hydrophic amino acid residues; and (2) on the cytoplasmic side of the membrane, a short C-terminal domain rich in arginine and lysine residues.

POLYMORPHISM. The most striking feature of MHC-I and MHC-II proteins is their great allelic diversity (polymorphism). There are at least 50 known allelic variants of the MHC-I K gene in mice (see H-2K^b, H-2K^d, etc., above), and there are probably as many for each of the other MHC-I and -II genes. In contrast, most other proteins are essentially monomorphic; that is, they have two or three allelic variants, if any. Hence, individuals chosen at random from, say, a human population may share one or a few

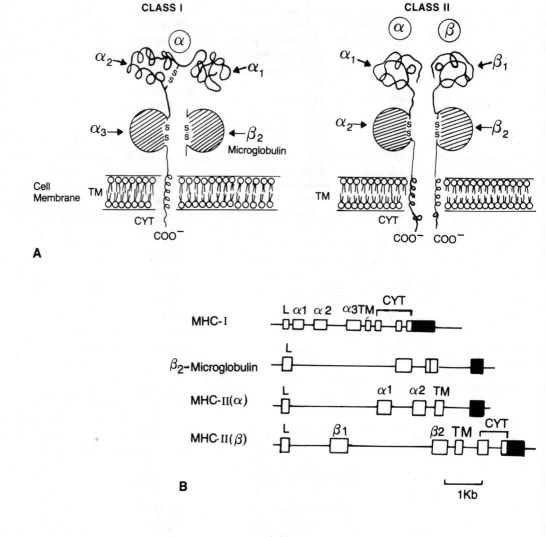

Figure 15–24. (*A*) Diagram of MHC class I (left) and class II (right) glycoproteins on the cell surface. The shaded domains have distinct amino acid sequence homology with Ig constant (C) domains. TM and CYT are transmembrane and cytoplasmic regions, respectively. (*B*) Exon–intron organization of the MHC-I and MHC-II genes. The β_2-microglobulin gene is on a different chromosome from the MHC-I and MHC-II genes. **L** encodes the signal (leader) peptide that guides the nascent polypeptide chains into the lumen of the endoplasmic reticulum. TM and CYT are exons that encode the transmembrane and cytoplasmic domains, solid rectangles are 3' untranslated sequences. (From Flavell RA et al: *Science* 233:437, 1986)

MHC genes, but they will almost never share a complete set. It must be understood, however, that MHC proteins are not clonally variable, as are Igs (on B cells) or TcR (on T cells); thus, within any particular individual, all cells express the same MHC-I proteins and all APC express the same MHC-II (and MHC-I) proteins.

The MHC allelic variants differ from one another by amino acid substitutions that are primarily in N-terminal domains (α1 and α2 domains of MHC-I proteins and α1 and β1 of MHC-II proteins; Fig. 15–25); and within these

"variable" domains, the substitutions tend to cluster in several "hypervariable" regions (Fig. 15–25). The other domains (α3 and β_2-microglobulin in MHC-I and α2 and β2 in MHC-II proteins) are "monomorphic": they have essentially the same sequence in all allelic variants. With murine MHC-II proteins (A and E), most of the variability is in the β chains (the Aα chain is less polymorphic, and the Eα chain is virtually invariant). In the most polymorphic MHC chains (i.e., α chains of MHC-I and β chains of MHC-II), the amino acid sequences of independent allelic variants differ by as much as 15% of the amino acid residues.

The amino acid sequence differences between different MHC-II alleles must be responsible for differences in their ability to present ("restrict") antigenic peptides to T-helper cells; that is, the amino acid substitutions must underlie the ability of a given epitope to elicit T-cell responses in some individuals (or inbred mouse strains) and not in others (the respective phenotypes of high-responder and low-responder Ir genes). Similarly, amino acid sequence differences in the $\alpha 1$ and $\alpha 2$ domain of diverse MHC-I alleles must underlie differences in their abilities to restrict Ag recognition by CTLs.

The genetic mechanisms responsible for the great allelic diversity of MHC genes are described below (see Gene Conversion).

COMPARISON OF MHC PROTEINS AND IMMUNOGLOBULINS. Each of the invariant extracellular domains of MHC-I and -II proteins resembles Ig domains in having about 110 amino acid residues, with two cysteines, about 20 residues from each end (or about 70 residues apart), forming an intradomain S–S bond. They also have distinct (but low) sequence homology with Ig constant domains.

An x-ray analysis of an MHC-I protein confirms that its $\alpha 3$ domain and β_2-microglobulin have the characteristic three-dimensional folding pattern of Ig constant domains (Ig-fold, see Chap. 14). But, strikingly, the variable

domains ($\alpha 1$ and $\alpha 2$) have a novel structure: seven β strands of the two domains form a platform on which two α-helical sequences are arrayed to form a remarkably clear view of a binding site that could obviously accommodate a peptide ligand of 10 to 20 amino acid residues (see Fig. 15–26). Indeed, in the crystals analyzed, some unidentified peptide or mixture of peptides seem actually to be occupying the site as though it (or they) remained associated with the MHC-I molecule as it was crystallized. It is likely that MHC-II proteins will prove to have a similar structure.

That the polymorphic, ligand-binding domains of MHC-I and -II proteins are not structurally homologous with Ig domains is not surprising because MHC proteins and Igs differ considerably in their ligand-binding properties. Thus, a given MHC-I or MHC-II protein can bind an enormous number of different peptides (i.e., they are far more cross-reactive or "degenerate" in their binding activity than any Ab); moreover, it will be recalled that the binding of ligands to Abs is characterized by very rapid association and slow dissociation (see Appendix, Chap. 13), whereas the binding of peptides to MHC-II proteins seems to be characterized by very much slower association and remarkably slow dissociation.

GLYCOSYLATION. Like most cell-surface proteins, MHC-I and -II molecules are glycoproteins with N-linked oligosaccharides (N-glycans) attached to the amide N of asparagine (Asn) in Asn–X–Y sequences, where Y is serine or threonine and X is any amino acid but not proline.

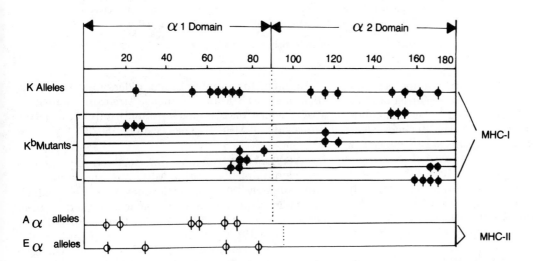

Figure 15–25. Distribution of sequence variability in polymorphic domains of murine MHC-I and MHC-II proteins suggestive of hypervariable regions. On the lines labeled "K alleles," "A_α alleles," and "E_α alleles," the marks indicate positions where various K alleles (K^b, K^a, etc.) or A_α or E_β alleles have different amino acids. Each of the lines labeled "K^b mutants" represents an independent mutant of the K^b allele; each mark represents an amino acid that differs from the one at that position in the wild type (K^b).

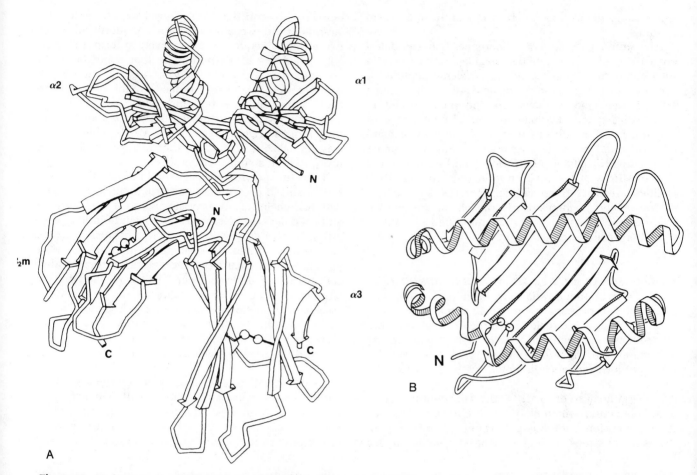

Figure 15–26. Structure of an MHC class I glycoprotein. *(A)* A side view of the HLA-A2 molecule showing its four domains. The heavy chain (α1, α2, and α3 domains) is normally anchored in the cell membrane, but in order to isolate the proteins, it was cleaned off by a proteolytic enzyme, thus removing the anchoring transmembrane and cytoplasmic domains. β_2-microglobulin, the fourth domain, is associated noncovalently with the heavy chain by multiple interactions with the α3 and α2 domains. The α3 and α2 domains form the putative binding site for peptide fragments of protein Ags. *(B)* A top view of the peptide-binding site. The base consists of a β sheet formed by eight antiparallel β strands, and the sides are formed by two γ-helical segments. (From Bjorkman B et al: Nature 329:590, 1987)

MHC GENES. As noted before, recombinations between congenic strains of mice indicated that the order of MHC loci is **K–A–E–S–D,** where **K** and **D** are class I, **A** and **E** are class II, and **S** represents several class III genes. More detailed analysis, especially with the aid of molecular gene cloning, has expanded the number of genes (see Fig. 15–13). Thus, most mouse strains have a third class I gene, termed **L** (next to **D**), and four class II genes, each encoding an MHC-II subunit: **Aα and Aβ encode the dimeric A molecule and Eα and Eβ the E molecule.** Humans have at least eight class II genes, each also encoding an α or β subunit for a heterodimeric MHC-II protein. In **S,** there are at least eight genes: several for complement proteins (see Chap. 17), and two for cytotoxic proteins, tissue necrosis factor (TNF) and lymphotoxin (LT) (also called TNF-α and TNF-β, respectively; see Chap. 19).

Although the number of loci differs from species to species or even from one mouse strain to another, all MHC-I genes have a characteristic exon–intron structure, as do all MHC-II genes (see Fig. 15–23).

Qa AND TLa LOCI. The most unexpected result of molecular cloning of the murine MHC was the discovery of approximately 30 additional genes that are strikingly similar in sequence to MHC-I genes. Located in three contiguous loci (Qa-2,3,T1a, and Qa-1) adjacent to the D,L end of the MHC (see Fig. 15–13), the polypeptide chains encoded by Qa and Tla genes are also expressed in association with β_2-microglobulin. But unlike MHC-I proteins, which are present on all cells, Qa and TL proteins are found only on various hematopoietic cells, including thymocytes of some strains and thymus leukemia cells (hence the term TL) of other strains.

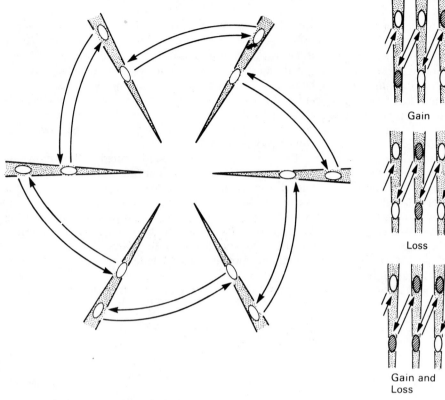

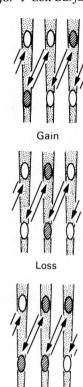

Gain

Loss

Gain and
Loss

Figure 15–27. Detection of mutations in histocompatibility (H) genes by exchange of grafts of tail skin. The mice are F1 hybrids (H-2$^{a/b}$) of H-2-different strains; because they have one copy of each H-2 haplotype, they permit the detection of mutations that result in the loss of an antigenic determinant. As is shown in the right panel, a mutant that gains an H antigenic determinant accepts grafts, but its donated grafts are rejected; a mutant that loses a determinant rejects grafts and its donated grafts are accepted; a mutant with both changes (gain and loss) rejects grafts, and its donated grafts are also rejected. *Open ovals,* accepted grafts; *shaded ovals,* rejected grafts. (Based on Bailey DW, Kohn HI: Genet Res 6:330, 1965)

Another difference is that the many Qa genes are extremely similar in sequence to each other, as are the TL genes. Perhaps in accord with this limited variability, the Qa and TL proteins do not restrict Ag recognition by CD8$^+$ T cells.

Although the function of Qa and Tla proteins is unknown, Qa and Tla genes are sources of nucleotide sequences that serve to diversify MHC-I genes by a process called gene conversion.

GENE CONVERSION. The extensive polymorphism of MHC-I and -II genes suggests that their mutation rates might be unusually high. Indeed, rejection of skin grafts exchanged among mice with the same (H-2^b) haplotype (Fig. 15–27) revealed a surprisingly high frequency (about 1 in 3000 mice) of mutations in the MHC-I K^b allele, making it possible to establish isogenic mouse strains (termed K^{bm1}, K^{bm2}, etc.) that differ from each other just in the K^b gene. By molecular cloning of cDNA, the variant K^{bm1} allele, for example, was found to differ from the unmutated allele by several nucleotides, resulting in three amino acid substitutions (in the variable α1 and α2 domains) (e.g., Fig. 15–25). A probe corresponding to the variant sequence then showed that it was identical to a block of about 50 nucleotides in one of the MHC-I-like genes in the Qa-2,3 locus. Other K^b mutants have also

been shown to have variant blocks of sequence that are identical to various nucleotide sequences in Qa-2,3 genes, and an MHC-II mutant similarly had a variant sequence that corresponded to one in a related gene. These observations suggest that the extreme **polymorphism of MHC-I and -II genes arises by intergenic exchanges of bits of DNA sequences between related but nonallelic genes,** a process termed gene conversion. (Similar exchanges are responsible for the diversity of Ig light chain genes in birds; see Chap. 14.)

MOLECULAR COMPLEMENTATION OF MHC-II PROTEINS. With two subunits (α, β) per MHC-II protein, and two (and often more) of these proteins on each APC, MHC-II molecules with various α–β chain combinations are possible. Combinatorial variations usually occur within a locus, like A or E, but not between loci. They increase the structural diversity of MHC-II molecules and hence the range of antigenic peptides that they can present to T cells. Thus, the F$_1$ hybrid progeny of a mating between A-different mice, say A^d × A^k, can have on their APC the two parental class II molecules (Aα^{d}Aβ^d and Aα^{k}Aβ^k) and also the two combinatorial variants (Aα^{d}Aβ^k and Aα^{k}Aβ^d). Some Ags can be presented by the combinatorial variants but not by the parental molecules.

TcR FOR ANTIGEN—MHC COMPLEXES

Although T cells have a striking propensity to react selectively with MHC-I and -II molecules, they can nevertheless distinguish sharply between such similar structures as 2,4-dinitrophenyl and 2,4,6-trinitrophenyl groups and between proteins that differ in only a few amino acid residues. It was therefore long suspected that T-cell Ag-specific receptors resemble Igs and differ from one T-cell clone to another. However, T cells lacked complete Ig heavy- and light-chain mRNA, and they did not convincingly react with Abs to Igs. Hence, the TcR was long known not to be an Ig, but its nature was an enigma.

The first clues to its identity came with the development of Abs, especially mAbs, to various T-cell clones. Each such clone-specific (**clonotypic**) Ab reacted with a similar cell-surface protein, but only from the clone of T cells against which the Ab had been produced. This protein was an S–S-linked heterodimer; that is, it was twice as large (80–95 Kd) under nonreducing conditions as under reducing conditions (40–45 Kd), and electrophoresis (in a pH gradient) separated an acidic (α) chain and a basic (β) chain. The clonotypic Abs also blocked Ag-specific responses of only the appropriate T-cell clone. Some of the peptides obtained by proteolytic cleavage of the α–β heterodimeric protein were shared by different T-cell clones, whereas other peptides differed between clones, as if the protein had constant domains and variable domains. These properties implied a clonally variable Ag-specific receptor, which thus has sometimes been referred to as **Ti** (for T idiotype, by analogy with the clonotypic Ig idiotype of B cell clones).

The α–β heterodimer was identified as the TcR when cDNA clones for the two subunits were eventually obtained from mouse and human T cells. The successful search for this cDNA in mouse T cells, illustrated in Figure 15–28, was based on two assumptions: that genes for the TcR subunits are transcribed in T cells and not in B (or other) cells; and that these genes, like Ig genes, are assembled from rearranged gene segments. Thus, cDNA prepared from mRNA of a mouse T-cell clone was hybridized ("subtracted") with RNA from B cells and then

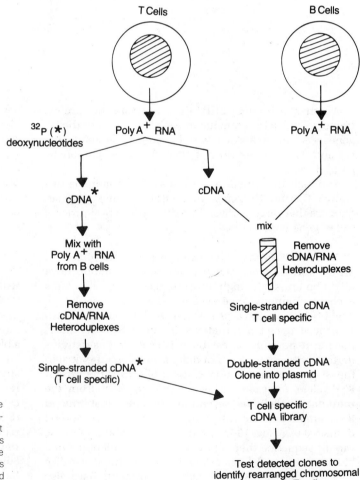

Figure 15–28. A ''T-minus-B subtractive'' cDNA library was the key to identifying subunits of clonotypic T cell Ag-specific receptors. The [32]P (*)-labeled T-cell–specific single-stranded cDNAs at **left** (from which cDNA shared with B cells was removed) served as probes to identify T-cell–specific cDNA clones in the subtractive library (at **right**). Probes prepared from the critical cDNA clones detected rearranged chromosomal genes in mature T cells. (Based on Hedrick S et al: Nature 308:149, 1984)

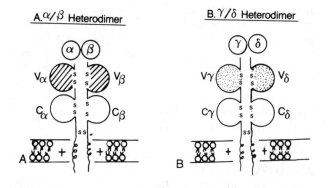

Figure 15–29. Diagram of the Ag-specific T cell receptors (TcRs). *(A)* The α–β heterodimer is expressed on CD8⁺ and CD4⁺ T cells. The V domain sequences (shaded) differ greatly from one T-cell clone to another. *(B)* Some T-cells with the γ-δ heterodimer are CD8⁺, but most of them are CD4⁻ CD8⁻ (double negatives). The V_γ domains and possibly the V_δ domains (dotted) are less clonally diverse than the V_α and V_β domains. Both α–β and γ–δ heterodimers are associated on the T-cell surface with CD3 molecules.

used to form a **subtracted (T minus B) library.** Rare cDNA clones in the library met all expectations for the putative TcR: (1) probes prepared from these clones hybridized to sequences of chromosomal DNA that were rearranged in the T cell from which the library was prepared but not in embryonic or other cells (B cells, kidney cells, etc.); (2) the probes hybridized to RNA from T cells (in Northern blots) but not to RNA from B cells or other cells. Finally, amino acid sequences deduced from these cDNA clones matched actual amino acid sequences of the α–β heterodimer and revealed each of the subunits to have unmistakable Ig-like variable (V), joining (J), and constant (C) domains (Figs. 15–29A and 15–30).

Finally, definitive evidence that the α–β heterodimer is the TcR was provided by transfecting the rearranged, functional α and β genes from one T-cell clone into a second T-cell clone, which then exhibited specificity of the donor cells for the Ag. As noted before (see Fig. 15–15, above), this finding also demonstrated formally that **the α–β heterodimer was sufficient for recognition of both Ag and the restricting MHC protein.**

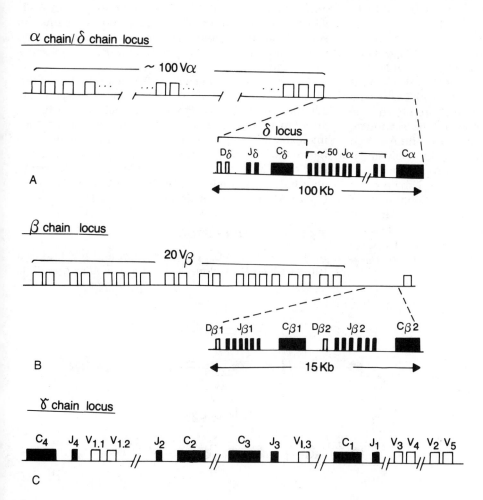

Figure 15–30. Organization of gene segments that encode the α, β, γ, and δ subunits of the mouse Ag-specific TcRs. The α–β heterodimer is the TcR on mature CD4⁺ T cells and CD8⁺ T cells. The γ–δ heterodimer is the TcR on many CD4⁻,CD8⁻ (double-negative) T cells. *(A)* The murine α-chain and δ-chain loci are interspersed on chromosome 14. For the α chain, there are about 100 V_α and 50 J_α gene segments and a single C_α gene segment. For the δ chain, there are at least two D_δ and two J_δ and a single C_δ gene segment. No D_α segments have been detected. *(B)* The murine β-chain locus. In the inbred mouse strain examined (BALB/c), there are 20 V_β gene segments (each shown as a rectangle) spread over 320 Kb. (Another V_β gene segment lies about 10 Kb 3' to the $C_{\beta2}$ gene segment, as shown.) The β-chain locus in the human has about twice as many V_β but fewer J_β gene segments. *(C)* The murine TcR γ-chain locus. Three of the V_γ gene segments (V1.1, V1.2, V1.3) have similar sequences and cross-hybridize; the other four V_γ gene segments are distinctive and do not cross-hybridize. Each of the four C_γ gene segments is associated with its own J_γ gene segment (as in the Ig lambda light-chain locus). *(A,* adapted from Chien Y et al: Nature 327:677, 1987; *B,* adapted from Chou HS et al: Science 238:545, 1987; *C,* adapted from Hayday AC et al: Cell 40:259, 1985 and Garman RD et al: Cell 45:733, 1986)

TcR β-CHAIN LOCUS. With cDNA clones for the α and β subunits as specific probes, the chromosomal TcR gene segments could be isolated and characterized. Their organization and assembly is remarkably similar to that of Ig genes. In the mouse, a cluster of approximately 20 V_β segments lies upstream of two almost identical clusters, each with one D_β, seven J_β, and one C_β segment (see Fig. 15–30*B*). The human β-chain locus is very similar but has more V_β segments and a few less J_β segments.

THE TcR α-CHAIN LOCUS. A striking feature of this locus (Fig. 15–30*A*) is its exceptionally large number (more than 50) of J_α gene segments spread out over a very large distance (more than 65 Kb). Upstream of all these J_α segments, there are probably more than 50 V_α segments.

Another unexpected feature is that between the arrays of V_α and J_α segments, there is an additional cluster of rearranging gene segments with little homology to TcR α or β sequences (see Fig. 15–30); these intervening segments rearrange to form the gene for a chain called δ, which pairs with still another Ig-like chain, γ, to form the TcR-like γ–δ heterodimer on a small subset of T cells (see The T-Cell γ–δ Receptor and also CD4⁻,CD8⁻ T Cells, below).

HEPTAMER AND NONAMER SIGNAL SEQUENCES. Separated by 12 or 23 nucleotide spacers, two highly conserved sequences of seven and nine nucleotides lie next to each V_β, D_β, and J_β segment, exactly as with each of the corresponding Ig-gene segments (see Chap. 14), and the same **12–23 spacer rule** that governs the rearrangement of Ig-gene segments determines that, within a given locus, only those TcR-gene segments with a dissimilar spacer length can be joined. Thus, as shown in Figure 15–31, the distribution of spacers in the β-chain locus predicts, as has been observed, that functional β genes can be formed by joining a V_β directly to a J_β segment or by joining a V_β, a D_β, and a J_β segment. Analysis of immature T cells in the thymus (and also of some T-cell tumors) indicates that when a V–D–J join occurs, the D_β–J_β occurs first and V_β then joins $D_\beta J_\beta$.

TcR–CD3 COMPLEX. As noted before, the TcR on the T-cell surface is closely associated with CD3, the marker present on all mature T cells. CD3 has about five subunits, and analysis of cDNA clones reveals that three of them are integral membrane proteins with unusual transmembrane (TM) sequences. Unlike most TM domains, those in three CD3 subunits (γ, δ, ε) have a centrally placed acidic residue (aspartic or glutamic acid), and because the TcR α and β subunits each have in their TM domains a centrally placed basic residue (lysine), salt bridges between the TM domains may help to stabilize the CD3–TcR complex.

The CD3 subunits also have unusually long cytoplasmic domains (81 residues in CD3-ε), suggesting that CD3 may transduce signals arising from binding of Ag (and MHC) to the TcR. Some evidence suggests that CD4 molecules may also be included in CD3–TcR complex.

DIVERSITY OF TcR α–β HETERODIMERS. Most of the mechanisms that generate Ig diversity can also account for TcR diversity. Thus, 50 V_α and 50 J_α gene segments can yield 2500 $V_\alpha J_\alpha$ sequences, and N-region addition and imprecision in V–J joining (see Chap. 14) can easily generate 100-fold more. The β-chain gene segments can similarly yield about 10^5 sequences. Thus, there could well be on the order of 10^{10} distinct α–β TcR molecules ($10^5 \alpha \times 10^5 \beta$).

However, unlike Ig genes, **TcR V regions do not undergo somatic mutations.** As we shall see (see Chap. 16), these mutations in Ig V regions make it possible for an Ag to selectively stimulate those B cells variants having high-affinity Igs. The absence of such mutations, and hence the lack of opportunity for selection of high-affinity T-cell clones by Ag, means that **TcR molecules probably have low intrinsic affinity for Ags,** like nonmutated IgM molecules of virgin B cells (see Chap. 16).

T-CELL γ–δ RECEPTOR

In the search for cDNA for the TcR α and β subunits, a third Ig-like cDNA clone, termed γ, was discovered. Its

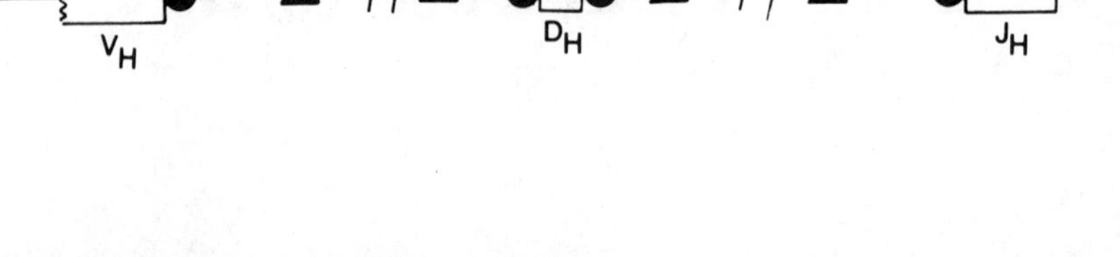

Figure 15–31. The 12–23 spacer rule that governs Ig-gene segment rearrangements also applies to gene segments for the Ag-specific T-cell receptor (TcR). In the Ig heavy (H)-chain locus, V_H and J_H can each join to D_H, but V_H–J_H joining is forbidden, because these gene segments have the same heptamer–nonamer spacer (23 nt). But in the TcR β-chain locus, V_β and J_β not only join to D_β but also can (infrequently) join directly to each other, because their spacers differ. ● = heptamer, ▲ = nonamer. The heptamer and nonamer sequence of the TcR gene segments are very similar to those of Ig gene segments (Chap 14, Fig 14–31).

TcR β – chain locus

Ig H-chain locus

deduced amino acid sequence was strikingly similar to TcR α and β and indicated that it also is an integral membrane protein with two extracellular domains having extensive sequence identity (20–25%) to Ig V, J, and C regions and a transmembrane sequence with a centrally placed lysine residue (see the TcR–CD3 Complex, above). In addition, an extra (fifth) cysteine suggested that the chain is linked by an S–S bond to another polypeptide chain (see Fig. 15–28). The γ-containing protein was subsequently identified on rare T cells (ca. 0.2% of murine adult thymus cells and ca. 0.2–10% of human peripheral blood cells) that are unusual in that they lack both CD4 (the T_H cell marker) and CD8 (the CTL marker) but possess a CD3–TcR complex. These CD4⁻,CD8⁻ (double-negative) CD3⁺ T cells express a heterodimer in which γ is S–S linked to the fourth T-cell-specific Ig-like chain, termed δ (see T α-Chain Locus, above). The tissue distribution of T cells having γ-δ receptors differ from those having α-β receptors. In virtually all organs and tissue where lymphocytes are found nearly all T cells have α-β receptors; but those in epithelial layers of skin (epidermis) and intestine have γ-δ receptors.

Compared to the TcR α- and β-chain loci (see above), the **TcR γ-chain locus** (Fig. 15–29) has relatively few V$_\gamma$ gene segments (seven have been identified in the mouse genome) and more C$_\gamma$ segments (four identified so far), each having on its upstream side a J$_\gamma$ segment, as in the Ig λ light-chain locus (see Chap. 14). The γ and δ chains of γ-δ T cells in mouse epidermis appear to be largely devoid of sequence variations: they are formed predominantly from single V, J, and C gene segments (for both γ and δ) and there seems to be little diversity at their respective V-J and V-D-J junctions. The γ subunits of γ-δ T cells of intestinal epithelium are formed predominantly from another V$_\gamma$ gene, but much sequence diversity at their V$_\gamma$-J$_\gamma$ junction is evident.

The Ags that are recognized by TcR γ–δ molecules are not yet established, but, as noted above, they might be the MHC-I-like proteins of limited variability (Qa and TL). The function of the double-negative T cell having these receptors is also unclear, although some of the γ–δ T cell clones grown in culture are cytolytic and CD8⁺ (CD4⁻, CD8⁺), like conventional CTLs.

CD4 AND CD8 GLYCOPROTEINS

As noted before, a mature T-cell's expression of either CD4 or CD8 almost always correlates with the cell's MHC specificity: CD4⁺ T cells are specific for MHC-II (self-MHC-II plus fragments of extrinsic protein Ags or nonself [allogenic] MHC-II), and CD8⁺ T cells are similarly specific for MHC-I. The correlation probably arises because the CD8 and TcR molecules on a given T cell cooperate in binding MHC-I molecules on another cell, with CD8

binding to invariable (monomorphic) epitopes and the TcR to variable or polymorphic epitopes (including associated peptides). Similarly, on CD4⁺ T cells, CD4 and the TcR could cooperate in binding to MHC-II molecules (with their associated peptides) on another cell.

Most thymocytes (about 80%) are double-positive (CD4⁺ and CD8⁺), and about half of them also contain the CD3–TcR complex; they may be precursors of single-positive (CD4 or CD8) cells. How the specificity of the TcR for MHC-I or -II comes finally to match a T-cell's expression of CD4 or CD8 is not understood.

CD4

The CD4 polypeptide chain has six domains, four of them extracellular (Fig. 15–32). The most N-terminal domain has distinct amino acid sequence homology with Igs, especially with L-chain V domains (28–35%). The next 270 amino acid residues are made up of three domains, none with sequence homology to any known protein except perhaps the Ig-like receptor for IgA (see Fig. 15–34). The transmembrane domain, which follows, is not unusual, but the cytoplasmic domain, at the C-terminus, is extremely long (40 amino acids) and conserved: for example, there is only a single amino acid difference between this domain in mouse and rat CD4. This conservation (and other observations) suggest that CD4 may function in signal transduction.

CD4 IN INFECTIONS WITH HIV. The severe immune deficiency that characterizes infections with the human immunodeficiency virus (HIV) arises because the cellular receptor for the virus is the CD4 glycoprotein, which specifically binds a glycoprotein (gp 120) on the viral envelope. Hence the virus's great propensity to infect T_H cells. Some Abs to CD4 block infections of these cells, and human fibroblasts become susceptible to HIV infection if they are transfected with and express the human CD4 gene.

HIV-infected T cells express gp 120 on the cell surface and readily fuse with uninfected CD4⁺ T cells but not with CD4⁻ T cells. Only a small fraction of T cells (about 1/50,000) in blood from infected individuals harbor HIV, and it is likely that CD4-mediated cell fusion facilitates the spread of virions from infected to uninfected T cells. The resulting T-cell syncytia are thought to be eliminated by macrophages, which might account for the striking depletion of CD4⁺ T cells that is characteristic of HIV-induced AIDS. (For more likely possibilities, see AIDS, Chap. 20.) Therefore, **the interaction of CD4 with the HIV viral envelope glycoprotein (gp 120) is the key to viral replication and pathogenesis of AIDS.** Although there is extensive polymorphism of the encoding sequences for gp 120 in different HIV isolates, it is likely that only a particular conserved segment of this protein

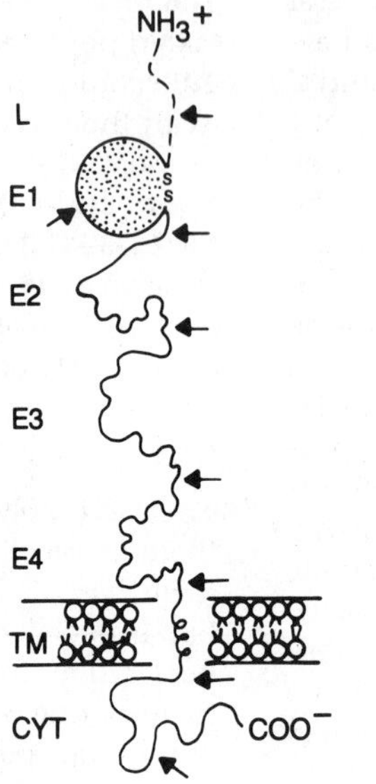

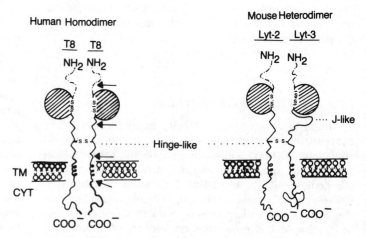

| % Amino Acid Sequence Homology | | |
Mouse vs. Human	Mouse vs. Rat	Mouse vs. Ig L Chain V Domains
54	59	
53	68	28-35
48	66	
58	77	
58	80	
38	66	
79	97	

Figure 15–32. Structure of the CD4 protein deduced from the sequence of cDNA. The leader (L) domain (dashed) is absent from the mature protein on the T-cell surface. The N-terminal extracellular domain (E1) (shaded) has marked amino acid sequence homology to Ig light L-chain V domains. Arrows mark introns in the coding region of the CD4 gene. Note the cytoplasmic (CYT) domain, which is extremely long and conserved in sequence, suggesting that it might be involved in transducing signals from the T-cell surface. (Based on Littman DR: Annu Rev Immunol 5:561, 1987)

interacts with CD4; this segment may prove the key to development of an effective vaccine.

CD4 is also expressed by human macrophages, neutrophils, and lymphoblastoid B-cell lines, which are all susceptible to HIV infection, and the dementia often seen in AIDS suggests that HIV can infect brain cells or other cells that infiltrate brain. CD4 mRNA has been found in human brain tissue; whether it encodes a functional brain protein is not known.

CD8

The cell surface CD8 molecule of human $CD8^+$ T cells consists of identical polypeptide chains, in dimers and higher multimers (Fig. 15–33). Each chain has at the N

terminus two extracellular domains, followed by a transmembrane domain and a C-terminal cytoplasmic domain rich in basic amino acids. The N-terminal extracellular domain has considerable sequence homology (30%) with V domains of Ig L chains. The following domain is rich in proline, serine, and threonine residues and resembles the hinge region of IgG proteins. Besides cysteine residues at positions that are characteristic of Ig domains, CD8 has additional cysteine residues in the hinge-like region and in the transmembrane and cytoplasmic domains that could form the S–S bonds that link multiple subunits.

Unlike the CD8 molecule of human $CD8^+$ T cells, on the corresponding cells of the mouse and rat, the CD8

Figure 15–33. Structure of the CD8 molecule deduced from cDNA nucleotide sequences. Human CD8 is a homodimer (two T8 subunits), whereas in the mouse and rat, CD8 is a heterodimer made up of Lyt-2 (the mouse homologue of human T8) and Lyt-3 (which is similar to Lyt-2). The leader (L) sequence in all subunits is dotted to indicate that it is cleaved from the nascent chain as it enters the endoplasmic reticulum. The N-terminal domain of the mature subunits is shaded to emphasize its amino acid sequence similarity to Ig light-chain V domains. In T8, Lyt-2, and Lyt-3, the sequence following the Ig V-like domain has amino acid sequence similarity to the Ig hinge region (Ch. 14). In Lyt-3, there is also a distinct Ig-J-like sequence between the V-like and hinge-like sequences. A homolog of mouse Lyt-3 has also been identified in human $CD8^+$ T cells. Termed CD8β, this chain pairs with the chain designated T8 at left (now termed CD8α). Both CD8α homodimers and CD8α/CD8β heterodimers are found on human $CD8^+$ T cells; whether they differ functionally is not clear. Arrows point to boundaries of exons in the T8 (CD8α) gene. (Based on Littman DR: Annu Rev Immunol 5:561, 1987)

polypeptide chain (termed **Lyt-2** in the mouse) is paired with another chain, called **Lyt-3** (see Fig. 15–32). The latter's amino acid sequence, deduced from a cDNA clone, is even more Ig-like than Lyt-2 (or CD8 on human cells): thus, the domain at the N terminus has 24% to 29% sequence homology with V domains of various Ig and TcR chains, and the sequence of the next domain is strikingly similar to the J regions of Ig and TcR molecules. Following the J-like region, the amino acid sequence resembles the hinge region of Ig γ chains.

ALTERNATIVE SPLICING OF CD8 GENE PRODUCTS. The exon–intron structure of the human CD8 genes is shown in Figure 15–33. In the mouse, alternative splicing of the primary transcript of the Lyt-2 gene results in a shortened form (called α'; the longer form is termed α). The shortened form is evident particularly in the thymus, and it may be regulated during T-cell development. In human CD8$^+$ T-cell leukemias, a different splicing variation removes the transmembrane domain and results in a secreted CD8 molecule.

CELL ADHESION MOLECULES (CAM)

T cells are highly motile: they change shape and can crawl relatively rapidly (approximately one cell diameter per min). When they make contact with another cell, they adhere to it, forming transient **conjugates** in which the T cell moves back and forth over the other cell's surface, as though searching for Ags (**immune surveillance**). The T-cell-surface molecules responsible for this adhesion have been identified primarily with the aid of Abs that block T-cell functions requiring conjugate formation (e.g., lysis of target cells by CTLs). The principal cell adhesion molecules (CAMs) are described below:

LFA-1 is a heterodimer made up of an α chain of 180 Kd noncovalently associated with a β chain of 95 Kd. It is present on many mouse and human cells of hematopoietic origin (T cells, granulocytes, monocytes, etc.). There may be several ligands for LFA-1, one of which has been identified as ICAM-1 (intercellular adhesion molecule-1), a cell-surface glycoprotein found on a great variety of cells. Two similar CAMs, on B cells, monocytes, and granulocytes, are termed **Mac-1** (which is also the receptor for a fragment of complement component 3) and **p150,95**. Each of the three CAMs has a distinctive α chain (180, 170, and 150 Kd), but they all share a common β subunit (95 Kd). (In the international nomenclature for cell-surface markers, the α chains are termed CD11 a, b, and c, and the β chain is CD18.)

The functional importance of these molecules is evident in human families with a heritable leukocyte adhesion deficiency (LAD) disease. Affected individuals have profound defects in adhesion properties of granulocytes and monocytes, in phagocytosis by granulocytes, and also in target-cell lysis by CTL. Hence, they are subject to recurrent life-threatening infections. The molecular basis for the disease is a defect in the β-subunit gene: various mutations result in undetectable or low levels of its mRNA or in β-chain precursors that are abnormally large or small. Severely affected individuals have less than 1%, and less-affected individuals have 5% to 10%, of the normal level of these cell-surface adhesion molecules. In some families, the β-chain precursors are normal in amount and size, but formation of the α–β molecule is still defective, probably because some critical mutation affects the ability of the β chain to pair with α chains.

The specific blocking effects of mAbs to **CD2** and **LFA-3** show that these molecules are involved in the adhesion of CTLs to target cells, T_H cells to APC, and thymocytes to thymic epithelium. CD2 (a single chain of 45–50 Kd) is present exclusively on T cells, whereas LFA-3 (a single chain of 55–70 Kd) is present on a great variety of cells: epithelial, endothelial, and connective tissue cells, as well as most blood cells, and even erythrocytes. Indeed, the homologue of human LFA-3 on sheep erythrocytes (E) is responsible for the distinctive adhesion of these cells to human T cells, forming the E-rosettes (see Fig. 15–10, above) that initially distinguished human T from B cells.

The binding of LFA-3 to CD2 may play a role in the Ag-driven activation of T cells that are adherent ("conjugated") to target cells or APC. Thus T cells are stimulated to proliferate and to secrete lymphokines by certain combinations of mAbs to CD2 and by certain of these Abs acting synergistically with Ab to CD3.

LFA-3 occurs on some cells as a typical integral membrane protein, with the customary transmembrane and cytoplasmic domains, and on others as a shortened chain from which the transmembrane and cytoplasmic domains have been eliminated. The short chain is anchored in the cell membrane by linkage at its C terminus to **phosphatidyl inositol (PI).**

cDNA clones of CD2 and LFA-3 have similar sequences, which resemble those of Ig domains. They also resemble neural cell-adhesion molecules (NCAMs), which, owing to alternative RNA processing, also exist on neural cells in two forms, one anchored in the cell membrane by transmembrane and cytoplasmic domains, and the other, which lacks these domains, by PI. Thy-1 is another T-cell protein that is anchored in the cell membrane by PI.

THE Ig SUPERFAMILY

The domain structure and amino acid sequences of many of the T-cell-surface proteins considered in this chapter resemble those of Igs (Fig. 15–34). Some of these proteins (the TcR α, β, γ, and δ subunits and the MHC-I and -II proteins) are also encoded by **multigene fami-**

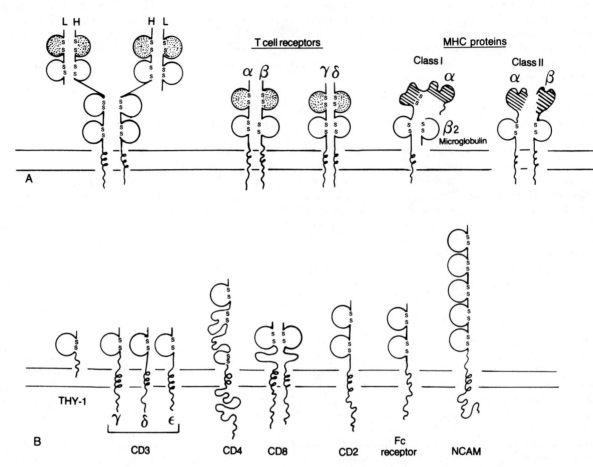

Figure 15–34. The Ig gene superfamily. Domains with the Ig fold are shown as circles closed by S–S bonds. *(A)* Molecules involved in Ag recognition. The subunits (chains) in all of these proteins (with the exception of β_2-microglobulin in the MHC-I molecules) are encoded by sets of many similar genes (multigene families). The shaded N-terminal domains (Ig H and L chains, TcR α, β, γ, and δ chains) differ in sequence from one B- or T-cell clone to another. The cross-hatched N-terminal domains of MHC-I and MHC-II proteins differ in sequence among individuals of the same species (highly polymorphic), but they are not clonally variable. *(B)* Cell-surface molecules encoded by single-copy genes; those shown are neither clonally variable nor polymorphic. They are representative of a much larger group. *NCAM,* neural cell-adhesion molecule. (From Williams A: Immunol Today 8:298, 1987; Hunkapiller T, Hood L: Nature 323:15, 1986)

lies, like those of Ig heavy and light chains; others are encoded by **single-copy genes** (e.g., CD3, CD4, and CD8). All members of this Ig gene superfamily share with Igs a **homology unit** of about 100 amino acid residues, in which an S–S bond between two cysteine residues separated by about 70 amino acids, links two β-pleated sheets (each formed by multiple antiparallel β-polypeptide strands) to form a stable domain with a characteristic shape, the Ig fold (see Figs. 14–23 and 14–24, Chap. 14). Some members of the family probably have paired homology units (like V_H–V_L domains of Igs and V_α–V_β in TcR molecules).

Many members of this family function as Ag-recognition molecules (Ig, TcR, MCH-I, MCH-II) and others as cell adhesion molecules (CD2, LFA-3, CD4, CD8). Other members of the family are expressed by neurons, and one is a developmentally regulated NCAM. All of these Ag-recognition and cell adhesion molecules share the fundamental ability to bind specific ligands, and their similarity in sequence suggests that all members of the family may have evolved from a primordial exon encoding an Ig-like domain that was involved in cell–cell recognition or adhesion.

Because so many proteins have retained the Ig-like

homology unit, it evidently confers considerable advantages, such as inherent stability and the ability to fold up rapidly into a stable shape during the protein's biosynthesis or when it is subjected to transient denaturing conditions (fast-folding kinetics). The finding of the characteristic Ig fold by x-ray analysis even in some proteins that have no amino acid sequence homology to Igs (superoxide dismutase; α-amylase inhibitor) provides further evidence for the exceptional advantages of the Ig homology unit.

Appendix
ANTIBODIES TO CELL-SURFACE ANTIGENS

Cells of the immune system are identified primarily by Abs to their surface Ags. The Abs are usually produced by injecting cells from one individual into other individuals of the same species (**alloimmunization**) or of other species (**xenoimmunization**). In alloimmunizations, cells that express a particular alloAg (call it X.1) are injected into individuals that lack X.1 (expressing, say, X.2 instead). The resulting alloantisera are especially reproducible when the donors and recipients of the injected cells are from mice (or rats) of different inbred strains: because all members of each strain are the same genetically, all of them either do, or do not, express any particular alloAg. For ethical reasons, humans cannot be subjected to such alloimmunization; but valuable alloAbs to human alloAgs are often obtained from those who receive multiple blood transfusions, and women with multiple pregnancies often produce such Abs to alloAgs (inherited from the father) of their fetuses.

Antisera resulting from xenoimmunization (e.g., injecting human cells into rabbits) are usually less useful, because the number of Ags that differ in such donor–recipient combinations is so large that an Ab response to any one of them is likely to be low. However, with mAb technology (see Chap. 13), and the ability to screen enormous numbers of hybridomas (e.g., from a population of spleen B cells from mice immunized with human lymphocytes), the rare ones that produce Abs to a cell-surface Ag of interest can be identified and expanded to produce essentially unlimited amounts of valuable mAb. Some of the most useful mAbs to human B and T cells have been developed in just this way (see anti-CD3, anti-CD4, anti-CD8, etc., above).

Valuable mAbs to cell-surface Ags of mouse lymphocytes have also been obtained by injecting these cells into rats or hamsters and fusing the immunized animal's spleen cells with mouse myeloma cells to yield **interspecific hybridomas** that secrete rat or hamster mAb to the mouse Ags.

Immunoprecipitation

Ags on the surface of intact cells are commonly labeled with ^{125}I through the use of the enzyme lactoperoxidase and H_2O_2 to convert ^{125}I-iodide ion into a short-lived reactive form (OI^-). The enzyme cannot penetrate into living cells; hence, only proteins on the cell surface are labeled. The labeled cells are disrupted with neutral detergents (to maintain integral membrane proteins in solution), and Abs to the Ag of interest are then added. The resulting immune complexes (^{125}I-Ag–Ab) are then specifically adsorbed (immunoprecipitated) in various ways: for instance, by staphylococci (Cowan strain) having a surface protein (**protein A**) that binds many Igs and Ab–Ag complexes, or by beads coated with purified protein A (see Chap. 13), or with Abs of the appropriate specificity (e.g., goat Abs to mouse Igs, if the first Ab added was of mouse origin). After washing the particles or precipitates free of extraneous proteins, the labeled Ag is eluted with sodium dodecyl sulfate (SDS, an anionic detergent) and subjected to polyacrylamide gel electrophoresis in SDS (the widely used acronym is SDS-PAGE).

Because SDS binds to virtually all peptide bonds, proteins dissolved in its presence acquire a uniform negative charge per unit mass and migrate toward the anode at a rate that is proportional to the **apparent mol. wt.** (M_r). The position of the ^{125}I-labeled Ag is identified by radioautography; i.e., by exposing the dried gel to an x-ray film. By carrying out the electrophoresis in the presence and absence of a reducing agent (such as 2-mercaptoethanol) that cleaves S–S bonds, the procedure can indicate whether the cell-surface Ag is a monomer or a multimer with S–S linked subunits.

Immunofluorescence

In this method, Abs are labeled with fluorescent groups, and cells with surface Ags that bind the Abs appear as bright objects in a microscope that is equipped with an ultraviolet light source to excite fluorescent groups. When excited, the commonly used groups emit green (500 nm; fluorescein) or red light (700 nm; Texas red or phycoerythrin).

To avoid denaturing Abs, only a few fluorescent groups can be attached per molecule, and to increase the fluorescent signal, fluorescent groups are often attached, not to the Ab (Ab no. 1) that binds to the Ag of interest, but rather to a second Ab (Ab no. 2) that binds to Ab no. 1 (e.g., goat anti-mouse Ig is Ab no. 2 if a mouse Ab is Ab no. 1). Because few Ab no. 1 molecules will bind to the Ag (often only one Ab per Ag molecule), whereas many molecules of Ab no. 2 can bind to each molecule of Ab no. 1, this amplifying procedure can focus many more fluorescent groups on the Ag.

The need for a second Ab can be circumvented by taking advantage of the extremely high affinity ($\sim 10^{15}$ liters/mole) of **avidin,** a protein in hen's egg white, or **streptavidin,** a similar protein from *Streptomyces griseus,* for **biotin,** a vitamin. Several biotin groups per Ab molecule are easily attached, and avidin can be made fluorescent; for example, by attaching to it fluorescein or an extremely fluorescent algal protein such as phycoerythrin (PE). Hence, a single preparation of, say, avidin–PE can serve as a general fluorescent reagent that specifically identifies any biotinylated Ab, regardless of the Ag it binds. The specificity and sensitivity of these reagents make it possible to detect as few as about 1000 surface Ag molecules per cell.

FLOW CYTOMETRY AND CELL SORTING

An instrument that measures the fluorescence of individual cells has transformed fluorescence microscopy from a useful but qualitative and subjective procedure into a quantitative one of great versatility and precision. The basic principles are illustrated in Fig. 15–35. Cells are

stained–for example, with a biotinylated Ab and then with fluorescent avidin (for instance avidin–PE)—and passed in linear array in a fine stream in front of an intense beam of laser light that activates the fluorescent group. Any fluorescent light emitted is picked up by a detector placed at 90° to the beam of exciting light. Exciting light that has passed through the stream of cells is also useful: by blocking the direct beam with a small solid object (obscuration bar), another detector can detect light that has been scattered by cells in the moving stream. This **low-angle forward scattering** serves both as a cell counter and a means for eliminating fluorescent signals from spurious sources such as debris and cell fragments. The information obtained from the two detectors, one detecting fluorescence and the other low-angle forward light scattering, can be analyzed and displayed in various ways, often as a histogram relating cell number to fluorescence intensity.

Flow cytometry can also be used to separate cells with a surface Ag of interest from those that lack it (**cell sort-**

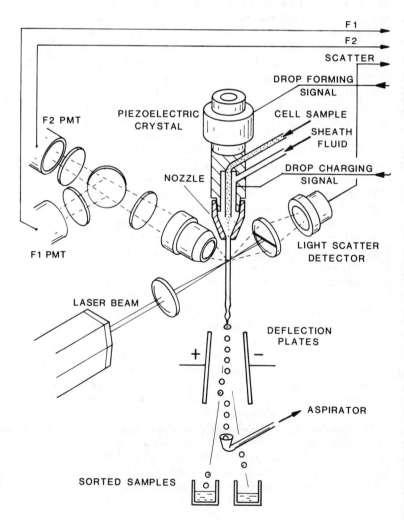

Figure 15–35. Sorting of fluorescein-antibody-tagged cells in a fluorescence-activated cell sorter. (From Parks D, Herzenberg LA: Methods in Enzymology 108:197, 1984)

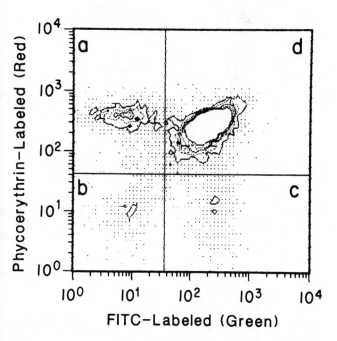

Figure 15–36. Two-color analysis of thymus cells by flow cytometry. The cells were stained with a mAb to CD4 coupled to phycoerythrin (PE, red) and a mAb to CD8 coupled with fluorescein isothiocyanate (FITC, green). **(a)** CD4⁺, CD8⁻ cells. **(b)** CD4⁻, CD8⁻ (double-negative) cells. **(c)** CD4⁻, CD8⁺ cells. **(d)** CD4⁺, CD8⁺ (double-positive) cells. (Kindly provided by Dr Cathryn Nagler–Anderson, Massachusetts Institute of Technology.)

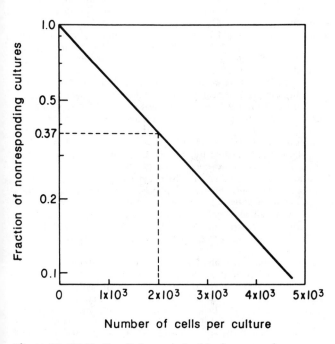

Figure 15–37. Limiting dilution analysis of the frequency of precursors of CTLs in mouse spleen.

ing). For this purpose, special devices break up the stream of cells before it passes through the beam of exciting laser light into tiny, negatively charged droplets containing 0 or 1 cell (rarely >1 cell). As droplets containing a fluorescent cell are detected and pass between two highly charged plates, they can be deflected and collected. Thus, with the thymus cell population illustrated in Fig. 15–36, it is possible to collect in separate vessels droplets containing a) CD4⁺ CD8⁻ cells or b) CD4⁻ CD8⁻ cells or c) CD4⁻ CD8⁺ cells or (d) CD4⁺ CD8⁺ cells. Separations can be carried out under sterile conditions, permitting the desired cells to be collected in culture medium and grown as purified subsets of the original heterogeneous population. Rare mutants can also be identified, isolated, and cultured if they have a distinctive surface Ag for which there is an appropriate Ab.

LIMITING DILUTION ANALYSIS

The frequency in a mixed cell population of cells with a particular function and specificity can be estimated by limiting dilution analysis. For instance, to measure the frequency in a suspension of spleen cells of precursors for CTLs that are specific for viral Ag X, graded numbers of the spleen cells are cultured in multiple replicas under conditions designed to stimulate the specific induction of cytolytically active anti-X CTLs from resting precursor T cells (pCTLs). The pCTLs must be present in limiting number (i.e., some cultures contain none of them), and the cultures must contain, or be supplemented with, an excess of any other cells needed for the response of interest (e.g., cells expressing viral Ag X and perhaps CD4⁺ T cells and macrophages as sources of lymphokines). For each cell dose, the fraction of nonresponding cultures is determined; by plotting this fraction on a logarithmic scale against the number of spleen cells on an arithmetic scale, (Fig. 15–37), a linear relation is obtained if the differentiated progeny of a single pCTL can be detected (e.g., by lysis of ⁵¹Cr-labeled virus X-infected target cells). From the Poisson distribution,* it follows that the cell dose that yields a fraction of nonresponding cultures of 0.37 (i.e., e⁻¹) contains a single anti-X pCTL, a frequency in the example shown of one per 2 × 10³ spleen cells. Such a frequency might be found in a secondary response; the frequency in a primary response is probably 1/100 to 1/1000 of this. Limiting dilution analyses are also useful for measuring the frequency of T_H cells and B cells.

---

* $P(k) = \dfrac{e^{-m} m^k}{k!}$, where $P(k)$ is the fraction of cultures with k pCTLs, m is the average number of pCTLs per cell dose, and e is the base of natural logarithms. Cultures with no cytolytic activity after 5 days are assumed to have had no pCTL at the start; when $m = 1$ the fraction of such cultures, $P(0)$, is e^{-m} (because $0! = 1$) or 0.37.

Selected Reading

BOOKS AND REVIEW ARTICLES

Fink PJ, Bevan M: The influence of thymic H-2 antigens on the specificity of maturing killer and helper T cells. Immunol Rev 42:3, 1978

Kronenberg M, Sui G, Hood LE, Shastri N: The molecular genetics of the T-cell antigen receptor and T-cell antigen recognition. Annu Rev Immunol 4:529–591, 1986

Greene WC, Leonard WJ: The human interleukin 2 receptor. Annu Rev Immunol 4:69–95, 1986

Klein J: The natural history of the major histocompatibility complex. New York, Wiley and Sons, 1986

Littman DR: The structure and function of CD4 and CD8 genes. Annu Rev Immunol 5:561–583, 1987

McDevitt HO, Benacerraf B: Genetic control of specific immune responses. Adv in Immunol 11:31, 1969

Nathenson SG, Geliebter J, Pfaffenbach GM, Zeff RA: Murine major histocompatibility complex class-I mutants: Molecular analysis and structure–function. Annu Rev Immunol 4:471–502, 1986

Paul WE, O'Hara J: B-cell stimulatory factor-1/interleukin 4. Annu Rev Immunol 5:429–459, 1987

Raulet DH: The structure, function, and molecular genetics of the γ/δ T cell receptor. Ann Rev Immunol 7:175, 1989

Sprent J: Role of H-2 gene products in the function of T helper cells from normal and chimeric mice measured in vivo. Immunol Rev 42:108, 1978

Springer TA, Dustin ML, Kishimoto TK, Marlin SD: The lymphocyte function-associated LFA-1, CD2, and LFA-3 molecules: Cell adhesion molecules of the immune system. Annu Rev Immunol 5:223, 1987

Toyonaga B, Mak TW: Genes of the T-cell antigen receptor in normal and malignant cells. Annu Rev Immunol 5:585–620, 1987

Unanue ER: Antigen-presenting function of the macrophage. Ann Rev Immunol 2:395, 1984

Weiss A, Imboden J, Hardy K, Manger B, Terhorst C, Stobo J: The role of the T3/antigen receptor complex in T-cell activation. Annu Rev Immunol 4:593–619, 1986

SPECIFIC ARTICLES

Allison J, McIntyre B, Block D: Tumor-specific antigen of murine T lymphoma defined with monoclonal antibody. J Immunol 129:2293–2300, 1982

Babbitt BP, Allen PM, Matsueda G, Haber E, Unanue ER: Binding of immunogenic peptides to Ia histocompatibility molecules. Nature 317:359–361, 1985

Buus S, Sette A, Colon SM, Jenis DM, Grey HM: Isolation and characterization of antigen-Ia complexes involved in T cell recognition. Cell 47:1071–1077, 1986

Cantor H, Boyse EA: Functional subclasses of T lymphocytes bearing different Ly antigens I: The generation of functionally distinct T-cell subclasses is a differentiative process independent of antigen. J Exp Med 141:1376, 1975

Ceredig R, Dialynas DP, Fitch FW, MacDonald HR: Precursors of T cell growth factor producing cells in the thymus: Ontogeny, frequency, and quantitative recovery in a subpopulation of phenotypically mature thymocytes defined by monoclonal antibody GK-1.5. J Exp Med 158:1654–1671, 1983

Chou HS, Nelson CA, Godambe SA, et al: Germline organization of the murine T cell receptor β chains. Science 238:545, 1987

Fowlkes BJ, Edison L, Mathieson BJ, Chused TM: Early T lymphocytes: Differentiation in vivo of adult intrathymic precursor cells. J Exp Med 162:802–822, 1985

Guillet J-G, Lai M-Z, Briner TJ, Buus S, Sette A, Grey HM, Smith JA, Gefter ML: Immunological self, nonself discrimination. Science 235:865–870, 1987

Haskins K, Kubo R, White J, Pigeon M, Kappler J, Marrack P: The major histocompatibility complex-restricted antigen receptor in T cells I: Isolation with a monoclonal antibody. J Exp Med 157:1149–1169, 1983

Hedrick SM, Cohen DI, Nielsen EA, Davis MM: Isolation of cDNA clones encoding T cell-specific membrane-associated proteins. Nature 308:149–153, 1984

Hedrick SM, Nielsen EA, Kavaler J, Cohen DI, Davis MM: Sequence relationships between putative T-cell receptor polypeptides and immunoglobulins. Nature 308:153–158, 1984

Kappler JW, Roehm N, Marrack P: T cell tolerance by clonal elimination in the thymus. Cell 49:273–280, 1987

Kappler JW, Skidmore B, White J, Marrack P: Antigen-inducible, H-2-restricted, interleukin-2 producing T cell hybridomas: Lack of independent antigen and H-2 recognition. J Exp Med 153:1198–1214, 1981

Lanzavecchia A, Roosnek E, Gregory T, et al: T cells can present antigens such as HIV gp120 targeted to their own surface molecules. Nature 334:530, 1988

Le Meur M, Gerlinger P, Benoist C, Mathis D: Correcting an immune response deficiency by creating Ea gene transgenic mice. Nature 316:38–42, 1985

Lindahl KF, Wilson DB: Histocompatibility antigen-activated cytotoxic T lymphocytes: Estimates of the frequency and specificity of precursors. J Exp Med 145:508–522, 1977

Meuer S, Fitzgerald K, Hussey R, Hodgdon J, Schlossman S, Reinherz E: Clonotypic structures involved in antigen-specific human T cell function: Relationship to the T3 molecular complex. J Exp Med 157:705–719, 1983

Mitchison NA: The carrier effect in the secondary response to hapten–protein conjugates II: Cellular cooperation. Eur J Immunol 1:18, 1971

Mossman TR, Cherwinski H, Bond MW, Geidlin MA, Coffman RL: Two types of murine helper T cell clone 1: Definition according to profiles of lymphokine activities and secreted proteins. J Immunol 136:2348–2357, 1986

Reichard RA, Gallatin M, Butcher EC, Weissman IL: A homing receptor-bearing cortical thymocyte subset: Implications for thymus cell migration and the nature of cortisone-resistant thymocytes. Cell 38:89–99, 1984

Saito H, Kranz DM, Takagaki Y, Hayday AC, Eisen HN, Tonegawa S: Complete primary structure of a heterodimeric T-cell receptor deduced from cDNA sequences. Nature 309:757–762, 1984

Shevach E, Rosenthal AS: Function of macrophages in antigen recognition by guinea pig T lymphocytes. J Exp Med 138:1213, 1973

Simonsen M: The clonal selection hypothesis evaluated by grafted cells reacting against their hosts. Cold Spring Harbor Symposium on Quantitative Biology 32:517–523, 1967.

Von Boehmer H, Schubiger K: Thymocytes appear to ignore class I major histocompatibility complex antigens expressed on thymus epithelial cells. Eur J Immunol 14:1048–1052, 1984

Yanagi Y, Yoshikai Y, Leggett K, Clark SP, Aleksander I, Mak TW: A human T cell-specific cDNA clone encodes a protein having extensive homology to immunoglobulin chains. Nature 308:145–149, 1984

Zinkernagel RM, Callahan GN, Althage A, Cooper S, Klein PA, Klein J: On the thymus in the differentiation of "H-2 self-recognition" by T cells: Evidence for dual recognition? J Exp Med 147:882, 1978

Zinkernagel RM, Doherty PC: H-2 compatibility requirement for T cell mediated lysis of target cells infected with lymphocytic choriomeningitis virus: Different cytotoxic T cell specificities are associated with structures coded for in H-2K or H-2D. J Exp Med 141:1427, 1975

16

Herman N. Eisen
Malcolm L. Gefter

Antibody Formation

The central problem of antibody (Ab) formation is to understand how an individual can form Ab molecules to an almost limitless variety of foreign antigens (Ags) but not to substances naturally found in the body (**self-Ags**). Previous chapters noted that the pool of Ab-forming B lymphocytes (close to 10^{12} in an adult human) consists of a great many clones, each derived from one B cell. The individuality of the Ig that distinguishes each clone derives from the singularity of its Ag-combining region, formed by the variable (V) domains of its heavy (H) and light (L) chains ($V_H + V_L$). Chapter 14 described how such a vast number of Ag-combining sites (estimated at approximately 10^9 per person) are formed by the seemingly random rearrangements of diverse gene segments, along with the introduction of additional short, variable sequences at the junctions of the linked segments (V and J segments for L-chain genes and V, D, and J segments for H-chain genes). In the vast majority of B cells, which are quiescent or "resting" cells, the Ig is an integral membrane protein, with its combining site exposed on the cell surface. The diversity of these receptors is so great that virtually any foreign Ag that gains entry into the body will be bound specifically (i.e., will be "recognized") by some B cells. However, although this recognition is necessary to activate resting B cells, it is rarely sufficient, and additional substances (lymphokines) provided by helper (CD4) T cells are required. The responding cells generally proliferate and differentiate into two kinds of daughter cells: **B lymphoblasts and plasma cells** are specialized to synthesize and secrete Igs at an enormous rate (up to about 20,000 molecules per minute in a plasma cell), whereas **memory B cells** remain in a resting state (G_0 in the cell cycle) poised to respond to future encounters with the same (or a cross-reacting) Ag. In contrast to these responses to foreign Ags, self-Ags normally elicit "tolerance" (i.e., unresponsiveness) rather than an immune response.

In this chapter, we will consider: (1) B-cell responses to Ags and lymphokines; (2) the development of B cells from precursor cells into Ig-secreting cells; and (3) the basis for tolerance to self-Ags.

Before encountering a foreign Ag, an individual's serum generally lacks the corresponding Abs (i.e., their concentration is below the limits of detection: <1–10 ng per ml). But several days to a few weeks after an encounter with the antigen, these Abs appear in serum, and they can increase in concentration a million-fold or more, reaching levels up to several mg per ml. The rate and magnitude of the increase, its persistence, and the isotypes and affinities of the Abs that are formed are dependent on many factors, including the chemical nature of the Ag (its size, polymeric state, etc.), its dose and route of administration, and the presence of enhancing substances (**adjuvants**). Many of these factors will be considered later in this chapter.

Antibody Responses to T-Dependent Antigens

Most Ags are proteins, and in the course of the immune response, the patterns of Abs that they elicit change with respect to H-chain isotype and affinity for the Ag. Because the changes depend on the lymphokines produced by activated T cells, these Ags are termed "T-dependent." In contrast, the Abs elicited by some other Ags, characteristically purified polysaccharides of bacterial origin, do not change and are not dependent on T-cell help; these "T-independent Ags" will be discussed later. The evolving nature of the responses elicited by T-dependent Ags is especially evident when the initial (**primary**) and subsequent (**secondary**) responses to an Ag are compared.

As indicated schematically in Figure 16–1, an organism's first encounter with a typical T-dependent protein Ag (injected, say, in saline) results in a transient rise in serum Abs. These early Abs are IgM molecules, and they are usually present at low levels (e.g., 1–50 μg per ml) and have low intrinsic affinity for their epitope (usually about 10^4 to 10^5 L/M for a typical haptenic group). The initial response usually subsides in about 1 to 2 weeks, and serum Abs again become undetectable, but the cells that responded do not return to their preimmune status. Instead, they persist as memory cells, **primed** to give a greatly enhanced secondary response to a subsequent encounter with the same Ab, even after a lapse of decades. In the secondary response, the Abs in serum appear earlier, increase more rapidly, and reach a higher peak level. Moreover, the Abs made in the secondary response are no longer IgM; they are predominantly IgG molecules, and they usually have much higher intrinsic affinity for the Ag (typically 10- to 1000-fold higher for haptens).

PRIMARY RESPONSE

In eliciting a primary response, the Ag initially encounters very few B and T cells that recognize it (or its peptide fragments in association with MHC-II proteins); hence, the immune response is very limited. However, the B and T cells that do respond proliferate and expand the size of the respective Ag-specific clones. Some of the progeny B cells differentiate into IgM-secreting cells, termed **lym-**

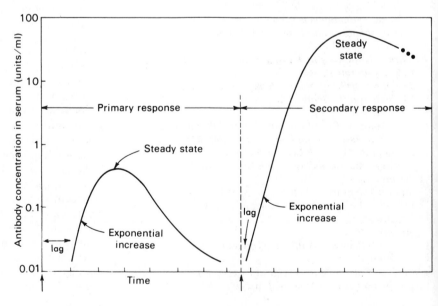

Figure 16–1. Comparison of serum Ab concentrations following the first (priming) and second (booster) injections of immunogen *(arrowheads)*. Note the logarithmic scale for Ab concentration. Time units are left unspecified to indicate the great variability encountered with different immunogens under different conditions.

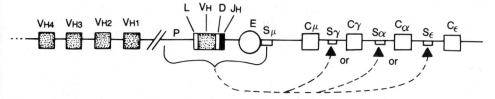

Figure 16–2. Functional heavy-chain gene showing the relocation (recombination, dashed lines) of its rearranged V-region sequence (L, V_H, D, J_H) from "switch" sequences (S) just upstream of the C_H gene segments for μ to homologous sequences (S_γ, S_α, S_ϵ) just upstream of C_H segments for γ, α, or ϵ. (P = promoter region; E = enhancer). For further schematic details see Chapter 14.

phoblasts, which have about twice the diameter of resting B cells. In resting cells, the RNA transcripts of the functionally rearranged μ-chain genes are cleaved and polyadenylated at a site that results in a membrane-anchored μ chain (with a transmembrane plus a cytoplasmic domain at its C terminus), but in the Ig-secreting cells, this process occurs further upstream, yielding the shorter μ chain of the pentameric IgM molecules found in serum (Chap. 14, Fig. 14–39).

SECONDARY RESPONSE: IMMUNOLOGIC MEMORY

As a result of the B- and T-cell proliferation that occurs in the primary response, the same Ag will encounter many more responsive B and T cells in a secondary response. Moreover, in the secondary response, T_H (CD4) cells can be stimulated by peptide–MHC-II complexes on B cells, as well as by these complexes on dendritic cells and macrophages, whereas in the primary response, it seems that only dendritic cells and macrophages can serve as Ag-presenting cells. (B cells, like the other Ag-presenting cells, can internalize and process the Ags that they bind and reexpress the peptide fragments in association with MHC-II proteins on the cell surface; see Chapter 15.)

Switching of Heavy-Chain Isotypes

Probably in response to lymphokines (see below), the H-chain gene in the responding memory B cell undergoes recombination: its V_HDJ_H assembly, initially next to the C_μ gene, switches to a corresponding position next to a downstream C_H gene, usually one of the C_γ gene segments (Fig. 16–2). As described in Chapter 14, this switch does not entail a change in V_HDJ_H sequence or in the L-chain gene; hence, the resulting Ab (IgG or, less often, IgA or IgE) has the same Ag-binding site as the IgM Ab made previously by that B cell.

The proliferating B cells in which the switch takes place also yields two kinds of progeny cells: (1) additional but different memory B cells, in which the new H-chain gene is expressed as the H chain of a new integral membrane protein (IgG or, less often, IgA or IgE); and (2) Ig-

secreting B cells in which the new H-chain gene's transcript is processed to yield mRNA for the shorter, secreted form. All of **these changes account for the enhanced secretion in the secondary response of IgG (or IgA or IgE) Abs.** On subsequent encounters of the expanded clones of switched memory B cell with the Ag, the same Abs are produced promptly and in large amounts. Further switching from a C_γ gene to another C_H gene located downstream can also occur on repeated exposure to the Ag (**hyperimmunization**).

Somatic Mutations and Affinity Changes

In addition to the switch in the H-chain's constant-region gene, a B-cell's H- and L-chain genes undergo critical changes in nucleotide sequence during the response to antigenic stimulation. These changes consist of **single-base substitutions** scattered throughout the sequences that encode the variable domains of the H and L chains. To a lesser extent, they are also found in the noncoding sequences on the upstream side of V and downstream side of J, but **they do not occur in encoding sequences for constant regions.**

Some of the resulting changes in amino acid sequence change the Ab's affinity for its Ag. **Because the Ag can be thought of as a growth factor for the B cell and the cell's surface Ig as a receptor for it, a B cell with increased affinity for the Ag will have a higher probability of binding that Ag and being stimulated to divide further. Hence, V-region mutations are probably responsible for the progressive increases in the average affinity of the serum Abs that appear during the secondary response to protein Ags and hapten–protein conjugates.** Sometimes termed **affinity maturation,** these changes depend on T-cell help: they are not seen in T-deficient animals or in responses to T-independent Ags (see below).

Low levels of Ag are expected to be particularly effective in preferentially stimulating B cells that make high-affinity Abs. Hence, the administration of small doses of Ag favors the early production of high-affinity Abs, and large doses delay their appearance (Table 16–1).

Although the nucleotide substitutions are found at

TABLE 16–1. Sequential Changes in Affinity of Anti-Dnp Abs (IgG Immunoglobulins) Made with Increasing Time After Immunization*

Group	Ag Injected Per Rabbit (mg)	Average Intrinsic Association Constants for Binding ε-Dnp-L-Lysine At		
		2 Weeks	5 Weeks	8 Weeks
I	5	0.86	14	120
II	250	0.18	0.13	0.15

* Immunogen was 2,4-dinitrophenyl bovine γ-globulin (Dnp–BγG). Values are averages for five animals per group and are given in liters mole × 10^6 (30°C).
(Eisen HN, Siskind GW: Biochemistry 3:966, 1964)

Igs, these substitutions also appear to be clustered in CDRs, reinforcing the view that selection by Ag favors the proliferation of B cells whose Ig V regions have amino acid replacements that confer high affinity for the Ag.

THE CLONAL FAMILY. The diversity of the Igs made by various B cells of a particular clone emphasizes that although a clone is, by definition, derived from a single progenitor cell, it can become diversified during an immune response. Nevertheless, all members of a clone (the "clonal family") share the same unique V_LJ_L and V_HDJ_H gene segment rearrangements and the same inserted N-region sequences at the junction of these segments (V_L–J_L and V_H–D–J_H) despite differences in H-chain isotype, allotype, idiotype, and affinity for Ag.

DURATION OF RESPONSES. The duration of primary and secondary responses varies with the dose and mode of administration of Ag. If administered simply in a buffered salt solution, the Ag is rapidly eliminated, and the primary response is short lived (e.g., a few days). Another injection of Ag is then required to elicit the secondary response. If, however, the Ag is retained for a long period, as when it is given in a water-in-oil emulsion (see Freund's Complete Adjuvant, below), Ab production continues at a high level for many months, and the transition from the production of IgM to IgG molecules and from low to high affinity occurs without the need for a second injection. When the prolonged response finally subsides, after many months, a subsequent injection of the same Ag promptly elicits the formation of high affinity IgG Ab molecules, like those made at the end of the earlier response (as though the immune system "remembers what it has learned").

HOW LONG CAN MEMORY B CELLS PERSIST? Ab responses to viral Ags suggest that memory cells probably can endure for the individual's life-time. This suggestion derives from the commonplace observation that a secondary response can sometimes be elicited with an immunogen that is not quite identical to the primary Ag: most of the Abs made will then react more strongly with the first than with the second immunogen. Formerly called **original antigenic sin,** this phenomenon was initially recognized in epidemiologic studies with cross-reacting strains of influenza virus. Each epidemic is caused by a different strain of virus. During a particular epidemic, serum Abs often react less strongly with the strain causing the current illness than with the strain that patients encountered in some previous epidemic. Evidently, the clones originally stimulated by the first strain are more abundant than the naive B cells responding for the first time, and they have higher affinity for the strain that initially stimulated them than for the new cross-reactive strain.

scattered positions throughout V, J, and D sequences, they have a distinct tendency to be clustered in complementarity-determining regions (Chap. 14, Fig. 14–36). In addition, whereas about 25% of random, single nucleotide substitutions are "silent" (i.e., they cause no change in the encoded amino acid), a smaller proportion of V-region substitutions are silent. **It appears, therefore, that immune responses to Ags select for B cells with amino acid replacements in CDRs of their Igs, probably because these changes confer increased affinity for the immunogen.**

Abs from a hyperimmunized mouse can contain as many as five (or even more) amino acid replacements per V region. Because replacements can occur at any of the approximately 40 positions within the CDRs of a V region and can consist of essentially any of the 20 amino acids, the number of possible sequence variations of a single V domain is enormous. For instance, with four replacements more than 10 million different sequences of a given V region can be generated. From the substitutions found at various times after immunization, it has been estimated that **the rate at which V-region sequences are altered approaches one nucleotide change per B cell division.** Thus, there is approximately one "mutant" and one parental sequence in the two daughter cells of nearly every B cell division cycle, providing a rich supply of variant daughter B cells for selection by Ag. (Of course, for most variants, the affinity will be lower or no different than in the parental sequence, and only a rare one will have higher affinity.)

The mechanism responsible for these "somatic mutations" in mammals is not known, but in chickens it appears that the sequence changes can be brought about by a process termed **gene conversion,** in which nucleotide replacements are introduced, in blocks as long as 100 residues, into a functional L-chain's V region gene by patchy recombination from donor V-gene segments that are defective ("pseudogenes"). Like those in mammalian

From the study of sera from elderly patients, it has thus been possible to identify strains of influenza virus that caused major epidemics in the past, as in 1918. Once a B-cell clone has been triggered by one Ag (X), it appears to persist for at least 70 years and then be restimulated by a cross-reacting Ag (X'). Whether these long-lived clones persist without any stimulation for 70 years, or whether their persistence depends on occasionally stimulation by various cross-reacting Ags, is unclear.

Lymphokines, Subsets of T-Helper Cells, and Ig Isotypes

Analyses of cultured clones of CD4 T cells show that the lymphokines they secrete have a profound influence on the Ig isotypes of B cells. As noted before (Chapter 15), mouse CD4 T cells, maintained as clones in cell culture, fall into two distinct subsets. The lymphokines secreted by both subsets promote B-cell proliferation, but they stimulate the formation of different Ig isotypes, as summarized in Table 16–2. (The same lymphokines also have various other effects on a variety of other cells; see Chapter 15). It is possible that the assignment of CD4 cells to the two subsets is obvious only with long-term cultured T-cell lines, whereas *in vivo*, individual CD4 T cells may be more diverse in the particular mix of lymphokines they secrete.

T_H2 cells (also called T_h cells) secrete IL-4, IL-5, and also IL-3. When added to stimulated, polyclonal populations of B cells, IL-4 strikingly enhances the production of IgE (about 100- to 1000-fold) and also of IgG1 (about 20-fold). In addition, IL-4 and IL-5, acting synergistically, enhance IgA production. The dramatic effect on IgE is exerted by IL-4 on the individual B cell, causing it to switch from producing IgM to IgE; the effects on the other isotypes may similarly reflect the specific induction by particular lymphokines of recombination of VDJ sequences to particular switching sequences in the H-chain locus (Fig. 14–41, Chap. 14). Because T_H2 clones also promote the proliferation and maturation of mast cells (via secreted IL-3 plus IL-4) and of eosinophils (via IL-5), the total effect of these CD4 cells would be to enhance immune defenses against infestations with parasitic worms (see IgE and Intestinal Parasitism, Chapter 18).

The other subset of cloned mouse **CD4 T cells, termed T_H1, secrete interferon-γ (IFN-γ) and IL-2.** These cells are also called T_{inf} to indicate their role in promoting the inflammation associated with delayed-type hypersensitivity (see Chapter 19). Resting B cells have low-affinity receptors for IL-2; when stimulated (e.g., by Ab to cell-surface Igs), they promptly express high-affinity IL-2 receptors, and in response to IL-2, they then proliferate vigorously and secrete IgM.

The IFN-γ suppresses the enhancing effect of IL-4 on IgE and IgG$_1$ production. It also increases IgG$_{2a}$ production and stimulates the expression by macrophages of Fc receptors, which have especially high affinity for the Fc of IgG$_{2a}$ molecules; hence these CD4 T cells, via IFN-γ, promote Ab-dependent cell-mediated cytotoxicity (ADCC). Some of these cells contribute further to Ag-induced inflammation by lysing the target cells they recognize: i.e., they are CTLs (see Chapter 19).

IL-6, sometimes referred to as **B-cell factor-2 (BSF-2),** is also produced by various CD4 T cells. It promotes the growth of B-cell hybridomas in culture and helps stimulate B cells to proliferate and secrete Igs; whether it is essential for responses of B cells *in vivo* is not clear.

COGNATE VERSUS NONCOGNATE COOPERATION. As pointed out previously (Chapter 15), T cells help B cells most efficiently when both recognize epitopes on the same Ag. In this situation, termed **cognate cooperation,** the B cell binds, internalizes, and processes the Ag and presents its peptide fragments, in association with the cell's MHC-II molecules, to the CD4 T cells. Generally, cooperating B and CD4 T cells recognize different epitopes on the same Ag molecule. As noted earlier, the reason is that T cells recognize linear sequences of amino acids in small (10–20 residue) peptides, whereas B cells usually recognize noncontiguous sequences of amino acids whose proximity to each other depends on the protein Ag's three-dimensional configuration. For optimal effectiveness, however, the T and B cell epitopes initially have to be part of the same Ag molecule, probably because the cooperating cells adhere to each other, just as in the conjugates formed by cytotoxic T lymphocytes with target cells (Chapter 19). Thus, if the Ag is termed X, it can be said that as an anti-X T cell adheres to

---

TABLE 16–2. Subsets of CD4$^+$ T-Cell Clones Produce Different Lymphokines

CD4 T Cells

Subsets*	Lymphokine†	Effect
T_H1	IFN-γ and IL-2	Stimulate production of IgG$_{2a}$
	IFN-γ	Increases expression of Fc receptor (high affinity for IgG2a) on macrophages
		Blocks IL-4 stimulated switching of IgM to IgE production
T_H2	IL-4	Greatly stimulates production of IgE
	IL-5	Stimulates eosinophil proliferation and maturation
	IL-4 and IL-5	Enhances production of IgA
	IL-3 and IL-4	Stimulates mast-cell proliferation and maturation

* T_H1 also termed T_{inf}; T_H2 also termed T_h.

† Some lymphokines act synergistically, e.g., IFN-γ and IL-2, IL-4, and IL-5.

an anti-X B cell and recognizes peptide–MHC-II complexes on that cell, the T cell is stimulated to secrete its lymphokines into the narrow synapse-like intercellular cleft between the adherent cells: this **polarized secretion focuses the T_H cell's secreted lymphokines on the B cell it helps.**

However, T and B cells can also cooperate when the epitopes they recognize are on different Ags. For instance, high doses of an Ag can activate many CD4 T cells (by means of peptide–MHC-II complexes on dendritic cells and macrophages), and the resulting release of relatively large amounts of lymphokines can promote the responses of nearby B cells that are specific for unrelated Ags. In this **noncognate** or **bystander cooperation,** the B cell does not function as an APC, and its MHC-II protein is irrelevant.

Antibody Responses to T-Independent Antigens

These Ags are generally protein-free high-mol.-wt. polymers made up of repeating epitopes; for example, type-specific pneumococcal capsular polysaccharides (such as Type III, made up of a repeating disaccharide, cellobiuronic acid [see Chap. 13, Fig. 13–14]) and also Ficoll (a polymer of sucrose), dextran sulfate, and lipopolysaccharides of gram-negative bacteria. The **multivalent binding of these Ags to Ig molecules on the surface of a B cell can stimulate secretion of IgM Abs** (Fig. 16–3). However, these Ags do not elicit T-cell responses, and thus they fail to trigger isotype switching and nucleotide substitutions in V-region sequences. Because the Abs elicited by these Ags have V regions with unmutated germ-line sequences, their intrinsic affinity for the repeating epitope is low (typically 10^4 to 10^5 L/M for a hap-

tenic group; see Chapter 13) and does not increase with time. Without T-cell participation and without memory effects, a second injection of these Ags elicits the same response as the first.

Why do T cells not respond to polysaccharides and other T-independent Ags? One possibility is that mammalian tissues lack enzymes for degrading these large polymers; another is that fragments (if produced) do not bind to MHC proteins. Abs generally have lower affinity for oligosaccharides than for proteins or peptides or aromatic haptens (Chapter 13), suggesting that polysaccharide Ags (or their fragments) are bound very poorly by MHC proteins and by Ag-specific receptors on T cells.

Although the response to a purified bacterial polysaccharide Ag amounts essentially to a protracted form of the transient primary response to a protein Ag, the Abs that are elicited can confer considerable protection against pneumococcal infections because bacteria coated with these Abs and with complement (see Chapter 17) have greatly enhanced susceptibility to be phagocytosed and destroyed by leukocytes. Hence, the elderly and other individuals at high risk for pneumonia infection are immunized with mixtures of purified type-specific pneumococcal polysaccharides, each from a prevalent pathogen (see Vaccination against Microbial Antigens, Appendix, this chapter).

Although purified polysaccharides elicit only limited IgM Ab responses, the same Ag in association with protein, as in pneumococcal cells or in vaccines prepared from killed bacteria, can elicit much more vigorous anti-polysaccharide responses, including the production of IgG Abs. The bacterial proteins probably act here as "carriers" and elicit cooperating T_H-cell responses. Under these circumstances, some bacterial polysaccharides can elicit enormous Ab responses (e.g., rabbits making up to 20 mg of Ab per ml of serum), as though B cells can

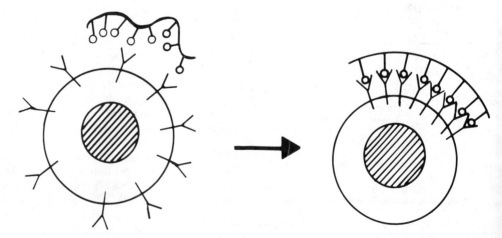

Figure 16–3. Multivalent binding of a T-independent Ag to surface immunoglobulin on a B cell can trigger limited cell proliferation and secretion of immunoglobulin.

make extraordinarily vigorous responses to the combined effects of lymphokines plus multivalent binding of Ag. As we shall see later (Vaccination against Microbial Antigens, below), in a recently introduced, highly effective vaccine against a polysaccharide from *Haemophilus influenzae*, the purified polysaccharide is chemically linked, like a hapten, to diphtheria toxoid, which serves as carrier protein: the resulting antipolysaccharide Abs are expected to have the properties of Abs elicited by a T-dependent Ag (H-chain isotype switching, higher affinity).

B-Cell Development

B cells develop from stem cells into Ig-secreting cells in two stages (Fig. 16–4). In the first, **Ag-independent, stage,** mammalian B cells develop in the fetal liver or adult bone marrow from stem cells into **virgin B cells,** which have surface IgM molecules. These cells migrate to the spleen and lymph nodes, where a cognate Ag can trigger the second, or **Ag-dependent, stage.** As described earlier, the second stage involves the proliferation and differentiation of the B cell into memory B cells and into Ig-secreting B lymphoblasts and plasma cells.

Normally, B cells do not grow and differentiate in culture, and little would be understood about their development were not B-cell tumors also available for study. Arrested at a fixed stage in the normal developmental pathway, each of these tumors is an immortalized clone that can be grown in culture or by animal passage. Many of them arise spontaneously: for instance, B-cell lymphomas (which grow *in vivo* as masses of malignant B cells) and B-cell leukemias (which grow *in vivo* as both massed and dispersed cells) correspond to virgin or memory B cells or B lymphoblasts (see below); and myeloma tu-

mors (also termed plasma cell tumors or plasmacytomas) are similar to normal plasma cells in appearance and in their ability to synthesize and secrete Ig molecules at an enormous rate.

Even more valuable are the tumor cell lines that are produced deliberately with the Abelson murine leukemia virus (A-MuLV, a replication-defective retrovirus). Specific for the immature B cells that abound in fetal liver and adult bone marrow of mice, this oncogenic virus transforms these cells in culture into tumor cell clones that correspond to pre-B and even earlier stages in B-cell development. In culture, some of these cell lines can continue to undergo normal differentiation events, including the rearrangement of Ig-gene segments and the recombination (switching) of H-chain genes. As will be seen below, these cells have shown that rearrangement of Ig-gene segments occurs in a highly regulated sequence.

TEMPORAL ORDER OF Ig-GENE SEGMENT REARRANGEMENTS

As described in Chapter 14, each of the Ig-gene V-region segments is flanked by a **recognition sequence** that consists of a **heptamer** that abuts directly on the joining end of the encoding sequence of each V, D, and J segment and a **nonamer,** with a **spacer** region between them. Both the heptamer and the nonamer have extremely conserved nucleotide sequences; the sequence of the spacer is not conserved, but its length is fixed at either 12 ($\pm$1) or 23 ($\pm$1) base pairs. According to the 12–23 spacer rule (see Chap. 14, Fig. 14–32), **only Ig-gene segments with dissimilar spacers can be joined.** The joining of two segments is termed **productive** when their translational reading frame is preserved (i.e., in-frame) and **nonproductive** when it is out-of-frame. With

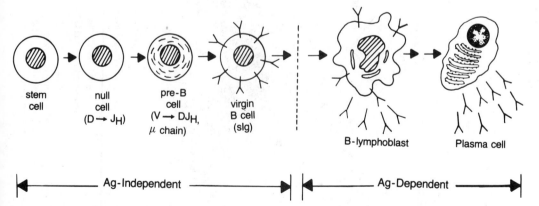

Figure 16–4. B-cell lineage. The Ag-independent steps occur in central organs (fetal liver, adult bone marrow in mammals; bursa of Fabricius in birds), whereas the Ag-triggered stage takes place in the periphery (spleen, lymph nodes, mucosa of intestines and respiratory tract, etc.). sIg in the virgin B cell is surface membrane Ig (mIg).

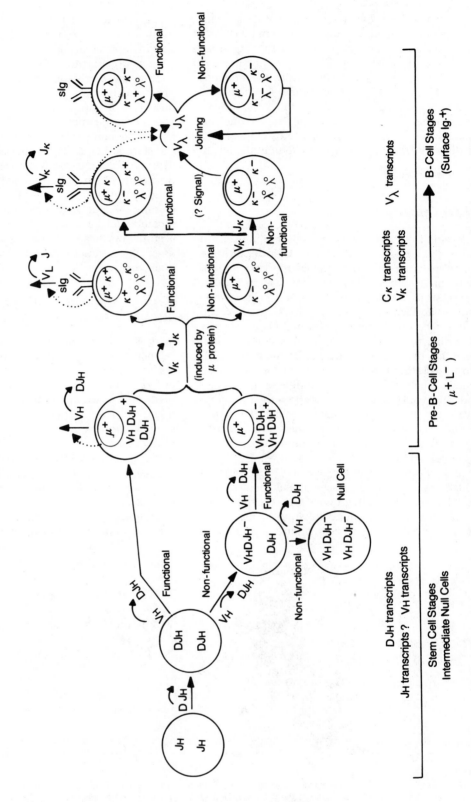

Figure 16–5. A model for allelic exclusion based on sequential regulated gene-segment rearrangement. 0, −, + superscripts refer, respectively, to unrearranged, nonproductively rearranged, and productively rearranged gene segments. **Dotted arrows** represent negative signals terminating further rearrangement of the indicated gene segments. Transcripts of unrearranged V_H, V_κ, V_λ, and C_κ gene segments, and of DJ_H, are indicated to suggest the accessibility of these segments to rearrangement. (Based on Yancopoulos GD, Alt FW: Annu Rev Immunol 4:339, 1986)

three nucleotides per codon and a random joining process, two out of three joins are expected to be nonproductive; the sequences downstream of such joins are marked by frequent nonsense (chain-terminating) codons.

The progressive development of B cells through the B lineage is marked by a series of Ig-gene segment rearrangements. The earliest recognizable cell in the lineage—termed a **null cell** because it lacks the distinctive markers of B or T cells—has the D $\rightarrow$ J$_H$ rearrangement, usually at both of its H-chain loci. Nonproductive DJ$_H$ assemblies are common, but they can be replaced by productive ones by joining an upstream D to a downstream J$_H$ and deleting the intervening out-of-frame DJ$_H$. (However, a nonproductive VDJ$_H$ cannot be similarly replaced, and a cell with two such nonproductive rearrangements cannot continue to develop: because such abortive B cells are not normally seen, they probably do not survive very long.)

Once a productive V$_H$–D–J$_H$ assembly is formed, the corresponding μ chain is synthesized, but it cannot be expressed on the cell's surface until it is paired with an L chain: in such **pre-B cells,** μ chains accumulate in the cytoplasm (see Fig. 16–4), where they appear to provide the signal for ceasing further rearrangements of H-chain gene segments and for beginning rearrangements of κ-chain gene segments (Fig. 16–5).

Once a productive V$_\kappa$ $\rightarrow$ J$_\kappa$ join occurs, κ chains are synthesized: they pair with μ chains, and the Ig ($\mu\kappa$) molecules become anchored in the cell membrane, yielding virgin B cells in which further Ig-gene segment rearrangements cease. If, however, a cell has two out-of-frame V$_\kappa$–J$_\kappa$ joins, its V$_\lambda$ gene segments undergo rearrangement. Because of this sequence, a B cell that produces a κ-containing Ig will have one or two V$_\kappa$–J$_\kappa$ rearrangements (if two, one is nonproductive), but it will have no V$_\lambda$–J$_\lambda$ rearrangements. In contrast, a B cell that produces a λ-containing Ig usually has two nonproductive V$_\kappa$–J$_\kappa$ joins, and perhaps one nonproductive V$_\lambda$–J$_\lambda$, in addition to its productive V$_\lambda$–J$_\lambda$ rearrangement (Fig. 16–5).

EXPRESSION OF Ig GENES IN IMMATURE AND MATURE B CELLS

As described in Chapter 14, each of the hundreds of V$_H$ gene segments in a B cell has a transcription-promoter region at the 5′ end of its encoding sequence. But in a mature B cell, the only transcriptionally active H-chain promoter is the one associated with the productive V$_H$DJ$_H$ assembly: the others, being too distant from the H-chain gene enhancer (located in the intron between J$_H$ and Cμ), are silent (see Chap. 14, Fig. 14–37). (Transfection of diverse cells with the H-chain enhancer linked to a marker gene has shown that this **enhancer is tissue-**specific; that is, **it is active only in B cells, evidently because only they produce the DNA-binding proteins that react specifically with it.)**

Despite the powerful effect of this enhancer, some enhancer-deficient B-cell lines can be stimulated by bacterial lipopolysaccharide (LPS) to express the enhancer-less H-chain gene, suggesting that there are additional enhancer sequences for H-chain genes. These auxiliary enhancers could account for the low-level transcription of unrearranged V$_H$-gene segments in immature B cells; the transcripts have an intact leader sequence, indicating that they can be translated, but whether the resulting truncated "V$_H$ polypeptides" have any function in the developing B cell is not clear. D-gene segments also have transcriptional promoters on their upstream (5′) side, and in some immature cells of the B lineage, DJ$_H$ assemblies yield mRNA and even short polypeptide "Dμ" chains.

Ig-SECRETING CELLS: B LYMPHOBLASTS AND PLASMA CELLS

Of all B cells, the Ig-secreting ones are the most mature. Their identity and morphology is evident on examining the cells that form clear areas of hemolysis ("plaques", Fig. 16–6) when spleen or lymph node cells from mice immunized with sheep red blood cells (SRBCs) are plated in agar with SRBCs and complement (see Chapter 17). The plaques (resembling those formed by lytic bacteriophage on a lawn of susceptible bacteria) have an Ab-secreting (plaque-forming) cell in the center (Fig. 16–6).

When cells from spleen and lymph nodes are sampled a few days after antigenic stimulation, the plaque-forming cells are **lymphoblasts;** when sampled later, they are **plasma cells.** The lymphoblasts are much larger than resting B cells and have abundant ribosome-rich cytoplasm (Fig. 16–7). The Igs they produce reflect their transitional status between resting B cells and plasma cells: thus, some of their Ig molecules have transmembrane and cytoplasmic domains and are anchored in the cell membrane (mIg), whereas others, with a shortened C terminus, are secreted (sIg) (see Chap. 14, Fig. 14–39). In contrast, plasma cells have the distinctive appearance of cells that are specialized to secrete large amounts of protein: their cytoplasm is loaded with lamellae of rough endoplasmic reticulum (Fig. 16–7), and virtually all of the Ig they synthesize is of the secreted form (sIg).

Whereas plaque-forming lymphoblasts produce sIg and mIg, other B lymphoblasts produce only mIg. This diversity is mirrored in human B-cell tumors: each B-cell lymphoma has a distinctive mIg, but some also secrete the Ig, which appears in the serum as a monoclonal protein (usually IgM) at low concentration (e.g., 0.1 mg per ml). In contrast, plasma-cell tumors have little or no detectable mIg and secrete enormous amounts of sIg,

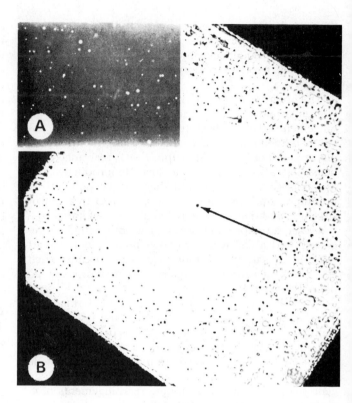

Figure 16–6. Hemolytic plaque assay for Ab-producing cells. *(A)* Multiple pin-head size circular areas of hemolysis ("plaques") in a Petri dish. (Courtesy of Dr. L. Claflin) (about ×15) *(B)* Single plaque with its central Ab-secreting cell **(arrow).** Representative plaque-forming cells (PFCs) are shown in Fig. 16–7.

with the monoclonal Ig (called a **myeloma protein;** see Chapter 14) attaining serum levels as high as 50 mg per ml.

Nearly all resting B cells, in tissues and blood, have mIgM, and only a small proportion (<10%) have mIgG. However, IgG is about 10 times more abundant in serum than IgM. The disparity suggests that once activated B cells switch to production of IgG, they differentiate rapidly into lymphoblasts and then into plasma cells. Plasma cells are terminally differentiated: they appear not to divide and to survive for only a few days; hence, in an ongoing Ab response to an Ag, these cells have to be continuously replenished by activated, differentiating B cells. B cells with surface IgA or IgE are found in substantial numbers primarily in association with exocrine glands of intestine, lungs, etc. (see Chapter 14), perhaps because T_H cells in these locations are predominantly those that produce the required lymphokines (see IL-4, IL-5, and T_H2 cells, above).

SYNTHESIS, ASSEMBLY, AND SECRETION OF Igs

Like secreted proteins in general, Igs are synthesized on polyribosomes attached to the rough endoplasmic reticulum. The chains are formed as larger precursors, with an additional N-terminal sequence of about 20 amino acids (the **leader**) that is cleaved in the course of transfer across the membrane into the lumen of the endoplasmic reticulum (see Leader, Chapter 14). The newly synthesized Ig molecules are secreted from the cells after a 20- to 30-min lag (Fig. 16–8), during which they pass through cisternae of the endoplasmic reticulum, traverse the Golgi apparatus, and then move toward the cell surface in secretory vesicles, which fuse with the surface membrane and release their Ig molecules. During this migration, the completed chains are assembled into molecules, the interchain S–S bonds are formed, and sugars are added successively by hexosetransferases to form the oligosaccharide groups of complete Ig molecules (Fig. 16–9).

The order of chain assembly has been studied primarily in myeloma tumors, in which various patterns have been deduced from the variety of incompletely assembled molecules found intracellularly. Complete molecules are usually made by joining two H–L half-molecules or by adding one L chain at a time to H-chain dimers (H_2). Interchain S–S bonds form slowly (2–20 min after the constituent chains are completed). In myeloma cells that make the polymeric IgA or IgM, the intracellular Ig seems not to progress beyond the four-chain monomer, although polymers are found in the culture

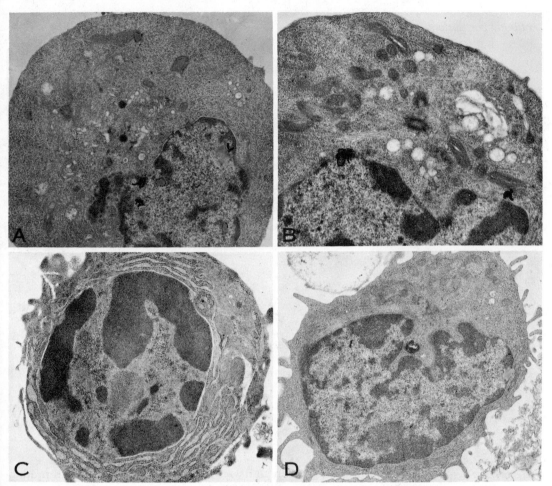

Figure 16–7. Electron micrographs of representative Ab-secreting cells (hemolytic plaque-forming cells, PFCs, as in Fig. 16–6). Cells in *A, B,* and *C* are from lymph nodes and spleen; the one in *D* is from efferent lymph emerging from an antigenically stimulated lymph node. Most PFCs from within lymph nodes and spleen are plasma cells *(C)*, except during the first few days after immunization when lymphoblasts *(A, B, D)* predominate. *(A* and *B,* Gudat FG et al: J Exp Med 134:1155, 1971; *C,* Gudat FG et al: J Exp Med 132:448, 1970; *D,* Hummeler K et al: J Exp Med 135:491, 1972)

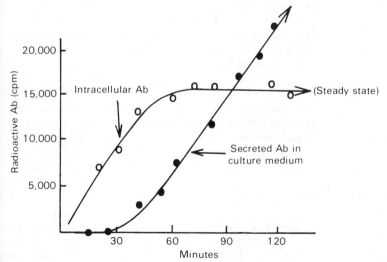

Figure 16–8. Lag in secretion of Abs. Labeled amino acid was added at zero time to a suspension of lymph node cells from an immunized rabbit, and cells and supernatant fluid were then assayed at intervals for newly synthesized Abs. (Based on Helmreich E et al: J Biol Chem 236:464, 1961)

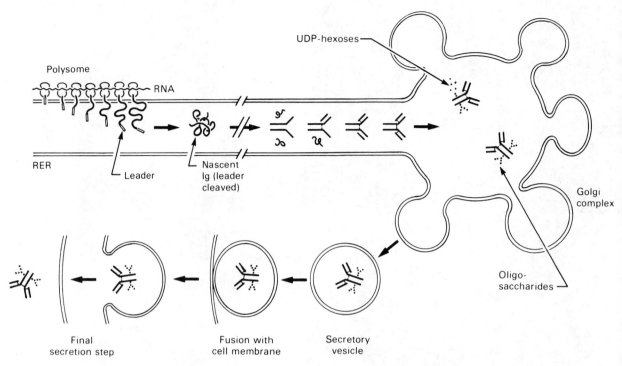

Figure 16–9. Secretion of Ig by a plasma cell. RER = rough endoplasmic reticulum with bound ribosomes. The diagram shows the secreted form of the Ig. In B cells or B lymphoblasts, the Ig has modified and extended C-terminal regions (transmembrane and cytoplasmic domains) that anchor it in the membrane of RER and, ultimately, in the cell's surface membrane. (Note that the leader marks the N-terminus of the growing Ig chain.)

medium. Evidently, the monomers associate with each other and with J chains (which are made in the same cells; see Chapter 14) as Ig molecules are secreted.

DEVELOPMENT OF THE B-CELL REPERTOIRE

How many different B-cell clones does an individual have? Total Ig, normally about 10 mg per ml of serum, is a pool of the Igs produced by the body's activated B-cell clones. Because prior to immunization with any particular Ag, the serum Abs that react with that Ag are usually below the level of detection, about 10^{-6} mg per ml of serum, it has long seemed evident that more than 10^7 different Abs are present in the serum pool, indicating that there are more than 10^7 B-cell clones.

A more direct estimate is provided by the **splenic focus assay,** in which a pool of mouse spleen B cells is injected intravenously into a lethally irradiated mouse. The recipient's spleen is removed the next day and cut up into many fragments, each of which is then cultured in a separate well along with an Ag. Because the recipients were irradiated, their own B lymphocytes cannot respond to the Ag, but the irradiated T cells can provide helper activity if the recipient was primed with the Ag before irradiation.

A single Ag-stimulated B cell can, with T-cell help,

yield in 10 days over 1000 daughter cells, each producing up to 20,000 Ig molecules per minute (see Lymphoblasts and Plasma Cells, above). Hence, a fragment containing one responsive B cell to start with can secrete enough Ab in 10 days to allow its characterization (Ag binding, H- and L-chain type, etc.). All the Ab molecules produced by an active fragment appear to have the same Ag-binding sites (idiotype) and hence probably come from one clone.

The number of fragments (clones) that produce Abs to Ag X divided by the number of B cells that have lodged in the spleen (estimated with radiolabeled cells) provides a measure of the frequency of anti-X B cells. The number of different B cells seems to be on the order of 10^7 in the adult mouse. For instance, about one B cell in 10,000 can make anti-Dnp Abs. Because independent estimates suggest that there are about 1000 different anti-Dnp Abs (distinguishable by isoelectric focusing electrophoresis), and each is presumably the product of a distinctive clone, the frequency of any particular anti-Dnp B cell is about 1 in 10^7. Roughly similar values have been found for B cells to some other epitopes.

SEQUENTIAL DEVELOPMENT. It has generally been assumed that V-gene segments rearrange randomly (to DJ_H or J_L gene segments; Chapter 14). Nevertheless, respon-

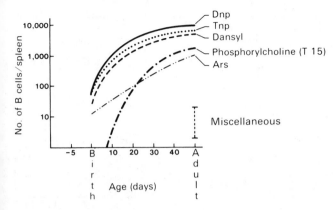

Figure 16–10. B-cell repertoire in the spleen of mice of various ages. B cells that react specifically with the haptens shown were counted by the splenic focus assay (this Ch.). (Based on Klinman NR et al: Cold Spring Harbor Symp Quant Biol 41:165, 1977)

TABLE 16–3. Placental Structure and Mode of Passive Transfer of Immunoglobulins to the Fetus*

Species	No. of Tissue Layers Between Maternal and Fetal Circulation at Term	Placental or Amniotic Transmission	Importance of Transmission Via Colostrum
Pig	6	–	+++
Ruminants	5	–	+++
Carnivores	3	±	+
Rodents	2	+ (yolk sac)	+
Man	2	+++ (placenta)	–

* In chickens, and presumably in other birds, β-globulins containing Abs are transmitted from hen to egg via follicular epithelium and are stored in the yolk sac, from which the proteins are absorbed into the fetal circulation shortly before hatching. (Good RA, Papermaster BW: Adv Immunol 4:1 1964; based on Vahlquist B: Adv Pediat 10:305, 1958)

siveness to some Ags appears at different times during development. For instance, the developing fetal lamb can respond to ferritin after 1 month's gestation and to diphtheria toxin a few months later, at the time of birth; and in the mouse, anti-Dnp B cells appear at the time of birth and anti-phosphorylcholine B cells about 7 days later (Fig. 16–10). Accordingly, the increase in size of the repertoire, from about 10^4 different clones in the newborn mouse to about 10^7 shortly afterward (Fig. 16–10), may result from a programmed developmental process rather than from stimulation by haphazardly encountered environmental Ags. Thus, in developing B cells in the fetal liver of the mouse, those V_H-gene segments closest to D-gene segments are the first to join DJ_H segments (see Ch. 14, Fig. 14–31).

SERUM IMMUNOGLOBULINS IN THE HUMAN NEWBORN

Although synthesis of Igs can be detected in mammalian fetuses, protective levels of Abs to common pathogens are not produced until some time after birth. The newborn would thus be vulnerable to many infections were it not for the maternal Abs it receives before or shortly after birth. In some species, the offspring receives these Abs only from colostrum, which is usually rich in IgA and IgG; in others, the Igs are transferred also *in utero* (Table 16–3).

In man and in higher primates, absorption from colostrum is probably of minor importance compared with transfer across the placenta. Maternal IgG, but not IgM, IgA, or IgE, is transmitted freely to the human fetus *in utero*, suggesting selective transport. Special sites on the Fc domain are evidently required: in rabbits, Fc fragments of γ chains are transferred as readily as intact IgG molecules and much more rapidly than Fab fragments.

Because of the selective transport, the newborn infant's blood contains high levels of IgG with the allotypes of the mother (Chapter 14), traces of IgM of fetal origin, and essentially no IgA. The IgG (and total Ig) declines until about 8 to 10 weeks of age, when it starts to rise as the neonate's biosynthesis becomes sufficiently active. Adult serum levels of IgM are reached at about 10 months of age, of IgG at about 4 years, of IgA at about 9 to 10 years, and of IgE at about 10 to 15 years (Figs. 16–11 and 16–12).

Tolerance

That immune responses are not made against self-Ags has been appreciated at least since 1900, when Ehrlich introduced the term **horror autotoxicus** to indicate that **one can form Abs to almost any substance except components of one's own tissues.** This discrimination is clearly evident in the cross-immunizations, described in preceding chapters, between mice of different congenic strains: **a mouse makes Abs to alloantigens that it lacks but not to those that it possesses.**

The occasional breakdown of this **self-tolerance** can result in serious autoimmune diseases (Chapter 20). Conversely, under certain conditions a foreign Ag acts as a **tolerogen,** establishing a state in which the later introduction of that Ag, even in optimally immunogenic form, fails to elicit Abs or T cells; study of these conditions has revealed some of the mechanisms that probably contribute to self-tolerance.

NATURAL TOLERANCE TO SELF-ANTIGENS

Most self-Ags are proteins and are therefore expected to be T dependent. Although unresponsiveness of either

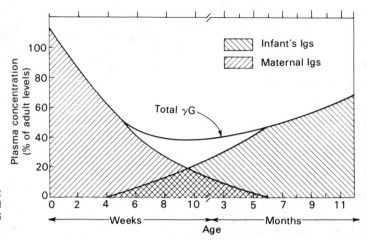

Figure 16–11. Changing plasma levels of Igs in the human infant during the first year. Maternal IgG, which accounts for almost all the infant's Igs at birth, has essentially disappeared by about 6 months. (Based on Gitlin D: Pediatrics 34:198, 1964)

the cognate B or T cells could account for the failure to produce Abs to these Ags, it appears that T cells are primarily responsible. Consider, for example, a pair of congenic mice that differ only in the gene for one of the complement serum proteins, complement factor 5, or C5 (see Chapter 17). In response to injected C5, Abs are produced by mice of the C5⁻ strain, which lack the gene and the protein, but not by those of the C5⁺ strain, which produce C5 and are tolerant of it. When irradiated C5⁻ mice receive B and T cells in various combinations from the two strains (see Adoptive Transfer of Immune Cells, Chapter 15) their production of Abs in response to injected C5 showed that C5⁺ mice **lack C5-responsive T cells, but they have B cells that are capable of making Abs to C5. In C5⁻ mice, both the T and the B cells can respond to C5.**

DELETION OF T CELLS THAT REACT WITH SELF-AGS. As described in Chapter 15, T cells that can respond to self-MHC proteins, or to other self-Ags that associate with self-MHC, seem to be purged from the body's pool of T cells as these cells mature in the thymus. It is thus possible that as C5 protein circulates in C5⁺ mice, it is taken up by APC in the thymus and presented to thymocytes as peptide fragments in association with MHC-II protein: the immature double-positive (CD4⁺,CD8⁺) T cells that recognized these complexes are then somehow destroyed. Whether the many noncirculating self-Ags found normally in cells of heart, adrenal, or muscle, etc., also find their way to the thymus to eliminate the corresponding developing T cells is not clear. This issue is considered further in connection with autoimmune diseases (Chapter 20).

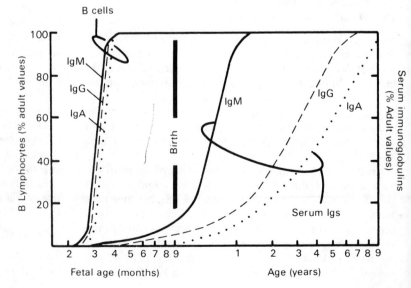

Figure 16–12. Maturation of B cells and serum Ig levels in man. With both cells and their secreted products, the ontogenetic order (IgM, IgG, IgA) recapitulates the presumptive evolutionary sequence of their appearance. (Based on Cooper MD, Lawton AR: Am J Pathol 69:513, 1972, from data of Lawton AR et al: Clin Immunol Immunopathol 1:104, 1972)

B-CELL TOLERANCE. In the model system described above, it is clear that although C5⁺ mice lack anti-C5 T cells and are thus solidly tolerant of C5, their cognate (anti-C5) B cells are perfectly capable of making anti-C5 Abs, at least when transferred with the proper T cells into (irradiated) mice. But are these B cells perfectly normal as they reside in the C5⁺ animal? Probably not, according to evidence provided by transgenic mice. These mice develop from fertilized ova that have been inoculated with a foreign gene (a "transgene") that becomes integrated into the cell's genome. When the transgene encodes hen's egg lysozyme (HEL), the resulting mice produce this protein. In other transgenic mice, carrying transgenes that encode H and L chains of Abs to HEL, a high proportion of the B cells produce these Ags constitutively; that is, without the mice having to be immunized against HEL. In hybrids made by mating transgenic mice that make HEL with those that make Abs to HEL, the HEL continued to be produced, but the B cells that make anti-HEL were altered: they had IgD on their surface, not IgM, and they did not secrete anti-HEL Abs. Thus, although the B cells that can make Abs to self-Ags are not physically eliminated, as are the corresponding T cells, they probably exist in an "anergic" or paralyzed state in the tolerant individual. However, as indicated below, when T_H-cell activity is provided, the anergic B cells can evidently change and respond normally to antigenic stimulation.

EXPERIMENTAL ABROGATION OF SELF-TOLERANCE. Despite tolerance of self-Ags, individuals sometimes produce Abs that react or cross-react with them (Chapter 20). These **autoreactive** Abs can be elicited experimentally by administering a self-Ag in a modified form, having some epitopes that are shared with the original Ag and others that are not. The persistence of cognate B cells (see above) provides an explanation. If the new epitopes are foreign, they can engage T_H cells and thereby help stimulate quiescent B cells that are specific for the original Ag. An example is seen in animals with natural tolerance to their own thyroglobulin (Tg): when immunized with denatured Tg, they produce Abs that react with native Tg (Fig. 16–13). Autoimmunity to self-Ags is discussed further in Chapter 20.

INDUCED TOLERANCE TO FOREIGN ANTIGENS. Many of the substances (soluble proteins, polysaccharides, haptenic groups, etc.) that elicit Ab formation can be administered under conditions that establish tolerance. As with other immune responses, **induced tolerance is specific and is directed to particular epitopes.** For instance, rabbits made unresponsive to the Fc fragment of human IgG can still respond to immunization with intact IgG, but they then form Abs only to Fab domains. Broadly speaking, tolerance and immunity are alternative responses. The circumstances under which tolerance is induced to foreign Ags are described later (see Appendix, this chapter). In general, the intravenous injection of high doses of soluble Ag in monomeric form tends to establish unresponsiveness to that Ag, whereas the subcutaneous, intramuscular, or intraperitoneal injection of the Ag in aggregated form enhances its immunogenicity.

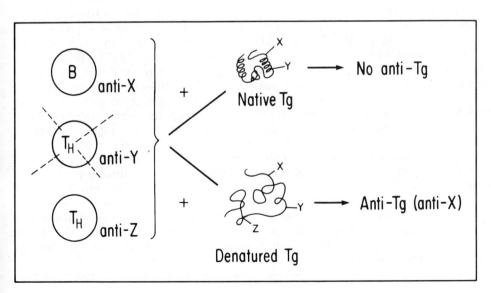

Figure 16–13. Abrogation of tolerance to a self-Ag (thyroglobulin, *Tg*). Native Tg has epitope X (recognized by anti-X B cells) and epitope Y (recognized by anti-Y T_H cells). Because anti-T_H cells are eliminated as they arise in the thymus, the B cells do not respond to Tg, and Abs to Tg are normally not made. However, altered or denatured Tg *(dTg)* exposes a new T-cell epitope (Z) while retaining epitope X; hence, the anti-X B cells can produce Abs that react with native Tg.

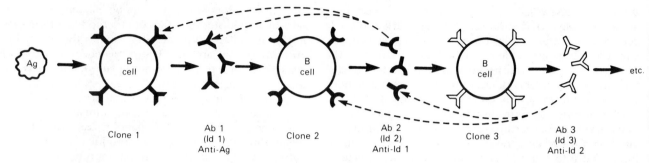

Figure 16–14. Schematic representation of a possible idiotype/anti-idiotype network. The Ag elicits Ab no. 1, which elicits Ab no. 2 directed to the idiotype (Id) of Ab no. 1. Besides stimulating or suppressing the clone that produces Ab no. 1, Ab no. 2 (anti-Id no. 1) elicits Ab no. 3, which is specific for the Id of Ab no. 2 and which can stimulate (or suppress) the clone producing Ab no. 2, as well as elicit Ab no. 4, specific for the Id of Ab no. 3 (etc.).
    The combining site of Ab no. 2 is said to be an **internal image** of an epitope of the Ag, because both are bound specifically and competitively by Ab no. 1. (Based on Jerne NK: Ann Immunol (Paris) 125:373, 1974) (see also Fig. 14–18, p 57.)

ID/ANTI-ID REACTIONS AND REGULATION OF B-CELL RESPONSES

Although Ags and lymphokines are the principal substances that control the proliferation of B cells and their differentiation into Ig-secreting cells, it has been suggested that additional "fine-tuning" controls are exercised by various regulatory circuits. One of these is based on the notion that T cells with suppressor activity can turn off B-cell responses. Another derives from Jerne's proposal that the immune system is a network formed by interactions between the combining sites (idiotypes) of some Igs (Ids) and the complementary (antiidiotype) combining sites of other Igs (anti-Ids). For instance, introduction of an Ag into the body elicits Ab no. 1 whose Id, acting as a surrogate Ag, elicits another Ab, no. 2, whose combining site is complementary (anti-Id) to the combining site of Ab no. 1. Besides stimulating (or suppressing) the clone that produces Ab no. 1, Ab no. 2 elicits still another Ab (Ab no. 3), which is specific for the Id of Ab no. 2 and which can stimulate (or suppress) the clone producing Ab no. 2, as well as elicit Ab no. 4, etc. (Fig. 16–14).

Panels of B-cell hybridomas from immunized mice have not yielded the Abs predicted by the hypothesis (Abs no. 2, 3, etc.), indicating that an Id/anti-Id network probably does not operate in normal immune responses. However, panels of B-cell hybridomas prepared from fetal liver have yielded pairs of hybridomas whose Igs interact as would an Id with an anti-Id. If mutually stimulatory, such interacting Id/anti-Id pairs may be responsible for maintaining the B cells that produce some "**natural Abs**"; these Abs are capable of reacting (or cross-reacting) with certain Ags in the absence of known immunization against them.

Appendix

FACTORS INFLUENCING ANTIBODY PRODUCTION IN THE WHOLE ANIMAL

The amounts and types of Abs formed vary widely with the conditions of immunization, some of which are reviewed in this section.

Route of Administration of Antigen

Natural Immunization. Lymphatic tissues are probably bombarded almost constantly with Ags from transiently invasive or indigenous microbes (normal flora of skin, intestines, etc.) and by those that enter the body by inhalation (e.g., plant pollens), by ingestion (e.g., foods, drugs), and by penetration of the skin (e.g., catechols of poison ivy plants). The resulting stimulation is probably responsible for the familiar histologic appearance of lymph nodes and spleen, for the normal concentration of Igs in serum (about 15 mg/ml), and perhaps also for **natural Abs**—those Igs that react or cross-react (one cannot be sure which) with Ags that have not been known to serve as immunogens in the individual under test. Animals reared under **germ-free** conditions synthesize Igs at about 1/500 the normal rate, have **exceedingly low serum Ig levels** (especially of IgG), and have small, poorly developed lymph nodes and spleen.

Deliberate Immunization. For this purpose, immunogens are usually injected into skin (intradermally or subcutaneously) or muscle, depending on the volume injected and the irritancy of the immunogen. Regardless of the route, most Ags eventually become distributed widely throughout the body via lymphatic and vascular channels.

Because most Ags are degraded in the intestines,

feeding is effective only under special circumstances, such as with attenuated poliomyelitis vaccine, which can invade the intestinal wall. Allergic responses to food are probably attributable to Ags that resist degradation by intestinal enzymes. **Inhalation** can also be used, such as aerosol administration of attenuated strains of *Pasteurella tularensis*. **Preferential synthesis of IgA Abs** occurs when immunogens are introduced into the respiratory or intestinal tract, many of whose B cells are committed to produce Igs of this class.

Adjuvants

The immunogenicity of soluble proteins is enhanced if they persist in tissues; for example, repeated small injections of diphtheria toxoid evoke a greater Ab response than the same total amount of toxoid given as a single injection. Accordingly, a widely used procedure involves the administration of inorganic gels (e.g., alum, aluminum hydroxide, or aluminum phosphate) with adsorbed, slowly released proteins. The term **adjuvant** is applied to any substance whose admixture with an injected immunogen increases the response.

The most effective adjuvants are the water-in-oil emulsions developed by Freund, particularly those in which living or dead mycobacteria are suspended (**complete Freund's adjuvant**). After a single subcutaneous or intramuscular injection (e.g., 0.5 ml in a rabbit), droplets of emulsion metastasize widely from the site of injection; Ab formation, detected as early as 4 or 5 days later, may continue for 8 or 9 months or longer (Fig. 16–15).

The intense, chronic inflammation around the deposits of emulsion precludes their use in man. However, emulsions without mycobacteria (**incomplete Freund's adjuvant**) are less irritating and have been used clinically; their enhancing effect is also less than that of complete Freund's adjuvant.

The adjuvant activity of the mycobacteria is due largely to a complex glycolipid, whose activity has been duplicated by a small, synthesized glycopeptide, **muramyl dipeptide** (MDP): (N-acetyl-muramyl-L-alanyl-D-isoglutamine). Like intact mycobacteria, this peptide also elicits local inflammation and causes fever, but a synthetic variant, with threonine in place of alanine (Fig. 16–16), is reported to have fewer side effects while retaining the adjuvant activity.

Most adjuvants act not only by increasing Ag persistence, but also by somehow **increasing macrophage and T_H activities.** Some other adjuvants are killed *Bordetella pertussis*, the lipopolysaccharide (LPS) of gram-negative bacteria, and large polymeric anions (e.g., dextran sulfate). A few adjuvants (LPS, dextran sulfate) are **polyclonal B-cell activators;** that is, they stimulate most B cells to proliferate and sometimes even to secrete IgM. Some adjuvants affect the Ab isotype, probably by affecting the subset of the T_H cells they stimulate (see Lymphokines, above). Thus, protein Ags adsorbed onto precipitated alum tend to elicit Abs of the IgG1 class.

Dose

Humans are normally injected (subcutaneously or intramuscularly) with relative small amounts of Ag; for example, about 10 μg of inactivated influenza virus vaccine. With widely used vaccines (see Table 16–4, below), this dose is sufficient to elicit protective Ab levels (although probably only a few μg of Ab per ml of serum). However, to raise large amounts of Abs, experimental animals are commonly injected with much larger doses, such as 0.1 to 1.0 mg of an Ag into a rabbit or 100 μg into a mouse. In

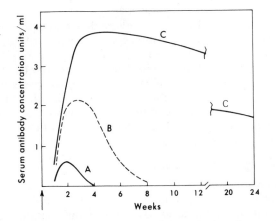

Figure 16–15. Influence of adjuvants: Schematic view of amounts of Ab produced by rabbits in response to one injection **(arrow)** of a soluble protein such as bovine γ-globulin in dilute salt solution *(A)*, adsorbed on precipitated alum *(B)*, or incorporated in a water-in-oil emulsion containing mycobacteria (Freund's complete adjuvant, *C*).

TABLE 16–4. Some Vaccines Commonly Used To Prevent Infectious Diseases in Man

Diphtheria	Diphtheria toxoid	⎫ injected
Tetanus	Tetanus toxoid	⎬ together
Pertussis	*Bordetella pertussis* (killed)	⎭
Poliomyelitis	Poliovirus (attentuated or killed)	
Measles	Measles virus (attenuated)	⎫ injected
Mumps	Mumps virus (attenuated)	⎬ together
Rubella	Rubella virus (attenuated)	⎭
Pneumococcal pneumonia	Mixture of purified capsular polysaccharides from the 12–14 most prevalent types of *Streptococcus pneumoniae*	
Haemophilus influenzae type b (infectious meningitis, septic arthritis, epiglottitis, etc.)	Purified capsular polysaccharide (Hib) given alone or as conjugate with diphtheria toxoid	
Influenza	Influenza virus (killed)	
Rabies	Rabies virus (killed)	

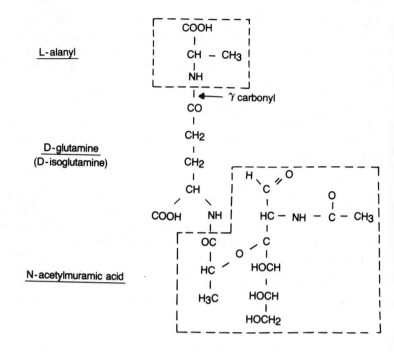

L-alanyl

D-glutamine
(D-isoglutamine)

N-acetylmuramic acid

γ carbonyl

N-acetylmuramyl-L-alanyl-D-isoglutamine
(muramyl dipeptide = MDP)

Figure 16–16. Structure of muramyl dipeptide (MDP): N-acetylmuramyl-L-alanyl-D-isoglutamine, the key component in the mycobacteria of Freund's complete adjuvant.

general, less Ag is required for previously primed than for immunologically "virgin" ("naive") animals. Moreover, a subthreshold dose can sometimes prime animals for a pronounced secondary response without actually eliciting detectable Abs in the primary response.

Aggregated versus Soluble Form. Protein Ags are more immunogenic when administered in aggregated than in soluble form. Thus chemically cross-linked protein molecules (e.g., by gluteraldehyde) and Ag-Ab complexes, prepared in slight Ag-excess (Fig. 13–7) are usually highly immunogenic. (When, however, the complexes are prepared in Ab-excess their immunogenicity is greatly reduced, probably in part because epitopes are blocked.)

Antibody Turnover and Distribution

The level of Ab in the serum reflects the balance between rates of synthesis and degradation. When the rates are equal, the serum Ab concentration is constant (**steady state**). The rate of synthesis probably depends largely on the total number of Ab-producing cells. By contrast, the rate of degradation (expressed as half-time, or $t_{1/2}$) is determined by the H-chain class: **IgM and IgA are normally broken down much more rapidly than IgG molecules.**

However, infusion of a trace amount of ^{125}I-labeled IgG into individuals with widely differing IgG levels (from agammaglobulinemia or multiple myeloma) revealed an inverse relation between the half-time for IgG degradation and the total concentration of this Ig class: at high and low levels, the $t_{1/2}$ was about 11 and 70 days, respectively, compared with 23 days at normal levels. Injected Fab fragments and light chains disappear rapidly ($t_{1/2} < 1$ day), but the Fc fragment has the same half-life as intact IgG. Analogy with some other serum proteins suggests that shortening of oligosaccharide branches, by random removal of terminal sialic acid or other residues by blood glycosidases, makes Ig molecules susceptible to uptake by the asialoglycoprotein receptor on liver cells, with resulting internalization and degradation of the Ig.

The actual serum concentration of Ig also depends on the volume in which the molecules are distributed. The total mass of IgG is about the same in blood and in extravascular fluid, and about 25% exchanges between the two compartments each day.

Fate of Injected Antigen

Following intravenous injection of a soluble Ag, the decline in its concentration in serum exhibits three sharply distinguishable phases: (1) a brief **equilibration phase** due to rapid diffusion into the extravascular space, (2) slow **metabolic decay** during which the Ag is degraded, and (3) rapid **immune elimination,** which identifies the onset of Ab formation; during this phase, the Ag exists largely as soluble Ab–Ag complexes, which are taken up and degraded by macrophages. Free Ab appears at the end of the immune elimination stage.

Extensively phagocytized particulate Ags, such as bacteria and red cells, do not diffuse into extravascular spaces and hence do not exhibit the initial equilibration phase of rapid decrease in serum concentration after intravenous injection. Trace antigenic fragments can persist in lymphoid tissues long after the Ag is no longer detectable in blood.

Antigenic Competition. The response to an Ag may be diminished if an unrelated Ag is injected at the same time or shortly before. For instance, rabbits injected with a foreign serum (say from horse) produce Abs to serum globulin but not to serum albumin, although serum albumin alone elicits antialbumin Abs. Similarly, poly-L-alanyl-protein probably elicits Abs to the L-polypeptide, but on coimmunization with poly-D-alanyl-protein, only the latter elicits Abs to its polypeptide. This **intermolecular antigenic competition** is important in practical immunization programs (see Vaccination against Microbial Antigens, below), which often involve giving several different Ags in one vaccine. Adjusting the amounts of the several components ("balancing") can overcome the competitive effect.

Different determinants on the same molecule can also compete (**intramolecular competition**): thus a protein with both D- and L-polyalanyl peptides substituted on the same molecule evokes synthesis only of Abs to the D-polyalanyl groups. Presumably, the available cell surface receptors for the two determinants differ in affinity, and one determinant becomes dominant because the corresponding cells bind the limited supply of Ag. The mechanism for intermolecular competition is obscure.

INDUCED TOLERANCE TO FOREIGN ANTIGENS

This chapter noted earlier (see Tolerance of Self-Ags) that many foreign Ags can be administered under conditions that elicit specific unresponsiveness to that Ag, rather than Ab and T-cell responses to it. These conditions are described below.

Dose and Form of the Antigen. Every Ag has an optimal immunogenic dose range. Much larger amounts elicit tolerance ("high-zone" tolerance). With some Ags, lower amounts (repeatedly injected) can also cause tolerance ("low-zone" tolerance).

Tolerance was first induced experimentally with pneumococcal capsular polysaccharide, a T-independent Ag. Mice injected with 0.01 μg–1.0 μg of a pneumococcal polysaccharide, say of type 2, become resistant to infection with type 2 pneumococci and produce Abs to the polysaccharide, but if given 1000 μg of the same substance, they fail to become resistant or to form detectable Abs. The unresponsiveness is specific: although no response to type 2 can be elicited, the mice react normally to immunogenic doses of other Ags, including other pneumococcal polysaccharides.

Another factor with many Ags is their **physical state:** generally, aggregation enhances an Ag's immunogenicity, whereas monomeric Ags tend to be tolerogenic. **It is thus difficult or impossible to establish tolerance to many particulate Ags (viruses, bacteria, etc.),** which are usually highly immunogenic.

Route of administration is another determinant. Soluble Ags tend to be immunogenic when injected into tissues but to be tolerogenic when given intravenously.

Newborn versus Adult. In the fetus, and also shortly after birth in species where the newborn is relatively immature, tolerance is more easily established than in the adult. One reason seems to be that immature B cells are more readily made unresponsive than mature B cells because of **modulation** (see Clonal Deletion, below). As described later (Chapter 20), the effect of immaturity was first recognized by studies of foreign tissue grafts.

B Cells versus T Cells. Tolerance to **T-independent Ags** derives from unresponsiveness of the corresponding B cells, and T cells are not involved; thus T-deficient (e.g., athymic) mice are as easily made tolerant as normal mice by excessive doses of these Ags.

As noted previously (earlier, this chapter and also Chapter 15), in individuals who are naturally tolerant of a self-Ag, the cognate T cells are probably absent, whereas the corresponding B cells persist in an unresponsive state. However, when tolerance to a foreign Ag is induced experimentally, both T and B cells become unresponsive, but **T cells are made tolerant much more readily than B cells.** The difference is evident when the prospective donors of T and B cells are treated with various doses of Ag at various times before the cells are separately transferred to irradiated adoptive hosts (Fig. 16–17): compared with B cells, unresponsiveness of T cells is established sooner, lasts longer, and can be initiated by much lower levels of Ag.

How foreign Ags administered under tolerizing conditions cause inactivation (or elimination) of T cells is obscure. For B cells, the loss of cell-surface IgM may be a critical event (see IgM Modulation, above).

As noted earlier (Modulation of B-Cell Surface Ig, this chapter), the binding of a multivalent Ag (or of Ab–Ag complexes) by a B cell causes the cell's surface Ig to aggregate in the plane of the membrane. The resulting internalization (or shedding) of the aggregates leaves the cell denuded of its surface Ig and thus unresponsive to Ag until the Ig is regenerated.

In most B cells of mature mice, the modulation of surface Ig is slow (requiring about 1 h) and is seldom complete, and regeneration occurs in a few days. However, in immature B cells (from fetal or newborn mouse liver or spleen), the disappearance is more rapid and is

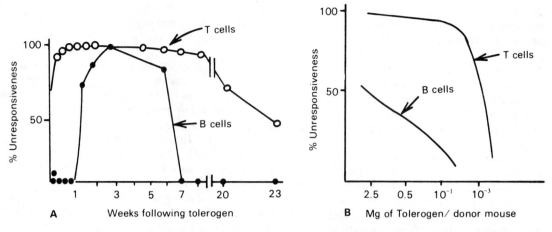

Figure 16–17. Induction of tolerance to a foreign Ag (bovine γ-globin, BγG). Thymus (T) and bone marrow (B) cells were removed at various times from mice rendered tolerant with various amounts of BγG and were tested, with complementary cells from normal donors, for the ability to cooperate in Ab formation when transferred to irradiated syngeneic mice. Results are given as percent of values in controls (untreated donors). In ***A***, tolerance was induced with 2.5 mg of BγG. In ***B***, the cells were removed 15–20 days after the doses of Ag shown (abscissa). Tolerance appeared sooner, lasted longer, and was established with lower Ag doses, in T than in B cells. (Chiller JM et al: Science 171:813, 1971)

complete, and regeneration may not occur at all. The difference suggests why experimental tolerance to foreign Ag is much more easily established in the fetus and newborn than in the adult. (The effect of immaturity on establishment of tolerance is discussed further in connection with Allograft Rejection, Chapter 20).

Persistence of Ag is necessary for the maintenance of tolerance. New B and T cells continue to be generated from stem cells, and once a tolerance-eliciting Ag disappears, responsiveness to it returns. Hence, the duration of tolerance depends on the amount of Ag injected, its rate of breakdown in tissues, and the rate at which new B and T cells of the appropriate specificity arise.

The duration of experimentally induced tolerance varies widely. Recovery is retarded by thymectomy (in the case of T-dependent Ags), and it is accelerated by the injection of lymphocytes from normally responsive syngeneic donors. Polysaccharides generally are not broken down in mammalian tissues (which lack the appropriate enzymes), and a single high dose of these Ags can establish life-long tolerance. Proteins, in contrast, are broken down readily; thus, a few weeks after tolerance to bovine serum albumin is established in mice, the declining level of Ag reaches an immunogenic range, causing a short burst of Ab (anti-BSA) synthesis.

VACCINATION AGAINST MICROBIAL ANTIGENS

Conventional vaccines are usually prepared from killed or attenuated microbes or from inactivated toxins (diphtheria and tetanus toxoids, Table 16–4): infectivity or tox-

icity is lost, while the epitopes that elicit protective Abs and/or T cells remain immunogenic. Given the effectiveness of these vaccines, the view that "Never in the history of human progress has a better or cheaper method of preventing illness been developed than immunization at its best" is probably justified. Nevertheless, serious side effects can be encountered, and although rare, they can be tragic (e.g., about 1 in 300,000 children immunized with *B. pertussis* suffers serious brain damage). To reduce these hazards and to increase immunogenicity, various strategies are used to produce new vaccines.

1. Subunit Vaccines. Some of these consist of individual viral proteins, or segments of a protein, produced by recombinant DNA technology; others consist of synthetic short peptides that encompass the epitopes that elicit protective Abs. Thus, an effective vaccine against hepatitis B virus consists of just the virus's envelope glycoprotein. In another one, a small synthetic peptide (12 amino acid residues), encompassing the key epitope of the infectious (sporozoite) form of malaria, is linked covalently to tetanus toxoid as carrier protein; Abs elicited by the conjugate protect mice against infection with malaria organisms.

2. Polysaccharide–Protein Conjugates. Vaccines consisting of purified polysaccharides from pneumococci and *Haemophilus influenzae* type b (Hib) elicit Abs that protect against infection by the corresponding bacteria. In an improved vaccine, Hib polysaccharide is linked covalently to a protein (tetanus toxoid), converting the T-independent Ag (polysaccharide alone) into a T-dependent one. The benefits are evident in young children, who are at especially high risk from infection by *H. influenzae*. With the older vaccine (polysaccharide alone), protective responses are not elicited in children below the age of about 24 months, but the Hib–tetanus toxoid conjugate elicits a high level of resistance to infection when administered to children as young as 3 to 6 months. Evidently, the expanded number of antipolysaccharide (Hib) B cells required for a protective response is not normally attained until about age 2 (probably because several infections with Hib have to be experienced), but the conjugate vaccine probably elicits the required number of cognate B cells in younger children because its carrier protein probably stimulates considerable T_H cell activity.

3. Internal Image Vaccines. The Ab (termed no. 1) elicited by an Ag can be used itself as an immunogen to elicit another Ab (no. 2). As noted in Figure 16–14, Ab no. 2 and the Ag can both bind to the combining site of Ab no. 1, and therefore the combining site of Ab no. 2 must resemble to some extent an epitope on the Ag; that is, it corresponds to the Ag's "internal image" (Fig. 16–14). A mAb that represents Ab no. 2 and appears to correspond to the internal image of a virus (reovirus) is being tested to determine if it can be used as a vaccine to protect against infection by that virus.

Selected Reading

REVIEW ARTICLES

Coffman RL, Seymour BWP, Lebman DA et al: The role of helper T cell products in mouse B cell differentiation and isotype regulation. Immunol Rev no. 102, 1988

Warren HS, Vogel FR, Chedid LA: Current status of immunological adjuvants. Annu Rev Immunol 4:369, 1986

Weill J-C, Reynaud C-A: The chicken B cell compartment. Science 238:1094, 1987

Yancopoulos GD, Alt FW: Regulation of the assembly and expression of variable-region genes. Annu Rev Immunol 4:339, 1986

SPECIFIC ARTICLES

Atchison ML, Perry RP: The role of the κ enhancer and its binding factor NF-κB in the developmental regulation of a κ gene transcription. Cell 48:121, 1987

Bliar PR, Bothwell ALM: A limited number of B cell lineages generates the heterogeneity of a secondary immune response. J Immunol 139:3996, 1987

Chua M, Goodgal SH, Karush F: Germ line affinity and germ line variable region genes in the B cell response. J Immunol 138:1281, 1987

Claflin JL, Berry J, Flaherty D, Dunnick W: Somatic evolution of diversity among anti-phosphorylcholine antibodies induced by *Proteus morganii*. J Immunol 138:3060, 1987

Ephrussi A, Church GM, Tonegawa S, Gilbert W: B lineage-specific interaction of an immunoglobulin enhancer with cellular factors *in vivo*. Science 227:134, 1985

Gearhart PJ, Johnson ND, Douglas R, Hood L: IgG antibodies to phosphocholine exhibit more diversity than their IgM counterparts. Nature 291:29, 1981

Gillies SD, Morrison SL, Oi VT, Tonegawa S: A tissue-specific transcription enhancer element is located in the major intron of a rearranged immunoglobulin-heavy chain gene. Cell 33:717, 1983

Goodnow CC, Crosbie J, Adelstein S et al: Altered immunoglobulin expression and functional silencing of self-reactive B lymphocytes in transgenic mice. Nature 334:676, 1988

Grosschedl R, Baltimore D: Cell-type specificity of immunoglobulin gene expression is regulated by at least three DNA sequence elements. Cell 41:885, 1985

Gurish MF, Ben-Porat T, Nisonoff A: The use of anti-idiotypic antibodies as vaccines. In Eibl MM, Rosen FS (eds): Primary Immunodeficiency Diseases, pp 217–227, 1986

Harris DE, Cairns L, Rosen FS, Borel Y: A natural model of immunologic tolerance: Tolerance to murine C5 is mediated by T cells and antigen is required to maintain unresponsiveness. J Exp Med 156:567, 1982

Hayakawa K, Hardy RR, Honda M, Herzenberg LA, Steinberg AD, Herzenberg LA: Ly-1 B cells: Functionally distinct lymphocytes that secrete IgM autoantibodies. Proc Natl Acad Sci USA 81:2494, 1984

Hirano T et al: Complementary DNA for a novel human interleukin (BSF-2) or IL-6 that induces B lymphocytes to produce immunoglobulin. Nature 324:73, 1986

Kawano M et al: Autocrine generation and requirement of BSF-2/IL-6 for human multiple myelomas. Nature 332:83, 1988

McKean D, Huppi K, Bell M, Staudt L, Gearhard W, Weigert MG: Generation of antibody diversity in the immune respone of BALB/c mice to influenza virus hemagglutinin. Proc Natl Acad Sci USA 81:3180, 1984

Schlomchik MJ, Avcoin AH, Pisetsky DS, Weigert MG: Structure and function of anti-DNA antibodies derived from a single autoimmune mouse. Proc Natl Acad Sci USA 84:9150, 1987

Sen R, Baltimore D: Inducibility of a κ immunoglobulin enhancer-binding protein NF-κB by a posttranslational mechanism. Cell 47:921, 1986

Tony H-P, Parker DC: Major histocompatibility complex-restricted polyclonal B cell responses resulting from helper T cell recognition of anti-immunoglobulin presented by small B lymphocytes. J Exp Med 161:223, 1985

Weigert MG, Cesari IM, Yonkovich SJ, Cohn M: Variability of the lambda light chain sequences of mouse antibody. Nature 228:1045, 1970

Wysocki L, Manser T, Gefter ML: Somatic evolution of variable region structures during an immune response. Proc Natl Acad Sci USA 83:1847, 1986

17

John P. Atkinson
Herman N. Eisen

The Complement System

The principal function of the immune system is to eliminate foreign antigens (Ags). For this to occur, the Ags must first be identified, and previous chapters were concerned largely with how they are recognized by antibodies (Abs), B cells, and T cells. In this chapter, we consider the complement system, a set of proteins that constitute the chief means for destroying Ags and Ag-bearing cells when they are recognized by Abs.

Complement was discovered in the 1890s, when it was recognized that a normal serum component contributes to host defenses by interacting with Ab–Ag complexes. Thus, cholera vibrios were rapidly lysed when added to serum from immunized animals. However, if the serum had been previously heated to 56°C for a few minutes or simply allowed to age for a few weeks, it lost its lytic activity, although its Abs were retained; and the addition of fresh **normal** serum to the inactivated antiserum restored its bacteriolytic capacity. Hence, lysis required **both** stable, specific Ab and a labile nonspecific factor present in normal (as well as in immune) serum. Originally called **alexin** (Gr. *alexein;* to ward off), the unstable serum factor was subsequently named **complement** (at first referred to as **C′** and now as **C**). Complement consists of 25 to 30 proteins, some in plasma, others membrane bound. Some react in an ordered sequence that terminates in lysis of Ag-bearing cells, whereas peptide fragments of others stimulate inflammation. Other C proteins serve as inhibitors that prevent excessive cell destruction and inflammation, and still others provide the chief mechanism for ridding the body of Ag–Ab complexes.

The C proteins constitute about 5% of the serum proteins of vertebrates. They are entirely unrelated structurally to Igs, and they are not increased in concentration by immunization. However, most of them are "acute-

385

phase" proteins; i.e., they are synthesized rapidly and appear at elevated levels in the serum during acute inflammatory responses. C eliminates Ags both by promoting their phagocytosis and by damaging the membranes of Ag-bearing cells, sometimes causing cell lysis.

Of the system's many effects, lysis of red blood cells (RBC; hemolysis) is especially easy to measure *in vitro* and has been widely used to analyze C proteins and their reaction mechanisms. Much less is known about how C destroys microbes, although the resulting protection against infection has probably constituted the main driving force in its evolution.

Complement (C) Proteins: General Concepts and Nomenclature

Complement was shown to consist of more than one substance: its activity could be restored when preparations inactivated in various ways were recombined. Table 17–1 summarizes the properties of 11 proteins of the classical pathway, three additional proteins of the alternative pathway, and six inhibitory proteins. Most are glycoproteins. In some, a single precursor chain is cleaved intracellularly to give a multichain structure that is held together by disulfide bonds, whereas in others, several distinct polypeptides are combined to form a single multichain molecule.

The C proteins react in two ordered sequences, a classic and an alternative pathway. The components in plasma are synthesized in the liver, although several migratory cells that accumulate at inflammatory lesions (such as macrophages and fibroblasts) can also synthesize many of them.

Most of what we know about the complement system derives from human C, on which the description that follows is largely based; guinea pig and mouse C are similar, and all vertebrates appear to possess both pathways. However, homologies among distantly related species are difficult to establish because of the large number of components involved and incompatibilities between those of different species. An activity like that of the alternative pathway appears to be present in invertebrates.

NOMENCLATURE. Components were mostly numbered in the order of discovery rather than in the order in which they react, but the only resulting inconsistency is that C4 reacts before C3. Some components in the alternative pathway (see below) are designated with the capital letter B, P, and D. Peptide fragments derived by proteolysis are described by the suffixes "a," "b," etc. (e.g., C3a, C3b). The "b" fragments are larger and may combine directly with a target membrane and continue to participate in the cascade, whereas the liberated smaller "a" fragments promote inflammatory responses. The acti-

TABLE 17–1. Serum Complement Proteins*

Components	Apparent Mol. Wt.†	No. of Chains Preactivation	Serum Concentration (µg/ml)
Early Components			
CLASSIC PATHWAY			
C1q	410,000	18 (6A + 6B + 6C)	70
C1r	90,000	2 (identical)	50
C1s	85,000	2 (identical)	50
C4	206,000	3 ($\alpha + \beta + \gamma$)	300
C2	117,000	1	25
C3‡	190,000	2 ($\alpha + \beta$)	1200
ALTERNATIVE PATHWAY			
C3‡	190,000	2 ($\alpha + \beta$)	1200
B	100,000	1	225
D	25,000	1	1
P	55,000	3 or 4 (identical)	25
Late Components (Both Pathways)			
C5	185,000	2 ($\alpha + \beta$)	85
C6	128,000	1	60
C7	120,000	1	55
C8	150,000	3 ($\alpha + \beta + \gamma$)	55
C9	79,000	1	60
Regulatory Components			
C1 INH	105,000	1	200
I	105,000	2 ($\alpha + \beta$)	200
H	150,000	1	500
C4bp	560,000	7 (identical)	250
S	84,000	1	500
Anaphylatoxin inactivator	310,000	6 ($2\alpha + 2\beta + 2\gamma$)	35

* Modified from Reid KBM: Essays Biochem 22:69, 1986.
† Including oligosaccharides.
‡ C3, like the late or terminal components, is a member of both pathways.

vated enzymatic state of a complement factor is often designated by an overbar; for example, $\overline{\text{C1}}$.

The Reaction Sequence Leading to Cell Lysis

The reaction sequence is illustrated in Figure 17–1, and individual steps are discussed below. In several of the early steps, the activating protein, a protease of the serine esterase type, cleaves the next reacting protein (Table 17–2). The larger of the resulting fragments then behaves as another activated proteolytic enzyme, cleaving and thereby activating the next protein. Unlike most proteases, **the C proteases are remarkably specific: each confines its attack to a particular bond in a particular C protein.** Some of the small proteolytic frag-

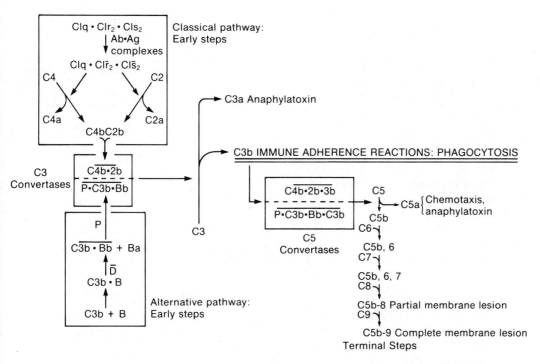

Figure 17–1. Reaction sequence of the complement system. The central role of C3 is emphasized. Bars over components indicate enzymatically active forms.

ments have "**phlogistic**" (Gr. *phlogistos*; burnt) activity; that is, they cause inflammatory tissue changes such as increased vascular permeability and attraction of polymorphonuclear leukocytes (**chemotaxis**).

AN OVERVIEW OF THE SEQUENCE

It is useful to distinguish early from late stages. In the early steps (up to cleavage of C3), there are two different pathways, the classic and the alternative (see Fig. 17–1).

In the **classic pathway,** C1, a complex of three proteins, binds to appropriate Ab–Ag complexes and is thereby triggered to become an active protease that cleaves and activates C4 and C2. These form an enzyme complex (**C3 convertase**) that specifically splits C3. The smaller of the resulting fragments (C3a) has potent phlogistic effects, and the larger (C3b) has a critical role in activating the remaining proteins in the sequence (C5–C9).

The **alternative pathway** does not require Ab for activation. Instead, many substances, especially on bacterial and fungal cell walls and on some parasite membranes and viral envelopes, engage and activate a separate set of serum proteins that cleave C3 into exactly the same fragments as the C3-splitting complex of the classic pathway.

The **late stages** of the C sequence are common to both the alternative and classic pathway. An enzyme complex involving the C3b fragment cleaves C5; the smaller fragment (C5a) has phlogistic effects, and the larger one forms the initial component of the large multimolecular complexes of the remaining "late" proteins (C6, C7, C8, and C9), which ultimately cause cell-membrane lesions and cell death.

TABLE 17–2. Serine Proteases of Complement System

Protease	Substrate	Remarks
CLASSIC PATHWAY		
C1r	C1s	Part of C1, Ca^{2+}-dependent enzyme complex ($C1q.C1r_2C1s_2$)
C1s	C4 and C2	As above. For efficient cleavage, C2 must be associated with C4b.
C2 (as C2b)*	C3	C4b positions C3
	C5	C3b positions C5
ALTERNATIVE PATHWAY		
D	B	B must be in association with C3b
B (as Bb)†	C3	First C3b positions B; second C3b
	C5	positions C5

* As C2b in the C4bC2b and C4bC2bC3b complexes that cleave C3 and C5, respectively.

† As Bb in the C3bBbP and C3bBbC3bP complexes that cleave C3 and C5, respectively.

EARLY STEPS

The Classic Pathway

ACTIVATION BY Ab–Ag COMPLEXES. The classic pathway is initiated by Ab–Ag complexes only if the Ab is of the appropriate class. Human IgM, IgG1, and IgG3 are effective; IgA and IgE are not. As noted below (One-Hit Theory), C can be activated by a single IgM molecule on a cell membrane, but a cluster of IgG molecules is required. Indeed, when Igs of the appropriate class are aggregated by mild heat or are cross-linked chemically, they also can activate the classic C pathway. Because close packing of IgG molecules is necessary, the **small complexes formed by these Abs with univalent haptens, or with multivalent Ags in great excess, are ineffective** (see Lattice Theory, Chapter 13).

Aggregated IgG1 or IgG3 remains active if they are missing just the H-chain's C_H3 domain but not if they lack both C_H2 and C_H3 domains. Thus F(ab)′$_2$ fragments (see Chap. 14, Fig. 14–6) of these Igs are inactive, and a critical site in the C_H2 domain appears to be required; it probably is exposed to C1 in aggregated Igs (of appropriate isotype), not in monomeric ones.

SEQUENTIAL STEPS LEADING TO CLEAVAGE OF C3. These are described chiefly in relation to lysis of erythrocytes (E), but they are similar for Ags on microbes and for soluble Ags. For simplicity, Abs are designated A in the following paragraphs.

E + A = EA. Lysis of E is initiated by the specific binding of one IgM Ab molecule or a pair of IgG molecules (A) (One-Hit Theory, below) to an antigenic site on the cell surface, forming a **sensitized cell.** The surface Ag need not be a natural constituent of the cell membrane: when soluble Ags or small haptens are chemically linked to the E membrane, the cells can be sensitized with the corresponding Abs.

The requirement for a pair of IgG molecules implies that the epitopes on the cell surface must be closely spaced. Many more IgG than IgM molecules must be bound per cell. If the epitopes are too far apart, C will not be activated, no matter how many IgG Ab molecules are bound: hence, Abs to some cell-surface Ags are unable to cause C-mediated lysis (for example, Abs to Rh and many other important Ags on human E).

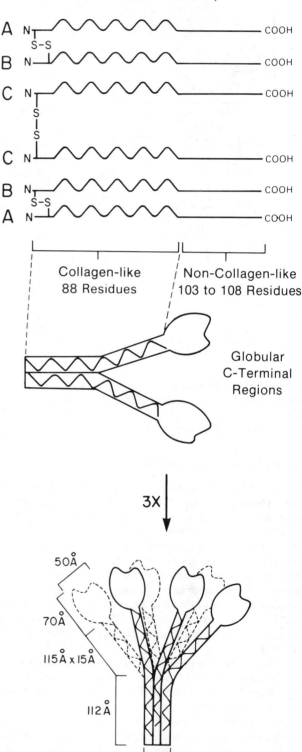

Figure 17–2. Proposed chain structure of human C1q. Wavy lines = triple-helix sections (collagen-like fibrils). In the N-terminal domain (88 residues), the chains have a typical collagen-like sequence: glycine occupies every third position, hydroxyproline and hydroxylysine are frequent, and a galactose–glucose disaccharide is attached to the hydroxyl of many hydroxylysine residues. Dimensions are from electron microscopy. (Porter RR, Reid KBM: Nature 275:699, 1978)

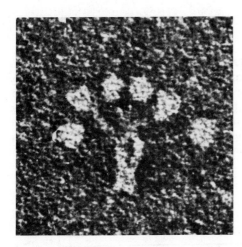

Figure 17–3. Electron micrograph of a human C1q molecule, showing a stalk and six terminal globular heads (each with a binding site for the C_H2 domain of γ chains in IgG1 and IgG3 and of μ chains in IgM). (Knobel HR, Villiger W, Isliker H: Eur J Immunol 5:78, 1975)

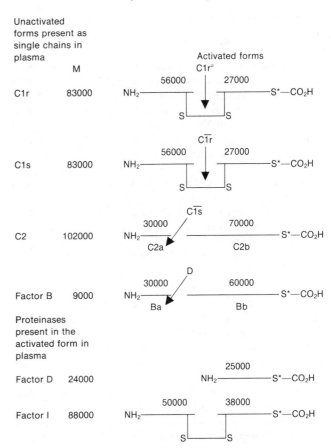

Figure 17–4. The serine proteases involved in the activation and control of the complement system. (*) denotes the active-site serine (S) residue, located about 50 residues from the C terminus of the catalytic chain of each protease. Note the striking similarities between C1r and C1s and between C2 and factor B. Arrows point to site of cleavage that transforms a proenzyme into an active enzyme. Note also the enzymes responsible for each of the cleavages. C1r° denotes a single-chain proenzyme form of C1r that is considered to cleave and activate C1r (to $C\overline{1}r$). (Reid KBM: Essays Biochem 22:29, 1986)

EA + C1 + Ca²⁺ = EAC1. C1 exists in serum as an aggregate of three proteins, C1q, C1r, and C1s, loosely associated noncovalently in a complex with Ca^{2+}. The binding of this aggregate to Ab–Ag complexes leads to a single proteolytic cleavage in C1r and in C1s (see below).

C1q lacks protease activity and serves as the recognition unit of C1. Its structure is unusual in that it combines collagen-like fibrils with globular domains: each of the molecule's six subunits has a globular domain at the end of a collagen-like fibril (Figs. 17–2 and 17–3). If the fibrils are digested with collagenase, the remaining globular heads retain the sites that bind aggregated IgG. However, the equilibrium binding (association) constant of the individual C1q globular fragments for Ig appears to be only about 1/100 to 1/1000 than that of intact C1q, suggesting that the stability of normal C1q–Ab–Ag aggregates is attributable to multivalent binding, with several globular domains of an intact C1q molecule bound to several of the Fc domains of an IgM molecule or to two or more IgG molecules in an Ab–Ag complex. C1q can, in fact, form a specific precipitate with many soluble Ab–Ag complexes, and this reaction has been used diagnostically to detect such complexes in serum in diseases where they are associated with severe inflammatory lesions (e.g., rheumatoid arthritis). In serum, as much as 30% of C1q may be free; the rest exists in readily dissociable **C1qC1r₂C1s₂** complexes that, by themselves, lack proteolytic activity. When the entire complex binds (via C1q) to the proper Ab–Ag complexes, a peptide bond in **C1r is cleaved, and it becomes an active proteolytic enzyme ($C\overline{1}r$) that splits C1s, its only known substrate.**

C1r and C1s are very similar. They have the same mol. wt. (83,000); in the cleavage-activation step, each is similarly split into two fragments (56,000 and 27,000 daltons) (Fig. 17–4) that remain linked by an S–S bond; they are both inhibited as proteases by diisopropylphosphorofluoridate (DFP), which reacts with a serine residue in the catalytic site of each molecule; and their amino acid sequences are similar to those of other proteases of the serine protease family, such as trypsin. Extensive nucleotide sequence similarity of their cDNA clones indicates that they arose by duplication of a common ancestral gene. **C4 and C2, the next C proteins that react in the C cascade, are substrates for activated C1s.**

The stability of the C1 complex (C1qC1r₂C1s₂) depends on **calcium ions (Ca^{2+}), which are thus essential for immune lysis of cells.** Chelating agents that bind Ca^{2+} cause C1–Ab–Ag complexes (or C1 by itself) to dissociate, leaving only C1q associated with Ab–Ag complexes.

EAC1 + C4 → EAC1,4b + C4a. The next protein to react, C4, has three chains per molecule (α,β and γ, see Table 17–1) held together by disulfide bonds. Activated C1s cleaves a small N-terminal fragment of about 9000 daltons (C4a) from the α chain (see Fig. 14–1). The remaining molecule, C4b, has an internal thioester bond in its α chain. This short-lived reactive site (designated C4b* or nascent C4b) forms covalent (amide and ester) bonds between a reactive glutamyl carboxyl group in C4b and amino or hydroxyl groups of many proteins, including Ig heavy chains (Fd segment; Chapter 14). Many C4b molecules thus bind to the membrane of E and a few to the bound Ab; more often, though, the thioester is promptly hydrolyzed, and the fragment (termed iC4b) loses its activity.

EAC1,4b + C2 + Mg^{2+} → EAC1,4b,2b + C2a. In this reaction (which requires Mg^{2+}), the C4b moiety of the EAC1,4b complex binds C2, which is then cleaved (by the activated C1s moiety) into two fragments. The larger one, C2b, remains bound to C4b, forming the next activated complex, C4b,2b, which is called **C3 convertase.**

The binding of C2 by EAC1,4b before C2 is cleaved minimizes the loss of C2b, which otherwise quickly deteriorates in solution. In the EAC1,4b,2b complex, the C2b is relatively unstable (half-life at 37°C is 10 min): it dissociates as an inactive fragment, but the remaining EAC1,4b complex can then bind and cleave additional C2, forming more EAC1,4b,2b.

C3 CLEAVAGE IN THE CLASSIC PATHWAY: EAC1,4b2b + C3 → EAC1,4b,2b,3b + C3a. In this critical step, each EAC1,4b,2b unit cleaves hundreds of C3 molecules, each of them at an arginine, 77 residues from the N terminus of its α chain. The smaller C3a fragment (mol. wt. 9000) has pronounced phlogistic activity (see Anaphylatoxins, below). The larger, C3b, contains a thioester bond like that in C4b, and transfer of the reactive acyl from the thioester to a hydroxyl or amino group binds C3b covalently to a cell membrane or an Ab heavy chain. Some C3b joins membrane-bound C4b,2b to form the next catalytic unit, C4b,2b,3b (termed **C5-convertase**), which cleaves C5 (see Fig. 17–5 and below).

The cell-bound C3b fragments are clustered around the antigenic site and mediate many of the biologic activities of complement. **For instance, C3b on the cell surface has powerful opsonic activity; that is, it greatly increases the cell's susceptibility to phagocytosis** (see Receptors for C3b Fragments as Phagocytic Cells, below). Also, although the C3b not associated with a C4b,C2b complex lacks catalytic activity, it can bind alternative

pathway components to form another C3-splitting enzyme (see below).

AMPLIFICATION IN THE C SEQUENCE. The tremendous **self-amplifying** capacity of the complement system is striking: one IgM molecule, binding to an epitope, binds one C1 molecule; the resulting activated C1s then cleaves approximately 100 C4 molecules, from which about 20 C4b fragments bind to the Ag (and Ab); although only about five of the approximately 100 C2b fragments that

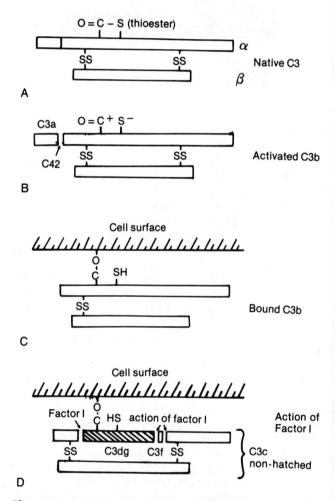

Figure 17–5. Diagram of the C3 molecule. **(A)** The native molecule with the thioester bond on the α chain. **(B)** Cleavage by a C3 convertase produces the small C3a peptide and the larger C3b fragment and results in activation of the thioester bond. **(C)** Combination of activated C3b with the target surface. **(D)** Degradation of C3b. The attached fragment is cleaved in several places by factor I to produce small fragments (C3f, the larger C3c, and C3dg still covalently attached to the target surface). C4b is similarly degraded. (Hughes-Jones NE: In Ross GD: Immunobiology of the Complement System. Orlando, Academic Press, 1986)

are then formed are captured to form C4b,C2b, this enzyme complex can cleave thousands of C3 molecules. Each of the resulting approximately 1200 C3b fragments that bind to the membrane can interact with alternative pathway components to form another C3 cleaving enzyme (see below). Thus, **the potential exists for the deposition of thousands of opsonizing C3b molecules around a single antigenic site to which one IgM Ab molecule is bound.**

The Alternative Pathway

In this pathway, as in the classic pathway, opsonic C3b fragments are produced and the late steps (C5–C9) of C-mediated cell lysis are activated (see Fig. 17–1). However, Ab–Ag complexes and the early C components (C1, C4, and C2) are not required.

The alternative pathway was discovered serendipitously when it was found that, on addition of a yeast cell wall polysaccharide (zymosan) to fresh serum, C3 was lost with negligible reduction in levels of C1, C4, and C2, and some antimicrobial activities appeared such as the ability to destroy *Shigella dysenteriae*. The effect was attributed to a novel protein, named **properdin** (L. *perdere;* to destroy). Properdin eventually turned out to be a member of a second complement pathway, one that recognizes a wide variety of microbes and deposits C3b on the microbial membrane in the absence of specific Ab.

The essential features of this system are best illustrated when diverse microbes are introduced into the serum of a **nonimmune** host or are placed in the presence of the purified alternative pathway components: a C3-splitting enzyme and large quantities of C3b became attached to the microbe's surface. As a result, it can be lysed by the terminal C complex (C5–C9) or destroyed by C3b-mediated phagocytosis. Thus, **the alternative pathway is an independent system with its own recognition and effector capabilities.** Because a similar pathway is found in some invertebrates, during evolution it probably preceded adaptive immunity attributable to Abs and T cells.

C3 CLEAVAGE IN THE ALTERNATIVE PATHWAY. This reaction sequence depends on the C3b fragment and three serum proteins that do not participate in the classic sequence: **properdin (P), Factor B (B), and Factor D (D).** (As in C3 cleavage in the classic pathway, Mg^{2+} is also required.)

B binds to C3b (analogous to C2 binding to C4b), forming a C3b,B complex from which D, an active protease in serum, splits off the small Ba fragment (about 30,000 daltons), leaving C3b,Bb. This complex (analogous to C4b,C2b) cleaves C3. **C3b,Bb readily dissociates and loses activity, but by binding serum P, it forms P,C3b,Bb, a relatively stable proteolytic complex** that cleaves C3 at precisely the same peptide bond as in the classic pathway and liberates the same C3a and C3b fragments. Thus, many C3b molecules become bound around the site where the initial C3b was attached. These, in turn, capture more B molecules, forming more of the C3-splitting enzyme (P,C3b,Bb), and so on. Amplification of C3b deposition is the end result.

INITIATION OF THE ALTERNATIVE PATHWAY. Diverse particles activate the alternative pathway, including: (1) various polysaccharides, especially of microbial origin (zymosan, inulin, lipopolysaccharide of gram-negative bacteria, teichoic acid of gram-positive bacteria, etc.); (2) various gram-negative and gram-positive bacteria; and (3) some parasites (e.g., *Schistosoma mansoni* larvae). Activation of this pathway is also enhanced by aggregated Igs of those classes that do not bind C1q and are thus ineffectual in the classic pathway (aggregated human IgG4 and IgA, and also aggregated F [ab]$_2$' fragments); these Igs may provide sites that are protected from regulatory proteins (see below).

The role of the microbial polysaccharides seems to be, not that of a conventional activator, but rather to provide a microenvironment in which spontaneously activated C3 convertases are shielded from inhibitory proteins. Thus, the pathway seems normally always to be active at a low level, but its amplification is prevented by a group of virtually ubiquitous regulatory proteins that are found in plasma and on mammalian cells and tissues but not on most microbes (bacteria, fungi). **The microbial polysaccharides (and other "activators" of the alternative pathway) serve as binding sites for C3b and block the inhibitory effects of the regulatory proteins** (see below). Not surprisingly, some microbes have acquired virulence factors that behave like the complement regulatory proteins: they bind and inactivate C3b and thereby inhibit complement activation.

In the first step of this pathway, C3b is paradoxically both part of the enzyme complex, C3b,Bb, and its product. What is the source of the C3b in the initial C3b,Bb complex? Although this question has not been settled, the evidence indicates that native C3 is unstable, and a small amount turns over each hour (C3 "tickover"). A form of C3 (called C3i or C3 [H_2O]) is functionally the equivalent of C3b: it has a thioester bond that (like the one in C3b and C4b fragments) can bind covalently to protein NH_2 and OH groups (Fig. 17–6). If it binds to B, it forms the "alternative pathway C3 convertase." Normally, this convertase is formed at low levels and is promptly inactivated by the regulatory proteins, but if it forms in the favorable, inhibitor-free environment of the surface polysaccharides on many bacteria and fungi, it is sufficient to activate the rest of the alternative pathway.

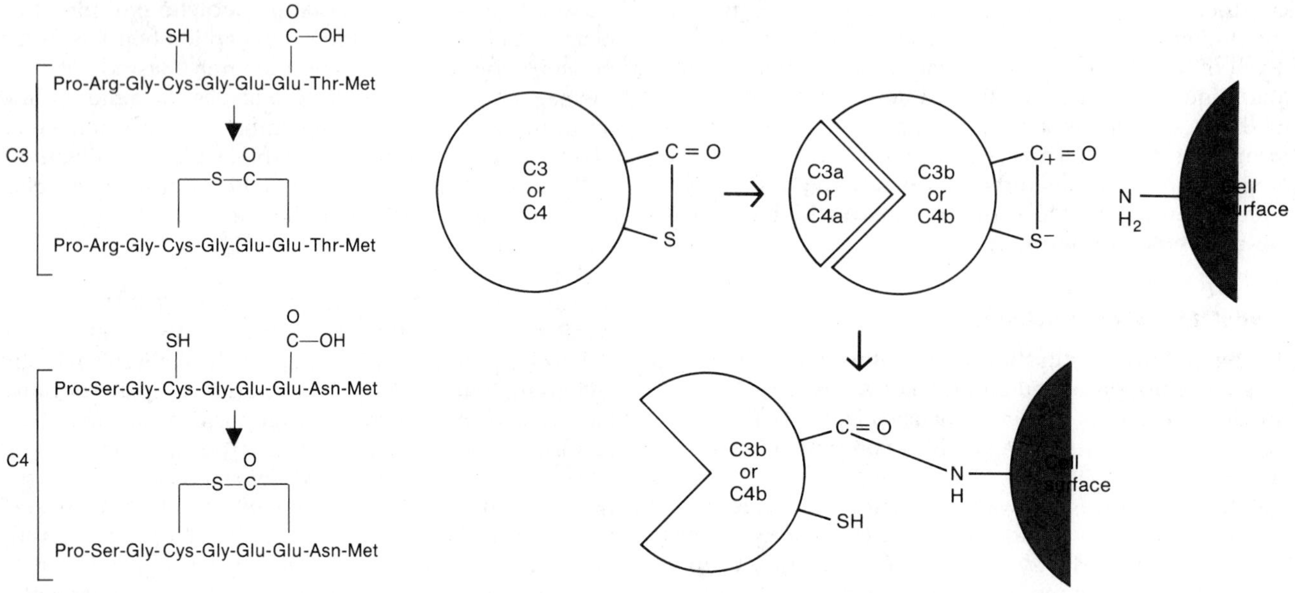

Figure 17-6. Formation of the thioester bond in C3b and C4b and the covalent bond it forms with an NH_2 group. The thioester bond also reacts with OH groups of proteins (presumably of a serine, threonine, or tyrosine residue) and of polysaccharides. (Hughes-Jones NE: In Ross GP: Immunobiology of the Complement System. Orlando, Academic Press, 1986)

LATE STEPS

C5 Cleavage

The C3-splitting enzymes of the classic (C4b,2b) and alternative (P,C3b,Bb) pathways can each combine with one or more C3b molecules to form C5-splitting enzymes or **convertases.** Like C3, which it resembles (Table 17-1), C5 is split by its convertases near the N-terminus of the α chain, yielding fragments C5a and C5b (Fig. 17-7). **C5a** (75 residues) and C3a (the corresponding fragment of the α chain of C3) have about 40% amino acid sequence homology and, as noted below, both have anaphylatoxin activity. In addition, C5a is a chemoattractant for polymorphonuclear leukocytes and macrophages. **C5b** initiates assembly of the terminal C proteins (C6–C9) into a "membrane-attack" complex that can cause cell lysis.

The Membrane-Attack Complex

Unlike the steps leading up to cleavage of C5, the remaining reactions involve the formation of progressively larger complexes without breaking peptide bonds. The C5b fragment is the nidus, cumulatively binding, in succession, C6, C7, C8, and finally C9. After binding C7, the complex, if in solution, transfers to the cell membrane. The key to effective cell destruction by C is C9: multiples of this protein, possibly as many as 18, are bound at each site and form transmembrane channels (see below).

MEMBRANE LESIONS. When assembled on a cell, the C5b–C9 complex impairs surface membrane permeability, allowing cations (Ca^{2+}, Na^+) and water to enter rapidly. RBCs swell and then burst **(osmotic lysis),** while nucleated cells become "leaky," losing first low- and then high-mol. wt. substances (e.g., initially K^+, later nucleotides, finally proteins). In addition, ionic dyes that are excluded by intact cells penetrate into the cytoplasm. Staining by trypan blue or eosin is thus often used to detect C-damaged nucleated cells.

How are the membrane lesions formed? The possibility of an enzymatic attack by C5b–9 has been virtually eliminated by the finding that activated C causes the same impaired permeability in **liposomes** (synthetic lipid vesicles) as in cells, and no covalent changes have been found in any of the liposome's chemically well-characterized constituents. A detergent-like action is also unlikely because with authentic detergents, lysis requires about 10^8 to 10^{10} molecules per RBC, whereas only one or a few C5b–9 units per cell is sufficient (see One-Hit Theory, below).

Instead, it appears that as soluble, monomeric C9 associates with cell-bound C5b–8 complexes, it undergoes a change in shape and inserts into the cell membrane as a circularly polymerized transmembrane channel. When polymerized *in vitro*, C9 forms similar structures, and channel size differs with the extent of polymerization. The largest channels may correspond to the doughnut-

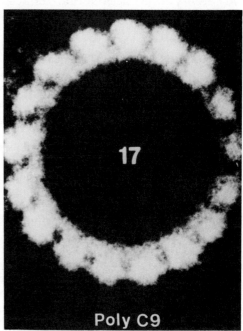

Figure 17–7. Homology between C3 and C5. The two proteins have the same mol. wt. and chain structure (Table 17–1), and each is split by its convertase at the same susceptible arginine bond (77 and 75 residues from the N-terminus of the α chain in C3 and C5, respectively). Carbohydrate (CHO) is present on this region of human C5 (and in C5a). Despite many structural similarities to C3 (and C4), C5 does not have a thioester bond (see Fig. 17–4). (Hugli TE: Contemp Top Mol Immunol 7:181, 1978)

shaped holes seen in electron micrographs of C-damaged cells (Fig. 17–8).

Because the proposed conformational changes in C9 are probably unstable, exposed hydrophobic sites would be expected to slip back promptly into the protein interior, unless they interact with cell membrane lipids. Hence, any C5b–9 complexes that form in solution quickly lose their cytotoxic activity. This instability, plus the presence of inhibitors in plasma and on most mammalian cells, explains why **cell lysis caused by C is**

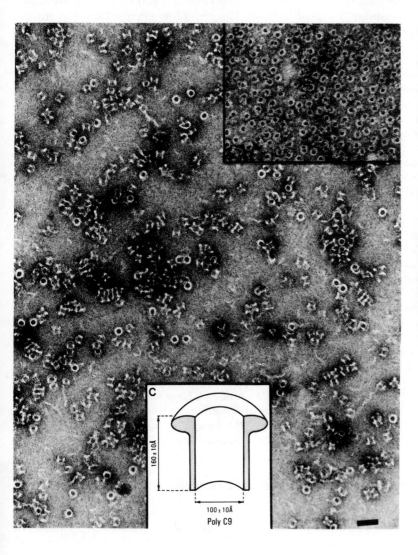

Figure 17–8. *(A)* Structures formed by purified C9 polymerized in solution (main panel) resemble the lesions formed in membranes of complement-lysed cells (inset, upper right). The lower inset shows a schematic view of a hypothetical transmembrane channel formed by polymerized C9, bisected along the channel's axis. *(B)* Top view of a polymerized C9 complex showing 17 clearly visible subunits. (Podack EP: In Ross GD: Immunobiology of the Complement System. Orlando, Academic Press, 1986)

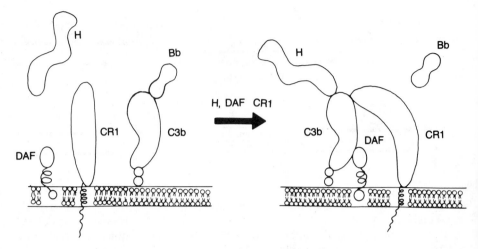

Figure 17–9. Inactivation of C3 convertase. Protein H, decay accelerating factor (DAF), and CR1 bind to cell-associated C3b; the result is that Bb dissociates, and the convertase is inactivated. The liberated C3b remains hemolytically active: it can capture another B molecule and continue the reaction sequence unless it is totally inactivated by proteolytic cleavage (see Fig. 17–7). Note that DAF is anchored in the cell membrane by phosphatidyl inositol. For complement receptor type 1 (CR1), see text.

sharply restricted to those cells on which the initiating events occur; neighboring "innocent bystander" cells, which lack the appropriate Ags, escape damage.

THE ONE-HIT THEORY. The quantitative relation between the extent of RBC lysis and the amount of C (Appendix, Fig. 17–14, this chapter) was previously interpreted to mean that lysis depends on the accumulation of many damaged sites per cell. However, lysis probably depends not on this accumulation but rather on one site per cell. This view is based on the finding that the average number of lytic lesions formed per RBC is linearly related to the concentration of C1, C4, or C2 (see Appendix, this chapter). Similarly, the activation and binding of C1 is linearly related to the concentration of IgM Abs (to RBC) or to the square of the concentration of the corresponding IgG Abs.

These linear relations indicate that **lysis of an erythrocyte can be caused by a single site, established by the binding of one IgM molecule or a pair of IgG Ab molecules, followed by one molecule each of C1, C4, and C2.** Such a site is evidently sufficient to activate and bind many molecules of C3 and the remaining C components, causing an RBC to undergo lysis. The situation is more complex with nucleated cells, where repair mechanisms may be able to eliminate and resynthesize segments of damaged membranes.

Comparison Between the Classic and Alternative Pathways

SIMILARITIES BETWEEN THE PATHWAYS. The proteins and the enzymatic reactions that lead to C3 and C5 cleavage are similar in the two pathways. Thus, C2 in the classic and B in the alternative pathway have about 70% identity in amino acid sequence. Each of them is also the respective active proteolytic component of C3 and C5

convertases, which cleave C3 and C5 at the homologous peptide bond. The genes that encode C2 and B are also near neighbors in the major histocompatibility complex (Fig. 17–13, below, and Chapter 15), and they have a similar exon/intron organization. They very likely arose from duplication of an ancestral gene.

C3 (which is active in both pathways) and C4 (active only in the classic pathway) constitute another homologous pair. Both have a reactive thioester bond, which is most unusual in proteins, and their major cleavage fragments, C3b and C4b, serve the same function in the two pathways: C3b in the alternative pathway binds covalently to the target and then interacts with and activates another protein (B) that becomes an active protease; C4b does the same (to C2) in the classic pathway.

DIFFERENCES BETWEEN THE TWO PATHWAYS. Although C1s and D are both serine proteases that cleave homologous proteins in the two pathways (C2 in the classic and B in the alternative), they do not appear to be closely related structurally. The unique aspect of the classic pathway is the requirement for triggering by Ab–Ag complexes, which depends on the linking or attachment protein, C1q; there is no comparable initiating factor or trigger for the alternative pathway. Properdin stabilizes the alternative pathway C3 convertase; there is no stabilizing analogue for the classic pathway's C3 convertase. Finally, although C3b and C4b have similar roles in both pathways, in the alternative one, C3b has an additional, virtually autocatalytic, function, for it is both part of an enzyme complex (C3b,Bb) and its product (Fig. 17–1, above).

Regulatory Proteins

The destruction of normal cells by excessive activity of C is prevented by a set of seven regulatory proteins: five

TABLE 17–3. Complement Regulatory Proteins

Component	Location	Target	Function
C1 INH	Plasma	C1r/C1s	Inactivates C1
S protein	Plasma	C5b67	Blocks soluble C5b-C9 complexes
Homologous restriction factor (HRF)	All peripheral blood cells except resting T cells	C8	Blocks action of C5b-C9 complexes on targeted cells
C4bp	Plasma	C4b*	Decay accelerating activity; cofactor activity
H	Plasma	C3b	Decay accelerating activity; cofactor activity
Decay accelerating factor (DAF)	On all peripheral blood cells; epithelial, mesenchymal, and endothelial cells	C4b/C3b†	Decay accelerating activity
Membrane cofactor protein (MCP)	On all peripheral blood cells (ex. RBC), epithelial, endothelial, and mesenchymal cells	C3b/C4b‡	Cofactor activity

* C4bp binds C3b as well as C4b; H is probably the major C3b binding protein of plasma.

† DAF appears to inactivate the convertases preferentially by displacing the proteases, C2 or B, from C4b or C3b.

‡ MCP has higher affinity for C3b than for C4b.

plasma proteins that primarily inactivate C complexes in solution ("fluid phase"), and two membrane proteins that inactivate C complexes on normal cells (Table 17–3). These proteins act by inhibiting the formation, accelerating the decay, or inactivating C3b and the C3 and C5 convertases. Some of their principal features are described briefly below.

REGULATORY PROTEINS IN PLASMA

C1 INH inhibits the activation of fluid-phase C1, when it is not associated with Ab–Ag complexes, by causing rapid dissociation of C1r and C1s from C1q. When the inhibitor reacts with C1 in an Ag–Ab–C1 complex, the time required to inactivate C1 completely (2–3 minutes) is sufficient for the next step in the pathway to be initiated. C1 INH is the only protease inhibitor in plasma that interacts with C1.

C4b-binding protein (C4bp) binds to C4b and acts as a cofactor for a serine protease, Factor I, which digests C4b, rendering it incapable of binding C2 and participating in the rest of the lytic pathway. It can also dissociate C2b that is already bound to C4b.

Factor H is analogous to C4bp but acts on C3b and the C3b-containing convertases. With H bound to it, C3b cannot bind B, thus preventing amplification of the alternative pathway. H also causes C3b to dissociate from Bb in both the C3 or C5 convertases (Fig. 17–9), and it likewise serves as a cofactor for the protease, Factor I, that cleaves and inactivates C3b (Fig. 17–10).

Factor I is a serine protease that cleaves and inactivates C4b and C3b, but only in the presence of the respective cofactors, C4bp and H (Fig. 17–10).

S protein combines with C5b,6,7 complexes in solution and prevents their insertion into cell membranes.

REGULATORY PROTEINS IN CELL MEMBRANES

Decay-accelerating factor (DAF) prevents the assembly of the two C3 convertases by promoting dissociation of C2b from C4b and Bb from C3b (Fig. 17–9). Found on the surface of all peripheral blood cells and many other cells, this protein is not an integral membrane protein but instead is anchored in the cell membrane by attachment at its C terminus to phosphatidyl inositol as in Thy-1 and some cell adhesion molecules (Chapter 15).

Membrane cofactor protein (MCP) is an integral

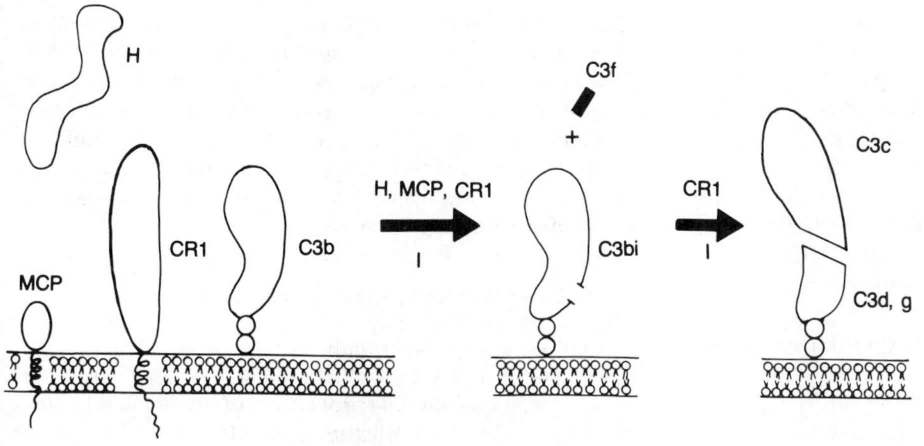

Figure 17–10. Protein H, membrane cofactor protein (MCP), and complement receptor-type 1 (CR1) serve as cofactors for the proteolytic inactivation of cell-associated C3b by the serine protease, I. The resulting fragments, C3bi and C3c, are no longer hemolytically active. CR1 plus I can further degrade C3bi to C3c and C3d,g, which contains the thioester and remains attached to the substrate (see Fig. 17–5).

membrane protein that serves as a cofactor for the pro-teolytic inactivation of C4b and C3b. Found on the same cells and tissue as DAF, it lacks decay-accelerating activity.

With different but complementary functions, DAF and MCP exhibit the same functional capabilities as the plasma proteins, C4bp and H. However, the primary targets of H and C4bp are C3b and C4b in solution, whereas the DAF and MCP molecules on a cell probably inactivate only the C3b and C4b that bind to that cell.

Homologous restriction factor (HRF) is also widely distributed on human peripheral blood and other cells. Like DAF, it is anchored in cell membranes through attachment of its C terminus to phosphatidyl inositol. Any fluid-phase C5b6,7 complexes that escape capture by S protein (see above) and adhere to a cell, independently of its Ags, are unlikely to complete the lytic sequence because cell-bound HRF blocks the establishment of effective C5b–C9 complexes by binding to C8. Together, S in solution and HRF on cells protect cells ("bystanders") from being inadvertently lysed as a result of specific Ab–Ag–C complexes that form on neighboring cells.

Cell Receptors for C Fragments

Receptors on cells bind some of the peptide fragments that result from activation and cleavage of C proteins. Some receptors are specific for the larger (b) fragments, especially those (termed **opsonins**) that coat particles and promote their uptake and ingestion by phagocytes (granulocytes, macrophages). Others are specific for the smaller (a) fragments, with phlogistic activities. The four types of receptors described below (Table 17–4) have been analyzed extensively in humans; little is known about them in other species.

COMPLEMENT RECEPTOR TYPE ONE (CR1): THE C3b/C4b RECEPTOR

This receptor is present on all types of human peripheral blood cells except platelets. There are few CR1 (about 500 per cell) on RBC and many (about 50,000 per cell) on granulocytes. However, because RBC are about 1000 times more numerous, more than 85% of CR1 in blood are on RBC, where they provide an important means for ridding the body of Ab–Ag–C complexes. In blood, these complexes bind rapidly to RBC (**immune adherence**) and are transported to the liver and spleen, where macrophages strip the complexes (and possibly the receptor as well) from the RBC.

Fc receptors on granulocytes and monocytes probably cooperate with CR1 to internalize Ab–Ag–C complexes: the CR1 receptors promote the initial binding, while Fc receptors more effectively signal internalization.

TABLE 17–4. Complement Receptors

Receptor	Apparent Mol. Wt.	Ligand	Distribution
CR1	190,000 to 280,000	C3b > C4b	Erythrocytes, neutrophils, monocytes/macrophages, B cells, 15% of T cells, eosinophils, kidney podocytes
CR2	140,000	C3d, C3bi > C3b	B cells, some T cells
CR3	165,000/95,000	C3bi > C3d	Monocytes/macrophages, neutrophils, some lymphocytes
CR4	150,000/95,000	probably C3bi, C3b	Same as for CR3
C3a-R	?	C3a	Mast cells, basophils, granulocytes
C5a-R	~70,000	C5a	Mast cells, basophils, granulocytes, monocytes/macrophages, platelets

The internalized complexes are degraded by lysosomal enzymes. CR1 on B cells and on a subpopulation (approximately 15%) of T cells may help trap C3b-coated Ag–Ab complexes in lymph nodes and spleen and thereby facilitate immune responses to the Ag.

CR1 has an unusual polymorphism, with four codominantly expressed allelic forms that differ markedly in mol. wt. (Two common ones are 220 and 250 Kd, and two rare ones are 190 and 280 Kd). All four have about the same affinity for C3b and bind the aggregated better than the monomeric form of this fragment.

The amino acid sequence deduced from cDNA for the common variant (220 Kd) indicates that CR1 is an integral membrane protein whose extracellular domain(s) have 30 short consensus repeats (SCR) of approximately 60 to 70 amino acids each (Fig. 17–11). These are grouped into four long homologous repeats, each with 7 SCRs. Striking sequence similarities (60% to 90%) among the long repeats of the allelic variants suggest that they arose by unequal crossing over with duplications or deletions of the consensus sequence.

COMPLEMENT RECEPTOR TYPE 2 (CR2): THE C3d RECEPTOR

CR2 binds C3 degradation fragments (termed C3d and C3dg; see Fig. 17–5). It is detectable on most (50% to 80%) B lymphocytes, but not on monocytes, granulocytes, or

```
  4    7         30  32  35        46  50  52    57  59
CYS—PRO————TYR—CYS—GLY————CYS—GLY—TRP— ALA –CYS
                PHE                            PRO
```

Conserved Residues in the repeating homology unit of C3b-C4b
binding proteins

Complement Proteins	No. of Homology Units/Chain	Interacts With
C1r	2	?
C1s	2	?
C2	3	C4b
Factor B	3	C3b
C4b-binding protein (7 identical chains)	8	C4b
Factor H (Mouse)	20	C3b
CR1 (C3b/C4b Receptor)	30	C3b, C4b
CR2	16	C3d
Decay Accelerating Factor	4	C3 convertases
Membrane Cofactor Protein	4	C3b, C4b

Figure 17–11. Repeating homology unit in proteins of the complement system, particularly those that bind C3b and C4b. Shown above are the unit's invariant amino acid residues. This unit has also been identified in some noncomplement proteins (IL-2 receptor, Factor XIII of the blood clotting system, and β_2-glycoprotein I). (Based on Reid KBM et al: Immunol Today 7:230, 1986)

RBC. It is also sparsely present on some cultured T-cell lines and on some peripheral blood T cells. **A distinct binding site for the Epstein–Barr virus (EBV) on this receptor accounts for the unique susceptibility of human B cells to EBV infection.**

Along with CR1, CR2 may help localize Ag–Ab–C complexes to B-cell-rich areas of the spleen and lymph nodes, and it may thus help promote Ag-driven activation of B cells. CR2 is also an integral membrane protein, with extracellular SCR sequences like those in CR1.

COMPLEMENT RECEPTOR TYPE 3 (CR3): THE C3bi RECEPTOR

Found on macrophages/monocytes and subpopulations of lymphocytes, this receptor is a heterodimer. Its α chain has a binding site for breakdown products of C3 (iC3b, C3b, C3d; see Fig. 17–5), and its β chain is identical to that of some heterodimeric cell adhesion molecules (CR3 is also termed Mac 1; see LFA-1 and Cell Adhesion Molecules, Chapter 15). Most infectious particles become covered with various combinations of C3b, C3bi, and C3dg and bind to the respective receptors of these fragments; CR3 is more effective than CR1 in triggering phagocytosis of these coated particles. Heritable deficiencies of CR3 secondary to defects in the gene for the β chain are associated with impaired phagocytic activity and recurrent infections (see Chapter 15, Cell Adhesion Molecules).

RECEPTORS FOR C3a, C4a, C5a

C3a (also termed anaphylatoxin; see below) binds to mast cells and basophils, causing them to release histamine and other vasoactive mediators (see Chapter 18). High concentrations of C4a elicit similar responses and appear to interact with the same receptor. Little is known about this receptor, but the one for C5a has been extensively characterized.

Found on granulocytes, the **C5a receptor** rapidly internalizes C5a and then recycles to the cell surface. On neutrophils, these receptors are abundant (10,000–50,000 per cell) and have high affinity for C5a (equilibrium dissociation constant, K_d, is 1–2 nM).

OTHER RECEPTORS

A **C1q receptor,** found on monocytes, B-lymphocytes, and neutrophils, specifically binds C1q in Ag–Ab–C complexes but not free C1q or C1. The C1q site that is recognized by the receptor seems to become exposed when C1 INH displaces C1r and C1s from C1q, and perhaps the role of this receptor is to enhance the binding of Ag–Ab–C1q complexes to cells. Indeed, a cell's Fc receptor and C1q receptor may cooperate in binding Ab–Ag–C complexes: thus, C1q's collagen-like region appears to bind to the C1q receptor, whereas its globular portion interacts with IgG, which binds to the cell's Fc receptor.

Binding sites for H protein are found on human B cells, monocytes, and neutrophils, but their function is unknown.

Complement and Inflammation

Although cell lysis has dominated the *in vitro* study of C, the most important and noticeable effects of activated C *in vivo* are related to cellular and tissue changes associated with inflammation (Table 17–5). Various effects are attributable to particular C components and fragments. These phlogistic activities are generated in the immediate vicinity of the immune complexes that activate C, and they lead to increased local concentrations of serum proteins (including Igs and C) and blood leukocytes (including activated phagocytes). The resulting destruction of pathogens by phagocytosis is of critical importance for host defenses, especially because gram-positive bacteria and viruses are not susceptible to the lytic action of C. Serious recurrent infections in individuals who are deficient in C3, but not in those deficient in C5, C6, C7, or C8 (see below), point to the overriding importance of C3, and to the early components leading to the activation of C3, rather than to the late cytolytic components, in host defense against infection.

TABLE 17–5. Principle Proinflammatory Activities of Activated Complement (C) Proteins and Their Fragments

Activity	C Protein or Fragment
IMMUNE ADHERENCE AND OPSONIZATION	
Adherence of Ab–Ag–C complexes to leukocytes, platelets (nonprimates), and erythrocytes (primates), leading to increased susceptibility of complexes to phagocytosis by granulocytes and macrophages.	C3b/C4b
MEMBRANE DAMAGE	
Nonspecific ion channels in target-cell membranes, causing lysis of RBC; impaired permeability of nucleated cells; lysis of gram-negative bacteria.	C8, C9
ANAPHYLATOXIN	
Releases histamine and other vasoactive mediators from mast cells and thereby increases permeability of capillaries.	C4a, C3a, C5a
CHEMOTAXIS/CHEMOKINESIS	
Attracts polymorphonuclear leukocytes and macrophages to sites of inflammation (chemotaxis) and increases their overall activity (chemokinesis).	C5a

ANAPHYLATOXINS. This term is derived from the old observation that guinea pigs undergo fatal shock, resembling anaphylaxis (Chapter 18), when injected with normal serum that has been incubated briefly with various substances (e.g., inulin, Ab–Ag complexes, talc) that are now known to activate C through either the classic or the alternative pathway. The effect was attributed to the appearance of "anaphylatoxins," which are now known to be the C4a, C3a, and C5a fragments cleaved from C4, C3, and C5 (see Fig. 17–1). They may also be cleaved from these C proteins by a variety of proteases, such as plas-

min, indicating that nonspecific formation of fragments also can initiate inflammatory responses.

C4a, C3a, and C5a promote smooth muscle contraction and vascular permeability (termed "spasmogenic" properties; Table 17–6). These effects arise from their binding to receptors on mast cells and basophils and stimulating these cells to secrete histamine and other mediators that act on smooth muscle and small blood vessels (Chapter 18). Thus, injection of C3a into human skin promptly elicits a response that duplicates the immediate-type hypersensitivity responses that are elicited by Ags ("wheal and erythema") and the effect can be specifically blocked by antihistamine drugs (Chapter 18). Although similar in origin and structure, C3a and C5a act on different mast-cell receptors: thus, isolated mast-cell-rich tissues that are treated repeatedly with C3a lose their responsiveness to it (**tachyphylaxis**) but still respond to C5a, and vice versa. Both peptides are active at extremely low concentrations (1×10^{-8} to 5×10^{-10} M).

C4a, C3a, and C5a are similar structurally. They have about the same number of amino acids (77 in C3a and C4a, and 75 in C5a), and their C-terminal residue is arginine, indicating that the serine protease cleavage that produces each of them has trypsin-like specificity. Anaphylatoxin activity is lost when this arginine residue is removed by a specific serum carboxypeptidase, called **anaphylatoxin inhibitor.** C3a and C4a are converted to the inactive des-Arg forms within seconds in human sera and hence probably exert their effects only locally. Although C5a is also a substrate for this enzyme, it is inactivated incompletely (approximately 5% appears to be resistant to cleavage, and C5a-des Arg retains some biologic activity), and it is found in the circulation under conditions associated with widespread complement activation (see Table 17–6).

C5a, but not C4a or C3a, has profound effects on granulocyte function (Table 17–7). These effects, exerted at

TABLE 17–6. Spasmogenic Properties of the Human Anaphylatoxins*

Biologic Response	Effective Dose (M/L)			
	C5a	des-Arg⁷⁴ C5a†	C3a	C4a
Smooth muscle contraction				
Ileum	5.0×10^{-10}	1.2×10^{-6}	1×10^{-8}	1.5×10^{-6}
Uterus	7.5×10^{-10}		1×10^{-8}	
Vascular permeability				
Guinea pig	$0.1–1.0 \times 10^{-13}$	1.0×10^{-10}	$0.01–1.0 \times 10^{-10}$	$0.01–1.0 \times 10^{-8}$
Human	$0.1–1.0 \times 10^{-13}$		$0.01–1.0 \times 10^{-10}$	

* From Chenoweth DE: In Ross GD: Immunobiology of the Complement System. Orlando, Academic Press, 1986.

† Formed by removing the C-terminal arginine of C5a.

TABLE 17-7. Leukocyte-Related Activities of Human C5a*

Target Cells	Cellular Responses
Neutrophils	Augmented adherence
	Cellular polarization
Monocytes	Chemotactic migration
	Degranulation and enzyme release
	Production of toxic oxygen metabolites
	Enhanced arachidonic acid metabolism
	Augmented expression of complement receptors
	Increased production of IL-1

* Taken from Chenoweth DE: In Ross GD: Immunobiology of the Complement System. Orlando, Academic Press, 1986.

concentrations as low as 10^{-10} M, suggest a central role for C5a as a mediator of acute inflammatory responses.

CHEMOTAXIS. In diffusion chambers divided by porous membranes (Fig. 17–12), C5a in one compartment attracts granulocytes from the adjacent compartment (**chemotactic** activity). Evidently granulocytes, through their C5a receptors, can detect a gradient in C5a concentration.

IMMUNE ADHERENCE AND OPSONIZATION. As noted above, Ab–Ag complexes with C3b bound to them adhere to receptors for C3b, particularly those on granulocytes and macrophages. Bacteria, viruses, and other particles that are coated ("opsonized") with Ab and C3b bind to these receptors, and are then ingested and degraded. This **opsonic activity** is probably one of the C system's most important functions. Also, as noted above, C3b receptors are also present on nonphagocytic cells: B lymphocytes, a subpopulation of T lymphocytes, and, especially, on primate RBC (and nonprimate platelets). By facilitating the transport of Ag–Ab–C complexes on RBC to liver and spleen, where they are degraded by macrophages, immune adhesion on RBC makes a critical contribution to the elimination of Ab–Ag–C complexes.

As we shall see below, if the classic pathway is deficient in any component up to and including C3, or if the activity of C3b receptors is reduced, the complexes do not bind to red blood cells, and they fail to be eliminated effectively in liver and spleen. Instead, **they are deposited in the lung and kidney,** which have only a limited capacity to degrade them; impaired pulmonary and renal function can follow.

The **C3b receptor clearance mechanism** probably evolved to eliminate the large quantities of Ag–Ab–C that form in association with many infections, especially those caused by certain parasites, such as malaria. The rarity of inflammatory illnesses of the kidney in most chronic parasitic infections suggests that this clearance system is usually highly effective.

LYTIC REACTIONS. Gram-negative bacteria coated with specific Ab can be lysed by C through the same reaction sequence as in RBC lysis, but gram-positive bacteria and mycobacteria are resistant. Their resistance probably stems from their cell wall, as protoplasts of gram-positive bacteria are readily lysed by C. Cells of metazoan parasites are also lysed by C.

TISSUE DESTRUCTION. C and Ab can damage host cells as well as microbes. Two mechanisms appear to be operative. In the first, C becomes activated with Abs (autoantibodies) that bind to self-Ags on cells (e.g., on red cells, platelets, and cells of muscle, thyroid, and pancreas). In the second mechanism, large quantities of Ab–Ag complexes become deposited or form specifically on small blood vessels, such as in the kidney, and then activate C, promoting inflammation and tissue injury (see Arthus Reaction, Chapter 18).

Genetic Deficiencies in Complement
IN HUMANS

Heritable deficiencies in C proteins (as in other proteins) provide powerful insights into their normal activity *in vivo*. Genetic defects have been recognized in humans for each of the C proteins of the classic pathway and for all but B of the alternative pathway (Table 17–8). Recovery of full activity following the addition of the missing compo-

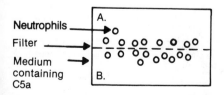

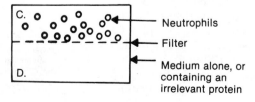

Neutrophils

Filter

Medium alone, or containing an irrelevant protein

Figure 17–12. A two-compartment chamber demonstrates **chemotaxis.** Neutrophils are introduced into one compartment; C5 or C5a into the other compartment. After several hours, the neutrophils have migrated to and through the filter. In control chambers (not shown), neutrophils do not migrate out of a compartment into which they are introduced together with C5a.

TABLE 17–8. Human Complement Deficiencies*

Component	Number of Individuals with Homozygous Deficiency	Number with Associated Diseases	
		Immune Complex Disease†	Infections
CLASSIC			
C1q	15	14	
C1r/C1s	8	6	} less than 20% with bacterial infections
C4	16	14	
C2	66	38	
ALTERNATIVE			
D	2	–	
B	0	–	} 5-*Neisseria*
P	4	–	
BOTH PATHWAYS			
C3	11	8	10 with severe bacterial infections
TERMINAL COMPONENTS			
C5	12	1	9-*Neisseria*
C6	17	2	10-*Neisseria*
C7	14	1	6-*Neisseria*
C8	14	1	8-*Neisseria*
C9	Many	None	None/healthy
REGULATORS			
C1 INH	>500	Few	Hereditary angio-edema
I	5	1	4-bacterial
H	2	1	1-bacterial

* Modified from Schifferli JA, Peters DK: Lancet 2:957, 1983.

† Immune complex-mediated diseases such as systemic lupus erythematosus (SLE), SLE-like syndromes, glomerulonephritis, vasculitis.

nent in purified form shows that a serum defect in C activity is secondary to the loss of a particular protein rather than to the appearance of an inhibitor.

Heterozygotes with a defective C allele have about half the normal serum level of the corresponding C protein, and they usually have no associated illness. But many of those with homozygous deficiency suffer from the disorder known as **systemic lupus erythematosus** (SLE) or from increased susceptibility to infection. SLE is characterized by the excessive deposition of Ab–Ag–C complexes in blood vessel walls: tissue injury follows, especially in the kidney. This disease has been observed in almost all individuals with homozygous defects in C1q, C1r, C1s, or C4. More than 100 individuals deficient in C2 have been described, and over 50% have SLE or a related illness, whereas the remainder are healthy. Two possibilities might account for this high frequency of what is a relatively uncommon disease in the general population.

(1) The lack of an early complement component could lead to inefficient complement activation and poor immune elimination of an infectious agent that causes or triggers the disease. (2) Reduced processing of even normal quantities of immune complexes could result, in deficient individuals, in widespread tissue injury, as is seen in SLE.

In the rare individuals with homozygous C3 deficiency, infections are severe, recurrent, and life-threatening and start soon after birth. In contrast, excessive infections in individuals with homozygous deficiency of the late components, C5, C6, C7, or C8, or of the alternative pathway (B and P), are caused primarily by one species of gram-negative bacteria (*Neisseria*), and these individuals are, for the most part, healthy. Lysis, requiring the late proteins, probably represents an important defense against *Neisseria*, but **the opsonic activity, not the lytic activity, of C apparently offers more protection against most pathogenic bacteria and viruses.**

IN LABORATORY ANIMALS

C4-DEFICIENT GUINEA PIGS. Guinea pigs without C4 were recognized through the observation that they formed Abs (anti-C4) in response to injections of guinea pig C4 (Self-tolerance; Chapter 20). Because these guinea pigs lack the classic pathway for activating the C cascade, they provided some of the most conclusive evidence for the importance of the alternative pathway. Isolated macrophages from normal guinea pigs synthesize C4, but those from the C4-deficient strain do not.

TABLE 17–9. Special Structural Features of Complement Proteins*

Structural Feature	Protein	Function
Collagen-like strands	C1q	Scaffolding for globular domains that interact with the Fc region of Abs
Serine proteases (with very limited substrate specificity)	C1r, C1s C2, B D	Cleave and thereby activate other complement components
Thioester bond	C4, C3	Covalent attachment to proteins
Homology unit with tandom repeats (~60 amino acids long)	C1r, C1s, C2, B H, DAF, MCP CR1, CR2, C4bp	Bind to domains of C3b and C4b
Hydrophobic domains	C5, C6, C7 C8, C9	Insert into cell membrane

* Many proteins with similar structural features probably arose by duplication of a common ancestral gene: C1r and C1s; C2 and B; C4 and C3; H, DAF, MCP, C4bp, CR1 and CR2; C6 and C7; and C8 and C9. See also Figures 17–4, 17–6, and 17–7.

C5-DEFICIENT MICE. Many inbred mouse strains lack C5 but appear healthy, probably because their alternative and classic pathways are intact through C3. However, when deliberately exposed to *Corynebacterium kutscheria*, a bacterium pathogenic for mice, they exhibit increased susceptibility. Like humans deficient in C5–C8, the defect in these mice is inapparent until they are challenged by a particular pathogen.

C6-DEFICIENT RABBITS. The inherited absence of C6 in some rabbits has been confirmed by their ability to produce anti-C6 Abs in response to injections of purified rabbit C6. The deficient animals have impaired serum bactericidal activity, but are healthy under laboratory conditions.

C3-DEFICIENT DOGS. A colony of C3-deficient dogs has been developed. Inherited as an autosomal codominant trait, the deficiency is associated with skin infections, a profound defect in clearance of immune complexes, renal disease (glomerulonephritis), impaired inflammatory responses, and multiple abnormalities in *in vitro* tests of serum for opsonic and chemotactic activity.

IN REGULATORY PROTEINS

The potential dangers of uncontrolled complement activity are evident in disorders associated with rare genetic defects in I and in C1 inhibitor (C1 INH), two serum proteins that inhibit C-activating proteins (see above). H deficiency has also been described.

DEFICIENCY OF C1 INHIBITOR (C1 INH). Individuals with a deficiency in C1 INH have **hereditary angioedema:** they experience periodic episodes of acute, painless local accumulations of interstitial edema fluid, typically lasting 48 to 72 hours. The swelling attacks are most often subcutaneous and cause primarily a cosmetic problem. However, the attacks can become life-threatening when the swelling is in the larynx, obstructing the airway, and painful when it involves the bowel wall, leading to partial obstruction.

Unlike heritable deficiencies of other C-regulatory proteins, disease secondary to C1 INH deficiency is inherited as an autosomal dominant (rather than recessive) trait; thus, heterozygotes are affected. Their serum level of C1 INH would be expected to be reduced by about half, but it is usually much lower (5% to 20%). The reason is unknown. There must be various genetic defects responsible for the deficiency, because about 15% of affected persons produce normal to increased quantities of an inactive C1 INH.

Serum obtained during attacks has increased C1s activity, leading to decreased C4 and C2. Injected into skin, the serum causes increased permeability of cutaneous blood vessels. (The responsible factor may be a small polypeptide, termed **C-kinin,** which is split from C2.)

I AND H. Because of the spontaneous turnover of C3, an individual without I would be expected to have virtually unchecked activity of the resulting C3b, leading to excessive breakdown of C3 by C3b,Bb complexes. Indeed, in I-deficient individuals, serum C3 is reduced to approximately $\frac{1}{20}$ of the normal level, and, as expected, the concentrations of B and C5 are also reduced; bactericidal activity for gram-negative bacteria, opsonic activity for Ab-coated pneumococci, and chemotactic activity are all diminished. Most affected individuals suffer from severe, recurrent infections with β-hemolytic streptococci or meningococci. In some, the syndrome resembles that seen in individuals with a homozygous defect in C3 itself (see above). The infusion of I corrects the deficit. Similar abnormalities are present in an H-deficient family.

DAF AND HRF. Paroxysmal nocturnal hemoglobinuria is an acquired hemolytic disorder characterized by spontaneous episodes of RBC lysis. *In vitro*, RBCs, leukocytes, and platelets from these patients have increased sensitivity to lysis by C. One cause is a deficiency of DAF and of HRF, two membrane-associated proteins that inhibit the activity of C. Both proteins are anchored in cell membranes by phosphatidyl inositol, and it is possible that the underlying anomaly is a defect in attachment of phosphatidyl inositol to the C terminus of these proteins. In some forms of the disease, the defect can be corrected *in vitro* by supplying DAF to cells. This disease clearly points up the critical role of DAF and HRF in preventing complement-mediated damage to normal cells.

DEPLETION OF COMPLEMENT

Because animals with genetic C deficiencies are not always available for experimental studies of C function *in vivo*, soluble Ab–Ag complexes formed *in vitro* have been injected into normal mice to deplete their C levels. The injection often has to be accompanied by the administration of antihistamines to prevent anaphylaxis caused by the production of anaphylatoxin and massive release of histamine (see Aggregate Anaphylaxis, Chapter 18).

The most selective and prolonged depletion (of C3) is brought about with venom from the cobra (*Naja haja*). The active component, cobra venom factor (CoF; mol. wt. 140,000), is homologous to C3b but is entirely resistant to the C3b-inhibiting activity of mammalian regulatory proteins; hence, it forms a stable P,CoF,Bb complex that cleaves C3. The released C3b, in turn, forms more C3-cleaving P,C3b,Bb. Through this sequence, intact C3 is eliminated, effectively eliminating the C system for 4 to 96 h. Antibodies soon develop to CoF, so its use is limited

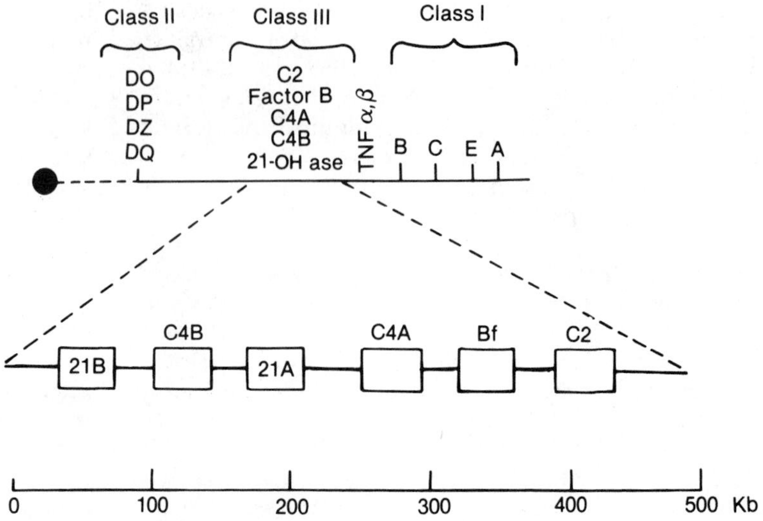

Figure 17–13. Map of major histocompatibility complex (MHC) on short arm of human chromosome 6, showing alignment in the class III region of complement genes C2, factor B, C4A, and C4B (centromere is at the left). The entire MHC spans about 3500 Kb. The proteins encoded by genes for steroid 21-hydroxylase A and B are not parts of the complement system or related to the MHC class I and class II proteins. TNFα is tissue necrosis factor; TNFβ is lymphotoxin (Chap. 19). ● = centromere. (Based on Carroll et al: Proc Natl Acad Sci 84:8535, 1987)

to one or two injections. As yet, there is no specific inhibitor that can be repetitively administered to mammals to block the C system *in vivo*.

Complement Genes

POLYMORPHIC VARIANTS

Genetic variants of most human C proteins have been identified by their altered electrophoretic mobilities. Perhaps because of their relatively high serum concentration, more variants (>20) of C3 and C4 (see Table 17–1) than of other C proteins have been recognized. Most C proteins are specified by autosomal codominant genes; an exception is P, whose expression is sex-linked.

Genes for several polymorphic C proteins (B,C2,C4) have been localized in the human HLA complex (Fig. 17–13) and in the homologous locus of the mouse H-2 complex (see Fig. 15–13, Chap. 15). Genes for six of the C receptor and regulatory proteins are located on chromosome 1 of humans and mice; they probably also have a common origin in evolution, because the proteins they encode share the 60 amino acid repeat that is common to most of the proteins that bind C3b or C4b (see Fig. 17–11).

Human C4 is encoded by two closely linked genes (C4A and C4B). Their products are more than 99% identical in sequence, and the few amino acid differences between them are concentrated near the site of the thioester group. Upon activation, C4A reacts better with amino and C4B better with hydroxyl groups; whether this difference is related to differences in the reactivity of C4 with Ig heavy chains of various isotypes is not clear. There are multiple alleles at both the C4A and C4B loci, and several have been shown to have altered hemolytic activity.

cDNA clones for all of the C-activating proteins, inhibi-

tors, and receptors (except those for C3a and C5a) have been isolated and sequenced. The deduced amino acid sequences have confirmed many of the previously suspected homologies, including C1r–C1s, B–C2, C3–C4–C5, C6–C7, C8–C9, and the C3b/C4b binding proteins.

Metabolism and Biosynthesis

Although monocytes, macrophages, and fibroblasts can synthesize some components (including C1q, C2, C3, C4, C5, B, D, and P), synthesis in the liver appears to account for most, if not all, of the C protein in serum. Thus, after a human recipient's diseased liver was replaced by a liver allograft from a donor with a different C3 allotype, the recipient's serum C3 soon became replaced by C3 of the donor's type.

Inflammation increases the synthesis of C proteins. A basis for the increase is suggested by the finding that interferon-gamma (γ-IFN) and interleukin-1 (normally released in inflammatory responses by activated T cells and macrophages, respectively) increase transcription of B and C3 (and presumably other C components as well) in a human hepatoma cell line.

During development, some C appears to be synthesized as early as the fifth intrauterine week, and the concentration of most components in newborn sera is about 50% of the adult levels; by 12 months, adult levels are reached. The catabolic rates of C components (1–3% per hr) are high compared with many other plasma proteins.

Summary

The complement (C) system consists of a series of sequentially acting proteins that: (1) promote phagocytosis and the degradation of Ab–Ag complexes; (2) elicit inflammation; and (3) in some instances cause the lysis of bacterial and animal cells. Nearly all of the C proteins exist in normal serum as inactive precursors; when activated, some of them are highly specific proteolytic enzymes whose substrate is the next protein in the sequential chain reaction. The entire C cascade can be triggered by either of two initiation pathways. In the classic pathway, appropriate Ab–Ag complexes (with Abs of the correct isotype and Ab–Ag in proper molar ratio) bind and activate C1, C4, and C2 to form a C3-splitting enzyme. In the alternative pathway, another set of sequentially reacting proteins (B, D, P) forms a different C3-splitting enzyme. Both C3-splitting enzymes act in precisely the same way to elicit the remaining (late) steps. The alternative pathway is not initiated by Ab–Ag aggregates; instead, its activity derives from the spontaneous low-grade turnover of the C3 protein, which continually deposits activated C3 indiscriminately on cell surfaces. Inhibitory proteins on most mammalian cells prevent further activity of the deposited C3, but most bacteria and fungi lack these inhibitors, and the active C3 deposited on them can then bind trace amounts of two other proteins (factor B and properdin), forming a C3-splitting enzyme and allowing the rest of the sequence to proceed.

Many of the inflammatory (phlogistic) effects of the C sequence can be accounted for by individual components or their active fragments: C3b on the surface of a cell (or virus) is a powerful opsonic agent, increasing susceptibility to phagocytosis by polymorphonuclear leukocytes and macrophages; C3a and C5a act through receptors on mast cells and stimulate the secretion of mediators that cause vasodilation and increase capillary permeability (anaphylatoxin activity); C5a attracts leukocytes (chemotactic activity); and C8 and, especially, C9, form nonspecific ion channels in cell membranes, resulting in the osmotic lysis of many cells (cytotoxic activity).

The opsonic and cytolytic effects of activated C are almost entirely confined to those cells that initiate the sequence. Neighboring host cells that lack the triggering immune aggregates or the initiating complexes of the alternate pathway are spared because of the instability of activated C proteins and their fragments and because of soluble and cell-bound inhibitory proteins.

The importance of the C system to host defenses against microbial pathogens and to the destruction of immune complexes is evident from the increased susceptibility to infections and to immune complex-mediated diseases in persons with rare genetic defects of C. Although the C system is largely beneficial, it can also cause damage to host tissues if autoantibodies are made or if quantities of Ab–Ag aggregates exceed its clearing capabilities. Thus, C can both amplify the protective effects of the humoral immune system and, in certain autoimmune responses, cause excessive tissue damage (hypersensitivity).

Appendix
MEASUREMENT OF COMPLEMENT

Because RBC lysis is easy to measure, it provides the basis for measurements of C activity. The standard reagents are sheep RBC and rabbit Abs (termed hemolysins) to these cells. When the cells are optimally coated with nonagglutinating amounts of the Abs, the addition of C (usually as fresh serum), in the presence of adequate concentrations of Ca^{2+} and Mg^{2+}, promptly causes the cells to lyse; the released hemoglobin is then measured after removing intact RBC and stroma by centrifugation. The proportion of sensitized RBCs that are lysed increases with the amount of C added (Fig. 17–14). Because 100% lysis is approached asymptotically, it is convenient to **define the hemolytic unit of complement (the CH_{50} unit) as that amount which lyses 50% of sensitized RBCs** under conditions that are arbitrarily standardized with respect to the concentration of sensitized RBCs, the concentration and type of sensitizing Ab, the ionic strength and pH of the solvent, the concentrations of Mg^{2+} and Ca^{2+}, and the temperature.

The dose–response curve of Figure 17–14 follows the von Krogh equation:

$$x = K\left(\frac{y}{1-y}\right)^{1/n}$$

in which x is the amount of C added (i.e., milliliters of guinea pig or other serum), y is the proportion of cells lysed, and n and K are constants. The curve described by this equation (which was arrived at empirically) is sigmoidal when $1/n < 1$; for fresh normal guinea pig serum, $1/n$ is usually about 0.2. In estimating the number of CH_{50} units per milliliter of serum, it is convenient to plot $\log x$

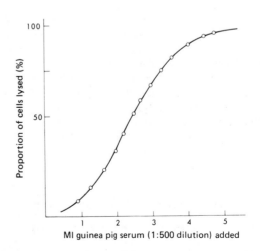

Figure 17–14. Dose–response curve of immune hemolysis. The curve follows the empiric von Krogh equation (see text).

versus log $(y/1 - y)$; the data fall on a straight line:

$$\log x = K + \left(\frac{1}{n}\right) \log \frac{y}{1 - y}$$

in which the intercept at 50% lysis $(y = 1 - y; \log y/1 - y = 0)$ gives the volume of serum that corresponds to one CH_{50} unit.

MEASUREMENT OF COMPLEMENT IN CLINICAL MEDICINE. Most hospital laboratories routinely measure C4, C3, B, and the whole complement titer (CH_{50}) or total hemolytic complement (THC). Abs to C3, C4, and B measure these proteins as Ags using various quantitative immunoassays (Chapter 13). Although these measurements do not assess function, there is generally a close correlation between the antigenic and hemolytic activities of complement proteins.

To measure total hemolytic complement activity, sheep RBC are coated with a rabbit Ab (hemolysin) and incubated with dilutions of human serum. The reciprocal of the dilution of serum that lyses 50% of the RBC is the total hemolytic complement activity or CH_{50}. A normal titer requires that all nine components of the classical pathway be present at approximately 50% or greater of their usual concentration. In individuals who lack C9, CH_{50} levels are low but not absent (because C8 can compensate to some extent). Complete deficiency of any one of the other components results in a very low or undetectable whole complement titer. A measure of the alternative pathway is not routinely used in the clinical setting.

THE ONE-HIT THEORY

As noted earlier in this chapter, the one-hit theory of RBC lysis by C depends on evidence for linear relations between the average number of lytic lesions per RBC and the concentration of C1, C4, and C2. For instance, with RBC coated with Abs, the average number of lytic lesions per cell varies linearly with the concentration of C1 (the other C components being present in excess). Similarly, with RBC coated with Abs and C1 or with Abs, C1, and C4, the average number of lytic lesions per cell varies linearly with the concentrations of C4 and C2, respectively. The average number of lytic lesions per RBC is calculated from the proportion of cells that are not lysed by applying the Poisson distribution.* The activation and

binding of C1 is likewise linearly related to the concentration of IgM Abs (anti-RBC), or to the square of the concentration of the corresponding IgG Abs.

These linear relations indicate that a single critical site is established by the binding of one IgM or one pair of IgG Ab molecules, followed by one molecule each of C1, C4, and C2. This is sufficient to activate and bind many molecules of C3 and the remaining C components and to cause lysis.

Selected Readings

Alper CA: Complement and the MHC. in Dorf ME (ed): The Role of the Major Histocompatibility Complex in Immunobiology, p 173. New York, Garland Press, 1981

Atkinson JP, Farries T: Separation of self from non-self in the complement system. Immunol Today 8:212, 1987

Bottger EC, Bitter–Suermann D: Complement and the regulation of humoral immune responses. Immunol Today 8:261, 1987

Colomb MG, Arlaud GJ, Villiers CL: Structure and activation of C1: Current concepts. Complement 1:69, 1984

Fearon DT, Wong WW: Complement ligand–receptor interactions that mediate biological responses. Annu Rev Immunol 1:243, 1983

Frank MM: Complement in the pathophysiology of human disease. N Engl J Med 316:1525, 1987

Holers VM, Cole JL, Lublin DM, Seya T, Atkinson JP: Human C3b- and C4b-regulatory proteins: A new multigene family. Immunol Today 6:188, 1985

Hugli TE: The structural basis for anaphylatoxin and chemotactic functions of C3a, C4a and C5a. Crit Rev Immunol 1:321, 1981

Joiner KA, Brown EJ, Frank MM: The role of complement in infectious diseases. Annu Rev Immunol 2:461, 1984

Mayer MM, Michales DW, Ramm LE et al: Membrane damage by complement. Crit Rev Immunol 2:133, 1981

Muller–Eberhard HJ: The membrane attack complex. Springer Semin Immunopathol 7:93, 1984

Pangburn MK, Muller–Eberhard HJ: The alternative complement pathway. Springer Semin Immunology 7:164, 1984

Porter RR, Lachmann PJ, Reid KBM (eds): Biochemistry and Genetics of Complement. London, The Royal Society, 1984

Reid KBM: Activation and control of the complement system. Essays Biochem 22:69, 1986

Reid KBM, Bentley DR, Campbell RD et al: Complement system proteins which interact with C3b or C4b: A superfamily of structurally related proteins. Immunol Today 7:230, 1986

Reid KBM, Porter RR: The proteolytic activation systems of complement. Annu Rev Biochem 50:433, 1981

Ross GD (ed): Immunobiology of the Complement System: An Introduction for Research and Clinical Medicine. Orlando, Academic Press, 1986

Ross SC, Densen P: Complement deficiency states and infection, epidemiology, pathogenesis, and consequences of neisserial and other infections in an immune deficiency. Medicine (Baltimore) 63:243, 1984

Ross GD, Medof ME: Membrane complement receptors for bound fragments of C3. Adv Immunol 37:217, 1985

Schreiber RD: Complement receptors. Springer Semin Immunopathol 7:221, 1984

Whaley K (ed): Methods in Complement for Clinical Immunologists. New York, Churchill Livingstone, 1985

---

*$P(k) = e^{-m}m^k/k!$, where $P(k)$ is the proportion of cells with k lytic lesions per cell, m is the average number of lytic lesions per cell, and e is the base of natural logarithms. Unlysed cells have no lytic lesions ($k = 0$); their frequency is e^{-m} (because $0! = 1$), and $m = -2.303 \log_{10}P(0)$.

18

Antibody-Mediated (Immediate-Type) Hypersensitivity

With the discovery of antitoxins and antimicrobial antibodies (Abs), the immune response appeared at first to be purely protective. However, it was soon found that immune responses also possess dangerous potentialities. For instance, during studies of the toxicity of extracts of sea anemones, it was observed that dogs given a second injection several weeks after the first often became acutely ill and died within a few minutes. The response was called anaphylaxis (Gr. *ana*, against; and *phylaxis*, protection), and, almost simultaneously, observers in the United States and in Germany noted that guinea pigs responded similarly to various nontoxic antigens (Ags). Later, when horse and rabbit antisera were used to treat various infectious diseases in man, diverse pathologic consequences of the immune response to the foreign proteins became commonplace.

To develop a coherent terminology, the term **allergy** (Gr. *allos* and *ergon*, altered action) was introduced to cover any altered response to a substance induced by previous exposure to it. Increased resistance, called **immunity,** and increased susceptibility, called **hypersensitivity,** were regarded as opposite forms of allergy. Usage has modified these definitions. **Allergy** and **hypersensitivity** are now synonymous: **both refer to the altered state, induced by an Ag, in which pathologic reactions can be subsequently elicited by that Ag, or by a structurally similar substance.**

In previous chapters, the administration of an **immunogen** (i.e., an Ag) to stimulate Ab formation was called **immunization.** In discussions of the allergic response, however, the immunogen is often referred to as the **allergen** or **sensitizer,** immunization as **sensitization,** and the immunized individual as **sensitive, hypersensitive,** or **allergic.**

TWO BASIC TYPES. Various allergic responses have different time courses, which reflect fundamental differences in the underlying mechanisms. **Immediate reactions,** mediated by IgE Abs, begin within minutes and subside after about half an hour. **Subacute reactions,** caused by IgG or IgM Abs, begin after about 1 to 3 hours and last for about 10 to 15 hours. **Delayed reactions,** mediated by T cells and macrophages, become evident only after 1 to 2 days and persist from several days to a few weeks. To emphasize these differences, the Ab-mediated reactions (immediate and subacute) are usually lumped and called **immediate-type hypersensitivity** ("type" means that "immediate" is not to be taken literally). The **delayed-type hypersensitivity** reactions are also often referred to as **cell-mediated hypersensitivity** (i.e., T-cell-mediated): they are part of a larger group of reactions, called **cell-mediated immunity,** in which similar mechanisms are also involved in resistance to many infectious agents and to neoplastic cells.

In this chapter, we consider the allergic reactions attributable to Ab molecules and in the next those attributable to T cells. Both reactions can be involved in autoimmune responses and will be discussed further in Chapter 20.

ANTIBODY-MEDIATED RESPONSES. The most important Ab-mediated responses are grouped in Table 18–1 on the basis of underlying mechanisms. The arrangement reflects the principle that a **combination of Ab and Ag is seldom damaging unless the immune complexes trigger certain cells to release various mediators,** which serve as the immediate causes of pathologic change. However, aberrations may follow directly from the combination of Abs (and complement) with certain cell-surface Ags, such as on red blood cells and platelets.

Anaphylaxis

Anaphylactic reactions are attributable to special Abs that bind with exceptionally high affinity to receptors on tissue mast cells and blood basophils. In man, these Abs are of the IgE class; in other species, they are IgE or, less effectively, a special class of IgG (see Homocytotropic Abs, below).

Injection of an Ag into a hypersensitive individual can cause an explosive response within 3 to 4 minutes. If the Ag is injected intravenously, the response, called **systemic** or **generalized anaphylaxis,** can lead to shock, vascular engorgement, and asphyxia secondary to bronchial and laryngeal constriction; if death does not follow promptly, recovery is complete within about 1 hour. If the Ag is injected into the skin, the same type of reaction occurs in miniature form at the local site: called **cutaneous anaphylaxis,** it is characterized by transient redness and swelling, with complete return to normal appearance in about 30 minutes. Both reactions can occur, not only in actively immunized individuals, but also in those who are **passively sensitized** with antiserum containing IgE Abs.

The basic mechanisms have been largely illuminated by studies of **passive cutaneous anaphylaxis,** which can be elicited simply and safely at multiple skin sites in the same individual, providing opportunities for controlled observations on the mediating Abs and Ags.

CUTANEOUS ANAPHYLAXIS IN HUMANS

The response begins 2 or 3 minutes after Ag is injected into the skin of a sensitive person: itching at the injected site is followed within a few minutes by a pale elevated, irregular wheal surrounded by a zone of erythema (**hive** or **urticarium**). This **wheal and erythema** response (Fig. 18–1) reaches maximal intensity about 10 minutes after the injection, persists for an additional 10 to 20 minutes, and then gradually subsides.

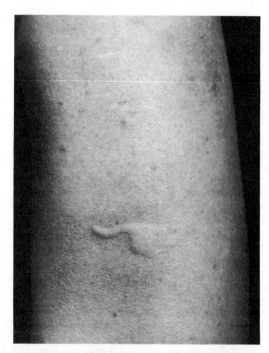

Figure 18–1. Cutaneous anaphylaxis (wheal and erythema response) in a human subject. At 15 minutes before the photograph was taken, the subject was injected intradermally with 0.02 ml containing about 0.1 µg protein extracted from guinea pig hair. Note the irregularly shaped wheal, with striking pseudopodia; the surrounding erythema is not easily visible. No reaction is seen at the control site, where 0.02 ml of buffer alone was injected.

TABLE 18–1. Antibody-Mediated Hypersensitivity Reactions

Prototype*	Examples	Isotype of the Triggering Antibodies	Mechanism	
			Activated Cells	Mediators Released
Anaphylaxis	Anaphylactic shock Wheal and erythema responses Hay fever Asthma (some forms) Hives	IgE	Mast cells; Basophils† (platelets in some species)	Histamine, leukotrienes
Immune complex disease	Arthus reaction Serum sickness syndrome Glomerulonephritis Subacute lupus erythematosus	IgG, IgM, etc.	Neutrophils†	Lysosomal enzymes, reactive oxygen intermediates
Reactions to transfused blood	Red cell incompatibilities (e.g., maternal–fetal, as in Rh disease) Autoantibodies to some self-Ags (Ch. 20; e.g., to platelets or to antihemophilic globulin) causing bleeding and purpura	IgM, IgG, etc.		

* Hypersensitivity reactions are sometimes classified into four types: Type I—anaphylaxis (i.e., attributable to Abs bound to mast cells and basophils), Type II—cytotoxic reactions attributable to Abs against autologous (self) Ags, as in blood transfusions, Rh incompatibility, etc., Type III—attributable to Ab–Ag (immune) complexes, as in serum sickness, Arthus reactions, etc., and Type IV—delayed-type reactions (i.e., mediated by T cells rather than by Abs).

† On the basis of affinity for dyes, polymorphonuclear leukocytes (granulocytes) are classified as neutrophils (>95%), basophils (about 1%), or eosinophils (about 1%).

ATOPY. Certain persons, constituting about 10% of the population in the United States, are especially prone to hypersensitive responses of the anaphylactic (IgE) type. These individuals readily become sensitive spontaneously (i.e., without deliberate immunization) to a variety of **environmental Ags,** such as allergens in airborne pollens of ragweed, grasses, or trees, or those in fungi, animal danders, house dust, or foods. As a class, these Ags are relatively resistant to proteolytic destruction. Nonetheless, the basic difficulty derives from the tendency of affected individuals to produce IgE Abs in response to extremely small amounts of certain Ags (for instance to ragweed pollen, see below). As a result, when they inhale or ingest the appropriate allergen, these persons promptly develop hives or the manifestations of hay fever and asthma. The tendency to develop this form of allergy, called **atopy** (Gr. *a* and *topis*, out of place), is heritable (see under Genetic Control of IgE Production). Many other persons, not atopic, can develop IgE Ab responses (and IgE-mediated anaphylaxis) to larger amounts of certain injected Ags (e.g., an Ag in bee venom; penicillin acting as a hapten and conjugating to proteins *in vivo*).

PASSIVE TRANSFER. The serum of an atopic person, even after extensive dilution (1000-fold or more), can passively sensitize the skin of normal persons. Passive sensitization is performed by injecting about 0.05 ml of dilute serum from the sensitive donor into the skin of a nonsen-

sitive recipient. After 1 day, and for as long as 4 weeks, injection of the corresponding Ag into the same skin site elicits the wheal and erythema response. To elicit the reaction, it is necessary to allow a **latent period** of at least 10 to 20 hours after the injection of serum.

This transfer response is called the **Prausnitz–Küstner (P-K)** reaction after those who first described it.* Patients are commonly tested for wheal and erythema responses to intradermal injections of extracts of plant pollens, fungi, food, animal danders, etc., to identify etiologic Ags. P-K tests were sometimes used to avoid direct skin tests on young children or on adults with disseminated skin disease, but they no longer are because of the possibility that hazardous viruses (hepatitis B, human immunodeficiency virus, etc.) might be transferred. Removal of IgE, but not of other immunoglobulin (Ig) classes, from human serum eliminates activity in P-K tests. For decades before IgE was discovered, the distinctive properties of these **skin-sensitizing Abs** were recognized: they were named **reagins** to distinguish them from other Abs.

* As described in 1921, Küstner was extremely sensitive to certain fish, but his serum gave no detectable reaction with extracts of these fish. Prausnitz injected a small amount of Küstner's serum into a normal person's skin and injected fish extract into the same site 24 h later: the immediate wheal and erythema response provided the basis for much of the clinical experimental work on allergy of succeeding decades.

IgE AND BLOCKING ANTIBODIES

If ragweed extract is injected repeatedly into nonatopic human volunteers, anti-ragweed Abs (predominantly of IgG class) appear in the serum and may be detected by conventional assays. However, these Abs are incapable of sensitizing human skin for wheal and erythema responses; instead, they combine with Ag and specifically **block** its ability to evoke this response in a sensitive person's skin or in a normal person's skin at a P-K site. These **blocking antibodies** differ substantially from the skin-sensitizing Abs (reagins) that cause the wheal and erythema reaction (Table 18–2).

Reagins, like IgE molecules in general, are heat labile and do not cross the human placenta, whereas blocking Abs, like IgGs in general, are heat stable and readily cross the placenta. Most important, **IgE Abs persist at passively prepared (P-K) skin sites for several weeks, whereas blocking Abs diffuse away completely within 1 to 2 days.** In addition to containing reagins, serum from atopic individuals usually contains some blocking Abs of the same specificity. Until the blocking Abs diffuse away, they can competitively inhibit the reaction of injected Ag with reagin at P-K sites. The latent period in the P-K reaction probably also reflects the time required for reagins to bind to tissue receptors (see IgE Receptors on Mast Cells and Basophils).

CUTANEOUS ANAPHYLAXIS IN GUINEA PIGS

Cutaneous anaphylaxis can also be elicited in actively or passively sensitized guinea pigs. **Passive cutaneous**

anaphylaxis (PCA) has been especially well developed by Zoltan Ovary into a valuable model system for evaluating the ability of various Abs and Ags to elicit anaphylactic responses. PCA is fundamentally the same as the human P-K reaction, but special measures are necessary to increase the visibility of the response in animal skin. Thus, several hours after an antiserum or purified Ab is injected intradermally, the corresponding Ag is injected intravenously along with a dye, such as Evans blue, that is strongly bound to serum albumin. Hence, as serum proteins rapidly leak into the dermis at the site of the reaction, the response appears as an irregular circle of stained skin; the area is an index of the reaction's intensity (Fig. 18–2). In guinea pigs, two kinds of Abs produce PCA reactions. Present at trace levels in serum (nanograms per milliliter), IgE Abs persist at injected skin sites for weeks, and their skin-sensitizing activity is destroyed by disulfide-reducing agents and by heat (56°C for 4 hours). In contrast, IgG1 molecules are present at much higher serum levels (several milligrams per milliliter), are stable to heat and S–S-splitting reagents, and persist at injected skin sites for only 1 to 2 days.

HOMOCYTOTROPIC ANTIBODIES. The Abs that mediate anaphylaxis are sometimes called **cytotropic** because they bind to mast cells and to circulating basophils. Because guinea pig IgE and IgG1 molecules bind to mast cells of the guinea pig but not of other species, they are termed **homocytotropic.** (The other major class of guinea pig IgG, called IgG2, is **heterocytotropic:** these Igs can sensitize mouse but not guinea pig skin, because they fortuitously bind with sufficient affinity to receptors on mouse mast cells.)

Many other species (rat, rabbit, dog, mouse) also have two classes of homocytotropic Abs: IgE and a class of IgG that binds much less persistently than IgE to receptors on mast cells and basophils, below. In man, only IgE molecules are homocytotropic. IgM and IgA Abs do not sensitize animals of the same or other species for anaphylactic responses.

GENERALIZED ANAPHYLAXIS

Systemic anaphylaxis in man is a rare event brought on occasionally in hypersensitive individuals by insect stings (especially bees, wasps, or hornets) or by injection of an Ag such as horse serum or (more commonly at present) penicillin. Because of this hazard, patients who receive foreign proteins (e.g., horse antitoxin) or penicillin are first questioned about previous allergic reactions and sometimes tested for wheal and erythema responses: when horse serum is used, greatly diluted serum (1000-fold or more) is injected, for even minute amounts of undiluted serum (e.g., 0.05 ml) can precipitate systemic anaphylaxis. (For more details, see Appendix, this chapter.)

TABLE 18–2. Comparison of Human IgE (Reagins) and Blocking Antibodies (Chiefly IgG) To Pollen Antigens*

	Reagins	*Blocking Antibodies*
Immunoglobulin class	IgE	IgG (predominantly)
Activity in Prausnitz–Küstner (P-K) test	Yes	No (inhibits)
Persistence in human skin (P-K test)	Up to about 4 weeks	Up to 2 days
Stability		
To heat (56°C, 4 h)	Labile	Stable
To disulfide reducing reagents	Labile	Stable
Transfer to fetus across human placenta	No	Yes
Carbohydrate†	12%	3%
Heavy chains	ε	γ (predominantly)
Light chains	κ,λ	κ,λ

* Highly purified protein Ags have been isolated from ragweed and grass pollen. As little as 10^{-4} μg of some ragweed fractions evoke specific wheal and erythema responses. Fatal anaphylaxis has been known to occur in response to skin tests with small amounts of crude extracts, and pollen Ag may be as potentially lethal (on a weight basis) for a pollen-sensitive person as botulinus toxin is for humans in general.

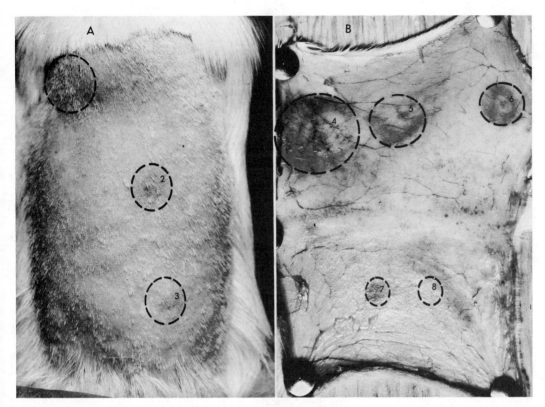

Figure 18–2. Passive cutaneous anaphylaxis in the guinea pig. In *(A)*, the guinea pig was injected intradermally at three sites with 0.1 ml saline containing 100 μg rabbit antichicken ovalbumin (EA) *(1)*, 10 μg anti-EA *(2)*, and buffered saline *(3)*. Four hours later, 1 ml containing 2 mg EA and 5 mg Evans blue was injected intravenously; the photo was taken 30 minutes later. Note blueing at *1* and at *2* and absence of blueing at the control site *(3)*. In *(B)*, a similar sequence was followed, but 30 minutes after the intravenous injection of EA, the animal was sacrificed and skinned; the photograph is of the skin's undersurface. The amount of rabbit anti-EA injected initially was 100 μg (at *4*), 10 μg (at *5*), 1 μg (at *6*), and 0.1 μg (at *7*). The control site, which did not turn blue *(8)*, had been injected with buffered saline. Another site (not shown) had been injected with 0.01 μg anti-EA; it also failed to react.

MAST CELLS AND BASOPHILS

IgE binds with high affinity (see below) to mast cells, which are nonmotile and localized in tissues, and to basophils, which circulate in blood (Fig. 18–3). Derived from different lineages of bone marrow stem cells, both cell types are characterized by prominent cytoplasmic granules that contain powerful low-mol. wt. mediators of anaphylaxis, as well as large amounts of basic (cationic) proteases and highly sulfated (anionic) proteoglycans (heparin or chondroitin sulfates). Some cationic dyes (such as toluidine blue) undergo a pronounced shift in absorption spectrum when they bind to the proteoglycans, accounting for the characteristic **metachromatic staining** properties of these cells.

Mast cells are ubiquitous in vascularized connective tissues. They are abundant near capillaries and lymph channels beneath epithelial cell layers of skin, lungs, gastrointestinal tract, nasal membranes, tongue, etc.; and

they are also found in the peritoneal cavity (of mice and rats). Two principal types are recognized. The **connective-tissue type** is found widely distributed in connective tissues (skin, etc.) and in peritoneal cavity; these mast cells have extremely high levels of histamine (approximately 15 pg per cell) and the proteoglycan they contain is heparin. The other, **mucosal, type,** found in the lining of the intestinal tract and elsewhere, has about one-tenth as much histamine and contains chondroitin sulfate, a less highly sulfated proteoglycan than heparin. Growth of the mucosal type, but not of the connective tissue type, is T-cell dependent: for instance, these cells are not found in nude mice unless the animals are recipients of a thymus graft. Nevertheless, both types appear to derive from a common precursor; thus, in the presence of a T-cell lymphokine (interleukin-3), bone marrow cells give rise to mucosal-type mast cells, but when these cells are injected into mice of a mast cell–deficient strain, the mast cells that turn up in skin, intestinal mu-

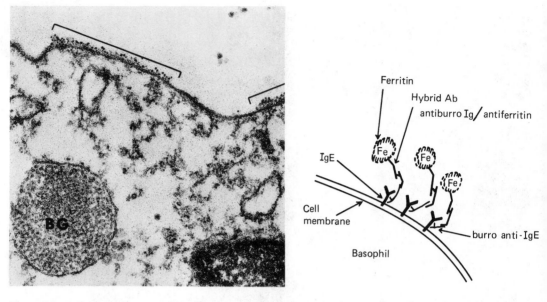

Figure 18–3. Human IgE on the surface of a human basophil. Washed white blood cells were incubated successively (with intervening washes) with human IgE (a myeloma protein), burro antihuman IgE, hybrid Abs in which one combining site was specific for burro Ig and the other for ferritin, and finally with ferritin—the iron-rich, electron-dense particles seen under *brackets* on the cell surface. Basophil granules (*BG* is a typical one) resemble the histamine-containing granules of tissue mast cells (Fig. 18–8). *Diagram* shows enlargement of the bracketed region. (Sullivan AL et al: J Exp Med 134:1403, 1971. Electron micrograph, ×77,500)

cosa, etc., have the features characteristic of the mast cells that are normally in that tissue. Hence, phenotypic differences among these cells seem to be determined by the microenvironment of the tissues in which they reside. **Both mast cell types have a high affinity Fc receptor for IgE** (see below).

Basophils derive from the bone marrow stem-cell lineage that gives rise to granulocytes. They are the least abundant granulocytes (normally about 1% of the total), and the only ones that have high-affinity receptors for IgE. They also contain histamine (although less per cell than mast cells) and other preformed mediators of anaphylaxis.

IgE RECEPTORS ON MAST CELLS AND BASOPHILS

Human skin sites can be sensitized for P-K reactions with serum having IgE levels as low as 0.2 μg/ml (10^{-9}M/L), implying that receptors on mast cells have high affinity for IgE (Fc domain, see below). The affinity has been measured directly on basophil leukemia cells, which have about 500,000 of the receptors per cell. (The number of receptors differs on basophils, the various mast cells, basophil leukemia cells, etc., but they all appear to express the same IgE receptor molecule.) For the reversible binding reaction with the receptor (R):

$$\text{IgE} + \text{R} \underset{k_d}{\overset{k_a}{\rightleftharpoons}} \text{IgE} \cdot \text{R}$$

the equilibrium constant (the measure of affinity, Chapter 13) is extremely high, about 10^{10}L/M. This value is the ratio of the association rate constant (k_a, about 10^5L/M per second) and the dissociation rate constant (k_d), which is less than 10^{-5} per second. The binding reaction appears to be a straightforward bimolecular reaction ($\text{A} + \text{B} \rightleftharpoons \text{A} \cdot \text{B}$), and the half-time ($t_{1/2}$) and the rate constant for dissociation are related as follows:

$$t_{1/2} = \frac{0.693}{k_d}$$

Therefore, it takes more than 27 h (i.e., over 10^5 seconds) for half the IgE molecules that are bound to a basophil or mast cell to dissociate from that cell. **This remarkable stability accounts for the long persistence of skin sensitization in passive cutaneous anaphylaxis (e.g., the P-K reaction).**

The basophil receptor (130,000 daltons), when isolated from the cell-surface membrane, forms 1:1 molar complexes with IgE. The receptors are evidently specific for the Fc$_\varepsilon$ region, as the Fc$_\varepsilon$ fragment of IgE molecules, but not the Fab$_\varepsilon$ fragments, can block P-K skin reactions (by competitively displacing intact IgE Abs from skin mast cells).

STRUCTURE OF THE HIGH-AFFINITY RECEPTOR FOR IgE.

On rat basophil leukemia cells, the high-affinity receptor (termed **Fc$_\varepsilon$R**) has been clearly shown to be a four-chain molecule: an α chain, which appears to bear the binding site for the IgE Fc domain, a β chain, and two identical disulfide-linked γ chains (Fig. 18–4). Thus monkey fibroblasts that are transfected with cDNA for each of the subunits acquire the ability to bind IgE with high affinity. The α, β, and γ chains are associated noncovalently and are readily separated by mild detergents.

An entirely different receptor for the Fc domain of IgE, present on B cells and monocytes, is discussed below (see Regulation of IgE Production).

CROSS-LINKING OF IgE RECEPTORS ACTIVATES MAST CELLS

Anaphylaxis is normally initiated by Ags that bind to IgE Abs while these Abs are associated with Fc$_\varepsilon$ receptors on mast cells, causing the receptors to aggregate. Thus, when a skin site is passively sensitized (with antihapten IgE Abs), multivalent haptens can elicit a wheal and erythema response, but univalent haptens are specifically inhibitory, just as they competitively block lattice formation in the precipitin reaction *in vitro* (Ch. 13). The following observations emphasize the key role of Fc$_\varepsilon$ receptor aggregation in anaphylaxis (Fig. 18–5).

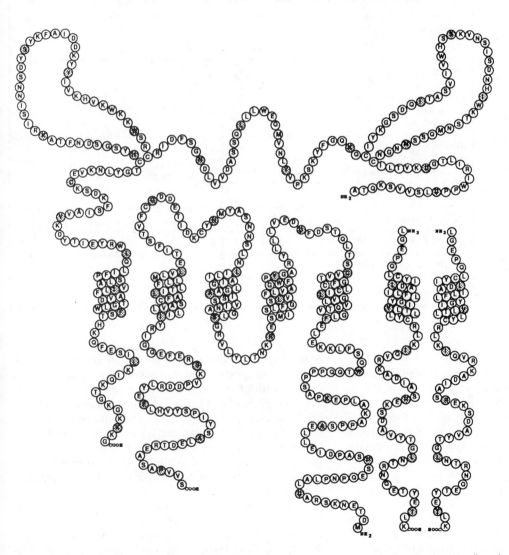

Figure 18–4. A model of the high-affinity tetrameric receptor for IgE (present normally only on mast cells and basophil). The α subunit is at left, oriented with its large, extracellular, putative IgE-binding domain at top; to its right is the β-subunit with 4 transmembrane domains; at the extreme right is the homodimer formed by a pair of γ subunits. (Courtesy of H. Metzger; from Blank et al: Nature 337:187, 1989)

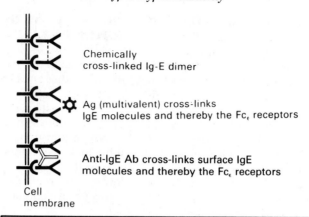

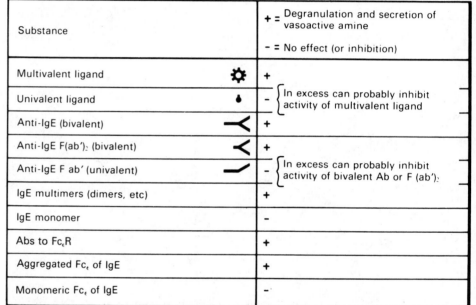

Figure 18–5. Degranulation of mast cells and basophils and secretion of vasoactive amines induced by cross-linking the cell surface receptors that bind the Fc_ε domain of IgE ($Fc_\varepsilon R$).

Substance		+ = Degranulation and secretion of vasoactive amine − = No effect (or inhibition)
Multivalent ligand	✿	+
Univalent ligand	●	− ⎱ In excess can probably inhibit activity of multivalent ligand
Anti-IgE (bivalent)	✓	+
Anti-IgE F(ab')₂ (bivalent)	✓	+
Anti-IgE F ab' (univalent)	╱	− ⎱ In excess can probably inhibit activity of bivalent Ab or F (ab')₂
IgE multimers (dimers, etc)		+
IgE monomer		−
Abs to $Fc_\varepsilon R$		+
Aggregated Fc_ε of IgE		+
Monomeric Fc_ε of IgE		−

1. Multimers of IgE (previously cross-linked chemically), but not monomeric IgE, cause basophils, in the absence of Ag, to release histamine; dimers of IgE suffice, but larger oligomers are more effective.

2. Abs of the IgG class produced against the isolated receptors (anti-receptor Abs), but not the Fab fragments of these Abs, can elicit both cutaneous anaphylaxis *in vivo* and histamine release *in vitro*. (These anti-receptor Abs are not "cytotropic;" they react with the $Fc_\varepsilon R$ via binding sites in their Fab domains, not via their Fc domain, as in the special case of IgE.)

3. Wheal and erythema skin reactions can be elicited by injecting anti-IgE Abs or their bivalent F(ab')₂ fragments but not their monovalent Fab' fragments. A similar effect is seen with aggregated Fc_ε fragments of IgE myeloma protein but not with the monomeric Fc_ε fragment (Fig. 18–5).

SERUM IgE. Concentrations of IgE in serum are measured by enzyme-linked or radioimmunoassay. For instance, anti-IgE Abs are attached covalently to particles of an inert adsorbent and mixed with a standard amount of ^{125}I-labeled IgE and variable amounts of the human serum to be tested. Unlabeled IgE in the test serum competitively reduces the specific binding of ^{125}I-IgE; hence, radioactivity associated with the washed particles decreases in proportion to the serum IgE concentration (Fig. 18–6A).

Another assay measures IgE Abs of a particular specificity, such as to dog dander (epithelial scales). Protein extracts of the dander are coupled to agarose particles, which are then trapped in small cellulose discs. The discs are incubated with about 0.05 ml of a patient's serum, washed, treated with radioactive (^{125}I) anti-IgE, washed again, and counted. A positive test (adherent ra-

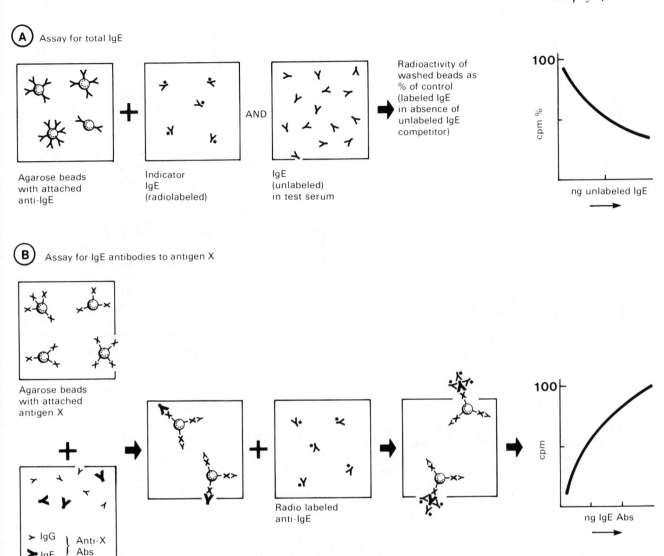

Figure 18–6. Assays for total IgE concentration in serum *(A)* and for IgE Abs of a particular specificity (anti-X) *(B)*. IgE molecules (in *heavy type*) function as Ag in the assay at top and as both Ag and Ab in the one below.

dioactivity) can detect a few nanograms per milliliter of IgE Abs of a particular specificity (Fig. 18–6B). In persons with severe atopic allergies, the IgE levels in serum are increased about two- to three-fold above normal, and levels are very much higher in some individuals who are chronically infected with intestinal parasites (see below).

REGULATION OF IgE PRODUCTION

IgE-producing plasma cells are not as rare as might be expected from the extremely low levels of IgE in the serum of normal persons (approximately 1/50,000 the con-

centration of IgG). They are easily detected by immuno-fluorescence in the mucosa of the intestinal and respiratory tracts and, particularly, in the mesenteric lymph nodes, where there are at least as many B-lymphocytes with surface IgE as with surface IgG. (IgE-producing plasma cells are also conspicuous in human surgical specimens of tonsils, adenoids, and bronchial and intestinal mucosa; they are rare in spleen and in peripheral lymph nodes. In the respiratory and intestinal tracts, IgE-producing cells are greatly outnumbered by IgA producers.) Hence, the very low IgE levels in serum suggest that IgE production is tightly regulated, as expected from

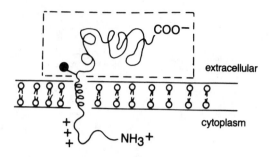

Figure 18–7. Receptor for Fc domain of IgE (Fc$_\varepsilon$R) on human B lymphocytes. Note the inverted arrangement, with the N-terminus intracellular and the C-terminus extracellular. The boxed extracellular region corresponds to a 25 Kd soluble form of the receptor. The ● symbol represents an oligosaccharide. (Based on Kikutani et al: Cell 47:657, 1986)

the hazards of anaphylaxis. How the regulation is achieved is not clear, but several possibilities are suggested by the following observations.

1. IgE production requires T-cell help: IgE is not detected in nude (athymic) mice, and T-independent Ags (Ch. 16) do not elicit IgE Abs. It is probable that only certain CD4$^+$ T cells can help B cells to produce IgE. For instance, the lymphokine IL-4, which stimulates B-cell production of IgE, is secreted by only a subset of CD4$^+$,CD8$^-$ T cells (T$_H$2 cells, see Ch. 15). Under the influence of IL-4, B cells shift from producing IgM to producing IgE. The change is due to the relocation of the VDJ gene segment assembly of the functional μ chain gene to a downstream (3′) position on the same chromosome close to the C$_\varepsilon$ gene (Chap. 14 and Chap. 16, Fig. 16-2). Hence a functioning ε chain gene replaces the functioning μ chain gene. Because the ε chain has the same V$_H$ domain as the preceding μ chain, and L chain production is unaffected by the switch, the resulting IgE has the same specificity for Ag as the IgM. Interferon-γ (IFN-γ) blocks this IL4-induced effect. IFN-γ and IL-4 are produced by different activated CD4$^+$ (CD8$^-$) T cells (T$_H$1 and T$_H$2 cells, respectively; see Chap. 15). Hence the proportions of these cells may regulate the amounts of IgE synthesized; what regulates their proportions is not clear.

2. IgE production seems to be more susceptible than IgG production to T-cell suppression. In mice, for example, low doses of x-rays or cyclophosphamide, which are thought to reduce suppressor T-cell (T$_s$) activity, enhance IgE more than IgG Ab responses. Conversely, high Ag doses, which are thought to increase T$_s$-cell activity, are much less effective than low doses in eliciting IgE.

IgE$^+$ B CELLS. B cells with surface IgE (IgE$^+$ cells) are the ultimate source of most serum IgE. Thus mesenteric lymph node cells produce IgE upon polyclonal activa-

tion of B lymphocytes with pokeweed mitogen (see Mitogens, Ch. 16) but not if the lymphocytes with surface IgE are first removed by binding them to a solid support coated with rabbit anti-IgE. In humans, most IgE$^+$ B cells also have surface IgM but not other Igs. It therefore seems likely that when (after stimulation with Ag and IL-4) the VDJ sequence of the B-cell's functional μ chain gene is translocated downstream to form a functional ε chain gene the intervening gene segments for γ and α constant domains are eliminated. The factors that are responsible for this switching, and their regulation, are, in a sense, the key to understanding IgE-mediated hypersensitivity and atopy.

IgE RECEPTOR ON B CELLS. An entirely different Fc$_\varepsilon$ from the one on mast cells and basophils (see above) is present on human B cells and on macrophage cell lines and may play a role in regulating the production or serum concentration of IgE. It binds IgE with lower affinity (about 10^{-7}M/L) than the receptor on mast cells (above 10^{-10}M/L, see above). The amino acid sequence of the B-cell receptor, deduced from the sequence of its cDNA, reveals an unusual "inverted" structure (Fig. 18–7): a single-chain integral membrane protein with an intracellular N-terminal region and a glycosylated extracellular C-terminal region. It probably becomes internalized with its bound ligand (IgE, which could be degraded in the cell's lysosomes).

The T-cell lymphokine IL-4 induces the expression of this IgE receptor on IgM$^+$/IgD$^+$ B cells but not on B cells that have switched to producing γ chains. (As noted above, IL-4 also helps induce IgE production by B cells when they are stimulated in culture with bacterial lipopolysaccharide).

A soluble form of this receptor has been found as a complex with IgE in serum of atopic patients, and relatively large amounts of a truncated form are released in culture from receptor-producing B-cell lines, probably by cleavage at the junction of the receptor's extracellular and transmembrane domains (Fig. 18–7). Whether this soluble fragment corresponds to an IgE-binding "factor" that is thought to be released from T cells and to regulate IgE Ab responses is not clear.

CORRELATIONS BETWEEN EXPERIMENTAL AND CLINICAL OBSERVATIONS. Ags that are clinically associated with high IgE Ab responses are also especially effective in eliciting such responses in mice and rats (e.g., purified proteins from ragweed pollen, extracts of *Ascaris* worm, and hen's egg albumin). When haptens are attached to them, these proteins also elicit considerable amounts of antihapten IgE Abs. Hence, it is possible that critical epitopes in these unusual "carrier" proteins are especially effective stimulators of those T_H cells that produce IL-4, rather than those that produce IFN-γ (see above).

Eventually, all of these experimental observations will have to be reconciled with the central clinical evidence for the selective ability of extremely small doses of certain proteins to elicit IgE Abs in atopic individuals. The effectiveness of unusually small amounts is strikingly emphasized by the Ag responsible for ragweed hayfever, one of the commonest clinical manifestations of IgE-mediated hypersensitivity: present in the pollen of ragweed plants, the amount of Ag inhaled has been estimated to be about 1 μg per person per year!

By contrast, in the injection schedules used routinely to elicit immunity to tetanus and diphtheria toxins, etc., the use of much higher Ag doses and appropriate adjuvants results primarily in the production of IgG Abs, with little or no IgE and with minimal (although not negligible) danger of anaphylaxis following repeated ("booster") Ag injections.

GENETIC CONTROL OF IgE PRODUCTION. As noted before, the tendency to produce IgE Abs in response to trace amounts of environmental Ags is heritable (see Atopy, above). Population studies suggest that serum IgE levels are regulated by a single genetic locus, not linked to the major histocompatibility (HLA) complex. Inbred mouse strains also differ in their ability to produce IgE Abs, especially in response to small Ag doses (e.g., 0.1 μg per mouse), and one strain (SJL) seems unable to form any IgE Abs although perfectly able to produce Abs of other classes.

Human IgE responses to certain purified pollen Ags seem also to be linked to particular major HLA haplotypes, suggesting that major histocompatibility complex class-II (MCH-II) glycoproteins may control the ability in humans to make IgE Abs of particular specificities.

Mediators of Anaphylaxis

When their Fc$_\varepsilon$ receptors are aggregated, mast cells are stimulated both to release preformed mediators from secretory granules and to synthesize and secrete several lipid mediators that are derived from arachidonic acid.

PREFORMED MEDIATORS

Secretory granules of human mast cells contain histamine, several basic (cationic) proteases, heparin (a proteoglycan), and chemotactic factors for eosinophils and neutrophils (Table 18-3). The granules of basophils have smaller amounts of these components, and their pro-

TABLE 18–3. Mediators of IgE-dependent Hypersensitivity Reactions (Anaphylaxis)

Mediators	Biologic Effects
STORED IN SECRETORY GRANULES OF MAST CELLS AND BASOPHILS	
Histamine	Vasodilatation, vasopermeability, pruritus, bronchospasm
Proteases	?
Heparin (mast cells)	Complexes with proteases and histamine
Chondroitin sulfate (basophils)	Complexes with proteases and histamine
Eosinophil chemotactic factors	Eosinophil chemotaxis
Neutrophil chemotactic factor	Neutrophil chemotaxis
SYNTHESIZED IN ACTIVATED MAST CELLS AND VARIOUS OTHER CELLS	
Cysteinyl-leukotrienes (LT–C$_4$, LT-D$_4$, LT-E$_4$)	Vasopermeability, bronchospasm
Prostaglandin D$_2$	Vasopermeability, bronchospasm
Platelet-activating factor(s)	Vasopermeability, bronchospasm, neutrophil chemotaxis, aggregation of platelets

teoglycans are both heparin and chondroitin sulfate (Fig. 18–8: mast cell granules.).

HISTAMINE. Except for special (enterochromaffin) cells in the gastric mucosa, mast cells and basophils are the only cells in the body that contain histamine. Formed by decarboxylation of L-histidine (Fig. 18–9), histamine makes up about 10% by weight of mast cell granules and, in the low pH environment of these granules, it is bound electrostatically to anionic groups (sulfate and other) of heparin–protease complexes. When mast cells are stimulated to release the granules, the higher pH of the extracellular medium causes histamine to dissociate. Increased plasma levels of histamine have been measured in persons undergoing anaphylactic shock and in episodes of bronchial asthma induced by exposure to Ag.

Histamine has inflammatory and noninflammatory effects. Both are exerted via two receptors found on many mammalian cells. Through **H$_1$ receptors,** it: (1) constricts smooth muscle, including that of bronchial airways and gastrointestinal tract; (2) increases the permeability of small blood vessels, especially venules; (3) stimulates nasal mucous secretion; and (4) causes pruritus and dilatation of cutaneous blood vessels. All of these effects are blocked by the classic antihistaminic drugs, which are antagonists of these receptors. By way of **H$_2$ receptors,** histamine causes many of the same effects, except for bronchodilation in place of bronchoconstriction. When histamine is injected into skin, its effects (redness, itching, and a wheal, as in Fig. 18–1) are

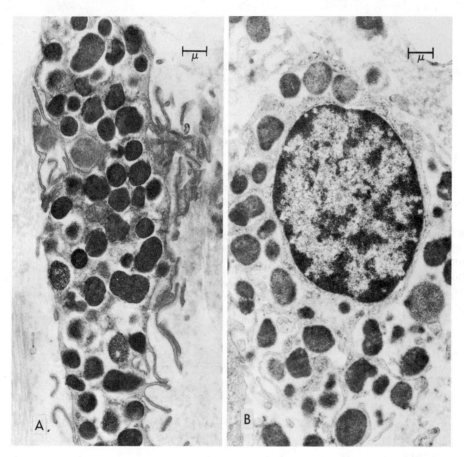

Figure 18–8. Electron micrographs of mast cells from rat dermis. The intact cell **(A)** contains small, dense granules, each about the size of a mitochondrion. Mitochondria, which are generally scarce in mast cells, are not visible. The nucleus also is not visible in this section. The degranulating cell **(B)** contains larger, paler granules. In the release of granules (associated with secretion of histamine), the membrane surrounding each granule fuses with the cell membrane, releasing the contents of the swollen granules into the extracellular space. (Courtesy of SL Clark, Jr; based on Singleton EM, Clark SL Jr: Lab Invest 14:1744, 1965. ×7000)

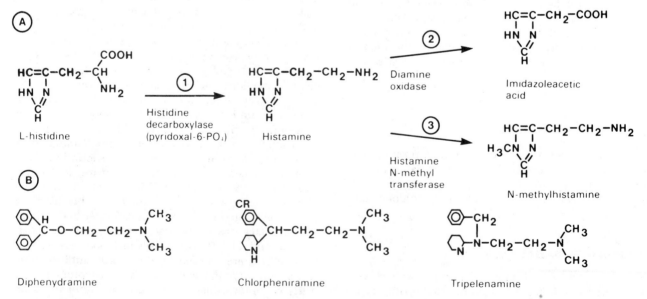

Figure 18–9. **(A)** Formation of histamine from L-histidine by histidine decarboxylase (with pyridoxal-6-phosphate as cofactor), an enzyme in mast cells and basophils. Once secreted, histamine is rapidly degraded to inactive derivatives by histaminase (diamine oxidase) and histamine N-methyl transferase. **(B)** Some antihistamines block H$_1$ receptors for histamine and are useful in the treatment of allergic reactions mediated by IgE Abs.

blocked completely by a combination of H_1 and H_2 antagonists but not by either alone. However, these antagonists are less effective against Ag-elicited anaphylaxis, because they do not block other more potent mediators of this response (see below).

PROTEASES. These proteolytic enzymes are present at extremely high levels, making up 50% of total granule protein in some species. They are highly positively charged (isoelectric point >9) and form stable complexes with the highly negatively charged (polysulfated) proteoglycans that are stored in the same granules. The most abundant one, **tryptase,** resembles trypsin in its preference for certain peptide bonds (it cleaves only the carboxyl side of lysine and arginine residues), and another one, **chymase,** is similar to chymotrypsin. They are maximally active at neutral pH (7–8) and inactive at the low pH (about 4) that prevails in the granules. Hence, they probably function only after the granules are released from the cells or if the pH within granules should rise as they are being released by exocytosis. Even outside the cell, at neutral pH, the proteases remain tightly associated with proteoglycan; and in this form, they are stable for a much longer time (several hours) than when isolated as free protein (several minutes). Their function and natural substrates are still unknown, but they probably have a role in IgE-mediated hypersensitivity, as some protease inhibitors antagonize the cutaneous manifestations of these responses. At least one of them is structurally similar to one of the proteases that is also present at high levels in the cytotoxic granules released by cytotoxic T lymphocytes when they destroy their target cells (Ch. 19).

PROTEOGLYCANS. These macromolecules have a protein core rich in serine–glycine sequences to which are attached covalently many oligosaccharides made up of sulfated disaccharide repeats. Because of the many sulfate groups (300–1000 per molecule of 100–200 Kd), they carry an enormous negative charge, accounting for the great stability of the complexes they form with the positively charged proteases and histamine that are present in the same granules. The proteoglycan in mast cells is heparin; in basophils, it is predominantly chondroitin sulfate, which differs from heparin in disaccharide composition and is less highly sulfated.

CHEMOTACTIC FACTORS. At tissue sites of IgE-mediated hypersensitivity responses, mast-cell degranulation is often accompanied by prominent infiltration with eosinophils, neutrophils, and lymphocytes. Among the identified chemotactic factors responsible for attracting these "secondary" cells, the most potent, for eosinophils, are the lipid mediators described below (a leukotriene, LTB_4, and platelet-activating factor); less potent are two tetra-

peptides (**Val–Gly–Ser–Glu** and **Ala–Gly–Ser–Glu**) that are preformed and stored in mast cell granules. These tetrapeptides also enhance the expression of complement receptors for C3b (see Ch. 17) on eosinophils and augment the Ab- and complement-dependent destruction of some parasites by eosinophils (see below). A large (600 Kd) protein that acts as an attractant for neutrophils seems also to be released by degranulating mast cells.

LIPID MEDIATORS

Unlike the stored, preformed mediators, the lipid mediators appear in mast cells and basophils only after these cells are activated (normally by $Fc_\varepsilon R$ aggregation); the most potent and best-characterized ones include leukotrienes and prostaglandins (both of them arachidonic acid derivatives), and a phospholipid derivative termed platelet-activating factor (PAF).

LEUKOTRIENES. As outlined in Figure 18–10, **arachidonic acid** is released in activated cells from membrane phospholipids by phospholipase A_2 or by phospholipase C and diacylglycerol lipase. The addition of oxygen at C5 by 5-lipoxygenase and some additional changes transform arachidonate into an unstable epoxide, termed leukotriene A_4 ($LT–A_4$); the latter can be either enzymatically hydrated to $LT–B_4$ or transformed by covalent attachment of glutathione (via its SH group) into $LT–C_4$. The subsequent elimination of the γ-glutamyl and then the glycine residues from $LT–C_4$ yields $LT–D_4$ and $LT–E_4$, respectively (Fig. 18–11).

The **cysteinyl-leukotrienes** ($LT–C_4$, $LT–D_4$, $LT–E_4$) are among the most powerful constrictors of human bronchioles known (they are 100- to 1000-fold more potent than histamine on a molar basis). They also increase the permeability of postcapillary venules and are potent stimulators of mucous secretion. In humans, they are the principal mediators of acute IgE-mediated bronchial asthma. Before their chemical identity was established, they were long studied as "slow-reacting-substance anaphylaxis" or SRS-A (Fig. 18–12).

$LT–B_4$ is a Ca^{2+} ionophore and acts primarily on leukocytes (neutrophils), attracting these cells and stimulating their production of superoxide anion (see Toxic Oxygen Intermediates, Ch. 19). Ags induce the release of leukotrienes from lung tissue of asthmatic patients, not only from their activated mast cells and basophils, but also from eosinophils, neutrophils, and alveolar macrophages, all of which also have the capacity to synthesize leukotrienes.

PROSTAGLANDINS. In an alternative metabolic pathway (see Fig. 18–10), cyclooxygenase acts on arachidonic acid to form various prostaglandins (PG), of which one, termed PGD_2, has effects on small blood vessels and

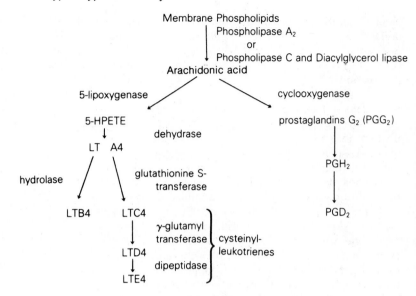

Figure 18–10. Synthesis of leukotrienes (LT) and prostaglandins (PG) from arachidonic acid, which is derived from membrane phospholipids of activated mast cells and various other cells (e.g., neutrophils, eosinophils, monocytes, keratinocytes). (Based on Samuelsson et al: Science 237:1171, 1987; Serafin WE, Austen KF: N Engl J Med 317:30, 1987)

bronchial airways like those of other mediators of IgE-dependent hypersensitivity. Mast cells, but not basophils, produced PGD_2 (although both produce the cysteinyl-leukotrienes). Injected into human skin in minute (nanomolar) quantities, PGD_2 elicits the same wheal and erythema responses as do Ag and histamines (see Fig.

18–1) but without the accompanying itching. When inhaled, it is a ten-fold more potent bronchoconstrictor than histamines, and it can be recovered from nasal fluids following Ag-induced responses in atopic individuals. Hence, PGD_2 is also a significant participant in immediate-type hypersensitivity.

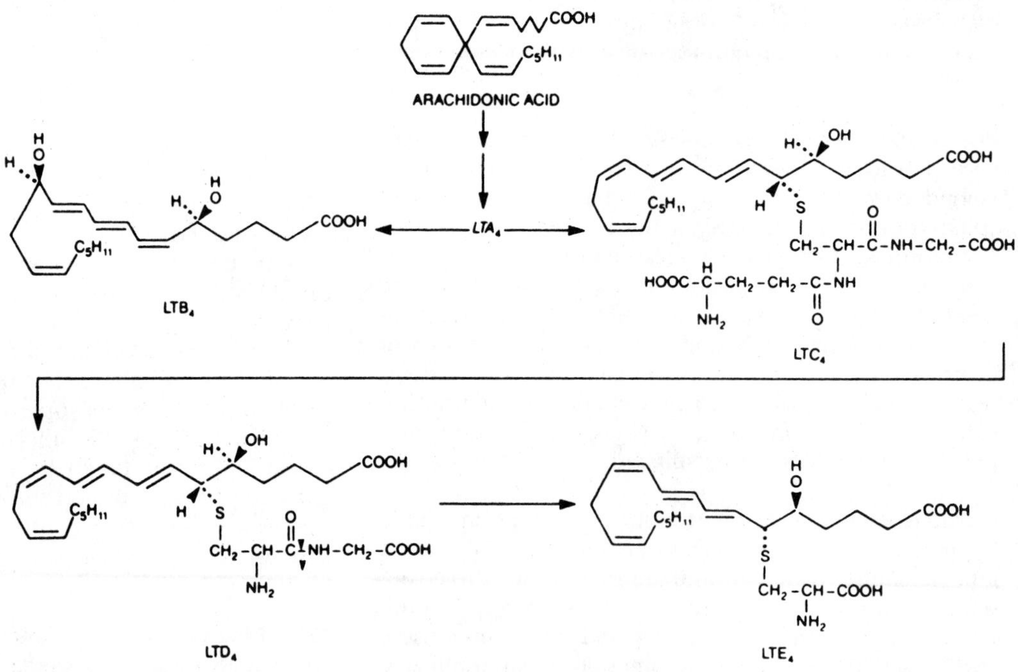

Figure 18–11. Structure of arachidonic acid and its leukotriene derivatives. (Redrawn from Rosen FS, Steiner LA, Unanue ER: Dictionary of Immunology. New York, Stockton Press, 1989)

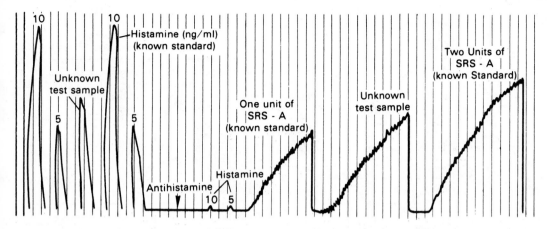

Figure 18–12. Assays for histamine and leukotrienes. Standards and test samples were added to an isolated strip of guinea pig ileum, whose contractile response was recorded. Antihistamines block the response to histamine. Note the slow response to leukotrienes (labeled in the diagram as *SRS-A,* for *slow-reactive substance of anaphylaxis,* the designation applied before the structure was elucidated) and the faster response to histamine. Time scale is about 30 seconds (vertical markers). (Based on Orange RP, Austen KF: In Good RA, Fisher DW (eds): Immunobiology. Stamford, Sinauer, 1971)

PLATELET-ACTIVATING FACTOR (PAF). Originally identified by its capacity to aggregate rabbit platelets, PAF (Fig. 18–13) has effects on a variety of other cells and is another mediator of anaphylaxis. When injected into skin, it is 1000-fold more potent than histamine in eliciting wheal and erythema responses; when inhaled, it causes severe bronchoconstriction (in baboons; it has not yet been tried on human volunteers), and it is a potent chemoattractant for neutrophils. It is produced by human mast cells, monocytes, and platelets but not by basophils.

RELEASE OF MEDIATORS. Only a few steps have been identified in the reaction sequence in mast cells (or basophils) that begins with aggregation of Fc_ε receptors and culminates in release of the mediators (1) initially, there is a rapid influx of Ca^{2+} ions; (2) from the inhibitory effect of diisopropylphosphorofluoridate (DFP), it is inferred that in one of the early steps, a critical serine protease is activated; (3) intracellular cyclic AMP (cAMP) levels drop; and (4) mediator-rich granules migrate to the cell's surface, fuse with the surface membrane, and are discharged to the cell's exterior (**exocytosis).** The discharge is secondary to secretion, not to cell lysis. Thus, the releasing cells remain impermeable to ionic dyes (which penetrate into dead cells). The level of cAMP in mast cells is crucial: as with many other secretory processes, **the rate and extent of granule release are enhanced when intracellular cAMP levels are low and are reduced when the levels are high.**

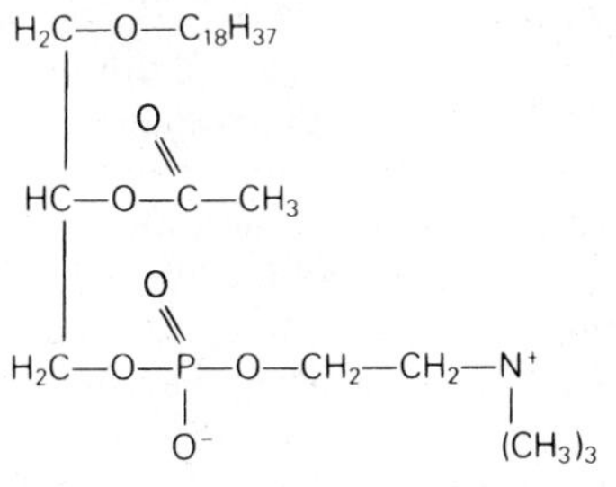

Drugs (isoproterenol, epinephrine, aminophylline) that either stimulate adenylcyclase, the enzyme that synthesizes cAMP, or inhibit the phosphodiesterase that degrades it result in increased cAMP levels and block the release of histamine and cysteinyl-leukotrienes. These drugs were used clinically for the control of anaphylaxis and allergic bronchospasm for many years before their mechanism of action was suspected. Another drug (cromolyn) is thought to prevent asthma by directly inhibiting granule secretion.

DEGRADATION OF MEDIATORS. Because the mediators are degraded rapidly (Table 18–4) and synthesized slowly, they do not accumulate extracellularly after being released. Hence, repeated, closely spaced injections of small doses of Ag are effective in depleting tissues of stored mediators (desensitization).

DESENSITIZATION

Various strategies are used to prevent or treat allergic reactions in humans due to IgE Abs.

$$H_2C-O-C_{18}H_{37}$$

$$HC-O-\overset{\displaystyle O}{\overset{\|}{C}}-CH_3$$

$$H_2C-O-\overset{\displaystyle O}{\overset{\|}{P}}-O-CH_2-CH_2-N^+$$
$$\underset{O^-}{|} \qquad \underset{(CH_3)_3}{|}$$

Figure 18–13. Platelet activating factor ($PAF_{acether}$: 1-alkyl-2-acetyl-glycero-3-phosphocholine) is produced by and acts on a variety of cells, and it exists in diverse forms, with saturated or unsaturated alkyl groups at C-1, various acyl substituents at C-2, and "head" groups other than phosphocholine at C-3.

TABLE 18–4. Degradation of Mediators

Mediators	Degrading Enzymes*	Inactive Derivatives
Histamine	Histaminase (diamine oxidase)	Imidazoleacetic acid (Fig. 18–8)
	Histamine N-methyl transferase	N-methylhistamine (Fig. 18–8)
Serotonin	Monoamine oxidase	5-Hydroxyindole acetic acid
Cysteinyl-leukotrienes ($LT-C_4$, $LT-D_4$, $LT-E_4$)	Peroxidases	Sulfones
ECF-A	Peptidases	?
LT–B4	20-lipoxygenase	20-OH $LT-B_4$
		20-COOH $LT-B_4$
$PAF_{acether}$	Deacetylase	Lyso-PAF

* Some are in eosinophils; others are in mast cells or basophils.

PROLONGED DESENSITIZATION. In addition to forming IgE Abs to an Ag, atopic individuals can form IgG Abs (termed "blocking" Abs) that competitively inhibit reactions between IgE Abs and the same Ag. In response to injections of Ag, blocking rather than IgE Abs are formed. Accordingly, atopic persons are sometimes treated (**desensitized**) by repeated injections of small amounts of allergen given in doses and at intervals that avoid systemic anaphylactic reactions. The level of blocking Abs, but not of IgE Abs, often rises considerably. However, therapeutic benefits are not always evident or regularly correlated with the titers of blocking Abs.

ACUTE DESENSITIZATION. Because the mediators are rapidly degraded and do not accumulate, the speed at which they are released (determined by the rate of reaction between Ag and mast-cell-bound Abs) determines whether anaphylaxis will occur. Shock can therefore be prevented by administering Ag slowly; for example, if 100 μg of a particular Ag (injected intravenously) provokes fatal shock in an experimental animal, the same quantity given in ten doses at 15-min intervals would not elicit shock. Moreover, if the full dose were then given all at once after the last small injection, shock would probably still not be elicited, because the reactive Abs and mast cells would have been depleted.

Desensitization by repeated, closely spaced injections of small doses of Ag is thus often resorted to clinically when it becomes necessary to administer a substance, such as penicillin or horse antiserum, to a person known or suspected to be intensely allergic to it. The procedure is effective but requires great care to avoid anaphylaxis, and it has only temporary value. Several weeks afterward, IgE-mediated hypersensitivity is likely to be fully restored, in contrast to the desensitization based on the formation of IgG (blocking) Abs.

Other Aspects of Anaphylaxis

IgE, EOSINOPHILIA, AND INTESTINAL PARASITISM

From the foregoing sections, the pathological effects of IgE Abs are clear. However, these Abs must also offer some advantages, because their wide distribution in mammalian species and perhaps in vertebrates generally implies that genes for ε chains have been preserved over a hundred million years of evolution. What survival benefits do they confer? An answer is suggested by their potency in stimulating eosinophils, and also monocytes, macrophages, and platelets, to exert cytotoxic effects on some common parasites. As outlined speculatively in Figure 18–14, IgE Abs to Ags of intestinal parasites are formed by IgE+ B cells in the intestinal mucosa, probably with help from neighboring CD4+ T cells that secrete IL-4. Mast cells in the vicinity bind these Abs, and subsequent interaction with the parasite's Ags activates these cells to secrete (among other mediators) chemotactic factors that attract eosinophils. Because these cells have their own Fc$_\varepsilon$ receptor, IgE Abs can bind at the same time to both the eosinophils (via the Ab's Fc$_\varepsilon$ domain) and the Ags on the parasite (via the Ab's Fab domains), triggering the eosinophils to release cytotoxic components that damage or destroy the parasite. The eosinophil-attracting tetrapeptides released by activated mast cells (see above) also enhance the eosinophil's IgE Ab-dependent cytotoxic activity (see Table 18–3). Similar reaction sequences could involve infiltrating macrophages and neutrophils as cytotoxic cells, as described in Chapter 19 (see Ab-Dependent Cell-mediated Cytotoxicity, ADCC).

Other observations also point to a relation between IgE, eosinophils, mast cells, and chronic infestation with intestinal parasites. For instance: (1) serum IgE levels are extremely high in African children with chronic intesti-

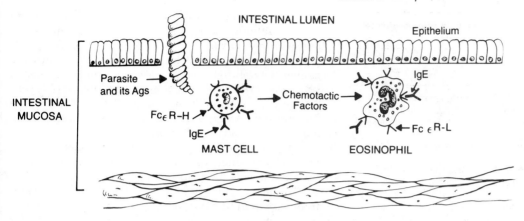

Figure 18–14. Diagram of possible relations between IgE, mast cells, and eosinophils. Fc$_\epsilon$R-H and Fc$_\epsilon$R-L are high-affinity and low-affinity receptors of Fc domain of IgE.

nal roundworm infections (up to 10,000 ng per ml or about 100-fold the level observed in uninfected individuals); (2) mast cells are unusually abundant in the intestinal mucosa of laboratory rats infected with intestinal parasites; and (3) eosinophilia characteristically accompanies many chronic parasitic infections.

Broadly viewed, therefore, IgE, mast cells, and eosinophils, acting in concert, appear to confer an important defense against common intestinal parasites. Although the prevalence of IgE-producing B cells in the intestine appears to offer certain benefits, the same cells in the respiratory tract (derived embryologically from the fetal gut) contribute to the reactions underlying allergic asthma and hay fever. Like many other immune reactions, IgE Ab responses can confer protective effects under some circumstances and pathological effects under others; while the pathological effects are clear, the protective effects are conjectural.

OTHER FORMS OF ANAPHYLAXIS

AGGREGATE ANAPHYLAXIS. Anaphylaxis can also be elicited with Abs (e.g., IgG) that do not bind to mast cells or basophils. The reaction involves large amounts of Ab–Ag complexes ("aggregates") that activate complement. The resulting C3a and C5a fragments are **anaphylatoxins** (Ch. 17): they cause mast cells to release their granules and mediators, hence the term **aggregate anaphylaxis.** Even some heat-aggregated Igs, without any Ag, can elicit cutaneous anaphylaxis, showing that the essential role of the Ag is simply to cross-link certain classes of Ab molecules and trigger the complement cascade. (Normal serum, lacking Ab–Ag aggregates, can become similarly toxic after it is incubated with suspensions of various particles—kaolin, talc, barium sulfate, insulin, agar—

that apparently activate the alternative complement pathway, again with formation of anaphylatoxin; see Ch. 17. The response to these incubated sera without Ag is sometimes called **anaphylactoid** shock.)

CYTOTOXIC ANAPHYLAXIS. This form of acute allergic reaction, called **cytotoxic anaphylaxis,** sometimes follows the injection of Abs to natural constituents of cell surfaces (see Table 18–1). For example, guinea pigs injected with rabbit Abs to the Forssman Ag, a glycolipid on many guinea pig cells, undergo acute shock. Acute hemolytic **transfusion reactions** in man (Ch. 20) are also sometimes associated with shock and could be considered a form of cytotoxic anaphylaxis. The mechanisms are obscure.

COMPLEMENT AND ANAPHYLAXIS. Aggregated IgE does not activate complement, and thus the complement system does not participate in IgE-mediated hypersensitivity. For instance, cutaneous anaphylaxis can be elicited in animals depleted of C3 by cobra venom factor (see Ch. 17). However, C activation is essential for aggregate anaphylaxis.

Immune Complexes and Subacute Hypersensitivity
ARTHUS REACTION

Shortly after the discovery of anaphylaxis, a different kind of Ab-dependent allergic reaction was recognized. When rabbits were inoculated subcutaneously at weekly intervals with horse serum, there was at first no noticeable response, but after several weeks, each injection

TABLE 18–5. Subacute Hypersensitivity in Lungs (Allergic Pneumonitis) Caused by Inhaled Antigens

Occupationally Related Disease	Antigen
Farmer's lung	Moldy hay (*Thermoactinomyces vulgaris*)
Mushroom worker's lung	Compost (thermophilic actinomycetes)
Pigeon breeder's lung	Pigeon dander and droppings (avian proteins)
Bagassosis	Moldy bagasse (thermophilic actinomycetes)
Malt worker's lung	Moldy barley (*Aspergillus clavatus*)
Wheat weevil disease	Infested flour (*Sitophilus granarius*)
Seqouiosis	Moldy sawdust (*Coraphium* and *Pullularia* species)
Cheese-washer's lung	Cheese castings (*Penicillin caseii* spores)

(Based on Barrett JT: Textbook of Immunology, 3rd Ed. St Louis, CV Mosby, 1978)

evoked a localized inflammatory reaction. Similar responses were soon observed in humans and were called **Arthus reactions** after the French physiologist who first described them. These reactions are not limited to the skin: they can take place wherever Ags are injected, such as into the pericardial sac or synovial joint spaces. **The principal requirement is the formation of Ab–Ag aggregates that activate complement (C); the resulting C fragments (C5a, etc.) attract polymorphonuclear leukocytes (neutrophils).** The lysosomal enzymes and other toxic agents (superoxide anion and other reactive oxygen intermediates) released by the infiltrating leukocytes cause tissue damage, characteristically with destructive inflammation of small blood vessels (**vasculitis**). Provided they can react with C *in situ*, Abs of any Ig class can mediate the reaction. Even the injection of Ab–Ag complexes formed in the test tube can evoke the response, although with less intensity than when the aggregates form *in situ*.

Patients with serum sickness or with certain forms of glomerulonephritis (below) develop similar lesions in small blood vessels and in kidney glomeruli, respectively. Similarly, persons with high serum levels of Abs to the thermophilic *Aspergillus* that thrives in decaying vegetation or to molds used to produce cheese, develop severe localized Arthus-type lung lesions when they inhale these fungi or fungal spores (farmer's lung, cheese-washer's lung, and other examples; Table 18–5).

The main features are illustrated by the **passive cutaneous form of the Arthus reaction**, in which an antiserum is first injected intravenously into a nonsensitive (naive) recipient and the corresponding Ag is then injected into the skin. Alternatively, to conserve antiserum, in the **reverse passive Arthus reaction**, the antiserum is injected in the recipient's skin and the Ag is then injected into the same dermal site or intravenously.

The passive Arthus reaction requires a large amount of Ab, about 10 mg when injected in a rabbit intravenously and about 100 μg when injected into the skin. In contrast, about 1/100,000 as much (i.e., 1 ng or less) of IgE Ab is sufficient for passive cutaneous anaphylaxis in humans (P-K reaction; see Passive Transfer, above).

TIME COURSE. After intradermal injection of Ag, the Arthus response becomes evident more slowly than cutaneous anaphylaxis and is more persistent. Local swelling and erythema appear after 1–2 hours followed by punctate hemorrhages. The changes are maximal in 3 to 4 hours and are usually gone in 10 to 12 hours; but severe reactions, with necrosis at the test site, subside more slowly (Table 18–6).

TABLE 18–6. Comparison of Immediate and Subacute Allergic Skin Reactions

Properties	Immediate (Anaphylactic) Reactions	Subacute (Immune-Complex) Reactions
Time course		
Onset	2–3 minutes	1–2 hours
Peak	10 minutes	3–4 hours
Disappearance	30 minutes	10–12 hours
Class of mediating Abs	IgE (or other cytotropic Igs)	IgG or any other complement-activating Ig
Amount of Ab necessary for passive sensitization of skin site	<0.001 μg	>10 μg
Latent period required between Ab and Ag injections	Yes	No
Complement participation	No	Yes
Major mediators	Histamine, cysteinyl-leukotrienes, platelet-activating factor, etc.	Lysosomal enzymes; reactive oxygen intermediates, C3a and C5a (anaphylatoxin)
Major cells involved	Mast cells, basophils (eosinophils)	Neutrophils (minor role for basophils)

HISTOPATHOLOGY. In anaphylaxis, the inflammatory changes are largely limited to vasodilatation and exudation of plasma proteins; inflammatory cells are not conspicuous. The Arthus response, however, is characterized by classic inflammation: blood flow through small vessels is markedly retarded; thrombi rich in platelets and leukocytes form within small blood vessels; erythrocytes escape into the surrounding connective tissue; and, after several hours, the skin site becomes edematous and heavily infiltrated with neutrophils (Fig. 18–15). Finally, localized patches of necrosis appear in the walls of the affected small blood vessels. As the lesion begins to subside, after 4 to 12 hours, neutrophils become necrotic and are replaced by macrophages and eosinophils. Within a few days, the phagocytized immune complexes are degraded and inflammation disappears.

The response in the cornea emphasizes the role of blood vessels. The injection of Ag into an immunized rabbit's normal cornea, which is devoid of functional blood vessels, can result in concentric opaque rings of Ab–Ag precipitates, like bands in gel precipitin reactions *in vitro* (Chap. 13), but little or no inflammation is observed. If, however, functional blood vessels are present (e.g., as a sequel of some earlier trauma to the cornea), then the Ag can elicit an Arthus response in the cornea, as in any other tissue.

ROLE OF COMPLEMENT AND GRANULOCYTES. At the site of the local reaction, immunofluorescence reveals Ab–Ag aggregates with C components (C3) localized in blood vessel walls between endothelial cells and the internal elastic membrane (Fig. 18–13). The aggregates are also evident within granulocytes in perivascular connective tissue. If an animal's C activity has been greatly reduced (e.g., by depleting C3 with cobra venom factor; Ch. 17), or if its level of circulating neutrophils has been depressed (e.g., by an anti-neutrophil serum), no inflammatory reaction appears even though the immune complexes form in blood vessel walls.

It appears therefore that the Arthus reaction depends on the following sequence: (1) Ag and Ab diffuse into blood vessel walls, where they form complexes and activate C; (2) some C fragments and complexes (C5a, C5b,6,7) are chemotactic attractants for neutrophils, and

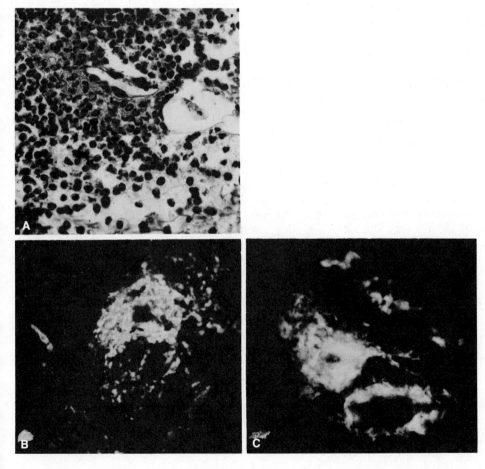

Figure 18–15. Passive Arthus reaction in a rat, showing localization of Ag and complement *(C)* in the wall of an affected blood vessel. The skin site was excised 2 to 3 hours after an intradermal injection of 300 μg of rabbit Abs to bovine serum albumin (anti-BSA) and an intravenous injection of 6 mg BSA. (The Ab was injected intradermally, and the Ag intravenously, to conserve Abs.) *(A)* Note intense neutrophil infiltration in and around the wall of a small blood vessel adjacent to skeletal muscle. *(B)* Section was stained with fluorescent rabbit Ab to a purified component of rat C (C3; see Ch. 20). *(C)* Section was stained with fluorescent anti-BSA to localize the aggregated Ag in the blood vessel wall and in the adjacent perivascular connective tissue. The same result would be obtained by staining the aggregated Ab (rabbit anti-BSA) with fluorescent anti-rabbit Ig. (Ward PA, Cochrane CG: J Exp Med 121:215, 1965)

other fragments (the anaphylatoxins C3a and C5a) probably cause the release of other leukocyte attractants from mast cells and basophils; (3) the accumulated neutrophils ingest the Ab–Ag complexes and release lysosomal enzymes; (4) the enzymes cause focal necrosis of the blood vessel wall and the other inflammatory changes. Because small peptides are released from radiolabeled Ags, it is evident that lysosomal enzymes also degrade the immune complexes, leading to subsidence of the inflammation.

Increased permeability of the blood vessel endothelium (caused, for example, by histamine and leukotrienes) probably aids the penetration of Ab–Ag complexes into blood vessel walls (see Serum Sickness Syndrome, below), but antihistamines do not block the development of Arthus lesions.

SERUM SICKNESS SYNDROME

From about 1920 to 1940, various bacterial infections were treated in humans by injecting large volumes of antiserum prepared in horses or rabbits. After a week or so, the recipients often developed a characteristic syndrome called **serum sickness.** The same syndrome is sometimes now encountered as an allergic reaction to penicillin and other drugs (Ch. 20), and it may be expected as an occasional response to the mouse Igs that are injected as mAbs for therapeutic and diagnostic purposes.

The syndrome includes fever, enlarged lymph nodes and spleen, erythematous and urticarial rashes, and arthritis. The disease usually subsides within a few days. In the few patients who have died at the height of the illness, autopsy has disclosed disseminated vascular and perivascular inflammatory lesions like those of the Arthus reaction.

The mechanisms have been analyzed in rabbits injected with large amounts of purified foreign protein. In addition, an opportunity to make detailed observations in humans arose in connection with attempts, during World War II, to use bovine serum albumin (BSA) as a plasma expander in the treatment of traumatic shock (Fig. 18–16).

MECHANISMS. The illness usually becomes evident 7 to 14 days after the initial injection of Ag. During this interval, the Ag level declines, but it is still high enough, after Ab production starts, to form the soluble Ab–Ag complexes (in Ag excess) that initiate focal vascular lesions in coronary arteries, glomeruli, and elsewhere (Fig. 18–17). Serum sickness is thus usually observed only after exceptionally large amounts of foreign proteins are injected, such as 25 g of BSA in a human or 1 g in a rabbit. However, in previously sensitized persons with accelerated (anamnestic) Ab responses (see Primary and Secondary

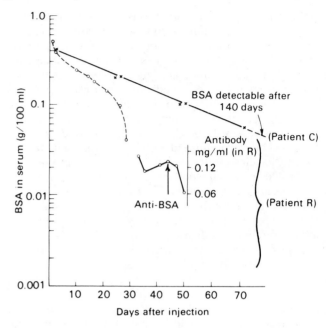

Figure 18–16. Serum sickness syndrome in a human subject following the injection of 25 g bovine serum albumin (BSA) at zero time. In patient R, BSA levels declined abruptly (o - - - o), anti-BSA Ab levels rose (o——o), and serum sickness became evident, days 24 to 31; patient C did not form Abs to BSA or develop serum sickness. (Data of FE Kendall; modified from Seegal B: Am J Med 13:356, 1962)

Responses, Ch. 16), the reaction has appeared earlier and required much less Ag: 3 or 4 days after 1 ml of horse serum, for example.

As the manifestations of serum sickness appear, soluble Ab–Ag complexes can be detected in the serum, and the decline in the level of free Ag is markedly accelerated (Fig. 18–16 and 18–18). Moreover, the Ab–Ag complexes activate C, and the serum C level is depressed at the height of the illness (Fig. 18–16); as in the Arthus reaction, the most abundant C component (C3) can be detected by immunofluorescence in immune aggregates within the focal blood vessel lesions (see Fig. 18–13). As the complexes disappear, free Abs become detectable, and inflammatory lesions regress.

VASOACTIVE AMINES. Increased vascular permeability probably facilitates the penetration of immune complexes from plasma through endothelium into the blood vessel wall. Vasoactive amines probably aid at this step, because in animals treated with antihistamines, the vascular deposition of injected preformed Ab–Ag complexes is diminished. The pathogenic steps may be summarized as follows:

1. Ab–Ag complexes activate C, resulting in C fragments (anaphylatoxins) that cause mast cells and basophils to release mediators of anaphylaxis.

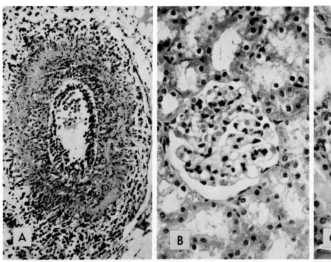

Figure 18–17. Representative cardiovascular and renal lesions in experimental serum sickness in the rabbit. The Ag was BSA (see Fig. 18–18). **(A)** Medium-sized coronary artery: endothelial cell proliferation, necrosis of media, neutrophils leukocyte infiltration through all layers, and mononuclear cells in the media and adventitia are evident. **(B)** Section through a normal glomerulus of a control rabbit. **(C)** An affected glomerulus showing increase in size, proliferation of endothelial and epithelial cells, and obliteration of capillary spaces. Note the much lower density of glomerular cells and patency of capillaries in **(B)**. (Dixon FJ: In Samter M (ed): Immunological Diseases. Boston, Little, Brown, 1965)

2. Permeability of vascular endothelium increases.

3. Ab–Ag complexes penetrate into blood vessel walls or form within the walls; C chemotactic factors (C5a) attract neutrophils.

4. Neutrophils penetrate into blood vessel walls, ingesting immune complexes and releasing lysosomal enzymes and toxic oxygen intermediates (see Ch. 19).

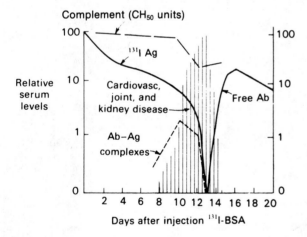

Figure 18–18. Serum sickness in the rabbit. Changes in serum levels of free Ag (^{131}I-labeled BSA), free Ab (anti-BSA), Ag–Ab complexes, and complement (C) activity (CH$_{50}$ units; see Chap. 17) following the injection of rabbits at zero time with 250 mg ^{131}I-BSA/kg of body weight. Ammonium sulfate at 50% saturation precipitates the ^{131}I-BSA–anti-BSA complexes but not free ^{131}I-BSA. *Ordinate* (log scale) refers to free ^{131}I-BSA in total blood volume, as % of amount injected; anti-BSA, measured as μg of Ag bound per ml of serum; and C activity, as % of normal serum. All animals had cardiovascular, joint, and kidney lesions (Fig. 18–15), shown by shaded area, on day 13. (Dixon FJ: In Samter M (ed): Immunological Diseases. Boston, Little, Brown, 1965)

5. Toxic components released by neutrophils damage neighboring cells and lead to more inflammation.

6. If immune complexes are formed in an acute episode ("one-shot" serum sickness), the lesions abate as complexes are degraded.

7. If immune complexes are formed repeatedly (when Ag is continuously present, as in persistent viremia, malaria, etc.), widespread chronic inflammatory disease can develop in small blood vessels (vasculitis) and in kidney glomeruli (glomerulonephritis).

RELATION TO OTHER ALLERGIC REACTIONS. Serum sickness has both Arthus and anaphylactic aspects. The focal vascular lesions and the requirement for immune complexes and for C suggest that the syndrome is essentially a disseminated form of the Arthus reaction, with the same injected substance, given in a large amount, serving first as immunogen and then as reacting Ag. However, mast-cell-activating Abs evidently play a larger role than in the Arthus reaction: urticarial skin lesions are also prominent in serum sickness, and a person who has recovered from the disease will generally show a wheal and erythema response to intradermal injection of the Ag. The released amines probably contribute also to the development of the focal vasculitis, as in the Arthus reaction.

IMMUNE-COMPLEX DISEASES
Glomerulonephritis

The pathogenesis of experimental Arthus lesions and serum sickness probably accounts for some forms of glomerulonephritis, a kidney disease in which obstructive inflammatory lesions of glomerular blood vessels can lead to renal failure. Immunofluorescence study of biopsies usually reveals lumpy deposits of Ig and C3 (probably complexed with some unknown Ag) beneath the glomerular endothelium (Fig. 18–19). The deposits resemble those of serum sickness, especially in the chronic experimental model in which Ag is administered almost daily for many weeks at a rate that approximates Ab synthesis and provides continuous production of immune complexes.

Ags have been identified in human glomerular lesions in special circumstances. *Plasmodium malariae* Ags have been recognized by immunofluorescence in kidneys of patients with the chronic nephritis associated with malaria, and Abs to malarial Ags have been eluted from kidney biopsies (at pH 2–3 to dissociate Ab–Ag complexes; see Appendix, Ch. 13). Similarly, Abs to single- and double-stranded DNA have been eluted from kidney tissue of patients with systemic lupus erythematosus; these patients often have high serum levels of Abs to nucleic acids and develop progressive glomerulonephritis with lumpy glomerular deposits containing Ig, C, and DNA (see Autoimmune Diseases, Ch. 20).

Most cases of human glomerulonephritis occur as a sequel to infection with β-hemolytic streptococci (especially type XII, the "nephritogenic" strain); but streptococcal Ags have not been detected consistently in the associated glomerular deposits of Ig and C, perhaps because reactive sites are covered by antistreptococcal Abs.

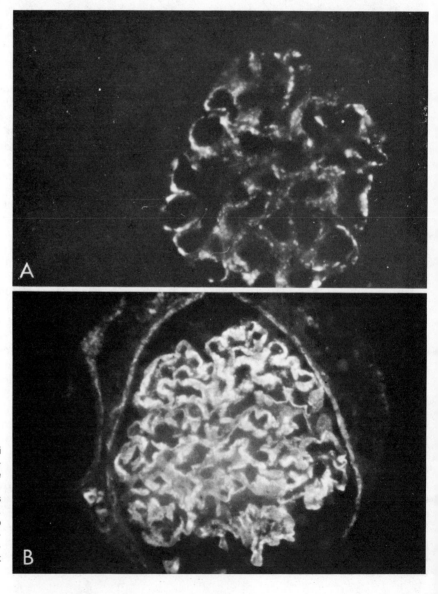

Figure 18–19. Immune complexes in glomeruli revealed by immunofluorescence. Kidney biopsies from patients with glomerulonephritis were stained with fluorescein-labeled Abs to human Igs. *(A)* Lumpy deposits of Abs–Ag–C in glomerulus from a patient with systemic lupus erythematosus. *(B)* Linear deposits of Igs attached specifically to the glomerular basement membrane (Goodpasture's syndrome; see Characteristics of Autoimmune Disease, Chap. 20). (Courtesy of Dr C Kirk Osterland)

VIRAL COMPLEXES. Chronic viral infection appears to be a source of immune-complex disease in mice. Animals infected at birth with lymphocytic choriomeningitis (LCM) virus become chronic carriers of the virus, producing large amounts of antiviral Abs that do not neutralize infectivity. Virus–Ab–C complexes in serum can be precipitated if antiserum to mouse Igs or to mouse C3 is added. The mice develop progressive renal disease associated with inflammatory vascular lesions and with lumpy glomerular deposits containing virus, antiviral Abs, and C.

Immune-complex disease with glomerulonephritis also occurs in mice as a result of neonatal infection with murine leukemia viruses, coxsackie B virus, and polyomavirus.

ANTIKIDNEY ANTIBODIES. In a rare form of human glomerulonephritis (Goodpasture's disease), immunofluorescence reveals not lumpy but linear glomerular deposits of Ig that follow the basement membrane continuously (Fig. 18–17). The pattern resembles that seen in the experimental nephritis produced with heteroantiserum to basement membrane (e.g., the so-called Masugi nephritis produced in rabbits with duck antiserum to rabbit kidney). Some monkeys have developed glomerulonephritis when inoculated with Igs eluted from human kidneys with linear deposits, suggesting that the human lesion could be caused by autoantibodies to glomerular basement membranes (see Characteristics of Autoimmune Diseases, Ch. 20).

Rheumatoid Arthritis

In this common chronic inflammatory disease of joints, the synovial fluid in joint cavities contains high levels of Ig (much of it synthesized locally in the synovial membrane) and C-activating aggregates of Igs, as well as granulocytes and C components that attract granulocytes (C5a). Hence, the joint fluids contain all the ingredients for an Arthus reaction. However, as in most human diseases that arise from immune complexes, the actual Ags remain unknown.

Some of the IgG in joint fluid probably functions as Ag for the characteristic **rheumatoid factors** of rheumatoid arthritis: IgM and IgG molecules that react specifically with antigenic determinants on Fc domains of various IgGs (see Human Allotypes, Ch. 14). The IgG–IgM and the IgG–IgG complexes could then initiate the C–granulocyte–reactive oxygen intermediates sequence that results in Arthus inflammation. Some Igs might also function as Abs that bind special Ags in affected joints, such as DNA (and probably other, unidentified, Ags); in this case, the rheumatoid factors would not be essential participants but would arise secondarily as Abs to new antigenic sites on conformationally altered IgG molecules in immune complexes. Indeed, **IgM molecules**

that behave like rheumatoid factors are found in diverse situations where Abs and immune complexes are present at high levels for protracted periods (e.g., experimental chronic serum sickness).

EVIDENCE FOR PERSISTENT SOLUBLE IMMUNE COMPLEXES. In rheumatoid arthritis, glomerulonephritis, systemic lupus erythematosus, and other chronic diseases in which immune complexes are probably pathogenic, their presence is often revealed by the formation of precipitates when serum (or joint fluid in rheumatoid arthritis) is simply stored at 4°C. These **cryoprecipitates** contain IgM (probably anti-Abs), IgG, and sometimes additional components that could represent Ags (e.g., single-stranded DNA in patients who form anti-DNA, Abs, as in those with systemic lupus or with rheumatoid arthritis; see Chap. 20).

The presence of soluble immune complexes can also be revealed by: (1) the appearance of breakdown products of C3 (recognized by immunoelectrophoresis with specific antisera); (2) precipitation by C1q, the first C component, which reacts specifically with soluble immune complexes if the Ab moiety of the complex belongs to certain Ig classes (e.g., IgG1 and IgM in man; Ch. 17); and (3) polyethylene glycol, which precipitates soluble immune complexes.

Appendix
EXPERIMENTAL ANAPHYLAXIS

Species Variations. Anaphylaxis in humans has been studied primarily as cutaneous responses to injections of minute amounts of Ags; systemic anaphylaxis can hardly be studied because it is nearly always an unanticipated, catastrophic episode, terminating quickly (e.g., in less than half an hour) in either recovery or death. Accordingly, much of what we know about these responses has been derived from experimental studies of other mammalian species. Guinea pigs have been preferred because they react uniformly and intensely. However, anaphylaxis can also be elicited in other vertebrates. The manifestations differ in different species and even when the Ag is injected by different routes. In a sensitized guinea pig, for example, intravenous injection leads to respiratory distress secondary to bronchial constriction, and at autopsy, the lungs appear bloodless and are greatly distended with air; in contrast, subcutaneous or intraperitoneal administration produces primarily hypotension and hypothermia, and death occurs after many hours, with engorged blood vessels in abdominal viscera as the main pathologic finding. These differences and the different manifestations of anaphylaxis among vari-

TABLE 18–7. *Species Variation in Tissue Levels and Susceptibility to Histamine and Serotonin*

Species	Lung Content (μg/g)		Bronchiolar Sensitivity (Minimal Effective dose in μg)	
	Serotonin	Histamine	Serotonin	Histamine
Cat	>0.2	34	0.01	2
Rat	2.3	5	0.01	>5
Dog	<0.1	25	0.05	0.3
Guinea pig	<0.2	5–25	0.4	0.4
Rabbit	2.1	4	>8	0.5
Man	<0.3	2–20	>20	0.2

(From various sources summarized in Austen KF, Humphrey JH: Adv Immunol 3:1, 1963)

ous species are probably attributable mostly to differences in the distribution or the reactivity of released pharmacologically active mediators (Table 18–7).

Mode of Administration of Antigen. Anaphylaxis depends not only on the **amount** but also on the **rate** of Ag–Ab complex formation, for the complexes act by causing the release of pharmacologically active mediators that are rapidly degraded (below). Hence, intravenous injection of Ag, or its inhalation in aerosols, can provoke fatal shock, whereas responses elicited by subcutaneous and intraperitoneal injections come on more slowly and are less often fatal.

Fixation of Antibodies. Only those Abs that bind to mast cells can mediate passive anaphylaxis. Less Ab is needed if a latent period intervenes between injection of antiserum and of Ag: for example, 180 μg of anti-egg albumin rendered guinea pigs uniformly susceptible to fatal shock when they were challenged 48 hours later, whereas about 100 times more was required if the Ag was injected immediately after the antiserum. **During the latent period, cytotropic Abs are bound to mast cells; in addition, the circulating level of unbound Ab, which competes with cell-bound Ab for the Ag, is reduced.**

Reverse Passive Anaphylaxis. Passive anaphylaxis can also be evoked by reversing the order of injections if the Ag is itself a foreign Ig of the type that is readily bound to mast cells. In that event, if the Ag is injected first and a latent period is allowed to elapse, the intravenous injection of specific antiserum (anti-Ig) can cause anaphylaxis. This procedure, reverse passive anaphylaxis, is not effective with other Ags because they do not bind to mast cells. **Reverse passive cutaneous anaphylaxis** is used occasionally to evaluate an Ig's ability to bind to mast cells: e.g., the Ig under test is injected into a normal guinea pig's skin, and then antiserum to the Ig (plus blue dye) is injected intravenously.

Quantities of Antibody and Antigen Required for Anaphylaxis. The levels of Ag required are substantially greater than those necessary for precipitation *in vitro*: guinea pigs sensitized with 180 μg of anti-egg albumin (anti-EA) require for a fatal response over 500 μg of EA, about 25-fold more than is usually needed for maximal precipitation of this amount of Ab in the EA/anti-EA precipitin reaction. Much of the injected Ag probably never has a chance to react with Abs *in vivo*, because it is taken up by phagocytic cells or excreted. Ags that form large complexes with circulating soluble Abs tend to be rapidly phagocytized and are also not efficient in provoking anaphylaxis. In fact, as suggested above, **high levels of circulating Abs may protect against anaphylaxis** because they compete with mast-cell-bound Abs for the Ag. Thus, when an animal is passively sensitized with a small amount of antiserum and then given a large dose of the same antiserum immediately before the Ag, fatal shock can be replaced by mild signs (see Desensitization).

ANAPHYLACTIC RESPONSES IN ISOLATED TISSUES

Many organs from sensitized animals respond to Ag *in vitro*. In the **Schultz–Dale reaction,** the isolated uterus from a sensitized guinea pig contracts promptly when

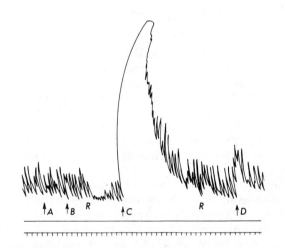

Figure 18–20. Smooth muscle contraction *in vitro* in response to Ag (Schultz–Dale reaction). A uterine horn was excised from a guinea pig 13 days after a sensitizing injection of a horse serum euglobulin (Ag) and was suspended in Ringer's solution. Various protein fractions from horse serum were added (*arrows*): at *A,* 1 mg pseudoglobulin; at *B,* 10 mg pseudoglobulin; at *C* and at *D,* 10 mg euglobulin (the immunogen). Following the specific response at *C,* the muscle was almost totally desensitized, either because the tissue-bound Abs were saturated with Ag or because the mediator content was depleted. Time scale markers at 30-sec intervals. *R* = changes of Ringer's solution. (Dale HH, Hartley P: Biochem J 10:408, 1916)

incubated with Ag, which evidently reacts with cytotropic Abs on tissue mast cells and causes the release of mediators (Fig. 18–20). Similar reactions are obtained with isolated segments of ileum, gallbladder wall, and arterial wall. These responses can also be elicited with tissues from passively sensitized animals and with isolated normal tissues that are sensitized simply by incubating them with antiserum. Because of the high affinity of IgE Abs for the mast-cell surface, the isolated tissues retain their reactivity after extensive washing.

In one of the simplest *in vitro* reactions, Ag elicits the release of histamine from washed leukocytes and the degranulation of basophils (demonstrated by staining smeared cells); extremely small amounts of Ag suffice (e.g., for purified ragweed Ag, 10^{-13} mg/ml). The degranulation has been used as a diagnostic assay for penicillin allergy. Human basophils can also be passively sensitized with atopic sera and with purified human IgE.

Selected Reading

REVIEW ARTICLES

Capron A, Dessaint JP: Effector and regulatory mechanisms in immunity to schistosomes: A heuristic view. Annu Rev Immunol 3:455, 1985

Galli SJ: New approaches for the analysis of mast cell maturation, heterogeneity, and function. Fed Proc 46:1906, 1987

Galli SJ, Dvorak AM, Dvorak HF: Basophils and mast cells: Morphologic insights into their biology, secretory patterns, and function. Prog Allergy 34:1, 1984

Metzger H, Alcaraz G, Hohman R, Kinet J-P, Pribluda V, Quarto R: The receptor with high affinity for IgE. Annu Rev Immunol 4:419, 1986

Samuelsson B, Dahlen S-E, Lindgren JA, Rouzer CA, Serhan CN: Leukotrienes and lipoxins: Structures, biosynthesis, and biological effects. Science 237:1171, 1987

Serafin WE, Austen KF: Mediators of immediate hypersensitivity reactions. N Engl J Med 317:30, 1987

Vane J, Botting R: Inflammation and the mechanism of action of anti-inflammatory drugs. FASEB J 1:89, 1987

SPECIFIC ARTICLES

Blank U, Ra C, Miller L, et al: Complete structure and expression in transfected cells of high affinity IgE receptor. Nature 337:187–189, 1989

Cochrane CG: Mechanisms involved in the deposition of immune complexes in tissue. J Exp Med 134:75S, 1971

Haba S, Nisonoff A: Induction of high titers of anti-IgE by immunization of inbred mice with syngeneic IgE. Proc Natl Acad Sci USA 84:5009, 1987

Ishizaka K, Ishizaka T, Okudaira H, Bazin H: Ontogeny of IgE-bearing lymphocytes in the rat. J Immunol 120:655, 1978

Kikutani H, et al: Molecular structure of human lymphocyte receptor for IgE. Cell 47:657, 1986

Nabel G, Galli SJ, Dvorak AM, Dvorak HF, Cantor H: Inducer T lymphocytes synthesize a factor that stimulates proliferation of cloned mast cells. Nature 291:332, 1981

Schlessinger J, Webb WW, Elson EL, Metzger H: Lateral motion and valence of Fc receptors on rat peritoneal mast cells. Nature 264:550, 1976

19

Cell-Mediated Immunity

Long before B and T cells were distinguished, it was realized that antigens (Ags) can elicit slowly developing tissue inflammatory reactions whose intensity is not correlated with the serum antibody (Ab) levels. Indeed, these **delayed-type hypersensitivity (DTH)** reactions could be elicited even in individuals who were almost totally devoid of Igs (e.g., children with X-linked agammaglobulinemia [Ch. 20] or mice depleted of B cells by having been treated from birth with Abs to μ chains). And because they could also be transferred from immunized donors to naive recipients with intact leukocytes (later shown to be lymphocytes) but not with antisera, they came to be called **cell-mediated immune reactions.** Similar responses were subsequently found to be responsible for a wide variety of protective as well as destructive reactions, such as (1) protection against many viral, bacterial, fungal, and protozoan infections; (2) resistance against many tumor cells; (3) inflammation associated with various microbial infections (bacterial, fungal, etc.); and (4) rejection of allografts (Table 19–1).

In all of these reactions, the triggering event is the recognition of an antigenic structure on a target cell by a T cell. The consequences depend on whether the T cell is a CD4+ or CD8+ cell. Generally, CD4+ cells respond by secreting lymphokines, some of which (e.g., γ-interferon; IFN-γ) stimulate macrophages to release substances that cause inflammation and the destruction of many bacteria and tumor cells, regardless of their Ags. CD8+ cells, in contrast, respond by destroying only those cells whose surface Ag they recognize. Although these differences are striking and characteristic, CD8+ cells also secrete some lymphokines, and some CD4+ cells can also cause Ag-specific lysis of target cells. We describe below some of the better-characterized cell-mediated

431

TABLE 19–1. Some Cell-Mediated Immune Responses

Delayed-type hypersensitivity
Lysis of target cells
Resistance to many infectious agents (especially intracellular pathogens)
Resistance to some tumors
Allergic contact dermatitis
Rejection of allografts
Graft-versus-host reactions
Some drug allergies
Some autoimmune diseases

immune reactions, beginning with delayed-type hypersensitivity (DTH).

Delayed-Type Hypersensitivity

The response to proteins of the tubercle bacillus, studied for almost a century, serves as a general model for DTH reactions.

TUBERCULIN HYPERSENSITIVITY

Koch observed in 1890 that filtrates of cultures of *Mycobacterium tuberculosis* elicit an inflammatory reaction many hours after injection into tuberculous animals but not into normal ones. The culture filtrate, concentrated by boiling, was called **tuberculin** (later **old tuberculin** or **OT**). The active material, called **purified protein derivative** or **PPD,** is now partly purified from autoclaved cultures by precipitation with ammonium sulfate and is a mixture of many protein fragments (average mol. wt. about 5000). The epitope(s) that trigger tuberculin-spe-

cific T cells are not known. Similar preparations from other bacterial and fungal cultures also elicit delayed-type responses in those infected with the corresponding organisms. These **responses to cutaneous injections have been used to identify infected individuals** and to screen large populations to determine the prevalence of certain infections (Table 19–2, Fig. 19–1). Such a test first revealed that calcified pulmonary lesions often result from infection by the fungus histoplasma, as well as from tuberculosis.

CUTANEOUS REACTION. After 0.1 μg of tuberculin is injected intradermally into a sensitized (i.e., previously immunized or infected) individual, no change is observed at the inoculated site for at least 10 hours. Erythema and swelling then gradually appear and increase; maximal intensity and size (up to about 5 cm diameter) are reached in 24 to 72 hours, after which the response subsides over several days.

In highly sensitive humans, 0.2 μg of tuberculin can cause necrosis, ulceration, and scarring at the inoculated site. In contrast, highly sensitized guinea pigs require more than 0.5 μg to elicit even a faint response; even more is necessary in cattle and rabbits, and in rats and mice, erythema is not discernible but local swelling provides a crude measure of the reaction's intensity. Why species vary so widely in responsiveness is not known.

COMPARISON BETWEEN ARTHUS AND DELAYED-TYPE SKIN REACTIONS. Arthus reactions, caused by Ab–Ag complexes (Ch. 18), sometimes look like DTH. However, several differences, summarized in Table 19–3, generally permit them to be distinguished, especially if it is possible to transfer the reactivity from a sensitive donor: **T cells transfer DTH, and Abs transfer Arthus reactions.**

TABLE 19–2. Some Delayed-Type Skin Reactions That Have Been Used for Diagnosis and Epidemiologic Surveys

Disease	Type of Etiologic Agent	Antigenic Preparation Used in Skin Test
Tuberculosis	Bacterium	Tuberculin
Leprosy	Bacterium	Lepromin
Brucellosis	Bacterium	Brucellin
Psittacosis	Bacterium	Heat-killed organisms
Lymphogranuloma venereum	Bacterium	Extract of chorioallantoic membrane of infected chick embryo
Mumps	Virus	Noninfectious virus from yolk sac of infected chick embryo
Coccidioidomycosis	Fungus	Concentrated culture filtrate
Histoplasmosis	Fungus	Concentrated culture filtrate
Blastomycosis	Fungus	Concentrated culture filtrate
Leishmaniasis	Protozoan	Extract of cultured *Leishmania*
Echinococcosis	Helminth	Fluid from hydatid cyst
Contact dermatitis	Simple chemical	Patch tests with simple chemicals

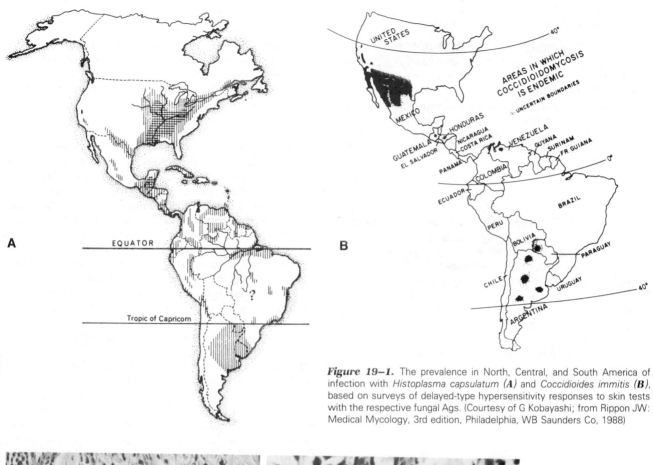

Figure 19–1. The prevalence in North, Central, and South America of infection with *Histoplasma capsulatum* (**A**) and *Coccidioides immitis* (**B**), based on surveys of delayed-type hypersensitivity responses to skin tests with the respective fungal Ags. (Courtesy of G Kobayashi; from Rippon JW: Medical Mycology, 3rd edition, Philadelphia, WB Saunders Co, 1988)

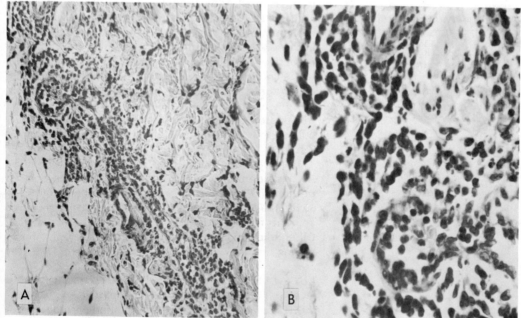

Figure 19–2. Delayed-type hypersensitivity reaction in guinea pig skin. The animal was sensitized by injecting 5 μg of hen's egg albumin (HEA) in complete Freund's adjuvant. Six days later, it was injected intradermally with 5 μg of HEA in saline. The skin site was excised 24 hours later, when induration and redness (which had probably first become evident at about 12 hours) were maximal. The infiltrating lymphoid cells appear, by electron microscopy and with special stains, to be lymphocytes and macrophages. (Coe JE, Salvin SB: J Immunol 93:495, 1964). (**A**, ×64; **B**, ×355)

433

HISTOLOGY. The response is characterized by the accumulation of inflammatory cells around postcapillary venules, first detected after 6 hours and maximal at 24 to 48 hours (Fig. 19–2). Some of these cells are lymphocytes, but most are monocytes that are presumed to differentiate later into macrophages. Basophils can also be prominent (see Cutaneous Basophil Hypersensitivity, below). Fibrin accumulates and probably accounts for the firmness of the lesion.

NONCUTANEOUS AND SYSTEMIC REACTIONS. Delayed responses can occur in tissues other than skin: for example, tuberculin can cause severe inflammation and necrosis in the cornea of sensitized guinea pigs. A systemic response, **tuberculin shock,** ensues when a sensitized guinea pig is injected intraperitoneally with a relatively large amount (e.g., 5 mg) of tuberculin. Prostration develops in 3 to 4 hours, body temperature falls, and death may follow in 5 to 30 hours. A systemic reaction (headache, malaise, prostration) that is only rarely fatal also occurs in highly sensitized persons who are injected with an excessive amount of tuberculin or who inhale it in aerosols in the laboratory.

When humans with tuberculosis are exposed to large amounts of tuberculin, they sometimes develop focal reactions in their tuberculous lesions, in the lungs and elsewhere, resembling histologically the responses elicited in the skin with tuberculin. Systemic responses have also been evoked with Ags of histoplasma, brucella, vaccinia, and pneumococci in persons with delayed-type sensitivity to these organisms.

SENSITIZATION. The time required for induction of tuberculin-specific T cells and for DTH is in general about the same as for the induction of effector lymphocytes from resting precursor cells, such as cytotoxic T lymphocytes (CTLs) from precursor cells (pre-CTLs) and Ab-secreting B cells from resting B cells, namely about 1 week after Ag is first administered. Small quantities of Ag on the surface of living cells are especially potent immunogens. Sensitization to tuberculin is most effectively induced by infection with virulent tubercle bacilli or with the attenuated Bacillus Calmette-Guérin (BCG) strain. Killed bacilli are less effective. Purified tuberculin is ineffectual unless given in appropriate adjuvants, as described below, but it can apparently stimulate a secondary response (i.e., enhance a declining DTH).

ADJUVANTS. Through efforts to improve immunogenicity, it was found that egg albumin injected into an animal's tuberculous lesions established intense DTH to this protein. This observation led to the development of Freund's complete adjuvant (water-in-mineral oil emulsions containing killed tubercle bacilli suspended in the oil phase and Ag in the water phase), the most potent adjuvant known for stimulating both Ab and T-cell-mediated immunity (Ch. 16). Too toxic for use in humans—because the mineral oil is not metabolized and the mycobacteria elicit an intense chronic DTH response—its use is confined to the laboratory. The active component of the tubercle bacillus is **muramyl dipeptide** (Ch. 16, Fig. 16–16, p. 138). A water-in-oil emulsion containing this peptide and tuberculin can establish DTH to tuberculin. How the peptide acts is poorly understood (Ch. 16).

Complete Freund's adjuvant also strongly enhances Ab formation (see Adjuvants, Ch. 16), but the dose of protein is very important: generally, small doses (e.g., 1–50 μg in a guinea pig) elicit intense DTH, whereas larger amounts tend to induce vigorous Ab formation, not DTH. Other adjuvants (such as alumina) promote only Ab formation and may even inhibit the induction of DTH.

CUTANEOUS BASOPHIL HYPERSENSITIVITY. Histamine levels are increased at sites of DTH reactions to tuberculin. This previously puzzling observation became understandable when it was found that the infiltrating leukocytes include many basophils, which contain high levels of histamine (Ch. 18). In the guinea pig, DTH to many proteins is readily induced by injecting the protein in complete Freund's adjuvant; if the same protein is given

TABLE 19–3. Comparison of DTH and Arthus Reactions

	DTH	Arthus
Ag recognition is due to	T-cell receptors (TcR)	Abs
Principal effector cells	Activated T cells; activated macrophages	Granulocytes
Time course of skin reaction to injected Ag*		
Onset	≈10 hrs	~2 hrs
Maximum intensity	24–48 hrs	2–4 hrs (but severe reaction can be evident 24 hrs or longer)
Histology	Intense infiltration with T cells, monocytes, macrophages (basophils)	Edema; mild infiltration initially with granulocytes, later also mononuclear cells
Ag-specific reactivity can be transferred from hypersensitive donor to naive recipient with T cells		Abs (or antiserum)

* Tuberculin can also be applied on human skin as a "patch test" (see Allergic Contact Dermatitis, this ch.) and probably penetrates into the skin via sweat ducts.

instead in saline, the allergic skin reaction that can be evoked a few days later (formerly called the Jones–Mote reaction) is also delayed-type, but distinctive: it follows the same time course as the classic DTH reaction, but it lacks fibrin and is less indurated. In this reaction, about 20% to 60% of the infiltrating inflammatory cells are basophils (which normally account for about 1% of the leukocytes in blood). The cutaneous basophil hypersensitivity reaction is transferable from a sensitized to a normal animal with T cells, and one of the lymphokines these cells secrete is thought to be chemotactic for basophils.

MECHANISMS

The mechanisms responsible for DTH to a soluble protein, such as tuberculin, can be visualized from the general principles described in Chapter 15 (Fig. 19–3). Taken up by dendritic cells and macrophages (and perhaps by B cells), the protein is fragmented into peptides that are expressed on the cell surface in association with MHC-II proteins. CD4$^+$ T cells that recognize the complexes become activated, very likely with the aid of cytokines, perhaps interleukin-1 (IL-1) and IL-6 acting synergistically. The activated cells secrete various lymphokines, and at

least one of them, γ-interferon, stimulates many changes in neighboring macrophages (see Activated Macrophages, below), including the release of toxic components (see below) that cause inflammation and destroy many bacterial and other cells. CD8$^+$ T cells are not activated by soluble Ags (in contrast to their response to Ag-bearing cells; see below), but when activated by Ag in association with MHC-class I proteins, they also secrete γ-interferon and thus can also contribute to macrophage activation.

A requirement for macrophages in DTH was first suggested by adoptive transfer studies with lethally irradiated mice, which develop DTH only when given, not only lymphocytes, but also bone marrow cells as a source of circulating monocytes and tissue macrophages. The blood-borne monocytes (immature macrophages) infiltrate into developing DTH skin lesions and differentiate into mature macrophages. Unlike the transferred lymphocytes, which have to be derived from a sensitized donor, the macrophages act nonspecifically, for they are equally effective whether they come from nonsensitized or from sensitized donors. Relatively few transferred T cells are needed to initiate the allergic response, and macrophages are much more abundant at the DTH reaction site.

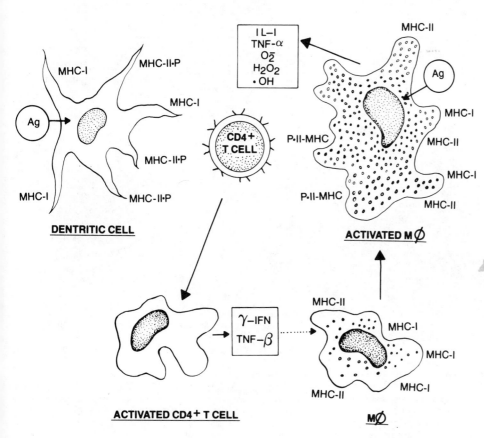

Figure 19–3. Cellular interactions underlying DTH reactions. P represents peptide fragments of Ag, formed by dendritic cells and macrophages (MØ) and expressed on the cell surface as an adduct of MHC-II glycoproteins. Because MHC-II is expressed only slightly on nonactivated MØ and much more on activated MØ, the CD4$^+$ T cells are probably initially stimulated by MHC-II complexes on dendritic cells and later by those on activated MØ. Note the secreted products of activated CD4$^+$ cells and activated MØ (boxed).

Activated Macrophages

In comparison with resting macrophages, activated macrophages are larger, express more MHC-II proteins on their surface, contain more lysosomes and lysosomal enzymes, and secrete a variety of substances, including IL-1, tissue necrosis factor (TNF-α), reactive oxygen intermediates, collagenase, and lysosomal enzymes (Figs. 19–3, 19–4). The activation process and some of the secreted products are discussed below.

ACTIVATION. Expression of MHC-II proteins appears to be constitutive in dendritic cells but inducible (by γ-interferon) in macrophages. Hence, a DTH reaction is probably initiated by the interaction of Ag-specific CD4$^+$ T cells with Ag–MHC-II complexes on dendritic cells (see Fig. 19–4). The resulting activation of the CD4$^+$ T cells and secretion of γ-interferon probably induces macrophages at the site to express MHC-II proteins. Thus **the ratio of MHC-II$^+$/MHC-II$^-$ macrophages increases at the tissue site of a response to antigenic stimulation.** The MHC-II$^+$ cells can present Ag and activate additional CD4$^+$ T cells; with the resulting increase in γ-interferon, additional MHC-II is produced, increasing the effectiveness with which antigenic peptides are presented to CD4$^+$ T cells.

A CD4$^+$ T cell's recognition of Ag–MHC-II complexes on macrophages is probably not sufficient to drive the T

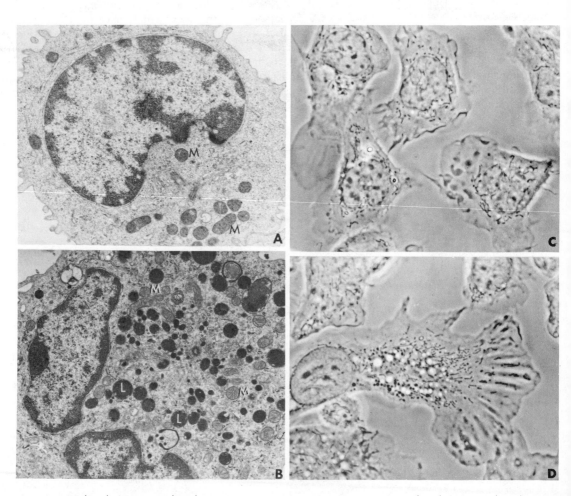

Figure 19–4. Comparison of resting *(A, C)* and activated *(B, D)* macrophages. All are peritoneal cells from normal *(A, C)* or infected *(B, D)* mice 14 days after injection of tubercle bacilli (BCG, Bacillus Calmette-Guérin). In the phase-contrast photographs *(C, D;* ×1900), the activated macrophages *(D)* are larger (the field is almost filled by half of a cell), are more spread out, and contain more organelles, especially lysosomes (dense spherical bodies); the translucent spherical bodies represent ingested culture medium (pinocytotic vesicles). In the electron micrographs *(A, B;* magnification uncertain) the dense spherical lysosomes *(L)* are abundant in activated cells and rare in resting cells, most of whose organelles are mitochondria *(M)*. *(AB:* Blanden RV et al: J Exp Med 129:1079, 1969; *C,D:* courtesy of DR GB Mackaness)

cell from the resting (G_0) stage into the cell cycle and to secrete lymphokines (see Fig. 19–2); IL-1 and IL-6 may also be required.

Independently of CD4$^+$ T cells, macrophages can also be activated by diverse microbial products such as the lipid A component of lipopolysaccharide (LPS) and muramyl dipeptide, the active component of the mycobacteria in Freund's adjuvant. As noted above and in Chapter 16, this peptide is a potent enhancer of Ab production. It also enhances development of DTH in response to immunization with soluble proteins.

It is likely that the phosphatidyl inositol–protein kinase C pathway, described below in connection with the activation of CTLs, is also responsible for the activation of macrophages, because phorbol myristate also stimulates their secretion of IL-1. Some secreted products of activated macrophages are described below.

IL-1

Human IL-1 consists of two proteins, IL-1α and IL-1β. Encoded by different genes (on the same chromosome), each is produced as a 31Kd protein that is processed intracellularly by serine proteases and is secreted as a 15- to 17-Kd single-chain protein. The two secreted proteins have only limited amino acid sequence similarity (identity at only 25% to 40% of their positions, depending on the species). IL-1β is the more abundant form, both at the level of mRNA and as a serum protein.

Produced in relatively large amounts by activated macrophages and monocytes, IL-1 is also synthesized by a variety of other cells, including keratinocytes, skin Langerhans cells, activated B cells, corneal epithelial cells, kidney mesangial cells, and large granular lymphocytes (that include natural killer [NK] cells, see below). A membrane-bound form (IL-1α) appears to be expressed by activated macrophages, and may account for IL-1's localized immunostimulatory effects, in contrast to its diverse systemic effects (see below).

IL-1 exerts its effects on T and B cells primarily as a costimulator. It acts synergistically with IL-6 to stimulate the secretion of IL-2 and expression of IL-2 receptors on T cells when they respond to Ags and mitogens. It also enhances the stimulatory effects of IL-4 and IL-6 on the growth and differentiation of B cells (Ch. 16).

The extensive effects of IL-1 on a wide variety of other cells and tissues accounts for many of the manifestations of acute and chronic infections and inflammation of immune origin. For instance, **it causes fever by stimulating release of a pyrogen from the brain (hypothalamus), induces somnolence, diminishes appetite, augments the catabolic effects of the cytokine termed cachectin (or TNF-α; see below), and stimulates proliferation of granulocytes** by inducing production of bone marrow colony-stimulating factors. In many of the diverse cells it affects, IL-1 enhances arachidonic acid breakdown into prostaglandins (via the cyclooxygenase pathway, Ch. 18) and, perhaps in some cells, into leukotrienes (via the lipoxygenase pathway, Ch. 18); hence, aspirin blocks IL-1-induced fever. The antiinflammatory effects of corticosteroids are probably attributable in part to their effect in blocking IL-1 production.

IL-1 receptors are present on diverse cells in a high-affinity (dissociation constant, K_D, of 5–50 pM and about 1000–4000 receptors per cell) and a low-affinity (K_D of about 400 pM; about 15,000 receptors per cell) form. The binding of IL-1 to the high-affinity receptor leads to rapid internalization (down regulation) of the receptor, suggesting a basis for the self-limiting effect of IL-1 on some cells.

TISSUE NECROSIS FACTOR (TNF)

Activated macrophages and monocytes release trace amounts of a highly potent cytotoxic protein, termed tissue necrosis factor or TNF. At concentrations as low as 10^{-11} M/L, this cytokine kills susceptible cells (e.g., many tumor cell lines and fibroblasts); the destruction takes place very slowly (over 48 to 72 hours) and by mechanisms that are still unknown.

TNF is very similar to **lymphotoxin (LT),** a cytotoxic protein released by activated CTLs. Both proteins are extremely hydrophobic, have a similar sequence and three-dimensional structure, and bind with high affinity (K_D of about 10^{-9}M/L) to the same receptors on cells. Their cytolytic activity is enhanced by IFN-γ, and both act similarly on neutrophils, augmenting phagocytic activity, superoxide anion (O_2^-) production (see below), and cytolytic activity in Ab-dependent cell-mediated cytotoxicity (ADCC; see below). Also termed **cachectin,** TNF has pronounced catabolic effects (e.g., breakdown of muscle protein).

The genes for TNF and LT are located in the MHC, where they are separated by less than 1 kilobase pairs. Their similar sequences suggest that they arose by duplication of a common ancestral gene, and their similarity in structure and function has led to the suggestion that they be designated TNF-α and TNF-β (for TNF and lymphotoxin, respectively) (see Fig. 15–13, p. 332).

REACTIVE OXYGEN INTERMEDIATES

The molecular oxygen in a cell is normally reduced almost completely to water, within mitochondria, by the regulated addition of electrons (four per O_2 molecule), but small amounts (2%–5%) are partially reduced (by addition of one, two, or three electrons) to give rise to two free radicals (the **superoxide anion** O_2^-, and the **hydroxyl radical** ·OH) and to **hydrogen peroxide** (H_2O_2, Fig. 19–5). Before they can do any damage (see below),

(1) $2O_2 + NADPH \xrightarrow{\text{"oxidase"}} 2\mathbf{O_2}^- + H^+ + NADP^+$

(2) $2\mathbf{O_2}^- + 2H^+ \xrightarrow[\text{dismutase}]{\text{superoxide}} \mathbf{H_2O_2} + O_2$

(3) $\mathbf{O_2}^- + \mathbf{H_2O_2} \xrightarrow{Fe^{2+}\ \text{salt}} \cdot\mathbf{OH} + OH^- + O_2$

(4) $\mathbf{H_2O_2} + 2\ GSH \xrightarrow[\text{peroxidase}]{\text{glutathione}} GSSG + 2H_2O$

(5) $GSSG + NADPH + H^+ \xrightarrow[\text{reductase}]{\text{glutathione}} 2GSH + NADP^+$

(6) $2\mathbf{H_2O_2} \xrightarrow{\text{catalase}} 2H_2O + O_2$

Figure 19–5. Toxic oxygen intermediates are derived from molecular oxygen (reactions 1–3) and eliminated by scavenger enzymes (reaction 2 and reactions 4–6). The toxic free radicals (superoxide anion, hydroxyl radical) and molecules (hydrogen peroxide) are in boldface. For the structures of the successive reduced states of oxygen, see Figure 19–6.

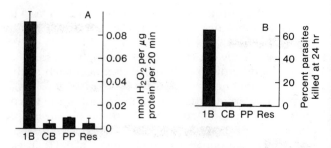

Figure 19–7. Correlation between release of H_2O_2 and destruction of phagocytized microbes (trypanosomes) by activated macrophages. Peritoneal macrophages were from four groups of mice: 1B—immunized with viable *Trypanosoma cruzi* and later boosted with heat-killed *T. cruzi;* CB—controls given the booster injection only; PP—controls injected with proteose peptone, which elicits inflammation and altered macrophages that look like lymphokine-activated cells but lack microbicidal activity; RES—untreated controls ("resident" macrophages from the normal peritoneal cavity). *(A)* H_2O_2 release. *(B)* Destruction of trypanosomes added to the isolated macrophages. (Nathan C et al: J Exp Med 149:1, 1979)

the free radicals (so named because each has an unpaired electron; see Fig. 19–6) and H_2O_2 are destroyed by endogenous scavenger enzymes (see below). However, in activated macrophages (and in activated polymorphonuclear leukocytes), a membrane-bound (NADPH-dependent) enzyme complex ("oxidase") rapidly generates larger amounts than the cell can destroy, leading to their transient accumulation and secretion. These reactive oxygen intermediates can damage proteins, lipids, DNA, and cell membranes; and they are responsible for the destruction of phagocytized bacteria and viruses within endosomes. Hydroxyl radicals are extremely short-lived, but O_2^- and H_2O_2 can escape from activated macrophages, and the extent to which they can be inactivated by neighboring cells determines how much local damage they cause. As shown in reaction 2 (see Fig. 19–5) **superoxide dismutase** catalyzes the conversion of O_2^- to H_2O_2, which can be destroyed by **catalase** (reaction 6) and by

peroxidases such as glutathione peroxidase (reaction 4). With the elimination of O_2^- and H_2O_2, hydroxyl radicals are not formed (reaction 3). At the site of an unusually intense DTH reaction, the amounts of O_2^- and H_2O_2 released from large numbers of activated macrophages can cause extensive destruction of normal cells and tissues, leading to ulceration and scarring. **Many tumor cells and parasites are killed by activated macrophages, probably because they are unusually susceptible to bursts of released toxic oxygen intermediates, not because they are phagocytized** (Figs. 19–7, 19–8).

Cytotoxic T-Lymphocytes

In contrast to the diverse inflammatory effects of activated CD4 T cells, which are expressed largely through the macrophages they stimulate, activated CD8 T cells are much more highly focused: they act primarily as CTLs, destroying only cells whose surface Ag–MHC–I complexes they recognize. However, the recognition of target cells also stimulates them to synthesize and secrete some IFN-γ, and thus they probably also contribute to some extent to macrophage activation.

Observed under the light microscope at 37°C, CTLs appear to be highly motile, changing shape and moving about almost like amebae (Fig. 19–9). When a CTL touches another cell, it dwells on it for a few minutes, moving back and forth and over and under it, as if exploring its surface for an Ag that the T-cell's receptor (TcR) can recognize. The principal adhesion molecules responsible for these **CTL–target cell "conjugates"** have been described earlier (see Chap. 15). If an Ag is not recognized, the CTL crawls away, leaving the explored

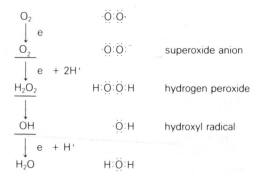

Figure 19–6. Stepwise reduction of molecular oxygen (e = electron). The toxic intermediates are underlined (Personal communication from JA Badwey)

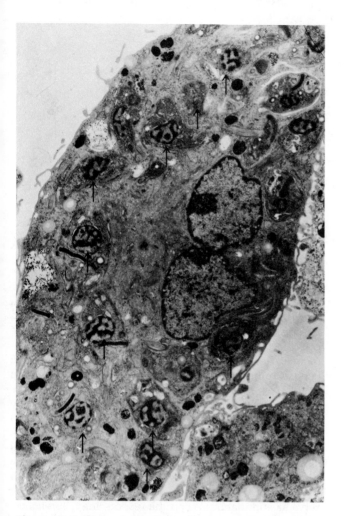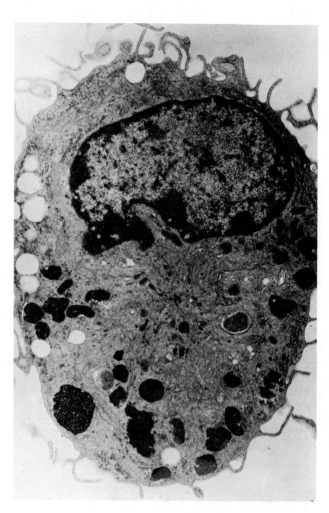

Figure 19–8. Phagocytosed microbes (*Trypanosoma cruzii*) are destroyed by the activated macrophage at *right* and not by the resting macrophage at *left*. The activated macrophage (*right*) had been stimulated in vivo by two successive injections (primary and secondary immunizations) of avirulent mycobacteria (*Bacillus calmette guerin*, BCG); note its dense, irregularly shaped lysosomes. (Courtesy of B Bloom; based on Kress Y, et al: Nature 257:394, 1975, and Kress Y, et al: Exp Parasit 41:385, 1977)

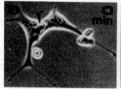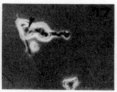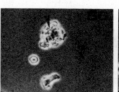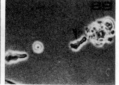

Figure 19–9. The lytic cycle in the attack of a CTL on a target cell. The adhesion of a CTL to the target cell ("conjugate formation") requires Mg^{2+} and involves specific interactions between the Ag-specific receptor on the CTL and Ag–MHC-I complexes on the target cell. Also required are Ag-independent interactions between adhesion molecules, such as between LFA-1 and LFA-2 (or T11 or CD2) on the CTLs with their ligands (ICAM and LFA-3, respectively) on the target cell, and between CD8 on the CTL and MHC-I (its probable ligand) on the target cell. For $CD4^+$ CTLs, the corresponding ligand is probably MHC-II on the target cell.

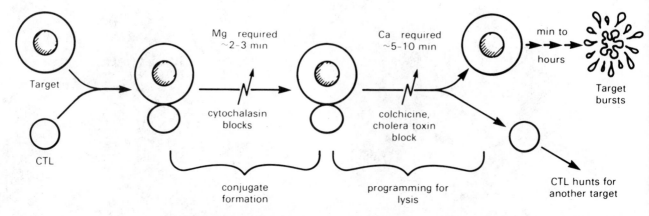

Figure 19–10. The lytic cycle in the attack of a CTL on a target cell.

cell undamaged, but if an Ag is recognized, the CTL is activated to release cytotoxic components. It then moves away to explore the surface of other cells, leaving the recognized cell to disintegrate (lyse) a few minutes later (Figs. 19–9 and 19–10). A CTL can repeat the process many times, killing one target cell after another while generally leaving undamaged neighboring ("bystander") cells that lack the recognized Ag.

In the following sections, we consider how CTLs arise from inactive precursors (**pre-CTLs or pCTLs**), recognize Ags, activate their cytocidal machinery, lyse target cells, and avoid killing themselves when they kill target cells.

INDUCTION. A pCTL whose TcR recognizes an Ag on another cell (the prospective target cell) is stimulated to proliferate and differentiate into mature CTLs (often termed "effector" cells) (Fig. 19–11). Additional signals, provided by IL-2 and IL-6 and perhaps by other lymphokines as well, are needed for an optimal response. The time required (4 to 6 days) is approximately the same *in vivo* as it is with cultured cells. *In vivo*, the same MHC-I is normally present on the responding CD8$^+$ pCTL and on the Ag-bearing stimulator cells, which are usually virus-infected cells or, less commonly, tumor cells with distinctive tumor-associated Ag. However, the stimulator

$$pCTL \xrightarrow[\text{(4-6 days)}]{\text{Induction}} CTL \xrightarrow[\text{(minutes)}]{\text{Activation}} CTL^* \leftrightharpoons \begin{array}{l}\text{Polarized secretion of}\\ \text{cytotoxic proteins,}\\ \text{serine protease(s),}\\ \text{proteoglycans, etc.}\end{array}$$

Figure 19–11. Ag-bearing prospective target cells induce a precursor CTL (pCTL) over a 4- to 6-day period to proliferate and differentiate into a clone of CTLs. When a CTL encounters a cell whose Ag it recognizes, the CTL is reversibly activated (to CTL*) to mobilize and release some of its cytotoxic components; it then dissociates from that target cell to search for another one, where the reversible activation is repeated if Ag is recognized.

cells can also be MHC-different (i.e., allogeneic), as in allografts of kidney, heart, or bone marrow. *In vitro*, these diverse Ag-bearing cells may be used to induce the pCTL → CTL transition, but for experimental convenience, the **mixed lymphocyte response** (MLR) is often used (Ch. 15). In this procedure, lymphoid cells from MHC-different individuals of the same species are coincubated: for example, murine spleen cells—principally lymphocytes, macrophages, and small numbers of dendritic cells—or mononuclear cells from human blood—principally lymphocytes and monocytes. The mutual stimulation of the MHC-disparate cells (**two-way reaction**) is usually made **one-way** by irradiating one cell population: these cells cannot divide, but they can still serve as stimulators. When the responding (alloreactive) lymphocytes are collected after about 6 days and separated into CD4$^+$ and CD8$^+$ T cells, the cytolytic activity is found to reside almost entirely in the CD8$^+$ population (Fig. 19–12), and it appears that virtually all of these cells are CTLs.

The induction of cytolytic T cells from noncytolytic precursors requires the coordinate expression of many genes. Cytokines from macrophages or monocytes are probably necessary, but it is clear that CD4 T cells are not required (as they are to activate Ig-secreting B cells; see Chs. 15 and 16). Thus, when spleen cells are depleted of CD4 cells by Abs to CD4, plus complement, the residual population can still be stimulated in MLR to yield CD8 CTLS. (CTLs of the CD4$^+$ phenotype can also be elicited in the MLR, especially when the reaction is initiated after CD8 cells are removed from the responder spleen-cell populations. Perhaps CTLs are normally more often CD8 than CD4 cells because precursor T cells of the CD8 phenotype (CD4$^-$, CD8$^+$) are especially effective in competing for a limited supply of essential cytokines.)

Once CTLs have been induced, they can be propagated from single cells (**cloned**) and grown for years as

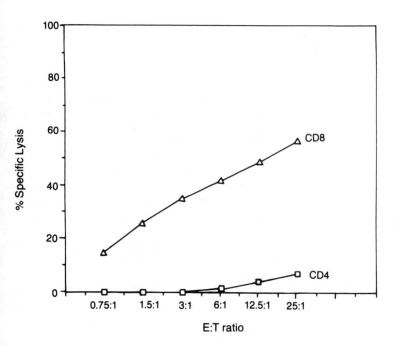

Figure 19–12. Induction of CTLs in a mixed lymphocyte culture. Spleen cells from mice of one strain (BALB/c; MHC type H-2^d) were incubated for 6 days with irradiated spleen cells from an MHC-different (allogeneic) mouse strain (BALB.B; MHC type H-2^b). The "responder" (BALB/c) cells were then divided into purified CD8$^+$ and CD4$^+$ T-cell populations, which were tested for their ability to kill ^{51}Cr-labeled H-2^b target cells using various ratios of "effector" cells (the population tested for killer cells) to target cells (effector to target, or E:T ratio). After 4 hours, ^{51}Cr released into the medium ("specific release") was determined as a measure of target-cell death. Note that virtually all the CTLs are in the C8$^+$ T-cell population. (Nagler–Anderson C et al: Immunol Rev 103:111, 1988)

cytolytically active CTL cell lines by providing them with lymphokines and stimulating them at intervals (e.g., 1–2 weeks) with the Ag-bearing (i.e., target) cells. (Unlike other cell lines that grow in cultures indefinitely, cultured T cells retain a normal karyotype and lack the characteristics of transformed, i.e. tumor, cells.)

ANTIGEN RECOGNITION BY CTLs. As emphasized previously (Ch. 15), the antigenic structures that are normally recognized by CTLs on target cells are fundamentally the same as those recognized by T-helper cells on Ag-presenting cells, namely, peptide fragments of proteins in association with self-MHC proteins, either MHC-I if the CTL is a CD8 cell or MHC-II if it is a CD4 cell. However, **besides recognizing a peptide–self-MHC complex, a CTL's Ag-specific receptor nearly always cross-reacts with one or more foreign (allogeneic) MHC proteins** (a CD8 CTL with a foreign MHC-I and a CD4 CTL with a foreign MHC-II). The propensity of these receptors to cross-react with allogeneic MHC proteins underlies the intensity of allograft rejection reactions (Chs. 15 and 20). It is possible that some CTLs recognize peptide–allogeneic MHC complexes, but that other CTLs recognize the allogeneic MHC proteins themselves, devoid of peptide adducts.

CTL ACTIVATION. On CTLs, as on other mature T cells, the Ag-specific receptor (TcR) is intimately associated with CD3, a complex of five membrane proteins. In contrast to the receptor's clonal variability, CD3 is invariant. **Ligands that bind and aggregate the TcR–CD3 com-**

plexes activate CTLs and stimulate them to secrete cytolytic molecules (see below). The importance of aggregation is evident from the ability of Abs to the TcR or CD3 moiety to substitute, as activating stimuli, for the TcR's natural ligand (peptide–MHC complexes on target cells). Thus particularly when these Abs are attached to the surface of another cell (any cell will do) or to synthetic beads or even when they are simply adsorbed on a plastic surface, they stimulate the CTLs to release serine proteases and other components of toxic granules (see below and Fig. 19–16). In contrast, as soluble monomeric Igs, the anti-receptor Abs have little, if any, stimulatory effect; instead, they usually block the activation of CTLs by their natural target cells.

Several distinct changes take place in CTLs after they become activated: (1) within 2 to 3 minutes, the intracellular Ca^{2+} concentration rises transiently (Fig. 19–13); (2) the CTL's microtubule organizing center and Golgi apparatus become oriented to the site where the CTL makes contact with the target cell; (3) secretory granules, which are normally dispersed throughout the CTL's cytoplasm, migrate to the site of contact with the target cell, fuse with the CTL surface membrane, and release their contents, which include a cytolytic protein (see below), into the narrow, synapse-like intercellular cleft at the CTL–target-cell junction (**exocytosis**) (Figs. 19–14, 19–15); and (4) transcription of the gene for IFN-γ is initiated, and, after a few hours, this protein is secreted (see below). The transduction of the signal from aggregated TcR–CD3 complexes probably depends on the same sequence of reactions, involving phosphatidyl inositol phosphates

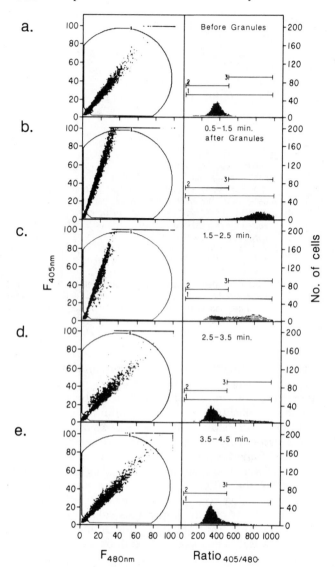

Figure 19–13. Intracellular (cytoplasmic) Ca²⁺ levels rise precipitously in target cells under cytolytic attack by CTLs or their isolated granules. Ca²⁺ concentration was measured with an intracellular dye (indo-1) whose fluorescence emission maximum shifts from 480 nm to 405 nm when it binds Ca²⁺. In the panels at *left* target cells loaded with the dye were examined at approximately minute-intervals after they were exposed to CTL granules. Each dot represents an individual cell (about 20,000 were analyzed at each time point) as it passes through a flow cytometer (Chap. 15, Fig. 15–35). Note the transient increase in fluorescence at 405 nm and decrease at 480 nm, indicating the transient increase (about 10-fold) in Ca²⁺ concentration; Ca²⁺ returned to normal levels (about 150 nm) as the cells recovered. (They were not lysed because a sublytic amount of granules was added.) In the panels at *right* the data are replotted with number of cells (y axis) versus their intracellular Ca²⁺ concentration (fluorescence ratio 405 nm/480 nm, x axis). (From Allbritton NL, et al: J Exp Med 167:514, 1988)

and protein kinase C, that underlies the activation of diverse cells by many different receptor–ligand interactions.

HOW CTLs LYSE TARGET CELLS. Target cells undergo two conspicuous changes when they are lysed by CTLs: (1) their intracellular Ca²⁺ concentration increases markedly and rapidly (more than ten-fold within a few minutes) (see Fig. 16–13); and (2) their DNA is cleaved into nucleosome-sized fragments (multiples of approximately 200 base pairs; see Fig. 19–16).

Dense lysosome-like secretory granules in mouse CTLs contain a protein that resembles C9, the last-acting protein of the complement cascade (Ch. 17, Fig. 19–17). When the granules are released at the CTL–target-cell junction (Fig. 19–14), this protein, known as perforin (or cytolysin), inserts into target cell membranes, where it polymerizes and creates transmembrane pores that act as **nonspecific ion channels.** By electron microscopy the lesions resemble those formed by activated C9 in complement-lysed red blood cells (Chap. 17, Fig. 17–7).

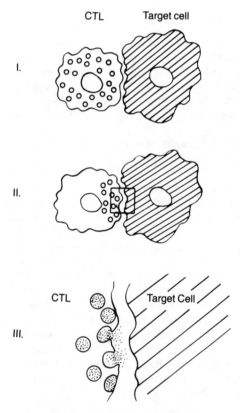

Figure 19–14. CTLs release toxic secretory granules when they recognize Ag-MHC-I complexes on target cells. The granules are normally dispersed throughout the cytoplasm (I). When the target cell's antigenic complexes are recognized by the CTL's T_cR, the granules migrate towards the target (II) and their contents are released into the synapse-like cleft between the adherent cells (III). Boxed area in II is expanded in III.

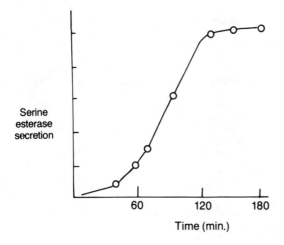

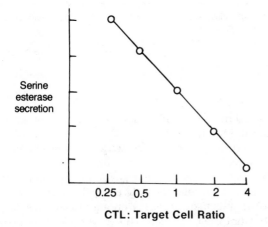

Figure 19–15. Serine esterase secretion, an indicator of secretory granule exocytosis, is triggered by cytolytic attack of CTLs on specific target cells. *(A)* Time course of secretion. *(B)* Influence of the ratio of CTL to target cells. When the ratio is one CTL to four target cells (0.25), essentially all CTLs are surrounded by target cells and are activated. When the ratio is four CTLs to one target cell (4), only a few CTLs are activated. (Based on Pasternack MS et al: Nature 314:743, 1985)

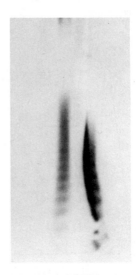

Figure 19–16. Fragmentation of DNA in target cells that are being subjected to cytolytic attack by CTLs. Target cell DNA was marked with radioactive iodine–labeled deoxyuridine (^{125}I-IUdR) and analyzed by electrophoresis in agarose gel. Cleavage of this DNA into a ladder-like series of fragments, differing in length by about 200 base-pairs, is evident when target cells were recognized and attacked by CTLs (*right*) or exposed to secretory granules isolated from CTLs (*left*). (Based on Russell JH: Immunol Rev 72:97, 1983, and Allbritton NL: J Exp Med 167:514, 1988)

The pore-forming perforin is a highly hydrophobic protein and appears to insert rapidly into target-cell membranes; hence, its diffusion is very limited and neighboring ("bystander") cells are spared.

Because the concentration of Ca^{2+} is normally about $1 \times 10^{-3}M$ extracellularly and about $1 \times 10^{-7}M$ intracellularly, the ion channels result in a rapid and massive influx of Ca^{2+}, raising the intracellular concentration to toxic levels. Other effects of the ion channels seem to be responsible for the breakdown of target-cell DNA, probably by activating endogenous endonucleases. However, although both CTLs and Ab-activated complement create nonspecific ion channels in membranes, the cytolytic processes they mediate are not entirely analogous be-

cause **fragmentation of target-cell DNA is seen in CTL-mediated lysis but not in complement-mediated lysis.**

OTHER GRANULE PROTEINS. In addition to perforin, the cytotoxic granules of mouse CTL cell lines contain a set of several (six to eight) proteins of the serine protease family, as well as proteoglycans and one or more proteins that resemble TNF (Fig. 19–17).

The **serine proteases** have the characteristic amino acids of this protein family at their active site (*viz*, noncontiguous serine, histidine, and aspartic acid residues). Present in large amounts in some CTLs (where the principal one accounts for about 1% of total cell protein), some of these proteins cleave synthetic lysine- or arginine-containing substrates (hence their resemblance to trypsin), but they do not cleave proteins in general, and their natural substrates and function are unknown. Because the pH optimum for their catalytic activity is in the 7 to 8 range, whereas the pH within granules is thought to be around 4 to 5, they probably do not function within the granules. Moreover, these highly positively charged proteins may be stabilized in the granules as complexes with the highly negatively charged **proteoglycans,** as in granules of mast cells (Ch. 18). Because they can be detected readily, the serine proteases are valuable indicators of granule maturation and of granule release when CTLs attack target cells (see Fig. 19–15).

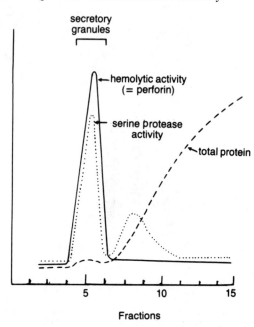

Figure 19–17. The high density of secretory granules makes it possible to separate them from other cytoplasmic components of CTLs. The CTLs were lysed under conditions that make it possible to separate cytoplasm from nuclei, and the cytoplasm was then subjected to centrifugation in Percoll, which establishes a density gradient during centrifugation (high density is at the left). Besides perforin and several serine proteases, the dense granules contain proteoglycans and probably also lymphotoxin (tissue necrosis factor β) and another lymphotoxin-like protein. (Based on Pasternack MS et al: Nature 314:743, 1985)

TABLE 19–4. Comparison between Tissue Necrosis Factor (TNF-α) and Lymphotoxin (TNF-β)

Properties	TNF-α	TNF-β
Principal cell source	Macrophages	Cytotoxic T-lymphocytes (CD8+ and CD4+)
No. of amino acids per molecule (one chain)	159	171
Approximate mol. wt. of the secreted protein	17,000	25,000*
No. of S–S bridges	1	0 (no cysteine)
Glycosylated	No	Yes (1 Asn-linked glycan)
Affinity (K_d) for cell receptors	ca 10^{-9}M/L	ca 10^{-11}M/L
No. of receptors per susceptible cell†	2000–3000	2000–3000
Potentiation of γ-interferon activity	Yes	Yes

* Some TNF-β molecules are smaller (approximately 20 Kd) and lack 23 amino acids at the N terminus.

† The same 70- to 90-Kd glycoprotein appears to be the cell receptor for both TNF-α and TNF-β. Abs to TNF-α block the activity of TNF-α, not of TNF-β, and vice versa with Abs to TNF-β.

CTLs also secrete TNF-β (also termed lymphotoxin; see above and Table 19–4), and another similar factor, both apparently also present in the secretory granules. But, in contrast to the rapid death caused by perforin, these cytotoxic proteins kill target cells very slowly (over 24–72 hours) and by mechanisms that are still unknown. They may be responsible for the limited bystander-cell death that is sometimes observed when CTLs are incubated for long periods with a mixture of Ag-bearing target cells and cells that lack that Ag.

PRIMARY CTLs. In contrast to cultured CTL cell lines, CTLs that have been stimulated *in vivo* and promptly isolated have only barely detectable levels of perforin. Nevertheless, the target cells that are lysed by these more natural CTLs exhibit the same increase in intracellular Ca^{2+} and the same fragmentation of DNA. Whether the cytolytic components of normal CTLs (*in vivo*) and of the cultured cell lines differ in their nature or only in their levels is not clear.

CTLs RESIST SELF-LYSIS. Because the cytolytic components released by CTLs at the CTL–target-cell junction can lyse virtually any target cell, how do CTLs escape

being lysed by the components they release? An answer is suggested by the finding that **CTLs are relatively resistant to their perforin-rich toxic granules.** The molecular basis for the resistance is unknown.

It has been suggested that at each encounter with a target cell, a CTL releases only a small proportion (perhaps 10%) of its toxic granules, enough to kill most target cells, but not the CTL itself. This leaves a sufficient supply of granules to kill many target cells in succession in a short time. If, however, a CTL is itself a recognized target and subjected to concerted attack by several ("aggressor") CTLs, as in a two-way MLR (see above), the recognized CTL can succumb because it would then be the recipient of all the granules unloaded at the same time by, say, three or four aggressor CTLs, but each of the aggressors would be spared because it would be exposed only to the limited number of granules it releases. Hence the observation that one-way recognition can lead to one-way killing.

SECRETION OF LYMPHOKINES. The contribution of CTL to defenses against virus infections, to rejection of allografts, and to other cell-mediated immune reactions is not limited to lysis of target cells. Ag recognition also stimulates CTL to synthesize and secrete IFN-γ and low levels of IL-2. Although this response does not promote lysis of target cells, the IFN-γ (also termed **immune interferon**) can contribute to immune defenses; e.g., it inhibits viral multiplication in infected cells, and, as noted above, it activates macrophages.

TABLE 19–5. Some Inhibitors of Target Cell Lysis by Cytotoxic T Lymphocytes (CTLs)

Inhibitor	Probable Mechanism
Monomeric Abs to Ag-specific receptors (TcR) of CTLs	Down regulation of the TcR–CD3 complexes
Monomeric Abs to CD3	Down regulation of the TcR–CD3 complexes
Protease Inhibitors	
Toxyl-lysine-chloromethylke- tone (TLCK)	?
Phenylmethylsulfonylthoride (PMSF)	Inactivates serine esterase(s)
Abs to CD8	Probably reduces CTL–target-cell adhesion by blocking the reaction between CD8 on a CTL with MHC class-I protein on the target cell
Abs to LFA-1*	Interferes with CTL–target-cell adhesion
Ethylenediaminetetraacetic acid (EDTA)	Removes Ca^{2+} from extracellular medium

* Abs to LFA-1 are potent inhibitors, blocking the cytolytic activity of nearly all CTLs; Abs to CD8 block the activity of only about half of cloned CTL cell lines, perhaps those with lower affinity of their receptors for Ag–MHC-I on target cells.

INTERFERENCE WITH THE CYTOLYTIC ACTIVITY. Besides interfering with the binding of target-cell Ags, Abs to the TcR–CD3 complex can cause these complexes to be removed from the CTL surface (termed **down regulation** or **modulation**), perhaps by **endocytosis.** Abs to several other CTL surface Ags, and several enzyme inhibitors, are also potent inhibitors of cytolytic activity, as shown in Table 19–5.

The lysis of target cells by CTLs can also be prevented by removing Ca^{2+} from extracellular medium (with ethylenediamine tetraacetic acid, a Ca^{2+}-chelating agent). The need for extracellular Ca^{2+} probably reflects its essential role in exocytosis and in the pore-forming activity of perforin, and perhaps also in raising the target cell's cytoplasmic Ca^{2+} concentration to toxic levels. However, **some CTLs can lyse some target cells in the virtual absence of extracellular Ca^{2+}, suggesting that there may be alternative cytolytic pathways,** possibly based on two other cytotoxic proteins in CTLs, lymphotoxin (tissue necrosis factor β) and a lymphotoxin-like protein.

Other Cytotoxic Cells

NATURAL KILLER CELLS

Among the lymphocytes in human blood and mouse spleen, there are some cytotoxic cells that lyse a variety of tumor cell lines, regardless of their MHC haplotype, and even lyse some cells that express **no** MHC proteins. Because prior immunization with susceptible target cells does not increase the level of this **MHC-nonrestricted** cytotoxicity, it is called **natural killer activity.** The responsible cells, termed natural killer or NK cells, **are defined by their ability to kill certain tumor cells without prior immunization and without restriction by MHC glycoproteins.** NK cells can also kill cells infected with some enveloped viruses, and they may have a role in defenses against some virus infections before Abs and CTLs appear.

NK cells have a lower buoyant density than other peripheral blood leukocytes and can be separated by density-gradient centrifugation through Percoll, a high-mol.-wt. polysaccharide. The separated cells are "**large granular lymphocytes**" with prominent secretory granules that contain cytotoxic components like those of CTLs; they probably also kill their target cells by exocytosis of these granules. The tumor cell lines that are lysed by NK cells are distinguished by unusual sensitivity to the isolated secretory granules (see perforin, above).

NK cells have several characteristic surface markers (termed NKH-1 and HNK-1), including a specific receptor (called $Fc_\gamma R$ or CD16) for the Fc domain of IgG. This receptor is responsible for the activity of NK cells in the process called Ab-dependent cell-mediated cytotoxicity (see ADCC, below). Some NK cells lack Ag-specific TcR, and those that have them are not prevented from killing target cells when these receptors are removed by anti-receptor Abs, underscoring the irrelevance of target-cell MHC for the killer activity of NK cells. Nonetheless, NK cells are stimulated to release secretory granules when they kill their targets, and so they probably have a unique receptor for a unique ligand on the target cells; neither the receptor nor its ligand has been identified.

Many cultured CTL clones can be stimulated by long exposure to high concentrations of IL-2 to exhibit NK activity (i.e., to kill the same targets as NK cells, unrestricted by MHC). This activity is expressed even after Ag-specific TcR–CD3 complexes have been removed (down regulated) by Abs to CD3. Thus, CTLs that express NK activity probably also express the distinctive receptor that characterizes NK cells in general.

ANTIBODY-DEPENDENT CELL-MEDIATED CYTOTOXICITY (ADCC)

As we have seen (Ch. 17), Abs can target Ag-bearing cells for lysis by complement. However, independently of complement Abs can also mediate cell lysis by triggering **ADCC.** In this process, Abs bind specifically via their Fab domains to surface Ags on target cells and via their Fc domain to receptors for Fc on diverse cytotoxic cells (Fig. 19–18). The resulting aggregation of these receptors (e.g., see Mast Cell Receptors for IgE, Ch. 18) probably provides

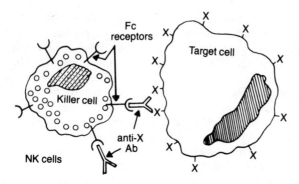

Figure 19–18. Ab-dependent cell-mediated cytotoxicity (ADCC). Abs to a cell-surface marker (x) on target cells is bound via the Fc domain to an Fc receptor (FcR) on natural killer (NK) or some other cytotoxic cells.

TABLE 19–6. Some Intracellular Pathogens*

Mycobacterium tuberculosis	
M. leprae	
Listeria monocytogenes	
Yersinia pestis	
Brucella species	Bacteria
Salmonella species	
Legionella pneumophilia	
Rickettsiae	
Chlamydiae	
Histoplasma capsulatum	Fungus
Trypanosoma cruzi	
Leishmania donovani	Protozoa
Toxoplasma	

* Nearly all the microorganisms listed can grow outside as well as inside host cells, i.e. their intracellular domicile is *facultative*. But for some the intracellular environment is *obligate* (e.g. Rickettsiae, Chlamydiae).

the stimulus to express cytolytic activity. NK cells and macrophages have Fc receptors and participate in ADCC; CTLs lack these receptors and do not.

Patients injected with mAbs to distinctive Ags on some tumor cells (melanoma, B-cell lymphoma, etc., see Ch. 20) sometimes experience extensive tumor destruction, and both ADCC and complement-mediated cytotoxicity are probably responsible. The mAbs are mouse Igs, and the isotypes with greatest effect are IgG3, IgG$_{2a}$ and IgG$_{2b}$, which have especially high affinity for Fc receptors on human macrophages. Target cells are probably destroyed by reactive oxygen intermediates secreted by activated macrophages.

Cell-Mediated Immunity and Disease

COMPARISON OF CELL-MEDIATED AND Ab-MEDIATED DEFENSES AGAINST INFECTIOUS AGENTS. Cell-mediated immune responses are at least as effective as Abs in combatting many infections, particularly those caused by viruses and other pathogens that multiply within host cells (Table 19–6). Thus, children who cannot produce Abs because of an inherited B-cell defect (Chs. 16 and 20) but who have normal T cells generally recover normally from measles, mumps, and other common viral infections of childhood, although they are subject to recurrent, life-threatening infections with common bacterial pathogens such as the pneumococcus and streptococcus.

The contribution of CD4 T cells to defenses against intracellular pathogens is triggered by recognition of the pathogen's Ag on MHC-II$^+$ cells (normally, macrophages, B cells, and dendritic cells but sometimes a variety of other cells [see Autoimmunity, Ch. 20]); the T cells then secrete IFN-γ and other lymphokines, thereby activating macrophages and helping B-cell responses. The power of CD8 T cells in conferring resistance derives from their

ability to recognize viral Ags on almost any infected cell, because virtually all cells express MHC-I proteins. Activated by this recognition, CD8 CTLs confer resistance in two ways: by secreting IFN-γ, and by destroying the virus-infected cells whose viral-encoded surface Ags the CTLs recognize. Because this lysis often occurs before mature virions are formed, CTLs offer the advantage of a "strategic" defense; in contrast, neutralizing Abs provide a "tactical" defense by blocking the infectivity of individual extracellular virions.

CTLs offer another advantage, based on the viral Ags they recognize. Neutralizing Abs are often specific for only one of many antigenic variants (serotypes) of envelope glycoproteins that are found among diverse isolates of some highly pathogenic viruses (e.g., influenza virus, human immunodeficiency virus [HIV]). Hence many viral antigenic variants escape the effects of neutralizing Abs. However, they are less likely to avoid the defenses conferred by CTLs, because these cells are more often specific for MHC-associated peptide fragments of diverse viral Ags, such as capsid nucleoproteins, that do not vary from one viral serotype to another.

The extent to which CTLs provide resistance against virus infections of humans is not easily measured, but indirect evidence suggests that they are protective. For example:

1. Among human volunteers infected with influenza virus, those with higher anti-virus CTL activity of their peripheral blood lymphocytes shed less virus in their nasal secretions.

2. Among bone marrow transplant recipients, individuals with nonlethal cytomegalovirus (CMV) infections have demonstrable CMV-specific CTLs, whereas those with a fatal outcome have far fewer such cells.

The protective effects of CTLs can be directly demonstrated in experimental infections of mice with influenza virus: the intravenous injection of cloned anti-viral CTLs increases survival and greatly reduces viral multiplication. Although most anti-influenza CTLs are specific for the influenza virus nucleoprotein (see above) and cross-protect mice infected with diverse strains of the virus, some CTLs recognize the strain-specific hemagglutinin, a surface glycoprotein on the virions and on virus-infected cells. In mice infected with several strains, the strain-specific CTLs inhibit multiplication only of the strain for which they are specific. If this protective effect were attributable to the secretion of IFN-γ, the strain-specific CTLs would have been effective against other strains as well. Thus, *in vivo*, the lysis of infected cells by CTLs seems clearly to be protective.

Because Abs do not penetrate into cells, cell-mediated immune responses are the principal means of combating infections caused by those bacteria, fungi, and protozoa that survive or even multiply within host cells. *Listeria monocytogenes* is the prototype for such infectious agents. When taken up by macrophages from a normal mouse, these bacteria escape from endocytic vesicles and multiply in the cytoplasm. They can also spread from one macrophage to another without going through an extracellular phase, and so Abs, not surprisingly, offer no protection. However, when mice that have been immunized with *Listeria* (e.g., by infecting and then curing them with an antibiotic) are reinfected, the reintroduced bacteria stimulate the *Listeria*-specific CD4+ T cells (which evidently recognize *Listeria* Ags on the surface of infected macrophages), causing the macrophages to become activated and to destroy their intracellular *Listeria*. Although Abs acting alone are not protective, together with complement, they can cooperate with CD4 T cells and macrophages by coating ("opsonizing") bacteria and

viruses, enhancing their uptake by phagocytic cells (Fig. 19–19) (Ch. 17).

CTLs can also lyse *Listeria*-infected cells (epithelial and others), presumably because these cells express on their surface *Listeria*-encoded Ags associated with MHC-I protein. And although the released bacteria cannot be killed by the CTLs (because bacteria lack MHC protein), they can be killed by neighboring activated macrophages. **Hence, CTLs and activated macrophages can cooperate in destroying bacteria that multiply in various cells.** How efficiently this cooperative killing operates *in vivo* is not clear.

Because the destructive molecules in activated macrophages are toxic oxygen derivatives, it is obvious that an activated macrophage can kill a wide variety of microorganisms and even susceptible tumor cells and extracellular parasites, regardless of the particular activating antigenic stimulus. But, because macrophage **activation depends upon Ag recognition by CD4+ T cells, it is Ag specific; and once activated, the macrophages kill diverse bacteria and other cells nonspecifically.**

The nonspecific antimicrobial activity of stimulated macrophages may account for the alleged benefits of some older forms of nonspecific **vaccine therapy,** such as immunization with typhoid vaccine to treat pneumococcal infections. Moreover, it is also possible that deliberately activated macrophages will prove to be therapeutically useful. Thus, in the progressive **lepromatous form of leprosy** skin lesions contain masses of non-activated macrophages that are packed with viable *M. leprae*, whereas in the quiescent, **tuberculoid** form of the disease, the lesions contain masses of activated macrophages but hardly any visible bacilli. The injection of IFN-γ into lepromatous nodules appears to activate the macrophages and convert the lesions within a few days into the tuberculoid form.

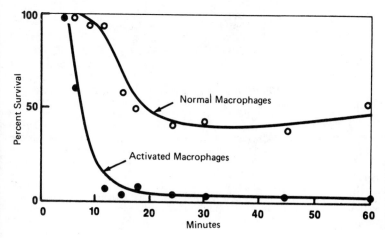

Figure 19–19. Increased bactericidal activity of activated macrophages. *Salmonella typhimurium* coated (opsonized) with anti-*Salmonella* Abs are ingested and killed more rapidly and in greater numbers (decreased percent survival) by activated than by normal macrophages. (Mackaness GB: Hosp Practice 73:1970)

***CELL-MEDIATED IMMUNITY IS SOMETIMES RESPONSI-
BLE FOR DISEASE.*** Not all infections are inherently pathogenic, and when an infection is benign, a cell-mediated
immune response to it may, in the form of DTH, actually
cause disease, sometimes with a fatal outcome. Some
examples follow.

Infection of the neural tissue of immunologically normal adult mice with lymphocytic choriomeningitis virus
usually has a fatal outcome, with extensive focal destruction of virus-infected cells. By contrast, in immunologically unresponsive mice (e.g., fetal or newborn, or adults
treated with irradiation), the virus multiplies and
spreads harmlessly, causing no apparent disease; but if
an immune response subsequently develops in these animals, death will ensue secondary to severe inflammatory and necrotic lesions (i.e., DTH reactions), especially
in neural tissues. In hepatitis virus infection, CTLs may
similarly be responsible for the death of infected cells.
And in a localized, quiescent tuberculous lesion in a
bronchus or in the meninges, a tuberculin-specific DTH
reaction can result in extensive inflammation and necrosis; and the resulting release of tubercle bacilli can cause
fatal disseminated infection in the bronchopulmonary
tree or meninges (tuberculous meningitis).

Thus, like Ab responses, cell-mediated immune responses can either protect against infection or cause benign infections to become devastating. In Chapter 20, we
shall consider some autoimmune diseases in which cell-
mediated immune responses to self-Ags can cause extensive tissue damage. In the following section, we consider the immune responses that are responsible for one
of the commonest skin disorders of humans. In this disorder—allergic contact dermatitis—low-mol.-wt. chemicals, acting as haptens, attach to skin proteins. By itself,
the chemical reaction with tissue protein is usually in-
consequential, but the T-cell response to the altered proteins can produce severe inflammatory reactions in the
skin.

Contact Skin Sensitivity

Contact skin sensitivity (also termed **allergic contact
dermatitis**) is induced, and its expression is elicited,
by contact of low-mol.-wt. chemicals (generally <1000
daltons) with intact skin. These include an enormous
variety of drugs, cosmetics, and other chemicals, ranging
from catechols of poison ivy plants to penicillin. The
reactions are mediated by T cells, most likely both CD4+
and CD8 cells.

Sensitivity is **induced** by contact of the chemical sensitizer with a limited area of skin (e.g., <1 cm²); and the
skin can even be bypassed altogether in experimental
studies in guinea pigs by injecting the sensitizer subcutaneously in complete Freund's adjuvant. Beginning 4 or

5 days after the initial exposure, an application of the
sensitizer almost anywhere on the skin surface elicits
delayed inflammation.

Guinea pigs are tested with a drop of dilute solution
on the skin after hair has been removed. Humans are
tested with a **patch test:** a piece of filter paper soaked
with a dilute solution of sensitizer is placed on the skin,
covered with tape, and left for 24 hours. The response,
confined to the area of contact, is scored for intensity a
few hours after the patch is removed and again the following day (Fig. 19–20). Because sensitizers react indiscriminately with most proteins and are potential irritants
(see below), they must be used at concentrations that
avoid nonspecific inflammation.

The **time course** is the same as that of the tuberculin
reaction; erythema and swelling appear at about 10 to 12
hours and increase to a maximum at 24 to 48 hours.

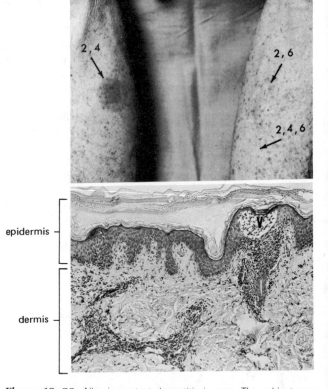

Figure 19–20. Allergic contact dermatitis in man. The subject was
sensitized to 2,4-dinitrofluorobenzene (DNFB) and then tested with 2,4-
dinitrochlorobenzene (*2,4*), 2,6-dinitrochlorobenzene (*2,6*), and 2,4,6-
trinitrochlorobenzene (*2,4,6*-TNCB). A positive response was evident at
24 hours and photographed *(Top)* at 72 hours. Specificity is shown by the
strong reaction to 2,4-dinitrochlorobenzene and the absence of reactions
to the 2,6 and 2,4,6 analogues. All the analogues tested form dinitrophenyl (or trinitrophenyl) derivatives of skin proteins *in vivo* (see Fig.
19–21). *(Bottom)* Histology of the skin reaction. Note the characteristic
intraepidermal vesicle (*V*). The dermis and epidermis are infiltrated by
many lymphocytes and macrophages. Epidermal cells around vesicles
generally have foamy cytoplasm (spongiosis).

Substituents (X)
on C-1 of

combine with protein in vivo

O_2N⬡X
NO_2

Substituents (X) on C-1 of	with ε-NH₂ of lysine residues	with SH of cysteine residues	Ability to induce and elicit contact skin sensitivity
X = -F	+	+	+
-Cl	+	+	+
-Br	+	+	+
-SO₃	−	+	+
-SCN	−	+	+
-SCl	−	+	+
-H	−	−	−
-CH₃	−	−	−
-NH₂	−		−

Figure 19–21. Correlation among the C-1-substituted 2,4-dinitrobenzenes between the ability to form 2,4-dinitrophenylated proteins *in vivo* and the ability to induce and to elicit contact skin sensitivity.

Unusually intense reactions produce necrosis, and, even without necrosis, complete recovery can take several weeks.

Histologically (see Fig. 19–20), the dermis at the site of contact is invaded by monocytes (macrophages), lymphocytes, and small numbers of basophils, as in DTH responses to tuberculin. But the more superficial epidermis differs: it is hyperplastic, invaded by monocytes and lymphocytes and, in addition, contains (in man, but not in the guinea pig) intraepidermal vesicles, or blisters, filled with serous fluid, granulocytes, and mononuclear cells (Fig. 19–19).

MECHANISMS. In accord with the general requirements for immunogenicity (Ch. 12), the actual immunogens are not the simple substances (haptens) themselves but the covalent derivatives they form with tissue (skin) proteins *in vivo*. Thus, among a group of 2,4-dinitrobenzenes, those that can form stable covalent derivatives of protein SH and NH₂ groups *in vivo* are effective sensitizers, whereas those that cannot form such derivatives are not (Fig. 19–21).

In addition to epithelial cells, the normal epidermis contains small numbers of special bone-marrow-derived Ag-presenting cells (APC) and T cells. Called **Langerhans cells,** the APC resemble dendritic cells and the T cells are CD4⁻, CD8⁻ (double-negative) cells with γ–δ, rather than α–β, Ag-specific TcR (see Ch. 15). It is likely, though not yet established, that the γ–δ receptors recognize different MHC class-I molecules than the α–β

receptors (of other T cells). Whether it is the indigenous γ–δ-bearing T cells or the CD4⁺ and CD8⁺ (single-positive) α–β-bearing T cells that infiltrate into the epidermis, or both, that are responsible for Ag recognition is not

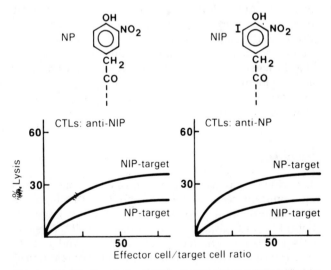

Figure 19–22. Specificity of CTLs against target cells modified by attachment of small haptenic groups, *NP* (3-nitro-4-hydroxyphenyl acetate) or *NIP* (its 5-iodo analogue). CTLs elicited by NP-cells lysed NP-target cells better than they did NIP-targets, whereas those elicited by NIP-cells lysed NIP-target cells better than NP-targets. CTLs elicited by NP-syngeneic cells do not lyse NP-target cells with different H-2K and H-2D alleles **(H-2 restriction).** (From Wall KA, personal communication)

clear. The nominal Ag that is recognized is clearly a skin protein derivative resembling the hapten–protein conjugates discussed earlier (e.g., Chs. 12 and 13). Whether it is recognized by T cells as a haptenated peptide in association with an MHC protein or as a haptenated MHC protein is unclear, but the haptenic group is critical. Thus, as shown in Figure 19–20, the contact skin responses of a laboratory worker who had become sensitized to 2,4-dinitrofluorobenzene were specific for the 2,4-dinitrophenyl group and not for 2,6-dinitrophenyl or 2,4,6-trinitrophenyl groups. Similarly, CTLs can distinguish between syngeneic cells whose surface proteins are substituted with either 3-nitro-4-hydroxyphenyl acetate (NP) or its 5-iodo analogue (NIP) (Fig. 19–22).

DESENSITIZATION. In contrast to the establishment of tolerance, where an Ag acts as "toleragen" before it has a chance to function as an immunogen, desensitization is established by administering an Ag *after* an individual has already been sensitized to it. It is possible that partial desensitization occurs when an individual with DTH is tested simultaneously at many skin sites with the same Ag: the reaction at each site is less intense than when a single test is applied, presumably because the number of Ag-specific ("sensitized") T cells is limiting. Similarly, in overwhelming infections such as miliary tuberculosis or disseminated fungal or protozoan infections, DTH skin responses usually cannot be elicited, perhaps because the large number of disseminated Ag-bearing cells saturates the sensitized T cells.

Comparable events occur with industrial workers, who sometimes develop and then lose skin sensitivity during prolonged and intense exposure to the sensitizer. However, deliberate desensitization of cell-mediated immune responses by repeated administration of Ag or simple sensitizers has been difficult to achieve regularly and frequently precipitates a severe allergic reaction. Moreover, any desensitization that is achieved is short-lived (e.g., 5 to 10 days).

Summary

The wide-ranging systemic and local effects of cell-mediated immune responses are triggered by T-cell recognition of protein Ags, presented as peptide fragments bound to MHC glycoproteins on diverse cells. Triggered CD4 T cells are activated to secrete IFN-γ (and TNF-β?), which induce nearby macrophages to become intensely phagocytic and bactericidal. These "angry" macrophages release: (1) small proteins (IL-1, TNF-α) that have diverse local and systemic effects (fever, increase in numbers of blood granulocytes) and (2) partially reduced, reactive oxygen intermediates (superoxide anion, hydroxyl radical, hydrogen peroxide) that act locally, killing phago-cytized bacteria and viruses, destroying tumor cells and parasites, and, when especially intense, damaging normal cells and tissues. Cytotoxic T-lymphocytes (CTLs, mostly CD8 and less often CD4 cells) act only on cells with which they are in contact, lysing them if they recognize their Ag–MHC complexes. All of these effects constitute a powerful source of defense against infections by viruses and other intracellular pathogens and against some tumors and parasites. However, they can also elicit harmful effects from some otherwise-benign infections and essentially harmless reactions of chemicals and drugs with tissue proteins; and they are also responsible for the severe consequences of some immune responses to autologous Ags (Autoimmune Disease, Ch. 20). Thus, like other immune responses, cell-mediated immunity can exert protective or damaging effects, depending on the eliciting agents and the circumstances.

Selected Reading

BOOKS AND REVIEW ARTICLES

Beutler B, Cerami A: Cachectin and tumor necrosis factor as two sides of the same biological coin. Nature 320:584, 1986

Burakoff SJ, Weinberger O, Krensky AM, et al: A molecular analysis of the cytotoxic T lymphocyte response. Adv Immunol 36:45, 1984

Davis MM, Bjorkman PJ: T-cell antigen receptor genes and T-cell recognition. Nature 334:395, 1988

Henkart PA: Mechanisms of lymphocyte-mediated cytoxicity. Ann Rev Immunol 3:31, 1985

Martz E, Howell DM: CTL: virus control cells first and cytolytic cells second? Immunol Today 10:79, 1989

Möller G (ed): Molecular mechanisms of T cell-mediated lysis. Immunol Rev 103, 1988

Nabholz M, MacDonald HR: Cytolytic T lymphocytes. Ann Rev Immunol 3:237, 1985

Ortaldo Jr, Herberman RB: Heterogeneity of natural killer cells. Ann Rev Immunol 2:359, 1984

Pasternack MS: Cytotoxic T lymphocytes. Adv Int Med, 1987

Stanley K, Luzio P: Perforin, a member of a family of killer proteins. Nature 334:475, 1988

Tirosh R, Berke G: Immune cytolysis viewed as a stimulatory process of the target. In: Mechanisms of Cell-Mediated Cytotoxicity II. Henkart P, Martz E (eds.). New York, Plenum Publishing Corp, 1985

Unanue ER, Allen PM: The basis for the immunoregulatory role of macrophages and other accessory cells. Science 236:551–557, 1987

SPECIFIC ARTICLES

Allbritton NL, Verret CR, Wolley RC, Eisen HN: Calcium ion concentration and DNA fragmentation in target cell destruction by murine cloned cytotoxic T lymphocytes. J Exp Med 167:514, 1988

Carswell EA, Old LJ, Kassel RL, Green S, Firoe N, Williamson B: An endotoxin-induced serum factor that causes necrosis of tumors. Proc Natl Acad Sci USA 72:3666, 1975

Clayberger C, Parham P, Rothbard J, Ludwig DS, Schoolnik GK, Krensky AM: HLA-A2 peptides can regulate cytolysis by human allogeneic T lymphocytes. Nature 330:763–765, 1987

Dennert G, Podack ER: Cytolysis by H-2 specific T killer cells: assembly of tubular complexes on target membranes. J Exp Med 157:1483, 1983

Gotch F, Rothbard J, Howland K, Townsend A, McMichael A: Cytotoxic T lymphocytes recognize a fragment of influenza matrix protein in association with HLA-A2. Nature 326:881–882, 1987

Kranz DM: Tonegawa S, Eisen HN: Attachment of an anti-receptor antibody to non-target cells renders them susceptible to lysis by a clone of cytotoxic T lymphocytes. Proc Natl Acad Sci USA 81:7922, 1984

Lichtenheld MG, Olsen KJ, Lu P, Lowrey DM, Hameed A, Hengartner H, Podack ER: Structure and function of human perforin. Nature 335:448, 1988

Lukacher AE, Braciale VL, Braciale TJ: In vivo effector function of influenza virus-specific cytotoxic T lymphocyte clones is highly specific. J Exp Med 160:814, 1984

Maryanski JL, Pala P, Corradin G, Jordan BR, Cerottini J-C: H-2-restricted cytolytic T cells specific for HLA can recognize a synthetic HLA peptide. Nature 324:578–579, 1986

Masson D, Tschopp J: A family of serine esterases in lytic granules of cytolytic T lymphocytes. Cell 49:679, 1987

Morrison LA, Lukacher AE, Braciale VL, Fan DP, Braciale TJ: Differences in antigen presentation to MHC class-I and class-II restricted influenza virus-specific cytolytic T lymphocyte clones. J Exp Med 163:903, 1986

Ostergaard H, Kane K, Mescher M, Clark WR: Cytotoxic T lymphocyte mediated lysis without release of serine esterase. Nature 330:71, 1987

Pasternack MS, Eisen HN: A novel serine esterase expressed by cytotoxic T lymphocytes. Nature 314:743, 1985

Poenie M, Tsien RY, Schmitt-Verhulst A-M: Sequential activation and lethal hit measured by [Ca^{2+}]$_i$ in individual cytolytic T cells and targets. EMBO J 6:22–33, 1987

Russell JH, Masakowski VR, Dobos CB: Mechanisms of immune lysis. I. Physiological distinction between target cell death mediated by cytotoxic T lymphocytes and antibody plus complement. J Immunol 124:1100, 1980

Russell JH, Masakowski VR, Rucinsky T, Phillips G: Mechanisms of immune lysis. III. Characterization of the nature and kinetics of the cytotoxic T lymphocyte-induced nuclear lesion in the target. J Immunol 128:2087, 1982

Shinkai Y, Takio K, Okumura K: Homology of perforin to the ninth component of complement (C9). Nature 334:525, 1988

Sprent J, Schaeffer M, Lo D, Korngold R: Properties of purified T cell subsets. II. In vivo responses to Class I vs. Class II H-2 differences. J Exp Med 163:998, 1986

Takayama H, Trenn G, Humphrey W, Bluestone JA, Henkart PA, Sitkovsky MV: Antigen receptor-triggered release of a trypsin-type esterase from cytotoxic T lymphocytes. J Immunol 138:566, 1987

Tirosh R, Berke G: T lymphocyte mediated cytolysis as an excitatory process of the target. I. Evidence that the target cell may be the site of Ca^{2+} action. Cell Immunol 95:113, 1985

Townsend ARM, Rothbard J, Gotch FM, Bahadur G, Wraith D, McMichael AJ: The epitopes of influenza nucleoprotein recognized by cytotoxic T lymphocytes can be defined by short synthetic peptides. Cell 44:959–968, 1986

Townsend ARM, Bastin J, Gould K, Brownlee GG: Cytotoxic T lymphocytes recognize influenza haemagglutin that lacks a signal sequence. Nature 324:575–577, 1986

Verret CR, Firmenich AA, Kranz DM, Eisen HN: Resistance of cytotoxic T lymphocytes to the lytic effects of their toxic granules. J Exp Med 166:1536, 1987

Zinkernagel RM, Doherty PC: Restriction of in vitro T cell-mediated cytotoxicity in lymphocytic choriomeningitis within a syngeneic or semiallogeneic system. Nature 248:701, 1974

20

Aberrant Immune Responses

As earlier chapters noted, immune responses not only confer powerful defenses against a wide variety of infectious agents but also can have pathological effects, as in immediate-type (Chap. 18) and cell-mediated (delayed-type) hypersensitivity (Chap. 19). In this chapter, we consider several other pathological conditions that arise from excessive, inappropriate, or defective immune responses: autoimmune diseases, reactions against allografts, immune responses to tumors, and some immunodeficiency disorders, including the acquired immune deficiency syndrome (AIDS) caused by the human immunodeficiency virus (HIV).

Autoimmune Responses

Clinical and experimental observations show that individuals sometimes produce Abs and T cells that react with Ags of their own cells and tissues. These exceptions to the principle of self-tolerance often appear to be responsible for disease. Under certain circumstances, however, they are the consequences of an underlying disease rather than its cause, such as the Abs to heart muscle protein that appear after a myocardial infarction or cardiac surgery. In other cases, Abs to self may not be associated with any pathology. It is thus necessary to distinguish between **autoimmune responses** to self-Ags and **autoimmune disease,** in which these responses cause or at least contribute to disease.

MECHANISMS

Some mechanisms that are likely to underlie autoimmune responses are summarized below.

ALTERED FORMS OF SELF-ANTIGENS. As noted in Chapter 16 (Tolerance to Self-Antigens), B cells to self-Ags are normally present but quiescent, presumably because the cognate anti-self T-helper cells are purged as they arise in the thymus (see Chaps. 15 and 16). However, if a self-Ag is altered (e.g., by mutation or post-translational modifications) it can acquire novel epitopes. Because the new epitope (E) is now part of a self-Ag (call it X), the altered Ag (E-X) can be taken up by Ag-presenting cells, including inactive anti-X B cells, and presented to anti-E T$_H$ cells (which would not have been subjected to thymic elimination because E is not normally present). Hence, the previously quiescent anti-X B cells would be stimulated to produce their Abs, which react with X. As an example, we considered earlier (Chap. 16, Fig. 16–13) how rabbit thyroglobulin (Tg), when chemically modified, elicits, in rabbits, Abs that react with native rabbit Tg and cause thyroiditis (see below).

ALTERED DISTRIBUTION OF A SELF-Ag. Some self-Ags, such as those of sperm, are confined to anatomic sites that are not ordinarily accessible to lymphocytes; hence, they do not establish tolerance, but they also do not normally elicit autoimmune responses. Such responses are readily produced experimentally by removing cells that produce these Ags and injecting them back into a site where they are accessible to lymphoid cells. Clinical incidents that release such Ags have the same effect, e.g. eliciting the Abs to heart muscle mentioned above and Abs to eye Ags after trauma to the eye. In these instances, **disease gives rise to the autoimmune response,** rather than the reverse. Nonetheless, **such responses can be self-perpetuating:** once the response is initiated, the resulting immune-mediated inflammation in the target organ can lead to contact of Ag with infiltrating lymphocytes and hence to further responses.

ANTIGENIC MIMICRY. The epitopes of many bacterial and viral proteins bear some resemblance to those of host proteins (Table 20–1), and the immune responses they elicit can cross-react with self-Ags. For example, a monoclonal Ab (mAb) to Coxsackie virus B4 cross-reacts with heart muscle; this virus has also been identified in individuals with myocarditis. In another example, a sequence of amino acids in myelin basic protein (MBP) of the central nervous system (CNS) resembles a sequence in hepatitis B virus polymerase; the viral peptide elicits Abs and T cells that react with native MBP and cause inflammation around the blood vessels of the CNS.

Such antigenic mimicry could underlie the brain damage (encephalopathy) that occurs as a rare event following immunization of humans with vaccinia virus, probably through a weak cross-reactions with MBP: the resulting tissue injury, causing release of this normally sequestered Ag, could induce a further immune response. In support of this hypothesis, peripheral blood mononuclear cells removed during certain acute virus infections proliferate in response to MBP. Infections with some viruses such as Coxsackie and cytomegalovirus are also associated statistically and temporally with the onset of myasthenia gravis and insulin-dependent diabetes mellitus, both probably autoimmune diseases; some Ags of these viruses have some sequence similarity to the acetylcholine receptor and the insulin receptor, respectively.

CHRONIC VIRAL INFECTION. Mice infected at birth with certain temperate viruses (e.g., lymphocytic choriomeningitis virus, lactic dehydrogenase virus, and others that also seem not to injure infected cells) become lifelong carriers, producing Abs that form virus–Ab complexes without neutralizing the infectivity of the virus (see Viral Complexes under Immune Complex Diseases, Chap. 18). Budding virions on infected cells, or viral Ags adsorbed on RBCs or other cells, simulate self-Ags: their combination with antiviral Abs (or perhaps T cells) can give rise to chronic disorders, such as hemolytic anemia. It is thus

TABLE 20–1. Antigenic Mimicry: Sequence Similarities between Microbial Proteins and Human Host Proteins

Protein	Position of Starting (N-Terminal) Residue	Sequence
Human cytomegalovirus IE2	79	PDPLGRPDED
Human lymphocyte antigen DR	60	VTELGRPDAE
Poliovirus VP2	70	STTKESRGTT
Acetylcholine receptor	176	TVIKESRGTK
Papilloma virus E2	76	SLHLESLKDS
Insulin receptor	66	VYGLESLKDL
Rabies virus glycoprotein	147	TKESLVIIS
Insulin receptor	764	NKESLVISE
Klebsiella pneumoniae nitrogenase	186	SRQTDREDE
Human lymphocyte antigen B27	70	KAQTDREDL
Adenovirus 12 E1B	384	LRRGMFRPSQCN
A-gliadin	206	LGQGSFRPSQQN
HIV p24	160	GVETTTPS
Human IgG constant region	466	GVETTTPS
Measles virus P3	13	LECIRALK
Corticotropin	18	LECIRACK
Measles virus P3	31	EISDNLGQE
Myelin basic protein	61	EISFKLGQE

From Oldstone MBA: Cell 50:819, 1987.

conceivable that some ostensibly autoimmune human diseases might be secondary to viral Ags formed as a result of unrecognized chronic viral infections.

DEFECTIVE PRODUCTION OF SUPPRESSOR T CELLS AND EMERGENCE OF ANTI-SELF T CELLS.

Although evidence for T cells that specifically suppress immune responses to certain Ags (T_s cells) is still controversial, such cells could play an important role in several autoimmune disorders. By inhibiting particular autoreactive T cells, T_s cells could be responsible for maintaining tolerance to some self-Ags; hence, defective production of these T_s cells could result in activating otherwise suppressed or quiescent autoreactive T cells.

CHARACTERISTICS OF AUTOIMMUNE DISEASES

ANTIBODY- VERSUS CELL-MEDIATED REACTIONS.

All of the mechanisms that cause allergic reactions to foreign Ags (see Table 18–1, Chap. 18) can participate in autoimmune diseases. **Auto-Abs** can lyse RBCs or platelets or injure cells of the thyroid gland (thyroiditis). They can also form **autoimmune Ab–Ag aggregates;** for instance, in systemic lupus erythematosus (SLE), large quantities of Ab–DNA–complement complexes lodge in kidney glomeruli and eventually lead to progressive local damage and renal failure (see Immune Complex Diseases, Chap. 18). Similarly, IgG molecules that function as auto-Ags combine with certain IgM (or IgG) molecules that serve as Abs, termed **rheumatoid factors,** that react specifically with these auto-Ags. The resulting aggregates are detectable in serum; they also are localized in synovial membranes, and contribute to the destructive inflammation of joints in rheumatoid arthritis (Chap. 18).

Striking mononuclear cell infiltrates in many autoimmune disorders (pancreatic islets of Langerhans in juvenile diabetes mellitus, atrophic gastritis in pernicious anemia, thyroiditis, allergic encephalomyelitis, etc.) suggest that **autoreactive T-lymphocytes are responsible.** Experimental studies provide stronger support. When bits of an animal's thyroid or brain or adrenal are removed, emulsified in Freund's adjuvant, and injected back into the same animal, mononuclear cell infiltrations appear after 1 to 2 weeks in the corresponding organ, and serum Abs to the organ's Ags become detectable. Moreover, viable T cells from the affected animals usually transfer the disease to normal, genetically identical recipients.

LOCALIZED VERSUS DISSEMINATED DISEASE.

Autoimmunity can affect almost every part of the body (Table 20–2). **Organ-specific** auto-Abs are directed to Ags that are found only in particular tissues or organs or even only in a particular cell type (e.g., the beta cells of the pancreatic islets of Langerhans in insulin-dependent di-

abetes mellitus or thyroid epithelial cells in thyroiditis). Other Abs are directed to widely distributed Ags and are associated with **disseminated** disease (e.g., Abs to nuclear Ags in systemic lupus erythematosus). In still other diseases, the responses are **intermediate** between these extremes: for instance, in **Goodpasture's disease,** characterized by chronic glomerulonephritis and pulmonary hemorrhages, Abs are deposited selectively on the basement membranes of kidney glomeruli (see Fig. 18, Chap. 18) and lung parenchyma, which have identical or crossreacting Ags.

TABLE 20–2. Some Autoimmune Disorders in Man

Organ or Tissue	Disease	Antigen
B cells of islets of Langerhans (Pancreas)	Insulin-dependent ("juvenile") diabetes mellitus	?
Thyroid	Hashimoto's thyroiditis (hypothyroidism)	Thyroglobulin
		Thyroid cell surface and cytoplasm
	Thyrotoxicosis (Graves' disease; hyperthyroidism)	Receptor for thyroid-stimulating hormone (TSH)
Gastric mucosa	Pernicious anemia (vitamin B_{12} deficiency)	Intrinsic factor (I)
		Parietal cells
Adrenals	Addison's disease (adrenal insufficiency)	Adrenal cell
Skin	Pemphigus vulgaris	Epidermal cells
	Pemphigoid	Basement membrane between epidermis and dermis
Eye	Sympathetic ophthalmia	Uvea
Kidney glomeruli plus lung	Goodpasture's syndrome	Basement membrane
Red cells	Autoimmune hemolytic anemia	Red cell surface
Platelets	Idiopathic thrombocytopenic purpura	Platelet surface
Skeletal and heart muscle	Myasthenia gravis	Acetylcholine receptor
Brain	Allergic encephalitis	Brain tissue
Spermatozoa	Male infertility (rarely)	Sperm
Liver (biliary tract)	Primary biliary cirrhosis	Mitochondria (mainly)
Salivary and lacrimal glands	Sjögren's disease	Many: secretory ducts, mitochondria, nuclei, IgG
Synovial membranes, etc.	Rheumatoid arthritis	Fc domain of IgG; other
	Systemic lupus erythematosus (SLE)	Many: DNA, DNA–protein, cardiolipin, IgG, microsomes, etc.

Based on Roitt I: Essential Immunology, Oxford, Blackwell, 1971.

***MULTIPLICITY OF RESPONSES.* An individual who makes one autoimmune response is likely to make others.** For instance, individuals with insulin-dependent diabetes mellitus produce Abs to insulin and to other constituents of pancreatic beta cells as well as T cells that react specifically with surface Ags of islet cells. Moreover, 10% of persons with autoimmune thyroiditis have pernicious anemia (another autoimmune disease; see below), which is present in only 0.2% of the population at large. Similarly, thyroid disease is found with excessive frequency in those who suffer from pernicious anemia, and 30% of those with autoimmune thyroiditis have Abs to gastric parietal cells, while 50% of those with pernicious anemia have Abs to thyroid Ags, although these Abs are entirely noncross-reacting. Similar associations are found among the disseminated group of autoimmune diseases: persons with SLE often have evidence of rheumatoid arthritis, autoimmune hemolytic anemia, or thrombocytopenia. All of these associations suggest an underlying abnormality in the mechanisms that are responsible for tolerance of some Ags.

The frequency of autoimmune responses increases with age. For unknown reasons, it is also higher in women than in men.

GENETIC FACTORS. The key role of genetic factors is suggested by the many inbred animal strains that suffer from a high frequency of certain autoimmune disorders. In the NOD (nonobese diabetes) mouse strain and the BB rat strain, almost all animals develop autoimmune inflammation and destruction of the pancreatic islet (beta) cells, and diabetes mellitus, by 6 months of age. All mice of the NZB strain (New Zealand black) eventually develop autoimmune hemolytic anemia, and most of the hybrids (B × W) made by crossing NZB with another inbred strain, New Zealand white (NZW), develop a syndrome that is strikingly similar to SLE in man. A genetic basis for these disorders is also suggested by their association in humans with certain histocompatibility Ags (see HLA and Autoimmunity, below).

TARGETED ANTIGENS. In only a very few instances has the molecular identity of the Ag responsible for an autoimmune disease been established. In myasthenia gravis, which is characterized by muscle weakness, the target Ag is the acetylcholine receptor, located at nerve–muscle junctions, and in Graves' disease (hyperthyroidism), the self Ag is the thyroid epithelial cell receptor for thyroid-stimulating hormone (TSH). In other instances, the Ag is identified more vaguely, for example, as an "RBC Ag" in autoimmune hemolytic anemia or a "platelet Ag" in thrombocytopenic purpura. More importantly, none of the Ags or peptide fragments recognized by autoreactive T cells have so far been identified.

HLA AND AUTOIMMUNITY

Certain haplotypes of the MHC complex (termed HLA in humans) are found much more frequently in individuals affected with particular autoimmune diseases than in healthy controls. The same correlations are observed in diverse ethnic groups, suggesting that they are attributable to particular MHC alleles, not merely to linked genes (which are expected to separate from the MHC during evolution). Nevertheless, the presence of one of these persistently associated MHC alleles is no guarantee that the disease will occur. For instance, more than 90% of Caucasians with insulin-dependent diabetes mellitus have one or two (out of many possible) MHC-II gene clusters, termed HLA-DR3 and HLA-DR4, yet most individuals with these haplotypes never develop diabetes. More strikingly, in about 50% of monozygotic twins in which one twin develops diabetes, the other also eventually develops the disease. This high level of concordance (100 times the frequency [0.5%] in unselected Caucasian populations) emphasizes the importance of the genetic basis for the disease, but the frequency of twins that fail to develop the disease (also about 50%) shows that other (environmental) factors (e.g., viral infections; see below) are also important determinants.

Besides these clear, positive associations with some MHC alleles, there are negative associations with other alleles at the same locus. These can be just as significant (e.g., insulin-dependent diabetes mellitus does not occur in persons who have the HLA-DR5 haplotype), but they are difficult to recognize in population studies because of the enormous polymorphism of MHC genes. Thus, the frequency of any particular MHC allele in an outbred population is likely to be very low to start with, and a further decrease in its frequency among affected individuals would be difficult to detect.

The significance of any of these correlations is not entirely clear, but they very likely reflect the critical role of peptide presentation by MHC proteins to T cells. For instance, a positively correlated MHC-II protein would be expected to be especially effective in binding and presenting a particular self-peptide to T_H cells. Alternatively, it has been suggested that a negatively correlated MHC allele (such as HLA-DR5 in diabetes) might have a sequence that resembles the critical peptide and therefore establishes tolerance to it, thereby preventing the autoimmune response even in individuals who have the allele that confers susceptibility.

Ly-1 B Cells and Autoimmunity

A special set of about 1% of all B cells in mice appear to be responsible for most of the Abs to self-Ags. These cells are relatively abundant in the peritoneal cavity but are rare in the spleen (where conventional B cells are abundant), and they are usually not detectable in lymph nodes. Besides having surface glycoprotein markers of conventional B cells (see Chap. 15), these cells have Ly-1, a T-cell marker that is absent on other B cells, and they also have five to ten times more surface IgM and only 5% to 10% of the surface IgD of conventional B cells.

In addition to reacting selectively with some self-Ags, the Igs on many Ly-1$^+$ B cells share a restricted set of common cross-reacting idiotypes (Ids). The explanation may be that only a few dozen of the many hundreds of V_H gene segments (the ones closest to the C_H gene segments of the Ig heavy chain locus; see Chap. 14, Fig. 14–30) are used to form the functional Ig H chain genes of most Ly-1$^+$ B cells.

Homologous B cells in humans have the Leu-1 surface Ag (which is structurally similar to murine Ly-1), and they also seem to be responsible for various auto-Abs (cold hemagglutinins, rheumatoid factors). Why Ly-1$^+$ (Leu-1$^+$) B cells are less readily rendered tolerant than conventional B cells to some self-Ags is not understood.

SOME AUTOIMMUNE DISEASES

Insulin-Dependent ("Juvenile") Diabetes Mellitus

Type I or juvenile diabetes results from selective destruction of insulin-producing cells, namely the beta cells in the islets of Langerhans of the pancreas. For several months before disease onset is recognized by its metabolic effects, affected individuals produce Abs to insulin and to cytoplasmic constituents of pancreatic beta cells, and their islets are infiltrated with T and B cells; by the time the disease becomes evident, nearly all of the islets are destroyed. A similar disease in an inbred mouse strain (NOD) and in a strain of rats (BB) can be transferred with T cells from affected to normal animals of the same strain.

The human disease appears to depend on CD4$^+$ T cells, as susceptibility to the disease is strikingly correlated with the MHC-II haplotype (see below). The key beta-cell Ag is unknown, but circumstantial evidence suggests that it might be of viral origin because the onset of disease is often preceded by infection with a Coxsackie B virus (B4). This virus, isolated at autopsy from the pancreas of a child shortly after the onset of diabetes, appears to have transferred the disease to susceptible mice.

Juvenile diabetes affects about 0.5% of the Caucasian population, and family studies show a much higher frequency of certain HLA-D alleles (notably **DR3** and **DR4**) in affected than in normal individuals. The D region includes several loci (**DR, DO, DP;** Fig. 20–1), and the correlation is with **DR** and **DO.** These loci are virtually inseparable in family pedigrees, but from analyses of DNA samples by restriction fragment-length polymorphisms (using restriction enzymes to cleave samples of DNA at rare deoxynucleotide sequences and testing the separated fragments with oligodeoxynucleotide probes for marker sequences), the correlation with *DQ* has emerged as particularly striking. Homozygotes for HLA-**DR3** and **DR4** (or **DR3/DR4** heterozygotes) have a high probability of developing juvenile diabetes, whereas those with **DR5** are statistically unlikely to have this disease even if they are heterozygous at this locus and the other haplotype is DR3 or DR4. Moreover, nucleotide sequences of the DQ

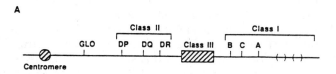

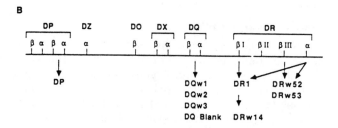

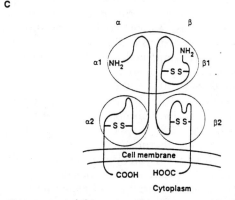

Figure 20–1. *(A)* A portion of the short arm of human chromosome 6 and location of the class I, II, and III genes. *(B)* Map of the class II genes of the human HLA-D region. The DR$_{\beta I}$ and DR$_\alpha$ gene products form a heterodimeric glycoprotein on the cell surface. This molecule reacts with the alloantisera that define the major serologic allotypes HLA-DR1 through DRw14. On the DR3 and DR4 haplotypes, the DR$_{\beta IIa15}$ gene is not expressed. The DQ$_\alpha$ and DQ$_\beta$ genes encode the DQ serologic specificities (DQw1, DQw2, DQw3, and DQ Blank). The DX$_\alpha$ and DX$_\beta$ and the second DP$_\alpha$ and DP$_\beta$ genes are not expressed, and the DO$_\beta$ and DZ$_\alpha$ genes are expressed only at low levels. *(C)* Schematic diagram for the structure of a class II molecule. As noted in Chap. 15, these cell surface glycoprotein molecules are organized into domains that correspond to the exon–intron structures of the genes. Their membrane proximal domains (α_2 and β_2) have structural homology with immunoglobulin constant region domains. It is possible that their α_1 and β_1 domains fold together to form an antigen-binding cleft like that of the class I molecule shown in Figure 15–25. (From Todd et al: Science 1988)

β-chain alleles have revealed consistent differences that distinguish susceptible from unsusceptible individuals: in a hypervariable region of this chain (β1 domain, see Fig. 15–15, Chap. 15), several amino acids at position 57 (serine, valine, or alanine) are correlated with susceptibility, whereas aspartic acid seems to confer protection against the disease.

Why this protection is dominant (DR5 haplotype) is not known; perhaps with Asp^{57} the DQ β chain resembles (and thus induces tolerance of) self or viral peptide, which in combination with the appropriate MHC-II protein would otherwise stimulate the disease-causing self-reactive T cells. That an amino acid at position 57 of the DQ β chain might directly affect the presentation of peptides to T cells is plausible in view of the probable structure of MHC-II proteins: in this structure, which is assumed to resemble that of an MHC-I protein (Fig. 15–25), the amino acid at position 57 is located in the protein's putative peptide-binding groove.

Rheumatoid Arthritis

In rheumatoid arthritis, many joints are affected by intense infiltration of synovial membranes (which enclose the joint spaces) by B- and T-lymphocytes, plasma cells, macrophages, and dendritic cells. In the thickened membranes (termed "pannus"), fibroblasts and capillaries are also present in profusion, and the lymphoid cells are organized into clusters resembling miniature lymph nodes, even to the extent of forming germinal centers (Fig. 15–5, Chap. 15). Large amounts of Ig are synthesized in these joints, and many of the infiltrating cells (macrophages, dendritic cells, and activated T cells) express large amounts of MHC-II protein.

"Rheumatoid factors" (RF) are the hallmark of this disease. These factors are Abs (usually IgM, but sometimes IgG) that react specifically with epitopes in the Fc domain of diverse Igs. (Many RF are specific for particular Ig allotypes, and they were instrumental in the discovery of these Ig variants [Chap. 14].) Many plasma cells in the affected joints probably produce RF, as they bind fluoresceinated Igs. The RF may be products of a special set of B cells. However, Igs resembling RF sometimes appear in laboratory animals that are intensively immunized to produce large amounts of Ab to conventional Ags, and it is possible that in rheumatoid arthritis, the prominent production of RF reflects intense polyclonal B-cell activation (especially in affected joints).

The latter explanation is also favored by studies of an inbred strain of mice (MLR) with a high spontaneous incidence of autoimmune disease. B-cell hybridomas from these mice produce Igs that resemble RF (i.e., they bind to certain other Igs). Their H-chain sequences suggest that the large number of hybridomas examined derive from a small number of B-cell clones that have many somatic mutations in their V_H domains, as if the clones

had undergone an enormous proliferation as the result of an intense (but otherwise conventional) immune response. The same may be true of RF in rheumatoid arthritis, but the responsible Ag (self or foreign) is unknown.

T cells are also prominent in affected joint membranes. Moreover, as in insulin-dependent diabetes, certain HLA haplotypes (e.g., DR4, DR1, DRw10) occur with much greater frequency in rheumatoid arthritis patients than in normal controls. Hence, it is likely that presentation of a self (or other) peptide by particular MHC-II alleles to CD4 T cells is a critical step in the development of this autoimmune disease.

Pemphigus Vulgaris

The essential lesion in pemphigus vulgaris is loss of cohesiveness between epidermal cells; the result is diffuse blistering of the skin and mucous membranes, with loss of epidermal cells. Serum IgG from affected individuals can duplicate the disease in transplanted human skin growing in nude mice (which accept xenografts; see Chap. 15). This Ig (presumably containing auto-Abs) can also cause similar changes in cultured explants of skin provided plasminogen is present in the culture medium. The need for plasminogen arises because the responsible auto-Ab appears to stimulate epidermal cells to secrete a protease (plasminogen activator) that selectively cleaves plasminogen to yield plasmin, a trypsin-like serine protease. The plasmin evidently cleaves the sticky protein molecules associated with desmosome processes that are responsible for the normal adhesion of epidermal cells to each other. Inhibitors that selectively block plasmin activity can thus overcome the ability of the auto-Abs to cause epidermal cells to separate from each other in cultured skin.

More than 90% of patients with this disease have the DR4 or DRw6 cluster of MHC-II alleles. Analyses of DNA from such individuals suggest, moreover, that susceptibility to the disease is associated with a particular DQ allele (which appears to be present in virtually all Israeli pemphigus patients but only rarely in Israeli controls). The product of this allele is probably the β subunit of an MHC-II protein that effectively presents a key peptide to the CD4 T cells that are required for the formation of the auto-Abs. The self-Ag recognized by these Abs appears to be present in epidermal cells.

Some patients with pemphigus also have myasthenia gravis, another autoimmune disease, or a thymoma (which often is found in individuals with myasthenia gravis; see below).

Acquired Hemolytic Anemia

In acquired hemolytic anemia, an individual's Abs react with his or her own red blood cells (RBCs). Such Abs are sometimes found in persons with other diseases that might alter self-Ags or introduce cross-reacting ones, such as mycoplasma pneumonia or infectious mononucleosis. More often, however, this disorder is unassociated with other diseases or with known exposure to agents toxic to RBCs.

Abs to the patient's red cells are usually demonstrated by rabbit antiserum to human Igs in two ways. In the **direct antiglobulin (Coombs) test,** the patient's washed RBCs are agglutinated by the antiserum. In the **indirect test,** RBCs from another person are incubated with the patient's serum, washed, and examined for clumping by the rabbit antiserum.

The anti-red cell Abs have no hemolytic activity *in vitro*, but they accelerate destruction of RBCs *in vivo*. The Ab-coated RBCs are phagocytized by macrophages, and their breakdown occurs especially in the spleen. Therapy includes nonspecific immunosuppressants and splenectomy.

Mice of the inbred NZB strain almost invariably develop hemolytic anemia as they age, and viable lymphocytes from older (affected) animals can transfer the disease to young, unaffected mice of the same strain. However, these mice are chronically infected from birth with a retrovirus, and it has been suggested that what looks like an autoimmune disease may be attributable to a conventional immune reaction to viral Ags adsorbed on RBCs.

Thrombocytopenic Purpura

In thrombocytopenic purpura, platelets can decline to about one-tenth the normal level, and bleeding occurs in many organs, including the skin, causing petechial rash and purpura. In the dramatic experiment that provided the first evidence of the immune nature of this disease, a human volunteer injected with a patient's plasma suffered a precipitous fall in platelets (Fig. 20–2) and extensive bleeding into internal organs and skin. A patient's serum can also cause normal platelets to clump and to lyse if complement (C) is present. Infants born to mothers with the disease may have transient thrombocytopenia and bleeding secondary to placental transmission of the maternal Abs.

Allergic Encephalomyelitis

When laboratory rats, guinea pigs, or monkeys are injected with suspensions of CNS tissue from individuals of the same or other species, they develop patchy areas of vasculitis and demyelination in the brain and spinal cord (Fig. 20–3). This response is readily evoked with a single injection of a small amount of brain or spinal cord tissue, even from the same animal, in Freund's adjuvant. The immune basis of the disease is indicated by the following. (1) Lesions appear 9 days or more after the primary injection, but the onset is more rapid in animals that have recovered and are then reinjected (secondary

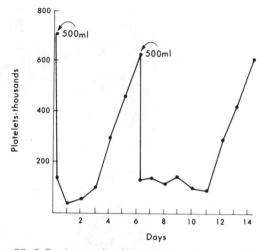

Figure 20–2. Passive transfer of thrombocytopenic purpura. The platelet count of a normal human volunteer dropped following transfusion *(arrows)* of blood from a patient with idiopathic thrombocytopenic purpura. Ig fractions from other donors with the disease produced similar results. Some of the recipients suffered bleeding in internal organs simulating the natural course of the disease. (Harrington WJ et al: J Lab Clin Med 38:1, 1951)

response). (2) The lesions are specific: they follow inoculation only of myelin-containing tissues and appear only in myelinated tissue, especially white matter of the brain. (3) Lymphocytes from inoculated animals produce cytopathic effects on myelinated brain tissue and glial cells in culture. (4) The lymphocytes can also cause specific neural lesions in nonsensitized syngeneic recipients. (5) Intradermal injection of myelinated tissue evokes a delayed-type skin response in affected animals. (6) Serum Abs that react with brain tissue can be demonstrated. However, they seem not to play a major role in the disease: the intensity of the lesions does not parallel Ab levels, and serum fails to produce lesions in recipient animals.

The responsible self-Ag is a small protein (18,000 daltons) that is heterogenetic (i.e., present in many species) and organ-specific (found only in the CNS) and constitutes at least 30% of the protein in myelin. As little as 0.1 μg in complete Freund's adjuvant is sufficient to elicit severe allergic encephalomyelitis in a guinea pig.

The protein's amino acid sequence is fully established. Of its many proteolytic fragments, the smallest with encephalitogenic activity is a nine-residue peptide (Phe-Ser-Trp-Gly-Ala-Glu-Gly-Gln-Lys) that contains the protein's only tryptophan residue. Modification of this residue by attaching 2-hydroxy-5-nitrobenzyl bromide

eliminates the protein's encephalitogenic activity.

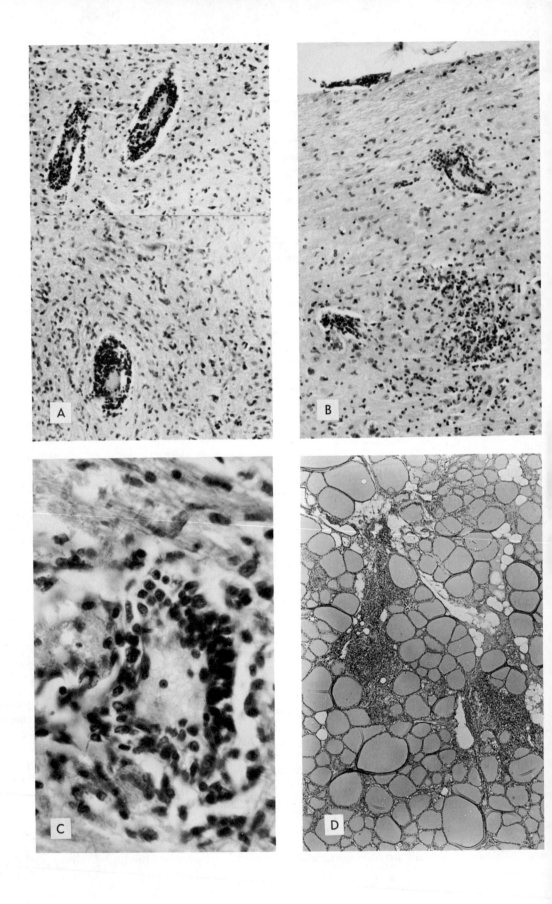

With this experimental evidence, it is understandable that encephalitis sometimes occurs in humans after immunization with what used to be the standard rabies vaccine, a suspension of infected rabbit brain. (Rabies vaccine is now prepared from virus grown in human cell lines [not nerve cells] or in duck embryo tissues that lack myelin.) The demyelinating encephalitis that occasionally follows infection with measles and vaccinia virus could arise from infection of the nervous system, bringing the encephalitogenic Ag into contact with inflammatory (lymphoid) cells. A similar mechanism is suspected for the characteristic focal demyelinating lesions of **multiple sclerosis,** but a role for a virus has not been established.

Myasthenia Gravis

In myasthenia gravis, which is characterized by severe muscle weakness, a defect in neuromuscular transmission has been traced to auto-Abs to the acetylcholine receptor on skeletal muscle. Many affected individuals also have an otherwise very rare thymic tumor (**thymoma**). Although the presence of two such rare disorders in the same individual suggests that they are somehow connected with each other, the basis for a connection is unknown.

It is possible that an Id–anti-Id reaction (see Chap. 16, Fig. 16–14) provides the stimulus for the production of Abs to the acetylcholine receptor. Thus, injection of Ab to an acetylcholine analogue stimulated rabbits to produce Abs to the Id of the injected Ab; these anti-Id Abs react with acetylcholine receptors and cause muscle weakness in rabbits.

Thyroiditis and Hyperthyroidism (Graves' Disease)

Patients with chronic inflammation of the thyroid (Hashimoto's disease) suffer destruction of its secretory cells and loss of thyroid function. Their serum contains some Abs that react in high titer with thyroglobulin (Tg) and others that react with Tg-free particulate fractions of thyroid (see Fig. 20–4). Moreover, in an inbred strain of chickens that spontaneously develops antithyroid Abs and thyroiditis (and finally hypothyroidism and obesity), the Abs appear to be causal, as neonatal bursectomy, but not thymectomy, prevents the anomalies. (Recall that in

chickens B cells mature in a special hind gut–associated organ, **the bursa of Fabricius** [Chap. 15, p. 320]; removing the bursa prevents B cell maturation.) However, the immunologic features of the experimental thyroiditis induced in other species by injections of Tg or thyroid tissue are very similar to those of experimental allergic encephalomyelitis (above). The suspicion therefore remains that cell-mediated, rather than (or in addition to) humoral autoimmunity is responsible for the human disease.

The interaction of Abs with Ags on cells sometimes causes cell proliferation and differentiation rather than destruction; for example, when anti-Igs react with B-lymphocytes (Blast Transformation; Chap. 15) or when appropriate Abs react with sea urchin eggs. Similar mechanisms may be involved in some patients with hyperplastic and hyperfunctional thyroid glands, who have auto-Abs to thyroid (often called **long-acting thyroid stimulators,** or LATS). If present during pregnancy, these autoimmune Abs cross the placenta and cause neonatal hyperthyroidism, which subsides within a few weeks of birth as the maternal IgG is degraded (Chap. 16). The **responsible auto-Ab appears to bind specifically to the cell-surface receptor for thyroid stimulating hormone (TSH) and to act as an agonist;** thus, its activity, like that of TSH, is potentiated by drugs, such as theophylline, which affect cellular levels of cyclic AMP.

Systemic Lupus Erythematosus

SLE is characterized by high levels of Abs to self Ags, especially those in cell nuclei. Large amounts of immune complexes formed by these Abs and Ags with C (Ab–Ag–C complexes) are deposited in the walls of small blood vessels and cause vasculitis in diverse organs. Deposits in kidney glomeruli are particularly damaging, leading to glomerulonephritis and renal failure.

The diversity of auto-Abs in affected individuals is extraordinary. Abs to double-stranded native DNA are especially prominent, and Abs (termed **anti-Sm**) to several polypeptides associated with **small nuclear ribonucleoproteins (snRPs)** are virtually SLE-specific: they are found in about one-third of SLE patients and in no other autoimmune disease. Other auto-Abs react with 15 to 20 other nuclear Ags, including single-stranded DNA, DNA–histone complexes, and topoisomerases. Sometimes Abs

---

Figure 20–3. Autoimmune allergic reactions. *(A–C)* Allergic encephalomyelitis in a rat sensitized adoptively with viable lymph node cells from a donor rat that had been immunized with rat spinal cord (injected in complete Freund's adjuvant). The recipient, which had severe ataxia and hind leg paralysis 5 days after receiving the donor's lymphocytes, was sacrificed at 7 days. Sections of brain show a focal inflammation with perivascular infiltration by mononuclear cells. H & E stain. *(D)* Thyroiditis in a rabbit that had been immunized repeatedly with hog thyroglobulin. A small proportion of the rabbit's Abs to the hog protein reacted also with rabbit thyroglobulin. Note intense focal infiltration of the immunized rabbit's thyroid with mononuclear cells. Similar lesions appear in animals injected with their own thyroglobulin or with homogenates of a bit of their own thyroid tissue. *(A–C:* Patterson PY: J Exp Med 111:119, 1960; *D:* Witebsky E, Rose NR: J Immunol 83:41, 1959). *A* and *B,* ×130 reduced; *C,* ×500 reduced; *D,* ×60 reduced.

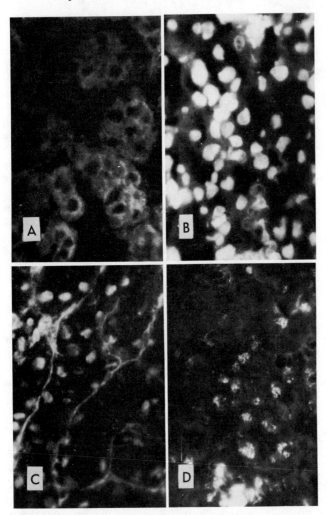

Figure 20–4. Variety of anti-tissue Abs in sera of different patients with SLE. Mouse kidney sections were incubated with the sera and, after washing, were stained with fluorescein-labeled rabbit antiserum to human IgG. Similar reactions occur with human tissues. *(A)* Normal human serum control. *(B)* Abs in a lupus serum react uniformly with all nuclei, giving homogeneous nuclear staining. *(C)* Abs react with nuclei and with basement membrane of renal tubules. *(D)* Abs react with selected parts of nuclei, giving speckled staining. (Courtesy of Drs E Tan and H Kunkel) ×250

to blood clotting factors and to Igs (RFs) are also formed, but not Abs to the self-Ags that are prominent in other autoimmune diseases, for example, not to thyroglobulin or to receptors for acetylcholine.

The origin of the SLE Abs is obscure. Native DNA is not immunogenic in experimental animals, even in those inbred mouse strains (see below) that are genetically prone to develop SLE-like disease. Abs to xenogeneic snRNPs can be elicited in mice, but only one strain (MLR), with a propensity to develop SLE spontaneously, produces Abs

to mouse snRNP. The anti-DNA Abs found in humans with SLE cross-react extensively with many polyanionic macromolecules, including some bacterial polysaccharides and fibrous proteins of the cytoskeleton; they also cross-react with cardiolipin. Thus, the identity of the natural ligand for these Abs is obscure. IgM molecules with these reactivities are also found at low levels in the serum of some normal individuals, but in SLE patients, the reactive Abs are IgG molecules, and they are present at high concentration, as though formed in response to conventional (but unknown) antigenic stimuli.

In certain inbred mouse strains, such as the NZB and NZW strains and their F1 hybrids, most animals succumb to an SLE-like disease by the time they reach a certain age. In MRL mice, the *lpr* gene (autosomal recessive) is associated with auto-Ab formation (e.g., anti-snRP) and autoimmune disease. The genetic determination of SLE in humans is less striking. Nevertheless, healthy relatives of patients with SLE often have low levels of serum Igs (IgM) that react with DNA and snRNP. Particularly striking is the 60% concordance rate of SLE among monozygotic twins, with both twins having the disease; but the 40% in which one twin escapes having the disease suggests that environmental factors are important also.

As noted in Chapter 17, the SLE syndrome is found in a high proportion of individuals with heritable defects in the early-acting C proteins. It is thus possible that most persons normally also form considerable amounts of circulating Ab–Ag complexes but that normal C-dependent clearing mechanisms get rid of them; with defects in C proteins, the clearance mechanism fails, and the complexes cause diffuse vasculitis.

Pernicious Anemia

Defective red cell maturation in pernicious anemia is the result of lack of vitamin B_{12}. Affected persons have atrophic gastritis; their poor absorption of ingested vitamin B12 is secondary to lack of intrinsic factor (IF), a protein that is necessary for this absorption and is secreted into the stomach by the parietal cells of the gastric mucosa. Most patients with the disease have Abs to parietal cells (revealed by immunofluorescence of gastric biopsies), and cell-mediated immunity to these cells may also be present. In addition, auto-Abs to IF itself may be involved, for large amounts of oral B12 (which ordinarily cure the anemia) are ineffective if fed together with serum from many patients, and the active serum contains Abs to IF. The inhibitory effect of anti-IF appears to be exercised within the stomach, for absorption of the fed vitamin (mixed with Abs to IF) remains unimpaired in normal human volunteers. In patients, their gastric Abs, produced by plasma cells in the gastric lesions, are able to function within the stomach (normally extreme acidic) because atrophy of the affected mucosa reduces the secretion of HCl. Thus, the autoimmune atrophic gastritis may cause B12 deficiency by decreasing production of both IF and HCl, and by secreting Abs to IF into the stomach lumen.

Transplantation Immunity: The Allograft Reaction

The clustered array of about 20 genes that make up the MHC was considered at length in earlier chapters because their protein products on cell surfaces play a central role in presenting peptide fragments of Ags to the Ag-specific receptors of T cells. The same MHC proteins, and to a variable extent some other ill-defined Ags, elicit the powerful immune responses that are responsible for rejecting organ (kidney, heart, lung, pancreas, liver) and bone marrow cell transplants from one individual to another. This section focuses on these responses.

Definitions

Tissue grafts fall into four classes:

1. **Autografts** are transplanted from one region to another of the same individual.

2. **Isografts** are transplanted from one individual to a genetically identical individual. These are possible only between monozygotic twins or between members of lines of mice and some other species that have been so highly inbred as to be **syngeneic;** i.e., identical in respect to histocompatibility genes (see below) or **isogeneic** (identical in all genes).

3. **Allografts** (formerly termed **homografts**) are transplanted from one individual to a genetically nonidentical one; i.e., an **allogeneic** individual of the same species.

4. **Heterografts** or **xenografts** (Gr. *xenos;* foreign) are transplanted from one species to another.

The donors are designated, respectively, as **autologous, isologous, homologous,** or **heterologous** with respect to the recipient.

THE ALLOGRAFT REACTION AS AN IMMUNE RESPONSE

Studies of tissue transplantation grew largely out of efforts to understand cancer by transplanting mouse tumors. These studies, beginning in the early 1900s, led to the development of inbred mouse strains and to the eventual realization that the results illuminated the general rules of transplantation—for normal as well as cancer cells—rather than the nature of the cancer cell.

Successful transfers of tumors between mice of an inbred strain, but not of different strains, showed that rejection of a graft is attributable to genetic differences between host and donor. More specifically, **autografts and isografts endure,** whereas **allografts and heterografts are rejected.** Especially illuminating were observations on the hybrid offspring mice of a cross between inbred parental strains (a/a × b/b). The a/b hybrids are tolerant of grafts from either parental strain, but the parental strains reject grafts from the hybrids. Thus a **graft is permanently accepted only when essentially all of its histocompatibility Ags are present in the recipient.** If a recipient lacks transplantation Ags that are present in the graft, it mounts immune responses to those Ags; the resulting reactions lead to the destruction (rejection) of the graft.

The mechanisms of the allograft reaction have been investigated most extensively with skin grafts because of their technical advantages: they are easy to prepare, their rejection is readily detected, and their survival time provides an estimate of the intensity of the host's immune response. The same principles are involved in grafts of other tissues and cells.

THE SECOND-SET REACTION. When an allograft of skin is placed on a recipient animal in a bed created by excising a slightly larger piece of skin, the graft at first becomes vascularized and its cells proliferate; but after about 10 days, it quite abruptly becomes the site of intense inflammation, withers, and is sloughed (**first-set reaction**). If a second graft is then made to the same recipient with another piece of skin from the same donor, it is rejected much more rapidly, perhaps in 5 to 6 days. This accelerated rejection, the **second-set reaction,** is specific for a particular donor: if, after the accelerated rejection, another donor, antigenically different from the first, provides skin grafts to the same recipient, first- and second-set reactions to successive grafts are again seen. Thus, **the capacity to reject an allograft (transplantation immunity) is specific and is acquired by virtue of exposure to the donor's transplantation Ags.** The shorter survival of the second graft results from persistence of the immunity acquired from the first graft or from an anamnestic response (see Primary and Secondary Responses, Chap. 16).

The second-set reaction to a skin graft can be induced, not only by prior skin grafts, but also by prior inoculation of virtually any tissue (including spleen cells). Mature RBCs are the exception: they have no MHC proteins.

HISTOCOMPATIBILITY GENES

Transplantation Ags are specified by histocompatibility (H) genes, and permanent graft acceptance (in the absence of immunosuppressive therapy) requires that essentially all of the donor's H alleles be present in the recipient. Hence when donor and recipient are drawn at random from an outbred population, such as humans, the probability of acceptance depends on (1) the number of H genes or loci in the species; and (2) the number of alleles at each locus and their frequencies in the population.

The H loci and their alleles were initially characterized most extensively in the mouse, because its many inbred strains permit detailed genetic analysis with skin grafts.

H Genes in the Mouse

The number of independent H loci at which two inbred strains differ can be estimated by mating them (AA × BB), crossing the F1 progeny (AB × AB), and using animals of the F2 generation as recipients for skin grafts from the purebred parental strains. As is illustrated in Figure 20–5, the number, n, of H loci is provided by the proportion (x) of F2 animals that accept grafts from one of the purebred parental strains: $x = (3/4)^n$. This method yields minimum values, because some H genes are linked to one another and behave as single rather than as multiple genes and because some inbred strains have certain H alleles in common.

A better estimate of the number of loci has been obtained through the use of **congenic mouse strains** produced by the mating protocols originally devised by Snell. As was shown in Chapter 15 (Fig. 15–15), a congenic strain A.B is identical genetically with its inbred partner A except for a chromosomal segment derived from strain B. If the chromosomal segment includes an H locus, grafts exchanged between A.B and A mice will be rejected in both directions. Many congenic lines can be derived from the progeny of a single A × B mating (Fig. 15–15), and grafts exchanged between different pairs of congenic lines (A.B[1], A.B[2], etc.) reveal whether they do or do not have the same H loci: the exchanged grafts are accepted if the loci are the same and rejected if they are different. This and other approaches have revealed more than 40 H loci, designated H-1, H-2, etc.

Other approaches demonstrate **multiple alleles at each locus;** for example, 12 at H-1, five at H-3, six at H-4, and four at H-7. At H-2, as noted in Chapter 15, polymorphism is extreme, with at least 50 alleles at H-2K and more than 50 at H-2D. The **number of alleles** at each H locus can be estimated by the **F-1 test,** which involves three strains: a congenic pair, A and A.B, and an entirely different inbred strain, C. Suppose that A and A.B differ at H-1, with A having the H-1^a allele and A.B the H-1^b allele; C has an unknown H-1 allele. A graft of A skin to an (A.B × C) F1 hybrid will be accepted if C has the H-1^a allele but rejected if C's H-1 allele is not a. On the other hand, a graft of A.B skin to an (A × C) hybrid will be accepted if C has the H-1^b allele but rejected if C's H-1 allele is not b. If the H-1 allele of C turns out to be not a and not b, then there must be **at least three alleles** at H-1. When many inbred strains were typed in this way, it could be estimated from the number of non-a and non-b strains that there are at least 12 alleles at H-1.

H-2 LOCUS. As was noted in Chapter 15, the transplantation Ags specified by H-2 elicit the most intense rejection reactions: allografts exchanged between mice that differ only at this locus are usually rejected in about 11 days (first-set rejection), whereas when the mice have the

Parental Strains Differ by One H Gene

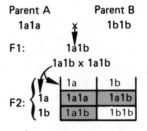

(¾)¹ or 75% of F2 progeny accept grafts from parent A or parent B

Figure 20–5. Estimate of the number of independent histocompatibility **(H)** genes at which two inbred strains of mice differ. **Shaded squares** correspond to progeny in the F₂ generation that accept a graft from parent A. (Courtesy of Dr RJ Graff)

Parental Strains Differ by Two Unlinked H Genes

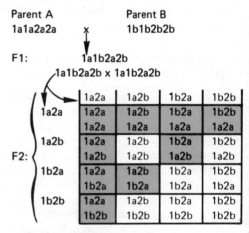

(¾)² or 56% of F2 progeny accept grafts from parent A or parent B

same H-2 alleles but differ at any one of the other H loci, the median survival times range from 20 to upward of 200 days. Indeed, skin allografts that differ only at certain H loci are usually not rejected at all unless the recipient is first immunized by several injections of cells from the prospective donor. Thus the first MHC discovered was the H-2 locus in the mouse. The non-H-2 loci are called **minor H loci;** the Ags they encode are termed "**minors.**"

Minor (Non-H-2) Transplantation Antigens ("Minors")

Although survival times are long (weeks or months) for graft exchanges between congenic lines that differ only at one non-H-2 locus, the cumulative effect of many non-H-2 differences can approximate that of an H-2 incompatibility and can lead to rapid allograft rejection. Various non-H-2 loci are associated with genetic markers on various linkage groups (i.e., chromosomes): for example, the H-1 locus is linked with albinism. One of the most interesting minors, termed **H-Y,** is associated with the Y sex chromosome: within an inbred strain, grafts (of skin, spleen, thyroid, etc.) from female to male are accepted permanently, but those from male to female are rejected (after long survival times). Male tolerance of female cells is attributable to the presence of the X chromosome in both sexes, but some product of the Y chromosome is evidently responsible for a minor transplantation Ag. (Because the H-Y Ag is weak, tolerance to it is readily established, for example, by transplanting an extra large piece of skin from male to female.)

T-CELL RECOGNITION OF MINORS IS MHC-RESTRICTED. Abs to H-2 (i.e., the mouse MHC) Class I and Class II proteins (MHC-I and MHC-II) are readily elicited, and, as we have seen, they played a significant role in the characterization of these proteins and their functions (Chap. 15). In contrast, efforts to elicit Abs to the minor Ags have consistently failed. Nevertheless, these Ags elicit specific T-cell proliferative responses, but only when they are associated with the appropriate MHC-I or MHC-II proteins. As explained in the following paragraph, this MHC restriction suggests that **minors are very likely peptide fragments of diverse allogenic proteins.**

As an example of minors, consider two strains of mice, BALB/c and DBA/2, that share the same H-2 haplotype (H-2^d) but differ in many minors and rapidly reject exchanged skin grafts. The rejection reaction is mirrored in test tube assays by lysis of BALB/c spleen cells by cytotoxic T-lymphocytes (CTLs) from DBA/2 mice that have been immunized against BALB/c cells (e.g., by a prior skin graft from BALB/c donor mice or simply by an injection of BALB/c spleen cells). Although the same CTLs do not lyse cells from the congenic BALB.B mice, which have the same minors as BALB/c but a different MHC

(H-2^b instead of H-2^d), they will lyse cells from a hybrid mouse (b/d) made by crossing BALB.B with DBA/2. The hybrid cells are recognized because their BALB minors can be presented in association with H-2^d MHC proteins.

TISSUE-SPECIFIC ALLOANTIGENS. As has been emphasized many times, MHC-I proteins are present on all cells except mature RBCs, whereas MHC-II proteins are limited to dendritic cells, activated macrophages, B cells, and various other cells (particularly when stimulated by interferon [IFN]-γ). Some minors are also expressed only on certain cells. For instance, when mice of one strain (X) are rendered tolerant (see below) of lymphocytes from an MHC-different strain (Y), they can still reject skin grafts from the Y strain, probably because some minors are expressed by epidermal cells and not by lymphocytes (other minors are probably expressed by lymphocytes and not by epidermal cells). The tissue variations probably explain why kidney grafts in mice tend to survive much longer than skin grafts.

REJECTION MECHANISMS

ADOPTIVE IMMUNITY. The transfer of lymphoid cells from immunized donors to naive recipients ("adoptive immunity") has helped clarify rejection mechanisms. For instance, the second-set reaction can be transferred by T-lymphocytes but not by serum. (When the donor is syngeneic with the recipient, the adoptive immunity can be enduring; when the donor is allogenic, the recipient's adoptive immunity is short-lived owing to an allograft reaction against the donor's lymphocytes.) In accord with this evidence for cell-mediated rejection, the site of an allograft undergoing rejection is intensely infiltrated with macrophages and lymphocytes; granulocytes and plasma cells are much less conspicuous.

It should be recalled from Chapter 15 that complexes of self-MHC proteins and Ags (or peptide fragments of Ag) are usually recognized by CD4$^+$ T cells when the MHC is Class II and by CD8$^+$ T cells when it is Class I. Similarly, the recipient's CD4$^+$ T cells respond to an allograft's MHC-II proteins and its CD8$^+$ T cells to the allograft's MHC-I. (Whether the allorecognition requires particular peptides to be associated with the allograft's MHC proteins is not clear.) Both CD4$^+$ and CD8$^+$ T cells appear to be involved in rejection. Thus clones of both kinds, grown out of a surgically removed human allograft undergoing rejection, react in culture against the donor's cells. And when mouse allografts differ from a recipient only in MHC-I, adoptive transfer of CD8$^+$ T cells from the immunized recipient's spleen can cause rapid rejection.

These relations are more readily analyzed in mixed lymphocyte reactions (MLR), an *in vitro* microcosm of the allograft reaction. The MLR is most intense when the MHC disparity is in both MHC-I and MHC-II, but it can also occur when the disparity is limited to certain MHC-I proteins. Thus, K^b and a variant MHC-I protein termed K^{bm1} differ only in three amino acid residues, and yet skin grafts exchanged between congenic mice whose only difference is K^b versus K^{bm1} are rejected.

(It should be recalled [Chaps. 15 and 19] that the maturation of $CD8^+$ CTLs from quiescent precursors probably requires cytokines that derive, directly or indirectly, from $CD4^+$ cells, which recognize MHC-II, not MHC-I, proteins. How is it possible, then, for an MHC-I disparity alone to elicit an alloreactive response? The most reasonable possibility is that MHC-I molecules, or fragments of them, are shed by allografts and presented in association with MHC-II of the recipient's Ag-presenting cells, thereby stimulating alloreactive, anti-MHC-II $CD4^+$ T_h cells to promote responses of the alloreactive, anti-MHC-I $CD8^+$ T cells. It is also possible that rare $CD4^+$ T cells react [or cross-react] with allogeneic MHC-I proteins and thus help responses of the alloreactive $CD8^+$ T cells.)

Regardless of how the recipient's alloreactive T cells are stimulated, the allograft is probably ultimately destroyed by two processes: $CD8^+$ T cells specifically lyse allogeneic cells, and $CD4^+$ T cells and activated macrophages generate severe delayed-type hypersensitivity reactions, in which nonspecific cytotoxic activity of the activated macrophages causes cell death. Some $CD4^+$ T cells also have cytolytic activity and probably lyse cells of the allograft.

Although Abs to the donor's MHC proteins are normally incapable of transferring a typical second-set reaction, antisera from some intensively hyperimmunized mice can specifically interfere with the healing-in of a fresh allograft and cause it to undergo unusually rapid rejection (the **white-graft reaction**).

PREVENTION OF ALLOGRAFT REJECTION

Two general procedures are used to enhance the survival of allografts: (1) selecting donors with few MHC mismatches from the recipients; and (2) subjecting recipients to immunosuppressive measures.

SEROLOGIC TYPING OF HLA. In "microcytotoxicity" assays, minute volumes $(1-2 \ \mu l)$ of human antiserum to HLA, normal rabbit or guinea pig serum as a source of C, and about 2000 lymphocytes from the prospective donor or recipient are incubated beneath mineral oil to prevent evaporation. Donor cells bearing HLA Ags recognized by the antiserum undergo membrane damage (Chap. 17) and thus can be stained by ionic dyes such as eosin or trypan blue. The typing sera are generally obtained from multiparous women, of whom about 30% have anti-HLA Abs produced against those offspring HLA Ags that are inherited from the father. Some HLA alleles can also be typed with monoclonal Abs (from mouse B-cell hybrido-

mas [Chap. 14, Fig. 14–3]). More than 50 HLA-A, -B, and -C alleles and about 25 HLA-D alleles can be typed serologically, but this is a lower limit for polymorphism at these loci because reagents for typing many more alleles are still lacking.

MIXED LYMPHOCYTE REACTIONS. As noted before (Chap. 15), the MLR is indicated by a T-cell proliferative response and can also be used for MHC typing. After incubation of peripheral blood lymphocytes from the prospective recipient with those from a prospective donor for about 5 days, ^{3}H-thymidine is added, and the next day, ^{3}H-labeled DNA is counted. The intensity of the response depends on MHC-II differences, i.e., at the HLA-D locus, which is homologous to the I region of the murine H-2 complex (see Chap. 15). Prior treatment of the donor cells with mitomycin C or x- or γ-irradiation to block DNA synthesis converts the MLR into a **one-way reaction,** limited to the recipient cells' proliferative response. When the cell population that responds in the one-way proliferation reaction is tested in a cytolytic assay (see Chap. 19, Fig. 19–11), it lyses ^{51}Cr-labeled cells from the "stimulator" (donor) population.

MLR responses are more discriminating than serologic reactions, and the human polymorphic variants they identify are termed **w subtypes.** For instance, a person whose MHC-II (HLA-D) haplotype is identified serologically as DR4 can be subtyped by MLRs against peripheral blood cells (monocytes particularly) from individuals of known Dw subtypes (see Fig. 20–1). (Minor Ags are not detected in these reactions unless the prospective recipient had previously been immunized against the donor's cells ["primed *in vivo*"].)

For grafts of heart, liver, and lungs, only organs from cadavers unrelated to the recipient are available; hence, HLA mismatches are usually extensive, and preventing allograft rejection depends largely on suppressing the recipient's immune system. But for kidney and bone marrow transplants, living, related donors are often available, and HLA typing to select the best-matched donors increases the probability of graft survival and diminishes (but does not entirely eliminate) the need for immunosuppression. Only when the donor is an identical (monozygotic) twin of the recipient or the recipient has severe combined immunodeficiency disease (SCID) and thus can make no immune responses at all are allografts successful without suppression of the immune system.

NONSPECIFIC IMMUNOSUPPRESSIVE REGIMENS. Various regimens are currently in use. In general, starting when a transplant is put in place, **corticosteroids** (e.g., **prednisolone** or **prednisone**) are administered in conjunction with a cytotoxic drug (either **azathioprine,** a purine analogue, or **cyclophosphamide**) or **cyclosporin,** or both. (Corticosteroids reduce inflammation;

the cytototoxic drugs block recipient immune responses by interfering with cell proliferation; and cyclosporin acts somehow to inhibit T_h-cell activity.) Sometimes the total Ig fraction from rabbit or horse antisera to human lymphocytes (**anti-lymphocyte globulin, ALG**) is given to reduce the number and activity of the recipient's lymphocytes (especially T cells). The skillful use of these agents has greatly increased the success rate, and organ transplantation has become a routine procedure in an increasing number of medical centers.

Nevertheless, Ag-nonspecific suppression of immune responses has serious consequences. The leading cause of death in transplant recipients is infection with opportunistic microbes, including bacteria such as *Legionella*, *Serratia*, *Listeria*, *Nocardia*, and atypical mycobacteria; fungi (*Aspergillus*, *Candida*, *Pneumocystis carinii*); protozoa (*Toxoplasma*); and viruses (herpes simplex and herpes zoster, cytomegalovirus). Perhaps as another consequence, some cancers are as much as 100 times more frequent in transplant recipients than in the rest of the population (see Tumor Immunology, below). These include a few of the common cancers (as of skin and uterine cervix), as well as less usual ones, such as lymphomas associated with Epstein–Barr virus infection. Additional serious side effects are attributable to particular drugs, such as renal damage and hypertension (cyclosporin) and liver damage (azathioprine).

SELECTIVE SUPPRESSION. In view of the serious side effects of nonspecific immune suppression, efforts to suppress selectively the responses to the graft's allo-Ags are being extensively explored through several approaches; some are described below.

1. **Elimination of MHC-II⁺ Cells from Allografts.** In addition to their specialized parenchymal cells, transplanted organs are normally infiltrated with the donor's "passenger" leukocytes, some of which (B-lymphocytes, monocytes, etc.) express MHC-II genes. Differences between these MHC-II proteins and those of the recipient elicit the vigorous CD4⁺ T-cell response that plays a significant role in the rejection of most allografts. The elimination of these passenger cells before a graft is put into place can greatly prolong graft survival (e.g., of islets of Langerhans in the treatment of experimental diabetes mellitus).

It is probably not feasible to eliminate all MHC-II⁺ cells from large organs (heart, kidney), but simply by culturing small grafts (such as islets of Langerhans) or by treating them with C and Abs to their MHC-II proteins, these cells can be largely eliminated. A potential difficulty, however, is that even a minimal CD4⁺ T-cell response to a few residual allogeneic MHC-II⁺ leukocytes, or a minimal CD8⁺ T-cell response, can lead to release of IFN-γ, which induces the expression of MHC-II genes in nonlymphoid cells. The graft's endothelial cells (and some other cells) can thus be induced to express allogeneic MHC-II proteins, which might then activate more host CD4⁺ T cells, leading to more IFN-γ, etc., amplifying the overall response.

2. **Total Lymphoid Irradiation (TLI).** High doses of total body x-irradiation (2000–3000 rads divided into doses of about 200 rads), administered in such a way as to protect bone marrow (by lead shielding of the sternum, upper humerus, upper femur, etc.), destroys most lymphoid cells of the lymph nodes and spleen while leaving intact the hematopoietic stem cells, which can regenerate new T and B cells. Before this regeneration, the irradiated individual is immunologically incompetent; like a newborn mouse, it will accept allografts and, indeed, become highly tolerant of their allogeneic MHC (see Tolerant Chimeras, below).

3. **Destruction of Activated T Cells.** T cells that respond to an allograft, like those responding to any other Ag, become activated and express high-affinity receptors (IL-2R) for interleukin (IL)-2. By covalently linking a mAb to IL-2R with the cytocidal β chain of diphtheria toxin, a toxic "heteroduplex" is formed: one element (Ab to IL-2R) targets the activated T cells and the other introduces a cytotoxic agent that can selectively kill these cells. Although it is effective in laboratory animals, the value of this approach in humans has still to be demonstrated.

TREATMENT OF GRAFT REJECTION CRISES. Despite thorough HLA typing and skillful immunosuppression, host allogeneic responses commonly reach an intensity that threatens total destruction of the graft. To cope with these crises, high doses of corticosteroids are administered with or without anti-lymphocyte globulin (see ALG, above). The administration of mAb to CD3 has particularly striking benefits, because it leads to a rapid decrease in the number and activity of mature T cells, all of which are CD3⁺ (see Chap. 15).

RESULTS OF HUMAN ALLOGRAFTS. More than 80,000 human kidney allografts have been carried out since the first ones were performed in the late 1950s. Currently, about 9000 kidney transplants are performed each year in the U.S., with an overall 2-year survival rate of more than 90% when donors are related to the recipients and approximately 80% when they are not (e.g., when cadaver kidneys are used) (Fig. 20–6). To an increasing extent, other organs are also being transplanted. In 1987, there were, in the U.S., about 1500 heart transplants and about 1200 liver transplants, as well as smaller numbers of lung and pancreas transplants.

Corneal allografts have been carried out since around 1905 and have a high success rate without benefit of HLA typing or immunosuppressing the recipient. The reasons are that the cornea may be a relatively privileged site (see below) and that only a small amount of

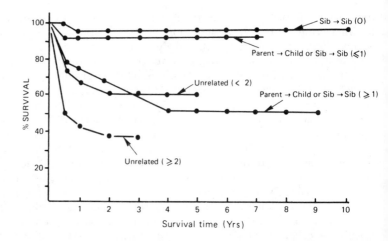

Figure 20–6. Correlation between HLA compatibility and survival of human kidney grafts. Number of incompatibilities, based on leukocyte typing, is given in parentheses. Every parent–child combination and half the sib–sib combinations have at least one haplotype in common. (Dausset J, Hors J: Transplant Proc 3:1004, 1971)

allogeneic tissue is transplanted; the antigenic load may thus be insufficient to elicit significant allogeneic responses.

ALLOGENEIC BONE MARROW TRANSPLANTATION. Early attempts to transplant bone marrow cells were successful only between monozygotic twins. Transplants of allogeneic bone marrow always failed despite extensive HLA matching and immunosuppression of recipients: if the recipient was not sufficiently suppressed, engraftment would fail, whereas if the recipient was thoroughly suppressed, mature allogeneic T cells in the transplanted cell population would react against the recipient's transplantation Ags, causing a **graft-versus-host (GVH) reaction** (see below). Even with HLA-identical bone marrow, in earlier years, this reaction developed in 30% to 70% of recipients, probably because of mismatched minor Ags (see Minors, above), and appeared to be responsible for the recipient's death. However, GVH reactions can now be prevented by eliminating mature T cells from the transplanted bone marrow.

GRAFT-VERSUS-HOST REACTIONS

The GVH reaction that proved initially to be such a stumbling block for bone marrow transplants occurs whenever allografts containing mature T cells are transplanted into immunologically incompetent hosts. Thus, this reaction was first recognized when newborn mice, whose immune system is immature, served as recipients for allogeneic spleen cells: as a result of the reaction of the donor's lymphocytes against the recipient's allo-Ags, the newborn host fails to gain weight normally, develops skin lesions and diarrhea, and usually dies within a few weeks (**runting syndrome).**

In human recipients, a GVH reaction is marked by skin rash, hepatitis, and diarrhea. It can be fatal or can resolve spontaneously or in response to treatment with high doses of corticosteroids and other drugs used to treat allograft-rejection crises (see above).

As noted before, eliminating mature T cells from bone marrow transplants can prevent the GVH reaction. To eliminate these cells, the bone marrow can be treated in various ways before being injected into recipients. First, mixing the bone marrow cells with sheep RBCs, which bind to T cells via their CD2 glycoprotein (see Chap. 15), agglutinates them into dense, rapidly sedimenting rosettes (see Fig. 15–10). Second, the addition of complement and mAb to CD3 will lyse virtually all mature T cells, which express CD3 proteins as part of their Ag-specific receptor complex. Third, "immunotoxins," formed by linking anti-CD3 mAb to the A chain of ricin (a highly cytotoxic plant toxin), specifically deliver that chain to CD3$^+$ T cells, which are selectively killed. As a result of these measures, allogeneic bone marrow cells can be successfully transplanted to treat a wide variety of disorders such as bone marrow aplasia, leukemia, and severe combined immunodeficiency disease (SCID, see below).

PRIVILEGED SITES

Even when immunosuppressive measures are omitted, allografts can flourish for long periods in a few special ("privileged") sites. These sites, in which lymphatic drainage is lacking and stimulation of host lymphocytes is thus minimal, include the meninges of the brain and the anterior chamber of the eye.

PREGNANCY. Histocompatibility Ags are formed early in embryonic life (by day 7 after fertilization in the mouse); many of those inherited from the father are foreign to the mother. Hence, in humans and other mammals, **the intrauterine fetus is actually an allograft in a privileged**

site. Its failure to evoke an allograft rejection response, even when the mother has previously been immunized against the father's H Ags, is not understood. One possible explanation is that mucinous secretions mask H Ags on the special fetal cell layer (trophoblast) at the placental interface with the maternal host.

INDUCED TOLERANCE TO ALLOGRAFTS

TOLERANCE CHIMERAS. Interest in immunologic tolerance (Chaps. 15 and 16) grew largely out of a crucial observation on nonidentical cattle twins, which frequently have *in utero* anastomoses of their placental blood vessels; hence, each twin ends up with two antigenically different kinds of RBCs. These persist to maturity, indicating that hematopoietic stem cells from each twin, transferred *in utero*, settle in the marrow of the other and then survive in genetically foreign soil through the animal's lifetime. Individuals with such mixtures of genetically different cells are called **chimeras,** after the monster in Greek mythology with a lion's head, a goat's body, and a serpent's tail. Rare blood group chimeras among nonidentical human twins have also been found. Such chimeras were found to accept skin grafts from each other without an allograft reaction. Tolerance could also be produced experimentally.

If embryonic or even newborn mice of inbred strain A were inoculated with spleen cells from mice of strain B, the inoculated animals, even after maturing, accept B skin grafts permanently, although they reject grafts from any other strain in a normal manner.

The newborn mouse appears to develop allograft tolerance with ease because its immune apparatus is immature, and it therefore cannot reject the foreign cells by an allograft reaction. Once established, the tolerance persists, allowing the foreign cells to remain and to proliferate. An individual rendered tolerant in this manner is a chimera: its spleen cells or white blood cells can induce, in a third strain, allograft sensitivity to both A and B cells.

The enduring chimerism implies that the two sets of cells are tolerant of each other. If allo-Ags of the donor's cells find their way to the thymus (Chap. 15), they might be recognized as self-Ags by the host's developing T cells. But why the graft's mature T cells become unresponsive to the host's transplantation Ags is obscure.

Tumor Immunology

Tumor immunology is based on two simple propositions: (1) that tumor cells have distinctive Ags (**tumor-associated Ags, TAAs**) that are present to only a negligible extent on normal cells, including those of the same histologic type as the tumor; and (2) that immune responses of the host to these Ags can destroy a tumor cell as though it were a virus-infected cell or an allograft. Hence, **immune surveillance** by lymphocytes (especially T cells) as they percolate normally through virtually all tissues of the body may be able to detect and eliminate tumors as they arise. Tumors that succeed in growing to the point where they become clinically evident and threaten the host's survival might thus be the result of (1) defects in the host's immune system; (2) selective growth of tumor cell variants whose TAAs have little or no immunogenicity; or (3) other mechanisms that enable them to escape immune destruction.

In the following sections, we consider TAAs, the responses they elicit, and some mechanisms that enable tumors to escape immune destruction. We shall also consider various immunologic strategies for treating tumors.

TUMOR-ASSOCIATED ANTIGENS

Convincing evidence that tumors have TAAs required the development of **inbred strains of mice and rats,** which permit a tumor arising in one animal (the **autochthonous host**) to be continuously propagated by serial transplantation in syngeneic recipients (i.e., with the same transplantation Ags; see Allograft Reaction as an Immune Response in this chapter). In an early classic study (Fig. 20–7), a sarcoma induced by methylcholan-

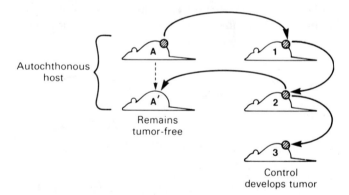

Figure 20–7. Immunity to a transplantable tumor. A methylcholanthrene-induced tumor is completely excised from the original (autochthonous) host *(A)*, "passaged" by serial transplantation through syngeneic mice *(1, 2)*, and then injected back into the surgically cured original host *(A')* and into normal control mice *(3)*. The original host, immunized ("primed") by its growing tumor cells, rejects the transplant (remains tumor-free), whereas the controls develop tumors that grow progressively and fatally. In the original study, the autochthonous host, after excision of the tumor, was injected repeatedly with irradiated tumor cells (to increase immunity), but this is not usually necessary: the excision of a small, growing tumor often leaves sufficient immunity to reject a subsequent inoculum of the same tumor. (Based on Klein G et al: Cancer Research 20:1561, 1960)

threne was excised and transplanted into syngeneic mice, while the surgically cured host was immunized with x-irradiated cells of its original tumor (x-irradiation blocks cell division by damaging chromosomes but leaves the cell Ags intact). The immunized animal could then reject a graft of its own tumor, and its resistance could be transferred to normal syngeneic recipients with its T cells. TAAs that elicit such transplantation-rejection responses are referred to as **tumor-specific transplantation Ags** (TSTAs).

As we shall see below, the many different tumors that can be induced by a given chemical carcinogen can differ greatly in their TSTAs. In contrast, the tumors induced by an oncogenic virus share TSTAs that are dependent on infection with that virus (although they are not necessarily components of the virion).

Antigens of Tumors Induced by Chemical Carcinogens

Many carcinogen-induced tumors have **individually distinctive ("private") TAAs.** For instance, mice immunized against a methylcholanthrene-induced tumor are resistant to transplanted cells from that tumor but not to cells from other tumors, including those of the same histologic type elicited by the same carcinogen in the same mouse strain. Indeed, methylcholanthrene painted on different skin areas of the same autochthonous host elicits multiple fibrosarcomas that exhibit little or no cross-immunity in transplantation-resistance tests. Resistance to these tumors can be transferred with T cells, and a tumor-specific clone of CTLs has been used to identify the gene that encodes one of the private TAAs. This gene has some remarkable properties: (1) it lacks a leader sequence, indicating that it is not a membrane protein; and (2) the only difference between it and the corresponding gene in other cells is a single nucleotide replacement leading to a single amino acid substitution (arginine to histidine). The tumor-specific CTLs evidently recognize this mutation, because they can kill specifically other cells (having the correct MHC Class I) to which the peptide is added (Fig. 20–8). **Thus, private TAAs in general may be peptides that derive from virtually any mutated gene, whether or not the gene product is membrane associated.**

Tumors induced by chemical carcinogens can differ widely in immunogenicity and in **latent period** (the interval before the appearance of the tumor). Tumors appearing after the longest latent periods are generally the least immunogenic, as though the host immune responses to a slowly growing clone of nonidentical tumor cells containing various TAAs selectively eliminate the most immunogenic variants. Such **immune selection** is also suggested by the gradual decrease in the immunogenicity of some tumors as they are passaged by transplantation through successive hosts. Perhaps for the same reason, the spontaneous tumors that arise sporadically in old mice also seem to lack TAAs. Whether the common human cancers (lung, breast, colon, etc.) also represent the end result of similar selective elimination of their most immunogenic variants is not known.

Other TAAs (**"public" TAAs), are shared by many tumors;** they sometimes represent **anomalous expression of normally silent genes.** An example is the **Forssman Ag** of human gastrointestinal cancer. This ceramide-pentasaccharide:

GalNAcα1 → 3GalNAcβ1 → 3Galα1 → 4Galβ1 → 4Gluceramide

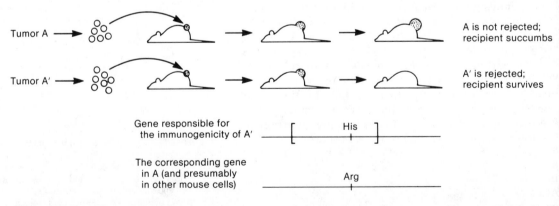

Figure 20–8. A peptide containing a somatic mutation can serve as a "tumor-specific transplantation antigen." Cells from tumor A were mutagenized and cloned to yield a series of immunogenic variant tumors, such as A'. Unlike transplants of tumor A, which grow progressively in syngeneic hosts and are lethal, transplants of A' are rejected. Cells of tumor A', but not those of tumor A, are killed by CTLs from the host that rejects A'. The gene responsible for the immunogenicity of A' contains a single mutation (Arg → His), and a synthetic 15-amino acid peptide containing the His mutation (enclosed in brackets) can convert cells of tumor A into targets for the anti-A' CTLs. Recognition of the His-peptide is restricted by an MHC-class I protein (L^d). Based on Lurquin C, et al: Cell, 1989, in press, and Boon T: Immunol Today 6:307, 1985.

is synthesized by many Forssman-positive (F⁺) species. Man has been considered to be Forssman-negative (F⁻), but the gastrointestinal mucosa in some persons is F⁺; hence, it is an allo-Ag in man. F⁻ humans make a precursor that lacks the terminal N-acetyl galactose (GalNAc) of the complete Ag. However, gastrointestinal cancers in such individuals produce the complete pentasaccharide; Abs to it appear to recognize primarily the terminal disaccharide (GalNAcα1 → 3GalNAc). The relationship between expression of the public TAA and gastrointestinal cancers in these individuals is not known. Some other public TAAs are expressed primarily on normal cells during fetal development (see Oncofetal Ags, below).

Oncofetal Antigens

Oncofetal Ags, expressed by various cells at certain stages of normal fetal development, are produced in normal adults only at trace levels, if at all. Because some of them also appear to be produced by certain tumors, as shared (public) TAAs, they have been termed "oncofetal" Ags. Abs detect two of them, α-fetoprotein and carcinoembryonic Ag, in the serum of individuals with certain forms of cancer and are used to monitor the clinical course in some cancer patients.

α-Fetoprotein (AFP) is synthesized in the fetal liver, yolk sac, and gastrointestinal tract. At its peak level (2–3 mg/ml) in the human fetus (third to sixth month of gestation), it amounts to about one-third of all serum proteins. At birth, the level drops about one million-fold, and only traces (about 5 to 25 ng/ml) are present in normal human serum. However, AFP was discovered to be greatly elevated in the serum of mice carrying transplanted hepatomas and in about two-thirds of patients with primary liver cancer (which is frequent in Asia and Africa, although rare in the U.S.). High levels are also found in patients with embryonal cell tumors and in some with cancers of the stomach and pancreas. The levels may also be high, but fluctuate more widely, in individuals with acute or chronic hepatitis or cirrhosis of the liver. After surgical excision of a tumor, the persistence of an elevated AFP level, or a later increase, suggests that tumor cells remain or that the tumor has recurred.

(AFP may represent a fetal form of serum albumin: it is a single polypeptide chain of 70,000 daltons showing some amino acid sequence similarity with albumin; like serum albumin, it also binds estrogens and a variety of anionic dyes. As with some other pairs of proteins showing partial amino acid sequence similarity, native human AFP does not cross-react with Abs to native human serum albumin, but the denatured molecules cross-react extensively.)

Carcinoembryonic antigen (CEA) was discovered by immunizing rabbits with surgically excised specimens of human colon cancer and then adsorbing the antisera with normal tissue from the same surgical samples. The residual Abs were found to react specifically with: (1) colon cancer cells from many patients; (2) some other human cancers of gastrointestinal origin; and (3) endodermal tissues from the normal human fetus but not from normal adults. For use as a radioactive ligand in radioimmunoassays (Chap. 13), the corresponding Ag, called CEA, is currently isolated from liver metastases of colon cancers.

CEA is generally present at trace levels (less than 5 μg/ml) in normal human serum. Elevated levels are found in the serum of most patients with cancer of the lower gastrointestinal tract and pancreas and, less frequently, in patients with cancer of other organs (breast, lung) or with certain chronic or recurrent inflammatory conditions (e.g., colitis or chronic bronchitis, heavy cigarette smokers). Many of these conditions have in common excess mucin production. The significance of elevated levels of CEA is complicated by the heterogeneity of the Ag and by difficulty in distinguishing it from substances that cross-react with anti-CEA Abs.

CEA is a glycoprotein (180,000 daltons) with more carbohydrate (65%) than protein. Immunofluorescence suggests that it is present in a mucinous layer (glycocalyx) that surrounds certain cells. Most Abs to CEA are probably directed to the protein moiety, because the association constant is high (10^{11} L/M), and serologic reactivity persists after removal of many of the sugar residues. However, some Abs to CEA probably react with oligosaccharide groups and account for low-level cross-reactivity with "blood group substances" (antigenic polysaccharides on RBCs).

SCREENING HUMAN POPULATIONS FOR CANCER. A major goal in the management of human cancer is the detection of the disease at early stages (when treatment is more effective) by testing large populations with sensitive, accurate, and inexpensive procedures. One approach is to use Abs to detect TAAs in serum. Such a test for CEA has been abandoned as a screening procedure, for although the levels in persons with colon cancer generally differ substantially from those in normal persons, the ranges in affected and normal populations overlap significantly. However, CEA levels are useful for following the course of individual patients; if the level drops after surgical excision of a colon cancer, its subsequent elevation strongly suggests recurrence.

MONOCLONAL ANTIBODIES TO TUMOR-ASSOCIATED ANTIGENS

To develop mAb to human TAAs, mice are immunized against cells from human tumors, and supernatant fluids from B-cell hybridomas prepared from these mice are screened for their ability to bind to a wide variety of cells, principally: (1) the tumor cells used as the immunogen;

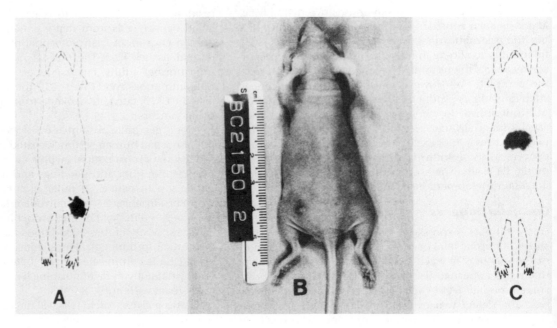

Figure 20–9. Specific localization of a radiolabeled (^{111}In) anti-tumor monoclonal antibody in a human B-cell tumor (lymphoma) grown in the hind leg of a nude mouse *(A, B)*. The control *(C)* shows the nonspecific accumulation in the liver of the same antibody radiolabelled under conditions in which the antibody was probably denatured. (From Rodwell JD et al: Proc Natl Acad Sci USA 83:2632, 1986)

(2) normal cells (leukocytes, fibroblasts) from the individual furnishing these tumor cells; and (3) large panels of other tumor cells of many different types from many other individuals. From extensive efforts carried out over the past 10 to 15 years, several dozen mAb that are highly specific for TAAs of melanomas and various carcinomas (i.e., epithelial cell cancers) of breast, colon, lung, and some other organs have been developed.

However, when subjected to detailed tests, these Abs have invariably been found to react (or cross-react) with Ags of some normal cells, indicating that these TAAs are not, strictly speaking, expressed exclusively by the tumor cells. Nevertheless, the extent to which they are present in normal tissue may be so limited (e.g., to some epithelial cells of some bile ducts) that for practical purposes, the cross-reactions can be ignored. Several of these mAbs are being tested clinically for their ability to locate and identify tumor masses (metastases of primary tumors) as small as 1 cm in diameter (using radiolabeled Abs, see Fig. 20–9) or for their ability to aid in the destruction of tumors (see Therapeutic Strategies, below).

HOST IMMUNE RESPONSES TO TUMORS

In the tumor-bearing host, TAAs elicit diverse immune responses, involving almost all classes of Abs and types of T cells. Under various experimental conditions, tumor cells can be destroyed by:

1. Antibodies, either with C or in antibody-dependent, complement-independent, cell-mediated cytotoxicity (ADCC);
2. CTLs;
3. Macrophages activated by lymphokines from Ag-stimulated T cells;
4. Natural killer (NK) cells.

For unknown reasons, tumor cells generally are more susceptible than normal cells to destruction by all of these effector mechanisms, especially by NK cells and CTLs and by the cytolytic secretory granules that can be isolated from these cells (Chap. 19, Fig. 19–17). Which (if any) of these mechanisms actually have a role *in vivo* in restraining the growth and spread of tumors is obscure. However, CD4$^+$ and CD8$^+$ T cells can readily be grown from surgically removed human tumors that are cultured in the presence of IL-2 (Chap. 15), and these T-cell populations are highly active in lysing ^{51}Cr-labeled cells from the tumor. Indeed, as described below, these **tumor-infiltrating T-lymphocytes (TIL)**, grown in culture to high cell densities and then injected back into the same patient, can bring about a substantial reduction in the mass of some tumors. As noted above, the TAAs recognized by these T cells are probably peptides associated with MHC proteins, although no such peptides have so far been identified in human tumors. The infiltration of a tumor by these cells probably represents a specific immune attack on the tumor cells.

Immune Surveillance

Individuals with a growing tumor often produce Abs and T cells that react with cells or cell-free components of the tumor. (As a "solid" tumor mass enlarges, the center usually becomes deprived of a blood supply and undergoes extensive necrosis; some of the released cell constituents are evidently immunogenic.) If these T cells and Abs destroy tumor cells or interfere with their growth and spread, as proposed by the immune surveillance concept, then the incidence of cancer ought to be increased in individuals who are chronically immunodeficient. As indicated below, this prediction is borne out clinically for some unusual tumors, but not for those that cause most of the death and morbidity of human cancer such as carcinomas of the lung, colon, breast, and pancreas.

1. Children with some primary immune deficiencies (see below) have an approximately ten-fold higher frequency of lymphosarcoma and reticulum cell sarcoma than age- and sex-matched controls, but they show no increase in the incidence of the most common tumors of childhood (retinoblastoma, neuroblastoma, Wilms' tumor) or of adulthood.

2. Individuals given long-term immunosuppressive therapy to prevent allograft rejection (see above) have an approximately 300-fold increase in the incidence of reticulum cell sarcomas and a higher than normal frequency of skin cancer, but they have no increased frequency of cancers of the lung, colon, or breast.

3. Individuals with AIDS (see below) often have Kaposi's sarcoma (ordinarily an extremely rare form of cancer) or B-cell lymphomas.

Immune responses can also control or prevent certain virus-induced tumors. For instance:

1. Viral lymphomas of chickens (Marek's disease) can be prevented by immunization with an attenuated form of a similar virus (herpesvirus of turkeys).
2. The frequency of primary liver cancer (hepatoma) in humans appears to be much reduced (in Asia and elsewhere where this form of cancer is common) by immunizing populations with hepatitis B vaccine, which prevents viral hepatitis, including the chronic form that is a forerunner of primary hepatoma.
3. Mice deprived of the T-cell immune system through neonatal thymectomy or administration of antilymphocytic serum are much more susceptible to tumor induction by polyoma virus and by murine leukemia virus.

In contrast, the tumors that account for more than 90% of human cancer deaths in the U.S. and Western Europe (carcinomas of the lung, colon, breast, etc.) are not increased in frequency in the chronically immunosuppressed individuals listed above or in certain others (nude mice, patients with the lepromatous form of leprosy). Finally, if immune defenses were the key controlling element, one would expect to see many more individuals with multiple forms of cancer.

Taken together, **the evidence argues for the ability of normal immune responses to reduce the frequency of certain rare tumors but not to control the more frequent forms of human cancer.**

ESCAPE FROM SURVEILLANCE. Why immunologic surveillance against tumors is not more effective is poorly understood. Some tumors have greatly **reduced amounts of cell-surface MHC-I protein.** In others, these proteins are **covered** by huge amounts of a polysaccharide or glycoprotein. Another possiblity is that immunologic surveillance, acting on a heterogeneous tumor cell population, eliminates those cells with the most immunogenic TAAs, leaving those with weak TAAs to proliferate.

ESCAPE MECHANISMS AND CONCOMITANT IMMUNITY. Tumors often grow progressively even though the hosts are making anti-TAA responses, demonstrable *in vitro*. However, when some of the tumor cells are reinjected into the same individual at a distant site, they are usually eliminated, although the main tumor continues to grow. This **concomitant immunity** may be responsible for a commonplace event in the natural history of most tumors: small clusters of cells frequently separate from a primary tumor mass and spread through blood and lymph to distant sites, but they only rarely succeed in establishing a metastatic tumor.

THERAPEUTIC STRATEGIES

Patients with malignant tumors are generally subjected to surgery to remove the primary tumor mass and then to x-irradiation and chemotherapy to destroy cells that might have spread from the primary mass to form satellite tumors (**metastases**) in distant organs. Most primary tumors can be successfully excised, and metastases are responsible for most cancer deaths. Various combinations of surgery, x-irradiation, and chemotherapy are curative in about half the patients with cancer (with the proportion varying widely among different cancers), but the severe toxicity of chemotherapy has stimulated a search for more focused agents, particularly those that take advantage of the specificity of mAbs and the specificity and cytotoxic activity of T cells. Some of the specific immunotherapeutic approaches now under development are outlined below.

Monoclonal Antibodies to Tumor-Associated Antigens

A tumor sometimes regresses after a patient is injected intravenously with mAbs to the tumor's Ags. The tumors formed by malignant B cells (B-cell lymphoma) have been most extensively studied in this way because the idiotype (Id) of the surface Ig on these cells is not present on normal B cells or on any other cells; hence, these Igs are, in a sense, tumor-specific Ags. The injection of mAbs to these Ids has caused complete regression of one patient's tumor and partial regression of these tumors in many other patients. The isotypes of the most effective mAbs (IgG_{2a} and IgG_{2b}) are particularly active in mediating ADCC (see Chap. 19) and C activation (Chap. 17), suggesting that these cytolytic mechanisms are probably responsible for the tumor regression.

However, the B-cell tumors that respond to anti-Id Abs usually recur, and the recurrent tumors do not react with the anti-Id mAbs used for the initial therapy. The reason is a change in amino acid sequences in the complementarity determining regions (CDR) of the V domains of the Igs in the recurrent tumors. The changes are attributable to nucleotide substitutions reminiscent of those that occur during normal immune responses (see Somatic Mutations and Affinity Changes during Immune Responses, Chap. 16). Because of the extremely high rate of mutation in gene segments for Ig V domains, this therapy has turned out to be of limited usefulness clinically. In effect these tumors evade therapy with mAbs by selection of natural variants, a mechanism similar to the antigenic variation observed in some infectious diseases (e.g., due to influenza virus).

The emergence of variant malignant B cells having different CDR sequences testifies to the ability of the injected mAb to destroy the original tumor cells. The results thus suggest that this approach might be more effective against tumors whose TAAs are less mutable than Igs. Another limitation of this approach is that most humans who receive mouse mAbs in therapeutic doses (a few hundred milligrams to perhaps one gram) develop Abs to the mouse Igs. To overcome this problem, novel **chimeric genes** for Abs have been constructed by replacing the nucleotide sequences of the CDRs of a gene for human Ig with the corresponding sequences from a mouse anti-tumor mAb. In these **chimeric Abs,** the amino acid sequences of V-domain framework regions and of C domains are of human origin, whereas the amino acid sequences that determine specificity for TAAs are of mouse origin. Preliminary trials indicate that these human–mouse hybrid molecules elicit a much lower anti-Ig immune response in human subjects than do conventional mouse mAbs.

IMMUNOTOXINS. Various toxic agents can be attached to Ab molecules to enhance their antitumor activity. These agents include radionuclides (^{131}I, yttrium, etc.), cytotoxic drugs (methotrexate, doxorubicin, etc.), and polypeptide chains from toxic plant and bacterial proteins (ricin, diphtheria toxin). The latter are generally heterodimeric proteins in which one polypeptide chain has lectin-like specificity, causing the protein to bind to glycoproteins on cell surfaces, and the other has highly cytotoxic activity once it enters a cell. Accordingly, **immunotoxins** are prepared by covalently attaching the isolated toxic polypeptide chain to the tumor-specific mAb: ideally, the Ab specifically targets the toxin to the appropriate tumor cells. To minimize nonspecific binding to other cells (e.g., via their Fc receptors), some immunotoxins are prepared by coupling just the Fab or $F(ab')_2$ fragment to a toxic polypeptide chain.

According to one protocol, an immunotoxin prepared from a mAb that is specific for all human B cells is used to eliminate these cells, including malignant ones, from a sample of the patient's bone marrow cells. Then, after total body x-irradiation is applied to destroy all of the patient's B lymphoma cells and, incidentally, all of his or her normal lymphocytes, the purged bone marrow cells are reintroduced as an autologous marrow transplant. Because it retains normal stem cells, this transplant can give rise to normal B (and T) cells and restore the treated individual's immune system.

Lymphokine-Activated Killer Cells

When cytotoxic lymphocytes are activated by IL-2 in culture and then injected intravenously into patients, they can reduce some tumor masses, especially metastases of melanomas and renal cell carcinomas. To obtain these killer cells, large numbers of peripheral blood lymphocytes (from 500–700 ml of blood) are collected from the patient, incubated for several days with IL-2 at high concentration (1000 Units/ml), and then reinjected. The process is repeated on four successive days and again after 2 weeks, while the patient is given enormous doses of IL-2 to maintain the injected T cells in an activated state. The surface markers and cytotoxic activity of these lymphokine-activated killer (LAK) cells are similar to those of natural killer (NK) cells (Chap. 19): in the test tube, they lyse many different kinds of tumor cells of any MHC haplotype. Because LAK cells have no demonstrable specificity, an enormous number are administered (more than 10^{11}, about 10% of the patient's total lymphocyte pool). Unfortunately, the high doses of IL-2 administered to the patients elicit life-threatening side-effects.

Tumor-Infiltrating Lymphocytes

What seems to be a more specific and safer procedure is based on the finding that many tumors are infiltrated by T cells *in vivo*. When the excised tumor is grown in culture in the presence of IL-2, the T cells proliferate readily, but the tumor cells die off (either because most freshly excised tumors do not readily adapt to culture or because they are killed by the T cells). Many of the proliferating T cells are specific CTLs (CD8+ and CD4+ CTLs; see Chap. 19): in test tube assays, they lyse ^{51}Cr-labeled cells of the tumor from which they are derived. After the T cells have multiplied in culture to about 10^{11} cells over 4 or 5 weeks, they are injected into the patient from whom they were derived. In the few patients so far tested, TIL have brought about marked shrinkage of metastatic masses of melanomas and renal carcinomas; toxic side effects have also been minimal because patients receive much less IL-2 than those given LAK cells.

Targeting Tumor Cells for Destruction by Cytotoxic Lymphocytes

Through the use of "heteroduplex" Ab conjugates, diverse cytotoxic lymphocytes, regardless of the Ags they normally recognize, can be specifically targeted to kill a chosen set of tumor cells. In one example, a mAb to the invariant (CD3) moiety of the Ag-specific T-cell receptor (CD3/TcR) is joined covalently to a mAb to a TAA (call it X). This bifunctional conjugate (anti-CD3–anti-X) specifically cross-links mature T cells (all of which express surface CD3/TcR receptor complexes) to tumor cells having surface Ag X. Those cross-linked T cells that happen to be CTLs will be activated (via aggregation of their CD3/TcR complexes) to express their cytolytic activity; hence, the CTLs are targeted to kill X-bearing tumor cells, for which the CTLs are not specific. In another kind of bifunctional conjugate, the anti-X mAb is replaced as the targeting moiety by a peptide hormone, melanocyte-stimulating hormone (MSH); the anti-CD3–MSH conjugate targets CTLs to kill melanoma cells which express receptors for MSH.

In a different bifunctional conjugate, the anti-CD3 Ab is replaced by a mAb to the Fc receptor (FcR), which is present on NK cells and binds the Fc domain of certain Ig isotypes (γ chains). In the presence of this conjugate (anti-FcR–anti-X), NK cells are targeted to kill cells with surface Ag X (Fig. 20–10). The efficacy of various bifunctional conjugates has been demonstrated *in vitro*, and some have been active in experimental animals, but none has been tested so far in human subjects.

Immunodeficiency Diseases

Some profound deficiencies of the immune system are heritable. Others are congenital or acquired later in life, often as a consequence of the destruction of hematopoietic stem cells by the drugs and ionizing radiation used to treat cancer. Since 1981, by far the most common immunodeficiency disease has been AIDS, which is associated with infection by human immunodeficiency virus (HIV).

ACQUIRED IMMUNE DEFICIENCY SYNDROME

The distinctive features of AIDS arise from the selective binding of the envelope glycoprotein (gp 160) of HIV to the CD4 glycoprotein on CD4+ T cells and on macrophages and some other cells (see below). The resulting infection of these cells by HIV eventually leads to a profound loss of many immune responses and to recurrent, life-threatening infections with **opportunistic microbes:** commonplace viruses, bacteria, and fungi of low virulence that are pathogenic virtually only for individuals whose immune defenses are profoundly impaired. Some examples are pneumonia caused by *Pneumocystis carinii* (probably a fungus), infections of the mouth and skin by yeast (monilia), chronic diarrhea caused by rotavirus, and disseminated infection by cytomegalovirus. Another feature is the high incidence of certain malignant tumors, principally Kaposi's sarcoma (a rare vascular neoplasm of skin ordinarily seen only above the age of 60) and B-cell lymphomas.

The isolation of HIV-1 (a retrovirus) from tissues of persons with AIDS, and the discovery of a T-cell line in which it could be propagated, led to large-scale production of the virus, Abs, and Ags for serologic diagnosis and to the production of nucleic acid probes for viral RNA and complementary DNA. These developments have made it possible to identify a large reservoir of latently infected individuals and to map the spread of the infection.

Transmitted primarily by infectious blood and semen, the disease was first recognized in male homosexuals in New York City and San Francisco, especially passive partners in anal intercourse. Currently, the spread in the U.S.

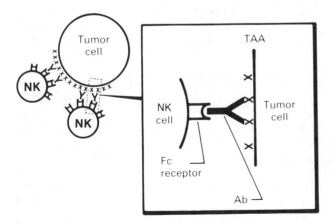

Figure 20–10. Ab molecules specific for TAAs (X) link target cells to natural killer (NK) cells via the latter's Fc receptor, resulting in destruction of the tumor target cell (Ab-dependent cell-mediated cytotoxicity, ADCC; Chap. 19).

is greatest among drug addicts who use needles contaminated with each other's blood. Also at risk in the past were the recipients of transfused blood (until a simple test for Ab in donors became available) and hemophiliacs receiving Factor VIII (which is now readily freed of virus by heating). In the U.S., between 1981, when the disease was first recognized, and mid-1988, approximately 65,000 AIDS victims had been reported, and it is estimated that there are now around 1.5 million infected individuals. The vast majority of these are expected eventually to die of AIDS unless effective therapy becomes available.

In those instances when the infection has been accurately timed, serum Abs to HIV appear after several weeks to several months, but the individuals usually remain free of disease for years. Eventually, nearly all infected individuals become overwhelmed by recurrent infections, and it is estimated that about 35% die of the disease within 8 years. HIV is therefore an extraordinarily lethal, although slow, virus.

Symptomatic disease appears in two forms. Persons with the **AIDS-related complex (ARC)** have generalized lymph node enlargement, low-grade fever, and pronounced loss of weight (perhaps as manifestations of excessive production of **IL-1,** which is also termed **cachectin**). In **full-blown AIDS,** these manifestations are accompanied by recurrent opportunistic infections (e.g. *Pneumocystis carinii* pneumonia), Kaposi's sarcoma, or both.

Immune Responses to HIV

Virtually all HIV-infected individuals become "seropositive": i.e., they develop Abs that react specifically with HIV epitopes. In culture, some of these Abs neutralize the virus: they block its ability to infect cultured CD4$^+$ T cells. Moreover, some Abs contribute to the destruction of infected cells by means of ADCC. (As described in Chap. 19, in ADCC, Abs bind specifically via their Fab domains to a target cell [e.g., an HIV-infected cell] and via their Fc domain to Fc receptors on NK cells, which are thereby stimulated to kill the target cells; see Fig. 19–16 and 20–10.

In addition to anti-HIV Abs, many infected individuals have CTLs that lyse ^{51}Cr-labeled cells that express HIV genes (provided these cells share HLA proteins with the CTLs, i.e., the reaction is MHC restricted). Virtually all of the CTLs are CD8$^+$ T cells, probably because there are relatively few CD4$^+$ cells in these individuals (see below). Because these CTLs are actively cytolytic on being removed from blood, without having to be stimulated by culturing them with HIV-infected cells, they are probably active killers *in vivo*.

EPITOPES. The HIV epitopes that are recognized by neutralizing Abs are remarkably variable. Thus, the Abs from any particular patient block the infectivity of only a few of the many HIV isolates now available. The reason is that these Abs are specific for the virus envelope glycoprotein (gp 160), and the amino acid sequences of parts of this protein are extraordinarily diverse, differing among HIV isolates that are derived from different individuals and even at different times from the same individual (Fig. 20–11). Indeed, each individual isolate, when molecularly cloned, turns out to be a mixture of genotypically distinguishable HIV variants that differ from each other in the sequence of the virus's gp 160 gene (and protein).

In contrast, CD4, the cell receptor for gp 160, does not vary in sequence, so the gp 160 site that interacts with it is expected to be similarly conserved. It is likely, therefore, that the variable neutralizing Abs do not bind to the conserved CD4-binding site but rather block it sterically, perhaps by binding to variable sequences that surround it.

The epitopes recognized by neutralizing Abs are clustered in a few "hypervariable" regions of gp 160, whereas those recognized in ADCC are dispersed all over gp 160. CTLs recognize an even wider range of epitopes, not only in gp 160, but also in the viral polymerase (reverse transcriptase).

There are interesting similarities between HIV's gp 160 and the hemagglutinin of the influenza virus envelope. Both proteins bind specifically to receptors on susceptible cells and are essential for virus entry into these cells; both are also extremely variable in sequence, because the respective genes are extraordinarily mutable; and both are targets for neutralizing Abs that block infectivity of only a few similar variants. Indeed, with both viruses, these Abs are probably the selective agents that promote the emergence of viral variants. But whereas influenza virus variants change from year to year, in any given outbreak of the disease viral isolates from different patients are the same. Hence, recurrent annual epidemics of influenza virus infections can be controlled by prophylactic vaccination, matching each year's vaccine to the prevalent viral variant. The development of similar vaccines for HIV is not feasible, because the number of variants is so enormous.

Immune Defects in AIDS

Despite the neutralizing Abs and CTLs in HIV-infected individuals, the infection persists and spreads progressively to involve more CD4$^+$ and other cells. The onset of symptomatic disease is marked by a profound decrease in the number of circulating CD4$^+$ cells, ultimately inverting the ratio of CD4$^+$/CD8$^+$ cells from about 2/1 (the normal value) to considerably below 1/1. As recurrent infections worsen, the Ab and CTL levels also decline (see CD8$^+$ Cells, below). The decreases could be secondary to worsening of the disease, but the reverse is also likely; and the growing immune deficiency is probably both a cause and an effect of advancing disease.

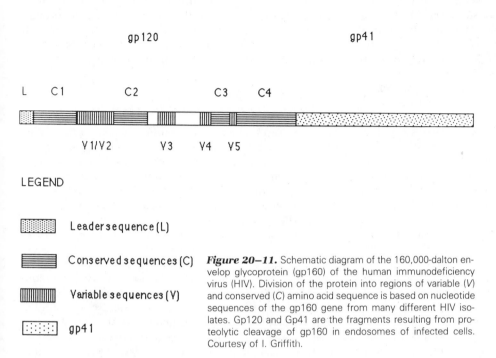

Envelope protein (gp160)

gp120　　　　　　　　　　　　　　gp41

L　C1　　　C2　　　C3　C4

V1/V2　　　V3　V4 V5

LEGEND

▦　Leader sequence (L)

▤　Conserved sequences (C)

▥　Variable sequences (V)

▨　gp41

Figure 20–11. Schematic diagram of the 160,000-dalton envelop glycoprotein (gp160) of the human immunodeficiency virus (HIV). Division of the protein into regions of variable (*V*) and conserved (*C*) amino acid sequence is based on nucleotide sequences of the gp160 gene from many different HIV isolates. Gp120 and Gp41 are the fragments resulting from proteolytic cleavage of gp160 in endosomes of infected cells. Courtesy of I. Griffith.

CD8⁺ Cells. Although the CD8⁺ T cells persist at normal levels until very late in the course of infection, their activity changes. Initially normal in function, these cells eventually become unresponsive to antigenic stimuli. The reason is probably that the cytokines required for their maturation derive in part from CD4⁺ T cells or macrophages (see Chaps. 15 and 19). With progressive disease, the CD8⁺ T cell population loses its responsiveness to viral Ags while retaining reactivity with allogeneic (MHC-different) cells, although eventually this responsiveness also declines. The reason for the delay may be that T cells reactive with cells having foreign MHC are far more frequent than T cells specific for other Ags (see T-Cell Repertoire, Chap. 15). The loss of CD8⁺ T cell function almost certainly further diminishes the ability of AIDS patients to cope with infections caused by viruses and other intracellular pathogens.

HYPERGAMMAGLOBULINEMIA. AIDS patients usually have a marked elevation of polyclonal serum Igs, involving diverse isotypes. Because CD4⁺ (helper) T cell activity is important for the production of all Ig isotypes except IgM, the elevated Ig level is puzzling. However, it is possible that even with a depleted pool of CD4⁺ T cells, the repeated infections, with the accompanying massive antigenic stimulation of B cells, accounts for the marked polyclonal increase in serum Ig levels.

BINDING OF HIV gp 160 TO CD4. As noted above, human cells with surface CD4 are selectively infected with HIV because this protein binds the envelope protein (gp 160) of the virus, leading to endocytosis of the virions. In endosomes, the gp 160 is cleaved to yield gp 120, a "fusogenic" protein that promotes fusion of the virions with the endosome's limiting membrane and hence transfer of the viral RNA into the host cell's cytoplasm. Reverse transcription by the viral polymerase then yields a DNA copy that becomes integrated as a "provirus" into the infected cell's genome. Some mAbs to CD4 block infection of CD4⁺ T cells in culture. Soluble CD4 (produced by recombinant DNA technology) can also inhibit infection, by competition, and it is being tested as a therapeutic agent to limit the spread of HIV from infected to uninfected cells.

DESTRUCTION OF CD4⁺ T CELLS. Although CD4⁺ T cells are readily infected by HIV in culture, in AIDS patients, only about 1 in 10⁵ to 10⁶ peripheral blood lymphocytes early in the disease, and about 1 in 10⁴ later on, expresses HIV genes or is infected latently (i.e., with viral genes integrated into the cell's genome but not expressed). Given this low frequency of infection, the massive decline in CD4 cells is puzzling. One possibility is that infected cells, having budding virions and gp 160 on their surfaces, can bind to CD4 molecules on uninfected CD4⁺ T cells, leading to cell fusion; the resulting **multinucleated giant cells** may be unstable and die.

Another possibility is that CD4$^+$ T cells, even when uninfected by HIV, are especially susceptible to destruction by anti-gp 160 CTLs. The reason is that when human CD4$^+$ cells are activated by any Ag, they express MHC Class II proteins and can thus serve as Ag-presenting cells. Accordingly, if these cells happen to bind soluble gp 160, shed, say, by infected cells, **they can be specifically lysed by gp 160-specific, MHC-II-restricted CD4$^+$ CTLs.** (Although most CTLs are CD8$^+$,CD4$^-$ T cells, some of them are CD8$^-$,CD4$^+$ T cells; see Chaps. 15 and 19.) Because individuals with AIDS suffer from frequent severe infections and are exposed to a heavy load of microbial Ags, many of their CD4$^+$ T cells are activated and probably express MHC-II proteins; hence, even though they are uninfected by HIV, they are at risk, if they bind soluble gp 160, of being destroyed by CTLs (Fig. 20–12).

CD4 is expressed not only by CD4$^+$ T cells but also, at lower levels, by macrophages, glial cells and neurons, and epithelial cells of the colon and vagina; hence these cells are also susceptible to HIV infection. CD4 molecules are difficult to detect by immunofluorescence on these susceptible non-T cells; it is likely that the virus is more active than the fluorescent Ab as a ligand. Whether macrophages are infected via endocytosis of virions that bind specifically to their CD4 molecules or by other means (e.g., phagocytosis of virions) is not clear.

Vaccines

The most effective immune response to an infectious agent is generally elicited by natural infection: individuals who recover are often solidly resistant to reinfection, even for a lifetime. Currently available vaccines, at their best, approach but rarely achieve this level of protection. With HIV, unfortunately, the antiviral Abs and CTLs that are formed in the natural infection appear to be incapable of eradicating it; and although vaccines involving various fragments of HIV proteins linked to various carriers are currently under development, whether any of them

will prevent or eradicate infection remains an open question. The difficulties in developing candidate HIV vaccines are especially complex because of the extremely high rate of mutation in the viral envelope glycoprotein. Moreover, the paucity of suitable animal models for HIV infection and AIDS means that vaccines may have to be evaluated almost exclusively in humans.

HERITABLE AND OTHER IMMUNOGLOBULIN DEFICIENCIES

Genetic and congenitally acquired defects in the ability to make immune responses have been recognized since the 1950s, when it became possible to prolong the survival of immunodeficient individuals through the use of antibiotics and of Igs transferred from normal donors. Several clinical patterns are recognized. Suspected subjects with recurrent severe infections or with close kinship to affected persons are evaluated by procedures listed in Table 20–3. It is important to avoid the use of live vaccines such as attenuated viruses (polio, vaccinia, measles, rubella, mumps) or bacteria (BCG: an attenuated tubercle bacillus), which can cause overwhelming infections in severely affected persons. By testing lymphocytes with isotype-specific anti-Ig Abs and with nucleic acid probes for gene segments of various Ig and TCR gene segments, some defects have been localized to particular steps in the development of B and T cells.

Infantile X-Linked Agammaglobulinemia

X-linked agammaglobulinemia is seen in very young male children or infants, who begin to suffer from recurrent bacterial (pyogenic) infections at about 9 to 12 months of age, when maternal Igs received transplacentally have disappeared (see Fig. 16–11). These patients form virtually no Abs or plasma cells following immunization, and serum Igs of all classes are almost entirely absent (IgG is reduced to less than 10% and IgA and IgM to about 1% or less of the normal level; Chap. 16, Fig. 16–12, Fig. 20–13). Family pedigrees show inheritance from

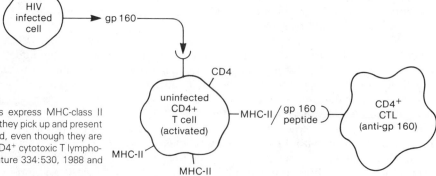

Figure 20–12. Activated human CD4 T cells express MHC-class II proteins and can serve as Ag-presenting cells. If they pick up and present gp160 from HIV-infected cells, they can be killed, even though they are not infected by HIV, by autologous anti-gp160 CD4$^+$ cytotoxic T lymphocytes (CTL). Based on Lanzavecchia A et al. Nature 334:530, 1988 and Siciliano RF et al. Cell, 54:561, 1988.

TABLE 20–3. Some Tests Used To Identify Individuals Suspected to Be Immunodeficient

Tests for B-cell functions	Serum Ig levels*
	Serum Ab levels†
	Biopsies examined for plasma cells by histologic methods and immunofluorescence‡
	Viable blood lymphocytes stained for surface Igs (also stained to test for regeneration of surface Igs after these are removed by treating the cells with trypsin)
Tests for T-cell functions	Skin tests for delayed-type hypersensitivity§
	Rosette formation with sheep red blood cells
	Lymphocyte proliferation induced by plant mitogens (phytohemagglutinin or concanavalin A) or by incubation with allogeneic lymphocytes¶

* Radial immunodiffusion (Ch. 3, Fig. 13–25) is preferred. It requires little serum (about 10 μl), and it is accurate ($\pm$10%), not too slow (24 hours), and relatively sensitive ($\geq$10 μg/ml): with radiolabeled anti-Igs, the sensitivity can be increased 1000-fold to where, for instance, 0.001 μg/ml of IgE can be detected. The distribution of Ig levels in the normal population is essentially bell-shaped and lacks the discontinuities that permit sharp definition of an Ig deficiency. By common agreement, deficient levels are <2 mg/ml for IgG and <10 μg/ml for IgA.

† Commonly measured are "natural" Abs to blood group substances A and B or to sheep RBCs or *E. coli* or Abs induced by immunization with potent, harmless, and potentially helpful Ags, such as diphtheria and tetanus toxoids and *Bordetella pertussis* (triple vaccine) or polysaccharides from pneumococci, or *Haemophilus influenzae* or *Neisseria meningitidis*.

‡ Plasma cells are sought in biopsies of lymph nodes that drain intracutaneous sites of injection of Ags or in biopsy of the rectal mucosa, whose lamina propria layer normally contains many plasma cells (IgA-containing).

§ The Ags injected intradermally are derived from prevalent microbes, such as mumps virus, tuberculin (from *Mycobacterium tuberculosis*), streptokinase–streptodornase from hemolytic streptococci, and culture media supernatants from various fungi (e.g., *Candida, Trichophyton, Coccidioides* [useful in California], or *Histoplasma* [useful in Mississippi Valley]; see Chap. 19, Fig. 19–1.). Skin patch tests are performed after deliberate skin sensitization with 2,4-dinitrochlorobenzene (Chap. 19, Fig. 19–21).

¶ Blast transformation can be evaluated by changes in cell morphology, by radioautography or by measuring the incorporation of ^{3}H-thymidine into DNA. For the mixed lymphocyte reaction, see Ch. 15.

the mother (hence the X-linked designation), but no genetic markers are yet known for heterozygous women, who transmit the defect to half their male progeny. Studies of DNA from diverse members of affected families (by analysis of restriction fragment-length polymorphisms)

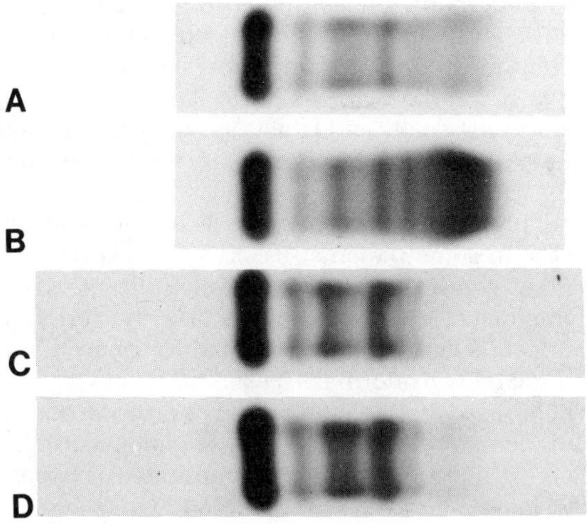

Figure 20–13. Agammaglobulinemia revealed by electrophoresis of human sera. *(A)* Normal serum. *(B)* Serum with elevated heterogeneous Igs (polyclonal hypergammaglobulinemia). *(C, D)* Sera from children with virtual absence of Igs. Serum albumin in the compact dark band at the left. Arrows point to immunoglobulin region. (Courtesy of Dr C K Osterland)

have localized the responsible gene(s) to the long arm of the X chromosome. In some families, male cousins of an affected patient have depressed serum Igs but not the virtual absence of Igs seen in the classically affected individual.

The underlying defect appears to be an inability to rearrange Ig V gene segments. Thus, affected individuals appear to have a normal number of bone marrow cells of the early B lineage; i.e., with truncated μ chains and short RNA transcripts having Cμ sequences. Whether only Cμ gene segments are transcribed, or whether the cells have D $\rightarrow$ J$_H$ rearrangements and produce "Dμ" chains (Chap. 16, Fig. 16–5) is not clear.

In contrast to the B cells, the T cells in affected children are normal in number, subset distribution, and function. **Because these children generally recover without difficulty from measles, mumps, and other viral diseases of childhood, it appears that resistance to most virus infections is attributable to T-cell-mediated immunity rather than to Abs.** However, defenses against some viruses evidently require Abs, for these patients are at risk of developing poliomyelitis from vaccination with live attenuated poliovirus, and they can have persistent gastrointestinal tract rotavirus infections. They can also have pneumonia caused by *Pneumocystis carinii*, an opportunistic fungus that often causes pneumonia in patients with AIDS (see above). Some individuals, now about 30 years of age, have been treated since infancy with periodic administration of pooled human Ig. Injected at approximately monthly intervals, the Ig is able to maintain serum Ig at approximately normal levels and largely to prevent recurrent bacterial infections.

Ig Deficiency with Increased IgM (and IgD)

In another heritable Ig deficiency (possibly also X-linked), serum levels of IgM, and sometimes of IgD, are elevated, but all other Ig classes are greatly depressed. It should be recalled (Chap. 16) that a shift from IgM to IgD synthesis entails alternative splicing of a rearranged H-chain gene's primary RNA transcript, whereas a shift from IgM to IgG and to all other H-chain isotypes requires translocation ("switching") of a rearranged V_HDJ_H assembly of gene segments (to a downstream position on the same chromosome next to one of the other C_H gene segments; Fig. 16–2, Chap. 16). The underlying defect could thus involve either an enzyme that is responsible for translocation of V_HDJ_H or the "switching" sequences that the enzyme recognizes (Fig. 14–40, Chap. 14). Affected individuals are subject to recurrent bacterial infections, but their T cells are normal in number and function, and their cellular immunity is intact. Why IgM (and IgD) are elevated is not clear.

Selective IgA Deficiency

About 1 in 700 persons is estimated to be deficient in serum IgA. Many are asymptomatic, but about half are said to be subject to recurrent infections or (surprisingly) to autoimmune diseases. As noted in Chapter 14, there are two IgA subclasses in humans; IgA1 predominates in serum and in bone marrow plasma cells, whereas IgA1 and IgA2 are about equally abundant in secretions and in plasma cells of the mucosa of intestine and various exocrine glands. Most IgA-deficient individuals lack both serum and secretory IgA, but some lack only serum IgA1. About half the patients with IgA deficiency are also deficient in IgE. From what is now known about the regulatory effects of IL-4 on IgE and IgA (Chap. 16), it seems possible that IgA deficiency is secondary to a defect in IL-4 secretion by T_H cells or in the B-cell receptor for this lymphokine.

Other Immunoglobulin Deficiencies

PARTICULAR ISOTYPES. In certain individuals, the serum level of total Ig is normal, whereas a particular isotype (either κ chain or IgG2 or IgG3 or IgG4) is greatly depressed or absent. The presence of chronic or recurrent infections in these individuals probably accounts for the careful study of their Igs; without such studies, a selective isotype defect would be easily overlooked. Hence, it is difficult to assess the overall prevalence of such disorders in the population.

TRANSIENT HYPOGAMMAGLOBULINEMIA OF INFANCY. Normally, total serum Ig levels in infants are at their lowest at about 6 months after birth, as maternally derived Ig becomes fully degraded and the infant's Ig biosynthesis is still poorly developed (Chap. 16, Fig. 16-11). By 1 year, serum IgM and IgG are about 20% of normal adult levels, and IgA is much lower. However, the onset of Ig production, particularly of IgG, is retarded for 1 to 2 years in some infants. Their B cells appear normal but are diminished in their response to lectin (pokeweed mitogen) stimulation of Ig production, possibly a result of retarded maturation. Some of these infants have recurrent infections. Spontaneous recovery is complete by 1 to 2 years of age.

COMMON VARIABLE Ig DEFICIENCY. A clinical syndrome occurring in males or females resembles X-linked agammaglobulinemia (see above), but it can occur at any age, and the patients have B cells. In some patients, these cells are not stimulated to develop into plasma cells when Ags or mitogens are added to peripheral blood cells, perhaps because their T_H cells are defective. The disease is often familial and associated with a high incidence of diverse autoimmune diseases (SLE, hemolytic anemia, idiopathic thrombocytopenic purpura) in close relatives; many of these patients have pernicious anemia (see Autoimmune Disease, this chapter). The basis for these associations is not understood.

T-CELL DEFICIENCIES
Severe Combined Immunodeficiency Disease (SCID)

Within a few months after birth, infants with SCID develop widespread cutaneous yeast (monilia) infections, severe pneumonia caused by *Pneumocystis carinii* (see also AIDS and X-linked agammaglobulinemia), and other recurrent infections with opportunistic microbes. Infections with common viruses (varicella, herpes, and cytomegalovirus) usually end fatally, as do mistaken attempts to induce immunity by injecting live vaccines such as BCG or vaccinia.

The number of circulating T cells is low, as are serum Ig levels. In some patients, T cells fail to express HLA-A, -B, and -C genes ("bare lymphocyte" syndrome). The underlying defect probably varies in severity, and in some patients, B cells have been reported to behave normally when mixed with normal T cells.

The disease in man is inherited as an autosomal or X-linked recessive trait. Many of these patients also have a deficiency in the **adenosine deaminase** enzyme (see below).

Untreated, this disease is fatal within a few years of birth. Although these patients are exquisitely sensitive to GVH disease (see Transplantation Biology, this chapter), bone marrow transplants have recently been highly successful in long-lasting restoration of the immune system. The success is attributable to the introduction of procedures for eliminating mature T cells from the transplanted populations of bone marrow cells (e.g., with Abs to CD3, plus C). This precaution has eliminated the need to limit bone marrow transplants to those situations in which donor and recipient are MHC identical. Indeed, parental bone marrow, which is only half MHC identical ("haploidentical"), has been successfully engrafted into affected children. With female donors and male recipients, the donor's cells can be identified in the light microscope by their Barr body formed from one of the two X chromosomes per female cell. This test has shown that such recipients are **permanent chimeras:** their lymphocytes are entirely of donor origin.

SCID with Adenosine Deaminase Deficiency

Severe combined immunodeficiency is inherited as either an X-linked or an autosomal recessive disorder. About half of those with the autosomal pattern of inheritance also lack the enzyme adenosine deaminase. Although this enzyme is present in all mammalian cells, its deficiency appears to be deleterious only for lymphocytes, and particularly for thymocytes.

These cells have an active kinase and readily accumulate levels of adenosine and deoxyadenosine mono, di, and triphosphates that are toxic, perhaps because they inhibit ribonucleotide reductase and block DNA synthesis. These purine nucleotides also inhibit enzymes in the pathway that generates S-adenosylmethionine for the transfer of methyl groups and methylation of DNA. Preliminary evidence suggests that high levels of adenosine, deoxyadenosine, and deoxyguanosine can activate an endogenous endonuclease in thymocytes, causing cell death with cleavage of DNA at the junction of nucleosomes (as in target cells that are killed by cytotoxic T lymphocytes or other means; see Chap. 19, Fig. 19–16.

The disease can be corrected by transplanting bone marrow from normal (partially HLA-matched) donors: a few patients treated in this way have remained healthy chimeras for more than 10 years with normal T and B cells of donor origin; other Ag-presenting cells are of recipient origin. Although donor and recipient cells are not HLA identical, they are mutually tolerant and cooperate in supporting normal immune responses.

SCID Mice

A similar heritable disease is found in certain mice (SCID mice), in which **the defect has been tracked to inability to rearrange both Ig and TCR gene segments; hence the absence of functional B and T cells.**

When injected with human peripheral blood lymphocytes, these mice develop a functional immune system that produces human Igs, and they even respond to immunization by producing human Abs. A more durable human immune system has been engrafted in these mice by transplanting into them bits of human fetal thymus, fetal liver (as a source of stem cells), and fetal lymph nodes. The mice eventually develop mature human T and B cells. With a functional human immune system, they may provide a valuable model for experimental study of HIV infection and AIDS as well as other immune reactions and potential therapies.

Selected Reading

AUTOIMMUNE DISEASE: REVIEWS

Davidson A, Shefner R, Livneh A, Diamond B: The role of somatic mutation of immunoglobulin genes in autoimmunity. Annu Rev Immunol 5:85, 1987
Eisenberg RA, Cohen PL: Mechanisms of autoantibodies in systemic lupus erythematosus. Clin Aspects Autoimmunity 2:8, 1988
Kofler R, Dixon FJ, Theofilopoulos AN: The genetic origin of autoantibodies. Immunol Today 8:374, 1987
Lindstrom J: Immunobiology of myasthenia gravis, experimental autoimmune myasthenia gravis, and Lambert–Eaton syndrome. Annu Rev Immunol 3:109, 1985
Oldstone MBA: Molecular mimicry and autoimmune disease. Cell 50:819, 1987
Rossini AA, Mordes JP, Like AA: Immunology of insulin-dependent diabetes mellitus. Annu Rev Immunol 3:289, 1985
Schwartz RS: Autoantibodies and normal antibodies: Two sides of the same coin. The Harvey Lectures Series 81:53, 1987
Singer KH, Mashimoto K, Jensen PJ, Morioka S, Lazarus GS: Pathogenesis of autoimmunity in pemphigus. Annu Rev Immunol 3:87, 1985
Todd JA, Acha–Orbea H, Bell JI et al: A molecular basis for MHC class II-associated autoimmunity. Science 240:1003, 1988

AUTOIMMUNE DISEASE: SPECIFIC ARTICLES

Chan EKL, Tan EM: Human autoantibody-reactive epitopes of SS-B/La are highly conserved in comparison with epitopes recognized by murine monoclonal antibodies. J Exp Med 166:1627, 1987
Dersimonian H, Schwartz RS, Barrett KJ, Stollar BD: Relationship of human variable region heavy chain germ-line genes to genes encoding anti-DNA autoantibodies. J Immunol 139:2496, 1987
Livneh A, Halpern A, Perkins D, Lazo A, Halpern R, Diamond B: A monoclonal antibody to a cross-reactive idiotype on cationic human anti-DNA antibodies expressing λ light chains: A new reagent to identify a potentially differential pathogenic subset. J Immunol 138:123, 1987
Schwartz RS, Stollar BD: Origins of anti-DNA autoantibodies. J Clin Invest 75:321, 1985
Shizuru JA, Taylor–Edwards C, Banks BA, Gregory AK, Fathman CG: Immunotherapy of the nonobese diabetic mouse: Treatment with an antibody to T-helper lymphocytes. Science 240:659, 1988
Shlomchik MJ, Marshak–Rothstein A, Wolfowicz CB, Rothstein TL, Weigert MG: Role of clonal selection and somatic mutation in autoimmunity. Nature 328:805, 1987

TRANSPLANTATION IMMUNITY: REVIEWS

Bach FH, Sachs DH: Transplantation immunology. N Engl J Med 317:489, 1987
Snell GD, Dausset J, Nathenson S: Histocompatibility. New York, Academic Press, 1976
Yunis EJ, DuPont B: The HLA system. In Nathans D, Oski FA (eds):

Hematology of Infancy and Childhood, 3rd ed, pp 1522–1548. Philadelphia, WB Saunders, 1987

TRANSPLANTATION IMMUNITY: SPECIFIC ARTICLES

Billingham RE, Brent L, Medawar PB: Actively acquired tolerance of foreign cells. Nature 172:603, 1953

Madsen JC, Superina RA, Wood KJ, Morris PJ: Immunological unresponsiveness induced by recipient cells transfected with donor MHC genes. Nature 332:161, 1988

Russell PS, Chase CM, Colvin RB, Plate JMD: Kidney transplants in mice: An analysis of the immune status of mice bearing long-term H-2 incompatible transplants. J Exp Med 147:1449, 1469, 1978

Sachs DH, Suzuki T, Sundt TM, Sykes M: A new approach to bone marrow transplantation across MHC barriers. In Gale RP, Champlin CR (eds): Bone Marrow Transplantation: Current Controversies, vol 91. New York, Alan R. Liss, (in press)

TUMOR IMMUNOLOGY: REVIEWS

Boon T: Tum⁻ variants: Immunogenic variants obtained by mutagen treatment of tumor cells. Immunol Today 6:307, 1985

Herlyn M, Koprowski H: Melanoma antigens: Immunological and biological characterization and clinical significance. Annu Rev Immunol 6:283, 1988

Schreiber H, Ward PL, Rowley DA, Strauss HF: Unique tumor-specific antigens. Annu Rev Immunol 6:465, 1988

Vitetta ES, Uhr JW: Immunotoxins. Annu Rev Immunol 3:197, 1985

TUMOR IMMUNOLOGY: SPECIFIC ARTICLES

Cleary ML, Chao J, Warnke R, Sklar J: Immunoglobulin gene rearrangement as a diagnostic criterion of B-cell lymphoma. Proc Natl Acad Sci USA 81:593, 1984

Cleary ML, Meeker TC, Levy S, Lee T, Treia M, Sklar J, Levy R: Clustering of extensive somatic mutations in the variable region of an immunoglobulin heavy chain gene from a human B cell lymphoma. Cell 44:97, 1986

Houghton AN, Mintzer D, Cordon–Cardo C et al: Mouse monoclonal IgG3 antibody detecting GD3 ganglioside: A Phase I trial in patients with malignant melanoma. Proc Natl Acad Sci USA 82:1242, 1985

Korsmeyer SJ, Bakhshi A, Siminovitch K, Arnold A, Waldmann T: Immunoglobulin genes in human leukemias and lymphomas as markers of clonality, differentiation, and translocation. In Fairbanks VF (ed): Current Hematology and Oncology, vol 4, p 39, 1986

Liu MA, Nussbaum SR, Eisen HN: Hormone conjugated with antibody to CD3 mediates cytotoxic T cell lysis of human melanoma cells. Science 239:395, 1988

Rayner AA, Grimm EA, Lotze MT, Chu EW, Rosenberg SA: Lympho-kine activated killer (LAK) cells: Analysis of factors relevant to the immunotherapy of human cancer. Cancer 55:1327, 1985

Real FX, Mattes MJ, Houghton AN, Oettgen HF, Lloyd KO, Old LJ: Class I (unique) tumor antigens on human melanoma: Identification of a 90,000 dalton cell surface glycoprotein by autologous typing. J Exp Med 160:1219, 1984

Tanaka K, Isselbacher KJ, Khoury G, Jay G: Reversal of oncogenesis by the expression of a major histocompatibility complex class I gene. Science 228:26, 1985

IMMUNODEFICIENCY DISEASES: REVIEWS

Kantoff PW, Freeman SM, Anderson WF: Prospects for gene therapy for immunodeficiency diseases. Ann Rev Immunol 6:581, 1988

Rosen FS, Cooper MD, Wedgwood RJP: The primary immunodeficiencies. The New England J Med 311:235, 300, 1984

IMMUNODEFICIENCY DISEASES: SPECIFIC ARTICLES

Clayton LK, Hussey RE, Steinbrich R, Ramachandran H, Husain Y, Reinherz EL: Substitution of murine for human CD4 residues identifies amino acids critical for HIV-gp120 binding. Nature 335:363, 1988

Lanzavecchia A, Roosnek E, Gregory T, Berman P, Abrignani S: T cells can present antigens such as HIV gp120 targeted to their own surface molecules. Nature 334:530, 1988

McCune JM, Namikawa R, Kaneshima H, Shultz LD, Lieberman M, Weissman IL: The SCID-Hu mouse: Murine model for analysis of human hematolymphoid differentiation and function. Science 241:1632, 1988

Mosier DE, Gulizia RJ, Baird SM, Wilson DB: Transfer of a functional human immune system to mice with severe combined immunodeficiency. Nature 335:256, 1988

Saag MS, Hahn BH, Gibbons J et al: Extensive variation of human immunodeficiency virus type I in vivo. Nature 334:440, 1988

Schwaber J, Molgaard H, Orkin SH, Gould HJ, Rosen FS: Early pre-B cells from normal and X-linked agammaglobulinemia produce C_μ without an attached V_H region. Nature 304:355, 1983

Sethi KK, Näher H, Stroehmann I: Phenotypic heterogeneity of cerebrospinal fluid-derived HIV-specific and HLA-restricted cytotoxic T-cell clones. Nature 335:178, 1988

Shearer GM, Bernstein DC, Tung KSK et al: A model for the selective loss of major histocompatibility complex self-restricted T cell immune responses during the development of acquired immune deficiency syndrome (AIDS). J Immunol 137:2514, 1986

Siliciano RF, Lawton T, Knall C et al: Analysis of host-virus interactions in AIDS with anti-gp120 T cell clones: Effect of HIV sequence variation and a mechanism for CD4⁺ cell depletion. Cell 54:561, 1988

Walker BD, Chakrabarti S, Moss B et al: HIV-specific cytotoxic T lymphocytes in seropositive individuals. Nature 328:345, 1987

Walker BD, Flexner C, Paradis TJ et al: HIV-1 reverse transcriptase is a target for cytotoxic T lymphocytes in infected individuals. Science 240:64, 1988

Part Three

Pathogenic Bacteria

21

Samuel C. Silverstein
Thomas H. Steinberg

Host Defense against Bacterial and Fungal Infections

Pathogenicity: Infection versus Disease

In utero, the mammalian fetus is bathed in sterile amniotic fluid and is protected against the microbial world by its mother's defense mechanisms. After birth, the skin, mucous membranes, and intestinal tract rapidly become colonized with large numbers of **nonpathogenic** microorganisms. These **commensals** (Chap. 42) live in favorable ecological niches within the host and under normal circumstances do not cause disease. They include lactobacilli, bacteroides, some strains of streptococci that inhabit the mouth, various enterobacteria, and *Candida*, as well as the potentially more pathogenic staphylococci and pneumococci. When a break in host defenses allows these organisms access to hitherto protected tissues or environments they may cause disease. In contrast, highly virulent pathogens usually produce disease whenever they colonize the host.

Most pathogens are eradicated completely at about the time that clinical manifestations of infection disappear, but with some organisms the host may remain persistently infected after recovery. Infections that may later relapse (e.g., with tubercle bacilli or the treponemes of syphilis) are called **dormant,** whereas hosts with nonrelapsing infections (e.g., with typhoid or diphtheria bacilli) are said to be **carriers** of the organism (see below). This text accepts the traditional practice of using the term "**infection**" in an ambiguous manner, as a synonym for either **colonization** or **disease.** Nevertheless,

485

the distinction is often fundamental for understanding pathogenesis and for evaluating reports from the diagnostic laboratory. For example, viridans streptococci colonize the throats of over 90% of humans, where they do not cause disease; but their repeated presence in the blood, which normally is sterile, signifies bacterial endocarditis, a life-threatening illness. In sites such as the throat or intestine, where the endogenous flora includes many different organisms, it is essential to understand which are part of the normal flora and which are likely to be causing disease.

THE BALANCE BETWEEN HEALTH AND DISEASE: AN ECOLOGICAL VIEWPOINT

Considering the huge number of organisms that inhabit our bodies (estimated to equal the number of our own cells), it is astonishing that they attack us so infrequently. The explanation lies in the many mechanical, chemical, cellular, and immunologic mechanisms that have evolved to prevent invasion. Modest impairment of one or more of these defense systems shifts the precarious balance existing with organisms of intermediate virulence, whereas severe impairment permits even nonpathogens to invade and cause disease. Infections that occur as a consequence of impaired host defenses are termed "**opportunistic.**" They have become increasingly commonplace as a result of immunosuppression by drugs, by radiation therapy, and by the disease AIDS. In addition, cytotoxic drugs and radiation impair mucosal barriers by inhibiting the regeneration of epithelial cells. Paradoxically, use of antibiotics also may lower host resistance by altering the competing normal bacterial flora on the skin and mucous membranes.

We tend to take a theatrical view of disease-causing organisms, casting the organisms as villains and our physiological defenses as heroes. Satisfying as this anthropomorphic view may be, the evolutionary biologist sees the host–parasite relationship in terms of ecological niches and long-standing adaptations. If an organism has no reservoir in the natural environment and has a narrow host range, overwhelming virulence would be a disadvantage; it would be selected against, because by rapidly eliminating the host, it would prevent further spread of the organism. Accordingly, we find that pneumococci, which are restricted to a small number of host species, exhibit a fine balance between growth and virulence: they colonize the oropharynx of normal individuals at a density sufficient for their transmission to others, and in this way, they persist. It is when they are aspirated into the lower respiratory tract in large numbers that they cause disease.

Occasionally, the same adaptations that facilitate an organism's survival in nature permit it to cause disease in man. An example is the capacity of the Leigonnaire's

disease bacillus to grow in human macrophages. In nature these bacteria grow in association with freshwater algae, and both are ingested by common soil amebae. However, unlike the algae, *Legionella* have evolved the capacity to escape the ameba's microbicidal and digestive armamentarium, so they also grow within the amebae and kill them. When the bacteria are aerosolized and inhaled by humans, they are phagocytosed by alveolar macrophages in the lower respiratory tree, and they grow in these cells just as they do in soil amebae. To these bacteria, the intracellular environment of the two hosts must appear similar.

Other organisms can adapt to many environments and hosts. For example, *Enterobacteriaceae*, a group of closely related species, are widely distributed in terrestrial habitats as well as in humans and other animals, although different species are adapted to different hosts or environments.

Those bacteria that are highly lethal for man usually have stable reservoirs, either in other animals, in carriers, or in the soil. The plague organism colonizes rats without killing them, and anthrax spores remain viable for many years in dry soil. With bacteria that live in both the intestine and the soil, the survival value of genes encoding toxins (e.g., tetanus toxin) is unknown.

A significant factor in the ecological interactions of bacteria and humans is the range of variation in resistance within the host species. Even the most devastating plagues have rarely eradicated all members of a community, and survival of the species may depend on the Darwinian lottery that makes some individuals genetically more resistant to some organisms and others to other organisms by a variety of mechanisms.

VIRULENCE

Whereas "**pathogenicity**" refers to the capacity of a microorganism to cause disease, the essentially synonymous term **virulence** is generally used to denote variations in degree. Virulence encompasses two features of an organism's disease-producing capacity: **infectivity** (i.e., the ability to colonize and invade a host) and **severity** of the disease that is produced. Virulence differs not only among microbial species but also among strains of the same species. **Virulence factors** are those components of an organism that determine its capacity to cause disease but do not affect its viability *per se*. Two principal classes have been characterized: **toxins** and **surface molecules.** For instance, the toxins secreted by diphtheria bacilli or by enteropathogenic *E. coli* are virulence factors but are not required for the growth of these organisms or for colonization of their hosts. The surface properties of bacteria can enhance their capacity to colonize, and so hence enhance their virulence, in two ways:

by promoting their **adhesion** to specific cells or by decreasing their attractiveness to **phagocytes.**

Virulence is a **polygenic** property of microorganisms: it can be affected by virtually any aspect of their physiology. This includes not only toxin production and surface properties, but also growth rate, nutritional requirements, efficiency of iron uptake, temperature sensitivity, and resistance to oxidant injury or to attack by enzymes. Moreover, as with higher organisms, the adaptation of a microorganism to its ecological niche depends on the **balanced interactions** (coadaptation) of its many genes and their products. Hence the insertion of a gene for a specific virulence factor into an unrelated nonpathogenic microbe cannot be expected to convert it into an effective pathogen. Gradual recognition of this fundamental evolutionary principle helped to still the controversy that arose in the 1970s over possible dangers from recombinant DNA technology.

Measurement of Virulence

The virulence of an organism, like the toxicity of a toxin or a drug, is usually expressed as the quantity of the organism that will infect or kill 50% of inoculated animals: this is expressed as the **infectious dose**$_{50}$ (ID_{50}) or the **lethal dose** (LD_{50}). The utility of these endpoints is illustrated in Figure 21–1, which compares the ID_{50} for outbred mice inoculated with *Salmonella enteritidis* via oral or subcutaneous routes. Notice that there is tremendous variability in the susceptibility of the mice to oral inoculation with this strain of salmonella: the relation between dose and infection is described by a shallow sigmoid curve, some mice being infected by as few as 1000 bacteria, whereas the least susceptible required

more than 100 million. The rate of change in infectivity with increasing dose was greatest at the inflection point of the sigmoid dose–response curve, which for a normally distributed population is given by the ID_{50}. Inbred strains of mice exhibit a much steeper curve, reflecting more uniform susceptibility.

Several factors had a profound influence on the efficiency of infection in this experiment. Efficiency was enhanced nearly 10,000-fold when the mice were inoculated subcutaneously rather than orally and nearly 100,000-fold when the normal intestinal flora was destroyed by treatment with the antibiotic streptomycin prior to oral inoculation. Other host factors that influence susceptibility include age, sex, genetic background, nutritional status, population density, and previous exposure to the organism.

LATENT INFECTIONS AND THE CARRIER STATE

In **latent (dormant)** infections, the offending microorganism is harbored within the body without causing evident pathology but can cause disease months or years later. Sometimes the reason for the emergence of the organisms is apparent: immunosuppressive or cytotoxic drugs can reactivate tuberculosis in an individual whose immunologic processes had been holding latent tubercle bacilli in check. Often, however, there is no obvious reason for reactivation.

A **carrier** of a disease-causing microorganism is a host that harbors the organism but is immune to the disease. This state is sometimes established without preceding illness. It is not known why some individuals but not others become carriers and continue to spread an

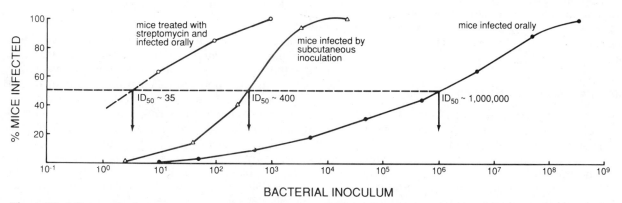

Figure 21–1. Percentage of mice infected after oral or subcutaneous inoculation with different numbers of *Salmonella enteritidis*. One group of mice was treated with streptomycin prior to oral inoculation. The ID_{50} for each condition is indicated. (Data from Miller CP and Bohnhoff M: J Inf Dis 111:107, 1962, and Bohnhoff M and Miller CP: J Inf Dis 111:117, 1962)

organism. Under epidemic conditions, the carrier rate may approach 100%, presumably because of continued reinfection.

The carrier state is often unstable, ending after a number of weeks (as after staphylococcal or beta-streptococcal infections). However, following some diseases, such as typhoid fever and gonorrhea (especially in women), individuals may remain carriers indefinitely, thereby providing a continual reservoir of infectious organisms. For instance, "Typhoid Mary," a cook who was a chronic carrier of *Salmonella typhi*, spread typhoid to more than 50 people.

Bacteria that form long-term associations with a carrier may be impossible to eradicate with antibiotic therapy alone. Carriers of *S. typhi* often harbor this organism in the gallbladder, and individuals with gallbladder stones who become carriers of *S. typhi* often cannot be cured of their carrier status without cholecystectomy. In an even more complex situation, adult schistosomes can harbor typhoid bacilli: in areas endemic for schistosomiasis, termination of an individual's typhoid carrier state may require eradication of the schistosome infestation.

Pathogenic Properties of Bacteria

Use of bacterial mutants and of modern methods in cell and molecular biology has revolutionized the study of pathogenicity. Specific pathways and gene products that permit various organisms to cause disease are rapidly being identified. The section that follows focuses on four specific pathogenetic mechanisms: **colonization of surfaces,** which may lead to local damage to cells; **invasion of tissues,** with consequent destruction of deeper cells and tissue architecture; **production of exotoxins and endotoxins,** which may act locally or at remote sites; and **elicitation of host inflammatory, allergic, and fibrotic reactions,** which may cause either temporary or permanent alterations in organ physiology. In addition, as indicated above, other factors influence adaptation to ecological niches within the host and within the environment.

COLONIZATION OF SURFACES

Virtually all moist surfaces provide fertile soil for microbial colonization. Because bacteria adhere well to organic materials that coat these surfaces it should be no surprise that they employ similar mechanisms when colonizing the mucous membranes and epithelia of animals. The factors responsible, **adhesins,** are better understood for pathogenic bacteria than for commensals. For instance, the fimbriae of some strains of *E. coli* that invade the urinary tract contain carbohydrate-specific receptors (**lectins**) that bind to mannose-containing oli-

gosaccharides on glycoproteins of bladder epithelium, thereby preventing the flow of urine from washing these organisms from the bladder. Similarly, surface glycosyl transferases on *Streptococcus mutans* promote its adherence to salivary glycoproteins adsorbed to the teeth, thereby promoting the formation of plaque and tooth decay.

The genetic make-up of the host can also affect susceptibility or resistance to bacterial colonization. For instance, *E. coli* serotypes K88 and K99 colonize the intestinal tract of some strains of piglets, but not of others or of other host species, which lack the **membrane receptors** to which these bacteria bind.

INVASION OF TISSUES

"Invasiveness" signifies the ability of an organism to penetrate into a tissue after it adheres to a cell surface. Most bacteria that adhere do not invade. However, many otherwise harmless bacteria can gain a foothold in tissues if mechanical or chemical injury allows them to penetrate the skin or intestine. Spread of these organisms may be aided by their secretion of enzymes such as collagenase (*Clostridia*) or plasminogen activator (streptococci).

Some bacteria can invade tissues in the absence of physical injury. Examples include *Neisseria meningitidis* in nasal epithelium, *Neisseria gonorrhoeae* in fallopian tubal epithelium, and salmonellae in intestinal epithelium. These organisms are endocytosed by epithelial cells, transported across these cells within vacuoles, and released into the submucosal space, from which they invade the underlying tissues (Fig 21–2). *Shigella* and enteroinvasive *E. coli* also are endocytosed by intestinal epithelial cells but do not penetrate the basement membrane. At least some of the genes determining invasiveness in enteropathogenic bacteria are carried by plasmids that encode bacterial surface proteins.

PRODUCTION OF TOXINS

Exotoxins

Table 21–1 lists some of the toxins secreted by bacteria commonly associated with human diseases. It is evident that the potency of these toxins varies enormously. Tetanus, botulinus, and shigella neurotoxins, which bind only to specialized cells, are among the most lethal molecules known; injection of 1 ng (about 10^7 molecules) is sufficient to kill a guinea pig. In contrast, much larger quantities of cholera and diphtheria toxins are needed to cause diarrhea and heart damage, respectively.

Despite detailed knowledge of the molecular anatomy and mechanisms of action of several of these toxins, their contributions to the success of the bacteria are not clear. The genes for some are located in **temperate bacteriophages** (diphtheria, botulinus, streptococcus erythrogenic toxin) or in **plasmids** (*E. coli* and staphylococcal

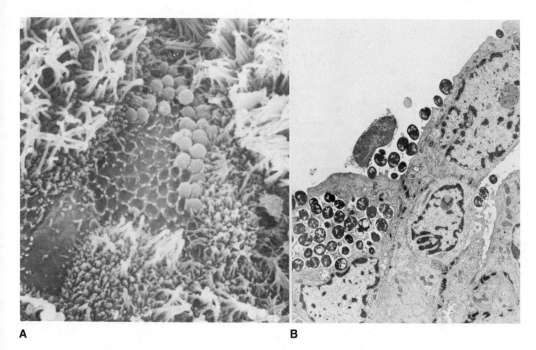

A   **B**

Figure 21—2. Role of nasal epithelial cells in the pathogenesis of meningitis. (Panel *A*) Scanning electron micrograph of *Neisseria meningitidis* adhering to human nasopharyngeal mucosal cells 6–8 hours after infection. (Panel *B*) Transmission electron micrograph of these cells phagocytizing the organisms 12–24 hours after infecton. The meningococci are transported across the epithelial cells within vacuoles and are released via exocytosis into the submucosal space, from which they invade the brain. Courtesy of DS Stephens, (From Stephens DS: J Inf Dis 148:369, 1983)

enterotoxins, staphylococcal exfoliatin), rather than in the bacterial chromosome. For these, the toxin probably has value for the survival of the phage or plasmid, as well as for the bacterium that harbors it.

Some toxins (botulinus, staphylococcal enterotoxin) are resistant to inactivation by gastric acid and intestinal proteases and are active when ingested. In fact, several types of botulinus toxin are converted to a more active form by intestinal proteases. Other toxins (tetanus, diphtheria) are inactivated by intestinal proteases; to cause disease, these toxins must be produced in or on the tissues. Chemical treatment of toxins (e.g., by formaldehyde) or mutation of their genes (e.g., by recombinant DNA techniques) converts them to **toxoids** (nontoxic but immunogenic molecules) that are used for prophylactic immunization. The genetic approach also lends itself to the development of live vaccines.

The toxins produced by various bacterial species can be grouped into classes on the basis of their mechanisms of action. The **neurotoxins,** such as tetanus and botulinus toxins, act by selectively binding to and blocking presynaptic terminals in the central nervous system. Tetanus toxin blocks inhibitory synapses, thereby causing unopposed activation of motor neurons and "tetanic" spasm of skeletal muscles.

Several unrelated bacterial species produce toxins that transfer ADP-ribose from NAD to host cell proteins. The initial cellular targets of these **ADP-ribosylating toxins** reflect the tissues infected by the bacteria that produce them. *Corynebacterium diphtheriae* infects the throat, and the initial lesion is toxin-mediated necrosis of the epithelium of the upper respiratory tract, followed by absorption of the toxin and intoxication of distant cells. With *Vibrio cholerae* and enterotoxigenic *E. coli*, the intestinal epithelium is the target.

Different toxins catalyze ADP-ribosylation of different proteins and exert distinct physiological effects. For example, the toxins that **block host-cell protein synthesis,** such as diphtheria and pseudomonas toxins, contain two peptide chains (called A and B) linked by disulfide bonds. The B chain promotes binding to receptors on host cells. Following this attachment these toxins are endocytosed, and acidification of the endocytic vacuole leads to transport of the A subunit across the vacuolar membrane into the host cell's cytoplasm. The A subunit is an enzyme that transfers ADP-ribose from NAD to elongation factor 2 (EF-2). The resulting block in protein synthesis is irreversible and highly efficient: a single toxin molecule can modify many EF-2 molecules and is sufficient to kill a susceptible cell.

TABLE 21-1. Bacterial Toxins

Toxin:	Structure*:	Gene Location:	Mechanism of Action:	Role in Disease:
Diphtheria toxin	A + B	Lysogenic phage	ADP-ribosylates and activates elongation Factor 2	Inhibits protein synthesis in animal cells
Cholera toxin	A + 5B	Bacterial chromosome	ADP ribosylates G proteins; stimulates adenylate cyclase	Promotes secretion of fluid and electrolytes in intestinal epithelium
Pertussis toxin	A + 5B	?	ADP ribosylates G proteins; blocks inhibition of adenylate cyclase	? Hypoglycemia
E. coli heat-labile toxin	A + 5B	Plasmid	ADP ribosylates G proteins; stimulates adenylate cyclase	Promotes secretion of fluid and electrolytes from intestinal epithelium
E. coli heat-stable toxin	A	Plasmid	Activates guanylate cyclase	Promotes secretion of fluid and electrolytes from intestinal epithelium
Botulinum toxin	A + B†	Phage	?	Inhibits neurotransmission in cholinergic synapses
Tetanus toxin	A + B	Plasmid	?	Inhibits neurotransmission in inhibitory synapses
Adenylate cyclases of *Bordetella pertussis* and *Bacillus anthracis*	A A + B	?	Increase cyclic AMP in phagocytes	? Inhibit phagocytosis by neutrophils

* A denotes peptide chain with enzymatic activity; B denotes peptide chain that mediates binding to the cell surface.

† There are eight immunologically distinct but structurally similar botulinum toxins.

The **enterotoxins,** such as those produced by *Vibrio cholerae* and enterotoxigenic *E. coli,* are composed of five B (binding) chains surrounding an A chain. Once within the cytoplasm of an epithelial cell, the A chain catalyzes the ADP-ribosylation of regulatory G proteins (which bind and hydrolyze GTP), and the resulting activation of adenyl cyclase* initiates a series of enzymatic reactions that cause profuse electrolyte and water secretion by the small intestine. Unlike diphtheria toxin, cholera toxin does not have to be endocytosed: its enzymatically active subunit enters its host cell's cytoplasm via direct penetration of the plasma membrane. *Bordetella pertussis* produces a toxin that also ADP-ribosylates G proteins, thereby affecting the generation of intracellular second messengers.

Childhood immunization against diphtheria, pertussis, and tetanus (the familiar DPT vaccine) is highly effective. The vaccine works by inducing the formation of Abs that neutralize the toxins produced by the bacteria.

Several common pathogens, such as clostridia, staphylococci, and streptococci, produce **hemolysins,** proteins that lyse red blood cells. Streptococcal hemolysins produce lesions in red cell membranes (see Fig. 24-8) that resemble the holes produced by the terminal components of the complement cascade (Chap. 17). Al-

though hemolysis itself is unlikely to be important in pathogenesis, these hemolysins can also destroy other host cells, including phagocytic leukocytes.

Endotoxins

Unlike the secreted exotoxins, endotoxins are **endoge**nous **toxic** components: the lipopolysaccharides (LPS) from the outer membranes of gram-negative bacteria (Chap. 2). Endotoxins exert a wide spectrum of effects on the host, the most dramatic of which are fever and the shock syndrome associated with gram-negative bacterial sepsis. Endotoxin exerts its effects both directly, by its actions on complement proteins and granulocytes, and indirectly, by the products it stimulates endothelial cells and macrophages to express and secrete. Some of the mechanisms are discussed below (see TNF/Cachectin).

The endotoxic activity of LPS resides in its lipid A moiety (but its biological potency is affected by the attached polysaccharide moiety). Lipid A is not destroyed by autoclaving; hence infusion of a sterile solution containing endotoxin can cause serious illness.

ADAPTIVE VARIATIONS IN VIRULENCE

It has long been recognized that the adaptation of bacteria to various environments can affect their virulence: For example, the ID_{50} of tubercle bacilli is lower for bacteria taken from an infected animal than for the same strain from a culture. However, only after several decades of study of gene regulation in nonpathogens (primarily *E.*

---

* Elevation of host-cell cAMP is a strategy also employed by *Bacillus anthracis* to evade host defenses. This bacterium releases an adenyl cyclase that penetrates leukocytes, increasing their cAMP 100- to 1000-fold and thereby paralyzing their phagocytic capacity.

coli) has this approach begun to be applied to problems of pathogenesis. It is clear that infecting pathogens adapt not only to presence in the host but also to variations in their location in that host (including the presence in phagocytes).

Observed adaptations that affect survival in a host (i.e., virulence) include changes in the formation of fimbriae and flagella, in the amount of other surface Ags, in porin formation, in the secretion of toxins and enzymes, in chemotaxis, and in the assimilation of various nutrients. Although most regulatory environmental factors are still largely unknown, **iron** has long been recognized to play a decisive role in regulating the formation of diphtheria toxin and several other toxins. **Temperature** has a marked effect on the formation of various surface proteins in *Yersinia pestis*, which has to adapt to grow either in lice or in mammals; and cultivation at 30°C rather than 37° strikingly decreases the virulence of *Shigella*.

Coordinate regulatory mechanisms in the bacteria are beginning to be identified: for example, in *V. cholerae*, a single gene, *toxR*, controls formation of toxin, fimbriae, and various outer membrane proteins. In addition to the mechanisms of gene regulation that influence the amounts of various gene products by immediately reversible induction or repression, **phase variation** (Chap. 7) gives rise to occasional changes in gene arrangement that cause cells to shift the nature of their surface Ags, and outgrowth of the variant then depends on selection by the host.

Antibacterial Defenses of the Host

The term "nonspecific" resistance has been used to describe the mechanical, chemical, and some of the humoral and cellular mechanisms that prevent colonization or infection of normal individuals with the sea of bacteria, yeast, fungi, and protozoa in the environment. In the sense that these defense mechanisms do not depend on specific immunologic responses to a microorganism, they are nonspecific. However, they are specific in the sense of being determined by the precise molecular characteristics of the host and of the microbe. A few truly are nonspecific: cilia mechanically "sweeping" particles from the bronchi, peristalsis emptying the intestine, tears washing the corneal epithelium, and urine flushing the urinary tract.

MICROBIAL ANTAGONISM

Our skin and mucous membranes are richly endowed with their own microbial flora. One of the most important host defenses against microbial pathogens is competition from the endogenous flora. The importance of this flora is well known to everyone who has experienced intestinal discomfort after antibiotic therapy. Changes in the composition of the endogenous flora create an ecological vacuum and hence an opportunity for overgrowth by other endogenous species of bacteria or for infection by exogenous bacteria. Thus *Clostridium difficile*, a minor endogenous species, has toxic effects on the colon when present at high concentration; and streptomycin treatment reduces by 10^5 the oral dose of *S. enteritidis* required to produce intestinal infection in mice (see Fig. 21–1).

The normal flora protects against colonization by potentially pathogenic bacteria in several ways. Besides competition for nutrients and effects on pH and pO_2, the streptococcal species that inhabit the oral cavity produce compounds that prevent the growth of most gram-negative and gram-positive cocci. *E. coli* in the gut produce colicins (Chap. 7) that are lethal to enteric pathogens such as *Salmonella* and *Shigella*, as well as organic acids that inhibit their growth.

Among the host factors that determine the quantity and quality of the "normal" microbial inhabitants of our bodies are the availability of oxygen, iron, and metabolizable nutrients such as glucose; the pH and temperature; and the chemistry of the various surfaces on which they grow. Similar factors determine the tissues and organs attacked by various pathogenic microorganisms and the routes they use to reach their targets. As with viruses, the mechanisms employed by the normal flora to bind to specific cells, and by pathogenic microorganisms to breach host defenses, all utilize receptors, cells, and pathways necessary for normal physiologic functions. Were this not so, natural selection would rapidly eliminate these receptors, cells, and pathways from the population.

Different microbial pathogens use various mechanisms to breach host defenses, and higher organisms therefore have developed a wide spectrum of defenses. These mechanisms, and the responses of the host, are detailed in the chapters describing specific pathogens. The rest of this chapter is devoted to a general overview of the cellular defenses and "nonspecific" humoral factors that microbes encounter as they attempt to invade mammalian hosts. Specific immunologic mechanisms have been discussed in Chapters 12 through 20.

SECRETORY AND HUMORAL MEDIATORS OF ANTIMICROBIAL DEFENSE

Bodily secretions, plasma, and interstitial fluids contain many proteins important in antimicrobial defense. The blood, interstitial fluids, and pulmonary secretions contain IgG and IgM Abs, C (complement) components, lysozyme, and fibronectin, whereas secretions in the gut contain IgA but not C or fibronectin. Binding of IgA to the bacterial surface inhibits attachment to mucosal surfaces, while Abs, C components, and fibronectin promote phagocytosis. In addition, C has microbicidal activity, and it may be viewed as the first line of defense. The ability of bacteria to survive encounters with these proteins is a critical determinant of their ability to cause disease.

Lysozyme

The enzyme lysozyme, which digests peptidoglycan (Chap. 2), is present in all body fluids, especially tears. Because it attacks most nonpathogenic gram-positive bacteria, it may be an important reason for their lack of pathogenicity. However, for lack of humans defective in this enzyme, its role has not been precisely defined.

Antibodies

The structure of Abs, and the mechanisms that control their formation, secretion, and function, have been described in earlier chapters.

Fibronectin

Fibronectin, a 220-Kd protein, is found both in plasma and as a component of extracellular matrices throughout the body. It binds to the surfaces of gram-positive cocci (staphylococci and streptococci) and promotes their adhesion to macrophages via this cell's fibronectin receptors. Its role in phagocytosis is discussed below.

Complement

The C system (Chap. 17) consists of some 14 structural proteins and five regulatory proteins. Two pathways for C activation are known. As indicated in Chapter 17, Ab complexed with Ag is a potent activator of the **classic pathway,** and Abs bound to the surfaces of bacteria also promote the deposition of C proteins. In addition, the surfaces of many microorganisms, such as the endotoxin-rich surfaces of unencapsulated gram-negative bacteria, directly activate the **alternative pathway.** The two pathways converge at the level of the third component, C3. Its activation leads to the deposition of C3b, which promotes lysis of gram-negative bacteria by assembly and insertion of the "late" components (C5–C9, the membrane-attack complex) into the outer membrane.

Hereditary deficiencies in various C components cause different patterns of increased risk for specific bacterial infections. For instance, deficiencies in the late-acting components (C5–C9) predispose individuals to disseminated infections with *Neisseria* but not with many other gram-negative bacteria. Given the requirement for these late components in bacteriolysis, it is surprising that the invasive potential of other bacterial strains is not increased. Perhaps this reflects the redundant nature of antibacterial defense mechanisms. Only in the rare instances when C3 is deficient is there a marked increase in susceptibility to many bacterial infections.

PHAGOCYTIC LEUKOCYTES

Phagocytic white blood cells are the primary line of cellular defense against microbial infection. In vertebrates,

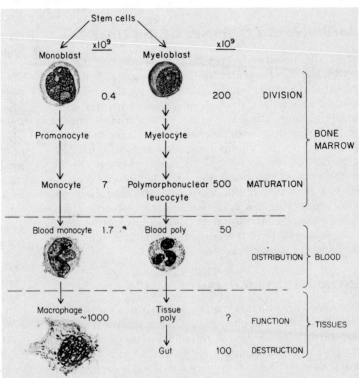

Figure 21–3. The development of mononuclear and polymorphonuclear phagocytes. Both cells are derived from stem cells in the bone marrow, which can form monoblasts or myeloblasts. After further differentiation, monocytes and polymorphonuclear leukocytes enter the blood, circulate, and migrate into various tissues.

there are two types: the polymorphonuclear phagocytes (neutrophils and eosinophils; also called **granulocytes**) and the **mononuclear phagocytes** (monocytes and macrophages). They have been termed "professional" phagocytes because eating is their principal occupation. Both polymorphonuclear and mononuclear phagocytes develop from a reservoir of precursor stem cells in the bone marrow (Fig. 21–3). **C**olony **s**timulating **f**actor 1 (CSF-1) promotes monocyte differentiation, **g**ranulocyte **c**olony **s**timulating **f**actor (G-CSF) promotes granulocyte differentiation (presumably by binding to a distinct stem-cell receptor), and **g**ranulocyte-**m**onocyte **c**olony **s**timulating **f**actor (GM-CSF) stimulates both granulocyte and monocyte differentiation.

We have little information about the factors that regulate **release** of monocytes and granulocytes from the bone marrow into the blood. The marrow contains nearly 10-fold the number of mature granulocytes found in the blood. Systemic infection with bacteria, but generally not with viruses, stimulates the release of both mature and immature granulocytes from the marrow into the circulation; hence the diagnostic value of assessing the number and maturity of circulating white blood cells. By contrast, most infections have little effect on the level of blood monocytes; but one exception, *Listeria monocytogenes*, causes a rise in blood monocytes in infected rabbits.

Granulocytes emerge from the marrow as **mature cells,** incapable of further replication and with a rela-

tively low capacity for synthesis of RNA and proteins. They circulate in the blood for 8 to 12 hours before migrating into the tissues, where they function for 1 or 2 more days and then die. In contrast, **mononuclear phagocytes** emerge from the marrow as **immature cells** called **monocytes,** which circulate in the blood for 2 to 4 days and then enter the tissues, where they mature into **macrophages** (Fig. 21–4). These cells are the **immobile phagocytes** that line the sinusoids of the liver (Kupffer cells) and spleen and are the principal phagocytic cells in lymph nodes, pulmonary alveoli, and serous cavities (pleural and peritoneal) of the body. They also are abundant in the brain (the microglia) and are present in large numbers in the connective tissues of the skin and intestinal tract and the synovial membranes of joints. Macrophages survive in each of these locations for weeks to months, ingesting many meals and, as described below, secreting many physiologically important substances. Collectively, they are termed the **mononuclear phagocyte system.**

The importance of granulocytes to health is dramatically illustrated by the disastrous effect of a spontaneous or iatrogenically induced reduction in their number. When there are fewer than 500 neutrophils per cubic millimeter of blood, bacterial infection and death are frequent. Moreover, genetic defects (see below) in the capacity of phagocytic leukocytes to emigrate from the blood into the tissues, or to kill bacteria, are associated with repeated bacterial and fungal infections.

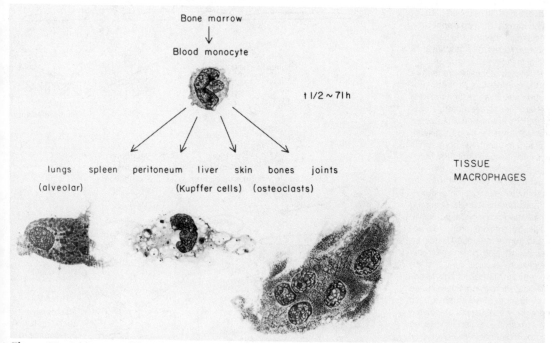

Figure 21–4. Monocyte differentiation. Morphologic characteristics of alveolar macrophages, Kupffer cells, and osteoclasts are shown.

Less widely appreciated are the roles of phagocytic leukocytes, primarily macrophages, in the turnover of cells. They engulf red blood cell nuclei extruded from maturing erythroid precursor cells in the bone marrow; they remove senescent red blood cells from the circulation; and they scavenge senescent cells, including neutrophils and lymphoid cells, in the tissues. The magnitude of this task is enormous. In the course of a year, the macrophages of an average adult ingest and digest more than 2.5 kg of senescent red blood cells alone.

Cellular Mechanisms of Antimicrobial Defense

THE HUNT

A phagocyte must find a bacterium before it can kill it. This is no small task, because phagocytes comprise a very small proportion of the total cells of the body. Their task is roughly analogous to that of a person trying to locate a few thousand rice grains scattered about a house. Fortunately, bacteria are not inert but produce chemical signals (**chemoattractants**) that draw phagocytic leukocytes. They also induce the host to produce chemoattractants and other factors that guide phagocytes from the blood to sites of infection in the tissues. Three independent pathways have evolved for this purpose, reflecting the importance for host survival of sensing microbial invasion.

Chemoattractants Formed by Bacteria

In contrast to animal cells, bacteria initiate synthesis of their proteins with N-formyl methionine; consequently, **N-formylated peptides** are byproducts of their secreted proteins. These small peptides diffuse freely within the intercellular spaces. Neutrophils and monocytes bear specific plasma-membrane receptors for N-formylated peptides such as N-formyl-methionyl-leucyl-phenylal-

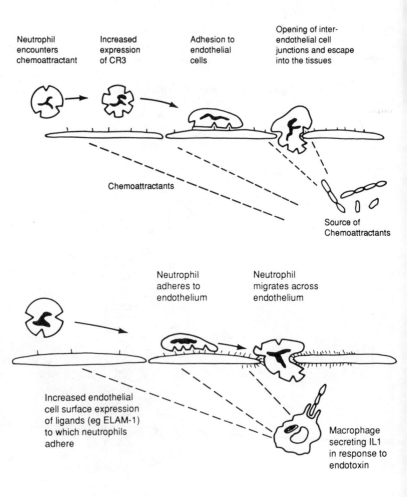

Figure 21–5. Polymorphonuclear leukocyte migration from the blood into the extravascular tissues in response to different types of stimuli. The **top panel** illustrates the effects of bacterial chemoattractants on neutrophils. Binding of these formylated peptides to specific neutrophil membrane receptors stimulates increased expression of leukocyte adhesion receptors (e.g., CR3) and activates these receptors, thereby promoting attachment of neutrophils to vascular endothelial cells. Formylated peptides also act as chemoattractants (within blood vessels) to regions containing a high concentration of chemoattractant (outside blood vessels). Guided by the chemoattractant gradient, the neutrophils crawl through the extravascular tissues until they reach the site of infection.

The **bottom panel** illustrates the effects of bacterial products (e.g., endotoxin) or cytokines (e.g., interleukin-1 or tumor necrosis factor) on endothelial cells. Depicted is a tissue macrophage ingesting gram-negative bacilli. Bacterial lipopolysaccharide (endotoxin) promotes secretion of interleukin-1 and tumor necrosis factor by macrophages. Both interleukin-1 and tumor necrosis factor induce endothelial cells to express new surface proteins, such as ELAM-1 (endothelial cell-leukocyte adhesion molecule 1). As indicated in the diagram these promote adherence and emigration of neutrophils from the vascular compartment in the absence of soluble chemoattractants. ELAM-1 expression also is induced by the interaction of endotoxin directly with endothelial cells.

anine (fMLP), whose binding stimulates neutrophils and monocytes to crawl from regions of low peptide concentration to regions of higher concentration. Neutrophils are able to sense a chemoattractant gradient of fMLP from the neutrophil's advancing lamellapodium to its tail end (Fig. 21–5).

Chemoattractants Formed by the Host

Many bacteria activate the complement pathway, thereby generating C5a, a cleavage product of the fifth C component. In addition, when suitably stimulated, neutrophils, monocytes, and macrophages synthesize and secrete **leukotriene B₄** (LTB₄, a metabolite of arachidonic acid). Both these products are chemoattractants for neutrophils and monocytes.

These chemoattractants also promote emigration of phagocytic leukocytes from the blood into the tissues (Fig. 21–6) by diffusing into the blood, binding to membrane receptors on neutrophils and monocytes, and thereby signalling in the number and the activity of adhesion-promoting surface receptors on these cells. Vascular endothelial cells express on their surfaces several molecules to which leukocyte adhesion receptors bind when they are activated, especially **ICAM-1** (**i**nter**c**ellular **a**dhesion **m**olecule). Adhesion is the first step in phagocyte movement into the tissues. The phagocytes migrate between endothelial cells, usually at the level of postcapillary venules, and then crawl into the tissues. Within the tissues they are guided toward sites of infection or tissue damage by the chemoattractant gradient, and the adhesion receptors also mediate attachment to epithelial cells and extracellular matrix components.

Phagocytes express at least three adhesion receptors on their surfaces: LFA-1 (**l**ymphocyte **f**unction **a**ntigen), CR3 (**c**omplement **r**eceptor), and p150/95. These **leukocyte adhesion receptors** are a family of heterodimeric molecules. Each receptor contains a unique alpha chain noncovalently bound to a common beta chain. In individuals with a genetic defect in beta chain formation the phagocytes exhibit markedly reduced or absent expression of all three receptors, and they are defective in their capacity to adhere to vascular endothelial cells, to emigrate from the vasculature, and to bind and ingest C-coated bacteria.

The interaction of chemoattractants with their receptors on neutrophils causes a marked increase in the number of leukocyte adhesion receptors, and it also activates their capacity to attach to endothelial cells. Chemoattractants also stimulate monocytes, but without increasing the number of their leukocyte adhesion receptors.

Postcapillary venules are the primary sites of phagocyte adhesion, opening of interendothelial cell junctions and emigration from the vascular compartment by crawling between the cells (Fig. 21–7). In general, neutrophils precede monocytes into damaged or infected tissues, but the factors that orchestrate this orderly procession have not been identified.

Cytokines

In addition to changes in the leukocytes, bacterial products can stimulate tissue macrophages to secrete locally acting hormones (**cytokines**) that increase adhesiveness of endothelial cells for neutrophils and monocytes. Bac-

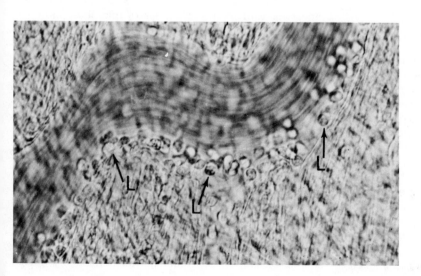

Figure 21–6. Unilateral sticking of leukocytes to the endothelium of the venule in the rabbit-ear chamber 30 min after injury. The leukocytes **(L)** are adhering to the endothelial surface nearest to the zone of injury, which is located below the vessel. (Allison F et al: J Exp Med 102:655, 1955) (×200)

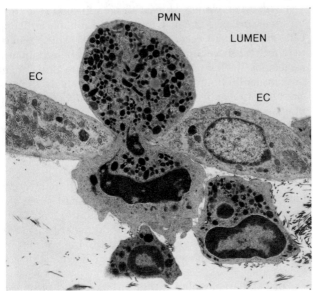

Figure 21–7. Electron micrograph of a PMN migrating from the luminal to the abluminal surface of a monolayer of endothelial cells in response to a gradient of chemoattractant. Note the close apposition between the PMN and the endothelial cells. (From Furie MB: J Cell Sci 88:161, 1987)

terial endotoxin stimulates macrophages to secrete **interleukin-1** (IL-1) and **tumor necrosis factor (TNF/cachectin*).** These cytokines induce endothelial cells to express a new class of surface receptors, called **endothelial–leukocyte adhesion molecules (ELAMs).** ELAMs facilitate the adhesion of phagocytes to the endothelium and their emigration from the vascular compartment, thus promoting the accumulation of phagocytes at sites of infection and inflammation, even in the absence of soluble chemoattractants.

PREPARING FOR A MEAL

Elie Metchnikoff, the father of cellular immunology, popularized the concept that engulfment of microbial pathogens by phagocytic cells plays an important role in host defense against infection. After a controversy with proponents of humoral immune mechanisms, such as von Behring and Ehrlich, the cellular and humoral theories of immunity began to converge in 1903, when Wright and Douglas reported that both heat-stable and heat-labile factors in plasma are required for optimal phagocytosis of bacteria by white blood cells. We now know that the principal heat-stable factors are Abs, the labile factors are C, and that these proteins promote bacterial engulfment by acting as **ligands** for receptors on the membranes of

* Tumor necrosis factor is also known as cachectin because of its capacity to block anabolic processes.

phagocytes. These proteins were called **opsonins** after the Greek word *opsonein* (to prepare for a meal). The three most important types are Abs of the IgM and IgG classes, proteins of the C cascade (especially C3), and fibronectin.

Many unencapsulated strains of bacteria bear surface oligosaccharides and lipids (endotoxin) that are ligands for receptors on phagocytes. Phagocytes ingest these bacteria in the absence of plasma opsonins. In general, such bacteria do not cause disease, but some are facultative intracellular pathogens (discussed below), such as the agents of tuberculosis, leprosy, and Legionnaires' disease.

Some common bacterial invaders are components of the normal flora of the skin or intestinal tract, and so the host is repeatedly immunized by their products. In contrast, the host may be first exposed to other organisms when they cause disease. In the absence of cross-reacting or natural Abs, it may take several days to more than a week until the immune system produces specific Abs against these organisms. Until then, the phagocytes will be unable to attack them: for example, encapsulated pneumococci, whose polysaccharide coat provides no ligands for receptors on phagocytes. However, once the host begins to produce Abs against the organisms, the phagocytes can begin to do their work.

Polymorphonuclear and mononuclear phagocytes do not have membrane receptors that recognize IgM. However, they have receptors for cleavage products of two of the principal complement components, C3 and C4, and IgM Abs directed against bacterial surface Ags promote binding of complement to those surfaces.

Receptors for Opsonins on Phagocytes

Phagocytic leukocytes express more than 40 different types of receptors on their plasma membranes. Those most relevant for phagocytosis of microbial pathogens are summarized in Table 21–2. Neutrophils, monocytes, and macrophages express two different receptors for C3: CR1 binds C3b and C4b, and CR3 binds C3bi, a proteolytic cleavage product of C3b. These phagocytes also express three different receptors (called **Fc receptors**) for the Fc portion of IgG. Macrophages, but not neutrophils or monocytes, have receptors for mannose-containing oligosaccharides, whereas fibronectin receptors are present on all three types of phagocytes.

In general, particles coated with oligomeric ligands bind to phagocytes much more efficiently than particles coated with monomeric ligands. Similarly, Ag–Ab complexes containing three or more IgG molecules are avidly ingested by phagocytes despite the vast molar excess of monomeric IgG in plasma. In both of these examples, it is the clustering of ligands, not a change in their conformation, that promotes their uptake by phagocytes.

TABLE 21–2. Macrophage Receptors

Receptor	Binds	Structure	Present on	Clinical Defect	Function
Fc receptor I (huFcγRI)	Monomers of IgG1 > IgG3 > IgG4 ≥ IgG2	72,000 M$_r$	Monocyte, macrophage	Subjects lacking FcRI appear to be healthy.	ADCC Phagocytosis ? Secretion†
Fc receptor II (huFcγRII)	Aggregates of IgG1, IgG3 > IgG2, IgG4	Transmembrane protein 42,000 M$_r$	Monocytes, macrophages, granulocytes, platelets		Clearance of immune complexes, phagocytosis, ? secretion†
Fc receptor III (huFcγRIII)	Aggregates of IgG1 = IgG3	Transmembrane/PI-anchored* 50–70,000 M$_r$	Macrophages, not monocytes, granulocytes, large granular lymphocytes		Clearance of immune complexes, phagocytosis, ? Secretion†
Mannose receptor	Oligosaccharides terminating in mannose, fucose, or N-acetyl-glucos-amine	175,000 M$_r$	Macrophages		Phagocytosis
Complement receptor 3 (CR3)	C3bi, fibrinogen factor X	αβ α-170,000 M$_r$ β-95,000 M$_r$	Monocytes, macrophages, granulocytes, large granular lymphocytes	⎫ Patients deficient in these three receptors have recurrent, severe bacterial and fungal infections ⎬	Adhesion, phagocytosis
LFA-1	ICAM-1	αβ α-180,000 M$_r$ β-95,000 M$_r$	Monocytes, macrophages, granulocytes, B and T lymphocytes		Adhesion
p150,95		αβ α-150,000 M$_r$ β-95,000 M$_r$	Monocytes, macrophages, granulocytes, large granular lymphocytes		Adhesion
Fibronectin receptor	Fibronectin oligomers	αβ α-160,000 M$_r$ β-130,000 M$_r$	Monocytes, macrophages	⎭	Adhesion, modulation of phagocytosis
f-Met-Leu-Phe receptor	fMLP	50,000–70,000 M$_r$	Monocytes, granulocytes		Chemotaxis, secretion†
C5a receptor	C5a	?	Monocytes, granulocytes		Chemotaxis, secretion†
LTB4 receptor	LTB4	?	Monocytes, granulocytes		Chemotaxis

* huFcγRIII on macrophages is a transmembrane protein. On neutrophils huFcγRIII does not have a membrane-spanning region; it is bound to the plasma membrane by a glycan phosphatidylinositol linkage.

† Secretion denotes generation of O$_2$ metabolites and arachidonate derivatives in addition to release of granular contents.

Phagocytosis

Phagocytes contact many different cells in the course of their travels around the body, but contact alone is not a signal for ingestion: the membrane receptors on the phagocyte also must transmit signals to the cytoplasm that cause pseudopod extension. The nature of these transmembrane signals is yet unknown. However, a great deal is known about the engulfment process itself.

Engulfment requires the sequential interaction of receptors on the surface of a phagocyte with ligands on the surface of a particle. This has been termed the "zipper" mechanism of phagocytosis (Fig. 21–8). Pseudopod extension is guided by the distribution of opsonic ligands (e.g., IgG or C) on a particle's surface. Receptors on the phagocyte bind to these ligands. Supporting this concept, spherical particles coated with ligands on only one hemisphere are not ingested; instead, the phagocyte adheres only to the particle's ligand-coated hemisphere.

The cytoplasmic motor that propels pseudopods around a particle appears to involve the actin-containing cytoskeleton. Thus, a dense meshwork of interconnected **actin filaments** is observed in the portion of a phagocyte's cytoplasm that is in contact with particles being engulfed; actin filament assembly is stimulated during phagocytosis; and drugs that block this assembly, such as cytochalasins, block engulfment.

The interaction of receptors on the surface of a phagocyte with opsonic ligands on the surface of a particle sends transmembrane signals to the phagocyte's cytoplasm. These signals initiate assembly of an interconnected meshwork of actin filaments, coordinate with the formation of pseudopods, in the segment of cytoplasm in contact with the particle. Receptors on the surface of the

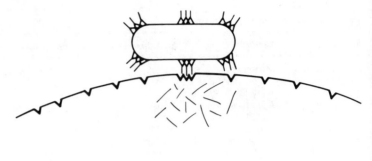

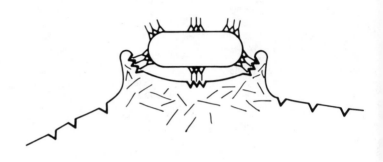

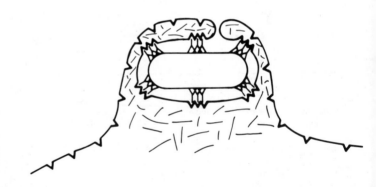

Figure 21–8. The "zipper" mechanism of phagocytosis. A bacterium opsonized with phagocytosis-promoting ligands (e.g., IgG) adheres to the phagocyte's Fc receptors. Engulfment of the bacterium proceeds via the sequential interaction of these ligands with these receptors. This interaction promotes the assembly of actin filaments in the cytoplasm underlying the forming phagosome.

advancing pseudopods bind to additional ligands on the particle's surfaces and the resulting additional series of signals stimulates further assembly of actin filaments and pseudopod extension. This process continues until the advancing pseudopods completely envelop the particle and fuse with one another to form a **phagocytic vacuole.**

Fc receptors, and receptors for mannose-terminated oligosaccharides, promote phagocytosis of particles coated with the corresponding ligands. Both receptors are constitutively active under all circumstances. In contrast, the **complement receptors** must be **activated** to promote phagocytosis. Regulation of their activity appears necessary, as receptor CR3 also participates in the

adhesion of neutrophils to the endothelium. Were these receptors constitutively active, neutrophils might always be adherent to the endothelium. **Chemoattractants** activate CR3 on neutrophils without promoting phagocytosis, thereby specifically promoting adhesion to endothelium and hence migration into tissues.

Fibronectin (see above), present as a soluble dimer in the plasma, also plays an important role in regulating complement receptors. It binds as an oligomer to the surface of many gram-positive bacteria (as well as to the basement membrane in various tissues). Unlike soluble fibrinonectin, these coated bacteria bind to fibronectin receptors on phagocytes, and this binding activates CR3 receptors to bind complement. With neutrophils and monocytes in the blood, this activation and the resulting binding of complement, like the activation by chemoattractants, does not result in phagocytosis, but with macrophages, it does so. Hence in the tissues fibronectin serves as an opsonin.

Digestion: Postphagocytic Microbicidal Processes

Although engulfment may be the most dramatic event in the encounter of an opsonized bacterial cell with a neutrophil or a macrophage, it is merely the first step in getting rid of a potentially lethal pathogen (Fig. 21–9). The events during and immediately after engulfment determine whether the bacterium lives or dies and ultimately perhaps whether the host survives.

The first detectable effect on bacterial physiology, occurring within minutes of engulfment, is loss of viability. The mechanism is unknown, but the importance to the host is evident. Simply stated, the bacterium can no

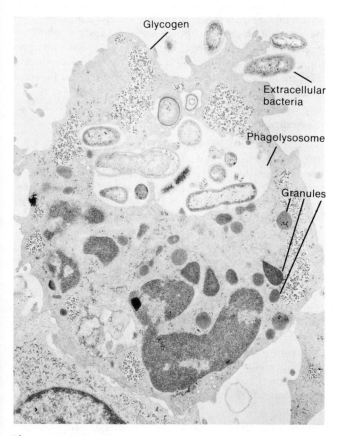

Figure 21–9. Electron micrograph of a PMN ingesting bacteria. The specimen was prepared for microscopy 10 min after the introduction of bacteria into the peritoneal cavity of a rabbit. Both intracellular and extracellular bacteria are shown. Some PMN granules have already released their contents into the large phagosome, which contains several bacteria; one of these is partially degraded. Courtesy of DF Bainton.

longer cause disease. Inhibition of macromolecule synthesis occurs later, followed ultimately by lysis and digestion of the bacterium by lysosomal enzymes. The microbistatic and microbicidal events that occur immediately after phagocytosis involve both oxygen-dependent and oxygen-independent systems.

Oxygen-Dependent Activity

Neutrophils and most types of tissue macrophages derive their metabolic energy primarily from anaerobic glycolysis, which suits their requirement to function in ischemic tissues. Liganding of Fc receptors* (on granulocytes, monocytes, and macrophages) and mannose receptors (on macrophages) markedly increases their O_2 uptake, a process termed **the "respiratory burst."** These receptors activate an NADPH–cytochrome b-dependent oxidase that reduces O_2 to **superoxide,** O_2^- (Chaps. 4 and 19), a potent oxidant and mutagen. Because the cytochrome b operates in an extremely low redox potential, it is able to scavenge oxygen even in poorly oxygenated or ischemic tissues.

Superoxide can be reduced to hydroxyl radical (OH·) or dismutated to hydrogen peroxide (H_2O_2), and these activated oxygen species also adversely affect a number of cellular structures, including membranes and nucleic acids. Thus these reactive oxygen intermediates have the capacity to damage bacteria directly, as well as to act in concert with neutrophil enzymes (see below).

The importance of reactive oxygen intermediates in host defense is illustrated by **chronic granulomatous disease,** an inherited defect in which the oxidase that reduces O_2 to O_2^- is decreased in amount or absent. These children suffer, and often die, from recurrent bacterial infections. Moreover, gamma interferon (IFN-γ), which enhances the capacity of neutrophils and monocytes to produce O_2^-, can ameliorate the disease in some patients.

Soon after its formation the phagocytic vacuole with its bacterial contents fuses with lysosomes and, in neutrophils, also with "specific" granules (see Table 21–3 for enzymes contained within lysosomes and specific granules). **Myeloperoxidase** is one of the lysosomal enzymes released into the phagocytic vacuole by this fusion. Myeloperoxidase uses H_2O_2, formed by the dismutation of superoxide generated during the respiratory burst, to catalyze the **halogenation** (primarily **chlorination**) of phagocytosed microbes. Halogenation is a potent mechanism for killing both prokaryotic and eukaryotic cells. However, individuals genetically deficient in myeloperoxidase do not show increased susceptibility to infection.

---

* Note that phagocytosis via C receptors does not activate a respiratory burst in either neutrophils or monocytes. See section on facultative intracellular pathogens, below, for further discussion.

TABLE 21–3. *Contents of Azurophil and Specific Granules of PMN*

AZUROPHIL GRANULES
Degradative lysosomal enzymes
Glycosidases
β-glucuronidase
Arylsulfatase
Proteinases
Cathepsin G
Elastase
Phosphatases
Acid phosphatase
5'-nucleotidase
Nucleases
Acid DNAse
Acid RNAse
Enzymes and proteins with antimicrobial activity
Myeloperoxidase
Lysozyme
BPI
Defensins
Azurocidin

SPECIFIC GRANULES
Vitamin B12 binding protein
Alkaline phosphatase
Lactoferrin
Collagenase
Lysozyme

Oxygen-Independent Activity

Neutrophil granules contain a variety of extremely **basic proteins** that strongly inhibit bacteria, yeast, and even viruses. These include **BPI** (**b**acterial **p**ermeability **i**ncreasing factor), the **defensins, azurocidin** (found only in azurophil granules), **cathepsin G,** and **elastase.** The microbicidal activity of cathepsin G and elastase is independent of their enzymatic activities. A few molecules of any one of these cationic proteins appear able to inactivate a bacterial cell, but, with the possible exception of BPI, their mechanism of action is unresolved.

Bacteria require a supply of **iron** for growth, and the **lactoferrin** released from specific granules into the phagocytic vacuole binds free iron. This process presumably deprives phagocytosed bacteria of an essential nutrient.

Once phagosome–lysosome fusion has occurred, the interior of the vacuole becomes acidic, creating an environment that is conducive to digestion of its contents by lysosomal enzymes. Digestion completes the destruction of the invading microbe, but it is not a significant defense factor.

THE MONONUCLEAR PHAGOCYTE SYSTEM

Monocytes from the blood migrate into virtually every organ of the body, where they develop into macrophages

(see Fig. 21–4). These cells comprise a large but relatively immobile reservoir of phagocytic cells, ready to defend the host against microbial pathogens. The earlier literature refers to these fixed phagocytes as the **reticuloendothelial system.** By 1972, it had become apparent that macrophages, and not the very different endothelial cells, carry out the activities attributed to this system, and so it was renamed the mononuclear phagocyte system.

Contrary to a common belief, most organisms are less capable of provoking disease when injected intravenously than when administered by any other route. This is because most bacteria that enter the blood stream are rapidly cleared by the mononuclear phagocyte system, primarily the macrophages in the liver and spleen. As Figure 21–10 shows, avirulent pneumococci are rapidly cleared from rabbit blood, but highly virulent pneumococci are not. The avirulent pneumococci fix complement and are readily engulfed by macrophages in the liver and spleen, but the virulent pneumococci have carbohydrate capsules that prevent these interactions. However, when previous infection or immunization has induced the host to produce Abs against a specific polysaccharide, liver macrophages rapidly clear virulent encapsulated pneumococci (Fig. 21–11), because Abs promote C deposition on the surfaces of the pneumococci, and macrophage receptors for IgG and C then promote phagocytosis.

Secretory Products

Monocytes and macrophages can secrete a large number of physiologically active substances (Table 21–4). The particular subset secreted by a cell varies with its stage of maturation, its previous exposure to cytokines and infectious agents, and the ligand or stimulus that elicits the secretory response. Only those secretory products that are clearly relevant to the interplay between bacteria and host are discussed below.

METABOLITES OF OXYGEN. O_2^-, H_2O_2, and OH· are essential mediators of the microbicidal activity of mononuclear phagocytes. The capacity to produce large amounts of these oxygen metabolites is a hallmark of the "activated," highly microbicidal macrophage (see below). **Gamma interferon** is a potent activator of this respiratory burst. Ligation of Fc or mannose receptors also activates the respiratory burst in macrophages; liganding of complement receptors does not.

NITROGEN OXIDES. Mononuclear phagocytes activated by IFN-γ or by endotoxin oxidize NH_2 of the guanidinium group of arginine to nitrogen oxides. These products mediate killing of tumor cells by activated macrophages, but their role in combatting microbial infections remains to be explored.

METABOLITES OF ARACHIDONIC ACID. Prostaglandins and **thromboxane** are potent vasoconstrictors. Prostaglandin formation may contribute to the increased vascular permeability that accompanies infection and inflammation. **Leukotriene B4** is a chemoattractant for neutrophils and monocytes, and its secretion by macrophages may be one mechanism by which these cells accumulate at sites of infection. Leukotriene C4 (**LTC₄**) promotes smooth muscle constriction and an increase in vascular permeability. Because macrophages secrete LTC4 when their Fc receptors are stimulated by immune complexes containing IgE or IgG, they may participate in immediate hypersensitivity reactions (asthma, anaphylaxis). However, C receptor-mediated phagocytosis does not cause secretion of arachidonate metabolites.

COMPLEMENT. Monocytes synthesize and secrete all components of the C pathways and their regulatory proteins. Thus they can produce opsonins and chemoattractants at the site of an infection.

INTERLEUKIN-1. Macrophages stimulated with endotoxin synthesize and secrete IL-1, which exerts a number of local and systemic effects relevant to bacterial infection. Locally, in the tissues where it is produced, it helps other cytokines (e.g., IL-6) to stimulate T-lymphocyte proliferation, thereby promoting the formation of lymphokines and Abs. It also enhances the adhesiveness of endothelial cells for neutrophils, thereby attracting neutrophils to sites of inflammation.

Systemically, IL-1 stimulates hepatocytes to secrete "acute-phase reactants" (e.g., fibrinogen C9), plasma proteins essential for clot formation and for bacteriolysis. It also stimulates the secretion of the hypothalamic releasing factor for ACTH, thereby increasing the plasma cortisol level. And it is an **endogenous pyrogen,** stimulating the thermoregulatory center in the anterior hypothalamus and thereby causing fever.

TNF/CACHECTIN. Endotoxin stimulates macrophages to synthesize and secrete TNF, which exerts many effects, both local and systemic; a few are described below.

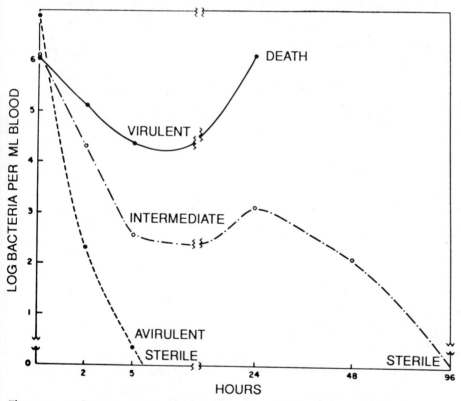

Figure 21–10. Comparison of the rates of clearance of three strains of *Streptococcus pneumoniae* from the bloodstream of rabbits. The avirulent strains express surface ligands that promote their attachment and ingestion by macrophages in the liver and spleen. In addition, their surfaces stimulate complement deposition, which further promotes their uptake by splenic and hepatic macrophages. (Redrawn from Rogers DE: Bacteriol Rev 24:41, 1960)

Some effects of TNF are similar to those of IL-1. For instance, TNF enhances the adhesiveness of endothelial cells for neutrophils, activates neutrophil adhesive mechanisms, and stimulates the production of GM-CSF. It also acts as an **endogenous pyrogen,** both through its direct effect on hypothalamic neurons and through the peripheral induction of IL-1 synthesis and secretion by endothelial cells throughout the body. Hence, administration of TNF to rabbits elicits a **biphasic febrile response:** an immediate increase in temperature secondary to the direct effect of TNF and a second, more sustained increase attributable to IL-1.

TNF is thought to be the principal physiological mediator of **endotoxic shock.** In this condition, neutrophil activation, uncontrolled intravascular coagulation, C activation, and a generalized increase in vascular permeability lead to a precipitous and often irreversible decline in blood pressure, culminating in death. These effects are mediated directly by the action of endotoxins on neutrophils and vascular endothelial cells and indirectly by stimulating macrophages to secrete TNF. In addition, TNF induces vascular endothelial cells to express procoagulant activity. Many of the shock-promoting effects of endotoxin can be blocked by administration of anti-TNF Abs, suggesting a novel approach to treating this life-threatening condition.

Facultative Intracellular Pathogens

Multicellular organisms evolved from single cells that foraged in the primordial sludge. These ancestral cells probably had the capacity to eat bacteria and algae, as do present-day amebae. Some bacteria, however, have developed ways to escape the amebae's bactericidal actions and to parasitize them. Thus it should not be surprising that some pathogenic bacteria have evolved mechanisms to parasitize the mononuclear phagocytes of higher organisms. Among these are *Mycobacterium tuberculosis* (the causative agent of tuberculosis), *M. leprae* (leprosy), *S. typhi* (typhoid fever), *Brucella abortus* (brucellosis), *Legionella pneumophila* (Legionnaires' disease), and *Listeria monocytogenes* (listeriosis). These facultative intracellular pathogens are capable of both extracellular and intracellular growth, in contrast to obligate intracellular pathogens such as viruses, rickettsiae, chlamydiae, and some protozoa. How do these intracellular pathogens escape macrophage antibacterial defenses?

L. pneumophila has developed a way to enter macrophages without activating their oxidant defenses: bind-

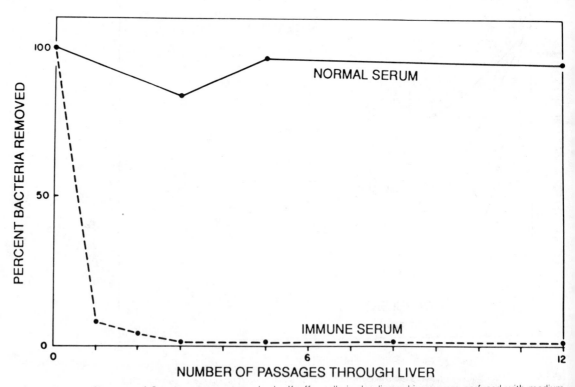

Figure 21–11. Clearance of *Streptococcus pneumoniae* by Kupffer cells in dog livers. Livers were perfused with medium containing bacteria and control or immune serum as indicated. Only the immune serum, which coats the bacteria with antibodies, promotes binding and ingestion of the bacteria by the macrophages (Kupffer cells) that line the sinusoids of the liver. This is an example of Fc receptor-mediated phagocytosis. (Redrawn from Rogers DE: Bacteriol Rev 24:41, 1960)

ing to macrophage C receptors, which promote engulfment but do not activate the respiratory burst. Thus even though the organism is sensitive to the bactericidal effects of oxygen metabolites, it evidently enters macrophages without being exposed to them. Whether other facultative intracellular bacteria use similar mechanisms to avoid oxidant injury is not known.

Many facultative intracellular bacterial pathogens, such as *M. tuberculosis* and *M. leprae*, grow within macrophage lysosomes and are evidently resistant to the digestive enzymes and antibacterial substances present within this compartment. Chlamydiae and *L. pneumophila* are sensitive to inhibitory substances in lysosomes and have evolved mechanisms to avoid entry into this cellular compartment. Chlamydiae prevent fusion of phagosomes with lysosomes, whereas *L. pneumophila* induces the macrophage to sequester it in a special membrane-bound, ribosome-studded compartment that is distinct from lysosomes. The mechanisms of these two special interactions are unknown.

Infection with a facultative intracellular bacterial pathogen is not necessarily fatal to the host. Mammals combat these wily opponents by "activating" their mononuclear phagocytes.

Macrophage Activation

The microbicidal activities of mononuclear phagocytes are markedly enhanced by lymphokines (hormones), principally **Gamma interferon (IFN-γ**, also known as macrophage-activating factor), produced by T cells when they encounter Ags (or antigenic peptides) on Ag-presenting cells such as macrophages. The CD4⁺ T cells are more effective producers than the CD8⁺ cells. IFNγ markedly enhances the capacity of macrophages to produce toxic oxygen metabolites and oxides of nitrogen. Moreover, it induces macrophages to express higher levels of Class II MHC Ags on their surfaces, and so they are more effective in presenting Ags to CD4⁺ T cells. IFN-γ also potentiates the capacity of mononuclear phagocytes to produce IL-1 and TNF (described above) in response to suitable stimuli.

Even in an immune host, it takes 24 to 48 hours for T cells to be recruited to a site of infection and to produce IFN-γ. For this reason, immune responses in which macrophages, T cells, and IFN-γ play a prominent role are termed **delayed-type immunity** (Fig. 21–12).

Mononuclear phagocytes treated with IFN-γ block the growth of intracellular pathogens whose growth they

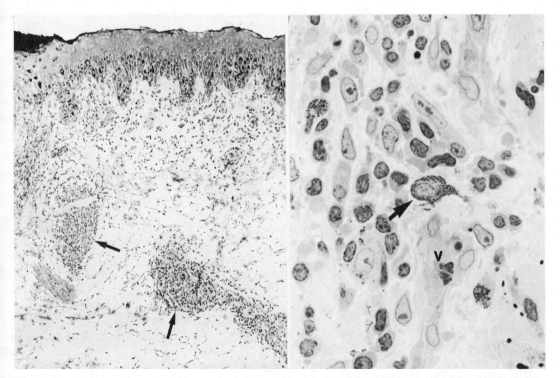

Figure 21–12. Delayed hypersensitivity reaction in human skin elicited by dinitrochlorobenzene, a skin-sensitizing hapten. **(Right panel)** shows perivascular collections of mononuclear cells *(arrows)* in the dermis. **(Left panel)**, at higher magnification, reveals a small dermal venule *(v)* surrounded by lymphocytes, macrophages, and a mast cell *(arrow)*. (Courtesy of HF Dvorak. Right panel reproduced from Colvin RB, Johnson RA, Mihm MC Jr, Dvorak HF: J Exp Med 138:686, 1973)

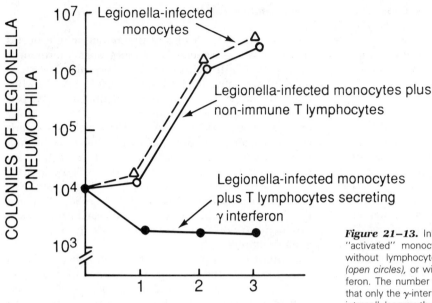

Figure 21–13. Inhibition of growth of *Legionella pneumophila* in "activated" monocytes. Monocytes were infected and incubated without lymphocytes *(triangles)*, with unstimulated lymphocytes *(open circles)*, or with stimulated lymphocytes that secreted γ-interferon. The number of viable *Legionella* was determined daily. Note that only the γ-interferon–treated monocytes were able to inhibit the intracellular growth of the bacteria. (Redrawn from Horwitz MA, Silverstein SC: J Exp Med 154:1618, 1981)

support in its absence (Figure 21–13). The mechanisms are uncertain; the recent discovery that these cells constitutively produce nitrogen oxides suggests at least one mechanism.

Transplantation of T cells from donor mice that are immune to *Listeria monocytogenes* into histocompatible naive mice renders them resistant to an otherwise lethal inoculum of this bacterium. IFN-γ evidently plays a major role, because treatment with Abs against it eliminates this transplanted resistance. There is abundant evidence that T-cell secretion of IFN-γ associated with delayed-type cellular immunity plays a similar role in controlling human infections with mycobacteria leprosy bacilli: for example, these infections are frequent after impairment of T-cell function in patients with AIDS.

COOPERATION BETWEEN CYTOTOXIC LYMPHOCYTES AND MACROPHAGES

As noted elsewhere (Chap. 19), cytotoxic T-lymphocytes **(CTLs)** form a major line of defense against many viral infections. However, they can probably also contribute to resistance to those bacteria, fungi, or protozoan pathogens that grow within phagocytic cells. For instance, when a macrophage contains intracellular pathogens such as *Listeria* or *Legionella*, some of the antigenic determinants of these bacteria are probably displayed on the macrophage surface in association with MHC molecules. CTLs that recognize these complexes are thus ex-

pected to attack and lyse the infected macrophages, releasing its enclosed pathogens. Once released, however, the pathogens would no longer be recognized by CTLs.

In the course of their cytolytic attack on infected macrophages, the CTLs also synthesize and release IFN-γ, which will activate neighboring macrophages, leading them to destroy the released bacteria. Experiments with infected cells in culture suggest that CTLs can cooperate with macrophages to eliminate some intracellular pathogens.

EXTRACELLULAR EFFECTS ON MICROORGANISMS

Many protozoa and filamentous fungi are too large to be ingested by a single phagocyte. In these instances, monocytes, macrophages, neutrophils, or eosinophils may attach to the organism's surface and kill it by secreting toxic substances onto it. Antibodies that coat the surface of these organisms may promote leukocyte attachment and vectorial secretion of antimicrobial effector substances onto the pathogen. Such effects are especially prominent in the interactions of **eosinophils** with **protozoa**.

Granulomas

Some facultative intracellular bacteria, such as *M. tuberculosis* and *Listeria monocytogenes*, induce macrophages and lymphocytes to form a granuloma. In this structure, macrophages cluster together to form a sphere, within which may lie bacteria and cellular debris. Lymphocytes generally cluster around the outside of the sphere. Some granulomas exhibit a high influx and turnover of monocytes and lymphocytes. Within such granulomas, bacterial growth is slowed but not entirely inhibited. Others become relatively static structures within which tubercle bacilli may remain dormant for many years. We have only rudimentary information about the factors that elicit and maintain granulomas.

The Constantly Changing Relations Between Host and Parasite

Each living species occupies a specific ecological niche. Human beings are unique in being able to change their environment deliberately and therefore to change the ecology within it. In so doing, people alter the number and types of microorganisms to which they are exposed. The emergence of several hitherto-unrecognized human diseases within the past 15 years shows that these changes in human ecology can have large effects on host–parasite interactions. For example, large-scale air-conditioning systems and cooling towers have provided a means for disseminating an otherwise innocuous and poorly infectious bacterium, *L. pneumophila*. Synthetic chemistry has created new types of vaginal tampons, a novel microenvironment within which staphylococci are induced to produce the toxin that causes toxic shock syndrome. Widespread use of antibiotics has greatly increased the incidence of human infections with drug-resistant bacteria. High-speed air transport, transmission of blood from person to person through use of contaminated needles, and relaxed sexual mores have facilitated the spread of HIV throughout the globe. At the same time, improved sanitation and water, vaccination, and antimicrobial therapy have nearly eradicated many infectious diseases.

In viewing host–parasite interactions, it is important to remember that the human being's relationship to the microbial world is constantly changing. The ecology of people and of the earth are in a state of flux. We continue to evolve, as do the microorganisms that inhabit our bodies and the surrounding earth. We must expect new diseases to evolve as old ones give way to vaccines, drugs, and evolutionary pressures. The battle between microbial invaders and host defenses is unending.

Selected Reading

Intracellular Bacteria. Curr Topics Microbiol Immunol 138, 1988

Bainton DF: Phagocytic cells: Developmental biology of neutrophils and eosinophils. In Gallin JL, Goldstein IM, Snyderman R (eds): Inflammation: Basic Principles and Clinical Correlates. New York, p 265, Raven Press, 1988

Clark SC, Kamen R: The human hematopoietic colony-stimulating factors. Science 236:1229, 1987

Cotran RS, Pober JS: Endothelial activation. Its role in inflammatory and immune reactions. In Simionescu N, Simionescu M (eds): Endothelial Cell Biology in Health and Disease. New York, Plenum Publishing, p 335, 1988

Gimbrone MA Jr, Bevilacqua MP: Vascular endothelium. Functional modulation at the blood interface. In Simionescu N, Simionescu M (eds): Endothelial cell biology in health and disease. New York, Plenum Publishing, p 255, 1988

Gordon S: Biology of the macrophage. J Cell Sci Suppl 4:267, 1986

Harlan JM: Leukocyte-endothelial interactions. Blood 65:513, 1985

Johnston RB: Monocytes and macrophages. N Engl J Med 318:747, 1988

Kaplan G, Cohn ZA: The immunobiology of leprosy. Int Rev Exp Pathol 28:45, 1986

Klebanoff SJ: Phagocytic cells: Products of oxygen metabolism. In Gallin JJ, Goldstein IM, Snyderman R (eds): Inflammation: Basic Principles and Clinical Correlates. New York, Raven Press, p 391, 1988

Klemm P: Fimbrial adhesins of *Escherichia coli*. Rev Inf Dis 7:321, 1985

Lehrer RI, Ganz T, Selsted ME, et al: Neutrophils and host defenses. Ann Int Med 109:127, 1988

McGee ZA, Gorby GL, Wyrick PB, et al: Parasite-directed endocytosis. Rev Inf Dis 10:S311, 1988

Middlebrook JL, Dorland RB: Bacterial toxins: Cellular mechanisms of action. Microbiol Rev 48:199, 1984

Miller JF, Mekalanos JJ, Falkow S: Coordinate regulation and sensory transduction in the control of bacterial virulence. Science 243:916, 1989

Mims CA: The Pathogenesis of Infectious Diseases. 3rd Ed. London, Academic Press, 1987

Morrison DC, Ryan JL: Endotoxins and disease mechanisms. Annu Rev Med 38:417, 1987

Moss J, Burns DL, Hsia JA, Hewlett EL, et al: Cyclic nucleotides: mediators of bacterial toxin action in disease. Ann Int Med 101:653, 1984

Murray HW: Interferon-gamma, the activated macrophage, and host defense against microbial challenge. Ann Int Med 108:595, 1988

Nathan CF: Secretory Products of Macrophages. J Clin Invest 79:319, 1987

Rotrosen D, Gallin JI: Disorders of phagocyte function. Annu Rev Immunol 5:127, 1987

Ruoslahti E: Fibronectin and its receptors. Ann Rev Biochem 57:375, 1988

Unkeless JC, Wright SD: Phagocytic Cells: Fc$_\gamma$ and Complement Receptors. In Gallin JI, Goldstein IM, Snyderman R (eds): Inflammation: Basic Principles and Clinical Correlates. New York, Raven Press, 1988

van Furth R: Phagocytic Cells: Development and Distribution of Mononuclear Phagocytes in Normal Steady State and Inflammation. In Gallin JI, Goldstein IM, Snyderman R (eds): Inflammation: Basic Principles and Clinical Correlates, New York, Raven Press, p 281, 1988

22

R. John Collier

Corynebacteria*

The corynebacteria are gram-positive, rod-like organisms, which often arrange themselves in palisades, possess club-shaped swellings at their poles, and stain irregularly. They appear to be related to the mycobacteria (Chap. 35) and nocardiae (Chap. 36), as the principal cell wall antigens of all three genera are closely related chemically and serologically. In the species that can cause diphtheria, *Corynebacterium diphtheriae*, lysogenization by a bacteriophage causes synthesis of a potent heat-labile protein toxin.

Corynebacterium Diphtheriae

No other bacterial disease of man has been studied as successfully as diphtheria. Its etiology and mode of transmission were established early, and a highly effective method of prevention—immunization with diphtheria toxoid—was subsequently developed. As a result of mass immunization, diphtheria has become rare in many countries, including the United States, and toxigenic strains of *C. diphtheriae* have virtually disappeared. Nevertheless, we shall discuss diphtheria in some detail as a prototype of toxigenic disease and as an example of successful control.

HISTORY

Diphtheria was not recognized as a specific disease until 1821, when Pierre Bretonneau proposed that the throat "distemper" could be differentiated from other afflictions of the throat by the formation in the respiratory tract of a false membrane (composed largely of fibrin, bacteria, and trapped leukocytes rather than true epithelium). He called the malady **diphtheritis** (Gr. *diphthera*, skin or

* The author gratefully acknowledges his debt to AM Pappenheimer, Jr., for material retained from earlier editions.

membrane). In 1883, the causative organism was described by Klebs in stained smears from diphtheritic membranes, and its etiologic role was proved a year later when Loeffler grew the organism on artificial media and produced fatal infections in experimental animals.

Loeffler was surprised to find that the diphtheria bacilli remained only in the local lesions at the site of inoculation of guinea pigs although damage was visible in the heart, liver, kidneys, adrenal glands, and other tissues. He concluded that the bacilli growing at the primary site must have produced a soluble poison, which was transported to remote tissues by the blood stream. In 1888, Roux and Yersin demonstrated a heat-labile toxin in the fluid phase of diphtheria bacillus cultures, whose injection into appropriate animals caused all the systemic manifestations of diphtheria. Two years later, von Behring and Kitasato succeeded in immunizing animals with toxin modified with iodine trichloride, and they demonstrated that the serum of such immunized animals protected susceptible animals against the disease. On Christmas night 1891, in Berlin, the antitoxin was first given to a diphtheritic child.

This caused severe local reactions when injected and therefore could not be used as an immunizing agent in man. In 1909, Theobald Smith suggested the use of toxin neutralized by an equivalent amount of antitoxin (**toxin–antitoxin**). Its use was greatly facilitated by Schick's discovery in 1913 of a practical test (see below) for distinguishing immune from nonimmune individuals by their reactions to an intradermal injection of a small dose of toxin. Finally, in 1923, Ramon introduced Formalin-treated toxin, or **toxoid,** which is noninjurious to tissues but is fully immunogenic; it is now used universally for active immunization against diphtheria.

In 1951, Freeman discovered that all toxigenic strains of *C. diphtheriae* are lysogenic; i.e., are infected with a temperate bacteriophage. If such strains lose their specific phage, they cease to produce toxin and become relatively avirulent.

MORPHOLOGY

Corynebacteria (Gr. *coryne*, club) are gram-positive, non–spore-bearing rods, tapered from their septal ends, without flagella or demonstrable capsules. They range from 2 to 6 μm in length and from 0.5 to 1 μm in diameter. Because of the way the individual bacilli divide, they tend, in stained smears, to form sharp angles with one another, making characteristic figures resembling Chinese letters. When grown on coagulated serum slants rich in phosphate (Loeffler's medium), they contain polyphosphate granules, called Babès–Ernst bodies, which stain metachromatically with methylene blue or toluidine blue. In some strains, well-defined polar bodies are discernible at the ends of each bacillus. These bodies are

most frequently seen in organisms growing slowly on suboptimal media; they are less prominent during rapid growth, especially on media containing potassium tellurite (K_2TeO_3). On Loeffler's medium and on blood agar, surface colonies are cream-colored or grayish white; on tellurite agar, they are dark gray or black because of intracellular reduction of the tellurite to tellurium.

Corynebacteria contain in their cell walls mycolic acids (very long-chain branched fatty acids), somewhat smaller (C28–C40) than those of mycobacteria (ca. C80: see Chap. 35).

CULTIVATION

C. diphtheriae is an obligate aerobe. Most strains grow as a waxy pellicle on the surface of liquid media. For primary isolation, Loeffler's coagulated serum medium is still useful, because it permits growth of diphtheria bacilli with characteristic morphology but does not support growth of the streptococci and pneumococci commonly present in the throat. Blood or chocolate agar with potassium tellurite to inhibit the growth of most other bacteria is an even better selective medium for *C. diphtheriae.*

Although the black colonies formed by the diphtheria bacilli are characteristic, other organisms found in the respiratory tract, particularly staphylococci and non-pathogenic corynebacteria (e.g., *C. pseudodiphtheriticum* [*C. hofmannii*]), may also form black colonies.

C. diphtheriae grows well on relatively simple media containing essential amino acids and an energy source such as glucose or maltose; most strains also require nicotinic acid, pantothenic acid, and biotin.

Diphtheria bacilli typically ferment glucose rapidly and maltose slowly, producing acid but no gas. A comparison of the fermentation reactions of the common corynebacteria is shown in Table 22–1.

DIPHTHERIA TOXIN

RELATION TO LYSOGENY. Only those strains of *C. diphtheriae* that are lysogenic for β-prophage or related temperate phages produce diphtheria toxin. The structural gene for the toxin (*tox*) resides on the phage genome and is expressed under certain nutritional conditions even in the absence of phage multiplication.

TABLE 22–1. Fermentation Reactions of Corynebacteria Commonly Cultured from Man

Corynebacteria	Glucose	Maltose	Sucrose
C. diphtheriae	+	+	–(+)
C. xerosis	+	–	+
C. hofmannii	–	–	–

Fragments of the *tox* gene coding for nontoxic portions of the toxin have been cloned in *E. coli* and sequenced, but regulations forbid cloning of the whole gene except under the most stringent containment conditions.

REGULATION OF TOXIN FORMATION. The expression of the *tox* gene is controlled by the metabolism and physiological state of the host bacterium. With an adequate supply of essential nutrients, including O_2, the most important factor is the inorganic iron (Fe^{3+}) concentration. Toxin is synthesized in high yield only after the exogenous Fe supply has become exhausted. There is evidence that Fe regulates transcription of *tox*, perhaps by interacting with a bacterial regulatory protein.

The classic Park–Williams strain (PW8) of *C. diphtheriae*, isolated in 1896, is still used as a source of toxin for the preparation of diphtheria vaccine (toxoid). Alterations in its metabolism, including inability to produce the siderophore, corynebactin, give it the unusual capacity to increase its bacterial mass five- to six-fold after depletion of the exogenous iron supply. During this period, toxin synthesis may reach 5% of the total protein synthesis.

TOXIN MODE OF ACTION. Diphtheria toxin (M_r 58,342) may be isolated from culture filtrates of *C. diphtheriae* as an iron-free, heat-labile protein. In highly susceptible species (rabbit, guinea pig), the pure toxin is lethal at 0.1 μg/kg or less, and in man, intradermal injection of 0.1 ng (one billion molecules) will produce a visible skin reaction. The toxin kills cultured cells from susceptible animals, but cells from insensitive animals (rats, mice) are affected only at very high toxin concentrations. Cell culture has provided a convenient system for assaying the toxin's activity and studying its mode of action.

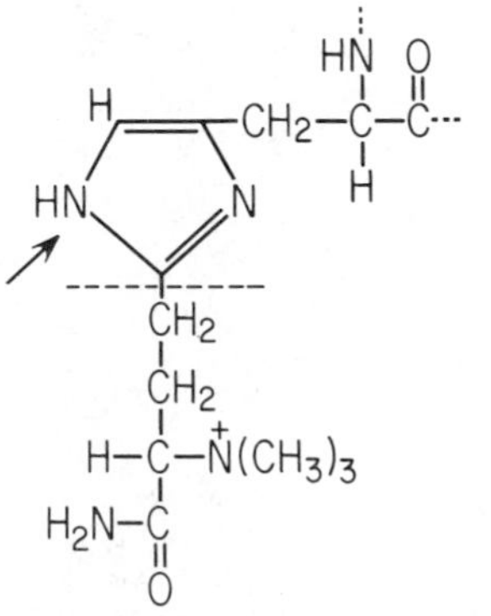

Figure 22–1. Structure of diphthamide residue on EF-2. A series of at least three enzyme-catalyzed reactions results in addition of the group shown below the *dashed line* to a specific histidine side chain of EF-2. The backbone and three methyl groups of the adduct are derived from methionine. Site of attachment of ADP-ribose by diphtheria toxin is indicated *(arrow)*.

Diphtheria toxin kills sensitive cells by **blocking protein synthesis.** It does so by being converted to an **enzyme** that inactivates EF-2, the elongation factor required for translocation of polypeptidyl-tRNA from the acceptor to the donor site on the eukaryotic ribosome. The inactivation involves transfer of the ADP-ribosyl group of NAD to a specific site on EF-2:

$$\text{NAD} + \text{EF-2} \rightleftharpoons \text{ADP-ribosyl–EF-2} + \text{nicotinamide} + \text{H}^+$$

The equilibrium lies far to the right, and the reaction is in effect irreversible under physiologic conditions. No way is known of rescuing a cell in which the toxin has ADP-ribosylated all the EF-2.

EF-2 is the only protein ADP-ribosylated by diphtheria toxin. EF-2 from all eukaryotic species tested, from yeasts and protozoa to higher plants and man, acts as substrate, whereas the prokaryotic translocation factor (EF-G) does not.* This specificity depends on the presence in EF-2 of a unique residue, **diphthamide** (Fig. 22–1), which is formed by post-translational modification of a single histidine side chain within the factor. Mutant cells unable to form diphthamide are resistant to diphtheria toxin, thus proving that the ADP-ribosylation of EF-2 is responsible for the toxin's lethal effect on cells.

The diphthamide residue may be involved in regulating protein synthesis under certain conditions, for there are recent reports that extracts of animal cells contain low levels of an enzyme that can specifically ADP-ribosylate EF-2. If such an enzyme is the evolutionary precursor of diphtheria toxin, it would represent an interesting example of capture of a eukaryotic gene by a prokaryote.

ADP-ribosylation reactions have been found with other bacterial toxins. *Pseudomonas aeruginosa* exotoxin A, like diphtheria toxin, acts by ADP-ribosylating EF-2. Cholera toxin and its close relative, *E. coli* heat-labile toxin, ADP-ribosylate a crucial arginine residue on the Ns subunit of adenylate cyclase. Pertussis toxin ADP-ribosylates a cysteine side chain on the Ni subunit of adenylate cyclase. Evolutionary relations among these toxins are obscure.

The selective advantage of diphtheria toxin production to a lysogen of *C. diphtheriae*, or to the temperate phage carrying the *tox* gene, is unknown. Mutant strains of β phage that encode various inactive forms of diphtheria toxin replicate normally, and toxin production does not affect the growth of lysogens in the laboratory. Toxin production may provide a selective advantage for *C. diphtheriae* in man by facilitating infection or bacterial

---

* Archaebacteria, a group of organisms distinct from both eukaryotes and eubacteria, do have an elongation factor that can be ADP-ribosylated by diphtheria toxin, albeit at a low rate, and there is evidence that diphthamide (or perhaps a precursor lacking the amide group) is present on their elongation factor. This and other characteristics of the archaebacteria suggest that they are direct descendants of early unicellular organisms that also gave rise to eukaryotes.

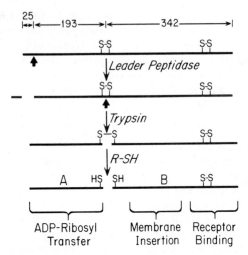

Figure 22–2. Sequential alterations believed to occur in diphtheria toxin during its action. Bacterial leader peptidase cleaves the 25-residue leader sequence from the primary translation product yielding mature toxin (535 residues), which is released from the bacterium. The toxin is subsequently cleaved by a trypsin-like enzyme, creating a "nicked" form containing two chains linked by a disulfide bridge. Reduction of the bridge after the toxin has contacted the cytosol permits the A chain, which is responsible for ADP-ribosyl transfer, to separate from the B chain, which is involved in receptor binding and membrane insertion of the toxin. The scale at the top gives the number of amino acid residues in the various fragments. *Heavy arrows,* proteolytic cleavage sites.

growth or conceivably by enhancing the rate of dissemination (e.g., by inducing coughing). The advantage is probably manifested in subclinical infections, which are more numerous and likely to be of greater ecological importance to the microbe than severe infections.

TOXIN STRUCTURE AND INTERACTION WITH MAMMALIAN CELLS. Diphtheria toxin is synthesized as a single polypeptide chain (560 residues), containing a 25-residue amino-terminal leader sequence that promotes secretion from the bacteria (Fig. 22–2). The leader is removed in secretion of the mature protein (535 residues). The complete primary structure of the toxin has been deduced from the nucleotide sequence of the *tox* gene. The toxin has been crystallized, and x-ray diffraction studies to determine its three-dimensional structure are under way.

The mature toxin must be covalently altered before it can ADP-ribosylate EF-2. Mild trypsin digestion nicks the toxin preferentially at arginine[193], within a disulfide loop, thereby cleaving the protein into two chains: A (amino-terminal, 193 residues) and B (carboxyl-terminal, 342 residues). Trypsin-like enzymes are believed to accomplish this *in vivo* either before or soon after the toxin binds to the cell surface. The A chain contains the catalytic center for ADP-ribosylation, which is active only after the disulfide bridge between A and B has been ruptured and the chains are separated. The A chain by itself is not toxic for cells or animals, however; the B chain is required for binding and entry. Mutant forms of the toxin, as well as isolated fragments, have been useful in localizing these functions (Table 22–2).

Before the toxin can block protein synthesis in cells, its catalytic center on the A chain must penetrate to the cytosolic compartment. The process by which the B chain binds the toxin to cells and mediates transfer of A into the cytosol is not yet fully understood, but a rational model has emerged from fragmentary information (Fig. 22–3):

1. **Attachment to receptors.** The receptor binding site on the toxin evidently lies on B near its carboxyl terminus, because a mutant toxin (CRM45) lacking the carboxy-terminal 149 residues does not bind to cell receptors. The receptor appears to be a high-molecular-weight glycoprotein and may correspond to an ion-transport protein.

2. **Endocytosis.** The entry of receptor-bound diphtheria toxin into the cytosol is believed to involve exposure to low pH (ca. 4–5) within endosomal vesicles. Weak bases such as NH_4Cl, which maintain the endosomal pH near neutrality, block intoxication of cells and maintain

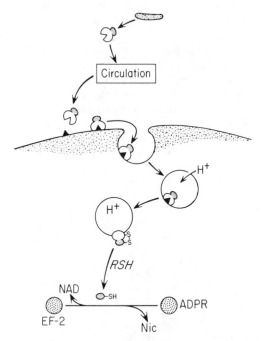

Figure 22–3. Events believed to lead to the inhibition of protein synthesis by diphtheria toxin in a sensitive cell. Circulating toxin attaches to cell-surface receptors *(dark triangles)* via a receptor binding site on the B moiety. The complex enters cell surface pits and is internalized into endosomes. Acidification of the endosomal lumen induces insertion of the B moiety into the endosomal membrane and transfer of A *(stippled)* to the cytosolic face. Reduction of the disulfide linking A to B permits release of A into the cytosol, where it catalyzes the ADP-ribosylation of EF-2, causing inhibition of protein synthesis.

TABLE 22–2. *Some Properties of Diphtheria Toxin and Related Proteins*

Protein	Approximate Mol. Wt.	Toxicity (MLD/µg)	Enzyme Activity (%)*	Binding†	Number of Half-Cystines
Toxin	58,000	25–30	100	(+)	4
Toxoid	58,000	0	0	−	4
Fragment A	21,000	0	100	−	1
Fragment B	37,000	0	0	+	3
CRM 45	45,000	0	100	−	2
CRM 176	58,000	ca. 0.1	8–10	+	4
CRM 197	58,000	0	0	+	4
$A_{45}B_{197}$‡	58,000	25–30	100	(+)	4

CRM = Serologically cross-reacting material.

* ADP-ribosylating activity after "nicking" and reduction, relative to fragment A as 100%.

† Ability to compete with toxin for specific membrane receptors.

‡ Toxic hybrid molecule formed by allowing a mixture of reduced, "nicked" CRM 45 and CRM 197 to reoxidize.

the toxin in an antitoxin-resistant compartment. Certain viruses, such as influenza virus, follow a similar pathway into the cytoplasm.

3. **Membrane insertion.** When the toxin is exposed to low pH, buried hydrophobic sequences within the B chain become exposed, and the toxin inserts into membranes. Also, when toxin bound to the cell surface is artificially exposed to acidic pH, protein synthesis is rapidly inhibited, implying that the A chain traverses the plasma membrane into the cytosol under these conditions. The B chain, inserted into artificial lipid bilayers, forms ion-conductive channels, and it has been proposed that the A chain traverses such channels in an unfolded or partially folded form. The A chain alone is unable to traverse membranes or kill cells.

4. **Release of A into the cytosol.** It is assumed that the disulfide bridge linking A to B is reduced (perhaps by glutathione) once it contacts the cytosol, permitting A to be released into the cytosol. Binding of cytosolic NAD to the active site stabilizes the A chain against proteolytic attack, permitting its survival for long periods within cells. One or two molecules of A can ADP-ribosylate all of the approximately two million EF-2 molecules within a cell over a period of hours to days.

PATHOGENICITY

EXPERIMENTAL MODELS. The only known natural reservoirs for toxigenic as well as nontoxigenic *C. diphtheriae* are the upper respiratory tracts of men and horses and the indolent cutaneous lesions of man that are seen in tropical climates. Natural infections have been observed only in man.

Although protein synthesis is blocked by activated toxin in extracts from all eukaryotes, the cells of certain animal species do not bind toxin. For this reason, rats and mice are more than 1000 times as resistant per unit body weight as humans, monkeys, rabbits, guinea pigs, pigeons, and chickens.

Subcutaneous injection of diphtheria toxin into a guinea pig is followed by death within 12 hours to several days, depending on the dose. Local swelling and apparent tenderness develop within a few hours, and at autopsy, edema, hemorrhage, and necrosis are noted at the site of injection together with congestion of the adrenal cortices and degenerative changes in the heart, liver, and kidneys. Sublethal doses of toxin may cause late paralyses similar to those observed in man. As was first recognized by Loeffler, when virulent bacilli are injected instead of the toxin, the end result is much the same.

HUMAN DISEASE. Diphtheria in man usually begins in the upper respiratory tract. When virulent diphtheria bacilli become lodged in the throat of a susceptible individual, they first multiply in the superficial layers of the mucous membrane. There, they elaborate toxin, which causes necrosis of neighboring tissue cells and establishes a nidus for further multiplication of the bacteria. The inflammatory response eventually results in the characteristic **diphtheritic pseudomembrane** which usually appears first on the tonsils or posterior pharynx and may then spread either upward into the nasal passages or downward into the larynx and trachea. In laryngeal diphtheria, mechanical obstruction may cause suffocation unless the airway is restored by intubation or tracheotomy.

In contrast to streptococcal pharyngitis (with which it may easily be confused), diphtheria of the upper respiratory tract tends to remain localized. Regional lymph nodes in the neck often become enlarged, but invasion of other tissues seldom occurs, and bacteremia is not seen. Redness and swelling of the mucous membranes in the pharynx are much less pronounced than in streptococcal infections. Fever is usually only moderate. In the tropics, indolent, ulcerative cutaneous lesions with a diphtheritic membrane and *tox*⁺ *C. diphtheriae* are common.

IMMUNITY AND EPIDEMIOLOGY

Newborn infants whose mothers are resistant acquire temporary immunity lasting a year or two, from transplacental antitoxin. Active immunity can be produced by a mild or inapparent infection in infants who retain some circulating maternal antitoxin and in susceptible adults infected with a strain of low toxigenicity. However, in areas where diphtheria is *not* endemic, most children, unless artificially immunized, become highly susceptible within a few months after birth. Artificial immunization at an early age is therefore universally advocated.

Persons who recover from diphtheria may continue to harbor the organism in the nose or throat for weeks or months. In the past, such healthy carriers spread the disease by droplet infection, and toxigenic bacteria were maintained among the population. The carrier rate for toxigenic *C. diphtheriae* in large cities was often 5% or higher, but it fell dramatically after the advent of universal immunization. Hence, the *tox* gene must have survival value both for *tox*⁺ phage and for its bacterial host under natural conditions.

SCHICK TEST. In the absence of circulating antitoxin the intradermal injection of 1/50 MLD* of diphtheria toxin will cause a local reaction characterized by a pigmented area of swelling and tenderness, reaching a maximum after 4 to 5 days. If, on the other hand, the blood stream contains a sufficient level of antitoxin, no reaction will occur. Thus, a positive Schick test indicates that little or no antitoxin is present (<0.01 U/ml).†

Persons who have become hypersensitive to the toxin or to other antigens in the toxin preparation, either as a result of naturally acquired infections or from artificial immunization with toxoid, will react allergically to the intradermally injected toxin. In order to distinguish these reactions from the primary action of the toxin, a control injection of toxoid (about 0.005 L‡) is administered intradermally in the opposite arm. If the individual is immune but is sensitive to antigens in the toxin prepa-

---

* One minimum lethal dose (MLD) was originally defined by Ehrlich as that amount of diphtheria toxin which, when injected subcutaneously into a 250-g guinea pig, causes death on the fourth or fifth day.

† Antitoxin titers in human serum are measured by comparison with a standard antitoxin in the rabbit intradermal test. Toxin itself loses toxicity during storage without a parallel loss of antitoxin-binding capacity.

‡ L stands for the Latin word *limes* (limit), and 1 Lf is that quantity of toxin or toxoid that flocculates most rapidly when mixed with 1 U of antitoxin.

ration, he or she will react to both the toxin and the toxoid. The allergic (delayed-type) **pseudoreactions**, however, usually reach a maximum within 48 to 72 hours and then fade, whereas the true positive Schick reaction persists for many days.

Reimmunization of adults and older children should be approached with caution in order to avoid serious local and systemic reactions in persons sensitive to toxoid. For anyone who shows a pseudoreaction in the Schick test, it is inadvisable to inject a full immunizing dose of toxoid, and the test itself will usually have served as a booster.

LABORATORY DIAGNOSIS

A definitive diagnosis of diphtheria can ordinarily be made only by isolating toxigenic diphtheria bacilli from the primary lesion. Exudate from the lesion, taken preferably from the membrane if present, should be immediately transferred to a Loeffler slant, a blood agar plate, and tellurite agar. After 24 hours, each culture should be carefully examined, and smears should be made from each type of colony that has grown out on any of the media. If growth appears on the blood agar plate but not on the tellurite plate, it may be tentatively concluded that no diphtheria bacilli are present. However, the tellurite plate should be reincubated for an additional 24 hours. Smears should immediately be made of any colonies appearing on the tellurite agar and should be stained with methylene blue. Corynebacteria should be readily detected in such smears, and they should be subcultured on a Loeffler's slant and tested for toxigenicity, either by an intradermal guinea pig virulence test or by the *in vitro* gel diffusion method (Fig. 22–4).

TREATMENT

Once circulating diphtheria toxin has gained entrance to susceptible tissue cells, it can no longer be neutralized by antitoxin. Accordingly, in suspected cases of diphtheria, **antitoxin therapy** must be implemented without delay. The time factor is so critical (Table 22–3) that the clinician is amply justified in giving antiserum without waiting for the results of the bacteriologic tests provided the circumstances of the infection and the clinical signs of the disease suggest diphtheria. To ensure the maximum intermediate therapeutic effect, the antitoxin should be injected intramuscularly in a single large dose. Because the antiserum used is derived from horses, the usual **skin test for sensitivity to horse serum proteins** should be performed first, and a syringe containing epinephrine should be available for immediate use in the event of an anaphylactic reaction. If the patient is sensitive to horse serum, the antitoxin should be given with caution, beginning with a small, highly diluted (e.g.,

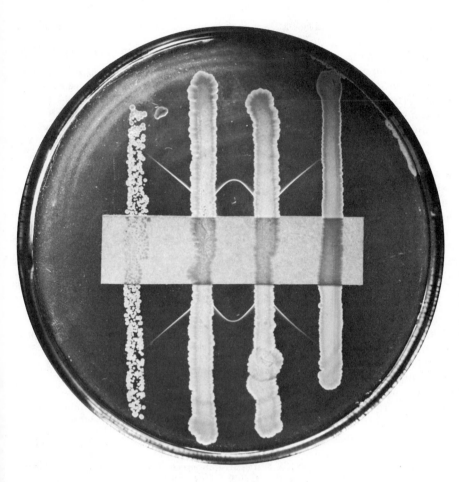

Figure 22–4. Gel diffusion test of toxigenicity. Outer strains are nontoxinogenic, whereas those streaked in center of plate produce toxin. The antitoxic serum used had been previously absorbed with nontoxic proteins obtained from a nontoxigenic culture and thus behaved as a **monospecific** antiserum. The intersection of the bands with the bacterial growth is removed some distance from the piece of filter paper impregnated with antiserum because horse antitoxin was employed, which inhibits the precipitin reaction in the region of Ab excess. Note that lines of precipitate generated by the two toxinogenic strains merge to form arcs, indicating that the toxins elaborated are immunologically identical. (King EO et al: Am J Public Health 39:1314, 1949)

1:10,000) subcutaneous dose, followed by gradually increasing doses administered intramuscularly until the full dose has been injected.

Although diphtheria bacilli are susceptible to penicillin, the tetracyclines, and erythromycin, antibiotic therapy alone should never be relied on in treating diphtheria. However, these drugs, in conjunction with antitoxin, may hasten the elimination of the organisms from the primary lesion.

TABLE 22–3. Relation of Case Fatality Rate to Time of Treatment with Antitoxin

Day of Disease Antitoxin Administered	Cases Treated	Case Fatality Rate (%)
1	225	0
2	1441	4.2
3	1600	11.1
4	1276	17.3
≥5	1645	18.7

PREVENTION

Because only man appears to be an important reservoir for *C. diphtheriae*, and because all strains elaborate the same antigenic type of toxin, it should be possible to eradicate the disease by immunization.

Diphtheria has become rare in certain areas of the world, including the U.S., where children are immunized at an early age and are given booster injections after 1 year and when they enter school. In other countries, however, where diphtheria immunization is rarely practiced, the disease is still prevalent. It is spread by droplet infection from active cases and asymptomatic carriers. Persons with cutaneous diphtheria or diphtheritic ulcers (who are invariably Schick-negative) also may transmit toxigenic *C. diphtheriae* by contact.

When diphtheria toxin is treated with dilute formaldehyde under suitable conditions, it is converted to toxoid. **Toxoid** is devoid of toxicity but is virtually indistinguishable antigenically from toxin. It is usually injected either as an alum precipitate or adsorbed on aluminum phosphate gel. Two doses of 10 Lf given 1 month apart are usually adequate for primary immunization. A booster injection is given about a year later.

It is common practice in the U.S. to immunize infants at 3 or 4 months of age with a combined vaccine containing diphtheria toxoid, tetanus toxoid, and pertussis vaccine: the pertussis exerts an adjuvant effect. The immunity ordinarily lasts for several years. It is important to administer several booster injections during childhood.

Although toxoid prepared with formaldehyde has served well as a vaccine, imperfect control has occasionally yielded toxoid that reverted to the toxic state, causing disastrous results. It is now possible to eliminate such errors by using a mutant, inactive form of the toxin as starting material for the toxoiding process. One company is preparing to manufacture toxoid from CRM197, a mutant toxin in which an amino acid substitution renders the A chain enzymically inactive.

Other Corynebacteria (Diphtheroids)

Corynebacteria are widely distributed in nature. Many species inhabit the soil, and a number cause disease in animals. Both *C. ulcerans* and *C. pseudotuberculosis* (*C. ovis*) cause infections in certain domestic animals (e.g., horses) and occasionally in man. Certain strains of both organisms produce diphtheria toxin and contain *tox* and non-*tox*-related DNA sequences that hybridize with β phage DNA. *C. kutscheri* causes disease in mice and commonly gives rise to latent infections.

Selected Reading

BOOKS AND REVIEW ARTICLES

Andrewes FW, Bulloch W, Douglass SR et al: Diphtheria: Its Bacteriology, Pathology and Immunity. London, HMSO, 1923

Collier, RJ: Diphtheria toxin: Mode of action and structure. Bacteriol Rev 39:54, 1975

Pappenheimer AM Jr: Diphtheria toxin. Annu Rev Biochem 46:69, 1977

Singer RA: Lysogeny and toxinogeny in *Corynebacterium diphtheriae*. In Bernheimer AW (ed): Mechanisms in Bacterial Toxinology, pp 31–51. New York, Wiley, 1976

SPECIFIC ARTICLES

Boquet P, Silverman MS, Pappenheimer AM Jr, Vernon WB: Binding of Triton X-100 to diphtheria toxin, CRM45 and their fragments. Proc Natl Acad Sci USA 73:4449, 1976

Carroll SF, McCloskey JF, Crain PF, Marschner TM, Collier RJ: Photoaffinity labeling of diphtheria toxin fragment A with NAD: structure of the photoproduct at position 148. Proc Natl Acad Sci USA 82:7237, 1985

Collier RJ: Effect of diphtheria toxin on protein synthesis. J Mol Biol 25:83, 1967

Collier RJ, Kandel J: Structure and activity of diphtheria toxin. J Biol Chem 246:1492, 1971

Freeman VJ: Studies on the virulence of bacteriophage infected strains of *Corynebacterium diphtheriae*. J Bacteriol 61:675, 1951

Gill DM, Pappenheimer AM Jr: Structure–activity relationships in diphtheria toxin. J Biol Chem 246:1492, 1971

Honjo T, Nishizuka Y, Kato I, Hayaishi O: Adenosine diphosphate ribosylation of aminoacyl transferase II by diphtheria toxin. J Biol Chem 246:4251, 1971

Kagan BL, Finkelstein A, Colombini M: Diphtheria toxin fragment forms large pores in phospholipid bilayer membranes. Proc Natl Acad Sci USA 78:4950, 1981

Moehring T, Danley DE, Moehring JM: In vitro biosynthesis of diphthamide, studied with mutant Chinese hamster ovary cells resistant to diphtheria toxin. Mol Cell Biol 4:642, 1984

Mueller JH: Nutrition of the diphtheria bacillus. Bacteriol Rev 4:97, 1940

Sandvig K, Olsnes S: Diphtheria toxin entry into cells is facilitated by low pH. J Cell Biol 87:828, 1980

Uchida T, Gill DM, Pappenheimer AM Jr: Mutation in the structural gene for diphtheria toxin carried by beta phage. Nature New Biol 233:8, 1971

Yamaizumi M, Mekada E, Uchida T, Okada Y: One molecule of diphtheria toxin fragment A introduced into a cell can kill the cell. Cell 15:245, 1978

23

Robert Austrian

Pneumococci

The bacteria to be discussed in this and the next three chapters are all pyogenic cocci, predominantly invasive pathogens that tend to produce purulent lesions: the streptococci and pneumococci, the staphylococci, and the neisseriae. All but the neisseriae are gram-positive. Functioning predominantly as extracellular parasites, they cause tissue damage when outside phagocytic cells. With the exception of some strains of staphylococci, pyogenic cocci are promptly destroyed once ingested by leukocytes. The diseases they cause are acute except when the organisms form abscesses or become lodged on heart valves. The organisms are generally susceptible to antimicrobial drugs, notably the beta-lactams, but they differ significantly in their tendencies to yield drug-resistant mutants: whereas penicillin-resistant variants of pneumococci are relatively uncommon and those of group A streptococci virtually unknown, strains resistant to benzylpenicillin are common among staphylococci and group D streptococci and fairly frequent among α-hemolytic and nonhemolytic streptococci and gonococci.

History

Elucidation of the properties of *Streptococcus pneumoniae* (pneumococcus, formerly *Diplococcus pneumoniae*) as an agent of disease has resulted in some of the most significant discoveries of biomedical science. Isolated first from saliva in 1880 by Sternberg in the United States and by Pasteur in France, the organism's relation to lobar pneumonia was established 6 years later. Recognition of serologically distinct types in 1910 led to the development of specific antisera, the first effective treatment for pneumococcal pneumonia. The observations of Dochez, Avery, Heidelberger, and Goebel on the chemical nature and structure of the capsular antigens led to elucidation of their roles in virulence and to the initial development of quantitative immunology. The discovery of the function of DNA in pneumococcal transformation in 1944 by Avery, MacLeod, and McCarty opened the door to molecular genetics and the subsequent revolution in biology.

Formerly a leading cause of death, pneumococcal pneumonia remains a common and serious illness, although it is usually responsive to prompt chemotherapy unless the patient is an infant, is over age 55, or has a chronic complicating illness. In a large study, uncomplicated bacteremic pneumococcal pneumonia in persons over age 12 treated with penicillin had a case fatality rate of 17%.

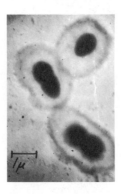

Figure 23–1. Electron micrograph of *Streptococcus pneumoniae,* type 1. The capsule has been reacted with type 1 Ab to accentuate its visibility (quellung reaction). (Mudd S et al: J Exp Med 78:327, 1943)

Morphology

Pneumococci, when isolated from an infected site, are typically encapsulated, gram-positive, lancet-shaped diplococci. In sputum, pus, serous fluid, and body tissues, they may be found in short chains and occasionally as individual cocci. Their tendency to form chains is exaggerated by an unfavorable medium for growth, by a low concentration of Mg^{2+}, or by the presence of type-specific antibody. Although gram-positive during the exponential phase of growth in laboratory media, more and more cells become gram-negative as the culture ages. If incubation is continued, the viable count falls, and the culture tends to clear. These changes are caused by autolytic enzymes, which first render the cell gram-negative and later bring about lysis. Autolysis is accelerated by surface-active agents such as bile, sodium deoxycholate, or sodium dodecylsulfate; and tests for "bile solubility" are useful in presumptively identifying pneumococci. These detergents activate an amidase that splits the tetrapeptide from muramic acid in peptidoglycan—a normal reaction in wall morphogenesis and cell division.

In liquid media, most strains of encapsulated pneumococci grow diffusely, tending to sediment only when the medium becomes acid; unencapsulated strains, particularly those growing in chains, exhibit granular growth, which results in relatively rapid sedimentation. Pneumococci are non-motile. On the surface of solid media (e.g., blood agar), encapsulated organisms form round, glistening, unpigmented colonies with a diameter of 0.5 to 1.5 mm after 24 to 36 hours of incubation. In general, the larger the capsule, the bigger and more mucoid are the colonies; those of type 3 and type 37 may reach a diameter of 3 mm. As surface colonies age, their centers autolyze, often giving rise to forms resembling checkers. Both surface and deep colonies become surrounded by a zone of α-hemolysis (see History and Classification, Chap. 25) but when grown anaerobically, no hemolysis or β-hemolysis may occur.

Pneumococcal capsules are demonstrable by suspending organisms in India ink or by treatment with homologous type-specific Ab, whose combination with the polysaccharide makes the capsule a more refractile gel. This **quellung** (Ger., swelling) reaction (Fig. 23–1) was described by Neufeld in 1902. Like other precipitin reactions, it is inhibited by excess Ag. In electron photomicrographs, pneumococcal capsules can be made out only in hazy outline (Fig. 23–2). They tend to become smaller in later phases of growth as the polysaccharide diffuses into the medium.

Pneumococcal L forms (Chap. 42), deficient in their cell walls, have been cultivated on hypertonic agar media containing penicillin.

Both lytic and temperate DNA bacteriophages have been isolated from pneumococci; they do not adsorb to encapsulated cells.

Nutrition and Growth

The pneumococcus is an obligate parasite with nutritional requirements resembling those of its hosts. It is classified among the lactic acid bacteria: facultative anaerobes that derive energy primarily from fermentation of carbohydrates to lactic acid. The ability to ferment inulin differentiates pneumococci from most α-hemolytic streptococci.

The most satisfactory media contain fresh beef heart infusion and may be supplemented with 10% serum or 5% defibrinated whole blood. Inclusion of reducing agents (cysteine, thioglycollate) permits the growth of small inocula and prevents the medium from becoming inhibitory after long exposure to air. Because pneumococci lack catalase, the H_2O_2 formed during growth causes loss of viability, but an exogenous source of catalase, such as RBCs, will enable their survival in broth cultures at 0° to 4°C for several months.

Synthetic media for the growth of pneumococci have been devised. Although too complex for routine use, they are suitable for recovering macromolecular fractions and products of pneumococci because their constituents are dialyzable. An uncommon growth requirement is **cho-**

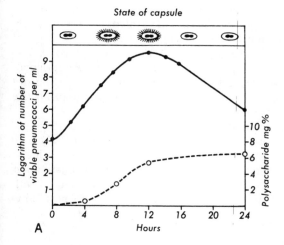

State of capsule

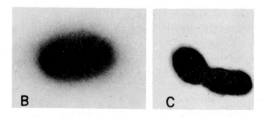

Figure 23–2. Relation of the growth of type 3 pneumococcus in broth culture to the state of the capsule and cumulative synthesis of capsular polysaccharide. *(A)* Electron photomicrographs of type 3 pneumococci from 4-hour *(B)* and 24-hour *(C)* cultures demonstrate loss of outer portion of capsule (slime layer) as culture ages and synthesis of capsular polysaccharide slows (note change in slope of broken curve in chart), (×6700; Wood WB Jr, Smith MR: J Exp Med 90:85, 1949)

line, which is incorporated into cell wall teichoic acid. It evidently plays a crucial role in the structure and functions of the cell wall, for substitution of ethanolamine for choline in a synthetic medium gives rise to several abnormalities: (1) the cells fail to divide normally and form long chains; (2) they are resistant to autolysis even when grown in the presence of penicillin, (3) they lose their ability to undergo transformation, and (4) they do not adsorb phages.

Antigenic Structure

Eighty-four serologic types of pneumococci have been recognized, distinguished by their capsular polysaccharides. Three classes of somatic Ags* have also been described. The C polysaccharide of the cell wall and a poorly defined R antigen are species-specific; the M protein is type-specific.

CAPSULAR ANTIGENS

Pneumococcal capsules are composed of large polysaccharide polymers, which form hydrophilic gels on the surface of the organisms. Some are linear, such as the chain of repeating glucose–glucuronic acid units of pneumococcus type 3, whereas others, with a larger number of units, have a branching structure. The pathway of biosynthesis of type 3 polysaccharide from uridine nucleotides has been elucidated (Fig. 23–3).

Some pneumococcal capsular polysaccharides cross-react with structurally related capsular Ags of other pneumococcal types (or of other bacterial species, including α-hemolytic and nonhemolytic streptococci,

klebsiellas, and salmonellae). For example, the cross-reacting polysaccharides of types 6A and 6B have the same constituent sugars but differ in having, respectively, a $1 \rightarrow 3$ and $1 \rightarrow 4$ rhamnosyl–ribitol bond; and the cross-reacting types 3 and 8 both contain residues of cellobiuronic acid.

PATHOGENETIC ROLE. The importance of the pneumococcal capsular Ags, which are devoid of toxicity, can be demonstrated in several ways. First, only encapsulated strains are pathogenic for man and susceptible laboratory animals, and active or passive immunization against a specific polysaccharide produces a high level of resistance to infection with pneumococci of the homologous type. Second, treatment of animals with an enzyme that depolymerizes type 3 capsular polysaccharide will protect them against infection with this pneumococcal type. Third, variants of type 3 that produce small capsules are less virulent than fully encapsulated strains but more virulent than unencapsulated variants. However the chemical structure of a capsular polysaccharide appears to be a more important determinant of virulence than the quantity produced.

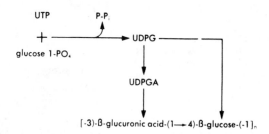

Figure 23–3. Metabolic pathway of type 3 capsular polysaccharide synthesis. *UTP*, uridine triphosphate; *UDPG*, uridine diphosphoglucose; *UDPGA*, uridine diphosphoglucuronic acid; *P-P$_i$*, inorganic pyrophosphate. (Austrian R et al: J Exp Med 110:585, 1959)

---

* The term "somatic antigen" is used to designate antigenic components of the body (Gr, *soma*) of a bacterial cell, exclusive of its capsule.

SOMATIC ANTIGENS

In 1930, Tillett, Goebel, and Avery isolated from pneumococcal cells a carbohydrate that is specific for species rather than type. This cell wall Ag, referred to as **C substance,** appears to be analogous to (although antigenically different from) the group-specific C Ags of hemolytic streptococci (see Cellular Antigens, Chap. 25). It also forms a portion of the pneumococcal Forssman antigen.

C polysaccharide consists of glucose, 2-acetamido-4-amino-2,4,6-trideoxygalactose, galactosamine, ribitol phosphate, and phosphorylcholine, the last being attached to the unacetylated galactosamine residue. The carbohydrate is linked to the peptidoglycan of the cell wall and has some properties of a teichoic acid. Some mutants produce soluble "C-like" (C_s) polysaccharide that may represent an early step in the evolution of the pneumococcal capsule, as each of its components is found in a capsular polysaccharide.

The C substance is precipitated in the presence of Ca^{2+} by a β-globulin sometimes present in serum, **C-reactive protein (CRP).** CRP is not an Ab but is a pentamer with a total molecular weight of approximately 110,000. In the presence of Ca^{2+}, it combines with phosphorylcholine and with phosphate monoesters. Complexes of CRP with the C substance can activate the complement pathway. CRP is detectable in blood during the acute phase of certain illnesses (not necessarily pneumococcal in origin) that are accompanied by inflammation, and its level has been used as a measure of "activity" in diseases such as rheumatic fever.

The **"R" antigen,** extracted initially from unencapsulated (R or "rough") pneumococci, is thought to be a protein on or near the surface of the cell. It has not been defined chemically.

Both capsulated and unencapsulated pneumococci possess a type-specific somatic protein Ag, **pneumococcal M protein,** with physicochemical properties similar to those of the M proteins of group A streptococci. The many different pneumococcal M proteins are independent of capsular type. They do not exert a significant antiphagocytic effect, and Abs to them are not protective as are those to streptococcal M Ags.

Immunization of rabbits with heat-killed unencapsulated pneumococci causes a slight increase in resistance to pneumococci of any capsular type, presumably due to Abs to the species-specific C polysaccharide and to other somatic Ags. This immunity is negligible compared with that mediated by Ab to the type-specific capsules, however.

Genotypic Variation

Noncapsulated mutants can be selected by serial passage in the presence of type-specific anticapsular serum, which agglutinates encapsulated cells and probably places them at a metabolic disadvantage. Conversely, in cultures of unencapsulated pneumococci, anti-R serum favors encapsulated back-mutants; and these enjoy an even greater selective advantage, because of their virulence, when a culture is injected into a mouse. Hence, passage of a strain through a mouse at frequent intervals is useful for maintaining maximal virulence.

The morphology of pneumococcal colonies on the surface of solid media is determined by two independent cellular properties: production of capsular polysaccharide, and completeness of cell separation after division. Cells that separate after division form dome-shaped

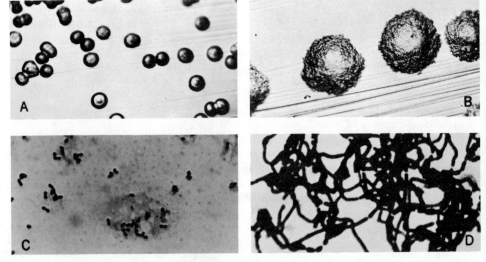

Figure 23–4. *(A)* Colonies of a nonfilamentous (fil⁻), unencapsulated (S⁻) variant (usual rough form) of pneumococcus type 2 on blood agar after 24 hours at 36°C. (×18) *(B)* Colonies of a filamentous (fil⁺), unencapsulated (S⁻) variant (very rough form) grown under same conditions. (×18) *(C)* Cells from colony of nonfilamentous variant. (Gram stain; ×900) *(D)* Cells of filamentous variant. (Gram stain; ×1100; Austrian R: J Exp Med 98:21, 1953)

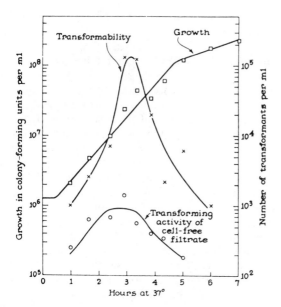

Figure 23–5. Development of transformability and release of transforming material by pneumococci growing in broth culture. The strain in the culture was sulfonamide resistant but streptomycin sensitive. Filtrates prepared from the culture at various intervals were used as donor material to transform a sulfonamide-sensitive strain **(transforming activity). Transformability** of the cultured strain was tested at various stages of the growth phase by adding purified DNA from a streptomycin-resistant culture. The cells from the original culture were exposed to the DNA for 30 minutes, and the reaction was terminated by DNase. (Ottolenghi E, Hotchkiss RD: J Exp Med 116:491, 1962)

colonies with entire edges, whereas cells that fail to separate form long chains (filaments) and give rise to colonies with rough surfaces and rugose margins (Fig. 23–4). These differences can be masked by large amounts of capsular polysaccharide. Filamentous variants are rarely, if ever, isolated from man.

Transformations of pneumococcal types by exogenous DNA have been discussed (Chap. 7). They have been demonstrated experimentally in mixed pneumococcal lesions in mice, and they may occur in nature. Cultures of pneumococci release transforming DNA maximally into the medium during the phase of growth when the cells are most responsive to added DNA (Fig. 23–5); Binary encapsulated pneumococci producing the polysaccharide Ags of two capsular types have been isolated from transforming reactions. Pneumococci also have been transformed with DNA from streptococci, with which pneumococci are now classified.

Pathogenicity

HOST RANGE. In addition to being pathogenic for man, most encapsulated strains of pneumococci will produce disease when inoculated into mice, rats, monkeys, or dogs. Cats and birds are relatively resistant. Pneumococcal infection occurs in cattle and horses and occasionally causes epizootics in monkeys, rats, and guinea pigs.

INCIDENCE AND SIGNIFICANCE OF TYPES. The nomenclature of Lund for pneumococcal capsular types is now widely accepted. With few exceptions, it groups chemically and immunologically related strains under an Arabic numeral, followed by a capital letter to designate individual types within a group. Not unexpectedly, the lower numerical groups, which were the first to be described, are responsible for the preponderance of infections (Table 23–1). Eighty per cent of bacteremic illnesses in the U.S. are caused by 22 of the 84 recognized types. The relative frequency of individual types may change with time and geographic area, but the more invasive types invariably predominate. In this country and in Northern Europe, types 2 and 5, formerly major causes of infection, have been encountered less frequently in recent years, although they persist in other areas of the world. The type 3 pneumococcus causes the highest fatality rate in man.

In children, types 6A, 6B, 14, 19F, 19A, and 23F account for more than half of all pneumococcal infections, including otitis media, in the first 6 years of life. The cross-reaction of type 14 capsular polysaccharide with the ABO blood group substances has been related to the occurrence of hemolytic anemia in some patients treated with type 14 antipneumococcal horse (but not rabbit) serum.

TOXICITY. The pneumococcus produces several toxic proteins, but there is no conclusive evidence that they play an important role in infection. Pneumolysin is a hemolysin related immunologically to the oxygen-labile O hemolysin of hemolytic streptococci, *Clostridium tetani*, and *Clostridium perfringens*. The pneumococcus

TABLE 23–1. Relative Frequency of Pneumococcal Types Isolated from 5797 Blood Cultures, 1967–1984, in the United States, All Ages

Type	% of Cases	Type	% of Cases
14	11.2	9V	4.0
4	10.1	12F	3.5
8	8.7	9N	3.0
6A + 6B*	7.5	19A	2.5
3	6.4	22F	2.1
23F	5.8	20	1.4
7F	5.3	5	1.3
18C	4.5	11A	1.0
1	4.3	16F	1.0
19F	4.1	Other	12.3

* Types combined because of their high degree of cross-reactivity.

also produces a neuraminidase, and during autolysis, the organism releases a purpura-producing principle that causes dermal and internal hemorrhages when injected into rabbits. Attempts to demonstrate a lethal toxin in the terminal stages of infection, analogous to that described in anthrax (Chap. 34), have been unsuccessful.

The type-specific capsular polysaccharides are essentially nontoxic; they contribute to virulence simply by protecting encapsulated pneumococci from phagocytosis. Late in infection, free polysaccharide promotes further bacterial invasion by diffusing into tissue fluids and neutralizing Ab there. In agranulocytic animals, unencapsulated pneumococci may cause progressive (and lethal) infection.

Intact killed unencapsulated pneumococcal cells can induce pulmonary leukostasis after intravenous injection and inflammatory changes in the subarachnoid space after intrathecal injection; they also activate the alternate complement pathway. However, 40 billion heat-killed pneumococci have been injected intravenously into man without significant untoward effect. How the pneumococcus causes death is still unknown.

PATHOGENESIS OF PNEUMOCOCCAL PNEUMONIA

DEFENSE BARRIERS OF THE RESPIRATORY TRACT. Colonization of the human upper respiratory tract with pneumococci may occur as early as the day of birth. Pneumococcal "adhesin," responsible for adherence of pneumococci to epithelial cells, is independent of the capsule; it may be a protein that attaches to a glycoprotein receptor of the host's cells. Between 40% and 70% of normal human adults carry one or more capsular types of pneumococci in their throats, yet epidemics of pneumococcal pneumonia are rare, and morbidity is estimated at one to five per 1000 persons per annum. Bacterial antagonism, primarily with α-hemolytic streptococci, tends to limit the growth of pneumococci in the pharynx. A pneumococcal protease hydrolyzes IgA_1, but its role in colonization of the respiratory tract is not established.

The extraordinarily efficient defense barriers of the lower respiratory tract include: (1) the epiglottal reflex, which prevents gross aspiration of food and infected secretions; (2) the sticky mucus to which airborne organisms adhere on the epithelial lining of the bronchial tree; (3) the cilia of the respiratory epithelium, which keep the mucus moving upward into the pharynx (see Mechanical Factors, Chap. 22); (4) the cough reflex, which aids the cilia in propelling accumulated secretions from the lower tract; (5) the lymphatics draining the terminal bronchi and bronchioles; and (6) the mononuclear alveolar macrophages ("dust cells"), which patrol the normally fluid-free alveoli.

PREDISPOSING FACTORS. Pneumococcal pneumonia develops most often during the course of viral infections of the upper respiratory tract, when the resulting increase in mucous secretions in the nose and pharynx enhances the likelihood of their aspiration. Once past the epiglottal barrier, the thin mucus, laden with bacteria, including encapsulated pneumococci, is carried by gravity, probably during sleep, to the farthest reaches of the bronchial tree, where it establishes the initial focus of pulmonary infection. Aspiration is promoted by factors that depress the epiglottal and cough reflexes, including chilling, alcoholic intoxication, morphine, and anesthesia.

Experiments in mice with infected aerosols have also revealed that an edematous lung is far more susceptible to pneumococcal infection than is the normally dry lung. Pulmonary edema fluid provides a suitable culture medium for aspirated pneumococci, and it interferes with the phagocytic activity of tissue macrophages—the first line of cellular defense in the alveoli. Factors that produce either local or generalized pulmonary edema, and hence predispose to pneumococcal pneumonia, include inhalation of irritating gases, aspiration of foreign material, viral infections of the lower respiratory tract (notably influenza), trauma to the thorax, cardiac failure, and pulmonary stasis resulting from long-term bed rest.

EVOLUTION OF THE LESION. Once infection has become established in a pulmonary segment, the pneumonic lesion spreads centrifugally (Fig. 23–6). In the edema zone, at the outer margin of the spreading lesion, the alveoli are filled with acellular serous fluid, which serves as a suitable culture medium. Following the outpouring of edema fluid and RBCs, polymorphonuclear leukocytes (PMNs) begin to accumulate in the infected alveoli and eventually fill them with a densely packed leukocytic exudate (consolidation). As they accumulate in sufficient numbers, the leukocytes phagocytize and destroy the infecting pneumococci. When the bacteria have been disposed of, macrophages replace the granulocytes in the exudate, and resolution of the lesion ensues. Thus, all stages of the inflammatory process are demonstrable simultaneously in the spreading pneumonic lesion, from the earliest stage in the peripheral edema zone to the subsiding inflammation in the central "burned-out" portion of the lesion.

When the alveoli underlying the pleura become involved, pleurisy develops, and the pleural cavity may become infected. If unchecked, pleural infections may develop into extensive intrapleural abscesses (empyema). The adjacent pericardium may also be affected (pericarditis).

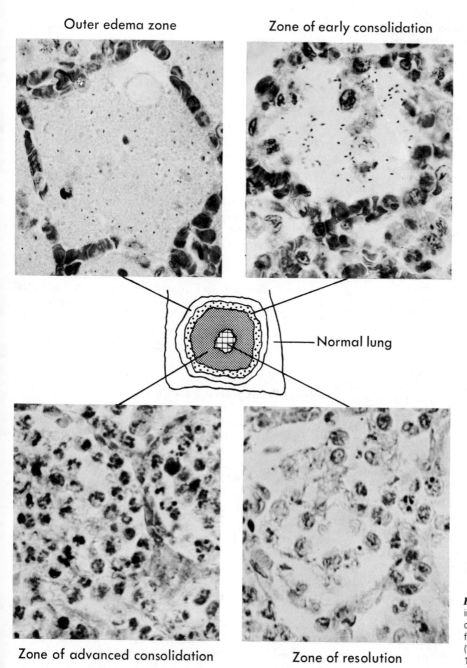

Outer edema zone

Zone of early consolidation

Normal lung

Zone of advanced consolidation

Zone of resolution

Figure 23–6. Schematic diagram of spreading pneumonic lesion *(center)* showing a characteristic microscopic field in each of its four histologically distinguishable zones. (Wood WB Jr: Harvey Lect 48:72, 1951–1952)

Pneumococcal pneumonia is often multilobar. Spread of the infection from one lobe to another results from the flow of infected edema fluid, propelled by the combined effects of respiration, coughing, and the force of gravity.

Although most of the pneumococci in the pulmonary lesion are destroyed by phagocytosis, some may be carried by the lymphatics to the regional lymph nodes at the hilus of the lung and thence, via the thoracic duct, to the blood stream. Once bacteremia has developed, or-

ganisms may settle on the heart valves or in the meninges or joints and occasionally can be cultured from the urine. In less serious cases, the primary pneumonic lesion resolves spontaneously without complications.

The phagocytic mechanisms that operate at the various lines of cellular defense have been described in Chapter 22. These mechanisms are relatively inefficient in fluid-filled cavities (subarachnoid space, pleura, pericardium, joints) and are incapable of destroying all pneumococci after an abscess has formed. Furthermore, type 3 pneumococci, which usually produce large capsules, are highly resistant to the surface phagocytosis that occurs even without homologous type-specific Ab, and they tend to reach considerably higher population densities than other types of pneumococci, resulting in irreversible tissue damage and abscess formation. Type 3 is virtually the only type that may cause lung abscesses in man.

Factors affecting the PMNs may worsen the course of pneumococcal pneumonia: granulocytopenia of any cause; glucocorticosteroid hormones, alcohol, and general anesthetics, which interfere with the migration of leukocytes from capillaries; and high levels of glucose (as in diabetes), which impede phagocytic activity.

OTHER PNEUMOCOCCAL DISEASES

Primary pneumococcal diseases of the upper respiratory tract include sinusitis and otitis media. The latter occurs most commonly in children and may spread to involve the mastoid. Progressive infections of the mastoid or paranasal sinuses sometimes extend directly to the subarachnoid space to cause pneumococcal meningitis. Secondary pneumococcal peritonitis, resulting from transient bacteremia following a primary respiratory infection, is observed most often in children with ascites secondary to nephrosis and in adults with cirrhosis or carcinoma of the liver. Pneumococcal bacteremia in the absence of an identifiable focus of infection occurs mostly in infants but has been recognized in adults.

Immunity

Immunity to pneumococcal infection depends on the presence of anticapsular Abs, which may be IgM, IgG, and IgA. Antibodies of both the IgM and IgG classes enhance phagocytosis and are protective. Although human Abs to pneumococcal capsular polysaccharides fix complement poorly *in vitro*, complement promotes Ab-mediated phagocytosis, both *in vitro* and *in vivo*. In immunization, purified capsular polysaccharides function as B-cell Ags, but when chemically linked to a protein they behave as T-cell Ags.

Patients with pneumococcal pneumonia usually develop a demonstrable increase in type-specific anticapsular Ab by the fifth or sixth day, when a spontaneous crisis, characterized by dramatic defervescence and subsidence of symptoms, may occur in a third of untreated patients. Recovery occurs in approximately 70% of untreated cases and may take place even in the "preantibody" stage of illness, as a result of the primary cellular defenses that operate in the lung (see Chap. 22). Following recovery, anticapsular Ab usually remains detectable in the patient's serum for months to years.

Type-specific antibody may be detected by precipitin tests, radioimmunoassay, or ELISA with the homologous polysaccharides or by agglutination, phagocytic, or quellung tests performed with homologous cells. Antibodies to those types virulent for the mouse may be assayed by protection tests in this species. Circulating Ab may be detected also by injecting homologous capsular polysaccharide intradermally (Francis' skin test). The interaction of Ab with the injected Ag causes an immediate wheal and erythema at the site of the injection.

Pneumococcal capsular polysaccharides may reach amounts in consolidated lung exceeding 1 g, and they remain in the tissues for relatively long periods. In experimental pneumonia, they have been demonstrated in alveolar macrophages many weeks after recovery from acute illness. The polysaccharide retained in the lung is released gradually and may be detected in the urine by precipitin tests as long as 3 months after recovery. Polysaccharide may be detected also, when present in the serum or in infected body fluids, by counterimmunoelectrophoresis.

Laboratory Diagnosis

A tentative diagnosis of pneumococcal pneumonia may be made most rapidly by examining the patient's sputum. Smears made from a fresh sample raised directly from the lower respiratory tract in the presence of the physician should be stained by the gram method to distinguish *S. pneumoniae* from *Klebsiella pneumoniae* and staphylococci, which also produce acute bacterial pneumonia. If typical lancet-shaped diplococci in large numbers are seen in the smear together with PMNs and alveolar macrophages, a presumptive diagnosis of pneumococcal pneumonia may be made and treatment begun. At the same time, the sputum should be cultured on blood agar incubated in 5% CO_2 for final identification (see below). When sputum cannot be obtained (e.g., from a small child or a comatose patient), a pharyngeal culture is used in the same fashion, or material may be obtained by transtracheal or lung puncture.

Rapid typing of pneumococci in sputum by the quellung reaction was formerly done routinely to permit prompt treatment of the patient with the correct antiserum. Although this procedure is now performed infrequently in diagnostic laboratories, if typical gram-positive diplococci are not seen in the sputum of a patient suspected strongly of having bacterial pneumonia, a sample of the sputum should be emulsified with a small amount of broth in a 1- or 2-ml syringe and injected intraperitoneally into a mouse. When virulent pneumococci are present, the mouse will usually die within 4 days, and the offending pneumococcus can then be recovered from the cardiac blood in pure culture and typed directly from peritoneal washings. The quellung reaction is especially useful for the prompt identification of pneumococci in body fluids such as spinal fluids. A reagent containing antibodies to 83 pneumococcal capsular polysaccharides (Omniserum) is most suitable for this purpose.

Because many healthy humans carry pneumococci in their throats, demonstration of the organism in sputum or a pharyngeal culture does not provide conclusive evidence of pneumococcal infection. Recovery of pneumococci from the patient's blood, on the other hand, is diagnostic. For this reason, blood should be obtained prior to antimicrobial therapy and cultured immediately in beef infusion or in trypticase soy broth. Bacterial counts in pour plates made with known volumes of blood are useful prognostically.

Fluids obtained from the pleural, pericardial, peritoneal, synovial, or cerebrospinal cavities should be cultured in the same way and also on blood agar, which should be incubated in an atmosphere containing 5% CO_2. At the same time, direct smears of gram-stained material should be examined. If organisms resembling pneumococci are present, they can be identified immediately as pneumococci by the quellung reaction. Capsular polysaccharide can sometimes be identified in the spinal fluid of a treated patient.

Pneumococci are morphologically similar to other streptococci of the viridans group (see α-Hemolytic Streptococci, Chap. 25), but they differ usually in being bile-soluble, virulent for mice, and sensitive to optochin (ethylhydrocupreine), an antibacterial compound relatively specific for pneumococci. The bile solubility test requires the use of live cells and is best done with deoxycholate and with saline suspensions of pneumococci; because proteins in liquid media inhibit the reaction, presumably by binding deoxycholate. A paper disc impregnated with optochin may be used to test for inhibition of bacterial growth on the surface of a blood agar plate.

Treatment

Type-specific antiserum is no longer available, and sulfonamides are not recommended. The drug generally used is benzylpenicillin, although resistance to this agent and to other antibiotics is found occasionally. Pneumococcal resistance to penicillin results from mutations in its penicillin-binding proteins. In uncomplicated pneumococcal pneumonia caused by a sensitive strain, treatment with penicillin is usually successful unless started too late.

Erythromycin or clindamycin may be used to treat pneumonia in patients with known hypersensitivity to penicillin, but the pneumococcal isolate should be tested for its sensitivity to the drug employed. Broad-spectrum antibiotics (e.g., the tetracyclines) may also be effective, although tetracycline-resistant strains are not rare. Chloramphenicol should be used only to treat pneumococcal meningitis in patients allergic to penicillin. Vancomycin is the drug of choice for pneumococcal strains resistant to multiple drugs.

Prevention

Although pneumococcal diseases usually respond to antimicrobial therapy, the case fatality rate of optimally treated bacteremic infection among those over 50 years of age and in individuals with underlying systemic illness exceeds 25%. Occasionally, in military, industrial, and custodial institutions, an epidemic will result when a significant proportion of the population lacks immunity to the pneumococcal types carried by its members. Accordingly, renewed interest in prophylaxis has arisen. Vaccines of 12 to 14 pneumococcal capsular polysaccharides prevent pneumococcal pneumonia and bacteremia caused by organisms of the corresponding types. A vaccine containing 23 capsular Ags is now available, and its administration to individuals at high risk of fatal infection and in epidemic situations is recommended.

Indiscriminate treatment of acute respiratory infections with antimicrobial drugs to prevent pneumonia should be discouraged, not only because of its inutility, but also because of the hazard of drug reactions and the selection of drug-resistant mutants of bacteria being carried by the host.

Ideally, every patient with pneumococcal pneumonia should be isolated. Although rules of isolation are often disregarded because of the relatively low rates of cross-infection, such patients should not be placed in crowded hospital wards in proximity to persons with congestive heart failure or other debilitating diseases.

Selected Reading
BOOKS AND REVIEW ARTICLES

Austrian R: Life with the Pneumococcus. Philadelphia, University of Pennsylvania Press, 1985

Heffron R: Pneumonia with Special Reference to Pneumococcus Lobar Pneumonia. New York, Commonwealth Fund, 1939*

White B: The Biology of Pneumococcus: The Bacteriological, Biochemical, and Immunological Characters and Activities of *Diplococcus pneumoniae*. New York, Commonwealth Fund, 1938*

* Although unrevised, these two monographs remain landmarks in the field. They were reprinted by the Harvard University Press in 1979.

Winkelstein JA: Complement and the host's defense against the pneumococcus. CRC Crit Rev Microbiol 11:187, 1984

SPECIFIC ARTICLES

Andersson B, Dahmén J, Frejd T, Leffler H, Magnusson G, Noori G, Eden CS: Identification of an active disaccharide unit of a glycoconjugate receptor for pneumococci attaching to human pharyngeal epithelial cells. J Exp Med 158:559, 1983

Austrian R: *Streptococcus pneumoniae* (Pneumococcus). In Lennette EH, Spaulding EH, Truant JP (eds): Manual of Clinical Microbiology, 2nd Ed, p 109. Washington, DC, American Society for Microbiology, 1974

Austrian R, Gold J: Pneumococcal bacteremia with especial reference to bacteremic pneumococcal pneumonia. Ann Intern Med 60:759, 1964

Beuvery EC, Von Rossum F, Nagel J: Comparison of the induction of immunoglobulin M and G antibodies in mice with purified pneumococcal type 3 and meningococcal group C polysaccharides and their protein conjugates. Infect Immun 37:15, 1982

Bornstein DL, Schiffman G, Bernheimer HP, Austrian R: Capsulation of pneumococcus with soluble C-like (C$_s$) polysaccharide. J Exp Med 128:1385, 1968

Brown EJ, Hosea SW, Hammer CH, Burch CG, Frank MM: A quantitative analysis of the interactions of antipneumococcal antibody and complement in experimental pneumococcal bacteremia. J Clin Invest 69:85, 1982

Francis T Jr, Terrell EE, Dubos R: Experimental type III pneumococcus pneumonia in monkeys II: Treatment with an enzyme which decomposes the specific capsular polysaccharide of pneumococcus type III. J Exp Med 59:641, 1934

Garcia-Bustos JF, Chait BT, Tomasz A: Altered peptidoglycan structure in a pneumococcal transformant resistant to penicillin. J Bact 170:2143, 1988

Jennings HJ, Lugowski C, Young NM: Structure of the complex polysaccharide C-substance of *Streptococcus pneumoniae*. Biochemistry 19:4712, 1980

Katzenellenbogen E, Jennings HJ: Structural determination of the capsular polysaccharide of *Streptococcus pneumoniae* type 19A (57). Carbohydr Res 124:235, 1983

Lund E: Laboratory diagnosis of *Pneumococcus* infections. Bull World Health Org 23:5, 1960

McDaniel LS, Briles DE: A pneumococcal surface protein (PspB) that exhibits the same protease sensitivity as streptococcal R antigen. Infect Immun 56:3001, 1988

Ottolenghi E, MacLeod CM: Genetic transformation among living pneumococci in the mouse. Proc Natl Acad Sci USA: 50:417, 1963

Rich AR, McKee CM: The pathogenicity of avirulent pneumococci for animals deprived of leukocytes. Bull Johns Hopkins Hosp 64:434, 1939

Robbins JB, Austrian R, Lee C-J et al: Considerations for formulating the second-generation pneumococcal capsular polysaccharide vaccine with emphasis on cross-reactive types within groups. J Infect Dis 148:1136, 1983

Ward J: Antibiotic-resistant *Streptococcus pneumoniae:* Clinical and epidemiologic aspects. Rev Infect Dis 3:254, 1981

24

Maclyn McCarty

Streptococci

History and Classification

Globular microorganisms growing in chains were first described by Billroth in 1874 in purulent exudates from erysipelas lesions and infected wounds. Similar organisms, eventually named streptococci (Gr. *streptos*, winding, twisted), were isolated from the blood in puerperal fever and from the throat in scarlet fever. It is now known that **a single streptococcal species may be responsible for a variety of diseases.** However, a number of different kinds of streptococci may be cultured from human patients and animals, and the first classifications were based on their capacities to hemolyze RBCs. In 1919, Brown introduced the terms **alpha, beta,** and **gamma** to describe the three types of **hemolytic** reactions observed on blood agar plates.

Primarily through the efforts of Lancefield in the early 1930s, the β-hemolytic streptococci were further differentiated into a number of **immunologic groups** designated by the letters A through O. Most strains causing human infections were found to belong to **group A.** That group, in turn, contains a variety of **antigenic types,** later demonstrated by precipitin tests (Lancefield) and by agglutination reactions (Griffith). The group-specific Ags were identified as carbohydrates and the type-specific Ags as proteins.

More than 55 types of group A β-hemolytic streptococci have been identified.

HEMOLYTIC CLASSES

β-Hemolytic streptococci produce a wide clear zone of complete hemolysis (Fig. 24–1*A*) in which no red cells are visible on microscopic examination. Two types of β-hemolysin are released. **Streptolysin O** is inactivated by atmospheric oxygen and is therefore demonstrable only in deep colonies. **Streptolysin S** is oxygen stable and is

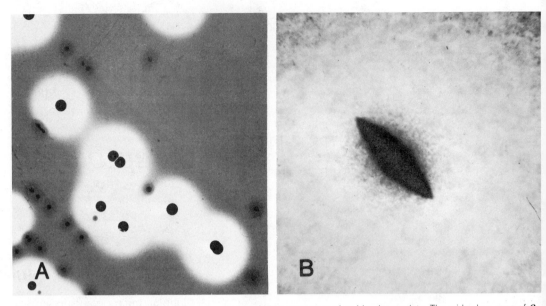

Figure 24–1. *(A)* Surface colonies of *S. pyogenes* and viridans streptococci on blood agar plate. The wide clear zone of **β-hemolysis** of the former is much more prominent than the latter's narrower dark zone of **α-hemolysis.** A few small viridans colonies can be seen to have grown within some of the zones of β-hemolysis (×4). *(B)* Higher-power (×50) view of a deep α-hemolytic colony on blood agar (note oblong shape) showing border of incomplete hemolysis about the colony. No such band of intact red cells is present in the much wider zones of β-hemolysis that surround comparable colonies of β-hemolytic streptococci. (Preparation by E. D. Updyke; photograph by courtesy of the Centers for Disease Control, Atlanta, GA)

responsible for surface colony hemolysis. Because most strains produce both S and O hemolysins, they can usually be recognized as β-hemolytic by their surface colonies. To be certain of the hemolytic characteristics of a certain strain, however, it may be necessary to examine the colonies located beneath the surface of a pour plate. Group A streptococci are commonly referred to as *Streptococcus pyogenes.*

α-Hemolytic streptococcus colonies are surrounded by a narrower zone of hemolysis, with unhemo-

TABLE 24–1. Group Classification of β-Hemolytic and Other Immunologically Related Streptococci

Group	Hemolysis	Usual Habitat	Pathogenicity
A	+	Man	Many human diseases
B	±	Man	Neonatal meningitis
	+	Cattle	Mastitis
C	±	Many animals	Many animal diseases
		Man	Mild respiratory infections
D	±	Dairy products, intestinal tract of man and animals (enterococci)	Urinary tract and wound infections; endocarditis
E	+	Milk	Unknown
		Swine	Pharyngeal abscesses
F	+	Man	?; Found in respiratory tract
G	+	Man	Mild respiratory infections
		Dogs	Rare genital tract infections
H	±	Man	?; Found in respiratory tract
K	±	Man	?; Found in respiratory tract
L	+	Dogs	Genital tract infections
M	+	Dogs	Genital tract infections
N	−	Dairy products	None
O	±	Man	Carried in upper respiratory tract; endocarditis

+ = All strains hemolytic; ± = some strains hemolytic, others nonhemolytic; − = all strains nonhemolytic.

(Modified from McCarty M: Hemolytic streptococci. In Dubos RJ, Hirsch JG (eds): Bacterial and Mycotic Infections of Man. Philadelphia, JB Lippincott, 1965)

lyzed RBCs persistent in an inner zone and complete hemolysis in an outer zone (Fig. 24–1*B*). (The mechanism responsible for sparing some of the red cells is not known.) Green discoloration of the hemolyzed zone, due to formation of an unidentified reductant of hemoglobin, frequently occurs, depending on the type of blood in the medium and the duration of incubation; hence the synonym term **viridans group.** *Streptococcus salivarius* is the most commonly encountered species of this category.

γ-Streptococci produce no hemolysis, either on the surface or within the agar. ~~*Streptococcus faecalis* is a typical nonhemolytic species.~~

This classification of streptococci based on hemolysis is not entirely reliable, because there is considerable strain variation. For example, certain members of antigenic groups B, C, D, H, and O are nonhemolytic, despite the usual classification of these groups in the β-hemolytic category (Table 24–1). Hemolysis remains a useful characteristic for the recognition of streptococci, but serologic grouping is required for accurate identification.

Because streptococcal disease in man is caused primarily by group A organisms, which produce β-hemolysis, most of this chapter will be devoted to this group.

β-Hemolytic Streptococci

MORPHOLOGY

Cell Division

β-Hemolytic streptococci (often simply called hemolytic streptococci), like all streptococci, are gram-positive and characteristically grow in chains; *in vivo*, they commonly occur as diplococci. The length of the chains tends to be inversely related to the adequacy of the culture medium: in actively spreading lesions within the tissues, diplococcal and individual coccal forms are common, whereas in purulent exudates from walled-off lesions and in artifi-

cial culture media, chain formation is the rule (Fig. 24–2). Prior to division, the individual cocci become elongated on the axis of the chain, eventually dividing to form pairs. When the dividing pairs of cocci do not separate, chaining results. The bridges between the individual cocci in the chain are composed of cell wall material that has not cleaved. Uncleaved cell walls are particularly striking in mutants with excessive chaining, which produce opaque colonies on clear agar (Fig. 24–3).

Factors tending to promote preservation of the intercoccal junctions and thus to exaggerate chaining include not only conditions that impair growth (unfavorable medium, cold, antimicrobial agents, etc.), but also the presence of Abs that react with cell wall Ags, especially the M protein surface Ag (see below).

Because streptococcal chains are difficult to disrupt without killing the organisms, it is customary to record streptococcal colony counts in **streptococcal units.** These values provide only a rough index of the number of cells, as they are obviously influenced by the degree of chaining.

Capsules and Colony Morphology

Many strains of hemolytic streptococci produce capsules, which in groups A and C are composed of hyaluronic acid. These capsules are demonstrable throughout the logarithmic phase of growth in liquid cultures, but after the onset of the stationary phase they dissolve rapidly into the medium.

On blood agar plates group A streptococci may form any one of three colony types, designated **mucoid, matt** (Ger. *matt*, dull), and **glossy.** Mucoid colonies are formed by strains that produce large capsules: the abundance of hyaluronic acid gel gives the colony a glistening, watery appearance. The flatter, rougher, matt colonies were originally thought to reflect the production of M protein (the designation M was based on this apparent relation), but they are simply dried out mucoid colonies; as Figure

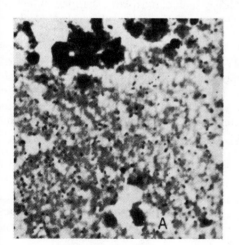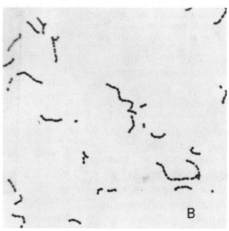

Figure 24–2. (*A*) Group A β-hemolytic streptococci in edema zone of experimental pneumonic lesion (rat). (See Evolution of Lesion, Chap. 27). Note diplococcal morphology (×600). (*B*) Chain formation characteristic of usual growth of streptococci in artificial media. Smear made from 24-hour culture in serum broth (×1000). (*A*, Glaser RJ, Wood WB Jr: Arch Pathol 52:244, 1951; Copyright © 1951 by the American Medical Association)

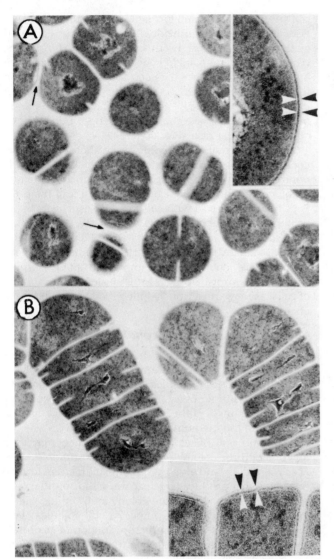

Figure 24–3. Thin-section electron micrographs of parent M⁻ strain of *S. pyogenes* (**A**) and a mutant (**B**) that produces opaque colonies. Whereas intercellular septa are completely cleaved in the parent strain to form individual cocci and diplococci, most of the septa of the mutant remain uncleaved so that the organism grows in long chains. The fine structure of the cell walls in the two strains appear to be identical, however (see *insets,* between *arrows*). (Swanson J, McCarty M: J Bacteriol 100:505, 1969)

24–4 shows, as the gel becomes dehydrated the surface of the colony shrinks and becomes roughened.

Glossy colonies are smaller; they are formed by cells that do not generate hyaluronate or do not retain it as a capsular gel. Groups F and G include **minute streptococci,** which produce not only smaller cells than other streptococci but also smaller colonies.

L FORMS AND PROTOPLASTS. L forms (Chap. 43) of group A streptococci, which lack most cell wall constituents, may be isolated from anaerobic cultures on hypertonic media containing penicillin. Complete removal of the wall to form protoplasts may be achieved by treating intact cells with a muralytic enzyme (e.g., the phage-associated mucopeptidase of group C streptococci). Unlike the protoplasts isolated from most other bacterial species, these will multiply and produce typical L form colonies in hypertonic agar medium. During growth they release cell wall M antigen, hemolysin, and deoxyribonuclease into the medium.

METABOLISM

Hemolytic streptococci are routinely grown in beef infusion media containing blood or serum. For the isolation of specific Ags and extracellular enzymes, a medium containing only the dialyzable components of the complex meat infusion peptone medium may be used, and recently a chemically defined medium has been devised that will serve this purpose. The growth requirements are very similar to those of pneumococci (see Metabolism, Chap. 23).

All streptococci are **lactic acid bacteria,** which derive their energy primarily from the fermentation of sugars, regardless of whether they are growing aerobically or anaerobically. Accumulation of lactic acid in media of high glucose content limits growth unless the pH is corrected.

CELLULAR ANTIGENS
Capsular Hyaluronic Acid

The hyaluronate of the capsule of groups A and C streptococci is a prominent surface constituent of the organism (see Fig. 24–6, below). It is chemically indistinguishable from the hyaluronate in the ground substance of connective tissue, which can explain its apparent lack of immunogenicity. Recent findings indicate that streptococci can induce Abs to hyaluronate, but there is no evidence that they have protective action. The hyaluronate capsule is retained only by growing streptococci or by cells that have been rapidly chilled while in the logarithmic phase. The process responsible for release of the capsule in the stationary phase is not known, and it cannot be attributed to the production of hyaluronidase by the organism.

Group-Specific C Antigens

As already indicated, the separation of β-hemolytic streptococci into immunologically specific groups (A to O) depends on the presence of group-specific **C carbohydrate Ags,** in most cases represented by a structural

Colony forms:
group A

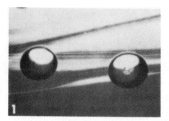

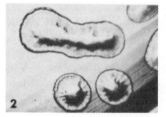

Mucoid

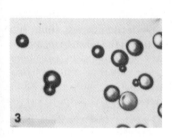

Matt

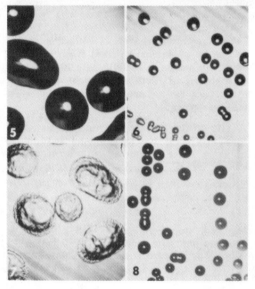

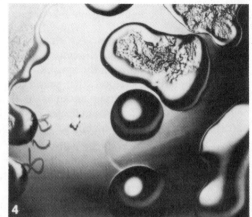

Glossy

Figure 24–4. Interrelations between mucoid, matt, and glossy colonies of group A hemolytic streptococci. *(1–3)* The three types of colonies that form on the surfaces of blood agar plates. *(4)* Conversion of mucoid to matt form as a result of aging (20 hours) and drying out of colonies (×6.8). *(5)* 19-Hour mucoid colonies of type 17 strain grown on Todd–Hewitt sheep blood agar. *(6)* Glossy colonies of same type 17 strain grown on the same medium containing hyaluronidase. *(7)* 24-Hour matt colonies of type 14 strain grown on Todd–Hewitt blood agar. *(8)* Glossy colonies of same type 14 strain grown on the same medium containing hyaluronidase *(5–8,* ×5.5). Note that the presence of hyaluronidase in agar prevents capsule formation and results in formation of glossy rather than mucoid (or matt) colonies. *(1–3,* Lancefield RC: Harvey Lect 36:251, 1942; *4–8,* Wilson AT: J Exp Med 109:257, 1959)

component of the protective cell wall. These insoluble Ags can be extracted by a number of techniques.

In the test used routinely in grouping streptococci, the cells are suspended in dilute HCl (pH 2) at 100°C for 10 minutes, neutralized, and centrifuged; the clear supernatant fluid contains the Ag. It may also be extracted by treatment with formamide at 150°C, by autoclaving, or by treatment with a cell wall-dissolving enzyme from *Streptomyces albus*.

The group-specific Ag reacts with antisera produced by immunizing rabbits with hemolytic streptococci of the same group. Precipitin reactions performed with appropriate sera permit the grouping of unknown strains. Although, as noted earlier, most streptococci that cause disease in man fall into group A, human disease can be caused by members of other groups.

The carbohydrate Ag of the cell wall makes up approximately 10% of the dry weight of the organism, and

in groups A and C its antigenic specificity depends largely on hexosamine side chains attached to the core rhamnose backbone. The determinant is β-linked N-acetyl glucosamine in the group A Ag, and a disaccharide of N-acetyl galactosamine in the group C Ag. Variant strains have also been described whose group-specific Ag lacks the hexosamine side chains; the specificity then appears to reside in the rhamnose polymer of the backbone.

Type-Specific M Antigens

Group A streptococci can be further distinguished as more than 55 immunologic types that differ in their cell wall M Ags. M protein is distributed on the surface of the cell associated with fimbriae (Fig. 24–5), which are lacking in most M⁻ strains (see Fig. 24–3). The M proteins may be extracted either by the relatively drastic acid treatment (boiling at pH 2) used to solubilize the C Ag or by lysis of the cell (in the absence of proteolysis) with cell

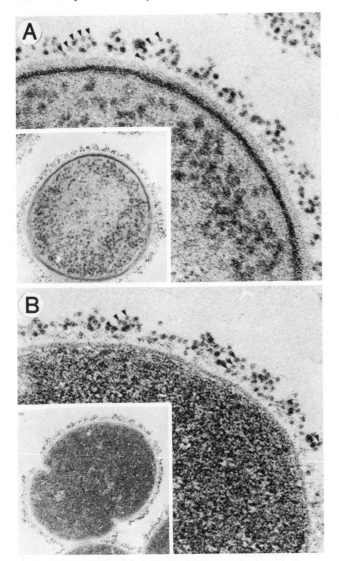

Figure 24—5. Electron micrographs of fimbriae on surface of group A β-hemolytic streptococci. The fimbriae have taken up homologous ferritin-conjugated anti-M Ab. The section of an intact cell shown in *(A)* is compared in *(B)* with a nitrous acid-extracted cell; this treatment removes most of the C polysaccharide and teichoic acid of the wall, leaving the M protein intact. The ferritin particles can be seen to have assumed a linear distribution *(arrows)* along the surfaces of the fimbriae. (×250,000; insets ×60,000; Swanson J et al: J Exp Med 130:1063, 1969)

wall-dissolving enzymes. Limited cleavage by pepsin at the suboptimal pH 5.8 also releases a serologically active fragment of the antigen.

Typing is usually done by precipitin tests with the extracted M protein and specific rabbit antisera that have been absorbed with cells of heterologous types to eliminate cross-reactions. Although streptococci may also be typed by agglutination tests, the precipitin method is preferred because of the effect of T Ags (see below) on the agglutination reactions.

The M protein appears to be anchored in the cell membrane and, after extending through the wall, projects from the surface of the cell as a fibrillar structure (fimbriae). It is therefore readily accessible to anti-M Ab even when the hyaluronate capsule is present. Furthermore, anti-M Ab is protective, showing that the M Ag is directly involved in streptococcal virulence; indeed, both the hyaluronate capsule and the M protein are antiphagocytic (see Pathogenicity, below). Finally, removal of the M Ag of intact cells with trypsin does not affect cell viability or remove the group Ag.

It is striking that the M Ags of the many different types, so distinctive in immunologic specificity, retain the common property of being antiphagocytic. Current research involving the amino acid sequencing, and cloning of the genes, of several M proteins is throwing light on structure–function relations. The M Ags have a coiled-coil structure, with a highly variable distal, amino-terminal portion and a more conserved proximal portion; the protective epitope(s) apparently occur at the external portion.

Other Cellular Antigens

Two other kinds of cell wall proteins participate in specific agglutination reactions but do not seem to influence virulence. The **T antigens** include a number of immunologically distinct proteins, also designated by numbers; their distribution is not parallel with that of the M proteins. The T antigens resist digestion with proteolytic enzymes but are readily destroyed by heat at an acid pH and hence are not present in the usual M-containing acid extract. Two different **R proteins** have thus far been identified: one (designated 3R) is destroyed by either pepsin or trypsin, the other (28R) only by pepsin.

A **nucleoprotein fraction (P antigen)** is antigenically similar in hemolytic and nonhemolytic streptococci and in pneumococci; it also cross-reacts with staphylococcal nucleoproteins. The **glycerol teichoic acids** (Chap. 2), which make up approximately 1% of the dry weight of the cells, act as the group-specific Ag in groups D and N but not in other groups. In group A strains the glycerophosphate polymer has no substituents other than ester-linked D-alanine and the Abs to this Ag reflect the glycerophosphate specificity and occasionally also the D-alanine specificity. In those groups in which teichoic acid serves as the group-specific Ag the specific determinants are sugar substituents in the glycerophosphate chain. When isolated with attached lipid (**lipoteichoic acid**), these Ags adsorb readily to RBCs and other mammalian cells; and surface lipoteichoic acid is involved in the attachment and colonization of streptococci on mucosal surfaces *in vivo*.

The **peptidoglycan,** which cross-reacts with those of

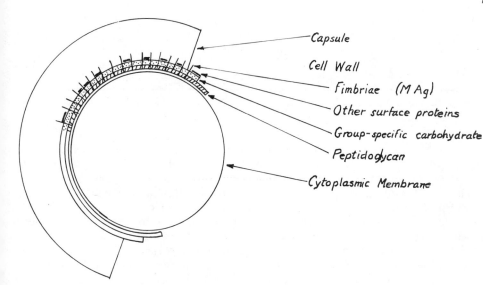

Figure 24–6. Schematic diagram of the surface components of group A hemolytic streptococcal cell. The general relations are shown, although the wall carbohydrate and peptidoglycan layers are probably less distinctly separate from one another than depicted here.

many other bacteria, produces many of the same biological reactions as the endotoxins of gram-negative bacteria (see Endotoxin, Chap. 27), such as fever, dermal and cardiac necrosis, lysis of RBCs and platelets, and enhancement of nonspecific resistance. The **cytoplasmic membranes,** prepared from osmotically shocked protoplasts, contain numerous protein Ags and exhibit distinctive antigenic differences when derived from streptococci of different immunologic groups.

Apparent Spatial Relations

In summary, virulent group A streptococci may possess, in addition to their polysaccharide capsules, at least three distinct protein antigens on their cell walls (Fig. 24–6). One of these, the type-specific M protein, is important because it is the dominant antiphagocytic component and therefore intimately concerned with virulence; the other two (T and R Ags) are unrelated to virulence. Among other surface proteins, not well defined as antigens, are a receptor for the Fc portion of IgG and a recently described enzyme that inactivates the chemotactic complement fragment, C5a.

The group-specific **C Ag is covalently linked to the peptidoglycan,** which is itself immunogenic. Other streptococcal Ags, ordinarily not exposed to the surface of the intact cell, include the lipoprotein Ags of the cell membranes and a nucleoprotein (P) Ag, in the cytoplasm. The glycerol teichoic acids appear to be attached to the membrane and not to the wall, although a small portion must be exposed at the surface of the cell where it participates in the attachment to host cells.

EXTRACELLULAR PRODUCTS

The exceptionally wide variety of human diseases caused by group A streptococci may well be related to the large number of extracellular products they produce. The best known of these enzymes and toxins are listed in Table 24–2. Analysis of the extracellular material indicates that there are still others as yet unidentified. By means of immunoelectrophoresis, for example, 20 different Abs that react with the extracellular Ags elaborated by one strain of group A streptococcus have been found in pooled human γ-globulin (Fig. 24–7). Of those Ags identified thus far, the following appear to be of greatest clinical significance.

ERYTHROGENIC TOXIN. The erythrogenic toxins are responsible for the rash in scarlet fever. Strains of group A streptococci that produce them are lysogenic, like toxigenic strains of *Corynebacterium diphtheriae* (see Lysogeny and Toxin Production, Chap. 22). Nontoxigenic strains can be converted to toxin producers by lysogenization with the appropriate phage.

TABLE 24–2. Some Extracellular Products of Group A β-Hemolytic Streptococci

	Stimulates Production of Inhibitory Antibody
Erythrogenic toxins (A, B, and C)	+
Streptolysin O	+
Streptolysin S	−
Diphosphopyridine nucleotidase	+
Streptokinases (A and B)	+
Deoxyribonucleases (A, B, C, and D)	+
Hyaluronidase	+
Proteinase	+
Amylase	?
Esterase	−

Figure 24–7. Diagrammatic representation of group A streptococcal extracellular Ags detectable by immunoelectrophoretic analysis performed with crude streptococcal concentrate and 16% solution of pooled human γ-globulin. (Halbert SP, Keatinge SL: J Exp Med 113:1015, 1961)

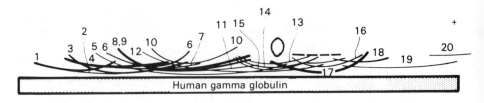

Human gamma globulin

The mode of action of erythrogenic toxin is not clear. When injected into the skin of susceptible children, it causes localized erythematous reactions, which reach a maximum at about 24 hours **(Dick test).** This erythrogenic effect is neutralized by Ab: during convalescence, when the patient's serum contains demonstrable antitoxin, the skin test becomes negative; and an injection of homologous antitoxin at the height of scarlet fever causes a local blanching of the rash **(Schultz–Charlton test).** Accordingly, a positive Dick test is interpreted as indicating an absence of circulating antitoxin and thus a state of susceptibility to scarlet fever.

There are at least three immunologically distinct forms of erythrogenic toxin (types A, B, and C), produced by different streptococcal strains. They are proteins that cause a number of toxic effects in animals, including pyrogenicity and enhancement of the action of gram-negative endotoxins. Certain strains of group C and group G hemolytic streptococci, as well as some staphylococci, produce erythrogenic toxins closely related to those of group A streptococci.

STREPTOLYSINS S AND O. The two hemolysins responsible for the zones of hemolysis around streptococcal colonies have already been mentioned. **Streptolysin S** is stable in air and is largely cell bound, indicating that it might more appropriately be classed as a cellular constituent. The designation "S" derives from the fact that it can be extracted from intact streptococcal cells with serum. This extraction depends on association with serum albumin as a macromolecular carrier, and other carriers (e.g., RNA) will similarly form a complex with the hemolysin. No Ab capable of neutralizing the hemolytic action of streptolysin S has been described, but this action is inhibited by serum lipoproteins. This cell-bound hemolysin appears to be responsible for the **leukotoxic** action of group A streptococci, manifested by the killing of a proportion of the leukocytes that phagocytize them.

Streptolysin O has been so named because it is reversibly **inactivated by atmospheric oxygen.** It gives rise to Abs that neutralize its hemolytic action. Because most strains of group A streptococci produce streptolysin O, patients recovering from streptococcal disease usually have antistreptolysin O Abs in their serum (see Tests for other Antibodies, below). As with other oxygen-labile bacterial exotoxins, the antigenicity of streptolysin O survives its detoxification by oxidation. Although its hemolytic activity is inhibited by cholesterol, the protein-bound cholesterol in normal serum does not have this effect and therefore does not interfere with the measurement of antistreptolysin O Abs.

Both the S and the O hemolysins **can injure the membranes of cells other than RBCs.** The mechanism of action of streptolysin O has recently been shown to be analogous to that of the membrane attack complex of complement and of staphylococcal α-toxin. In binding to cholesterol-containing membranes, the soluble molecules of streptolysin O assemble into oligomeric curved rod structures that form rings and arcs penetrating the apolar domain of the lipid bilayer (Fig. 24–8). These generate slits and pores in the membrane that allow leakage of cellular contents. In the macrophage and the granulocytic leukocyte, the membranes of the nucleus and cytoplasmic granules are breached, presumably by the same mechanism, with severe damage to the cell and release of lysosomal enzymes.

NADase (NICOTINAMIDE ADENINE DINUCLEOTIDASE). Streptococcal cultures contain an NADase that liberates nicotinamide from DPN. Strains of nephritogenic type 12 are particularly prone to produce this enzyme, but there is no evidence that it plays a role in the pathogenesis of glomerulonephritis. Antibodies that inhibit its action are frequently found in the serum of patients convalescing from streptococcal disease.

STREPTOKINASES. A substance in streptococcal culture filtrates that promotes the lysis of human blood clots was first termed "streptococcal fibrinolysin." It was later shown to catalyze the conversion of plasminogen to plasmin, and so it was renamed **streptokinase.** Two species of streptokinase (A and B), differing in antigenicity and electrophoretic mobility, have been isolated from group A strains; and there are reports of still other variants of this kinase. They are immunogenic and induce antistreptokinase Abs in the course of most diseases caused by group A streptococci. Although their action has often been assumed to prevent the formation of effective fibrin barriers at the periphery of streptococcal lesions, there is no conclusive evidence to support this attractive hypothesis. In fact, the invasiveness of strepto-

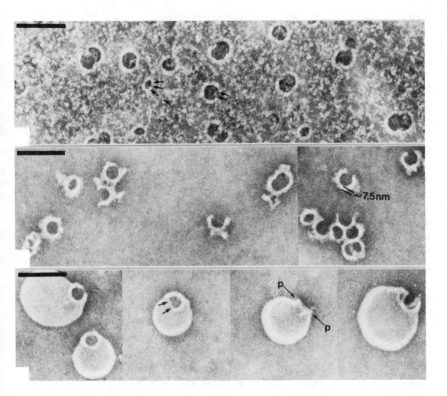

Figure 24–8. Mechanism of action of streptolysin O. *(A)* Negatively stained erythrocyte membrane lysed by streptolysin O showing numerous 25- to 100-nm-long and approximately 7.5-nm broad, curved rods of 13- to 16-nm inner radius of curvature. Most rods are approximately semicircular, often joined in pairs at their ends. Dense accumulations of stain are seen at the concave side of the rods. When these do not form closed profiles, the stain deposit is partly bordered by a "free" edge of the erythrocyte membrane *(arrows)*. *(B)* Negative staining of isolated streptolysin O oligomers, showing numerous curved rod structures identical to those found in toxin-treated membranes. *(C)* Purified streptolysin O complexes reincorporated into cholesterol-free lecithin liposomes. The toxin oligomers create holes in the liposomes. Part of the circumference of such holes appear bordered by a "free" edge of liposomal membrane *(unlabeled arrows)*. Arrows marked p, a lesion seen in profile. (Scale bars indicate 100 nm in all frames; sodium silicotungstate used as negative stain; Bhakdi S, Tranum–Jensen J: Phil Trans Roy Soc Lond B 306:311, 1984)

cocci appears to be uninfluenced by antistreptokinase Abs.

DEOXYRIBONUCLEASES. Group A streptococci also elaborate enzymes that degrade DNA (DNases). Four immunologically and electrophoretically distinct types (A, B, C, and D) have been found. Because these enzymes do not penetrate the plasma membranes of living mammalian cells, they are not cytotoxic. However, they are capable of depolymerizing the highly viscous DNA that accumulates in thick pus as a result of the disintegration of polymorphonuclear leukocytes. Enzyme preparations containing both streptokinase and streptococcal deoxyribonuclease (streptodornase) were introduced clinically by Tillett to liquefy purulent exudates (enzymatic debridement) in such diseases as pneumococcal empyema.

Hyaluronidase is of particular interest. Its substrate occurs in the streptococcal capsule. However, only certain group A strains (those of types 4 and 22) produce the enzyme *in vitro*, and they never form capsules; other strains fail to produce the enzyme *in vitro*, even after prolonged growth and complete loss of capsules. Nevertheless, most patients recovering from streptococcal disease have Abs to the type 4 and 22 hyaluronidase; hence all group A streptococci may well produce a related protein, at least *in vivo*.

Originally termed **"spreading factor"** because of its striking lytic effect on the ground substance of connective tissue, hyaluronidase has long been thought to play a role in the characteristic tendency of streptococci to spread rapidly through mammalian tissues. How important its action really is in this regard has not been determined.

Streptococcal proteinase is capable of destroying another cell factor involved in pathogenesis, the M protein, and possibly also other extracellular proteins such as streptolysin O and streptokinase. It is activated by sulfhydryl compounds, and it is released initially from the cells in the form of an inactive zymogen, which is activated autocatalytically under reducing conditions. Both the zymogen and the active enzyme have been obtained in crystalline form. The possible pathogenic role of the enzyme is unknown.

GENOTYPIC VARIATIONS

Genetic variations in hemolytic streptococci have been demonstrated to affect numerous traits, including elaboration of hemolysins, colonial morphology (capsule formation), production of M protein, synthesis of other cell wall antigens (including alterations in C polysaccharides), and resistance to antimicrobial drugs. The most thoroughly studied variants are those related to colony formation. When repeatedly cultured on artificial media many mucoid strains become glossy, and on passage through mice glossy variants revert to the mucoid form. Similarly, strains producing the M antigen (M$^+$ strains), which are carried in the throat after an attack of streptococcal pharyngitis, may eventually lose their M antigens. When such M$^-$ strains are passed through mice, they frequently revert to M$^+$. Both these variations affect virulence.

Mutants of group A streptococci resistant to sulfonamides and to tetracyclines have been encountered. Following mass prophylaxis with sulfonamides in military personnel during World War II, sulfonamide-resistant mutants became prevalent, but the introduction of penicillin promptly suppressed their spread. No significant change in the sensitivity of naturally occurring hemolytic streptococci to penicillin has occurred. Even in the laboratory, it is extremely difficult to obtain penicillin-resistant streptococci, and those resistant mutants that have been isolated have been found to lack virulence.

PATHOGENICITY

S. pyogenes causes both suppurative diseases and nonsuppurative sequelae. The first group includes acute **streptococcal pharyngitis** (with or without scarlet fever) and all its suppurative complications, including cervical adenitis, otitis media, mastoiditis, peritonsillar abscesses, meningitis, peritonitis, and pneumonia. It also includes postpartum infections of the uterus (**puerperal sepsis**), **cellulitis** of the skin, **impetigo, lymphangitis,** and **erysipelas.** The principal diseases of the nonsuppurative category are **acute glomerulonephritis** and **rheumatic fever.**

SUPPURATIVE DISEASE. The pathogenesis of suppurative streptococcal disease is fairly well understood. The factors that determine invasiveness are particularly important. Because hemolytic streptococci ingested by phagocytic cells are almost all killed within minutes, their antiphagocytic properties play a critical role in invasiveness. These properties, in turn, depend on the hyaluronic acid capsule and the M protein. In human infections, **the M protein appears to be of primary importance** because of the presence in human serum of a poorly defined factor that neutralizes the antiphagocytic effect of the capsular hyaluronate. On the other hand, the importance of both antiphagocytic components has been demonstrated in infections of experimental animals and confirmed in *in vitro* experiments, as illustrated in Table 24–3.

Although nearly all phagocytized streptococci are promptly killed, an occasional organism will escape un-

TABLE 24–3. *Relative Antiphagocytic Effect of the Hyaluronate Capsule and the M Protein of a Fully Virulent Strain of Group A β-Hemolytic Streptococcus**

Treatment of Organism	State of Capsule†	Amount of M Protein†	% Phagocytosis‡
None	+++	+++	3 (± 1.8)
Trypsin	+++	0	49 (± 5.4)
Hyaluronidase	±	+++	41 (± 2.8)
Trypsin and hyaluronidase	±	0	64 (± 0.85)

* Type 14.

† Number of plus signs indicates approximate size of envelope, as seen in India ink preparations, or amount of M protein demonstrable by quantitative precipitin tests. Figures in parenthesis are standard deviations. The phagocytic tests were performed in the absence of serum (i.e., surface phagocytosis).

(Foley MJ, Wood WB Jr: J Exp Med 110:617, 1959)

harmed. One mechanism is egestion, in which the engulfed organism is ejected from the cell. This event occurs only rarely *in vitro*, and there is no evidence that it is frequent enough *in vivo* to influence the course of the infection. A second escape mechanism results from the elaboration of a **leukotoxic factor,** identified as the cell-bound streptolysin S.

Scarlet fever occurs as a complication of pyogenic streptococcal disease when the infecting strain produces erythrogenic toxin in a susceptible patient (usually a child). It has long been a matter of controversy, however, whether the rash is secondary to a direct action of the circulating toxin or to a generalized cutaneous hypersensitivity reaction. In favor of the latter possibility is the observation that infants under the age of 2 rarely have the disease and do not show positive Dick reactions, regardless of the immune state of the mother. For reasons that are not clear this disease has become very uncommon in recent decades.

NONSUPPURATIVE SEQUELAE. Acute glomerulonephritis results from infections caused by a limited number of types of group A streptococci. Many **nephritogenic strains** belong to type 12; others have been identified as types 4, 18, 25, 49, 52, and 55. The manner in which these strains cause acute glomerulonephritis is not fully understood, but several findings are consistent with a reaction to an **immune complex.** Thus, the characteristic symptoms of hematuria, edema, and hypertension do not appear until a week or more after the onset of the acute pyogenic infection, usually of the pharynx or skin; the serum titer of complement often falls during an attack; and immunoglobulin, the third component of complement (C3), and streptococcal Ags have been demonstrated by immunofluorescence in glomerular lesions.

An extracellular protein that is produced by streptococcal strains associated with nephritis but rarely by other strains has been identified recently as a **streptokinase** that differs immunologically from those previously described. Its role in the disease is under investigation.

The pathogenesis of **rheumatic fever** is even more obscure, because it may follow pharyngeal infection with practically any type of group A streptococcus. The latent period between the onset of acute streptococcal pharyngitis and the symptoms and signs of rheumatic fever is usually 2 or 3 weeks. Antistreptococcal Abs are consistently found in the serum of patients with acute rheumatic fever, and following a streptococcal epidemic, most patients who develop rheumatic fever (roughly 3%) have higher titers of antistreptococcal Abs in their serum than do those who escape the disease. Nevertheless, it is far from clear how **immunologic hyperreactivity** to streptococcal products could cause the recurring cardiac, joint, and skin lesions that characterize rheumatic fever. Nor is it clear what particular streptococcal products may be involved, although many have been implicated in animal experiments. For example, streptolysin O has been shown to be cardiotoxic; streptococcal proteinase injected intravenously causes subendocardial lesions (as do proteases from other sources); and cell wall fragments, composed of group-specific carbohydrate and peptidoglycan, are capable of causing cardiac and joint lesions. Moreover, immunologic cross-reactions have been described between streptococcal Ags and tissue Ags of cardiac muscle and between the group A carbohydrate and a structural glycoprotein of heart valves. Suggestive as these findings are, there is still no convincing evidence to support the implication of any one streptococcal product in the pathogenesis of rheumatic fever.

Although **erythema nodosum** occurs in association with a variety of diseases (tuberculosis, coccidiomycosis, sarcoidosis), there is both clinical and experimental evidence that it may also be a poststreptococcal illness. Intradermal injection of the same kind of cell wall fragments mentioned above produce in rabbits chronic remittent skin lesions that resemble erythema nodosum in man. There is evidence that the peptidoglycan portion exerts the primary toxic effect. The relation of this model to the human disease remains to be determined.

The possibility that **streptococcal L forms** are involved in the pathogenesis of rheumatic fever and glomerulonephritis has been investigated, but there is no clear evidence for the participation of these penicillin-resistant forms.

GROUP B STREPTOCOCCI

Streptococci of this group were first isolated from bovine mastitis, and they were only occasionally encountered in association with disease in man. However, during the past two decades, they have assumed special importance in **neonatal infections.** They are a common cause of circumscribed epidemics of **meningitis** and **septicemia** in newborn nurseries.

Several serologic types of Group B streptococci are known. In contrast to group A, **type specificity** in this group is dependent on **capsular polysaccharides,** which are the principal determinants of virulence. As with pneumococci, Abs to the polysaccharides are protective. There is evidence that, at least with some types, Abs against certain surface proteins of the organisms can also be protective in experimental mouse infections. In view of their association with meningitis, it is of interest that group B streptococci share with meningococci the property of having sialic acid as an important component of the polysaccharides.

Of the types of group B that have been defined, all have been found associated with neonatal infections, although type III strains are the most common offenders. Susceptibility of the newborn appears to be related to the lack of protective Abs, as affected infants have inadequate levels of maternally transmitted Abs.

DISEASE CAUSED BY STREPTOCOCCI OF OTHER GROUPS

Group C and group G streptococci are not uncommonly recovered as the predominant organism in cases of pharyngitis. However, these infections are generally milder than group A infections, and they are not known to initiate nonsuppurative sequelae.

Streptococci of other groups may also be encountered in man (see Table 24–1), most often in the respiratory tract, but only rarely do they cause overt disease. Nonhemolytic strains of group D (*S. faecalis*) are common inhabitants of the human gastrointestinal tract (see Nonhemolytic Streptococci, below).

IMMUNITY

Of the many varieties of Abs that are generated in response to group A hemolytic streptococcal disease, **only anti-M** is known to protect the host against the invasiveness of the organisms. In acute streptococcal disease this Ab ordinarily becomes detectable in the serum within a few weeks to several months, and it usually persists for 1 to 2 years; in some individuals it may still be present after 10 to 30 years. Inasmuch as there are more than 55 serologic types of group A streptococci, no individual is likely to become fully immune to group A streptococcal infections in general.

On the other hand, only a relatively few types of group A streptococci are nephritogenic; therefore, persistence of anti-M Abs to one of these types may account for the observation that an initial attack of acute glomerulonephritis greatly decreases the probability of a subsequent attack. No such protective effect occurs in rheumatic fever because of the wide variety of streptococcal types that may cause the disease. There is no information yet on the possible role of antibodies to the streptokinase associated with nephritogenic strains.

Immunity to **scarlet fever** is associated with the presence of **erythrogenic antitoxin** in the serum, although this affords no protection against streptococcal pharyngitis. Because there are at least three immunologic types of erythrogenic toxin, occasional second attacks of scarlet fever may be expected.

LABORATORY DIAGNOSIS

IDENTIFICATION OF GROUP A ORGANISMS. The techniques used to culture, group, and type hemolytic streptococci have already been described, and the need to employ pour plates to be certain of detecting β-hemolysis has been emphasized. A simple method of recognizing *S. pyogenes* (group A) depends on the particular sensitivity of group A strains **to bacitracin;** an agar plate test using paper discs impregnated with bacitracin is useful.

TESTS FOR ANTI-M ANTIBODIES. Tests for type-specific streptococcal Abs in patients' sera based on precipitation, agglutination, or complement-fixing techniques are often misleading because of cross-reacting Ags. The most widely used technique, based on the bactericidal properties of whole blood, is more specific: it measures indirectly the opsonizing action of the homologous anti-M Ab. The mouse protection test depends on the same principle. A somewhat simpler but less sensitive method depends on the tendency of group A streptococci to grow in long chains when cultured in the presence of homologous type-specific Ab.

TESTS FOR OTHER ANTIBODIES. Serologic tests for Abs to extracellular products are much easier to perform and are widely used to obtain evidence for recent streptococcal infection. The **antistreptolysin test** measures Abs against streptolysin O. Techniques to measure Abs against streptokinase, hyaluronidase, or DNase B may be similarly employed. The antistreptolysin test is used routinely in most diagnostic laboratories, but in streptococcal skin infections the response to this Ag tends to be low, and the DNase B test is more reliable.

TREATMENT

β-Hemolytic streptococci are among the most susceptible of all pathogenic bacteria to the action of antimicrobial drugs. The sulfonamides readily suppress growth both *in vitro* and *in vivo*, but because they are only bacteriostatic, their use will not eliminate the organisms from the upper respiratory tract, nor will it significantly modify the Ab response of the host. Penicillin is bactericidal and hence is far more effective. When used in adequate dosage for a sufficient length of time, it will often rid the pharynx of hemolytic streptococci. Persistence usually indicates a suppurative complication such as intratonsillar abscess or purulent sinusitis. When given early in the course of acute streptococcal pharyngitis, penicillin will also depress the patient's Ab response, and such treatment of susceptible individuals greatly reduces the rate of rheumatic attacks.

Other antibiotics, such as erythromycin, may also be used in the treatment of group A streptococcal infections, particularly in patients who have a history of hypersensitivity to penicillin. Many strains are now resistant to the tetracyclines, which are therefore no longer generally recommended.

PREVENTION

Penicillin is often given continually in small doses to rheumatic patients to prevent streptococcal infections (**chemoprophylaxis**) and hence a recurrence of rheumatic fever. Prophylactic therapy of this kind is possible only because group A streptococci do not generate mutants that are significantly resistant to penicillin. Prevention of rheumatic fever with continuous sulfonamide treatment has also been reasonably successful, but because these drugs are not bactericidal and occasionally cause severe reactions (e.g., periarteritis nodosa), penicillin is usually preferred.

The earlier custom of isolating scarlet fever patients but not patients with acute streptococcal pharyngitis was based on the erroneous view that the two diseases were basically dissimilar. From an epidemiologic standpoint, there is no justification for such a distinction.

Immunization of the general population against group A streptococcal infections has not proved practical because of the very large number of types. Efforts to devise suitable M protein vaccines for special purposes have continued.

EPIDEMIOLOGY

The incidence of streptococcal infections varies widely in different geographic regions and appears to be related to climate. Streptococcal diseases are most common in cold, relatively dry areas and occur most often in the winter and spring. Endemic rates in the U.S. are particularly high in the Rocky Mountain states such as Colorado and Wyoming. Although overt streptococcal **disease** is less prevalent in the southern states, culture surveys and

Ab studies reveal that streptococcal **infections** are not uncommon.

Group A streptococcal **carrier rates** ordinarily run well below 10%. Just before an epidemic, however, they become much higher. Infection is transmitted from the respiratory tract of one person to that of another by relatively intimate contact. The epidemiologic studies of Rammelkamp and coworkers have shown that group A streptococci in the air, in dust, on blankets, etc., are far less infectious than the moist secretions ejected from the respiratory tract during speech, coughing, and sneezing. Nasal carriers disseminate many more streptococci into their environments than pharyngeal carriers do. The source of puerperal sepsis has often been traced to the upper respiratory tract of the obstetrician or of someone else in the delivery room. Milkborne epidemics of streptococcal disease are now uncommon because of the effectiveness of pasteurization. Isolated outbreaks attributable to infected food still occur on rare occasions.

Other Streptococci

α-HEMOLYTIC STREPTOCOCCI

The α-hemolytic streptococci are often referred to collectively as the **viridans group;** their classification depends largely on culture characteristics rather than serologic analysis. A number of immunologic varieties have been recognized by antigenic analysis, but only a few of these seem to fall into the Lancefield groups (A to O). One of the most common species is *S. salivarius.*

The viridans streptococci colonize the human upper respiratory tract within the first few hours after birth; rarely does a carefully performed throat culture fail to reveal their presence. They have a very low degree of pathogenicity compared with pneumococci, which also are α-hemolytic and are often cultured from the throat. Unlike pneumococci, however, viridans streptococci are neither bile-soluble nor sensitive to ethylhydrocupreine (optochin). (The oral streptococci and the role of *S. mutans* in dental caries are discussed under Oral Microbiology in Chap. 42.)

The principal significance of α-hemolytic streptococci in clinical medicine relates to **subacute bacterial endocarditis.** This serious illness results from infection of an endocardial surface already damaged by either rheumatic fever or congenital heart disease. Because α-hemolytic streptococci are continually present in the throat and about the teeth, even minor trauma such as that caused by vigorous chewing may result in their entry into the blood stream. The transient bacteremias that follow dental extraction and tonsillectomy may initiate subacute bacterial endocarditis in patients with abnormal valves. The seriousness of this type of infection is greatly increased by the frequency of drug-resistant strains.

In order for viridans streptococci to gain a permanent foothold on the endocardium, the organisms must be trapped in a suitable nidus on the surface, usually provided by a tiny fibrin clot over an area of endocardial trauma. Dogs with artificially induced arteriovenous aneurysms in the peripheral circulation regularly develop microscopic clots of this kind on the endocardium. Similar endocardial lesions have been produced in rats by exposing them to prolonged anoxia, which also causes a hyperkinetic circulatory response. The remarkable frequency of bacterial endocarditis in such animals illustrates the importance of existing endocardial damage in the pathogenesis of the disease.

Histologic examination of the vegetations on the heart valves in both naturally acquired and experimentally induced viridans endocarditis reveals that the organisms grow in large colonies embedded in a fibrinous, relatively acellular exudate. The avascularity of the heart valves accounts for the paucity of phagocytic cells in the lesions and explains why an organism so easily phagocytized *in vitro* can survive and multiply in the valvular vegetations. As the organisms continue to multiply at the periphery of the lesion, they break off and are carried away in the blood. Quantitative blood cultures, taken at repeated intervals over long periods in patients with subacute bacterial endocarditis, show that the organisms are shed from the vegetation at a surprisingly constant rate. Thrombotic lesions, resulting in the formation of petechiae, commonly develop and constitute a hallmark of the disease.

NONHEMOLYTIC STREPTOCOCCI

The term "**nonhemolytic streptococcus**" is confusing because it is often used to include any streptococcus that is not β-hemolytic and because many nonhemolytic species (including a particularly common one, *S. faecalis*) possess the same group-specific cell wall Ags as certain hemolytic streptococci.

The organisms that fall in the nonhemolytic group are generally of low pathogenicity for man and, like α-hemolytic streptococci, are of concern to physicians primarily as causative agents of subacute bacterial endocarditis. *S. faecalis*, often referred to as the **enterococcus** because of its frequent presence in the gastrointestinal tract, is an exceptionally hardy microorganism. Its ability to grow in the presence of 0.05% sodium azide is often used in the laboratory to separate it from other streptococci. Enterococci also tend to be relatively resistant to heat (62°C for 30 minutes) and will multiply in media containing 6.5% sodium chloride. Many strains encountered in clinical practice are highly resistant to antimicrobial drugs, making the treatment of enterococcal endocarditis especially difficult.

ANAEROBIC STREPTOCOCCI

All the varieties of streptococci thus far considered are facultative anaerobes. Obligate anaerobic (or microaerophilic) streptococci do exist, however, and may also cause human disease. They are usually nonhemolytic and are smaller than other streptococci. Although a number of different species have been described, they have not been systematically classified.

Because anaerobic streptococci are normal inhabitants of the female genital tract, they occasionally give rise to intrauterine infections. However, their virulence for humans, as well as for other animals, is low, and they tend to multiply only in necrotic or frankly gangrenous lesions. When growing in purulent exudates, they produce a fetid odor; hence, their presence in lung abscesses is often suggested by the foul odor of the sputum. Although most anaerobic streptococci are susceptible to the action of antimicrobial drugs, the lesions in which they are found often require surgical drainage as well.

Selected Reading

BOOKS AND REVIEW ARTICLES

Fox EN: M proteins of group A streptococci. Bacteriol Rev 38:57, 1974

Kuttner AG, Lancefield RC: Unsolved problems of the non-suppurative complications of group A streptococcal infections. In Mudd S (ed): Infectious Agents and Host Reactions. Philadelphia, WB Saunders, 1970

McCarty M: The streptococcal cell wall. Harvey Lect 65:73, 1971

Patterson MJ, Hafeez AEB: Group B streptococci in human disease. Bacteriol Rev 40:774, 1976

Rammelkamp CH Jr: Epidemiology of streptococcal infections. Harvey Lect 51:113, 1957

Read SE, Zabriskie JB (eds): Streptococcal Disease and the Immune Response. New York, Academic Press, 1980

Uhr JW (ed): The Streptococcus, Rheumatic Fever, and Glomerulonephritis. Baltimore, Williams & Wilkins, 1964

SPECIFIC ARTICLES

Beachey EH, Ofek I: Epithelial binding of group A streptococci by lipoteichoic acid on fimbriae denuded of M protein. J Exp Med 143:759, 1976

Cromartie WJ, Craddock JG, Schwab JH, Anderle SK, Yang C: Arthritis in rats after systemic injection of streptococcal cells or cell walls. J Exp Med 146:1585, 1977

Fischetti VF, Jones KF, Manjula BN, Scott JR: Streptococcal M6 protein expressed in *Escherichia coli:* Localization, purification, and comparison with streptococcal-derived M protein. J Exp Med 159:1083, 1984

Freimer EH, McCarty M: Rheumatic fever. Sci Am 213:6, 1965

Goldstein I, Halpern B, Robert L: Immunological relationship between streptococcus A polysaccharide and the structural glycoprotein of heart valve. Nature 213:44, 1967

Johnston KH, Zabriskie JB: Purification and partial characterization of the nephritis strain-associated protein from *Streptococcus pyogenes*, group A. J Exp Med 163:697, 1986

Kaplan MH, Svec KH: Immunologic relation of streptococcal and tissue antigens III: Presence in human sera of streptococcal antibody cross-reactive with heart tissue: Association with streptococcal infection, rheumatic fever, and glomerulonephritis. J Exp Med 119:651, 1964

Lancefield RC: Current knowledge of type-specific M antigens of group A streptococci. J Immunol 83:307, 1962

Lancefield RC, McCarty M, Everly WN: Multiple mouse-protective antibodies directed against group B streptococci. J Exp Med 142:165, 1975

Tillett WS: Studies on the enzymatic lysis of fibrin and inflammatory exudates by products of hemolytic streptococci. Harvey Lect 45:149, 1952

Wannamaker LW: Differences between streptococcal infections of the throat and of the skin. N Engl J Med 282:23, 1970

Zabriskie JB: The role of temperate bacteriophage in the production of erythrogenic toxin by group A streptococci. J Exp Med 191:761, 1964

Zabriskie JB: The relationship of streptococcal cross-reactive antigens to rheumatic fever. Transplant Proc 1:968, 1969

25

Richard P. Novick

Staphylococci

As Koch recognized in 1878, distinct diseases are produced by gram-positive cocci that have different patterns of growth: in pairs, chains, or clusters. The last group, the staphylococci, are non-motile, facultatively aerobic, glucose-fermenting gram-positive cocci, distinguished by growth as irregular clusters (Gr. *staphyle*, bunch of grapes; see Figs. 25–1 and 25–2) and by a pentaglycine cross-bridge in their peptidoglycan. Most species are natural inhabitants of the mammalian skin and mucous membranes and have no other important habitat.

Classification

Staphylococci were classified until recently as two species: the pathogenic *S. aureus*, whose colonies are golden yellow, and the generally nonpathogenic *S. albus*, whose colonies are characteristically white. Other groups of gram-positive cluster-forming cocci are characterized in Table 25–1. The peptococci and the related but chain-forming peptostreptococci are strictly anaerobic inhabitants of the animal body.

Although these organisms have long been grouped in the family Micrococcaceae on morphological grounds, members differ strikingly in nucleic acid base composition (Table 25–1) and are fundamentally unrelated, so that "Micrococcaceae" is an invalid taxon and should be discarded. Nucleic acid sequence analysis has shown that staphylococci are related more closely to the bacilli than even to the streptococci (Fig. 25–3), whereas micrococci, with a much higher G + C content, are closely related to arthrobacter and the actinomycetes.

Because pathogenicity has been found to correlate better with the ability to produce coagulase than with pigmentation, all **coagulase-positive staphylococci** of human origin are now grouped as *S. aureus*. These or-

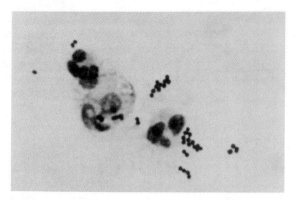

Figure 25–1. Gram stain of exudate containing intracellular and extra-cellular staphylococci. (White A, Brooks GF. In Hoeprich PD ed: Infectious Diseases, 2nd ed. Hagerstown, Harper & Row, 1977) (×650)

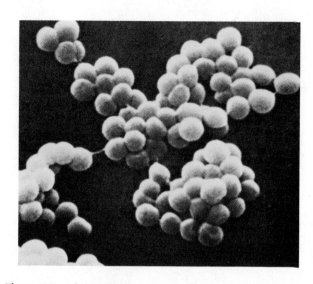

Figure 25–2. Scanning electron photomicrograph of *S. aureus* in serum–salts broth. (Kunakorn W: Infect Immun 4:73, 1971)

ganisms cause a wide variety of suppurative disease in humans, including superficial and deep abscesses, wound infections, and infections of various internal organs. In addition, they cause several toxinoses, including food poisoning, toxic epidermal necrolysis, and the toxic shock syndrome (TSS). *S. aureus* is also an important pathogen for domestic animals, being the principal cause of bovine mastitis. Two groups of animal-specific, coagulase-variable strains have been granted species status, *S. intermedius* and *S. hyicus*.

Coagulase-negative staphylococci show much greater heterogeneity than the coagulase-positive, and as the tools of modern taxonomy have been applied, the number of biotypes that can arguably be regarded as separate species has increased from two in the 1974 edition of *Bergey's Manual* to 20 in a 1984 listing. Differentiation of these species on the basis of biochemical characteristics is consistent with the oligonucleotide patterns of the 16S RNA. Nevertheless, there is far from general agreement on the speciation of staphylococci.

Although most coagulase-negative species are nonpathogenic or are opportunistic pathogens for man, *S. epidermidis* (*sensu strictu*) is by far the most frequent cause of infection from intravascular catheters and prostheses; additionally, some strains can cause many of the types of infections formerly considered to be the province of *S. aureus*. Although such strains could be genotypically *S. aureus* that do not produce coagulase, one well-defined coagulase-negative species, *S. saprophyticus*, is an important cause of urinary infection in young women. Other coagulase-negative species are important as animal pathogens.

Biotyping of S. Aureus

Individual *S. aureus* isolates differ widely in their patterns of exoprotein production, antibiotic resistance, surface antigens, phage sensitivity, and other variable traits. The species is thus composed of a large number of individual biotypes, for which there are various typing schemes. The most important of these is phage typing: the determination of sensitivity to an internationally

TABLE 25–1. Genera of Gram-Positive Cluster-Forming Cocci

	Staphylococcus	Micrococcus	Planococcus	Peptococcus; Peptostreptococcus
Typical form	Irregular clusters	Tetrads or cubical packets	Tetrads	Irregular clusters, short chains
Habitat	Animal body	Saprophytic	Saprophytic (marine)	Animal body
Motility	–	–	+	–
Metabolism	Facultative anaerobe	Strict aerobe	Strict aerobe	Strict anaerobe
Glucose fermentation	+	–	–	+
Catalase	+	+		–
Pentaglycine bridge	+	–	–	–
% G + C	30–35	66–75	39–52	33–37

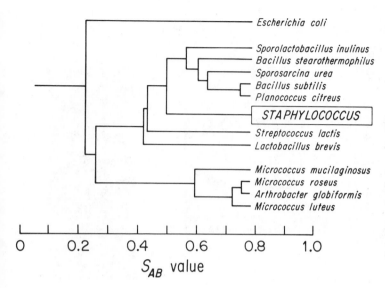

Escherichia coli

Sporolactobacillus inulinus
Bacillus stearothermophilus
Sporosarcina urea
Bacillus subtilis
Planococcus citreus
STAPHYLOCOCCUS
Streptococcus lactis
Lactobacillus brevis
Micrococcus mucilaginosus
Micrococcus roseus
Arthrobacter globiformis
Micrococcus luteus

0   0.2   0.4   0.6   0.8   1.0

S_{AB} value

Figure 25–3. Dendrogram of phylogenetic relationships based on homologies of 16S ribosomal RNA. The scale represents the similarity coefficient (the percentage of shared oligonucleotides in T1 nuclease digests; see Chap. 1). (Ludwig W et al: J Gen Microbiol 125:359, 1981

standardized set of bacteriophages, divided into three principal host-specificity groups (I, II, and III). The phages all adsorb to the same receptor located in the peptidoglycan–teichoic acid complex; differences in susceptibility are thus related to postadsorption phenomena including restriction-modification systems and host-, plasmid-, or prophage-mediated blockage of phage development. Certain biotypes are specifically associated with particular disease states. Thus exfoliatin is produced largely by strains sensitive to group II phages, and the toxic shock toxin, TSST-1, by group I-sensitive strains. Other biotypes are associated with local or widespread hospital epidemics, and phage typing can trace their spread and assess their prevalence.

During the 40 years that phage typing has been in use, an increasing proportion of the clinical *S. aureus* isolates have been found insensitive to any of the phages and are thus **nontypable.** This problem has been partially solved by the local introduction of new phages, which are generally considered experimental and have not been added to the standard set. Other phages are used for animal isolates, which tend to be quite distinct from human isolates. However, no standard set of phages of limited size will be useful for all strains. Additionally, because the phage typing system is not based on any uniform principle, phage types may be genetically labile for reasons that are often difficult to determine. For these and other reasons, several other biotyping schemes have been developed, which are generally applied only in special circumstances. An extensive **serotyping** system is based on variability of surface antigens, particularly teichoic acid. **Reverse phage typing** involves evaluating **lysotypes**—the lytic activities of phages released from the test strain against a set of standard indicator strains. This evaluation has good precision and reproducibility,

and because most naturally occurring *S. aureus* strains are lysogenic, it bypasses the problem of nontypability.

Antibiotic resistance patterns and molecular characterization of plasmids and other mobile genetic elements are also epidemiologically useful. Plasmids can be analyzed in terms of overall content and size (Fig. 25–4A and B) or by restriction enzyme fingerprinting of isolated plasmid DNA (Fig. 25–4C). Plasmids tend to be structurally labile, however, and the constancy of their restriction patterns may be eroded by time and distance. Chromosomal transposons, analyzed by blot hybridization (Fig. 25–5), provide a particularly reliable indication of epidemiologic relatedness, as they tend to be highly stable.

Morphology

The diameter of individual cocci is 0.7 to 1.2 μm. Cells in old cultures, or those ingested by phagocytes, may be gram-negative. The characteristic **cell clustering** (see Fig. 25–2) is most striking on solid media; it arises because staphylococci divide in three successive perpendicular planes, and the daughter cells do not separate completely. The formation of irregular aggregates is attributable to attachments eccentric to the plane of division, as well as to actual movement of cells from the centric position. In liquid media, short chains are common, but, unlike streptococci, staphylococci rarely form chains containing more than four members.

Growth and Metabolism

Growth is usually more luxuriant under aerobic than under anaerobic conditions; multiplication of some

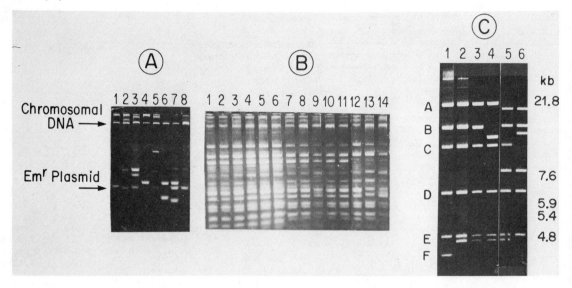

Figure 25–4. Plasmid analysis by gel electrophoresis. *(A)* Whole-cell lysates of epidemiologically unrelated erythromycin-resistant clinical *S. aureus* isolates. *(B)* Whole-cell lysates of erythromycin-resistant isolates from swine housed in a common pen and given tylosin-containing feed (tylosin and erythromycin are closely related antibiotics). *(C)* Restriction endonuclease EcoRI digests of a set of 53- to 57-Kb conjugative plasmids, all of which carry resistance to gentamicin, kanamycin, neomycin, penicillin, and quaternary amines. Although the intact plasmids are electrophoretically indistinguishable, the restriction digests reveal that only two of the six are the same *(track 2 and 3)*; the others are subtly but definitely different. In panels *A* and *B*, each band represents a different plasmid; in panel *C*, each band represents a different EcoRI subfragment of a single large plasmid. (*A* and *B*, unpublished experiments by S. Carleton and R. Novick; *C*, Holly, Goering and Ruff In Jeljascewicz J (ed): The Staphylococci, Berlin, Springer Verlag 1985, p 625)

strains is enhanced by increased CO_2 tension. Individual colonies on nutrient agar are opaque, sharply defined, round, convex, and 1 to 4 mm in diameter. The classic golden yellow color of *S. aureus* colonies is caused by carotenoids. Pigmentation is usually apparent after 18 to 24 hours of growth at 37°C but is more pronounced

when cultures are held at room temperature for a further 24 to 48 hours; it is also enhanced if the medium is enriched with glycerol monophosphate or monoacetate. Pigment is not produced during anaerobic growth or in liquid culture. There is marked variation, from white to deep orange, among strains and even among individual

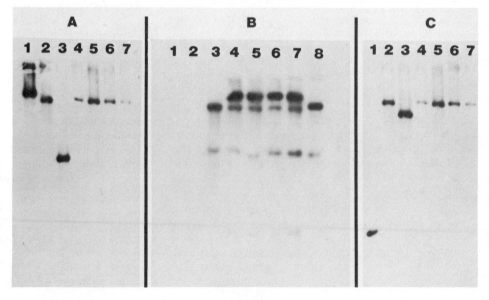

Figure 25–5. Southern blotting with probes for chromosomal transposons. Tracks 4–7 in each panel contain ClaI restriction digests of chromosomal DNA from TSS-causing *S. aureus* strains that are epidemiologically related. Tracks 1–3 contain digests of chromosomal DNA from epidemiologically unrelated TSS strains. Probe in *A* is specific for the β-lactamase gene; that in *B,* for Tn554; that in *C,* for the TSST-1 gene. (Kreiswirth BN et al: Ann Intern Med 105:704, 1986)

TABLE 25–2. Accessory Genetic Traits in S. aureus

Trait	Location			
	Plasmid	Phage	Chromosomal Transposon or HI*	Chromosomal
RESISTANCE				
Penicillin (β-lactamase)	x		x	
Methicillin			x	
Tetracycline	x		x	
MLS	x		x	
Streptomycin	x			
Spectinomycin			x	
Kanamycin-neomycin	x			
Gentamicin	x		x	
Chloramphenicol	x			
Ethidium bromide	x			
Mercury	x		x	
Arsenate	x		x	
Cadmium	x		x	
EXOPROTEINS AND TOXINS				
α-Hemolysin				x
Staphylokinase		x		
Exfoliatin A				x
Exfoliatin B	x			
TSST-1			x	
Enterotoxin A		x		
Enterotoxin B			x	

* HI, inserted DNA segment of heterologous origin.

colonies of a single strain. Staphylococcal colonies are readily differentiated from those of streptococci by their opacity.

On blood agar, a clear zone of hemolysis (**β-hemolysis**) is frequently seen around colonies. Because *S. aureus* can produce four distinct hemolysins, with interstrain variability and with different RBC species specificities, the hemolytic pattern depends on both the staphylococcal strain and the source of the blood.

Most strains will grow readily in a chemically defined medium containing glucose, salts, 14 amino acids, thiamine, and nicotinic acid. On meat digest media, they grow well over a wide range of pH (4.8–9.4). Under aerobic conditions, catalase is produced, and acid is formed from glucose, mannitol, xylose, lactose, sucrose, maltose, and glycerol. *S. aureus* is the only *Staphylococcus* species that ferments mannitol anaerobically. *S. aureus* has a high **salt tolerance,** and media containing 7.5% to 10% NaCl permit its selective growth.

Staphylococci are among the hardiest of all non–spore-forming bacteria. They remain alive for months on the surface of sealed agar plates stored at 4°C and may be cultured from samples of dried pus many weeks old. Some strains are relatively resistant to heat (withstanding 60°C for 30 minutes) and to most disinfectants.

Genetics

The staphylococcal genome consists of a chromosome of 1.6×10^6 nucleotide pairs plus various accessory genetic elements including **plasmids, transposons, prophages,** and uncharacterized chromosomal insertions of heterologous DNA. Table 25–2 lists the remarkable assemblage of nonessential, **variable traits** that are carried by accessory genetic elements and collectively determine the uniqueness of the genus and the individuality of particular strains of any one species. These traits include resistance to antibiotics and other substances and formation of extracellular enzymes, toxins, and other proteins that are involved in pathogenicity.

ANTIBIOTIC RESISTANCE. Soon after antibiotics were introduced into clinical medicine, resistant strains of *S. aureus* appeared among clinical isolates, and the organism has continued to respond in this manner to the introduction of new drugs. Resistance to penicillin, mediated by a powerful β-lactamase, appeared in the early 1950s and was rapidly followed by resistance to macrolide antibiotics, aminoglycosides, and tetracyclines. During the succeeding years, the frequency of resistant strains increased rapidly, and in many clinical settings multiple antibiotic resistance is now the rule. The determinants of these resistances have probably always existed in natural population of staphylococci and other bacteria—which could account for the rapidity with which the resistant organisms became prevalent. For example, some 5% to 10% of stored pre-antibiotic-era *S. aureus* isolates show β-lactamase-mediated penicillin resistance. The introduction of "penicillinase-resistant" penicillin derivatives such as methicillin around 1960 was again followed shortly by the emergence of resistant strains, and these are now one of the principal causes of therapeutic failure in hospital-acquired infections. As with other bacteria, individual staphylococcal strains tend to accumulate multiple determinants of resistance even under conditions where they are exposed to only a single antibiotic. Although plasmids and transposons are certainly involved, the actual evolutionary mechanism underlying this phenomenon has yet to be explained; one of its consequences has been the emergence of epidemic hospital strains of *S. aureus* resistant to virtually all useful antibiotics, including methicillin, but thus far excepting vancomycin. These strains are currently a significant cause of nosocomial infections in many parts of the world.

Plasmids are the primary carriers of antibiotic resistance in staphylococci. Three major types have been identified. One consists of small multicopy plasmids ranging in size from 2.5 to 5 Kb and in copy number from 10 to 50. Each contains a single resistance determinant for tetracycline, streptomycin, chloramphenicol, macrolides, kanamycin, or cadmium salts. These plasmids can replicate in other gram-positive species, and relatives are found in *Bacillus* and *Streptococcus* species. A second type consists of larger plasmids, 25 to 35 Kb in size and about five copies per cell. These typically carry resistance to penicillin and inorganic ions; they have not been observed to replicate in other genera. Recently, a third type, related to the second, has been identified: still larger (40–60 Kb) conjugative plasmids, typically carrying resistance to gentamicin, penicillin, neomycin, quaternary ammonium compounds such as ethidium bromide, and sometimes trimethoprim.

As in gram-negative bacteria, many of the antibiotic resistance genes of staphylococci are carried by **transposons** and therefore can exist either on plasmids or integrated into the chromosome. Included are determinants of resistance to erythromycin, spectinomycin, penicillin (β-lactamase), and gentamicin and probably also methicillin. A widespread nosocomial strain of phage type 88 carries multiple antibiotic resistance genes that seem to be clustered in the chromosome and are likely to represent a transposon complex. Other accessory genes are also carried by variable genetic elements; the staphylokinsae and enterotoxin A structural genes are located on **temperate phage** genomes, and the gene for TSST-1

seems to be carried by a transposon. Two accessory genes, encoding lipase and β-hemolysin, are inactivated by lysogenization, because the phage integration site is within the gene.

Staphylococci participate in several different types of **genetic exchange,** including generalized transduction, DNA-mediated transformation of either intact cells or protoplasts, plasmid-mediated conjugation, and protoplast fusion. Conjugative transfer has been demonstrated for plasmid but not for chromosomal markers. Staphylococci also exchange plasmids with *Bacillus* species and streptococci.

Cellular Antigens

CAPSULES. A few laboratory strains of *S. aureus* have capsules, often composed of glucosaminuronic acid. Capsules may be present *in vivo* more often than is appreciated but lost on cultivation. The prototype encapsulated strain (the Smith strain) gives rise reversibly to nonencapsulated variants, implying the existence of a genotypic switch that could be related to the apparent loss on cultivation.

POLYSACCHARIDE A. Species-specific surface carbohydrate Ags of *S. aureus* and *S. epidermidis* (polysaccharides A and B, respectively) have been identified as teichoic acids. Polysaccharide A is a linear ribitol teichoic acid with N-acetylglucosamine attached at C-4 of ribitol and D-alanine at approximately 50% of the C-2 atoms. The antigenic determinant is the glucosamine residue, which may be in either α or β glycosidic linkage. Most strains have teichoic acids with both anomers, but some have only one; hence, tests for species identification and for Ab require antisera and teichoic acids, respectively, with both specificities. A glycerol lipoteichoic acid is also present.

PROTEIN A. Virtually all *S. aureus* strains possess as a surface component the 42-Kd protein A, mostly linked covalently to the peptidoglycan; some is also released extracellularly. Protein A can induce specific Abs and will react with their Fab portion. In addition, **protein A, on the bacterial surface or in solution, interacts nonspecifically with the Fc portion of immunoglobulins of virtually all mammalian species.** All subclasses of human IgG except IgG3, and some IgM and IgA2 samples, are adsorbed by staphylococci—a useful procedure for quantitating Ag–Ab complexes.

Protein A–Fc interactions *in vivo* have a variety of biological effects: local and systemic anaphylaxis in animals; wheal-and-flare reactions in humans; Arthus reactions; activation of complement by both the alternate and classic pathways with generation of chemotactic factors; inhibition of opsonic antibody activity because of competition with the Fc receptors of phagocytes; induction of histamine release from leukocytes; and proliferation of human B, but not T, lymphocytes.

CLUMPING FACTOR (BOUND COAGULASE). Most nonencapsulated strains of *S. aureus* clump when suspended in plasma or in fibrinogen solutions. It is believed that the clumping factor is a surface coagulase.

ADHESINS. Like other bacteria, staphylococci have specific surface proteins (adhesins) that enable them to bind to matrix proteins such as laminin, fibronectin, and collagen and to host cellular surfaces. These binding activities are thought to be involved in colonization of the intracellular matrix, in the invasion of tissue cells, and in resistance to phagocytosis. A fibronectin binding protein of M_r 197,000 has been purified and is distinct from protein A and clumping factor.

Extracellular Proteins

Staphylococci, especially *S. aureus*, produce a wide variety of immunogenic exoproteins. Some are toxins, and others contribute to pathogenicity by attacking the intercellular matrix as well as the tissue cells. These are mostly accessory proteins which, during optimal growth in rich media, are synthesized at the end of exponential growth or in early stationary phase. Under suboptimal conditions such as Mg^{2+} deficiency, which may be present in infected tissue, they may be synthesized throughout the exponential phase.

COAGULASE. Culture filtrates of *S. aureus* clot the plasma of many animal species, as a result of production of the clotting factor, coagulase: the standard marker for *S. aureus*. However, a few wild-type strains (identifiable by DNA hybridization), as well as mutants, are coagulase-negative. Antigenically distinct coagulases occur; moreover, a **metalloproteinase** with coagulase-like activity is produced by some coagulase-negative strains and may interfere with their identification. DNA hybridization or other taxonomic criteria could be used for speciation in such cases.

Clotting requires interaction with a **coagulase-reacting factor (CRF)** in plasma, which is probably a derivative of prothrombin: a coagulase–CRF complex converts fibrinogen to fibrin. Although the same fibrinopeptides are released as with thrombin, the process differs from normal clotting in that the multiple accessory factors, including Ca^{2+}, are not required, and the clot is more friable and does not retract.

HYDROLASES. **Staphylokinase,** like streptokinase and urokinase, causes clot dissolution by activating conversion of the proenzyme plasminogen to the fibrinolytic enzyme plasmin. Its gene resides on a phage. The **nuclease** of *S. aureus* has both endonuclease and exonuclease activity on both DNA and RNA, producing $3'$ nucleotides. The **lipases** are assayed by testing for the ability to produce opacity on egg yolk agar or to split Tween detergents. Lipase production appears to contribute to survival of the organism on skin. Most *S. aureus* strains produce **hyaluronidase** and one or more proteases; three have been identified. A recently discovered enzyme detoxifies staphylocidal fatty acids by linking them to cholesterol. **Lysostaphin,** a lytic enzyme produced by a strain of *S. simulans*, attacks the pentaglycine bridge between peptidoglycan chains and is thus specific for staphylococci. It is used for diagnostic as well as for research purposes.

HEMOLYSINS. Four different protein hemolysins of *S. aureus* are now recognized; all produce clear β-hemolysis, but they differ in RBC species specificity and in their mechanism of action. A single strain may produce more than one. Tissue cells may also be damaged: some of the hemolysins produce local necrosis and are lethal for experimental animals.

1. *α-Hemolysin (α-toxin)* is the principal hemolysin of human strains of *S. aureus*. It is most active against rabbit RBCs; human RBCs are not susceptible, but human platelets and tissue culture cells are affected. In experimental animals, α-hemolysin causes dermal necrosis after local injection and is lethal when given systemically; the main effect appears to be spasms of vascular smooth muscle. The specific receptor on the erythrocyte membrane is a sialoglycoprotein. α-Hemolysin is secreted as a water-soluble monomer of 34,000 daltons, which rearranges, on contact with a membrane receptor, to form a cylindrical hexamer that penetrates the membrane. As Figure 25–6 shows, this cylinder not only traverses the membrane but projects above the surface. Negative staining reveals a pore of 2 to 3 nm on the surface, but its diameter within the membrane is not known. This structure resembles the lytic C5b-9(m) complex of complement.

2. *β-Hemolysin* is produced commonly by animal strains but by only 10% to 20% of human isolates. It is a "hot–cold" hemolysin: its lytic effects are not fully developed unless mixtures with blood (or blood agar cultures) are placed at low temperature following incubation at 37°C. β-Hemolysin is a sphingomyelinase C, of M_r 30,000, that is activated by Mg^{2+} but not by Ca^{2+}; it splits sphingomyelin into N-acylsphingosine and phosphorylcholine. Sheep, human, and guinea pig RBCs, in that order, contain decreasing amounts of sphingomyelin and are decreasingly sensitive. The β-hemolysin is cyto-

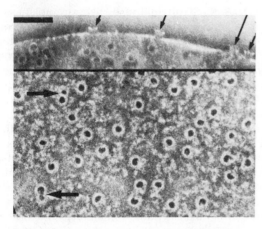

Figure 25—6. Negatively stained fragment of rabbit erythrocyte lysed with *S. aureus* α-toxin. Numerous 10-nm ring-shaped structures with a 2- to 3-nm pore are seen in a surface view of the membrane, whereas the view of an edge *(above)* shows the projection of the cylinders above the membrane. (Bhakdi S, Tranum—Jensen J: Phil Trans Roy Soc Lond B 306:311, 1984)

toxic for a variety of tissue culture cells, and large doses are toxic for experimental animals.

3. **γ-Hemolysin** consists of two basic proteins acting in concert. Rabbit, human, and sheep RBCs are susceptible, whereas horse and fowl RBCs are not. Agar and other sulfated polymers inhibit γ-hemolysin, and so it is not active on blood agar plates. Cholesterol and many other lipids are also inhibitory.

4. **δ-Hemolysin** is produced by most human strains of *S. aureus* and occurs as heterogeneous aggregates of subunits of M_r 5000. It acts, possibly as a direct surfactant, on various cell types including RBCs, leukocytes, cultured mammalian cells, and bacterial protoplasts and is not species specific.

PYROGENIC EXOTOXINS. *S. aureus* strains elaborate a series of toxins that have in common several pathogenic activities: they are pyrogenic, at least partly as a consequence of interleukin-1 induction; they are immunosuppressive owing to potent mitogenicity for suppressor T-lymphocytes; they dramatically enhance the toxicity of gram-negative endotoxin by blockading the clearance function of the reticuloendothelial systems; and they cause erythroderma by evoking delayed hypersensitivity. They are generally not serologically cross-reactive, but an individual sensitized by any one of them will show delayed hypersensitivity to each of the others. Included in this group are staphylococcal **pyrogenic exotoxins A and B,** staphylococcal **enterotoxins** (of which there are five distinct serotypes), and **TSST-1,** the cause of toxic shock syndrome. A large majority of the TSST-1 producing strains have a characteristic biotype, which includes sensitivity to typing phage 29, 52, or both and the

presence of chromosomally located resistances to Cd^{2+}, AsO_4^{2-}, and penicillin. Some 50% of *S. aureus* isolates produce one or more enterotoxins, 15% produce TSST-1, and a smaller fraction produce pyrogenic exotoxin A or B.

Some of these toxins have specific pathogenic properties. Staphylococcal enterotoxins evoke emesis and diarrhea on oral administration. Staphylococcal enterotoxin B is closely related to streptococcal pyrogenic exotoxin A (erythrogenic toxin), which causes specific heart damage and is implicated in rheumatic fever.

OTHER EXOTOXINS

Panton—Valentine (P-V) leukocidin, produced by most *S. aureus* strains, acts only on human and rabbit polymorphonuclear cells and macrophages. It has two components (F and S): component S first binds to ganglioside GM_1 (the cholera toxin receptor) and activates an endogenous membrane-bound phospholipase A_2. The products then bind component F, inducing a K^+-specific ion channel in the membrane and hence cytolysis.

Exfoliatin (epidermolytic toxin, ET) causes a variety of dermatologic lesions (see Toxinoses, below). This relatively heat-stable and acid-labile protein of M_r 24,000 is produced by approximately 5% of *S. aureus* strains, mostly of phage group II. It occurs as two antigenic variants: ETB, occurring primarily in strains of phage group II, is plasmid-coded; ETA, produced by strains of various phage types, is chromosomal. Many strains produce both types. The toxin acts by cleaving the stratum granulosum of the epidermis, probably by splitting desmosomes that link the cells of this layer.

Pathogenesis of Invasive Disease

COLONIZATION. The skin and nares of infants are colonized by *S. aureus* within a few days after birth; the carrier rate then drops, only to increase during childhood to the adult rate of approximately 30%. The organisms are most commonly found in the anterior nares and on skin and mucous membranes; coagulase-negative staphylococci prefer skin and coagulase-positive ones prefer mucous membranes. Colonization represents a stable association that presumably involves an interaction between specific staphylococcal **adhesins** and cellular receptors. Organisms resident in the nares are probably the principal cause of endogenous infections.

DISEASE. Suppuration is the hallmark of staphylococcal disease, and the most frequent lesion is a cutaneous abscess or boil (furuncle), which begins as an infection of sebaceous glands or hair shafts. At full development, the center of the abscess shows liquefaction necrosis (pus) consisting of dead bacteria, phagocytes, and fluid, surrounded by a firm wall of fibrin, inflammatory cells, and viable bacteria. Sometimes a series of interconnected abscesses occurs (carbuncle). In addition to skin infections, which are usually self-limiting, serious, often life-threatening deep-seated infections occur, including abscesses of various organs, osteomyelitis, pyelonephritis, pneumonia and empyema, meningitis, purulent arthritis, and septicemia and endocarditis (often with metastatic abscesses). Although *S. aureus* is probably the most common cause of bacterial infection in humans, most infections are minor and superficial; serious infections occur much more commonly in association with a predisposing condition than spontaneously. Newborns are particularly susceptible, as are persons with traumatic or operative wounds, burns, or other serious skin lesion or chronic debilitating disorders such as diabetes mellitus, cancer, or cystic fibrosis. It is therefore not surprising that serious staphylococcal disease is most often the result of hospital-acquired (nosocomial) infections.

The relative avirulence of *S. aureus* for normal persons has been demonstrated in human volunteer experiments. Large numbers of organisms injected under the skin may cause no more than a barely discernible lesion. On the other hand, suppurative lesions invariably result from inserting a silk suture contaminated with a small number (fewer than 100) of cells: the foreign body permits the organisms to gain a foothold, perhaps by providing sites of bacterial multiplication inaccessible to phagocytes.

Special mechanisms of pathogenesis operate in the **mammary gland.** *S. aureus* is the commonest cause of **mastitis** in domestic livestock as well as in humans. An inoculum of 10^2 or 10^3 organisms infused into the bovine udder can cause typical mastitis, which involves adherence of the organism to the glandular epithelium followed by erosion, local invasion, and a diffuse exudative inflammatory reaction accompanied by systemic symptoms.

DETERMINANTS OF PATHOGENICITY. Although the precise roles of individual bacterial factors in staphylococcal disease have not been clearly defined, virtually all of the toxic and enzymatic products have been implicated. α-Toxin is lethal for animals and seems likely to play a role in overwhelming septicemic disease; δ-hemolysin and P-V leukocidin both destroy human polymorphonuclear leukocytes (which may be why *S. aureus* are killed less efficiently than coagulase-negative organisms by phagocytosis); lipase may be important in the development of boils; other enzymes detoxify bactericidal fatty acids released from lipids in response to the infection; coagulase probably contributes to the localization and persistence of the lesions by walling them off from phagocytic cells (although a fibrin coating on individual bacteria does not impede their phagocytosis). Other factors would seem to enhance the spread of lesions: hyaluronidase breaks down interstitial hyaluronic acid, proteases degrade collagen and elastin, and staphylokinase causes clot lysis, antagonizing the action of coagulase.

Consistent with such differential effects are observations that strains isolated from boils are high in lipase and low in hyaluronidase, whereas the reverse is true of those isolated from spreading lesions such as bullous impetigo. On the other hand, strains that lack one or more of these several substances have been isolated from lesions, and similar mutants appear to be no less virulent in experimental infections.

The role of bacterial surface Ags is also unclear. The rare constitutively encapsulated strains are more virulent for animals (no data are available for humans), probably because encapsulated staphylococci are relatively resistant to phagocytosis. There is suggestive evidence that other strains form capsules only *in vivo*, so that capsule formation may be more important in pathogenesis than is currently appreciated. Protein A, despite the wide variety of biological effects of its interactions with Igs (particularly inhibition of phagocytosis), has not been shown to be a primary virulence factor. Surface proteins (adhesins), which enable the organisms to bind to various tissue components and cell surfaces, may impede phagocytosis and may also be involved in invasiveness. Data linking them specifically to virulence are not yet available.

Because no single factor is decisive, virulent and avirulent strains of *S. aureus* cannot be defined sharply, as can rough and smooth pneumococci, or *tox*$^+$ and *tox*$^-$ strains of *Corynebacterium diphtheriae*. Even epidemic strains (e.g., 80/81) demonstrate no qualitative or quantitative difference in presumed virulence factors and indeed may be less virulent for animals than conventional strains.

Humoral Abs are a critical line of defense, as agammaglobulinemic individuals are highly susceptible to invasive staphylococcal disease. Adult humans normally have high levels of circulating Abs to staphylococci and most of their products; presumably, those directed at surface components (teichoic acids, capsular Ags) are the most important, because they facilitate phagocytosis. It is known that anticapsular Abs are protective whereas Abs against most of the exoproteins (with the exception of TSST-1) are not.

In addition, **delayed hypersensitivity** to *S. aureus* can result from repeated skin infections, and in experimental animals, it is associated with more severe although more localized disease. Accordingly, delayed hypersensitivity may conceivably participate in the pathogenesis of staphylococcal disease, both positively and negatively, much as it does in tuberculosis.

In summary: *S. aureus* coexists with man in a semistable equilibrium, which can be shifted in favor of either organism by a variety of circumstances. Because the interacting bacterial and host factors are so multiple, their individual roles cannot be easily identified by experimental manipulation. Whereas most strains of staphylococci produce primarily invasive disease, some strains form potent exotoxins (described in an earlier section) that cause characteristic distant lesions.

Toxinoses

STAPHYLOCOCCAL FOOD POISONING. S. aureus is one of the commonest causes of food poisoning, which is due to preformed enterotoxin in the food. Nausea, cramps, vomiting, and, usually, diarrhea appear abruptly 1 to 6 hours after ingestion of contaminated food. Recovery generally occurs within 24 hours; rarely, death occurs in infants and the elderly. Foods commonly implicated are pastries, custards, salad dressing, sliced meats, and meat products, usually contaminated by food handlers. **Staphylococcal enterotoxins are heat-stable** (100°C for 30 minutes); it is therefore essential to prevent multiplication of the organisms by refrigerating food before as well as after cooking.

EXFOLIATIVE SKIN DISEASE. **Exfoliatin** causes a variety of syndromes: **generalized exfoliative dermatitis** in newborns (Ritter's disease); a form of **toxic epidermal necrolysis** in children and occasionally adults; bullous **impetigo;** and **staphylococcal scarlatina,** which, unlike streptococcal scarlatina, spares the tongue and palate. The group of entities is collectively termed the **staphylococcal scalded-skin syndrome** (SSSS). Recovery is usual because the lesion is in the stratum granulosum, leaving a sufficient layer of epidermis to avoid massive fluid loss and to protect against secondary deep skin infection.

The organisms are sometimes found at the site of the skin lesions but often are at distant sites, with or without evidence of a primary focus of infection. The most severe form of the human disease is mimicked in newborn mice following injection of purified exfoliatin or of organisms producing it. Exfoliatin is antigenic; the variation in the clinical picture and the rarity of the severe syndrome in adults may reflect various degrees of antitoxic immunity.

Toxic shock syndrome is a recently described symptom complex attributable primarily to local infection with TSST-1-producing organisms. The full-blown syndrome includes shock, high fever, nausea, vomiting, diarrhea, thrombocytopenia, renal and hepatic dysfunction, and a scarlatiniform rash followed by desquamation, particularly of the palms and soles. The mortality rate in uncomplicated cases is about 2%; however, TSS complicating influenza can have a mortality rate in excess of 50%. Some 80% of cases occur in association with

menstruation, during which there seems to be a heightened susceptibility to the toxin. Additionally, certain types of menstrual tampons may play an important accessory role by providing trapped O_2 and by depleting Mg^{2+}, both of which stimulate production of staphylococcal exoproteins including TSST-1 *in vitro*. In keeping with the ability of TSST-1 to enhance endotoxin toxicity, most severe and fatal cases of TSS occur in association with a gram-negative infection in which endotoxin gains access to the circulation. Some 20% of TSS cases occur in association with postoperative and other local *S. aureus* infections at various sites. Whereas virtually all of the menstrual isolates produce TSST-1, some 40% of the extravaginal isolates do not, and enterotoxin B may be the causative agent in at least some of these cases.

Toxic shock is the clearest example of a staphylococcal disease that is determined by immunity. Some 99% of human adults are immune to TSST-1 and are not susceptible to TSS, and some TSS victims seroconvert. Others, however, do not seroconvert and suffer repeated bouts of the syndrome. The hypoimmunity shown by these individuals is focal—their response to other Ags, including staphylococcal Ags, is normal.

Neonatal necrotizing enterocolitis is a life-threatening condition affecting primarily premature infants. It is caused by **coagulase-negative** staphylococci that grossly overproduce **δ-hemolysin:** the toxin can readily be recovered from the feces, and it causes similar pathology in a rat intestinal loop model. Only when overproduced in the unnatural environment of the sterile, relatively aerobic premature intestine does this weakly toxic protein have its devastating effect; in the anaerobic bowel an inactive variant is produced.

Laboratory Diagnosis

The finding of gram-positive cocci in stained smears of purulent exudates provides only suggestive information, because staphylococci cannot be differentiated from other gram-positive cocci on purely morphological grounds. Specimens should be inoculated directly onto sheep blood (or preferably rabbit blood) agar plates and into thioglycollate broth. If contamination with other organisms is likely, mannitol-salt agar or phenylethyl alcohol agar should also be used. Blood cultures should be inoculated into blood agar pour plates as well as in broth.

Identification of *S. aureus* is suggested by colony morphology, pigment production, hemolysis, mannitol fermentation, and growth of the organisms at a high salt concentration, but these properties are variable, whereas a positive coagulase test certifies the diagnosis. Although the presence of clumping factor (bound coagulase) often correlates with free coagulase production, testing for free coagulase is preferred.

The **coagulase test** is performed by adding a loopful of a colony from an agar plate, or 0.1ml of a broth culture, to 0.5 ml of citrated rabbit plasma and incubating the mixture at 37°C. Most positive strains cause clot formation within 4 hours and many within 1 hour, but tubes are observed for 24 hours before being considered negative.

Enterotoxins in suspected food are demonstrated by immunologic techniques such as gel diffusion. Diagnoses of SSSS and TSS are usually made on clinical grounds and by the isolation of the causative organism. Phage typing is helpful, but definitive identification is immunologic.

Treatment

Minor lesions do not generally require antimicrobial treatment. Localized suppurative lesions such as abscesses must be drained; antibiotics are useful primarily to inhibit dissemination. Systemic disease must be treated vigorously with an appropriate antibiotic in addition to establishing drainage, if possible. *S. aureus* without β-lactamase is exquisitely sensitive to penicillin, minimal bactericidal concentrations of 0.01 to 0.02 μg/ml being typical. Penicillin is far and away the drug of choice if the organism is known to be sensitive. If the patient is allergic to penicillin, erythromycin should be used. The therapeutic problem posed by drug-resistant staphylococci is self-evident. Because of the prevalence, particularly in hospital populations, of staphylococci resistant to penicillin and other antimicrobials, it is essential to determine the drug sensitivity of the infecting organism. In the absence of sensitivity information, treatment is normally started with a semisynthetic penicillinase-resistant penicillin such as methicillin or oxacillin. In certain hospital settings throughout the world, serious nosocomial epidemics are caused by *S. aureus* strains resistant to all antibiotics save vancomycin, which is, therefore, the initial drug of choice in life-threatening nosocomial staphylococcal disease in these settings. A less toxic drug may be substituted later on the basis of susceptibility tests.

Control

Because of the high level of antistaphylococcal immunity in the population at large, staphylococcal infections outside the hospital are not ordinarily considered to be contagious; most often, infection is caused by an endogenous strain. In the community, control is therefore attempted only for individuals with chronic or recurrent conditions and is directed toward treatment of the infections plus disinfection of the skin and local environment. An exception is a food handler who is a carrier of or has an open infection with an enterotoxin-producing strain of *S. aureus*. As such individuals have been implicated in outbreaks of food poisoning, they should not be permitted to handle food until active dissemination of the organism has stopped. Replacement of an endogenous strain by another of lower virulence is sometimes effective in controlling the carrier state or in the treatment of conditions such as chronic furunculosis (see below).

In the hospital setting, where susceptibility to staphylococcal infection may be much greater, cross-infection is an extremely serious problem. The organism is most commonly transferred between patients by direct contact or by hospital personnel who may themselves be chronic carriers. Patients with open staphylococcal infections should be isolated, those attending them should use vigorous disinfection procedures, and contaminated materials should be sterilized as rapidly as possible.

EPIDEMIOLOGY. A general increase in our ability to prolong life by measures that compromise resistance to infection, plus a seemingly inexorable increase in the prevalence of multi-resistant bacteria, have combined to make hospital epidemics a significant source of morbidity and mortality. *S. aureus* has always played a major role and will doubtless continue to do so; however, the prevalence of nosocomial *S. aureus* infections has fluctuated widely both in space and in time, and different strains emerge and recede with a temporal rhythm that has defied understanding. Thus, in the 1950s and 1960s, a worldwide epidemic of hospital infections was caused by the notorious phage type 80/81 *S. aureus*. As these organisms had the unusual ability to attack healthy individuals through the unbroken skin, they were an important exception to the rule that *S. aureus* infections are not highly contagious in the community. In the late 1960s, the 80/81 strains were largely replaced globally by a new group, susceptible to phages 83/84/85 or some subset of these. These strains did not show the extreme virulence of the 80/81 strains. The 1980s have seen a new worldwide hospital epidemic involving multiply antibiotic-resistant strains of phage type 88. It is not known whether displacing strains are variants of previously prevalent strains with new phage types or are entirely different strains.

A major aspect of any epidemiologic control program is the ability to identify strains accurately so as to trace their spread. Classical biotyping, involving the determination of serotypes, of phage types and lysotypes, and of antibiograms have recently been supplemented with molecular methods based on variable gene systems, as shown in Figures 25–4 and 25–5. One can now document with great precision the flow of organisms and of plasmids and other unique genetic elements that are transmitted from strain to strain, sometimes undergoing rearrangements. Such information on genotypic relations should reveal the biological mechanisms underlying global shifts in the biotypes of epidemic strains.

BACTERIAL INTERFERENCE. In addition to the standard measures used to control staphylococcal spread, deliberate colonization with an *S. aureus* strain of low virulence (502A) has proved effective in aborting nursery outbreaks and in controlling furunculosis in adults. Its effectiveness is based on the inability of a superinfecting bacterium to colonize an individual who is already colonized by another strain of the same species. Usefulness is limited because 502A cannot usually displace an existing organism and because it may itself cause infections.

Selected Reading

BOOKS AND REVIEW ARTICLES

Easmon CSF, Adlam C: Staphylococci and Staphylococcal Infections. London, Academic Press, 1983

Jeljaszewicz J: The Staphylococci. Proceedings of the Vth International Symposium on Staphylococci and Staphylococcal Infections. Stuttgart, Gustav Fischer Verlag, 1985

Lacey RW: Antibiotic resistance plasmids of *Staphylococcus aureus* and their clinical importance. Bacteriol Rev 39:1, 1975

Lyon, BR, Skurray R: Antimicrobial resistance of *Staphylococcus aureus*: genetic basis. Microbiol Rev 51:88, 1987

Martin WJ: Anaerobic cocci. In Lennette EH, Spaulding EH, Truant JP (eds): Manual of Clinical Microbiology, 2nd Ed, p 381. Washington, DC, American Society for Microbiology, 1974

Rogolsky M: Nonenteric toxins of *Staphylococcus aureus*. Microbiol Rev 43:320, 1979

SPECIFIC ARTICLES

Betley MJ, Mekalanos JJ: Staphylococcal enterotoxin A is encoded by phage. Science 229:185, 1985

Cox HU, Newman SS, Roy AF, Hoskins JD: Species of staphylococcus isolated from animal infections. Cornell Vet 74:124, 1984

Fussle R, Bhakdi S, Sziegoleit A, et al: On the mechanism of membrane damage by *Staphylococcus aureus* α-toxin. J Cell Biol 91:83, 1981

Garbe PL, Arko RJ, Reingold AL et al: *Staphylococcus aureus* isolates from patients with nonmenstrual toxic shock syndrome. JAMA 253:2538, 1985

Gudding R, McDonald J, Cheville NF: Pathogenesis of *Staphylococcus aureus* mastitis: Bacteriologic, histologic, and ultrastructural pathologic findings. Am J Vet Res 45:2525, 1984

Johnson LP, L'Italien JJ, Schlievert PM: Streptococcal pyrogenic exotoxin type A (scarlet fever toxin) is related to *Staphylococcus aureus* enterotoxin B. Mol Gen Genet 203:354, 1986

Kreiswirth BN, Lofdahl S, Betley M et al: The toxic shock syndrome exotoxin structural gene is not detectably transmitted by a prophage. Nature 305:709, 1983

Lee CY, Iandolo, JJ: Lysogenic conversion of staphylococcal lipase is caused by insertion of the bacteriophage L54a genome into the lipase structural gene. J Bacteriol 166:385, 1986

Lofdahl S, Guss B, Uhlen M, Philipson L, Lindberg M: Gene for staphylococcal protein A. Proc Natl Acad Sci USA 80:697, 1983

Martin-Bourgon C, Berron S, Casal J: Hospital infection caused by non-typable *Staphylococcus aureus*: Application of reverse typing. J Hyg Camb 94:201, 1985

Melish ME, Glasgow LA: The staphylococcal scalded-skin syndrome: Development of an experimental model. N Engl J Med 282:1114, 1970

Novick RP, Morse SI: In vivo transmission of drug resistance factors between strains of *Staphylococcus aureus*. J Exp Med 125:45, 1967

Novick R, Edelman I, Schwesinger M, Gruss A, Swanson E, Pattee PA: Genetic translocation in *Staphylococcus aureus*. Proc Natl Acad Sci USA 76:400, 1979

Schaberg DR, Clewell DB, Glatzer L: Conjugative transfer of R-plasmids from *Streptococcus faecalis* to *Staphylococcus aureus*. Antimicrob Agents Chemother 22:204, 1982

Scheifele DW, Bjornson GL, Dyer RA, Dimmick JE: Delta-like toxin produced by coagulase-negative staphylococci is associated with neonatal necrotizing enterocolitis. Infec Immun 55:2268, 1987

Schlievert PM: Enhancement of host susceptibility to lethal endotoxin shock by staphylococcal pyrogenic exotoxin C. Infect Immun 36:123, 1982

Smith RM, Parisi JT, Vidal L, Baldwin JN: Nature of the genetic determinant controlling encapsulation in *Staphylococcus aureus* Smith. Infect Immun 17:231, 1977

Speziale P, Raucci G, Visai L, Switalski LM, Timpl R, Hook M: Binding of collagen to *Staphylococcus aureus* Cowan 1. J Bacteriol 167:77, 1986

Stahl ML, Pattee, PA: Computer-assisted chromosome mapping by protoplast fusion in *Staphylococcus aureus*. J Bacteriol 154:395, 1983

Tierno PM, Hanna BA, Matias J: TSS *S. aureus*, endotoxin, and tampon induced death in a mouse model. Proc Int Conf Antimicrob Agents Chemother 25:678, 1985

Todd J, Fishaut M: Toxic-shock syndrome associated with phage-group-1 staphylococci. Lancet 2:1116, 1978

Tzagaloff H, Novick RP: Geometry of cell division in *Staphylococcus aureus*. J Bacteriol 129:343, 1977

26

Emil C. Gotschlich

Neisseriae

The Genus Neisseria

This group of gram-negative pyogenic cocci includes two species that are pathogenic for man, the **meningococcus** (*Neisseria meningitidis*) and the **gonococcus** (*Neisseria gonorrhoeae*). Several other, nonpathogenic, *Neisseria* species colonize the upper respiratory tract and may be confused with meningococci.

 Meningococcal meningitis was recognized as a contagious disease early in the nineteenth century and occurs in both an endemic and an epidemic form. The causative organism was first isolated in 1887 by Weichselbaum from the spinal fluid of a patient.

 Gonorrhea, the sexually transmitted disease (**STD**) caused by the gonococcus, was described in antiquity by Chinese, Hebrew, and Egyptian writers (i.e., the Ebers papyrus, ca. 1550 BC). The term "gonorrhea"—"flow of seed"—is attributed to Galen (130 AD), but Maimonides (1135–1204 AD) recognized that the discharge was not semen. Syphilis and gonorrhea were not clearly distinguished until the nineteenth century. The celebrated English physician John Hunter contributed to the confusion because he believed he had proved, by a self-inoculation experiment, that a single agent was responsible. Unfortunately, the donor had both diseases. *N. gonorrhoeae,* the causative agent, was described by Neisser in 1879 and first cultivated by Leistikow and Loeffler in 1882. Despite the wide use of highly effective antibiotic therapy, gonorrhea may still (with the exception of tuberculosis) be the most prevalent communicable bacterial disease.

MORPHOLOGY

The *Neisseriae* are nonmotile gram-negative cocci, most often growing in pairs but occasionally in tetrads or clusters. The individual cocci are small (about 0.8 μm), and

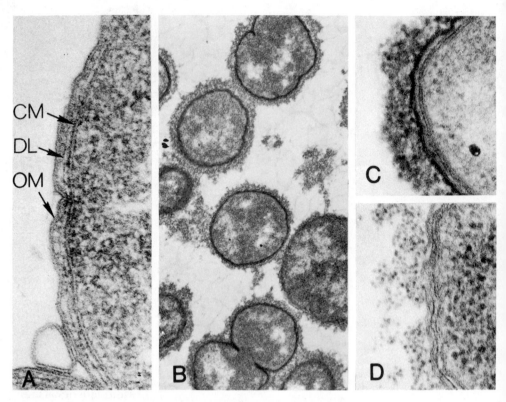

Figure 26–1. *(A)* Thin-section electron micrograph of a gonococcus. Note the location of the cell membrane *(CM)*; the dense layer *(DL)*, which consists at least in part of the peptidoglycan; and the outer membrane *(OM)* containing the endotoxic lipopolysaccharide. (×160,000) *(B–D)* Cells labeled with purified Ab against the group A meningococcal polysaccharide conjugated with horseradish peroxidase or ferritin. *(B)* Group A meningococci stained with peroxidase-conjugated antibody. The polysaccharide forms a capsule around the organisms. (×25,000) *(C)* Higher magnification (×120,000) showing an intensely opaque region immediately external to the cell wall and a less densely staining peripheral zone. *(D)* Appearance of the capsule of the group A meningococcus stained with ferritin-conjugated Ab. (×120,000) (Electron micrographs by John Swanson)

their shape may be distorted by partial autolysis. The cell envelope is typical of a gram-negative organism (Fig. 26–1). Meningococci or gonococci freshly isolated from patients bear pili. Meningococci isolated from blood or spinal fluid have a polysaccharide capsule.

METABOLISM

Neisseriae grow best aerobically in an atmosphere containing 5%–10% CO_2; hence cultures are usually incubated in a candle jar. Gonococci and some strains of meningococci grow anaerobically if supplied with NO_2^-. All members of the genus are oxidase-positive; i.e., the colonies turn pink and then black when flooded with a 1% dimethyl- or tetramethyl-p-phenylenediamine solution. A positive **oxidase test** indicates only that the isolate is part of the genus *Neisseria*, as the commensal organisms also react.

Table 26–1 presents the culture characteristics used to differentiate the principal species in the genus *Neisse-*

ria. The pathogenic species (and *N. lactamica*) are unable to grow at room temperature; also, each species exhibits a characteristic **sugar fermentation pattern.**

The growth of gonococci and meningococci is sensitive to free fatty acids contaminating the medium, but

TABLE 26–1. Principal Differential Characteristics of Common Species of the Genus Neisseria

Species	Growth at 22°C	Fermentation			
		Glucose	Maltose	Sucrose	Lactose
N. meningitidis	−	+	+	−	−
N. gonorrhoeae	−	+	−	−	−
N. lactamica	−	+	+	−	+
N. catarrhalis*	+	−	−	−	−
N. sicca	+	+	+	+	−
N. flavescens	+	−	−	−	−

* Now *Branhamella catarrhalis.*

added starch or blood can eliminate the inhibition. Blood heated at 80° to 90°C to form **chocolate agar** is particularly suitable for their growth. Defined media have been developed, and in classifying gonococcal strains variations in nutritional requirements have been useful (**auxotyping**).

The pathogenic neisserias are exceptionally sensitive to unfavorable conditions; they are autolytic, and cultures may die out in a few days, especially at refrigerator temperature. Strains are best preserved by freezing or lyophilization.

PATHOGENESIS

Studies of pathogenesis have been limited by the absence of animal models that closely mimic human infection. The pathogenic *Neisseriae* can invade human mucosal tissue (Fig. 26–2). The organisms attach to the mucus-secreting cells, but not to ciliated cells. The initial attachment, by the pili, is followed by extensive membrane-to-membrane contact. The epithelial cells then actively engulf the bacteria, rapidly transport the vesicles containing them to the basement membrane, and egest the organisms into the submucosal space. Thus, the first breach of tissue integrity is achieved by subverting functions of the epithelial cells to the advantage of the microbe. It is notable that a few other microbes elicit similar events; i.e., *Yersiniae*, *Shigellae*, enteroinvasive *E. coli* in intestinal mucosa, and *Chlamydia trachomatis* in ocular or genitourinary epithelial cells.

It is important to recognize that the mucosal invasion by the meningococcus generally occurs in the nasopharynx and is asymptomatic. With the gonococcus, the most common site is the genitourinary epithelium, and the infection frequently causes considerable discomfort. However, gonococcal pharyngitis (like the meningococcal infection at the same site) is most often asymptomatic.

ANTIGENIC STRUCTURE AND GENETIC VARIATION

The gonococcus and the meningococcus can be **transformed with DNA** as long as the organisms are piliated. Gonococci may contain three classes of **plasmids:** (1) a 24.5-Md conjugative plasmid able to mobilize other plasmids but not chromosomal genes; (2) a 2.6-Md plasmid of unknown function; and (3) resistance plasmids causing production of β-lactamase. The latter group are quite prevalent, particularly in the Far East and Africa. In meningococci, plasmids have only very rarely been found, and penicillin resistance has so far not been a problem. Curiously, no phages infective for gonococci or for meningococci have been found.

Various chromosomally mediated drug resistances, especially sulfonamide resistance, are frequent in both species. Tetracycline resistance is increasing among gonococcal isolates.

CAPSULES. Most meningococci have a **polysaccharide capsule,** which is the basis for **serogroups.** N-acetyl neuraminic acid, a common constituent in eukaryotes, has been found in bacteria only in meningococcal capsules and in the chemically related capsule of *E. coli* K1 (see Table 26–2). Group A strains have caused most of the major epidemics. Group B and C strains generally cause

TABLE 26–2. *Structures of the Polysaccharide Antigens of N. meningitidis*

Serogroup	Repeating Unit	Linkage	O-Acetyl Content*	Location of O-Acetyl Groups
A	2-Acetamido-2-deoxy-D-mannopyranosyl phosphate	$1 \rightarrow 6$-α	0.7	C-3 of mannosamine
B	D-N-Acetylneuraminic acid	$2 \rightarrow 8$-α	None	–
C1⁺	D-N-Acetylneuraminic acid	$2 \rightarrow 9$-α	1.3	C-7 and C-8 of sialic acid
C1⁻	D-N-Acetylneuraminic acid	–	None	–
W-135	4-O-α-D-Galactopyranosyl-N-acetylneuraminic acid	$2 \rightarrow 6$-α	None	–
X	2-Acetamido-2-deoxy-D-glucopyranosyl phosphate	$1 \rightarrow 4$-α	None	–
Y	4-O-α-D-Glucopyranosyl-N-acetylneuraminic acid	$2 \rightarrow 6$-α	1.1	Not specifically located
Z'	7-O-α-D-2-Acetamido-α-deoxy-galactopyranosyl-2-keto-3-deoxy-D-octulosonic acid	$2 \rightarrow 3$-β	1.0	C-4 and C-5 of keto-deoxyoctonate
Z	Unknown	–	–	–

* Expressed in moles per mole of repeating unit.

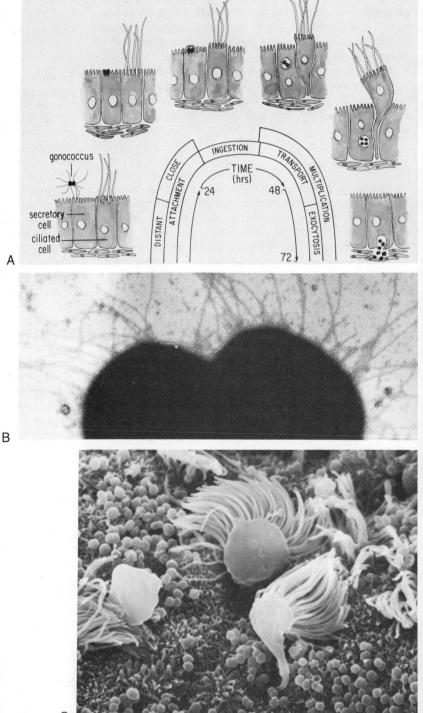

Figure 26–2. *(A)* Schema summarizing the fallopian tube mucosal infection seen in organ cultures. The initial step, attachment at a distance by means of pili, converts to a close attachment. Thereafter, the epithelial cells actively ingest the gonococci and transport them to the basement membrane. Note that the organisms attach and invade only the mucus-secreting cells; the ciliated cells, however, exhibit toxic changes (ciliostasis) and are then pushed out of the epithelium. The series of events requires 48 to 72 hours. *(B)* Electron micrograph of negatively stained gonococci showing pili emanating from their surfaces. *(C)* Scanning electron micrograph of infected fallopian tube mucosa. Note the many spherical gonococci adherent on the nonciliated cells. Note also the expulsion of ciliated cells from the mucosa. (Electron micrographs by John Swanson and Zell McGee; drawing by Kenneth H. Johnston)

endemic disease but on occasion cause an epidemic outbreak. Other serogroups less frequently cause disease but are quite commonly found in nasopharyngeal cultures. Meningococci also produce a high-molecular-weight **polyphosphate,** which is loosely adherent to the surface. Its function is unknown.

Gonococci also produce polyphosphate but no polysaccharide capsule.

PILI. Both species, when freshly isolated from patients, carry pili on their surfaces: helical aggregates of identical protein subunits, called pilin, ranging in molecular weight from 17,000 to 21,000. *In vitro* gonococci can lose the ability to produce pili, and such strains are easily recognized by the altered appearance of the colonies (Fig. 26–3). Nonpiliated gonococci can regain the production of pili (phase variation), sometimes with a shift in antigenic type.

The **variability of pilin sequence** resides primarily in the carboxy-terminal half of the molecule, for which the genome contains many incomplete sequences. **Gene conversion** recombines these into the copy that is being expressed, and if the new pilin can be assembled into pili, an antigenic variant is produced. The frequency *in vitro* is high (10^{-3} per cell division) under some circumstances: transforming DNA, released from lysing cells, can recombine efficiently with partly homologous regions. Gonococci have thus evolved sophisticated means for varying the antigenic specificity of their pili, and similar variation probably also exists in meningococci.

The amino-terminal 50 residues remain unaltered in the phase variation of pilin. This constant region is widely distributed: it is nearly identical in *Moraxella spp., Pseudomonas aeruginosa, Vibrio cholerae,* and even the anaerobe *Bacteroides nodosus.*

PROTEINS. The **outer membrane antigens** of the gonococcus and the meningococcus are quite similar; their nomenclature is outlined in Table 26–3. The most prominent are the porins (Chap. 2), and their genes have been sequenced. Two principal antigenic forms are recognized in gonococci (IA and IB, of mol. wt. 32,000 and 37,000) and in meningococci (proteins 2 and 3, of mol. wt. 37,000 and 41,000). Meningococci have an additional class 1 protein, whose sequence suggests that it is also a porin. Antigenic variations in these proteins are useful in **serotyping.**

All meningococci also form **protein 4** (mol. wt. 33,000), and gonococci form the antigenically similar **protein III** (mol. wt. 31,000). These Ags exhibit no serological variation among strains, and they are similar in sequence to OmpA proteins of enterobacteria. Human complement-fixing IgG Abs to these proteins can block bacteriolysis *in vitro* dependent on Ab and complement; the relevance of these **blocking Abs** in disease is not known.

Both species express in their OM the H.8 antigen, a remarkable protein of unknown function consisting almost entirely of 13 or 14 repeats of the pentapeptide Pro-Ala-Ala-Glu-Ala, with slight variations. The amino-terminal residue is a lipid-substituted cysteine, as in *E. coli* lipoproteins (see Fig. 2–23).

Gonococci can also form a variable **protein II.** Most forms cause the growing cells to adhere to each other, which makes the colonies opaque to transmitted light. These adherent proteins probably also interact with the epithelial cell surface.

The genome contains 8 or more protein II genes, whose expression is controlled by a unique mechanism. Shortly after the initiation codon the mRNA contains 7 to 28 repeats of CTCTT, which codes in repeats for Leu, Ser,

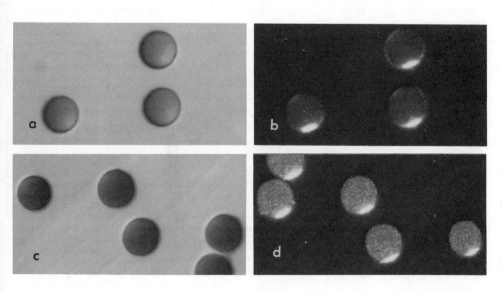

Figure 26–3. Appearance of gonococci as seen through a colony microscope ($\times 60$). Two modes of substage lighting are used: light reflected from a ground-glass diffuser (*a, c*) or transmitted from a mirror (*b, d*). Panels *a* and *b* show heavily piliated transparent organisms, panels *c* and *d*, heavily piliated opaque gonococci. Note the sharply defined borders (*a, c*) and the highlight on the edge of the colony (*b, d*), both indicative of profuse piliation and lacking in colonies of nonpiliated gonococci. The opacity to transmitted light is seen in (*d*). For an illustration of pili, see Figure 26–2B. (Photomicrographs by John Swanson)

TABLE 26–3. *Comparison of the Surface Components of N. gonorrhoeae and N. meningitidis*

	Meningococcus	Gonococcus	Pathogenic Function and Other Importance
Capsules	Polysaccharides (Table 26–3)	Not isolated or chemically defined	Probably antiphagocytic. Basis of serogroup classification
Polyphosphate	+	+	Unknown
Pili	+	+	Adhesin. May also have antiphagocytic effect. Required for DNA uptake. Antigenically highly variable
Main OM proteins*	Class 1	Not described	Probably porins; define certain meningococcal serotypes
	Class 2 and 3	PIA and PIB	Porins; define gonococcal and meningococcal serotypes
	Class 4	P III	Unknown; noncovalently associated with porins. No antigenic variation
	Class 5	P II	Implicated in attachment to human cells. Antigenically highly variable
LPS/LOS	12 Serotypes†	6 Serotypes	Endotoxic component of cells

* Note that roman numerals are used for gonococcal and arabic numerals for meningococcal OM proteins.

† Note that with meningococci "serogroup" refers to the capsule and "serotype" to the OM proteins or LOS.

and Phe (appropriate for a signal sequence). The number of repeats is varied by a mechanism independent of homologous recombination, and, depending on the number, the initiation codon will be in or out of frame with the remainder of the gene. Hence, although transcription is always occurring, the protein gene is translated only when a correct number of repeats are present. Its expression is gained or lost at a rate of about 10^{-3} per cell division, in vitro (and also frequently in natural infection), and between zero and three protein IIs may be expressed by a gonococcus at one time. Meningococci possess analogous highly variable OM proteins (**class 5 proteins**), except these do not lead to opaque colonies.

Both the meningococcus and the gonococcus secrete an **IgA protease** that cleaves the heavy chain of monomeric or polymeric human IgA of the **IgA₁ isotype** in the **hinge region.** Its role in pathogenesis is not understood, but it is noteworthy that the pneumococcus (Chap. 23) and *Haemophilus influenzae* (Chap. 31) produce an analogous enzyme, and DNA hybridization suggests a common origin.

Metabolic conditions such as anoxia or starvation can affect protein composition of the OM. Iron limitation (as occurs *in vivo*) enhances the expression of several proteins.

LPS. The OM also contains LPS. Unlike the polysaccharide of the enterobacterial LPS, which generally contains multiple repeating units (Ch. 2), the LPS of *Neisseria* has short sugar chains and hence is now called **lipooligosaccharide (LOS).** There are six known serotypes among gonococci and a dozen among meningococci. The LOS contain glucose, galactose, 3-keto-2-deoxyoctanoic acid, glucosamine, galactosamine, and ethanolamine in different ratios, depending on the serotype, and their structures are subject to rapid antigenic variation.

The sera of normal human beings often contain IgM Abs to LOS capable of causing complement-dependent bacteriolysis.

Meningococcal Disease

EPIDEMIOLOGY

The meningococcus most often inhabits the human nasopharyngeal area without causing any symptoms. This **carrier state** may last for a few days to a few months; it provides the reservoir for the meningococcus and enhances the immunity of the host. In the general population, the carrier rate tends to be appreciable at all times, and in military populations, it may exceed 90%. When individuals without adequate immunity acquire the meningococcus, usually through contact with a healthy carrier, the nasopharyngeal infection may lead rapidly to bacteremia, ordinarily followed by acute purulent meningitis.

Meningococcal disease occurs with an **endemic incidence** of approximately 2/100,000 per annum or less. More than half the cases occur in children below the age of 5 years, with the highest incidence in the first year. During the first 3 months, however, there still are sufficient maternal antibodies to confer protection. Rates in an **epidemic** may exceed the endemic rate by more than 100-fold, and the incidence above 2 years of age increases disproportionately. Epidemics occur in the winter months, and contributing factors include a large number of nonimmune individuals in the population and crowding and stress (as exemplified by the unusual susceptibility of military recruits). However, the causes that initiate an outbreak are not precisely known.

The **mortality** of meningococcal meningitis is approximately 85% without treatment, but in young adults, such as military recruits, it can be less than 1% if vigorous antibiotic and supportive therapy is provided early. It is approximately 10% in the general population. Mercifully the rate of permanent **neurologic sequelae** is low, in contrast with the other prevalent meningitides.

Infrequently, **meningococcemia** does not progress to meningitis but causes thromboembolic lesions containing cultivable meningococci in the skin, joints, lungs, middle ear, or adrenal glands. **Acute adrenal insufficiency (Waterhouse–Friderichsen syndrome)** occurs in fulminant cases and is commonly associated with bilateral hemorrhagic adrenal cortical necrosis. This lesion has a striking resemblance to that produced in rabbits by intravenous LPS after the adrenals have been stimulated by ACTH or a prior injection of LPS (general **Schwartzman reaction**). Very rarely, meningococcemia becomes **chronic,** persisting for weeks as a fever of unknown etiology.

IMMUNITY

Antibodies, present in the sera of most adults, play a role in preventing meningococcal disease. Thus, in a study of 15,000 military recruits followed, serum bactericidal activity against this organism was initially present in only three of the 54 who contracted group C meningococcal disease but in the majority of those who did not contract the disease. Moreover, the newborn very rarely contracts the disease until after the loss of maternal Abs.

Protective Abs are evoked within a week by the meningococcal carrier state. They are directed not only against the capsular group-specific polysaccharides but also against other surface antigens, including LOS and OM proteins. Low-level immunity may explain why young children rarely contract disease on their first contact with a potentially virulent meningococcus. The immunity might result from prior contact with a nonencapsulated strain, or with an encapsulated strain of low virulence, or with a related nonvirulent organism (such as the *Neisseria lactamica* frequently found in nasopharyngeal cultures of children), or even with **cross-reactive polysaccharide** from other sources. Thus, in the United States, the majority of children and young adults have Abs to the group A capsular polysaccharide, although group A meningococci have only rarely been encountered since 1950. Organisms that produce polysaccharides cross-reactive with group A have been identified (some strains of *Bacillus pumilis* and of group D *Streptococcus*). Furthermore, the *E. coli* capsular antigen K92 cross-reacts with group C polysaccharide and that of *E. coli* K1 is indistinguishable from the group B polysaccharide. Curiously, strains carrying the K1 antigen cause 75% of *E. coli* neonatal meningitis.

Multiple attacks of meningococcal meningitis appear to be associated frequently with **deficiencies of late complement components C5, C6, C7, and C8.** These patients also show increased susceptibility to systemic infection with gonococci but not with other organisms.

LABORATORY DIAGNOSIS

In cases of suspected meningococcal diseases, stained specimens of blood, spinal fluid, and nasopharyngeal secretions should be examined for *N. meningitidis*. When heavy bacteremia is present, a diligent search may reveal gram-negative diplococci in routine blood smears. In addition, smears made from the petechial lesions of the skin occasionally reveal the organism.

The accepted **blood culture** procedure is to add 10 ml of blood to 100 ml of a suitable liquid medium (e.g., tryptose phosphate broth) and also to spread 0.1 ml of blood on the surface of a blood (or chocolate) agar plate. Both cultures are incubated at 37°C in a candle jar and are inspected daily for 7 days before being discarded.

Spinal fluid may be permitted to drop directly from the lumbar puncture needle onto the surface of agar plates, and a tube of broth should also be inoculated. In addition, a sample of the spinal fluid by itself should be incubated in a candle jar at 37°C and later subcultured; this procedure will occasionally reveal meningococci when the original drop cultures are negative. Smears of spinal fluid that are to be stained for bacteria must be fixed promptly to prevent autolysis. **Capsular antigen,** which is generally present in the spinal fluid, may be demonstrated rapidly by countercurrent immunoelectrophoresis; appropriate antisera are commercially available. The number and kind of leukocytes should be determined: as a rule, polymorphonuclear leukocytes will predominate. Spinal fluid should also be tested for low glucose and elevated protein.

Nasopharyngeal cultures are best performed on specimens obtained with a cotton swab from the posterior nasopharyngeal wall behind the soft palate, taking care to avoid touching the tongue. The secretions should be cultivated on selective media containing antibiotics to inhibit the predominant normal flora. A positive nasopharyngeal culture detects meningococcal carriers but does not prove meningococcal disease.

Neisseria colonies may be tentatively recognized by the oxidase test. To identify meningococci requires fermentation and serologic tests.

TREATMENT

Because it is imperative that treatment be started as soon as the provisional diagnosis of bacterial meningitis is made and before the agent is identified, the regimen employed initially is that recommended for *Haemophilus influenzae* meningitis, in which penicillin resistance is common (Chap. 31). Once the meningococcal etiology has been established, the drug of choice is penicillin administered intravenously. Although this drug does not penetrate the normal blood–brain barrier, it does so readily when the meninges are acutely inflamed. If a history of anaphylactic reactivity to penicillin contraindicates its use, combined therapy with erythromycin and chloramphenicol is recommended. The success of antimicrobial treatment is much greater if therapy is started as soon as the specimens for bacteriologic diagnosis have been obtained. If signs of adrenal insufficiency develop, corticosteroids, pressor amines, and parenteral fluids are required.

PREVENTION

Two methods for preventing meningococcal disease exist: chemoprophylaxis and immunoprophylaxis. **Chemoprophylaxis** with sulfonamides was first used in World War II among military recruits. The meningococcal carrier rate and the incidence of the disease were very effectively lowered, but by the early 1960s, this measure was no longer applicable because of the prevalence of resistant meningococci. At present, **rifampin** and **minocycline** are used, but because they have several disadvantages, they should be considered only for individuals in **close contact** with a case, such as those living in the same household or participating in mouth-to-mouth resuscitation. There is no evidence that classroom contact or the usual hospital personnel contact entails a significant added risk.

Vaccines consisting of the purified group A and C **capsular polysaccharides** are nontoxic, and wide use under epidemic conditions in several countries has shown them to be highly effective in preventing meningococcal disease. The group B polysaccharide is a poor AG. Combined vaccines that include polysaccharides A, C, Y, and W-135 are also available, and vaccines using other surface Ags are under development.

As with other polysaccharide Ags, the immune response of infants and young children is weak: group C especially provides no significant protection below 18 months, but group A may be effective at 6 months. The Ab response to vaccine administered above 7 years of age may last for several years, but it is shorter in young children. Because of the low incidence of the disease in the U.S. today (1 : 100,000 per annum) the vaccines are recommended only for epidemic control.

Gonococcal Disease
EPIDEMIOLOGY

It is estimated there are **2 million cases a year of gonorrhea in the U.S.** In heterosexual men, the most commonly infected site is the anterior urethra, producing symptoms in 90% of cases. In homosexual men rectal and pharyngeal infections are common. The later infections are usually asymptomatic. The **asymptomatic infections** (although a minority) represent an important **reservoir** of the disease, because usually they are not treated, and the infection therefore lasts for months. In women, the most commonly infected site is the endocervix; the urethra, the rectum, the periurethral glands, and Bartholin's ducts are also sites of infection. Perhaps as many as 50% of infected women have insufficient symptoms to seek treatment.

The most common complication is ascending infection of the fallopian tubes, **acute pelvic inflammatory disease (PID),** which occurs in about 15% to 20% of infected women, usually within a week of the onset of the first menses following infection. Acute gonococcal PID frequently necessitates hospitalization and can lead to scarring of the oviducts, resulting in **sterility or ectopic pregnancies.** The scarred fallopian tubes can also become superinfected with a number of bacterial species leading to chronic PID, which often requires surgical treatment. In men receiving current treatment, local extension of the infection is uncommon, but in developing countries, epididymitis, prostatitis, and other local complications remain common in untreated males.

In 1% to 3% of infected men or women, the gonococcus invades the blood stream, leading to **disseminated gonococcal infection (DGI).** Patients may present with either of two syndromes: polyarthralgias, tenosynovitis, and dermatitis or purulent arthritis. Very rarely, additional complications such as perihepatic abscess, endocarditis, or meningitis occur.

IMMUNITY

It is not unusual for an individual to acquire gonorrhea repeatedly, even from the same consort, which has led to the view that natural immunity does not exist. However, this view is incorrect, because in the preantibiotic era, uncomplicated gonorrhea as well as PID usually did resolve spontaneously, although the course could span several months. There is also epidemiologic evidence for immunity to second attacks of PID with the same serotype. The reason for the difficulty in detecting natural immunity probably lies in the remarkable antigenic variability of both pili and protein IIs.

LABORATORY DIAGNOSIS

In acute gonococcal disease, **stained smears of fresh exudate** will often reveal the presence of **intracellular gram-negative diplococci.** This finding, together with a convincing clinical history, may permit the physician to make the provisional diagnosis of acute gonorrhea and to institute antibiotic therapy. Whenever possible, the exudate should be cultured for gonococci before treatment is begun. The diagnosis is definitively established by recovery of typical gram-negative oxidase-positive diplococci that ferment glucose but not maltose, sucrose, or lactose (see Table 26–1). Rectal cultures are sometimes positive when urethral and cervical cultures are negative. Because gonococci are not hardy, specimens should be cultured immediately or placed in special transport media. The culture medium of choice usually contains antibiotics that inhibit the contaminating flora, and incubation must be in the presence of CO_2. Rapid simple tests for Ag in the exudate or urine are likely to become available soon.

TREATMENT

The sulfonamide drugs provided the first effective therapy, but resistant mutants rapidly became predominant. Penicillin replaced sulfonamides and also was extremely effective at very low doses. Over the years, gonococci developed partial resistance to penicillin, so that now, rather large doses are often required. To compound the problem, in 1976, **plasmids** coding for **β-lactamase** production appeared in gonococci, and these are now prevalent in many parts of the world. Nevertheless, penicillin remains a drug of choice. In the presence of penicillin resistance, spectinomycin has been recommended. Some consider tetracycline the drug of choice because it is also effective against *Chlamydia trachomatis* infection, which frequently is acquired at the same time. The treatment of DGI is intravenous penicillin.

PREVENTION

Although treatment of gonococcal disease is extremely effective, the morbidity rates are of pandemic proportions. Because the incubation period of symptomatic gonorrhea is short, ranging from 2 to 7 days, **tracing and treating the recent sexual contacts** lessens the spread of the disease. However, at least 10% of males and 50% of females with recently acquired gonorrhea have insufficient symptoms to seek treatment, and unfortunately, immunologic tests are not a cost-effective method for identifying them. Greater mobility, greater sexual freedom, and replacement of the condom by other birth control measures make containment of the disease next to impossible. Vaccines are being sought, but none are now available. For the individual, the best preventive measures remain discretion and the condom.

The time-honored method of preventing ophthalmia neonatorum (the **Credé procedure**) consists of dropping 1% silver nitrate solution into the infant's eyes immediately after birth. Generally, this irritating material has been replaced with penicillin ointment.

Other Neisseriae

Nonpathogenic species of *Neisseria* may be mistaken for meningococci or gonococci. For example, *N. catarrhalis* (*Branhamella catarrhalis*) and *N. sicca* (see Table 26–1), and *N. lactamica* (as mentioned earlier), are frequently present in secretions of the normal pharynx, and other nonpathogenic species occasionally inhabit the female genital tract. The first two occasionally cause bacterial endocarditis.

Several other species of **gram-negative diplococci** may be confused with *Neisseria*. An **anaerobic group,** of the genus *Veilonella*, inhabit the mouth and gastrointestinal tract of humans and certain animals and have been found in dental abscesses and in chronic urinary tract infections. An **aerobic group,** of the genus *Acinetobacter* (formerly *Mima* and *Herellea*), including a species originally named *Bacterium anitratum*, are tiny aerobic coccobacilli that may simulate gonococci in morphology and are occasionally cultured from the genitourinary tract. The Morax–Axenfeld bacillus (genus *Moraxella*) is sometimes cultured from patients with conjunctivitis.

Selected Reading

BOOKS AND REVIEW ARTICLES

Blake MS, Gotschlich EC: Functional and immunological properties of pathogenic neisserial surface proteins. In Inouye M (ed): Bacterial Outer Membranes as Model Systems, pp 377–400. New York, John Wiley and Sons, 1986

Britigan BE, Cohen MS, Sparling PF: Gonococcal infection: A model of molecular pathogenesis. N Engl J Med 312:1683–1694, 1985

Frasch CE: Immunization against *Neisseria meningitidis*. In Easmon CSF, Jeljaszewicz J (eds): Medical Microbiology, pp 115–144. New York, Academic Press, 1983

Holmes KK, Mårdh PA, Sparling PF, Wiesner PJ: Sexually Transmitted Diseases. New York, McGraw-Hill Book Company, 1984

Jennings HJ: Capsular polysaccharides as human vaccines. In Tipson RS, Horton D (eds): Advances in Carbohydrate Chemistry and Biochemistry, pp 155–208. New York, Academic Press, 1983

Meyer TF: Molecular basis of surface antigen variation in *Neisseria*. Trends Genetics 3:319, 1987

Morse SI: The biology of the gonococcus. CRC Crit Rev Microbiol 7:93–136, 1980

Poolman JT: Gonococci and Meningococci. Dordrecht, Kluwer Academic Publishers, 1988

Schoolnik GK: The Pathogenic Neisseriae. Washington DC, American Society for Microbiology, 1985

SPECIFIC ARTICLES

Carbonetti NH, Simnad VI, Seifert HS, So M, Sparling PF: Genetics of protein I of *Neisseria gonorrhoeae:* construction of hybrid porins. Proc Nat Acad Sci USA 85:6841–6845, 1988

Gotschlich EC, Seiff M, Blake MS: The DNA sequence of the structural gene of gonococcal protein III and the flanking region containing a repetitive sequence. Homology of protein III with enterobacterial OmpA proteins. J Exp Med 165:471–482, 1987

Haines KA, Yeh L, Blake MS, Cristello P, Korchak H, Weissman G: Protein I, a translocatable ion channel from *Neisseria gonorrhoeae*, selectively inhibits exocytosis from human neutrophils without inhibiting O_2 generation. J Biol Chem 2630:945–951, 1988

James JF, Swanson JL: Studies on gonococcus infection. XIII. Occurrence of color/opacity colonial variants in clinical cultures. Infect Immun 19:332–340, 1978

Koomey M, Gotschlich EC, Robbins K, Bergstrom S, Swanson JL: Effects of *recA* mutations on pilus antigenic variation and phase transitions in *Neisseria gonorrhoeae*. Genetics 117:391–398, 1987

Mandrell RE, Griffiss JM, Macher BA: Lipooligosaccharides (LOS) of *Neisseria gonorrhoeae* and *Neisseria meningitidis* have components that are immunochemically similar to precursors of human blood group antigens. Carbohydrate sequence specificity of the mouse monoclonal antibodies that recognize crossreacting antigens on LOS and human erythrocytes. J Exp Med 168:107–126, 1988

Mauro A, Blake M, Labarca P: Voltage gating of conductance in lipid bilayers induced by porin from outer membranes of *Neisseria gonorrhoeae*. Proc Nat Acad Sci USA 85:1071–1075, 1988

McGee ZA, Robinson EN Jr: Molecular mechanisms by which pathogenic bacteria interact with host mucosal cells. In Jackson GG, Thomas H (eds): The Pathogenesis of Bacterial Infections, pp 8–16. Springer-Verlag, 1985

McKenna WR, Mickelsen PA, Sparling PF, Dyer DW: Iron uptake from lactoferrin and transferrin by *Neisseria gonorrhoeae*. Infect Immun 56:785–791, 1988

Meyer TF, Haas R: Phase and antigenic variation by DNA rearrangements in procaryotes. In Kingsman AJ, Kingsman SM, Chater KF (eds): Transposition, pp 193–219. Cambridge, Cambridge University Press, 1988

Olyhoek T, Crowe BA, Achtman M: Clonal population structure of *Neisseria meningitidis* serogroup A isolated from epidemics and pandemics between 1915 and 1983. Rev Infect Dis 9:665–692, 1987

Pohlner J, Halter R, Beyreuther K, Meyer TF: Gene structure and extracellular secretion of *Neisseria gonorrhoeae* IgA protease. Nature 325:458–462, 1987

Rice PA, Vayo HE, Tam MR, Blake MS: Immunoglobin G antibodies directed against protein III block killing of serum resistant *Neisseria gonorrhoeae* by immune sera. J Exp Med 164:1735–1748, 1986

Rothbard JB, Fernandez R, Wang L, Teng NNH, Schoolnik GK: Antibodies to peptides corresponding to conserved sequence of gonococcal pilins block bacterial adhesion. Proc Natl Acad Sci USA 82:915–919, 1985

Saukkonen K, Abdillahi H, Poolman JT, Leinonen M: Protective efficacy of monoclonal antibodies to class 1 and class 3 outer membrane proteins of *Neisseria meningitidis* B:15:P1.16 in infant rat infection model: new prospects for vaccine development. Microbiol Pathogenesis 3:261–267, 1987

Stern A, Meyer TF: Common mechanism controlling phase and antigenic variation in pathogenic neisseriae. Molec Microbiol 1:5–12, 1987

Stromberg N, Deal C, Nyberg G, Normark S, So M, Karlsson KA: Identification of carbohydrate structures that are possible receptors for *Neisseria gonorrhoeae*. Proc Natl Acad Sci USA 85:4902–4906, 1988

Swanson J, Koomey JM: Mechanisms for variation of pili and outer membrane protein II in *Neisseria gonorrhoeae*. In Berg DE, Howe MM (eds), Mobile DNA. Washington, American Society for Microbiology (in press)

Swanson JL, Goldschneider I: The serum bactericidal system: ultrastructural changes in *Neisseria meningitidis* exposed to normal rat serum. J Exp Med 129:51–79, 1969

Swanson JL, Robbins K, Barrera O, Corwin D, Boslego J, Ciak J, Blake MS, Koomey JM: Gonococcal pilin variants in experimental gonorrhea. J Exp Med 165:1344–1357, 1987

27

Stanley Falkow
John Mekalanos

The Enteric Bacilli and Vibrios*

The Enteric Organisms

Stool cultures incubated under **aerobic** conditions yield primarily members of the family *Enterobacteriaceae:* gram-negative, non–spore-forming, facultatively anaerobic bacilli with simple growth requirements. These organisms (Table 27–1) are found mostly in the vertebrate intestine as normal flora or as pathogens, although some genera include saprophytes and plant parasites. *Escherichia coli* is the predominant facultative organism in stool, and its presence (along with other **coliforms:** *Klebsiella, Enterobacter,* and *Citrobacter*) is used by public health departments as presumptive evidence of fecal contamination of water. One genus of the *Enterobacteriaceae, Yersinia,* will be considered with the genus *Pasteurella* in Chapter 30.

The *Enterobacteriaceae* (or **enterobacteria**), together with the gram-negative **vibrios,** are also frequently referred to as **enteric bacilli** or **enterics.** The term "enterics" has sometimes been extended loosely to include other aerobic gram-negative rods occasionally found in the gut, such as *Pseudomonas.* Members of this genus have become increasingly important in opportunistic infections outside the gut; they will be considered in Chapter 29. Chapters 30 through 32 will discuss other, highly pathogenic gram-negative bacilli (*Francisella, Brucella, Haemophilus,* and *Bordetella*), which have complex growth requirements and are not normally found in the gut. Facultative gram-positive organisms may also be present in the gut: enterococci (chiefly *Streptococcus faecalis,* Chap. 24), lactobacilli, and, under some circumstances, staphylococci (Chap. 25).

* The authors acknowledge the contributions of the late Alex C. Sonnenwirth to parts of the present chapter that have been retained from the third edition of this text.

TABLE 27–1. Principal Genera of Enterobacteriaceae

Genera	Pathogenicity
Shigella	Bacillary dysentery
Escherichia*	Pathogenic only under special circumstances; certain types produce diarrheal or invasive (dysenteric) disease
Edwardsiella	Can cause gastroenteritis and other salmonellosis-like diseases
Salmonella ⎫ Arizona ⎭	Gastroenteritis, septicemia, enteric fever
Citrobacter† ⎫ Klebsiella ⎪ Enterobacter‡ ⎪ Hafnia ⎬ Serratia ⎪ Proteus ⎪ Providencia ⎭	Pathogenic only under special circumstances ("opportunistic," "secondary" pathogens)
Yersinia	Plague§; enterocolitis, mesenteric lymphadenitis¶
Erwinia ⎫ Pectobacterium ⎭	Plant pathogens or saprophytes**

* *E. coli;* includes alkalescens–dispar organisms, formerly in *Shigella.*

† Formerly *Escherichia freundii;* includes Bethesda–Ballerup "paracolon" organisms.

‡ Formerly *Aerobacter.*

§ *Y. pestis* (Chap. 30).

¶ *Y. pseudotuberculosis* and *Y. enterocolitica.*

** Not medically significant; one species isolated from animal and human hosts.

(Nomenclature based on Ewing WH: Differentiation of *Enterobacteriaceae* by Biochemical Reactions, rev ed. Atlanta, Centers for Disease Control, 1973; *Yersinia* added according to Buchanan RE, Gibbons NE (eds): Bergey's Manual of Determinative Bacteriology, 8th ed. Baltimore, Williams & Wilkins, 1974)

ANAEROBES. Although conventional aerobic cultures reveal the important enteric pathogens, they do not detect the bulk of the gut flora (amounting to some 10^{11} bacteria per gram of feces), as more than 95% are **obligate anaerobes** with complex growth requirements. Gram-negative rods (*Bacteroides,* Chap. 28) predominate, but obligately anaerobic gram-positive organisms, including *Bifidobacterium,* anaerobic lactobacilli, anaerobic streptococci (Chap. 24) and clostridia (Chap. 34), are usually also present.

TESTS. The several groups of facultative and aerobic gram-negative rods are differentiated by a variety of criteria, listed in Table 27–2. The initial division between **fermenters** of sugars (*Enterobacteriaceae, Vibrionaceae*) and **nonfermenters** (i.e., either **oxidizers** or **nonutilizers** of sugars) is conveniently made by growth in two tubes of **oxidation–fermentation (O-F) medium,** one aerobic (open) and the other anaerobic (sealed with mineral oil). Fermenters produce acid in both tubes, oxidizers only in the open tube, and nonutilizers in neither.

Fermentation of specific sugars is of special value in differentiating enterobacterial species.

Because *Vibrio cholerae* is a significant cause of enteric disease, the vibrios are included in this chapter, but genetically they are widely separated from *Enterobacteriaceae,* as shown by the difference in their **GC/AT ratio** (Table 27–2), their polar rather than peritrichous **flagella,** and their positive **oxidase** test (in which cytochrome oxidase oxidizes *p*-phenylenediamine to a colored product).

MEDICAL IMPORTANCE

Accurate identification of organisms causing serious enteric disease is of great value for choosing appropriate antimicrobial agents, for prognosis, for recognizing potential danger to contacts, and for epidemiologic investigation of the sources of infection (Table 27–3).

The former scourges of typhoid fever (*Salmonella typhi*), bacillary dysentery (*Shigella*), and cholera (*V. cholerae*) are now largely controlled in the Western world through public health measures, but in underdeveloped countries, they are still serious and periodically recurring problems. However, in developed countries milder forms of infectious diarrhea, caused primarily by certain strains of *E. coli,* are second in incidence only to respiratory infections; they include sporadic cases, institutional outbreaks, and "traveler's diarrhea" caused by *E. coli* strains to which the local population has evidently acquired immunity. Moreover, in underdeveloped countries acute gastroenteritis caused by these organisms is widespread among malnourished small children and is the principal cause of death in this age group.

The **gastroenteritis** caused by enteric bacteria has an incubation period of 12 hours to days, during which the organisms multiply in the gut. In **food poisoning,** the gastrointestinal disturbances occur within a few hours of ingestion of preformed toxins of various organisms, including staphylococci and bacilli as well as enterobacteria.

Whereas the severe enteric infections have been declining in the developed countries, various kinds of extraintestinal disease are increasingly associated with ordinarily harmless enteric organisms (*E. coli, Klebsiella, Enterobacter, Serratia, Pseudomonas, Bacteroides*) as a result of the suppression of other organisms by antibiotics, the use of immunosuppressive and cytotoxic agents, and the survival of patients with impaired immune responses. Enteric organisms have always been the most common agents of urinary tract infections, but they are now also the predominant etiologic agents in various **endogenous** systemic infections (those caused by indigenous organisms) and **nosocomial** infections (i.e., hospital-acquired, such as surgical wound infections, pneu-

TABLE 27–2. Some Differential Characteristics of Enteric Bacilli and Nonfermenting Gram-Negative Bacteria

Family, Genus, or Species	Ox/F*	Oxidase	Growth on MacC	Growth on SS	Motility	Nitrate to Nitrite	Nitrate to Gas	Ly-sine†	Argi-nine‡	Orni-thine†	DNA Base Composition (% G+C)
Enterobacteriaceae	F	−	+	+	+or−	+	−	d§	d§	d§	39–58¶
Yersinia***	F	−	+	+,−	−,+#	+	−	−	−	+or−	46–47
Vibrio	F	+	+	−§	+	+	−	+	−	+	40–50
Aeromonas hydrophilia	F	+	+	+	+	+	−	−	+	−	57–63
Pasteurella	F	+	−§	−	−	+	−	−	−	d	36–43
Pseudomonas	Ox	+**	+	+	+	−	+or−	+	+	−	57–70
								(NC	NC	NC)	
Achromobacter	Ox	−	d	d	+(−)	+or−	−	−	+,−	−	40–70
Acinetobacter											
anitratum (Herellea)	Ox	−	+	−§	−	−	−	NC	NC	NC	40–46
A. Iwoffi (Mima)	In	−	+	−§	−	−	−	NC	NC	NC	40–46
Moraxella	In	+	−or+	−	−	−or+	−				41–43
Flavobacterium	Ox or In	+(−)	+(−)	−	+(−)	−	+or−	NC	NC	NC	30–42
Alcaligenes	In	+	+	(+)−	+	+	+or−	NC	NC	NC	58–70

F, Fermentative; Ox, oxidative; In, inactive (in O-F medium; see text); MacC, MacConkey agar; SS, Salmonella–Shigella agar.

+, Positive reaction or growth; −, no reaction or growth; (+), delayed positive reaction or poor growth; d, different reactions: +, (+), or −; NC, no change; +(−), majority positive, occasional strain negative.

* Based on reactions in Hugh and Leifson's O-F medium (0.2% peptone, 1.0% glucose, 0.5% NaCl, 0.03% K_2HPO_4, 0.2% agar, and a pH indicator). Glucose can ordinarily be used if any sugar can.

† Decarboxylases.

‡ Dihydrolase.

§ Rare strains grow.

Motility, when present, demonstrable at 20°–25°C but not at 37°C.

** Except P. maltophilia.

¶ Range of DNA base composition of practically all Enterobacteriaceae is 50–58 moles % of G+C, except for Proteus–Providencia organisms, with a value of 39–53, and Yersinia, with 46–47.

*** Yersinia is now included in the family Enterobacteriaceae.

monia, and septicemia). These two classes of infection now represent a large proportion of the serious bacterial diseases in Western countries, especially since staphylococcal, streptococcal, and pneumococcal infections have been declining in importance. The treatment of gram-negative infections is often difficult because of drug resistance and also because of the presence of underlying serious diseases or impaired host defenses.

Enterobacteriaceae

The Enterobacteriaceae are a family of gram-negative, facultatively anaerobic bacilli (2–3 × 0.4–0.6 μm) that ferment glucose with the production of acid, reduce nitrate to nitrites, and do not produce cytochrome oxidase. Except for Shigella and Klebsiella, they are motile, with **peritrichous flagella.** Glucose fermentation is generally by the mixed acid pathway (Chap. 4) but sometimes by the butanediol pathway. A wide array of other carbohydrates are also attacked, and variations in the pattern

TABLE 27–3. Infectious Gram-Negative Bacterial Agents That Commonly Cause Diarrhea and/or Dysentery

DIARRHEA*
  Salmonella†‡
  Shigella†‡
  Enterotoxigenic E. coli
  Vibrio cholerae
  "Noncholera" vibrios
  Vibrio parahaemolyticus
  Yersinia enterocolitica
  Campylobacter fetus
DYSENTERY§
  Shigella†‡
  Salmonella typhi†#
  Salmonella, other†‡
  Enteroinvasive E. coli
  Yersinia enterocolitica

* Profuse, watery diarrhea, no blood in stool.

† Fecal leukocytes present.

‡ Predominant leukocytes: polymorphonuclear.

§ Abdominal cramps, tenesmus, usually blood in stool.

Predominant leukocytes: mononuclear.

have classically formed an important basis for species identification (Table 27–4).

The cell envelopes have a prototypic gram-negative structure (see Chap. 2). In addition to flagella, many species produce fimbriae (pili), capsules, or both, which often are important virulence determinants. These organisms grow well on simple artificial media, both aerobically and anaerobically. Some strains (mostly virulent) are hemolytic on blood agar.

Members of the family can be found in a variety of hosts, including vertebrates, invertebrates, and higher plants. The *Enterobacteriaceae* of medical importance grow chiefly in the lower gastrointestinal tract of humans and animals, but many can survive in bodies of water in nature. In healthy individuals, *E. coli* and several other enteric species are transiently found on the skin, and some may colonize the female genital tract. In humans with defective resistance, they may cause opportunistic infections.

ISOLATION AND CLASSIFICATION

A variety of special **differential** and **selective** media are utilized in the isolation and preliminary characterization of enteric bacteria from clinical specimens. Typically, such media contain inhibitors of gram-positive organisms (bacteriostatic dyes such as brilliant green or surface-active compounds such as bile salts), an acid–base indicator (e.g., neutral red), and one or more fermentable carbohydrates. Selective media containing such substances (e.g., **MacConkey agar, deoxycholate agar**) greatly facilitate the isolation of enteric bacilli from cultures of feces. Shigellae and salmonellae are less sensitive than the coliform organisms to inhibition by citrate (which may depend on chelation of divalent metal ions). **SS** (*Salmonella–Shigella*) **agar,** containing both citrate and bile salts, is used for selective cultivation of pathogenic species, although it inhibits some strains of shigellae.

Although the *Enterobacteriaceae* have been separated into genera and species on the basis of their genetic, serologic, and pathogenic properties, in the clinical laboratory, they are still identified by and large on the basis of a series of biochemical tests. Early taxonomic schemes relied heavily on lactose fermentation by *Escherichia* and *Klebsiella* but not by the major pathogenic members, *Salmonella* and *Shigella*. Although these media are still of considerable utility, more recent formulations no longer focus on lactose fermentation. Other tests are for oxidase, nitrate reduction, motility, fermentation of various carbohydrates, utilization of other substrates (e.g., citrate), and production of characteristic end products (e.g., indole from tryptophan). Some tests are restricted largely to the identification of a single genus or species (e.g., urease production by *Proteus*). Clinical laboratories now rely on commercial identification systems with a fixed set of differential tests.

Table 27–4 lists the biochemical reactions of the *Enterobacteriaceae* that are most important in human infections or that are frequently isolated from clinical specimens. Faced with this array, it is important to note that from 80% to 95% of the isolates seen in a general hospital will belong to three species: *E. coli, Klebsiella pneumoniae,* or *Proteus mirabilis.* More than 99% will belong to the 23 species listed in Table 27–4.

TYPING. Supplemental tests distinguish strains within the same species that have particular properties useful in tracing the source and the progress of an epidemic. Most useful traits are antigenic determinants on the cell surface, including lipopolysaccharide (**O** Ag), flagella proteins (**H** Ag), and polysaccharide capsule or fimbrial proteins (**K** Ags) (see Antigenic Structure, below).

For some species, further **typing** is based on strain variation in sensitivity to lysis by specific **bacteriophages** or in the production of (or susceptibility to) specific **colicins,** bacteriocins active against many enterobacteria (Chap. 7). For example, 72 subtypes of *S. typhi* have been distinguished by their distinct patterns of sensitivity to various phages (these include host-range mutants and host-modified variants; see Host-Induced Restriction and Modification, Chap. 8). Similarly, although *Shigella sonnei* (discussed below) is homogeneous according to phage typing and antigenic analysis, 15 types have been detected by typing with colicins.

It is also possible to identify some species or substrains by **hybridization tests,** utilizing a **diagnostic nucleic acid probe** to detect a complementary DNA sequence in the genomic DNA of a newly isolated strain. This class of tests has the advantage that the presence or absence of certain organisms in clinical samples (stool, urine, blood, etc.) can be established within a few hours without cultivation or isolation of the suspect organisms.

Evolutionary Relations

As a result of more than a decade of intensive biochemical, genetic, and molecular studies, together with computer analyses, the 12 genera and 26 species in the family of *Enterobacteriaceae* in 1972 have become 22 genera and 69 species. This extensive differentiation reflects both the widespread interest in this group and the use of DNA–DNA hybridization as a classification tool. In general, organisms are considered to be of the same species if they show more than 70% similarity by **DNA–DNA hybridization** under a defined set of conditions. The resulting genealogic relations among the genera of *Enterobacteriaceae* (Fig. 27–1) are reasonably consistent with the traditional classification schemes (Table 27–4). This consistency supports the conclusion that transfer of chromosomal genes (i.e., recombination and stable pro-

TABLE 27–4. Biochemical Reactions of the Enterobacteriaceae That Are Most Important in Human Infections or That Are Frequently Isolated from Clinical Specimens*

Species	Indole Production	Methyl Red	Voges–Proskauer	Citrate (Simmons')	Hydrogen Sulfide (TSI)	Urea Hydrolysis	Phenylalanine Deaminase	Lysine Decarboxylase	Arginine Dihydrolase	Ornithine Decarboxylase	Motility (36°C)	Gelatin Hydrolysis (22°C)	D-Glucose, Gas	Lactose Fermentation	Sucrose Fermentation	D-Mannitol Fermentation	Dulcitol Fermentation	Adonitol Fermentation	D-Sorbitol Fermentation	L-Arabinose Fermentation	Raffinose Fermentation	L-Rhamnose Fermentation	D-Xylose Fermentation	Melibiose Fermentation	DNase, 25°C	ONPG†
Escherichia coli	98	99	0	1	1	1	0	90	17	65	95	0	95	95	50	98	60	5	94	99	50	80	95	75	0	95
Shigella serogroups A, B, and C	50	100	0	0	1	0	0	0	5	1	0	0	2	0	0	93	2	0	30	60	50	5	2	50	0	2
Shigella sonnei	0	100	0	0	0	0	0	0	2	98	0	0	0	2	1	99	0	0	2	95	3	75	2	25	0	90
Salmonella, most serotypes	1	100	0	95	95	1	0	98	70	97	95	0	96	1	1	100	96	0	95	99	2	95	97	95	2	2
Salmonella typhi	0	100	0	0	97	0	0	98	3	0	97	0	0	1	0	100	0	0	99	2	0	0	82	100	0	0
Salmonella paratyphi A	0	100	0	0	10	0	0	0	15	95	95	0	99	0	0	100	90	0	95	100	0	100	0	95	0	0
Citrobacter freundii	5	100	0	95	80	70	0	0	65	20	95	0	95	50	30	99	55	0	98	100	30	99	99	50	0	95
Klebsiella pneumoniae	0	10	98	98	0	95	0	98	0	0	0	0	97	98	99	99	30	90	99	99	99	99	99	99	0	99
Enterobacter aerogenes	0	5	98	95	0	2	0	98	0	98	97	0	100	95	100	100	5	98	100	100	96	99	100	99	0	100
Enterobacter cloacae	0	5	100	100	0	65	0	0	97	96	95	0	100	93	97	100	15	25	95	100	97	92	99	90	0	99
Hafnia alvei	0	40	85	10	0	4	0	100	6	98	85	0	98	5	10	99	0	0	0	95	2	97	98	0	0	90
Serratia marcescens	1	20	98	98	0	15	0	99	0	99	97	90	55	2	99	99	0	40	99	0	2	0	7	0	98	95
Proteus mirabilis	2	97	50	65	98	98	98	0	0	99	95	90	96	2	15	0	0	0	0	0	0	1	98	0	50	1
Proteus vulgaris	98	95	0	15	95	95	99	0	0	0	95	91	85	2	97	0	0	0	0	0	1	5	95	0	80	5
Providencia rettgeri	99	93	0	95	0	98	98	0	0	0	94	0	10	5	15	100	0	100	1	1	5	70	10	5	0	5
Providencia stuartii	98	100	0	93	0	30	95	0	0	0	85	0	0	2	50	10	0	5	1	1	7	0	7	0	10	10
Morganella morganii	98	97	0	0	5	98	95	0	0	98	95	0	90	1	0	0	0	0	0	0	0	0	0	0	0	5
Yersinia enterocolitica	50	97	2	0	0	75	0	0	0	95	2	0	5	5	95	98	0	0	99	98	5	1	70	1	5	95
Yersinia pestis	0	80	0	0	0	5	0	0	0	0	0	0	0	0	0	97	0	0	50	100	0	1	90	20	0	50
Yersinia pseudotuberculosis	0	100	0	0	0	95	0	0	0	0	0	0	0	0	0	100	0	0	0	50	15	70	100	70	0	70

* Each number gives the percentage of positive reactions after 2 days of incubation at 36°C. The vast majority of these positive reactions occur within 24 hours. Reactions that become positive after 2 days are not considered.

† ONPG, o-Nitrophenyl-β-D-galactopyranoside.

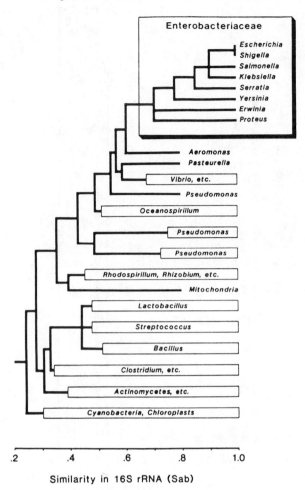

Figure 27–1. Phylogenetic relationships among eubacteria. The main dendrograph is based on partial nucleotide sequences of 16S ribosomal RNAs from eubacteria, chloroplasts, and mitochondria. The coefficient Sab is an indirect measure of the extent of sequence homology between molecules where Sab = 1 denotes complete homology. (From Ochman H, Wilson AC: Evolutionary history of enteric bacteria. In Neidhardt FC, et al (eds): *Escherichia coli* and *Salmonella typhimurium*: Cellular and Molecular Biology, vol. 2. Washington, DC, American Society for Microbiology, 1987)

liferation) is rare in natural populations of enterobacteria. Thus, most enterobacterial species, particularly those associated with specific disease states, each comprises a fairly limited number of independently evolving lineages or clones.

At first view, this conclusion may seem to contradict the ease of gene transfer among these organisms in the laboratory by conjugation, transduction, transformation, and transposition of mobile genetic elements and the rapid flow of R-plasmids among the *Enterobacteriaceae* (and many other gram-negative bacteria). Part of the ex-

planation is that most genes in the bacterial chromosome are essential for reproduction of the cell and are not easily replaced. Successful recombination between species is further limited by differences in chromosomal gene order and by DNA sequence divergence within genes. In contrast, extrachromosomal DNA confers traits that are of transient evolutionary significance but can often provide benefits to diverse species. Thus, different species of *Enterobacteriaceae* often carry the same **determinant of pathogenicity** encoded on a plasmid, transposon, or phage. These virulence properties probably represent recent additions to the genetic repertoire of an organism, giving it access to a new ecological niche.

Antigenic Structure

Although the principal varieties of enteric bacilli can be identified by their reactions in differential media, final identification of many species, as well as of strains, is based on antigenic structure. However, strains with the same antigenic pattern may exhibit different metabolic reactions (fermentative variants or **biotypes**).

As is shown in Figure 27–2, three kinds of surface Ags (H, O, and K or Vi)* determine the organism's reaction with specific antisera. Formaldehyde treatment preserves the labile Ags of the flagella, and the cells are agglutinated by specific antiflagellar (anti-H) Abs, forming a light, fluffy precipitate; the numerous peritrichous flagella also sterically prevent agglutination by anti-O Ab. On the other hand, when flagella are absent, or are denatured by heat (100°C, 20 min), acid, or alcohol, the somatic O Ag at the surfaces of adjacent bacilli can be linked by anti-O Abs, resulting in closely packed, granular clumps.

The polysaccharide **Vi Ag** in certain species is usually too thin to be seen as a capsule, and it does not cover the O Ag completely as it allows adsorption of anti-O Abs. However, it does inhibit O agglutination unless it is destroyed (along with H Ag) by boiling for 2 hours. The Vi Ag of *S. typhi* is a homopolymer of N-acetylgalactosaminuronic acid. Other Vi Ags are found in other salmonellae.

The O Ags in **smooth (S)** strains cover the underlying **R Ag** (the LPS core, Chap. 2), which becomes accessible to Ab in **rough (R) mutants.** The change from S to R may take place without the loss of flagellar or of Vi Ags. Rough

---

*The designation H (Ger. *hauch*, breath) was first used to describe the growth of *Proteus* bacilli on the surfaces of moist agar plates: the film produced by the swarming of this highly motile organism resembles the light mist caused by breathing on glass. The designation O (Ger. *ohne*, without), first applied to nonswarming (i.e., nonflagellated) forms, is now used as a generic term for the lipopolysaccharide somatic Ags of all enteric bacilli and, more specifically, for their polysaccharide components. Capsular Ags are called **K** Ag (Ger. *Kapsel*), and a specific capsular Ag of *S. typhi* is called **Vi** because of its role in virulence. **Fimbrial antigens** (e.g., K88 and K99) also became designated as K Ags before their structure was recognized, and they now bear descriptive names (e.g., CFA: colonization factor Ag).

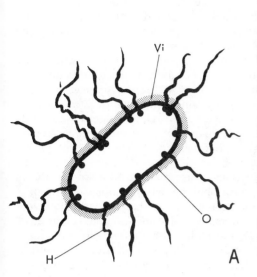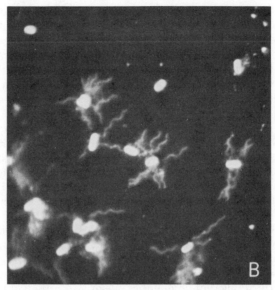

Figure 27–2. *(A)* Schematic diagram of cellular locations of H, O, and Vi antigens of enteric bacilli. *(B)* *S. typhi* stained with fluorescein-labeled immune serum containing anti-H, anti-O, and anti-Vi Abs. Note that the flagella of different bacilli have in some cases become agglutinated with one another. Note also, however, that the presence of the flagella has prevented the bodies of the bacilli from coming close enough together to agglutinate, despite the presence of the antisomatic (Vi and O) Abs in the serum. The interflagellar agglutinate is, therefore, understandably less densely packed than if the flagella had been absent and intersomatic agglutination had occurred. (×3500, reduced) (From Thomason BM, et al: J Bacteriol 74:525, 1957)

strains tend to agglutinate spontaneously unless suspended in media of proper ionic strength.

Specific antisera, reacting with individual surface Ags in agglutination tests, are prepared by **selective adsorption.** For example, anti-H Ab may be removed by suspensions of homologous flagella (mechanically removed) or by suspensions of mutant cells possessing the immunogenic cells' flagella but neither their Vi nor O Ags. Similarly, anti-O or anti-Vi Abs may be selectively removed by appropriate cell fractions.

KAUFFMANN–WHITE CLASSIFICATION OF SALMONELLA.
The antigenic complexities of the enteric bacilli have been most thoroughly documented in the genus *Salmonella*. Largely as a result of the studies of Kauffmann in Denmark and White in England, a system has been developed for distinguishing a wide variety of serotypes by exhaustive cross-adsorption and cross-reaction tests, as in the following example.

Assume that two strains of *Salmonella*, a and b, have been isolated from separate outbreaks. Antisera prepared against them (anti-a and anti-b) are first reacted with suspensions of each strain (standardized to the same density), and the intensity of the reactions is recorded in roughly quantitative terms (see below). Each serum also is adsorbed with the heterologous strain (i.e., anti-a with b, and vice versa) and then reacted with the homologous suspensions. The observed agglutination reactions are as follows:

ANTISERA	ORGANISMS	
	a	b
Anti-a, unadsorbed	4+	2+
Anti-b, unadsorbed	2+	4+
Anti-a, adsorbed with b	2+	0
Anti-b, adsorbed with a	0	2+

Thus, it can be concluded that a and b have both unique and shared antigenic determinants. Using an arbitrary numbering system, type a might be said to possess determinants (or factors) 1,2 and type b determinants 2,3. If, on the other hand, strains a and b are equally effective in removing all the agglutinating Ab from the two antisera, they would be considered antigenically identical. Every new strain isolated would be similarly tested with the existing antisera (anti-a and anti-b, both adsorbed and unadsorbed) and with antiserum to the new strain itself, before and after adsorption. Whenever a new determinant was detected, it would be given a new number.

Application of this technique to O, H, and Vi agglutination reactions has resulted in the identification of more than 1500 *Salmonella* "species" (serotypes), often named after the city where they were found. Only large *Salmonella* typing centers (Copenhagen, London, Atlanta, etc.) have the necessary collections of specific antisera for such typing. In most diagnostic laboratories, *Salmonella* strains are merely **grouped** by means of fermentation tests and by agglutination reactions performed with group-specific antisera.

O AND H ANTIGENIC DETERMINANTS. Each *Salmonella* O Ag has two or three **determinants (factors),** each given a number; Ags that share some but not all of a particular set exhibit **cross-reactions,** noted above. O Ags that share a major determinant are classified as a serogroup; the first 26 were designated by letters (A–Z) and subsequent ones by numbers (50, 51, etc.). The members of each O group may be differentiated still further into serotypes on the basis of additional minor determinants as well as flagellar (H) Ags.

A given strain may form at different times either one of two kinds of H Ag. The first, **phase 1 Ags,** are shared with only a few other species of *Salmonella;* the second, **phase 2 Ags,** are less specific. Although the organisms in a given culture may be entirely in one phase (monophasic culture), they frequently give rise to variants in the other phase (diphasic culture), especially if the culture is incubated for more than 24 hours. Such **phase variation,** which depends on a reversible DNA rearrangement (see Phase Variation, Chap. 8), can be accentuated by growing the organisms in serum containing Abs to their flagellar Ags, thereby favoring the growth of mutants with the alternative (allelic) Ag that does not react with the antiserum.

CHEMISTRY OF THE O ANTIGENIC DETERMINANTS. As described in Chapter 2, the O Ags and their associated endotoxin have the following overall structure: **O-specific chains,** consisting of **repeating** (oligosaccharide) **units,** are attached to a basal **core polysaccharide,** which in turn is attached to **lipid A;** the whole forms a **lipopolysaccharide (LPS).** The structure of the core (see Fig. 2–25) is identical or very similar in all salmonellae but differs somewhat in other genera. The serologic specificity of each LPS is determined by the O-specific chains, whose variations form the main basis for classification of salmonellae.

A total of 18 different sugars (monosaccharides) have been identified in various *Salmonella* LPSs; some species have as many as 9. Among the 5 "basal" sugars of the core, a heptose (L-glycero-D-mannoheptose) and **KDO (ketodeoxyoctonate,** 1-keto-3-deoxy-D-mannooctonic acid) are unique to bacterial LPS (KDO linking the core to lipid A). The core is responsible for the serologic specificity of R (rough) mutants, which are blocked in the synthesis of the repeating units: R_a mutants contain the

complete core, whereas R_e have lost all their sugars except KDO. This minimal (R_e) core (KDO plus lipid A) appears to be identical (except for slight differences in the lipid) in all *Enterobacteriaceae* studied.

Despite the layer of O side chains on S organisms, antigenic determinants of the core have been detected on their surface. Moreover, Ab to such Ags (e.g., anti-lipid A) protects animals against challenge by various gram-negative bacilli or by endotoxin and reduces the severity of bacteremia in humans. These recent findings suggest the possibility to general immunoprophylaxis of enterobacterial infection.

Dideoxyhexoses contribute to the specificity of many major group-defining determinants (see Immunologic Determinants, below). The characteristic sequences of several *Salmonella* groups are listed in Table 27–5. Groups A, B, D, and E all contain a repeating mannose–rhamnose–galactose unit, but their linkages and substituents differ. These differences include: (1) changes of position of the glycoside linkages, e.g., 1–4 versus 1–6; (2) altered anomeric configurations, i.e., α versus β linkage; (3) attachment of additional monosaccharides, such as glucose; (4) presence or absence of acetyl groups; and (5) deletion of, or substitution for, one of the monosaccharides in the basic trisaccharide unit. **The length of a determinant is less than that of a repeating unit,** so a given sugar can contribute to more than one determinant; i.e., **different determinants in a given sequence can overlap.**

Alteration of the O Ag can also occur by **lysogenic conversion** (Chap. 8), in which a prophage encodes an enzyme (usually a glycosyl transferase) that modifies the side chain. In *Shigella* species, plasmids encode critical modifications of the O Ag that enhance virulence.

ENDOTOXIN. The biological activities of endotoxin (LPS) have been discussed (Chap. 21). All enterobacteria have endotoxin, but the pathological consequences are seen only in disease caused by invasive organisms such as *S. typhi* and *Y. pestis.* In addition, there is evidence that LPS contributes to the capacity of *Salmonella* species to adhere and enter host cells.

Endotoxin in blood can be measured by gelation of extracts of blood cells of the horseshoe crab (*Limulus polyphemus*). Because high levels in patients with systemic enterobacterial disease coincide with their most severe symptoms, endotoxin is evidently at least partially responsible for the pathophysiological effects.

ESCHERICHIA COLI

The alimentary tract of most warm-blooded animals typically is colonized within a few hours or days of birth by *E. coli* from ingested food or water or directly from other individuals. Most *E. coli* strains can adhere to the mucus

TABLE 27–5. Simplified Structures of O Repeat Units of Some Salmonella Serogroups*

Serogroup	Species	O Antigen	Structure
A	*S. paratyphi* A	1,2,12	Par OAc Glc ↓ ↓ ↓ Man → Rha → Gal
B	*S. typhimurium*	1,4,5,12	OAc-Abe Glc ↓ ↓ Man ⟶ Rha → Gal →
C₁	*S. choleraesuis*	6,7	Glc ↙ ↘ Man → Man → Man → Man → GlcNac
C₂	*S. newport*	6,8	Abe OAc-Glc ↓ ↓ Rha ⟶ Man → Man → Gal →
D₁	*S. typhi*	9,12	Tyv OAc-Glc ↓ ↓ 2α-Man ⟶ Rha → Gal →
E₁	*S. anatum*	3,10	OAc ↓ 6α-Man → Rha — Gal →
E₂	*S. newington*	3,15	6β-Man → Rha → Gal
E₂	*S. minneapolis*	(3),(15),34	Glc ↓ 6β-Man → Rha → Gal

Par, Paratose; OAc, acetyl; Glc, glucose; Abe, abequose; Tyv, tyvelose; Man, mannose; Rha, rhamnose; Gal, galactose.

* Only those type-linkages and anomeric positions of sugars that may explain differences between groups are included.

(Modified from Roantree RJ: In Kadis S, Weinbaum G, Ajl SJ (eds): Microbial Toxins, vol 5, p 18. New York, Academic Press, 1971. Reprinted with permission of Verlag Chemie GMBH, Weinheim, Germany)

overlying the surface of the large bowel and distal small bowel. It has been estimated that the doubling time of *E. coli* within the intestine is about 40 hours. This species is normally the most common facultative anaerobe in the large bowel.

Once an *E. coli* strain becomes established within a host, it may persist for months or years. Other *E. coli* are constantly introduced, but most persist for only a few days or weeks. Resident strain(s) usually shift over a long period, but much more rapidly after enteric infection or antimicrobial therapy. *E. coli* of the normal flora provide protection against colonization by harmful microorganisms.

E. COLI *DIVERSITY*. *E. coli* **O, K,** and **H** Ags are usually determined by chromosomal genes. Fortunately, not all of the 10^6 theoretically possible O/H/K combinations are found; in one study of more than 14,000 isolates, some 708 distinct O/H combinations were identified. Although the serotypes do not necessarily provide an index of overall genetic similarity among strains, the correlation with pathogenicity is high, and serotyping has been of extraordinary importance in distinguishing the small number of strains that actually cause disease.

Pathogenesis: Extraintestinal Diseases

The pathogenic traits expressed by specific strains of *E. coli* are a microcosm of those seen for other members of the *Enterobacteriaceae* and so will be described in some detail. The three principal kinds of disease, each depending on a specific array of pathogenic determinants, are urinary tract infections, neonatal meningitis, and intestinal (diarrheal) diseases. Mechanistically, these diseases depend on combinations of bacterial properties: adherence to specific host receptors, elaboration of specific exotoxins, and penetration (invasion) of host cells. Other bacterial factors, although not playing as direct a role in disease pathology, enhance the virulence of pathogenic *E. coli* causing different diseases. For example, capsules are antiphagocytic, and they inhibit the opsonizing and lytic activities of complement by blocking the alternate (Ab-independent) pathway of complement activation. Also, synthesis of iron-chelating siderophores (Chap. 4), and of their corresponding membrane transport systems, enables the organism to obtain iron for growth in host tissues, thus neutralizing the inhibitory effect of host iron-binding proteins (transferrin in serum, lactoferrin in secretions).

Urinary Tract Infection

E. coli is responsible for almost 90% of infections in anatomically normal, unobstructed urinary tracts. The **uropathogenic** strains are present in the stool and subsequently colonize the vaginal and periurethral region. This colonization sets the stage for the ascent of bacteria into the bladder; females suffer more urinary tract infection (UTI) than males, perhaps because of their shorter urethra. A single catheterization causes UTI in about 1% of ambulatory patients, and infection will develop within 3 or 4 days in essentially all patients who have indwelling catheters. **Host receptors** also play a role in susceptibility, as uropathogenic bacteria can adhere in larger numbers to uroepithelial cells from patients with recurrent UTI than to cells from normal individuals.

In the bladder, colonization of the uroepithelium leads to the appearance of larger numbers of bacteria in the urine (**bacteriuria**) than the normal background count. Symptoms arise when invasion of the mucosa, cell death, and inflammation occur (cystitis). The invading bacteria may also pass up the ureters to multiply in the renal pelvis and parenchyma (pyelonephritis).

A UTI was long assumed to be caused by whatever strain was most prevalent in the host's fecal flora. It is now clear, however, that uropathogenic strains usually belong to a restricted set of serogroups that possess a constellation of virulence factors (see below).

FIMBRIAL ADHESINS. Most *E. coli* strains possess proteinaceous fimbriae (pili) that bind the bacteria to each other and to a variety of animal cell surfaces. **Type 1 or common fimbriae** are **mannose sensitive** in that their binding to host receptors is inhibited by D-mannose (see Chap. 2). These fimbriae appear to anchor *E. coli* to mucus in the large intestine. The less common **mannose-resistant** fimbriae bind neutral glycolipids of the globoside series; among these, the P or **Pap (pyelonephritis-associated pili)** fimbriae bind to globotetraosylceramide and trihexosylceramide, which are Ags of the human P blood group system. Other, less well-defined adhesins, **X adhesins,** are also found on pyelonephritogenic *E. coli* strains. Either Pap pili or X adhesins are expressed by almost all pyelonephritis *E. coli* isolates, about 50% of cystitis isolates, and less than 10% of fecal isolates. Animal experiments with genetically defined strains have demonstrated that both type 1 and Pap-specific adhesion may promote bladder colonization, but only Pap fimbriae are associated with renal colonization.

Other factors contributing to uropathogenicity include the elaboration of a cytolytic hemolysin, resistance to the inhibitory properties of normal human serum, and enhanced iron sequestration.

Genetic and molecular analysis of pilus biosynthesis

has shown that type 1 and Pap pilus biosynthesis and assembly involve at least seven different gene products. The adhesin that recognizes the receptor present on uroepithelial cells is a minor component of the pilus, bound to its tip. Some X adhesins are not associated with any observable pilus structure and are probably surface proteins similar to the tip adhesins.

Although no vaccine currently exists for *E. coli* UTI, purified Pap pili have demonstrated protective efficacy in animal models, and immunization of women suffering from recurrent urinary tract infections is being studied.

Laboratory diagnosis of UTI involves microscopic examination of the urine for leukocytes, red blood cells, and bacteria. Clean-catch midstream urine that yields 10^5 bacteria per ml in culture can be considered evidence of true bacteriuria, and together with symptoms (frequency, urgency, and dysuria) is diagnostic of UTI. Treatment of urinary tract infection ranges from nonspecific therapy by the maintenance of low urinary pH (through the ingestion of large quantities of cranberry juice or mandelic acid) to administration of antimicrobial agents.

Neonatal Meningitis

E. coli is the most common cause of neonatal bacterial meningitis, affecting about 1 in 2000 to 4000 infants. Approximately 80% of the isolates synthesize the **K1 capsular polysaccharide** (this Ag is also common in strains associated with septicemia and UTI). *E. coli* K1 strains are found in the colonic flora of 20% to 40% of all individuals. It is assumed that neonates acquire the strains from their mothers through the nasopharynx or, more probably, the intestine, after which the organisms invade the blood stream and are carried to the meninges.

K1 is a homopolymer of **sialic acid.** It is antiphagocytic and provides at least partial resistance against the usual sensitivity of *E. coli* to complement in the absence of Ab. It has been suggested that the host immunologic mechanisms do not respond to the invading microorganism because of the similarity of K1 to sialic acid polymers found in mammalian embryonic neuronal membranes. Genetic and biochemical studies have suggested that there are **six** widespread **clonal groups** of K1 bacteria. Not all are equally virulent.

Whereas genetic and immunologic studies have shown that K1 is a critical determinant in the capacity of *E. coli* to cause meningitis, other virulence properties must also contribute. A frequent one in K1 isolates, as in strains associated with pyelonephritis, is one or another **siderophore**-based iron uptake system. The genes for these systems may be located either on plasmids or on the chromosome and are usually associated with a transposable element.

E. coli meningitis is best treated with a beta-lactam antibiotic. Immunization of mothers would theoretically provide passive protection of the neonate, but no vaccine exists. The meningococcus Group B capsule and *E. coli* K1 polysaccharides are chemically and immunologically identical, so a vaccine might provide protection against both agents.

Intestinal Diseases

Four classes of *E. coli* that cause diarrheal disease can be distinguished: enterotoxigenic (ETEC), enteropathogenic (EPEC), enteroinvasive (EIEC), and the recently recognized enterohemorrhagic strains. Each class manifests distinct features in pathogenesis, clinical syndrome, and epidemiology, and each falls within a different set of serogroups (Table 27–6).

Enterotoxigenic E. Coli (ETEC)

Enterotoxigenic strains are an important cause of diarrhea in infants and travelers in less developed countries, in some villages causing about three episodes per child in the first year of life. This disease is rare in infants in industrialized countries. The disease ranges from minor discomfort to severe cholera-like purging of liters of fluid per day, leading to severe dehydration, particularly in children. The ETEC are acquired by the ingestion of contaminated food and water, and adults in endemic areas are evidently usually immune. Ordinarily, large numbers of organisms (10^8) must be consumed to cause disease in a susceptible individual. The process requires intestinal colonization as well as the elaboration of one or more enterotoxins. Both of these traits are **encoded on plasmids.**

ADHESINS. Fimbrial adhesins cause ETEC cells to adhere to specific receptors on enterocytes of the proximal small bowel. These adhesins tend to be host-species specific. Thus, the K88 fimbrial Ag is found on strains from piglets and the K99 Ag on those from calves and lambs. In human ETEC, three **colonization factors** (fimbrial adhesins) are found: CFA-1, CFA-2, and E8775; others undoubtedly exist.

ENTEROTOXINS. Bacteria that synthesize only a colonization factor but no toxin may cause a mild diarrheal disease, because their adhesion to the small bowel in large numbers causes a malabsorption syndrome. However, true ETEC synthesize one or both of two plasmid-mediated **enterotoxins: heat-stable (ST)** or **heat-labile (LT).** Either causes net secretion of fluid and electrolytes into the lumen of the bowel. ETEC strains usually possess two distinct plasmids, one encoding a colonization factor, and another encoding one or two enterotoxins; but the LT and ST genes may reside on separate plasmids.

LT, an 86,000-dalton protein, is structurally and functionally very similar to cholera toxin, as described below

TABLE 27–6. *A Comparison of Four Classes of* E. coli *That Cause Diarrhea*

| Class of E. coli | Clinical Syndromes | Epidemiologic Syndromes | Most Common O Serogroups | Pathogenesis | | |
				Relation to Enterocytes	Bacterial Toxins Elaborated	Plasmid Involvement (Size)
Entero-toxigenic	Watery diarrhea	Infant diarrhea in less developed countries; adult travelers' diarrhea	O6, O8, O15, O20, O25, O27, O63, O78, O80, O85, O115, O128, O148, O159	Attach by means of fimbriae; no morphologic changes	Heat-labile and/or heat-stable enterotoxins	Yes (30–75 Md)
Enteroinvasive	Dysentery; diarrhea	Usually adults affected; some foodborne outbreaks	O28, O112, O124, O136, O143, O144, O147, O152, O164	Invade and multiply within enterocytes; polymorphonuclear infiltration	? *Shigella* toxin	Yes (140 Md)
Entero-hemorrhagic	Bloody diarrhea; hemorrhagic colitis	One foodborne outbreak	O157	Do not invade	*Shigella* toxin	Yes (70 Md)
Entero-pathogenic	Acute and chronic infant diarrhea	Outbreaks of diarrhea in infant nurseries; both sporadic and epidemic infant diarrhea in communities; rarely adult diarrhea	O26, O55, O86, O111, O114, O119, O125, O126, O127, O128, O142	Bacteria adhere tightly to enterocytes resulting in loss of microvilli and cupping of enterocyte membrane around the bacteria (seen on electron microscopy)	*Shigella* toxin	Yes (55–65 Md)

in Fig. 27–7 and the accompanying text. Both toxins are composed of an **enzymatically active (A) subunit** surrounded by five identical **binding (B) subunits.** In the crypt cells, the enzymatic unit initiates a cascade of events involving **cAMP** that results in a profuse watery, noninflammatory diarrhea (see Cholera Enterotoxin, below).

ST, of which there are several types, are **small polypeptides,** ranging in size from 18 to 50 amino acids. Sequence analysis has shown that all STs are structurally related, with a large number of disulfide bonds that may account for their heat stability. It is not clear how ST binds to small-bowel enterocytes, but it stimulates guanylate cyclase, and the resulting intracellular accumulation of **cGMP** has a net secretory effect. Unlike LT, ST does not stimulate an immune response in infected individuals. Some ST genes reside on a transposon.

At least half of the cases of traveler's diarrhea are caused by ETEC that elaborate only one toxin. In general, strains that produce both LT and ST cause the most severe disease.

Identification of ETEC strains is a formidable task. Individual colonies of *E. coli* isolated from stool can be tested with antisera specific for fimbrial Ags or for the enterotoxins. Biological assays for LT utilize tissue culture lines (e.g., Y1 adrenal cells or Chinese hamster ovary cells) that respond to increased cAMP with morphological changes. Biological assays for ST involve difficult fluid accumulation assays in suckling mice and are therefore seldom used. Specific DNA diagnostic probes are available to detect bacteria harboring most LT and ST genes within mixed cultures from clinical specimens. These methods have been used primarily for epidemiologic and other research investigations but promise eventually to have an impact on clinical identification.

THERAPY AND PREVENTION. The current therapy of ETEC infections is the simple restoration of fluid balance by intravenous or oral glucose and electrolytes and the use of pharmacologic agents to reduce diarrhea. Antimicrobial therapy in travelers has proved to be of little value.

Because ETEC do not penetrate the intestinal mucosa, protection is thought to be afforded by IgA. In the veterinary field, immunization of cows and sows with purified colonization factor Ag and the B subunit of LT has yielded promising results in protecting newborns through Ab in maternal colostrum. Although a multivalent vaccine for human use based on recombinant living strains or purified components seems promising, none is yet available.

Enteropathogenic E. coli (EPEC)

In the 1940s the application of serotyping detected certain serotypes (e.g., O111 and O125) more frequently from infants with diarrhea than from healthy controls. However, not until 1978 was a causal relation unequivocally demonstrated in studies in human volunteers. Although these strains induce a watery diarrhea not unlike that seen with ETEC strains, EPEC do not produce either LT or ST, nor do they possess the same colonization factors as ETEC.

EPEC-induced diarrhea in the rabbit is correlated with a histopathologic lesion identical to that seen in biopsies from infected babies (Fig. 27–3). The EPEC cells adhere tightly to the surface of intestinal epithelial cells (in either a diffuse or clustered pattern), indenting the enterocyte membrane and causing localized destruction of the microvilli but without overt invasion of the cells.

The capacity of EPEC strains to adhere tightly to cultured human cells is frequently associated with a plasmid. The precise nature of the **EPEC adherence factor** (EAF) is not known; it does not appear to be fimbriae. The genes associated with EAF have been cloned, and their use as a DNA probe showed that they were restricted to serotypes implicated in worldwide EPEC outbreaks (O55, O111, O119, O127, and O128).

EPEC strains have also been found to elaborate a **cytotoxin** that is **enterotoxic** and similar to a toxin synthesized by some *Shigella*. Evidently, the pathogenesis of EPEC involves a specialized adhesion followed by synthesis of sufficient cytotoxin to have an enterotoxic effect.

Like ETEC, EPEC is not currently diagnosed in the clinical laboratory. Colonies of *E. coli* cultured from the stools can be tested for membership in an EPEC serogroup, and a diagnostic DNA probe has been described.

There is no current vaccine. Oral nonabsorbable antibiotics such as neomycin or gentamicin are used, together with the maintenance of fluid and electrolyte balances.

Enteroinvasive E. coli (EIEC)

Members of the serologically distinct enteroinvasive class of *E. coli* closely resemble *Shigella* in their pathogenic mechanisms and the kind of clinical illness they produce. Moreover, like *Shigella*, they are characteristically nonmotile and lactose-negative, cross-react with certain *Shigella* O Ags, and possess a large (140-Md) plasmid that confers the capacity to invade human epithelial cells. This plasmid is similar but not identical to plasmids seen in *Shigella* species. It and the virulence properties of these strains will be further considered under *Shigella*, below. Suffice it to say that EIEC penetrate and multiply within epithelial cells of the distal ileum and colon of primates, causing widespread cell destruction. The organisms rarely enter the blood stream in individuals who are adequately nourished. The clinical syndrome is identical to shigella dysentery, as is its treatment and prevention.

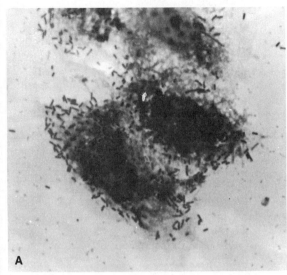

A

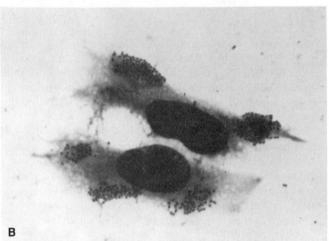

B

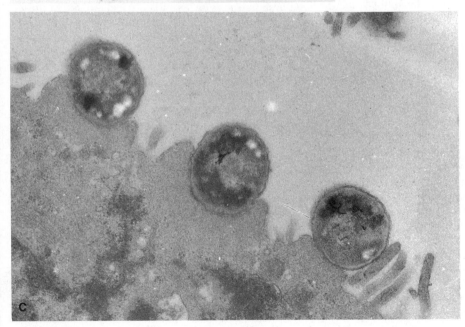

C

Figure 27–3. (*A*) and (*B*) Light micrographs showing two different enteropathogenic strains of *E. coli* (EPEC) adhering to cultured HEp-2 cells (*A*, diffuse adherence; *B*, localized adherence). (*C*) Electromicrograph showing an EPEC strain attached to the membrane of CaCo-2 cells. This attachment is characterized by effacment (disruption) of microvilli and formation of pedestals that cup the bacteria cells. Micrographs kindly supplied by Drs. Ben Hall and James Kaper.

Enterohemorrhagic E. coli

Worldwide, a single strain of *E. coli* serotype O157 : H7 has caused a diarrheal syndrome distinct from the bacillary dysentery caused by *Shigella* and EIEC, in that the bloody discharges are copious rather than scanty and there is no fever. A frequent life-threatening complication is a toxic effect on the kidneys (hemolytic uremic syndrome). The strain does not elaborate LT or ST nor invade epithelial cells. It does, however, possess a 60- to 70-Md plasmid that is associated with virulence. This strain also produces a cytotoxin, apparently identical to Shiga toxin (see below), that is likely responsible for its pathogenicity. The toxin is encoded by bacteriophages, and its production is enhanced by cultivation in media of low iron concentration.

Opportunistic Infections

The *Enterobacteriaceae* are responsible for about half the hospital-acquired (nosocomial) infections in the United States, and fully one-quarter of these are caused by *E. coli.* It is an important cause of bacteremia, surgical infections, and lower respiratory tract disease, generally in patients whose normal defense mechanisms have been breached. Moreover, the hospital environment often selects for strains that are resistant to many drugs (via R plasmids), so their eradication may be difficult.

The *E. coli* strains that have the capacity to cause opportunistic infection generally produce one or more of the virulence determinants discussed above for strains associated with urinary tract infection: hemolysin, serum resistance, and enhanced iron-uptake systems.

After a long history as a model organism for studying bacterial genetics, physiology, and molecular biology, *E. coli* has also become valuable in studying microbial pathogenicity. Virtually all pathogenesis exhibited by *E. coli* strains depends on a plasmid or transposable element, thus emphasizing the special role played by extrachromosomal determinants in the adaptive evolution of bacteria.

SHIGELLA

The *Shigella* species are the principal agents of bacterial **dysentery.** Unlike the noninflammatory diarrheal disease seen with enterotoxigenic **E. coli,** this disease produces a smaller volume of feces, but with blood, mucus, and inflammatory cells; and **as few as 100 organisms can lead to infection** (in contrast to 10^4 to 10^8), even in a well-nourished individual. Hence, these organisms are the most communicable bacterial agents of diarrheal disease. Only humans and higher apes serve as the natural host and reservoir.

In developed countries, bacillary dysentery is primarily a disease of children from 6 months to 10 years of age, although it can affect susceptible individuals at any age who are subject to poor sanitation. In underdeveloped countries, the disease is uncommon in breast-fed infants, but it later takes on monumental public health importance, approaching an average of two attacks in the first 3 years of life. In industrialized countries, the incidence is much lower (50 cases per 100,000 per year), but some populations (e.g., day care centers for preschool children) are endemic centers, and at institutions for mentally retarded children, with poor sanitary conditions, the incidence may be as high as 35,000 per 100,000. Nearly every long military campaign, at least since the Peloponnesian War through many modern conflicts, has produced epidemics of dysentery, often causing a heavier toll of mortality and morbidity than have weapons.

Classification

The genera *Shigella* and *Escherichia* are much closer in DNA sequence than many strains within other species, and, as noted, EIEC *E. coli* causes an indistinguishable illness. All shigellae are **nonmotile** and **lactose-negative** (except that *Sh. sonnei* is weakly positive), and they do not produce gas from fermentable carbohydrates.

The genus *Shigella* is subdivided into four groups on the basis of their biochemical and serologic reactions. Group A, designated *Sh. dysenteriae*, fails to ferment mannitol and falls into ten distinct serotypes. Groups B and C, which ferment mannitol, are termed respectively *Sh. flexneri*, with six serotypes, and *Sh. boydii*, with 15 serotypes. Group D, *Sh. sonnei*, is represented by a single mannitol-fermenting serotype.

Sh. dysenteriae **type 1** holds a special place in public health because it causes **especially severe infections** that may occur in explosive epidemics and even pandemics. This disease was rare after the early part of this century until a widespread outbreak in Central America in 1968–1970. Subsequently, large-scale epidemics have occurred in many areas of the world, including Bangladesh (1971–1974), Central Africa (1980–1982), and South Asia (1984–present). These organisms harbored an R plasmid encoding resistance to several antibiotics. The current pandemic strain in South Asia is resistant to sulfonamides, tetracycline, chloramphenicol, ampicillin, and trimethoprim, leaving relatively few therapeutic options.

Although there are more than 30 recognized *Shigella* serotypes, only a few predominate in any geographic area. *Sh. sonnei* (which causes relatively mild disease), as well as *Sh. flexneri* 2a and 3, are responsible for virtually all the dysentery seen within the US. In industrialized nations, *Sh. sonnei* is predominant. *Sh. flexneri* is the most common cause of endemic diarrheal disease in underdeveloped countries.

Pathogenesis

Shigellosis is acquired by ingestion. Because of its high infectivity, person-to-person spread is of great significance, and, at least in industrialized societies, food and water take on a lesser role. *Shigella* organisms survive gastric acidity: they can be recovered from the stomach as long as 20 hours after ingestion. Within 12 hours, virulent organisms begin multiplying within the small bowel, reaching concentrations approaching 10^9 per ml of luminal contents in 24 to 36 hours. At this point the patient begins to suffer from abdominal pain, cramps, and fever. If diarrhea is present, it is often watery. The critical step in pathogenesis occurs with colonization of the colon and invasion of the colonic epithelium by the pathogen. The capacity of *Shigella* to invade epithelial cells can be detected by the keratoconjunctivitis they cause in rabbits or guinea pigs (the **Sereny test**). Penetration of cultured mammalian cells also provides a useful invasion model.

How *Shigella* cells penetrate the intestinal mucus to reach the surface of the epithelium is still a mystery; **they do not appear to have a well-defined adhesin,** as seen with the enteropathogenic *E. coli*, although some have fimbriae. Once at the surface of the cell, however, the organism disrupts the brush border and is engulfed in an invagination of the host cell membrane, which becomes an intracellular vacuole. Shortly thereafter the organism is found free in the cytoplasm, where its rapid multiplication leads to cell death and the infection of adjacent epithelial cells. Repetition of this process leads to local destruction of the epithelial layer and the formation of microabscesses; these coalesce to form large abscesses, leading to **mucosal ulcerations.** However, invading bacteria that reach the underlying lamina propria evoke an intense inflammatory reaction, which efficiently destroys them. Diarrhea may occur because the colon is unable to absorb fluid entering from the small bowel.

VIRULENCE FACTORS. The penetration of epithelial cells and the subsequent intracellular multiplication of the microorganism depends on a plasmid of approximately 140 Md, which is present in all virulent *Shigella* strains as well as enteroinvasive *E. coli* strains. It encodes **outer membrane proteins** that mediate attachment to the epithelial cell and initiation of parasite-induced phagocytosis. Other plasmid-encoded proteins then break down the membrane of the endosome, allowing bacteria to multiply within the cytoplasm.

In *Sh. sonnei*, another plasmid of 120 Md encodes enzymes involved in the biosynthesis of another virulence factor, type-specific LPS; its loss results in avirulent rough variants. The structure of these oligosaccharide repeat units is apparently an essential factor in bacteria–host cell interactions, possibly responsible for the preference of shigellae for primates.

In addition to the plasmid-encoded factors, chromosomal genes confer virulence traits, including the capacity to multiply subsequent to cellular invasion, to elicit an intestinal secretory response, and to produce Shiga cytotoxin.

SHIGA TOXIN. It has been known for many years that the exceptionally virulent *Sh. dysenteriae* type 1 elaborates a potent exotoxin, which causes paralysis when injected into small animals and is cytotoxic to tissue cultures. It is composed of an enzymatically active **A subunit** (32,000 daltons) and several identical receptor-binding **B subunits** (7700 daltons). The toxin irreversibly **inactivates the mammalian 60S ribosomal subunit** by cleavage of a single adenine base from 18S ribosomal RNA, leading to cessation of protein synthesis and death of the susceptible cell. Other *Shigella* species, EPEC, and enterohemorrhagic *E. coli* elaborate structurally related cytotoxins (referred to as Shiga-like toxins), but usually in smaller amounts.

The analysis of bacterial mutants in macaque monkeys has suggested a specific role for Shiga toxin in the pathogenesis of shigellosis. Although toxin-negative mutants of *Sh. dysenteriae* can still invade the epithelium, they do not induce a bloody inflammatory diarrhea; hence, Shiga toxin is probably responsible for the severe colonic vascular damage and resulting polymorphonuclear inflammatory response seen in bacillary dysentery. Other sequelae of severe dysentery (e.g., hemolytic uremic syndrome), which are also seen after *E. coli* hemorrhagic colitis, are probably secondary to systemic effects of Shiga toxin.

Diagnosis, Prevention, and Treatment

In contrast to pathogenic *E. coli*, shigellae are easily identified in the clinical laboratory. In the first few days of disease, the stool usually contains large numbers, whereas in the later stages, lower counts may render isolation more difficult. When shigellosis is suspected, a fecal sample is cultured on differential media that inhibit the growth of gram-positive microorganisms and that also distinguish between most pathogenic and nonpathogenic enteric species (e.g., MacConkey agar). Suspect colonies are picked to other differential media and subjected to a battery of biochemical tests. Isolates that are identified as *Shigella* may be further identified with appropriate antisera.

As in all diarrheal disease, the cardinal consideration is to maintain fluid and electrolyte balance. Because the disease is self-limiting, most experts consider antibiotic treatment only for the young: it reduces the average duration of the illness from 5 days to 3 and reduces excretion of viable organisms in the stool. *Shigella* frequently acquire R plasmids and become resistant to many common antibiotics. Where the sensitivity is known ampicillin or tetracycline is effective, but when susceptibility is unknown or resistance is common, trimethoprim–sulfamethoxazole is usually used.

Shigellosis can be most effectively controlled by adequate disposal of feces and by ensuring a potable water supply. The disease in the underdeveloped world is commonly one of "feces, flies, food, and fingers." Education on hygienic practices and food preparation is of high value. Frequent handwashing alone has a significant impact, even in highly endemic areas. Because of the high infectivity of shigellae, steps must be taken to minimize transmission from patients to family members and to other members of the community.

Although clinical and subclinical infections induce **immunity** to the same type of organism, there is no vaccine. However, continued identification of the critical determinants of pathogenicity offers promise.

SALMONELLA

Members of the genus *Salmonella* are ubiquitous pathogens found in humans and their livestock, wild mammals, reptiles, birds, and even insects. As noted above, antigenic analysis has distinguished well over 1500 serotypes. The precise naming of members of the genus *Salmonella* is still controversial. The least confusing system artificially treats *Salmonella* serotypes as if they were species (which they clearly are not), thus avoiding cumbersome long names.

In addition, it is useful to group the *Salmonella* on the basis of host preference, as follows:

1. **Salmonella serotypes highly adapted to humans.** The prototype is the typhoid bacillus, *S. typhi*, although *S. paratyphi* A, *S. paratyphi* B, *S. paratyphi* C, and *S. sendai* are also highly adapted for human infection. These *Salmonella* have no known reservoir outside of humans.
2. **Salmonella highly adapted to specific hosts other than humans.** For example, *S. pullorum* and *S. gallinarum* affect avian hosts, *S. dublin* cattle, *S. abortusequi* horses, and *S. choleraesuis* swine. Some, such as *S. choleraesuis*, can also cause infection in humans; others, such as the avian-adapted ones, rarely cause significant disease in other species.
3. **Salmonella with a broad host range.** Most *Salmonella* belong to this category, and they cause most of both human and nonhuman infection. Acute gastroenteritis is the usual response, but the spectrum ranges from asymptomatic carriage to systemic disease.

About 10 of the 1500+ serotypes make up most of the human isolates in a given year. A single serotype, *S. typhimurium*, is the most frequently isolated cause worldwide of *Salmonella* gastroenteritis, bacteremia, and asympto-

matic carriage. It also causes disease in many animal species. Other common human serotypes are *S. enteritidis*, *S. newport*, *S. infantis*, and *S. heidelberg*, their relative frequency varying with time and geographic locale.

Several other enterobacterial species resemble *Salmonella* in pathogenesis, including *Y. pseudotuberculosis* and *Y. enterocolitica* (Chap. 30), *Arizona hinshawii*, and *Citrobacter* species.

The clinical pattern of salmonellosis can be divided into gastroenteritis, enteric fever (typhoid-like disease), bacteremia with or without focal extraintestinal infection, and the asymptomatic carrier state. Virtually any *Salmonella* serotype can cause any of these manifestations under appropriate conditions (e.g., in a compromised host) and can persist afterward. However, certain serotypes are likely to be associated with a particular clinical syndrome: for example, *S. typhimurium*, *S. enteritidis*, and *S. newport* with gastroenteritis; *S. typhi* and the paratyphoid species with enteric fever; and *S. choleraesuis* with bacteremia and focal infection without antecedent gastrointestinal disturbance.

Gastroenteritis

Salmonella gastroenteritis usually follows the ingestion of food or drinking water contaminated by feces and accounts for almost 15% of foodborne infection in the US. Typically, the episode begins 12 to 48 hours after the ingestion, with nausea and vomiting, followed by, or concomitant with, abdominal cramps and diarrhea. Diarrhea persists as the prominent symptom for 3 or 4 days and is usually gone within a week. Fever (<102°F) is present in about half the patients. The spectrum of disease ranges from a few loose stools to severe cholera-like or even dysentery-like syndromes. The disease is likely to be most severe in infants and in adults over the age of 50.

The ingestion of 10,000 or more *Salmonella* bacilli can cause illness in 25% of healthy volunteers. Individuals with achlorhydria or those taking antacids can be infected with considerably smaller inocula. *Salmonella* that survive passage through the stomach probably replicate within the bowel lumen before penetrating the epithelial cells of the distal small bowel, cecum, and proximal large bowel.

How salmonellae enter host cells is not known, but the process appears to be induced only by viable bacterial cells. The invading bacteria replicate intracellularly but cause little mucosal damage or inflammation. They pass rapidly through the epithelial barrier and eventually proliferate in the lamina propria, resulting in a superficial inflammatory response with infiltration by polymorphonuclear leukocytes.

Although some strains of *Salmonella* produce a LT (cholera toxin-like) enterotoxin, the diarrhea associated with salmonellosis is thought to be associated primarily with the inflammatory response, which stimulates local prostaglandin synthesis. The resulting activation of the adenylate cyclase system increases the secretion of fluid and electrolytes into the bowel lumen. In addition, many *Salmonella* produce a potent **cytotoxin,** which may cause local cell death and necrosis. Ordinarily, local host defense mechanisms, particularly the polymorphonuclear leukocytes and macrophages, prevent access of the invading *Salmonella* to the lymphatics and systemic circulation, so that infection with nontyphoidal strains is usually mild and self-limiting.

However, serious sequelae, and every death, may occur in hosts impaired in humoral or in cell-mediated immunity or with a compromised reticuloendothelial system (e.g., from sickle cell disease or Hodgkin's disease). *Salmonella* bacteremia may be the first manifestation of AIDS.

Salmonella typhi *and Typhoid Fever*

The early pathogenesis of typhoid fever is similar to that of other *Salmonella* infections, but the Peyer's patches of the terminal ileum are thought to be the portal of entry of the bacillus. Experimental evidence indicates that the M cell, which is the outermost layer of Peyer's patches and lymphoid follicles, is the principal site of entry, which is followed by proliferation and local destruction of the underlying lymphoid and adjacent epithelial cells.

During the first 7 to 10 days of infection individuals are mostly asymptomatic, and typhoid bacilli disappear from the stool. In severe typhoid fever, there are hyperplastic changes during this period in Peyer's patches and solitary lymphoid follicles of the cecum. Unlike the polymorphonuclear leukocyte response seen in acute salmonella diarrhea, *S. typhi* infection evokes a more intense mononuclear response, with hyperplastic mesenteric lymph nodes. Fever and other symptoms of endotoxemia accompany the spread of bacilli from the infected cells of the reticuloendothelial system into the blood stream. The liver and biliary tree become infected, resulting in reinvasion of the intestinal tract. **Rose spots** (2–4-mm maculopapular erythematous lesions) appear on the abdomen, and splenomegaly becomes apparent (typhoid belly).

The **systemic manifestations** of typhoid include suppurative and nonsuppurative infection of several organ systems. The most common complications are **intestinal perforation** and **hemorrhage,** usually in the ileum. Clinical improvement of untreated patients usually begins in the third week following infection, coincident with the development of humoral and, particularly, cell-mediated immunity.

Typhoid fever is a severe disease. When untreated, there is an average of 30 days of fever, during which about 20% of patients die; an additional 10% suffer a relapse of fever or intestinal hemorrhage or peritonitis. Fortunately, typhoid fever can usually be managed effectively by antimicrobial agents (see below).

Because typhoid is a systemic disease, in the early stages the organism should be sought by **culture of the blood** and not the stool. When the disease becomes established, both materials will be culture-positive, as is the urine in about one-quarter of the cases. During the convalescent phase 4 to 5 weeks after infection, the blood will return to sterility, but the stool may remain culture-positive in about half of patients. More than three-fourths of patients will have high titers of circulating Ab against O and H Ags. Those who recover, whether or not on chemotherapy, may continue to excrete the organism for long periods of time. **Chronic carriers** may be of extraordinary importance as reservoirs of infection (e.g., the famous cook "typhoid Mary").

Extraintestinal Infection

The acute gastroenteritis caused by many *Salmonella* serotypes is also associated with transient bacteremia, but a persistent bacteremia and frank sepsis is seen in those with a compromised reticuloendothelial system. In humans, *S. choleraesuis* often presents as a focal infection without any obvious gastrointestinal manifestations; in persons with sickle cell anemia, skeletal infection is common. Moreover, with *S. choleraesuis, S. typhimurium,* and a few other serotypes, gastroenteritis may lead to infection of distant sites: the endothelium of large arteries or endocarditis, mostly in older patients and those with arterial plaque or aneurysm; or meningitis, in patients less than 2 years of age.

CARRIERS. Almost one-half of infected persons continue to excrete salmonellae 1 month after the symptoms have disappeared, and 1 in 20 still do so 5 months later. An individual who continues to excrete the organism after 1 year is considered a carrier: the rate following typhoid is about 3% and 0.5% following nontyphoidal salmonellosis. An unknown fraction of people become carriers after asymptomatic infection; the median carriage rate of *Salmonella* among healthy persons in developed countries is 0.13.

More than 40,000 *Salmonella* isolates are reported in the US each year, but these may represent only 1% to 10% of the actual cases. More than 18,000 hospitalizations and 500 deaths are associated with this disease each year.

Determinants of Pathogenicity

TOXINS. *Salmonella* infection occasionally causes a profuse cholera-like diarrhea, and a heat-labile enterotoxin, similar to cholera toxin and *E. coli* LT, has been reported from a *S. typhimurium* strain. During *Salmonella* gastroenteritis, there are cytopathic changes, probably attributable to a cytotoxin associated with the outer membrane fraction of the bacteria, although its precise structure and role in disease remain undefined.

Lipopolysaccharide (LPS) is the most extensively characterized virulence determinant of *Salmonella*. The lipid A (endotoxin; see Chaps. 2 and 21) can activate macrophages, resulting in pyrogenicity, leukocytosis, and hypotension (shock). There is no doubt that the general picture of systemic *Salmonella* infection is **attributable largely to the toxic moiety of LPS,** but it is not clear whether these pathophysiological responses benefit the microbe.

SURFACE ANTIGENS. Specific O Ags are important for the virulence of salmonellae: by decreasing the susceptibility to phagocytosis and the ability to activate the alternative complement pathway. Experimental shift of *S. typhimurium* from O-6,7 to O-4,12 Ag decreases virulence, whereas rough variants lacking O-specific side chains are avirulent. With *S. typhi* strains, the Vi capsular antigen also contributes to virulence. It is not certain whether O or Vi Ags act by preventing phagocytosis (through inhibition of complement-mediated opsonization) or by preventing subsequent destruction within macrophages.

ADHESION AND MOTILITY. The localization of *Salmonella* in the terminal ileum suggests that these organisms adhere to the intestinal epithelium. *Salmonella* synthesize common mannose-sensitive type 1 fimbriae, but the role of these structures in virulence appears to be minimal. A mannose-resistant adhesin is found in some serotypes associated with gastroenteritis, but its role remains undefined.

Flagella appear to be important virulence factors, as shown by mutants that have lost them. Surprisingly, the critical effect of this loss seems to be a decreased capacity for survival and growth in macrophages.

ENTRY AND PENETRATION OF HOST CELLS. Invasion of the gastrointestinal mucosa is an essential step in *S. typhimurium* pathogenesis. The mechanisms are not fully understood. In tissue culture models, entry (invasion) and penetration through polarized epithelial cells (transcytosis) involve specific bacterial surface proteins (**invasion factors**), which are synthesized in response to interaction with the brush border of epithelial cells. This **parasite-induced phagocytosis** is seen in Figure 27–4.

INTRACELLULAR SURVIVAL AND MULTIPLICATION. After entry, *Salmonella* multiply in membrane-limited vacuoles, with a division time of about 50 minutes. *Salmonella* species survive within many cells, but most importantly macrophages. Mutations that destroy this capacity include loss of LPS and certain auxotrophic and regulatory defects.

PLASMID GENES. Most *Salmonella* species (but not *S. typhi*) contain a large (50–100-Kb) plasmid that is essential for virulence. Strains that have lost the plasmid enter epithelial cells and macrophages normally but do not persist. The nature of the plasmid-encoded virulence property is unknown.

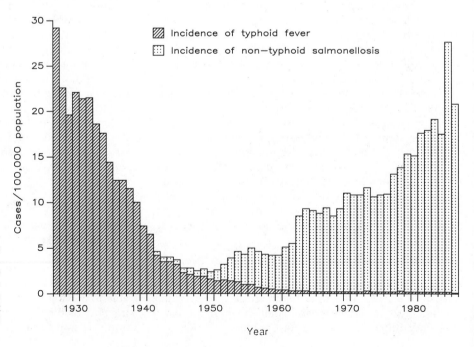

Figure 27–4. Reported incidence of typhoid fever and nontyphoid salmonellosis in the United States from 1934 to 1984. The large spike in 1985 was due to a large outbreak of milk-associated *S. typhimurium* infections in Chicago. (Data from Morbididity and Mortality Weekly Report *35*:55, 1986, and figure kindly provided by Dr. Robert Tauxe)

Epidemiology

Typhoid fever and nontyphoidal salmonellosis are reported to public health laboratories. In recent years, studies of the epidemiology of salmonellosis employed not only serotyping but also antibiotic susceptibility testing, bacteriophage typing, and comparison of plasmids.

The incidence of salmonellosis has changed dramatically since the middle of this century (Fig. 27–5). In the developing world, typhoid is still a major cause of disease, but in the US only about 500 isolates are reported annually. The incidence of nontyphoidal salmonellosis, however, has increased markedly, reflecting changes in animal husbandry, the mechanization of food processing (particularly of eggs), and the mass distribution of food.

Diagnosis, Treatment, and Prevention

Salmonella can be isolated on any of the common enteric media. During the acute phase of gastroenteritis, large numbers of bacilli are usually present in the stool, but in enteric fever, the organism must be cultured from blood.

Historically, rising serum Ab titers against *Salmonella* O and H Ags (the **Widal test**) were employed to diagnose typhoid, other enteric fevers, and systemic salmonellosis. Ab responses to *Salmonella* gastroenteritis or the carrier state are not consistent.

In uncomplicated *Salmonella* gastroenteritis patients should be monitored for fluid and electrolyte balance, as in any diarrheal disorder. Antimicrobial therapy does not reduce the duration and severity of symptoms and may in fact prolong convalescence and intestinal carriage of the infecting microorganism. However, some physicians treat infants and elderly persons who have acute gastroenteritis, to prevent complications.

Patients with bacteremia, meningitis, enteric fever, or other extraintestinal infections require antimicrobial treatment. Chloramphenicol is especially effective for treating typhoid, and the incidence of resistance has been low. Various beta-lactams or trimethoprim–sulfamethoxazole is also used.

Because of the large number of *Salmonella* serotypes, no general vaccine seems likely soon. However, considerable effort has been made to develop a vaccine against *S. typhi*. The present procedure consists of two subcutaneous injections of a saline suspension of acetone-killed cells given 4 to 8 weeks apart. Local discomfort is the rule, sometimes accompanied by fever. The vaccine offers about 70% protection for 3 years against infection by low numbers of ingested organisms. A 1988 field trial with purified Vi Ag produced similar levels of protection after 1 year, with essentially no immunization side effects.

A promising approach to the prevention of typhoid and other salmonellosis involves the use of **orally administered attenuated strains.** The most widely used is a strain of *S. typhi*, Ty21a, which is a Vi⁻, *gal*E mutant that can safely be fed to humans. Immunization with this strain affords excellent protection against disease in endemic areas where the incidence is low. Auxotrophic strains (e.g., *aroA*) also seem promising.

OTHER IMPORTANT ENTEROBACTERIA
Klebsiella–Enterobacter–Serratia

The genera *Klebsiella*, *Enterobacter*, and *Serratia*, in the tribe Klebsiellae, can be identified by biochemical tests, including decarboxylase reactions (Table 27–4). Most strains of *Klebsiella* and *Serratia* can also be typed serologically. Members of the group are second to *E. coli* as causes of gram-negative bacteremia, which sometimes results from their ready proliferation in contaminated intravenous solutions containing glucose. The necessity for differentiating these three genera from each other and from other enteric bacilli is underlined by their wide differences in antibiotic sensitivity and in pathogenicity. *Klebsiella* predominates in clinical isolates and as a primary pathogen and usually produces more severe illness; the other two are opportunistic pathogens.

In testing water supplies, it is important to distinguish *E. coli*, which is an index of fecal contamination, from *Enterobacter* (formerly *Aerobacter*) *aerogenes*, which is found widely on plants. Accordingly, biochemical tests for this purpose were developed early. Some of these are based on the fact that *E. coli* carries out the **mixed acid fermentation** whereas *Klebsiella* and *Enterobacter* carry out the **butylene glycol fermentation** (Chap. 4), which forms large quantities of this neutral product (CH₃-CHOH-CHOH-CH₃) and hence forms less acid.

Four metabolic tests (indole, methyl red, Voges–Proskauer, and citrate utilization), collectively referred to as the **IMViC tests,** were originally used to distinguish *Enterobacter aerogenes* from *E. coli*. Only the latter produces **indole** in media containing tryptophan. The **methyl red** test distinguishes heavy and light production of acid, because this indicator shifts from yellow to red below pH 4.5, and in glucose–peptone broth cultures incubated for 48 hours, only the mixed acid fermentation produces enough acid to turn the indicator red. The **Voges–Proskauer** reaction is a color test for acetoin, a product of the butylene glycol type of fermentation. **Citrate** can serve as the sole carbon source for *En. aerogenes* but not for *E. coli*.*

The three genera are differentiated by a combination of tests, primarily for motility, lactose utilization, decar-

---

* These tests are standard procedures in the study of *Enterobacteriaceae*. The IMViC formula for *E. coli* is ++−−, for *En. aerogenes* and *En. cloacae*, −−++. All 16 possible combinations of the IMViC test results have been found.

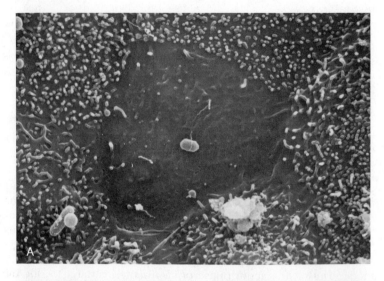

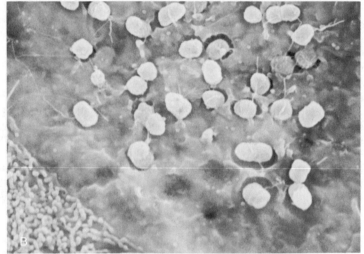

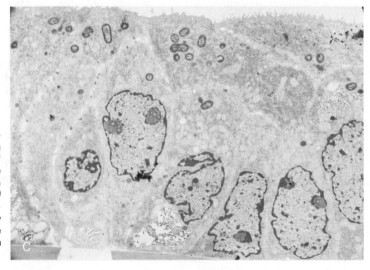

Figure 27–5. Entry of salmonellae into polarized MDCK epithelial cells by parasite-induced phagocytosis. *(A)* Scanning electron micrograph of salmonellae adhering to the surface of the epithelial cells. Initial contact is with microvilli (seen on the edges of this micrograph), but eventually these disappear from the MDCK cells, producing a smooth membrane *(center)*. *(B)* After 2 to 4 hours salmonellae can be seen entering the epithelial cells through an endocytic process involving the now smooth membrane. *(C)* After 6 hours the salmonellae are present in the cytoplasm of the MDCK cells surrounded by a phagocytic membrane.

boxylases, Voges–Proskauer reaction, fermentation of several carbohydrates, and urease production.

KLEBSIELLA. *Klebsiella pneumoniae* (Friedländer's bacillus) is the most important human "pathogen" of the *Klebsiella* group. It forms a capsule and hence produces large, moist, often very mucoid colonies. A total of five O Ags and 72 capsular (K) polysaccharide Ags have been identified. Type-specific (K) antisera are useful in determining the epidemiology of hospital-acquired *Klebsiella* infections, which represent about two-thirds of all infections caused by these organisms.

K. pneumoniae is found in the respiratory tract and the feces of 5% to 10% of healthy subjects and is frequently a secondary invader in the lungs of patients with chronic pulmonary disease. It causes approximately 3% of all acute bacterial pneumonias, and it is the second most common urinary tract pathogen. Its invasive properties depend on the antiphagocytic effect of its capsule: unencapsulated (R) strains are avirulent. Pneumonia caused by *K. pneumoniae* is characterized by thick, gelatinous sputum and a high bacterial population density in the edema zones of the active lesions and by destructive action of the unphagocytized organisms on the pulmonary tissue, often resulting in lung abscesses requiring surgical resection.

Although *Klebsiella* has been found in acute diarrhea in children, its enteric pathogenicity has been questioned. However, strains isolated from patients with **tropical sprue** elaborate an **enterotoxin** that resembles *E. coli* ST enterotoxin. *Klebsiella* species have been implicated in chronic inflammatory diseases of the upper respiratory tract: *K. ozaenae* in **ozena,** a progressive fetid atrophy of the nasal mucosa, and *K. rhinoscleromatis* in **rhinoscleroma,** a destructive granuloma of the nose and pharynx.

In acute, uncomplicated urinary tract infections, oral sulfonamides, nalidixic acid, ampicillin, and tetracyclines are usually effective; in recurrent or chronic infection, sensitivity tests are needed for selection of effective agents. In life-threatening infections, aminoglycosides, cephalosporins, and chloramphenicol are the drugs of choice. Most strains of *Klebsiella*, unlike *Enterobacter* and *Serratia*, are sensitive to cephalothin.

ENTEROBACTER. Organisms in the *Enterobacter* group occur in soil, dairy products, water, and sewage, as well as in the intestinal tract of man and animals. Enterobacters are frequently isolated from sputum (often after antibiotic therapy), urinary tract infections (often hospital-acquired), blood, and wound infections. They are usually considered **secondary pathogens** (i.e., superinfecting underlying primary infection), **opportunistic** (e.g., in urinary tract infections following catheterization), or **commensals** (i.e., not causally associated with disease).

In this genus, the most common species in man is *En. cloacae*, followed by *En. aerogenes* and *En. hafniae* (now renamed *Hafnia alvei*). *En. agglomerans* (formerly *Erwinia*) achieved notoriety, together with *En. cloacae*, in a nation-wide epidemic of septicemia caused by contaminated intravenous products, and it is now increasingly recognized as an opportunistic pathogen in a wide variety of settings. *En. agglomerans* includes both aerogenic (gas-producing) and anaerogenic organisms; more than half of both groups produce yellow pigment, useful in identification.

Enterobacters are susceptible to aminoglycosides, chloramphenicol, the tetracyclines, trimethoprim–sulfamethoxazole, nalidixic acid, and nitrofurantoin (the latter three being used in urinary tract infections).

SERRATIA. Cultures of *Serratia marcescens* have been used for many years by bacteriologists for demonstration purposes (e.g., to demonstrate bacteremia after dental extraction) because the bright red pigment of some strains is so easily observable.* The organism was long considered a harmless saprobe, but since 1960, it has been isolated with increasing frequency in human, mostly in nosocomial, infections (often severe). The earlier incidence is not known, as many nonpigmented strains were probably included with other slow lactose fermenters as paracolon organisms. *Ser. marcescens* is the most common species in clinical practice.

Serratiae are motile. Unlike most other coliforms, most strains do not ferment lactose or do so slowly. Although the organisms may produce a red pigment (**prodigiosin**), especially at room temperature, at least three-fourths of strains isolated at present are nonpigmented. Fifteen O Ags and 16 H Ags of *Ser. marcescens* have been identified.

Serratiae usually infect patients with debilitating disorders, or under treatment with broad-spectrum antibiotics, or subjected to instrumentation such as tracheostomy tubes or indwelling catheters. Outbreaks have occurred in nurseries, intensive-care units, and renal dialysis units. Serratiae can cause endocarditis, osteomyelitis, septicemia, and wound, urinary tract, and respiratory tract infections.

Aminoglycosides (especially amikacin), chloramphenicol, and carbenicillin are useful. In urinary tract infections, nalidixic acid and trimethoprim–sulfamethoxazole are possible alternatives; sensitivity testing is required. Drug-resistance plasmids have been demonstrated.

---

* Instances of the "miraculous" appearance of "blood" on communion wafers and other foods were most likely caused by strains of *Ser. marcescens.*

Edwardsiella–Citrobacter

The genus *Edwardsiella* includes a group of motile, H_2S-producing, lacose-negative organisms that resemble salmonellae in some biochemical features (Table 27–4) and sometimes in pathogenicity. *Ed. tarda* has been isolated from a variety of mammals and reptiles. It is occasionally also found in the human intestinal tract, especially in acute gastroenteritis, and it has been associated with meningitis, septicemia, and wound infections. A total of 49 O Ags and 37 H Ags have been identified. Kanamycin, ampicillin, cephalothin, and chloramphenicol are the drugs of choice.

The *Citrobacter* group (tribe Salmonelleae) is composed of *Enterobacteriaceae* previously designated as *Escherichia freundii* and the Bethesda–Ballerup group of paracolon organisms. Many strains ferment lactose, but this is frequently delayed. They are differentiated from salmonellae by their possession of β-galactosidase and lack of lysine decarboxylase.

Citrobacter strains are found infrequently in normal feces; they have been associated with diarrhea, with secondary invasion in compromised patients, and occasionally with severe primary septic processes. They are susceptible to chloramphenicol, gentamicin, kanamycin, and colistin, but strains vary in sensitivity to ampicillin, carbenicillin, and cephalothin.

Proteus–Providencia

The lactose-negative, motile bacilli of the *Proteus–Providencia* group are unusual among *Enterobacteriaceae* in being able to deaminate phenylalanine* and lysine. **Rapid** and **abundant urease production** distinguishes *Proteus* from *Providencia*.

PROTEUS. *Proteus* are commonly found in soil, sewage, and manure. They are found with some frequency in normal human feces but often in much increased numbers in individuals receiving antibiotic therapy or during diarrheal diseases caused by other organisms. *Proteus* organisms are frequent causes of urinary tract infection and are also involved in other, often serious infections.

The antigenic structure of *P. vulgaris* is of particular medical interest because strains possessing certain O Ags (OX2, OX19, and OXK) are agglutinated by the serum of patients with various rickettsial diseases (Weil–Felix reaction; see Laboratory Diagnosis, Chap. 40). These particular O Ags seem to be fortuitously related to antigenic determinants of rickettsiae.

P. vulgaris and *P. mirabilis* form a thin spreading growth (swarm) on the surface of moist agar media. To obtain isolated colonies, the swarming is prevented by cultivation on the relatively dry surface of 5% agar or on

ordinary 1% to 2% agar containing 0.1% chloral hydrate. They also produce abundant H_2S and liquefy gelatin; *P. rettgeri* and *P. morganii* do not possess these characteristics. Fermentation of most *Proteus* strains is of the mixed acid type.

Gentamicin is active against all four species, but only the most commonly occurring, indole-negative *P. mirabilis* is sensitive to ampicillin, several aminoglycosides, cephalothin, trimethoprim–sulfamethoxazole, and often penicillin G.

PROVIDENCIA. Organisms in the genus *Providencia* are closely related to *P. morganii* and *P. rettgeri*. Members of the group have been isolated from human feces during outbreaks of diarrhea but also occur in normal individuals. They are primarily associated with urinary tract infections; *Providencia stuartii* has recently emerged as a major agent in burn infections, displaying marked resistance to many antibiotics, while *Prov. alcalifaciens* is less frequently encountered and is more susceptible.

Vibrionaceae

The *Vibrionaceae* family of gram-negative curved rods share many biochemical and physiologic properties with the *Enterobacteriaceae*. Their natural habitats include fresh- and saltwater environments, where they exist free-living or in normal or pathogenic association with aquatic life. The most important human pathogens of the group are members of the genus *Vibrio*, but species in the genera *Campylobacter*, *Aeromonas*, and *Plesiomonas* also occasionally cause human disease.

Vibrios (L. *vibrare*, to vibrate) are curved, highly motile bacilli with a **single polar flagellum** (Fig. 27–6). They grow on simple media, and their metabolism is facultative. Other differentiating characteristics are given in Table 27–2. *V. cholerae*, the agent of cholera, is most important worldwide, whereas *V. parahaemolyticus* has been increasingly implicated in seafood-associated gastroenteritis and extraintestinal infection. Other occasionally pathogenic members are *V. vulnificus*, *V. alginolyticus*, and the group F vibrios (*V. fluvialis*, *V. hollisae*, *V. damsela*, and *V. furnissi*).

VIBRIO CHOLERAE

Cholera is a severe diarrheal disease caused by *V. cholerae*. This organism has a curved, **comma** shape (hence its earlier name, *V. comma*) and displays high motility in wet mount preparations. These distinctive characteristics allowed Pacini to describe the organism almost 30 years before it was isolated in pure culture by Robert Koch in 1883.

---

* The product, phenylpyruvic acid, develops an intense green color on addition of $FeCl_3$.

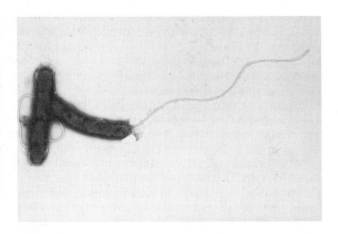

Figure 27–6. Electron micrograph of *Vibrio cholerae*. Each comma-shaped cell carries a single long polar flagellum. Pili can also be seen as much thinner filaments closer to the bacterial cell and near the attachment point of the flagellum.

V. cholerae strains can be divided into two main groups or **biotypes: classic** and **El Tor,** which can be distinguished by various tests (e.g., El Tor strains tend to lyse sheep erythrocytes and are resistant to polymyxin) and by phage typing. The El Tor biotype, first isolated in 1901 from healthy pilgrims at the El Tor cholera quarantine station on the Gulf of Suez, was originally thought to be nonpathogenic, but it was later isolated in epidemics of cholera.

Endemic in the Bengal region of India and Bangladesh for centuries, cholera has spread across the world seven times since the beginning of the 19th century, usually beginning in India. The last of these great **pandemics** started in Indonesia in 1961, swept north to China, through Thailand into India, and across the Asian continent to Africa. Within a decade, it had travelled to Europe, Japan, and the US. The first six pandemics were caused by the classic biotype but the most recent by the El Tor biotype. Since 1986, the classic biotype has been isolated from patients in Bangladesh and India with increasing frequency, suggesting the beginning of yet another cholera pandemic.

Characteristics

In many characteristics *V. cholerae* is very similar to the *Enterobacteriaceae*. It can ferment a variety of carbohydrates, producing acid but (like *Shigella*) no gas. It utilizes lactose slowly and is generally scored as negative for this sugar. It can grow (albeit slowly) on most selective media for gram-negative enterics, including those containing bile salts, bismuth sulfite, tellurite, and toxic dyes. However, *V. cholerae* differs from the *Enterobacteriaceae* in that fresh isolates show a **curved rod (vibrio)** morphology and high motility, a single **polar flagellum,**

a positive oxidase test, good growth in **alkaline** (pH 9–9.6) media but no growth below pH 6.5, and agglutination by anti-O and anti-H Abs that do not cross-react with other common enteric species.

Pathogenesis of Cholera

Cholera is characterized by a profuse, watery diarrhea containing flecks of mucus ("rice-water stools") but no blood or inflammatory cells. The disease starts about 2 to 5 days after infection by the oral route, with nausea, vomiting, abdominal cramps, and diarrhea. In extreme cases, the loss of fluid from diarrhea can exceed 20 liters per day. However, even at moderate rates of fluid loss (10 liters per day), hypovolemic shock can cause death within a few hours of the onset of symptoms, particularly in young children. Because the cholera stool contains about the same concentration of sodium, twice the concentration of bicarbonate, and about five times the concentration of potassium as normal plasma, the cholera victim suffers from electrolyte deficiency (especially hypokalemia) and metabolic acidosis. In the absence of appropriate therapy, the mortality rate can reach 60%, but it is reduced to less than 1% by replacement of lost fluids and electrolytes.

Human volunteers and animal models for cholera have been very helpful in defining other aspects of cholera pathogenesis. For example, in healthy volunteers, oral administration of up to 10^{11} bacteria rarely produces any signs of infection, but after neutralization of stomach acid with bicarbonate, 10^4 organisms can cause disease. The low pH of gastric juice is thus an important nonspecific defense mechanism against *V. cholerae*.

When *V. cholerae* does survive the acid barrier of the stomach, it colonizes the small intestine mucosa by adhering to epithelial cells. The infection remains localized on the surface of the small intestine, with no invasion of the epithelium or the blood stream. Once the diarrhea begins, the organism is shed in large numbers (10^8/ml) in stool.

The organism elaborates a powerful enterotoxin that causes most of the secretory diarrhea. Cholera is thus much like diseases caused by enterotoxigenic *E. coli* but usually more severe. Indeed, **cholera enterotoxin** (choleragen, cholera toxin) is closely related to the LT of *E. coli* (see below).

VIRULENCE DETERMINANTS. The reduced virulence of mutants lacking motility or chemotaxis suggests that the presence of these properties enables the organism to swim deep into the intestinal crypts and penetrate the mucous gel coating the epithelium. Proteases and neuraminidase produced by the organism may also play a role in mucous gel penetration as well as provide substrates for bacterial growth by hydrolyzing glycoproteins.

Adhesion to the brush border of intestinal epithelial cells is mediated by fimbrial adhesins produced by *V. cholerae* (much as was described above for enterotoxinogenic *E. coli*), especially a colonization factor called TCP (for *toxin coregulated pilus*). Another colonization factor, called ACF, also seems important and may be a second type of pilus. A single regulatory gene (*toxR*) for cholera enterotoxin, TCP, and ACF, assures their coordinate production during the infection cycle.

CHOLERA ENTEROTOXIN. Cholera enterotoxin is clearly the principal cause of the secretory diarrhea seen in cholera. For example, human volunteers who ingested less than 10 μg of the purified toxin purged more than 20 liters of diarrhea in a 2-day period. The toxin activates the membrane-bound adenylate cyclase of target enterocytes. The elevated levels of cAMP in the mucosal cells of the small bowel cause a cascade (probably involving cAMP-activated protein kinases) that ultimately results in hypersecretion of chloride and bicarbonate into the intestinal lumen, and hence a net osmotic efflux of water.

Cholera toxin and the immunologically related LT enterotoxin of *E. coli* are composed of one A subunit and five B subunits, totalling about 84,000 daltons. The B subunits have a high affinity for GM_1 ganglioside receptors on the surface of target cells; Abs against these subunits block this binding and neutralize the toxin. After binding of the holotoxin, the A subunits enter the cytoplasm, where they catalyze transfer of the ADP-ribose moiety of NAD to, and thus activate, a membrane-associated regulatory protein called G_s. As described in Figure 27–7, this activated G_s stimulates adenylate cyclase by a mechanism that involves GTP. The resulting increase in cAMP increases the secretion of fluid and electrolytes into the bowel lumen by crypt cells and decreases absorption of fluid by cells at the villus tip. The net result is a profuse watery, noninflammatory diarrhea.

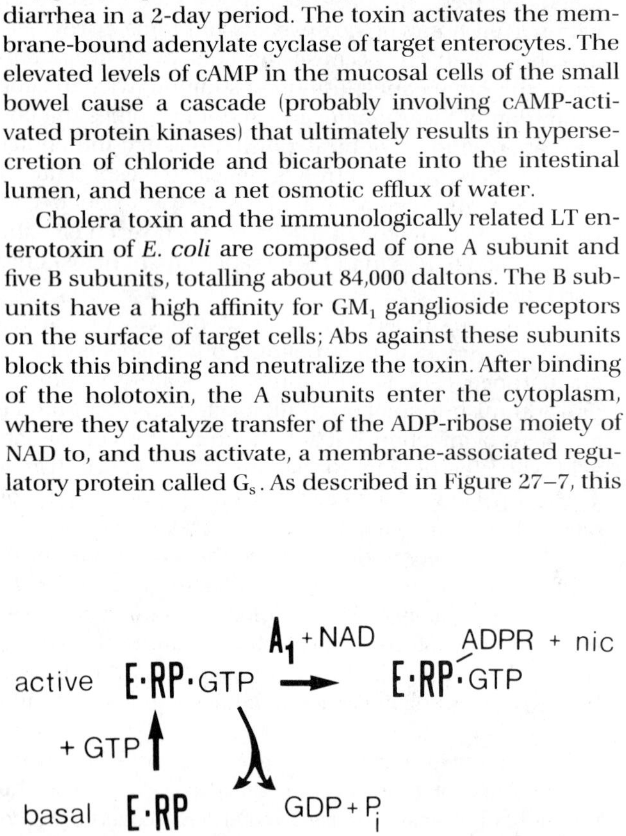

In contrast to the plasmid-encoded LT of *E. coli*, the genes encoding the two enterotoxin subunits of *V. cholerae* are located on the chromosome. Strains can possess one or more copies of the cholera toxin genes, which appear to be associated with a large transposable genetic element.

Mutants of *V. cholerae* that lack the enterotoxin still cause diarrhea, although to a lesser extent, in human volunteers. The cause in these cases may be a **Shiga-like toxin** that is produced, along with cholera enterotoxin, by several strains of *V. cholerae*. It is related immunologically to the cytotoxin produced by *Sh. dysenteriae*.

Laboratory Diagnosis

V. cholerae is easily isolated and identified if the laboratory is aware of the potential for cholera in the community. Dark-field microscopic observation of stool should reveal numerous comma-shaped organisms, with rapid motility, that are subsequently agglutinated and immobilized by specific antisera. Organisms of the O antigen group 1 are most often involved in overt disease (see Non-O1 Vibrios, below). They can be divided into three serotypes (Ogawa, Inaba, and Hikojima), but these cross-react; polyvalent antisera are of the most value in rapid diagnosis.

The organism can be best isolated by streaking on thiosulfate–citrate–salt–sucrose agar (**TCBS**), on which it forms yellow colonies. Although it will grow on some of the usual enteric media, they are not optimal. Enrichment can be performed by inoculating alkaline peptone water (pH 8.4) with stool followed by incubation and streaking on any rich medium having bile salts and an alkaline pH. Positive identification depends on testing isolated colonies serologically and biochemically (i.e., anti-O1 agglutination, a positive oxidase test, the acid reaction with no gas in triple-sugar–iron stabs, and positive lysine and ornithine decarboxylase tests).

Figure 27-7. Activation of adenylcyclase by cholera toxin. The toxin, a complex of an A polypeptide (mol wt 29,000) and 5 copies of B polypeptide (each 11,500), binds to **ganglioside GM₁** receptors on host cells; the binding is very tight because of the cooperative action of the 5 B chains. Cleavage of the A chain and SS reduction separates it into polypeptides A₁ and A₂, and A₁ enters the cell. There it transfers adenosine diphosphate ribose *(ADPR)* from NAD to covalent linkage with regulatory protein RP, which is complexed with the cellular enzyme adenylcyclase *(E)*. This complex has little enzymatic activity unless it binds GTP, and the steady-state of this binding is normally low because the complex also hydrolyzes GTP. However, this reaction is blocked by the attachment of ADPR to RP. The adenylcyclase is thereby stabilized in an active conformation, and the resulting increase in the level of cAMP in intestinal cells stimulates secretion of ions (and fluid) into the intestinal lumen.

Treatment

Like other severe diarrheal disease, cholera is treated by replacement of fluid and electrolytes. Even victims in hypovolemic shock will improve dramatically when given sterile intravenous replacement fluid (containing in mEq/liter 133 Na^+, 13 K^+, 99 Cl^-, and 48 HCO_3^- ions). Oral rehydration therapy can also be successful because glucose-facilitated sodium uptake is not impaired. Oral rehydration solution consists of 3.5 g of sodium chloride, 2.5 g of sodium bicarbonate, 1.5 g of potassium chloride, and 20 g of glucose per liter of potable water. Once dehydration and electrolyte imbalances are corrected, cholera is a self-limiting disease lasting only a few days. Treatment with tetracycline or other suitable antibiotics shortens the period of shedding of infectious organisms and also reduces fluid loss.

Epidemiology and Prevention

Cholera is spread primarily by food and water contaminated with the material of infected individuals. In endemic areas, asymptomatic carriers undoubtedly play a significant role in disseminating the disease, but not by person-to-person contact because of the very large doses required for infection. The breakdown of adequate sewage control (as after flooding or a tropical rainy season) can suddenly expose large numbers of potential victims to the threat of the disease. Accordingly, good sanitation is the most effective means of cholera control. Once cholera has broken out, an attempt must be made to isolate patients and disinfect their stools. Stool cultures should also be done on contacts, and infected individuals should be treated with antimicrobials.

Sporadic outbreaks of cholera have occurred repeatedly in certain well-defined geographic regions that are not typically considered cholera-endemic areas. For example, since 1973, the Gulf Coast of the US (including the states of Texas and Louisiana) has experienced several outbreaks involving more than a dozen individuals. Epidemiologic investigations have shown that raw or improperly cooked seafood (shellfish, shrimp, and crabs) was the source; a single atypical El Tor strain, carrying genes for both TCP fimbrae and cholera enterotoxin, was the cause over the 13-year period.

Although "environmental" strains of *V. cholerae* can be isolated from US coastal waters such as the Chesapeake Bay, they have never been associated with diarrheal disease, probably because they lack the structural genes for cholera enterotoxin and TCP adhesin. Thus, although *V. cholerae* has the ability to survive in aquatic environments, perhaps in association with shellfish, only the persistence of toxigenic, adherent strains carries the threat of cholera.

There is evidence that the production of cholera toxin and TCP is under osmotic control: levels are lowest in media of high salt concentration and highest in media that approximate the osmotic conditions of mammalian hosts. In addition, the severity of the disease varies widely. It is not clear how much of this variation is attributable to bacterial factors or to variation in the host, but an association between the O blood group and increased suceptibility to cholera has been noted.

IMMUNITY. Human volunteer studies have shown that convalescence from cholera imparts solid immunity to homologous serotypic challenge for at least 3 years. Moreover, in cholera-endemic areas, the attack rate is low in older individuals, who probably have developed some level of immunity during subclinical infections or environmental exposure to *V. cholerae*. Parenterally administered, killed whole-cell vaccines (containing both the Ogawa and Inaba serotypes) are capable of inducing some short-lived immunity to cholera.

Because immunity to cholera is thought to be mediated by intestinal secretory IgA Abs against bacterial and toxin Ags, an oral vaccine has been sought. Three types are being considered. A combined vaccine composed of cholera toxin B subunit mixed with killed *V. cholerae* cells of both the Ogawa and Inaba serotypes provided 65% protection for at least 1 year. Several stably attenuated strains of *V. cholerae* that carry deletions in the gene for cholera toxin A gene have induced greater than 90% protection in human volunteers but do cause some mild reactions. A killed whole-cell vaccine genetically engineered to express large amounts of the cholera B subunit and the TCP colonization factor is currently being tested.

RELATED ORGANISMS
Other Vibrios

NONCHOLERA VIBRIOS (NCV or NON-O1). The noncholera vibrios are very similar biochemically and morphologically to El Tor *V. cholerae* but are not agglutinated by cholera polyvalent O1 antiserum; they are agglutinated by their homologous antisera. They are found in surface waters and in shellfish throughout the world, and various strains cause a mild diarrhea or a frank cholera-like disease; they have been responsible for epidemics in Czechoslovakia, Malaysia, and Sudan and for rare cases in the US. Some strains possess cholera enterotoxin genes, but most lack genes for the TCP colonization factor.

VIBRIO PARAHAEMOLYTICUS. The **halophilic** *V. parahaemolyticus* (which requires 2%–7% NaCl for growth) is found in marine water and marine fauna throughout the world. It has been recovered from seafoods, especially mollusks and crustaceans, and is found with increasing frequency in cases of **food poisoning** in various countries, including the US. In Japan it accounts for about half the cases of bacterial food poisoning. The disease ranges from the usual moderate, short-term illness to severe cases necessitating hospitalization. Because the organism often can be recovered from stool, the disease probably involves primarily gastroenteritis as well as some immediate toxicity attributable to preformed toxins. *V. parahaemolyticus* infections of the extremities, eyes, and ears, as well as of the blood stream, have also recently been recognized in the US, usually in persons scratched by the sharp edges of clams or oysters.

The organism does not grow on most routine enteric media but can be cultured by simple addition of NaCl (5%). It is positive for oxidase, lysine and ornithine decarboxylase, and indole formation; it ferments glucose, mannitol, and mannose and utilizes citrate as the sole source of carbon. Most strains isolated from diarrheal stools are β-hemolytic on a special blood agar (**Kanagawa phenomenon**), whereas most marine isolates are not. Some strains also have peritrichous flagella that are immunologically distinct from the cell's single polar flagellum.

Antibiotics are used only in protracted or dysentery-like cases. The organism is sensitive *in vitro* to tetracycline, chloramphenicol, penicillin, ampicillin, and aminoglycosides.

V. VULNIFICUS, V. ALGINOLYTICUS, *AND GROUP F VIBRIOS.* These organisms are halophilic vibrios that on occasion cause extraintestinal disease in man after exposure to seawater or contaminated seafood. *V. vulnificus* has been the cause of wound infections and frequently fatal septicemia in compromised patients. *V. alginolyticus* can cause ear and wound infections. Group F vibrios cause opportunistic infections that often result in bloody diarrhea. All these species produce several potent cytotoxins and enterotoxins.

Aeromonas

Organisms of the *Aeromonas* group (aeromonads) are found in natural water sources and soil and are frequent pathogens for cold-blooded marine and freshwater animals. *A. hydrophila* and *A. (Plesiomonas) shigelloides* may easily be mistaken for *E. coli* because of their similar reactions; some strains ferment lactose. However, aeromonads are **oxidase-positive** and possess a **single polar flagellum,** like the pseudomonads (Chap. 28) and the vibrios. Enterotoxic, cytotoxic, and hemolytic exotoxins have recently been detected in *A. hydrophila*. These organisms have been associated in man with septicemia, pneumonia, and moderate to severe gastroenteritis. Their recognized incidence in serious human disease has been steadily increasing, and many isolates are probably misidentified as coliforms. The organisms have also been isolated from urine, sputum, feces, and bile without evident pathogenic significance.

Most strains are sensitive to gentamicin, the tetracyclines, polymyxin, and trimethoprim–sulfamethoxazole.

Campylobacter

Among the species of *Campylobacter*, *C. jejuni* and the closely related *C. coli* are common causes of gastrointestinal disease characterized by bloody diarrhea with abdominal pain and fever. Infections are recognized with increasing frequency in infants and children (especially those with pet dogs), in the aged (particularly in individuals suffering from debilitating disorders), and in homosexual men, where the infection is associated with proctitis. Organisms can be isolated not only from stool and, rarely, blood (5%), but also from the placenta and spinal fluid.

A third, newly recognized species, *C. pylori*, colonizes the stomach and causes a chronic gastritis. *C. intestinalis* most often causes serious systemic infections in immunocompromised hosts and can usually be isolated from blood or spinal fluid but infrequently from feces. *C. fetus* (previously *Vibrio fetus*) infections in cattle, sheep, and goats result in abortions and sterility. The biological and molecular basis of the invasive properties of *Campylobacter* is unknown.

Campylobacter are easily missed during routine culture because they are **microaerophilic:** they grow best, albeit slowly, at 42°C in an atmosphere containing 5% oxygen and 10% CO_2 but not in ordinary air. They ferment components of peptone but not carbohydrates. Most *Campylobacter* strains are susceptible to erythromycin and quinolones.

Selected Reading

BOOKS AND REVIEW ARTICLES

Achtman M, Pluschke G: Clonal analysis of descent and virulence among selected *Escherichia coli*. Annu Rev Microbiol 40:79, 1986

Bagg A, Neilands JB: Molecular mechanism of regulation of siderophore-mediated iron assimilation. Microbiol Rev 51:509, 1987

Betley MJ, Miller VL, Mekalanos JJ: Genetics of bacterial enterotoxins. Annu Rev Microbiol 40:577, 1986

Butzler JP (ed): Campylobacter Infections in Man and Animals. Boca Raton, Florida, CRC Press, 1984

Clerc P, Baudry B, Sansonetti PJ: Molecular mechanisms of entry, intracellular multiplication and killing of host cells by Shigellae. Curr Top Microbiol Immunol 138:3, 1988

Ewing WH: Edwards and Ewing's Identification of *Enterobacteriaceae*, 4th ed. New York, Elsevier Science, 1986

Falkow S, Small P, Isberg R, Hayes SF, Corwin D: A molecular strategy for the study of bacterial invasion. Rev Infect Dis 9 (suppl 5):S450, 1987

Finkelstein RA, Sciortino CV, McIntosh MA: Role of iron in microbe–host interactions. Rev Infect Dis 5 (suppl 4):S759, 1983

Finlay BB, Faklow S: Virulence factors associated with *Salmonella* species. Microbiol Sci 5:324, 1988

Freter R, Jones GW: Models for studying the role of bacterial attachment in virulence and pathogenesis. Rev Infect Dis 5 (suppl 4):S647, 1983

Gaastra W, DeGraaf FK: Host-specific fimbrial adhesins of noninvasive enterotoxigenic *Escherichia coli* strains. Microbiol Rev 46:129, 1982

Jann K, Jann B: Polysaccharide antigens of *Escherichia coli*. Rev Infect Dis 9 (suppl 5):S517, 1987

Klemm P: Fimbrial adhesions of *Escherichia coli*. Rev Infect Dis 7:321, 1985

Levine MM: *Escherichia coli* that cause diarrhea: Enterotoxigenic, enteropathogenic, enteroinvasive, enterohemorrhagic and enteroadherent. J Infect Dis 154:377, 1987

Maurelli AT, Sansonetti PJ: Genetic determinants of *Shigella* pathogenicity. Annu Rev Microbiol 42:127, 1988

Miller JF, Mekalanos JJ, Falkow S: Coordinate regulation and sensory transduction in the control of bacterial virulence. Science 243:916, 1989

Miller VL, Finlay BB, Falkow S: Factors essential for the penetration of mammalian cells by *Yersinia*. Curr Top Microbiol Immunol 138:15, 1988

Mooi FR, DeGraaf FK: Molecular biology of fimbriae of enterotoxigenic *Escherichia coli*. Curr Top Microbiol Immunol 118:119, 1985

Moulder JW: Comparative biology of intracellular parasitism. Microbiol Rev 49:298, 1985

Reid G, Sobel JD: Bacterial adherence in the pathogenesis of urinary tract infection: A review. Rev Infect Dis 9:470, 1987

Riley LW: The epidemiologic, clinical and microbial features of hemorrhagic colitis. Annu Rev Microbiol 41:383, 1987

Silver RP, Aaronson W, Vann WF: The K1 polysaccharide of *Escherichia coli*. Rev Infect Dis 10 (Suppl 2):S282, 1988

Sperber SJ, Schleupner CJ: Salmonellosis during infection with human immunodeficiency virus. Rev Infect Dis 9:925, 1987

Timmis KN, Boulnois GJ, Bitter SD, Cabello FC: Surface components of *Escherichia coli* that mediate resistance to the bactericidal activities of serum and phagocytes. Curr Top Microbiol Immunol 118:197, 1985

Uhlin BE, Baga M, Goransson M, et al: Genes determining adhesin formation in uropathogenic *Escherichia coli*. Curr Top Microbiol Immunol 118:163, 1985

SPECIFIC ARTICLES

Abraham SN, Sun D, Dale JB, Beachey EH: Conservation of the D-mannose-adhesion protein among type 1 fimbriated members of the family *Enterobacteriaceae*. Nature 336:682, 1988

Baldini MM, Kaper JB, Levine MM, Candy DCA, Moon HW: Plasmid-mediated adhesion in enteropathogenic *Escherichia coli*. J Pediatr Gastroenterol Nutrition 2:534, 1983

Beltran P, Musser JM, Helmuth R, et al: Toward a population genetic analysis of *Salmonella*: Genetic diversity and relationships among strains of serotypes *choleraesius, derby, dublin, enteritidis, heidelberg, infantis, newport,* and *typhimurium*. Proc Natl Acad Sci USA 85:7753, 1988

Blaser MJ, Rellen LB: *Campylobacter* enteritis. N Engl J Med 305:1444, 1981

Clerc P, Sansonetti PJ: Entry of *Shigella flexneri* into HeLa cells: Evidence for directed phagocytosis involving actin polymerization and myosin accumulation. Infect Immun 55:2681, 1987

Farmer JJ III, Davis BR, Hickman–Brenner FW, et al: Biochemical identification of new species and biogroups of *Enterobacteriaceae* isolated from clinical specimens. J Clin Microbiol 21:46, 1985

Fields PI, Swanson RV, Haidaris CG, Heffron F: Mutants of *Salmonella typhimurium* that cannot survive within the macrophage are avirulent. Proc Natl Acad Sci USA 83:5189, 1986

Finlay BB, Heffron F, Falkow S: Epithelial cell surfaces induce *Salmonella* proteins required for bacterial adherence and invasion. Science 243:940, 1989

Finlay BB, Gumbiner B, Falkow S: Penetration of *Salmonella* through a polarized Madin–Darby canine kidney epithelial cell monolayer. J Cell Biol 107:221, 1988

Finlay BB, Falkow S: Comparison of the invasion strategies used by *Salmonella cholerae-suis, Shigella flexneri* and *Yersinia enterocolitica* to enter cultured animal cells: Endosome acidification is not required for bacterial invasion or intracellular replication. Biochimie 70:1089, 1988

Giannella RA, Washington O, Gemski P, Formal SB: Invasion of HeLa cells by *Salmonella typhimurium:* A model for study of invasiveness of *Salmonella*. J Infect Dis 128:69, 1973

Gorbach SL (ed): Infectious diarrhea. Inf Dis Clin North Am 2:557, 1988

Gulig PA, Curtiss R III: Plasmid-associated virulence of *Salmonella typhimurium*. Infect Immun 55:2891, 1987

Hale TL, Formal SB: Genetics of virulence in *Shigella*. Microbial Pathogen 1:511, 1986

Israele V, Darabi A, McCracken GHJ: The role of bacterial virulence factors and Tamm–Horsfall protein in the pathogenesis of *Escherichia coli* urinary tract infection in infants. Am J Dis Child 141:1230, 1987

Labigne RA, Falkow S: Distribution and degree of heterogeneity of the afimbrial–adhesin-encoding operon (*afa*) among uropathogenic *Escherichia coli* isolates. Infect Immun 56:640, 1988

Lund B, Marklund BI, Stromberg N, et al: Uropathogenic *Escherichia coli* can express serologically identical pili of different receptor binding specificities. Mol Microbiol 2:255, 1988

Maurelli AT, Baudry B, dHauteville H, Hale TL, Sansonetti PJ: Cloning of plasmid DNA sequences involved in invasion of HeLa cells by *Shigella flexneri*. Infect Immun 49:164, 1985

Miller VL, Taylor RK, Mekalanos JJ: Cholera toxin transcriptional activator *toxR* is a transmembrane DNA binding protein. Cell 48:271, 1987

Minion FC, Abraham SN, Beachey EH, Goguen JD: The genetic determinant of adhesive function in type 1 fimbriae of *Escherichia coli* is distinct from the gene encoding the fimbrial subunit. J Bacteriol 165:1033, 1986

Norgren M, Normark S, Lark D, et al: Mutations in *E. coli* cistrons affecting adhesion to human cells do not abolish Pap pili fiber formation. EMBO J 3:1159, 1984

Sansonetti PJ, Ryter A, Clerc P, Maurelli AT, Mounier J: Multiplication of *Shigella flexneri* within HeLa cells: Lysis of the phagocytic vacuole and plasmid-mediated contact hemolysis. Infect Immun 51:461, 1986

Selander RK, Musser JM, Caugant DA, Gilmor MN, Whittam TS: Population genetics of pathogenic bacteria. Microbial Pathogen 3:1, 1987

Stocker BA: Auxotrophic *Salmonella typhi* as live vaccine. Vaccine 6:141, 1988

Taylor RK, Miller VL, Furlong DB, Mekalanos J: Use of *phoA* gene fusions to identify a pilus colonization factor coordinately regulated with cholera toxin. Proc Natl Acad Sci USA 84:2833, 1987

28

Stanley Falkow, Ph.D.

Bacteroides and Fusobacterium

The classic anaerobic infections described in the medical literature—tetanus, botulism, and gas gangrene—are caused by gram-positive, spore-forming bacteria of the genus *Clostridium*, which all produce potent exotoxins (Chap. 34). However, with advances in the methods for transporting, culturing, and identifying anaerobic bacteria, we have come to appreciate that gram-negative anaerobes, mostly members of the genus *Bacteroides*, are the most frequent cause of the anaerobic infections seen in clinical practice, even though these organisms do not form potent toxins. These obligately anaerobic, non–spore-forming, non-motile, gram-negative bacilli are also prevalent in the indigenous flora and in the gut on mucosal surfaces; and when there is significant necrosis or impaired oxygenation of the tissues, various members contribute to mixed infections.

The importance of *Bacteroides* in mixed human infection may be related to their **relaxed anaerobiosis:** they can survive exposure to oxygen for long periods, although they do not grow in its presence. Some species produce catalase; *B. fragilis* also produces superoxide dismutase (SOD; see Chap. 4). The oxygen tolerance of *Bacteroides* stands in sharp contrast to the exquisite susceptibility of many other anaerobes.

Bacteroides Species

Bacteroides accounts for as much as 30% of all fecal isolates. The most numerous *Bacteroides* of the colon (total 10^{10} per gram dry fecal weight), all **bile resistant,** are *B. vulgatus, B. distasonis,* and *B. thetaiotaomicron.* The principal pathogenic species, *B. fragilis,* is a relatively minor member of the gastrointestinal flora (ca. 10^4–10^5/g).

589

The oropharynx and upper gastrointestinal tract in healthy individuals are devoid of colonic species but contain a group of **bile-sensitive** species, including another common pathogen, *B. melaninogenicus*, as well as *B. oralis*, *B. asaccharolyticus*, and *B. ruminicola*. The vaginal flora also contains *Bacteroides* species, predominantly *B. melaninogenicus*, *B. bivius*, *B. disiens*, and occasionally *B. fragilis*.

B. fragilis is the most important of all anaerobic species because of its frequency in clinical infection and its growing resistance to antimicrobial agents. It is an irregularly staining, pleomorphic, gram-negative rod with rounded ends that grows well on ordinary blood agar under anaerobic conditions. It is resistant to and may even be stimulated in its growth by bile; indeed, most strains can conjugate bile salts. Glucose and a number of carbohydrates are fermented via the glycolytic pathway. The resulting endproducts—acetate, propionate, and succinate—have proved important for taxonomic studies utilizing gas-liquid chromatography.

B. melaninogenicus and *B. asaccharolyticus* are short to coccoid rods that produce a heme-derived pigment, yielding distinctive brown to black colonies on blood agar. Most strains require vitamin K as well as heme for growth.

Bacteroides appear to be responsible for much of the polysaccharide digestion that occurs in the human colon. This carbohydrate includes both dietary and host-derived polysaccharides that cannot be digested by the host enzymes in the upper bowel. Indeed, *Bacteroides* species that degrade cellulose have been isolated from human feces. *Bacteroides* species also attack the host-derived mucins.

A role for *Bacteroides* in the etiology of colon cancer, and also in other noninfectious disease of the bowel (e.g., ulcerative colitis), has been suggested but is not established. There is evidence that certain *Bacteroides* species produce mutagenic substances within the lumen of the bowel, but they also can inactivate mutagenic substances.

CELL ENVELOPE. *Bacteroides* are unusual in their lipid composition: about half of their extractable lipids are sphingolipids and ceramides. In addition, the lipopolysaccharide (LPS) lacks the 3-keto-2-deoxyoctanoic acid and heptose found in the LPS of other gram-negative bacteria, and it is far less toxic than the classic LPS of the *Enterobacteriaceae*.

B. fragilis, unlike other *Bacteroides* species, possesses a specific polysaccharide **capsule** that is easily seen in the electron microscope. The main components are L-fucose, D-galactose, DL-quinovasamine and D-glucosamine. As in some other pathogens, the capsule appears to be a critical virulence factor: unencapsulated strains are far less virulent in animal models of intra-abdominal abscess formation, and *B. fragilis* is more resistant to phagocytosis than are other *Bacteroides* species.

Fusobacterium Species

Members of the anaerobic genus *Fusobacterium* are also important in both the normal flora and infection. These pale-staining, slender, gram-negative bacilli with tapered ends (hence the name) grow readily on ordinary blood agar with a characteristic "fried egg" colony. They weakly ferment glucose and other carbohydrates, and their principal metabolic endproduct, in contrast to *Bacteroides*, is butyric acid. This difference can be exploited for identification of clinical isolates by gas-liquid chromatography. Some species possess LPS with typical components found in enteric bacteria. They are not encapsulated.

Six species are common inhabitants of the oral cavity, gastrointestinal tract, and genital tract. In dental plaque they may represent as much as 4% of all anaerobic isolates. They are minor components of the colonic flora but are sometimes a major component of the vaginal flora. The most frequent isolates in human clinical infection are *F. necrophorum*, in liver abscesses, and *F. nucleatum*, in anaerobic pleuropulmonary infections.

Clinical Features and Pathogenesis

Anaerobic infection generally results when a deficit in the normal host defense network from antecedent infection, tissue destruction, or compromised blood supply leads to a local reduction in oxidation–reduction potential, coupled with opportunistic seeding with nearby normal flora. The source of most anaerobic bacteria in human infection is the patient's own normal flora that have spread beyond the mucocutaneous barrier of their normal site in the oropharynx, gastrointestinal tract, or genital region (Table 28–1). Anaerobic infections are thus characteristically polymicrobial, with **aerobic and anaerobic components acting in concert.** Certain members of the normal flora, especially *B. fragilis*, may predominate because they possess determinants that add to their virulence.

Anaerobic bacteria resident in the upper airways, particularly *B. melaninogenicus* and *F. nucleatum* together with peptostreptococci, may move into normally sterile structures to cause deep infection of the head and neck. Fully 85% of **brain abscesses** yield anaerobes, which probably arise from antecedent infection of the paranasal sinuses and the middle ear. Similarly, anaerobic bacteria are implicated in almost 90% of **aspiration pneumonias** and in **lung abscess.**

TABLE 28–1. Infections Commonly Associated with Anaerobes

Site	Likely to Involve Anaerobes	Unlikely to Involve Anaerobes

Head and Neck	Chronic sinusitis
	Chronic otitis media
	Periodontal abscess
	Space infections
		Acute infections of:
		  Sinuses
		  Nasopharynx
		  Middle ear

CNS	Brain abscess (nontraumatic) Subdural empyema	Meningitis
Pulmonary	Aspiration pneumonia Necrotizing pneumonia Abscess Adult empyema	Bronchitis Lobar pneumonia
Intra-abdominal	Peritonitis and abscess Liver abscess Cholangitis	Peritonitis (spontaneous or "primary") Cholecystitis Pancreatitis

Female genital	Salpingitis and pelvic
	  peritonitis
	Tuboovarian abscess
	Vulvovaginal abscess
	Septic abortion and
	  endometritis
		Cystitis
		Pyelonephritis
		Urethritis

Skin, bone, and muscle	Crepitant cellulitis Myonecrosis Necrotizing fasciitis Synergistic cellulitis	Septic joints Osteomyelitis

Intra-abdominal sepsis (peritonitis and abscess) following perforation of the bowel usually involves several species of anaerobes together with facultative organisms: *B. fragilis* is the predominant anaerobic species in 80% of infections, and it is also the organism most commonly isolated in subsequent positive blood cultures.

B. fragilis, B. bivius, and *B. diseus,* as well as peptostreptococci and clostridia, can be responsible for serious infections of the upper female genital tract. The involvement of obligate anaerobes in **pelvic abscess** is particularly noteworthy, because in about one-third of patients these organisms are found in the absence of facultative species.

Anaerobic infection of the **skin and soft tissues** is commonly secondary to trauma, surgery, or restricted circulation. *B. fragilis,* along with other anaerobes, aerobes, and facultative organisms, is universally associated with decubitus ulcers and is frequent in diabetic foot ulcers.

In all of the infectious processes involving *Bacteroides* and *Fusobacterium,* **abscess formation** and **tissue destruction** are characteristic. Hence, once these organisms are introduced into a site under conditions favorable to their multiplication, these processes maintain the anaerobic environment, often aided by the growth of associated facultative species.

With the exception of the capsule of *B. fragilis,* none of the non–spore-forming anaerobes has precisely defined determinants of pathogenicity, although the myriad of enzymes produced by some of these species may play a role. Thus, *B. melaninogenicus* possesses high collagenase activity, and it and other *Bacteroides* produce neuraminidase. Similarly, many *Bacteroides* produce hyaluronidase, deoxyribonuclease, fibrinolysin, and phosphatase. *B. fragilis* synthesizes a heparinase that may contribute to intravascular clotting. *F. necrophorum* produces a potent leukocidin and hemolysin.

Mixed infections with only a few species generally evolve after inoculation of a vast array of normal flora, owing to selection of strains endowed with virulence factors that facilitate their multiplication within the host's tissues. Precise analysis of these factors must await the development of genetic tools. It is not clear whether the polymicrobial nature of most so-called anaerobic suppurative processes reflects an important microbial synergy or obscures a central pathogenic mechanism.

Laboratory Diagnosis

The possibility of an anaerobic infection may be suggested by location adjacent to a mucosal surface. A **foul-smelling discharge is pathognomonic,** although its absence does not exclude the diagnosis. Other indices include gas in the tissues, severe tissue necrosis, abscess formation, and gangrene—especially if the gram stain of infected material shows many organisms that do not emerge on routine aerobic culture and if the infection fails to respond to antimicrobials, such as the aminoglycosides, that are not active against anaerobes.

The collection of specimens for anaerobic culturing takes into account the lethal effect of atmospheric oxygen, and special gassed, stoppered collection tubes have been devised for this purpose. Appropriate media inoculated with clinical material are incubated under anaerobic conditions. Because infecting anaerobic organisms originate from the normal flora of the mucocutaneous surfaces, it may be impossible to distinguish pathogen from commensal in contaminated specimens. Appropriate clinical samples include blood and abscess contents.

Several **anaerobic culture systems** are available. The most common system utilizes a plastic jar and a commercially available chemical mixture, which, in the presence of water, generates H_2 that is catalytically converted together with any O_2 into water. Alternatively, specially prepared prereduced sterilized media can be employed. The most flexible system is the anaerobic glovebox, consisting of a contained vinyl plastic chamber with an airlock and gloves or sleeves to permit the manipulation of media and cultures within the chamber, which is kept anaerobic by the same catalytic principle just described. The advantages of the isolator chamber are that detailed studies can be done using standard bacteriological procedures, and media can be prepared conventionally and reduced in the chamber. Additionally, the chamber can be easily maintained at 37°C to act also as an incubator.

The primary cultivation of anaerobic species from clinical material usually involves an all-purpose solid medium, such as blood agar, to ensure the recovery of fastidious and nonfastidious organisms alike, together with a selective solid medium, usually incorporating antibiotics, to facilitate the rapid isolation of certain pathogens, particularly *B. fragilis* or pigmented *Bacteroides* species, from the polymicrobial flora so typical of anaerobic infections. A broth medium, typically thioglycollate, is also utilized to enhance the growth of anaerobic pathogens that may be present in low numbers within a clinical sample.

Species are identified by gram stain, resistance to bile, fermentation patterns, pigment production, antimicrobial susceptibility patterns, and analysis of the fatty acid endproducts of glucose metabolism. Some of these methods are time-consuming, and complete identification of anaerobic species can be prohibitively expensive.

Therapy and Antimicrobial Susceptibility

The treatment of anaerobic infection entails surgical drainage and the use of appropriate antibiotics. Surgery is often essential to achieve the drainage of pus and the removal of necrotic tissue, and in uncomplicated cases it may be curative. In most severe infections, however, antibiotics are also required. This is not a simple matter, because, as already noted, such infections are usually polymicrobial. Definitive diagnosis rests on demonstrating and culturing the organisms from the infection, but a gram stain alone can be helpful, because the *Bacteroides* and fusobacteria each display distinctive morphologies. Direct gas-liquid chromatography of clinical specimens may also be useful; a large amount of butyric acid points to *Fusobacterium*, and succinic acid to *Bacteroides*. The clinician is often forced to rely initially on empiric antimicrobial therapy, so knowledge of the anaerobes (and other microbial species) generally associated with the various types of infection is valuable.

The selection of antimicrobials depends on whether the infection is **above or below the diaphragm.** Infections of the head and neck, lungs and pleura, and the brain are usually associated with the anaerobes of the **oral flora.** These bacteria (*Fusobacterium*, peptostreptococci, and *B. melaninogenicus*) are ordinarily susceptible to penicillin G, and for many years this was considered

the drug of choice, with clindamycin and chloramphenicol as secondary alternatives. In recent years, however, there has been a steady rise in the incidence of penicillin-resistant *B. melaninogenicus*, so some of the newer cephalosporins are increasingly useful.

For infections below the diaphragm, including intra-abdominal, pelvic, and soft tissue infections, the predominant pathogen is *B. fragilis*. Not only is this species the most virulent of the anaerobes, but many strains have become resistant to tetracycline, penicillins, and many cephalosporins. The emergence of clindamycin resistance has also been documented, and there are scattered reports of resistance to chloramphenicol and metranidazole. However, cefoxitin, piperacillin, and moxalactam have proved to be effective. Anaerobes are resistant to the aminoglycosides because electron transport is needed for effective uptake (Chap. 10). Most of the emerging resistance within the *Bacteroides* group is attributable to plasmids, as will be described below.

In infections below the waist, a successful regimen must also cover the common accompanying aerobic and facultative species. Accordingly, the treatment of these mixed infections employs a combination of an aminoglycoside and an antibiotic with an anaerobic spectrum. The choice is critical, as different regimens in *Bacteroides* bacteremia have yielded mortality rates ranging from 12% to 60%.

Genetics

Genetic studies of anaerobic bacteria, beginning with the mechanisms of antibiotic resistance, promise to increase our understanding of their physiology and their interactions with the host in health and in disease. In 1979 transmissible clindamycin resistance was discovered in *B. fragilis*, subsequently shown to be classic macrolide–lincosamide–streptogramin resistance (MLS[r]) mediated by a methylase affecting 23S rRNA (see Chap. 10). This resistance determinant shows striking similarity to *MLS* genes from staphylococcal and streptococcal plasmids and transposons as well as from erythromycin-producing *Streptomyces*. A conjugative plasmid carrying MLS[r] can transfer it to other species of *Bacteroides*. Plasmid-linked chloramphenicol acetyltransferase has also been reported in the *Bacteroides*.

In the early 1960s nearly all *B. fragilis* isolates were susceptible to tetracycline, but nearly two-thirds of isolates are now resistant, and tetracycline is no longer of therapeutic value in anaerobic infections. The mechanism is a decreased net uptake of the drug. Transfer of tetracycline resistance (Tc[r]) by *B. fragilis* has been demonstrated. A surprising finding is that this transfer is not associated with plasmid DNA, yet it appears to be conjugative (DNase-resistant, requiring cell-to-cell contact); hence the "tet transfer element" appears to be chromosomal, like the transferable element called a conjugative transposon (see Chap. 7) found in *Streptococcus faecalis*. The transfer of Tc^r to *Bacteroides* recipients is stimulated by growth in subinhibitory concentrations of the antibiotic, which evidently induces synthesis of an apparatus for chromosome transfer.

Most clindamycin-resistant *Bacteroides* are also Tc^r, and transfer of the two resistances is often linked. Similar Tc^r transfer has been described in *Clostridium perfringens* and *C. difficile*.

Transfer of genes has been observed between *B. fragilis* and *E. coli*. With the ability to clone *Bacteroides* DNA in *E. coli* and transfer it back again, the powerful methods of recombinant DNA technology can now be applied to anaerobic bacteria.

Selected Reading

Finegold SM: Anaerobic Bacteria in Human Disease. New York, Academic Press, 1977

Finegold SM, George WL, Rolfe RD (eds): International Symposium on Anaerobic Bacteria and Their Role in Disease. Rev Infect Dis 6(Suppl 1), March–April, 1984

Smith L, Williams BL: The Pathogenic Anaerobic Bacteria, 3rd Ed. Springfield, Ill, Charles C Thomas, 1984

Salyers AA: *Bacteroides* of the human lower intestinal tract. Annu Rev Microbiol 38:293–313, 1984

Tally FP, Bieluch VM, Cuchural GJ: Malamy MH: Antimicrobial resistance in *Bacteroides*. Drugs Exp Clin Res 10:149–154, 1984

29

Stephen Lory

Pseudomonads and Other Nonfermenting Bacilli*

The nonfermenting gram-negative rods, a heterogeneous group, are incapable of fermenting a variety of sugars, in contrast to the *Enterobacteriaceae* that are often isolated from the same source. Most species are strict aerobes, but a few can ferment compounds other than sugars. These organisms are abundant in natural reservoirs such as soil, water, and the normal flora of humans. Some can cause serious infections in man, primarily in immuno-compromised patients. The most important clinically (more than 70% of those isolated in clinical laboratories) are members of the genus *Pseudomonas*, followed by a small group of opportunistic pathogens, including *Acinetobacter*, *Moraxella*, *Alcaligenes*, *Flavobacterium*, and *Achromobacterium*. All of these may be nosocomial pathogens, so rapid identification and epidemiologic characterization are important in tracking hospital out-breaks. The related *Rhizobium* and *Agrobacterium* are important in agriculture but are not human pathogens.

Pseudomonas

Like *Enterobacteriaceae*, members of the genus *Pseudomonas* are motile, gram-negative rods capable of growing on simple laboratory media. Unlike *Enterobacteriaceae*, however, they have **polar** rather than peritrichous **fla-gella,** are oxidase positive, are obligate aerobes, and me-

* The contributions of the late Dr. Alex C. Sonnenwirth, from the preced-ing edition, are gratefully acknowledged.

tabolize sugars via the 2-keto-deoxygluconate (Entner–Doudoroff) pathway (Chap. 4) rather than by glycolysis. Some strains can utilize nitrate as a terminal electron acceptor, which may account for the occasional isolation of pseudomonads from anaerobic environments.

The genus *Pseudomonas* has been assigned to an unusually broad range of organisms, with the G + C content of their DNA from 56% to 70%. Nucleic acid hybridization analysis leads to subdivision into the Fluorescent, Pseudomallei, Acidovorans, Diminuta, and Xanthomonas groups, with little cross-hybridization. Human pathogens are almost exclusively of the first two subgroups.

FLUORESCENT GROUP: PSEUDOMONAS AERUGINOSA AND RELATED FORMS

DISTRIBUTION. *P. aeruginosa* can be found in most moist environments and occasionally in the normal intestinal or skin flora. In hospitals, sinks, respiratory therapy equipment, and humidifiers can be important sources. The ability to use simple organic molecules as a carbon and energy source allows multiplication of these organisms in solutions that would not support most bacterial growth, such as weak antiseptic, saline, and soap solutions. In addition, patients may be infected systemically by their own normal flora.

Because of its ubiquitous presence, *P. aeruginosa* can be found in clinical samples as a contaminant without any relation to disease. The underlying condition of the patient is important in assessing the clinical relevance of an isolation, as this organism rarely infects healthy, nonhospitalized individuals. However, *P. aeruginosa* is re-sponsible for some of the most serious and lethal infections of immunocompromised individuals. It exhibits unusually high levels of resistance to many antibiotics; hence, the introduction of broad-spectrum antibiotics, suppressing other flora, has resulted in its emergence as a significant nosocomial pathogen.

Laboratory Identification

P. aeruginosa grows on most rich media employed for primary isolations of aerobic bacteria, forming flat spreading colonies with irregular edges. Strong hemolysis is noticeable on blood agar plates, especially on longer incubation. Like other members of the fluorescent pseudomonad subgroup, *P. aeruginosa* produces a fluorescent, water-soluble greenish-yellow pigment called **pyoverdin** and a second, blue, nonfluorescent phenazine pigment termed **pyocyanin.** These pigments diffuse around colonies and aid in the initial identification. Colonies from initial isolation plates are confirmed as oxidase-positive microorganisms, capable of oxidizing glucose, xylose, fructose, and galactose but not lactose or maltose. They produce arginine dihydrolase, indophenol oxidase, and proteases. Ability to grow at 42°C distinguishes *P. aeruginosa* from other fluorescent pseudomonads. The most important biochemical reactions are listed in Table 29–1.

Typing sera, bacteriophage or bacteriocin typing systems, and DNA hybridization techniques are used primarily for epidemiologic studies of nosocomial outbreaks. The presence of a large number of serologically nontypable strains reflects the diversity of the cell-surface structures found in this organism.

TABLE 29–1. Some Differential Characteristics of Nonfermentative Gram-negative Bacilli

	Pseudomonas aeruginosa	*P. fluorescens*	*P. pseudomallei*	*P. mallei*	*P. cepacia*	*P. maltophilia*	*P. stutzeri*	*P. acidovorans*	*Acinetobacter anitratum (Herellea)**	*A. lwoffi (Mima)†*	*Flavobacterium spp.*	*Alcaligenes faecalis*
Fluorescein	+	+	–	–	–	–	–	–	–	–	–	–
O-F medium	O	O	O	O	O	O	O	O	O	N	O/F	N
MacConkey agar	+	+	+	–	+	+	+	+	+	+	+/–	+
Motility	+	+	+	–	+	+	+	+	–	–	–	+/–
Oxidase	+	+	w+	w+	+	–	+	+	–	–	+	+
Growth: 42°C	+	–	+	+	+/–	+/–	+/–	–	+	+/–	–	+/–
Growth: 4°C	–	+	–	–	–	–	–	–	–	–	–	?
Gluconate oxidation	+	+/–	–	–	–	–	–	–	–	–	–	–
Glucose (O-F)	+	+	+	+	+	–	+	+	+	–	+/–	–
Gelatinase	+	+	+	–	+/–	+	–	–	–	+/–	+	–
Arginine dihydrolase	+	+	+	+	–	–	–	–	–	–	–	–

† No acid from 10% lactose medium.

O = oxidative; N = nonoxidative; F = fermentative; ? = not determined; +/– = variable; + = positive; – = negative; w = weak.

* Acid from 10% lactose medium.

Pathogenicity

Whereas *P. aeruginosa* rarely causes disease in healthy individuals, it can be a serious pathogen of patients with immunodeficiencies or neutropenic malignancies. Children and young adults suffering from **cystic fibrosis** invariably become colonized in their respiratory tract by **highly mucoid variants.** Invasive surgical procedures, long-term catheterization, and severe trauma such as burns and wounds can also lead to serious infections.

Several cell-surface components play a role in pathogenesis. The **endotoxin** of *P. aeruginosa* can elicit responses similar to those of enterobacteria but is several orders of magnitude less toxic. **Fimbriae** found on most *P. aeruginosa* strains have been shown to be attachment and colonization factors, as with *Neisseria gonorrhoeae* (Chap. 26). There are many different, non–cross-reactive fimbrial serotypes.

ALGINATE CAPSULE. Many bacteria are surrounded by a layer of exopolysaccharide sometimes called the capsule, slime layer, or glycocalyx, depending on its relative affinity for the bacterial cell. The mucoid layer is particularly evident on fresh isolates of *P. aeruginosa* from the sputum of **cystic fibrosis patients,** where the quantity by weight may exceed that of the entire bacterial cell (Fig. 29–1); subsequent subculture results in their reversion to more typical, non-mucoid forms. The exopolysaccharide allows bacteria to adhere to each other, forming micro-

colonies in the lungs of patients with *P. aeruginosa* pneumonia; and the surrounding anionic matrix also protects the large bacterial mass from phagocytes and from the action of antibodies and complement.

The exopolysaccharide resembles that produced by certain marine algae; hence its name "alginate." It is a polymer of acetylated D-mannuronic and L-guluronic acids (Fig. 29–2), but, unlike many bacterial capsules, these components are not arranged as orderly repeating disaccharide units. Instead, alginate contains homopolymer domains of one or the other residue. This arrangement presents a complex antigenic picture to the host, and despite an active immune response to the polysaccharide, the antibodies provide little protection against repeated infections.

EXOTOXIN A. An extracellular toxic protein, exotoxin A, is produced by more than 90% of *P. aeruginosa* isolates. Like diphtheria toxin, it is induced by iron limitation, as is found in most tissues. It is excreted as a 66,000-dalton polypeptide that is highly toxic when administered to susceptible animals (the LD_{50} in mice is 100 ng). Exotoxin A exerts its lethal action by binding to receptors on a variety of cells and entering the cytoplasm, where it catalyzes the covalent modification of elongation factor 2 (EF-2), like diphtheria toxin (Chap. 22), by ADP-ribosylation of a unique amino acid, diphthamide.

Despite an identical molecular mode of action, exotoxin A differs considerably from diphtheria toxin. The amino acid sequences have little homology. Like diphtheria toxin, exotoxin A is released from bacteria as a cytotoxic but enzymatically inactive polypeptide; but instead of being cleaved into an enzymatically active fragment A and a fragment B that binds to the target-cell receptor, exotoxin A undergoes activation by unfolding, which results in exposure of the carboxy-terminal catalytic domain. Moreover, it enters via different receptors from those utilized by diphtheria toxin. Consequently, the relative toxicities of the two toxins for various animals is quite different. Trace amounts of exotoxin A completely inhibit protein synthesis in rodent cell lines, whereas cultured cells from humans or primates are considerably more resistant. In contrast, diphtheria toxin is highly toxic to cultured human cells, but mouse and rat cells are completely refractory.

Despite its low toxicity for human cells, exotoxin A appears to play a role in human disease, as a fatal outcome is correlated with a poor antitoxic Ab response. Moreover, strains of *P. aeruginosa* that do not synthesize exotoxin A are avirulent in several animal models.

Interestingly, some *P. aeruginosa* strains produce an ADP-ribosyltransferase distinct from exotoxin A. This enzyme, termed **exoenzyme S,** modifies several eukaryotic proteins other than EF-2. Strains of *P. aeruginosa* that do not produce exoenzyme S are less virulent in animal

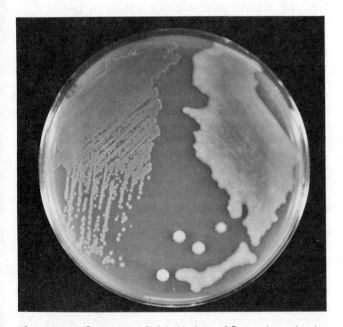

Figure 29–1. Comparison of clinical isolates of *P. aeruginosa* showing differences in production of alginate exopolysaccharide. Strain streaked on the *left* side of the plate was isolated from a wound infection; strain on the *right* was isolated from a patient with cystic fibrosis.

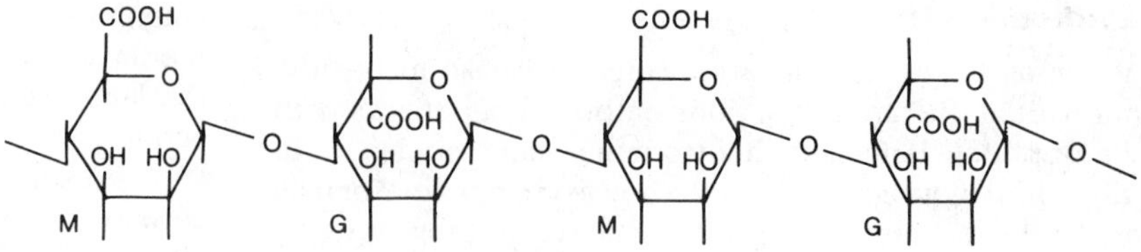

Figure 29–2. Structure of alginate exopolysaccharide of *P. aeruginosa*. The alternating sugars of D-mannuronic acid *(M)* and L-guluronic acid *(G)* are joined via a β (1–4) linkage. Carboxyl groups of mannuronic acids are occasionally acetylated.

models than strains that do. The physiological process that this enzyme affects in the infected host has not been delineated.

P. aeruginosa also produces a number of distinct **extracellular proteases** during infection. In addition to facilitating invasion and dissemination of the organisms, these enzymes make nutrients available by breakdown of host tissues, and they destroy Igs and complement. One of the proteases, an **elastase,** destroys the elastin lining of blood vessels, and it has been implicated in the hemorrhagic and necrotic lesions of the lung and skin that characterize *P. aeruginosa* septicemia and in the rapid destruction of the cornea during eye infections.

Other virulence factors obtained from clinical isolates of *P. aeruginosa* include a protein hemolysin with a phospholipase C activity, a glycolipid hemolysin, a leukocidin, and an enterotoxin. Although these have been purified and extensively characterized, their roles in virulence are poorly understood.

Infections Caused by *P. aeruginosa*

Infections of healthy individuals with *P. aeruginosa* are rare and usually mild. Cutaneous infections acquired in swimming pools or hot tubs are usually brief and self-limited.

Serious *Pseudomonas* infections nearly always involve immunocompromised or chronically debilitated patients, and the nature of the underlying condition generally determines the outcome. In cystic fibrosis patients, the respiratory tract is colonized by *P. aeruginosa* late in the disease, and death often results from pulmonary complications of the chronic infection. Patients suffering from hematologic malignancies such as leukemia, or with neutropenia from immunosuppressive therapy, are also at risk, with bacteremic pneumonia being the most common infection. Similarly, long-term intravenous or urinary catheterization, invasive surgical procedures, and severe burns can allow the organism to circumvent the protective layers of the skin and colonize various tissues, often leading to septicemia. *Pseudomonas* endocarditis is occasionally encountered in intravenous drug users, as well as in patients with complications from open heart surgery. Highly destructive ocular infections may be caused by *P. aeruginosa* originating from contaminated ophthalmologic solutions or following severe fa-

cial burns. *Pseudomonas* osteochondritis may result from severe trauma or occasionally from puncture wounds through contaminated clothing. *P. cepacia* can cause a similar range of diseases (see below).

Therapy

Most strains of *P. aeruginosa* are resistant to relatively high levels of most antibiotics in use, for two reasons. First, entry of antibiotics into the periplasmic space and further into the cytoplasm is considerably more restricted than in other gram-negative bacteria, because the porins of the outer membrane, under the influence of divalent cations, limit the passage of water-soluble molecules. Second, high-level resistance mechanisms are present and include production of several β-lactamases and aminoglycoside-inactivating enzymes, acetylation of chloramphenicol, and efficient expulsion of tetracycline. Both plasmid and chromosomal genes are involved. The plasmids are often transmissible, not only within the genus, but to other gram-negative pathogens as well.

Acute, life-threatening infections are treated by injecting a **combination** of tobramycin and an antipseudomonal β-lactam (e.g., azlocillin, piperacillin, or ceftazidime). Oral quinolones (e.g., ciprofloxacin) have proved effective in chronic or milder infection, including those of the eyes, urinary tract, or bones and joints.

Polyvalent vaccines appear to be promising for patients who are at special risk of infection with *P. aeruginosa*. Prophylactic therapy with human monoclonal antibodies against cell-surface Ags is being developed as well.

OTHER MEMBERS

P. fluorescens and *P. putida* are found predominantly in soil and water but can be isolated from hospital environments and contaminated food. Clinical specimens sometimes contain low numbers of these organisms as part of the normal or transient bacterial flora. The pathogenic potential of these species is limited to opportunistic infections in immunocompromised patients. However, the LPS of *P. fluorescens* contains an extremely toxic lipid A moiety, causing a severe **endotoxic shock** following intravenous administration of contaminated solutions. Unlike *P. aeruginosa*, these organisms are relatively sensitive to a wide range of antibiotics.

PSEUDOMALLEI GROUP

The Pseudomallei group includes several opportunistic pathogens: *P. mallei*, *P. pseudomallei*, *P. cepacia*, and *P. pickettii*.

P. mallei is the only non-motile member of the genus *Pseudomonas*. It is the causative agent of **glanders,** a severe infection of horses that is transmitted occasionally to animal handlers. Glanders is extremely rare in Western countries but occurs in parts of Asia, Africa, and South America. The disease is characterized by pneumonia and by necrosis of mucous membranes, skin, and lymphatics. Systemic invasion and septicemia can occur and is usually fatal. Trimethoprim–sulfamethoxazole, chloramphenicol, kanamycin, and tetracycline are used in treatment.

P. pseudomallei is found in the soil and water in tropical areas. It is the causative agent of **melioidosis,** a disease endemic in tropical parts of Asia. The organism is usually inhaled and may remain dormant for several month or even years. Chronic pneumonia, resembling tuberculosis, may then develop. The organism can also cause an acute suppurative infection in traumatized skin lesions and can progress to septicemia. Patients usually respond to chloramphenicol, tetracycline, or trimethoprim–sulfamethoxazole.

P. cepacia has long been recognized as a pathogen of plants, but in recent years it has also been associated with outbreaks in a number of hospitals throughout the world. Environmental reservoirs include contaminated solutions or medical instruments. It can cause the same range of diseases as *P. aeruginosa*, including pulmonary disease in cystic fibrosis patients. It also is resistant to a variety of antimicrobial agents. Infections are treated with chloramphenicol or trimethoprim–sulfamethoxazole and with some cephalosporins.

Other Nonfermenters

ACINETOBACTER. The genus *Acinetobacter* includes a single species, *A. calcoaceticus*. Two variants can be distinguished: *A. calcoaceticus* var. *anitratus* oxidizes glucose with production of acid, whereas var. *lwoffi* lacks this trait. These organisms are short gram-negative rods, frequently found in pairs; they are non-motile (hence the name). They grow only aerobically but are oxidase-negative. *Acinetobacter* can be found widely distributed in the environment and in the normal flora in approximately 10% of healthy individuals. Nosocomial outbreaks of *Acinetobacter* pneumonia and bronchitis have been reported. Intravenous catheterization sometimes leads

to septicemia. Infections are usually treated with carbenicillin, trimethoprim–sulfamethoxazole, colistin, gentamicin, or kanamycin.

FLAVOBACTERIUM. The flavobacteria are non-motile, slender gram-negative rods that form yellow colonies on most solid media. Flavobacteria are widely distributed in nature. *F. meningosepticum* can be highly virulent for the newborn infant, especially the premature; it has been the causative agent in epidemics of septicemia and meningitis with a high fatality rate. Although these infections are usually attributed to contaminated hospital equipment and solutions, the organism has recently been isolated from the female genital tract. Bacteremia caused by *F. meningosepticum* also occurs in postoperative patients, in whom the illness is much milder. Infants with flavobacterial meningitis sometimes have temperatures below normal, whereas adults with septicemia usually have a high fever and recover rapidly. Because many *F. meningosepticum* strains cannot grow at 38°C, it has been suggested that body temperature is an important factor in the difference between the adult and infant responses.

This organism has an unusual antibiotic sensitivity pattern for a gram-negative bacillus: it is resistant to aminoglycosides and penicillins but susceptible to erythromycin, novobiocin, rifampin, trimethoprim–sulfamethoxazole, and vancomycin.

MORAXELLA. Members of the genus *Moraxella* are similar to *Acinetobacter* but are oxidase-positive and highly sensitive to penicillin. Most of these organisms are nutritionally exacting and do not utilize carbohydrates. Because of their microscopic appearance and positive oxidase reaction, they are easily confused with *Neisseria*. *Moraxella lacunata* is a rare cause of conjunctivitis and corneal infections. *M. osloensis*, *M. nonliquefaciens*, and *M. phenylpyruvica* are members of the normal flora of man and may be involved in serious infections.

ACHROMOBACTER. *Achromobacter xylosoxidans*, a motile, oxidase-positive organism first described in 1971, occurs in lower animals as well as free-living in nature. It has been associated with a variety of human illnesses, including meningitis, septicemia, and otitis media.

ALCALIGENES. *Alcaligenes faecalis* is oxidase-positive and usually motile. It does not metabolize usual carbohydrates but does oxidize organic acids and amino acids, making the medium more alkaline. It may be encountered in feces or sputum as a harmless saprophyte, but it has been associated with serious infections. As a contaminant of irrigation fluids and intravenous solutions, it has caused epidemics of urinary tract infections and postoperative septicemia.

Selected References

BOOKS AND REVIEW ARTICLES

Bodey GP, Bolivar R, Fainstein V, Jadeja L: Infections caused by *Pseudomonas aeruginosa*. Rev Infect Dis 5:279, 1983

Brown MRW (ed): Resistance of *Pseudomonas aeruginosa*. New York, John Wiley, 1975

Deretic V, Gill JF, Chakrabarty AM: Alginate biosynthesis: A model system for gene regulation and function in *Pseudomonas*. Biotechnology 5:469, 1987

Doggett RG (ed): *Pseudomonas aeruginosa:* Clinical Manifestations of Infection and Current Therapy. New York, Academic Press, 1979

Gilardi GL (ed): Nonfermentative Gram-Negative Rods: Laboratory Identification and Clinical Aspects. New York, Marcel Dekker, 1984.

Holloway BW, Morgan AF: Genomic organization in *Pseudomonas*. Annu Rev Microbiol 40:79, 1986

Sabath LD (ed): *Pseudomonas aeruginosa:* The Organism, the Diseases It Causes and Their Treatment. Bern, Hans Huber Publishers, 1980

Sokatch JR (ed): The Bacteria, vol. 10: The Biology of *Pseudomonas*. New York, Academic Press, 1986

Pier GB: Pulmonary disease associated with *Pseudomonas aeruginosa* in cystic fibrosis: Current status of the host–bacterium interaction. J Infect Dis 151:575, 1985

Woods DE, Iglewski BH: Toxins of *Pseudomonas aeruginosa:* New perspectives. Rev Infect Disease 5:S715, 1983

SPECIFIC ARTICLES

Cross AS, Sadoff JC, Iglewski BH, Sokol PA: Evidence for the role of toxin A in the pathogenesis of infection with *Pseudomonas aeruginosa* in humans. J Infect Dis 142:538, 1980

Iglewski BH, Kabat D: NAD-dependent inhibition of protein synthesis by *Pseudomonas aeruginosa* toxin. Proc Natl Acad Sci USA 72:2284, 1975

Lam J, Chan R, Lam K, Costerton JW: Production of mucoid microcolonies by *Pseudomonas aeruginosa* within infected lungs in cystic fibrosis. Infect Immun 28:546, 1980

Woods DE, Strauss DC, Johanson WG Jr, Berry VK, Bass JA: Role of pili in adherence of *Pseudomonas aeruginosa* to mammalian buccal epithelial cells. Infect Immun 29:1146, 1980

30

Morton N. Swartz

Yersinia, Francisella, Pasteurella, and Brucella

Zoonoses

Zoonoses are infections that are naturally transmitted between lower vertebrates and man. This chapter will describe the agents of several important members of this group: plague and other yersinioses, tularemia, brucellosis, and less common infections produced by various pasteurellae. Several other groups of bacteria also cause zoonoses. The gram-negative members include salmonellae and vibrios (Chap. 27), pseudomonads of glanders and melioidosis (Chap. 29), and *Streptobacillus moniliformis* (Chap. 41). The gram-positive members include the bacilli of anthrax (Chap. 33), listeriosis, and erysipeloid (Chap. 41). Others are the spirochetes of leptospirosis, relapsing fever, and one form of rat-bite fever (Chap. 37); the rickettsiae (Chap. 38); some chlamydiae (Chap. 39); and the agents of bovine and avian tuberculosis (Chap. 35).

The organisms described in this chapter are all gram-negative facultative or aerobic rods. Except for *Brucella*, which is distinctive in its chemical properties and pathogenicity, all were assigned until recently to the genus *Pasteurella*.

Yersin named this genus after his teacher when he (and Kitasato independently) discovered the agent of plague in 1894. However, this organism (*Pasteurella pestis*) and *P. pseudotuberculosis* have been shifted to the new genus *Yersinia* and *P. tularensis* to the new genus *Francisella*. Yersiniae, in contrast to *Francisella* and *Brucella*, have simple growth requirements and are not intracellular parasites. This genus is now included in the family Enterobacteriaceae (Chap. 27), but because of the prominence of animal hosts it is retained in this chapter.

Yersinia Pestis

No infectious disease has created greater havoc in the world than plague.* The first adequately described pandemic, in the sixth century AD, is believed to have killed more than 100 million people in its 50-year rampage. In the fourteenth century plague again assumed catastrophic proportions, presumably because of a vicious cycle of deteriorating social conditions that drove rats closer to humans. This pandemic, known as the **black death** because of the severe cyanosis of the terminally ill, destroyed approximately a quarter of the population of Europe and spread into the Middle and Far East. With improvement in living conditions the disease receded in Europe, but serious epidemics recurred elsewhere. The last pandemic developed in China at the close of the nineteenth century.

Plague declined worldwide in the first half of the twentieth century, with occasional outbreaks in Asia and Africa and sporadic cases in South America and the southwestern United States. From 1925 to 1950 an average of one human case was reported annually in the U.S. However, since 1960, there has been a gradual increase, with a recent resurgence; 40 human cases in the U.S. in 1983 and 31 in 1984, indicating an increased incidence of rodent plague or increased exposure of humans to infected animals.

Urban (domestic) plague, the **epidemic** form of the disease, is transmitted by fleas from domestic rats to man (and from rats to rats), as was established in 1906 by the British Plague Research Commission in Bombay. Meyer later discovered **sylvatic (wild) plague,** epizootic among squirrels, prairie dogs, rabbits, and pack rats. This reservoir leads to sporadic cases in man and also constitutes a potential source of future epidemics. In the U.S. sylvatic plague exists in some 15 western states.

THE ORGANISM

Among the three pathogenic *Yersinia* species, *Y. pestis* shares about 90% overall DNA sequence homology with *Y. pseudotuberculosis* and about 50% homology with *Y. enterocolitica*. These species will be described in a later section.

---

* The term as used here refers to the specific disease caused by *Y. pestis;* it is also often applied generically to any epidemic disease with a high mortality rate.

MORPHOLOGY AND CULTIVATION. *Yersinia pestis* is a non-motile, short, non–spore-forming ovoid bacillus. Its tendency to stain in a **bipolar** "safety pin" fashion in preparations from tissues, from buboes, and to a lesser extent from cultures, is best demonstrated by Wayson's stain (methylene blue and carbolfuchsin) but can also be seen with a Giemsa's or gram stain. Freshly isolated virulent strains produce a generous capsule (Fig. 30–1). Colonies on blood agar are nonhemolytic and often "fried egg-like."

Unlike most pathogenic species, *Y. pestis* **multiplies rapidly at 28°C** (temperature optimum). Glucose and mannitol are fermented without gas production; lactose, sucrose, and rhamnose are not attacked. *Y. pestis* requires L-methionine and L-phenylalanine for growth. The organism is susceptible to *Y. pestis* bacteriophage at both 35° and 25°C. *Y. pestis* **may remain viable for weeks** in dry sputum or in flea feces at room temperature.

ANTIGENS. *Y. pestis* strains produce a number of antigenic components (Table 30–1). A heat-labile protein–lipid–polysaccharide capsular Ag is known as **Fraction 1 (F1).** The **VW Ag** system is made up of a cytoplasmic protein V (M_r 38,000) and a lipoprotein W (M_r 145,000) excreted into the medium.

Several **plasmid-coded outer membrane proteins (POMPs)** are produced during infection (as shown by Ab formation), and in cells grown in an intraperitoneal capsule.

The **murine toxin** is located in the cell envelope, is independent of endotoxin, and is not released until cell

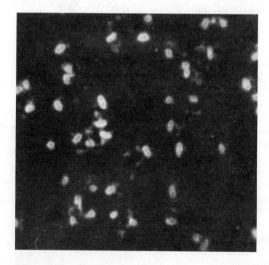

Figure 30–1. Capsules of smooth-phase *Yersinia pestis* stained by the indirect fluorescent Ab technique. (×1200; Cavanagh DC, Randall R: J Immunol 83:348, 1959. Copyright © 1959 by The Williams & Wilkins Co, Baltimore)

TABLE 30–1. Virulence Factors of Yersiniae

Gene Location	Phenotype	Function	Presence of Phenotype			Effect of Loss of Function on Virulence
			Y. Pestis	Y. Enterocolitica	Y. Pseudotuberculosis	
Plasmid (72 Kb)	Vwa					Profound reduction
		Ca²⁺ requirement	+	+	+	
		Synthesis of V Ag	+	+	+	
		Synthesis of W Ag	+	+	+	
		Synthesis of POMPs	+*	+	+	
		Production of surface fibrillae	nk†	+	+	
		Mannose-resistant hemagglutination	nk	+	+	
		Autoagglutination; surface hydrophobicity	−	+	+	
		Resistance to serum bactericidal action	−	+	−	
		Cytotoxicity for macrophages	+	+	+	
		Adhesion to epithelial cells	−	+	+	
		Resistance to phagocytosis by macrophages	+	+	nk	
Plasmid (9 Kb)	Pst					Major reduction
		Synthesis of pesticin, coagulase, and fibrinolysin	+	−	−	
Plasmid (~100 Kb)		Synthesis of murine toxin (probable)	+	−	−	
Chromosome						
	Fra	Synthesis of capsular Ag (F1)	+	−	−	Minor reduction in guinea pigs but not in mice
	Pgm	Storage of exogenous hemin	+	−	−	Major reduction
	Inv	Capacity to invade epithelial cells in culture	nk	nk	+	Only assayed *in vitro*
		Synthesis of heat-stable enterotoxin	nk	+	nk	None

Ca^{2+}

* Not synthesized on growth in culture; synthesized during infection *in vivo*.
† nk, not known.

autolysis occurs. It consists of two active polymeric proteins made up of five (toxin A) or ten (toxin B) subunits, each of 24,000 mol. wt. The toxin is lethal for the mouse (intravenous LD_{50} <1 μg) and rat.

A lipopolysaccharide **endotoxin** is also produced, similar in pharmacologic action to those produced by the enteric bacilli. The organism also shares an extractable Ag with all other Enterobacteriaceae, designated as **common enterobacterial antigen** or Kunin antigen (see Antigenic Structure, Chap. 27).

The antigens will be further discussed below (Virulence Factors of Yersiniae).

PATHOGENICITY

Plague is a natural disease of both domestic and wild rodents. **Rats** are the primary reservoir: they usually die acutely, with a high-grade bacteremia, but they occasion-

ally develop a more chronic form of infection. The disease is transmitted by the bites of **fleas** (e.g., *Xenopsylla cheopis*, the rat flea) that have previously sucked blood from an infected animal. The ingested bacilli proliferate in the intestinal tract of the flea and eventually block the lumen of the proventriculus. The hungry flea, upon biting another rodent, regurgitates into the wound a mixture of plague bacilli and aspirated blood. If its host dies the flea promptly seeks a replacement. If no rodent is available, it will accept a **human host, an accidental intruder** in the **rat → flea → rat** transmission cycle.

A small pustule may be present at the portal of entry in the skin, but more often there is no discernible lesion. The bacilli enter the dermal lymphatics and are transported to the regional lymph nodes, usually in the groin, where they cause the formation of enlarged tender nodes called **buboes.** In severe **bubonic plague** the regional lymph nodes fail to filter out all the multiplying bacilli; organisms that gain entrance to the efferent lymphatics disseminate via the circulation (septicemic plague) to the spleen, liver, lungs, and, sometimes, the meninges. The parenchymatous lesions produced are hemorrhagic; disseminated intravascular coagulation may occur. In the terminal stages, bacteremia is often intense.

When metastatic pneumonia develops, the sputum may become heavily contaminated, and infection may then be transmitted by way of respiratory droplets. **Pneumonic plague,** particularly under conditions of crowding in cold climates, is relatively contagious, and because the inoculum of virulent bacilli in the infected droplets tends to be large, this form of the disease is extraordinarily malignant.

The incubation period of bubonic plague, the commonest form of the illness in humans (80% to 90% of cases), ranges from 1 to 6 days, depending on the infecting dose. Onset is usually abrupt, with high fever, tachycardia, malaise, and aching of the extremities and back. Simultaneously or within the next day, a painful, tender **bubo** is noted, often with prominent overlying edema. If the disease progresses to the fulminant bacteremic stage, it causes prostration, shock, and delirium; death usually occurs within 3 to 5 days of the first symptoms. The course of plague pneumonia is even more fulminant; untreated patients rarely survive longer than 3 days. Pulmonary signs may be totally lacking until the final day of illness, making early diagnosis particularly difficult. Late in the disease, copious bloody, frothy sputum is produced.

The occurrence of asymptomatic cases is suggested by serologic studies in areas where the disease is endemic, and by the finding in Vietnam of a pharyngeal carrier rate of about 10% in family members of plague patients.

IMMUNITY. Recovery from plague appears to confer relatively solid immunity, but rare reinfections have occurred. The Abs primarily involved are those to the antiphagocytic Ag F1 and to the VW complex. In addition, Abs to several of the POMPs are present in convalescent sera of plague patients and in humans immunized with plague vaccine. Antitoxic sera are not protective.

LABORATORY DIAGNOSIS

Rapid preliminary diagnosis is of paramount importance, in view of the swift progression of the untreated disease. Because of the **danger of serious laboratory infections,** great care must be exercised in handling specimens suspected of containing *Y. pestis.* Smears of sputum or of fluid aspirated from lymph nodes should be stained by the gram method and also with either methylene blue or Wayson's reagent to identify bipolar

staining. **Fluorescent Ab** provides rapid, specific identification of *Y. pestis* in bubo aspirates or sputum. Aspirates from buboes, sputum, throat swabs, and autopsy materials should be cultured on blood agar and in infusion broth containing blood or 0.025% sodium sulfite. Blood samples should be placed in infusion broth and spread on plain extract agar. Cultured organisms are identified by colony characteristics, stained appearance, fluorescent Ab staining, lysis with specific bacteriophage, agglutination by specific antiserum, biochemical characteristics (for differentiation from other yersiniae), and animal inoculation (usually lethal in mice or guinea pigs, with typical lesions). On solid media containing Ab to F1 Ag *Y. pestis* colonies (in mixed culture), treated with chloroform vapor, release the Ag and form a precipitin ring around each colony.

Diagnostic serologic tests are of only retrospective value.

TREATMENT

The case fatality rate in untreated bubonic plague is 50% to 75% and in plague pneumonia approaches 100%. Fortunately, *Y. pestis* is responsive to streptomycin (and probably gentamicin), chloramphenicol, and tetracyclines.

If instituted early, antimicrobial therapy markedly alters the course of plague. In the past decade, the mortality rate in the U.S. was 11% in bubonic and 33% in septicemic (bacteremia without significant lymphadenopathy) plague. **Time is of the essence,** particularly in pneumonic plague, which can rarely be controlled after 12 to 15 hours of fever.

PREVENTION

While it is clear that plague is initially transmitted to man primarily by the **rat flea,** epidemiologic studies have revealed that in epidemics of bubonic plague person-to-person transmission also occurs, the principal vector being the **human flea,** *Pulex irritans.*

Prevention of the disease is difficult, because elimination of the animal reservoir through rodent control is virtually impossible. Indeed, wholesale poisoning of rats may accentuate an epidemic by forcing infected fleas to leave the dying rats and seek human hosts. However, insecticides (e.g., DDT) properly directed against human fleas may lower the transmission rate in epidemics. All patients with plague should be strictly isolated initially. After 48 hours of treatment, if plague pneumonia does not develop, wound precautions suffice.

Immunization with killed or attenuated vaccines, or with antigenic fractions of the bacilli, appears to provide short-term relative immunity. **Formalin-treated** (whole-organism) **vaccine** is recommended for persons involved in high-risk activities in plague-endemic areas and for laboratory personnel working with *Y. pestis*. Close contacts of patients with pneumonic plague should be treated prophylactically with tetracycline.

OTHER YERSINIAE

Besides *Y. pestis*, the genus *Yersinia* contains two other species that can produce human disease, *Y. enterocolitica* and *Y. pseudotuberculosis*, as well as several species (*Y. frederiksenii*, *Y. kristensenii*, and *Y. intermedia*) that are generally avirulent. *Y. enterocolitica* and *Y. pseudotuberculosis* are relatively large gram-negative coccobacilli. Both organisms have an extensive **reservoir** in domestic mammals (especially swine) and in wild mammals and birds, both as healthy carriers and in large epizootic outbreaks. They have also been isolated from streams and lakes, where their broad metabolic capabilities promote growth.

Y. enterocolitica and *Y. pseudotuberculosis* grow on the usual media for enteric pathogens, either in air or anaerobically, more slowly than other enterobacteria. Both are **motile at 22°** to 28°C **but not at 37°C,** which helps to distinguish them from the non-motile *Y. pestis* and from other *Enterobacteriaceae*. *Y. enterocolitica* and *Y. pseudotuberculosis* can be distinguished from each other by biochemical tests (Chap. 27), by susceptibility of the latter to *Y. pestis* phage, and by agglutination with specific antisera. On initial isolation, *Y. enterocolitica* is easily mistaken for certain other *Enterobacteriaceae* (*Proteus*, *Providencia*, and *Shigella*).

YERSINIA ENTEROCOLITICA

METABOLISM AND IDENTIFICATION. *Y. enterocolitica* is readily isolated from usually sterile body areas and blood, but isolation from feces requires additional techniques because the organism grows slower at 37°C than do other enteric organisms. **Cold enrichment** of the stool (refrigeration in isotonic saline at 4°C for 1 to 3 weeks, with weekly culture) markedly enhances isolation but hardly contributes to rapid bacteriologic diagnosis. Isolation has been improved recently by the use of a selective, antibiotic-supplemented CIN (cefsulodin, irgasan, novobiocin) medium, which is inoculated (and incubated at 29°C) either directly with a fecal specimen or from a selenite broth that has been incubated for 3 days.

In contrast to *Y. pestis*, *Y. enterocolitica* shows little or no bipolarity (a "safety pin" appearance). On triple sugar iron (TSI) agar, its reactions are those of anaerogenic *E. coli* (see Table 27–4). Many tests show a marked **temperature dependence:** motility, β-galactosidase production, maltose fermentation, and acetoin production are usually positive at 22° to 25°C but negative at 37°C.

ANTIGENS AND ANTIBODY RESPONSE. On the basis of O Ags, about 50 serotypes have been recognized. Serotype 8 predominates in isolates from humans in the U.S. and types 3 and 9 in Europe, Africa, Japan, and Canada.

Antibodies, demonstrable by agglutination or hemagglutination, peak during convalescence. Marked cross-agglutination reactions have been noted between serotype 9 and *Brucella abortus*. Remarkably, patients with autoimmune thyroid disease (Graves' disease, Hashimoto's disease) have circulating Abs that act as agglutinins against *Y. enterocolitica*, because Ags on the latter cross-react with a binding site (on thyroid cells) for human thyrotropin.

PATHOGENICITY. Transmission of *Y. enterocolitica* to humans occurs principally through **food and water,** including milk (in which the organism can grow at refrigeration temperatures). Raw pork has been implicated in the majority of European cases. The occurrence of infections within families and in hospitals suggests person-to-person transmission as well.

Y. enterocolitica is increasingly recognized as a pathogen, because of improved isolation techniques and perhaps an increase in incidence. In Australia, it was isolated from 0.8% of 4100 fecal specimens from children with diarrhea. (*Campylobacter jejuni* was present in 4.7%; *Salmonella* species in 3.7%; and *Shigella* species in 0.2%).

The commonest clinical infection caused by *Y. enterocolitica* is an acute self-limited **gastroenteritis** or an **enterocolitis,** occurring mainly in **children** and indistinguishable from that caused by *Salmonella* or *Shigella*. *Y. enterocolitica* often also causes acute **mesenteric lymphadenitis** and, less often, **terminal ileitis,** occurring mostly in older children and young adults; the symptoms mimic those of acute appendicitis.

Exudative **pharyngitis** caused by *Y. enterocolitica* occurs in **adults** without accompanying diarrhea. Bacteremia caused by this organism occurs uncommonly, usually in patients with iron overload (cirrhosis, hemochromatosis, hemolytic anemias), diabetes mellitus, malignancy, and advanced age. Bacteremia has followed blood transfusion from an asymptomatic donor; *Y. enterocolitica* can grow at 4°C, in banked blood. Patients with thalassemia, suffering marked iron overload as a result of transfusion dependence, are particularly vulnerable when they are treated with the chelating agent desferrioxamine, a siderophore from a *Streptomyces* species. By increasing the **availability of Fe^{3+} in tissues,** in competition with natural chelators (transferrin, lactoferrin), it contributes to invasiveness. Bacteremic patients may develop hepatic or splenic abscesses, meningitis, or osteomyelitis. Nonsuppurative complications of *Y. enterocolitica* infections include a "reactive" polyarthritis, Reiter's syndrome, and erythema nodosum.

In mice oral infection with virulent *Y. enterocolitica* produces a localized suppurative infection of Peyer's patches and the mesenteric lymph nodes. The organisms usually persist in feces for weeks, although strains lacking a 72-Kb virulence plasmid (see next section on Virulence Factors) disappear after a few days. With a larger inoculum, infection can extend to involve the liver, spleen, and other organs in a fatal infection. As with *Y. pestis*, organisms grown at 37°C are less infectious for mice (by oral challenge in the case of *Y. enterocolitica*) than those grown at 25°C.

TREATMENT. *Y. enterocolitica* bacteremia or metastatic infections require antibacterial treatment; *in vitro* clinical isolates are usually susceptible to tetracycline, chloramphenicol, trimethoprim–sulfamethoxazole, and gentamicin. Gastroenteritis and mesenteric adenitis syndromes are often self-limited and may not require antimicrobial therapy unless they are severe or prolonged or occur in a high-risk population.

YERSINIA PSEUDOTUBERCULOSIS

Y. pseudotuberculosis is very similar to *Y. enterocolitica* in growth characteristics, epidemiologic features, virulence factors, and clinical features of the illnesses it produces, but it is a much less frequent human pathogen. Infections have been noted much more often in Scandinavia than elsewhere. The reservoir is principally wild and domestic animals and fowl. Transmission to humans is probably through poorly cooked infected meat, foods contaminated by animal excreta, or possibly direct contact with infected animals. Most cases are sporadic. In contrast with *Y. enterocolitica*, *Y. pseudotuberculosis* is most commonly associated with mesenteric adenitis and a pseudoappendicitis syndrome and only rarely with acute gastroenteritis.

Six main serotypes, based on combinations of O Ags, are known; type 1 is responsible for about 90% of human cases. Several Ags cross-react serologically with *Y. enterocolitica* and some salmonellae. Antibodies (agglutination, indirect hemagglutination, or enzyme-linked immunosorbent assay [ELISA] tests) are normally demonstrable at the onset of illness but wane or disappear in 1 to 4 months.

Y. pseudotuberculosis is generally susceptible *in vitro* to ampicillin, tetracycline, chloramphenicol, and aminoglycosides.

VIRULENCE FACTORS OF YERSINIAE

A subcutaneous injection of fewer than 10 cells of a fully virulent strain of *Y. pestis* into a mouse or guinea pig is lethal. The factors responsible for virulence are multiple and complex. Some are also found in *Y. enterocolitica* and *Y. pseudotuberculosis* and others only in *Y. pestis*.

Some virulence factors are encoded on a plasmid and others on the chromosome (Table 30–1).

The initial descriptions of virulence factors among yersiniae were in *Y. pestis*, the most dramatically invasive of these species. Subsequently, most investigations have involved *Y. enterocolitica* (and *Y. pseudotuberculosis* to a lesser extent), because plasmids encoding certain virulence factors are common to all three species, *Y. enterocolitica* is now a much more frequent human pathogen than *Y. pestis*, and *Y. pestis* is a more dangerous pathogen with which to work. In common, many of the virulence factors and other phenotypic properties of these species are **temperature dependent.**

Yersinia Pestis

A **72-Kb plasmid** specifies a requirement for greater than 2.5mM Ca^{2+} for growth at 37° but not at 26°C: without it, the organisms become pleiomorphic and cease growth and may lyse. In addition, a low calcium medium (simulating the low level found intracellularly in leukocytes), at 37°C, induces synthesis of the V and W antigens. What specific role Ca^{2+} dependence plays in pathogenesis is unknown, but it may adapt the organism to intracellular conditions. V Ag appears to be an important virulence factor, for anti-V Ab provides passive protection against infection in experimental animals, and injection of V Ag enhances the survival in mice of avirulent yersinia mutants lacking the 72-Kb plasmid.

Cytotoxicity for macrophages is plasmid-dependent and is expressed only at 37°C; V and W Ags are probably not involved, as this property is not influenced by Ca^{2+} concentration.

Table 30-1 also lists virulence factors determined by other plasmids. Among these a bacteriocin (**pesticin**) exerts its antibacterial action on strains of *Y. enterocolitica*, *Y. pseudotuberculosis*, and *E. coli* through its N-acetylglucosaminidase activity, converting the cells to spheroplasts.

Chromosomal genes control additional virulence-associated factors in *Y. pestis*. The **capsular or fraction 1 Ag** is present on *Y. pestis* grown *in vivo* (but not at 28°C *in vitro*) and renders the organism resistant to phagocytosis by neutrophils and monocytes. The **pigment-binding surface component (Pgm⁺)** adsorbs exogenous hemin and thus provides a mechanism to store iron. Although Pgm⁻ *Y. pestis* mutants continue to use hemin as a source of iron and accumulate Fe^{3+} by an inducible, siderophore-independent cell-associated transport system, they suffer a significant defect in iron accumulation and loss of virulence.

The different temperatures in the two hosts, flea and mammal, have led to very different patterns of gene expression in *Y. pestis*, resulting in increased virulence on transfer from flea to man. The bacilli contained in the gut of the rat flea possess neither capsular nor VW Ag; consequently, they are promptly ingested and destroyed by polymorphonuclear leukocytes (PMNs). How, then, does the flea serve as an effective vector? **The virulence of the bacilli in the flea is masked by the low temperature (about 25°C) at which they have proliferated.** When such bacilli are phagocytized at 37°C by monocytes (in contradistinction to neutrophils), they survive, produce VW Ag, and subsequently multiply intracellularly; they then emerge as fully virulent organisms possessing both the F1 antiphagocytic factor and the VW Ag.

Yersinia Enterocolitica (and Y. Pseudotuberculosis)

The 72-Kb plasmid in *Y. enterocolitica* is associated with a variety of cell-surface properties, in addition to the Ca^{2+} dependence and V Ag production common to all three disease-producing yersiniae. It specifies at least 16 polypeptides that are formed at 37° but not at 25°C; at least five of these are POMPs and variably require low-Ca^{2+} medium for expression. The POMPs are responsible for increased hydrophobicity of the cell surface at 37°C. The presence of a particular POMP, P_1, correlates with the production of **fibrillae** (a lawn of fine fibers external to the OM), autoagglutination, and mannose-resistant hemagglutination of guinea pig erythrocytes.

Activity of the plasmid at 37°C is also responsible for resistance to the bactericidal activity of serum, cytotoxicity for cell cultures, resistance to phagocytosis, and capacity for intracellular proliferation within macrophages.

Chromosomal factors also play roles in invasiveness and virulence. A single genetic locus (*inv*) isolated from chromosomal DNA of *Y. pseudotuberculosis* converts an innocuous *E. coli* K12 into a HeLa cell-invasive organism.

Under conditions of iron starvation many bacteria release siderophores (high-affinity iron chelators) that transport Fe^{3+} into the bacterial cell via specific membrane receptors (Chap. 4). *Y. enterocolitica* **has receptors but lacks siderophores.** In the intestinal tract, it can use the abundant siderophores of other bacteria. Systemic infection with *Y. enterocolitica* is uncommon, probably reflecting the difficulty in obtaining iron from the tissues. In mice, administration of a siderophore, desferrioxamine, reduces the median lethal dose of intraperitoneally administered *Y. enterocolitica* more than 100,000-fold.

At 25°C *Y. enterocolitica* forms LPS with a full array of O side chains, but at 37°C the O side chains are defective, the colonies have a "rough" appearance, and the POMPs, no longer masked by side chains, produce cell surface changes that promote virulence.

GASTROINTESTINAL VIRULENCE FACTORS. With orally ingested *Y. enterocolitica* cells adhesion to the columnar epithelial cells is the initial step in establishing infection. In epithelial cell tissue cultures adhesion appears to be a plasmid-linked property, and it is more extensive for organisms grown at 25° than at 37°C. The normally pathogenic strains (serogroups O : 3, O : 8, O : 9) then invade the cells but do not appear to multiply within them. *In vivo*, the intracellular bacteria are exocytosed into the lamina propria, where they induce an inflammatory response.

At 26°, but not above 30°C, *Y. enterocolitica* produces in vitro a heat-stable chromosomally-determined **enterotoxin (ST)** demonstrable by its effects on infant mice. It appears to have little role in pathogenicity.

Francisella Tularensis

The history of **tularemia** is less dramatic and shorter than that of plague. While attempting to culture plague bacilli from ground squirrels in Tulare County, California, in 1912, McCoy and Chapin isolated a new bacterial species, which became known as *Bacterium tularense*. The human illness caused by this organism was described 2 years later. In an extraordinary series of field, laboratory, and clinical investigations in Utah in 1919, Francis proved that **jack rabbits** are an important source of human tularemia, and that the disease may be transmitted to man by the bite of a **deer fly. Ticks** were subsequently shown to be important also, not only as vectors but also as reservoirs, as they can transmit the organism transovarially.

While bites of flies and ticks are a significant mode of transmission to man, **direct contact** with the tissues of infected **rabbits** is more common. A major outbreak in 1968 resulted from handling infected muskrats. In some parts of the world, water polluted by carcasses of infected rodents is an important source. The organism may gain entrance through an abrasion in the skin (including an animal bite) or through the conjunctivae or by ingestion of improperly cooked meat or inhalation of aerosols. A very small dose is infectious. These features make the organism exceptionally dangerous in the laboratory.

Tularemia has been reported throughout North America; in many parts of Europe (particularly Scandinavia); in the USSR; and in Japan; it seems to be a disease of the northern hemisphere. In the United States, from 1978 to 1986, 150 to 300 cases were reported annually.

THE ORGANISM

MORPHOLOGY AND CULTIVATION. *F. tularensis* is a short, non-motile, unencapsulated (by light microscopy) bacillus. In young cultures, its morphology is relatively uniform, but in older cultures it is markedly pleomorphic, exhibiting bean-shaped, coccoid, bacillary, and filamentous forms. The organism is very small, stains poorly with bipolar prominence, and does not grow on ordinary media. Minute coccoid forms are visible in hepatic cells of experimental animals, but identifiable organisms are only rarely observed in tissues of humans dead of the disease.

Although not visible by routine microscopy, extracellular material (capsule?) is seen on virulent organisms by electron microscopy; older, decapsulated organisms have lost virulence. Capsular material contains lipid as well as protein and carbohydrate and is nontoxic for guinea pigs.

Colonies are slow to grow on primary inoculation, taking 2 to 10 days even on appropriate media. The colonies are minute, transparent, and easily emulsified (smooth phase) even though the cells lack an obvious capsule. Rough (R) mutants are readily recognized by their granular colonial morphology. They are generally less virulent and less immunogenic than smooth (S) strains.

The outstanding growth characteristic of *F. tularensis* is its **requirement for cysteine** (or other sulfhydryl compounds) in amounts exceeding those usually present in nutrient media. It grows best on cysteine–glucose–blood agar and on coagulated egg yolk medium (both rarely available in a clinical laboratory) and less well in thioglycollate broth. It can be recovered on charcoal yeast extract, Thayer–Martin, or supplemented chocolate agar. Multiplication is most rapid at 37°C. Although a facultative anaerobe, the organism grows best under aerobic conditions.

Although serologically homogeneous, isolates can be divided into two categories. Type A is commonly associated with rabbits and tick vectors, is more virulent, and is found only in North America, where it is responsible for about 80% of human cases. Type B is usually associated with rodents, water, or aquatic animals and is less virulent. The types can also be distinguished biochemically: only type A ferments glycerol and has the enzyme citrulline ureidase.

ANTIGENS. Only a **single immunologic type** of *F. tularensis* has been identified. The immunizing Ags appear to reside in the cell wall. Several kinds of Ags have been extracted: (1) a polysaccharide that causes an immediate wheal-and-erythema reaction when injected into the skin of patients convalescing from tularemia; (2) a protein Ag that cross-reacts with agglutinating Ags of the genus *Brucella;* and (3) an endotoxin whose role in pathogenesis appears to be similar to that of *S. typhi* endotoxin. No exotoxin has been identified.

PATHOGENICITY

The factors responsible for the pathogenicity of *F. tularensis* are poorly defined. The general correlation of virulence with colonial morphology suggests that surface components of the bacterial cell are involved. Inoculation of as few as one to five cells intraperitoneally in guinea pigs is lethal within 5 to 10 days.

The organism behaves primarily as an **intracellular parasite,** surviving for long periods in monocytes and other body cells. The long intracellular survival helps to explain the persistent immune response (see below) and the occasional tendency of the disease to relapse and to remain chronic. Cell-mediated immunity appears to be the dominant defense. Opsonizing Ab is required for phagocytosis and intracellular killing by PMNs but does not appear early in infection. However, a small role for opsonizing Ab and PMNs later in infection is suggested when responses to an attenuated and a wild strain are compared: although the wild strain is only slightly less efficiently phagocytosed than the attenuated one, it is much less readily killed, apparently because of decreased susceptibility to the hypochlorous acid generated by the H_2O_2-myeloperoxidase-chloride antimicrobial system of PMNs. The mechanism of this resistance is unknown.

At the site of primary lodgment in the skin or mucous membrane an ulcerating papule often develops. The organisms are carried by the lymphatics to regional lymph nodes, which become enlarged and tender and may suppurate. Further penetration to the blood stream causes transitory bacteremia in the acute phase of the illness and results in spread to parenchymatous organs, particularly the lungs, liver, and spleen. The characteristic lesions are granulomatous nodules in the reticuloendothelial system, which may caseate or form small abscesses.

The **ulceroglandular** and the **oculoglandular** forms of the disease result from primary infection of the skin or the conjunctivae, respectively. **Oropharyngeal** tularemia mimics nonexudative pharyngitis and results from inhalation of large infected droplets or from ingestion of contaminated food or water. **Pneumonic** tularemia, produced by inhalation of infected droplets, is apt to occur in laboratory workers, but, as in plague, it may also result from hematogenous dissemination from local infection elsewhere. **Typhoidal** tularemia follows ingestion of the organism; it resembles typhoid fever, with gastrointestinal manifestations, fever and toxemia.

The incubation period in tularemia ranges from 3 to 10 days and is followed by headache, fever, and general malaise. If specific treatment is not instituted, the course of the disease is usually protracted; delirium and coma may develop. The case fatality rate in untreated ulceroglandular tularemia is about 5%, and in the typhoidal and pulmonary forms it approaches 30%.

IMMUNITY. Naturally acquired immunity to tularemia is usually permanent. Agglutinins are usually demonstrable in the serum by the second or third week of illness and persist for many years after recovery. Opsonizing Abs appear slightly earlier. The tendency of the disease to progress and even to relapse, despite high titers of serum Abs, is undoubtedly due to the ability of the organism to survive within cells of the host. Cell-mediated immunity, detectable by skin test and by specific *in vitro* lymphocyte stimulation, appears earlier than agglutinins. However, these tests remain positive for years and do not discriminate between recent and remote infection.

LABORATORY DIAGNOSIS

A definitive diagnosis of tularemia from exudate smears requires specific **fluorescent Ab.** Cultures must be made with **special media** (e.g., cysteine–glucose–blood agar), and they should be incubated for 3 weeks before being discarded as negative. If an organism grows in the special medium, and not in ordinary media, it may well be *F. tularensis*. Its identity should be established by staining with fluorescent Ab or by an **agglutination test.** In all laboratory work with *F. tularensis*, great care must be taken to avoid infection.

Serologic tests are of diagnostic value. **Agglutinins** (and hemagglutinins) appear within 8 to 10 days of the onset of illness, continue to rise for as long as 8 weeks, and may be detectable for years after the disease. The demonstration of a rising titer is confirmatory evidence of recent infection. *Brucella* Abs cross-react, but they may be distinguished by comparative titers with Ags of both organisms.

ELISAs distinguish IgA, IgG, and IgM Abs; they become positive slightly earlier than the agglutination test. Because IgM and IgA Abs are long-lasting after tularemia, their presence does not establish the diagnosis, which still requires demonstration of a rise in titer.

TREATMENT AND PREVENTION

Because of its bactericidal properties, **streptomycin** (alternatively, gentamicin) is the drug of choice in the treatment of tularemia. The bacteriostatic tetracyclines and chloramphenicol are also effective, but relapses tend to occur when treatment is discontinued prematurely. Even when streptomycin is used, relapses occasionally occur, probably because of the failure of the drug to affect many of the intracellularly located organisms. Appropriate antibiotic therapy reduces the overall case fatality rate to approximately 1%, but the rate is higher with tularemic pneumonia.

Precautions include wearing of gloves while skinning and dressing rabbits. An attenuated live **vaccine** is available, and its use is indicated in laboratory workers and other individuals who are likely to be exposed to *F. tu-*

larensis. It causes a local reaction on intradermal administration, but it affords significant protection against respiratory (although not against cutaneous) challenge. Cell-mediated immunity is demonstrable for years after vaccination.

Pasteurellae

Organisms in the genus *Pasteurella* are primarily animal pathogens, but they are also responsible for a variety of syndromes in man ranging from localized abscesses to septicemias. The organisms are non-motile, ovoid or rod-shaped bacilli, frequently with bipolar staining. On stained smears of exudates, they can be very pleomorphic, suggesting, in cerebrospinal fluid, mixtures of *Haemophilus* and *Neisseria*; capsules may be evident. They grow best on media containing blood, and in contrast to yersiniae and francisellas, they are oxidase-positive.

Pasteurella multocida is the species most often encountered in human infections. It was described by Pasteur as the cause of fowl cholera, and it is the cause of hemorrhagic septicemia in a variety of animals. The organism is frequently carried in the respiratory tract of healthy domestic animals, swine, and rats. Human infections with *P. multocida* fall into three general groups: (1) **local infections resulting from animal** (most commonly cat) **bites** (cellulitis, abscess, or osteomyelitis); (2) **respiratory tract infections** (pneumonia, empyema, lung abscess) or colonization; and (3) **systemic infections** (bacteremia, peritonitis, meningitis).

When resistance in animals is lowered, as when herds of cattle are shipped, or on exposure to an intercurrent viral infection, the organisms may become invasive, producing fulminating septicemia or pneumonia (**shipping fever**) and spreading to other animals. Killed or attenuated vaccines are used to protect cattle from shipping fever and to control **fowl cholera** in areas where the disease is endemic.

Four capsular serotypes (A–D) have been identified in strains producing animal disease. The mucoid capsule (largely hyaluronic acid in Type A) is important for virulence and appears to serve as a protective Ag and to inhibit phagocytosis and the intracellular protein halogenation involved in the bactericidal action of PMNs; it is lost on subculturing. An early stage in respiratory tract infection of animals involves adhesion of *P. multocida* to pharyngeal epithelial cells, probably mediated by fimbriae. In experimental infections, nonadhesive strains are less pathogenic than adhesive strains (assayed on HeLa cells) isolated from respiratory pasteurellosis of rabbits. Specific virulence factors have not been characterized in human isolates of *P. multocida*.

Diagnosis depends on the isolation and identification

of *P. multocida*. It forms small, nonhemolytic, gray colonies on blood agar. Smooth variants and mucoid variants exhibit marked pathogenicity in mice, in contrast to rough variants. The organism cannot grow on MacConkey agar. It produces acid, but no gas, from glucose, sucrose and mannitol but not from lactose or maltose. It also produces H_2S, catalase, ornithine decarboxylase, and usually indole, but not urease. At least 16 O antigen serotypes are known.

Most strains of *P. multocida* are susceptible to penicillin; this serves in its rapid laboratory differentiation from other gram-negative bacilli. Tetracycline and chloramphenicol are also effective.

Pasteurella pneumotropica causes respiratory infections and abscesses in various animals, and it also occurs in the mouth of healthy dogs: following dog or cat bites, it occasionally is involved in human disease, with a few fatal cases recorded. *P. ureae* is occasionally found in the sputum of patients with chronic bronchitis and bronchiectasis, but its pathogenicity has not been demonstrated.

Brucellae

The brucellae are gram-negative coccobacilli. The genus contains three principal species pathogenic for man, originally differentiated on the basis of their major animal sources: goats and sheep for *B. melitensis*, cattle for *B. abortus*, and swine for *B. suis*. This speciation has since been supported by metabolic and antigenic differences. Three other species (*B. ovis*, *B. neotomae*, and *B. canis*) have been described more recently, of which only the last appears to have any role in human disease.

Brucellae were first isolated in 1887 by Bruce from the spleens of British soldiers dying on the island of Malta from a disease known as **Malta fever.** The source of the organism was discovered in 1904, when it was cultured from milk and urine of goats. When the consumption of raw goat's milk was stopped, the incidence of the disease declined sharply. The second organism of the group was isolated in Denmark by Bang in 1897 from cattle suffering from infectious abortion (**Bang's disease),** and the third was cultured in the U.S. in 1914 from the fetus of a prematurely delivered sow.

All brucellae are obligate parasites capable of causing acute or chronic illness or inapparent infection. The chronicity depends on the marked capacity for multiplication in phagocytic cells, which is opposed by the development of cellular immunity. In their natural animal reservoirs, brucellae show a striking propensity to localize in the pregnant uterus (frequently causing abortion) and in the mammary glands; **apparently healthy animals may shed brucellae in their milk for years.**

Man becomes infected through the ingestion of unpasteurized milk or cheese or through contact with the tissues of infected animals. Human brucellosis may be an acute or relapsing febrile illness, a chronic illness, or a subclinical infection. Unlike its counterpart in animals, it does not tend to localize in the genital tract but rather involves the reticuloendothelial system.

THE ORGANISM

Brucella organisms are nonmotile coccobacilli or short rods. Colonies are small, convex, smooth, moist-appearing, nonhemolytic, and translucent. Growth is slow, particularly on initial cultivation, and colonies are not usually visible for 2 days or more. As a rule, *Brucella* isolates recovered from tissues form smooth (S) colonies, and in freshly isolated strains small capsules can be demonstrated with appropriate staining.

The brucellae are aerobes; no growth occurs on usual laboratory media under strict anaerobiosis. Their nutritional requirements are relatively complex. They may be cultivated on trypticase soy plain (or blood) agar, in trypticase soy broth, or in synthetic media containing a variety of amino acids and vitamins. *B. abortus* differs from the other species infecting man in requiring, on primary isolation, an atmosphere containing 5% to 10% CO_2. All produce catalase and variably decompose urea; sugars are not fermented. Various differences, presented in Table 30–2, form the basis for the metabolic differentiation of the six species. However, they are often difficult to distinguish.

Brucellae may survive for many weeks in discarded infected fetal tissues. They are killed by pasteurization, and in cheese, they may be killed within a few days by the accumulated lactic acid.

GENETIC VARIATION. When serially grown on laboratory media, the smooth (S) form of *Brucella* isolated from infected tissues tends to be replaced by rough (R) forms, which are less virulent and also exhibit less specific and more nonspecific agglutination. The selection responsible for this "dissociation" is attributable to the greater resistance of R cells to alterations of the medium produced by the S cells, including accumulation of D-alanine and lowering of pO_2. Intermediate (I) and mucoid (M) forms, exhibiting reduced virulence, may also emerge.

ANTIGENIC STRUCTURE. Antisera from animals immunized with a smooth strain agglutinate the three principal *Brucella* species. Two shared determinants (A and M) have been proposed to account for these cross-reactions. Abortus (A) Ag is the major surface determinant in both *B. abortus* and *B. suis* and is a minor determinant (a) in *B. melitensis*, whereas the M Ag predominates in the latter and is a minor Ag (m) in the others. By adsorbing anti-Am (*B. abortus* or *B. suis*) Abs with *B. melitensis* organisms (aM), in an amount that will remove all the minor (m)

TABLE 30–2. Differential Characteristics of Brucella Species*

Species	CO_2 Requirement	H_2S Production	Hydrolysis of Urea	Growth on Dye† Media		Agglutination in			Lysis by Phage	
						Mono-specific Antisera to		Antirough Sera‡		
				Thionin	Basic Fuchsin	A	M		RTD†	$10^4 \times$ RTD
B. melitensis	−	−	Slow	+	+	−	+	−	−	−
B. abortus	+¶	+	Slow	−	+	+	−	−	+	+
B. suis	−	+	Rapid	+	−	+	−	−	−	+
B. canis	−	−	Rapid	+	−	−	−	+‡	−	−
B. ovis	+	−	Neg.	+	+	−	−	+‡	−	−
B. neotomae	−	+	Rapid	−	−	+	−	−	−	+

* To accommodate significant intraspecies heterogeneity, the classification scheme has been expanded to include species variants as biotypes (not shown here): three biotypes of *B. melitensis;* nine of *B. abortus;* four of *B. suis.* The properties listed in this table are those of reference strains and are generally characteristic of the majority (but not all) of the biotypes of each species.

† Species differentiation is obtained on tryptose agar with thionin at 1 : 50,000, basic fuchsin at 1 : 100,000.

‡ *B. canis* (and also *B. ovis*) grows as "rough" colonies on primary isolation and appear to be deficient in somatic O antigen of the cell wall. Only antisera to *B. canis* (or *B. ovis*) will produce agglutination of the homologous cells; the same antisera will not produce agglutination when tested with the usual type of brucella antigen prepared from "smooth" cells of *B. abortus* (employed in the diagnostic laboratory).

§ Lysis by reference brucella phage, *Tbilisi* (Tb) phage, at routine test dilution (RTD) and at $10^4 \times$ that concentration. (Other brucella phages have recently been described that are lytic for *B. suis* and *B. neotomae.* None of the phages are lytic for *B. melitensis, B. ovis,* or *B. canis.*)

¶ *B. abortus* has a need for increased CO_2, especially on primary isolation. An attenuated strain (*B. abortus* strain 19), widely employed as a living vaccine in cattle, does not require added CO_2 for growth.

agglutinin but only a small fraction of the major (A) agglutinin, it is possible to prepare monospecific serum to A Ag. Monospecific anti-M serum may be prepared similarly. These sera are useful in diagnosis (Table 30–2). Monospecific serum fails to agglutinate the species with the corresponding minor Ag.

PATHOGENESIS

Although each of the three principal *Brucella* species has preferred hosts, all are pathogenic in a wide range of mammals; experimental infections are readily produced in guinea pigs, rabbits, mice, and monkeys.

In naturally acquired brucellosis, the organisms gain entrance via the broken skin, the conjunctivae, the alimentary tract, or possibly the aerosol route. At the site of lodgment in the skin or mucous membranes, the organisms are ingested by polymorphonuclear cells, multiply within them, and are carried (mostly in these cells) via the lymphatics to the regional lymph nodes. There the bacteria enter and multiply within mononuclear cells; some of these cells die, and the released bacteria and cell contents stimulate local mononuclear cell activation and proliferation. The outcome of this confrontation determines whether the invasive infection is contained. If not, PMNs and mononuclear cells carrying the bacteria reach the blood and soon accumulate in the sinusoids of the liver. These focal aggregations of Kupffer cells containing large numbers of organisms develop and after another few days form typical small granulomas. Similar lesions appear in spleen, bone marrow, and kidney (Fig. 30–2). In certain mammals other than man (cattle, swine, sheep, goats, etc.), brucellae also accumulate in the mammary glands (causing infection of the milk), in the genital organs, and in the pregnant uterus (often resulting in abortion).

ERYTHRITOL. In **bovine infectious abortion,** the organisms are found mostly in the fetal portion of the placenta, the birth fluids, and the chorion. This remarkable **viscerotropism** depends on the presence of **erythritol.** This 4-C polyhydric alcohol ($HOCH_2$–$CHOH$–$CHOH$–CH_2OH) was found to be the factor in bovine allantoic and amniotic fluids that stimulates the growth of *B. abortus.* It is present in appreciable quantities only in the placenta of animals prone to infectious abortion (cows, sheep, pigs, goats, and dogs) but not in the human placenta, which is not a site of localization of the infection. Erythritol is not a necessary determinant of *Brucella* infection: there is none in macrophages, yet the reticuloendothelial system is commonly involved in chronic brucellosis.

SURVIVAL IN CELLS. No exotoxins or antiphagocytic capsular or cell wall constituents have been detected among *Brucella* species. Instead, **intracellular** events largely determine the course of the disease. PMNs readily ingest *Brucella* organisms, and are likely to be the first phagocytic defenses. Smooth strains of *B. abortus* are more resistant to intracellular killing than are rough strains. The usual stimulation of oxidative metabolism accompanying phagocytosis does not occur. *B. abortus* also appears to **inhibit neutrophil degranulation** (phagosome–lysosome fusion) and its attendant release into the phagosome of granule enzymes, including myeloperoxidase. As a consequence, the antibacterial activity of PMNs is suppressed. Components responsible for this inhibition are of low molecular weight (less than 1000 daltons) and appear to include adenine and 5'-guanosine monophosphate.

A possible **virulence factor made only *in vivo*** appears to enhance intracellular survival. Thus virulent *B. abortus* from cultures of monocytes or from infected bovine placenta survives better than the same strain grown on artificial media, and cell walls from organisms obtained from the bovine placenta, but not after growth on artificial media, inhibit the normal intracellular destruction of an avirulent (R) strain by mononuclear cells.

CLINICAL FEATURES. The incubation period in human brucellosis is long, often several weeks or even months. The onset of symptoms is usually insidious, with malaise, chills, fever, sweats, weakness, myalgia, and headache. Fever may be remittent, particularly with *B. melitensis* (**undulant fever**). Vague gastrointestinal and nervous symptoms are common. The acute illness may be associated with enlarged lymph nodes, spleen, and

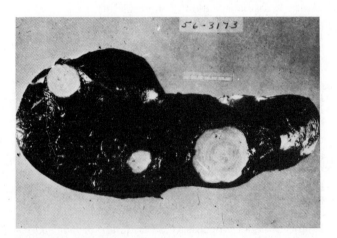

Figure 30–2. Longitudinal section of the spleen of a patient with chronic *B. suis* infection, showing splenomegaly and scattered large, partially calcified areas of caseation.

liver and with localized vertebral spondylitis. Bacteremia is present in more than 20% of cases. Meningoencephalitis, osteomyelitis, endocarditis, and interstitial nephritis with focal glomerular lesions sometimes occur in the course of the acute disease. Epididymoorchitis occasionally occurs with *B. melitensis* infection. In the later stages of the disease the persistence of vague complaints often suggests a psychoneurosis. The establishment of a definitive diagnosis at this "chronic" stage is especially difficult.

Hepatic involvement is common in human brucellosis, in the form of an acute diffuse hepatitis with focal necrosis, or chronic small noncaseating granulomas (observed in liver biopsies). *B. suis* infection may cause chronic suppurative abscesses and large areas of caseation in the liver and spleen, which usually calcify after some years (Fig. 30–2).

IMMUNITY

Circulating Abs are usually detectable from the time the first signs and symptoms of the disease develop (see Laboratory Diagnosis, below), but their presence does not prevent bacteremia or reinfection (which is common). However, relative immunity to brucellosis may be acquired: seropositive abattoir workers are less likely to develop clinical brucellosis than previously noninfected workers.

Cellular immunity plays a critical role in this disease: the survival of brucellae is shorter in cultured macrophages from immunized animals, owing to a nonspecific activation. The mechanism and its relation to hypersensitivity, are discussed in Chapter 19.

A **hypersensitivity reaction** to suddenly released brucella Ags is presumed to be responsible for the **Herxheimer**-like reaction that sometimes follows vigorous chemotherapy. Similarly, severe systemic as well as local reactions are observed after accidental inoculation of previously infected veterinarians with a vaccine strain.

LABORATORY DIAGNOSIS

The patient with brucellosis commonly presents with an unexplained fever. The diagnosis is usually suggested by the combination of clinical and epidemiologic considerations. It may also be suspected when liver biopsy reveals noncaseating granulomas.

The establishment of a definitive diagnosis requires **cultivation** of the organism from the blood or from a biopsy of bone marrow, liver, or lymph node; blood should be cultured repeatedly in all suspected cases. Specimens should be incubated in trypticase soy broth under 10% CO_2. (The Casteñada bottle, containing both solid and liquid media, is often used.) At 4- to 5-day intervals, or when visible growth is first noted, a sample is removed for staining and for subculture on blood trypticase soy agar under 10% CO_2. The primary cultures should be incubated for at least 4 weeks before being discarded. Because the number of viable bacilli present in specimens is usually small, cultivation is often difficult. Species are identified on the basis of the tests summarized in Table 30–2. Fluorescent Ab is useful for genus identification.

Owing to the increased use of antibiotics prior to obtaining cultures, the majority of cases of brucellosis are now diagnosed **serologically.** Because of the long incubation period, **Abs** are frequently demonstrable by the time the disease is first recognized. The initial response is the appearance of IgM, followed shortly by IgG. **Agglutination** tests are performed with phenolized suspensions of heat-killed smooth (S) bacilli. A standard, avirulent strain of *B. abortus*, no. 456, is generally used; it detects Abs to all three principal species equally well. Titers above 1:80 are usually considered indicative of either past or present infection, and four-fold or greater rise in titer during the course of the illness is strong evidence for the diagnosis. However, Serum containing Abs to *F. tularensis*, *Yersinia enterocolitica*, or *Vibrio cholerae* can cross-react in the *Brucella* agglutination test.

The titer remains elevated (as high as 1:640 to 1:2560) during the active phases of the disease and usually declines as the patient improves. High titers of **IgM agglutinins** can persist after recovery from infection and in the absence of overt disease; they may even be found with no history of clinical disease, usually in individuals who have been exposed to farm animals or unpasteurized dairy products. In contrast, the persistence or recrudescence of chronic active brucellosis is usually associated with the presence of **IgG**. In a **symptomatic patient** the finding of 2-mercaptoethanol-resistant (IgG) agglutinins, even at low titers (less than 1:100), is suggestive of active brucellosis; their absence is also significant in evaluating possible chronic brucellosis.

Occasionally, in chronic brucellosis particularly, the Abs are of the incomplete, or blocking, type. They may be detected by diluting sera to at least 1:1280 (in 5% sodium chloride or albumin solution) in the agglutination test, or by adding the Coombs reagent (anti-human-immunoglobulin serum) to the test for agglutinating Abs.

An ELISA has been developed for direct measurement of the IgG and IgM Abs individually in brucellosis. A recent modification utilizes the major OM proteins of *B. melitensis* as Ag. In addition to detecting Abs to *B. abortus*, *B. melitensis*, and *B. suis*, it is sensitive to the Ab response to infections with *B. canis*; the latter Abs are undetectable in the agglutination test because *B. canis* lacks somatic O Ag. (A specific agglutination test with *B. canis* cells is available only in veterinary centers.)

TREATMENT

Most strains of *Brucella* are sensitive *in vitro* to the tetracyclines and streptomycin, but streptomycin does not reach organisms sequestered within mononuclear phagocytes. Tetracycline alone, or in combination with streptomycin in severe infections, is usually effective, often within a few days. However, relapse commonly occurs unless therapy is prolonged for at least 3 to 4 weeks. The difficulty in eradicating the organisms undoubtedly arises because an intracellular location protects them from both drugs and Abs. Trimethoprim–sulfamethoxazole and rifampin also show activity against *Brucella* strains.

EPIDEMIOLOGY AND PREVENTION

B. abortus infects cattle almost worldwide, including the U.S. *B. suis* infects cattle as well as swine. Goats are important as sources of *B. melitensis* in Mexico and in Mediterranean countries, but this organism is rarely isolated from cases in the U.S.

An attenuated **live vaccine** (*B. abortus* strain 19) has been used **in calves** to decrease the incidence of brucellosis in cattle; it produces a limited infection, followed by reasonable immunity. Infected cattle can be identified by an agglutination test (on serum or milk), or by direct fluorescent Ab testing of bovine abortion material.

Through the use of public health measures (testing of cows followed by segregation or slaughter, vaccination of calves, pasteurization of milk products), the incidence of human brucellosis in the U.S. has decreased in the past 45 years from 6300 to 130 cases annually. Most cases now occur in workers in meat-packing plants (90% of cases related to slaughtering of hogs), in livestock raisers, and in veterinarians. About 10% of cases are due to ingestion of raw milk or imported cheeses.

The identification of epidemic disease caused by *B. canis* in dogs has revealed yet another reservoir for brucellosis. The infection may produce little evidence of illness, even though bacteremia may be demonstrable for months or years. A few cases have occurred in man.

Although active immunization of humans at high risk is practiced in the Soviet Union, public health authorities in the U.S. have been reluctant to use the currently available vaccines because of their potential pathogenicity for man.

Selected Reading

BOOKS AND REVIEW ARTICLES

Bahmanyar M, Cavanaugh DC: Plague Manual. Geneva, World Health Organization, 1976

Brubaker RR: The Vwa⁺ virulence factor of Yersiniae: The molecular basis of the attendant nutritional requirement for Ca⁺⁺. Rev Infect Dis 5:S748, 1983

Buchanan TM, Faber LC, Feldman RA: Brucellosis in the United

States, 1960–1972 I: Clinical features and therapy. Medicine 53:403, 1974

Buchanan TM, Hendricks SL, Patton CM, Feldman RA: Brucellosis in the United States, 1960–1972 III: Epidemiology and evidence for acquired immunity. Medicine 53:427, 1974

Buchanan TM, Sulzer CR, Frix MK, Feldman RA: Brucellosis in the United States, 1960–1972 II: Diagnostic aspects. Medicine 53:415, 1974

Cornelis G, Laroche Y, Balligand G, Sory M-P, Wauters G: *Yersinia enterocolitica*, a primary model for bacterial invasiveness. Rev Infect Dis 9:64, 1987

Elberg SS: Immunity to brucella infection. Medicine 52:339, 1973

Evans ME, Gregory DW, Schaffner W, McGee ZA: Tularemia: A 30-year experience with 88 cases. Medicine 64:251, 1985

Kelly MT, Brenner DJ, Farmer JJ III: *Yersinia* species. In Lennette EH, Ballows A, Hausler WJ Jr, Shodomy HJ (eds): Manual of Clinical Microbiology, 5th Ed, p 273. Washington, DC, American Society for Microbiology, 1985

Montie TC: Properties and pharmacological action of plague murine toxin. Pharmacol Ther 12:491, 1981

Oberdorfer TR: Characteristics and biotypes of *Pasteurella multocida* isolated from humans. J Clin Microbiol 13:566, 1981

Portnoy DA, Martinez RJ: Role of a plasmid in the pathogenicity of *Yersinia* species. Curr Top Microbiol Immunol 118:29, 1985

Reed WP, Palmer DL, Williams RC Jr, Kisch AL: Bubonic plague in the southwestern United States: A review of recent experience. Medicine 49:645, 1970

Spink WW: The Nature of Brucellosis. Minneapolis, University of Minnesota Press, 1956

Weaver RE, Hollis DG, Bottone EJ: *Francisella tularensis*. In Lennette EH, Ballows A, Hausler WJ Jr, Shadomy HJ: Manual of Clinical Microbiology, 4th Ed, p 316. Washington, DC, American Society for Microbiology, 1985

Weaver RE, Hollis DG, Bottone EJ: *Pasteurella* species. In Lennette EH, Balows A, Hausler WJ Jr, Shadomy HJ (eds): Manual of Clinical Microbiology, 4th ed. p 321. Washington, DC, American Society for Microbiology, 1985

Weber DJ, Wolfson JS, Swartz MN, Hooper DC: *Pasteurella multocida* infections: Report of 34 cases and review of the literature. Medicine 63:133, 1984

Young EJ: Human brucellosis. Rev Infect Dis 5:821, 1983

SPECIFIC ARTICLES

Bertram TA, Canning PC, Roth JA: Preferential inhibition of primary granule release from bovine neutrophils by a *Brucella abortus* extract. Infect Immun 52:285, 1986

Butler T: A clinical study of bubonic plague: Observations on the 1970 Vietnam epidemic. Am J Med 53:268, 1972

Canning PC, Roth JA, Deyoe BL: Release of 5′ guanosine monophosphate and adenine by *Brucella abortus* and their role in the intracellular survival of the bacteria. J Infect Dis 154:464, 1986

Hull HF, Montes JM, Mann JM: Septicemic plague in New Mexico. J Infect Dis 155:113, 1987

Isberg RR, Falkow S: A single genetic locus encoded by *Yersinia pseudotuberculosis* permits invasion of cultured animal cells by *Escherichia coli* K-12. Nature 317:262, 1985

Kay BA, Wachsmuth K, Gemski P, Feeley JC, Quan TJ, Brenner DJ: Virulence and phenotypic characterization of *Yersinia enterocolitica* isolated from humans in the United States. J Clin Microbiol 17:128, 1983

Keppie J, Williams AE, Witt K, Smith H: The role of erythritol in the tissue localization of the brucellae. Br J Exp Pathol 46:104, 1965

Lofgren S, Tarnvik A, Thore M, Carlsson J: A wild and an attenuated strain of *Francisella tularensis* differ in susceptibility to hypochlorous acid: A possible explanation of their different handling by polymorphonuclear leukocytes. Infect Immun 43:730, 1984

Marriott DJE, Taylor S, Dorman DC: *Yersinia enterocolitica* infection in children. Med J Austral 143:489, 1985

Polt SS, Dismukes WE, Flint A, Schaefer J: Human brucellosis caused by *Brucella canis*: Clinical features and immune response. Ann Intern Med 97:717, 1982

Portnoy DA, Blank HF, Kingsbury DT, Falkow S: Genetic analysis of essential plasmid determinants of pathogenicity in *Yersinia pestis*. J Infect Dis 148:297, 1983

Portnoy DA, Wolf–Watz H, Bolin I, Beeder AB, Falkow S: Characterization of common virulence plasmids in *Yersinia* species and their role in the expression of outer membrane proteins. Infect Immun 43:108, 1984

Robins–Browne RM, Tzipori S, Gonis G, Hayes J, Withers M, Prpic JK: The pathogenesis of *Yersinia enterocolitica* infection in gnotobiotic piglets. J Med Microbiol 19:297, 1985

Ryu H, Kaeberle ML, Roth JA, Griffith RW: Effect of type A *Pasteurella multocida* fractions on bovine polymorphonuclear leukocyte functions. Infect Immun 43:66, 1984

Sikkema DJ, Brubaker RR: Resistance to pesticin, storage of iron, and invasion of HeLa cells by Yersiniae. Infect Immun 55:572, 1987

Sperry JF, Robertson DC: Inhibition of growth by erythritol catabolism in *Brucella abortus*. J Bacteriol 124:391, 1975

Une T, Brubaker RR: Roles of V antigen in promoting virulence and immunity in Yersiniae. J Immunol 133:2226, 1984

Wolf–Watz H, Portnoy DA, Bolin I, Falkow S: Transfer of the virulence plasmid of *Yersinia pestis* to *Yersinia pseudotuberculosis*. Infect Immun 48:241, 1985

31

Stephen I. Morse†
Porter Anderson

Haemophilus

Hemophilus are small, gram-negative, non-motile, non–spore-forming bacilli with complex growth requirements. Species of the genus *Haemophilus* require growth factors provided by blood (Table 31–1). *H. influenzae* is a major cause of bacterial meningitis in children, *H. aegyptius* causes conjunctivitis, and *H. ducreyi* causes chancroid. The morphologically similar organism *Bordetella pertussis*, which causes whooping cough, is described in the next chapter.

Haemophilus Influenzae

The widely distributed *H. influenzae*, first isolated by Pfeiffer during the influenza pandemic of 1890, was erroneously thought to be the cause of the disease and was named accordingly. Influenza is now known to be caused by a virus; but *H. influenzae* was probably an important secondary invader in some epidemics, as it was often the predominant bacterium cultivated from the lungs at autopsy. Moreover, an interaction between *Haemophilus* and viruses was demonstrated by Shope's discovery that swine influenza requires infection with both swine influenza virus and *H. suis*, and a synergism between human influenza virus and *H. influenzae* has been observed in chick embryos and in infant rats.

H. influenzae is the leading cause of bacterial meningitis in children under 4 years of age (Fig. 31–1). The organism is sometimes isolated from lesions in adults during exacerbations of chronic bronchitis, from children with obstructive bronchiolitis, and from as many as 25% of children with otitis media. However, its etiologic role in those diseases is not certain.

Although gram-negative, *H. influenzae* shares important pathogenic properties with the pneumococcus.

† Deceased.

TABLE 31–1. *Differential Characteristics of Species of* Haemophilus

Species	Growth Factor		Hemolysis	Increased CO₂ Requirement
	X	V		
H. influenzae	+	+	−	−
H. aegyptius	+	+	−	−
H. suis	+	+	−	−
H. haemolyticus	+	+	+	−
H. ducreyi	+	−	Slight	+
H. aphrophilus	+	−	−	+
H. parainfluenzae	−	+	−	−
H. parahaemolyticus	−	+	+	−

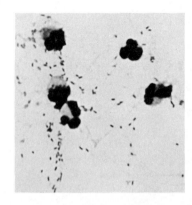

Figure 31–2. Gram-stained smear of exudate from spinal fluid of patient with *H. influenzae* meningitis. ×1000; courtesy of R. Drachman)

Both organisms are primarily invasive rather than toxigenic, they are inhabitants (commensal as well as pathogenic) of the respiratory tract, and they have antiphagocytic polysaccharide capsules.

MORPHOLOGY

Organisms seen in pathologic specimens such as cerebrospinal fluid are generally small, gram-negative, encapsulated coccobacilli ($1–1.5 \times 0.3\ \mu m$; Fig. 31–2), but short chains are often found. Improper decolorization in the gram stain may lead to mistaken identification as pneumococcus or streptococcus. Capsules may be identified by the quellung reaction. Unencapsulated strains tend to be pleomorphic and filamentous. Rarely, isolates

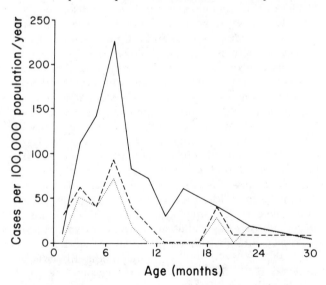

Figure 31–1. Age-specific incidence of meningitis caused by *H. influenzae (solid line)*, *N. meningitidis (broken line)*, and *S. pneumoniae (dotted line)* in children under 30 months of age. (Fraser DW et al: J Infect Dis 127:271, 1973)

from the nasopharynx are **piliated.** Most strains appear to have the genetic capacity for forming pili but express it only in a small proportion of the bacilli. Highly piliated populations can be obtained by culturing piliated bacilli selected by adherence to human red cells (or mucosal cells) *in vitro*.

On solid medium encapsulated virulent strains appear as small "dewdrop" colonies, and on transparent medium, such as Levinthal agar, these are characteristically iridescent in obliquely transmitted light. After 24 to 48 hours the capsules and iridescence disappear, and autolysis and a variable gram-stain reaction occur. Both the autolysis and the capsular destruction are apparently caused by activation of endogenous enzymes. Similarly, in liquid medium the capsules disappear early in culture.

Even in early cultures a few noniridescent colonies containing unencapsulated variants of *H. influenzae* are always demonstrable. It is evident, therefore, that the rate of spontaneous smooth to rough (S → R) mutation is relatively high. When cultural conditions are suboptimal R variants will often predominate. Such S → R shifts have been observed in the upper respiratory tracts of patients recovering from influenzal meningitis.

Transformation mediated by DNA from *H. influenzae*, extensively studied by Alexander, has included drug resistance and specific capsular antigen synthesis; interspecific transformation occurs. The demonstration of transformation between pneumococci in host tissues suggests that it may also take place with *Haemophilus*. Restriction endonucleases from *Haemophilus* species are widely used in the analysis and cloning of DNA (see Chap. 8).

GROWTH AND METABOLISM

H. influenzae is a facultative anaerobe that requires two growth factors present in blood, the heat-stable X and

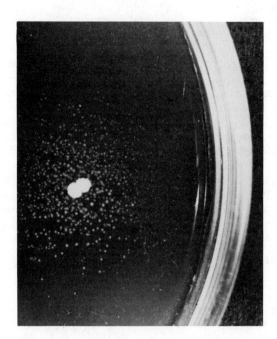

Figure 31–3. Satellite phenomenon: heavily seeded colonies of *H. influenzae* growing only in vicinity of staphylococcal colonies on autoclaved blood agar. Autoclaving destroys V factor but not X factor. (Courtesy of PH Hardy and EE Nell)

the labile V (Table 31–1). X factor can be replaced by hemin, which is a precursor for the prosthetic groups of the respiratory enzymes. (Under anaerobic conditions, the X factor requirement is usually reduced.) V factor can be replaced by NAD or NADP, both of which are destroyed by excessive heat. It can be supplied by other microorganisms, such as staphylococci, growing in the immediate vicinity; this **satellite phenomenon** is illustrated in Figure 31–3.

H. influenzae grows slowly in blood broth or on blood agar containing rabbit, horse, or guinea pig blood. Fresh human and sheep blood inhibit growth but can be used in the preparation of **chocolate agar,** on which *H. influenzae* grows profusely. Chocolate agar is prepared by adding blood to an agar base at 80°C and maintaining the temperature at 50° for approximately 15 minutes or until a brown color appears. The mild heat releases X and V factors from RBCs and also destroys inhibitors of V factor without inactivating V factor itself.

Growth is optimal at pH 7.6, and in liquid media, it may be stimulated by aeration. On primary isolation, some strains grow best in the presence of 5% CO_2. Defined media have been devised for use in biochemical and genetic studies. Most strains can utilize nitrate as an electron acceptor in the absence of oxygen.

Fermentation reactions of *Haemophilus* organisms are too variable to be of differential value. A biotyping scheme is based on the production of urease, ornithine decarboxylase, and indole.

ANTIGENIC STRUCTURE

As with the pneumococcus, the capsular polysaccharides of *H. influenzae* evoke protective Abs. **Six types,** designated types a to f, have been described; these are serologically identified by agglutination, precipitation, or quellung tests performed with specific antisera.

In type b, the most important pathogen for humans, the polysaccharide contains ribose, ribitol, and phosphate, linked as shown in Figure 31–4. In type a, the ribose is replaced by glucose. The structures of the other four types are less closely related.

Cross-reacting polysaccharides are common in other organisms and may contribute to the formation of natural Ab (see Immunity, below). Cross-reactions of type b with strains of pneumococci, streptococci, *Bacillus subtilis*, and *Staphylococcus aureus* may be based on ribitol phosphate in their teichoic acids, while cross-reacting *E. coli* strains have both ribitol and ribose in their Ags.

Somatic Ags include a lipopolysaccharide (LPS) and several outer membrane proteins (OMP). The lipid component of the LPS resembles that of enterobacteria in toxicity and other biological properties, but the saccharide component is small and has little antigenic heterogeneity. Six quantitatively major and 20 minor OMP differing in antigenic specificity and molecular weight, have been found in different strains. Molecular weight profiles (by gel electrophoresis) are used to type and subtype isolates. Abs to the LPS and OMP are found in patients and in animals infected with type b; their ability to react with encapsulated cells is under investigation.

PATHOGENESIS

Naturally acquired disease caused by *H. influenzae* seems to occur only in man. Experimental bronchopneumonia and meningitis have been produced in monkeys and fatal peritonitis in mice, but the most useful experimental model is the infant rat, in which bacteremia and meningitis follow intranasal or intraperitoneal

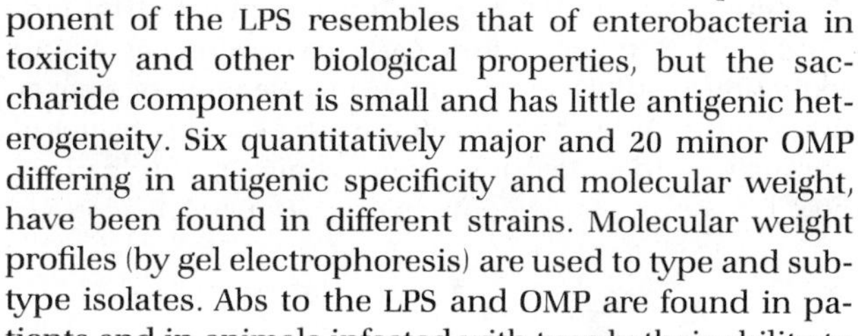

Figure 31–4. Structure of repeating unit of type b capsular polysaccharide. (Crisel RM et al: J Biol Chem 250:4926, 1975)

inoculation with type b *H. influenzae*. Diseases caused by *H. influenzae* are common in young children but rare in neonates and adults. The reason is explained under Immunity, below.

The organisms produce no demonstrable exotoxin, and **virulence** is directly related to **capsule formation**. The role of the endotoxin is not clear. Virtually all severe infections are caused by type b, whose polysaccharide is relatively ineffective in activating complement by the alternative (Ab-independent) pathway.

The organism may reside in the respiratory tract without causing trouble. Carrier rates in children may be as high as 50%, but these organisms are usually unencapsulated. Encapsulated strains are mostly type b, and they are rarely encountered in healthy adults. **Pili** increase the adherence to human mucosal cells *in vitro*, but their role in colonization and in disease remains to be defined. The Anton Ag (as defined in red cells) appears to be the receptor for the pili. Most type b strains secrete a protease that cleaves IgAl, but its function likewise is unclear.

Disease caused by *H. influenzae* usually begins as a nasopharyngitis, probably precipitated by a viral infection of the upper respiratory tract. The resulting coryza may be followed by sinusitis or otitis media and may lead to pneumonia; the latter is often complicated by empyema. Bacteremia occurs early in severe cases and frequently results in metastatic involvement of one or more joints or in the development of acute bacterial meningitis—the most important clinical entity caused by *H. influenzae*. Indeed, in children, *H. influenzae* is the commonest cause of bacterial meningitis (Fig. 31–1) except during epidemics of meningococcal meningitis. The clinical signs are like those of other forms of acute bacterial meningitis. Unless vigorously treated, the patient rarely recovers.

A less common but even more serious disease caused by *H. influenzae* type b is **epiglottis** and **obstructive laryngitis.** The onset is sudden and the course fulminating, often ending fatally within 24 hours. Infection starts in the pharynx and spreads to the epiglottis, which becomes cherry red and grossly edematous. Laryngeal obstruction ensues. The patient should be immediately hospitalized when the clinical diagnosis is made, for survival may require prompt tracheotomy. Bacteremia is usually a feature of the disease.

IMMUNITY

The incidence of *H. influenzae* meningitis as a function of age is inversely related to the titer of Ab in the blood (Fig. 31–5), whether passively acquired from the mother or actively formed. In children aged 2 months to 3 years, Ab levels are minimal; thereafter, Ab increases, and the disease becomes much less common.

Like other gram-negative bacilli, *H. influenzae* is susceptible to lysis by Ab and complement. But although the immunologic test used in the studies in Figure 31–5 primarily measures bacteriolysis, immunity is not necessarily attributable to this action. Thus anticapsular Ab, which promotes phagocytosis as well as bacteriolysis, is

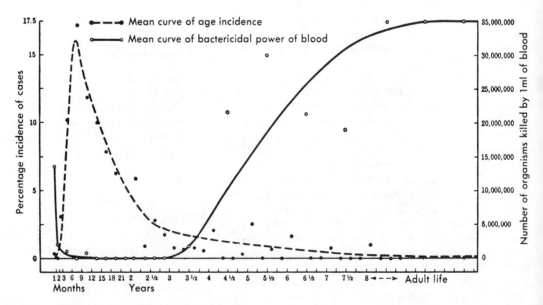

Figure 31–5. Relation of the age incidence of *H. influenzae* meningitis to bactericidal Ab titers in the blood. (Fothergill LD, Wright J: J Immunol 24:281, 1933. Copyright © 1933 by The Williams & Wilkins Co, Baltimore)

known to be the main factor in serum correlated with protection; phagocytosis is prominent in the meningeal lesions; complement is rarely detectable in the spinal fluid of patients with bacterial meningitis. Phagocytosis is thus evidently an important defense mechanism in influenza bacillus meningitis.

LABORATORY DIAGNOSIS

In all cases of suspected bacterial meningitis, a sample of blood, as well as of spinal fluid, should be cultured. A smear of the spinal fluid, or, preferably, a smear made with the sediment from a centrifuged specimen, should be stained by the gram method. The detection of small, pleomorphic, gram-negative bacilli warrants a provisional diagnosis of influenza bacillus meningitis. If exposure of the organisms in the spinal fluid to specific antiserum results in a positive quellung reaction (see Fig. 23–1), the diagnosis is established. The specimen of spinal fluid should be streaked on chocolate agar and incubated in a candle jar. Organisms suspected of being *H. influenzae* should be subjected to the quellung test. If the results are negative, the requirement of the organism for X and V factors (Table 31–1) is determined by adding commercially available filter paper strips impregnated with each factor onto a culture seeded on nutrient agar. Detection of free capsular Ag in the spinal fluid by countercurrent immunoelectrophoresis with type b antiserum or by agglutination of Ab-coated latex particles is exceedingly sensitive and provides rapid, accurate diagnosis.

TREATMENT AND PREVENTION

Virtually all patients treated early in the course of influenza bacillus meningitis can now be cured. Ampicillin and chloramphenicol are effective, and ampicillin has been the drug of choice. However, approximately 20% of strains are now resistant to ampicillin because of a plasmid-mediated β-lactamase. At present, therefore, initial therapy consists of a cephalosporin or of both ampicillin and chloramphenicol; ampicillin alone is continued if the organism is sensitive. Ampicillin resistance is conveniently and rapidly assessed by testing for β-lactamase formation. A few chloramphenicol-resistant strains of *H. influenzae* have been isolated, but combined ampicillin-chloramphenicol resistance has not been found.

The mortality rate of treated *H. influenzae* is less than 10%, and most children acquire effective immunity by age 10. Nevertheless, *H. influenzae* meningitis causes 1500 to 2000 deaths/year in the United States, mostly in young children. Moreover, a significant proportion, perhaps 30%, of those who recover have **residual neurologic defects;** about 5% must be institutionalized. For these reasons, efforts to develop a vaccine were undertaken about 1970.

Initially the type b capsule was evaluated as a vaccine. Like other polysaccharides, it elicits a long-lived Ab elevation, but with little induction of memory; moreover, responsiveness begins at a later age than with proteins. By 18 months of age, however, the Ab response is adequate for protection in most children. Because vaccination at this age could prevent about one-third of the cases of meningitis and most of the cases of epiglottitis, it was recommended by the American Academy of Pediatrics in 1985. Three years later the polysaccharide vaccine was replaced by "conjugate vaccines," in which it was coupled to protein. These can induce memory-type Ab responses in children, and they seem likely to be effective in younger infants, who are at higher risk for the disease (see Fig. 31-1).

Widespread outbreaks of *H. influenzae* meningitis are rare, although secondary cases do occur in families and in child-care facilities. In such settings prophylaxis with rifampin is recommended for contacts of the susceptible age.

Other Haemophilus *Species*

H. ducreyi causes **chancroid** (soft chancre), a sexually transmitted disease whose paragenital ulcerative lesions lack the indurated margins of syphilitic chancres. The organism is found in gram-stained smears from ulcerated areas. Response to sulfonamides and various antibiotics is usually prompt.

H. aegyptius (the Koch–Weeks bacillus) may cause endemic or epidemic purulent conjunctivitis. *H. haemolyticus*, a nonpathogenic inhabitant of the oral cavity, produces β-hemolytic colonies that may be mistaken for those of streptococci if the colonies are not smeared and stained. *H. aphrophilus* and some related species occasionally inhabit the oral cavity or dental plaque and, rarely, cause bacterial endocarditis. Some differential properties of these organisms are summarized in Table 31–1.

Selected Reading

BOOKS AND REVIEW ARTICLES

Kilian M: A taxonomic study of the genus *Haemophilus*, with the proposal of a new species. J Gen Microbiol 93:9, 1976

Robbins JB, Schneerson R, Pittman M: *Haemophilus influenzae* type b infections. In Germanier R (ed): Bacterial Vaccines, p 290. New York, Academic Press, 1984

Turk DC: The pathogenicity of *Haemophilus influenzae*. J Med Microbiol 18:1, 1984

SPECIFIC ARTICLES

Eskola J et al: Efficacy of *Haemophilus influenzae* type b polysaccharide-diphtheria toxoid conjugate vaccine in infancy. N Engl J Med 317:717, 1987

Insel RA, Anderson PW: Oligosaccharide–protein conjugate vaccines induce and prime for oligoclonal IgG antibody response to the *Haemophilus influenzae* type b capsular polysaccharide in human infants. J Exp Med 163:262, 1985

Pittman M: Variation and type specificity in the bacterial species *Haemophilus influenzae*. J Exp Med 53:471, 1931

Sell SHW, Merrill RE, Doyne ED, Zemsky EP Jr: Long-term sequelae of *Haemophilus influenzae* meningitis. Pediatrics 49:206, 1972

Sutton A, Schneerson R, Kendall–Morris S, Robbins JB: Differential complement resistance mediates virulence of *Haemophilus influenzae* type b. Infect Immun 35:95, 1982

32

John B. Robbins
Margaret Pittman

Bordetella

Bordetella Pertussis

Bordetellae are minute, aerobic, gram-negative bacteria that uniquely localize on **cilia** of the mammalian respiratory epithelium (Fig. 32–1); they do not invade tissues. *B. pertussis*, the agent of **pertussis (whooping cough),** was isolated in 1906 by Bordet and Gengou. It is a pathogen for humans, and possibly for high primates under certain conditions; no other reservoir is known. Infection is spread by aerosols and is higly communicable. Although the disease is mild in adults, it has a significant mortality rate in infants, and until immunization was introduced in the 1930s pertussis was one of the most frequent and severe diseases of infants and children in the United States.

MORPHOLOGY, GROWTH, VARIATION

B. pertussis is a gram-negative coccobacillus about 0.5 μm in diameter and 0.5 to 2 μm in length. The cells may be arranged singly or in pairs, and, rarely, in chains. Its nutritional requirements are simple, and it does not utilize sugars. It is extremely sensitive to fatty acids, survives poorly without protective factors, and does not grow in the usual diagnostic media. It is usually grown in Bordet–Gengou agar, which does not contain sugar. The albumin in the blood in this medium binds fatty acids; in some other media, charcoal or β-methylcyclodextrin provides this function.

Fresh isolates require 3 to 4 days to form colonies. On Bordet–Gengou medium, these are small, convex, raised, and nearly transparent, surrounded by an indefinite narrow zone of hemolysis. Repeated passages yield flat, more rapidly growing colonies whose cells are less virulent and exhibit structural alterations (Phase 4). Intermediate Phases (2 and 3) are not well defined.

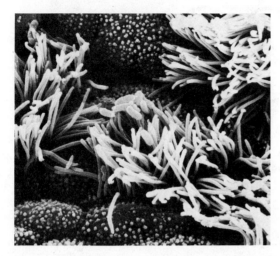

Figure 32–1. B. pertussis adhering only to ciliated cells of hamster tracheal rings in culture. Note cluster of six bacilli on tips of cilia in center of photograph. (Muse KE et al: In O Jahari, RP Becker [eds]: Scanning Electron Microscopy, Vol. II, Chicago, IIT Research Institute, 1977, p 263) (5000)

PATHOGENESIS

Pertussis has two phases. The first, **colonization,** is an upper respiratory disease with fever and coughing; the malaise gradually increases in intensity for about 10 days. Following these nonspecific symptoms the second, **toxemic,** stage gradually ensues, with prolonged and paroxysmal coughing that often ends in an inspiratory gasp (**whoop**). The coughing may be so severe as to provoke vomiting and aspiration. During the first stage, the organism, adherent to the cilia of the respiratory epithelium, can be recovered from pharyngeal swabs, and the severity and duration of the disease can be reduced by antimicrobial treatment. During the second stage, *B. pertussis* rarely can be recovered, and antimicrobials do not affect the course.

During the toxemic stage, there is a distinctive peripheral **lymphocytosis,** and there may be **hypoglycemia.** Loss of cilia, and subepithelial necrosis of the mucosa, may result from the coughing or the action of the toxins. The coughing and aspiration may also lead to pulmonary complications, including pneumonia, atelectasis, or pneumothorax. The greater severity of the disease in infants is probably attributable to their comparative inability to clear secretions, and to maintain adequate nutrition, during the paroxysmal coughing. Secondary pulmonary infections with other bacteria are common.

Central nervous system dysfunction is common: seizures occur in about 10% of infected infants, and **encephalopathy,** resulting in residual central nervous injury or in death, in about 0.1%. These are presumably effects of pertussis toxin, possibly aggravated by fever and by the hypoxia induced by the prolonged coughing and vomiting.

Because *B. pertussis* is localized exclusively to the cilia of the respiratory epithelium, and because systemic effects appear in distant tissues after the organism is no longer present, Pittman proposed that pertussis is a toxin-mediated disease. Several toxins have been identified, of which the most important is known as pertussis toxin (PT).

Pertussis Toxin

B. pertussis organisms or culture filtrates injected into laboratory animals exert diverse effects, which were previously attributed to various hypothetical products (lymphocytosis-promoting factor, histamine-sensitizing factor, islet-activating protein, protective Ag, and pertussigen). On purification, however, these effects were all accounted for by PT. Like many other bacterial toxins, PT is composed of A (active enzyme) and B (binding) subunits. The A subunit, a polypeptide of 25 Kd also designated **S1,** is an **ADP-ribosyl transferase.** The B subunit, composed of at least three different polypeptides, binds to specific carbohydrates on cell surfaces and on serum glycoproteins.

Following binding of the B subunit to various cells, the A subunit enters. It transfers the ADP-ribosyl moiety of NAD to a membrane-bound regulatory GTP-binding protein (called G_i or N_i) that normally **inhibits** adenyl cyclase, and the resulting inactivation of G_i **stimulates adenyl cyclase.** (Cholera toxin [see Ch. 26] stimulates cAMP synthesis by a parallel but opposite mechanism, ADP-ribosylating and thus **activating** a **stimulatory** GTP-binding protein, called G_s or N_s.

PT also affects several **hormonal actions.** Most prominently, it causes **hypoglycemia;** in particular, in infected mice epinephrine stimulates insulin production (whereas it normally inhibits adenylate cyclase and hence insulin production). PT also increases sensitivity to histamine and increases capillary permeability—effects that may contribute to shock. The relation of these findings to the pathogenesis of pertussis and to the development of encephalopathy is still unclear; the hypoglycemia may play a role in the CNS manifestations.

PT also has several effects on the **immune system** in experimental animals. It reduces the migratory and phagocytic activities of macrophages, and also responses of neutrophiles and macrophages to the chemotactic peptide fMet–Leu–Phe (aggregation, superoxide generation, and lysozyme release). It also stimulates the release of B and T cells from the bone marrow, spleen, and lymph nodes, which explains the clinically obvious **lymphocytosis** of pertussis; but while these cells are morphologically normal, they have lost the ability to return to lymphoid tissues and have diminished ability to elicit delayed hypersensitivity reactions. PT also either enhances or suppresses Ab responses, depending on the dose and the timing of administration. These several effects no doubt contribute to the high frequency of **secondary bacterial infections** during pertussis.

Other Toxins

B. pertussis not only stimulates host adenyl cyclase via PT: it also **secretes** its own **adenylate cyclase,** which enters mammalian cells. (*Bacillus anthracis* produces a similar enzyme.) This product reduces the phagocytic activity of macrophages, which may help the organism to initiate infection.

B. pertussis also produces a highly **lethal toxin** (formerly called dermonecrotic toxin), which causes local necrosis when injected intradermally. In the pathogenesis of the disease, it is thought to cause inflammation adjacent to the sites where *B. pertussis* is located. Another factor, called **tracheal cytotoxin,** is toxic for ciliated respiratory epithelium; its structure and immunopathologic role have not been defined.

The lipopolysaccharide of *B. pertussis* does not seem to have an imporant pathogenetic role.

ADHESION MECHANISMS. A **filamentous hemagglutinin (FHA)** and **fimbriae** both appear to play a role in the adhesion of *B. pertussis* to cilia, because Abs to each can inhibit adhesion to mammalian cells *in vitro.* (FHA assumes a filamentous structure only when isolated.) The suggested role of PT also as an adhesin is less clear.

REGULATION. The formation of virulence factors, including both adhesins and toxins, is subject to two kinds of regulation: reversible phenotypic alterations in response to changes in the environment (e.g., temperature, $MgSO_4$) level and phase variation, a reversible genetic shift. These mechanisms can act through a regulatory locus (*vir*) whose product has a coordinate effect on multiple virulence factors. In addition, the individual factors, whose genes are scattered on the chromosome, are subject to environmental influences. It has been speculated that shifts in the properties of the organism during the course of an infection may influence the ability to establish the carrier state and the ease of release from adhesion and transmission to other individuals.

IMMUNITY

Convalescence after pertussis is slow. Most patients develop serum Abs, in high titer, to PT, FHA, and fimbriae. The Abs to PT, but not those to FHA, remain elevated into adulthood and are correlated with the long-term immunity conferred by convalescence. In contrast, immunity induced by immunization wanes, so that adults immunized in infancy are often vulnerable to contracting per-

tussis. There is no evidence for asymptomatic infection or for a carrier state.

There is no established method for predicting whether an individual is immune to pertussis. PT Abs appear to be essential for immunity, but the role of Ab or other immune responses to other components of the organism, especially FHA, is still conjectural.

Vaccines

In the 1930s, convalescent serum was found to confer passive immunity, and pertussis vaccines were then developed following the principles set forth by Pasteur: identify and inactivate the causative organism. These **cellular vaccines** have been effective in reducing the incidence, morbidity, and mortality rate of the disease, although they have the disadvantage of containing not only protective moieties but also other components that produce adventitious reactions.

Reactions to the vaccine result rarely in permanent and even fatal sequelae, but the benefits of mass vaccination far outweigh the disadvantages. Nevertheless, public attention to the reactions has markedly decreased the use of the vaccine in some countries, with a resulting increase in the disease. This opposition has also raised the problem of how to allocate financial responsibility for the statistically inevitable reactions to a procedure that confers net benefit.

Purified PT and FHA have both been studied as potentially more specific vaccines. Immunization of mice with **inactivated PT** (toxoid), or passive immunization with either polyclonal or monoclonal PT Abs, confers immunity against both pulmonary and intracerebral challenge with *B. pertussis*. Moreover, treatment of infected mice with PT Abs both neutralizes the systemic effects of the PT and accelerates the clearance of the organisms.

Most patients develop FHA Abs of the IgM, IgA, and IgG isotypes within 4 weeks after the onset of pertussis. Cellular vaccines, in contrast, elicit high levels only of IgM and IgG. Accordingly, a rise of IgA Ab to FHA has diagnostic value, but with the limitations that not all patients develop Abs and that mild upper respiratory infections with *B. parapertussis* may also stimulate FHA Abs.

LABORATORY DIAGNOSIS

Nasopharyngeal mucus, collected by careful swabbing, should be cultured on Bordet–Gengou or Regan–Lowe medium, containing cephalexin to select against other organisms. *B. pertussis* is recovered in about 80% of cases in the first 2 weeks or in the early paroxysmal stage but only rarely after 4 weeks of symptoms. Direct immunofluorescence tests of secretions are of limited value, for false-negative or false-positive results are common. Lymphocytosis and a rising IgA Ab titer to FHA or PT provide valuable presumptive evidence.

TREATMENT AND PREVENTION

Erythromycin given in the initial stage is effective in reducing the symptoms. Supportive care, including parenteral fluids and assisted breathing, may be necessary in young infants during the paroxysmal stage. Although antibiotic treatment decreases the morbidity and mortality, pertussis continues to be highly communicable and dangerous in infants and young children. Cases should be promptly reported to state health departments.

Injection of **DTP** (diphtheria and tetanus toxoids and pertussis vaccine) is recommended at 2, 4, and 6 months for primary immunization, with boosters at 18 months and before entering the first grade. Active immunization of adults is effective in containing an outbreak in closed populations such as hospital personnel. Erythromycin is also useful as a prophylactic agent during outbreaks if given shortly after contact with a patient.

Immunization confers both individual and "herd" immunity. The latter has been demonstrated in the United Kingdom and Japan where public reaction to the rare severe or fatal complications reduced the use of pertussis vaccine from about 90% to 50% of infants: the result was re-emergence of epidemics after decades of negligible rates of the disease.

Immunity induced by cellular pertussis vaccines wanes after 5 to 10 years in most individuals, so adults may become susceptible again. Moreover, this reservoir is easily overlooked, because the disease in previously immunized adults may not elicit the characteristic "whooping." Nevertheless, adults may have prolonged coughing with secondary complications, and they transmit the organism.

Cellular pertussis vaccines elicit a high frequency of both local reaction and fever, likely secondary to their content of LPS. About 1 in 2000 injections induces a seizure or other central nervous system signs in infants. It has therefore been recommended that the P component of DTP vaccine be omitted for infants with a seizure disorder or nervous system disease or those who have had an earlier serious reaction to DTP.

Acellular vaccines are under investigation. Inactivated PT (pertussis toxoid) will probably be essential, but FHA and pili are also candidates. Serologic data alone cannot be used to justify replacement of the cellular vaccine, because there is no agreement about which Ags and host immune components are important in protection. Furthermore, animal models do not reproduce the disease: only clinical trials can provide conclusive data on the effectiveness of the new vaccines.

Other Bordetella Species

B. parapertussis closely resembles *B. pertussis* but does not form PT. It is frequently isolated along with *B. pertussis* from patients, suggesting that it may be a mutant strain, defective in formation of PT. By itself, it can cause a respiratory disease that is much milder than pertussis.

B. bronchiseptica is a closely related organism that causes atrophic rhinitis in swine and kennel cough in dogs.

Selected Reading

BOOKS AND REVIEW ARTICLES

Editorial: Whooping cough in infants. Lancet 2:496, 1988

Manclark CR, Hill JC (eds): International Symposium on Pertussis. Washington DC, US Department of Health, Education and Welfare, 1979. Publ. no. 79-1830

Masure HR, Shattuck RL, Storm DR: Mechanisms of bacterial pathogenicity that involve production of calmodulin-sensitive adenyl cyclases. Microbiol Rev 51:60, 1987

Pittman M: Pertussis toxin: The cause of the harmful effects and prolonged immunity of whooping cough: A hypothesis. Rev Infect Dis 1:401, 1979

Pittman M: The concept of pertussis as a toxin-mediated disease. Pediat Infect Dis 3:467, 1984

Sekura RD, Moss J, Vaughan M (eds): Pertussis Toxin: A Symposium. New York, Academic Press, 1985

SPECIFIC ARTICLES

Burnette WN, Cieplak W, Mar VL, et al: Pertussis toxin S1 mutant with reduced enzyme activity and a conserved protective epitope. Science 242:72, 1988

Cherry JD, Brunell PA, Golden GS, Karzon DT: Pediatrics 81:939, 1988

Granstrom M, Blenow M, Askelof P, Gillenius P, Olin P: Antibody response to pertussis toxin in whooping cough and pertussis vaccination. J Infect Dis 157:646, 1985

Imaizumi A, Suzuki Y, Ono S, Sato H, Sato Y: Effect of heptakis (2,6-dimethyl)β-cyclodextrin on the production of pertussis toxin by *Bordetella pertussis*. Infect Immun 41:1138, 1983

Meade BD, Kind PD, Ewell JB, McGrath P, Manclark CR: In-vitro inhibition of murine macrophage migration by *Bordetella* lymphocytosis-promoting factor. Infect Immun 45:718, 1984

Miller JF, Mekalanos JJ, Falkow S: Coordinate regulation and sensory transduction in the control of bacterial virulence. Science 243:916, 1989

Munoz JJ, Arai H, Cole RL: Mouse-protecting and histamine-sensitizing activities of pertussigen and fimbrial hemagglutinin from *Bordetella pertussis*. Infect Immun 32:243, 1981

Nicosia A, Bartoloni A, Perugini M, Rappuoli, R: Expression and immunological properties of the five subunits of pertussis toxin. Infect Immun 55:963, 1987

Sato H, Ikto A, Chiba J, Sato Y: Monoclonal antibody against pertussis toxin: Effect on toxin activity and pertussis infections. Infect Immun 46:422, 1984

Sato Y, Kimura M, Fukumi H: Development of a pertussis component vaccine in Japan. Lancet 1:122, 1984

Weiss AA, Hewlett EL: Annu Rev Microbiol 40:661, 1986

33

Morton N. Swartz

Aerobic Spore-Forming Bacilli

The genus *Bacillus* is composed of large gram-positive rods that form spores and grow best under aerobic conditions. Most species are saprobic and are found on vegetation and in soil, water, and air. The only species that is highly pathogenic for man is *B. anthracis*, which causes **anthrax,** a disease primarily of domestic livestock. Human anthrax is rare in the United States: it has occasionally been contracted from infected livestock by farmers, veterinarians, and slaughterhouse workers (**agricultural** anthrax), but it now occurs almost exclusively in workers at plants processing imported goat hair, wool, or hides (**industrial** anthrax). Anthrax remains an important human disease in undeveloped countries. (For example, more than 6000 cases occurred during a 6-month period in 1979–80 in Zimbabwe, accompanying war-associated breakdowns in veterinary and public health services.)

Bacillus Anthracis

The anthrax bacillus is unusually large and was the first bacterium shown to cause a disease. As early as 1850 it was seen in the blood of sheep dying of anthrax, and in 1877 Robert Koch grew it in pure culture, demonstrated its ability to form spores, and produced experimental anthrax by injecting it into animals.

In 1881, at the celebrated field trial at Pouilly-le-Fort, Pasteur vaccinated 24 sheep, one goat, and six cows with a culture of the bacillus attenuated by growth at 42°C, and after two weeks the animals, and unvaccinated controls, were injected with a virulent culture. Two days later the unvaccinated sheep and goat died and the unvaccinated cows were obviously ill, while all the vaccinated animals were well . This dramatic demonstration provided a potent stimulus to the development of immunology.

MORPHOLOGY

B. anthracis is a large gram-positive, non-motile, spore-forming rod, 1 to 1.5 μm in width and 4 to 10 μm in length. In smears from infected tissues, it appears singly or in short chains, and its capsule is readily demonstrable by McFadyean stain or with fluorescein-labeled anticapsular Ab. It does not form spores in the living animal. Spores are formed under conditions unfavorable for continued multiplication of the vegetative form; the mechanism is described in Chapter 2.

The organism grows well on blood agar, where it rarely causes hemolysis (in contrast to its saprobic relatives). Surface colonies of virulent strains are large, gray-white, and rough, with comma-shaped outgrowths; when viewed under a hand lens or colony microscope, they usually exhibit the "medusa head" or "curled hairlock" appearance illustrated in Figure 33–1. In the presence of high CO_2, the organisms form capsules, and the colonies are smooth and mucoid. Spores begin to appear at the end of the logarithmic phase of growth and are numerous after 48 hours. The oval spores are clearly visible in the centers of the bacilli in specially stained smears (Fig. 33–2).

METABOLISM

The anthrax bacillus is readily cultivated on ordinary nutrient media, and although it grows best aerobically, it will also multiply under anaerobic conditions. Aerobic conditions are required for sporulation but not for germination.

The nutritional requirements include thiamine and certain amino acids. Uracil, adenine, guanine, and manganese stimulate the growth of many strains. Glucose, sucrose, and maltose, but not mannitol, are fermented in most cultures.

Anthrax spores are relatively resistant to heat and to chemical disinfectants. They are usually destroyed by boiling for 10 minutes and by dry heat at 140°C for 3 hours. They may remain viable for months in animal hides and for years in dry earth.

ANTIGENIC STRUCTURE

Two major groups of Ags are associated with *B. anthracis:* (1) **cellular (somatic) Ags** and (2) **components of the complex exotoxin.**

CELLULAR ANTIGENS. In addition to a cell wall polysaccharide (containing equimolar quantities of N-acetyl glucosamine and D-galactose) the organism forms a single antigenic type of **capsular α-polypeptide of D-glutamic acid.** Capsule formation by virulent strains occurs in infected tissues; in culture it is enhanced by incubation in bicarbonate- and serum-containing medium under increased CO (which may stimulate glutamate formation from glucose; Chap. 4); the resulting colonies are mucoid. In the absence of CO_2 enrichment, the same organisms produce rough-appearing colonies. Smooth (S) and rough (R) variants of *B. anthracis* occur, and the S → R transition is associated with the selection of mutants that have lost the ability to synthesize capsular polypeptide. Encapsulated (S) strains may be selected for in cultures of unencapsulated (R) strains by addition to the medium of W_α phage, which attacks only the unencapsulated cells. Capsule production depends on a 60-megadalton plasmid (pXO2); its transfer to unencapsulated *B. anthracis*, via transduction or mating, produces the encapsulated phenotype.

The capsule is antiphagocytic, protects the organism from lytic antibody, and appears to play an important role in pathogenicity, as nonencapsulated mutants (even when grown under increased CO_2) are avirulent. However, this role appears to be limited to the establishment of the infection, whereas the terminal phase of the disease is much more closely linked to *in vivo* toxin production and toxemia.

EXOTOXIN COMPONENTS. Smith and Keppie first demonstrated an exotoxin in *B. anthracis* in 1954: in guinea pigs dying of experimental anthrax a toxic material was found in all infected tissues and exudates; it was most concentrated in edema fluid and plasma. This crude toxin produces extensive edema when injected subcutaneously in guinea pigs or rabbits and is lethal when injected intravenously in mice; it is also immunogenic. The same toxin is produced *in vitro*, but it is present in the culture medium only for a short time, when the cell density is about 1×10^8 chains/ml.* Bicarbonate ion is required for its production and possibly later for its release from the cell.

Production of anthrax toxin is mediated by a temperature-sensitive **plasmid** pXO1, of 110 megadaltons. The toxin consists of a mixture of three immunogenic proteins: (1) **edema factor (EF)**, M_r 89,000; (2) **protective antigen (PA)**, M_r 85,000 and capable of inducing protective antibodies; and (3) **lethal factor (LF)**, M_r 83,000. None of these proteins exhibits biological activity alone, but intravenous injection of PA and LF together causes death

---

* The delayed discovery of the anthrax toxin illustrates how the existence of a toxin may escape detection because of unfavorable conditions of artificial cultivation.

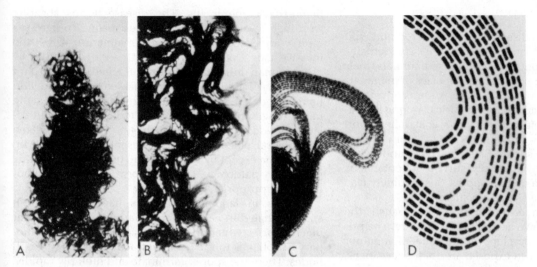

Figure 33–1. Basis of "medusa head" appearance of surface colonies of virulent strains of *B anthracis*. Organism grown on nutrient agar and stained with methylene blue. *(A)* Whole colony. (×45, reduced) *(B–D)* Border of colony. (×145, 400, and 1600, all reduced; Stein CD: Ann NY Acad Sci 48:507, 1947)

of rats, mice, or guinea pigs; injection of PA with EF into the skin of rabbits or guinea pigs causes local edema.

PA is thought to bind to cell receptors, rendering them capable of binding EF and facilitating its transfer to the cytoplasm. EF contains an **adenylate cyclase** that requires activation by tissue calmodulin. Local extracellular edema, a feature of cutaneous anthrax, may be the outcome of increased local intracellular concentrations of cAMP, analogous to the fluid and electrolyte loss in the intestine caused by cholera toxin (Chap. 27).

No enzymatic activities have been ascribed to LF.

GENETIC VARIATION

Mutants derived from wild-type strains of *B. anthracis* exhibit variations in virulence, in nutritional requirements, and in sensitivity to antimicrobial drugs, bacteriophages, and lysozyme. When repeatedly subcultured on laboratory media at elevated temperatures (42.5°C), wild-type strains become avirulent, and they no longer contain plasmid pXO1; transformation with purified plasmid DNA restores toxic activities.

Pasteur's famous heat attenuation likely decreased the proportion of cells containing pXO1 but did not eliminate the plasmid, and hence the toxin, from the culture; inoculation could then produce subclinical infection, evoking a protective immune response. Pasteur, in fact, had restored virulence through serial guinea pig passage.

For some time, the relation of **capsule formation** to virulence was confusing, for in growth under ordinary laboratory conditions some attenuated strains form capsules and many virulent strains do not. Further studies revealed that the latter strains generate capsular envelopes *in vivo*, and when grown on appropriate media with added CO_2. In contrast, avirulent mutants, although encapsulated when cultured, are incapable of forming capsules *in vivo*. Only those strains that produce **both capsules and toxin in the infected host** are highly pathogenic.

Sporulation and virulence are unrelated, for many nonsporulating mutants are still virulent.

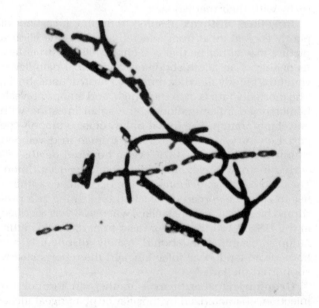

Figure 33–2. Anthrax bacilli from 48-hour plate culture stained with crystal violet. Spores are unstained and clearly visible. (×1200, reduced; Burrows W: Textbook of Microbiology. Philadelphia, WB Saunders, 1963)

PATHOGENICITY

Anthrax is primarily a disease of domesticated and wild animals. Humans become infected only incidentally, when brought into contact with diseased animals, their hides or hair, or their excreta. Many species of mammals and birds acquire the natural disease. Anthrax epizootics still occur in wildlife sanctuaries in Africa. Among laboratory animals, mice, guinea pigs, rabbits, goats, sheep, and monkeys are all highly susceptible. The LD_{50} for mice, for example, is about five spores. Rats, cats, dogs, and swine, on the other hand, will usually survive subcutaneous injections of at least a million spores. Susceptibility also varies widely with the site of inoculation.

The most common form of anthrax in humans is the cutaneous variety known as **malignant pustule.** The primary lesion usually develops at the site of a minor scratch or abrasion on an exposed area of the face, neck, or upper extremities into which anthrax spores have been accidentally inoculated. The spores germinate, and after an incubation period of 2 to 5 days, an inflamed papule develops, later becoming a vesicle. Eventually, the vesicle breaks down and is replaced by a black eschar (Fig. 33–3). A striking "gelatinous" nonpitting edema surrounds the eschar for a considerable distance. At no stage is the lesion particularly painful. In severe cases of cutaneous anthrax the regional lymph nodes become enlarged and tender, and the blood stream is eventually invaded. Lesions about the neck or face may produce mediastinal edema and respiratory distress. The systemic form of the disease is frequently fatal.

Inhalation anthrax (woolsorters' disease) results most commonly from exposure to spore-bearing dust where animal hair or hides are being handled. It not uncommonly leads to hemorrhagic mediastinitis and to hemorrhagic meningitis. The disease begins abruptly with high fever, dyspnea, and chest pain; it progresses rapidly and is often fatal before treatment can halt the invasive aspect of the infection.

In human inhalation anthrax tracheobronchial and mediastinal lymph nodes are markedly enlarged and hemorrhagic. The striking finding is an extensive acute hemorrhagic mediastinitis characterized by marked gelatinous edema. Focal hemorrhagic pulmonary edema and pleural effusion may be present, but there is no pneumonia except in a rare patient, usually with existing pulmonary pathology. Thus, the term "anthrax pneumonia" is inappropriate.

Studies in laboratory animals have revealed that spores inhaled in aerosols are phagocytized by alveolar macrophages, which in turn are carried via the pulmonary lymphatics to the regional tracheobronchial lymph nodes. There the spores germinate and multiply rapidly. Although many of the vegetative bacilli are destroyed by the cellular defenses of the lymph nodes, some escape and are carried by efferent lymphatics to the blood stream. Subsequently, they are rapidly cleared by the reticuloendothelial system (particularly the spleen), but they soon overgrow this defense system and establish a massive, fatal bacteremia.

To produce a fatal pulmonary infection it is necessary to introduce a relatively large number of spores. The LD_{50} for the guinea pig is approximately 20,000 spores. Moreover, because only particles (droplets) less than 5 μm in diameter are likely to penetrate to the alveoli, the average particle size in the aerosol is critical: the LD_{50} varies directly with their median size.

Intestinal anthrax results from the ingestion of poorly cooked meat from infected animals. The clinical picture may either be that of a cholera-like gastroenteritis or that of an acute abdomen (abdominal pain, fever, vomiting, bloody diarrhea, intestinal obstruction, shock). The mortality rate is extremely high, and autopsy reveals hemorrhagic inflammation of the small intestine with bowel perforation. The **intestinal tract** is commonly the portal of entry in cattle but rarely in man in developed countries. However, in 1979, over a hundred deaths occurred in an outbreak in Sverdlovsk in the Soviet Union. The outbreak was attributed by the U.S. military authorities to airborne spread of infection originating at a presumed biological warfare facility, whereas it was ascribed in the U.S.S.R. to ingestion of meat from diseased cattle. Autopsy examination should readily distinguish airborne from foodborne infection, and the reports clearly supported the latter.

Oropharyngeal anthrax is another rare form of this infection, characterized by tonsillar or pharyngeal ulceration and pseudomembrane formation (resembling diphtheria), difficulty in swallowing, and respiratory compromise.

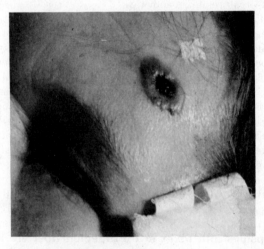

Figure 33–3. Cutaneous anthrax, 3- to 4-day-old lesion. Note black eschar in center surrounded by rim of edema. (Gold H: Arch Intern Med 96:387, 1955. Copyright © 1955 by the American Medical Association)

LETHAL TOXIN. Anthrax toxin may play a role in early stages of infection through a direct harmful effect on phagocytes. When virulent bacilli are injected subcutaneously into the susceptible host, the organisms proliferate freely and appear to resist phagocytosis by polymorphonuclear leukocytes, which accumulate in the lesion. Moreover, species with leukocytes more sensitive to toxin tend to be more susceptible than species with highly resistant leukocytes. Anthrax toxin (either PA plus LF or PA plus EF: see above) prevents the normal oxidative response [superoxide ion (O_2^-) release] to stimuli such as endotoxin; the combination of PA and EF also increases intracellular cAMP of neutrophiles and inhibits bacterial phagocytosis; and PA plus LF is lethal to macrophages. Toxin enters via an acidic endocytic vesicle, like diphtheria toxin and some viruses.

The level of lethal toxin in the circulation increases rapidly quite late in the disease, and it closely parallels the concentration of organisms in the blood. The primary site of action of the toxin is still unknown. Death frequently occurs suddenly and unexpectedly. Cardiac failure, increased vascular permeability, shock, hypoxia, and respiratory failure have all been implicated. Respiratory failure is regularly seen and may be due to cardiopulmonary changes (pulmonary capillary thrombosis), a central nervous system depression, or mediastinal edema.

Animal species vary in susceptibility to anthrax. Some are resistant to establishment of anthrax, and others to the toxin.

IMMUNITY

Animals surviving naturally acquired anthrax are resistant to reinfection; second attacks in humans are likewise extremely rare. Nevertheless, vaccines composed of killed bacilli produce no significant immunity, and anticapsular Ab is protective only in certain species, such as mice. Also, some descendant "Pasteur strains" in the U.S., which have totally lost the toxin plasmid pXO1, no longer produce PA, LF, and EF and do not provide protective immunity, while other strains were sufficiently virulent to cause serious disease. Although the Pasteur vaccine was later replaced by a safer nonencapsulated toxigenic strain for use in livestock, in the U.S. no attenuated spore vaccine has ever been considered to be satisfactory for human use. The best vaccine for humans now appears to be an alum-precipitated preparation of the protective Ag (PA) of the lethal toxin. Frequent boosters are necessary to maintain resistance.

Acquired immunity to anthrax seems, then, to be due to Abs both to the thermolabile toxin and to the capsular polypeptide. Their relative importance appears to differ widely in different species of hosts.

LABORATORY DIAGNOSIS

Anthrax bacilli may be seen in stained smears of the exudate from skin lesions in the vesicular stage and may be tentatively identified by their characteristic morphology. As the lesion ages, their demonstration becomes increasingly difficult.

A specimen should always be obtained for culture prior to the administration of antimicrobial therapy. The organism is encapsulated when grown under CO_2 on a rich bicarbonate-containing medium, and the cells form long chains, giving a bamboo-like appearance with gram stain. Unlike many other, saprobic members of the genus *Bacillus*, *B. anthracis* is nonhemolytic on sheep blood agar. It is also non-motile, unlike *B. subtilis* and many strains of *B. cereus*.

In pulmonary anthrax sputum cultures are rarely positive, because the inhaled spores usually do not germinate and multiply until they have reached the mediastinal lymph nodes. Whenever anthrax is suspected, the blood should be cultured. Because other aerobic spore-forming bacilli, such as *B. cereus*, may sometimes be cultured from the skin, respiratory tract, and even the blood, organisms thought to be anthrax bacilli should be definitively characterized (Table 33–1).

TABLE 33–1. *Properties Differentiating* Bacillus anthracis *from* B. cereus

	B. anthracis	*B. cereus*
Comma-shaped outgrowths in colonies on blood agar	Many	Few or more
Colonies on bicarbonate medium (CO_2)	Raised, mucoid	Flat, dull
Hemolysis (sheep RBCs)	None or weak	Usually β-hemolytic
Motility	−	+
Capsule (fluorescent Ab or McFadyean stain)*	+ or −	−
Agglutination by soybean lectin	+	−
Susceptibility to penicillin	+	−
Enhanced hydrolysis of p-nitrophenyl-α-D-glucoside in presence of 1% Triton X-100	+	−
Lysis by gamma bacteriophage	+	−

* In evaluation of smears obtained from lesions of patients or of isolates grown in appropriate medium for capsule production.

TREATMENT

Penicillin G is the drug of choice; tetracycline is an alternative for the patient who is allergic to penicillin. Most strains of *B. anthracis* are also sensitive to erythromycin and chloramphenicol. Antiserum, presumably containing antitoxin, was formerly used in the treatment of human anthrax, but has been superseded. Antimicrobial therapy is usually effective in cutaneous anthrax, although the toxin in the primary lesion often causes the formation of an eschar despite early treatment. In respiratory anthrax it is usually ineffective, because the disease is rarely recognized before bacteremia has developed; hence the mortality rate is extremely high. Treatment with both antibiotics and antitoxin might be advocated for the rare pulmonary form of anthrax.

PREVENTION

Anthrax still causes heavy loss of livestock, particularly in the Middle East, Africa, and Asia. In the U.S. the disease is endemic in cattle in Louisiana, Texas, South Dakota, Nebraska, and California. It is transmitted primarily through the ingestion of contaminated forage or from the carcasses of infected animals. Spores may remain viable in the soil for many years. Epidemiologic evidence indicates that in suitable soils anthrax bacilli can survive ecologic competition with other organisms and can maintain an organism → spore → organism cycle for years without infecting livestock. Whether the organism also grows saprobically is not known.

Animal anthrax can be at least partially controlled by immunization with attenuated vaccines. The disease has been virtually eliminated in South Africa by this means. The carcasses of animals dying of anthrax should be disposed of either by cremation or by deep burial.

No more than five cases of human anthrax have been reported annually over the past two decades in the U.S., but the disease is much more prevalent in some other countries.

In the U.S. industrial anthrax was formerly most common among textile workers employed in plants that processed goat hair imported from the Middle East. Its control poses many practical problems. Economically feasible methods of disinfecting hides without damaging them are difficult to devise. Industrial workers at high risk should probably be immunized with the protective Ag, as should veterinarians practicing in "anthrax districts" and laboratory workers who have contact with *B. anthracis*. It is important to continue to enforce hygienic measures at plants (clothing changes, etc.), to keep the incidence of disease at its current low level.

Other Aerobic Spore-Forming Bacilli

Many saprobic species of aerobic spore-forming bacilli are hard to distinguish from *B. anthracis* except on the basis of pathogenicity. The most commonly encountered are *B. cereus*, *B. subtilis*, and *B. sphaericus*. *Bacillus* species other than *B. anthracis* occasionally are responsible for infections in man: pulmonary and disseminated infections in immunologically compromised hosts; bacteremia in patients undergoing hemodialysis; meningitis after ventricular shunting for hydrocephalus; endocarditis in drug addicts; endophthalmitis associated with intravenous drug abuse or following penetrating eye injuries; wound infections; and crepitant myonecrosis following trauma, mimicking gas gangrene. *B. cereus* is involved as such an opportunistic invader more often than other *Bacillus* species. Several properties serve to differentiate it from *B. anthracis* (Table 33–1).

Unlike *B. anthracis*, *B. cereus* is resistant to penicillin and the cephalosporins by virtue of production of extracellular penicillinase and cephalosporinase. It is susceptible to vancomycin, clindamycin, and gentamicin.

Products of various *Bacillus species* have found roles in medicine, laboratory research, and agriculture: bacitracin, an antibiotic; penicillinase (from *B. cereus*); restriction endonucleases for DNA cloning; parasporal crystal glycoproteins (from *B. thuringiensis*), as potent insecticides; and relatively heat-resistant spores (*B. stearothermophilus*) for monitoring sterilization procedures.

FOOD POISONING

B. cereus (present on many grains, vegetables and dairy products) can cause outbreaks of food poisoning. These result from **toxins elaborated by germinating spores** consequent on improper refrigeration and subsequent reheating of cooked foods (e.g., refried rice). There are two forms of *B. cereus* food poisoning. The **diarrheal syndrome** (less than 24 hours' duration), with an incubation period of 10 to 12 hours, is caused by a **heat-labile enterotoxin** (produced during late exponential growth), which causes fluid accumulation in ligated rabbit ileal loops and alters vascular permeability of guinea-pig skin. The **emetic syndrome** (1 to 5 hours' duration), with an incubation period of 1 to 5 hours, is associated with a **heat-stable enterotoxin** (produced during sporulation and present preformed in food), which can be assayed only by its ability to induce vomiting on feeding to monkeys.

Selected Reading

BOOKS AND REVIEW ARTICLES

Lincoln RE, Fish DC: Anthrax toxin. In Montie TC, Kadis S, Ajl SJ (eds): Microbial Toxins, vol III. New York, Academic Press, 1970

Smith H: The use of bacteria grown in vivo for studies on the basis of their pathogenicity. Annu Rev Microbiol 12:77, 1958

Turnbull PCB: *Bacillus cereus* toxins. Pharmacol Ther 13:453, 1981

SPECIFIC ARTICLES

Albrink WS: Pathogenesis of inhalation anthrax. Bacteriol Rev 25:268, 1961

Brachman PS: Anthrax. Ann NY Acad Sci 174:577, 1970

Brachman PS: Inhalation anthrax. Ann NY Acad Sci 353:83, 1980

Friedlander AM: Macrophages are sensitive to anthrax lethal toxin through an acid-dependent process. J Biol Chem 261:7123, 1986

Green BD, Battisti L, Koehler TM, Thorne CB, Ivins BE: Demonstration of a capsule plasmid in *Bacillus anthracis*. Infect Immun 49:291, 1985

Ivins BE, Ezzell JW Jr, Jemski J, Hedlund KW, Ristroph JD, Leppla SH: Immunization studies with attenuated strains of *Bacillus anthracis*. Infect Immun 52:454, 1986

Leppla SH: Anthrax toxin edema factor: A bacterial adenylate cyclase that increases cyclic AMP concentrations in eucaryotic cells. Proc Natl Acad Sci USA 79:3162, 1982

Mikesell P, Ivins BE, Ristroph JD, Dreier TM: Evidence for plasmid-mediated toxin production in *Bacillus anthracis*. Infect Immun 39:371, 1983

O'Brien J, Friedlander A, Dreier T, Ezzell J, Leppla S: Effects of anthrax toxin components on human neutrophils. Infect Immun 47:306, 1985

Spira WM, Goepfert JM: Biological characteristics of an enterotoxin produced by Bacillus cereus. Can J Microbiol 21:1236, 1975

Thorne CB: Capsule formation and glutamyl polypeptide synthesis by *Bacillus anthracis* and *Bacillus subtilis*. Symp Soc Gen Microbiol 6:68, 1956

Uchida I, Hashimoto K, Terakado N: Virulence and immunogenicity in experimental animals of *Bacillus anthracis* strains harboring or lacking 110 MDa and 60 MDa plasmids. J Gen Microbiol 132:557, 1986

Wright GG, Mandell GL: Anthrax toxin blocks priming of neutrophils by lipopolysaccharide and by muramyl dipeptide. J Exp Med 164:1700, 1986

34

Morton N. Swartz

Anaerobic Spore-Forming Bacilli: the Clostridia

General Properties

The anaerobic spore-forming bacilli belong to the genus *Clostridium*. (L. *clostridium*, spindle). Their natural habitat is the soil and the intestinal tracts of animals and man. A few of these saprobes are also human pathogens under appropriate circumstances, causing six very different diseases: **botulism, tetanus, anaerobic cellulitis and gas gangrene, clostridial bacteremia, pseudomembranous colitis,** and **clostridial gastroenteritis.** The pathogenicity of these organisms depends on the release of powerful exotoxins or highly destructive enzymes. How soil organisms benefit from producing specific neurotoxins is not clear.

MORPHOLOGY AND GROWTH

The clostridia are relatively large pleomorphic, gram-positive, rod-shaped organisms. Filamentous forms are common. In 48-hour cultures, many of the bacilli may be gram-negative. All species form spores but with considerable variation in the required conditions. The highly refractile spores (Fig. 34–1) are oval or spherical and usually wider than the parental cell; they may be terminal or subterminal in the cell. Most species of clostridia possess peritrichous flagella and are motile (Fig. 34–2). A few (e.g., *C. perfringens*) are encapsulated (Fig. 34–3). Colony forms are variable; hemolysis on blood agar is frequent.

Clostridia lack the cytochromes required for electron transport to O_2. They contain flavoprotein enzymes that

633

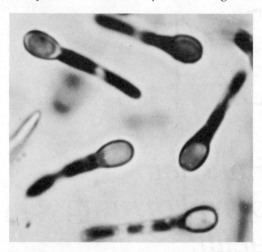

Figure 34–1. Terminal clostridial endospores in stained wet-mount preparation. (×3600; courtesy of CF Robinow)

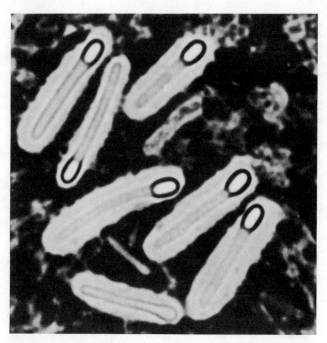

Figure 34–3. Nigrosin preparation of *C. pectinovorans* showing both capsules and endospores. (×3600; courtesy of CF Robinow)

reduce O_2 to H_2O_2 and to superoxide (O_2^-; Chap. 4), and they lack the catalase, peroxidases, and superoxide dismutase that would destroy these toxic products; hence their obligate anaerobiosis. Not all clostridia are equally oxygen-sensitive: *C. tetani* requires strict anaerobic conditions; *C. perfringens* is much less fastidious; and *C. histolyticum* and *C. tertium* may grow on aerobic blood agar plates. Clostridial spores not only are resistant to heat and disinfectants but survive long periods of exposure to air; they germinate only under strongly reducing conditions. Specimens for anaerobic culture should be collected carefully, transported in "gassed-out" (evacu-

ated) tubes, inoculated promptly on prereduced media, and incubated anaerobically by one of the methods previously described (Chap. 31).

METABOLISM AND CLASSIFICATION

Most clostridia produce large amounts of gas (mainly CO_2 and H_2) in butyric fermentation (Chap. 4). The fermentation of various sugars is of value in differentiating species. Other biochemical tests include reactions in milk, the liquefaction of gelatin, and the production of indole from tryptophan (Table 34–1). The characteristic "stormy fermentation" of milk by *C. perfringens* is the result of formation of a clot that becomes torn by the accumulating gas. Some clostridia are predominantly proteolytic and others saccharolytic.

A wide variety of **enzymes** have been identified in the filtrates of clostridial cultures, including collagenase, other proteinases, hyaluronidase, deoxyribonuclease, lecithinase, and neuraminidase. Some of these act as toxins in the animal host; other potent protein exotoxins are **botulinum toxins** and **tetanus toxin;** *C. perfringens* and *C. difficile* produce enterotoxins. Many species produce hemolysins. Abs to some of these products may be of use in identifying individual clostridial species. Nontoxigenic mutants of various species occur.

The somatic and flagellar Ags of clostridia are varied

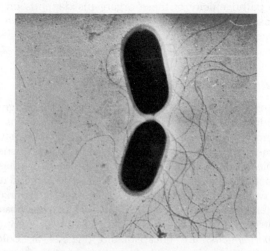

Figure 34–2. Electron photomicrograph of *C. tetani* showing cell wall and peritrichous flagella. (×11,000, reduced; courtesy of Stuart Mudd)

TABLE 34–1. Properties of Common Species of Pathogenic Clostridia

Disease and causative species	Aerobic growth	Spores	Motility	Lecithinase	Toxicity (mice)	Milk	Gelatinase	Lactose	Glucose	Maltose	Sucrose	Indole	Toxin neutralization for specific identification	Organic acids detected by GLC*
Botulism														
C. botulinum	–	ST	+	–	+	V	+	–	A	V	–	–	+	
Tetanus														
C. tetani	–	T	+	–	+	NC	+	–	–	–	–	V	+	A,P,B
Gas gangrene														
C. perfringens	–	ST†	–	+	V	CG	+	A	A	A	A	–		A,B
C. novyi	–	ST	+	+	V	V	+	–	A	V	–	–	+	A,P,B
C. septicum	–	ST	+	–	+	NC	+	A	A	A	–	–		A,B
C. histolyticum	+	ST	+	–	V	CD	+	–	–	–	–	–		A,L
C. tertium	+	T	+	–	–	V	–	A	A	A	A	–		A,B,L
C. bifermentans	–	ST	+	+	–	D	+	–	A	A	–	+		A,P,IB,IV,IC
C. sporogenes	–	ST	+	–	–	CD	+	–	A	A	A	–		A,IV,B
Pseudomembranous enterocolitis														
C. difficile	–	ST	+	–	V	NC	V	–	A	–	–	–	+	A,P,IB,B,IV,V,IC

A, acid; C, coagulated; D, digested; G, gas; NC, no coagulation; ST, subterminal; T, terminal; V, variable.

* Gas liquid chromatography: A, acetic acid; B, butyric acid; IB, isobutyric acid; IV, isovaleric acid; IC, isocaproic acid; L, lactic acid; P, propionic acid; V, valeric acid.

† Spores are only rarely seen in direct smears from wounds or cultures but can be demonstrated on growth in special media.

but have not provided a practical system for the identification of species.

Botulism

Botulism is usually **not an infectious disease** in adults but an **intoxication:** it results from the ingestion of food contaminated by preformed botulinum toxin rather than from multiplication (and toxin production) of *C. botulinum* in the gastrointestinal tract. In this respect, it resembles staphylococcal food poisoning. Uncooked meat or sausage (L. *botulus*) was formerly one of the commonest sources of the disease; currently, in the United States, the principal vehicles are improperly canned fruits and vegetables (usually home-processed), condiments, and fish products. From 1970 to 1977, there were 108 outbreaks (averaging 33 cases annually) of foodborne botulism in the U.S. Rarely (30 cases in the U.S. since 1950), wound contamination with *C. botulinum* has been associated with noninvasive infection and *in vivo* toxin formation, producing clinical **wound botulism.**

Infrequently, ingested *C. botulinum* colonizes the gastrointestinal tracts of infants (and very rarely of adults), where it elaborates toxin. More than 500 cases of **infant botulism** have been recorded since the entity was first described in 1976, and it has become the predominant form of botulism recognized in this country.

Botulinum toxin acts on the nervous system, producing a life-threatening illness with cranial nerve impairment and symmetric weakness or paralysis.

THE ORGANISM AND ITS TOXIN

C. botulinum is widely distributed in the soil, in the silt of lake and pond bottoms, and on vegetation; hence the intestinal contents of mammals, birds, and fish occasionally contain the organism. **Eight types** (A, B, C_1, C_2, D, E, F, G) have been recognized; each elaborates an **immunologically distinct form of toxin.** All the toxins except one (C_2) are neurotoxins. The C_2 toxin (botulinum binary toxin) is unique in structure (composed of separate, unlinked heavy and light chains) and pharmacologic action (increased vascular permeability). In the U.S. only types A (51% of cases), B (21%), and E (12%), have been significant causes of human botulism; and the geographic distribution of cases is in keeping with the isolation of various toxin types from regional soil samples: type A, from the West; type B, trom the Northeast and Central states; type E, from the Pacific Northwest, Alaska, and the Great Lakes area (particularly in marine sediments). Type F is rare; C and D are usually associated with botulism in fowl and mammals; G has been isolated from soil and has recently been found in several humans.

For convenience, *C. botulinum* can be divided into four groups by cultural characteristics: Group 1 (proteolytic) includes toxin-producing strains of type A, B, or F; Group II (nonproteolytic) includes toxin-producing strains of type B, E, or F; group III (weakly proteolytic or nonproteolytic) includes toxin-producing strains of type C_1, C_2, or D; and group IV (proteolytic but nonsaccharolytic) includes toxin-producing strains of type G. Growth of vegetative cells is required for toxin production, but little toxin appears in the medium until late in growth, when it is **released by cell lysis.** Toxin of group II cultures requires activation by trypsin for expression of maximum toxicity, whereas toxin in culture filtrates of group I is already active, as a result of selective "nicking" by proteolytic enzymes of the organism.

These are the **most powerful biological toxins known;** 1 μg contains 200,000 minimal lethal doses (MLD) for a mouse and is nearly a lethal dose for man.

Although most strains synthesize only one type of toxin, there are exceptions. Strains designated C_α can produce toxins C_1, C_2, and D; type D strains can produce C_1 and D toxins; one strain produces both type F and some type A; and some strains are nontoxigenic.

Toxin production in **some** strains depends on the presence of specific **prophages.** Cultures of types C and D cured of their prophages stop producing their dominant toxins (but still produce low levels of C_2) and become indistinguishable. Such cured strains can be converted to either type C or D toxin production by infection with the appropriate phage. The relation between the host bacteria and the phage is unstable (pseudolysogeny), which may account for the occasional isolation of nontoxigenic *C. botulinum* in areas where types C and D are prevalent. A role for phage infection has not been demonstrated for other botulinum toxin types. Moreover, most type A strains contain plasmids, but none of these have been correlated with toxigenicity.

Infection of a cured strain of *C. botulinum* type C by phage NA_1 (from *C. novyi* type A) can induce production of the α-toxin of *C. novyi*. The resultant organism would then be identified as *C. novyi* type A. Evidently, a prototype clostridial organism may be identified as one or another species, depending on the resident phage. This phenomenon might account for rare cases of infant botulism caused by *C. butyricum* or *C. barati* strains producing a botulinum toxin.

Botulinum neurotoxin is synthesized as a single chain polypeptide ($M_r \sim 150,000$) that contains at least one intrachain disulfide bond and is only weakly active. When nicked by endogenous proteases (or by trypsin in the intestine), it is converted to a dichain polypeptide consisting of a heavy (H) chain ($M_r \sim 100,000$) and a light (L) chain ($M_r \sim 50,000$) and becomes fully active. The **binding domain** of the molecule appears to be in the carboxyl terminus of the H chain; a **channel-forming domain,** which is likely to play a role in toxin insertion into membranes, is posited for the amino terminus of the H chain; the **poisoning** domain resides in the light chain. The individual domains lack neurotoxicity. No enzymatic activity has been found in any of the botulinum neurotoxins.

Binary toxin (C_2) also has an H chain ($M_r \sim 100,000$) and an L chain ($M_r \sim 50,000$), but these are not linked by a disulfide bond. Neither chain alone shows much activity, but when combined, they increase vascular permeability and have enterotoxic and cytopathic effects but no neurotoxic ones. The H chain mediates binding. The L chain is an enzyme that can **ADP-ribosylate nonmuscle actins** from various cells.

The **spores** of *C. botulinum* are relatively heat-resistant, and pressure sterilization is necessary to ensure their destruction. Effective sterilization is routine in the canning industry; home-canned foods, especially "low-acid" vegetables (pH above 4.5), have been the source of most outbreaks of botulism in this country. In the past, tomatoes have been sufficiently acid to inhibit production of *C. botulinum* toxin but "low-acid" tomatoes are now available and are a potential source of botulism in home-canned products.

In contrast to the spores, botulinum toxin is relatively heat-labile, being completely inactivated in 10 minutes at 100°C; hence **boiling just prior to ingestion renders home-canned vegetables or processed fish safe.** Care should be exercised in handling suspect food samples in the laboratory, because the toxin may be absorbed from fresh wounds and mucosal surfaces. Most outbreaks in the U.S. now involve types A or B in home-canned vegetables. During the last decade, type E and occasionally A in commercial smoked fish became more frequent.

PATHOGENESIS

Botulism results from the ingestion of uncooked foods in which contaminating spores have germinated and elaborated toxin. **Food that is not visibly fermented or spoiled to taste may still contain botulinum toxin** (produced by nonproteolytic strains).

The toxin is not inactivated by gastric acid or by the proteolytic enzymes of the stomach and upper bowel. In fact, crude toxin of *C. botulinum* type E can be potentiated 10- to 1000-fold by partial proteolysis (e.g., limited trypsin treatment). Because toxin-containing sera from patients with botulism do not show such activation, the toxin may have already undergone proteolysis in the gastrointestinal tract.

After absorption from the gastrointestinal tract, the toxin reaches susceptible **neuromuscular junctions and peripheral autonomic synapses,** by way of the blood. Botulinum neurotoxin also binds to isolated synaptosomes. The H chain of the holotoxin is responsible for binding, and free H chains prevent neurotoxicity of intact toxin. The molecular receptor has not been identified, but it is known that the neurotoxin interacts with **gangliosides** (particularly GT1b) found in nerve tissue, and it is inactivated in the process.

Histologic and neuropharmacologic evidence indicates that botulinum neurotoxin requires internalization to produce its neurotoxic effects. Receptor-mediated endocytosis (as in the case of diphtheria toxin) appears to be the mechanism by which it crosses the plasma membrane of cholinergic nerves. Subsequently, passage through the membrane of the endocytic vesicle into the cytoplasm (a presumed prerequisite for neurotoxicity) appears to occur. As with diphtheria toxin, proton-pump-mediated lowering of vesicular pH confers on botulinum toxin the capacity to insert into membranes and form channels.

Electrophysiologic and electron microscopic studies show that botulinum toxin **blocks both spontaneous quantal and nerve-stimulus-induced exocytosis of acetylcholine-containing vesicles.** In neuromuscular transmission, nerve depolarization is coupled to release of acetylcholine by Ca^{2+} entry into presynaptic nerve terminals. Botulinum toxin does not appear to act by directly blocking Ca^{2+} uptake. Because the number of vesicles far exceeds the number of toxin molecules, an as-yet-unidentified enzymatic function appears more likely than a stoichiometric action.

In addition to action at the neuromuscular junction, botulinum toxin paralyzes postganglionic parasympathetic and sympathetic transmission mediated by acetylcholine.

Although the various types of botulinum neurotoxin appear to have the same pharmacologic action, their potency varies with the test species. The ratio of the lethal doses for mice and fowl, for example, is 1/15 for type A, 1/2000 for type C, 1/100,000 for type D, and 1/25 for type E. The differences may well be of epidemiologic significance.

CLINICAL FEATURES. Symptoms in man usually begin 18 to 36 hours after ingestion and are the result of cholinergic blockade. Weakness, dizziness, constipation, and severe dryness of the mouth and pharynx are early manifestations; nausea and vomiting are common with type E disease. Fever is absent. Neurologic features soon develop: blurring of vision, dilatation of pupils, inability to swallow, difficulty in speech, urinary retention, generalized descending weakness of skeletal muscles, and respiratory paralysis. Sensory abnormalities are absent.

A curious neurophysiologic response, a facilitated muscle action potential after repetitive nerve stimulation, is typical of patients with botulism.

The fatality rate has been extremely high but has declined to 16% in this country during 1970 to 1977. Fortunately, the disease is much less common in man than in animals.

Wound botulism (type A) should be considered in an isolated case when characteristic neurologic abnormalities develop but no food source is implicated. However, *C. botulinum* spores do not germinate readily in tissue. Chronic drug abusers, even with only minor infections at injection sites, represent a newly recognized high-risk group.

Infant botulism, secondary to **infection,** is characterized by constipation, weak sucking ability, cranial nerve deficits, generalized weakness, and sudden apneic episodes. The infants, 2 to 36 weeks of age, have usually developed the disease after they had been exposed to some solid foods. In a few instances, honey and environmental dust and dirt have been implicated epidemiologically as the source. This "infection–intoxication" is essentially a disease of infants, probably because of their less well-established competing intestinal flora. *C. botulinum* organisms as well as toxin have been found in the stools for as long as 160 days after the onset of symptoms but not in the stools of healthy infants or adults. All reported patients have recovered, usually without administration of specific antiserum. The possible role of infant botulism in a few cases of the sudden infant death syndrome has been suggested by the finding of *C. botulinum*, its toxin, or both in the bowel contents of several infants who died suddenly and unexpectedly.

In adults, *C. botulinum* is also present in stool of 60% of patients with foodborne (intoxication) botulism, having been ingested along with the preformed toxin. However, in six such cases, the incriminated food source lacked preformed toxin. In these cases of **adult infection,** achlorhydria, intestinal surgery, and antibiotic therapy were contributing factors, reducing the normal gastric barrier or changing the intestinal flora.

LABORATORY DIAGNOSIS

In cases of suspected botulism mice should be injected intraperitoneally with the patient's serum (up to 1.0 ml) and with aqueous cell-free extracts of stool and of the implicated food. Heat-treated samples should also be inoculated to serve as controls. Trypsin treatment of a portion of stool and food samples may enhance toxin activity (particularly type E) and make detection easier. If significant amounts of toxin are present, the mice will develop paralysis and will succumb within 1 to 5 days; neutralization of toxin by type-specific antiserum provides protection. Because toxin is detected infrequently in the serum of patients with infant botulism, the diagnosis is established by detection of toxin or *C. botulinum* or both in stool.

Samples of the suspected food should also be cultured anaerobically, with heat (or alcohol) treatment of part of the sample to select for spores. Because only vegetative cells or relatively heat-sensitive spores (type E) may be present, part of the sample should be incubated without heating. If an anaerobic gram-positive bacillus is recovered from food, or stool, it should be characterized by growth and metabolic properties. *C. sporogenes* cannot be differentiated by such testing from proteolytic group I strains of *C. botulinum*. A fluorescent Ab reagent for identifying group I strains can provide presumptive identification of *C. botulinum*. For definitive identification, cultures should be tested for toxin production. The cultural approach is generally less useful than direct tests for the toxin.

TREATMENT AND PREVENTION

The toxins that cause botulism in man are each specifically neutralized by its antitoxin. Botulinum toxin, as toxoid, is a good Ag; as little as 1 μg will induce high levels of protective Ab in the mouse. Clinical botulism, however, does not induce demonstrable Ab because an amount of toxin sufficient to induce an immune response would be lethal.

Once toxin has become "fixed" at susceptible nerve endings, its harmful action is unaffected by antitoxin. With type A botulism, antitoxin does not appear to alter the clinical course once neurologic symptoms have occurred, but beneficial results have followed the use of antitoxin in type E botulism. To neutralize any circulating or "unfixed" toxin, equine **polyvalent antiserum (types A, B, and E) should be given intravenously in suspected cases at once,** without awaiting the results of laboratory tests. The usual precautions should be taken against hypersensitivity reactions to the foreign serum.

Because most infants with botulism do not have toxin in their serum and are no longer acutely ill when the condition is diagnosed, antitoxin is rarely administered.

Enemas, cathartics, and gastric lavage are employed to facilitate elimination of unabsorbed toxin providing bowel paralysis is not present. Penicillin therapy is used in wound botulism and sometimes in foodborne botulism on the possibility that toxin may be released *in vivo* by germinating spores. In infant botulism, antibiotics may be detrimental by inducing rapid cell lysis (and

toxin release) and by allowing persistence of *C. botulinum* through altering competing intestinal flora.

Other individuals known to have ingested the same food as the patient should also be treated, even if they are asymptomatic.

As already mentioned, boiling of any improperly canned or processed food for at least 10 minutes will destroy botulinum toxin. Sodium nitrite is extensively used as a preservative in cured meats. Its antibotulinum properties stem from its capacity to react with iron–sulfur proteins (e.g., ferredoxin, essential in electron transport in anaerobes).

A pentavalent toxoid evokes a good Ab response, but human use is justified only in frequently exposed laboratory workers. Toxoids have been successful in immunizing cattle in areas where the disease is endemic.

Tetanus

Tetanus is an acute, often fatal bacterial disease in which the clinical manifestations stem, not from invasive infection, but from a potent neurotoxin (**tetanospasmin**) elaborated when spores of *C. tetani* germinate after gaining access to wounds. The disease develops in the setting of penetrating trauma, chronic skin ulcers, infections about the umbilical stump in the newborn (**neonatal tetanus),** obstetrical procedures (**postabortal tetanus),** and infected injection sites in narcotics addicts. The disease is of particular importance in military medicine. Because only **one antigenic type of toxin** is involved, an effective **monotypic toxoid** has been possible. Because of its widespread use for prophylactic immunization, fewer than 100 cases of tetanus occur annually in the U.S. (an 11-fold decrease over the past four decades). However, the disease remains a serious problem worldwide (approximately 300,000 cases a year), particularly in developing countries.

THE ORGANISM AND ITS TOXIN

C. tetani is a strict anaerobe without a capsule; spherical terminal spores give a characteristic "drumstick" appearance (Fig. 34–1). It is found in the soil and in feces of farm and domestic animals. In humans, fecal carrier rates are usually low but variable (0–25%), suggesting that the organism is a transient whose presence depends on its ingestion.

Tetanus toxin is only slightly less potent than type A botulinum toxin; as little as 1 ng/kg injected into a laboratory animal produces spastic paralysis. It also is produced by growing cells and released only on cell lysis: hence, the disease appears only when spores of *C. tetani* germinate after gaining access to wounds.

The structural gene for toxin production is on a 75-Kb plasmid. Tetanus toxin ("intracellular" or "progenitor" toxin) is produced initially as a single polypeptide chain ($M_r \sim 150,000$). As with *C. botulinum*, the **toxicity** of autolysates **can be increased by** autologous or trypsin-induced **proteolysis.** Such "nicked" ("extracellular") toxin molecules, like botulinum toxin, consist of an H chain ($M_r \sim 100,000$) and an L chain ($M_r \sim 50,000$) held together by a disulfide bond. They can be separated by disulfide bond reduction; individual chains are nontoxic, but reconstituted holotoxin regains toxicity. Digestion by papain of the nicked (but still disulfide-bonded) molecule yields two fragments; each of these can immunize animals against tetanus, reacts with antitoxin, and is nontoxic. The C fragment ($M_r \sim 50,000$) contains the carboxy-terminal portion of the H chain which mediates receptor binding; the B fragment ($M_r \sim 100,000$) consists of the remainder of the toxin.

Tetanus toxin is produced *in vitro* in amounts up to 5% to 10% of the bacterial weight, but it serves no known useful function for the bacillus.

Animals differ widely in their susceptibility to tetanus toxin: mammals are most sensitive, and birds are relatively resistant (e.g., the pigeon is 24,000 times as resistant as the guinea pig).

In addition to its neurotropic toxin, *C. tetani* produces an oxygen-labile hemolysin, antigenically similar to streptolysin O, known as **tetanolysin.** There is no evidence that it plays a significant role in pathogenesis.

Nontoxin-producing strains of *C. tetani* are not pathogenic. A related species, *C. tetanomorphum*, does not produce tetanus toxin.

Immunity to tetanus involves Ab to toxin: Abs to somatic Ags are not protective. Tetanus toxoid is an excellent immunogen in man, but **clinical tetanus does not induce immunity** because so little toxin is released. Actively immunizing all patients on recovery from tetanus is therefore extremely important.

PATHOGENESIS

Most cases result from small puncture wounds or lacerations; the infection remains localized to the traumatized tissue at the site of entry, usually with a minimal inflammatory response. Mixed infection with other organisms or the presence of a foreign body may induce more marked inflammation (and lower the oxidation–reduction potential locally), promoting the growth of *C. tetani*. However, in 5% to 10% of cases, the initial injury is so trivial as to have been forgotten by the patient and to have left no residual.

Access of tetanus spores to open wounds does not necessarily result in disease. *C. tetani* sometimes can be cultured from wounds of patients without tetanus, for in clean wounds, where the blood supply is good and the oxygen tension remains high, germination will rarely occur. In necrotic and infected wounds, on the other hand, the anaerobic conditions will permit germination, which may occur rapidly. Spores occasionally remain dormant in healed human wounds for months (a latent period as long as 10 years has been recorded); trauma to the area may then cause germination and disease.

The importance of tissue necrosis is readily demonstrable in laboratory experiments. Mice inoculated intramuscularly with heavy suspensions of tetanus spores fail to develop the disease unless necrotizing chemicals, such as $CaCl_2$ or lactic acid, are injected with the spores.

TOXIN ACTION. Tetanus toxin action proceeds via four steps: (1) **extracellular binding;** (2) **initial translocation across cell membranes;** (3) **intra-axonal and trans-synaptic transport to sites of toxic action;** and (4) **intracellular poisoning of specific neurotransmitter release processes.** Toxin is initially bound to nerve terminal membranes at neuromuscular junctions, then is internalized and migrates to its ultimate sites of action in the central nervous system primarily via retrograde axonal transport. Radiolabeled toxin has been used to trace this migration, which parallels axonal transport of other proteins (e.g., nerve growth factor). Once toxin has reached the spinal cord, it ascends within it. Some toxin may also travel via the blood, particularly in generalized tetanus with a short incubation period. However, because the toxin cannot penetrate the blood–brain barrier, it is less likely to enter the spinal cord by this route.

A component of nerve tissue exhibiting receptor-like features for tetanus toxin has been identified. When tetanus toxin is mixed with brain emulsion or with subcellular fractions rich in synaptosome membranes, a comparatively large dose can be injected into a susceptible animal without causing damage (**Wassermann–Takaki phenomenon).** The substances responsible for this binding of toxin are **gangliosides** (GD1b and GT1b), complex glycolipids containing *N*-acetyl neuraminic acid (sialic acid). Tetanus toxin binds to isolated neural gangliosides or to tissues (or tissue fractions) containing surface gangliosides. Binding is prevented *in vitro* by treatment with neuraminidase, which cleaves sialic acid residues from gangliosides.

Available evidence suggests that **translocation** of tetanus toxin at the neuromuscular junction occurs by receptor-mediated endocytosis, as has been described for botulinum toxin. The B fragment of tetanus toxin forms channels in artificial phospholipid vesicles at low pH. By analogy with diphtheria toxin, the hydrophobic region of this fragment may create pores *in vivo*, allowing transport of the toxic L chain into the cytosol.

Intra-axonal **retrograde transport** of tetanus toxin

occurs within smooth vesicles, and when these reach the dendrites of the neurons, the toxin is transferred trans-synaptically to its site of action, the abutting nerve terminals. The spasmogenic effect of the toxin has been shown by Eccles to be the result of its action on poly-synaptic reflexes involving two types of inhibiting inter-neurons in the spinal cord. It **blocks the normal inhibition of spinal motor neurons** following afferent impulses postsynaptically by **preventing the release of inhibitory transmitters glycine** and **γ-aminobutyric acid.** The resulting sensitivity to excitatory impulses, unchecked by inhibitory mechanisms, produces the generalized muscular spasms characteristic of tetanus.

The biochemical mechanism by which tetanus toxin blocks the release of inhibitory neurotransmitters is not known, but by analogy with diphtheria toxin and the binary toxin of *C. botulinum*, it seems reasonable to postulate an enzymatic role for the L chain of tetanus toxin.

CLINICAL PATTERNS. The incubation period of tetanus may range from several days to many weeks; an incubation period of less than 4 days is associated with a very high mortality rate. Although the portal of entry is most commonly a puncture wound or laceration, other foci of infection include burns, skin ulcers, compound fractures, operative wounds, and sites of subcutaneous injection of adulterated narcotics by addicts.

Generalized tetanus, the usual form of the disease, is characterized by severe, painful spasms and rigidity of voluntary muscles. The usual sequence is local injury followed after some days by mild intermittent muscular contractions near the wound, the trismus ("lockjaw," spasm of the masseter muscles), generalized rigidity, and violent spasms of the trunk and limb muscles. Spasm of the pharyngeal muscles causes difficulty in swallowing. Death ordinarily results from interference with the mechanics of breathing. The patient's sensorium remains clear. Fever is not seen except with increased metabolism (in patients with severe spasms), complicating infection, or autonomic nervous system complications. Occasional patients with severe tetanus show manifestations of sympathetic dysfunction (hypertension, tachycardia, fever, hypotension), probably from disinhibition of sympathetic reflexes.

Local tetanus is a much rarer form of the disease, usually occurring in individuals with partial immunity or as the result of minor wounds containing only a few organisms. It is characterized by localized twitching and spasm in muscles near the wound. It may persist for weeks or months and then subside; mild trismus may follow, or it may progress to generalized tetanus within a few days.

Generalized tetanus can readily be reproduced in experimental animals by intravenous injection of toxin and local tetanus by intramuscular injection of small amounts. Local tetanus is apparently caused by early involvement of anterior horn cells at the level of initial entrance of the toxin.

LABORATORY DIAGNOSIS

The diagnosis of tetanus is usually based on clinical findings alone. Although attempts should be made to culture *C. tetani* from all suspicious lesions, antitoxin should not be withheld for the 2 to 3 days needed to identify the organism.

The organism is cultured from an infected focus in only about 30% of cases; moreover, its isolation does not necessarily establish a clinical diagnosis of tetanus. The tetanus bacillus may be provisionally recognized by its round terminal spores, the narrow zone of hemolysis on blood agar incubated anaerobically, and the granular gray surface colonies surrounded by an area of swarming.* However, because other gram-positive anaerobic spore-forming bacilli may be cultured from infected wounds,† positive identification requires the demonstration of production of toxin and its neutralization by specific antitoxin. A mouse protection test is commonly used for this purpose.

TREATMENT AND PREVENTION

Antitoxin should be promptly administered in all cases of suspected tetanus to neutralize accessible toxin; it is ineffective against toxin already fixed in the central nervous system and does not reverse existing manifestations of neurotoxicity. **Tetanus immune globulin (TIG,** prepared from persons who have been hyperimmunized with tetanus toxoid) has supplanted conventional equine antitoxin: the risk of sensitivity reactions is minimal, and Abs persist longer (half-life of 3–4 weeks). A dose of 3000 to 6000 U‡ should be administered intramuscularly.

If human TIG is not available, equine antitoxin should be administered in a dose of 100,000 U, half given intravenously and half intramuscularly. This amount is far in excess of that needed to neutralize all the preformed or subsequently elaborated toxin. It is essential to test for immediate-type hypersensitivity to horse serum before

---

* Staining with fluorescent Ab to the somatic O Ag will probably prove the best method for rapid identification.

† About 30% of war wounds, for example, become contaminated with various *Clostridia*.

‡ An American unit of antitoxin is defined as 10 times the smallest amount needed to protect, for 96 hours, a 350-g guinea pig inoculated with a standard dose of toxin furnished by the National Institutes of Health.

injecting antitoxin and to take appropriate precautions if the result is positive (see Serum Sickness Syndrome). Local injections of antitoxin, totaling 10,000 to 20,000 U, may also be made around the suspected primary lesion.

Careful surgical debridement of the lesion and removal of any foreign bodies present should be carried out only after the TIG or antitoxin has been given. Penicillin should also be administered to prevent the germination of spores and further bacterial multiplication (and toxin production) in infected tissue; but chemotherapy alone should never be relied on.

Supportive measures to minimize spasm and aid breathing are of the utmost importance. These measures may be needed for one or more weeks, because fixed toxin in the central nervous system decays slowly. About 25% of patients with severe generalized tetanus die despite intensive treatment.

Because the spores of *C. tetani* are so widely disseminated, the only effective way to control tetanus is by **prophylactic immunization. Tetanus toxoid,** in combination with diphtheria toxoid and pertussis vaccine **(DPT),** is usually given during the first year of life. Three injections of adsorbed (DPT) toxoid should be administered in the initial course of immunization. A single booster injection of DPT should be given about a year later and again on entrance to elementary school. Subsequent booster immunization with a single dose of adult-type tetanus and diphtheria toxoid is recommended at 10-year intervals for persons at relatively high risk. A protective level of Ab is considered to be 0.01 IU (0.005 American units)/ml or greater.

Whenever a previously immunized individual sustains a potentially dangerous wound, a booster of toxoid should be injected. (Booster injections may be effective even after 10 to 20 years, inducing protective levels of Ab within 1–2 weeks.) Seriously wounded subjects who have not previously been immunized, on the other hand, should be given prophylactic human TIG (250 U), because the Ab response to an initial toxoid injection is too slow to be useful. Prompt, thorough surgical debridement of wounds is also essential in tetanus prophylaxis.

Intensive programs of prophylactic immunization with toxoid in both civilian and military populations* have led to a striking reduction in the incidence of tetanus.

Though naturally acquired immunity to tetanus had been thought not to exist, protective Ab levels have been found recently in some members of isolated, unimmunized populations.

---

* Of 231 cases of non-neonatal tetanus reported in the U.S. from 1982 to 1984, only six were in individuals who had previously had four or more tetanus toxoid injections; 56 occurred in unimmunized individuals, and the remainder occurred in individuals who had not received a full course of immunization or whose immunization status was unknown. The reliability of active immunization is clear.

Histotoxic Clostridial Infections

A variety of species of *Clostridium* are associated with invasive infection in humans (listed under gas gangrene in Table 34–1). They are not highly pathogenic when introduced into healthy tissues; but in the presence of tissue injury, particularly damaged muscle, they can cause a rapidly progressive, devastating infection characterized by the accumulation of gas and the extensive destruction of muscle and connective tissue (**clostridial myonecrosis** or **gas gangrene**). *C. perfringens*, the species most commonly involved, is also found in other kinds of infection. It is widely distributed in soil and sewage, is normally a commensal in the lower gastrointestinal tract of animals and humans, and is frequently isolated from contaminated skin surfaces or clothing.

THE TOXINS

Invasive strains of clostridia produce, during active multiplication, exotoxins with necrotizing (cytolytic), hemolytic, or lethal properties. In addition, enzymes such as collagenase,† proteinase, deoxyribonuclease, and hyaluronidase, elaborated by the growing organisms, cause accumulation of toxic degradation products in the tissues. Eleven or more soluble antigens elaborated by *C. perfringens*, referred to as toxins (Table 34–2), are produced in various patterns by the five types. Some strains have lost the ability to produce certain toxins. Little is known about the genetic control of toxin production; proteinase (caseinase) is mediated by a small non–self-transferable plasmid, and β-toxin by a 75-megadalton plasmid.

The **alpha (α) toxin** is a calcium-dependent **phospholipase-C** produced by all five types of *C. perfringens*, but in greatest quantities by type A strains; it is lethal and necrotizing. These actions, which can be neutralized by antilecithinase serum, are attributable to splitting of **lecithin in cell membranes** (Fig. 34–4). (This enzyme also hydrolyzes cephalin and sphingomyelin.) Because lecithin is present in the membranes of many different kinds of cells, the toxin can cause extensive damage in many tissues. The paucity of leukocytes in the exudate of gas gangrene may be due in part to this effect. This toxin may also cause platelet aggregation and lysis and local capillary thrombosis.

The **theta (θ) toxin** (or perfringolysin O) is **hemolytic** but has no phospholipase-C activity. It is a reversibly oxygen-labile (SH-activated) protein that is irreversibly inactivated by cholesterol, and its action starts with binding to membrane cholesterol. It cross-reacts immunologically with both streptolysin O and tetanolysin.

---

† Collagen, unless denatured to gelatin, is not digested by the usual proteases.

TABLE 34–2. *Toxins and Toxigenic Types of C. perfringens*

Toxins†	Bacterial types*				
	A‡	B	C	D	E
α (Lethal, lecithinase, necrotizing)	+	+	+	+	+
β (Lethal, necrotizing)	−	+	+	−	−
ε (Lethal, necrotizing)	−	+	−	+	−
ι (Lethal, necrotizing)	−	−	−	−	+
θ (Lethal, hemolytic)	+	+	+	+	+

* *C. perfringens* is classified into five types (A–E) by the ability of antisera to neutralize the lethal toxins. For example, antiserum to type A (containing antitoxin to α) will protect mice against toxin-containing filtrates from type A organisms but not against those of other types (e.g., type B). Antiserum to type B (containing antitoxin to α, β, and ε) will protect mice against toxin-containing filtrates of types B,A,C, and D, but not type E.

† Other toxins (δ, λ [proteinase], κ [collagenase], μ [hyaluronidase], ν [deoxyribonuclease], neuraminidase) are elaborated as well to various degrees by the different types of *C. perfringens*.

‡ Type A is the principal type involved in human disease; type C is implicated in enteritis necroticans in man; types B, D, and E produce enteritis and enterotoxemia in sheep and cattle.

Studies with inhibitors (EDTA, blocking phospholipase-C; heat treatment, blocking hemolytic activity), and with purified preparations, indicate that the initial action of the θ-toxin on RBC membranes exposes buried phospholipid groups to subsequent phospholipase-C action. This combined action may account for the intravascular hemolysis associated with *C. perfringens* bacteremia.

The **epsilon (ε) toxin** is of principal interest in veterinary medicine, as it causes a rapidly fatal **enterotoxemia** of sheep. Multiplication of the organism occurs in the intestine, accompanied by activation of inactive protototoxin by clostridial proteases (and intestinal trypsin). The **nu (ν) toxin,** a DNase, is produced by all five types of *C. perfringens;* it is a **leukocidin** and, with α-toxin, probably accounts for the absence of a local leukocytic response in gas gangrene. The **iota (ι) toxin,** produced only by type E strains, causes enterotoxemias in calves, lambs, and guinea pigs. It is a binary toxin consisting of

two unlinked polypeptides that are inactive alone but in combination act synergistically (lethal effect, dermonecrosis). One of the polypeptides can **ADP-ribosylate poly-L-arginine,** but the physiologic acceptor for ADP-ribose is unknown.

PATHOGENESIS: HISTOTOXIC (CYTOLYTIC)

WOUND INFECTIONS. There are three types of clostridial wound infection: wound contamination, anaerobic cellulitis, and true myonecrosis (gas gangrene). From 80% to 90% of isolations of *C. perfringens* from hospitalized patients represent simple saprobic **wound contamination,** especially of operative wounds, skin ulcers, etc., and usually in association with other organisms; it does not herald invasive infection.

Anaerobic cellulitis is a clostridial infection that does not involve the muscles and is much less aggressive than gas gangrene. It begins with the introduction of spores into an open wound. Severe wounds, such as those acquired in automobile accidents and military combat, grossly contaminated with soil or fecal matter and harboring a mixture of organisms, are particularly likely to contain clostridial spores. Germination occurs in devitalized tissue where damage to the blood supply and the presence of foreign material has lowered the redox potential. The vegetative bacilli multiply, and anaerobic cellulitis usually develops after several days and extends widely, spreading in the fascial planes; the marked gas formation is detectable by the resulting crepitus. The infection rarely produces intense local pain, toxemia, or invasion of healthy muscle.

Gas gangrene is an intensely aggressive, highly lethal infection, primarily of muscle. After the germination of clostridial spores in injured muscle, bacterial multiplication and toxin production occur. A self-perpetuating cycle of progressive tissue injury ensues. The onset of the disease is usually sudden, following an incubation period of 6 to 72 hours after injury or abdominal surgery. The involved area is edematous, and the skin has a bronze discoloration. Thin dark fluid is exuded, often in

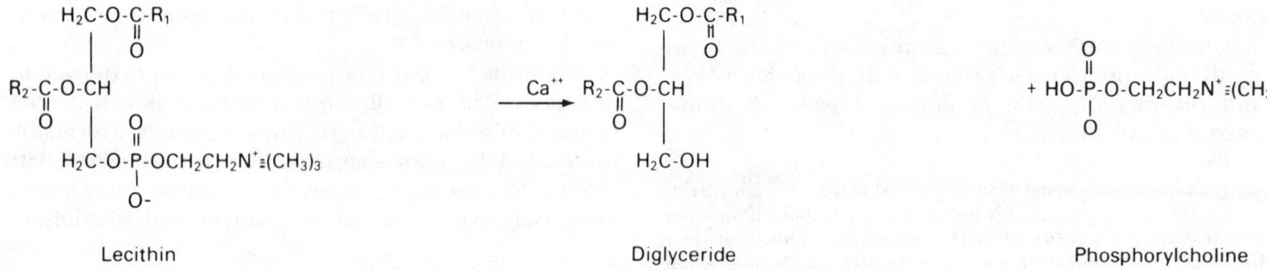

Figure 34–4. Action of *C. perfringens* α-toxin (lecithinase; phospholipase C) on lecithin (choline phosphoglyceride).

tense blebs; aspiration reveals many clostridia and a few polymorphonuclear leukocytes. Gas is present in the subcutaneous tissue and muscles.* Exploration of the wound reveals the muscle involvement: swollen, grayish or purple, and ischemic. Gas and fluid accumulation in tissue spaces confined by fascial compartments produces additional pressure, which in turn causes further muscle necrosis and ischemia, allowing rapid spread of the organism from one group of muscles to the next and rapidly leading to irreversible shock.

Only six clostridial species (all those, except *C. tertium*, listed under gas gangrene in Table 34–1) are capable on their own of producing gas gangrene in man, although other toxigenic and nontoxigenic species can sometimes be isolated from the lesions of gas gangrene (particularly in war wounds) caused by one or more of the six principal species. *C. perfringens* is the cause of more than 90% of gas gangrene in the U.S. It is widely distributed in soil and excreta and is often present on skin and clothing, and it frequently (4%–40%) contaminates major traumatic wounds. However, the incidence of gas gangrene in such wounds is less than 2%, indicating the importance of the type of wound and the circumstances of initial treatment in the genesis of clostridial myonecrosis.

UTERINE INFECTION. *C. perfringens* is present in the genital tract of about 5% of women. After septic abortion, or uncommonly after prolonged labor, it may invade the uterine wall, producing extensive necrosis, high fever, and circulatory collapse. **Severe bacteremia** is characteristic of this process.

BACTEREMIA. Bacteremia caused by *C. perfringens*, or by nonhistotoxic clostridia (e.g., *C. sporogenes, C. difficile, C. tertium*), occasionally occurs also in patients with leukemia, malignant tumors, gastrointestinal bleeding, bowel necrosis, gangrenous extremities, or decubitus ulcers. In patients with ulcerative lesions of the bowel prior treatment with aminoglycoside antibiotics may favor the overgrowth of clostridial species and predispose to enterogenous bacteremia. *C. septicum* infections occur in patients with intestinal malignancy and can evolve rapidly as **cryptogenic** gas gangrene, i.e. in the absence of traumatic wounds.

Bacteremia occurs in 15% of patients with gas gangrene and in most uterine clostridial infections. Occasionally it is intense, and intravascular hemolysis develops rapidly, leading to acute renal shutdown.

UNUSUAL LOCALIZED INFECTIONS. *C. perfringens* may cause necrotizing pneumonia and empyema, or meningitis, after a penetrating injury.

* The gas that accumulates is predominantly hydrogen, which is less soluble than CO_2 (see Butyric Fermentation, Chap. 4).

PATHOGENESIS: ENTEROTOXIC

THE ENTEROTOXIN. The toxin, quite distinct from the histotoxic and hemolytic toxins, is produced by certain strains of *C. perfringens* type A, which cause **acute food poisoning** in man. Unlike other *C. perfringens* toxins, this heat-labile protein is produced only during sporulation and not during vegetative growth. It appears to be a spore-coat protein that is produced in excess and accumulates in a parasporal inclusion body, constituting up to 10% of the total cellular protein just prior to spore release.

The enterotoxin causes a net secretion of fluid and electrolytes into ligated rabbit ileal loops and erythema (and increased capillary permeability) on injection into the skin of guinea pigs. The primary site of action in the intestine appears to be the microvillus membrane of epithelial cells on villus tips, which develop blebs and desquamate. The enterotoxin is also toxic to cultured Vero (African green monkey kidney) cells.

FOOD POISONING. From 1970 to 1981 in Great Britain, *C. perfringens* type A was responsible for 17% of cases of food poisoning. It produces a self-limited gastroenteritis, lacking constitutional symptoms, about 12 hours after the ingestion of heavily contaminated food. The incriminated food is usually meat that had been cooked and then held before reheating and serving: spores survive the cooking and later germinate during cooling, in a medium from which oxygen had been driven. A large number of viable organisms must be ingested to cause the disease (10^5/g) and 10^5–10^6/g are subsequently found in the feces. Healthy individuals normally carry 10^3 to 10^4 organisms/g in feces.

Serotyping (based on capsular Ags) and bacteriocin typing have been of value in the epidemiologic investigation of food-borne outbreaks.

ENTERITIS NECROTICANS. This much more serious form of clostridial enteric infection occurred in epidemic form in an undernourished population in Germany at the close of World War II, and it is currently seen among the natives of New Guinea. It is caused by strains of *C. perfringens* type C that produce a necrotizing β-**toxin.**

The disease develops a day after persons on a low-protein diet have a large meal of meat (usually pork), and it is characterized by abdominal pain, vomiting, and diarrhea (often bloody). The organism, present either in the meat or already in the small intestine, proliferates and produces large amounts of β-toxin. This toxin is susceptible to intestinal proteases, but if their level has been reduced by a low-protein diet it may not all be destroyed. The toxin then causes patchy necrosis of the upper small intestine, leading to intestinal obstruction. The "**pig-bel**" in New Guinea may also be promoted by trypsin inhibitors in the dietary staple, sweet potato. Immunization with a recently developed toxoid has dramatically reduced the incidence of the disease in New Guinea children.

ANTIBIOTIC-ASSOCIATED DIARRHEA. C. difficile has been found in 25% of cases of moderate diarrhea resulting from treatment with antibiotics, especially clindamycin, ampicillin, or cephalosporins. Rarely, the overgrowth is of enterotoxigenic strains of *C. perfringens* rather than *C. difficile;* the clinical picture is indistinguishable.

In the more severe reaction called **pseudomembranous enterocolitis** *C. difficile* is found in over 95% of cases. This occasionally fatal illness is characterized by diarrhea, multiple small colonic plaques, and toxic megacolon. The antibiotic selects for overgrowth of organisms that produce a **heat-labile toxin:** fecal filtrates from patients with enterocolitis, and supernatant fluids of cultures of *C. difficile* from these patients, are cytotoxic in tissue culture and cause enterocolitis when injected intracecally in hamsters. Normally this organism is found in only about 3% of adults, but in about 10% to 50% of neonates, who suffer no ill effects.

The enterotoxicity of *C. difficile* is primarily due to two **toxins, A and B,** each of Mr about 300,000. In animal models protection is provided by immunization against both but not against either alone. This toxin A, unlike *C. perfringens* toxin A, is not a spore coat constituent, nor is it produced during sporulation. It causes fluid accumulation and mucosal damage in rabbit ileal loops, and it appears to increase the uptake of toxin B by intestinal mucosa. Toxin B does not cause intestinal fluid accumulation but is 1000-fold more toxic than toxin A to tissue culture cells, causing membrane damage.

LABORATORY DIAGNOSIS

The bacteriology of gas gangrene is complicated, because most of the infections are mixed (aerobes and anaerobes). Furthermore, the **presence of gas in the tissues does not necessarily incriminate clostridia,** for klebsiellae, bacteroides, *E. coli,* and anaerobic streptococci may also cause the accumulation of enough gas to be detectable by palpation or roentgenography. The finding of many plump, blunt-ended, gram-positive bacilli but few granulocytes in smears of exudate from crepitant wounds, adjacent bullae or the uterine cervix suggests clostridial infection; *C. perfringens* rarely forms spores in infected wounds. In wound smears *C. septicum,* the cause of about 10% of war-time cases of gas gangrene and the usual cause of nontraumatic (cryptogenic) gas gangrene, sometimes appears as chains of elongated cells or as rods with large subterminal spores. Smears of the peripheral blood (or of the buffy coat) from patients

with intense bacteremia occasionally show the bacilli, providing a rapid diagnosis.

Exudate for anaerobic culture should be obtained if possible (using a needle and syringe from which all air has been expelled) and processed promptly. Solid media (enriched blood agar; or selective media such as kanamycin–vancomycin–laked blood agar or phenethyl alcohol blood agar if mixed bacterial populations are likely) should be incubated aerobically and anaerobically, and liquid media (chopped meat–glucose or supplemented brain heart infusion broth available as prereduced medium; thioglycollate medium) should also be employed. If gram-positive spore-bearing bacilli are found in the liquid media, and if colonies of such bacilli appear on the blood agar incubated anaerobically but not on that incubated aerobically, the genus *Clostridium* should be suspected.

The identification of individual clostridial species is based primarily on the biochemical tests listed in Table 34–1. *C. perfringens* can be recognized by its failure to show spores in direct smear or culture, by double-zone hemolysis around colonies on blood agar, and by the **Nagler reaction** (formation of a visible opacity secondary to **lecithinase** action around colonies grown on egg yolk agar; Fig. 34–5); type A antitoxin in the agar prevents this opacification without inhibiting growth. In a **wound specimen from a patient with gas gangrene,** isolation and definition of *C. perfringens* may be hastened by primary anaerobic plating on neomycin–egg yolk (NEY)

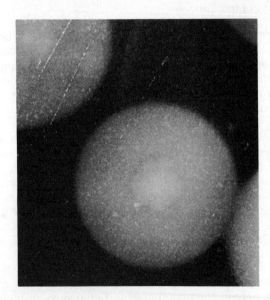

Figure 34–5. Colonies of *C. perfringens* grown on egg yolk medium. The halo of precipitate about the colonies is caused by splitting of lecithin by lecithinase released by the organisms; the diglyceride released is insoluble. (×5, enlarged; McClung LS, Toabe R: J Bacteriol 53:139, 1947)

agar, where lecithinase activity can be identified by the Nagler reaction and proteolysis by a zone of translucent clearing around the colonies. Other properties helpful in distinguishing *C. perfringens* are capsule formation, lactose fermentation, and lack of motility. With other clostridia found in wounds the demonstration of histotoxin production in animals, and its neutralization with specific antitoxin, is useful.

In patients with pseudomembranous enterocolitis, yellow patches of pseudomembrane are visible on the rectosigmoid mucosa on endoscopic examination. A selective medium (cefoxitin–cycloserine–egg yolk–fructose agar) has been developed for the isolation of *C. difficile*. However, diagnosis is more accurate by cytotoxin assay, because assuring proper handling of stool specimens for culture is difficult, and nontoxigenic strains of *C. difficile* are encountered. Toxin B is identified by the cytopathic effect of diluted stool filtrates on tissue culture cells, and its neutralization by antitoxin. Latex particle agglutination tests for *C. difficile* Ags and enzyme-linked immunosorbent assay (ELISA) for toxins A and B have been developed.

TREATMENT AND PREVENTION

Prompt surgical debridement of dirty wounds is the most effective means of preventing anaerobic cellulitis and gas gangrene; antibiotic therapy alone does not suffice. Established clostridial wound infection requires surgical debridement as promptly as possible. It is important to distinguish between anaerobic cellulitis and gas gangrene, as the former requires wide excision and debridement whereas the latter requires complete extirpation of involved muscle (usually amputation of a limb). Penicillin is administered in large doses to prevent or treat bacteremia and to inhibit further bacterial multiplication in the wound. Clindamycin (occasional strains are penicillin-resistant), chloramphenicol, and metronidazole are also useful. (However, the recent observation of conjugative plasmid-mediated resistance in *C. perfringens* to tetracycline and chloramphenicol, and to erythromycin and clindamycin, portends future problems in the use of these antimicrobial agents.) **Hyperbaric oxygen** at 3 atm in a compression chamber, to raise the oxygen tension in healthy tissue, may have a place in therapy, especially in gas gangrene of the trunk, where complete debridement may be precluded.

Polyvalent equine antitoxin prepared against toxic filtrates of *C. perfringens*, *C. novyi*, *C. septicum*, and *C. histolyticum* has been used in the prophylaxis and treatment of gas gangrene. Its efficacy has never been established, and it is no longer available for clinical use.

In antibiotic-associated diarrhea and pseudomembranous enterocolitis, oral vancomycin (or metronidazole), as well as omission, if possible, of the predisposing antimicrobial agents(s), is effective. Prevention of *C. difficile* diarrhea involves avoidance of unnecessary antimicrobial usage and the preferential employment of a narrow- rather than broad-spectrum agent.

Selected Reading

BOOKS AND REVIEW ARTICLES

Allen SD: Clostridium. In Lennette EH, Balows A, Hausler WJ Jr, Shadomy HJ (eds): Manual of Clinical Microbiology, 4th Ed., p 434. Washington, DC, American Society for Microbiology, 1985

Bizzini, B: Tetanus toxin. Microbiol Rev 43:224, 1979

Bleck TP: Pharmacology of tetanus. Clin Neuropharmacol 9:103, 1986

Finegold SM: Anaerobic Bacteria in Human Disease. New York, Academic Press, 1977

Maclennan JD: The histotoxic clostridial infections of man. Bacteriol Rev 26:177, 1962

McDonel JL: *Clostridium perfringens* toxins (type A, B, C, D, E). Pharmacol Ther 10:617, 1980

McFarland LV, Stamm WE: Review of *Clostridium difficile*-associated diseases. Am J Infect Control 14:99, 1986

Simpson LL: The origin, structure and pharmacological activity of botulinum toxin. Pharmacol Rev 33:155, 1981

Simpson LL: Molecular pharmacology of botulinum toxin and tetanus toxin. Ann Rev Pharmacol Toxicol 26:427, 1986

Sugiyama H: *Clostridium botulinum* neurotoxin. Microbiol Rev 44:419, 1980

Van Heyningen S: Tetanus toxin. Pharmacol Ther 11:141, 1980

SPECIFIC ARTICLES

Aktories K, Bärmann M, Ohishi I, Tsuyama S, Jakobs KH, Habermann E: Botulinum C2 toxin ADP-ribosylates actin. Nature 322:390, 1986

Arnon SS: Infant botulism. Annu Rev Med 31:541, 1980

Ball AP, Hopkinson RB, Farrell ID et al: Human botulism caused by *Clostridium botulinum* type E. The Birmingham outbreak. Q J Med 83:473, 1979

Bartholomew BA, Stringer MF: Clostridium perfringens enterotoxin: A brief review. Biochem Soc Trans 12:195, 1984

Bartlett JG: Virulence factors of anaerobic bacteria. Johns Hopkins Med J 151:1, 1982

Bartlett JG: Treatment of antibiotic-associated pseudomembranous colitis. Rev Infect Dis 6:S235, 1984

Boquet P, Duflot E: Tetanus toxin fragment forms channels in lipid vesicles at low pH. Proc Natl Acad Sci USA 79:7614, 1982

Brooks VB, Curtis DR, Eccles JC: The action of tetanus toxin on the inhibition of motorneurones. J Physiol (Lond) 135:655, 1957

Centers for Disease Control: Botulism in the United States, 1899–1977: Handbook for Epidemiologists, Clinicians and Laboratory Workers. Issued May 1979

Critchley DR, Habig WH, Fishman PH: Reevaluation of the role of gangliosides as receptors for tetanus toxin. J Neurochem 47:213, 1986

Eklund MW, Poysky FT, Meyers JA, Pelroy GA: Interspecies conversion of *Clostridium botulinum* type C to *Clostridium novyi* type A by bacteriophage. Science 186:456, 1974

Finn CW Jr, Sylver RP, Habig WH, Hardegree MC, Zon G, Garon CF: The structural gene for tetanus neurotoxin is on a plasmid. Science 224:881, 1984

Helting TB, Parschat S, Engelhardt H: Structure of tetanus toxin: Demonstration and separation of a specific enzyme converting intracellular tetanus toxin to the extracellular form. J Biol Chem 254:10728, 1979

Lawrence G, Cooke R: Experimental pigbel: The production and pathology of necrotizing enteritis due to *Clostridium welchii* type C in the guinea-pig. Br J Exp Pathol 61:261, 1980

Staub GC, Walton KM, Schnarr RL et al: Characterization of the binding and internalization of tetanus toxin in a neuroblastoma hybrid cell line. J Neurosci 6:1443, 1986

Stiles BG, Wilkins TD: Purification and characterization of *Clostridium perfringens* iota toxin: Dependence on two nonlinked proteins for biological activity. Infect Immun 54:683, 1986

Wilkins T, Krivan H, Stiles B, Carmen R, Lyerly D: Clostridial toxins active locally in the gastrointestinal tract. Ciba Found Symp 112:230, 1985

35

Emanuel Wolinsky

Mycobacteria

The mycobacteria are a group of non-motile rods that are defined on the basis of a distinctive staining property: they are relatively impermeable to various basic dyes, but once stained, they retain dyes with tenacity. Specifically, they resist decolorization with acidified organic solvents and are therefore called **acid-fast.** This property, and their relatively slow growth, are attributable to the presence of a lipid-rich cell wall. Mycobacteria range from widespread innocuous saprobic inhabitants of soil and water to the organisms that are responsible for **tuberculosis** and **leprosy.**

In both these chronic diseases, intracellular infection, delayed hypersensitivity, and cellular resistance play important roles, and slowly evolving granulomatous lesions result in extreme tissue destruction. Leprosy largely involve the skin, sometimes with shocking disfigurements, while tuberculosis is usually confined to internal organs. Moreover, the contagious nature of leprosy was recognized in Biblical times, whereas tuberculosis, although even more contagious, was not recognized as such until the last century. Hence the leper became a social outcast, but in Europe a century or two ago tuberculosis was regarded romantically as a source of enhanced esthetic sensitivities.

The leprosy bacillus, discovered by Hansen in 1879, was the first bacterium shown to be associated with human disease. It is strikingly adapted to man: it has been difficult to transfer to any other host, and it has not been grown on artificial culture media. In contrast, the agents of human tuberculosis (*Mycobacterium tuberculosis* and the closely related *M. bovis*) are readily cultivated on simple media and are pathogenic for various lower animals, especially guinea pigs and mice. With the decreasing prevalence of tuberculosis, it has been recognized that similar but generally milder infections are caused by a variety of mycobacterial species, previously ignored because they do not cause progressive disease in these test

647

animals. These organisms have **reservoirs in the environment** or in lower animals rather than in man.

Tuberculosis

Pulmonary tuberculosis (**consumption, phthisis**) has been recognized as a widespread and grave clinical entity for many centuries, and its incidence was probably increased by the social consequences of the Industrial Revolution. However, its communicable nature was not recognized until Villemin produced a similar disease in rabbits, in 1868, by injecting material from tuberculous lesions of man; and in 1882, Koch discovered the tubercle bacillus, impressively fulfilling the criteria he had developed (Koch's postulates) for identifying the etiologic agent of an infectious disease. Since then, tuberculosis has been one of the most intensively studied infectious diseases. Not only has it been a significant cause of death and prolonged disability, but until recent times, it usually struck people at the age of greatest vigor and promise.

PROPERTIES OF MYCOBACTERIUM TUBERCULOSIS

The mycobacteria are considered transitional forms between eubacteria and actinomycetes (Chap. 36): some of the latter, of the genus *Nocardia*, are weakly acid-fast, whereas some mycobacteria may exhibit branching. Accordingly, the mycobacteria have been classified in the order Actinomycetales.

Morphology

ACID-FASTNESS. To stain the tubercle bacillus in smears or in tissues, methods must be used that promote penetration of the dye. In the widely used Ziehl–Neelsen method, the smeared specimen is heated to steaming for 2 to 3 minutes in carbolfuchsin (a mixture of the triphenylmethane dyes rosaniline and pararosaniline in aqueous 5% phenol). Subsequent washing in 95% ethanol–3% HCl (acid alcohol) decolorizes most bacteria in a few seconds, whereas acid-fast organisms retain the stain much longer. The mechanism of acid-fastness will be discussed below, under Lipids.

Mycobacteria may appear to be gram-positive, but they take up the stain weakly and irregularly and without requiring iodine treatment to retain it.

Other acid-fast objects include some bacterial and fungal spores and a substance known as ceroid (found in the liver in certain states of nutritional deficiency). These materials, however, do not require the presence of phenol (or aniline) in the staining solution. The acid-fast nocardiae are more easily stained and more easily decolorized than are mycobacteria.

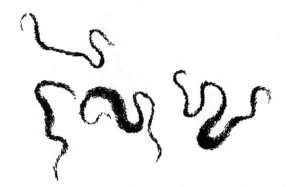

Figure 35–1. Tubercle bacilli in stained smear from colony. Note parallel growth in "cords." From original drawing of Koch. (Courtesy of Robert Koch-Institut, Berlin)

STRUCTURE. Tubercle bacilli in the animal are typically slightly bent or curved slender rods, about 2 to 4 μm long and 0.2 to 0.5 μm wide. The rods may be of uniform width but more often appear beaded, with irregularly spaced, unstained vacuoles or heavily stained knobs. In culture media, the cells may range from coccoid to filamentous. Strains differ in their tendency to grow as discrete rods or as aggregated long strands, called **serpentine cords** (Fig. 35–1).

The walls of mycobacteria contain a peptidoglycan with diaminopimelate, and the cells can be converted to spheroplasts by lysozyme. The walls have a remarkably high lipid content (up to 60%), much of which is attached to polysaccharide; the polysaccharides, which include glucan, mannan, arabinogalactan, and arabinomannan, are also found in culture filtrates. The glycolipids and protein are located in a firmly attached outer layer of the wall (Fig. 35–2), and the external location of the lipid accounts for the hydrophobic character of the cells.

Electron microscopy reveals a rather thick wall, and large lamellar mesosomes are common. Glycogen granules and polymetaphosphate (volutin) bodies are also seen: the latter stain metachromatically with cationic dyes. These inclusion bodies contribute to the frequently beaded, irregular staining of tubercle bacilli.

Growth

Unlike most other pathogenic bacteria, which are facultative aerobes or anaerobes, the tubercle bacillus is an **obligate aerobe.** It can grow in **simple synthetic media,** with glycerol or other compounds as the sole carbon source and ammonium salts as the nitrogen source; asparagine or amino acid mixtures are usually added to promote the initiation and improve the rate of growth.

In ordinary synthetic liquid media, the bacilli grow in adherent clumps that form a **surface pellicle.** (This "moldlike" property is responsible for the name *Myco-*

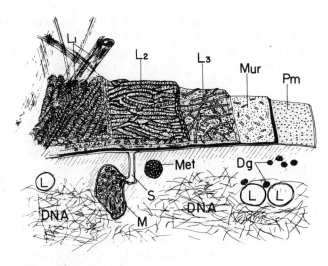

Figure 35–2. Mycobacterial cell wall as diagrammed from electron micrographic data. *Dg,* Dense granules; *L,* lipoidal bodies; *L1,* surface glycolipid; *L2* and *L3,* fibrous rope-like structures; *M,* mesosome; *Met,* metachromatic granule; *Mur,* murein or peptidoglycan; *Pm,* plasma membrane; *S,* septum. (Barksdale L, Kim K-S: Bacteriol Rev 41:217, 1977)

bacterium.) Nonionic detergents, such as Tweens,* cause the bacilli to grow in more dispersed form, although still not as single cells.

Mycobacteria generally show a marked nutritional preference for lipids; egg yolk has been a prominent constituent of the rich media used for diagnostic cultures. Thus, although the tubercle bacillus is very sensitive to inhibition by long-chain **fatty acids,** it is stimulated by them at very low concentrations. A satisfactory concentration is maintained by adding to the medium **serum albumin,** which binds the fatty acids with sufficient affinity to maintain a low free concentration.

Mycobacteria produce iron chelators (**mycobactins**), whose competition with host chelators (transferrins) may play a role in pathogenesis and resistance.

Growth of tubercle bacilli in culture media (and in animals) is characteristically slow: **the shortest doubling time observed, in rich media, is about 12 hours.** Saprobic mycobacteria grow more rapidly, but not so rapidly as most other bacteria (which have doubling times as short as 20 minutes). In harmony with the slow growth, the ribosomes of *M. tuberculosis* translate *in vitro* only 1/10 as rapidly as those of *E. coli.*

Genetic Variation and Virulence Tests

Human tubercle bacilli freshly isolated from pulmonary lesions produce progressive disease in guinea pigs,

which die within 1 to 6 months after infection, depending in part on the size of the inoculum. Tuberculous skin lesions, called **lupus vulgaris,** often yield less virulent organisms, as do lung lesions from some patients in India and Africa. As with other pathogenic bacteria, virulence varies quantitatively: serial passage through artificial culture media selects indirectly for less virulent mutants, whereas animal passage of large inocula of such strains selects directly for mutants with restored virulence. One attenuated bovine strain,† carried through several hundred serial cultures on unfavorable (bile-containing) media, is known as **Bacille Calmette-Guérin (BCG).** This strain, which is used to immunize humans against tuberculosis (see Immunization), has remained avirulent for more than 60 years.

Most virulent strains produce rough colonies, whereas many avirulent laboratory strains produce less rough colonies (called smooth, although the cells lack capsules). Thus, the correlation between colonial morphology and virulence, although not highly consistent, is the reverse of that seen with many other bacteria.

VIRULENCE TESTS. In contrast to pneumococci, virulent strains of tubercle bacilli cannot be distinguished reliably from avirulent strains by cellular or colonial morphology or by serologic tests; and the direct test for virulence in animals is slow and inconvenient. However, virulent strains grow, on the surface of liquid or on solid media, as intertwining **serpentine cords,** in which the bacilli aggregate with their long axes parallel (Fig. 35–1), whereas most avirulent strains grow in a more disordered manner. Growth in cords can be correlated with the content of a surface lipid (cord factor, described below). Nonionic detergents (e.g., Tween 80) reduce cord formation (but not virulence), presumably by coating the cell surface. Another property that is lost in many avirulent mutants is binding of the dye **neutral red.**

The failure to find a reliable virulence test is not surprising: because virulence is a multifactorial property, a given bacterial component may be necessary, but it cannot be sufficient to make an organism virulent.

BACTERIOPHAGE TYPING. With a set of four main and six auxiliary phages, we can now recognize eight main types and 64 subtypes of *M. tuberculosis.* The technique has been used for epidemiologic investigations.

Lipids

The most striking chemical feature of the mycobacteria is the abundance of lipids in the cell wall (up to 60% of its dry weight). This property accounts for the hydrophobic

---

* Polyoxyethylene ethers of sorbitol, or of other polyhydric alcohols, esterified to long-chain fatty acids.

† A strain is considered **attenuated** for a given host if it multiplies in that host to only a limited extent, causing, at most, minor transient lesions.

character of the organisms and probably also for some of the other unusual properties of mycobacteria, such as their relative impermeability to stains, acid-fastness, unusual resistance to killing by acid and alkali, and resistance to the bactericidal action of Abs plus complement.

Various lipid fractions are defined by the conditions used for their extraction from dried organisms. Among the lipids extracted with neutral organic solvents are **true waxes** (esters of fatty acids with fatty alcohols) and **glycolipids** (**mycosides:** lipid-soluble compounds with covalently linked lipid and carbohydrate moieties).

MYCOLIC ACIDS. Although many different fatty acids are found in mycobacteria, the **mycolic acids** appear to be unique to the cell walls of these organisms, nocardiae, and corynebacteria. These very large, saturated, α-alkyl, β-hydroxyl fatty acids (Fig. 35–3) are found in both waxes and glycolipids. A large arabinogalactan (mol. wt. 31,000), covalently attached to the peptidoglycan and to about 30 mycolic acid residues, forms a bridge between the rigid layer and the outer, lipophilic layers of the cell wall.

Three classes of mycolic acids have been found in *M. tuberculosis*, with cyclopropane, methoxy, or keto groups, and with slight variation in the chain length (mostly C_{78} and C_{80}). Mycolyl acetyl trehalose is a precursor of wall mycolic acid (and probably of cord factor, described below); the disaccharide solubilizes the very hydrophobic, unusually long-chain fatty acid.

CORD FACTOR. This factor, extracted from virulent cells by petroleum ether, has been identified as a mycoside, 6,6'-dimycolyltrehalose (Fig. 35–3). Several lines of evidence relate it to virulence. First, its extraction renders cells phenotypically nonvirulent (although they remain viable). Second, it is toxic: it inhibits migration of normal polymorphonuclear leukocytes *in vitro* (as do virulent tubercle bacilli), and 10 μg given subcutaneously will kill a mouse. Third, it is more abundant in virulent strains. Fourth, tubercle bacilli recovered from animals or from young cultures are more virulent, and they have a higher content of cord factor, than cells of the same strain from older cultures. Finally, mice have been protected against tuberculous infection by active immunization with a complex of cord factor and methylated bovine serum albumin or by passive transfer of rabbit anti–cord-factor serum. The toxicity of cord factor has been related to profound disturbances of microsomal enzymes, mitochondria, and lipid metabolism in the livers of mice.

A **sulfolipid** (trehalose-2'-sulfate esterified with long-chain fatty acids) also shows a correlation, but not with complete consistency, between its concentration and virulence.

WAX D AND THE IMMUNE RESPONSE. Another mycoside of interest is the high-molecular weight **wax D**, which is not a true wax but contains mycolic acids and a glycopeptide. It is apparently extracted from the basal wall

Mycolic acids

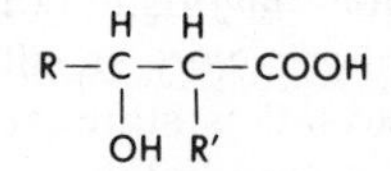

$$R - \overset{\overset{\displaystyle H}{|}}{C} - \overset{\overset{\displaystyle H}{|}}{\underset{\underset{\displaystyle R'}{|}}{C}} - COOH$$
$$\overset{|}{OH}$$

Human and bovine tubercle bacilli: $R' = C_{24}H_{49}$

Avian and saprophytic bacilli: $R' = C_{22}H_{45}$

R has about 60 C atoms, 1 or 2 O atoms

6, 6'-Dimycolyltrehalose (cord factor)

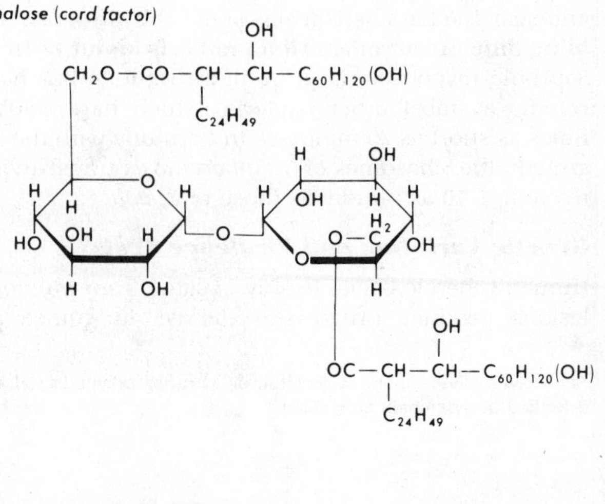

Figure 35–3. Structures of some distinctive mycobacterial lipids. Trehalose is D-glucose-α-1,1'-D-glucoside.

layer, as the peptide contains the characteristic amino acids of that layer, linked to a polymer of hexoses and hexosamines. In a water-in-oil emulsion (**Freund's adjuvant**), this fraction, like whole tubercle bacilli, **enhances the immunogenicity** of a variety of added antigens (see Chap. 16). Moreover, a mixture of wax D and proteins of the tubercle bacillus **induces delayed-type hypersensitivity** to tuberculin, whereas the protein alone is poorly immunogenic.

The **crude phosphatide** fraction has the interesting property of evoking a **cellular response resembling tubercle formation,** including caseation necrosis (see Pathogenesis). Rather large amounts must be injected, and comparable fractions from saprobic mycobacteria are also effective.

ACID-FASTNESS. After exhaustive extraction of the above-described lipids by organic solvents, the residual ghosts remain acid-fast, and they retain **firmly bound lipids** largely in the wall fraction. These lipids are removed by hot acid, which also destroys the acid-fastness. Because this property is also lost on sonic disruption of normal cells, it appears to depend on the integrity of the cell wall, including certain lipids.

Presumably because of their lipid layer, tubercle bacilli are unusually resistant to acid and alkali, and this property is exploited in their diagnostic isolation (see Laboratory Diagnosis, below). They are also relatively insensitive to cationic detergents but no more resistant than other nonsporulating bacteria to heat, ultraviolet irradiation, or phenol.

Numerous polysaccharide and protein antigens have been identified in culture filtrates and cell extracts of mycobacteria (Fig. 35–4). Young and his colleagues, utilizing gene cloning and monoclonal Ab probes, have isolated DNA sequences of *M. tuberculosis* that specify polypeptide components.

IMMUNE RESPONSE TO INFECTION

Acquired Immunity

THE KOCH PHENOMENON. Shortly after isolating the tubercle bacillus, Koch demonstrated that it induces an altered response to superinfection. In the original study, bacilli were injected subcutaneously into a guinea pig, and 10 to 14 days later, the inoculation site developed a nodule, which then became a persistent ulcer. In addition, the bacilli spread to the regional lymph nodes, causing them to enlarge and then become necrotic. When a similar injection was then made at another site, the response was faster and more violent, but also more circumscribed: a dusky, indurated lesion appeared in 2 to 3 days and soon ulcerated; but the ulcer healed promptly, and the regional lymph nodes remained virtually free of infection. Koch later showed that a similar second response could be obtained with culture filtrates of the organism (see Tuberculin Test).

The superinfecting bacilli are evidently better localized than the initial inoculum, and they multiply more slowly in the tissues. The infected animal has thus acquired increased resistance (i.e., partial immunity). But

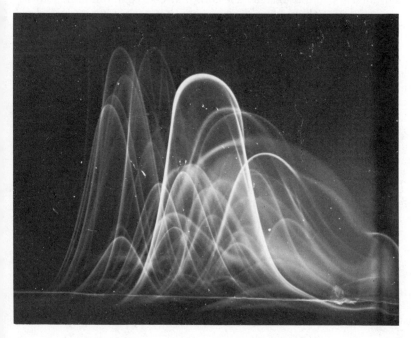

Figure 35–4. Two-dimensional immunoelectrophoresis illustrating the multiplicity of mycobacterial antigens. A sonicate of *M. tuberculosis* strain H37RV was analyzed with a WHO standard burro anti-Erdman strain serum. (Courtesy of SD Chaparas)

although this immunity may lead to elimination of the bacilli of superinfection, it cannot accomplish the same for the primary lesion, which has developed a denser bacterial population and a different histologic pattern. Evidently, the immunity acquired in the guinea pig is limited, and it can be overcome by local factors in the lesion.

NONHUMORAL IMMUNITY. Serum Abs do not account for this immunity. Thus, although the tubercle bacillus enhances formation of Abs to a wide variety of immunogens, Abs to proteins and polysaccharides of the tubercle bacillus itself are generally found only in low titers in tuberculous individuals, and the levels observed have no prognostic value. Moreover, these Abs are not bactericidal *in vitro*, even in the presence of complement; and although they promote phagocytosis of tubercle bacilli *in vitro*, the organisms multiply within the phagocytes. Finally, increased resistance to infection along with delayed-type hypersensitivity to tuberculin, can be transferred with viable lymphoid cells but not with serum.

Activated Macrophages and Hypersensitivity

Although tubercle bacilli flourish in macrophages of normal animals, they are destroyed more effectively in "activated" macrophages, from animals infected with tubercle bacilli or with various other bacteria (such as *Listeria*) that also can survive in macrophages. This increased bacteriolytic activity extends to a wide variety of microbes. Although the enhanced activity of altered macrophages is thus nonspecific, Mackaness has shown that it is induced by lymphocytes specifically interacting with the infecting organism (see Macrophage Activation, Chap. 21).

In macrophage activation, T cells (primarily T helpers) recognize microbial Ags (or processed Ags) on their Ag-specific surface receptors. This interaction causes them to secrete γ-interferon (formerly known as macrophage-activating factor), which stimulates differentiation into "activated macrophages." These cells are increased in their phagocytic activity, the number of lysosomes, and the production of "reactive oxygen species" (O_2^- [the superoxide anion], H_2O_2, and hydroxyl free radicals). The activated cells not only destroy ingested microbes, but the secreted reactive forms of oxygen also can kill nearby susceptible cells (e.g., many tumor cells: see Chap. 19). The activated macrophages also produce interleukin-1 (IL-1), a small protein, whose action on temperature-regulatory centers of the central nervous system causes the fever associated with tuberculosis and many other chronic microbial diseases.

Although tuberculin sensitivity attributable to tuberculin-specific T cells is associated with an increase in host defenses, under some circumstances, the response can exacerbate symptoms and promote tissue break-down, which can increase spread of the bacteria. For example, in sensitive individuals, the administration of a large amount of tuberculin can provoke severe systemic responses, including chills, fever, and increased inflammation around existing lesions. This effect was reluctantly recognized by Koch, who enthusiastically injected tuberculin in tuberculous patients in the hope of enhancing immunity.

Tuberculin sensitivity is clearly a double-edged sword: it is associated with increased resistance, but under some circumstances, the response can also exacerbate symptoms, augment tissue necrosis, and increase spread of the bacteria.

PATHOGENESIS

The consequences of inhaling or ingesting tubercle bacilli depend on both the **virulence** of the organism and the **resistance** of the host (as well as the size and the location of the inoculum). At one extreme, organisms with little virulence for the particular host disappear completely, leaving no anatomic trace behind. At the opposite extreme (e.g., in guinea pigs inoculated with human tubercle bacilli), the bacilli flourish in macrophages as well as extracellularly, are disseminated widely, and cause death within a few months.

Humans exhibit a range of responses. The initial infection in a tuberculin-negative individual most often produces a self-limited lesion, but sometimes the disease progresses, presumably because of low resistance or a large inoculum. Because of the delicate balance of resistance, involving local as well as systemic factors, healing and progressing lesions may coexist in the same individual, and the disease often has a chronic, cyclic course (especially without chemotherapy). This pattern stands in marked contrast to the acute course of those infections that instigate well-defined humoral immunity.

Histologically, the tubercle bacillus evokes two types of reaction. **Exudative** lesions are seen in the initial infection or in the individual in whom the organism proliferates rapidly without encountering much host resistance. Acute or subacute inflammation occurs, with exudation of fluid and accumulation of polymorphonuclear leukocytes around the bacteria. "**Productive**" (**granulomatous**) lesions form when the individual becomes hypersensitive to tuberculoprotein. The macrophages then undergo a dramatic modification on contact with tubercle bacilli or their products, becoming concentrically arranged in the form of elongated **epithelioid cells,** to form the **tubercles** characteristic of this disease. In the center of the tubercles, some of these cells may fuse to form one or more **giant cells,** with dozens of nuclei arranged at their periphery and viable bacilli often visible in their cytoplasm. Outside the multiple layers of epithelioid cells is a mantle of lymphocytes and prolifer-

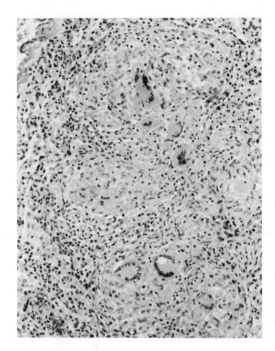

Figure 35–5. Section of a tubercle, showing several giant cells containing a peripheral ring of nuclei, epithelioid cells, and mononuclear cells toward the periphery of the lesion. (×180, reduced; courtesy of BW Castleman)

ating fibroblasts (Fig. 35–5), leading eventually to extensive fibrosis. The subsequent development of caseation necrosis, and its various fates, are noted below.

In early lesions, tubercle bacilli are localized primarily within macrophages, in which they multiply (at least for a time). In more advanced lesions, only extracellular bacilli are prominent, probably because the activated macrophages destroy the intracellular bacilli more efficiently.

Primary Infection

After inhalation of tubercle bacilli, the initial lesion appears as an area of nonspecific pneumonitis, usually located in a well-aerated peripheral zone. It is only after delayed hypersensitivity develops, in 2 to 4 weeks, that granulomatous inflammation supervenes and the characteristic **tubercles** (L. *tuberculum*, small lump) are formed. In the meantime, bacilli are carried to the draining lymph nodes and then, by way of the lymph and blood, throughout the body of the host. The pulmonary focus and the granulomatous lesion in the hilar lymph node together are known as the **primary complex.** The next stage in the inflammatory response consists of **caseation necrosis** (L. *caseus*, cheese), in which the necrotic centers of tubercles remain semisolid rather than softening to form pus, presumably because the enzymes that usually liquefy dead cells and tissue are inhibited.

Primarily tuberculosis in children usually stabilizes and heals. Caseous lesions heal by **fibrosis** and **calcification,** which may result in extensive scar formation and shrinkage. The healed and frequently calcified primary complex lesions are referred to as the **Ghon complex,** which may be recognized in chest radiographs for the remainder of the person's life. In a small proportion of individuals, however, the infection is not brought under control, and the primary lesions become progressively larger, coalesce, and **liquefy.** When this material is released, a **cavity** is formed in the lung, and there may be extension of the disease via the bronchi.

Reactivation Disease

Most tuberculosis in adults is secondary to reactivation of long-dormant foci remaining from the primary infection. The foci are located mostly in the posterior apical or subapical portions of the lung, whose persistent infection, after hematogenous spread, may be attributable to the high pO$_2$ resulting from their favorable ventilation–perfusion ratio. Viable tubercle bacilli are rarely found in the healed lesions of the primary complex.

By the time disease is recognized, liquefaction of the caseous lesion usually has occurred, and a cavity has provided a favorable site for the rapid proliferation of the bacilli. These may then be transmitted to other individuals via droplet nuclei produced by aerosols of infected sputum and to other parts of the lungs by bronchogenic spread. Almost every organ of the body may be the site of **extrapulmonary** tuberculosis. The most common locations are the genitourinary system, bones and joints, lymph nodes, pleura, and peritoneum. Extrapulmonary disease commonly develops as a result of reactivation of dormant lesions seeded during the primary infection. **Disseminated,** or **miliary,** tuberculosis may follow the rupture of a caseous lesion into a pulmonary vein.

The concept of reactivation disease is based on the following evidence: (1) phage types of bacilli isolated from multiple sites are usually identical; (2) in contrast to healed primary lesions, apical residuals are apt to contain viable tubercle bacilli; (3) it is unusual to find a source case to explain apparently new disease of the reactivation type, whereas in adults with primary type infection an index case often can be identified; (4) tuberculin sensitivity persists for a lifetime, and this sensitivity is occasionally eliminated by chemotherapy; (5) most suggestively, there has been a striking upward shift in the age of peak mortality ever since the total incidence of the disease began declining around 1870.

Because the present group of elderly tuberculin reactors had a high risk of acquiring initial infection at an earlier age and would then have remained tuberculin-positive, their frequent development of active tuberculosis is best explained as a reactivation of dormant foci acquired much earlier in life. It is thus no longer advantageous to be tuberculin-positive as a result of an earlier inapparent infection: although the hypersensitive state partially protects against the production of disease by a fresh infection, the level of exposure to such an infection is now so low that this advantage is outweighed by the possibility of progression or activation of the previous infection.

Although most cases of adult disease can be attributed to reactivation, exogenous reinfection has also been demonstrated by phage type and by drug resistance.

Variations in Host Resistance

Among persons infected with the tubercle bacillus, as detected by a positive tuberculin test (see below), only a small proportion develop overt disease, and even before the advent of chemotherapy, only about 10% of these progressed to fatal disease. The transition from **infection** to mild or to severe **disease** depends strongly on various factors besides the presence of the bacilli; hence, in an earlier era, when nearly everyone eventually became tuberculin-positive, tuberculosis could almost be regarded as one of the "endogenous diseases."

Although many of the observed variations in the response to infection may involve differences in the size, the site, or the virulence of the inoculum, there is also no doubt that resistance in man varies more strikingly with tuberculosis than with most infectious diseases. Thus in a tragic accident in Lübeck, Germany, in 1930, 251 children (tuberculin-negative, and hence without acquired immunity) received identical inocula of a virulent strain instead of an attenuated vaccine: 77 developed fatal disease, 127 developed radiologically detectable lesions that healed, and 47 showed no signs of disease. Such variations in resistance involve both genetic and nongenetic (physiologic) factors.

GENETIC DIFFERENCES. The importance of genetic factors in host resistance has been unequivocally established by Lurie's development of inbred lines of rabbits with a high or a low tendency to acquire progressive tuberculosis from experimental infection. Multiple factors are evidently involved: some lines are most resistant to **initiation** of disease by small inocula, whereas in others the resistance primarily influences the **rate of progress** of the disease.

In humans, it seems likely that there are similar **racial differences** in resistance associated with different lengths of exposure of the race to the selective pressures of an environment with widespread tuberculosis. Thus, in the U.S., the incidence of tuberculosis and the ratio of deaths to cases are especially high among American Indians, Eskimos, and blacks. These races may have had little or no exposure to tuberculosis until the last two or three centuries, in contrast with descendants of a European population. However, the evidence is complicated

by the concomitant differences in environmental and socioeconomic factors. Environmental factors, however, were relatively equalized in two kinds of studies. In the U.S. Army (from 1922 to 1936), the case fatality rate was four times higher among black soldiers than among whites. In a study of twins, the frequency of the disease in both members of the pair, compared with that in one member, was three times higher among monozygotic than among dizygotic pairs.

Search for genetic markers linked to susceptibility to tuberculosis has not yet produced dramatic results. Studies of the human HLA system have reported increased frequency of BW15 in tuberculous black patients and DR2 in India.

PHYSIOLOGIC FACTORS. Epidemiologic evidence on the frequency of tuberculosis in various populations has long suggested that **malnutrition, overcrowding,** and **stress** decrease resistance to the disease; but this kind of evidence does not firmly establish a causal relation because these conditions are generally also associated with a high rate of infection. However, the ability of one or more of these factors to overcome innate resistance is well illustrated by the experience of inmates of Nazi concentration camps during World War II. Tuberculosis was exceedingly prevalent in this population, which was subjected to extreme stress and prolonged starvation; yet many seemingly moribund persons with far-advanced disease exhibited a remarkable recovery when liberated from the camps and renourished. In contrast, before the era of chemotherapy, many persons who entered a sanatorium with minimal tuberculosis progressed inexorably to a fatal outcome despite good nutrition and general care. The most specific evidence on the effect of starvation has been obtained in experimental infections in mice: reduced **protein** consumption increased susceptibility, whereas variations in vitamin and total caloric intake had no demonstrable effect.

The significance of **hormonal** factors is suggested by the striking variations in resistance with **age** and, to a smaller extent, with **sex.** Tuberculosis is apt to be very severe in infants, perhaps because of the immaturity of the immune mechanisms. It then decreases rapidly in both incidence and severity with increasing age, and **between 3 and 12 years of age, progressive disease is almost unknown,** even in children heavily infected by exposure to a tuberculous parent. Susceptibility increases rapidly at adolescence, and among young adults, tuberculosis is more frequent in females. Curiously, in experimental animals, no marked influence of age on susceptibility has been noted.

Administration of **cortisone,** in humans and in experimental animals, decreases resistance to tuberculosis and tends to mask its symptoms and diminish reactivity to tuberculin. Hence in the therapy of other diseases with this hormone, the arousal of dormant tuberculosis is occasionally a serious and readily overlooked complication. Increased secretion of cortisone may also well be involved in the presumptive role of stress, noted above.

SILICOSIS. Tuberclosis is notoriously frequent among miners and others exposed to dust containing silica. Moreover, in guinea pigs that have inhaled silica suspensions, even the avirulent BCG strain produces fatal tuberculosis. The decrease in resistance appears to be due to damage to phagocytic cells: phagocytized silica particles cause rapid disruption of lysosomes, followed by cell lysis; and because the particles are never digested, they can attack cell after cell. Silica is exceedingly insoluble, and it is believed to act by direct contact with lysosomal membranes.

LABORATORY DIAGNOSIS

A provisional diagnosis of tuberculosis is usually made by demonstrating acid-fast bacilli in stained smears of sputum or of gastric washings (containing swallowed sputum). For rapid screening of smears, some laboratories employ fluorescence microscopy following staining with the fluorochrome dye mixture rhodamine–auramine.

Whether the smear is positive, the material should be cultured, for several reasons: (1) cultivation can detect fewer organisms; (2) cultural characteristics distinguish human tubercle bacilli from other acid-fast bacilli, including avirulent contaminants, other pathogenic mycobacteria (see below), and *Nocardia* (Chap. 36); and (3) tests for drug sensitivities may be initiated. During chemotherapy, frequent sputum smears and cultures provide a rapid, objective index of the response.

Sputum is prepared for culture by exploiting the unusual resistance of tubercle bacilli to strong alkalis and acids. For example, the material may be shaken at 37°C in 0.1N NaOH. The resulting liquefaction permits concentration of bacteria by centrifugation; and more rapidly growing bacterial contaminants are mostly destroyed by this treatment, whereas a fraction of the mycobacterial cells remain viable (and virulent). The centrifuged sediment should be smeared and stained as well as cultured.

Solid culture media are preferred for primary isolation; they often contain egg yolk to promote growth of macroscopic colonies from small inocula. However, oleic acid–albumin agar medium, which is transparent, allows detection of smaller colonies than those required on an opaque egg medium. These media contain malachite green or an antibiotic at levels that selectively suppress growth of pyogenic contaminants. A positive culture usually grows out in 2 to 4 weeks. The same methods are used to process body fluids and exudates not likely to be free of pyogenic organisms, but normally sterile fluids such as cerebrospinal fluid may be planted directly on culture media.

A selective liquid medium with a radiolabeled carbon substrate allows automated detection of growth several days sooner than with conventional culture, by recognition of radioactive carbon dioxide. Contamination with secondary organisms is kept to a minimum by the use of concentrated and digested sputum and the addition of selective inhibitors. In other approaches, specific Ags in the sputum and body fluids can be recognized by radioimmunoassay, and specific genetic markers by the use of DNA probe technology. Serologic tests have not proved useful in diagnosis, but promising results have recently been described with the use of the ELISA technique to measure antibody to PPD or to Daniel's antigen 5.

Tuberculin Test

SIGNIFICANCE. Delayed-type hypersensitivity to tuberculin is highly specific for the tubercle bacillus and closely related mycobacteria. Reactivity appears about 1 month after infection in man and persists for many years, often for life; hence the frequency of reactors in the population increases cumulatively with age. **A positive test thus reveals previous mycobacterial infection; it does not establish the presence of active disease.** Its persistence probably depends on persistence of bacilli in dormant foci, and reactivity may disappear following chemotherapy of recent infections.

The tuberculin skin test is a useful diagnostic and epidemiologic tool. Conversion from negative to positive provides good evidence for a recent infection, which should set in motion investigation of contacts and possible source cases, as well as a clinical evaluation of the converter. However, approximately 5% to 10% of patients with nondisseminated tuberculosis have negative initial tests, and the frequency is higher in miliary and extrapulmonary disease, probably related to an excess of Ag.

This **anergy** may be specific for tuberculin or nonspecific (including negative cell-mediated reactions to other Ags such as mumps and candida, to which most normal adults react). It may be caused by severe malnutrition, chronic renal failure, lymphoma, advanced age, acute stress, the administration of steroids, viral infection, vaccination with live viral agents, and certain bacterial infections. Suggested mechanisms of nonreactivity are defective chemotaxis, compartmentalization of tuberculin-reactive lymphocytes, and T-lymphocyte depression by circulating immune complexes. Many of these patients will regain positive reactions 2 or 3 weeks after drug treatment is started. Anergy may be tuberculin-specific or it may include many other antigens to which most healthy adults react, such as Candida and mumps.

Recall of a previously positive reaction may also occur within a week or two following a negative test, mainly in older people whose hypersensitivity has waned. This "booster" phenomenon should not be confused with a recent infection.

PREPARATION OF TUBERCULIN. Tuberculin as originally described by Koch, known as **old tuberculin (OT),** is prepared by autoclaving or boiling a culture of tubercle bacilli, concentrating it 10-fold on a steam bath, filtering off the debris, and adding glycerol as a preservative. In this impure product, the active constituent is a protein remarkable for its heat stability: after being autoclaved, it remains soluble and retains specific determinants of the protein in the infecting bacilli. Stock solutions retain full potency for years when stored at 5°C.

A slightly more refined tuberculin, called **purified protein derivative (PPD),** is prepared by precipitation several times with 50% saturated ammonium sulfate. The product is mostly a mixture of small proteins (average mol. wt. 10,000).

TESTING PROCEDURES. Tuberculin hypersensitivity is best evaluated by **intradermal** injection of 0.1 ml of an appropriate dilution of standardized PPD into the most superficial layers of the skin of the forearm (**Mantoux test**). The average diameter of **induration** (and not simply erythema) at the injected site is measured at 48 hours, and reactions of 10 mm or more are generally considered to be positive. Persons infected with cross-reacting mycobacteria (see Other Pathogenic Mycobacteria, below) frequently exhibit weak reactions (4–9 mm in diameter). Ordinarily, however, the population is quite sharply divided into tuberculin-positive or -negative.

In epidemiologic work, the standard test dose generally used is 5 tuberculin units (TU) of PPD (0.1 μg) in 0.1 ml, corresponding to OT 1/2000. In children suspected of having tuberculosis, a five-fold lower concentration is first used (**first strength**) to avoid a severe reaction, and if there is no response within 2 to 3 days, the standard strength is used. **Second-strength** PPD, containing 20 to 50 times the standard dose, may be used in those patients with negative or doubtful standard tests but still suspected of infection with tubercle bacilli or with cross-reacting mycobacteria.

Other commonly used methods of skin testing involve multiple punctures of the skin by means of various mechanical devices. These methods are less accurate than the Mantoux test, and positive or doubtful results should be checked by the intradermal technique.

THERAPY

Until the discovery of streptomycin in 1945, the treatment of tuberculosis was limited to rest, good nutrition, and artificial collapse of the lung. Unfortunately, the value of streptomycin was restricted by its toxicity to the eighth cranial nerve and by the frequent emergence of resistant tubercle bacilli during therapy. Some principles of drug therapy were learned rapidly: (1) long-term treatment was necessary to minimize the rate of relapse; (2) combinations of two or more drugs delayed the emergence of resistant organisms; (3) some combinations worked better than others; and (4) important drug characteristics included the ability to penetrate macrophages and kill mycobacteria in their acidic environment.

The older drug regimens included streptomycin (SM), para-aminosalicylic acid (PAS), isoniazid (INH), ethambutol (EMB) replacing PAS, or rifampin (RMP), in various combinations. These regimens were usually continued for 18 to 24 months. More rapid action of the newer regimens has been ascribed to special ability of pyrazinamide (PZA) to kill tubercle bacilli in the acid environment of macrophages; excellent intracellular penetration of INH, RMP, and PZA; and the rapid bactericidal activity of RMP during the periodic bursts of metabolic activity of otherwise-dormant bacilli. Dormant bacilli are not susceptible to killing by any available drug.

The most popular regimens now are INH/RMP for 9 months, often supplemented by EMB during the first 2 or 3 months. If it is desired to complete treatment in 6 months (especially for noncompliant patients), it is best to give INH/RMP/PZA, with or without the addition of SM for the first few months. The suspicion of bacillary drug resistance is the usual indication for adding SM. Modern chemotherapy should provide a cure for well over 95% of patients on initial treatment; most failures are the result of poor cooperation. Arrangements for supervised and intermittent (twice-weekly) drug treatment may be necessary to assure compliance. Ethionamide, cycloserine, and capreomycin are available as reserve drugs for instances of drug intolerance or bacillary resistance.

DRUG RESISTANCE AND COMBINATION THERAPY. The selection of drug-resistant mutants in patients with tuberculosis is favored by several features of the disease: the numerous bacteria in the lesions, especially in the walls of cavities; their further multiplication during the required long periods of therapy; and the limited degree of host resistance, which provides the rare mutant cell with a good opportunity to proliferate before being eliminated by host defenses. Hence, specifically resistant strains often appear in patients treated with any one of the drugs used singly. The rationale for preventing the emergence of resistant strains by **combined therapy** with two or more drugs has been presented in Chapter 10.

The INH-resistant mutants isolated from treated patients lack catalase and peroxidase activity, grow more slowly, and are much less virulent for guinea pigs. However, they retain virulence for man, and they may continue to be shed in sputum over months and even years.

Strains resistant to various antimicrobial agents (most often streptomycin or INH) not only arise during treatment but may be transmitted. The rate of such resistant primary infections varies in different populations in this country from 3% to 15%, being highest among Asians and Hispanics and in children. The overall rate has declined from 13% in 1975 to 7% in 1982.

EPIDEMIOLOGY

The human tubercle bacillus is spread principally by droplets and sputum from individuals with open pulmonary lesions. Small droplets produced by coughing are probably the most effective vehicles, as they rapidly dry in the air to yield droplet nuclei of less than 5 μm diameter, which can reach the alveoli. The organism can survive in moist or dried sputum for up to 6 weeks, but it is killed by a few hours' exposure to direct sunlight.

The incidence of tuberculosis may be estimated by tuberculin test surveys as well as from reports of active cases or of deaths. The frequency is higher in impoverished urban groups that live under crowded conditions and in certain nonurban groups (American Indians and Eskimos) that probably have a high genetic susceptibility. Socioeconomic conditions undoubtedly affect both host resistance and incidence of infection. With the progressive decline over the past century, the peak incidence has shifted from young adulthood, with a preponderance of females, to elderly, impoverished men, living alone in city slums and often alcoholic and malnourished.

The worldwide decline of tuberculosis over the past century probably reflects general social and economic improvement. In addition, death rates in the U.S. have declined especially sharply as a result of effective chemotherapy: in 1982, the rate was approximately 0.8 per 100,000 but was twice as high in large cities as in other areas. The incidence of new cases has dropped from 52 per 100,000 in 1953 to 9 in 1985. Thus, there are still about 1800 deaths and 20,000 new cases per year. The tuberculosis problem in this country today is largely one of reactivation of dormant lesions, for more than 90% of the population now reaches adulthood without infection. Nevertheless, although tuberculosis is no longer the "white plague" of previous centuries, in the world at large, it is estimated that more than a million die of the disease annually. In addition, the steadily declining case rate leveled off from 1984 to 1988 because of the association of tuberculosis with AIDS.

PREVENTION

The principal strategies for controlling tuberculosis are: (1) identification and prompt treatment of active cases; (2) investigation of the contacts of active cases, both to recognize newly infected individuals and to determine the source of the infection; (3) preventive drug treatment for recently infected but not diseased persons; and (4) immunization.

Case-finding schemes based on mass surveys with skin testing and chest films now have such a low yield that they have been abandoned except in certain localized areas of high incidence. Additional cases are uncovered by examination of the home and school contacts of recent tuberculin converters and newly recognized tuberculosis cases.

Chemoprophylaxis, or preventive treatment, is one of the mainstays of tuberculosis control in North America but has not been popular elsewhere. Isoniazid daily for 9 to 12 months is effective and well tolerated for this purpose. Prophylaxis is recommended for all young tuberculin reactors (less than 20 to 30 years of age); for recent skin-test converters (within the past 2 or 3 years) regardless of age; for household contacts, especially children, of sputum-smear-positive cases (3 months is considered a sufficient duration of therapy if repeated skin tests remain negative); and for previously untreated inactive cases with residual scars on radiographs.

Immunization with a live vaccine, the BCG strain (see Genetic Variation, above), may protect effectively against overt tuberculosis, although not necessarily against infection, for at least 5 to 10 years. Several well-controlled studies have demonstrated a protection rate of 70% or better. However, others have reported little or no protection. One reason for the difference may be the difficulty in demonstrating protection against an infection unless the natural rate is high. Although the matter remains controversial, it has lost its urgency, for a more effective approach to prevention today is recognition and prophylactic treatment of the recent tuberculin converter—and vaccination has the serious disadvantage of eliminating the usefulness of the tuberculin test. Accordingly, in countries with low or moderate prevalence of the disease there is little justification for widespread vaccination, and even vaccination of medical personnel is no longer recommended.

MYCOBACTERIUM BOVIS

M. bovis causes tuberculosis in cattle and is also highly virulent for man; unpasteurized milk (and occasionally other dairy products) from tuberculous cows has been responsible for much human tuberculosis. The ingested organisms presumably penetrate the mucosa of the oropharynx and intestine (although without apparent damage), giving rise to early lesions in the **cervical lymph nodes (scrofula)** or in the **mesenteric nodes.** Subsequent dissemination from these sites principally infects **bones and joints;** such infection of vertebrae was largely responsible for the hunchbacks of previous generations. When inhaled (e.g., by dairy farmers), the organism can also cause pulmonary tuberculosis indistinguishable from that caused by *M. tuberculosis.*

The conquest of bovine tuberculosis, through the widespread pasteurization of milk and the virtual elimination of tuberculosis in cattle, vividly illustrates the effectiveness of public health legislation when the reservoir of a disease can be controlled. In 1917, the U.S. Department of Agriculture, with widespread support from veterinarians, undertook an audacious program: tuberculin testing of all cattle and **the slaughter of all positive reactors.** As a result, the proportion of tuberculin reactors in American cattle has been reduced from 5% to 0.5% (most of which now have no visible lesion at autopsy and may be cross-reactors).

Koch maintained that all mammalian tuberculosis was caused by the same organism. However, largely through Theobald Smith's work, *M. bovis* and *M. tuberculosis* were clearly distinguished. *M. bovis* is a bit shorter and plumper than *M. tuberculosis;* the former is highly pathogenic in rabbits, whereas the latter is much less so; and in cultures, *M. bovis* tends to grow more slowly and cannot tolerate as high a concentration of glycerol. *M. bovis* also differs from *M. tuberculosis* in being niacin-test–negative, in not reducing nitrate, and in being resistant to pyrazinamide. Serologic tests and skin tests do not distinguish between the two organisms, however.

M. africanum, an organism isolated from tuberculosis patients in Africa, resembles *M. bovis* in its slow growth and in several biochemical reactions. The question of species status has not been decided.

OTHER PATHOGENIC MYCOBACTERIA

In addition to the mammalian tubercle bacilli described above, various other acid-fast bacilli occasionally have been cultured from respiratory secretions of apparently tuberculous individuals, but because they possessed little or no virulence for guinea pigs or rabbits, they were long considered contaminating saprobes. Recognition of the role of the "atypical" mycobacteria in human disease was crystallized in the 1950s by the repeated recovery of such organisms from the sputum and **directly from diseased tissue** in the absence of classic tubercle bacilli. Moreover, as the incidence of tuberculosis decreases, the relative importance of disease attributable to nontuberculous mycobacteria is increasing.

In certain areas of the world, including a few communities in the U.S., as much as 20% of newly diagnosed mycobacterial pulmonary disease is caused by these organisms. The proportion is even higher in soft-tissue and disseminated disease. Conditions that result in pulmonary destructive lesions and scarring (silicosis, bullous emphysema, bronchiectasis, and healed tuberculosis) predispose to pulmonary mycobacteriosis.

Table 35–1 presents a simplified scheme for the classification and differentiation of mycobacteria commonly cultured from human material. A more detailed description and illustrations may be found in the Centers for Disease Control publication by Kent and Kubica.

MYCOBACTERIUM AVIUM COMPLEX. The *M. avium* complex includes ***M. avium,*** which was recognized as a distinct species prior to 1900, and the more recently described ***M. intracellulare.*** The avian tubercle bacillus causes tuberculosis in chickens, pigeons, and other birds and in swine. There are many well-documented cases of human disease caused by this organism, mostly in farmers or their children and in men with silicosis.

The avian bacillus is readily distinguishable from *M. tuberculosis* and *M. bovis.* The individual cells are smaller; the colonies are smooth; it grows optimally at about 41°C (at which human and bovine bacilli will not grow); it is resistant to most of the antituberculosis drugs; and it is pathogenic for chickens and rabbits but not for guinea pigs. Antigenic differences are also readily demonstrated.

M. intracellulare (formerly known as the Battey bacillus) is generally less thermophilic than *M. avium,* and most strains are not pathogenic for birds or animals. Some, however, have intermediate virulence (as is also true of some *M. avium* strains). In seroagglutination tests, the avian strains are included in *M. avium* complex serotypes 1, 2, and 3, and the other recognized 25 serotypes are *"intracellulare"* types. The two species of the complex are not readily distinguishable by other routine laboratory procedures. Bacilli of serotypes 1, 4, and 8 are frequent agents of disseminated infection in patients with AIDS.

MYCOBACTERIUM SCROFULACEUM. *M. scrofulaceum* is a common cause of lymphadenitis in children. Seroagglutination has revealed three or four types, but some Ags are shared with the *M. avium* complex. Colonies are usually yellow-orange even when grown in the dark **(scotochromogenic).** Some strains derived from human material and from the environment have intermediate biochemical and pigment characteristics; they are usually resistant to antituberculosis drugs *in vitro.*

MYCOBACTERIUM KANSASII. *M. kansasii* and *M. avium-intracellulare* together account for most of the human mycobacterial disease attributable to acid-fast organisms other than mammalian tubercle bacilli. *M. kansasii* is

TABLE 35–1. Some Characteristics of Nontuberculous Mycobacteria Commonly Encountered in Human Material

Species	Clinical Significance*	Optimal Growth Temperature (°C)	Pigment†	Catalase 25–38°	Catalase 68°	Nitrate	Tween Hydrolysis	Urease	Iron Uptake	Growth Rate
M. avium-intracellulare	+	37	– or S	Weak	+	–	–	–		Slow
M. kansasii	+	37	P	Strong	+	+	+	+		Slow
M. xenopi	+	42	S	Weak	+	–	–	–		Slow
M. scrofulaceum	+	37	S	Strong	+	–	–	+		Slow
M. simiae	+	37	P(weak)	Strong	+	–	–	+		Slow
M. szulgai	+	37	S‡	Strong	+	+	±	+		Slow
M. gordonae	±	30–37	S	Strong	+	–	+	–		Slow
M. flavescens	±	30–37	S	Strong	+	+	+	+	–	Intermediate
M. terrae-triviale	±	30–37	–	Strong	+	+	+	–		Slow
M. gastri	–	30–37	–	Weak	–	–	+	+		Slow
M. marinum	+	30	P	Weak	+	–	+	+		Intermediate
M. fortuitum	+	30–37	–	Strong	+	+	±	+	+	Fast
M. chelonae	+	30–37	–	Strong	+	–	–	+	–	Fast
M. smegmatis	–	25–45	–	Strong	+	+	+	+	+	Fast

* +, May be pathogenic for hosts without general immune suppression; ±, documented pathogen only for hosts with abnormal local and/or general defense mechanisms.

† P, photochromogenic; S, scotochromogenic.

‡ Scotochromogenic when grown at 37°C but variably photochromogenic at 25°C.

photochromogenic; the overnight change of the colonies to yellow is followed by the formation of red crystals of β-carotene on exposure to light for several more days. Most strains are sensitive to rifampin and to several other drugs, and the disease responds well to treatment.

MYCOBACTERIUM ULCERANS. *M. ulcerans*, found mainly in Africa and Australia, **will grow only below 33°C.** It causes chronic, deep **cutaneous ulcers** in man, and in mice and rats, it produces lesions in the cooler parts of the body. Its usual drug sensitivity pattern—resistance to INH and ethambutol and susceptibility to streptomycin and rifampin—is unique. Human disease responds poorly to drug treatment, and extensive excision followed by skin grafting is often necessary. Although rare, the disease is of considerable theoretical interest, as the low temperature range of the organism provides a simple explanation for its unusual pathogenetic properties.

MYCOBACTERIUM MARINUM. *M. marinum* (synonyms: *M. balnei, M. platypoecilus*) also grows best at 30° to 33°C and relatively poorly at 37°. It causes a tuberculosis-like disease in fish and a chronic skin lesion, known as **"swimming pool (or fish tank) granuloma,"** in humans. Infection acquired by injury of a limb around a home aquarium or a marine environment also can lead to a series of ascending subcutaneous abscesses not unlike the lesions of sporotrichosis. *M. marinum* resembles *M. kansasii* in being photochromogenic, but it can be differentiated by the optimum growth temperature, negative nitrate test, agglutination with specific antisera, and distinctive drug sensitivity pattern (resistance to INH, sensitivity to the other major antituberculosis drugs).

MYCOBACTERIUM FORTUITUM COMPLEX. Most of the fast-growing disease-associated mycobacteria are members of this complex, which may be divided into two accepted species, *M. fortuitum* and *M. chelonae*. They abound as saprobes in soil and water. The spectrum of disease caused by these organisms includes soft-tissue abscesses, sternal wound infections after cardiac surgery, prosthetic valve endocarditis, disseminated and localized infection in hemodialysis and peritoneal dialysis patients, pulmonary disease, traumatic wound infection, and disseminated disease often with cutaneous lesions. Some of these strains, especially *M. chelonae*, are resistant to most antimicrobial drugs.

OTHER SPECIES. *M. xenopi*, first isolated in 1959 from a South African toad, has been reported to cause pulmonary infection in several areas of the world, most prominently in England. Contaminated hot water tanks may serve as a reservoir for infection, especially in institutions that care for patients with chronic lung disease. The organisms are thermophilic, scotochromogenic, and relatively sensitive to INH, rifampin, and streptomycin. Stained cells from cultures are long, fusiform, and palisaded. *M. szulgai* is a distinct species with a potential ability to produce chronic lung disease, as well as infection of lymph nodes and bursae. Almost all strains are scotochromogenic at 37°C, but many are photochromogenic at 25°. *M. simiae* was first recovered from monkeys in Budapest. Only a few documented cases of human lung disease have been reported. *M. haemophilum* is a distinctive species with a growth requirement for iron and with an optimum growth temperature of 25° to 30°. Reported cases of infection with this organism have included renal transplant patients with cutaneous nodules and abscesses and one child with lymphadenitis. *M. malmoense*, recently described as the cause of pulmonary disease in Sweden, is difficult to differentiate from strains of the *M. avium* complex except by lipid analysis and seroagglutination. It grows slowly even at its optimum temperature of 30° to 32°.

A group of acid-fast bacilli with little or no pathogenicity for man or animals may be found in human specimens and mistaken for established pathogens. *M. gordonae* is a scotochromogen resembling *M. scrofulaceum*; *M. gastri* and *M. terrae-triviale* are nonchromogenic; and *M. flavescens* is a scotochromogen with a moderately rapid growth rate. Even these species may cause human disease under the proper circumstances; local, generalized, and pulmonary infections have been attributed to strains of *M. gordonae, M. terrae,* and *M. flavescens.*

A summary of the nontuberculous mycobacterial diseases of humans is presented in Table 35–2.

EPIDEMIOLOGY. Many of these species (*M. scrofulaceum, M. avium-intracellulare,* and *M. fortuitum-chelonae*), including serotypes causing human disease, are found in dust, soil, water, and the tissues of domestic animals. *M. kansasii* and *M. xenopi* have been isolated from water taps and water storage tanks. Local soft-tissue infections (*M. marinum, M. scrofulaceum, M. fortuitum-chelonae*) may result from skin or mucous membrane contamination originating from the environment.

However, in pulmonary and disseminated disease, it often is not clear how the bacilli enter the human host or whether the disease in adults represents reactivation of dormant lesions or a new infection. Person-to-person transmission rarely, if ever, occurs.

The skin test Ags (**sensitins**) prepared from various mycobacteria show both specificity and cross-reactivity; hence patients with disease caused by nontuberculous mycobacteria may or may not respond to a standard tuberculin test. A large-scale epidemiologic study by the U.S. Public Health Service revealed that in general, humans infected with various mycobacteria react most intensely to the PPD from the homologous organism (Fig. 35–6). This approach revealed a high level of **inapparent infection** with nontuberculous mycobacteria in certain areas. In a study of more than 200,000 U.S. Navy recruits, only 8.6% reacted to the tuberculin of *M. tuberculosis,* whereas 35% reacted to the sensitin of *M. intracellulare.* The PPDs of several other mycobacteria, including some from soil, also caused reactions with striking frequency, and cross-reactions among various strains were frequent. Moreover, comparative studies with several Ags have provided strong evidence that **in some regions, the bulk of the weak reactions to tuberculin PPD are cross-reactions.** Hypersensitivity to the Ags of *M. scrofulaceum* and *M. avium* complex organisms is especially frequent in the southeastern part of the U.S. The nontuberculous acid-fast bacilli, with their ineradicable reservoir, may eventually become the major residue of the problem of mycobacterial infection.

Guinea pigs inoculated with various nontuberculous mycobacteria isolated from humans show some degree of protection against subsequent challenge with *M. tuberculosis.* Hence it seems quite possible that **inapparent human infection with these organisms may serve as a sort of natural vaccination against tuberculosis,** much as exposure to cowpox was noted, in Jenner's day, to protect against smallpox.

TABLE 35–2. Nontuberculous Mycobacterial Diseases of Man

Disease	*Common Associated Species*	*Other Associated Species*
Chronic cavitary lung disease in adults	MAI, *M. kans.*	*M. xenopi, szulgai, simiae, malmoense, scrof., fort.*
Local lymphadenitis in children	MAI, *M. scrof.*	*M. kans., M. fort.*
Arthritis, tenosynovitis, and osteomyelitis, including hand infection	MAI, *M. kans.*	*M. fort., M. terrae, M. marinum, M. xenopi*
Bursitis	*M. kans.*	*M. szulgai*
Skin nodules and abscesses	*M. marinum, M. haemophilum, M. fort.*	*M. kans., MAI, M. fort., M. szulgai*
Buruli or Bairnsdale ulcer	*M. ulcerans*	
Disseminated disease	MAI, *M. kans.*	*M. scrof., M. fort.*
Leprosy	*M. leprae*	

Abbreviations: MAI, *M. avium-intracellulare;* M. fort., *M. fortuitum-chelonae;* M. scrof, *M. scrofulaceum;* M. kans., *M. kansasii.*

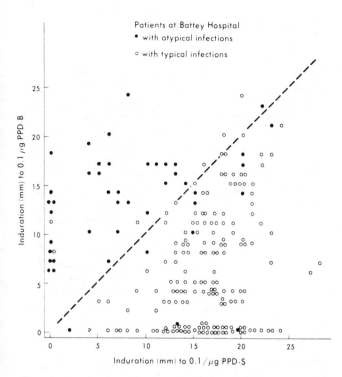

Patients at Battey Hospital
- • with atypical infections
- ○ with typical infections

Induration (mm) to 0.1/μg PPD-B

Induration (mm) to 0.1/μg PPD-S

Figure 35–6. Correlation of sizes of reactions of sanatorium patients with proved typical or atypical mycobacterial infections to standard tuberculin *(PPD-S)* and to comparable preparation *(PPD-B)* from a strain of *M. intracellulare* isolated from a patient in the same sanatorium. (Edwards LB et al: Acta Tuberc Scand Suppl 47:77, 1959. Copyright © 1959 by Munksgaard International Publishers Ltd, Copenhagen, Denmark)

The delayed recognition of the other pathogenic mycobacteria illustrates the absence of a sharp, testable distinction between pathogens and nonpathogens among the mycobacteria. On the one hand, most of the nontuberculous pathogens are probably saprobes that can become pathogenic under appropriate conditions; and although they are much less virulent than *M. tuberculosis,* they occasionally cause chronic and even life-threatening disease (just as do many saprobic fungi; see Chap. 43). On the other hand, the most frequent fate of the tubercle bacillus after infecting an individual is to persist for a lifetime without causing disease.

MYCOBACTERIA NOT ASSOCIATED WITH MAN

In spite of their sluggish growth, the mycobacteria are extremely widespread in nature, not only as saprobes but as parasites throughout the animal kingdom.

The **vole bacillus** (*Mycobacterium microti*) produces an epizootic chronic disease resembling tuberculosis in the field mouse. The bacillus is indistinguishable from *M. tuberculosis* in morphology, staining, and cultural behavior. In guinea pigs, it produces an infection that spon-

taneously regresses and establishes increased resistance to subsequent infection with virulent tubercle bacilli; it has therefore been used as a vaccine in man.

Mycobacterium paratuberculosis causes an often fatal enteritis of cattle and sheep, called **Johne's disease,** which is characterized by chronic infiltration of the intestinal mucosa and the mesenteric lymph nodes. The lesions resemble those caused by tubercle bacilli except that they are less localized and lack caseation. Infected cattle give delayed-type reactions to intradermal injections of culture filtrates (called johnin). The organism does not grow on the media used to cultivate other mycobacteria; it was initially cultivated by the ingenious expedient of enriching the medium with killed tubercle bacilli, and this special requirement can now be satisfied by mycobactin, an iron-complexing sideramine obtained from a mycobacterium. Recent DNA hybridization studies indicate that *M. paratuberculosis* is a member of the *M. avium* complex.

Mycobacterium lepraemurium causes an epizootic chronic disease of wild rats known as rat leprosy; the organism is observed within macrophages in lesions. The disease may be transmitted to mice, guinea pigs, and white rats by inoculation of infected tissue, but the organism, like that of human leprosy, has not been cultivated. Histologically, the lesions resemble those of human leprosy, but rats are not susceptible to infection with the human leprosy bacillus.

SAPROBIC MYCOBACTERIA. A number of acid-fast bacilli found chiefly on plants and in soil and water grow more rapidly than tubercle bacilli in culture; their role in nature is primarily concerned with the degradation of lipids. These organisms have not been established as pathogens. They include *M. phlei* (the timothy hay bacillus), and *M. smegmatis,* found in smegma and butter; both organisms are also found in dust, soil, and water.

Leprosy

MYCOBACTERIUM LEPRAE

Although *M. leprae* (**Hansen's bacillus**) has never been cultivated in the test tube, it has long been recognized as the etiologic agent of human leprosy, for the organism is readily demonstrated, often in great numbers, in stained smears of exudates of persons with leprosy and in tissue sections from lesions, whereas no other organism has been consistently identified in these preparations. Moreover, *M. leprae* is virtually indistinguishable in morphology and staining properties from *M. tuberculosis,* and leprosy has many clinical features in common with tuberculosis.

The failure to cultivate *M. leprae* has hampered its investigation and has made it difficult to test strains for drug sensitivity. The absence of an animal host presented another obstacle. However, in 1960, Shepard discovered that the bacilli could be propagated, although slowly, in the relatively cool environment of the **foot pads of mice.** This experimental model has made it possible to study the effects of various drugs and also the properties of the bacilli obtained from patients with various forms of leprosy. More recently, the nine-banded **armadillo** was found to develop disseminated disease, and it has yielded enough material for the production of a skin-test Ag.

LEPROMIN. Although *M. leprae* cannot be cultivated, an antigenic bacillary preparation for skin testing was developed by Mitsuda in 1919 by boiling human lepromatous tissue rich in bacilli. This material, called lepromin, is now standardized to contain 160×10^6 acid-fast bacilli/ml. Preparations from infected armadillo tissues have given comparable skin reactions.

A positive **Mitsuda reaction** consists of the slow development of a papule at the intradermal injection site, which, when biopsied at 2 to 4 weeks, reveals a hypersensitivity granuloma (not merely a granuloma of the foreign-body type). The test is not very helpful in diagnosis because of false-positive reactions in tuberculosis and in apparently healthy individuals, but it is useful in determining the prognosis and the phase of the disease (see Pathogenesis, below). Because lepromin also contains some soluble material, an earlier reaction (24 to 48 hours), typical of delayed hypersensitivity, is often also seen (the **Fernandez reaction**).

PATHOGENESIS

M. leprae causes chronic granulomatous lesions closely resembling those of tuberculosis, with epithelioid and giant cells, but without caseation. The organisms in the lesions are predominantly intracellular and can evidently proliferate within macrophages, like tubercle bacilli.

Leprosy is distinguished by its chronic, slow progress and by its mutilating and disfiguring lesions. These may be so distinctive that the diagnosis is apparent at a glance; or the clinical manifestations may be so subtle as to escape detection by any except the most experienced observers armed with a high index of suspicion. The organism has a predilection for skin and for nerve. In the **cutaneous** form of the disease, large, firm nodules (lepromas) are distributed widely, and on the face they create a characteristic leonine appearance. In the **neural** form, segments of peripheral nerves are involved, more or less at random, leading to localized patches of anesthesia. The loss of sensation in fingers and toes increases the frequency of minor trauma, leading to secondary infections and mutilating injuries. Both forms may be present in the same patient.

PHASES OF THE DISEASE. In either form of leprosy, three phases may be distinguished. First, in the **lepromatous** or **progressive** type, the lesions contain many **lepra cells:** macrophages with a characteristically foamy cytoplasm, in which acid-fast bacilli are abundant (Fig. 35–7). When these lesions are prominent, the lepromin test is usually negative, presumably owing to desensitization by massive amounts of endogenous lepromin, and the cell-mediated immune reactions to specific and nonspecific stimuli are markedly diminished. The disease is then in a progressive phase, and the prognosis is poor. Second, in the **tuberculoid** or **healing** phase of the disease, in contrast, the lesions contain few lepra cells and bacilli, fibrosis is prominent, and the lepromin test is usually positive. Third, in the **intermediate** type of disease, bacilli are seen in areas of necrosis but are rare elsewhere, the skin test is positive, and the long-range outlook is fair. Shifts from one phase to another, with exacerbation and remission of the disease, are common.

INTERFERON. The tuberculoid form of leprosy is a reaction to a partial immune response, associated with delayed-type hypersensitivity and macrophage activation. **Patients with the lepromatous form are anergic** and deficient in production of the macrophage activator, INF-γ. This material may have therapeutic promise, as its injection into lepromatous lesions converts them to the tuberculoid form.

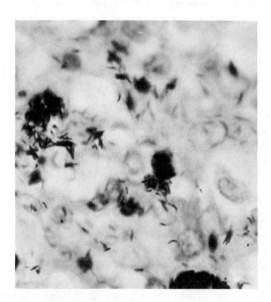

Figure 35–7. Leprosy bacilli in cells in section of human tissue. Acid-fast stain, methylene blue counterstain. (×1200; courtesy of CH Binford, Leonard Wood Memorial)

Hansen's bacillus may be widely distributed in the tissues of persons with leprosy, including the liver and spleen. Nevertheless, no destructive lesions or disturbance of function are observed in these organs. Most deaths of leprous patients are caused, not by leprosy itself, but rather by intercurrent infections with other microorganisms—often tuberculosis. A serious complication is **amyloidosis,** which is characterized by huge waxy deposits in kidneys, liver, spleen, and other organs. This curious disorder also occurs as a sequel to a variety of other chronic diseases with extensive necrosis and suppuration or to prolonged, intensive immunization of animals with diverse Ags, especially some bacterial toxins. The waxy deposits contain abundant precipitates of fragments of immunoglobulin light chains.

DIAGNOSIS AND TREATMENT

Bacteriologic diagnosis is accomplished by demonstrating acid-fast bacilli in scrapings from ulcerated lesions, or in fluid expressed from superficial incisions over nonulcerated lesions. Also useful is the skin test with lepromin in the tuberculoid phase. No useful serologic test is available, but patients with leprosy frequently have a false-positive serologic test for syphilis. The characteristic inflammatory response, including peripheral nerve involvement, and the presence of noncultivable acid-fast bacilli may be recognized by histologic study of biopsied lesions.

Therapy with **dapsone (diaminodiphenylsulfone)** or related compounds usually produces a gradual improvement over several years and is continued for a long period after apparent clinical remission. However, the emergence of both primary and acquired resistance to the sulfone drugs dictated the addition of rifampin and clofazimine (a phenazine) to the treatment regimens. For patients with widespread lepromatous disease, it is recommended that all three drugs be given for at least 2 years. Treatment results may be evaluated by counting the acid-fast bacilli in serial biopsies and skin scrapings.

Cloning of the genes encoding the major protein Ags and synthesis of specific epitopes offer promise for specific diagnosis and for vaccination.

The WHO, in 1987 reported a rapid serodiagnostic test for leprosy using gelatin particles coated with the chemically synthesized trisaccharide segment of a phenolic glycolipid from *M. leprae.*

EPIDEMIOLOGY

Leprosy is apparently transmitted when exudates of mucous membrane lesions and skin ulcers reach skin abrasions; it is not highly contagious, and patients need not be isolated. Young children appear to acquire the disease on briefer contact than adults. The incubation period is estimated to range from a few months to 30 years or more. Apparently, *M. leprae* can lie dormant in tissues for long periods. The prophylactic use of BCG vaccine or dapsone for contacts has not been successful, although immunologic tests with lepromin (lymphocyte transformation, leukocyte migration inhibition) suggest that inapparent infection is common among intimate contacts.

In ancient times, leprosy was rampant throughout most of the world, but for unknown reasons, it died out in Europe in the sixteenth century and now occurs there only in a few isolated pockets. In the U.S., leprosy occurs usually in persons from Puerto Rico, the Philippines, Mexico, Cuba, or Samoa. Several hundred patients are cared for at the national leprosarium in Carville, Louisiana. Recent estimates place the number of lepers in the world at large at about 10 million, with the greatest density in central Africa and in parts of Asia.

Selected Reading

BOOKS AND REVIEW ARTICLES

Arnason BG, Waksman BH: Tuberculin sensitivity. Adv Tuberc Res 13:1, 1964

Barksdale L, Kim KS: Mycobacterium. Bacteriol Rev 41:217, 1977

Binford CH, Meyers WM, Walsh GP: Leprosy. JAMA 247:2283, 1982

Chaparas SD: The immunology of mycobacterial infections. CRC Crit Rev Microbiol 9:139, 1982

Chaparas SD: Immunologic tests for the diagnosis of tuberculosis. Indian J Tuberc 32:3, 1985

Chapman JS: The Atypical Mycobacteria and Human Mycobacteriosis. New York, Plenum Medical, 1977

Daniel TM, Janicki BW: Mycobacterial antigens: A review of their isolation, chemistry, and immunological properties. Microbiol Rev 42:84, 1978

Dubos RJ, Dubos J: The White Plague. Boston, Little, Brown, 1952

Eickhoff TC: The current status of BCG immunization against tuberculosis. Annu Rev Med 28:411, 1977

Glassroth J, Robins AG, Snider DE: Tuberculosis in the 1980s. N Engl J Med 302:1441, 1980

Godal T: Leprosy immunology—some aspects of the role of the immune system in the pathogenesis of disease. Lepr Rev 55:407, 1984

Good RC: Opportunistic pathogens in the genus *Mycobacterium*. Annu Rev Microbiol 39:347, 1985

Goren MB: Mycobacterial lipids: Selected topics. Bacteriol Rev 36:33, 1972

Grange JM: Mycobacterial Diseases. New York, Elsevier, North Holland, 1980

Kent PT, Kubica GP: Public Health Mycobacteriology; a Guide for the Level III Laboratory. Atlanta, Centers for Disease Control, 1985

Kubica GP, Wayne LG (eds): The Mycobacteria: A Sourcebook. New York, Marcel Dekker, 1984

Lurie MB: Resistance to Tuberculosis. Cambridge, MA, Harvard University Press, 1964

Ratledge C, Stanford J (eds): The Biology of the Mycobacteria. New York, Academic Press, Vol 1, 1982; Vol 2, 1983

Rich AR: The Pathogenesis of Tuberculosis, 2nd Ed. Springfield, Charles C Thomas, 1951

Shepard CC: Leprosy today. N Engl J Med 307:1640, 1982

Skamene E: Genetic control of resistance to mycobacterial infection. Curr Top Microbiol Immunol 124:49, 1986

Wayne LG: The "atypical" mycobacteria: Recognition and disease association. CRC Crit Rev Microbiol 12:185, 1985

Wolinsky E: Nontuberculous mycobacteria and associated diseases. Am Rev Respir Dis 119:107, 1979

Young DB: Structure of mycobacterial antigens. Br Med Bull 44:562, 1988

SPECIFIC ARTICLES

Bailey WC, Byrd RB, Glassroth JL, Hopewell PC, Reichman LB: Preventive treatment of tuberculosis. Chest 87(suppl):128S, 1985

Barclay R, Ewing DF, Ratledge C: Isolation, identification, and structural analysis of mycobactins. J Bacteriol 164:896, 1985

Bloom BR, Godal T: Selective primary health care: Strategies for control of disease in the developing world V: Leprosy. Rev Infect Dis 5:765, 1983

Chapman JS: The ecology of the atypical mycobacteria. Arch Environ Health 22:41, 1971

Clemens JD, Chuong JJH, Feinstein AR: The BCG controversy: A methodological and statistical reappraisal. JAMA 249:2362, 1983

Coates ARM, Allen BW, Hewitt J, Ivanyi J, Mitchison DA: Antigenic diversity of *Mycobacterium tuberculosis* and *Mycobacterium bovis* detected by means of monoclonal antibodies. Lancet 2:167, 1981

Daniel TM, Debanne SM, van der Kuyp F: Enzyme-linked immunosorbent assay using *Mycobacterium tuberculosis* antigen 5 and PPD for the serodiagnosis of tuberculosis. Chest 88:388, 1985

Daniel TM, Gonchoroff NJ, Katzman JA, Olds GR: Specificity of *Mycobacterium tuberculosis* antigen 5 determined with mouse monoclonal antibodies. Infect Immun 45:52, 1984

Fox W: Whither short-course chemotherapy? Br J Dis Chest 75:331, 1981

Jones WD Jr, Good RC, Thompson NJ, Kelly GD: Bacteriophage types of *Mycobacterium tuberculosis* in the United States. Am Rev Resp Dis 125:640, 1982

Kato M, Miki K, Matsunaga K, Yamamura Y: Biologic and biochemical activities of "cord factor" with special reference to its role in the virulence of tubercle bacilli. Am Rev Respir Dis 77:482, 1958

Lederer E: The mycobacterial cell wall. Pure Appl Chem 25:135, 1971

Lurie MB: The fate of tubercle bacilli ingested by phagocytes derived from normal and immunized animals. J Exp Med 75:247, 1942

Mackaness GB: The immunological basis of acquired cellular resistance. J Exp Med 120:105, 1964

Nathan CF, Kaplan G, Levis WR, et al: Local and systemic effects of intradermal recombinant interferon-gamma in patients with lepromatous leprosy. N Engl J Med 315:6, 1986

Public Health Service Advisory Committee on Immunization Practices: BCG vaccines. Morbid Mortal Weekly Rep 28:241, 1979

Singh SPN, Mehra NK, Dingley HB, Pande JN, Vaidya MC: Human leukocyte antigen (HLA)-linked control of susceptibility to pulmonary tuberculosis and association with HLA-DR types. J Infect Dis 148:676, 1983

Snider DE, Cohn DL, Davidson PT, Hershfield ES, Smith MH, Sutton FD Jr: Standard therapy for tuberculosis 1985. Chest 87(suppl):117S, 1985

Waters MFR: The treatment of leprosy. Tubercle 64:221, 1983

Young RA, Bloom BR, Grosskinsky CM, Ivanyi J, Thomas D, Davis RW: Dissection of *Mycobacterium tuberculosis* antigens using recombinant DNA. Proc Natl Acad Sci USA 82:2583, 1985

Young RA, Mehra V, Sweetser D et al: Genes for the major protein antigens of the leprosy parasite *Mycobacterium leprae*. Nature 316:450, 1985

36

George S. Kobayashi

Actinomycetes: The Fungus-Like Bacteria

General Characteristics

The actinomycetes are gram-positive organisms that tend to grow slowly as branching filaments. In some genera, the filaments readily segment during growth and yield pleomorphic, club-shaped cells that resemble corynebacteria and mycobacteria; some are acid-fast.

Because the filamentous growth leads to mycelial colonies, and because some actinomycetes cause chronic subcutaneous granulomatous abscesses much like those caused by fungi, the actinomycetes (Gr. *aktino*, ray, and *mykes*, mushroom or fungus) were long regarded as fungi. (The term "ray" refers to the characteristic radial arrangement of club-shaped elements seen in microcolonies in infected tissues.) However, finer analysis showed that the actinomycetes are typical prokaryotes in terms of nucleoid and cell wall structure, antibiotic sensitivity, motility by means of simple flagella, genetic recombination via merozygotes rather than zygotes, absence of sterols, and presence of anaerobic and chemoautotrophic forms. Their long filaments have the diameter (1 μm) of bacteria (whereas fungal hyphae are larger), and they readily segment into bacillary and twig-like forms.

Actinomycetes are the most abundant organisms in the soil. They break down proteins, cellulose, and other organic matter (including paraffins); their cultures often have the odor of freshly turned over soil.

We will follow the practice of using the term "actinomycete" to refer to all members of the order *Actinomycetales* except the mycobacteria. Among the many genera, three are of particular medical interest. *Actinomyces* organisms grow as branching filaments when freshly culti-vated, but in older cultures and in lesions, an increased septation leads to fragmentation into bacillary and even coccoid elements indistinguishable from diphtheroids. Many *Nocardia* organisms are acid-fast and contain my-colic acids, like mycobacteria. *Streptomyces* organisms are more fungus-like, forming aerial mycelia and chains of asexual spores.

On primary isolation, actinomycetes can usually be identified to the genus level on the basis of morphologic features alone, but organisms that have been repeatedly transferred in culture may not retain the typical morpho-logic features and therefore require biochemical meth-ods for classification (Table 36–1). Serologic methods are also used, but cross-reactions among actinomycetes are extensive.

Actinomycosis was long assumed to arise from exog-enous infection by soil organisms. However, it is now clear that the bulk of the infections are endogenous, aris-ing from normal inhabitants of the oral cavity. Rather similar diseases resulting from inhalation of soil organ-isms are referred to as **nocardiosis.** With both groups (as with many fungi), local extension through successive adjacent layers of tissue is slow and inexorable, reflecting a poor immune response.

An allergic pneumonitis called **farmer's lung** occurs among agricultural workers who have inhaled dust from moldy plant material; it has been traced to at least three thermophilic actinomycetes, *Thermopolyspora poly-spora, Micromonospora vulgaris,* and *Micropolyspora faeni.* A similar disease is caused by allergens produced by various species of fungi, particularly in the genus *As-pergillus.*

Actinomyces

Several species of *Actinomyces* have been implicated as the cause of actinomycosis in humans and animals. *A. israelii* is usually responsible for the disease in man and *A. bovis* in cattle. These organisms are anaerobic or mi-croaerophilic and require rich media (e.g., containing blood or brain–heart infusion); growth is stimulated by CO_2 and is poor at temperatures below 37°C. Differences in cell wall composition, metabolic products, and toler-ance to oxygen distinguish several additional, less com-mon causes of the disease: *A. naeslundii, A. odontolyticus, A. viscosus,* and the related organisms *Arachnia pro-pionica.*

Most strains of *A. israelii* form rough colonies on agar and grow at the bottom of broth tubes as discrete aggre-gated clumps ("bread crumbs"; Fig. 36–1). A few strains, however, and most strains of *A. bovis*, form smooth colo-nies and tend to grow more diffusely in broth, and some strains of both species form intermediate colonies. In anaerobic cultures on brain–heart agar, macroscopic colonies commonly mature in about 7 days. Gram stains of cultures reveal highly pleomorphic, irregular, club-shaped, gram-positive rods. Occasional cells appear as branched twigs, but long branching filaments are not observed (Fig. 36–1).

PATHOGENESIS

Because most actinomycetes are found in soil, and be-cause human and bovine actinomycosis often affects the jaw and face, this disease was long held to arise from chewing straw and grass. However, *A. israelii* is not

---

TABLE 36–1. Major Constituents in Cell Wall Preparations of Important Actinomycetales*

Cell Wall Type	LL-DAP†	Meso-DAP	Lysine	Ornithine	Aspartic Acid	Glycine	Arabinose	Galactose	Xylose	Madurose (3-O-methyl-D-galactose)
I. *Streptomyces*	+					+				
II. *Micromonospora*		+				+	+		>+	
III. *Thermoactinomyces*		+						+		≥
IV. *Nocardia* Corynebacterium Mycobacterium		+					+	+		
V. *Actinomyces* (*israelii* type)			+	+						
VI. *Actinomyces* (*bovis* type)			+		+					

* All preparations contain significant amounts of glucosamine, muramic acid, alanine, and glutamic acid.

† DAP, 2,6-diaminopimelic acid.

(Modified according to suggestions of HA Lechevalier, from Lechevalier HA, Lechevalier MP: Annu Rev Microbiol 21:71, 1967). Reproduced with permission from the Annual Review of Microbiology, Vol. 21. © 1967 by Annual Reviews Inc).

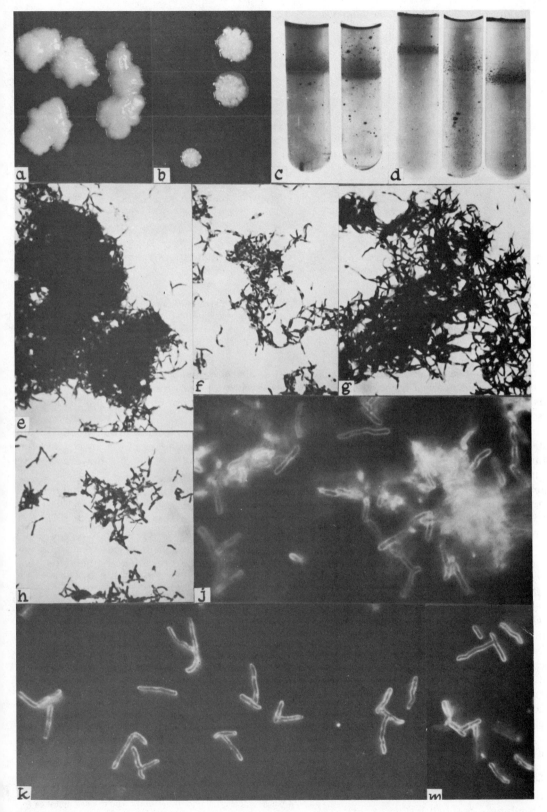

Figure 36–1. *Actinomyces israelli.* **(A,B)** Rough colonies grown anaerobically on brain–heart agar. **(C,D)** Shake cultures incubated anaerobically; note growth in a layer below the surface. **(E–H)** Gram-stained smears, showing masses of filaments. (× 750, reduced). **(J–M)** Unstained wet films under dark-field illumination; note distinct branching and twig-like forms. (× 1200, reduced). (Rosebury T et al: J Infect Dis 74:131, 1944)

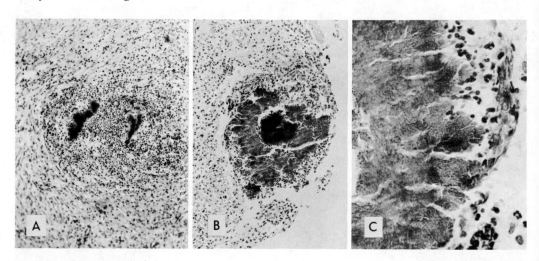

Figure 36–2. *(A)* Colonies of *A. israelli* (sulfur granules) in a lung abscess. A higher magnification of the periphery of the granule in *B* is reproduced in *C,* showing characteristic radial club-like structures. (Hematoxylin–eosin; *A* and *B,* ×130, reduced; *C,* ×600, reduced; *A,* Emmons CW et al: Medical Mycology. Philadelphia, Lea & Febiger, 1963; *B* and *C,* courtesy of AC Sonnenwirth)

present in soil or on vegetation but can be cultured from the majority of human tonsils and is nearly always found in scrapings of gums and teeth. Its fastidious growth requirements are in accord with this parasitic (or saprobic) existence. Like many respiratory pathogens, it is much more frequently commensal than pathogenic. *A. bovis* is a similar commensal of cattle.

The conditions that lead the organism to become invasive are not definitely known but may involve trauma (including dental surgery), aspiration of a heavily contaminated tooth or detached bits of dental tartar, or, rarely, human bites. In general, actinomycotic infections are accompanied by a mixed flora of gram-negative bacteria (*Actinobacillus actinomycetom-comitans, Eikenella corrodens, Fusobacterium,* and species of *Bacteroides*). It has been speculated that these organisms exert a synergistic action.

Actinomycosis is characterized by chronic, destructive abscesses of connective tissues. In one series of patients in the United States, about 50% of the infections involved the abdomen, particularly the cecum and appendix; 20% the lungs and chest wall; and 30% the face and neck. In a larger series in England, 60% of all cases involved the cervicofacial area. The incidence of cervicofacial disease has declined precipitously, presumably as a result of more effective oral hygiene.

Wherever the lesions occur, they are basically the same. Abscesses expand into contiguous tissues and eventually form burrowing, tortuous sinuses to the skin surface, where they discharge purulent material. Penetration into mucous membranes is much less frequent. Connective and granulation tissues tend to form a wall around the abscess. Histologically, the lesions are not distinctive except for the presence of the organisms as small colonies ("sulfur granules"; Fig. 36–2) described under Diagnosis, below.

Actinomycotic lesions of cattle are characteristically large, bone-destroying abscesses of the lower jaw, often referred to as "lumpy jaw." In humans, however, lesions of bone are infrequent.

Like most diseases caused by organisms that ordinarily are saprobes, actinomycosis is not transmissible from person to person or from animals to man. It is, in fact, difficult to establish the infection in laboratory animals. The actinomycetes isolated from abscesses are no more effective in establishing experimental infections than those isolated from the normal mouth.*

DIAGNOSIS

When pus from an abscess or infected sputum is examined carefully, yellow **sulfur granules,** named for their color, are occasionally seen. These small clusters of colonies of actinomycetes range from barely visible to several millimeters in diameter. Detection of granules is not required to establish a diagnosis of actinomycosis, but their presence facilitates identification of the organism. The granules, made up of one or more colonies embed-

* *Streptobacillus moniliformis* (Chap. 41), one of the causes of rat-bite fever, may be mentioned here because it is a normal inhabitant of the mouth of rats, is also pleomorphic, and often grows in filamentous form, and so it has been called *Actinomyces muris.* The disease that it causes in man, however, is an acute, self-limiting septicemia, with rash and arthritis.

ded in a matrix of calcium phosphate, consist of a central filamentous mycelium surrounded by club-shaped structures in a characteristic radial arrangement (Fig. 36–2). When granules are crushed and stained, the organisms appear as gram-positive bacillary and diphtheroid forms. Branched filaments are not readily discerned, and the club-shaped elements are gram-negative.

Actinomycotic abscesses are almost invariably mixed infections, like many other abscesses; even the washed sulfur granules may contain colonies of fusiform bacilli, anaerobic streptococci, and a tiny anaerobic gram-negative bacillus that bears the formidable name *Bacterium actinomycetemcomitans*. The accompanying bacilli may secrete collagenase and hyaluronidase and thus facilitate extension of the lesion.

EPIDEMIOLOGY

Actinomycosis is worldwide in distribution but is relatively rare. Its incidence is higher in men than in women, and in persons over 20; in older reports, it was much more frequent in rural than in urban areas. The allegedly greater incidence among farmers is not readily reconcilable with the prevailing view that the disease arises from invasion by an indigenous organism.

Actinomycosis occurs in a variety of wild and domesticated animals besides man and cattle.

TREATMENT

A. israelii is sensitive to tetracyclines, chloramphenicol, and streptomycin; penicillin is reported to be most effective clinically. Surgical drainage of abscesses and resection of damaged tissue are important adjuncts to chemotherapy. The cure rate is now about 90% for cervicofacial actinomycosis but somewhat less for abdominal and thoracic actinomycosis.

Nocardia

In contrast to *Actinomyces*, species of *Nocardia* are inhabitants of soil rather than commensals in animals, and they are aerobic, grow readily over a wide temperature range, and grow on relatively simple media.

When grown on agar, the colonies of *Nocardia* species may be smooth and moist or rough with a velvety surface due to a rudimentary aerial mycelium. However, when smeared and stained, the filaments fragment into bacillary and coccoid bodies. Examination of liquid cultures, especially slide cultures, may be helpful in identifying branching filaments. Growth in liquid media usually produces a dry, waxy surface pellicle, as with mycobacteria.

Nocardia species are gram-positive, and the two species most often pathogenic in man, *N. asteroides* and *N.*

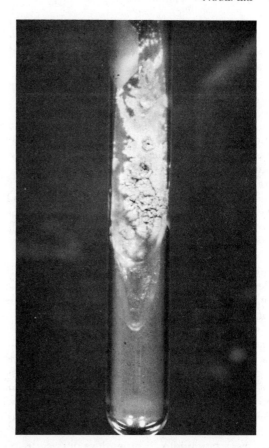

Figure 36–3. Colonies of *Nocardia asteroides* after 4 weeks on Sabouraud's glucose agar. Note the typical heaped-up, irregularly folded appearance. (Courtesy of Dr. AC Sonnenwirth)

brasiliensis, are also somewhat acid-fast: they are more easily stained with fuchsin and retain the stain less tenaciously than mycobacteria,* and their cell wall contains components characteristic of mycobacteria and corynebacteria (Table 36–1), including mycolic acid residues (very long-chain, branched fatty acids).

N. asteroides also resembles mycobacteria in being resistant to dilute alkali and to some of the dyes (such as brilliant green) used to inhibit the growth of rapidly growing gram-positive bacteria; hence they may grow on the same medium and after the same manipulations as used for routine selective isolation of tubercle bacilli from sputum and exudates (see Laboratory Diagnosis, Chap. 35). Moreover, the colonies formed by nocardiae resemble those of saprobic mycobacteria (Chap. 35 and Fig. 36–3). Finally, extensive serologic cross-reactions (in agglutination and complement fixation) are observed

---

* The acid-fast nocardiae are readily stained with basic fuchsin without heating, and to test for acid-fastness, 1% H_2SO_4 without ethanol is used, as acid plus alcohol is too effective as a decolorizing solvent.

with antisera to mycobacteria and to nocardiae. However, it is not difficult to distinguish between the two groups: nocardiae grow more rapidly, are less acid-fast, and tend to branch.

PATHOGENESIS

There are two common modes of infection by *Nocardia*. **Pulmonary** nocardiosis arises from inhalation of the organisms, whereas chronic subcutaneous abscesses (**mycetomas**) arise from contamination of skin wounds, usually on the feet and hands of laborers.

Infections with *Nocardia* are hard to establish in laboratory animals. Guinea pigs inoculated with suspensions of the organisms in gastric mucin regularly develop abscesses and occasionally succumb.

PULMONARY NOCARDIOSIS. In pulmonary nocardiosis, the lesions may be scattered through the lung parenchyma, simulating miliary tuberculosis or histoplasmosis, or they may take the form of larger, confluent, partially excavated abscesses, which superficially resemble the cavities of chronic pulmonary tuberculosis. The lesions are characterized histologically by suppuration, with granulation and fibrous tissue surrounding the areas of necrosis. Neither the characteristic granulomas of tuberculosis nor the burrowing sinuses of *Actinomyces* abscesses are seen. *N. asteroides* lie scattered through the abscesses in the form of tangled, fine, branching filaments: aggregation into granules does not occur, in contrast to the lesions of *A. israelii* or *A. bovis*.

In histologic sections, the bacterial filaments are not seen with hematoxylin–eosin stains. When examined with bacterial stains, the organisms (which tend to fragment during staining) appear as gram-positive, weakly acid-fast diphtheroid and bacillary forms, which may easily be mistaken for tubercle bacilli.

N. asteroides often spreads from pulmonary lesions by way of the blood and establishes metastatic abscesses, usually in subcutaneous tissues and in the central nervous system. Lesions in the brain and the meninges are usually fatal.

When *N. asteroides* is identified consistently in sputum from patients with chronic pulmonary disease, a presumptive diagnosis of pulmonary nocardiosis is warranted, but isolation in a solitary specimen may reflect its presence as a saprobe in the upper respiratory tract.

MYCETOMA CAUSED BY NOCARDIA. Different species of *Nocardia* are associated with mycetomas in different parts of the world, such as *N. brasiliensis* in Mexico. These chronic subcutaneous abscesses are clinically very similar to those attributable to *Streptomyces* and to various fungi. The abscesses spread locally by direct extension, destroy soft tissue and bone, and form burrowing sinus tracts. As with *Actinomyces*, colonial aggregates (granules) of the causative microorganism are often present in the abscesses and in their purulent discharge, and they help in the isolation and identification of the etiologic agent.

Table 36–2 lists properties that distinguish *N. asteroides* from *N. brasiliensis*.

EPIDEMIOLOGY

Nocardiae are widely distributed throughout temperate and tropical climates. The diseases it causes are seen frequently in association with immunosuppression or underlying chronic diseases such as Hodgkin's disease, leukemia, carcinoma, and chronic granluomatous disease of childhood. Once nocardiosis becomes clinically evident, it tends to be progressive and fatal; even with aggressive therapy, about 50% of patients succumb. It is noteworthy that in cases of obstructive lung disease, the isolation of nocardiae may indicate simply transient colonization.

TABLE 36–2. Some Aerobic Organisms That Cause Actinomycotic Mycetomas in Man

Species	Microscopic Appearance	Hydrolysis of Casein	Hydrolysis of Starch	Pathogenicity in Mouse and Guinea Pig
Nocardia asteroides	Partially acid-fast	0	0	Abscesses without granules; frequently causes death
Nocardia brasiliensis	Partially acid-fast	+	0	Abscesses with granules caused by some strains
*Streptomyces madurae**	Not acid-fast	+	+	Not pathogenic
*Streptomyces pelletierii**	Not acid-fast	+	0	Not pathogenic

* Sometimes placed in genus *Nocardia* rather than *Streptomyces*. In complement-fixation tests, they react with antisera to various mycobacteria, nocardiae, and streptomycetes.

TREATMENT

Various antibacterial drugs are used in the treatment of experimental nocardiosis, but sulfonamides are reported to be most effective. Draining of abscesses is an important adjunct. The distinction from fungal mycetomas is essential because entirely different chemotherapeutic agents are indicated.

Streptomyces

Streptomyces species are characterized by the stability of their filaments and by the formation of spores on the aerial mycelia that project above the surface of the culture medium. Mutants that lose the ability to form aerial mycelia and spores are difficult to distinguish from nocardiae.

With increasing appreciation of the distinction between nocardiae and streptomycetes (Table 36–2), it has been realized that both cause actinomycotic abscesses. Because streptomycetes are ubiquitous in soil, infection is attributed to contamination of scratches and penetrating wounds. Mycetomas caused by streptomycetes are indistinguishable clinically from those of other actinomycetes. Identification of these organisms is important, as they are not generally susceptible to antimicrobial agents, and surgical removal by excision or amputation of the affected area must be considered.

Since the isolation by Waksman of actinomycin in 1940, and streptomycin in 1943, the streptomycetes have received a phenomenal amount of attention. Innumerable isolates from soil samples, taken from all parts of the world, have been systematically scrutinized, and they have yielded more than 90% of the therapeutically useful antibiotics. Because of interest in improving antibiotic production, genetic studies in streptomycetes (especially *S. coelicolor*) are quite advanced, including analysis of fertility agents and bacteriophages.

Selected Reading

BOOKS AND REVIEW ARTICLES

Allen SD: Gram positive, nonsporeforming anaerobic bacilli. In EH Lennette, Balows A, Hausler WF Jr, Shadomy HJ (eds): Manual of Clinical of Clinical Microbiology, 4th Ed. Washington, DC, American Society for Microbiology, 1985

Bradley SG: Significance of nucleic acid hybridization to systematics of actinomycetes. Adv Applied Microbiol 19:59, 1975

Brownell G, Goodfellow M, Serrano J (eds): The Biology of the Nocardiae. New York, Academic Press, 1976

Chater KF, Hopwood DA, Kieser T, Thompson CJ: Gene cloning in *Streptomyces*. Curr Top Microbiol Immunol 96:619, 1982

Georg LK: Diagnostic procedures for the isolation and identification of the etiologic agents of actinomycosis. In Proceedings, International Symposium on Mycoses. Scientific Publ No. 205, p 71. Washington, DC, Pan-American Health Organization, 1970

Gordon MA: Aerobic pathogenic Actinomycetaceae. In EH Lennette, Balows A, Hausler EF Jr, Shadomy HJ (eds): Manual of Clinical Microbiology, 4th Ed. Washington DC, American Society for Microbiology, 1985

Hopwood DA, Wright HM: Recent advances in *Streptomyces coelicolor* genetics. Bacteriol Rev 37:371, 1973

Rosebury T: Microorganisms Indigenous to Man. New York, McGraw-Hill, 1962

Simpson GL, Stinson EB, Egger MJ, Remington JS: Nocardial infections in the immunocompromised host: A detailed study in a defined population. Rev Infect Dis 3:492, 1981

Smego RA Jr, Gallis HA: The clinical spectrum of *Nocardia brasiliensis* infection in the United States. Rev Infect Dis 6:164, 1984

Waksman S: The Actinomycetes, Vols 1, 2, 3 (with Lechevalier HA). Baltimore, Williams & Wilkins, 1962

SPECIFIC ARTICLES

Beaman BL: Structural and biochemical alterations of *Nocardia asteroides* cell walls during its growth cycle. J Bacteriol 123:1235, 1975

Black CM, Beaman BL, Donovan RM, Goldstein E: Intracellular acid phosphatase content and ability of different macrophage populations to kill *Nocardia asteroides*. Infect Immun 47:375, 1985

Cummins CS, Harris H: Studies on the cell-wall composition and taxonomy of Actinomycetales and related groups. J Gen Microbiol 18:173, 1958

Edwards JH: The isolation of antigens associated with farmer's lung. Clin Exp Immunol 11:341, 1972

Felice GA, Beaman BL, Remington JS: Effects of activated macrophages on *Nocardia asteroides*. Infect Immun 27:643, 1980

Hardisson C, Manzanal MB: Ultrastructural studies of sporulation in Streptomyces. J Bacteriol 127:1443, 1976

Jordan HV, Kelly DM, Heeley JD: Enhancement of experimental actinomycosis in mice by *Eikenella corrodens*. Infect Immun 46:367, 1984

Lechevalier MP, Horan AC, Lechevalier HA: Lipid composition in the classification of nocardiae and mycobacteria. J Bacteriol 105:313, 1971

Palmer DL, Harvey RL, Wheeler JK: Diagnostic and therapeutic considerations in *Nocardia asteroides* infection. Medicine 53:391, 1974

Redshaw PA, McCann PA, Sankaran L, Pogell BM: Control of differentiation in streptomycetes: Involvement of extrachromosomal deoxyribonucleic acid and glucose repression in aerial mycelial development. J Bacteriol 125:698, 1976

37

Joel B. Baseman

The Spirochetes

GENERAL CHARACTERISTICS

Spirochetes are motile, unicellular, spiral-shaped organisms, morphologically quite different from other bacteria. Certain structural features are shared by all spirochetes (Fig. 37–1), but in physiology, they range from obligate anaerobes to aerobes and from free-living forms to obligate parasites. Many are not yet cultivable.

Three genera are pathogenic for man. The genus *Treponema* includes the pathogens that cause syphilis (*T. pallidum*), yaws (*T. pertenue*), and pinta (*T. carateum*). The genus *Borrelia* includes the causative agents of epidemic and endemic relapsing fever and Lyme disease. The genus *Leptospira* includes a wide variety of small spirochetes that cause mild to serious systemic human illness (Fig. 37–2). In the United States, syphilis remains a disease of high incidence: approximately 27,000 cases of early infectious syphilis were reported in 1986, which may be less than one third of the actual cases. Only approximately 100 new cases of leptospirosis are reported in the U.S. yearly and fewer of classic borreliosis. Lyme disease, recently identified as a borrelia infection, is much more frequent.

Spirochetes (Gr. *spira*, coil, and *chaete*, hair) are relatively long, slender, flexible organisms, and most appear as helical coils, resembling a spring, or as undulating waves of varying amplitude. Many are too slender to be seen by ordinary light microscopy. They can be observed by **dark-field microscopy*** (Fig. 37–3) or by staining with special reagents such as silver salts. When examined by dark-field illumination, spirochetes have a characteristic motility, including apparent rotation around

---

* Dark-field microscopy requires the use of a special substage condenser that throws the light across rather than directly through the field. Only light that is reflected, refracted, or diffracted by an object in the field reaches the eye. Hence, observed objects are light, and the background is dark (Fig. 37–3).

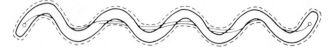

Figure 37–1. Schematic representation of a spirochete. *Broken line* represents the outer envelope; *solid heavy line,* adjacent to the broken line, delimits the protoplasmic cylinder. *Thin solid lines* represent axial fibrils (also termed periplasmic flagella or endoflagella), one of which is inserted at each end of the protoplasmic cylinder. (Canale–Parola E: Bacteriol Rev 41:181, 1977)

their long axis, flexion, and a boring corkscrew motion. Species differ somewhat in motility, a fact that may be useful in diagnosis. **Spirochetal motion persists at high viscosities** that block the flagellar motion of ordinary bacteria; this finding suggests a possible basis for the evolution of the complex structure of spirochetes.

All spirochetes contain a central protoplasmic cylinder consisting of cytoplasmic and nuclear regions surrounded by a cytoplasmic membrane and a closely adherent cell wall. This wall is a peptidoglycan similar to that of other bacteria, containing either lysine, diaminopimelic acid, or ornithine. The peptidoglycan, when isolated, retains a helical configuration, indicating that it influences the shape of the cell. Structures resembling microtubules can be seen in the cytoplasm of most treponemes. Their function and relation to the microtubules of eukaryotic cells are unknown.

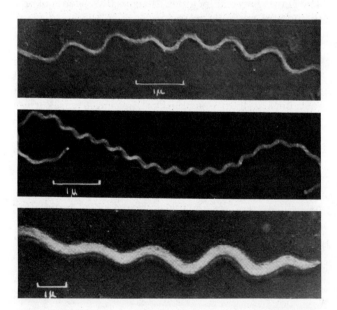

Figure 37–2. Electron microscopic study of the morphology of pathogenic spirochetes. *Top, Treponema pallidum* from exudate of infected rabbit. (×16,500) *Middle, Leptospira interrogans* serotype *icterohaemorrhagiae* from broth culture. (×17,000) *Bottom, Borrelia duttonii* from the blood of an infected mouse. (×8500) (Swain RHA: J Pathol Bacteriol 69:117, 1955)

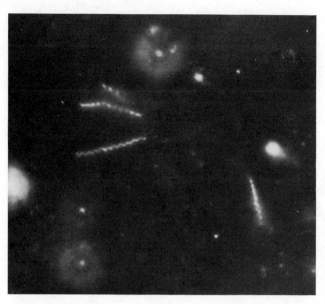

Figure 37–3. *T. pallidum* in a dark-field preparation (× about 2000). (From Pelczar MJ, Reid RD: Microbiology. Copyright © 1958, McGraw-Hill. Used with permission of McGraw-Hill Book Company)

Between the protoplasmic cylinder and the outer envelope are one or more filamentous structures, termed **axial fibrils** or periplasmic flagella or **endoflagella,** which on isolation, appear wavy or coiled. These structures are similar to the flagella of other bacteria, both in appearance under the electron microscope (Figs. 37–4 and 37–5) and in chemical content. The endoflagella are attached subterminally by characteristic organelles to either end of the protoplasmic cylinder and extend along the body of the organism, frequently overlapping in the center. They probably play a role in motility, as nonmotile mutants of *Leptospira* possess periplasmic flagella that are straight rather than coiled. It has been suggested that rotation of these flagella forces an opposing movement of the outer membrane and body cylinder and propels the spirochete.

The outer envelope is a membrane similar in structure to the outer membrane of gram-negative bacteria. Large spirochetes stain gram-negative, but there is no clear evidence for endotoxin in any spirochetes.

Syphilis

HISTORY

During the last decade of the fifteenth century syphilis became rampant in Western Europe. The story that it was brought from the West Indies by members of Columbus' crew is probably apocryphal. Records indicate, however, that the disease in Europe, in its acute phase, was

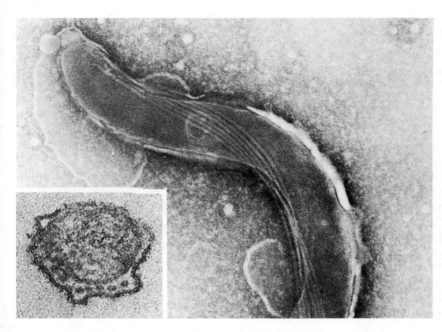

Figure 37–4. Electron photomicrograph of the cultivable Reiter treponeme (negative staining technique) showing axial fibrils arising in end bulb at tip of organisms. Outpouchings of periplastic membrane are probably an artifact. (×50,000). Cross-section *inset* (thin section) reveals spatial relations between outer envelope, axial fibrils, and central protoplasmic cylinder. (×120,000). (Ryter A, Pillott J: Ann Inst Pasteur 104:496, 1963)

extraordinarily malignant for about 60 years, beginning in the 1490s; thereafter, it became milder, although its late consequences remained serious. It now exists endemically in nearly all parts of the world.

Starting with the poem in which the early epidemiologist Fracastorius (1530) named the disease after a mythical shepherd, syphilis has been the subject of an extensive and colorful literature. The causative agent was discovered by Schaudinn and Hoffmann in 1905, and the "Wassermann reaction" for detecting antisyphilitic antibodies was described by Wassermann, Neisser, and Bruck in 1906. Widespread treatment of syphilis in the U.S. with penicillin beginning in the mid-1940s led to a decline of more than 85% in the incidence of early cases,

but after 1955 newly acquired infections increased again. This resurgence has been attributed to relaxation of control measures and to increased sexual promiscuity, but a decrease in the indiscriminate use of penicillin for minor ailments is probably also a significant factor.

MORPHOLOGY

T. pallidum, which is morphologically indistinguishable from other pathogenic treponemes, is an extremely slender spiral organism measuring 5 to 20 μm in length and less than 0.2 μm in thickness. It has 4 to 14 spirals that appear uniform near the center of the cell but frequently increase in periodicity and decrease in amplitude toward the ends, thus giving the cell a tapered appearance. Dark-field illumination is best for recognizing the organism, for it permits observation of the characteristic motility of live spirochetes.

In aqueous media, young treponemes demonstrate seemingly random vigorous movements. However, in a more viscous environment or on surfaces, they achieve sufficient traction to propel themselves in a snakelike fashion; in tissues, they exhibit remarkable flexibility as they adapt themselves to the intercellular spaces. Recent observations indicate that adhesion in tissue is mediated by treponemal adhesins that recognize the sequence Arg–Gly–Asp–Ser of fibronectin.

T. pallidum and other noncultivable pathogenic treponemes all contain three axial fibrils inserted at each end of the protoplasmic cylinder, overlapping in the midregion of the organism. The pathogenic treponemes are pointed at each end, unlike nonpathogens, which have

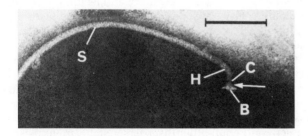

Figure 37–5. Axial fibril released from Nichols strain of *T. pallidum*, negatively stained with 1% ammonium molybdate. *Bar* represents 100 nm. Shaft *(S)* is sometimes seen to be surrounded by a sheath, not easily visible here. The fibril terminates in a hook *(H)*, collar *(C)*, and basal knob *(B)*, which are used for attachment to the protoplasmic cylinder. Remarkable physical and chemical similarities exist between the axial fibril and bacterial flagella. (×160,000). (Hovind–Hougen K: Acta Pathol Microbiol Scand B 80:297, 1972)

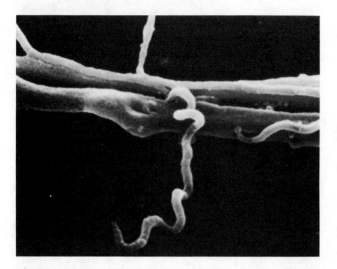

Figure 37–6. Scanning electron micrograph demonstrating the specific attachment of *T. pallidum* to rabbit testicular cells in monolayer. Note the orientation of the treponemes as mediated by their tapered ends and apparent terminal disclike organelle. (×28,000). (Hayes NS et al: Infect Immun 17:174, 1977)

blunt rounded ends; the pointed ends may be used for attachment to host cells mediated by interactions between specific treponemal proteins and host fibronectin (Fig. 37–6). There is suggestive evidence for a "slime" layer outside the outer envelope of *T. pallidum*, composed partly of bound host macromolecules, which could explain the serologic nonreactivity of freshly isolated treponemes and may contribute to their virulence.

METABOLISM

The pathogenic treponemes can be propagated *in vivo* in laboratory animals but only poorly, if at all, *in vitro*. Results in tissue culture have been marginal and inconsistent, and attempts in chick embryos have also failed. Many nonpathogenic treponemes (e.g., some oral species and the cultivable strains such as Reiter, Noguchi, and Kazan) have been grown in a variety of artificial media; they divide by binary fission. All cultivable strains are anaerobic and grow slowly, with division times ranging from 4 to 18 hours.

Recent studies have challenged the concept that *T. pallidum* is an obligate anaerobe. The presence of O_2 considerably enhances *in vitro* protein and RNA synthesis and glucose degradation during short-term experiments. Incomplete oxidation of glucose proceeds via the Embden–Meyerhof and the hexose monophosphate shunt pathways, with terminal electron transport to O_2 mediated by flavoproteins and specific cytochromes but without a complete Krebs cycle. *In vitro*, survival and retention of motility and virulence are improved by coincubation with certain tissue cell lines under low O_2 concentrations.

The cultivable treponemes utilize glucose or other fermentable carbohydrates as the primary energy source, and they have complex nutritional requirements, including multiple amino acids, purines, and pyrimidines. Many strains also need bicarbonate and one or more coenzymes, and all require exogenous fatty acid, usually supplied as protein-bound lipid in a serum supplement to the growth medium.

Suspensions of treponemes can be kept viable for years when frozen at temperatures below −70°C in the presence of glycerol or other cryoprotective agents. Of practical importance for the problem of transfusion-associated syphilis is the fact that in blood, serum, or plasma stored at refrigerator temperatures, viable *T. pallidum* organisms have not been recovered after 48 hours.

ANTIGENS

WASSERMANN ANTIGEN. The first serologic test for syphilis was a complement-fixation (CF) reaction—the so-called Wassermann test. In its original form, this test used as Ag an extract of liver, containing many treponemes, from human fetuses with congenital syphilis. However, the specific ligand involved was later found to be present in alcoholic extracts of normal liver and other mammalian tissues as well. It was subsequently isolated from cardiac muscle and identified as a phospholipid, **diphosphatidylglycerol** (designated earlier as **cardiolipin**).

Many modifications and variations of the Wassermann test have been devised in the hope of increasing specificity. In contrast to the original CF reaction, most of the later tests are flocculation reactions. These are analogous to precipitin reactions, but instead of a soluble Ag, they use cardiolipin in an aqueous suspension finely dispersed with the aid of cholesterol and lecithin. The anticardiolipin tests are designated **serologic tests for syphilis (STS),** to distinguish them from the antitreponemal tests developed in recent years.

Because cardiolipin is a normal constituent of host tissue, there arose a controversy about whether the primary antigenic stimulus for Wassermann Ab (anticardiolipin) comes from the invading organism or from the host, in an autoimmune response. The appearance of Wassermann Ab in other disorders, notably in lupus erythematosus, supports the autoimmune theory.

To serve as an immunogenic stimulus for Wassermann Ab, free cardiolipin, a hapten, must be attached to a suitable carrier. The lipid composition of cultivable treponemes depends to a large extent on the lipids in the growth medium; and because pathogenic treponemes growing *in vivo* have access to a great deal of cardiolipin, they might incorporate it. With the microbial cell as a foreign carrier, the bound cardiolipin could serve as an effective immunogenic determinant.

TREPONEMAL ANTIGENS. Two classes of Ags have been recognized in treponemes: those shared by many different serotypes, and those restricted to one or a few species.

Characterization of treponemal Ags has been impeded greatly by the inability to grow pathogenic treponemes free of animal cells or tissue. The Reiter treponeme, a spirochete once reputed to be a cultivable, nonvirulent, variant of *T. pallidum*, was formerly used in a diagnostic test, but DNA hybridization has now shown the two organisms to be only slightly related.

Specific treponemal Ags have been detected by a variety of serologic procedures. In the ***T. pallidum* immobilization (TPI) test,** a complement-dependent bactericidal reaction, treponemes obtained from syphilitic lesions in rabbits are mixed with a patient's serum and fresh guinea pig serum, and after anaerobic incubation for 18 hours at 35°C the mixture is examined microscopically. In a positive reaction more than half the organisms are immobilized (i.e., killed). In a parallel reaction with heat-inactivated complement to control for nonspecific effects the treponemes should remain motile.

The TPI test is highly specific for the detection of syphilis, yaws, and other treponematoses, but it cannot distinguish among these diseases. Evidently, the responsible Ag is shared by the various pathogenic species but is not present in indigenous organisms. The TPI test is expensive and difficult, and it has been replaced in the U.S. by other treponemal tests. With the advent of sensitive radioimmunoassays and Western blotting techniques, immunodominant treponemal protein Ags have been identified by using acute and convalescent sera. It is likely that these Ags will provide new, highly specific serodiagnostic assays.

GENETIC VARIATION

Because only *in vivo* methods are available for studying variations of *T. pallidum*, little is known about its mutations. Tests of cross-immunity and pathogenicity are crude and have yielded only fragmentary information. Usually, rapid passage in rabbits detectably increases virulence for rabbits. Some treponemal strains obtained by primary isolation from patients with yaws produce the typically mild lesions of experimental yaws, but after repeated passage in rabbits, they cause the malignant lesions of experimental syphilis. Such changes may involve the *in vivo* selection of mutants.

No penicillin-resistant *T. pallidum* strains have been reported.

PATHOGENICITY
Human Syphilis

Syphilis is ordinarily transmitted by sexual contact. In heterosexual men, the offending organisms either are present in lesions on the penis or are discharged from deeper genitourinary sites along with the seminal fluid. In women, the infectious lesions are most commonly located in the perineal region or on the labia, vaginal wall, or cervix. Homosexual men account for a large proportion of early syphilis cases in many cities; the infectious lesions in these individuals commonly occur in or about the rectum. Primary infection may also occur in the mouth or other areas.

The organism penetrates mucous membranes but seems to enter the skin only through small breaks. Multiplication at the site of entrance results, within 10 to 60 days, in the formation of a characteristic **primary** inflammatory lesion known as a **chancre,** which begins as a papule and breaks down to form a superficial ulcer with a clean firm base. The predominant inflammatory cells in the lesion are lymphocytes and plasma cells. Although the chancre heals spontaneously, organisms escaping from it at an early stage invade the regional lymph nodes, forming "**satellite buboes,**" and eventually reach the blood stream, where they establish a systemic infection.

Two to twelve weeks after the appearance of the primary lesion, a generalized skin rash (Fig. 39–7) usually appears, which also often involves the mucous membranes. During this systemic **secondary** stage of the disease, patients usually experience low-grade fever and a generalized enlargement of the lymph nodes. Lesions may develop in the bones, liver, kidneys, central nervous system, or other organs. The pathogenesis of the renal lesion in some instances is deposition of immune complexes. Tissue damage in other organs may be the result of local proliferation of treponemes. No treponemal toxins are known.

Secondary lesions often contain large numbers of spirochetes, and so they are highly infective. In time, they subside spontaneously, and once they have healed, the patient is no longer dangerous to others except for transplacental transmission.

Little is known concerning the mechanisms that bring about the destruction of the myriads of treponemes contained in the primary and secondary lesions. It is likely that the host defense in syphilis includes cellular immune mechanisms, as well as immobilizing and opsonizing (treponemicidal) Abs: the late primary and secondary stages of the illness are frequently accompanied by a temporary depression of T-lymphocyte responsiveness to certain treponemal Ags and common mitogens. Electron microscopy reveals *T. pallidum* organisms within a variety of host tissue cells, but there is no evidence that the organisms survive there.

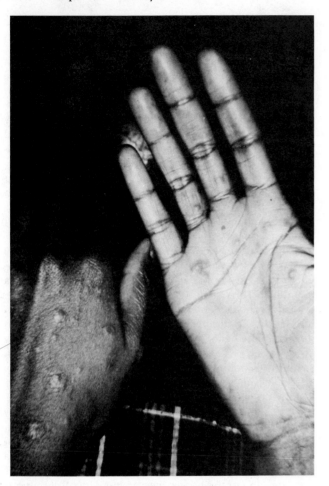

Figure 37–7. Typical papulosquamous lesions on palms and other skin surfaces during secondary syphilis.

In approximately one-third of untreated patients, enough treponemes persist in the tissues to give rise to the **late,** or **tertiary,** lesions of the disease several years after the primary infection. (Rarely, the primary and secondary stages go unrecognized, only to be followed by the late tertiary lesions.) In about another third of untreated cases, the disease remains asymptomatic (**latent**) and is recognized only by the detection of Abs in the serum; in the remaining third, the primary and systemic lesions heal so completely that even the STS become negative.

Tertiary lesions often contain very few organisms but frequently result in necrosis, scar formation, and extensive tissue damage, probably involving a **delayed hypersensitivity response** to products of the small number of persisting organisms. Among tertiary lesions, **gummas** of the skin or bones may cause relatively little trouble (gummas are now rare). However, serious manifestations usu-

ally result from lesions in the central nervous system (**general paresis** or **tabes dorsalis**), in the cardiovascular system (damage to the aortic valves or formation of aortic aneurysms), and in the eyes (possible permanent blindness).

Because *T. pallidum* readily passes the placenta, a syphilitic mother may transmit the disease to her child. The lesions of **congenital syphilis** resemble, in general, those of acquired syphilis of comparable duration. In infants who fail to survive for more than a few weeks or are stillborn, the syphilitic process is usually acute and is characterized by extensive invasion of nearly all body tissues.

Experimental Syphilis

Although humans are the only known natural host of *T. pallidum,* experimental infections may be produced in a variety of laboratory animals. The experimental disease in rabbits, monkeys, and chimpanzees simulates the early course of the natural disease in humans, but late lesions are rarely encountered. However, in infected rabbits, viable organisms persist for life and can be readily isolated from the lymph nodes.

Rabbits may be experimentally infected by inoculation of organisms into the eye, skin, testis, or scrotum. A single viable organism injected intratesticularly is said to be infectious. From the lag with different infecting doses, it can be estimated that the time required for the organisms to divide *in vivo* is about 24 to 36 hours.

In both experimental and human infections *T. pallidum* tends to proliferate at sites of trauma. In the rabbit, treponemes multiply best at peripheral tissue sites in which the temperature is several degrees below that of the internal tissues. Artificial cooling of the skin, for example, may strikingly increase the number of skin lesions that develop in the systemic phase of the infection. (Induced fever was formerly used successfully as a treatment of human syphilis.) Pretreatment of rabbits with the anti-inflammatory agent cortisone causes the formation of enlarged cutaneous syphilomas, which contain excessive amounts of hyaluronic acid and increased numbers of motile treponemes.

IMMUNITY

Resistance to reinfection, as determined both in human volunteers and in experimentally infected rabbits, usually begins about 3 weeks after appearance of the primary lesion. The persistence of a latent infection then maintains resistance, but if the disease is eradicated in the early stages by adequate treatment, the host may again become fully susceptible to infection. However, treatment late in the course of the disease does not result in loss of resistance to reinfection. Immunity to *T. pallidum* in rabbits shows considerable strain specificity.

It is clear that good stimulation of humoral immunity accompanies infection, yet treponemes are not completely eliminated, and the disease can progress through its characteristic stages. Passive transfer of large amounts of antitreponemal Ab to uninfected rabbits prior to challenge with virulent *T. pallidum* attenuates the disease, but it does not provide complete protection. Circulating immune complexes have been observed in syphilis, but their pathogenetic role is unclear.

It appears that both humoral and cellular components are necessary for acquired resistance to treponemal infection. Prospects for an effective human vaccine depend on the identification of virulence determinants and immunoprotective molecules. In rabbits, various treponemal Ags have yielded partial protection, such as delayed or atypical lesions.

LABORATORY DIAGNOSIS
Detection of T. pallidum in Lesions

In its primary and secondary stages, syphilis can often be diagnosed by **dark-field examination** of fresh exudate fluid obtained from open or abraded lesions. Because occasionally the exudates from nonsyphilitic lesions also contain spiral organisms, particularly near the gingival crevices and rectum, dark-field observations must be interpreted with care. An experienced observer can often differentiate *T. pallidum* from other spiral organisms on the basis of its characteristic morphology and motility. Negative dark-field examinations, on the other hand, do not necessarily exclude the diagnosis of syphilis, as lesions in the later stages of the disease may contain relatively few organisms.*

T. pallidum may also be identified in fluid from active lesions by **immunofluorescent staining** with *T. pallidum* Abs freed of cross-reacting treponemal Abs by absorption with cultivable treponemes. Monoclonal or polyclonal Abs to surface components of pathogenic treponemes can also be used.

Serologic Tests

Flocculation tests for Wassermann Abs are of great value in the presumptive diagnosis of syphilis. The standard is the Venereal Disease Research Laboratory (VDRL) test. A wide variety of other diseases, including malaria, lupus erythematosus, leprosy, and other infections, yield a **biological false-positive** (BFP) **reaction,** but in general, Wassermann Ab is present in a much higher titer in syphilis than in nontreponemal disorders. The Ab is usu-

ally first detected 1 to 3 weeks after the primary lesion appears and reaches a maximum during the secondary stage of infection. Subsequently, this Ab may remain at an elevated level, or it may disappear from the serum. It is positive in about 75% of patients with late (tertiary) stages of the disease; thus a **negative VDRL test does not exclude late syphilis of the heart or central nervous system.**

Tests for treponemal Abs, such as the TPI test (see Treponemal Antigens, above), are more specific but are not generally available. In the widely performed fluorescent treponemal antibody (FTA) test, *T. pallidum* cells extracted from animal lesions are exposed first to the patient's serum and then to fluorescein-labeled Abs to human immunoglobulins. In its simplest forms, the FTA test also detects cross-reactive and *T. pallidum*-specific Abs. Several modifications have therefore been devised in an attempt to increase specificity. One of these, the fluorescent treponemal antibody absorption (FTA-ABS) test, uses an extract of the Reiter treponeme to absorb or competitively inhibit cross-reacting Abs, but this procedure does not achieve complete immunologic specificity. This test is positive in only about 80% of patients with primary syphilis but in almost all patients with secondary or tertiary syphilis. It therefore should not be used as a screening test. A hemagglutination test for treponemal Ag (TPHA) is similar to the FTA-ABS in its sensitivity and specificity.

Antitreponemal Abs decline more slowly than Wassermann Ab after treatment, and positive reactions may persist for years. Positive serologic tests after therapy thus are not necessarily evidence of continuing disease. However, Wassermann Abs in the spinal fluid ordinarily reflect active central nervous system syphilis, as serum Abs do not penetrate the normal blood–brain barrier.

TREATMENT

When penicillin superseded arsenicals, bismuth, and mercury, the treatment of syphilis was greatly simplified and improved. Patients in the early stages of the disease can be treated adequately by a single injection of long-acting benzathine penicillin G, which provides treponemicidal serum levels of penicillin for several weeks. Alternatively, procaine penicillin (which is more rapidly excreted than benzathine penicillin) may be given by daily injection for at least 10 days.* Only rarely is a second course of treatment necessary.

In the late stages of the disease, penicillin is less effec-

---

* It must be remembered that each oil-immersion field in the usual cover slip preparation contains only about 10^{-6} ml of fluid. Accordingly, there must be approximately 10^6 organisms/ml of fluid under the cover slip for the observer to find an average of one per field. Despite the obvious insensitivity of the method, the spirochetes in early lesions are usually present in sufficient numbers to be detected.

* Within 6 to 10 hours after the start of treatment in early syphilis, transient (2 to 4 hours) fever and a brief exacerbation of the visible lesions (**Herxheimer reaction**) often occur, apparently caused by an immunologic response to Ags released by the organisms being killed in the tissues. In addition, some of the products released may have the properties of endotoxins.

tive, owing to the irreparable damage already sustained by the tissues. In addition, it has been suggested that penicillin occasionally fails to eradicate treponemes from the central nervous system and other sites in late syphilis.

PREVENTION

Many patients with early syphilis are unaware that they have the disease; in women, especially, the early lesions may be symptomless and unnoticed. In addition, a single promiscuous person may transmit the organism to many sexual partners. Hence, control of the spread of syphilis is extremely difficult. When the diagnosis of early syphilis is established in an individual all known sexual contacts should be examined. Most authorities recommend antibiotic treatment of all recently exposed contacts of patients with infectious (primary or secondary) syphilis.

Prophylaxis by thorough cleansing of the genitalia and adjacent areas with soap and water is often ineffective unless applied early and with great diligence. The prophylactic use of a single dose of medium- to long-acting penicillin is probably highly effective, because such therapy is known to cure early incubating syphilis. However, prophylaxis is best achieved by the use of condoms and by avoidance of sexual contact with persons likely to be infectious.

RELATED DISEASES
Yaws (Frambesia)

T. pertenue, which causes the **nonvenereal tropical disease** known as yaws, is virtually indistinguishable from *T. pallidum*, except for the character of the lesions it produces. Both organisms induce the formation of Wassermann Abs and serologically identical antitreponemal Abs, and a striking degree of cross-resistance has been demonstrated in both man and laboratory animals. A similar disease has been found among apes in central Africa, and the responsible spirochete is indistinguishable from *T. pertenue*.

The **mother yaw,** the primary lesion in the human disease, usually appears 3 to 4 weeks after exposure. It begins as a painless red papule surrounded by a zone of erythema, often referred to as a **frambiose** (Fr., raspberry). Eventually, it ulcerates, becomes covered with a dry crust, and heals. Generalized secondary lesions of a similar character make their appearance 6 weeks to 3 months later and commonly occur in successive crops over a period of months or even several years; on the soles of the feet, tender, hyperkeratotic lesions known as **crab yaws** often appear. The late, tertiary lesions are generally restricted to the skin and bones; gummatous nodules and deep chronic ulcerations may disfigure the nose and face and are often disabling. However, the disease is not as grave as syphilis, as it **rarely involves the viscera,** and congenital yaws is very uncommon.

Experimental yaws also differs from experimental syphilis. Intracutaneous inoculation of *T. pertenue* in hamsters ordinarily causes a local lesion, whereas *T. pallidum* usually does not.

EPIDEMIOLOGY. Yaws occurs in the tropics, where the combination of high temperatures, high humidity, and poor hygiene promotes the persistence of open skin lesions and thus facilitates nonvenereal transmission by direct contact. Children often become afflicted at an early age. In areas of high endemicity, more than 75% of the population may acquire the disease before the age of 20. Flies that feed on open lesions are thought by some investigators to act as vectors.

TREATMENT. Like syphilis, yaws responds dramatically to treatment with penicillin, often requiring only a single injection of a long-acting drug. However, yaws occurs primarily in areas where medical services are too limited for general application of this effective control measure.

Pinta

Pinta also occurs primarily in the tropics, especially Central and South America. The causative organism, *T. carateum*, is morphologically indistinguishable from *T. pallidum* but differs in being difficult to propagate in laboratory animals. An infection similar to the human disease, although less severe, has been produced in chimpanzees.

The human disease, which may be contracted at any age, is usually transmitted by nonvenereal person-to-person contact, although flies have been implicated as possible vectors. The primary lesion is nonulcerating and is followed within 5 to 18 months by successive crops of flat, erythematous skin lesions that first become hyperpigmented and then, after several years, depigmented and hyperkeratotic. They are most often seen on the hands, feet, and scalp. Late visceral manifestations are extremely rare.

Experimental pinta has been produced in syphilitic patients, and although subjects with pinta regularly develop Wassermann and treponemal Abs, they occasionally contract syphilis. These results suggest significant differences in host responses and in antigenic properties of *T. carateum* compared with other pathogenic treponemes.

Penicillin is effective.

Other Treponematoses

Endemic treponemal diseases occur in many areas of the world where people live under relatively unhygienic conditions. Transmitted by direct contact, these afflictions are often given local names, such as **bejel** in Syria and **siti** in West Africa. All resemble yaws and are not readily distinguishable from one another.

A venereal form of treponematosis also occurs naturally in **rabbits.** The causative organism, *T. paraluis-cuniculi,* is morphologically indistinguishable from *T. pallidum* and shares antigenic determinants. Its natural occurrence in rabbits may complicate experimental studies on treponemes pathogenic for man.

T. hyodysenteriae, an anaerobic spirochete implicated in swine dysentery, is currently the only consistently cultivable potentially pathogenic treponeme.

Borreliosis
RELAPSING FEVER

Spirochetes of the genus *Borrelia* are usually longer than the treponemes, **their spirals are more loosely wound** and more flexible, and they are thick enough to be readily visible when stained with ordinary aniline dyes (see Fig. 37–2). They usually contain 12 to 15 axial fibrils inserted at each end. They can be propagated in young mice and rats, but host susceptibility differs from one strain to another. Some *Borrelia* strains may also be grown in chick embryos, and some can be grown under microaerophilic conditions in a complex medium. The organisms have an average division time of 18 hours and retain animal pathogenicity through numerous subcultures.

In man, spirochetes of this genus cause **relapsing fever,** in an epidemic and an endemic form. The **epidemic** form, caused by *B. recurrentis,* is transmitted only from person to person, by the human body louse. There is no animal reservoir, and lice do not transmit the organism transovarially. The **endemic** form, caused by various species of *Borrelia,* is spread from various **animal reservoirs** (often rodents) to man; each species is named for the species of *Ornithodorus* tick that transmits it to man.

After an incubation period of 3 to 10 days, there is a sudden onset of fever, which ordinarily lasts for about 4 days: during this time, large numbers of organisms may be demonstrated in the blood and urine and, rarely, in the spinal fluid. The fever then declines, and the borreliae disappear from the blood. As they decrease in number, they become less motile, assume pleomorphic forms, and agglutinate, often in **rosettes.** During the ensuing afebrile period, the blood is not infectious, but after 3 to 10 days, it again teems with organisms, and the fever returns. The ensuing febrile attacks usually number from three to ten and become progressively less severe until they subside altogether.

Although the case fatality rate is less than 5% for the endemic disease, it may exceed 50% in severe louse-borne epidemics, presumably owing to increased adaptation to the human host in person-to-person transmission. There is evidence that circulating endotoxin is present during the height of symptomatic relapsing fever. Autopsy usually reveals miliary necrotic lesions containing large numbers of organisms, particularly in the spleen and liver. Gross hemorrhagic lesions may also be prominent in the gastrointestinal tract and kidneys. Transplacental transmission has been reported.

Experimental infections may be produced in monkeys, mice, rats, and guinea pigs. The experimental disease in monkeys follows the characteristic relapsing course of the illness in man.

MECHANISM OF RELAPSE. The most remarkable feature of this disease is its tendency to relapse at regular intervals. The pathogenesis of the sequential relapses is unique: the **organisms in each successive attack show antigenic differences,** and circulating Abs specific for the organisms of each onset appear in the blood. These Abs are responsible for the agglutination, and presumably for the subsequent disappearance, of the spirochetes; the next relapse depends on the outgrowth of antigenically distinct mutants, against which the host then elaborates new Abs. The rapidity and the regularity of the successive relapses imply that the mutation rates involved are high and that a reproducible and limiting sequence of antigenic variation exists. DNA rearrangements affecting the variable major protein are responsible for these defined shifts.

DIAGNOSIS. The diagnosis is usually made by microscopic examination of blood samples obtained during a febrile attack. The organisms can be identified by darkfield microscopy or in stained smears. Because of the numerous antigenic variants encountered, serologic tests are of little diagnostic value. Animal inoculation may help when direct microscopic examinations are negative: infected blood injected into young white rats will usually result in a readily demonstrable spirochetemia within 24 to 72 hours.

TREATMENT. Relapsing fever responds well to penicillin. Tetracyclines and chloramphenicol are also effective.

PREVENTION. In the U.S., sporadic cases are encountered in the South and the West. Infected ticks* are plentiful in endemic areas and are thought to be the principal vector, both from animal to animal and from animal to man. Relapsing fever may also be louse-borne and is not uncommonly associated with typhus epidemics. Tick- and louse-control measures are the most effective means of prevention.

---

* Transovarial infection occurs in ticks.

OTHER HUMAN BORRELIA INFECTIONS. Ulcerative lesions of the skin, mucous membranes, and lungs, occurring most commonly in debilitated individuals, often contain *Borrelia* organisms; their etiologic significance is uncertain.

LYME BORRELIOSIS

The etiologic agent of Lyme borreliosis or Lyme disease is a recently discovered spirochete, *Borrelia burgdorferi*, that is harbored by **ticks of the *Ixodes* species** and transmitted to man usually during the spring and summer seasons. The disorder is named after a unique cluster of manifestations observed in 1975 in patients in and around Lyme, Connecticut, including characteristic skin lesions (erythema chronicum migrans), flu-like symptoms, and sequelae such as arthritis, carditis, and neuritis. *B. burgdorferi* was isolated from *Ixodes dammini* ticks and from individuals with Lyme disease, and the latter were observed to form Abs to the organism. The spirochete has also been isolated from the *Ixodes pacificus* tick in the western U.S. and from the **white-footed mouse** and **white-tailed deer,** which are naturally infested with this tick. *Ixodes ricinus* and *Ixodes persulcatus* are the tick vectors of Lyme borreliosis in Europe and the Soviet Union.

In human beings the disease is a multisystem inflammatory disorder. After an incubation period of 1 to 4 weeks, a red macular or papular lesion develops at the site of the tick bite, and it expands into a distinctive large, annular lesion with partial central clearing. This important diagnostic sign may occur in any part of the body and resolves in about 3 weeks. It is frequently accompanied by fever, headache, stiff neck, myalgia, fatigue, and malaise. Arthritis, neurologic disorders, or involvement of the heart may occur after weeks or months. Associated immune abnormalities include elevated levels of serum IgM, cryoglobulins, and immune complexes and a delayed specific IgG response. In untreated cases, recurring attacks of arthritis have been observed for several years. In Europe, where symptoms of the disease in its various forms were first described in the early 1900s, arthritis is much less frequent than in the U.S., possibly owing to a difference in strain.

DIAGNOSIS. The unusual clinical and epidemiologic features of Lyme disease, highlighted by a history of tick bites, travel in endemic areas, and development of the migratory ring-like skin lesion, are important diagnostic indicators. High or rising antibody titers against *B. burgdorferi* are also meaningful. Observation of spirochetes in clinical specimens and direct culture are also diagnostic but infrequently successful even in definite cases.

TREATMENT. Tetracycline and penicillin are effective and can interrupt and prevent subsequent manifestations of the disease, but the chronic stage requires intensive treatment. Patients treated early do not develop protective immunity.

PREVENTION. Lyme borreliosis is an important cause of morbidity in endemic areas such as northeast, midwest, or western U.S., and other geographic locations where wildlife are hosts for *Ixodes* ticks. It is the **most common arthropod-borne disease** in North America and Europe. At present, individual precautions to prevent tick bites in endemic areas are the most appropriate control measure. Poisons in a form that the mice carry to their nests are also helpful.

Leptospirosis

The first human leptospiral disease to be described was a severe febrile illness characterized by jaundice, hemorrhagic tendencies, and involvement of the kidney. Known as **Weil's disease,** it was shown in 1915 by Inada to be caused by *Leptospira interrogans* serotype *icterohaemorrhagiae* (Gr. *leptos*, thin), transmitted to man from infected rats.

It has since been learned that many immunologically different strains of leptospiral organisms cause a variety of human illnesses, most of which are not associated with jaundice. Each also seems to have a different natural host. Thus, *L. interrogans* serotype *icterohaemorrhagiae* is most commonly found in rats, serotype *canicola* in dogs, and serotype *pomona* in swine. All the common species are pathogenic for man (except for the saprobic *L. biflexa*, found in small streams, lakes, and stagnant water). Each species can be identified by specific immunologic reactions, but there is considerable antigenic overlap, and so absorbed sera must be used for species identification.

Current classifications consider all pathogenic leptospires to belong to a single complex, which can be subdivided into 19 serogroups and approximately 200 serotypes. On the basis of G + C content of DNA and of DNA hybridization, the leptospires have also been divided into four distinct genetic groups, which bear little relation to groupings based on antigenic structure.

MORPHOLOGY

All the leptospires are characterized by **extraordinarily fine spirals,** wound so tightly as to be barely distinguishable under the darkfield microscope (see Fig. 37–2). The cells range in length from 4 to 20 μm. The fine structure is basically similar to that of other spirochetes. Motility results from rotational, flexing, and translational movements of the organism, one or both ends of which are often bent into a hook. Because the tightly coiled spirals are so difficult to recognize, diagnoses made solely on the basis of direct microscopic examination of the blood are unreliable. Tiny strands extending from the surface of RBCs in blood preparations are often mistaken for leptospires.

CULTIVATION

Leptospires are obligate aerobes and can be readily grown in a variety of artificial media supplemented with 10% heat-inactivated (56°C, 30 minutes) rabbit serum. They can also be grown in a synthetic medium containing inorganic salts, fatty acids, and vitamin B_{12}. Growth is stimulated by thiamine and is best at pH 7.2, at 25° to 30°C, and at a slightly increased pCO_2. Pathogenic leptospires cannot synthesize long-chain fatty acids *de novo*. These compounds (at least 15 carbon atoms long, and both saturated and unsaturated) are essential for growth, being a major energy source, and they must be supplied in the medium in a bound form. In contrast, certain aquatic leptospires can grow in a defined medium with acetate as the sole source of carbon and energy. The lipid content of leptospires as well as of the other spirochetes is high (about 20% of the cell dry weight), and it largely reflects the fatty acid composition of the environment. On solid media, leptospires produce a variety of subsurface colonies, some of which may be difficult to see unless stained with oxidase reagent.

Saprobic leptospires can be differentiated from the pathogenic types by several cultural differences: they produce more oxidase, and their requirements for environmental CO_2 are less. Neither type of leptospire incorporates exogenous pyrimidine; hence, cultivation in the presence of fluorouracil permits selective growth of leptospires from material contaminated with other microorganisms.

ANTIGENICITY AND GENETIC VARIATION

All leptospires possess a common somatic Ag (lipopolysaccharide), but antigenic types differ in their surface (agglutinating) Ag. Differences in surface Ags are most readily demonstrated by agglutination of suspensions of either living or formalin-killed organisms; CF and precipitin procedures are also sometimes employed. Mutations affecting virulence, morphology (nonhooked forms), motility, hemolysin production, and colony formation have also been noted. No leptospiral toxins other than a hemolysin and lipase have yet been described.

PATHOGENICITY

LOWER ANIMALS. Leptospirosis is primarily a zoonosis, wild rodents and domestic animals providing the princi-

pal reservoirs. The disease can be produced experimentally in many species of rodents; the young of the guinea pig and the Syrian hamster are particularly susceptible. When injected with *L. interrogans* serotype *icterohaemorrhagiae*, they develop fever within 3 to 5 days followed by jaundice and hemorrhages into the skin, subcutaneous tissues, and muscles. Death usually occurs in less than 2 weeks. At necropsy, the tissues are jaundiced and hemorrhagic, the liver and spleen are enlarged, and leptospires are recoverable from the blood, cerebrospinal fluid, and urine.

In contrast, in species that are naturally infected with leptospires (e.g., wild rats), the infection is usually mild, often lifelong, and characterized by chronic involvement of the kidneys. The more or less continuous shedding of organisms in the urine is often responsible for transmission of leptospirosis to man. Because the organisms will not survive long in an acid medium, the urine is usually infectious only when alkaline or excreted into alkaline water.

HUMANS. Different serotypes cause a similar pattern of illness after an incubation period of 8 to 12 days. The onset is abrupt, often with chills followed by high fever. Headache, photophobia, and severe muscular pains, particularly in the back and legs, are prominent symptoms. The most constant physical sign is conjunctivitis. The classic icterohemorrhagic picture is rarely seen: albuminurea is common, but jaundice occurs in fewer than 10% of clinically recognizable cases. Lymphocytic meningitis is often present. In some patients, meningitis occurs as the second phase of a biphasic illness, suggesting that immune mechanisms play a pathogenetic role. The acute illness ordinarily lasts for 3 to 10 days. The mortality rate in clinically recognized cases is approximately 5% to 10%, but serologic surveys in heavily endemic areas indicate that **subclinical cases are extremely common.**

During World War II a novel disease called **pretibial fever,** characterized by an erythematous rash most frequently over the shins, was encountered among soldiers stationed at Fort Bragg, North Carolina. The agent, obtained from the blood of a patient, was maintained for years by passage in guinea pigs and hamsters on the assumption that it was a virus, but nearly a decade later, it was identified as *L. interrogans* serotype *autumnalis,* a leptospiral species previously isolated in Japan. Subsequently, paired acute and convalescent sera saved from the Fort Bragg epidemic uniformly showed a rise in titer of specific agglutinins for the same organism.

Human convalescent serum protects guinea pigs against otherwise-fatal inoculations of homologous leptospires. These protective (and agglutinating) Abs persist in the patient's serum for many years.

LABORATORY DIAGNOSIS

A diagnosis based on direct microscopic examination of blood should be made only by experienced observers. Leptospiremia may be detected by culturing the blood, preferably at 30°C, in broth or agar media enriched with 10% serum or by inoculating it intraperitoneally into young guinea pigs or hamsters.

Serum Abs usually appear during the second week of illness and reach a maximum titer during the third or fourth week, but they are not easily identified because of the numerous antigenic types encountered. However, agglutination tests may be done with suspensions of killed leptospires pooled to contain the most common antigenic strains. A broader serologic test, for hemolysis, involves incubation of serum and complement with RBCs previously sensitized by **genus-specific antigen** extracted from the nonpathogenic *L. biflexa*.

TREATMENT

Penicillin, the tetracyclines, and chloramphenicol all are effective against leptospires *in vitro* and also, if given early, against experimental infections in animals. Nevertheless, the treatment of leptospirosis is relatively unsatisfactory, in part because the disease is generally recognized late. Penicillin and tetracycline appear to be the drugs of choice.

PREVENTION

Man usually acquires leptospirosis from infected animals through contact with water contaminated with their urine or through direct contact with their tissues. Workers in rat-infested slaughterhouses and fish-cleaning establishments, miners, farmers, sewer workers, and swimmers in stagnant ponds and canals run the greatest risk. Dogs vaccinated for leptospirosis may carry leptospires in their urine; they have been the source of urban outbreaks. Because the natural reservoir in wild animals is far too vast to be attacked directly, and because of the many serotypes, preventive measures must be directed at diminishing the chances of contact with contaminated water. The organisms are believed to gain entrance through abrasions in the skin and through the mucous membranes of the conjunctiva, nose, and mouth. Because of the acidity of the gastric juice, infection via the intestinal tract is probably rare.

Rat-Bite Fever (Sodoku)

Spirilla are spiral organisms distinct from spirochetes, for their motility depends on conventional polar flagella rather than on flexion. *Spirillum minor*, a short, rigid, spiral organism, is commonly carried by rats and causes one of the two forms of rat-bite fever in man. (The other is caused by *Streptobacillus moniliformis;* Chap. 41). From the primary rat-bite lesion, the organism invades the regional lymph nodes and eventually the blood stream, causing lymphadenitis, rash, and relapsing fever.

S. minor has never been cultivated on artificial media; its isolation from human patients depends on animal inoculation. Guinea pigs and mice are susceptible; when infected, they harbor in their blood large numbers of organisms, which are often visible in Wright-stained smears. The disease occasionally causes a false-positive serologic test for syphilis. Penicillin, streptomycin, and the tetracyclines are all effective.

Selected Reading

BOOKS AND REVIEW ARTICLES

Canale–Parola E: Physiology and evolution of spirochetes. Bacteriol Rev 41:181, 1977

Holt SC: Anatomy and chemistry of spirochetes. Microbiol Rev 42:114, 1978

Johnson RC (ed): The Biology of Parasitic Spirochetes. New York, Academic Press, 1976

Schell RF, Musher DM (eds): Pathogenesis and Immunology of Treponemal Infection. New York, Marcel Dekker, 1983

Southern PM Jr, Sanford JP: Relapsing fever: A clinical and microbiological review. Medicine 48:129, 1969

SPECIFIC ARTICLES

Baker–Zander SA, Hook EW, Bonin P et al: Antigens of *Treponema pallidum* recognized by IgG and IgM antibodies during syphilis in humans. J Infect Dis 151:264, 1985

Barbour AG: Laboratory aspects of Lyme borreliosis. Clin Microbiol Rev 1:399, 1988

Barbour AG, Barrera O, Judd RC: Structural analysis of the variable major proteins of *Borrelia hermsii*. J Exp Med 158:2127, 1983

Barbour AG, Burgdorfer W, Grunwaldt E, Steere AC: Antibodies of patients with Lyme disease to components of *Ixodes dammini* spirochete. J Clin Invest 72:504, 1983

Baseman JB, Hayes EC: Molecular characterization of receptor binding proteins and immunogens of virulent *Treponema pallidum*. J Exp Med 151:573, 1980

Baseman JB, Nichols JC, Hayes NS: Virulent *Treponema pallidum*: Aerobe or anaerobe. Infect Immun 13:704, 1976

Berman SJ, Tsai C-C, Holmes K et al: Sporadic anicteric leptospirosis in South Vietnam: A study in 150 patients. Ann Intern Med 79:167, 1973

Charon NW, Daughtry GR, McCuskey RS, Franz GN: Microcinematographic analysis of tethered *Leptospira illini*. J Bacteriol 160:1067, 1984

Fehniger TE, Walfield AM, Cunningham TM et al: Purification and characterization of a cloned protease-resistant *Treponema pallidum*-specific antigen. Infect Immun 46:598, 1984

Hanff PA, Bishop NH, Miller JN, Lovett MA: Humoral immune response in experimental syphilis to polypeptides of *Treponema pallidum*. J Immunol 131:1973, 1983

Joseph R, Canale–Parola E: Axial fibrils of anaerobic spirochetes:

Ultrastructure and chemical characteristics. Arch Microbiol 81:146, 1972

Magnuson HJ, Thomas EW, Olansky S et al: Inoculation syphilis in human volunteers. Medicine 35:33, 1956

Pavia CS, Niederbuhl CJ: Adoptive transfer of anti-syphilitic immunity with lymphocytes from *Treponema pallidum*-infected guinea pigs. J Immunol 135:2829, 1985

Peterson KM, Baseman JB, Alderete JF: *Treponema pallidum* receptor binding proteins interact with fibronectin. J Exp Med 157:1958, 1983

Schell RF, Lefrock JL, Chan JK et al: LSH hamster model of syphilis infection. Infect Immun 28:909, 1980

Schiller NL, Cox CD: Catabolism of glucose and fatty acids by virulent *Treponema pallidum*. Infect Immun 16:60, 1977

Steere AC, Grodzicki RL, Kornblatt AN et al: The spirochetal etiology of Lyme disease. N Engl J Med 308:733, 1983

Thomas DD, Baseman JB, Alderete JF: Fibronectin tetrapeptide is target for syphilis spirochete cytadherence. J Exp Med 162:1715, 1985

38

Charles L. Wisseman, Jr.

Rickettsiae

Introduction to the Intracellular Bacteria

With one exception (*Rochalimaea*), the **rickettsias** and **chlamydias,** described in this and the following chapter, are **obligate intracellular parasites.** Moreover (except for *Coxiella*), they can grow, unlike the optional intracellular bacteria (e.g., *Mycobacterium*, *Brucella*), in nonphagocytic cells. This attribute requires special mechanisms for attachment to and entry into host cells, for growth in specific intracellular sites (that differ for different species), and for release. Because of the protected intracellular habitats, both types of microorganisms often persist in the face of an immune response. The organisms are generally smaller than other pathogenic bacteria; they have a longer generation time; and some depend in part or wholly on host cell ATP for energy.

Chlamydias have a complex life cycle, with different forms for intracellular multiplication and for intercellular transmission; they are usually transmitted by contact or by the airborne route. In contrast, **rickettsias retain a bacillary form,** and their transmission between hosts usually depends on arthropod vectors.

Comparison of rRNA sequence has related a rickettsia to the intracellular plant pathogens and symbionts, *Agrobacter* and *Rhizobacterium*. Chlamydias are of different origin, and they lack a peptidoglycan layer.

General Characteristics of Rickettsiae

Four genera of the family **Rickettsiaceae** contain organisms known to cause human disease: *Rochalimaea, Coxiella, Ehrlichia,* and *Rickettsia* (Table 38–1). All but *Rochalimaea* are obligate intracellular parasites. The dominant type of host cell parasitized by each genus influences the nature of the resulting disease.

TABLE 38–1. Rickettsial Agents Causing Human Disease: Some Host Cell Interactions

Genus/Group/Species	Genome Mol. Wt. ($\times 10^{-9}$)	%G+C	Cell Association Entry	Localization	Optimal pH
Rochalimaea			Surface adhesion	Pericellular	7
R. quintana	1.03	39			
Coxiella			Endocytosis	Phagolysosome	4.5
C. burnetii	1.04	43			
Ehrlichia			Endocytosis	? Phagosome	—
E. sennetsu	—	—			
E. canis	—	—			
Rickettsia			"Active" transmembrane passage	Free in cytoplasm (no vacuolar membrane)	7
Typhus Group					
R. prowazekii	1.10	29			
R. mooseri (= *R. typhi*)	1.08	29			
R. canada	1.49	29		+ Intranuclear	
Spotted Fever Group				+ Intranuclear	
R. rickettsii	1.30	33			
Multiple species					
Scrub Typhus Group					
R. tsutsugamushi	—	—			
Multiple serotypes					

HISTORICAL PERSPECTIVE

Louse-borne typhus fever, best known in its devastating epidemic form, has played a large role in human affairs for centuries, commonly associated with war and its consequences and often more decisive in military campaigns than the battles. As Zinsser remarked in *Rats, Lice and History,* Napoleon's retreat from Moscow "was started by a louse." Between 1918 and 1922, typhus caused about 3,000,000 deaths in Eastern Europe and the Soviet Union, and during World War II, millions of cases occurred in prison camps and Eastern Europe. Now confined to remote primitive areas in Africa and mountainous regions of South America and Asia, the disease lies in its deceptively innocuous endemic form like a sleeping giant, stirring now and then to cause local outbreaks and occasional epidemics. **Murine typhus,** first differentiated from louse-borne typhus in the 1930s, and **Q fever,** whose broad geographic distribution began to be appreciated in World War II, occur over large parts of the world.

Rocky Mountain spotted fever, a devastating disease with a mortality rate as high as 40% to 80% among early settlers of certain western states of the United States, is now known throughout much of the western hemisphere, and its relatives are present on all continents. **Scrub typhus,** known since ancient times in Asia (where persisting religious harvest ceremonies of ancient origin include placations for protection against the vector mite), came sharply to the attention of the western world during World War II; it is now recognized as a leading cause of fevers in large endemic areas of Southeast Asia. Rickettsial diseases thus continue as significant world health problems. The name honors Howard Taylor Ricketts, who discovered the agent of Rocky Mountain spotted fever in the early 1900s and later died of typhus fever while investigating its etiology.

MORPHOLOGY AND METABOLISM

Rickettsias are gram-negative bacterial parasites of similar small size ($\sim 0.3 \times 1$ μm) and shape (coccobacillary to bacillary). They stain poorly with the standard gram stain and require special stains for good viewing by light microscopy (e.g., a strong red by the Gimenez stain in thin smears). Electron microscopy reveals a typical prokaryotic structure.

In most rickettsias, the envelope is similar to that of gram-negative bacteria, with a peptidoglycan layer between the outer (OM) and the inner membrane (IM). External to the OM in some are a microcapsular layer and a more voluminous slime layer (Fig. 38–1). In addition, surface proteins participate in the immune response. Lipopolysaccharide (LPS) has been demonstrated in many rickettsias, but in *R. tsutsugamushi* it is absent.

What rickettsias can perform with their own enzymes and what their host cells contribute are still poorly understood. ATP can be produced from glutamate (but not from glucose) via the citric acid cycle; additional ATP may be imported by an ATP–ADP translocator mecha-

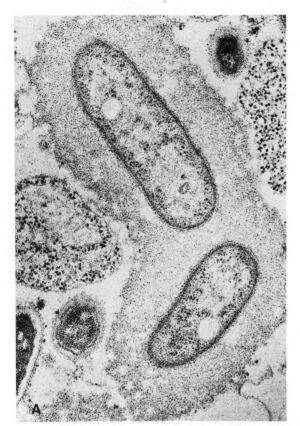

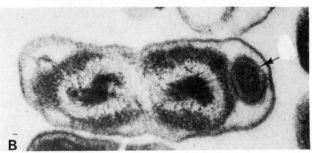

Figure 38–1. Selected structural features. *(A)* R. prowazekii embedded in abundant slime layer, which was stabilized by disrupting the infected host cell in the presence of antibody. *(B)* Dividing bacillary *C. burnetii* containing two nucleoids with visible DNA strands and with a developing small dense terminal spore-like form *(arrow)* within the OM. The small dense forms are highly resistant to adverse environmental conditions and can pass through some bacterial filters, hence the early designation as *Rickettsia diaporica*. (*A*, Silverman DJ, Wisseman CL Jr: Infect Immun 22:233, 1978; *B*, McCaul TF, Williams JC: J Bacteriol 147:1063, 1981)

nism. A limited amount of protein synthesis, but no multiplication, may occur in *R. prowazekii* outside the host cell under special conditions.

The size of the rickettsial genome is about 40% of that of *Escherichia coli*. The mole percent G + C of the DNA is unusually low (~28%–33%) for *Rickettsia* spp., but not for *Rochalimaea* or *Coxiella*. To date, plasmids have been found only in *C. burnetii*.

GROWTH IN HOST CELLS

Rickettsias multiply by binary transverse fission. Different genera are adapted to grow within subcellular compartments with very different kinds of chemical environment (Table 38–1; Fig. 38–2). The generation time is long (8–12 hours), and the optimal growth temperature is 33° to 35°C. *Rochalimaea* spp. are the only rickettsias capable of growth on acellular media, and *in vivo*, they grow on the surface of cells.

GROWTH IN MEMBRANE-BOUND VACUOLES. *C. burnetii* enters the host macrophage/histiocyte passively by endocytosis and grows in the highly acid environment within the membrane-bound **phagolysosomes,** where it may form huge colonies occupying much of the host cell cytoplasm. It resists degradation by lysosomal enzymes. The growth cycle may include the formation of very small, dense, highly resistant spore-like forms (Fig. 38–1).

On the other hand, *Ehrlichia canis*, which enters blood monocytes similarly, evidently inhibits lysosomal fusion and thus grows in a **phagosome** devoid of lysosomal enzymes and possibly at a more neutral pH. During growth, it forms characteristic inclusions (morulae).

GROWTH "FREE" IN THE CYTOPLASM. *Rickettsia* spp. attach to the host cell plasma membrane and pass through it directly into the cytoplasm, a process requiring active metabolic participation by both the rickettsia and the host cell and involving phospholipase A activity. The bacteria replicate free in the cytoplasm, not surrounded by any type of vacuolar membrane; in addition, the spotted fever group rickettsiae may also pass through the nuclear membrane and grow within the nucleus in a small proportion of infected cells. Metabolic activity is optimal near the pH of the host cell cytoplasm (~pH 7).

During intracytoplasmic growth, *R. prowazekii* accumulates to very large numbers with minimal overt cytopathology before the host cell plasma membrane breaks down to release the organisms. In contrast, *R. mooseri* and the spotted fever group organisms begin to escape through the host cell plasma membrane, without apparent damage, in the early stages of infection, thus producing a more rapidly spreading type of infection. *R. mooseri* may later accumulate to large numbers before host cell integrity is lost, whereas *R. rickettsii* (Fig. 38–2*B*) is highly cytotoxic and causes marked damage to host cell organelles and cell breakdown before large numbers of organisms accumulate.

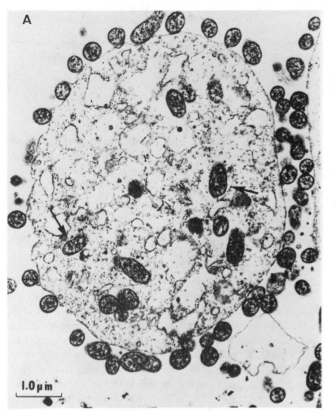

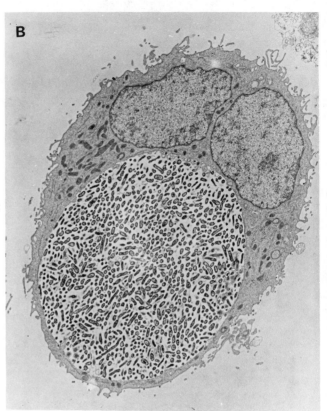

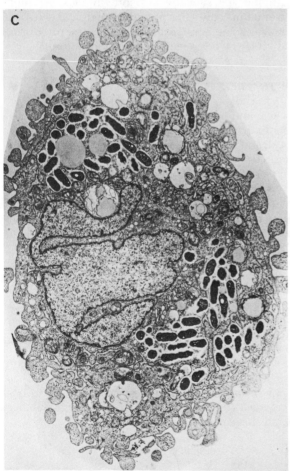

Figure 38–2. Types of rickettsia–host cell associations in cell cultures. *(A)* Pericellular attachment and localization of *Rochalimaea quintana*. In nature, this organism grows on the luminal surface of the midgut cells in its vector, the human body louse. *(B)* C. *burnetii* within membrane-bound phagolysosome. *(C)* R. *prowazekii* ''free'' within cytoplasm, not surrounded by vacuolar membrane. Note the clear zone surrounding intracytoplasmic organisms and the paucity of visible cytopathology. *(A,* Merrell BR et al: J Bacteriol 135:633, 1978; *B,* Burton PR et al: Infect Immun 21:556, 1978; *C,* Silverman DJ, Wisseman CL Jr, unpublished)

PATHOGENESIS AND IMMUNITY

In susceptible hosts infected by natural routes, various rickettsias grow mainly on or within characteristic kinds of cells (Table 38–2). The type of cell parasitized (e.g., endothelial cell, macrophage) determines in large part the nature of the basic pathologic lesion (e.g., focal endovasculitis, microscopic granulomas; Fig. 38–3); and it also influences the nature of the disease process, including the presence or absence of rash. Most rickettsias produce acute, self-limited febrile diseases in man, ranging in severity from subclinical or benign to fulminating and lethal.

Specific immunity against disease caused by the infecting species or serotype tends to be strong and long-lasting, but organisms persist in tissues. The mechanism of latent infection is unknown, and some rickettsias may cause overt recurrent disease. Immunity consists of both humoral Ab and cell-mediated components, the latter being the more important in controlling intracellular rickettsial growth. Certain rickettsial surface proteins elicit protective immunity.

Details of immune mechanisms, where known, follow similar general patterns but do differ at certain points with the type of rickettsia–host cell interaction described above. Thus, rickettsias grow freely in nonactivated macrophages but are killed by immune interferon (IFN-γ)-activated macrophages. They are not killed, but are opsonized, by Ab and complement. However, whereas opsonized *Rickettsia* spp. are then killed within the phagolysosome of nonactivated macrophages, *C. burnetii*, as noted above, may survive and grow in phagolysosomes.

Cell-mediated mechanisms are responsible for killing rickettsias replicating within their natural host cells. Thus, rickettsia-specific cytotoxic T-lymphocytes may lyse infected cells on contact. (T-lymphocytes with suppressor activity are produced under some circum-stances, but their role remains to be elucidated.) Moreover, IFN-γ, produced by immune T-lymphocytes on stimulation with specific rickettsial Ag, induces killing of both intraphagolysosomal and intracytoplasmic rickett-sias and also lysis of some infected cells. These actions are modulated by other lymphokines and monokines.

NATURAL HISTORY

Rickettsias occur under natural conditions (Table 38–3) not only in mammals but also in blood-sucking **arthro-pods**—either insects (lice, fleas) or arachnids (ticks, mites)—and may alternate between mammal and arthropod in their natural cycle. Some are transmitted from one generation of ticks or mites to the next through the eggs (i.e., **vertical** or **transovarial** transmission), an important **reservoir** mechanism. Except for Q fever, arthropod vectors are the primary means of transmission to man. However, when airborne, rickettsias are notoriously infectious for man. Except for louse-borne typhus and trench fever, most rickettsioses are **zoonoses;** i.e., infections of lower animals, with man only an incidental intruder into the natural enzootic cycle.

LABORATORY DIAGNOSIS

Laboratory diagnosis of rickettsial diseases may be accomplished by the following general methods: (1) isolation of the organisms by inoculation of susceptible laboratory animals or tissue cultures; (2) microscopic demonstration of the organisms in monocytes (ehrlichiosis) in stained blood smears, or in sections of skin biopsy or postmortem tissues stained with specific fluorescein-labeled Abs; and, most commonly; (3) specific Ab response, usually detected by the indirect fluorescent Ab (IFA) test. The capacity to measure different immuno-

TABLE 38–2. Some Features of Human Rickettsial Infections

Disease	Dominant Target Cell	Basic Lesion	Clinical Manifestations
Typhus-like fevers			
Typhus group	Endothelial	Vasculitis	Acute, self-limited fever, rash
Scrub typhus	Endothelial	Vasculitis	Acute, self-limited fever, rash
Spotted fever group	Endothelial + smooth muscle	Vasculitis	Acute, self-limited fever, rash
Q fever	Monocytes, macrophages, pneumocytes, ? other	Granulomas	Acute, self-limited fever, "atypical pneumonia"; subacute hepatitis; subacute to chronic endocarditis
Trench fever	Unknown	Unknown	Recurring febrile episodes
Ehrlichioses			
Sennetsu fever	Monocytes	Unknown	Acute, self-limited fever; lymphadenopathy*

* Peripheral blood lymphocytes, and some monocytes and neutrophils, were parasitized in a human patient naturally infected by *E. canis,* a monocytic *Ehrlichia* of dogs. *E. risticii,* the cause of Potomac horse fever, causes transiently reduced immune responsiveness and lymphoid depletion in mice.

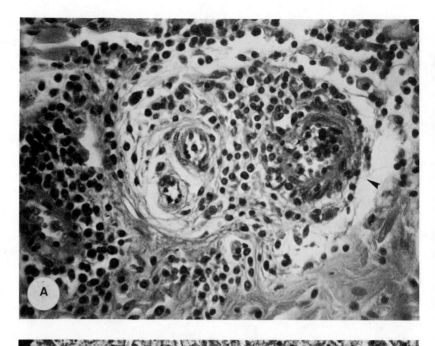

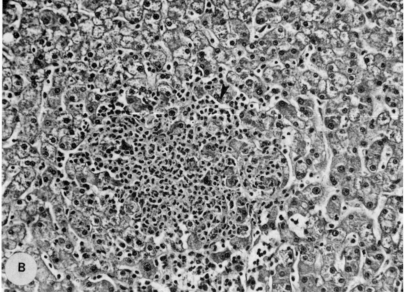

Figure 38–3. Basic histopathologic lesions of some rickettsioses in man. *(A)* Focal endovasculitis in fatal louse-borne typhus. Note the damaged endothelial layer, the intravascular deposition of cells and fibrin, and the perivascular mononuclear cell accumulation (mainly monocytes, macrophages, and lymphocytes). The lesions of murine typhus and scrub typhus are similar. Those of Rocky Mountain spotted fever involve in addition the smooth muscle layer of the blood vessel and tend to have more pronounced intravascular thrombosis. *(B)* Microscopic granuloma in liver biopsy of patient with Q fever (*Coxiella burnetii* infection). (*A,* Wisseman CL Jr, unpublished; *B,* Dupont HL et al: Ann Int Med 74:198, 1971)

globulin classes (IgM, IgG, IgA) permits the use of this test for the diagnosis of acute and chronic infections and for epidemiologic surveillance. Cross-reactions among related species make special procedures necessary when species-specific diagnoses are required.

The previously favored complement fixation (CF) test still has special uses, especially in Q fever and in the differentiation between louse-borne and murine typhus.

A wide variety of other tests using rickettsial Ags, such as microagglutination, ELISA, dot ELISA, latex agglutination, etc., have special uses. Unfortunately, specific rickettsial Ags are generally not available commercially, but they are available through state health departments, the Centers for Disease Control (CDC) in Atlanta, GA, and from certain WHO reference laboratories. A time-honored nonspecific **Weil–Felix test** depends on serologic cross-reactions between some members of the genus *Rickettsia* and *Proteus* OX2, OX19, or OXK strains, but it has serious limitations.

TREATMENT

The early acute infections respond well to the rickettsia-static tetracyclines and chloramphenicol. The new quinolone, ciprofloxacin, shows promise. Because organisms persist, prevention of relapse depends on an adequate immune response before treatment is terminated. For different reasons, late (more than 5 days) severe acute Rocky Mountain spotted fever and chronic Q fever endocarditis respond poorly.

Specific Diseases Caused by Rickettsiae

Tables 38–2 and 38–3 summarize the main features of the rickettsial diseases of man. Typhus, spotted fever, and scrub typhus follow a similar general pattern: (1) an incubation period of roughly 1 to 2 weeks; (2) a febrile period of about 1 to 3 weeks; (3) a rash beginning in the first week of disease; (4) disseminated focal vasculitis of small blood vessels resulting from selective infection of endothelial cells and associated with increased capillary permeability and hypotension; (5) an Ab response 1 to 2 weeks after onset of disease; (6) rickettsemia from the onset to the end of the febrile period, coexisting with the mounting serum Ab titer in the late febrile period; and (7) a strong, persistent specific delayed hypersensitivity.

TYPHUS GROUP

"Typhus" refers to two diseases that are similar clinically but differ markedly in epidemiologic features: the "louse-borne" typhus complex caused by *R. prowazekii* and murine typhus caused by *R. mooseri* (= *R. typhi*). The organisms show strong serologic cross-reactions, bearing group-specific as well as species-specific epitopes on a major envelope protein. Convalescence from either infection is accompanied by strong and long-lasting immunity against the infecting species and substantial cross-immunity to the other.

TABLE 38–3. Important Epidemiologic Characteristics of Rickettsial Diseases

Disease	Agent	Geographic Occurrence	Usual Mode of Transmission to Man	Reservoir
Typhus group				
Primary louse-borne typhus	*R. prowazekii*	Worldwide	Infected louse feces rubbed into broken skin or as aerosol to mucous membranes	Man
Brill–Zinsser disease	*R. prowazekii*	Worldwide	Recrudescence months or years after primary attack of louse-borne typhus	
Flying squirrel typhus	*R. prowazekii*	Eastern U.S.	Unknown	Squirrel
Murine typhus	*R. mooseri* (*R. typhi*)	Scattered pockets world wide	Infected flea feces	Rodents
Spotted fever group				
Rocky Mountain spotted fever	*R. rickettsii*	Western hemisphere	Tick bite	Ticks/rodents
Tick typhuses (boutonneuse)	*R. conorii**	Mediterranean, Caspian and Black Sea littoral, Africa, South Asia	Tick bite	Ticks/rodents; dogs
Rickettsialpox	*R. akari*	U.S., Russia, Korea	Mite bite	Mites/mice
Scrub typhus	*R. tsutsugamushi*	Japan, SE Asia, W & SW Pacific	Mite bite	Mites/rodents
Q Fever	*Coxiella burnetii*	Worldwide	Inhalation of infected particles from environment of infected animals	Ticks/mammals
Trench fever	*Rochalimaea quintana*	Europe, Africa, Mexico, South America	Infected louse feces	Man
Sennetsu fever	*Ehrlichia sennetsu*	Japan	Unknown	Unknown

* In addition, in Australia *R. australis* (Queensland tick typhus) and in North Asia *R. sibirica* (Siberian tick typhus) are antigenically and geographically distinct entities.

Louse-borne Typhus Complex

Louse-borne typhus, caused by *R. prowazekii*, has two forms: primary (epidemic) and recrudescent.

CLINICAL MANIFESTATIONS. Primary louse-borne typhus fever usually begins abruptly, after a 9- to 12-day incubation period, with fever, headache, generalized myalgia and prostration, progressive clouding of the sensorium, hypotension, and a macular to maculopapular rash toward the end of the first week. The untreated patient either dies or recovers in 2 to 3 weeks. The mortality rate, low for children, may reach 50% in persons over 50 years of age.

Immunity following recovery is long-lasting but not eradicative. Accordingly, months to many years after primary infection, the latent infection breaks out in occasional individuals as **recrudescent typhus (Brill–Zinsser disease).** The Ab response is accelerated (mostly IgG), and the disease generally is milder than primary typhus. However, if such a patient harbors lice, he or she may initiate an epidemic of the more severe form of the disease.

TREATMENT. The mortality rate is negligible in properly treated patients (see above). A single 100-mg dose of doxycycline, a lipophilic, long-acting tetracycline, is curative.

TRANSMISSION AND EPIDEMIOLOGY. Classic louse-borne typhus, a disease of poverty or catastrophic events (war, famine, natural disasters), is maintained in a transmission cycle between the human body louse vector *Pediculus humanus humanus* and man. The lice live and breed in clothing, become infected by feeding on the blood of a rickettsemic patient, and excrete rickettsias in the feces that infect susceptible persons through breaks in the skin or through the ocular or respiratory mucosa. The louse dies of infection in a week or two, without transmitting the organisms to the next generation; hence, when transmission is interrupted, the disease dies out until the organism is reintroduced into a susceptible lousy population, either from external sources or from local Brill–Zinsser disease.

Humans are thus the primary interepidemic reservoir. The human–louse–human transmission cycle can give rise to local outbreaks (villages, refugee and concentration camps, prisons, etc.), massive epidemics, or smoldering endemicity. Louse-borne typhus is now confined to eastern and central Africa and mountainous regions of Central and South America and Asia.

In contrast, the recently recognized **flying squirrel typhus** in the eastern U.S., caused by an organism with minor differences in DNA, is a **zoonosis** that involves the common flying squirrel, *Glaucomys volans*, and its lice. Sporadic human cases have occurred in occupants of houses whose attics harbor overwintering flying squirrels. The mode of transmission to man is unknown. Flying squirrel typhus could presumably initiate louse-borne typhus.

PREVENTION AND CONTROL. Control of classic louse-borne typhus involves: (1) control of the louse vector; and (2) immunization of the population at risk. Control of typhus outbreaks and epidemics through louse control can be very effective in the short term by the application of insecticides, such as DDT, malathion, lindane, carbamates, etc., to the clothing of infested persons. Long-term louse control in endemic situations is more difficult and complex because of the development of insecticide resistance and, even more, the difficulty in correcting the socioeconomic and environmental factors that underlie chronic lousiness.

Vaccines consisting of killed whole organisms offer partial protection against disease and significantly reduce the mortality rate. Vaccines composed of purified or recombinant immunogenic peptides are under test. An attenuated living vaccine (Madrid E strain) protects against disease during epidemic spread of typhus.

Murine Typhus

Murine typhus fever, caused by *R. mooseri* (*R. typhi*), resembles louse-borne typhus clinically and pathologically but is milder. Although the untreated disease has a low mortality rate (less than 5%), it can be debilitating and entail a long convalescence. It responds promptly to treatment with antirickettsial drugs.

TRANSMISSION AND EPIDEMIOLOGY. Murine typhus, a zoonosis, exists in nature as an infection of rats and certain other small mammals and is transmitted among these by fleas (*Xenopsylla cheopsis*, others) and rat lice. Fleas acquire infection of the midgut epithelial cells by feeding on rats during the transient rickettsemia of acute infection and then excrete rickettsiae in the feces for their natural lifespan. Neither rat nor flea is adversely affected by the infection.

Endemic foci are often concentrated in rat-infested buildings where man becomes infected from fleas. Such foci are widely distributed throughout the tropical and temperate zones of the world, coincident with the spread of *Rattus rattus* (black rats) and *Rattus norvegicus* (brown rats) to port cities and along roads, rivers, and railroads, such as in Asia, the Middle East, Africa, southern Europe, and the Americas south of the U.S. border. Fewer than 100 cases per year are reported in the U.S. In many developing countries murine typhus may be a substantial source of febrile disease.

PREVENTION AND CONTROL. Control measures for murine typhus consist of first reducing the flea population with insecticides applied to rat runs and then reducing the rodent population (rodenticides, rat-proofing buildings). Killed whole-organism vaccines have been prepared but are unevaluated. Immunogenic peptide vaccines are under study.

SPOTTED FEVER GROUP

The several species of tick-borne spotted fever (SF)-group rickettsias are transmitted by the bite of various species of hard (ixodid) **ticks.** The ticks maintain the infection in two ways: vertical transmission through the egg and an enzootic tick–mammal–tick cycle. These rickettsias are widely distributed over the world, with presumably a single species dominant over large, sometimes continental, areas.

Rocky Mountain Spotted Fever

Rocky Mountain spotted fever (**RMSF**) is a dangerous acute infectious disease of the western hemisphere caused by *R. rickettsii* and transmitted by various species of hard ticks.

CLINICAL MANIFESTATIONS. Although generally similar to typhus and scrub typhus fevers, RMSF differs in important ways. The incubation period is shorter, averaging 5 to 7 days. The rash usually begins on the extremities and then involves the trunk. The smooth muscle layer of small blood vessels is infected in addition to the endothelial cell layer, causing a more severe vasculitis. Although early RMSF responds promptly to antirickettsial chemotherapy, severe RMSF rapidly (±5–6 days after onset) enters a phase of severe physiological derangements, myocarditis, and intravascular coagulation abnormalities not directly responsive to antimicrobial or other therapies. The continuing approximately 5% case mortality rate is largely attributable to delay in instituting specific antirickettsial therapy. Because the disease may present as an undifferentiated fever, therapy must often be started on a presumptive diagnosis based on the history of a tick bite or potential exposure in an endemic area. An early presumptive diagnosis may be verified by finding the organisms in skin punch biopsy sections stained with specific fluorescent Ab. Antibody response, usually detectable later, serves a retrospective confirmatory role.

TRANSMISSION AND EPIDEMIOLOGY. The dominant vector tick differs with the geographic region—e.g., *Dermacentor variabilis* (eastern U.S.), *D. andersoni* (western U.S.), *Amblyomma cajanensis* (Mexico). People usually acquire infected ticks in infested suburban, rural, or wilderness areas during recreational or occupational activities, although dogs may carry ticks from such areas into the house or yard. Recently, several cases of RMSF were traced to foci of infected ticks in two parks in New York City. Cases have been reported in the U.S. in every month of the year, but most occur during the spring and early summer, coincident with maximum tick activity. About 800 to 1000 cases have been reported annually in recent years.

Although originally recognized in the Rocky Mountain area, cases have been reported from all 48 contiguous states, with most now occurring in the **eastern and south central states.** RMSF extends into South America. The mortality rate increases with age to exceed 60% in untreated persons over 50 years old.

PREVENTION AND CONTROL. Prevention of RMSF is largely a personal matter: avoidance of tick-infested endemic areas; protective clothing and repellents (e.g., permethrin); and periodic inspection of the body and removal of ticks. Area control of ticks is difficult. Conventional killed whole-organism vaccines, no longer available, are only partially effective. Recombinant surface proteins with protective action in animals offer promise.

Tick Typhus Fevers

Other tick-borne SF-group rickettsial diseases are widely distributed in the eastern hemisphere. *R. sibirica* (Siberian tick typhus, north Asian tick-borne rickettsiosis) is widely distributed in the Soviet Union and northern Asiatic regions. *R. australis* causes Queensland tick typhus. The SF group rickettsiae causing newly recognized human disease in Southeast Asia, Japan, and China are under current study; both *R. sibirica* and *R. conorii* have been found among them.

R. conorii (and presumed *R. conorii*) infections, under numerous local names (e.g., boutonneuse fever, Mediterranean spotted fever, Kenya tick typhus, Indian tick typhus), are distributed around the Mediterranean littoral and extend to southern Africa and South Asia. In Europe and North Africa, *R. conorii* is transmitted by the brown dog tick, *Rhipicephalus sanguineus*, which, brought in by dogs, may establish infestation of houses and compounds.

Strains from various areas are being reexamined by modern, more discriminating methods to determine if, indeed, all are a single immunologic type or species. The disease resembles RMSF with some differences. There is often an ulcerated primary lesion (**tache noire,** eschar) at the site of the infected tick bite, the rash tends to be more nodular, and the disease is generally milder, although recently, fatalities have been reported with increasing frequency. It responds readily to antirickettsial antibiotics. A noneschar-producing, *Rhipicephalus sanguineus*-transmitted strain that produces severe disease in Israel differs from classic *R. conorii* in serologic tests.

RICKETTSIALPOX. Rickettsialpox, caused by *R. akari*, has been recognized in the U.S. and the Soviet Union. Originally, *R. akari* was found associated with house mice and transmitted by the mouse mite, *Allodermanyssus sanguineus*. However, a more complex natural history is suggested by its isolation from field rodents in Korea and from rats in the Soviet Union. The disease is relatively mild and responds rapidly to specific chemotherapy. There is an eschar at the infection site and a strongly papular rash with pronounced vesiculation, superficially resembling that of chickenpox.

SCRUB TYPHUS (TSUTSUGAMUSHI DISEASE)

Scrub typhus is an acute typhus-like febrile disease of Asia caused by multiple serotypes of *R. tsutsugamushi*. It is transmitted by the bite of the **larvae** (**chiggers**) of certain species of **trombiculid mites.**

CLINICAL MANIFESTATIONS. Primary scrub typhus fever resembles louse-borne typhus in many ways. However, a lesion, the **eschar,** accompanied by regional lymphadenopathy, frequently develops at the site(s) of the infected chigger bite(s) during the roughly 9- to 12-day incubation period, and generalized lymphadenopathy develops in the latter part of the disease. Immunity against the infecting serotype is long-lasting, but against **heterologous serotypes,** it is transient (1–2 months). Thus, more than one attack of scrub typhus can occur. Postprimary attacks may be modified—for example, absent eschar and rash—and may not be recognized without specific laboratory diagnostic methods.

The mortality rate of untreated disease ranges from very low to very high (40%–60%), depending on a variety of known and unknown factors. Response to chemotherapy is prompt and life-saving. A single dose of doxycycline is often curative.

TRANSMISSION AND EPIDEMIOLOGY. **Trombiculid mites** (e.g., *Leptotrombium deliense*, *L. akamushi*, others) are both vectors and reservoirs of *R. tsutsugamushi*. The organism is maintained by efficient vertical transmission from one generation of mites to the next through the egg. Only the larval stage is parasitic. It feeds only once on field rodents and other small mammals, to which it may transmit the rickettsias, as well as to humans who enter a focus of infected chiggers. Foci tend to occur in the transitional vegetation along trails, roads, and streams and in the scrub vegetation overgrowing previously cleared areas.

The disease is best known from outbreaks that occur when large groups of nonimmune people enter endemic areas, as in military operations, road building, and clearing of land for agriculture. However, through the help of specific laboratory diagnostic methods, which detect both classic and atypical disease, scrub typhus has also been shown to be the leading cause of hospitalization for febrile disease among the indigenous people in some endemic Southeast Asian areas.

Scrub typhus is distributed from northern Japan and the Kamchatka Peninsula of the U.S.S.R. south through the islands of the western Pacific and parts of China and southeast Asia to northern Austrialia and west at least to Pakistan and Tadjikistan. Mite activity is a function of both temperature and ground moisture. In tropical zones, its occurrence is often correlated with rainfall and, in temperate zones, with the warmer seasons. However, *L. scutellare*-transmitted winter scrub typhus occurs in parts of Japan.

PREVENTION AND CONTROL. Vaccine development has been hampered by the multiple serotypes that can coexist even in small foci. Chemoprophylaxis is possible with long-acting doxycycline. Repellent treatment of clothing and exposed skin, although awkward, protects against chigger bites. Area control of vectors is feasible usually for only limited sites.

Q FEVER

Q fever is an infectious disease of worldwide distribution caused by *C. burnetii*. Unlike other rickettsias, *C. burnetii* produces a small, dense, highly resistant **spore-like form,** whose stability in the environment is important for transmission.

CLINICAL MANIFESTATIONS. Three clinical forms are recognized. **Uncomplicated** Q fever is an acute, self-limited febrile disease (9–14 days), readily responsive to chemotherapy. Radiologic evidence of interstitial pneumonitis is often present. Some patients develop a **granulomatous hepatitis** with a longer course, more slowly responsive to chemotherapy. Finally, even years postinfection, the rare patient develops a **subacute to chronic endocarditis,** with *C. burnetii* demonstrable in the blood and vegetations. Routine blood cultures are negative. Long-term antimicrobial therapy and valve replacement are not very satisfactory. Antibodies in ordinary acute infections are best detected with phase 2 (an avirulent phase, akin to rough forms) antigens. Clues to active persistent infections are elevated phase 1 (virulent) CF and IgA class Abs.

TRANSMISSION AND EPIDEMIOLOGY. Although the organism occurs in many arthropods (including ticks) and wild animals, human beings usually acquire infection from domestic animals (sheep, cattle, goats) by inhaling **airborne organisms.** Infected animals shed large numbers of organisms in milk, urine, feces, and, especially, placenta ($\pm 10^9$ ID50/g) which, presumably as the resistant spore-like form, readily disseminate as airborne dust.

Placentas and milk of infected women may also contain organisms.

PREVENTION AND CONTROL. A vaccine consisting of Formalin-killed phase 1 organisms protects against disease after a single small dose (20–30 μg). Its tendency to produce severe chronic granulomatous local reactions in some previously infected or vaccinated persons requires their exclusion by a prevaccination skin test. Chloroform–methanol-extracted vaccines under study may reduce reactions, but their capacity to induce long-lasting immunity is unproved.

OTHER RICKETTSIAL DISEASES

TRENCH FEVER. Trench fever, a nonlethal infection with unusual and unexplained host–parasite interactions, occurred in epidemic form in Europe during both world wars, and it persists as an unrecognized infection in several parts of the world where body louse infestation is common. The agent, *Rochalimaea quintana*, is transmitted by human body lice, which remain infected over a normal lifespan without transovarial transmission. The disease is maintained in a man–louse–man cycle, with no known extrahuman reservoirs. The 14- to 30-day incubation period is followed by sudden onset of fever of a few days. About half of the patients have **multiple relapses** over months to years; organisms may persist in the blood at least for months even in the absence of overt disease. Ab titers are low.

Unlike other rickettsias, the organisms **form small colonies** on a modified blood agar incubated in an atmosphere containing 5% CO_2. Tetracycline is effective treatment, but it is not known if it eradicates the organisms and prevents relapses. Control is directed at the louse vector (see louse-borne typhus above).

HUMAN EHRLICHIOSES. Sennetsu fever, caused by *Ehrlichia sennetsu* (formerly *R. sennetsu*), is an infectious mononucleosis-like disease of western Japan characterized by fever, lymphadenopathy, and an increase in peripheral lymphocytes, many atypical. It responds to tetracycline. The mode of transmission is unknown.

Recently, *Ehrlichia canis*, the cause of canine ehrlichiosis transmitted by ticks, has been found to cause a naturally acquired human disease in the U.S.

Selected Readings

BOOKS AND REVIEW ARTICLES

Baca OG, Paretsky D: Q fever and *Coxiella burnetii*: A model for host–parasite interactions. Microbiol Rev 47: 127, 1983

Burgdorfer W, Anacker RL (eds): Rickettsiae and Rickettsial Diseases. New York, Academic Press, 1981

Moulder JW: Comparative biology of intracellular parasitism. Microbiol Rev 49:298, 1985

Strickland GT (ed): Hunter's Tropical Medicine, III; Rickettsial and Chlamydial Infections, 6 Ed, pp 198–228. Philadelphia, W.B. Saunders, 1984

Tigertt WD, Benenson AS, Gochenour WS: Airborne Q fever. Bacteriol Rev 25:285, 1961

Traub R, Wisseman CL Jr, Farhang-Azad A: The ecology of murine typhus—A critical review. Trop Dis Bull 75:237, 1978

Weiss E: The biology of rickettsiae. Annu Rev Microbiol 35:345, 1982

Weiss E, Dobson ME, Dasch GA: Biochemistry of rickettsiae: Recent advances. Acta Virol 31:271, 1987

Wisseman CL Jr: Selected observations on rickettsiae and their host cells. Acta Virol 30:81, 1986

Wisseman CL Jr: Rickettsiae: Diversity in obligate intracellular parasitism. In Schlessinger D (ed): Microbiology—1983, p 375. Washington, DC, American Society for Microbiology, 1983

Wolbach SB, Todd JL, Palfrey FW: The Etiology and Pathology of Typhus. Cambridge, MA, Harvard University Press, 1922

WHO Working Group on Rickettsial Diseases: Rickettsioses: A continuing disease problem. Bull WHO 60:157, 1982

Zinsser H: Rats, Lice and History. Boston, Little, Brown, 1955

SPECIFIC ARTICLES

Atkinson WH, Winkler HH: Permeability of *Rickettsia prowazekii* to NAD. J Bacteriol 171:761, 1989

Carl M, Ching W-M, Dasch GA: Recognition of typhus group rickettsia-infected targets by human lymphokine-activated killer cells. Infect Immun 56:2526, 1988

Carl M, Robbins F-M, Hartzman RJ, Dasch GA: Lysis of cells infected with typhus group rickettsiae by a human cytotoxic T cell clone. J Immunol 139:4203, 1987

Clements ML, Wisseman CL Jr, Woodward TE, et al: Reactogenicity, immunogenicity and efficacy of a chick embryo cell-derived vaccine for Rocky Mountain spotted fever. J Infect Dis 148:922, 1983

Crist AE, Wisseman CL Jr, Murphy JR: Characteristics of lymphoid cells that adoptively transfer immunity to *Rickettsia mooseri* in mice. Infect Immun 44:55, 1984

Khavkin T, Tabibzadeh SS: Histologic, immunofluorescence, and electron microscopic study of infectious process in mouse lung after intranasal challenge with *Coxiella burnetii*. Infect Immun 56:1792, 1988

Li H, Jerrells TR, Spitalny GL, Walker DH: Gamma interferon as a crucial host defense against *Rickettsia conorii* in vivo. Infect Immun 55:1252, 1987

Maeda K, Markowitz N, Hawley RC et al: Human infection with *Ehrlichia canis*, a leukocytic rickettsia. N Engl J Med 316:853, 1987

McDonald GA, Anacker RL, Mann RE, Milch LJ: Protection of guinea pigs from experimental Rocky Mountain spotted fever with a cloned antigen of *Rickettsia rickettsii*. J Infect Dis 158:228, 1988

Ormsbee R, Peacock M, Gerloff R, Tallent G, Wike D: Limits of rickettsial infectivity. Infect Immun 19:239, 1978

Osterman JV: Rickettsiae and hosts. Acta Virol 29:166, 1985

Silverman DJ, Santucci LA: Potential for free radical-induced lipid peroxidation as a cause of endothelial cell injury in Rocky Mountain spotted fever. Infect Immun 56:3110, 1988

Winkler HH: Rickettsial permeability: An ADP–ATP transport system. J Biol Chem 251:389, 1976

Winkler H: Rickettsiae: Intracytoplasmic life. ASM News 48:184, 1982

Winkler HH: Early events in the interaction of the obligate intracytoplasmic parasite, *Rickettsia prowazekii*, with eucaryotic cells: Entry and lysis. Ann Inst Pasteur Microbiol 137(A):333, 1986

Woese CR: Bacterial evolution. Microbiol Rev 51:221, 1987

Woodward TE, Pedersen CE Jr, Oster CN et al: Prompt confirmation of Rocky Mountain spotted fever: Identification of rickettsiae in skin tissues. J Infect Dis 134:297, 1976

39

Julius Schachter

Chlamydiae

General Characteristics

TAXONOMY

The genus *Chlamydia* comprises two species, *C. trachomatis* and *C. psittaci*. They are obligate intracellular bacteria that have been placed in their own order and family (*Chlamydiales, Chlamydiaceae*). These organisms are differentiated from other bacteria by their morphology, by a common group antigen, and by a unique developmental cycle involving two morphologic forms—one adapted to extracellular survival and the other to intracellular multiplication.

Because chlamydiae are small and multiply only within susceptible cells, they were long thought to be viruses. However, their cellular organization, mechanisms of macromolecule synthesis and cell division, and antibiotic susceptibility are typically bacterial. Chlamydiae can be seen, without detail, in the light microscope: the genome (660×10^6 daltons) is about one-third the size of the *E. coli* genome and slightly larger than that of mycoplasma.

Many different strains have been isolated from birds and from man and other mammals. They have been classified in two species on the basis of properties listed in Table 39–1. There is strong homology of DNA within each species but surprisingly little between the two, suggesting long-standing evolutionary separation. Within each species different biovars and serovars can be distinguished on the basis of host range, disease pattern, and Ag composition.

The two species differ markedly in distribution. **C. trachomatis specifically parasitizes humans** and has no known animal reservoirs (except for a few rodent strains, which have not been shown to infect humans). It can be divided into three biovars, associated with different diseases and differentiated serologically and by invasive properties. The **lymphogranuloma venereum**

TABLE 39–1. Division of Chlamydiae into Species

Property	C. trachomatis	C. psittaci
Susceptibility to sulfonamides	Sensitive	Resistant
Type of inclusion produced	More compact	More diffuse
Presence of glycogen in inclusion	Yes	No
% G + C	~44%	~41%
Principal hosts	Man	Birds and mammals
Diseases induced	Trachoma Inclusion conjunctivitis Lymphogranuloma venereum Urethritis Cervicitis Salpingitis Mouse pneumonitis	Ornithosis, psittacosis Many diseases and subclinical infections of mammals and birds

(Adapted from Gordon FB, Quan AL: J Infect Dis 115:186, 1965.)

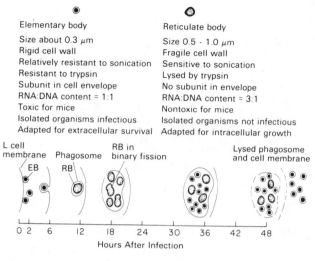

Figure 39–1. Schematic representation of the infectious cycle of chlamydiae, with characteristics of the two developmental forms of the organism.

(LGV) biovar can infect cultured cells efficiently, whereas the **trachoma** biovar requires mechanical assistance, such as centrifugation of the inoculum. In naturally occurring disease, the LGV biovar appears to infect endothelial and lymphoid cells, while the trachoma biovar infects squamocolumnar cells. The third, murine biovar is represented by the mouse pneumonitis agent.

In contrast, **C. psittaci is virtually ubiquitous among avian species** and is a common pathogen of mammals. It is known to infect humans only as zoonoses. The human being is a dead-end host, but there is some evidence for strains circulating among humans. No systematic schema for differentiating the many biovars and serovars has been developed.

A third species, **C. pneumoniae,** has been proposed to include those organisms that had been called the TWAR strains of *C. psittaci*. They are associated with **human respiratory disease** and have no known animal reservoir. These organisms can be distinguished from other chlamydiae on the basis of morphology (infectious particles are pear shaped, rather than coccoid) and lack of DNA relatedness.

Microorganisms morphologically similar to chlamydiae have been seen in electron micrographs of cells from invertebrates. They have not been cultured, and the taxonomic relations are not clear.

DEVELOPMENTAL CYCLE

The developmental cycle alternates between two forms. The **elementary body (EB),** 300 nm in diameter, is specialized for survival when released from the cell, and the **reticulate body (RB),** up to 1000 nm, is engaged in intracellular multiplication (Figs. 39–1 through 39–3). RBs are not infectious. The two forms, and the intermediate forms, all stain readily with Giemsa, Macchiavello, Castaneda, and Gimenez stains.

The first step in the infectious process involves attachment of the EB to a susceptible host cell. Attachment seems to involve a heat-labile surface component on the chlamydiae and a trypsin-sensitive receptor on the host cells, but those molecules have not been identified. Restrictions in host cell spectrum may be a function of available attachment sites. (Uptake of chlamydiae by

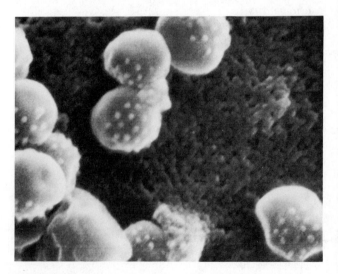

Figure 39–2. Elementary body of *C. trachomatis,* showing the hemispheric surface projections found on one pole of the cell.

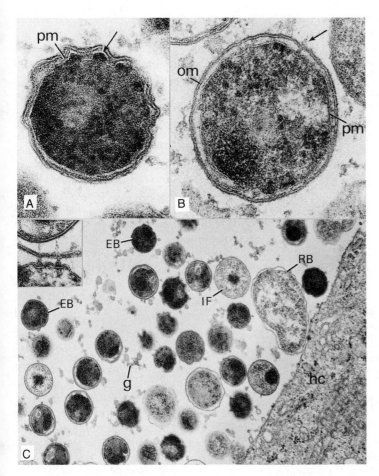

Figure 39–3. *(A)* Section of elementary body of *C. trachomatis*, showing that the hemispheric projections *(arrow)* are specializations of the plasma membrane *(pm)*. (×150,000) *(B)* Intermediate form, showing another kind of surface projection *(arrow):* a thin, needle-like spike extending from a depression of the plasma membrane *(pm)* across the periplasmic space and through the outer membrane *(om)* and tapered at the tip. (×150,000) *(C)* Part of an inclusion in an L929 mouse fibroblast 50 hours after inoculation with *C. trachomatis* (LGV biovar). All stages of chlamydial development can be seen: elementary bodies *(EB)*, intermediate forms *(IF)*, and reticulate bodies *(RB)*. *g*, glycogen particles; *hc*, host cell cytoplasm. (×33,500) *(Inset)* The spike-like projections in a slightly disrupted intermediate form. The root of the spike inside the protoplast and the segment crossing the periplasmic space are thicker than the part projecting beyond the outer membrane (×150,000) (Nichols BA et al: New view of surface projections of *Chlamydia trachomatis*. J Bacteriol 164:344, 1985)

macrophages or granulocytes apparently does not depend on such specific attachment mechanisms.)

In the next stage, the penetration of the EB into the host cell, it appears that chlamydiae induce nonphagocytic host cells to specifically phagocytize the organism. When presented to susceptible cells along with other bacteria or with inert particles, EBs are preferentially ingested by the cell, in a process called "parasite-specified endocytosis." Electron micrographic studies suggest that entry may be via clathrin-coated pits by a mechanism analogous to receptor-mediated endocytosis.

The EB enters the cell within an endosome, often termed a **phagosome.** Like some other obligate intracellular parasites, the organism inhibits phagolysosomal fusion, and the rest of the life cycle takes place within the expanding endosome. Within a few hours after entry, the EB undergoes profound changes in its cell envelope, and the characteristic central condensate begins to disperse, to form a more homogeneous cytoplasm in which strands of nucleic acid and ribosomes are seen. The resulting RB continues to grow, and 10 to 15 hours after infection, binary fission begins.

At 20 to 30 hours after infection, some of the RBs develop central condensation of cytoplasmic contents, decrease in size, and become typical EBs. When the transition from RBs to EBs begins, many of the RBs continue to multiply until the host cell cytoplasm is almost filled by the colony. The mechanism of release of organisms is not well understood. In cell culture, most host cells autolyze 40 to 60 hours after infection, but some host cells produce uninfected daughter cells, while others appear to survive the infection by extruding the intact endosome.

The intracellular particles can be seen by light microscopy. The early students of chlamydial disease described these colonies of bacteria as inclusions, which led to such terms as **inclusion conjunctivitis** and **inclusion urethritis.**

STRUCTURE

The EB is a spherical particle with projections of the envelope (of unknown function) on one hemisphere (Fig. 39–2). Electron microscopy reveals an outer and an inner membrane. There is no peptidoglycan layer with muramic acid, but the presence of penicillin-binding proteins suggests the presence of a related cross-linked structure.

The EB envelope is rigid and resistant to sonic treatment and is relatively impermeable to macromolecules. The outer membrane contains lipopolysaccharide and hemagglutinin and has a **major outer membrane protein (MOMP)** of 39,000 to 45,000 daltons, which represents approximately 60% of the weight of the outer membrane; it apparently functions as a porin and is synthesized throughout the growth cycle. The structural rigidity of the EB appears to depend on disulfide cross-linking of MOMP molecules with each other and with other cysteine-rich proteins (which appear late in the growth cycle, when EBs are formed). An inner layer of the OM is composed of hexagonally arranged subunits.

Soon after the EB enters the phagosome, its envelope loses its rigidity, and the subunit layer is disrupted and disappears. This reorganization to the more flexible and fragile structure of the RB probably involves reduction of the cross-linked disulfide bonds. The RB cell envelope is highly permeable; it contains no hemagglutinin. The RB is less dense (Fig. 39–3), and intermediate forms have occasional spike-like projections of unknown significance (Figs. 39–2, 39–3 *inset*).

METABOLIC PROPERTIES AND NUCLEIC ACIDS

Chlamydiae have been termed **"energy parasites"** because they do not generate their own ATP. In a sense, the endosome containing them functions as a reverse mitochondrion, taking in host cell-produced ATP and releasing ADP. The dependence on host cells is even greater than that of rickettsiae (Chap. 38), which make at least some of their ATP by oxidative phosphorylation. Typically, chlamydiae require well-nourished host cells for their replication. They inhibit host cell macromolecule synthesis and then use the pool of host cell metabolites for their own synthesis.

As expected from their metabolic activity, RBs have a much higher RNA/DNA ratio than do the EBs. Ribosomes appear similar to those of other bacteria. All human *C. trachomatis* serovars contain a cryptic plasmid of approximately 4×10^6 daltons. Morphologic evidence suggests that chlamydiae have bacteriophages.

ANTIGENS

All chlamydiae contain a serologically identical lipopolysaccharide (LPS). It is quite similar to the LPS of such gram-negative bacteria as *Acinetobacter calcoaceticus* and Re mutants of *Salmonella typhimurium*. Heat-labile genus-specific Ags also exist.

There are also species- and serotype-specific Ags. The human *C. trachomatis* pathogens can be divided into 15 serovars by a microimmunofluorescence test. The A, B, Ba, and C serovars are associated with hyperendemic blinding trachoma, while the D through K serovars are commonly associated with sexually transmitted disease; the L1, L2, and L3 serovars represent the lymphogranuloma venereum biovar. Ags of species, serogroup (closely related serotypes), and serotype specificity can be found on the MOMP molecule. The genes encoding the MOMP molecules of several serovars have been cloned and sequenced. They have four variable and five conserved sequences (the latter containing the cysteine residues).

Although no specific toxin (other than LPS) has been identified, large numbers ($>10^9$) of infectious EBs inoculated intravenously into young mice cause death within 24 hours secondary to damage to the vascular endothelium. Moreover, infection of cultured cells at high multiplicity (several hundred EBs per cell) results in their death without a productive infectious process. The toxic effect can be prevented by Ab, which prevents entry of chlamydiae into the host cells. Neutralization of infectivity or of toxicity is usually type-specific.

IMMUNITY

Diseases caused by chlamydiae tend to run chronic and relapsing courses: without treatment, the same serotype of *C. trachomatis* can be found in the eye or genital tract of an individual patient for 2 to 5 years or longer, which implies continued infection rather than reinfection. This chronicity in turn implies that chlamydiae do not usually evoke a thoroughly effective immune response. Nevertheless, the natural history of trachoma, as well as some early vaccine trials, indicate that short-lived protective effects can be induced. Infection or immunization results in abundant humoral, secretory, and cell-mediated immune responses, but their role in resistance is not clear. Lymphokines, particularly gamma interferon, restrict chlamydial replication. Infections with the trachoma biovar typically take place at mucous membranes, and immunity has been correlated with the level of secretory Ab.

The immune response can also be deleterious, as more severe disease can be seen after reexposure. A Triton-soluble extract of chlamydial EBs has been shown to be capable of inducing ocular disease in previously infected animals.

In primates, infection of the eye with *C. trachomatis* can induce quite solid immunity of a few months' duration. In birds and mammals, *C. psittaci* infections induce only partial protection; an immune response occurs, but it can be overwhelmed by large challenge doses or by adverse conditions.

Clinically inapparent infections occur with virtually all chlamydial infections. Healthy **carriers** can be important in spread of infection.

CHEMOTHERAPY

In general, tetracyclines are considered the drugs of choice for all chlamydial infections, and erythromycins are the alternative for those who cannot tolerate tetracyclines (pregnant women, young children). Penicillins show some antichlamydial effect in cell culture, but they are not useful for therapy. Aminoglycosides, which do not penetrate host cells, and the newer cephalosporins show no antichlamydial activity. The former are often used in collection media to kill unwanted bacteria. Sulfonamides are active against most *C. trachomatis* strains but not against most *C. psittaci* strains. Rifampin is the most active antibiotic in cell culture, but it is not used clinically because resistance develops quickly. Quinolones are active but have not had clinical trials.

Trachoma

History and Epidemiology

Trachoma is one of the oldest known human diseases, having been well described in ancient Egyptian and Chinese writings. Once common throughout the world, it is now a major problem only in certain developing countries. Still, trachoma is the world's leading preventable cause of blindness, with more than 400 million people affected and several millions blinded. Trachoma is a disease of poverty, associated with poor environmental sanitation and personal hygiene. In the hyperendemic area, trachoma is a disease of young children, and virtually all will be infected before the age of 2 years. Active inflammatory disease usually disappears by 10 years or earlier. Blindness develops later in life, in up to 25% of those more than 60 years old. Endemic trachoma is associated with *C. trachomatis* serovars A, B, Ba, and C.

Clinical Description

Although onset can be insidious, the disease begins as a mucopurulent conjunctivitis, developing into a follicular keratoconjunctivitis. Over time, some of the follicles necrose, resulting in scarring of the conjunctivae. The scars may slowly contract, distorting the eyelid and causing an inturning of the eyelashes so that they abrade the cornea. This complex represents the blinding lesions of trachoma, called trichiasis and entropion. Trachoma often occurs in areas of the world where seasonal outbreaks of bacterial conjunctivitis make the disease worse. It is likely that severe ocular damage depends on repeated reinfection—the associated hypersensitivity probably contributes to the severity of the disease. Severe lid deformity may not develop until 20 or 30 years after active disease has waned.

Diagnosis

Diagnosis of trachoma is based mainly on clinical findings: identification of follicular reaction, papillary hypertrophy, scars within the conjunctiva, and vascularization (pannus) of the cornea. Laboratory diagnosis is often based on demonstration of typical chlamydial inclusions or EBs in stained conjunctival smears. Fluorescent Ab methods are more sensitive than the classic Giemsa stain for this purpose. Chlamydiae may be readily isolated from active cases in cell culture systems. This is the most sensitive laboratory test.

Serologic tests are not useful for diagnosing individual cases. In hyperendemic areas, the great majority of individuals have serum Abs to *C. trachomatis*. Abs in tears correlate with intensity of the disease.

Prevention and Treatment

Experimental vaccines have induced a short-lived immune response, but some vaccinees developed more severe disease, suggesting hypersensitivity to the organism. Trachoma control is currently based on mass treatment of all affected individuals within a village setting with topical tetracycline ointment and on surgical intervention to correct lid deformities. These efforts are aimed at preventing blindness, not at eradication of trachoma. Improved living conditions provide the most effective control.

GENITAL TRACT INFECTIONS BY C. TRACHOMATIS

In industrialized society, *C. trachomatis* is now considered to be the **most common sexually transmitted pathogen.** In the United States, it is estimated that more than 3 million new infections occur each year (compared with 1.8 million gonococcal infections and approximately 500,000 genital infections with *Herpesvirus hominis*). These infections are also important in the developing countries.

The recognized clinical spectrum of chlamydial infection has expanded greatly since tissue culture methods for isolating chlamydiae came into broad use in the 1970s. Before then the most common diseases attributed to *C. trachomatis* in industrialized society were inclusion conjunctivitis in adults or neonates (see below); its origin by inoculation of infective genital tract discharges into the eye was recognized only later.

Clinical Description

In the male, *C. trachomatis* is recognized as the cause of 35% to 50% of cases of nongonococcal urethritis (NGU). NGU has an incubation period of 1 to 3 weeks and usually causes a mucopurulent discharge and dysuria. Ascending infections can occur, resulting in epididymitis.

C. trachomatis is now recognized as the leading cause of epididymitis in sexually active young men. Chlamydial proctitis is relatively common among homosexual males.

In the female, the most commonly affected site is the cervix, where the organism can cause a mucopurulent endocervicitis. This condition is characterized by a mucopurulent endocervical discharge. Urethral infections occur and can cause a "sterile" pyuria in young women. Ascending genital infection is common. *C. trachomatis* is found in the endometrium or fallopian tubes of approximately 25% of cases of acute salpingitis in the U.S. Chlamydiae are also an important cause of infertility and ectopic pregnancy as a result of tubal damage. Unfortunately, the preceding chlamydial salpingitis can be clinically mild or even inapparent.

Pathogenesis and Transmission

These chlamydial infections are sexually transmitted. The highest risk groups appear to be sexually active adolescents, particularly in lower socioeconomic groups. Approximately one in six sexually active adolescent females has a chlamydial infection, usually inapparent. Infection with *C. trachomatis* is similar to infection with *Neisseria gonorrhoeae* in transmission and in clinical outcome, although typically less acute. Approximately 20% of heterosexual men, and 40% of women, with gonorrhea have concomitant chlamydial infections. Successful treatment of gonococcal infection with penicillins will often be followed by postgonococcal urethritis or cervicitis secondary to persistent chlamydial infection. It is therefore recommended that drugs active against *C. trachomatis* be included in the treatment of gonorrhea.

Diagnosis

Definitive diagnosis is made by isolation of the agent in cell culture systems. Serology does not play a role in diagnosing uncomplicated genital tract infections, although the higher Ab levels seen by the micro-IF test in complications (epididymitis, salpingitis, etc.) may provide some support for a clinical diagnosis. Ag detection, based on the use of fluorescein-conjugated monoclonal Abs or enzyme immunoassay, is simpler and less expensive but also less sensitive than cell culture. Some chlamydial diseases can be treated on a presumptive basis. Urethritis in men can be easily managed without a specific diagnosis, on the basis of a gram stain (exclusion of gonorrhea by failure to demonstrate gram-negative diplococci in polymorphonuclear leukocytes). Women with mucopurulent endocervicitis or salpingitis should be automatically treated for chlamydial infection. Treatment of sex partners is always indicated.

Prevention and Treatment

No program for prevention of sexually transmitted chlamydial infection has been presented. Use of barrier contraceptives will reduce transmission. Treatment of uncomplicated genital tract infection with 2 g tetracycline/day for 7 days results in cure rates in excess of 95%. Upper genital tract infections call for longer courses of therapy. Short-term therapy plays no role in the management of chlamydial infections.

NEONATAL INFECTIONS

Approximately 60% to 70% of infants born through a chlamydia-infected birth canal show serologic evidence of infection. About one in three of the exposed infants develops **inclusion conjunctivitis of the newborn** (ICN). ICN has an incubation period of 5 to 21 days and usually resolves in a few months without treatment.

Approximately one in six exposed infants develops a characteristic **pneumonia syndrome.** The incubation period is usually between 2 and 12 weeks. The infants often have a prodrome of rhinitis, and many will have conjunctivitis. Affected infants are usually afebrile, are markedly tachypneic and occasionally apneic, and have a staccato cough. There are long-term consequences of this disease. Most infants with chlamydia pneumonia develop chronic respiratory tract disease. Vaginal and gastrointestinal tract infections also occur but have no known clinical consequences.

Diagnosis

Conjunctivitis may be diagnosed readily by any of the cytologic tests. Giemsa stain is adequate in diagnosing severe cases, and the fluorescent-Ab techniques are quite sensitive. The agent may be readily isolated.

A specific diagnosis for pneumonia may be more difficult because of sampling problems, but the organism can usually be isolated from the nasopharynx or tracheobronchial aspirates. Infants with chlamydial pneumonia almost always develop high IgM Ab levels, and because of their defined exposure (at birth), the diagnosis may be readily established on the basis of a single-point determination of specific antichlamydial IgM Ab exceeding 1:32 in the micro-IF test.

Prevention and Treatment

Chlamydial infection in the infant calls for systemic therapy with erythromycin (50 mg/kg in divided doses each day), 7 to 14 days for conjunctivitis and 14 to 21 days for pneumonia. Topical therapy is not recommended for ICN because of the relatively high failure rates and the need to eradicate extraocular infection and prevent subsequent development of pneumonia.

Ocular prophylaxis with erythromycin given soon after birth appears to prevent the development of ICN but not the development of pneumonia. *C. trachomatis* is a far more common pathogen in the U.S. than is *N. gonorrhoeae.* Thus, it seems reasonable to recommend routine ocular prophylaxis be based on use of **erythromycin** or **tetracycline** ointment, which appears to be effective against *N. gonorrhoeae* and *C. trachomatis*, instead of silver nitrate (standard Credé prophylaxis), which is active against the gonococcus but not chlamydia. This recommendation, however, should not carry over into areas where antibiotic-resistant *Neisseriae* are a problem until further studies determine efficacy.

Pregnant women can be screened for chlamydial infection; erythromycin treatment of those found to be infected will prevent perinatal transmission.

LYMPHOGRANULOMA VENEREUM

Lymphogranuloma venereum has been known for 200 years, but it is not a well-studied entity. It is caused by a **special (LGV) biovar** of *C. trachomatis* that includes several serovars. Although worldwide in distribution, LGV is more common in Southeast Asia, India, and Africa. In contrast with infections with the other *C. trachomatis* biovar, which seems to be restricted to growth in squamocolumnar cells, infections are systemic and typically involve endothelial and lymphoid cells. LGV is transmitted sexually, and it is probably far more common than is reported.

Clinical Description

The incubation period is variable (usually 1 to 3 weeks, but it may be much longer). The first manifestation of the disease appears to be a primary lesion—a painless superficial ulcer or vesicle on the genitals. In tropical countries, the ulcerative form of the disease appears to be quite important. Within 1 to 3 weeks, regional lymphadenopathy (the secondary stage of the disease) is typically seen in young men. (Women probably have primary implantation of the organism within the vagina, where the draining lymph nodes will be retroperitoneal rather than inguinal; they usually do not develop inguinal lymphadenopathy.) The lymph nodes will ultimately heal with scarring, but the infection can persist and cause late destructive lesions involving the gastrointestinal tract and genitalia. Scarring can result in obstruction, and fistulae are common. Primary implantation within the rectum can result in a severe proctocolitis, not an uncommon condition among homosexual men in some parts of the U.S.

Diagnosis

LGV results in relatively high complement-fixing Ab levels, which may be used to support a diagnosis. The micro-IF test can be used the same way. Chlamydiae can be isolated from ulcers, lymph node aspirates, rectal swabs, or biopsies. A delayed hypersensitivity skin test (Frei test) is no longer used in the U.S. because of problems with sensitivity and specificity; it is still available in some other countries.

The treatment of choice appears to be at least 2 weeks of tetracycline at 2 g/day.

Psittacosis (Ornithosis)

Human psittacosis is a disease contracted from exposure to avian species infected with *C. psittaci*. The term "ornithosis" is also used because the infection in birds is not restricted to psittacines. The organism is ubiquitous among avian species, usually infecting the intestinal tract. It is also common in domestic mammals, but they are seldom a source of human infection. This zoonosis is relatively uncommon, with only a few hundred cases occurring each year in the U.S.

Pathogenesis and Transmission in Birds

Infected birds may be totally asymptomatic or may be severely ill, with some flocks of birds suffering fatality rates in excess of 50%. The birds often have diarrhea, shedding copious amounts of organism, and they may have respiratory tract infection and conjunctivitis. Asymptomatic shedders can still provide sufficient environmental contamination to effect transmission. *C. psittaci* can remain viable in dust and cage litter for months.

Human Infection

Human psittacosis usually occurs in either a **respiratory** or a **typhoidal** form. Respiratory disease can be a mild influenzal disease, or it can develop into a severe and fatal (if untreated) pneumonia. The incubation period is typically 1 to 3 weeks. Fever, chills, and severe headache usually occur. Radiographs may show more extensive lung involvement than is expected from the respiratory difficulty.

The typhoidal form of the disease involves a general toxic febrile state without respiratory findings. Person-to-person transmission is uncommon but has occurred.

Serologic surveys indicate that most human infections with *C. psittaci* from domestic mammals are subclinical. However, several case reports suggest that *C. psittaci* causing abortions in lower mammals may also cause abortions in humans.

Diagnosis

Clinical signs are not pathognomonic. The clinician's index of suspicion (asking questions about potential exposure to birds) is usually crucial to arriving at a diagnosis. Serodiagnosis is generally considered to be the method of choice, because isolation of the agent is seldom achieved. Rising Ab levels can be demonstrated by CF or micro-IF tests.

Prevention and Treatment

Human psittacosis is considered an occupational hazard for those in the poultry or pet bird industries. Chemoprophylaxis for exotic birds is available, and clean premises can be maintained by avoiding introduction of untreated birds. Tetracycline, 2 g/day for at least 2 weeks, is considered the treatment of choice, with erythromycin being the alternative drug.

Chlamydia pneumoniae Infections

Recent findings suggest a distinct group of chlamydiae circulating among the humans. Serosurveys indicate that these "TWAR" strains have a worldwide distribution (TW from Taiwan, reflecting geographic locale of the first isolate; AR for acute respiratory, reflecting disease association of the second isolate). Abs to these organisms are first detected in children less than 5 years old and prevalence rates may exceed 45% by age 30 to 40. The organism is probably spread by the respiratory route. It has been associated with epidemics of mild pneumonia in young adults. Severe, even fatal pneumonias have been seen in debilitated adults and young children. These organisms are susceptible to tetracyclines and erythromycins.

Selected Reading

BOOKS AND REVIEW ARTICLES

Becker Y: The chlamydia: Molecular biology of procaryotic obligate parasites of eucaryocytes. Microbiol Rev 42:274, 1978

Darougar S (ed): Chlamydial Disease. Br Med Bull 39(2), 1983

Holmes KK: The chlamydia epidemic. JAMA 245:1718, 1981

Mårdh P-A, Holmes KK, Oriel JD, Piot P, Schachter J (eds): Chlamydial Infections. Amsterdam, Elsevier Biomedical Press, 1982

Moulder JW: The Psittacosis Group as Bacteria. New York, John Wiley, 1964

Moulder JW: Comparative biology of intracellular parasitism. Microbiol Rev 49:298, 1985

Oriel JD, Ridgway GL: Genital Infection by *Chlamydia trachomatis*. London, Edward Arnold Ltd, 1982

Schachter J: Chlamydial infections. N Engl J Med 298:428; 490; 540, 1978

Schachter J, Caldwell HD: Chlamydiae. Annu Rev Microbiol 34:285, 1980

Schachter J, Dawson CR: Human Chlamydial Infections. Littleton, MA, Publishing Sciences Group, 1978

Schachter J, Grossman M: Chlamydial infections. Annu Rev Med 32:45, 1981

SPECIFIC ARTICLES

Beem MO, Saxon EM: Respiratory-tract colonization and a distinctive pneumonia syndrome in infants infected with *Chlamydia trachomatis*. N Engl J Med 296:306, 1977

Berger RE, Alexander ER, Monda GD et al: *Chlamydia trachomatis* as a cause of acute "idiopathic" epididymitis. N Engl J Med 298:301, 1978

Dawson CR, Daghfous T, Messadi M et al: Severe endemic trachoma in Tunisia. Br J Ophthalmol 60:245, 1976

Holmes KK, Handsfield HH, Wang S-P et al: Etiology of nongonococcal urethritis. N Engl J Med 292:1199, 1975

Mårdh P-A, Ripa T, Svensson L, Westrom L: *Chlamydia trachomatis* infection in patients with acute salpingitis. N Engl J Med 296:1377, 1977

Moulder JW: Looking at chlamydiae without looking at their hosts. ASM News 50:353, 1984

Schachter J, Holt J, Goodner E et al: Prospective study of chlamydial infection in neonates. Lancet 2:377, 1979

Sweet RL, Schachter J, Robbie M: Failure of beta lactam antibiotics to eradicate *Chlamydia trachomatis* in the endometrium despite apparent clinical cure of acute salpingitis. JAMA 250:2641, 1983

40

Wallace A. Clyde, Jr.
Robert M. Chanock,
Joseph G. Tully

Mycoplasmas

General Characteristics

Contagious bovine **pleuropneumonia,** a fatal disease of cattle that created considerable economic loss, was first recognized in Germany in 1693 and reached the United States in 1843. Pasteur suggested that the cause was a specific ultramicroscopic agent, as bacteria could not be seen in serous exudate capable of producing the disease. The causative agent was cultivated by Nocard and Roux, in 1898, in a collodion sac filled with serum-broth in the peritoneal cavity of a rabbit and then on a serum-enriched medium. The organisms were difficult to detect—the colonies were very small, the individual organisms did not take up most stains—and they were too small to be defined morphologically at that time.

A number of similar microorganisms were isolated from animals and sewage between 1920 and 1940 and were termed **pleuropneumonia-like organisms (PPLO).** These organisms, now termed mycoplasmas, are the smallest free-living cells known. They lack the rigid peptidoglycan cell wall of eubacteria, yet they contain the minimal macromolecular constituents for replication in a cell-free environment. For this reason, and because their membrane is readily accessible, they are of considerable interest to molecular biologists.

Mycoplasms are closely related in rRNA sequence to clostridia and hence appear to have evolved from that group by degeneration of the capacity to form peptidoglycan. Their genome is only about one-third as large as that of most eubacteria, suggesting that their slow replication has allowed them to dispense with genes, not only for wall formation, but also perhaps for regulatory mechanisms that improve metabolic efficiency.

More than 70 organisms belonging to this group have now been recognized, including 12 species that infect man. They include important pathogens of animals, plants, and insects; they are also a significant part of the normal microbial flora of most animals; and they include saprobes. *Mycoplasma pneumoniae* has been established as the etiologic agent of primary atypical pneumonia, and mycoplasmas also appear to be involved in some cases of nongonococcal urethritis and pelvic inflammatory disease.

Mycoplasmas resemble chlamydiae, rickettsiae, and viruses in passing through 450-nm filters, but they differ in being able to grow (although slowly) on artificial media. They often appear as contaminants during the passage of viruses (in animals, chick embryos, or tissue cultures), and many mycoplasmas were initially mistaken for viruses. Their filterability is attributable, not only to their small size, but also to the flexibility of their cell envelope.

Because mycoplasmas are bounded only by a membrane, they have been designated as the class *Mollicutes* (L. *mollis* and *cutis*, soft skin). We shall follow the traditional practice of referring to all members of the class as mycoplasmas, one genus being *Mycoplasma*. Taxonomic divisions (Table 40–1) are based on nutritional requirements (particularly involving sterols), biochemical activities, genome size, morphology, and serologic characteristics.

L FORMS OF BACTERIA. Mycoplasmas were long confused with the L-phase variants of various eubacteria, which also lack a rigid cell wall and hence resemble them in cellular and colonial morphology, filterability, and slow growth. However, the loss of wall in L forms is often reversible. These variants are discussed in Chapter 41.

TABLE 40–1. Taxonomy of the Mycoplasmas

Class: Mollicutes
    Order: Mycoplasmatales
        Family I: Mycoplasmataceae
            Sterol required for growth
            Genome size about 5×10^8 daltons
            NADH oxidase localized in cytoplasm
            Genus I: *Mycoplasma* (over 60 species)
                Do not hydrolyze urea
            Genus II: *Ureaplasma* (2 species with serotypes)
                Hydrolyze urea
        Family II: Acholeplasmataceae
            Sterol not required for growth
            Genome size about 10^9 daltons
            NADH oxidase localized in the membrane
            Genus I: *Acholeplasma* (8 species)
        Family III: Spiroplasmataceae
            Helical organisms during some phase of growth
            Sterol required for growth
            Genome size about 10^9 daltons
            NADH oxidase localized in cytoplasm
            Genus I: *Spiroplasma* (4 species)
Genus of uncertain taxonomic position
    Anaeroplasma (2 species)

MORPHOLOGY

Electron microscopy has shown that in cellular morphology, the mycoplasmas are extremely variable and pleomorphic, even within a pure culture. Some organisms assume a predominantly spherical appearance (300–800 nm in diameter), whereas others may form **filaments** of uniform diameter (100–300 nm) that range in length from 3 μm to more than 150 μm. Most mycoplasmas stain gram-negative. The **spiroplasmas** vary over a range that includes pleomorphic spherical cells (200–300 nm in diameter), helical filaments (Fig. 40–1), and branched, nonhelical filaments.

Variations in the size and shape of mycoplasmas, as well as their poor staining, can be ascribed to their lack of a cell wall. Also, preparative techniques used in electron microscopy may distort the organisms. Thin sections reveal a simple ultrastructure consisting of a cell membrane and cytoplasm, including ribosomes and the characteristic prokaryotic nucleoid.

Some mycoplasmas have a specialized **terminal structure** that appears to play a role in attachment. These include *M. gallisepticum* (a respiratory pathogen of birds; Fig. 40–2) and *M. pneumoniae* (Fig. 40–3). These species exhibit a type of **gliding motility,** which may also involve the specialized terminal organelles.

Spiroplasmas also exhibit motility but of a different type, characterized by a rotary or "screwing" motion of the helix accompanied by flexional movements. Because they lack flagella and axial filaments, their movement may depend on intracellular contractile elements.

COLONIAL MORPHOLOGY. On solid medium, most mycoplasmas form very small colonies (50–600 μm in diameter), which can be seen only with a hand lens or under the low power of a microscope. Some of the acholeplasmas, however, may yield visible colonies (up to 5 mm). The classic "**fried-egg**" appearance of the usual colony is the result of an opaque, granular central zone of growth down into the agar (whose fibers may help cell division) and a flat, translucent peripheral zone of growth on the surface (Fig. 40–4A). Not all mycoplasmas produce "fried-egg" colonies (Fig. 40–4B), and variations in colonial morphology, such as size and the extent of the central zone, are frequently dependent on the constituents and the hydration of the medium and on aerobiosis. Ureaplasmas were designated earlier as tiny or **T-strains** because they form only 15-μm to 30-μm colonies on unbuffered medium.

MODE OF REPRODUCTION

Mycoplasmas usually divide, like other prokaryotes, by binary fission, but genomic replication and cytoplasmic division are not precisely synchronized and are easily

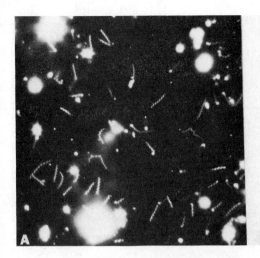

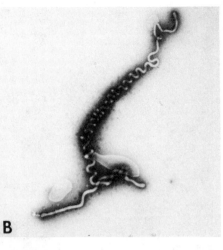

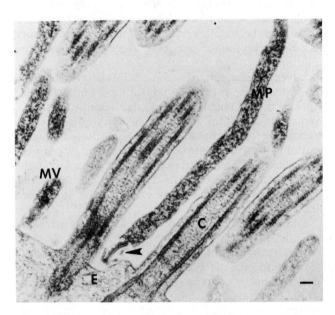

Figure 40–1. (A) Helical morphology of a spiroplasma (suckling mouse cataract agent) observed by dark-field microscopy. Photograph of the chorioallantoic fluid of embryonated hen's egg 4 days after yolk sac inoculation with spiroplasmas. (×2800) (B) Electron photomicrographs of a helical filament of *Spiroplasma citri* negatively stained with ammonium molybdate. Note sac-like blebs emerging from main helical body. *Bar* represents 1.0 μm. (A, Tully JG et al: Nature 259:117, 1976; B, courtesy of RM Cole)

dissociated. A lag in cytoplasmic division yields multinucleated filaments, which subsequently form chains of coccoid cells and then fragment into individual cells. Cells less than about 300 nm, like the "minicells" of certain mutant eubacteria, probably do not receive a complete genome. Fission by budding is observed in some species.

Mycoplasmas have a circular genome of doublestranded DNA, one-fifth to one-half as large as that in

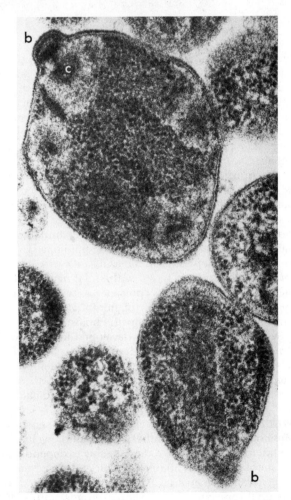

Figure 40–2. Electron photomicrograph of thin section of *Mycoplasma gallisepticum* showing specialized terminal structures. The densely stained structures consist of a "bleb" *(b)* and its infrableb core *(c)*. (×70,000; Maniloff J, Quinlan DC: Ann NY Acad Sci 225:181, 1973)

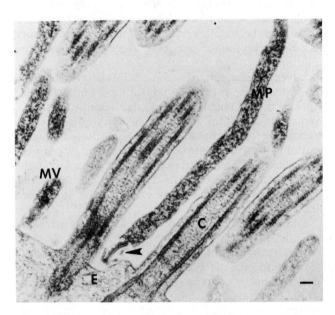

Figure 40–3. Electron photomicrograph of *Mycoplasma pneumoniae* infection of a hamster tracheal organ culture. Note filamentous structure of the organism *(MP)* with its specialized tip *(arrow)* in close apposition to the epithelial surface *(E)*. Also note proximity of several cilia *(C)* and a microvillus *(MV)*. The tip has a dense central core and is separated by a lucent space from the limiting unit membrane of the organism. *Bar* represents 0.1 μm. (Courtesy of AM Collier)

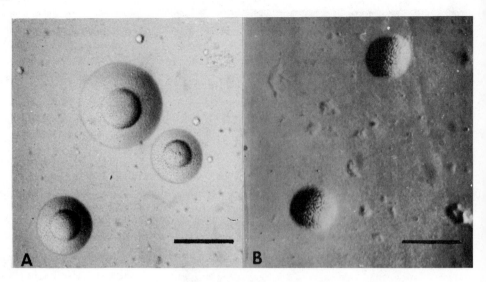

Figure 40–4. (**A**) Mycoplasma colonies (*Acholeplasma axanthum*) on the surface of solid medium. Note the classic "fried egg" appearance produced by central penetration of growth into the agar and peripheral growth on the surface. *Bar* represents 100 μm. (**B**) Morphology of *Mycoplamsa pneumoniae* colonies on agar medium. Note the "mulberry-like" appearance of colonies and absence of a peripheral halo. *Bar* represents 100 μm. (Chanock RM et al: Proc Natl Acad Sci USA 48:41, 1962)

most bacteria. This is evidently the smallest genome that can code for all the products needed for self-reproduction at the expense of the foodstuffs in an artificial medium. DNA hybridization has demonstrated relatedness among different mycoplasmas of the same serotype.

Mycoplasma genomes have a low G + C content (23–45 moles %). The G + C of their rRNA (43%–48%) is outside the range of eubacteria (50%–54%), indicating much evolutionary separation. Their lipids are also unusual: more than 50% contain glucose. Both lytic and temperate **bacteriophages** have been recovered from mycoplasmas.

Mycoplasmas generally grow more slowly than bacteria, with a mean generation time of 1 to 3 hours; for a few species it is so long (6–9 hours) that visible growth may require 1 to 2 weeks. *Acholeplasma laidlawii* is unusual in producing visible turbidity in 18 to 24 hours in broth cultures enriched with serum. The optimum temperature for growth of all *Mycoplasma* and *Ureaplasma* species is 37°C, but spiroplasmas and acholeplasmas (found in plants or as saprobes) have a wide temperature range (22°–37°C).

Many mycoplasmas utilize either glucose (fermentative) or arginine (nonfermentative) as a major source of energy; those that utilize arginine convert it to ornithine via a three-enzyme system. Ureaplasmas require urea and convert it to ammonia by the action of a urease. These properties are useful in classification. Most mycoplasmas are facultatively anaerobic, but growth of some is enhanced by incubation in air with 5% CO_2. Mycoplasmas of the human oral cavity generally prefer an anaerobic environment (95% N_2 + 5% CO_2).

NUTRITION. Mycoplasmas have exacting nutritional requirements, especially for lipids needed for synthesis of the plasma membrane. The most frequently employed medium is heart infusion broth (with peptone) supplemented with 0.5% glucose, 0.2% arginine, 10% fresh yeast extract, and 20% horse serum. Additional substances are used to demonstrate pH change (phenol red), to inhibit bacterial growth (penicillin and/or thallium acetate), or to provide a solid medium (0.6%–0.8% washed or purified agar).

The nutritional requirement of many mycoplasmas for a **sterol** is unique among prokaryotes. It is usually met by animal serum, which contains cholesterol bound to a lipoprotein. **Acholeplasmas** do not need exogenous cholesterol but synthesize lipids that substitute for it in maintaining fluidity of the membrane lipid bilayer. However, some acholeplasmas, such as *A. laidlawii*, will incorporate cholesterol (up to 8% of the total membrane lipids) when grown in its presence. Sterol-containing mycoplasmas are lysed by digitonin and other substances that form complexes with cholesterol.

Selective media have been developed for isolation of *M. pneumoniae* and the ureaplasmas from clinical materials. Media for the latter must be supplemented with urea; liberation of NH_3 from urea during growth results in a change in color of the phenol red pH indicator.

INHIBITORS. Mycoplasmas are generally not sensitive to inhibitors of cell wall synthesis (penicillin, cycloserine, bacitracin). Polyenes have variable effects depending on the sterol content of the cell membrane. Mycoplasmas are generally sensitive to tetracycline, aminoglycosides, and erythromycin, but individual strains and species vary.

Strains of several *Mycoplasma* species (*M. hyopneumoniae* and *M. flocculare*) are inhibited by benzylpenicillin, and ampicillin is used instead for their isolation. Thallium acetate at 1:2000 is selectively inhibitory for gram-negative bacteria and for aerobic sporeformers, but it also inhibits ureaplasmas and should be omitted from the medium used for their recovery.

IMMUNOLOGIC CHARACTERISTICS

The principal antigenic determinants of mycoplasmas are membrane proteins and glycolipids. Capsulelike Ags, including galactan and a hexosamine polymer, have been reported in a few mycoplasmas. The protein Ags have not been well characterized.

The **glycolipids** of *M. pneumoniae*, which contain glucose and galactose, have received special attention, because they are suspected of playing a role in autoimmunity in humans. They are haptens, losing immunogenicity when separated from membrane protein. Their surface location is confirmed by agglutination of the organism, and by complement-dependent lysis by rabbit Abs to the homologous glycolipid. These Abs cross-react with glycolipids of similar structure found in certain other mycoplasmas and also in human brain and in many plants.

Species classification of mycoplasmas is based primarily on **serologic** reactions. Tests that are carried out with whole cell extracts (complement fixation [CF], immunodiffusion) tend to show group relations. Tests that detect membrane Ags (growth inhibition, metabolism inhibition, and immunofluorescence) are more specific. The direct identification of mycoplasma colonies on agar by **immunofluorescence** (Fig. 40–5) is rapid and specific, and it has the additional advantage of detecting a mixture of mycoplasmas of different serotypes in the same culture—an important feature, as clinical material frequently contains more than one species.

In the **growth inhibition** (GI) test, growth of the organism on agar is inhibited in a zone around a filter paper disc saturated with specific antiserum. The **metabolism inhibition** test is based on inhibition of growth by specific Ab, as indicated by the inhibition of a metabolic activity (glucose fermentation, hydrolysis of arginine or urea, or reduction of tetrazolium). This technique has also been applied to the measurement of specific Abs.

The ureaplasmas of human origin represent a special problem in classification. At least eight serotypes have been distinguished; they are temporarily designated as a single species, *Ureaplasma urealyticum*, with numbered serotypes. Ureaplasmas from nonhuman hosts may represent additional species and types.

MYCOPLASMAL FLORA OF MAN

At least 12 serologically and biologically distinct mycoplasmas have been found in man (Table 40–2). A majority of those recovered from the **oral cavity** are commensals, which do not appear to play a role in disease; *M. orale* and *M. salivarium* are found in almost every healthy adult. The reported frequency of *M. hominis* and ureaplasmas range from 0 to 9%, and others are found in less than 0.1% of various population groups.

In the genital tract, *M. hominis* and the ureaplasmas are present in a large proportion of sexually active adults, whereas *M. fermentans* and *M. primatum* have been recovered infrequently. Genital mycoplasmas colonize 20% to 30% of newborns at the time of birth but usually only transiently. Following puberty, colonization occurs primarily as a result of sexual activity: these organisms can be recovered from only 5% to 10% of nuns and other sexual virgins, whereas in women attending venereal disease clinics, ureaplasma recovery rates as high as 75% to 80% have been observed. In the asymptomatic man, mycoplasmas may be present in the urine, semen, and distal urethra. The asymptomatic female may have organisms present over the entire genital mucosa, but not the bladder, uterus, or fallopian tubes.

Mycoplasmal Pneumonia

IDENTIFICATION OF THE ORGANISM

In the late 1930s, a group of nonbacterial pneumonias was first recognized and was given the name **primary atypical pneumonia** to distinguish them from typical (pneumococcal) lobar pneumonia. This syndrome was found to have a multiple etiology; viruses could be dem-

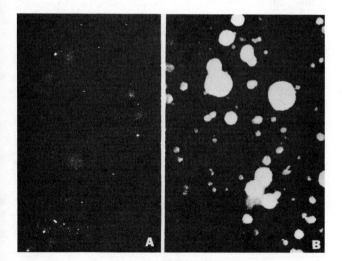

Figure 40–5. Colonies of *Mycoplasma pneumoniae* stained by the indirect immunofluorescence technique using acute-*(A)* and convalescent-*(B)* phase sera from a patient with mycoplasmal pneumonia. (Chanock RM et al: Proc Natl Acad Sci USA 48:41, 1962)

TABLE 40–2. *Properties of Mycoplasmas That Infect Man*

| Mycoplasma | Primary Site of Colonization | | Metabolic Substrate | | | Aerobic Growth (in vitro) | Hemadsorption of Guinea Pig RBCs |
	Respiratory Tract	Genitourinary Tract	Glucose	Arginine	Urea		
M. salivarium	+	−	−	+	−	−	−
M. orale	+	−	−	+	−	−	−
M. buccale	+*	−	−	+	−	−	−
M. faucium	+*	−	−	+	−	−	−
M. pneumoniae	+†	−	+	−	−	+‡	+
M. lipophilum	+*	−	−	+	−	−	−
Acholeplasma laidlawii	+*	−	+	−	−	+‡	−
M. hominis	+*	+	−	+	−	+‡	−
M. primatum	−	+*	−	+	−	−	−
M. fermentans	−	+*	+	+	−	−	−
M. genitalium	−	+	+	−	−	+‡	+
Ureaplasma urealyticum	+*	+	−	−	+	−	−§

* Rare.

† Does not colonize; rather, produces acute or subacute infection.

‡ Also grow anaerobically.

§ Serotype 3 hemadsorbs guinea pig red cells.

onstrated in some patients, but not in an additional large group, who developed cold agglutinins (which agglutinate certain RBCs at low temperature). Attempts to isolate the etiologic agent were unsuccessful until Eaton reported that a filterable organism could be passaged serially in embryonated eggs: there were no discernible changes (**"blind passage"**), but tissue extracts and extra-embryonic fluids from these eggs (like the original filtrate) produced pneumonia in cotton rats and hamsters. Confirmation was delayed for years, but the subsequent development of an immunofluorescence test, with sections of infected chick embryo lung as Ag, facilitated detection of the organism and measurement of the corresponding Abs. The tiny organisms were later seen as coccobacillary bodies, after Giemsa staining, on the surface of the bronchial epithelium of infected chick embryos.

The Eaton agent was considered to be a virus, but a problem arose when it was shown to be inhibited by tetracycline or streptomycin. (This feature of bacteria might have been recognized earlier in patients, but the results were inconsistent because the syndrome included viral infections.) The organism was finally cultivated on a cell-free medium in 1962 by Chanock, Hayflick, and Barile, identified by immunofluorescence with convalescent serum (Fig. 40–5), confirmed as an etiologic agent in human volunteers, and designated *Mycoplasma pneumoniae*. It forms circular colonies partially embedded in the agar, with a granular, "mulberry" surface (Fig. 40–4*B*) but without the light peripheral zone observed with many other mycoplasmas.

The colonies cause **β-hemolysis,** large enough to be seen without magnification, when overlaid with guinea pig RBCs (Fig. 40–6). This reaction is caused by the organism's production of hydrogen peroxide in larger amounts than other human mycoplasmas (which produce a slow, α-type hemolysis).

PATHOGENESIS

Unlike other mycoplasmas that inhibit the respiratory tract, *M. pneumoniae* can attach to the surface of the respiratory epithelium, its tip binding to neuraminic acid receptors (see Fig. 40–3). The organism does not enter host cells, nor does it penetrate beneath the epithelial surface. In tracheal organ cultures, its attachment leads to direct damage of the epithelium, with ciliostasis, loss of cilia, and finally cell death. This cell damage may be produced by the hydrogen peroxide released by the organisms; there is no evidence for the production of a protein exotoxin.

Because children 2 to 5 years of age often possess mycoplasmacidal Abs, while the disease appears most often at age 5 to 15, it has been suggested that the pathogenic effects of *M. pneumoniae* may include an **immunopathologic reaction** in a host sensitized by prior infection. Reinfection occurs with appreciable frequency, and second attacks of *M. pneumoniae* pneumonia have been documented. Additional support for the sensitization hypothesis is provided by the observation that thymic ablation preceding experimental infection of hamsters prevents the development of characteristic pulmonary

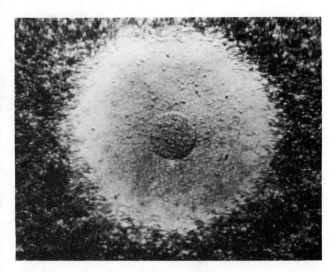

Figure 40–6. β-Hemolytic plaque produced by a 5-day colony of *Mycoplasma pneumoniae* overlaid with guinea pig RBCs in agar and reincubated for 48 hours. Mycoplasma colony is the small circular structure in the center of the plaque. (Chanock RM et al: Am Rev Resp Dis [Suppl]:223, 1963)

infiltration by mononuclear cells. However, it is not certain that this type of infiltrate is responsible for the symptoms experienced by patients with *M. pnemoniae* disease.

An immunopathologic basis of *M. pneumoniae* disease represents an intriguing possibility. Suggestive evidence is the prolonged asthenia, which is out of proportion to the limited lung consolidation. In addition, some patients develop neurologic symptoms, without demonstrable *M. pneumoniae* in the cerebrospinal fluid but usually with serum Abs to brain tissue; and these Abs can be adsorbed by *M. pneumoniae* or its surface glycolipids. (However, the pathogenetic role of Abs reacting with brain remains unsettled, because these Abs also develop in most patients with mycoplasmal pneumonia who do not exhibit central nervous system symptoms.) Finally, *M. pneumoniae* produces other distant effects, whose mechanism is also obscure and could be immunologic.

CLINICAL MANIFESTATIONS. In man, *M. pneumoniae* causes inapparent infection, or mild upper respiratory tract disease, more often than it causes pneumonia. The onset of pneumonia is generally gradual, and the symptoms are mild or moderately severe, with early complaints referable to the lower respiratory passages. Because the areas of consolidation are small, x-ray examination frequently reveals pneumonia before physical signs are apparent. Involvement is usually interstitial or bronchopneumonic and limited to one of the lower lobes. The organism can also cause bronchitis, tracheo-

bronchitis, laryngitis, otitis media, and bullous myringitis.

The course of the pneumonia is variable, with remittent fever, cough, and headache lasting for several weeks. Convalescence is prolonged, often extending for 4 to 6 weeks even in the absence of complications. Few fatal cases have been reported. Illness is usually limited to the respiratory tract, but other areas may be involved.

Complications most often affect the central nervous system (Guillain–Barré syndrome, polyradiculitis, encephalitis, aseptic meningitis, or acute psychosis may occur); occasionally, pericarditis or pancreatitis is seen. These sequelae may be related to immunopathology, as noted above. An infrequent complication is hemolytic anemia with crisis, brought about by the cold agglutinins in serum.

IMMUNOLOGIC RESPONSE. Infection with *M. pneumoniae* induces the development of IgM Abs and later IgG Abs that are detectable by CF, growth inhibition (GI), or cell lysis in the presence of complement. These serum Abs do not appear to provide effective protection against infection or disease: in one longitudinal study, more than two-thirds of the individuals possessed a moderate to high titer of mycoplasmacidal Ab prior to becoming infected and developing pneumonia. IgA Ab also is found, in respiratory secretions, and it appears to play a role in host resistance. Finally, cell-mediated immunity to *M. pneumoniae* has been detected by skin test reaction, lymphocyte transformation, and inhibition of macrophage migration.

Glycolipids are the predominant antigenic determinants inducing circulating Ab, whereas a polysaccharide–protein fraction seems to be the component involved in cell-mediated immunity. As was noted, circulating Ab often develops within the first few years of life, but whether it has been induced by *M. pneumoniae* or by related glycolipids found in many plants and eubacteria is not clear.

M. pneumoniae can perturb immune responsiveness. In one direction, tuberculin anergy occurs and may persist for weeks into convalescence, and the mycoplasmas themselves may escape initial recognition. Conversely, during infection, Abs to unrelated infectious agents may increase in level and Abs to tissue components appear in some patients. *In vitro*, the organism similarly causes nonspecific stimulation of lymphocytes, in addition to specific stimulation of cells forming Ab to itself.

EPIDEMIOLOGY. An unusual feature of mycoplasmal pneumonia, as we have noted, is its peak incidence in individuals 5 to 15 years of age. *M. pneumoniae* accounts for as much as 15% to 50% of all pneumonias observed among school children and young adults. The incubation period is relatively long (2–3 weeks). *M. pneumoniae* infection is endemic in most areas. Infections occur throughout the year, with a predilection for late summer and early fall. Intensive exposure to infected persons appears to be required for transmission: spread of the organism from person to person is quite slow and generally occurs within a closely associated group rather than by casual contact. The organism is usually introduced into a household by a school-aged child.

TREATMENT AND PREVENTION

Tetracycline and erythromycin are effective in mycoplasmal pneumonia. Elimination of symptoms, however, is not accompanied by eradication of the organism.

Although these antibiotics are effective in reducing the morbidity of *M. pneumoniae* pneumonia, prevention through **vaccination** is a more logical means for control, particularly in populations where the risk of disease is high. In field trials, the efficacy of experimental inactivated *Mycoplasma pneumoniae* vaccines in preventing pneumonia has ranged from 45% to 67%. In the hamster, prior infection with *M. pneumoniae* induces greater resistance to disease than does parenteral inoculation of inactivated organisms: hence, a live attenuated mutant might provide more effective protection than an inactivated vaccine. However, efforts in this direction must proceed with caution because of the possible role of immunopathology in *M. pneumoniae* disease.

LABORATORY DIAGNOSIS

M. pneumoniae infection is diagnosed by isolating the organism or by demonstrating a rise in serum Ab titer. Nasopharyngeal secretions are inoculated into a selective diphasic medium that contains mycoplasma broth on top of agar, supplemented with glucose and phenol red. When *M. pneumoniae* grows in this medium, it produces acid, thereby changing the color of the medium from red to yellow. Broth from the diphasic medium should be subcultured to mycoplasma agar when a color change occurs, or at weekly intervals for a minimum of 8 weeks. Isolates are identified as *M. pneumoniae* by staining colonies directly with fluorescein-conjugated Ab or by demonstrating that specific Ab inhibits growth on agar.

The Ab response in mycoplasmal pneumonia is most easily demonstrated by CF. Because a relatively high Ab level may persist for a year or more after infection, only a rise during convalescence (four-fold or more) is considered indicative of recent infection. The test for cold agglutinins is less useful: these Abs develop in only one-half of patients with mycoplasmal pneumonia, and they are also induced by several other diseases.

M. pneumoniae can occasionally be recovered from the oropharynx for 1 to 2 months after subsidence of fever and for a shorter period in silent infections.

Mycoplasmas in Genital Tract Disease

M. hominis and *U. urealyticum* are common inhabitants of the genital tract, acquired primarily through sexual contact. They usually behave as commensals. However, on rare occasion either appears to be capable of causing pelvic inflammatory disease (tuboovarian abscess, salpingitis).

M. hominis has been recovered from the blood of a small proportion of women who develop fever postpartum or after abortion, but its etiologic significance is not clear, because 3% to 5% of women have a transient invasion of the blood by mycoplasmas at the time of parturition.

There has been considerable dispute concerning the role of genital mycoplasmas in **nongonococcal urethritis (NGU).** Although most *U. urealyticum* infections are silent, this organism appears to be one of the several causes, as the disease could be produced in volunteers by inoculating ureaplasmas intraurethrally. Moreover, ureaplasma-positive NGU patients who were free of chlamydiae (another etiologic agent of NGU) shed more ureaplasmas than did chlamydia-positive patients or healthy carriers of *U. urealyticum*. There is no evidence for an etiologic role of *M. hominis*.

A newly described species, *M. genitalium*, was initially isolated from two males with urethritis, but the organism has subsequently been found with greater frequency in throat specimens, accompanying infections by *M. pneumoniae*. The two organisms are difficult to distinguish, for they cross-react in the usual serological tests, and *M. genitalium* is difficult to recover because its growth is especially fastidious and slow. Its identification depends on recognition of a unique 140Kd adhesin protein, on use of monoclonal antibodies for unique epitopes, or on probes for unique parts of the genome. Its pathogenetic significance is unknown.

Other Interactions of Mycoplasmas
ANIMAL DISEASES

Contagious bovine pleuropneumonia (*M. mycoides* subsp. *mycoides*), the first mycoplasma infection recognized, has been eradicated from most countries by the application of strict control and vaccination programs, although the disease remains endemic in some tropical areas. However, other mycoplasmas in cattle, sheep, goats, poultry, and swine cause serious economic loss in most parts of the world. Mycoplasmas are also indigenous to common pets and laboratory animals (mice, rats, dogs, and cats), commonly causing respiratory or neuro-logic disease or arthritis. Chronic respiratory disease produced by *M. pulmonis* in laboratory mice or rats often complicates long-term studies with these animals.

The clinical and histopathologic features of arthritis produced by mycoplasmas in many animal species closely resemble those of human rheumatoid arthritis, but there is no evidence to support this etiology of the human disease.

SPIROPLASMAS AS PATHOGENS. Recently, helical, wall-free prokaryotes were recovered from diseased plants and suspected insect vectors, and were termed spiroplasmas (Table 40–1). A filterable "suckling mouse cataract agent," initially recovered from a rabbit tick, was later shown to possess similar characteristics (Fig. 40–1A); it is pathogenic for several vertebrate hosts. In rodents, various strains produce cataracts, central nervous system disease, or stunted growth.

TISSUE CULTURE CONTAMINATION

Mycoplasmas frequently contaminate animal cell cultures, producing alterations in cell metabolism, chromosomal aberrations, and inhibition of lymphocyte transformation. Because these effects may appear without morphologic alterations or loss of viability of the cells, and because tests for bacterial contamination fail to detect mycoplasmas, their presence has often not been recognized, and their effects have been misinterpreted as spontaneous genetic or epigenetic changes in the cells.

Many mycoplasmas adsorb readily to the surface of tissue cells (Fig. 40–7) and derive part of their nutritional needs from the cell. They do not appear to penetrate cells, except for phagocytosis under appropriate conditions. However, the association of mycoplasma and tissue cell may be quite intimate. Recently, it was shown that T-lymphocyte and H-2 histocompatibility Ags of a lymphoblastoid cell line were transferred to *M. hyorhinis*, which had established a persistent infection in a culture of these cells. Abs specific for *M. hyorhinis* were cytotoxic for the lymphoblastoid cells, providing additional evidence for a close relation between host cell and mycoplasma membranes. These types of interactions may have relevance to tissue damage and autoimmune phenomena seen in *M. pneumoniae* pneumonia.

Certain mycoplasmas that grow rapidly in cell culture can destroy cells by depleting the medium of arginine or by producing excess acid. Mycoplasmas can also drastically decrease the growth of DNA viruses that require arginine by depleting this amino acid, and they can enhance viral replication by suppressing interferon production.

Mycoplasmal contamination occurs most often in continuous-passage cell lines. Commercial bovine serum

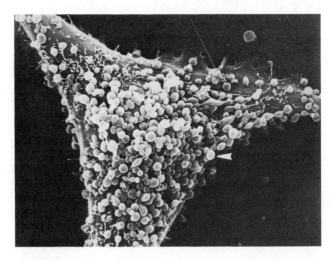

Figure 40–7. Scanning electron photomicrograph of a mouse tissue culture cell line (A9) infected with *Mycoplasma hyorhinis*. Note numerous mycoplasma cells *(arrow)* adsorbed to surface of tissue cell. (Courtesy of DM Phillips)

is the principal source, but human oral mycoplasmas are also frequent contaminants. Contamination is usually detected by direct culture. However, *M. hyorhinis*, a common contaminant, often cannot grow on artificial media and is identified by immunofluorescence.

Selected Reading

BOOKS AND REVIEW ARTICLES

Barile MF, Razin S (eds): The Mycoplasmas, Vol 1: Cell Biology. New York, Academic Press, 1979

Cassell GH, Cole BC: Mycoplasmas as agents of human disease. N Engl J Med 304:80, 1981

Clyde WA Jr: Mycoplasma pneumonia. Semin Infect Dis 5:81–82, 1983

Clyde WA Jr, Fernald GW: Mycoplasmas: The pathogens' pathogens. Cell Immunol 82:88, 1983

Maniloff J, Das J, Christensen JR: Viruses of Mycoplasmas and Spiroplasmas. Adv Virus Res 21:343, 1977

McCormack WM, Taylor–Robinson D: The Genital Mycoplasmas. In Holmes KK, Mårdh P-A, Sparling PF, Wiesner PJ (eds): Sexually Transmitted Diseases, pp 408–418. New York, McGraw-Hill, 1984

McGarrity GJ, Murphy DG, Nichols WW (eds): Mycoplasma Infection of Cell Cultures. New York, Plenum Press, 1978

Razin S: The Mycoplasmas. Microbiol Rev 42:414, 1978

Razin S: Molecular biology and genetics of mycoplasmas (Mollicutes). Microbiol Rev 49:419, 1985

Razin S, Barile MF (eds): The Mycoplasmas, Vol 4: Mycoplasma Pathogenicity. New York, Academic Press, 1985

Razin S, Tully JG (eds): Methods in Mycoplasmology, Vol 1: Mycoplasma Characterization. New York, Academic Press, 1983

Smith RF: Lipoglycans from mycoplasmas. CRC Crit Rev Microbiol 11:157, 1984

Tully JG, Razin S (eds): Methods in Mycoplasmology, Vol 2: Diagnostic Mycoplasmology. New York, Academic Press, 1983

Tully JG, Whitcomb RF (eds): The Mycoplasmas, Vol 2: Human and Animal Mycoplasmas. New York, Academic Press, 1979

SPECIFIC ARTICLES

Baseman JB, Dallo SF, Tully JG, Rose DL: Isolation and characterization of *Mycoplasma genitalium* strains from the human respiratory tract. J Clin Microbiol 26:2266, 1988

Bowie WR, Alexander ER, Floyd JF et al: Differential response of chlamydial and ureaplasma-associated urethritis to sulfafurazole (sulfisoxazole) and aminocyclitols. Lancet 2:1276, 1976

Chanock RM, Hayflick L, Barile MF: Growth on artificial medium on an agent associated with atypical pneumonia and its identification as a PPLO. Proc Natl Acad Sci USA 48:41, 1962

Fernald GW, Collier AM, Clyde WA Jr: Respiratory infections due to *Mycoplasma pneumoniae*. Pediatrics 55:327, 1975

Ford DK, Henderson E: Non-gonococcal urethritis due to T-mycoplasmas (*Ureaplasma urealyticum*) serotype 2 in a conjugal sexual partnership. Br J Vener Dis 52:341, 1976

Hopps HE, Meyer BC, Barile MF, Del Giudice RA: Problems concerning "non-cultivable" mycoplasma contaminants in tissue cultures. Ann NY Acad Sci 225:265, 1973

Taylor–Robinson D, Csonka GW, Prentice MJ: Human intra-urethral inoculation of ureaplasmas. Q J Med 46:309, 1977

Taylor–Robinson D, Tully JG, Barile MF: Urethral Infection in male chimpanzees produced experimentally by *Mycoplasma genitalium*. Br J Exp Path 66:95, 1985

Tully JG, Taylor–Robinson D, Rose DL, Cole RM, Bove JM: *Mycoplasma genitalium*, a new species from the human urogenital tract. Int J Syst Bacteriol 33:387, 1983

41

Morton N. Swartz

Other Pathogenic Microorganisms; L-Forms

Other Pathogenic Microorganisms

LEGIONELLA

In the summer of 1976 an outbreak of pneumonia (**Legionnaires' disease**), with 182 cases and 29 deaths, occurred among about 5000 persons who had attended an American Legion convention in Philadelphia. Epidemiologic investigation showed that the focus was the lobby of a hotel, the organism evidently being spread by air contaminated with water from a cooling tower (as shown in subsequent outbreaks). Cultures and staining of pulmonary lesions failed to reveal the agent. In the search for a virus the causative bacteria were eventually isolated by blind intraperitoneal passage through guinea pigs (which did not become severely ill) and then into yolk sacs of embryonated hens' eggs (which died with bacilli visible by Giménez stain). These previously undescribed bacteria, initially called Legionnaires' Disease bacilli and now designated *Legionella pneumophila*, slowly formed small colonies on enriched Mueller–Hinton agar with added hemoglobin (1%) but did not grow on routine media (blood, chocolate, or MacConkey agar). Their role in the disease was further established by indirect immunofluorescent staining with Abs that developed in the patients.

More than 40 outbreaks of *L. pneumophila* have now been reported, varying in severity; five of these occurred prior to 1976 and were identified retrospectively by testing stored sera. From 1983 to 1986 between 750 and 850 cases of **legionellosis** were reported annually in the United States, the majority sporadic.

MORPHOLOGY AND METABOLISM. Legionella are small, poorly staining or nonstaining **gram-negative rods** when examined on smears of infected secretions or in tissue, but they become pleomorphic, including long filamentous forms, and stain more readily after growth on culture plates. They are aerobic, unencapsulated, non-spore-forming bacilli with one or two monopolar flagella. **Cysteine and a high concentration of Fe²⁺** are required for growth. They use amino acids, but not sugars, as carbon and energy sources. The lipid composition is unique for a gram-negative organism in that **branched-chain fatty acids predominate.**

GENETIC RELATIONS. There are 23 known *Legionella* species, which can be differentiated by phenotypic properties (Table 41–1) but more definitively by DNA hybridization. More practical speciation is performed using specific absorbed antisera. Ten of the species (including *L. pneumophila, L. micdadei, L. bozemanii, L. dumoffii, L. wadsworthii,* and *L. longbeachae*) have caused human disease; the others have been isolated from environmental sources. *L. pneumophila* is responsible for 80% of cases of Legionella pneumonia and *L. micdadei* for 7%. All legionellas are classified in one genus because of their common cultural requirements, capacity to produce indistinguishable pulmonary infections in experimental animals, and susceptibility to the same antimicrobials. However, DNA hybridization data, phenotypic properties, and 16S rRNA oligonucleotide cataloguing have suggested two additional genera, *Tatlockia* (*L. micdadei*) and *Fluoribacter* (*L. bozemanii, L. dumoffii, L. gormanii*).

ANTIGENIC STRUCTURE. Ags specific to each *Legionella* species can be recognized by absorbed antisera utilizing either agglutination or immunofluorescent techniques. *L. pneumophila* consists of 12 antigenically distinct **serogroups** based on the **lipopolysaccharide** (LPS); other

Legionella species consist of one or two serogroups, totalling 38. About 50% of cases of Legionnaires' disease are caused by *L. pneumophila* serogroup 1.

PATHOGENICITY. *L. pneumophila* (and other disease-producing *Legionella* spp.) may cause a severe pneumonia, particularly in older individuals and patients with underlying diseases. The pneumonia is more frequent in the summer and causes a nodular or lobar consolidation with high fever, headache, nonproductive cough, and mild leukocytosis. Untreated, the mortality rate is about 15%. A **second form** of illness produced by *L. pneumophila* is **"Pontiac fever,"** usually occurring in outbreaks among healthy individuals and consisting of fever, headache, and myalgia (but without pneumonia and with no deaths). Characteristically, the incubation period of Pontiac fever is shorter and the attack rate among exposed persons is higher (up to 95%). Paradoxically, these features suggest exposure to a larger infecting inoculum or a more virulent strain, yet Pontiac fever is a milder disease.

The pathologic hallmark of Legionnaires' disease is an intra-alveolar exudate of both polymorphonuclear leukocytes (PMNs) and macrophages. Bacteremia occurs in as many as 38% of patients. Occasionally, the *L. pneumophila* pneumonia has been complicated by lung abscess or empyema caused by the same organism. In the absence of pneumonia, legionellas have, rarely, produced other types of infection (prosthetic valve endocarditis, sinusitis, wound infections).

L. pneumophila is primarily an **intracellular pathogen,** capable of multiplying within alveolar macrophages and monocytes. Phagocytosis of this organism by these cells, and by PMNs as well, takes an unusual form; i.e., instead of the usual extension of pseudopods about the organism from several sides, the bacillus is engulfed by a single coiled pseudopod (a response that can be blocked by Ab, suggesting mediation by a surface component). Once phagocytosed by macrophages, *L. pneumophila* are enclosed in phagosomes, within which an unusual

TABLE 41–1. Identification of Selected Legionella Spp. by Phenotypic Characteristics

Species	Urease	Nitrate Reduction	Browning of Tyrosine-Containing Yeast Extract Agar	Oxidase	Gelatinase	Hippurate Hydrolysis	β-Lactamase	Autofluorescence
L. pneumophila	−	−	+	+/−*	+	+	+	−
L. micdadei	−	−	−	+ʷ†	−	−	−	−
L. bozemanii	−	−	+	+/−	+	−	+	+ (blue-white)
L. dumoffii	−	−	+	−	+	−	+	+ (blue-white)
L. wadsworthii	−	−	−	−	+	−	+	−

* +/−, weakly or not always positive.

† ʷ, weakly positive.

mechanism permits virulent strains to survive and multiply: the phagosomes become coated with a layer of ribosomes, which inhibits fusion with lysosomes.

L. pneumophila LPS exhibits only limited toxicity compared with the endotoxicity of conventional gram-negative bacilli. *L. pneumophila* produces several extracellular products: a hemolysin (phospholipase-C activity), several proteinases with collagenase activity, and a **heat-stable polypeptide cytotoxin** of ~1300 daltons that kills embryonated hen's eggs and several types of tissue culture cells. This toxin selectively impairs activation by phagocytosis of superoxide generation and halogenation in PMNs, thus reducing bacterial killing.

IMMUNITY. Humoral immunity has only a limited role in host defense against *L. pneumophila*. The organisms are resistant to killing by complement even in the presence of Ab, and by PMNs in the presence of serum and Ab. Indeed, by promoting phagocytosis by monocytes, Ab may enhance infection, because the organisms can multiply more readily inside the phagosome than extracellularly.

Cell-mediated immunity plays a major role in the host's defense against *L. pneumophila*. Activated alveolar macrophages inhibit multiplication of the organisms. Guinea pigs sublethally infected with *L. pneumophila* via aerosol develop delayed hypersensitivity, are able to clear the organisms from the lungs, and are protected against subsequent lethal aerosol challenge.

EPIDEMIOLOGY. Person-to-person transmission does not occur. Rather, outbreaks and sporadic infections appear to result from **inhalation of small-particle aerosols** of legionellas produced by water cooling towers, air-conditioning systems, water faucets and shower heads, humidifiers, and contaminated respiratory therapy equipment. In the first outbreak of Pontiac fever water from the evaporative condenser of an air conditioner was later shown to have leaked into the air ducts of a new building. Contaminated water cooling towers have since been associated with several outbreaks, which were controlled by chlorination. Serious outbreaks have occurred in hospitals, where immunocompromised patients have been particularly at risk; legionnaires' disease accounts for about 4% of fatal nosocomial pneumonias in the U.S. Outbreaks due to contaminated showers and tap water have been stopped by intermittent or continuous heating of water to 60° to 70°C, along with continuous chlorination.

The natural habitat of legionellas is the aqueous environment, whence the organism can be transferred to artificial reservoirs in cooling towers or tap-water supplies. In fresh-water ponds legionellas can grow extracellularly, but they have a special **intracellular niche** within **amoebae,** where they can multiply and resist biocides;

algae in cooling tower water contribute to their nutrition. This behavior may explain why these organisms, so fastidious in culture, can thrive in cooling towers when biocides are not supplied.

LABORATORY DIAGNOSIS. *Legionella* infection is most reliably diagnosed by isolation of the causative organism from a tracheal aspirate or lung biopsy on buffered charcoal–yeast extract (BCYE) agar. Supplemented (cysteine, purines, vitamins) chocolate agar, or Mueller–Hinton agar with added hemoglobin and cysteine, are less satisfactory. Growth from clinical specimens takes 3 to 4 days. Isolation from blood is best accomplished by plating centrifuged, lysed blood on BCYE agar. Selective media (with vancomycin, polymyxin B, and anisomycin) can be used to isolate legionellas from polymicrobial clinical (sputum) or environmental specimens. The most rapid means of diagnosis available is direct fluorescent Ab staining for legionellas in a lung biopsy or bronchial washing.

Because seroconversion may take 7 to 9 weeks, and because Abs may persist for months or years after infection, serodiagnosis is of greater value for retrospective diagnosis and epidemiologic studies than for diagnosis during an acute illness. It can employ indirect fluorescent Ab procedures, microagglutination, or enzyme-linked immunosorbent assays (ELISA). Antigenuria, detected by ELISA or radioimmunoassay, can be used for diagnosis.

In epidemiologic studies, environmental isolates of *L. pneumophila* can be matched clonally to clinical isolates of the same serogroup by alloenzyme analysis, by plasmid profile, and by restriction endonuclease pattern of whole-cell DNA.

TREATMENT. Although *Legionella* species are susceptible to a variety of antibiotics *in vitro*, in animal models and human disease many are not effective because they do not penetrate mononuclear cells. Erythromycin is most commonly used; rifampin is added if the response is unsatisfactory. The newer quinolone drugs are active in animal models, but clinical experience is limited.

LISTERIA MONOCYTOGENES

Listeria monocytogenes is an important pathogen in veterinary medicine, causing abortion and encephalitis in sheep and cattle and a variety of diseases in other mammals, birds, and fish. Its descriptive epithet arose from the peripheral blood monocytosis observed in infected rabbits and guinea pigs. Injection of a lipid extract of the organism produces similar hematologic changes in rabbits. Although *List. monocytogenes* was first identified as a blood isolate from a human with a "mononucleosis-like" illness, the organism almost never produces such a clinical picture. It behaves as an **intracellular parasite;** it has been used in experimental models to study macrophage activation.

The incidence of sporadic listeriosis in humans in the U.S. is 2 or 3 per million population per year.

THE ORGANISM. *List. monocytogenes* is a short, **gram-positive,** aerobic to microaerophilic, nonspore-forming rod; it exhibits a peculiar end-over-end **tumbling motility at 20°** to 25°C but often not at 37°. In semisolid motility media it produces an umbrella-like subsurface colony at 30°C.

The organism grows well on blood or nutrient agar and in conventional blood culture broths. On blood agar the colonies usually are surrounded by a narrow band of β-hemolysis, and if the organism is not carefully examined in stained smears and tested for motility at 20° to 25°C, it may be mistaken for a hemolytic streptococcus. Because it often shows palisades on microscopic examination and also grows well on potassium tellurite agar, it is frequently mistaken for a diphtheroid (see Other Corynebacteria, Chap. 22) and discarded as a contaminant. It may also be confused with an enterococcus because of its growth on bile-esculin agar.

Detection of *List. monocytogenes* in contaminated specimens (food, environmental, fecal), where it is outnumbered by other organisms, can be accomplished by **cold enrichment** (storage in broth at 4°C for 2 to 8 weeks). Selective enrichment media containing antimicrobials (polymyxin, acriflavine, and nalidixic acid) also enhance isolation.

List. monocytogenes ferments glucose, producing principally lactic acid without gas (Table 41–2). It elaborates catalase, hydrolyzes esculin, and produces acetoin

(Voges–Proskauer test). Instillation into the conjunctival sac of a rabbit produces a purulent conjunctivitis in 3 to 6 days, followed by keratitis (**Anton test**).

On the basis of somatic (O) and flagellar (H) Ags, 17 serotypes have been described; serotypes 1a, 1b, and 4b account for more than 90% of clinical isolates. Serotyping and phage typing can be helpful in defining common-source outbreaks of listeriosis. **Serologic diagnosis** (microagglutination, complement fixation) is unreliable, because the test lacks sensitivity and cross-reacts with enterococci, *Staphylococcus aureus,* and other gram-positive bacteria.

Many closely related but nonhemolytic environmental isolates are nonpathogenic and appear to be of little epizootic or epidemiologic importance.

EPIDEMIOLOGY. *Listeria* are primarily psychrophilic or mesophilic bacteria found widely in nature. In domestic animals listeriosis is primarily of foodborne origin. *Listeria* are found in poor silage (neutral or slightly alkaline), which allows their growth at low temperatures. Wild birds feeding on infected sewage may serve as reservoirs and vectors.

Disease in animals is characterized by septicemia and the formation of multiple visceral abscesses; meningoencephalitis and involvement of the uterus and fetus occurs in domestic animals. Contact with infected cows has caused **skin infections** in veterinarians. Large numbers of organisms are discharged in the milk of cows with *Listeria* **mastitis.**

Most human infections are probably **food-borne.** *List. monocytogenes* is a gastrointestinal "transient" present in the stool of 5% of the population. Diarrhea (with numerous fecal *List. monocytogenes*) is occasion-

TABLE 41–2. Listeria and Erysipelothrix: *Comparison With Some Common Gram-Positive Bacteria*

	Shape*	β-Hemolysis	Catalase	Motility	Nitrate Reduction	Esculin Hydrolysis	Acid Production†		Keratoconjunctivitis
							Glucose	Mannitol	
Listeria monocytogenes	R	+	+	+	−	+	+	−	+
Erysipelothrix rhusiopathiae	R	−	−	−	−	−	+	−	−‡
Streptococcus pyogenes	C	+	−	−	−	−	+	−	−
Streptococcus faecalis	C	−/+	−	−	−	+	+	+	−
Corynebacterium	R	−+	+	−	+/−	−	+/−	+/−	−
Lactobacillus	R	−	−	−	−	−	+	+/−	−

* R, rod; C, coccus.

† Acid only; no gas. Some *Lactobacillus* species produce gas.

‡ Conjunctivitis but no keratitis.

(Based in part on Buchner L, Schneirson SS: Am J Med 45:904, 1968)

ally an early symptom of systemic listeriosis, accompanying or preceding bacteremia and meningitis. Epidemics have occurred as a consequence of epizootic disease. Cabbage fertilized by manure from sheep (several of which had died from listeriosis) and subsequently stored at 4°C (at which *List. monocytogenes* grows slowly) was incriminated in one outbreak. Others have been associated with contaminated cheese and milk. These outbreaks have been due to serotype 4b. Since surrounding sporadic cases were caused by other serotypes this serotype may have greater pathogenicity or transmissibility.

PATHOGENESIS. Individuals with impaired cellular immunity are particularly vulnerable to this intracellular pathogen: about 70% of patients with *Listeria* infection have **underlying immunosuppression.** Drugs that reduce gastric acidity may predispose to infection. Patients with cirrhosis or hemochromatosis and those undergoing long-term hemodialysis and requiring frequent transfusions are at increased risk, presumably related to iron overload. Under normal circumstances, iron acquisition by *List. monocytogenes*, necessary for its growth, is limited by Fe^{3+} binding to circulating transferrin.

Human infection most commonly (60%) involves the central nervous system. **Meningitis** accounts for almost all these cases; rarely, an encephalitic form occurs, with multiple focal abscesses in the brain stem. In the U.S. *List. monocytogenes* is the fifth most common cause of bacterial meningitis: in the past several decades, it has increased four- to five-fold in relative frequency, reflecting an increase in the number of immunosuppressed individuals at risk. In these cases the organism can usually be isolated from the spinal fluid and often from the blood.

The other major forms of listeriosis include primary **bacteremia, focal infections, and perinatal sepsis.** In the pregnant woman, bacteremic infection can cause **abortion, stillbirth,** or **premature birth** of an infected infant; transplacental infection produces disseminated abscesses or granulomas in multiple organs (**granulomatosis infantiseptica);** and neonatal meningitis, bacteremia, or both may result from perinatal bacteremia in the mother or from infection acquired during vaginal delivery.

List. monocytogenes produces a sulfhydryl-dependent **hemolysin,** which is antigenically related to streptolysin O, and, like the latter, binds to cholesterol and causes lysis of eukaryotic cells. The hemolysin appears to be associated with virulence: nonhemolytic mutants and environmental isolates are avirulent.

Ampicillin or penicillin are the drugs of choice: a synergistic combination of one of these β-lactams with gentamicin is sometimes used in immunocompromised or neutropenic patients. Trimethoprim–sulfamethoxazole is an alternative in the penicillin-allergic patient.

ERYSIPELOTHRIX RHUSIOPATHIAE

E. rhusiopathiae (*E. insidiosa*) is a **gram-positive,** nonsporulating, aerobic to microaerophilic bacillus that in culture forms delicate bacillary chains and filaments. It is similar to *List. monocytogenes* except for differences listed in Table 41–2; also, unlike *List. monocytogenes* and most other pathogenic gram-positive bacteria, it produces H_2S in triple sugar iron agar slants.

The organism causes **swine erysipelas** (a disease of economic importance) and is a parasite in fish, crustaceans, rodents, and a number of domestic animals (swine, sheep, turkeys, ducks). It is also found in decomposing organic matter. The organism enters the human skin through minor abrasions following contact with fish, shellfish, meat, or poultry and produces a disease known as **erysipeloid.** This disease is therefore an occupational hazard of fish and meat handlers, veterinarians, and housewives; epidemics have been reported among crab handlers. The localized cutaneous form of the disease is characterized by a spreading, painful, erythematous skin eruption, usually on the fingers and hands; the lesions exhibit sharp margins, extend peripherally, and clear centrally. The organisms are rarely seen on stained smears or cultured from swabs of skin lesions; bacteriologic diagnosis often requires culture of a skin biopsy specimen. Less commonly, the disease appears in a severe generalized cutaneous form or in a septicemic form (often followed by endocarditis). The organism is sensitive to penicillin, cephalosporin, clindamycin, and erythromycin.

STREPTOBACILLUS MONILIFORMIS

S. moniliformis is a facultatively anaerobic, **gram-negative,** pleomorphic bacillus named because of its tendency, in older cultures and on solid media, to form filaments and chains of bacilli with prominent yeast-like swellings (Fig. 41–1). It grows only in media enriched with blood, serum, or ascitic fluid. In young broth cultures and in infected tissues the organisms grow as typical bacilli, and on solid media the L-form (see below) is often demonstrable (Fig. 41–1 inset). Under the crowded conditions in surface colonies the organism has a tendency to form defective cell walls, thus leading to the growth of L-forms. All strains appear to be antigenically the same.

S. moniliformis is a normal inhabitant of the upper respiratory tract of wild and laboratory rats (as well as squirrels and weasels). It is the causative agent of one form of human **rat-bite fever,** the other being caused by *Spirillum minor* (see Rat-Bite Fever, Chap. 37). Clinically, the two diseases are similar, except that arthritis is more common in the *Streptobacillus* variety. Endocarditis, either acute or subacute, may also occur. The organism

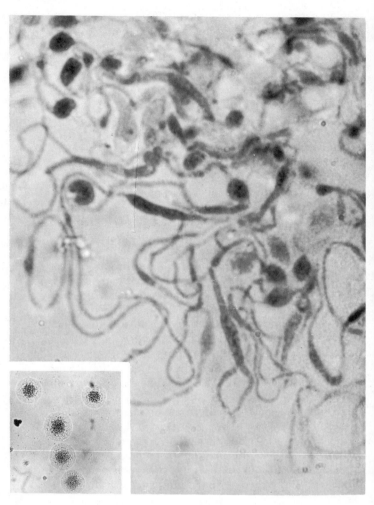

Figure 41–1. Many irregular filaments of *Streptobacillus moniliformis* with yeast-like swellings growing on solid medium. (× about 2520) *(Inset)* Unstained colonies of L-forms derived from bacillary form. (×80; courtesy of L. Dienes)

can usually be recovered, after 3 to 8 days' incubation, from blood cultures, where it grows on the surface of the sedimented blood cells in the form of "fluff balls." Growth of some strains of *S. moniliformis* is inhibited by sodium polyanethol sulfonate (present in many blood culture media to neutralize the antibacterial effect of fresh human blood).

In untreated *Streptobacillus* rat-bite fever the mortality rate is approximately 10%. Penicillin is the antimicrobial choice; cefuroxime, tetracycline, and erythromycin are also active.

Streptobacillus disease may also be acquired through chance infection of skin abrasions or by ingestion of contaminated food. When unassociated with a rat bite, the disease is often referred to as **Haverhill fever,** after a milkborne epidemic that occurred in Haverhill, Massachusetts, in 1929. This disease is characterized by an abrupt onset of fever, headache, rash (particularly about hands and feet), joint pains, and sore throat.

In the absence of isolation of the organism from blood cultures, the diagnosis can be made retrospectively by demonstration of a rising agglutinating Ab titer.

CALYMMATOBACTERIUM (DONOVANIA) GRANULOMATIS

Granuloma inguinale is an indolent, granulomatous, ulcerative disease caused by a short, plump, encapsulated **gram-negative bacillus** without flagella that is antigenically similar to, but not identical with, *Klebsiella pneumoniae* and *K. rhinoscleromatis* (Chap. 27). It is thought to be transmitted during coitus but is not highly communicable. The initial lesion commonly appears on or about the genital organs, beginning as a painless nodule. It soon breaks down, forming a sharply demarcated ulcer, which spreads by direct extension and often destroys large areas of skin in the groins and about the anus and genitalia. Occasionally, extragenital lesions oc-

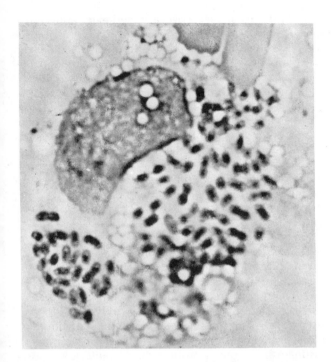

Figure 41–2. Donovan bodies within large macrophage in film stained with pinacyanole technique. (× about 8000; Greenblatt RB, Dienst RB, West RA: Am J Syph 35:292, 1951)

cur on the face and neck or in the mouth and throat; metastatic lesions in bones, joints, and viscera have also been reported. Histologic examination of the friable granulomatous tissue that forms the base of the coalescing ulcerative lesions reveals a heavy infiltration with mononuclear and plasma cells and lesser numbers of PMNs.

Granuloma inguinale is common in the tropics (India, Africa, New Guinea), but only about 50 cases are reported annually in the U.S.

In Wright- or Giemsa-stained smears of scrapings from the lesions, the causative organism can often be seen within the pathognomonic large mononuclear cells (Fig. 41–2); they are referred to as **Donovan bodies.** On electron microscopy intact bacilli are seen within phagosomes. These bacilli were first cultivated in the yolk sacs of chick embryos. They cannot be cultured on artificial media when first isolated, but they can be adapted to media containing egg yolk and even to beef heart infusion agar. Diagnosis rests with demonstration of Donovan bodies in stained spreads of granulation tissue or in the pathognomonic cells in biopsy material stained with hematoxylin and eosin or Dieterle silver impregnation.

Tetracycline or trimethoprim–sulfamethoxazole is the antimicrobial of choice in treatment. Chloramphenicol and gentamicin are reserved for resistant cases or areas where resistant cases have occurred.

BARTONELLA BACILLIFORMIS

Inhabitants of the Andes mountains in Peru, Colombia, and Ecuador have long been known to suffer from two different clinical manifestations of the same bacterial infection, collectively designated as **Carrión's disease:** a severe, febrile, **hemolytic anemia (Oroya fever)** and a relatively benign eruption of hemangioma-like **skin nodules (verruga peruana).** The causative agent is *Bartonella bacilliformis*, a small, motile, unencapsulated, gram-negative coccobacillus with flagella at one end. The organism is remarkable in its **geographic restriction** and its **tropism for RBCs.**

B. bacilliformis grows at either 28° or 37°C, in semisolid nutrient agar containing 10% fresh rabbit serum and 0.5% hemoglobin. The growth first appears just below the surface of the medium after about 10 days. There is apparently only a single antigenic type. It produces neither acid nor gas from any of the usual sugars.

Bartonellosis is transmitted from man to man by **sandflies** (*Phlebotomus*) indigenous to the region where the disease is endemic. No other reservoirs of the organism have been found, although monkeys can be infected experimentally. After an incubation period of 2 to 3 weeks patients exhibit intermittent fever and severe constitutional symptoms (including myalgia, nausea, vomiting, diarrhea, and headache), followed by increasingly severe signs and symptoms of **anemia.** Wright- or Giemsa-stained blood films usually reveal many organisms, either in or on the RBCs, and blood cultures are positive. More than 90% of RBCs may be parasitized. This initial stage of infection is frequently complicated by *Salmonella* superinfection. Among untreated patients, the mortality rate averages 40%, salmonellae being responsible for many of the deaths; in those who recover, convalescence is slow, and blood cultures may remain positive for many months.

Adhesion of actively motile *B. bacilliformis* occurs on a glycolipid site on the RBC and is dependent on energy generated by the organism's respiration. Binding produces invaginations of the RBC membrane, which result in the formation of intracellular vacuoles containing the bacteria ("forced endocytosis"). The severe anemia of Oroya fever is not due to direct intravascular destruction of RBCs but more likely results from sequestration and destruction of infected erythrocytes by macrophages in the enlarged liver and spleen.

The severe anemic stage of the disease may be followed in 2 to 8 weeks by a **cutaneous** stage, characterized by multiple eruptions of **hemangioma-like nodules (verruga),** which often ulcerate before healing. This form of the disease also occasionally develops without any obvious preceding anemia; it causes virtually no systemic manifestations and is not fatal. In this stage, the organism is not seen in the blood, the basic pathologic process being **endothelial proliferation** with new vessel formation. Very few intact bacteria are seen in verruga lesions, but numerous endothelial-cell phagocytic vacuoles contain digested bacillary remnants.

Treatment with penicillin, tetracycline, or chloramphenicol is effective, even in the severe anemic phase. Chloramphenicol is often preferred because of its efficacy against the accompanying salmonella infections as well. Control measures, including the use of DDT, are directed against the sandfly.

L-Forms

Some bacteria, during regular growth, produce **L-forms** (see Chap. 2) that replicate as **spherical structures** with partial or complete loss of cell wall architecture. They were first noted in agar cultures of *Streptobacillus moniliformis*, were found capable of reverting to bacillary form, and were initially named L$_1$ (L for Lister Institute). Ultrastructurally similar forms of *Neisseria gonorrhoeae* and several other pathogens have been observed in tissue and organ cultures. L-forms can be induced in many other bacterial species (gram-positive and gram-negative; cocci or bacilli) when peptidoglycan synthesis is interrupted (e.g., by penicillin or muralytic enzymes); hypertonic medium also supports their formation.

L-forms are either **stable** or **unstable.** The latter are capable of regenerating their cell walls and reverting to their antecedent bacterial form; the former, in contrast, are capable of indefinite growth in the wall-less state even after removal of agents inhibiting cell wall biosynthesis. L-forms pass through bacterial filters by virtue of their flexibility rather than their small size. Additional characteristics include considerable variation in cell size, irregular cell division, absence of typical mesosomal structures, lower growth rates than the parent bacteria, and resistance to inhibitors of cell wall biosynthesis but at least as great a susceptibility to inhibitors of protein synthesis (tetracyclines, aminoglycosides) as comparable bacterial cells.

Although L-forms resemble protoplasts and spheroplasts (see Chap. 2) and exhibit similar osmotic fragility, they have effected compensatory alterations that reinforce their cell membrane in several ways. Growth in the presence of certain of the fatty acids in human tissues may assist in this process. Lipopolysaccharide synthesis and assembly within the cell membrane is defective in L-forms, producing more hydrophobic molecules (with short O side chains) and thus increasing membrane stability. At the same time, phospholipids in L-forms have a lower content of long-chain saturated fatty acids and a higher content of short-chain fatty acids, enhancing membrane fluidity. In this way, some L-forms, even though lacking a wall, can grow at the osmolality of se-

rum. Surface colonies have a "**fried-egg**" appearance (Fig. 41–3), thickened in the center (where organisms have burrowed into the agar) with mainly dead cells in the periphery. The agar appears to assist division by pinching the growing L-form between strands of the gel.

In the past, L-forms have been confused with mycoplasmas (Chap. 40), because they both lack a cell wall, have similar cellular and colonial morphology, exhibit slow growth, and are filterable. However, mycoplasmas are distinctive, as judged by biochemical and immunologic criteria and DNA homology, and they lack penicillin-binding proteins. **Unlike mycoplasmas, many L-forms can revert to normal bacterial cells.**

RELATION TO DISEASE

Convincing evidence of a role of L-forms in human disease is lacking. They have been isolated from occasional cases of pyelonephritis, endocarditis, meningitis, osteomyelitis, and pneumonia. However, such isolations alone are insufficient to prove that the L-forms were present as such in the patient rather than emerging on cultivation. Because their granular and vesicular forms cannot be distinguished from necrotic debris in infected lesions, examination of stained smears is not helpful in diagno-

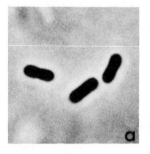
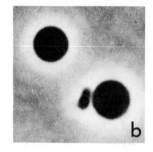
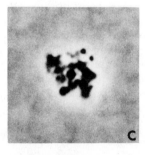
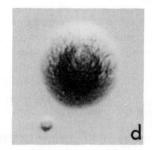

Figure 41–3. Variant phases. *Proteus mirabilis* is seen by phase contrast in identical media, and at the same magnification (×3400), as *(A)* vegetative cells, *(B)* spheroplasts, and *(C)* a clump of L-phase variants. *(D)* "Fried egg" colony of L-phase variants. (×150). (After McGee ZA et al: J Infect Dis 123:433, 1971)

sis. Because some of the reported clinical isolates of L-forms have been from patients receiving antimicrobials, their presence may have represented only transient drug effects on bacillary wall synthesis.

Cultivation in hypertonic media (e.g., with 0.6M sucrose) sometimes permits the outgrowth of typical bacteria from tissues while ordinary media yield no organisms: presumably organisms with damaged cell walls initiate growth in a hypertonic medium and then revert to the vegetative phase.

Although in culture L-forms produce the same exotoxins and endotoxins as the parent bacteria, in experimental animals they have not been shown to cause significant tissue damage, although they can persist for long periods. A possible exception is a murine model of *Nocardia caviae* pulmonary infection. Although infection is initiated with conventional bacillary forms, only L-forms (induced within alveolar macrophages) can be recovered from the lungs of many of the mice dying of pneumonia, suggesting an active role for these wall-less organisms in the disease.

Because Koch's postulates do not apply to an unstable form, it is particularly difficult to ascribe an etiologic role in human disease to L-forms: **they may be important largely as dormant forms,** resistant to antibiotics that act on wall synthesis and able to revert and cause a relapse after therapy ceases.

Host responses to L-forms may modulate any potential pathogenic role. The organisms stimulate an Ab response, and immunosuppression increases their persistence. They are **susceptible to killing by Ab plus complement,** but they are less susceptible to phagocytosis by neutrophils than their bacterial parents.

Because the role of L-forms in the pathogenesis, persistence, or relapse of infections remains speculative, the use of the currently complex methods to isolate such wall-less bacteria from clinical specimens is not indicated. In the rare patient with impressive clinical evidence suggesting bacterial infection yet negative cultures, it may be reasonable to employ hypertonic sucrose-containing blood culture media to try to isolate transient revertible forms. However, isolation of bacteria from such hypertonic media (and not from routine blood culture media) does not prove the presence or *in vivo* multiplication of wall-less forms: classic bacteria also occasionally grow more readily in such hypertonic media.

Selected Reading: Other Pathogenic Microorganisms

BOOKS AND REVIEW ARTICLES

Hart G: Donovanosis. In Holmes KK, Mårdh P-A, Sparling PF, Wiesner PJ (eds): Sexually Transmitted Diseases, p 393. New York, McGraw-Hill, 1984

Krier JP, Ristic M: The biology of hemotrophic bacteria. Annu Rev Microbiol 35:325, 1981

McDade JE, Shepard CC, Fraser DW et al: Legionnaires' disease: Isolation of a bacterium and demonstration of its role in other respiratory disease. N Engl J Med 297:1197, 1977

Nieman RE, Lorber B: Listeriosis in adults: A changing pattern—Report of eight cases and review of the literature, 1968–1978. Rev Infect Dis 2:207, 1980

Pollock SS, Pollock TM, Harrison MJG: Infection of the central nervous system by *Listeria monocytogenes:* A review of 54 adult cases. Q J Med 53:331, 1984

Stamm AM, Dismukes WE, Simmons BP et al: Listeriosis in renal transplant recipients: Report of an outbreak and review of 102 cases. Rev Infect Dis 4:665, 1982

Thornsberry C, Balows A, Feeley JC, Jakubowski W (eds): *Legionella.* Proceedings of the 2nd International Symposium, American Society for Microbiology, Washington, DC, 1984

SPECIFIC ARTICLES

Brenner DJ: Classification of *Legionellaceae:* Current status and remaining questions. Isr J Med Sci 22:620, 1986

Cowart RE, Foster BG: Differential effects of iron on the growth of *Listeria monocytogenes:* Minimum requirements and mechanism of acquisition. J Infect Dis 151:721, 1985

Edelstein PH: Laboratory diagnosis of infections caused by legionellae. Eur J Clin Microbiol 6:4, 1987

Fleming DW, Cochi SL, MacDonald KL et al: Pasteurized milk as a vehicle of infections in an outbreak of listeriosis. N Engl J Med 312:404, 1985

Fraser DW, Tsai TR, Orenstein W et al: Legionnaires' disease: Description of an epidemic of pneumonia. N Engl J Med 297:1189, 1977

Glick TH, Gregg MB, Berman B et al: An epidemic of unknown etiology in a health department I: Clinical and epidemiologic aspects. Am J Epidemiol 107:149, 1978

Horwitz MA: The legionnaires' disease bacterium (*Legionella pneumophila*) inhibits phagosome–lysosome fusion in human monocytes. J Exp Med 158:2108, 1983

Kathariou S, Metz P, Hof H, Goebel W: Tn916-induced mutations in the hemolysin determinant affecting virulence of *Listeria monocytogenes.* J Bacteriol 169:1291, 1987

Kuberski T, Papadimitriou, Phillips P: Ultrastructure of *Calymmatobacterium granulomatis* in lesions of granuloma inguinale. J Infect Dis 142:744, 1980

Lochner JE, Bigley RH, Iglewski BH: Defective triggering of polymorphonuclear leukocyte oxidative metabolism by *Legionella pneumophila* toxin. J Infect Dis 151:42, 1985

Muder RR, Yu VL, Zuravleff J: Pneumonia due to the Pittsburgh pneumonia agent: New clinical perspective with a review of the literature. Medicine 62:120, 1983

Ognibene FP, Cunnion RE, Gill V et al: *Erysipelothrix rhusiopathiae* bacteremia presenting as septic shock. Am J Med 78:861, 1985

Rowbotham TJ: Current views on the relationships between amoebae, legionellae and man. Isr J Med Sci 22:678, 1986

Schlech WF III, Lavigne PM, Bortolussi RA et al: Epidemic listeriosis: Evidence for transmission by food. N Engl J Med 308:203, 1983

Shanson DC, Midgley J, Gazzard BG et al: *Streptobacillus moniliformis* isolated from blood in four cases of Haverhill fever. Lancet 2:92, 1983

Selected Reading: L-Forms

BOOKS AND REVIEW ARTICLES

Dienes L, Weinberger HJ: The L-forms of bacteria. Bacteriol Rev 15:245, 1951

Guze LB (ed): Microbial Protoplasts, Spheroplasts and L-Forms. Baltimore, Williams & Wilkins 1967

Madoff S (ed): The Bacterial L-Forms. Microbiology Series No. 17. New York, Marcel Dekker, 1986

SPECIFIC ARTICLES

Gumpert J, Taubeneck U: Characteristic properties and biological significance of stable protoplast type L-forms. Experientia 46(Suppl):227, 1983

McGee ZA, Wittler RG, Gooder H, Charache P: Wall-defective microbial variants: Terminology and experimental design. J Infect Dis 123:433, 1971

Leon O, Panos C: Adaptation of an osmotically fragile L-form of *Streptococcus pyogenes* to physiologic osmotic conditions and its ability to destroy human heart cells in tissue culture. Infect Immun 13:252, 1976

Rousset A, Nguyen–Distèche, Minck R, Ghuysen J-M: Penicillin-binding proteins and carboxypeptidase/transpeptidase activities in *Proteus vulgaris* P18 and its penicillin-induced stable L-forms. J Bacteriol 152:1042, 1982

Wittler RG, Malizia WF, Kramer PE et al: Isolation of a corynebacterium and its transitional forms from a case of subacute bacterial endocarditis treated with antibiotics. J Gen Microbiol 23:315, 1960

42

Morton N. Swartz
Ronald Gibbons
Sigmund Socransky

Indigenous Bacteria; Oral Microbiology

Indigenous Bacteria

At birth the infant is bacteria-free, but during the first few days of life those areas of the body directly accessible to the environment become colonized. Various bacterial species (called **indigenous** or **autochthonous**) establish residence on superficial tissues or on the surface of the alimentary tract. This microbial flora is conveniently categorized as permanent (**resident**) or **transient.** The latter are organisms that may be present only temporarily in a given area in a minority of individuals (e.g., *Staphylococcus aureus* on the normal skin of 20% of individuals secondary to seeding from nasal carriage; *Pseudomonas aeruginosa* in stools of 3% to 24% of persons as a result of ingestion of raw vegetables).

The principal sites of the indigenous flora are the skin, the oral cavity, and the gastrointestinal and female genital tracts. In these areas the organisms usually are symbiotic and benefit the host. However, if systemic natural defenses are compromised, such as by neutropenia or various defects in cell-mediated immunity, or if local anatomic barriers are breached, such as by instrumentation or penetrating trauma, then the organisms may cause disease. Because many types of therapy now reduce resistance in these ways, **endogenous infections** have become a substantial fraction of the acute bacterial diseases seen in practice.

DISTRIBUTION

The cutaneous and mucosal surfaces of the body (nasopharyngeal and oral cavities; vagina) and the gastrointes-

TABLE 42–1. Bacteria Most Commonly Found on Surfaces of the Human Body

Bacteria	Skin	Conjunctiva	Nose	Pharynx	Mouth	Lower Intestine	External Genitalia	Vagina
Staphylococci	+	±	+	±	±	±	±	+
Pneumococci		±	±	+	+			
Streptococci								
viridans	±	±	+	+	+	+	+	+
β-Hemolytic				±	±			
S. faecalis	±			±	+	+	+	+
Anaerobic					+	+	+	±
Neisseriae			±	+	+	±	+	±
Veillonellae				±	+	±	+	
Lactobacilli					+	+		+
Corynebacteria	+	+	+	+	+	+		+
Clostridia					±	+	±	
Haemophilus		+	+	+	+			
Enteric bacilli				±	+	+	+	
Bacteroides				+	+	+	+	
Actinomycetes				+				
Spirochetes				+	+	+	+	
Mycoplasmas				+	+	+	±*	+

+, Common; ±, rare.

* Prevalence related to sexual activity.

(Modified from Rosebury T: Microorganisms Indigenous to Man. New York, McGraw-Hill, 1962.)

tinal tract are colonized by a variety of bacteria (Table 42–1) and in some cases by fungi and protozoa.

THE SKIN. The bacterial flora differs among three major regions of the skin: (1) exposed areas such as the face, neck, and hands, where the bacterial density is higher, where *Staph. aureus* is found more frequently, and where transients from the oropharynx may be carried; (2) moister areas of the body such as the axillae, perineum (commonly reflecting fecal soilage), and toe webs, where gram-negative bacilli (particularly *Acinetobacter*) are more numerous; and (3) covered dry areas such as the trunk, upper arms, and legs. Although scrubbing with soap and water or other disinfectants temporarily removes most surface bacteria, organisms within hair follicles and sweat glands soon restore the normal flora to its usual numbers (10^2–10^4 aerobes and anaerobes per cm^2). *Staphylococcus epidermidis*, uniformly found on the skin (in contrast to *Staph. aureus*), and anaerobic corynebacteria (*Propionibacterium*) comprise the majority of the resident flora. Micrococci, aerobic corynebacteria, and anaerobic streptococci are present in somewhat smaller numbers and less frequently.

THE PHARYNX. The airway below the larynx is normally sterile owing primarily to the efficient cleansing action of the mucociliary "blanket" that lines the bronchi (see Mechanical Factors, Chap. 21). The oropharynx, however, is regularly colonized by aerobic and facultative bacteria (viridans streptococci, *Branhamella catarrhalis*, *Neisseria* spp.) and anaerobic species (*Bacteroides melaninogenicus*, *Bacteroides oralis*, anaerobic streptococci). The nose is colonized chiefly by staphylococci (*Staph. aureus* in only about one-third of the population) and corynebacteria (*diphtheroids*).

GASTROINTESTINAL TRACT. At birth the intestinal tract is sterile. Within a few days, particularly in breast-fed infants, anaerobic lactobacilli and bifidobacteria appear and predominate (10^9–10^{11} per gram) in feces, along with fewer coliforms and enterococci. With broadening of the diet, coliforms become more numerous and are joined by *Bacteroides* and *Clostridium* spp.

In the adult, the esophageal mucosa contains only the bacteria ingested with food and saliva. Because of the low pH of gastric juice, few bacteria (mainly lactobacilli) are found in the normal fasting stomach. The **jejunum** has a sparse (10^4–10^5/ml of fluid), predominantly grampositive flora, the principal components being lactobacilli and various streptococci. The concentration of the microflora in the **ileum** increases (10^4–10^7), with the appearance of coliforms and anaerobes. The **colon** contains the greatest number of organisms (10^{11}–10^{12} per gram of feces); obligate anaerobes (*Bacteroides fragilis* and other *Bacteroides* spp., anaerobic streptococci, *Clostridium* spp., *Bifidobacterium*) outnumber coliforms and other facultative bacteria by as much as 1000 to 1.

THE VAGINA. Soon after birth, the vagina becomes colonized with lactobacilli, followed later by various cocci and bacilli. During the childbearing years, the predominant flora consists of *Staph. epidermidis*, lactobacilli, streptococci, corynebacteria, anaerobic gram-positive cocci, and various *Bacteroides* spp. Less frequently present are *Gardnerella* (formerly *Haemophilus*) *vaginalis*, group B streptococci, and coliforms. Anaerobes equal or slightly exceed facultative organisms in concentrations.

The female urethra may contain small numbers of contaminants from the mucosa of the external genitalia or perineum. *E. coli* from the latter may thus gain access to the bladder, where it is the commonest cause of bladder infections.

BENEFICIAL ACTIONS

COLONIZATION RESISTANCE. The indigenous flora in various sites can play a major role in preventing certain bacterial diseases through colonization resistance, also called **bacterial antagonism.** In the gastrointestinal tract it is manifested by the larger oral inoculum needed to colonize conventional mice (e.g., with 10^9 *E. coli* of a new, marked strain) compared with that needed to colonize germ-free animals (10^2).

The principal element in intestinal colonization resistance appears to be the anaerobic flora. When certain antibiotics (ampicillin, tetracycline, clindamycin) are administered in high dosage for many days potentially pathogenic organisms (e.g., *Clostridium difficile* or *P. aeruginosa*) may overgrow and produce, respectively, an enterocolitis or an invasive bacteremic infection. Other organisms besides anaerobic species may also contribute to colonization resistance: in mice, a single oral dose of streptomycin (which is ineffective against anaerobes) reduces by about 10^5 the oral dose of *Salmonella enteritidis* required to induce infection.

The concept of colonization resistance has led to current attempts at **selective intestinal decontamination** in patients at high risk for alteration of intestinal flora, particularly by *P. aeruginosa.* Thus, in patients who are neutropenic as a result of cancer chemotherapy and who are therefore likely to receive antibiotics for subsequent febrile episodes, prophylactic oral nalidixic acid, trimethoprim–sulfamethoxazole, or polymyxin can markedly reduce the gram-negative aerobic flora while maintaining the anaerobic flora.

Colonization resistance may also involve competition for nutrients and for mucosal attachment sites, accumulation of volatile fatty acids, and alterations in pH or oxidation–reduction potential. In addition, production of specific **bacteriocins** (Chap. 7) may be important in preserving a balanced distribution of species.

IMMUNITY. The indigenous flora stimulates the immune system. Animals reared in a **germ-free** environment have underdeveloped and relatively undifferentiated lymphoid tissues and low concentrations of serum immune globulins, and they exhibit a primary response rather than the usual secondary response to certain immunogens. Such animals are particularly susceptible to challenge with pathogenic microorganisms. Defects both in specific immune responsiveness and in nonspecific resistance (cellular activation) induced by endotoxin (Chap. 21) may account for their lowered resistance.

NUTRITION. Indigenous bowel bacteria **synthesize certain vitamins** in excess of their own metabolic needs. Vitamin K, which can be synthesized by coliforms, is required by germ-free, but not conventional, animals. Long-term use of broad-spectrum antibiotics in humans can contribute to vitamin K deficiency. Other vitamins produced by bacteria in excess of their own needs include folate, pyridoxine, pantothenate, biotin, and riboflavin; whether these vitamins are absorbed from their presumed colonic sites of synthesis in humans is not certain.

DETRIMENTAL ACTIONS

The indigenous bacterial flora may also act adversely on the host. **Bacterial synergism** may allow a strain to become pathogenic where otherwise it is not. For example, injection of a *Bacteroides melaninogenicus* strain alone failed to cause infection in an experimental animal, whereas when mixed with a diphtheroid producing vitamin K (necessary for growth of the *Bacteroides*), cross-feeding transformed the strain into an invasive pathogen. In another type of synergism, gonococci in the urethra may be protected against the action of penicillin by penicillinase-producing staphylococci, which do not themselves cause urethritis.

The usual harmful effects of **endotoxin** in the host may be caused in part by **hypersensitivity** induced by endotoxin Ags from intestinal flora, because germ-free animals are highly resistant to injections of endotoxin. The addition of **antibiotics to feed** for poultry and cattle suppresses the growth of many normal components of the intestinal flora as well as low-grade pathogens, and it enhances animal growth rate and food yield. The specific shifts in flora that are responsible have not been defined. On the debit side, such use of antibiotics can select for antibiotic-resistant organisms, especially *Salmonella*, that may be transferred by foodstuffs to humans (see Chap. 10).

OPPORTUNISTIC PATHOGENS. Under conditions of lowered general or local host resistance, bacteria of the resident flora may cause disease. For example, *Strepto-*

coccus mitis and *S. salivarius*, the most common aerobic species in the oropharynx, may cause transient bacteremia after dental extraction, tonsillectomy, or even vigorous mastication. If the heart valves are deformed by congenital defects or damaged by rheumatic fever, these usually bland streptococci may infect these altered sites (see α-Hemolytic Streptococci, Chap. 24) and cause **subacute bacterial endocarditis.** Similarly, *Bacteroides* may produce a life-threatening infection if introduced into the peritoneal cavity by a ruptured appendix or an abdominal knife wound, *E. coli* may infect the obstructed urinary tract, and *P. aeruginosa* may infect burns.

Various alterations in other host defenses can affect certain protective components of the normal flora and thus allow colonization, multiplication, and subsequent invasive infection by ordinarily transient but more pathogenic organisms. More than 60% of **hospital-acquired pneumonias** are caused by facultative and aerobic **gram-negative bacilli** (*Klebsiella*, *E. coli*, *Proteus*, *Pseudomonas*). Such pneumonia is much more likely to occur in patients whose upper airway has already been colonized by these organisms, which are isolated infrequently from the respiratory tracts of healthy individuals but frequently from seriously ill patients. Ordinarily, fibronectin on the surface of the oropharyngeal epithelium serves as an important receptor for adhesion to, and subsequent colonization of, the mucosa by a variety of streptococci (*S. mutans*, *S. sanguis*, *S. pyogenes*, groups C and G streptococci), but it inhibits the binding of gram-negative bacilli; removal of fibronectin from the cells markedly increases their binding capacity for *E. coli* and *P. aeruginosa*. Activation of salivary proteases in as yet undefined ways in seriously ill patients may contribute to fibronectin depletion in the oropharynx and the resulting shift of the predominant flora. Further selection would be encouraged by the use of antibiotics that are active primarily on gram-positive organisms. Microaspiration of upper respiratory secretions at this juncture could be followed by pneumonia caused by a species of colonizing gram-negative bacilli.

Host defense defects allow transients in the **intestinal flora** to invade, particularly when the normal competing flora has been reduced by antimicrobial use. For example, in neutropenic patients, *P. aeruginosa* bacteremia may develop. In an individual with defective cellular immunity *Listeria monocytogenes*, present as a transient from contaminated food stuffs in the stool of about 5% of adults, may cause invasive infection, including stillbirth or neonatal invasive infection.

ENDOGENOUS BACTERIAL DISEASES

A general knowledge of the normal bacterial flora of the human body is essential not only for interpreting the results of bacteriologic findings, but also because of the increasing incidence of **endogenous** bacterial diseases. Involving bacteria that are indigenous* yet potentially pathogenic, these diseases are "caused" by factors that lower the resistance of the host, either generally or at specific tissue sites. Such factors include radiation damage, treatment with cytotoxic drugs, long-term use of corticosteroid hormones, severe malnutrition, shock, debilitation from other diseases (particularly those involving the bone marrow or lymphoid tissues, such as leukemia), superinfection resulting from antimicrobial therapy, obstruction of excretory organs, introduction into the body of foreign materials (e.g., catheters or prostheses), interference with bacterial clearance from the respiratory tract (e.g., by narcotics), and predisposing lesions of unrelated etiology (see Chap. 21).

Unlike **exogenous** bacterial disease, those of **endogenous** origin have no definable incubation period, are not communicable in the usual sense, do not result in clinically recognizable immunity and tend to recur or to progress slowly for years, and involve bacteria found in the normal flora. These organisms characterized by low intrinsic pathogenicity, cause disease when they appear either in unusual body sites or in enormously increased concentration in or near their usual sites.

As the lives of more patients with serious illnesses are prolonged by improved methods of treatment, and as more infections caused by exogenous pathogens are controlled by effective antimicrobial drugs, **endogenous bacterial diseases have become a major proportion of the serious bacterial diseases encountered in clinical practice** (see Chaps. 27 and 28).

Oral Microbiology†

ORAL ECOLOGY

In the oral cavity distinct collections of indigenous bacteria colonize the surfaces and crypts of several sites: the teeth, the tongue dorsum, the buccal mucosa, and the gingival crevice. On the dental surfaces bacteria accumulate in large masses. Such **dental plaques** contain more than 10^{11} bacteria/g wet weight. In contrast, only 10^8 bacteria/ml are found in saliva (having been washed off the oral surfaces, and only about 10 to 100 are present on individual buccal epithelial cells and 100 to 150 on a cell of the tongue dorsum, because desquamation limits their numbers.

Nutrients available to the wide spectrum of bacterial species within the oral cavity include constituents of the

---

* Dormant or latent infections (Chap. 21) with exogenous pathogens (e.g., *Mycobacterium tuberculosis*) may also give rise to disease that is in a sense endogenous but is usually not classified as such.

† Contributed by Ronald Gibbons and Sigmund Socransky.

diet, gingival crevice fluid (a serous transudate), salivary components, and metabolites synthesized by associated organisms. The differences in the types of organisms found in various sites appear to be attributable largely to their selective **attachment** to different oral surfaces. Bacterial attachment is the first essential step for colonization because of the flow of oral fluids and the exposure of new epithelial surfaces by desquamation. Therefore, the species of bacteria initially colonizing tooth and oral epithelial surfaces is determined mainly by their **adhesiveness** for a particular surface and by their numbers, in saliva, available for attachment. On teeth, the first colonizing bacteria then provide new surfaces for attachment of additional species, and such distinct **epiphytic** formations are common (Fig. 42–1). Thus, population shifts occur, changing the composition and complexity of dental plaques.

Tooth mineral consists primarily of a complex calcium phosphate salt, hydroxyapatite, which readily adsorbs glycoproteins. Adsorbed salivary components, including blood-group–reactive salivary mucins, anionic proteins, and lysozyme, form a thin film termed the **enamel pellicle** on teeth. The **adsorbed** salivary constituents are thought to serve as **bacterial receptors,** whereas in the membranes of oral epithelial cells, blood-group–reactive glycoproteins serve as similar receptors. **Unadsorbed** mucins and other salivary constituents mimic bacterial receptors and hence serve as potent **inhibitors of bacterial attachment;** they also promote the desorption of adherent organisms. This probably explains the cleansing action of saliva.

Abs (secretory IgA predominating in saliva) and IgG in gingival crevices) may limit bacterial colonization by binding to surface Ags of the organisms and interfering with attachment. Whether the IgA-cleaving enzyme of *Streptococcus sanguis* reduces such potential inhibition of its attachment to dental surfaces *in vivo* is unclear. Abs to a wide range of indigenous species are commonly found in serum and saliva. However, antigenically shifting populations of *Streptococcus salivarius* colonize the dorsum of the tongue in spite of an Ab response by the host.

ACQUISITION AND NATURE OF THE ORAL FLORA. The oral cavity is sterile at birth, but bacteria are quickly introduced via food and other contacts. By 3 to 5 days of age, the buccal epithelial cells permit bacterial attachment, and increased populations of organisms such as *S. salivarius* are found. The eruption of teeth at 6 to 9 months of age leads to colonization by organisms that require a nondesquamating surface, such as *S. sanguis* and *Streptococcus mutans.* With the creation of the gingival crevice area anaerobes such as *Fusobacterium, Actinomyces,* and *Veillonella* are found. The complexity of the oral flora increases, and black-pigmented *Bacteroides* spp. and spirochetes colonize around puberty. Conversely, loss of all teeth results in the elimination of *S. sanguis, S. mutans,* and many anaerobic species from the mouth. (They can reappear when dentures are replaced.) The distribution of organisms commonly found in various sites of the mouth is listed in Table 42–2.

Oral streptococci have their individual niches: *S. mutans* and *S. sanguis* on the dental surfaces; *S. mitior* on the teeth and buccal mucosa; and *S. salivarius* on the tongue.

EFFECTS OF THE ORAL FLORA. The indigenous oral flora contributes to host **nutrition** through the synthesis of vitamins. Although a much larger mass of indigenous bacteria is found in the lower bowel, the greater efficiency of nutrient absorption in the small intestine increases the effective contribution of the oral flora.

Indigenous organisms (strains of *S. mitior* and *S. sanguis,* for example) may contribute to **immunity** by inducing low levels of circulating and secretory Abs that cross-

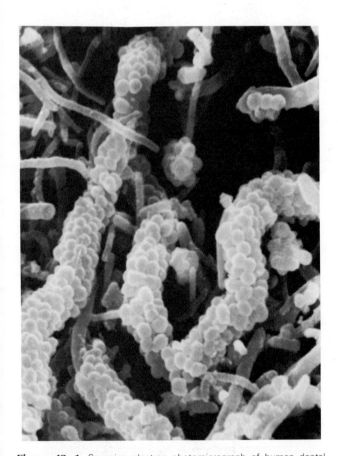

Figure 42–1. Scanning electron photomicrograph of human dental plaque showing cocci colonizing the surface of filamentous forms. These epiphytic arrangements have been referred to as "corn cobs." (Courtesy of Z Skobe, Forsyth Dental Center)

TABLE 42–2. *Distribution of Frequently Encountered Oral Bacteria in Different Sites of the Mouth*

	Supragingival Plaque Associated With			Subgingival Plaque Associated With				
	Pits & Fissures of Teeth	Smooth Tooth Surfaces	Gingivitis	Periodontosis	Periodontitis	Saliva	Cheek	Tongue
Gram-positive cocci								
Strep. sanguis	++	++	++	0	+	+	+	+
Strep. mutans	++	+	0	0	0	0	0	0
Strep. sobrinas	+	+	0	0	0	0	0	0
Strep. mitior-milleri	+	++	++	0	+	+	++	+
Strep. salivarius	0	0	0	0	0	++	+	++
Staph. epidermidis	0	+	+	0	0	+	+	+
Peptostreptococcus spp.	0	+	+	0	+	+	0	+
Gram-negative cocci								
Neisseria spp.	0	+	+	0	0	+	0	+
Veillonella spp.	+	+	+	+	+	++	0	++
Gram-positive rods								
Bacterionema matruchotii	+	+	+	0	0	0	0	+
Actinomyces viscosus	+	++	++	+	+	+	+	+
A. naeslundii	+	++	++	+	+	+	+	+
A. israelii	+	++	++	+	++	+	+	+
Other Actinomyces spp.	+	+	+	+	+	+	+	+
Lactobacillus spp.	+	0	0	0	0	0	0	0
Propionibacterium acnes		+	+	0	++	+	0	+
Rothia dentocariosa		+	+	0	0	+	0	+
Eubacterium spp.		0	0	0	++			
Gram-negative rods								
Black-pigmented Bacteroides								
B. melaninogenicus	0	0	+	+	+	0	0	0
B. intermedius	0	0	+	++	++	0	0	0
B. gingivalis	0	0	+	+	++	0	0	0
B. oralis	0	+	+	+	+	+	0	+
B. forsythus	0	0	0	0	+	0	0	0
Eikenella corrodens		0	+	++	++	0	0	0
Fusobacterium nucleatum	0	+	++	++	++	+	0	+
Capnocytophaga spp.		0	+	++	+	0	0	0
Haemophilus spp., including								
H. parainfluenzae	+	+	+	0	+	+	0	+
H. segnis; H. aphrophilus	0	+	+	0	+			
A. actinomycetemcomitans	0	0	0	++	+	0	0	0
Campylobacter concisus	0	0	+	+	++	0	0	0
Wolinella recta	0	0	+	+	++	0	0	0
Selenomonas sputigena	0	0	+	+	++	0	0	0
Small treponemes (Treponema macrodentium, T. orale, T. denticola)	0	0	+	+	+	0	0	0
Intermediate & large spirochetes	0	0	0	0	++	0	0	0

++, Frequently encountered in high proportions; +, frequently encountered in low to moderate proportions; 0, sometimes encountered in low proportions or not detectable.

react with some pneumococci. The oral flora also exerts microbial **antagonism** against certain pathogens. Thus when the indigenous bacterial flora has been suppressed by antibiotics the yeast *Candida albicans,* a frequent minor inhabitant of the mouth, may overgrow and cause lesions.

DISEASES INITIATED BY THE ORAL FLORA

Some members of the oral flora possess pathogenic potential. When dental plaque or saliva is injected subcutaneously into experimental animals, transmissible purulent abscesses are formed. Oral organisms gaining

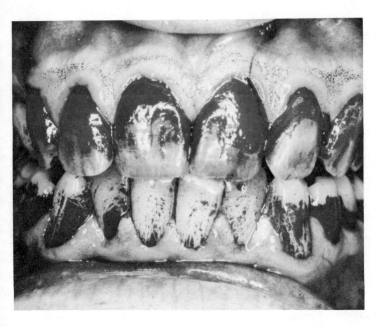

Figure 42–2. Accumulation of bacterial dental plaque 3 days after cleaning. Stained with beta rose.

entrance into tissues may cause abscesses of the alveolar bone or of the lung, brain, or extremities. Such infections usually contain mixtures of bacteria, with black-pigmented *Bacteroides* often playing a dominant role. Other residents of the oral cavity associated with distant infections are *Eikenella corrodens* (abscesses), *Actinomyces* and *Arachnia* spp. (actinomycosis), and *S. sanguis*, *S. mutans*, and *Actinobacillus actinomycetemcomitans* (subacute endocarditis). In patients with subacute bacterial endocarditis, it is important that *S. mutans* be distinguished from enterococci, because eradication of the latter requires both penicillin and gentamicin.

Dental plaque consists of mixed colonies of bacteria, which may reach a thickness of 300 to 500 cells on the more protected surfaces of teeth (Fig. 42–2). Bacterial cells make up 60% to 70% of plaque and are embedded in a matrix of bacterial and salivary polymers and remnants of epithelial cells and leukocytes. Streptococci and *Actinomyces* species predominate in supragingival plaque, whereas anaerobes (*Bacteroides*, *Fusobacterium*, *Actinomyes*, *Selenomonas*, *Treponema*) and *Eikenella corrodens* are the principal components of subgingival plaque. Some segregation of *S. mutans* and *S. sanguis* occurs in plaque on tooth surfaces. Whereas the latter is always present on smooth surfaces when plaque formation begins and then rapidly proliferates, the former's preferred niche is on occlusal fissures. These accumulations expose the teeth and gingival tissues to high concentrations of bacterial metabolites, which result in dental diseases.

DENTAL CARIES. Dental caries is the destruction of the enamel, dentin, or cementum of teeth by bacterial action (Fig. 42–3). The mechanisms appears to be a direct demineralization caused by lactic and other organic acids produced from dietary carbohydrates by the overlying bacteria. Although many bacteria can produce high concentrations of acid *in vitro*, only a few species are associated with dental caries in humans. Organisms of the *S. mutans* group are associated with the initial development of enamel lesions in humans; they are also highly cariogenic in monkeys, hamsters, and rats, as well as in **gnotobiotic (germ-free)** rats (Fig. 42–4). These organisms preferentially colonize occlusal fissures and the contact points between teeth; they are less frequently isolated from buccal or lingual tooth surfaces. This pattern correlates with the incidence of decay on these surfaces.

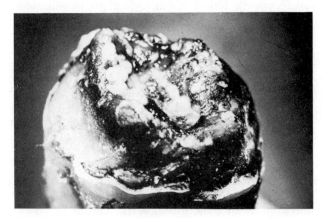

Figure 42–3. Crown of a human tooth with dental caries. Note the colonies of adherent bacteria associated with the decay.

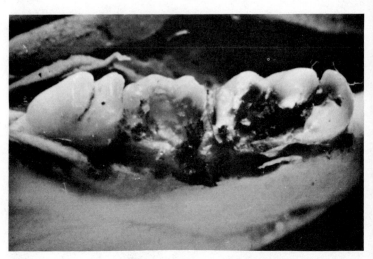

Figure 42–4. Dental caries in a gnotobiotic rat monoinfected with *Streptococcus mutans* for 90 days.

The high cariogenic potential of *S. mutans* is partly attributable to its ability to accumulate on teeth through the formation of **extracellular glucans** (dextran) synthesized specifically from **sucrose** (see Polysaccharides, Chap. 4): predominantly α-1,6- and α-1,3-linked polymers, which are formed from one-half the sucrose molecule by glycosyl transferases on the organism's surface. This effect of sucrose partially explains its well-known cariogenicity. Such extracellular polymers in colonies of *S. mutans* also reduce diffusion and promote accumulation of metabolic acids. Thus they attain higher acidity than colonies of other oral organisms, which is another important determinant of pathogenicity.

S. mutans appears to be important in the initiation of enamel caries, but it is probably not the only cause of dental decay. *Actinomyces* species also produce cemental and occasionally enamel carious lesions in experimental animals. Both lactobacilli and *Actinomyces* are commonly found in human carious dentin, which suggests they may also be common secondary invaders contributing to progression of lesions.

PERIODONTAL DISEASE. Diseases that affect the supporting structures of teeth (i.e., the gingiva, cementum, periodontal membrane, and alveolar bone) are collectively referred to as periodontal disease. The most common form, **gingivitis,** is a localized inflammatory condition associated with accumulations of bacterial plaque in the gingival crevice area. Its association with increased populations of *Actinomyces* suggests its etiology.

Another form, **acute necrotizing ulcerative gingivitis (ANUG)** (also known as **trench mouth** or Vincent's infection), is an acute infection that causes necrosis of the interdental papillae and leads to the formation of ulcerated "craters" between the teeth. This periodontal disease is the only type in which bacterial invasion of tissues is a predominant feature. Since the turn of the century, observations of gram-stained smears of scrapings have implicated the combination of a spirochete (*Borrelia vincentii*) and fusiform bacilli (principally *Fusobacterium nucleatum*) in the etiology of ANUG. Another intermediate-sized spirochete (uncultivatable and morphologically different from *B. vincentii*) has been observed in tissues (up to 300 μm from the crevicular surface) and is thought more likely to be responsible for this disease.

Diseases confined to the gingiva do not lead to loss of teeth. However, other types of periodontal disease commonly affect the periodontal membrane and alveolar bone, resulting in tooth loss. The commonest cause of tooth loss in a adults is a group of diseases known collectively as **destructive periodontitis.** Microorganisms colonizing the gingival crevice area often cause swelling of the gingiva and apical migration of the gingival epithelium attached to the tooth surface. The resulting space between the tooth and gingiva is termed a **periodontal pocket.** Bacteria accumulate in this protected niche, and its progress toward the apex of the root eventually destroys alveolar bone and periodontal membrane, causing tooth loss. Bacteria may also be found within gingival tissues.

The structure of **subgingival plaque** in periodontitis is complex. Microscopic observations reveal a dense layer consisting of *Actinomyces* and other gram-positive organisms attached to the cemental and root surfaces, a zone of gram-negative organisms between this layer and the pocket epithelium, and spirochetes and other motile forms at the base of the pocket. Large numbers of polymorphonuclear leukocytes (PMNs) are also present in the crevicular epithelium and pocket. The gram-positive

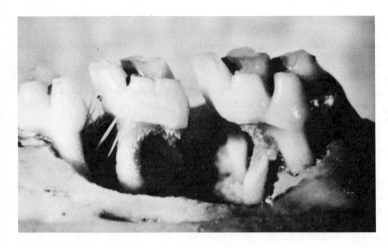

Figure 42–5. Periodontal destruction and root caries in gnotobiotic rat monoinfected with *Actinomyces naeslundii* for 90 days.

organisms consist of *Actinomyces, Peptostreptococcus, Propionibacterium, Eubacterium,* and streptococci; the gram-negatives include spirochetes, *Selenomonas sputigena, Wolinella recta, B. gingivalis, B. intermedius, B. forsythus, Fusobacterium nucleatum,* and *E. corrodens.*

Another periodontal disease, **periodontosis** (juvenile periodontitis), is a distinctive infectious process characterized by a rapid destruction of alveolar bone around the first molars and incisors of adolescents, often with minimal bacterial accumulations and gingival inflammation. The main associated organism is *A. actinomycetemcomitans.* Also frequently encountered are *Capnocytophaga* spp., *E. corrodens,* and *B. intermedius.* Patients frequently exhibit a defect in PMN chemotaxis and elevated serum Ab levels to *A. actinomycetemcomitans.*

The pathogenic potential of organisms associated with different forms of periodontal disease has been assessed in **gnotobiotic animals.** Not all organisms elicit disease. Gram-positive species, including *Actinomyces* and *S. mutans,* accumulate in large masses and lead to alveolar bone destruction and carious lesions on the root surfaces (Fig. 42–5). Gram-negative organisms, including *Capnocytophaga, E. corrodens, F. nucleatum, H. actinomycetemcomitans, B. gingivalis, B. intermedius,* and *S. sputigena,* do not form massive accumulations or carious root lesions, but they lead to extensive alveolar bone destruction characterized by large numbers of osteoclasts (Fig. 42–6).

The mechanisms of tissue destruction have not been clearly delineated in human periodontal disease. Invasion of gingival tissues has been observed, but its role in pathogenesis is unclear. Hydrolytic enzymes (e.g., collagenase of *B. melaninogenicus*), endotoxins, and other bacterial toxic products have been suggested as the agents that lead to destruction of the intercellular matrix of periodontal connective tissues; they may also interfere with the metabolism of local tissue cells. Destruction

may also result from the host's response to the organisms, involving inflammatory (releasing PMN collagenase and lysosomal enzymes) or hypersensitivity reactions.

CONTROL OF DENTAL DISEASES. The problem of controlling dental infections is unique in that the responsible organisms are widespread in the population and are accompanied by benign indigenous organisms. Dental caries can be controlled by stringent mechanical removal of the bacterial accumulations on teeth. However, such procedures have not been widely successful because few individuals can be adequately motivated or possess the requisite skill.

The most effective practical measure for the control of dental caries is the administration of **fluoride** in drinking water or as a dietary supplement during the period of

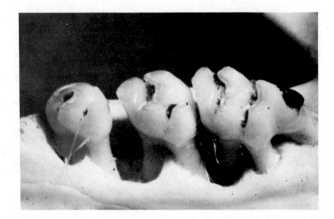

Figure 42–6. Periodontal disease involving extensive loss of alveolar bone in gnotobiotic rat monoinfected with *Eikenella corrodens.* Note the absence of root surface carious lesions in contrast to those which develop in the presence of *Actinomyces* (Fig. 42–5).

tooth formation. Such procedures reduce the incidence of decay by more than half. Topically applied fluorides are less effective. It is thought that systemically administered fluoride results in the formation of fluoroapatite, which resists acid dissolution. Topically applied fluorides may affect bacterial attachment to teeth or may be directly antibacterial.

Dental caries has decreased dramatically over the past decade in the U.S. and in Europe, probably owing to the use of fluorides and to the liberal use of antibiotics by the medical profession.

Reducing sucrose ingestion can also reduce decay, but this is not generally practiced. **Vaccines,** consisting of *S. mutans* cells or glycosyl transferase preparations, have reduced colonization and dental caries development in experimental animals. However, the effectiveness of such vaccines in human dental decay has not been assessed. Treatment with antibiotics and disinfectant agents is being explored, but total elimination of the organisms is difficult to achieve because of their inaccessibility, in fissures or in carious lesions, to topically or systemically administered agents, and because of their slow growth. In addition, such host defense mechanisms as phagocytosis, inflammatory responses, and desquamation are not operative in dental caries.

The frequent removal of gingival plaque by tooth brushing and using dental floss or by professional dental personnel will completely control gingivitis and destructive periodontitis, but these methods have not proved practical. The daily use of powerful antiseptic agents, such as chlorhexidine, can control gingivitis, but the teeth often become stained. Acute gingival infections such as ANUG are controlled by systemic treatment with penicillin and metronidazole, whereas rapidly destructive forms of periodontitis and periodontosis have responded favorably to tetracycline.

Selected Reading

BOOKS AND REVIEW ARTICLES

Beachey EH: Bacterial Adherence. New York, Chapman and Hall, 1980

Clarke RTJ, Bauchop T (eds): Microbial Ecology of the Gut. New York, Academic Press, 1977

Hill GB, Eschenbach DA, Holmes KK: Bacteriology of the vagina. In Mårdh PA, Taylor–Robinson D (eds): Bacterial Vaginosis, p 23. Stockholm, Almqvist and Wiksell 1984

Mackowiak P: The normal microbial flora. N Engl J Med 307:83, 1982

Noble WC, Somerville DA: Microbiology of Human Skin. Philadelphia, WB Saunders, 1974

Rosebury T: Microorganisms Indigenous to Man. New York, McGraw-Hill, 1962

Savage DC: Microbial ecology of the gastrointestinal tract. Annu Rev Microbiol 31:107, 1977

Skinner FA, Carr JG (eds): The Normal Microbial Flora of Man. New York, Academic Press, 1974

Williams REO: Benefit and mischief from commensal bacteria. J Clin Pathol 26:811, 1973

SPECIFIC ARTICLES

Abraham SN, Beachey EH, Simpson WA: Adherence of *Streptococcus pyogenes*, *Escherichia coli*, and *Pseudomonas aeruginosa* to fibronectin-coated and uncoated epithelial cells. Infect Immun 41:1261, 1983

Bartlett JG, Polk BF: Bacterial flora of the vagina: Quantitative study. Rev Infect Dis 6:S67, 1984

Dzink JL, Tanner ACR, Haffajee AD, Socransky SS: Gram negative species associated with active destructive periodontal lesions. J Clin Periodontol 12:648, 1985

Finegold SM, Attebery HR, Sutter VL: Effect of diet on human fecal flora: Comparison of Japanese and American diets. Am J Clin Nutr 27:1456, 1974

Finland M: Changing ecology of bacterial infections as related to antibacterial therapy. J Infect Dis 122:419, 1970

Gibbons RJ: Adhesion of bacteria to surfaces of the mouth. In Berkely, Lynch, Melling et al (eds): Microbial Adhesion to Surfaces, p 351. London Society of Chemical Industry, 1980

Liljemark WF, Gibbons RJ: Suppression of *C. albicans* by human oral streptococci in gnotobiotic mice. Infect Immun 8:846, 1973

Loesche WJ: Chemotherapy of dental plaque infections. Oral Sci Rev 9:65, 1976

Loesche WJ: Role of *Streptococcus mutans* in human dental decay. Microbiol Rev 50:353, 1986

McGhee JR, Michalek SM: Immunobiology of dental caries: Microbial aspects and local immunity. Annu Rev Microbiol 35:595, 1981

Miller CP, Bohnhoff M: Changes in the mouse's enteric microflora associated with enhanced susceptibility to salmonella infection following treatment with streptomycin. J Infect Dis 113:59, 1963

Morrison AJ Jr, Wenzel RP: Epidemiology of infections due to *Pseudomonas aeruginosa*. Rev Infect Dis 6:S627, 1984

Socransky SS, Haffajee AD, Listgarten MA: Microbiology of periodontal diseases. In Grant, Stern, and Everett (eds): Orban's Periodontics. St. Louis, CV Mosby, 1986

Sprunt K, Redman W: Evidence suggesting importance of role of interbacterial inhibition in maintaining balance on normal flora. Ann Intern Med 86:579, 1968

Sutter VL: Anaerobes as normal oral flora. Rev Infect Dis 6:S62, 1984

Van der Waaij D, Berghuis deVries JM, Lekkerkerk–van der Wees JEC: Colonization resistance of the digestive tract in conventional and antibiotic-treated mice. J Hyg (Camb) 69:405, 1971

Van Houte J: Bacterial specificity in the etiology of dental caries. Int Dent J 30:305, 1980

Woods DE, Straus DC, Johansson WG, Bass JA: Role of fibronectin in the prevention of adherence of *Pseudomonas aeruginosa* to buccal cells. J Infect Dis 143:784, 1981

Zambon JJ: *Actinobacillus actinomycetemcomitans* in human periodontal disease. J Clin Periodontol 12:1, 1985

43

George S. Kobayashi

Fungi

Characteristics of Fungi

The fungi (L. *fungus*, mushroom) have traditionally been regarded as "plant-like." Most species grow by continuous extension and branching of twig-like structures. In addition, they are mostly immotile; their cell walls resemble those of plants in thickness and, to some extent, in chemical composition and ultramicroscopic structure; and their cells are eukaryotic. However, they lack chlorophyll, are heterotrophic, and are now classified as a separate kingdom (Chap. 1).

Fungi grow either as single cells, the **yeasts,** or as multicellular filamentous colonies, the **molds** and **mushrooms.** The multicellular forms have no leaves, stems, or roots and are thus much less differentiated than higher plants, but they are much more differentiated than bacteria. However, fungi do not possess photosynthetic pigments, and so they are restricted to a saprobic (Gr. *sapros*, rotten; *bios*, life) or a parasitic existence. A single uninucleated cell can yield filamentous multinuclear strands, yeast cells, fruiting bodies with diverse spores, and cells that are differentiated sexually (in many species). Moreover, a few species form remarkable traps and snares for capturing various microscopic creatures.

Fungi are abundant in soil, on vegetation, and in bodies of water, where they live largely on decaying leaves or wood. Their ubiquitous airborne spores are frequently troublesome contaminants of cultures of bacteria and mammalian cells. In fact, just such a contaminant led to the discovery of penicillin.

Although we shall be concerned mainly with those few fungi that cause diseases of man, other fungi have had an even more adverse effect on human welfare as causes of plant diseases: for example, the potato blight led to death from starvation in Ireland alone of over 1 million persons in the period 1845 to 1860. More recently, *Aspergillus flavus* contaminating peanut meal was

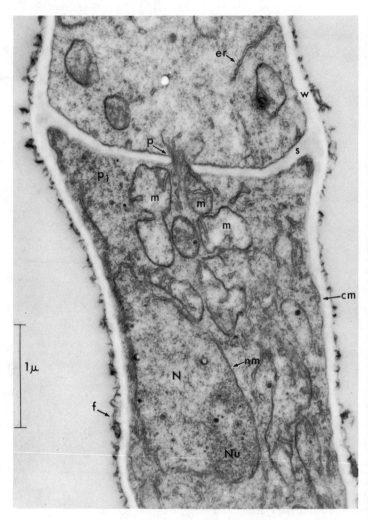

Figure 43–1. The coenocytic nature of hyphae. Electron micrograph of a longitudinal section through two cells of *Neurospora crassa* partially separated by a septum *(s).* Note the streaming of mitochondria *(m)* through the septal pore *(p).* Other labeled structures are cell wall *(w),* outer frayed coat of the cell wall *(f),* cell membrane *(cm),* nucleus *(N),* nucleolus *(Nu),* nuclear membrane *(nm),* ribosomal particles *(p₁),* and endoplasmic reticulum *(er).* Fixed with OsO_4 and stained with uranyl nitrate. (×47,000, reduced; Shatkin AJ, Tatum EL: J Biophys Biochem Cytol 6:423, 1959)

found to produce powerful carcinogens, called **aflatoxins.** On the other hand, fungi make essential contributions to the geochemical cycle; they are used in industrial production (e.g., penicillin, corticosteroids, citric acid); and they have long been used for the production of bread, alcoholic beverages, and certain cheeses.

STRUCTURE AND GROWTH

MOLDS. The principal element of the growing or vegetative form of a mold is the **hypha** (Gr. *hyphe,* web), a branching tubular structure, about 2 to 10 μm in diameter; i.e., much larger than bacteria. As a colony, or **thallus,** grows, its hyphae form a mass of intertwining strands called the **mycelium** (Gr. *mykes,* mushroom). Hyphae grow by elongation at their tips (apical growth) and by producing side branches.

Those hyphae that penetrate into the medium, where they absorb nutrients, are known collectively as the **veg-**

etative mycelium, whereas those that project above the surface of the medium constitute the **aerial mycelium;** because the latter often bear reproductive cells or spores, they are also referred to as the **reproductive mycelium.** Most colonies grow at the surface of liquid or solid media as irregular, dry, filamentous mats. Because of the intertwining of the filamentous hyphae, the colonies are much more tenacious than those of bacteria. At the center of mycelial colonies, the hyphal cells are often necrotic, owing to deprivation of nutrients and oxygen and perhaps to accumulation of organic acids.

In most species, the hyphae are divided by cross-walls called **septa** (L. *septum,* hedge, partition; Fig. 43–1). However, the septa have fine, central pores; hence even septate hyphae are **coenocytic;** i.e., their many nuclei are embedded in a continuous mass of cytoplasm.

YEASTS. Yeasts are unicellular oval or spherical cells, usually about 3 to 5 μm in diameter. Sometimes, yeast cells and their progeny adhere to each other and form chains or "pseudohyphae."

CYTOLOGY. Yeasts and molds resemble cells of plants and animals, with multiple chromosomes, a nuclear membrane, mitochondria, an endoplasmic reticulum, and various membrane-bound organelles. Moreover, their membranes contain sterols.

CELL WALL

Fungus cell walls appear thatched (Fig. 43–2). In many molds and yeasts, the principal structural macromolecule is **chitin,** which is made up of *N*-acetyl glucosamine residues linked by β-1,4-glycosidic bonds like the glucose residues in cellulose, the main cell wall material in higher plants.

and nitrogen as NH_4^+ or NO_3^-. Thermophilic species can grow at temperatures as high as 50°C and above; some species can flourish in the high-salt media of cured meats and others in highly acidic media. Some fungi can hydrolyze the complex organic substances in wood, bone, tanned leather, chitin, waxes, and even synthetic plastics.

The regulatory mechanisms for controlling enzyme synthesis and activity appear similar to those in bacteria. However, the structural genes for a given metabolic pathway are much more scattered in the genome than are those of bacteria. Because yeast cells are the simplest eukaryotes, and because they can be cultivated and cloned as easily as bacteria, they are increasingly used as model systems for studying the cell biology and molecular genetics of eukaryotes (Chap. 11).

Chitin also makes up the principal structural material of the exoskeleton in crustaceans. Yeasts also contain an insoluble **glucan,** made up of β-1,6-linked D-glucose residues with β-1,3-linked branches at frequent intervals and a soluble **mannan,** an α-1,6-linked polymer of D-mannose with α-1,2 and α-1,3 branches.

The walls of a number of yeasts contain complexes of polysaccharide with proteins rich in cystine residues, and the reversible reduction of -S–S- bonds has been implicated in the formation of buds. In some yeasts, lipids containing phosphorus and nitrogen are also abundant in the wall.

Fungus cell walls can be digested by enzymes contained in the digestive juices of the snail *Helix pomatia* or in certain soil bacteria. As with bacteria, digestion of the walls of yeasts or molds in hypertonic solution yields viable **protoplasts.** Protoplasts are also produced by growth in media, or by mutations, that inhibit cell wall synthesis.

METABOLISM

Most fungi are obligate aerobes, but yeast forms, able to grow in the depths of fluids, are often facultative. Except for the absence of autotrophs or obligate anaerobes, the fungi as a group exhibit almost as great a diversity of metabolic capabilities as the bacteria. Many species can grow in minimal media, given an organic carbon source

REPRODUCTION

In addition to growing by apical extension and branching, fungi reproduce by means of sexual and asexual cycles and also by a parasexual process. We shall consider asexual reproduction and the parasexual process in particular detail, as the vast majority of fungi that are pathogenic for man lack sexuality.

Asexual Reproduction

The vegetative **growth** of a coenocytic mycelium involves nuclear division without cell division, the classic process of mitosis ensuring transmission of a full complement of chromosomes to each daughter nucleus. The further step of cell division leads to asexual (vegetative) **reproduction;** i.e., the formation of a new clone without involvement of gametes and without nuclear fusion. Three mechanisms are known: (1) sporulation, followed by germination of the spores; (2) blastospore formation (budding); and (3) fragmentation of hyphae.

Asexual spores are classified in Table 43–1. They are sometimes all referred to as **conidia,** but more often, this term is reserved (as in this chapter) for those spores that form by a process akin to budding at tips of specialized hyphae, called **conidiophores.**

Other asexual spores (**chlamydospores** and **arthrospores**) develop **within hyphae.** The spores germinate when planted in a congenial medium, and, if destined to become a mold, they send out one or more germ tubes

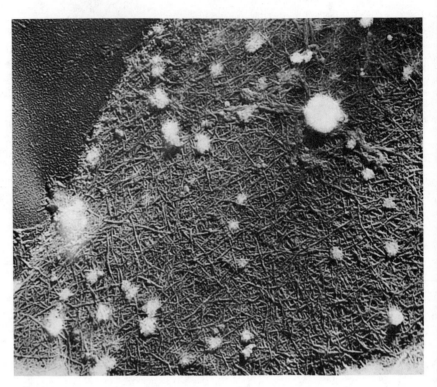

Figure 43–2. Microfibrillar structure of the wall of a species of phycomycete. Chemical analysis and x-ray diffraction showed the thatched fibrils to be chitin. Electron micrograph shadowed with palladium–gold. (×30,000, reduced; Aronson JM, Preston RD: Proc R Soc Lond [Biol] 152:346, 1969)

TABLE 43–1. Asexual Spores Formed by Certain Fungi

Conidia (Gr. *konis,* dust)	Sometimes used generically for all asexual spores, sometimes more specifically for spores borne singly or at tips of specialized hypal branches **(conidiophores).** Highly diversified in shape, size, color, and septation
Aleuriospores (Gr. *aleuron,* wheaten flour)	Spores that resemble conidia but develop on short lateral branches or directly on the hyphae rather than on specialized condiophores
Arthrospores (Gr. *arthron,* joint)	Cylindrical cells formed by double septation of hyphae, individual spores are released by fragmentation of hyphae; i.e., by disjunction
Blastospores (Gr. *blastos,* bud, shoot)	Buds that arise from yeast-like cells
Chlamydospores (Gr. *chlamy,* mantle)	Thick-walled, round spores formed from terminal or intercalated hyphal cells
Sporangiospores (Gr. *angeion,* vessel)	Spores within sac-like structures **(sporangia)** at ends of hyphae or of special hyphal branches **(sporangiophores).** Characteristically formed by species of *Phycomyces*

(see Fig. 43–8, below), which elongate into hyphae. **Chlamydospores,** which can be formed by many fungi, are thick-walled and unusually resistant to heat and drying; they are probably formed, like bacterial spores, by true endosporulation, and they similarly promote survival in unfavorable environments. In contrast, arthrospores and conidia are not unusually resistant; they probably function to promote aerial dissemination.

Spores differ greatly in color, size, and shape; they may contain more than one nucleus. Their morphology and mode of origin constitute the main basis for classifying fungi that lack sexuality. Some species produce only one kind of spore and others as many as four. Various common asexual spores are illustrated in Figures 43–3 and 43–4. They should not be confused with sexual spores (see Sexual Reproduction).

Budding is the prevailing asexual reproductive process in yeasts, although some species divide by fission **(fission yeasts).** Whereas in fission (the usual reproductive process of almost all bacteria) a parent cell divides into two progeny of essentially equal size, in budding the progeny cell is initially much smaller than the parent cell. As the bud bulges out from the parent cell, the nucleus of the latter divides, and one nucleus passes into the bud; cell wall material is then laid down between

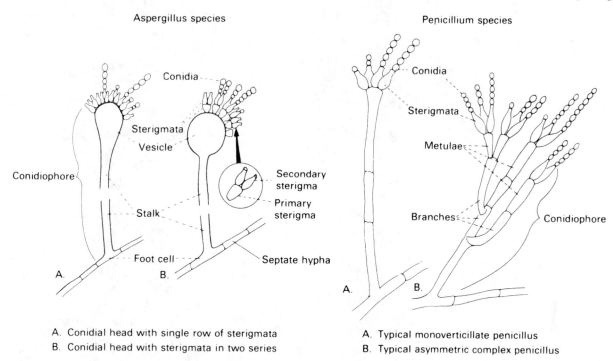

Aspergillus species

Penicillium species

A. Conidial head with single row of sterigmata
B. Conidial head with sterigmata in two series

A. Typical monoverticillate penicillus
B. Typical asymmetric complex penicillus

Figure 43–3. Diagram of some representative filamentous fungi and their asexual spores (conidia). (Ajello L et al: Laboratory Manual for Medical Mycology, USPHS Publ. No. 994. Washington, DC, Government Printing Office, 1963)

bud and parent cell, and the bud eventually breaks away (Fig. 43–5). A **birth** scar on the progeny cell's wall, and a **budding scar** on the parent wall, are visible in electron micrographs (Fig. 43–6). As a result of repeated budding, old yeast cells bear many budding scars, but they have only a single birth scar.

Fragments of hyphae (e.g., formed by teasing a mycelium) are also capable of forming new colonies. This capacity is often exploited in the cultivation of fungi, but it is probably not important in nature.

Sexual Reproduction

Fungi that carry out sexual reproduction go through the following steps. First, a haploid nucleus of a donor cell penetrates the cytoplasm of a recipient cell. Second, the donor and recipient nuclei fuse to form a diploid zygotic nucleus. Third, by meiosis, the diploid nucleus gives rise to four haploid nuclei, some of which may be genetic recombinants. In most species, the haploid condition is the one associated with prolonged vegetative growth and the diploid state is transient, but in other species, as in higher animals, the opposite is true.

In **homothallic** species, the cells of a single colony (arising from a single nucleus) can engage in sexual reproduction. In some homothallic species (hermaphro-

dites), donor and recipient cells are anatomically differentiated, but in others, they are indistinguishable. In **heterothallic** species, the cells that engage in sexual reproduction must arise from two different colonies of opposite mating type. The reproductive cells of some heterothallic species are anatomically distinguishable as donor and recipient, whereas those of others are only functionally differentiated into sexually compatible mating types. Among fungi with a sexual stage, the anatomy of sex organs and the mating procedures are characteristic for any particular species; hence they are important for taxonomy. The process of sexual reproduction in fungi, and the basis for homothallism, are described in Chapter 11.

The four haploid cells resulting from the meiosis remain together in the same sac (**ascus**); and in *Neurospora* (although not in all Ascomycetes) before the ascus is fully matured, each cell divides mitotically into two identical spores. In the ascus, which is shaped like a narrow pod, the eight resulting **ascospores** are held in a linear array whose order reflects the meiotic segregation of their chromosomes. This property has been valuable in studying the mechanism of genetic recombination, because the products of the recombination occurring during meiosis can be directly identified by genetic anal-

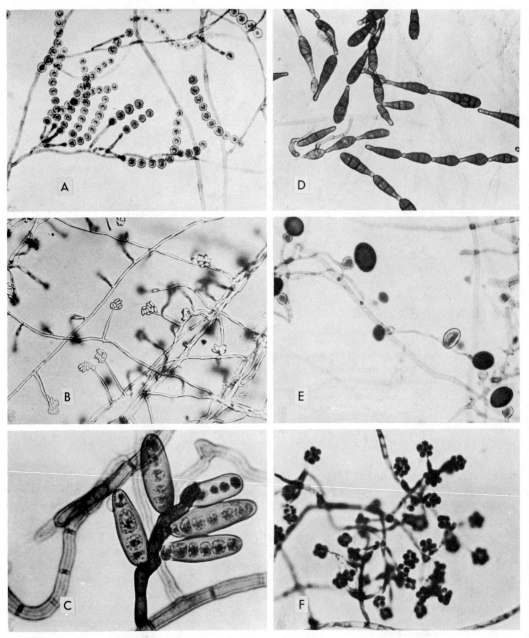

Figure 43–4. Slide cultures of some representative molds showing diverse forms of asexual spores (conidia), which aid in identifying species, particularly with members of the class Fungi imperfecti (Deuteromycetes). (Ajello L et al: Laboratory Manual for Medical Mycology, USPHS Publ. No. 994. Washington, DC, Government Printing Office, 1963)

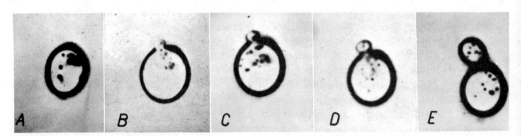

Figure 43–5. Budding in a yeast cell *(Saccharomyces cerevisiae)*. Wall-less bud in *B* was extruded in the 20-second interval between the photos in *A* and *B*. Subsequent photos were taken at approximately 15-minute intervals. Bud in *E* is nearly mature. (Nickerson WJ: Bacteriol Rev 27:305, 1963)

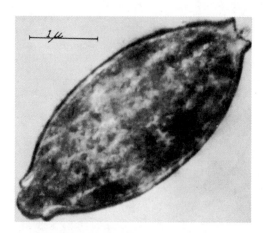

Figure 43–6. Thin section of an OsO₄-fixed yeast cell *(Saccharomyces cerevisiae)*, showing the concave birth scar at one pole and a convex bud scar at the other. (×29,000, reduced; Agar HD, Douglas HC: J Bacteriol 70:247, 1955)

ysis of the four adjacent pairs of spores in the same ascus (tetrad analysis; Chap. 11). In higher organisms, one can only deduce the recombinants from the statistical distribution of genetic markers among the progeny.

Parasexual Cycle (Mitotic Recombination)

Some fungi go through a cycle that imparts some of the biological advantages of sexuality (e.g., recombination of parental DNA) without involvement of specialized mating types or gametes. This process of parasexuality, first demonstrated by Pontecorvo with *Aspergillus*, involves the following steps (Fig. 43–7): (1) by **hyphal fusion**, different haploid nuclei come to coexist in a common cytoplasm. The **heterokaryon** thus formed can be stable, the two sets of nuclei dividing autonomously at about the same rate. (2) Rare **nuclear fusion** will yield heterozygous diploid nuclei. These are usually greatly outnumbered by the haploid nuclei, but once formed, they tend to divide at about the same rate as the latter, and stable diploid strains may be isolated. (3) Although homologous chromosomes are usually arranged independently on the equatorial plane in the mitosis of a diploid cell, rarely (about 10^{-4} per mitosis) sufficient **somatic pairing** will occur to permit crossing over, as in meiosis.

The result of such mitotic recombination between heterozygous homologous chromosomes is to make the products **homozygous for genes distal to the exchange point.** Thus, two diploid progeny with different properties result, each homozygous for some alleles for which the diploid parent cell is heterozygous (Figure 43–7). From this figure, it can also be projected that when these new diploid strains yield haploid progeny, half of these will be parental in genetic composition and half will be recombinant.

Mitotic recombination has provided unique opportunities for genetic analysis of asexual molds, and it has been extended to the study of the genetics of somatic diploid cells, such as human cells in tissue culture.

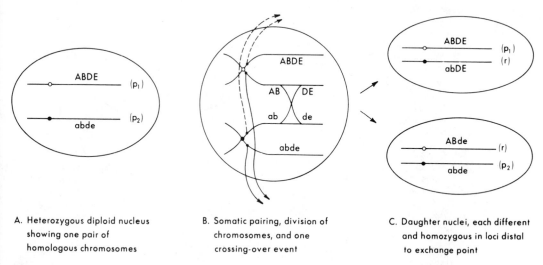

A. Heterozygous diploid nucleus showing one pair of homologous chromosomes

B. Somatic pairing, division of chromosomes, and one crossing-over event

C. Daughter nuclei, each different and homozygous in loci distal to exchange point

Figure 43–7. Somatic pairing and mitotic recombination in the parasexual cycle of fungi. After fusion of genetically different hyphae to form a heterokaryon, the unlike haploid nuclei occasionally fuse to yield the heterozygous diploid nucleus depicted in *(A)*. Rare somatic pairing *(B)* and recombination give rise, through the daughter nuclei depicted in *(C)*, to partially homozygous lines of diploid cells, as shown. These occasionally also segregate haploid strains, half of which are recombinant (compared with the original haploid parents) in respect to loci dD and eE. *p*, parental chromosome; *r*, recombinant chromosome.

TABLE 43–2. Classes of Fungi

Class	Asexual Spores	Sexual Spores	Mycelia	Representative Genera or Groups
Phycomycetes	Endogenous (in sacs)	Anatomy variable	Nonseptate	*Rhizopus, Mucor,* watermolds (aquatic)
Ascomycetes	Exogenous (at ends or sides of hyphae)	Ascospores, within sacs or asci	Septate	*Neurospora, Penicillium, Aspergillus,* true yeasts
Basidiomycetes	Exogenous (at ends or sides of hyphae)	Basidiospores, on surface of basidium	Septate	Mushrooms, rusts, smuts
Deuteromycetes (Fungi imperfecti)	Exogenous (at ends or sides of hyphae)	Absent	Septate	Most human pathogens

TAXONOMY

The four major classes of true fungi are summarized in Table 43–2.

The **Deuteromycetes (Fungi Imperfecti)** include the vast majority of human pathogens. Because no sexual phase has been observed, they are often referred to as imperfect fungi. The hyphae are septate, and conidial forms are very similar to those of the ascomycetes; they have therefore long been suspected of being **special ascomycetes** whose sexual phase is either extremely infrequent or has disappeared in evolution. Indeed, typical ascomycetous sexual stages have now been observed in

TABLE 43–3. Some Pathogenic Imperfect Fungi Discovered to Have a Sexual (Perfect) Stage

Name of Imperfect (Anamorphic) Species	Perfect (Teleamorphic) Form
Microsporum gypseum	*Nannizia incurvata* *N. gypsea*
M. fulvum	*N. fulva*
M. nanum	*N. obtusa*
M. cookei	*N. cajetana*
M. vanbreuseghemii	*N. grubia*
M. canis	*N. otae*
M. persicolor	*N. persicolor*

Trichophyton mentagrophytes	*Arthroderma benhamiae*
	   A. ciferri
	   A. vanbreuseghemii

T. simii	*A. simii*
T. ajelloi	*A. uncinatum*
T. simii	*A. simii*

The species listed are dermatophytes: they infect the epidermis, nails, and hair of mammals. Only the asexual (imperfect) form is found in infected skin. Conversion to the sexual (perfect) form was facilitated by growth on sterilized soil enriched with keratin (e.g., hair, feathers). The perfect stages were then identified as Ascomycetes by observing production of fruiting bodies when compatible "imperfect" forms were mated (e.g., + and − strains). (A fruiting body contains many asci with their enclosed ascospores.)

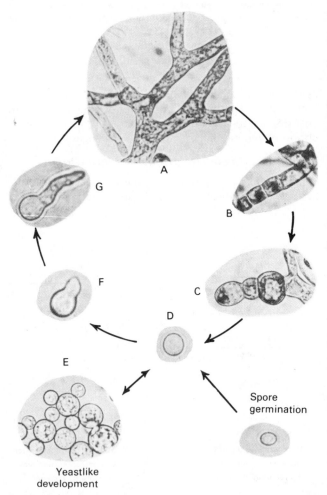

Figure 43–8. Mold–yeast dimorphism in *Mucor rouxii*. Note absence of septa, typical of phycomycetes, in hyphae of the mold at (**A**). Arthrospores are being formed in (**B**) and (**C**). At (**D**), an isolated arthrospore is shown developing into yeastlike cells (**E**), or into a mold (**A**) by outgrowth of a filamentous tube (**F** and **G**). (Bartnicki–Garcia S: Bacteriol Rev 27:293, 1963)

several species, and in some cases what has been considered a single species has been found to include the imperfect stage of two or more different species of ascomycetes (Table 43–3). The reversible change from sexual to asexual form superficially resembles phase variation in bacteria, and the imperfect fungi appear to be mutants in genes that regulate this process.

Pneumocystis carinii, a major cause of pneumonia in patients with AIDS, has long been classified as a protozoon. However, recent sequencing of its rRNA shows much greater similarity to various fungi than to any protozoa. Because its taxonomy awaits clarification the organism will not be described in this chapter.

DIMORPHISM

Some species of fungi grow only as molds and others only as yeasts. Many species, however, can grow in either form, depending on the environment. This capacity is known as **dimorphism.** It is important clinically, because most of the more pathogenic fungi (in man) are dimorphic: they usually appear in infected tissues as yeast-like cells but in cultures as typical molds (Figs. 43–8 and 43–9).

Dimorphism can be controlled experimentally by modifying cultural conditions, a single factor sometimes being decisive. For example, the human pathogen *Blastomyces dermatitidis* grows as a mycelium at 25°C but as yeast cells at 37°. In general, the mycelial forms, leading to aerial dissemination of asexual spores, are a response to unfavorable conditions, whereas the yeast forms are favored by rich nutrition.

COMPARISON WITH BACTERIA

Fungi resemble bacteria in their role in the biosphere, the methods used for their isolation and cultivation, their capacity to cause infectious diseases, and the applications of their fermentations to industrial processes. As eukaryotes, however, they differ greatly from bacteria (Table 43–4). As we shall see, the human diseases caused by fungi are much less common and less varied than those caused by bacteria.

Genetic, biochemical, and antigenic differences have been studied much less among fungi than among bacteria, and the genetics of the medically important fungi remains virtually unexplored.

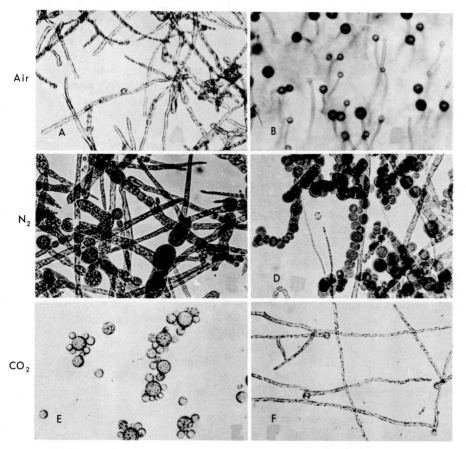

Figure 43–9. Mold–yeast dimorphism in *Mucor rouxii*, growing in yeast extract–peptone–glucose medium. Gaseous phase for incubation is shown at left. **(A)** Filamentous growth in submerged culture. **(B)** Surface growth with active spore formation. **(C)** Filamentous growth at low concentration of glucose (about 2%). **(D)** Arthrospore formation stimulated by high concentration of glucose (10%). **(E)** Yeastlike cells. **(F)** Inhibition of yeast-like growth by a chelating agent (diethylene-triamino-pentaacetic acid). All the forms shown can develop under appropriate conditions from a single uninucleated cell (Fig. 43–11). (Bartnicki-Garcia S: Bacteriol Rev 27:293, 1963)

TABLE 43–4. Contrast Between Fungi and Bacteria

Property	Fungi	Bacteria
Cell volume (μm^3)	Yeast 20–50 Molds: Not definable because of indefinite size and shape and coenocytic form, but much greater than yeast	1–5
Nucleus	Eukaryotic (well-defined membrane)	Prokaryotic (no membrane)
Cytoplasm	Mitochondria, endoplasmic reticulum	No mitochondria or endoplasmic reticulum
Cytoplasmic membrane	Sterols present	Sterols absent (except for *Mycoplasma* grown on sterols)
Cell wall	Glucans; mannans; chitin, glucan– and mannan–protein complexes No muramic acid peptides, teichoic acids, or diaminopimelic acid	Muramic acid peptides; teichoic acids; some have diaminopimelic acids residues No chitin, glucans, or mannans
Metabolism	Heterotrophic; aerobes or facultative anaerobes; no known autotrophs or obligate anaerobes	Obligate and facultative aerobes and anaerobes; heterotrophic or autotrophic
Sensitivity to chemotherapeutic agents	Sensitive to polyenes and griseofulvin (dermatophytes); not sensitive to penicillins, tetracyclines, chloramphenicol, streptomycin	Often sensitive to penicillins, tetracyclines, chloramphenicol, streptomycin; not sensitive to griseofulvin or polyenes
Dimorphism	A distinguishing feature of many species	Absent (except spore-formers)

General Characteristics of Fungus Diseases

Because fungi are larger than bacteria, they were recognized earlier as agents of disease. However, of the estimated 50,000 to 200,000 species of fungi, only about 100 are known to cause infectious disease (**mycoses**) in man. A few of these, with a special predilection for epidermal structures, seem to depend on parasitic growth in animal tissue, some only in man. In addition, the yeast *Candida albicans* is part of the normal flora of the oral mucosa and the gastrointestinal tract. All other fungi that cause disease are only accidental pathogens, acquired from soil or decaying vegetation. They cause problems when they breach the natural barriers (skin, lungs), sometimes aided by compromised immune mechanisms.

TYPES OF MYCOSES

It is useful to divide the mycoses into four groups, differing in the level of the infected tissue (Table 43–5). (1) The **systemic** or **deep mycoses** primarily involve internal organs and viscera. They are often widely disseminated and involve many different tissues. (2) The **subcutaneous mycoses** involve skin, subcutaneous tissue, fascia, and bone. (3) The **cutaneous mycoses** involve epidermis, hair, and nails. The responsible fungi are known as **dermatophytes** (Gr. *phyton*, plant) and the diseases as **dermatophytoses** or **dermatomycoses**. (4) The **superficial mycoses** involve only hair and the most superficial layer of epidermis.

The natural history of the diseases in these groups will now be summarized, and the following section will describe some representatives of each group.

The **systemic** or **deep mycoses** are caused by saprobic fungi in soil, through **inhalation of spores.** As will become evident, these infections resemble clinically the chronic bacterial infections caused by mycobacteria and actinomycetes. The earliest lesions are usually pulmonary, and the initial acute, self-limited pneumonitis is easily overlooked or ascribed to bacteria or viruses. The subsequent chronic form (which is usually much less frequent) begins insidiously, progresses slowly, and is characterized by suppurative or granulomatous lesions. These sometimes form pulmonary cavities and often spread by direct extension, such as into contiguous soft tissues such as the pleurae. These fungi are also prone to spread by way of the blood stream, yielding metastatic abscesses or granulomas in almost any organ including the skin. Prior to the development of effective antifungal chemotherapy, these disseminated mycotic diseases were almost invariably fatal. They are not contagious.

The **subcutaneous mycoses** are also caused by saprobes in soil and on vegetation. Infection occurs by **direct implantation of spores or mycelial fragments,** commonly in scratches caused by thorns. Hence, these diseases tend to be especially prevalent in rural and tropical regions, such as in jungle terrain. The diseases begin insidiously, progress slowly, and are characterized by localized subcutaneous abscesses and granulomas that spread by direct extension, often breaking through the skin surface to form chronic, draining, ulcerated, and crusted lesions. Extension may also occur via lymphatics, leading to suppurative, granulomatous lesions in the regional chain of lymph nodes. These diseases are often extremely disfiguring and not infrequently fatal, although dissemination to the viscera is rare.

Those localized subcutaneous abscesses that are particularly invasive and destructive of soft tissues, fascia, and bone are known as **mycetomas.** They are characterized by burrowing, tortuous sinus tracts that open onto the skin surface. The purulent discharge and the abscesses frequently contain "granules," which are bits of colonies of the responsible microorganism. Clinically indistinguishable abscesses, caused by *Nocardia* and *Streptomyces* (Chap. 36), are known as **actinomycotic mycetomas.** (The fungal mycetomas are sometimes referred to as **maduromycetomas.**)

The fungi that cause **cutaneous mycoses** have a striking predilection for growth in epidermis, hair, and nails. Only a few pathogenic species have been found in soil, and only one (*Microsporum gypseum*) with any frequency. The many other dermatophytes are found only in mammalian skin; they appear to be obligate parasites of man and other animals, transmitted by direct contact or by bits of infected hair or desquamated epidermal scales. The diseases they cause tend to be chronic, and the inflammatory response, mostly confined to the skin at the site of infection, is not especially destructive.

The dermatophytes acquired by man from contaminated soil (*M. gypseum*) or from animals (e.g., *M. canis* from dogs and cats) tend to produce relatively intense but transitory inflammatory lesions in human skin, whereas those that are indigenous in man, and apparently are obligatory parasites, usually evoke only trivial reactions. It would appear that man is immunologically more tolerant of the indigenous dermatophytes than of alien species.

The fungi that cause **superficial mycoses** are localized along hair shafts and in the more superficial, nonviable, cornified epidermal cells. The pathologic lesions are of minor importance.

Certain widespread fungal saprobes almost never establish infections in healthy humans but can cause serious illness in those with various conditions that lower their resistance. The diseases caused by these **opportunistic** fungi may be widely disseminated or they may be localized in the respiratory tract or the mucous membranes and skin.

DIAGNOSIS

The fungal origin of a disease is usually first suspected on the basis of its clinical behavior and the appearance of the lesion. Serologic reactions with Ags of the suspected fungus and delayed allergic skin reactions may provide supporting evidence, but as in infections with bacteria that are abundant in man's environment, these tests are usually not conclusive. The most convincing diagnostic evidence is usually provided by **detection of the fungus** in lesions and exudates by direct microscopic examination and by isolation and cultivation. With some fungous diseases, transmission of the infection to experimental

---

TABLE 43–5. Grouping of Most Frequently Encountered Human Pathogenic Fungi in the U.S. to Tissue Involved and Dimorphism

| Type of Mycotic Disease | Representative Fungus | Morphology in | | Dimorphism? |
		Infected Tissue	Room Temperature Culture	
Systemic	*Cryptococcus neoformans*	Yeast (encapsulated)	Yeast (encapsulated)	No*
	Coccidioides immitis	Spherules	Mycelia	Yes
	Histoplasma capsulatum	Yeast	Mycelia	Yes
	Blastomyces dermatitidis	Yeast	Mycelia	Yes
Systemic, and particularly opportunistic	*Candida* (especially *C. albicans*)	Yeast and hyphae	Yeast and hyphae	Yes
	Aspergillus (most often *A. fumigatus*)	Mycelia	Mycelia	No
	Phycomycetes (*Mucor*, *Rhizopus* spp.)	Mycelia	Mycelia	No
Subcutaneous	*Sporothrix schenckii*	Yeast	Mycelia	Yes
Cutaneous	*Microsporum* spp.	Mycelia	Mycelia	No†
	Trichophyton spp.	Mycelia	Mycelia	No†
	Epidermophyton floccosum	Mycelia	Mycelia	No†

* Except during sexual phase.

† The fungi that parasitize epidermis, nails, and hair (dermatophytes) all appear alike in infected skin, but in culture they develop a variety of specialized hyphae and spore structures that differentiate diverse genera and species; in a sense, they do exhibit a certain amount of dimorphism.

animals by inoculation of tissue suspensions or exudates facilitates isolation, and the lesions in the test animal may also aid in identification (e.g., *Histoplasma capsulatum* in mice, and *Coccidioides immitis* in mice and guinea pigs; see below).

FINDING OF FUNGI IN TISSUES. In one of the simplest procedures, scrapings of the lesion or bits of exudate (e.g., sputum, pus) are warmed on a slide in 10% NaOH or KOH (see, for example, Fig. 43–23). Proteins, fats, and many polysaccharides are extensively solubilized (hydrolyzed and saponified), and the tissues become optically clear; but the cell walls of most fungi remain largely intact and visible because of their alkali-resistant glucans and chitin. With some fungi, particularly small yeast cells, the visibility of the alkali-resistant cell wall is aided by warming tissue in a mixture of KOH and a suitable alkali-stable dye (e.g., 10% KOH in Parker Super Quick blue-black ink clarified by centrifugation).

One of the most widely used staining procedures is based on the periodic acid–Schiff reaction (PAS stain). Periodate cleaves vicinal hydroxyl groups and forms dialdehydes; subsequent reaction of the aldehydes with fuchsin leukosulfonate (Schiff's reagent) forms colorful quinonoid dyes. Nearly all fungus walls are stained an intense red or magenta by this reaction, because a large number of aldehyde groups is produced on periodate oxidation of their insoluble glucans and mannans. Chitin does not stain, however, owing to the absence of vicinal hydroxyls (see Cell Wall, above). The reaction is not, of course, specific for fungi, and some tissue polysaccharides (glycogen, hyaluronic acid) are also stained, although not as intensely.

CULTIVATION OF FUNGI. Fungi grow much more slowly than bacteria. Cultures must therefore be maintained for long periods, and it is essential to inhibit growth of bacterial contaminants, for example, by drugs or by maintaining low pH and low temperatures (25°C), which inhibit bacteria more than fungi. (For this reason, contaminating fungi often overgrow bacterial cultures stored in the refrigerator.)

Sabouraud's agar is the most widely used medium for cultivating fungi. Devised by a nineteenth century dermatologist for dermatophytes, it is useful for virtually all fungi.

With glucose and peptone as the sole nutrients, this medium was originally devised with a pH of 5 to discourage bacterial growth. At present, the medium is adjusted to neutral pH (which is more favorable for the growth of must fungi), and chloramphenicol (40 μg/ml) and cycloheximide (500 μg/ml) are added to reduce the growth of bacteria and saprobic fungi. However, cycloheximide inhibits *Cryptococcus neoformans* and some species of *Candida*, and chloramphenicol inhibits the yeast forms of some dimorphic fungi, so cultures are often prepared both with and without these drugs.

The anatomy of fungal spores and the manner in which they are produced are important determinative characteristics. With dimorphic forms, which generally grow in infected tissues or in rich media as yeasts, sporulation can be stimulated by cultivation under suboptimal nutritional conditions (e.g., rice medium, cornmeal agar). Mycelia are usually white and fluffy at first and then become colored as they develop pigmented spores.

Intact colonies may be examined directly under a dissecting microscope, or fragments of colonies may first be teased gently in media containing a dye such as Poirrier's blue, lactic acid, and phenol (**lactophenol cotton blue**). Fungi are gram-positive.

CHEMOTHERAPY

In view of the substantial physiologic differences between fungi and bacteria, it is not surprising that they respond to different drugs. Effective antifungal chemotherapy began late, with the development of griseofulvin and the polyene agents (Fig. 43–10).

GRISEOFULVIN. Griseofulvin, synthesized by several species of *Penicillium*, causes hyphal distortions in cultures of dermatophytes and other fungi. Its direct application to infected skin lesions has only a limited effect, but when given orally over a period of time, it is highly effective. It does not sterilize the structures already infected at the start of therapy, but it accumulates in newly formed keratinous structures (cornified layers of epidermis, hair, and nails) and renders them resistant to infection. Treatment must therefore be long-term (weeks or months), especially with infected nails. Fortunately, griseofulvin has only minimal toxicity, even on long-term administration. As might be expected from its specialized location, griseofulvin is ineffective in the deep mycoses, but it may have value in one of the subcutaneous mycoses, sporotrichosis.

Although little is known about the antifungal mechanism of griseofulvin, in animal cells it causes disorientation of the mitotic spindle and inhibits the movement of chromosomes at anaphase (much like colchicine and vinblastine, which bind to receptors on tubulin subunits). The microtubules in fungal cells therefore may be the site of action of griseofulvin.

POLYENES. The polyene antibiotics are fungicidal at sufficiently high concentration in growing cultures; they are effective against many systemic mycoses but not in the superficial and cutaneous mycoses. The most widely used member, **amphotericin B,** must be given intravenously for weeks, and it frequently has toxic side effects.

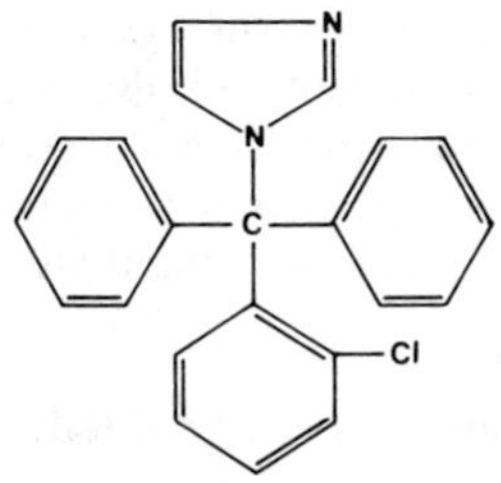

clotrimazole

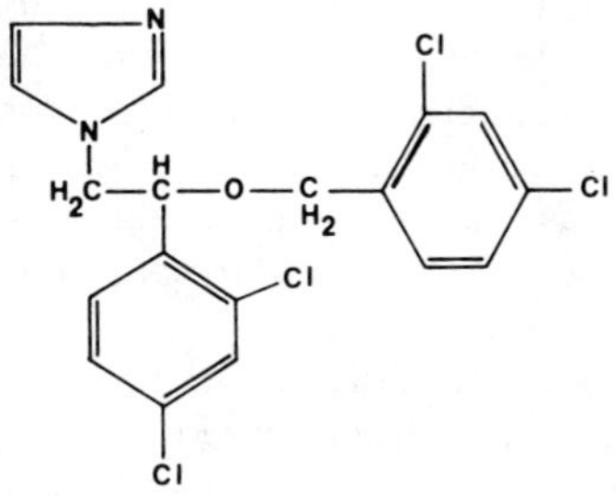

miconazole

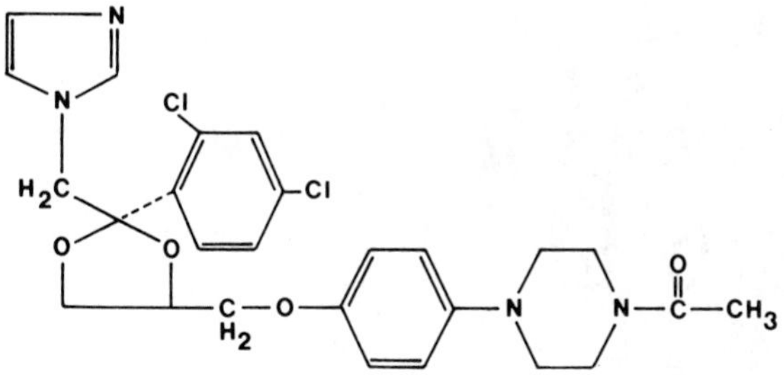

ketoconazole

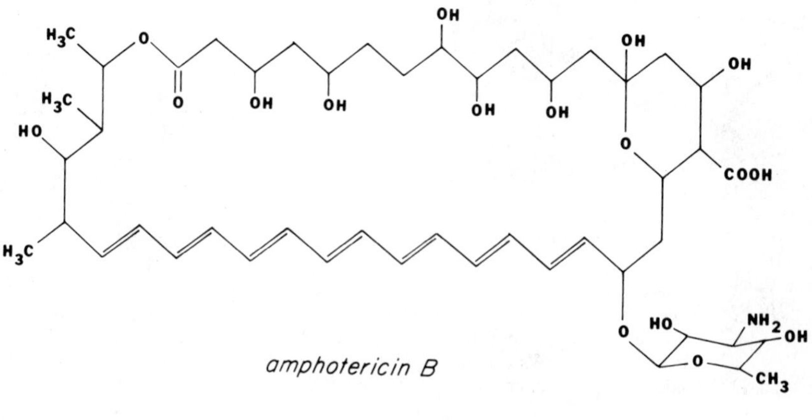

amphotericin B

Figure 43–10. Some antifungal agents. Griseofulvin, first isolated from *Penicillium griseofulvum*, is produced by several species of *Penicillium*. Various polyenes are produced by different species of *Streptomyces* (e.g., nystatin by *S. noursei*, pimaricin by *S. natalensis*). Nystatin and pimaricin are tetraenes; i.e., have four alternating double bonds; amphotericin B and candicidin are heptaenes.

Nystatin (named for its discovery in a New York State laboratory) is used topically for *Candida* infections.

Bacteria are not susceptible to the polyenes, because their cell membranes lack **sterols.** Red blood cell membranes contain sterols, and polyenes cause hemolysis *in vitro* and occasional hemolytic anemia.

FLUCYTOSINE (5-FLUOROCYTOSINE). The synthetic compound flucytosine is effective, taken orally, in the treatment of candidiasis, cryptococcosis, and chromomycosis. Fungi sensitive to this compound (but not man) deaminate it to yield fluorouracil, which is incorporated into RNA. Fungi rapidly develop resistance to flucytosine, but its combined use with amphotericin B appears to be better than amphotericin B alone.

IMIDAZOLES AND TRIAZOLES. Imidazole derivatives are active against dermatophytes, dimorphic fungi, yeasts, parasites, and several gram-positive bacteria. They inhibit ergosterol synthesis in fungi by interfering with the microsomal cytochrome P450-dependent lanosterol demethylase system. At high concentrations, these drugs also inhibit fatty acid synthesis. Miconazole and clotrimazole are used as topical agents in the treatment of dermatophyte infections. Ketoconazole, itraconazole, and fluconazole are effective orally against paracoccidioidomycosis and histoplasmosis. Derivatives in which the imidazole ring is replaced by the related 1,2,4-triazole ring have a similar spectrum of activity.

Some Pathogenic Fungi and Fungus Diseases

SYSTEMIC MYCOSES
Cryptococcus Neoformans (Cryptococcosis)

Fungi of the genus *Cryptococcus* appear as spherical cells that look like true yeasts (ascomycetes), but when two compatible isolates are crossed on sporulation medium, the cells conjugate and develop structures that identify them as basidiomycetes (Fig. 43–11). The only pathogen in the group, *C. neoformans*, is now placed in the genus *Filobasidiella*.

In rapidly growing cultures of the yeast phase, the buds separate from their parent cells precociously; hence, suspensions often exhibit unusually large variations in cell diameter, from about 4 to 20 μm (Fig. 43–12).

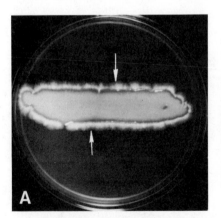
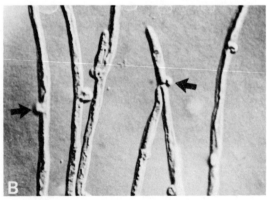
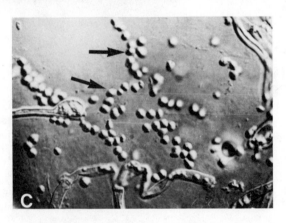

Figure 43–11. *Filobasidiella neoformans,* the sexual state of *Cryptococcus neoformans.* **(A)** Mated culture of yeast cells characterized by the production of dense white mycelium along the margin of yeast growth *(arrows).* (×10) **(B)** Hyphae with clamp connections *(arrows).* (×1200) **(C)** Terminal basidium from which subglobose to elliptical, finely roughened basidiospores, 1.8 μm–2.5 μm in diameter *(arrows),* are produced in chains by budding from four points on the apex of the basidium. (×1200). (Courtesy of KJ Kwon-Chung)

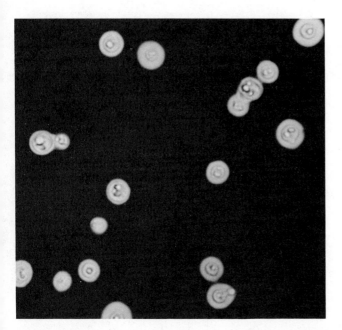

Figure 43–12. *C. neoformans* suspended in India ink. Note budding, thick capsules, and variations in cell diameter. In fresh spinal fluid, without India ink, the yeast cells are easily mistaken for lymphocytes (×450, reduced)

All strains produce capsules, some much thicker than the enclosed cells. About 12 species have been defined on the basis of antigenic and morphologic characteristics. *C. neoformans* is readily differentiated from nonpathogenic species by its virulence for mice. In infected tissues and ordinary cultures *C. neoformans* appear only as encapsulated yeast cells. It grows readily on Sabouraud's agar at 37°C.

The capsule of *C. neoformans*, its most distinctive feature, is easily seen in India ink suspensions of the cells (Fig. 43–12). It is composed of a polysaccharide containing xylose, mannose, and glucuronic acid, and it cross-reacts with antisera to the capsular polysaccharides of types 2 and 14 pneumococci. Although *C. neoformans* evokes only a feeble immune response in infected humans, hyperimmunized rabbits yield capsule-specific antisera that differentiate four strains, called A, B, C, and D. When suspended in homologous antiserum, the cells undergo a quellung reaction like encapsulated bacteria (Chap. 23).

PATHOGENESIS. The disease caused by *C. neoformans* is called **cryptococcosis.*** Inhalation of yeast cells is as-

* In the European literature, cryptococcosis is still referred to as **European blastomycosis,** the term "blastomycosis" formerly being used for any disease resulting from infection with yeast-like cells. In the U.S., *C. neoformans* was previously named *Torula histolytica*, and the disease was called **torulosis.**

sumed to initiate pulmonary infection, with subsequent hematogenous spread to other viscera and the central nervous system, especially in immunosuppressed individuals. It seems likely that silent infections of the lung are common and that only a very small proportion become disseminated.

In the chronic, disseminated form of the disease, the brain, lungs, other viscera, skin, and bones may be involved. The lesions may simulate tuberculous meningitis, brain abscess, or brain tumor. Pulmonary lesions are usually inapparent clinically but are almost always found at autopsies. In a few individuals, chronic pneumonitis is the most conspicuous clinical manifestation.

The microorganism appears in tissues as masses of budding encapsulated yeast cells. There is often little or no surrounding inflammatory reaction, but sometimes granulomatous lesions are formed, with multinuclear giant cells. The yeast cells may be observed within macrophages, particularly when the periodic acid–Schiff stain is used.

DIAGNOSIS. The diagnosis is usually established either by observing *C. neoformans* in spinal fluid (the India ink technique being particularly useful; Fig. 43–12) or by cultivating it from spinal fluid or pus or other exudates. Cycloheximide is inhibitory and should be omitted from the medium. The capsular Ag can be identified in spinal fluid, serum, or urine by the precipitin reaction with hyperimmune rabbit serum or by a particle agglutination test using latex beads coated with anticryptococcal rabbit Ab. A control test uses particles coated with normal rabbit serum to rule out false-positive reactions caused by rheumatoid factor, or the spinal fluid can be heated to denature the protein factor while leaving the reactive polysaccharide.

THERAPY. Cryptococcosis involving the central nervous system, with or without disseminated visceral lesions, formerly was invariably fatal, but amphotericin B (alone or in combination with 5–fluorocytosine) has cured the infection even when first administered in an extremely ill person.

EPIDEMIOLOGY. Cryptococcosis occurs sporadically throughout the world. The organism has been isolated from soil, particularly soil enriched with pigeon droppings. It is also found in pigeon roosts and nests far removed from the soil; for example, on window ledges and towers of urban buildings. Small outbreaks of acute pulmonary infection have occurred among workers demolishing old buildings.

Because the fungus remains viable in dried material for many months, contaminated materials are a potent source of airborne infection. Pigeon droppings are often highly contaminated: 5×10^7 viable organisms per gram were found in one study. These organisms are evidently attributable, not to intestinal infections of pigeons, but to airborne contaminants that find a particularly fertile medium in the droppings. Thus *C. neoformans* is unable to grow at the normal body temperature of birds (40°–42°C), and birds are highly resistant to cryptococcal infection; mice infected with *C. neoformans* have been observed to survive longer when maintained at 35°C than at 25°.

Blastomyces Dermatitidis *(Blastomycosis)**

B. dermatitidis grows as yeast cells in infected tissues or in cultures at 37°C and as a mold at 25°C. The mycelia are white at first, darken with age, and have characteristic spherical conidia, about 3 to 5 μm in diameter, borne directly on the sides of hyphae or at the tips of sort, slender lateral branches. The spore walls also darken with age and resemble chlamydospores.

B. *dermatitidis* is readily isolated on Sabouraud's medium. Conversion from yeast to *mycelial* growth, and vice versa, is readily accomplished simply by altering the temperature. In the sexual stage (called *Ajellomyces dermatitidis*), the fungus is a heterothallic ascomycete.

In sections of infected tissues (and in sputum or in pus expressed from skin lesions), *B. dermatitidis* appears as unusually thick-walled, multinucleated spherical cells, 8 to 15 μm in diameter, without a capsule (Fig. 43–13). Buds, attached to the parent cell by a broad base, are characteristically **unipolar;** i.e., there is not more than one bud per parent cell at any time.

PATHOGENESIS. Infection apparently begins in the lungs and spreads hematogenously to establish focal destructive lesions in bones, skin, prostate, and other viscera; the gastrointestinal tract is spared. The skin lesions are often particularly conspicuous; they may arise as metastases from the primary pulmonary lesion that break through the skin surface and establish spreading, ulcerated, crusted lesions. These are characterized by granulomatous inflammation, microabscesses, and extensive tissue destruction. The yeast cells are visible within the abscesses and granulomas (Fig. 43–13). Calcification is rare.

Persons with blastomycosis often give a complement-fixation (CF) reaction with intact *B. dermatitidis* yeast cells or soluble Ags prepared from them and a delayed-type skin response to **blastomycin,** a crude filtrate of mycelial culture. However, cross-reactions with *Histoplasma capsulatum* or *Coccidioides immitis* diminish the diagnostic value of either reaction. These reactions may be negative in far-advanced illness.

---

* Paracoccidioidomycosis, formerly referred to as South American blastomycosis, is caused by *Paracoccidioides brasiliensis*, discussed later in this chapter.

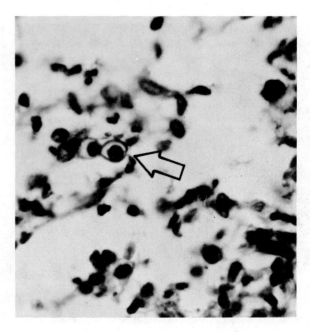

Figure 43–13. *Blastomyces dermatitidis* in a tissue section; a thick-walled yeast cell *(arrow)* with bud. The broad connection between parent cell and bud (dumbbell shape), and the single bud per parent cell, are both characteristic of *B. dermatitidis* (compare with *Paracoccidioides brasiliensis*, Fig. 43–22). (Hematoxylin–eosin stain; ×450, reduced)

DIAGNOSIS AND THERAPY. The demonstration of nonencapsulated, thick-walled, multinucleate yeast cells in pus, sputum, or tissue sections, and their isolation by culture, establish the diagnosis of blastomycosis. The yeast form of *B. dermatitidis* grows at 37°C and is inhibited by chloramphenicol or cycloheximide. Inoculation of mice intraperitoneally with pus or sputum is occasionally helpful; the fungus is usually readily cultivated from the localized abscesses that appear in the peritoneal cavity in 3 or 4 weeks.

Amphotericin B is the drug of choice.

EPIDEMIOLOGY. The disease caused by *B. dermatitidis*, **blastomycosis,** is largely confined to Canada and the U.S. It is most often encountered in the Mississippi valley. Autochthonous cases have also been encountered in various parts of Africa. Infections also occur sporadically in dogs, presumably from inhalation.

B. dermatitidis is thought to be a soil saprobe and has been cultivated in the laboratory on sterilized soil. However, the many attempts to isolate it from soil have rarely been successful.

Histoplasma Capsulatum *(Histoplasmosis)*

H. capsulatum appears in infected tissue as small (1–3 μm in diameter) oval yeast cells usually localized within macrophages and reticuloendothelial cells (Fig. 43–14).

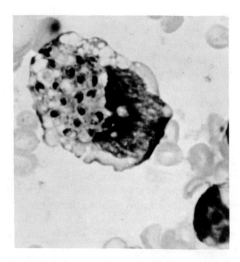

Figure 43–14. Yeast cells of *H. capsulatum* in a macrophage; an impression smear of liver from an infected mouse. (Wright's stain; ×1250)

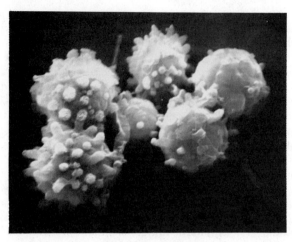

Figure 43–15. Characteristic thick-walled spores with spiny projections (tuberculate chlamydospores) in a culture of *H. capsulatum* at room temperature (×4,000; scanning electron photomicrograph courtesy of Robert G. Garrison)

Budding is only rarely observed in tissues, because buds separate readily from parent cells. The organism is dimorphic; when cultivated at room temperature, it forms slowly growing mycelial colonies. These are white at first, become tan with aging, and have fine, silky aerial mycelia. The conidia are small or large spheres with characteristic regularly spaced, spiny projections (Fig. 43–15). The sexual stage of *H. capsulatum* has been designated *Ajellomyces capsulata* and is classified as an ascomycete.

Hyphae are readily converted to yeast cells *in vitro* by enrichment of the medium with blood or yeast extracts, an increase in the temperature to 37°C, and the presence of adequate moisture. Hyphae become constricted at the septa and then fragment into elongated cells, which become oval and multiply by budding. The conversion to yeast also occurs when mycelial fragments are serially passed through animal cell cultures (e.g., HeLa cells) or inoculated into mice.

The reverse conversion (yeast to mold) is brought about simply by decreasing the incubation temperature of yeast cultures from 37° to 25°C.

PATHOGENESIS. *H. capsulatum* is present in soil, and inhalation of conidia leads to pulmonary infection. Miliary lesions appear throughout the lung parenchyma, and hilar lymph nodes become enlarged. The initial infection is mild. It may pass unnoticed or may appear as a self-limited respiratory infection. With healing, the pulmonary lesions become fibrotic and calcified and give rise to the characteristic roentgenographic pattern of healed histoplasmosis, formerly confused with healed primary tuberculosis (see Epidemiology below).

In a very small number of infected individuals, the infection becomes progressive and widely disseminated, with lesions in practically all tissues and organs. Fever, wasting, and enlargement of liver, spleen, and lymph nodes occur, and the disease may closely simulate miliary tuberculosis. In fact, this severe disseminated form of histoplasmosis often coexists in individuals who have tuberculosis or some other severe generalized disease, such as leukemia or Hodgkin's disease. Histoplasmosis is occasionally seen as a chronic pulmonary disease with cavitation, simulating pulmonary tuberculosis.

The tissue lesions are characterized by granulomatous inflammation similar to that in tuberculosis, with epithelioid cells, occasional giant cells, and even caseation necrosis. The characteristic features, however, are swollen fixed and wandering macrophages containing many small, oval yeast cells (Fig. 43–14). These are readily seen in tissue sections or cell smears treated with Wright's, Giemsa's, or the periodic acid–Schiff stain.

IMMUNE RESPONSE. Precipitation and agglutination reactions with filtrates of mycelial or yeast-phase cultures or with heat- of Formalin-killed yeast cells are observed in mild histoplasmosis. With more advanced disease, CF Abs also appear and are regarded as having some prognostic significance. Cross-reactions are seen with culture filtrates of *Blastomyces dermatitidis* and *Coccidioides immitis*, and unfortunately, the clinical manifestations of these three mycoses may be indistinguishable, particularly in early infections confined to the lungs.

Persons previously infected with *H. capsulatum* regularly give delayed-type skin responses to intradermal injection of **histoplasmin**, a crude, sterile culture filtrate of mycelia grown in synthetic medium. Cross-reactions also occur with coccidioidin (from *C. immitis*) and with blastomycin (from *B. dermatitidis*).

DIAGNOSIS. A provisional diagnosis of histoplasmosis is based on clinical manifestations, serologic tests, and a positive skin response to histoplasmin. The latter has, of course, virtually no value in those localities where the fungus is so prevalent that most persons react to histoplasmin (see Epidemiology). For a definitive diagnosis, it is necessary to identify *H. capsulatum* in tissues or exudates and to isolate it by culture. Staining of blood cells, sputum, and tissue biopsies with Wright's or Giemsa's stain often reveals monocytes or macrophages with characteristic intracellular small yeast cells; and the yeast has even been found in the urinary sediment of persons with progressive histoplasmosis. Cultivation is readily accomplished on Sabouraud's agar and a variety of other media.

Intraperitoneal inoculation of mice with sputum to which penicillin, streptomycin, and chloramphenicol are added can detect as few as 10 yeast cells. Autopsy of the mice 2 to 6 weeks later generally reveals the characteristic yeast within reticuloendothelial cells in smears of spleen cells; and culture of the tissues on Sabouraud's agar at room temperature yields characteristic mycelial growth.

THERAPY. Disseminated histoplasmosis was formerly invariably fatal, but it can be treated effectively with amphotericin B.

EPIDEMIOLOGY. Histoplasmosis provides a striking example of the value of epidemiologic analysis in the discovery of agents of disease. After the spherical yeast cells were first observed in 1906 in tissues taken postmortem, a few additional cases, all fatal, were reported in scattered parts of the world. But in the 1940s, an enormous background of mild or inapparent infection was discovered. At that time, pulmonary calcification was considered to be almost invariable the endproduct of old tuberculosis, and tuberculin-negative persons with such lesions (revealed by roentgenography) were assumed to have lost their previous tuberculin hypersensitivity. However, a survey of tuberculosis in student nurses in different parts of the U.S., undertaken by the U.S. Public Health Service, unexpectedly revealed that pulmonary calcification without tuberculin sensitivity was rare in eastern U.S. cities but common in some midwestern communities. This finding strongly suggested that some disease other than tuberculosis was producing pulmonary calcification. Skin testing with culture filtrates of several organisms revealed that histoplasmin sensitivity was much more prevalent in the regions where the aberrant calcifications were found and was regularly present

in the tuberculin-negative persons with these healed lesions.

H. capsulatum was then isolated from soil, particularly where contaminated heavily with droppings of birds and bats. Bird droppings enrich the soil as a culture medium, but birds do not carry the organism, which does not thrive at their high body temperature. Bats are naturally infected.

Mass surveys, with chest roentgenograms and histoplasmin skin testing, have now revealed that infection is extremely widespread. In some areas in the Ohio and Mississippi valleys, about 80% of all adults, and more than 97% of those with calcified pulmonary lesions, react positively to histoplasmin. Domesticated and wild animals are also naturally infected; in one area of Virginia, 50% of the dogs in a large sample were found at necropsy to have histoplasmosis.

Infection occurs by inhalation of airborne conidia. The yeast cells in sputum and other exudates are less stable and are readily killed by drying, freezing, or heating. Transmission from man to man, and from animal to man, has not been established.

Coccidioides Immitis (*Coccidioidomycosis*)

Like *H. capsulatum*, *C. immitis* was first observed in postmortem tissue, and almost 40 years elapsed before it was recognized that *C. immitis* likewise could cause an acute, benign respiratory infection as well as a fatal chronic systemic disease.

In infected tissues, *C. immitis* appears as spherules or sometimes as a mixture of spherules and hyphae. The **spherules** are thick-walled structures that may be as small as 5 μm in diameter but at maturity are usually 20 to 60 μm (Fig. 43–16). They are filled with a few to several hundred globular or irregularly shaped **endospores,** from 2 to 5 μm in diameter. When the large spherules rupture, the individual endospores are released and in turn develop into spherules: they enlarge, acquire thickened walls, and form multiple endospores.

Growth of *C. immitis* is not inhibited by chloramphenicol or by cycloheximide.

When the spherules are cultivated on Sabouraud's agar or other simple media, even at 37°C, fluffy white mycelia appear within about 5 days. A characteristic feature of the hyphae are the cask-shaped **arthroconidia,** which alternate with smaller, clear hyphal cells (Fig. 43–17). The hyphae of older cultures fragment easily and release huge numbers of arthroconidia, which are easily airborne and highly infectious. Unusual care is therefore required in handling the cultures.

The mycelial (saprobic) form is readily converted into the spherule (parasitic) form by inoculating mycelial fragments or arthroconidia intraperitoneally into mice or guinea pigs. Several days after inoculation, some arthroconidia become enlarged, spherical, and thick-walled,

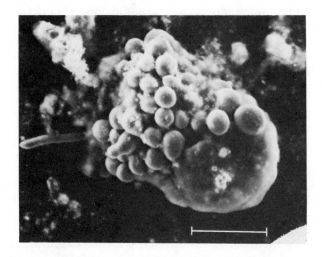

Figure 43–16. A ruptured spherule of *Coccidioides immitis* releasing endospores; *bar* represents 10 μm. (Scanning electron photomicrograph courtesy of SH Sun)

and by 1 week, when they are about 40 μm in diameter, radial partitions appear and subdivide the nascent spherule into cells that subsequently become endospores.

In vitro enrichment of cultures with ascitic fluid, serum, or blood and incubation at 37°C favor the conversion of mycelia into spherules, but hyphae persist, and some of the developing spherules remain linked to form hyphal chains.

PATHOGENESIS. *C. immitis* grows as a saprove in desert soils of the southwestern U.S. and northern Mexico. Infection is established by inhalation of airborne spores, and the disease is known as **coccidioidomycosis.**

During World War II, the establishment of military bases in areas of the U.S. where the disease is endemic provided a unique opportunity to observe its evolution in large numbers of freshly exposed persons. In about 60% of infected persons, infection is revealed only by acquisition of delayed-type hypersensitivity to Ags of *C. immitis.* In about 40%, however, acute pneumonitis develops, often with pleurisy. Various skin eruptions may also occur, such as erythema multiforme and erythema nodosum: sterile skin lesions that probably represent allergic responses to fungal Ags or perhaps fungus-modified tissue Ags. (Similar sterile skin eruptions appear in some other infections, such as with *Mycobacterium tuberculosis* and β-hemolytic streptococci.) About 5% of infected persons ultimately develop chronic pulmonary cavitary disease resembling pulmonary tuberculosis and occasionally leading to calcification. In less than 1%, dissemination occurs, with granulomatous lesions in the skin, bones, joints, and, particularly, the meninges.

The lesions of acute pneumonitis caused by *C. immitis* are histologically like those caused by pyogenic bacteria, whereas in the chronic pulmonary disease and in the disseminated lesions, the inflammation is granulomatous and is characterized by abundant histiocytes, giant cells, and caseation necrosis. Small spherules are found within macrophages or giant cells, and the larger, more mature spherules lie freely in tissue spaces (Fig.

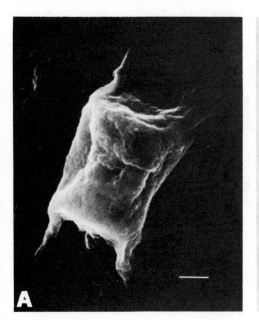

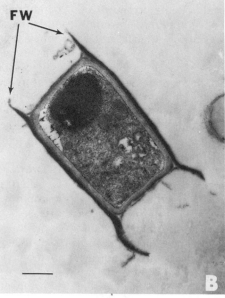

Figure 43–17. Arthroconidia of *C. immitis* as seen by *(A)* scanning and *(B)* transmission electron microscopy. The fragmented walls *(FW)* are characteristic of these infectious particles. *Bar* represents 1 μm. (Courtesy of SH Sun)

43–16). The spherules are readily seen with a number of special stains, such as the periodic acid–Schiff stain. In the walls of pulmonary cavities, **both** forms of this dimorphic fungus (spherules plus hyphae) may be seen, as in enriched cultures.

IMMUNE RESPONSE. Coccidioidin, a crude filtrate of a mycelial culture, is used in precipitin reactions, CF assays, and skin tests. The skin reaction is of the delayed type. During the first week, with overt symptoms, 80% of patients in one extensive study had positive coccidioidin skin tests, whereas only 50% and 10% gave positive precipitin and CF reactions, respectively. In those with self-limited disease (spontaneously cured), precipitins in the serum gradually diminished and were not detectable 4 to 5 months later. The CF Abs tended to appear later and to persist longer. Cross-reactions may occur with culture filtrates of *B. dermatitidis* and *H. capsulatum.*

A decrease in intensity of the skin response will often, but not invariably, occur in clinically well persons who move away from areas where *C. immitis* is endemic; their skin reaction may become entirely negative within 12 months. Hypersensitivity may, however, persist indefinitely in others, owing to survival of viable endospores within healed, walled-off scars. In experimental animals, viable organisms have been found in fibrotic and calcified scars as long as 2 to 3 years after infection.

Coccidioidin is often injected repeatedly in the same individuals during clinical and epidemiologic studies. Fortunately, repeated injections in humans, in the amounts used in routine skin tests, have not induced delayed-type hypersensitivity.

Coccidioidin, blastomycin, and histoplasmin at high concentrations may elicit cross-reacting skin responses in persons with any of the three corresponding diseases, and even non-specific responses due to the preservative in the test solution. At lower concentrations, however, coccidioidin seems to provide a relatively specific test.

DIAGNOSIS. A provisional diagnosis of coccidioidomycosis is usually based on epidemiologic considerations, clinical manifestations, the skin response to coccidioidin, and the detection of Abs. However, definitive diagnosis requires that the spherules be identified in sputum, exudates, or tissue sections.

Cultivation of *C. immitis in vitro* for this purpose is hazardous, because cultures release large numbers of airborne arthroconidia; it is best carried out by experienced personnel with access to ventilated hoods. Transmission of *C. immitis* to laboratory animals is, however, a relatively simple and safe procedure. Sputum or exudate is treated with penicillin, streptomycin, or chloramphenicol, and centrifuged; the sediment is injected either in the testes of guinea pigs or intraperitoneally in mice. If *C. immitis* is present, mice develop disseminated disease,

and the testes and the mouse tissue fluids should contain characteristic spherules; moreover, CF Abs may appear in the guinea pig.

THERAPY. When confined to the lungs, coccidioidomycosis usually heals with scarring, but the disseminated disease was invariably fatal until the polyene antibiotics became available. Treatment with amphotericin B is moderately successful.

EPIDEMIOLOGY. The fungus has a predilection for growth in desert soils, especially after winter and spring rains. Windborne arthroconidia readily infect man and also other mammals (wild rodents, dogs, and cattle). Skin testing of large human populations, and examination of animals, has established that coccidioidomycosis is prevalent in the southwestern U.S.: central California (especially in the San Joaquin valley), Arizona, New Mexico, western Texas, and southern Utah. In some of these areas, 50% to 80% of the population reacts to coccidioidin. The organism has also been found in northern Mexico, parts of Argentina, and Paraguay.

Paracoccidioides Brasiliensis (Paracoccidioidomycosis)

P. brasiliensis was thought to be similar to *C. immitis,* hence its name. It is probably a soil saprobe. The disease it causes has been reported mainly in Brazil but also in most other South and Central American countries.

The fungus appears in infected tissues as large (10–30 μm, even 60-μm) spherical or oval yeast cells. Characteristically, multiple buds sprout from a single parent cell and remain attached to it by narrow constricted bands (Fig. 43–18). When the buds are about the same size and all quite small, their distinctive arrangement around the parent cell is often referred to as a **pilot's wheel.** The buds may also be equal in size to the parent cell and remain attached as **satellite cells.** Chains of budding cells are also seen.

P. brasiliensis is dimorphic. In culture at room temperature on Sabouraud's medium, it grows as a mycelium with chlamydospores. Conversion to yeast cells is induced by enrichment of the medium (e.g., with brain–heart infusion), adequate moisture, and increase in incubation temperature to 37°C.

PATHOGENESIS. The disease produced by *P. brasiliensis* is called **paracoccidioidomycosis, paracoccidioidal granuloma,** or **South American blastomycosis.** The disease is primarily pulmonary, where it may remain inapparent or subclinical, like histoplasmosis. In progressive disseminated disease, lesions arise in the mucous membranes of the mouth or nose and spread by direct extension; for example, over the mucocutaneous borders to involve the face. Dissemination also occurs, with fre-

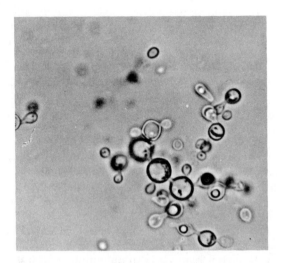

Figure 43–18. Budding of yeast cells in a culture (37°C) of *Paracoccidioides brasiliensis.* Multiple buds, attached to their parent cell by constricted tubes, are characteristic. Compare with the broad-based, unipolar buds characteristic of *Blastomyces dermatitidis* (Fig. 43–17). (×450, reduced)

quent involvement of lymphoid tissue, including the spleen. In the intestinal tract, lesions begin in submucosal lymphoid tissue and may lead to ulceration and even perforation. Subcutaneous abscesses can appear, and by extension to the skin surface, they form large, unsightly crusted and ulcerated lesions.

Histologically, skin lesions appear as pyogenic abscesses and granulomatous inflammation with epithelioid cells, giant cells, and necrotic centers. Large spherical or oval yeast cells with multiple circumferential buds (pilot's wheel or satellite forms) may be observed in routine hematoxylin–eosin stains of tissue sections but are more clearly brought out with the periodic acid–Schiff reaction. The yeast cells sometimes appear as chains and may be found within giant cells.

DIAGNOSIS. Detection of *P. brasiliensis* in tissue sections or in exudates, and cultivation as yeast and mycelial forms, establish the diagnosis. Chloramphenicol and cycloheximide are added to Sabouraud's medium, and the cultures are maintained as mycelia at room temperature, as these antibiotics inhibit the growth of the yeast cells but not the mycelia of this fungus. Transmission to laboratory animals is possible but is not often resorted to as a diagnostic procedure.

THERAPY. Long-term treatment with sulfonamides has been used effectively to control infections, but with cessation of therapy, the disease returns. Amphotericin B is highly effective but toxic. Recent clinical trials have shown ketoconazole to be highly effective, and it is currently the drug of choice in South America.

MYCOSES CAUSED BY OPPORTUNISTIC FUNGI

A number of fungi that are not pathogenic in healthy humans may be virulent in those suffering from a variety of disorders (e.g., malignant lymphomas, severe diabetes, AIDS) or being treated with broad-spectrum antibacterial drugs or with immunosuppressive measure. The frankly opportunistic fungi are mostly species of *Candida, Aspergillus, Rhizopus,* and *Mucor.* The clinical impression of the role of lowered resistance has been supported by experimental observations. For example, mice given cortisone are unusually susceptible to lethal infection with *C. albicans.*

In addition, among the pathogenic fungi discussed above, *Cryptococcus neoformans, H. capsulatum, B. dermatitidis,* and possibly even *Coccidioides immitis* are somewhat opportunistic, causing progressive infections more frequently under debilitating conditions.

Candida albicans *(Candidiasis)*

C. albicans is dimorphic. At the surface of a rich agar medium, it grows as oval budding yeast cells, but deeper in the medium, hyphae are found. Both forms are characteristically seen in infected tissues and in most cultures. Some hyphae, called **pseudohyphae,** have recurring constrictions, as though a chain of sausage-shaped cells were joined end to end (Fig. 43–19).

C. albicans is readily grown on conventional media at room temperature or at 37°C. In cultures on agar, the early colonies are smooth, creamy, and bacteria-like, but the older, larger colonies may appear furrowed and rough. Cultivation on cornmeal agar stimulates the formation of characteristic thick-walled **chlamydospores,** which distinguish *C. albicans* from other candidae (Fig. 43–19). On the basis of colonial morphology, sugar utilization patterns, and serologic reactions, several less frequent species of *Candida* from human lesions have been distinguished. These include *C. krusei, C. parakrusei,* and *C. parapsilosis.*

PATHOGENESIS. Species of *Candida* are frequently present on the normal mucous membranes of the mouth, vagina, and intestinal tract. When they become invasive, under the special circumstances mentioned previously, they establish a variety of acute or chronic, localized or widely disseminated, lesions. The following are some examples usually caused by *C. albicans.*

1. **Thrush (oral candidiasis)** consists of discrete or confluent white patches, composed of hyphae and yeast cells, on the mucous membranes of the mouth and pharynx. They occur particularly during the first few days of life (resulting from infection during birth) and in persons in the terminal stages of a wasting disease, such as carcinomatosis or AIDS.

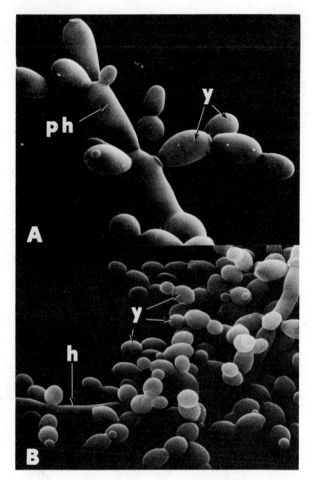

Figure 43–19. Multiplicity of structural forms in a culture of *Candida albicans.* *(A)* Pseudohyphae *(ph)* are elongated cells linked end to end. (×5060) *(B)* True hyphae (h) and yeasts (y). (×2690). (Scanning electron photomicrograph courtesy of GT Cole)

2. Vaginal mucous membranes are occasionally invaded (**vulvovaginal candidiasis**) during pregnancy and in diabetes.

3. Invasion of bronchial and pulmonary tissues (**bronchopulmonary candidiasis**) is usually secondary to chronic bronchial obstruction with impaired drainage of secretions (e.g., from bronchial carcinoma or bronchiectasis).

4. Infections in skin areas that are continuously wet and macerated (**intertriginous candidiasis**) are common in the perineum and inframammary folds and on hands subject to prolonged immersion in water.

Endocarditis caused by *Candida* is occasionally seen in drug addicts and in patients with intravascular tubes or cardiac prostheses. The organisms are most often *C. albicans* and *C. parapsilosis.*

Some individuals with candidiasis develop sterile vesicular or papular skin lesions, called **monilids** (because the genus *Candida* was formerly called *Monilia* and candidiasis was called **moniliasis**). These lesions, presumably allergic, resemble the dermatophytids observed in dermatophyte infections (see below).

DIAGNOSIS. It is not surprising that many normal human sera (15%–30% in one study) specifically agglutinate cells of *Candida* species, as these organisms are so commonly found on normal mucous membranes; and although agglutinin titers tend to be higher in those with frank candidiasis, serologic tests are of little diagnostic value. Similarly, skin tests with aqueous extracts of *C. albicans* (**oidiomycin**) are positive in most normal persons. A presumptive diagnosis of candidiasis is usually made by microscopic demonstration of abundant hyphae and yeast cells in scrapings of lesions, and the diagnosis is supported by isolation of the organism in cultures. However, *Candida* is so ubiquitous that it is often difficult to decide whether it is the causative agent. The response to therapy aids in arriving at a decision.

THERAPY. Polyene antibiotics are effective: nystatin is generally applied locally to accessible lesions, and amphotericin B is administered in the treatment of severe visceral infections. Ketoconazole is also used effectively, but in chronic mucocutaneous candidiasis (a disease associated with a T-cell defect), the lesions return when therapy is stopped.

EPIDEMIOLOGY. Usually, candidiasis is the result of increased susceptibility to a normal commensal. The underlying mechanisms are obscure, but defects in cell-mediated immunity have been implicated in chronic mucocutaneous candidiasis. Infection of the newborn by *C. albicans* from the birth canal is one of the few instances in which a fungus infection is clearly transmitted from one person to another.

Aspergillus fumigatus (*Aspergillosis*)

Many species of *Aspergillus* have been recognized in nature, and seven have been associated with human disease (**aspergillosis**). *A. fumigatus* accounts for more than 90% of all infections. Most aspergilli, including *A. fumigatus,* are **not dimorphic:** they grow only in mycelial form.

Colonies grow well over a wide temperature range, and *A. fumigatus* can thrive up to 50°C. Growth is inhibited by cycloheximide. In culture, the mycelia are powdery and have a dark bluish-green cast, hence the name **fumigatus** (L., smoky). Conidiophores are as much as 500 μm long; each bears a dome-shaped vesicle (about 20–30 μm in diameter) with a single row of sterigmata (see Fig. 43–3) arranged about the distal half. From these, green conidia (2–5 μm in diameter) grow in parallel linear chains, thus accounting for the generic name (L. *aspergillus,* brush).

As suggested earlier, most fungi that abound in the environment of birds do not grow well at their high body temperatures (e.g., *Cryptococcus neoformans*, *Histoplasma capsulatum*). Birds are, however, highly susceptible to fatal infection with various thermophilic species of *Aspergillus* (especially *A. fumigatus*).

Airborne species of aspergilli are ubiquitous, and because these fungi thrive at elevated temperatures, they tend to be particularly abundant in damp, decaying vegetation heated by bacterial fermentations. In compost piles, most microorganisms cease to grow as the temperature rises, and under these conditions, aspergilli can become almost a pure culture.

PATHOGENESIS. Farmers and others who handle decaying vegetation are often heavily exposed to spores of *Aspergillus*. These spores are also disseminated from humidifiers and from air conditioner filters and ducts that have accumulated moisture. Hypersensitivity pneumonitis, asthma, and rhinitis secondary to allergy to Ags of these spores are common.

In addition, progressive infection can be established under predisposing conditions, including not only those previously mentioned but also chronic pulmonary diseases with impaired ciliary activity in the bronchi (e.g., bronchiectasis, pulmonary tuberculosis, and bronchial neoplasms).

Most initial infections are pulmonary, following inhalation of spores. These germinate, and hyphae grow and penetrate contiguous tissues by direct invasion (Fig. 43–20). They tend particularly to invade blood vessel walls, producing angiitis and thromboses; severe hemoptysis is conspicuous and life-threatening in pulmonary aspergillosis. Infected emboli may also establish widespread metastatic granulomatous lesions in various organs.

Severe local infection can also arise by direct implantation of *Aspergillus* spores in the nasal sinuses, with resulting cellulitis of the sinuses and face; in the eye, especially during local treatment with corticosteroids; and in the external ear canal, in the presence of concomitant chronic inflammatory disease.

DIAGNOSIS. Because *Aspergillus* frequently contaminates cultures, the pathogenic significance of a single isolate is not clear. In general, if a species of *Aspergillus* is consistently isolated from a particular patient in repeated cultures of sputum, exudates, or scrapings of infected tissues, it is presumed to be significant. A definitive diagnosis is established by demonstrating hyphae, which are often abundant, in tissue sections. The hyphae are easily seen on hematoxylin–eosin and on Gram stains: they are 3 to 4 μm in diameter, exhibit dichotomous branching, and are septate (Fig. 43–20).

THERAPY. The prognosis in pulmonary aspergillosis is grave, but encouraging therapeutic results have been obtained with amphotericin B.

Phycomycetes (Phycomycoses)

Several genera of the class Phycomycetes, especially *Rhizopus*, are occasional causes of human disease. The disease produced was formerly referred to as **mucormycosis,** but the generic term **phycomycosis** is more appropriate. Phycomyces, like *Aspergillus*, is **not dimorphic:** growth is mycelial in both infected tissues and cultures.

PATHOGENESIS. Infection occurs by inhalation of spores, and, rarely, by their traumatic implantation in broken skin or mucous membranes. Severe infections of the central nervous system occur in poorly controlled diabetes. Widely disseminated visceral lesions have been described as complications of severe malnutrition, uremia, and hepatic insufficiency, as well as in persons receiving corticosteroids or broad-spectrum antibacterial drugs.

Hyphae are abundant in infected tissues. They grow by direct extension through contiguous tissues and tend to invade blood vessel walls, producing angiitis, thrombi, and ischemic necrosis; in addition, emboli establish metastatic infections in many organs. Acute inflammation is characteristically present at sites of infection.

DIAGNOSIS. Distinctive hyphae are seen in infected tissues stained with hematoxylin–eosin. In contrast to the hyphae of *Aspergillus*, those of *Phycomyces* are huge (up

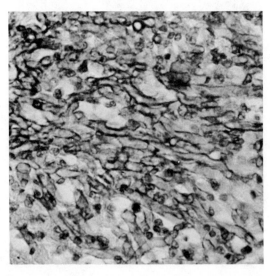

Figure 43–20. Hyphae of *Aspergillus fumigatus* in the wall of a pulmonary cavity (Hematoxylin–eosin stain; ×600)

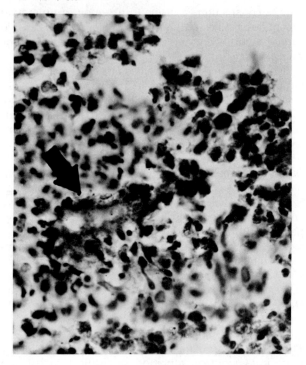

Figure 43–21. Phycomycosis caused by *Basidiobolus haptosporus*. The hyphae in the tissue section are unusually wide (about 15 μm) in diameter; see *arrow*), lack septa, and are surrounded by an intense leukocytic infiltrate, including many eosinophils. (Hematoxylin–eosin stain; ×450, reduced)

to 15 μm in diameter), lack septa, and branch haphazardly (Fig. 43–21; see also Fig. 43–8).

Because their walls are rich in chitin and probably correspondingly poor in glucans and mannas, phycomycetes stain poorly with the periodic acid–Schiff stain.

RHIZOPUS. Species associated with phycomycosis grow rapidly on Sabouraud's medium and form coarse and woolly mycelia, which are initially white but subsequently become peppered with black and brown fruiting structures (sporangia). Asexual reproductive elements consist of long, unbranched stalks (sporangiophores), which arise directly from a cluster of rhizoids (root-like structures) and are each topped by a spherical sac (sporangium). The latter are dark and when mature are filled with spores. The species isolated most often from human phycomycosis are *R. oryzae* (most frequently), *R. arrhizus*, and *R. nigricans*.

MUCOR. Cultures of these species grow rapidly on Sabouraud's medium and form fluffy mycelia that are initially white and subsequently are gray to brown. Sporangiophores, which do not originate from rhizoids, form thick upright tufts. Some are branched, and each termi-

nates in a spherical sporangium. The species most often identified in human infections is *M. pusillus*).

Phycomycosis is also occasionally caused by species of *Absidia*, *Mortierella*, and *Basidiobolus*.

SUBCUTANEOUS MYCOSES

Subcutaneous mycotic infections are usually initiated by penetration of the skin with contaminated splinters, thorns, or soil. Once established, these infections tend to remain localized in subcutaneous tissues and to be extremely persistent. The diseases are classified as **sporotrichosis**, **chromomycosis**, and **maduromycosis**.

Sporothrix schenckii (*Sporotrichosis*)

Sporotrichosis is characterized by an ulcerated lesion at the site of inoculation, followed by multiple nodules and abscesses along the superficial draining lymphatics. Only rarely is there dissemination to the meninges. In infected tissues, the organism appears as cigar-shaped, budding yeast cells (Fig. 43–22); these cells are usually scarce but may sometimes be recognized by the periodic acid–Schiff stain or with fluorescein-labeled Abs.

S. schenckii is dimorphic. When pus or curettings from skin lesions are cultured on Sabouraud's medium at room temperature (with chloramphenicol and cycloheximide), the fungus grows rapidly in mycelial form as a flat, moist colony. Hyphae are slender (about 2 μm in diameter) and septate, and conidia are individually at-

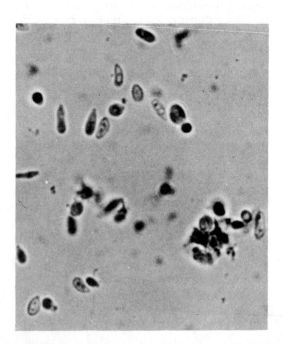

Figure 43–22. Cigar-shaped budding yeast cells of *Sporothrix schenkii* in culture at 37°C. (×450)

tached by sterigmata to a common conidiophore (see Fig. 43–3). Pigmentation of the conidia accounts for the dark color of the mycelium. The pigment is allegedly melanin, and tyrosinase has been identified in mycelia.

Identification of yeast cells is also of diagnostic value, because they are usually difficult to see in human lesions. Hyphae are converted to yeast forms by cultivation at 37°C, at slightly increased pCO_2 in media enriched with proteins, thiamine, and biotin. This change is also brought about by inoculating mycelial fragments into the testes of mice; pus withdrawn after 2 to 3 weeks contains abundant characteristic yeast cells.

S. schenckii has been isolated from soil and plants, and can apparently grow in wood. Penetration of skin by contaminated splinters and thorns is the principal means of introducing infection. The disease is usually sporadic among farmers and gardeners, but a few industrial outbreaks have occurred among workers exposed to batches of heavily infected timbers and plants.

Chromomycosis

A group of slowly growing, dimorphic fungi produce the subcutaneous mycoses known as chromomycosis. Although the first case was reported in Boston, the disease occurs primarily in the tropics. The infection is seen mostly on the legs of bare-legged laborers, and lesions appear as warty, ulcerating, cauliflower-like growths.

In draining lesions, the fungus appears as thick-walled, round, brown cells, about 6 to 10 μm in diameter. Their color gives the disease its name. These yeast cells apparently multiply by fission rather than by budding. In cultures on Sabouraud's medium at room temperature, darkly pigmented mycelial colonies are formed slowly.

Several species have been distinguished on the basis of conidial arrangements, but their classification is unsettled. According to one terminology, they are *Fonsecaea pedrosoi*, *F. compacta*, *Cladosporium carrionii*, and *Phialophora verrucosa*.

Eumycotic Mycetoma

Mycetoma is the generic term for localized destructive granulomatous and suppurative lesions that usually affect the foot or hand and involve skin, subcutaneous tissues, bone, and fascia. Mycetomas usually originate with injuries that break the skin. They are especially prevalent in the tropics.

Lesions are characterized by multiple burrowing sinus tracts that extend through soft tissues and penetrate to the skin surface. The draining pus contains granules (small pieces of colonies of the causative microorganism), which differ in texture, color, and shape, depending on the microorganism, and also in size (from about 0.1 to 2 mm).

The microorganisms that cause mycetomas are either fungi or actinomycetes; the fungal mycetomas are often referred to as **maduromycosis.** Diagnosis is based on demonstration of fungus cells directly in KOH-treated granules and pus, and by culture. At least 13 species of fungi have been identified, including *Madurella mycetomi*, *M. grisea*, *Allescheria boydii*, *Phialophora jeanselmi*, and *Aspergillus nidulans*.

Surgical drainage is an important adjunct to therapy. Polyenes, which have not yet been tried extensively, may prove of value, as the causative agents are susceptible *in vitro*.

CUTANEOUS MYCOSES (DERMATOMYCOSES)

The dermatophytes are fungi that infect only epidermis and its appendages (hair and nails); i.e., structures in which keratin is abundant. The ensuing skin lesions are usually roughly circular, tend to expand equally in all directions, and have raised serpiginous borders. They were therefore thought in ancient times to be caused by worms or lice, and they are still called **ringworm** or **tinea** (L., worm or insect larva). The names are usually qualified by the area of the skin involved: ringworm of the scalp (**tinea capitis**), of the body (**tinea corporis**), of the groin ("jock itch," **tinea cruris**), and of the feet (athlete's foot, **tinea pedis**).

Dermatophytes are not dimorphic. In infected skin lesions, they all look alike, with septate hyphae and arthroconidia (Figs. 43–23 and 43–24). However, additional differentiated structures appear in cultures and provide the basis for identification.

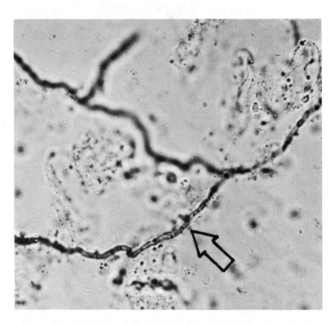

Figure 43–23. Skin scraping treated with 10% KOH to show hyphae *(arrow)* of a dermatophyte among epidermal debris from a human skin lesion. (×450, reduced)

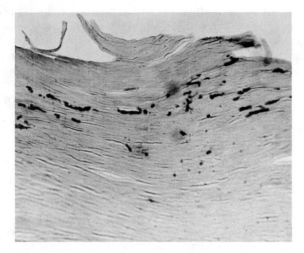

Figure 43–24. Periodic acid–Schiff stain of skin section of a human lesion showing a dermatophyte in the stratum corneum. (×100, reduced)

Attack on Keratin

The predilection of dermatophytes for epidermis, firmly established by clinical observations, is also demonstrable experimentally. For example, when conidia or mycelial fragments are injected intravenously into guinea pigs, no lesions develop; but if an area of skin is abraded at the time of the injection, dermatophyte infection appears in the scarified skin a few weeks later.

In view of the evident affinity of dermatophytes for keratin-rich tissues, one might expect these fungi to have an unusual capacity to degrade and utilize keratin. In fact, however, they do so at only a low rate *in vitro*. Evidently, the pathogenicity of dermatophytes depends on more than their ability to attack keratin.

Keratin is a fibrous and very insoluble protein, stabilized by the disulfide groups of frequent cystine residues. In its native state it is resistant to most proteolytic enzymes, but an enzyme preparation of *Streptomyces* cleaves disulfide bonds effectively and digests keratin.* *Microsporum gypseum*, on the other hand, one of the few dermatophytes often isolated from soil and more keratinolytic than the others, does not cleave keratin disulfides and digests this protein to only a limited extent. Nevertheless, many dermatophytes can be cultured on sterile hair, and they dissolve localized segments of hair fibers.

Although dermatophytes are epidermal parasites, most species grow well in simple media, with ammonium salts and glucose as the sole sources of nitrogen,

carbon, and energy. However, growth is more vigorous in media enriched with proteins or amino acids.

INVASION OF HAIR. In infection of hairs, hyphae grow first from the epidermis into hair follicles and then into the hair shafts. In the **endothrix** type of infection, the hyphae then grow only **within** the hair shaft, where they form long, parallel rows of arthrospores (Fig. 43–25). In **ecothrix** infections, they grow both **within and on the external surface** of the hair shaft (Fig. 43–26).

Epidemiology

About 15 species of dermatophytes are found primarily in human skin (**anthropophilic**). Many others are indigenous in domesticated and wild mammals (**zoophilic**); and a few may be free-living saprobes, as they are isolable from soil (**geophilic**) (e.g., *M. gypseum*, *Trichophyton mentagrophytes*, and *T. ajelloi*). Infection is transmitted, although with difficulty, from man to man, or animal to man or vice versa, by direct contact or by contact with infected hairs and epidermal scales (e.g., from barber shop clippers, shower room floors, etc.). The reservoir of animal infection is huge: about 30% of dogs and cats in the U.S. are infected with *Microsporum canis*, a frequent cause of ringworm of the scalp in children.

The incidence of different dermatomycoses varies with age. For example, intertriginous infection of the feet (athlete's foot) is common in adults but rare in children, whereas the opposite is true for ringworm of the scalp. The resistance of adults to scalp infection has been linked to the increased secretory activity of the seba-

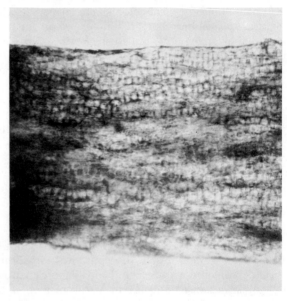

Figure 43–25. Endothrix hair infection with *Trichophyton tonsurans*. Chains of arthrospores are localized within the hair shaft. (×450, reduced)

---

* This keratinase is used industrially to remove hair from hides in the preparation of leather.

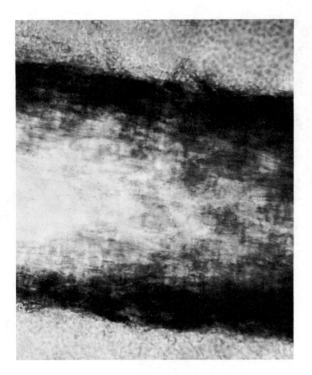

Figure 43–26. Ectothrix infection of hair by *Microsporum audouini*. Spores are clustered on the surface of the hair shaft. (×450, reduced)

ceous glands at puberty and the antifungal activity of the C-7 to C-11 saturated fatty acids in sebum.*

Most dermatophytes have a worldwide distribution, but a few species are restricted geographically. With increased travel in the past 25 years, even the localized species are becoming more widely distributed. For example, *Trichophyton tonsurans*, endemic in Mexico, has become common in the U.S.

Immunity

Human resistance to some dermatophytes is emphasized by the low incidence of conjugal infections; for example, in one study of 60 *T. rubrum*-infected persons, followed up for 1 to 20 years, not one spouse acquired active infection. This natural human resistance is probably not attributable to conventional immune reactions: circulating Abs are not, as a rule, demonstrable in the serum of persons with dermatomycosis. However, a fungistatic factor, which seems not to be an immunoglobulin, is demonstrable even in normal serum and may well be responsible for the limited penetration of dermatophyte infections. We do not understand the balance of forces that causes these infections to be so widespread yet difficult to transmit deliberately and so often self-limited yet difficult to cure.

* Undecylenic acid, an unsaturated C-11 fatty acid, is widely used for topical therapy of some dermatomycoses.

HYPERSENSITIVITY. Persons with dermatophytosis sometimes have **dermatophytids:** sterile vesicles, symmetrically distributed on the hands. These skin lesions are believed to represent an allergic reaction to fungal Ags that spread from the site of infection.

Hypersensitivity to dermatophytes appears in the course of infection and is usually persistent. Trichophytin, a crude culture filtrate, elicits delayed cutaneous responses and sometimes also wheal-and-erythema responses. However, as with tuberculin, these responses do not distinguish current from prior infection; they have little diagnostic or prognostic value.

Treatment

Many infections are eradicated by griseofulvin, but the response varies with the thickness of the keratin and the rate of its replacement. Infections of the scalp and smooth skin are usually cured after several weeks of therapy, but infections of the feet, especially of toenails, require many months of continuous treatment. Traditional forms of local therapy with keratinolytic agents are therefore still widely used, as well as topical treatment with miconazole or clotrimazole.

Classification

In identifying specific dermatophytes, the form and arrangement of macroconidia is especially important. Additional determinative characteristics are: (1) the form and pigmentation of mycelia; (2) the quantity and disposition of microconidia; (3) the development of special hyphal structures; for example, racket-shaped ends of some hyphae (racket mycelia), helically coiled hyphae (spirals), and tightly coiled, twisted hyphae (nodular bodies); (4) the presence of arthroconidia and chlamydospores; and (5) some physiologic characteristics such as growth in culture on sterile hair.

Identification of dermatophytes is hindered by their **pleomorphism**—a word used in mycology in a special sense, to describe the frequent loss of pigmentation and conidia formation during laboratory cultivation. The resulting nondescript mycelia resist identification. However, transfer on a medium that stimulates conidiation (e.g., potato–glucose agar) reduces the frequency of this conversion. In order to maintain sporulating cultures, frequent transfer (about once every 10 days) or else storage at −20°C is usually necessary.

Genetic crosses have shown that pleomorphic conversion is the result of one or more gene mutations. Thus, pleomorphism in dermatophytes resembles phase variation in bacteria, in which culture conditions select for a frequent, reversible inversion.

Dermatophytes fall into three genera: in general, *Microsporum* attacks hair and skin but not nails; *Trichophyton* attacks hair, skin, and nails; and *Epidermophyton* infects skin and occasionally nails, but not hair. From

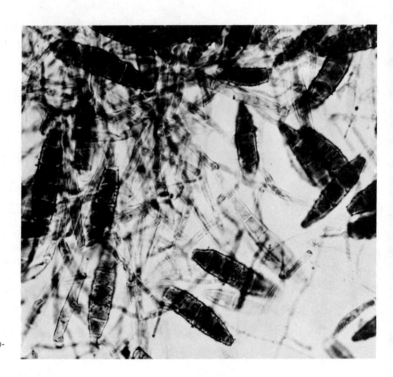

Figure 43–27. Macroaleuriospores in a culture of *Microsporum gypseum.* (×450, reduced)

20 to 100 species, depending on the classification, cause human infection. A few representative species will be discussed briefly.

MICROSPORUM. Hair infections are of the ectothrix type (Fig. 43–26), with spores packed closely on the external hair surface in a mosaic pattern. In culture, the genus is characterized by the production of rough-walled multicellular macroconidia (Fig. 43–27).

M. audouini is primarily a human pathogen and used to be the most frequent cause of epidemics of ringworm of the scalp in children in the U.S. Adults are only rarely infected, and animals are highly resistant. When the scalp is irradiated with ultraviolet light (366 nm), infected hairs emit a bright yellow-green fluorescence. This property makes possible the rapid diagnostic screening of large populations of children and also facilitates the selection of infected hairs for culture.

M. canis is primarily a parasite of domesticated and wild animals, and children commonly acquire infections from cats and dogs. An intense but localized inflammatory reaction (called a **kerion**) develops in the skin and subsides spontaneously after several weeks; it may represent an allergic response. Hairs infected with *M. canis* resemble those infected with *M. audouini* and also fluoresce in ultraviolet light.

M. gypseum is abundant in soil but is an infrequent cause of human infections. Infected hairs are not fluorescent. Arthrospores appear on the surface of infected hairs and are larger than those of other *Microsporum* spp. Sexual forms, with typical asci, have been isolated from cultures (Table 43–3).

TRICHOPHYTON. Species of *Trichophyton* usually produce smooth-walled macroconidia in culture, but classification is difficult because spores are often sparse or lacking.

T. schoenleinii is a major cause of **favus,** a severe form of chronic ringworm of the scalp, with destruction of hair follicles and permanent loss of hair. It was the first microbial pathogen of man to be identified (1843), isolated, and established as a pathogen through experimental infection of an animal host. In culture, hyphae are coarse and have knobby, broadened ends and many short lateral branches: these structures, reminiscent of reindeer horns, are called favic chandeliers.

T. violaceum causes endothrix infection in hair and may also cause favus. It is a common cause of ringworm of the scalp and body in the Mediterranean area.

T. tonsurans causes endothrix infections of hair. With a large influx into the U.S. of persons from Latin America, ringworm of the scalp in large cosmopolitan centers is now more frequently caused by *T. tonsurans* than *M. audouini*. Early diagnosis of infection is difficult, however, because unlike *M. audouini*-infected hairs, those infected with *T. tonsurans* do not fluoresce.

T. mentagrophytes and *T. rubrum* are common causes of athlete's foot and of infections of smooth skin and nails. *T. mentagrophytes* can also cause endothrix infections of hair (scalp and beard).

EPIDERMOPHYTON. The genus *Epidermophyton* is represented by a single species, *E. floccosum,* and is found only in man. It grows in epidermis (especially in intertriginous areas, as between toes) but does not invade hair.

SUPERFICIAL MYCOSES

Fungi that produce superficial infections are limited to invasion of the uppermost layers of the skin and hair. Four superficial mycoses are fairly common.

TINEA VERSICOLOR (PITYRIASIS VERSICOLOR). The disease is common in all parts of the world but is most frequently seen in warm climates. The infected lesions appear as white or tanned scaly areas on the trunk, and lesions are chronic but asymptomatic. The etiologic agent, *Malassezia furfur,* can be seen readily in clinical specimens (treated with 10% KOH) as clusters of round budding cells (3–8 μm in diameter) and mycelial elements. The yeast-like fungi that constitute this genus require long-chain fatty acids for their growth. *Pityrosporum ovale,* which morphologically resembles *M. furfur,* is frequently isolated from sebaceous glands and hair follicles but is not pathogenic and is considered to be part of the normal flora of the skin.

A similar disease, **erythrasma,** is caused by a corynebacterium, *C. minutissimum.*

TINEA NIGRA. The lesions of this infection are largely confined to the palms, where they appear as irregular, flat, darkly discolored areas. Infection is particularly prevalent in the tropics and is rare in the U.S. The fungus that causes the disorder is *Exophiala werneckii.* It appears in scrapings of skin lesions as branched hyphae, and it grows slowly on agar as greenish-black colonies with numerous dark, budding cells.

WHITE PIEDRA. The fungus that causes white piedra (*Trichosporon cutaneum*) grows on scalp or beard hair. Soft, pale nodules appear on the hair shafts; they consist of hyphae and oval arthrospores. On agar, this fungus grows as soft, creamy colonies that become wrinkled and gray with age, and its septate hyphae fragment easily into arthrospores.

BLACK PIEDRA. In the tropical disorder of black piedra, an ascomycete, *Piedraia hortai,* forms hard, dark nodules on the shafts of infected scalp hairs. The nodules contain oval asci with two to eight ascospores. On agar, the organism forms greenish-black mycelia that bear chlamydospores.

Selected Reading

GENERAL MYCOLOGY

Ainsworth GC, Sussman AS (eds): The Fungi: An Advanced Treatise. New York, Academic Press, 1965 (Vol I), 1966 (Vol II), 1968 (Vol III), 1973 (Vols IVA and IVB)

Cole GT: Models of cell differentiation in conidial fungi. Microbiol Rev 50:95, 1986

Cole GT, Kendrick B: Biology of Conidial Fungi (two volumes). New York, Academic Press, 1981

Fincham JRS, Day PR, Radford A: Fungal Genetics, 4th Ed. Berkeley, University of California Press, 1979

Hamilton–MIller JMT: Fungal sterols and the mode of action of the polyene antibiotics. Adv Appl Microbiol 17:109, 1974

Lemke PA (ed): Viruses and Plasmids in Fungi. New York, Marcel Dekker, 1979

Rose AH, Harrison JS (eds): The Yeasts. New York, Academic Press, 1969 (Vol I), 1971 (Vol II), 1970 (Vol III)

Smith JE, Berry DR (eds): The Filamentous Fungi. New York, John Wiley and Sons, 1975 (Vol I), 1976 (Vol II), 1978 (Vol III)

Smith JE, Pateman JA (eds): Genetics and Physiology of *Aspergillus.* London, Academic Press, 1977

Van Den Ende H: Sexual Interactions in Plants: The Role of Specific Substances in Sexual Reproduction. New York, Academic Press, 1976

Villanueva JR, Garcia–Acha I, Gascon S, Uruburu F (eds): Yeast, Mould and Plant Protoplasts. New York, Academic Press, 1973

MEDICAL MYCOLOGY

Campbell CC: Serology in the respiratory mycoses. Sabouraudia 5:240, 1967

Chu FS: Mode of action of mycotoxins and related compounds. Adv Appl Microbiol 22:83, 1977

Edman JC, Kovacs JA, Masur H, Santi DV, Elwood HJ, Sogin ML: Ribosomal RNA sequence shows *Pneumocystis carinii* to be a member of the fungi. Nature 334:519, 1988

Howard DH (ed): Fungi Pathogenic to Humans and Animals, Parts A and B. New York, Marcel Dekker, 1983

Kaufman L, Reiss E: Serodiagnosis of fungal diseases. In EH Lennette, Balows A, Hausler WF Jr, Shadomy HJ (eds): Manual of Clinical Microbiology, 4th Ed. Washington, DC, American Society for Microbiology, 1985

Medoff G, Brajtburg J, Kobayashi GS, Bolard J: Antifungal agents useful in therapy of systemic fungal infections. Annu Rev Pharmacol 23:303, 1983

Odds FC: Candida and Candidosis. Baltimore, University Park Press, 1979

Rebell G, Taplin D: Dermatophytes: Their Recognition and Identification, Rev. Ed. Miami, University of Miami Press, 1970

Rinaldi MJ: Invasive Aspergillosis. Rev Infect Dis 5:1061, 1983

Rippon JW: Medical Mycology: The Pathogenic Fungi and the Pathogenic Actinomycetes, 2nd Ed. Philadelphia, WB Saunders, 1982

Roberts SOB, Hay RJ, Mackenzie DWR: A Clinician's Guide to Fungal Disease. New York, Marcel Dekker, 1984

Rotrosen D, Calderone RA, Edwards JE Jr: Adherence of *Candida* species to host tissues and plastic surfaces. Rev Infect Dis 8:73, 1986

Stevens DA (ed): Coccidioidomycosis. New York, Plenum, 1980

Szaniszlo PJ (ed): Fungal Dimorphism with Emphasis on Fungi Pathogenic to Humans. New York, Plenum, 1985

Part Four

Virology

Renato Dulbecco
Harold S. Ginsberg

44

The Nature of Viruses

Viruses, as infectious agents responsible for many diseases in humans, animals, and plants are of great medical and economic importance. They were recognized at the end of past century as infectious agents smaller than bacteria ("filterable agents"). Transmission by a cell-free filtrate was demonstrated in 1898 for foot-and-mouth disease, for fowl leukosis in 1908, and for chicken sarcoma in 1911. The discovery of viruses affecting bacteria, made in 1917, made available an important model system for investigations of basic virology.

Distinctive Properties

Passage through the usual bacterial filters, and multiplication only as obligatory parasites in living cells, proved inadequate to distinguish viruses from the smallest bacteria (e.g., rickettsiae). Viruses are distinguished from other microbes in more fundamental ways: their simple organization and their characteristic mode of replication. In addition, animal viruses produce characteristic effects on host cells: death, fusion, or transformation into cancer cells.

The free viral particles, called **virions,** are made up of two essential constituents: a **genome,** which can be DNA or RNA, associated with proteins or polyamines; and a protein coat (**the capsid**), sometimes surrounded by a membranous **envelope.** In addition, some virions have enzymes that are needed in the initial steps of replication of the genome. They may also contain other minor constituents (see below). So a virion is relatively simple: it is little more than a block of genetic material enclosed in a coat. Capsid and envelope protect the genome from the nucleases present in the environment, and they facilitate

769

its attachment and penetration into the cell in which it will replicate.

Viruses have a unique method of multiplication. Whereas in the replication of other microbes all the constituents are made within the cell envelope, finally causing the microbe to undergo binary fission, virions lack the machinery for using and transforming energy and for making the proteins specified by the viral genes. Accordingly, after the viral genome is released from the coat, it uses the machinery of the host cell to make the constituents of viruses in the cell's cytoplasm or nucleus. Progeny virions are then assembled from these constituents. Although all viruses have this basic mechanism of replication in common, they differ considerably in such characteristics as size and shape, chemical composition of the genome (Fig. 44–1), and the type of cells they infect.

HOST RANGE

Viruses are subdivided into **animal viruses, bacterial viruses (bacteriophages),** and **plant viruses.** Within a class each virus is able to infect only cells of a certain species or of a certain type. The host range is determined in part by the specificity of attachment to the cells, which depends on properties of both the virion's coat and specific receptors on the cell surface. It also depends on the availability of cellular factors required for the replication or transcription of the genome. The host range is broader in **transfection:** infection by the naked nucleic acid, the entry of which does not depend on specific receptors. Limitations determined by intracellular factors, however, persist.

Are Viruses Alive?

When Stanley crystallized tobacco mosaic virus in 1935, there followed extensive debates on whether it was a living being or merely a nucleoprotein molecule. As Pirie pointed out, these discussions showed only that some scientists had a more teleologic than operational view of the meaning of the word *life*. Life can be viewed as a complex set of processes resulting from the actuation of the instructions encoded in the genes; those of viral genes are actuated after the viral genome has entered a susceptible cell; hence, viruses may be considered alive when they replicate in cells. Outside cells, virions are metabolically inert chemicals. Thus, depending on the context, viruses may be regarded both as exceptionally simple microbes and as complex chemicals.

Viruses are then not organisms in the usual sense: they are parasitic genomes, related to plasmids (see Chap. 8). Moreover, some viral genomes, like certain plasmids, become integrated into the DNA of their host cells,

exercising the same form of parasitism displayed by movable DNA elements and by certain repeated sequences abundant in the DNA of eukaryotic cells.

The Viral Particles

GENERAL MORPHOLOGY

Viruses of different families have virions of different morphologies, which can be readily distinguished by electron microscopy. This relationship is useful for diagnosing viral diseases and especially for recognizing new viral agents of infection. For instance, the wheel-shaped virions of rotaviruses in feces of infants with diarrhea could readily be distinguished from other viruses also present in feces, and recognition of paramyxovirus nucleocapsids in thin sections of the brains of patients helped to reveal the viral origin of subacute sclerosing panencephalitis (SSPE).

However, different classes of viruses within the same family have virions of similar morphology. The identification can be refined by the binding of specific antibodies to virions, which is also recognizable by electron microscopy (see Immuno-Electron Microscopy in Chap. 50).

Virions belong to several morphological types (Fig. 44–2 and Table 44–1).

1. **Icosahedral virions** resemble small crystals. Extensive studies, especially by Klug and Caspar, have shown that these virions have an **icosahedral** protein shell (**the capsid**) surrounding a core of nucleic acid and proteins. The capsid and the core form the **nucleocapsid.** Examples are picornaviruses, adenoviruses, papovaviruses, and bacteriophage ϕX174 (Fig. 44–3A).

2. **Helical virions,** of which tobacco mosaic virus (see Fig. 44–3B) and bacteriophage M13 are examples, form long rods. The nucleic acid is surrounded by a **cylindrical capsid,** in which a helical structure is revealed by high-resolution electron microscopy.

3. **Enveloped virions** contain lipids. In most cases the nucleocapsid—in some viruses icosahedral, in others helical—is surrounded by a membranous **envelope.** Most enveloped virions are roughly spherical but highly **pleomorphic** (i.e., of varying shapes) because the envelope is not rigid. Herpesviruses and togaviruses are examples of **enveloped icosahedral** viruses (see Fig. 44–3C). In **enveloped helical** viruses, such as orthomyxoviruses (see Fig. 44–3D), the nucleocapsid is coiled within the envelope.

4. **Complex virion** structures belong to two groups. Those illustrated by poxviruses (see Fig. 44–3E) do not possess a clearly identifiable capsid but have several coats around the nucleic acid, while certain bacteriophages (see Fig. 44–3F) have a capsid to which additional structures are appended.

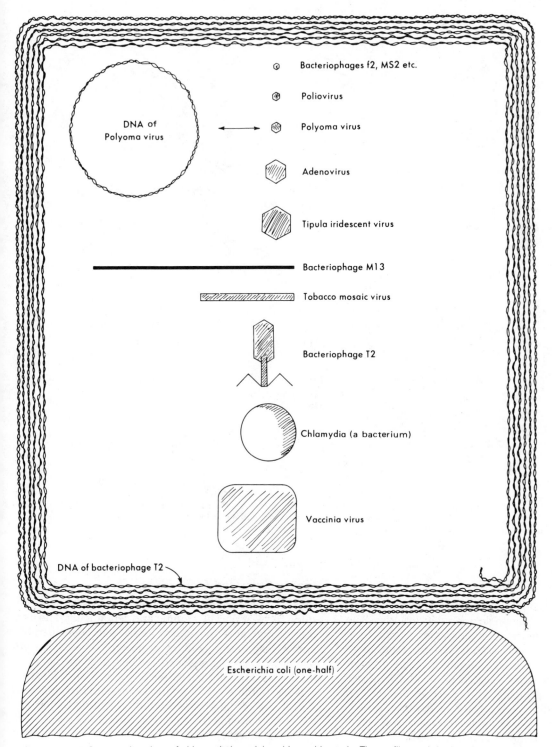

Figure 44–1. Comparative sizes of virions, their nucleic acids, and bacteria. The profiles and the lengths of the DNA molecules are all reproduced on the same scale.

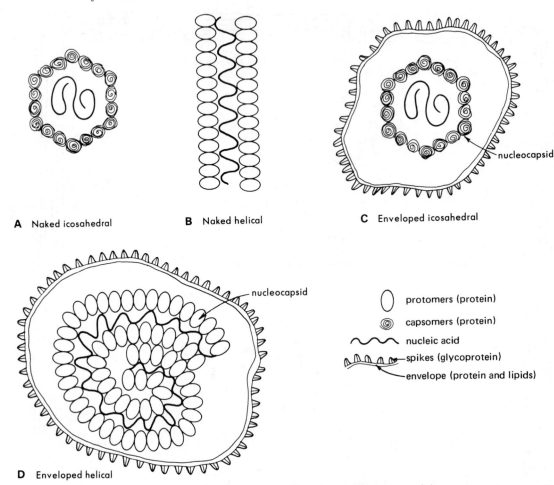

A Naked icosahedral   **B** Naked helical   **C** Enveloped icosahedral

nucleocapsid

D Enveloped helical

nucleocapsid

○ protomers (protein)
◎ capsomers (protein)
∿ nucleic acid
ⱭⱭⱭ spikes (glycoprotein)
— envelope (protein and lipids)

Figure 44–2. Simple forms of virions and of their components. The naked icosahedral virions *(A)* resemble small crystals; the naked helical virions *(B)* resemble rods with a fine regular helical pattern in their surface. The enveloped icosahedral virions *(C)* are made up of icosahedral nucleocapsids surrounded by the envelope; the enveloped helical virions *(D)* are helical nucleocapsids bent to form a coarse, often irregular coil within the envelope.

VIRAL GENOMES

In a given virus the genome may consist of either DNA or RNA, which may be either single or double stranded. The amount of genetic information per virion varies from about 3 to 300 kilobases (Kb). If 1 Kb is taken as the size of an average gene, small viruses contain perhaps three or four genes, and large viruses several hundred. The diversity of virus-specific proteins synthesized in the infected cells varies accordingly. With the exception of retroviruses (see Chap. 65), virions contain only a single copy of the genome; that is, they are **haploid.** The virions of some plant viruses contain only a fraction of the genome, and several virions, collectively containing the whole genome, must enter the same cell for viral multiplication to take place.

Double-Stranded Viral DNA

Table 44–2 gives the lengths of various viral DNAs, obtained in great part by cloning and sequencing. The base composition and the codon usage vary considerably: some viruses even contain **abnormal bases.** For instance, cytosine is replaced by 5-hydroxymethyl-cytosine in T-even coliphages (see Chap. 45), and substitutions for thymine are found in *Bacillus* and *Pseudomonas* phages. These differences from the host cells allow the viral DNA to escape the action of cellular nucleases or to be selectively recognized by virus-specified enzymes.

Many viral DNAs have **special features** related to their methods of replication. These features avoid the difficulty of complete replication of the ends of a linear molecule from an internal initiation (see Fig. 45–10). To

TABLE 44–1. Characteristics of Viruses

Morphological Class	Nucleic Acid*	Example Virus Family	Virus	Size of Capsid (nm)	No. of Capsomers	Size of Virions (Enveloped Viruses) (nm)	Special Features
Helical capsid							
Naked	DNA	Coliphage f1, M13		5 × 800			Single-stranded cyclic DNA
	RNA	Many plant viruses	Tobacco mosaic	17.5 × 300			
			Beet yellow	10 × 1200			
Enveloped	RNA	Orthomyxoviruses	Influenza	9 (diameter)		90–100	Segmented RNA
		Paramyxoviruses	Newcastle disease	18 (diameter)		125–250	
		Rhabdoviruses	Vesicular stomatitis			68 × 175	Bullet shaped
Icosahedral capsid							
Naked	DNA	Parvoviruses	Adeno-associated	20	12		Single-stranded linear DNA
		Coliphage φx174		22	12		Single-stranded cyclic DNA
		Papovaviruses	Polyoma	45	72		Cyclic DNA
			Papilloma	55	72		Cyclic DNA
		Adenoviruses		60–90	252		
	RNA	Coliphage F2 and others		20–25			
		Picornaviruses	Polio	28	32		
		Many plant viruses	Turnip yellow	28	32		
		Reoviruses		70	92		Segmented; double-stranded RNA
Enveloped	DNA	Herpesviruses	Herpes simplex	100	162	180–200	
		Hepadnaviruses	Hepatitis B	27	42		
Capsids of binal symmetry (i.e., some components icosahedral, others helical)							
Naked	DNA	Large bacteriophages	T2,T4,T6	Modified icosahedral head: 95 × 65; helical tail: 17 × 115			
Complex virions	DNA	Poxviruses	Variola } Vaccinia			250 × 300	Brick shaped
			Contagious pustular dermatitis of sheep			160 × 260	

* DNA double stranded, RNA single stranded, unless specified in last column

this purpose some viral DNA are **cyclic,** and therefore without ends, whereas others are made to become cyclic after entering cells. Others have **terminal redundancies,** which enable incompletely replicated molecules to complete each other by recombination. Some viral DNAs have **palindromes** or **terminal proteins** at the ends, which act as primers during replication. These characteristics and their roles will be considered in greater detail together with DNA replication in Chapter 50 and in the Chapters on specific viruses (45, 46, 52–65).

Some viral DNAs have features that show their **relatedness to transposons** (see Chap. 8), such as **terminal repeats.** The DNAs of some herpesviruses are made up of two unequal transposons joined together, each with its own terminal repeats (see Chap. 53); each transposon undergoes frequent inversion independently of the other, so a population of virions contains four, equally frequent, kinds of DNA: ⟶ →, ⟵ →, ⟶ ←, ⟵ ←. Some DNAs have single-strand nicks at characteristic places, which define special genomic segments during

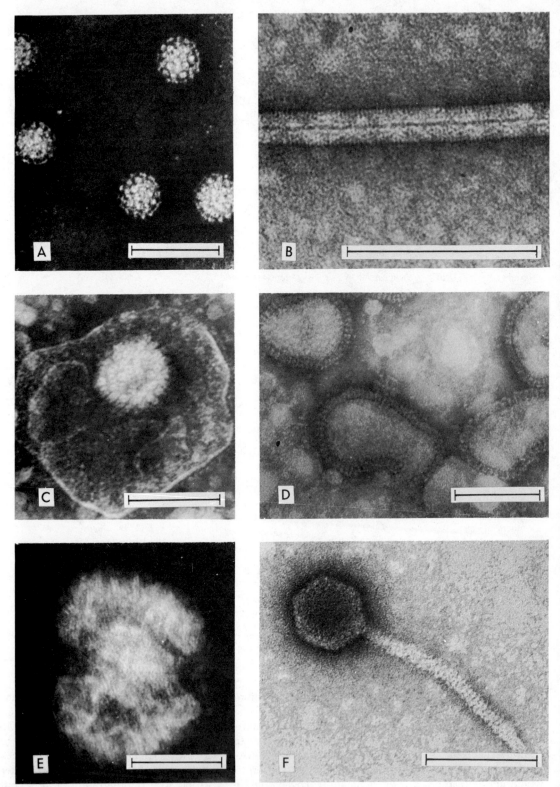

Figure 44–3. Electron micrographs of representative virions were obtained by negative staining; that is, suspending the virions in an electron-opaque salt solution so that structures are transparent on a dark background. Markers under each micrograph are 100 nm. *(A)* Naked icosahedral: human wart virus (papovavirus, Chap. 65). *(B)* Naked helical: segment of tobacco mosaic virus. *(C)* Enveloped icosahedral: herpes simplex virus (herpesvirus, Chap. 53). *(D)* Enveloped helical: influenza virus (orthomyxovirus, Chap. 56). *(E)* Complex virus: vaccinia virus (poxvirus, Chap. 54). *(F)* Coliphage λ (Chap. 46). *(A,* Noyes WF: Virology 23:65, 1964; *B,* Finch JT: J Mol Biol 8:872, 1964. Copyright by Academic Press, Inc. [London] Ltd.; *C,* courtesy of P. Wildy; *D,* Choppin PW, Stockenius W: Virology 22:482, 1964; *E,* courtesy of R. W. Horne; *F,* courtesy of F. A. Eiserling)

TABLE 44–2. Characteristics of Viral Nucleic Acids

Type of Nucleic Acid	Representative Virus	Mol. wt. (in 10^6 daltons)	Kilobases per Strand*	No. of Segments	Polarity
DNA, DOUBLE STRANDED					
Hepatitis B (cyclic)		1.6	2.5		
Papovavirus (cyclic)	Polyoma	3.5	5.0		
	Papilloma	6	9		
Pseudomonas phage PMS2 (cyclic)		6	9		
Adenovirus	Types 12,18	21	32		
	Types 2,5	23	35		
Coliphages T3,T7		25	38		
Coliphage Mu		26	39		
Coliphage λ		31	47		
Coliphage T5		77	117		
Herpesvirus	Herpes simplex	100	151		
Coliphages T2,T4,T6		110	167		
Bacillus subtilis phage SP8		130	197		
Poxvirus	Vaccinia	160	242		
DNA, SINGLE STRANDED					
Parvovirus	Adeno-associated†	1.5	4.5		
Coliphage φx174 (cyclic)		1.7	5.2		
Coliphage M13 (cyclic)		2.4	7.3		
RNA, DOUBLE STRANDED					
Rotaviruses		15^3	23	10	
Rice dwarf virus		15^3	23	10	
Cytoplasmic polyhedrosis of silkworms		15^3	23	10	
RNA, SINGLE STRANDED					
Satellite necrosis virus†		0.4	1.2	1	
Coliphage R17		1.3	4	1	+
Tobacco mosaic virus		2	6	1	+
Turnip yellow mosaic virus		2	6	1	+
Picornavirus	Polio	2.5	7.5	1	+
Bunyavirus		3‡	9	3	−
Retrovirus§	Rous sarcoma virus	3.5	10.5	1	+
Alphavirus	Sindbis	4	13	1	+
Rhabdovirus	Vesicular stomatitis virus	4	13	1	−
Orthomyxovirus	Influenza	6‡	18	8	−
Paramyxovirus	Newcastle disease	6	18	1	−

+, positive; −, negative

* A kilobase (1000 bases) corresponds to a molecular weight of about 700,000 for double-stranded and 350,000 for single-stranded nucleic acid; it can specify about 33,000 daltons of protein. The number of genes is approximately equal to the number of kilobases; φx174 has fewer kilobases because **some genes overlap each other** (see Chap. 45).

† These viruses are defective and multiply only in cells infected by a helper virus (adenovirus or tobacco necrosis virus, respectively). They probably specify only their own capsid, perhaps with another small protein.

‡ This value, as for other virions with segmented genomes, is the aggregate of all fragments.

§ Retroviruses have diploid virions.

entry into cells (Phage T5; see Regulation of Transcription in Chap. 45).

Control Elements of DNA Viruses

Genes contained in viral DNAs are controlled essentially like the genes of the host cells, and they have the corresponding characteristic sequences. DNAs of bacterial viruses, like bacterial genes, have promoters, operators, and ribosome-binding sites. DNAs of eukaryotic viruses have control regions comparable to those of eukaryotic genes, enhancers (see Chap. 64), and a TATA box for locating the exact initiation of the transcripts; they also have poly(A) addition sites at their 3′ ends where the messengers terminate. In poxviruses, however, the transcription signals do not conform to those of the host cells and are recognized by enzymes specified by viral genes. The structure of the genome is suitable for polycistronic transcription in bacterial viruses and for monocistronic transcription in eukaryotic viruses. The DNA of eukaryotic viruses encodes intervening sequences, whereas those of bacterial viruses usually do not. (For an exception in bacteriophage T4, see Posttranscriptional Regulation in Chap. 45.)

Single-Stranded Viral DNA

The DNA is single-stranded and cyclic in some very small bacteriophages (the icosahedral φX174 and the helical f1 and M13) and in one family of animal viruses (parvoviruses). The phages have DNA molecules of the same polarity in all virions; parvoviruses have strands of both polarities, but in different virions. Parvoviruses have also inverted terminal repeats that can form hairpins, important for replication.

Viral RNAs

Some RNA viral genomes are **double stranded** (in reovirus, in a phage, and in some viruses of lower animals, insects, yeasts, and plants). Other genomes are **single stranded.** Single-stranded genomes belong to two classes: **positive-strand** genomes that, on entering the cells, can directly act as messengers for protein synthesis; and **negative-strand** genomes that are not of messenger polarity and must be transcribed into messengers. Positive-strand RNAs of eukaryotic cells have the general organization of eukaryotic mRNAs: they have a cap at the 5′ end, and they end with a poly(A) chain at the other end. Picornaviruses are an exception: they do not have a cap but have a small protein covalently linked to the 5′ terminal uridylate. Negative-strand RNAs do not have caps, but each is terminated at the 5′ end with a nucleoside triphosphate.

Of these viruses, the retroviruses are closely related to transposons: their genome is flanked by two repeats, and it integrates into the cellular DNA where it is flanked by two short repeated cellular sequences. It is propagated by reverse transcriptions (RNA → DNA), like transposons of Drosophila and yeast.

Segmentation of the Genome

The genomes of double-stranded RNA viruses, and of those of some negative-strand viruses, have a peculiarity: they are made of separate segments. For instance, the double-stranded reoviruses have ten segments, and the negative-stranded orthomyxoviruses have eight. The segmentation of the genome is probably a mechanism for avoiding polycistronic messengers, because eukaryotic cells rarely initiate protein synthesis internally in a messenger. A segment, however, may specify two proteins.

Control Sequences for RNA Viruses

Control sequences in RNA genomes have the function of interacting with the replication or transcription apparatus, with initiation factors for protein synthesis and ribosomes, and with the capsid. Short sequences with these functions, present near the ends of genomes and at the ends of genes, are recognized because they are conserved among related viruses.

Exceptional arrangements are found in some viral genomes. For instance, the positive-strand phage MS2 lacks a ribosome entry site for a lysis gene. This gene uses ribosomes that translate the upstream coat gene, with which it partly overlaps but in a different phase. Ribosomes that accidentally go out of phase in the coat gene can enter the lysis gene. This arrangement ensures that the lysis protein is made in much smaller amounts than the coat protein, so that the cells lyse only after enough virus is made. The polymerase gene of retroviruses has a similar arrangement. These are examples of gene overlap with regulatory function.

Origin of Viral Genomes

Because viral genomes could not have evolved readily except by replication within cells, it is logical to assume that viral genomes are ultimately derived from the genomes of host cells. A step in this evolution may be the incorporation of cellular genes into the genomes of transducing bacteriophages (see Chap. 46) and retroviruses (see Chap. 65). The evolutionary separation, however, is long, for homologies between viral genomes and cellular genes are rare. One is found in vaccinia virus, which has a gene with some homology with a cellular gene for a growth factor.

More stringent evidence for a cellular origin is found in positive-strand RNA viruses, the genomes of which resemble cellular messengers. The RNAs of some plant viruses terminate at the 3′ end with sequences that fold into the tertiary structure of tRNAs and can be aminoacylated by specific tRNA aminoacylases. At its 5′ position this cistron is connected to a poly(A) sequence from a cistron with all the features of a cellular mRNA. These genomes were evidently derived from the recombination of a cellular mRNA with a tRNA-like polynucleotide.

THE VIRION'S COATS
The Capsid

The study of the organization of the capsid is important because it uncovers the principles by which biological macromolecules assemble into complex structures. The capsid encloses the genome and gives the virions their characteristic shapes. It accounts for a large part of the virion's mass and is made up of protein molecules, which are specified by viral genes. Since viruses have small genomes, they cannot afford too many genes for specifying capsid proteins; hence, the capsid must be formed by the association of many protein units of a single kind or of relatively few kinds (**protomers**). For instance, poliovirus RNA (7 Kb) can specify at most 250,000 daltons of protein altogether; some of the proteins must be used for replication. Yet the poliovirus capsid weighs about 6×10^6 daltons. In fact, it contains only four unique proteins. The shape and dimensions of the capsid depend on characteristics of the constituent protomers and, for helical capsids, on the length of the viral nucleic acid.

The repeated protomers forming the capsid must be arranged in a regular architecture that utilizes bonds between the same pairs of chemical groups. This goal is attained in different ways in the icosahedral and helical capsids, as shown by extensive x-ray crystallographic studies.

ICOSAHEDRAL CAPSIDS. The icosahedral shape of many viruses is of considerable interest because the only closed shell that can be made with identical protomers is icosahedral. The simplest icosahedron is a regular solid with 12 vertices and 20 triangular faces (Fig. 44–4). To

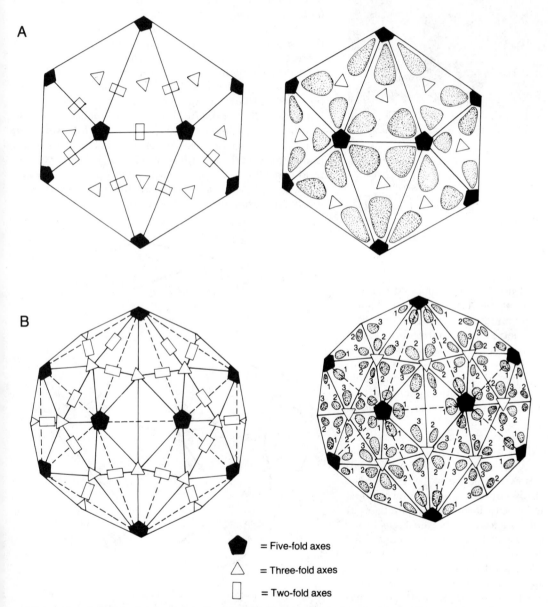

⬠ = Five-fold axes

△ = Three-fold axes

▢ = Two-fold axes

Figure 44–4. (**A**) The basic icosahedron. The drawing at left shows the triangular faces, with pentons at each vertex; the drawing at right shows the positions of the monomers around the fivefold axis. (**B**) A derived icosahedron (T = 3; see Appendix). Each triangular face of the icosahedron shown in **A** is subdivided into six half-triangles. The corners of the inscribed faces are solid lines; those of the basic faces are dashed lines. Monomers are arranged in pentons around the fivefold axes and in hexons around the threefold axes. *1*, *2*, and *3* indicate quasi-equivalent monomers.

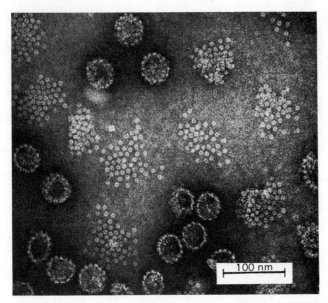

Figure 44–5. Preparation of rabbit papilloma virus (papovavirus) containing mostly empty capsids, i.e., devoid of nucleic acid. Some of the capsids have disintegrated during the preparation of the specimen for electron microscopy, each producing a small puddle of capsomers (some of the capsomers of the original capsid have been lost). The angular polygonal shape of the capsomers is evident, but it is not possible to differentiate hexamers from pentamers. (Breedis C et al: Virology 17:84, 1962)

THE SIMPLEST VIRIONS. Only the smallest and simplest virions have capsids made up of 60 identical protomers. One is that of the satellite tobacco necrosis virus. Enclosed in its capsid is a short RNA (about 1600 bases) with just one gene, that for the protomer of the capsid. Because of this simplicity this virus multiplies only in cells infected by the tobacco necrosis virus, which provides the proteins needed for its replication (hence the name satellite). Under suitable conditions the protomers of this virus can spontaneously assemble first into pentons, which then join to form the icosahedral capsids (**self-assembly**).

QUASI-EQUIVALENCE. Most other icosahedral viruses have more than 60 protomers per virion. They cannot form rigorous icosahedrons but form approximate ones, in the following way. In an icosahedron the triangular faces can be subdivided into a number of smaller triangles, generating **modified icosahedrons.** The smallest possible number of inscribed triangles per face is 3, followed by 4, 7, 9, 12, and so on (see Appendix). These figures are known as the **triangulation numbers (T)** of the various modified icosahedrons. Because each inscribed triangle must again have three protomers, their number in each modified icosahedron is 60 × T.

make a shell there must be sixty protomers—three per face, each located at one of the vertices (see Fig. 44–4A) and all connected to one another in the same way. The five protomers around each vertex together form knobs recognizable by electron microscopy, known as **capsomers,** and, more specifically, **pentons.** The bonds between protomers in a capsomer are usually more stable than those between capsomers, so the capsomers tend to persist after the capsid is disrupted under mild conditions (Fig. 44–5).

To enclose space, asymmetric units with identical bonding must be related to one another by rotational symmetry. This is easily seen by considering the two-dimensional case, as shown in Figure 44–6. Accordingly, the icosahedron has **only rotational symmetry;** that is, it is brought to coincide with itself after rotation of an appropriate angle around certain axes (see Fig. 44–4A). The icosahedron has axes of three kinds: fivefold axes through the vertices (coincidence is achieved five times in a full turn), threefold axes through the centers of the faces (three coincidences), and twofold axes through the middle of each corner (two coincidences). For this reason it is said to have a 2–3–5 rotational symmetry. In a perfect icosahedron all protomers are therefore related to one another in exactly the same way.

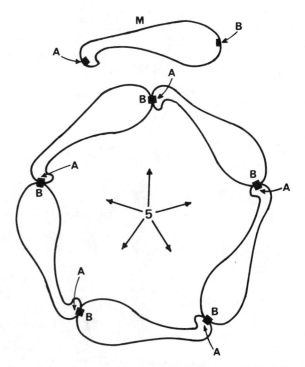

Figure 44–6. Formation of a closed ring by five asymmetric protomers (*M*), in which group B can form a bond with group A. Since the distance between successive A–B bonds and the angle of the A–B bonds to the axis of the monomer are constant, a closed ring having fivefold rotational symmetry around an axis through its center is formed.

For the basic icosahedron with 20 faces, T = 1. The simplest of the more complex viruses are alphaviruses and some plant viruses, for which T = 3; this icosahedron has 60 faces (see Fig. 44–4B). These capsids contain 180 protomers made up of identical polypeptide chains but with three **different configurations** (indicated by 1, 2, and 3 in Fig. 44–4B) that depend on the location of each protomer with respect to the axes of the icosahedrons. In all protomers the polypeptide chains have a tight boxlike structure, but with tails that establish connections between them. In Figure 44–4B all protomers No. 1 form **pentons** around the fivefold axes, whereas Nos. 2 and 3 protomers are regularly arranged in groups of six around the threefold axes (**hexons**). The relationships among protomers in hexons and pentons must be different, but the differences are small and can be taken care of by configurational differences of the same peptide chain (principle of quasi-equivalence).

HIGHER-ORDER CAPSIDS. In more complex viruses the capsids have a higher number of protomers and capsomers. Then the two types of capsomer are made up of different proteins, with arrangements that at times deviate from the basic icosahedral scheme. For instance, in adenoviruses (T = 25; Fig. 44–7), hexons contain three instead of six protomers, still retaining the ability to make contacts each with six other capsomers. This arrangement is compatible with icosahedral symmetry, be-

cause the axes going through the hexons have a threefold, not sixfold, symmetry (see Fig. 44–4B). In the construction of these capsids the hexons, which are the most abundant capsomers, often join together to form **complex structural units** with a closely packed hexagonal lattice. These units then assemble into capsids. The configuration of the polypeptide chains must still be different, depending on each hexon in the final assembly, whether at the center of a face of the basic icosahedron, at a corner, or adjacent to a penton.

These complex capsids cannot form by self-assembly. In principle, the hexons are capable of making, by self-assembly, flat sheets or cylinders; cylindrical forms are indeed found in cells infected by some viral mutants that are unable to make a complete capsid (Fig. 44–8). In con-

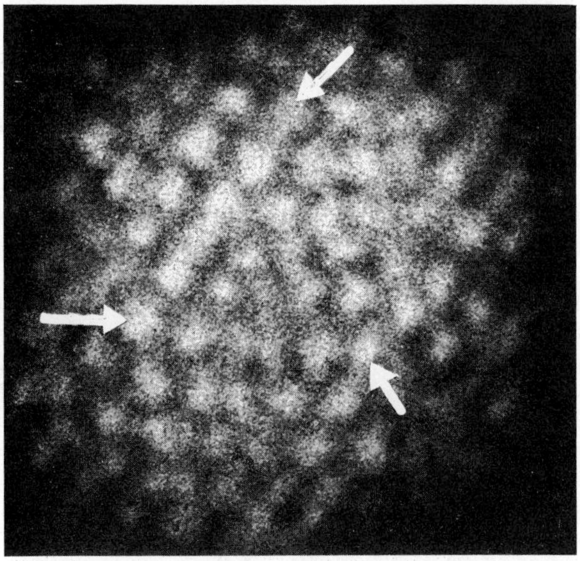

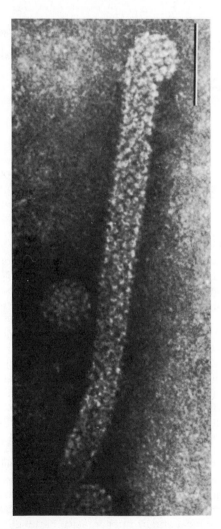

Figure 44–8. A very long filament of human wart virus (papovavirus) hexons, together with a regular virion. The filament, of a diameter close to that of the virions, is made up of hexagonal capsomers. (Noyes WF: Virology 23:65, 1964)

62.5 nm

Figure 44–7. Electron micrograph of GAL virus (chicken adenovirus) by negative staining, showing the capsomer structure. The arrowed capsomers are situated on the fivefold axis. (Wildly P, Watson JD: Cold Spring Harbor Symp Quant Biol 27:25, 1962)

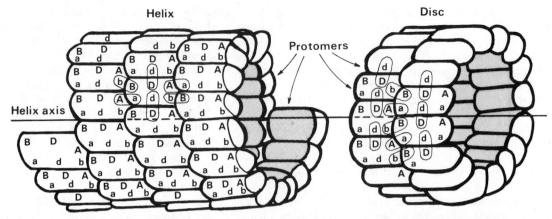

Figure 44–9. Constitution of the helical capsid. All protomers are identical and establish regularly repeated bonds with their neighbors between chemical groups indicated by letters. Since each protomer is staggered with respect to its lateral neighbors, it forms bonds with the two of them on each side along the helix axes. This confers considerable stability on the capsid. The protomers assemble first to constitute flat nonhelical discs containing two rings of protomers, with the staggered arrangement found in the finished helix. Under physiologic conditions, when the protomers of the discs associate with the RNA, they shift slightly to produce a helix. The helix grows in length by the addition and assimilation of discs.

trast, pentons make vertices; in combination with hexons, which make the flat faces, they allow the formation of a closed shell, approximately icosahedral, with the pentons at the axes of fivefold symmetry and the hexons in between. Large viruses, such as phage T4 or adenovirus, use **scaffolding proteins** as a mold for the capsid. The mold determines the dimensions of the capsid and the number of hexons, whereas the number of pentons remains fixed at 12. This principle explains how oblong capsids of variable length can be assembled.

An unusual arrangement is found in the **geminiviruses,** which cause important diseases in plants. The capsid is formed by two incomplete icosahedrons (T = 1) attached to each other, and it contains two different cyclic single-stranded DNAs, which are both required for infectivity.

HELICAL CAPSIDS. The roughly cylindrical helical capsid (Fig. 44–9) has the simplest organization. The identical protomers are bound end-to-end by identical bonds to form a ribbonlike structure, which is wound around the axis of the helix. The protomers in two successive turns of the ribbon each form bonds with two protomers of adjacent turns. This pattern confers great stability on the structure. The straight line in the center of the cylinder is an axis of rotational symmetry.

The diameter of the helical capsid is determined by the characteristics of its protomers, while the length is determined by the length of the nucleic acid it encloses. The tail of some bacteriophages (see below) is also helical but does not contain nucleic acid: its length is determined by the length of a filiform **tape protein** around which it assembles.

The capsids of naked helical viruses (e.g., tobacco mosaic virus) are very tight (see Fig. 44–3*B*). In contrast, the capsids of enveloped helical viruses (such as paramyxoviruses) are very flexible, because the whole capsid—and not only the nucleic acid—has to coil within the envelope. Often the turns of the helices are visible in electron micrographs (Fig. 44–10), suggesting a loose structure; in these viruses the envelope rather than the capsid may provide the required barrier to nucleases.

ORGANIZATION OF THE GENOME WITHIN THE CAPSID. In **icosahedral capsids** the nucleic acid is tightly packed, with attendant important topologic and thermodynamic problems, especially for stiff double-stranded DNA. In conjunction with certain basic proteins or with polyamines, DNA often forms a central **core** of parallel loops; folding is accompanied by some denaturation of the double helix. In some animal viruses, such as polyomaviruses, DNA folds tightly around cellular histones to form a **chromatinlike structure,** much like cellular chromatin in condensed chromosomes. Neither DNA nor RNA has a highly regular arrangement within the capsid, as deduced from absence of an orderly pattern in x-ray crystallography.

The highest level of organization is that of adenovirus DNA, which, in conjunction with virus-specified proteins, forms twelve equal balls, each located under one of the vertices of the icosahedral capsid. This arrangement is secondary to that of the capsid, because the DNA enters a preformed capsid.

In **helical capsids** the RNA is located in a helical groove between the protomers (Fig. 44–11), to which it is attached by multiple weak bonds, irrespective of sequences.

Capsids without nucleic acid—**empty capsids**—are found in most preparations of the icosahedral viruses. Electron microscopy reveals an external capsomeric

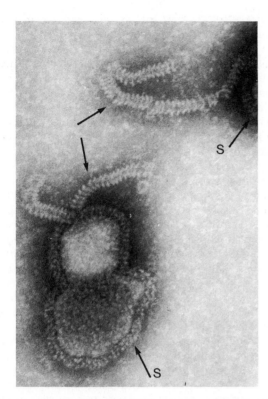

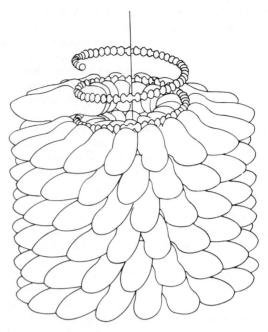

Figure 44–11. Drawing of a segment of tobacco mosaic virus showing the helical nucleocapsid. In the upper part of the figure two rows of protein monomers have been removed to reveal the RNA. This drawing is based on results of x-ray diffraction studies. (Klug A, Caspar DLD: Adv Virus Res 7:225, 1960)

Figure 44–10. The helical capsid of a paramyxovirus with negative staining. Two particles of the simian paramyxovirus SV5 are seen: segments of the helical capsid protrude from both particles (*arrows*), probably owing to rupture of the envelope. Note the loose arrangement of the protomers and the hollow along the axis of the helix. The envelopes are covered by the characteristic spikes (*S*). (Choppin PW, Stockenius W: Virology 23:195, 1964)

44–5). Their existence shows that the nucleic acid is not essential for the assembly of many kinds of capsids.

The Envelope

Envelopes, like cellular membranes, contain lipid bilayers and proteins with special functions. The presence of lipids makes enveloped viruses sensitive to disinfection or damage by lipid solvents, such as ether. The proteins of the envelope are of two kinds: one or more **glycoproteins** and a **matrix** protein.

configuration similar to that of normal virions (Fig. 44–12). However, these capsids may lack some capsid proteins. Empty capsids are less stable than the capsids of virions, and during preparation of specimens for electron microscopy they disintegrate more readily (see Fig.

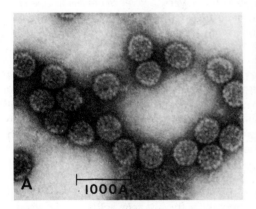

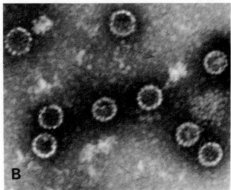

1000A

Figure 44–12. Electron micographs with negative staining of purified polyoma virus, a papovavirus. (*A*) The full virions are not penetrated by the stain and show only the pattern on the surface of the capsid. (*B*) The empty capsids are penetrated by the stain.

GLYCOPROTEINS. Individual glycoprotein molecules are **transmembrane** proteins, with a large external domain and a small cytoplasmic domain. The two domains are connected to each other by a stretch of hydrophobic amino acids (**anchor sequence**), usually close to the carboxyl terminus, which anchors the protein to the lipid bilayer of the membrane. Some glycoproteins (e.g., the influenza hemagglutinins) are anchored at both the carboxyl and the amino ends, forming a loop. In these cases the hydrophobic sequence at the amino end corresponds to the **signal sequence,** which is usually cut off after it has guided the protein through the membrane.

Glycoproteins have oligosaccharide residues, in the form of either N- or O-glycosylation. In many viruses glycoproteins have one or two molecules of a **fatty acid** (palmitate or myristilate), of uncertain function, attached to the carboxyl end in the cytoplasmic domain.

Small groups of glycoproteins (up to four) form the **spikes** or other knoblike structures protruding at the surface of enveloped virions (see Figs. 44–3*D* and 44–10). Each virion has several hundred spikes; their number generally does not correspond to that of the capsid protomers. Glycoproteins, although functionally essential, may not be required for the formation of the envelope: some paramyxovirus mutants, which lack a glycoprotein, form virions with otherwise normal morphology, though they are noninfectious.

Glycoproteins perform important functions: they cause the attachment of virions to cell surfaces and the penetration of their genomes into cells. The rabies virus glycoprotein may also mediate the neurotoxic effect of the virus by binding to the acetylcholine receptors at the neuromuscular junction. These functions of the glycoproteins in attachment and penetration are reflected in the ability of virions of several viral families to cause **hemagglutination,** that is, the bridging of red blood cells. Some glycoproteins cause the **fusion** of the viral membrane with the cell's membrane; they may also cause **hemolysis.**

With orthomyxoviruses and paramyxoviruses hemagglutination is carried out by **hemagglutinins** that bind to the terminal N-acetylneuraminic (sialic) acid present on oligosaccharides of the cellular surface, which act as **receptors** for the viruses. Fusion is carried out by **fusion proteins** with a hydrophobic amino acid sequence at its amino terminus; this sequence penetrates into the cell's lipid bilayer, destabilizing it and causing it to form a single membrane with the virion's envelope.

Some viruses (e.g., influenza and parainfluenza) also possess glycoproteins with **neuraminidase** activity on their surfaces, which cleaves the terminal sialic acid from cellular oligosaccharides. This function is important when progeny virus is released from the cells, to free it from entrapment by oligosaccharides.

MATRIX PROTEINS (M PROTEINS). Matrix proteins are usually not glycosylated. Some are transmembrane proteins with multiple stretches of hydrophobic amino acids, which traverse the membrane; others are held to the inner side of the membrane by hydrophobic amino acids. These proteins reinforce the envelope, connect the nucleocapsid to the glycoproteins, and perform a crucial function during the formation of the virions (see Chap. 48).

In many enveloped viruses the liquid state of the lipid bilayer, and the absence of connections among the proteins of the envelope, prevent the formation of a rigid structure, leading to pronounced **pleomorphism** of the virions. However, in other viruses a firm connection between envelope and nucleocapsid confers on the virions characteristic shapes. Thus, the alphavirus virions are icosahedral, but, surprisingly, the symmetries of the envelope (T = 4) and that of the capsid (T = 3) do not coincide; the glycoproteins form different contacts with proteins of the capsid. Rhabdoviruses are **bullet shaped,** with the helical nucleocapsids coiled under the outer layer (Fig. 44–13).

The major proteins of the envelope are, like those of the capsid, specified by viral genes. They constitute the major **antigens** of the virions, which are important in the immune response and in virion identification. Some virions contain also, as a minor component, glycoproteins derived from the surface of the cells in which they are produced. This is typical for vesicular stomatitis virions, which contain 10% to 20% of such adventitious protein molecules. The proteins thus incorporated do not represent a random sample of those present at the cell surface; preferentially incorporated are glycoproteins of other enveloped viruses infecting the same cell.

Complex Virions

POXVIRUSES. The poxvirus virions, brick-shaped or ovoid, hold the viral DNA, associated with protein, in a **nucleoid** shaped like a biconcave disc and surrounded by several lipoprotein layers. A layer of coarse fibrils near the outer surface gives the virions a characteristically striated appearance in negatively stained preparations (see Fig. 44–3*E*; see also Chap. 54).

LARGE BACTERIOPHAGES. Some bacteriophages, such as coliphages T2, T4, and T6 (**T-even coliphages**) have very complex structures (see Fig. 44–3*F*), including an icosahedral head and a helical tail. They are said to have **binal symmetry** because they have components with different kinds of symmetry within the same virion.

Other Virion Components

In addition to the structural proteins found in the coats or in association with the nucleic acids, some virions contain **enzymes,** which perform functions essential to

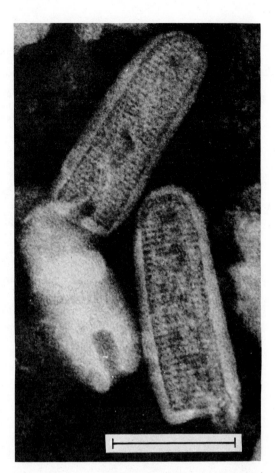

Figure 44–13. Virions of vesicular stomatitis virus (a rhabdovirus) with negative staining. The helical filament, present in a deeper layer, is visible in two particles. (Howatson AF, Whitmore GF: Virology 16:466, 1962)

the initial stages of viral multiplication (Table 44–3). Typical examples are enzymes transcribing the virion RNA into mRNA (in virions with a negative-strand RNA genome), those transcribing double-stranded RNA (in virions with such a genome), enzymes transcribing RNA into DNA (in retroviruses), and those that generate capped leaders for viral messengers by transferring them from cellular messengers (in orthomyxoviruses). Enzymes of these various types are not present in cells; they are specified by viral genes and are brought into the cells by the virions themselves. Virions of some viruses contain a variety of other enzymes, which often duplicate functions performed by the cellular enzymes. Their presence in virions may reflect specific needs of the virus. For instance, the vaccinia virions, which replicate in the cytoplasm, contain enzymes for the transcription of double-stranded DNA that recognize initiation and termination signals specific to vaccinia virus DNA.

DEFECTIVE VIRUSES

Viruses incapable of autonomous replication can arise by mutation of regular viruses; for multiplication they require a wild-type **helper virus,** coinfecting the same cells to provide the defective function. **Satellite viruses** are by nature defective; that is, they do not have a related replication-competent virus. These viruses are present only in cells infected by another unrelated virus, which acts as helper. Among satellite viruses the adeno-associated viruses, with a single-stranded DNA genome, require coinfecting adenovirus as helper. The satellite genome encodes only a few proteins, among which is the protein of its capsid. An important satellite virus associated with hepatitis B virus, the **δ agent** increases the severity of the disease. It has a cyclic RNA genome, resembling that of viroids (see below), and forms particles surrounded by hepatitis B surface antigen.

VIRUS-RELATED AGENTS
Viroids

Viroids, which are responsible for serious diseases of many plants, share with viruses some fundamental properties, such as a simple organization. However they are naked RNA, neither containing nor coding for any protein. Each viroid particle is a **cyclic single-stranded RNA molecule** containing between 250 and 400 nucleotides, depending on the strain. They resist enzymatic destruction because they have no free ends and because they have a very tight secondary structure (owing to self-complementary sequences), which makes them resemble small, compact rods.

All viroid strains, in spite of the different lengths of the RNAs, have similar characteristics. Their genome can be considered a double-stranded RNA, with many unpaired short "bubbles." The most striking feature is the lack of initiation codons for protein synthesis (AUG), or of their complements (in case the RNA is of the negative-strand type); there is no evidence that these RNAs are translated. They are replicated in the nucleus of infected cells by host enzymes through oligomeric double-stranded intermediates. Replication is blocked by alpha-amanitin, which inhibits RNA polymerase II, the enzyme that generates the transcripts of cellular genes destined to become mRNAs.

The base sequences of viroids have repeats, both direct and inverted, which suggest a relatedness to transposing elements (see Chap. 8). Moreover, they possess a sequence similar to that used by retroviruses—which are also closely related to transposing elements (see Chap. 65)—for initiating reverse transcription. Unlike retroviruses, however, viroids are not transcribed into DNA, and no sequences homologous to viroids are found in the DNA of the infected cells. DNA complementary to

TABLE 44–3. *Characteristics of Virion Enzymes*

Enzyme	Virus	Product of Function
ENZYMES AFFECTING INTERACTION OF VIRIONS WITH THE HOST CELL SURFACE		
Neuraminidase	Orthomyxovirus, paramyxovirus	Splits off NANA from surface polysaccharides
Endoglycosidase	*E. coli* K bacteriophages	Breaks down surface polysaccharides
Fusion factor*	Paramyxovirus	Alters lipid bilayer
ENZYMES TRANSCRIBING THE VIRAL GENOME INTO MESSENGER RNA		
DNA-dependent RNA polymerase	Poxvirus, polyhedrosis viruses of frogs, bacteriophages N4, SP02	Single-stranded mRNA
Double-stranded RNA transcriptase	Viruses with double-stranded RNA	Single-stranded mRNA
Single-stranded RNA transcriptase	Viruses with single-stranded RNA (negative strand)	Single-stranded mRNA (positive strand)
ENZYMES ADDING SPECIFIC TERMINAL GROUPS TO VIRAL mRNA MADE IN VIRIONS		
Nucleotide phosphohydrolase	Viruses synthesizing mRNA in virions (e.g., poxviruses, reoviruses)	Converts terminal 5'-triphosphate to diphosphate as prelude to guanylylation
Guanylyl transferase	Viruses synthesizing mRNA in virions (e.g., poxviruses, reoviruses)	Adds guanylyl residue to 5'-end diphosphate in mRNA
RNA methylases	Viruses synthesizing mRNA in virions (e.g., poxviruses, reoviruses)	Methylate guanylyl residue at 5'-end of mRNA and some riboses in 2' position
Poly(A) polymerase	Viruses synthesizing mRNA in virions (e.g., poxviruses, reoviruses)	Synthesizes poly(A) tail at 3' end of mRNA
ENZYMES INVOLVED IN COPYING VIRION RNA INTO DNA		
RNA-dependent DNA polymerase (reverse transcriptase)	Retroviruses	DNA–RNA hybrids; double-stranded DNA
RNase H (in association with reverse transcriptase)	Retroviruses	Breaks down RNA strand in RNA–DNA hybrids
Polynucleotide ligase	Retroviruses	Closes single-strand breaks in double-stranded DNA
ENZYMES FOR NUCLEIC ACID REPLICATION OR PROCESSING		
DNA-dependent DNA polymerase	Hepatitis B	Synthesizes double-stranded DNA
Deoxyribonucleases (exo- and endo-)	Poxviruses, retrovirus	Break DNA chains and crosslinks
Endoribonuclease	Viruses with single-stranded mRNA (e.g., poxvirus)	Processing of mRNA
OTHER ENZYMES		
Protein kinases	Hepatitis B	Phosphorylate proteins

NANA, N-acetylneuraminic acid

* No enzymatic activity known

viroid RNA is also infectious, and in cells it is transcribed into regular infectious viroid molecules.

A striking feature of viroid RNA is the presence of sequences highly homologous to some of the small nuclear RNAs, U_1 and U_3, which are involved in the splicing of introns in animal cells, and presumably also in plant cells. This finding suggests that viroids originated from introns and that their pathogenicity might be due to interference with the normal splicing of introns in the cell. Related to viroids are the **virusoids,** which are satellites of certain plant viruses and are encapsidated with their helper RNAs in the virions. A candidate for a viroidlike organism in humans is the δ agent (see Defective Viruses, above), which is much larger (1678 base pairs) and surrounded by a coat.

Agents of Slow Infections

The etiology of several transmissible slow diseases of humans (such as Creutzfeldt-Jakob disease and Kuru) or animals (scrapie) has defied characterization. The agents are like viruses in size and infectivity; no virus, however, has been isolated from the infected tissues. These contain a characteristic protein, which is also present in normal tissues. It has been suggested that the agent is of a novel type, not containing nucleic acid (**prion**); the nature of the agent, however, remains obscure (see Chap. 51).

Assay of Viruses

The methods used for the assay of viruses reflect their dual nature as both complex chemicals and living microorganisms. Viruses can be assayed by chemical and physical methods, by immunologic techniques, or by the consequences of their interaction with living host cells, i.e., their **infectivity.** Assays carried out by different techniques can differ vastly in their significance.

CHEMICAL AND PHYSICAL DETERMINATIONS
Counts of Physical Particles

Virions can be clearly recognized in the electron microscope; if a sample contains only virions of a single type, their number can be determined unambiguously. Virions are counted by mixing the sample with a known number of polystyrene latex particles, viewing droplets of the mixture in the electron microscope, and counting the two types of particles present in the same droplet. Simple arithmetic then yields the number of virions in the total sample (Fig. 44–14). This technique does not distinguish between infectious and noninfectious particles.

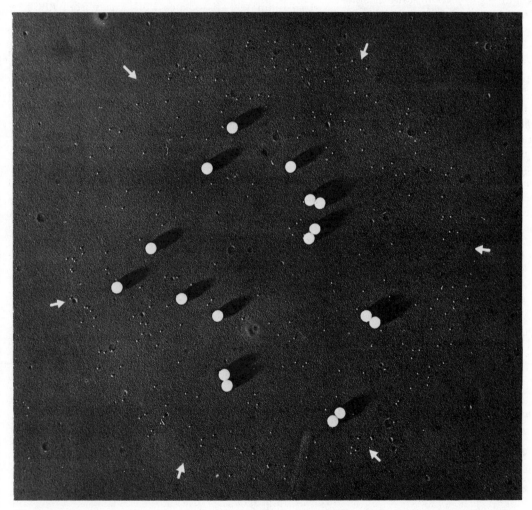

Figure 44–14. Counting of particles of poliovirus (a picornavirus) mixed with polystyrene latex particles. The mixture was sprayed in droplets on the supporting membrane, dried, and shadowed. The micrograph shows a droplet, the outline of which is partly visible (*arrows*). The small particles are virus, the large ones latex. There are 220 viral and 17 latex particles in the droplet. Since the latex concentration in the sample was 3.2×10^{10} particles/ml, the concentration of viral particles is $220/17 \times 3.2 \times 10^{10} = 4.1 \times 10^{11}$/ml. The precision of the assay based on this one droplet is only about $\pm 50\%$ (see Appendix), owing to the small number of latex particles counted. To obtain a greater precision, pooled counts from many similar drops would have to be used. (Courtesy of the Virus Laboratory, University of California, Berkeley)

Hemagglutination

Many viruses, both small and large, can agglutinate red blood cells (RBCs). This important property, discovered independently for influenza virus by Hirst and by McClelland and Hare in 1941, affords a simple, rapid method for viral titration. Hemagglutination is usually caused by the virions themselves; in some cases, however, as with poxviruses, it is caused by lipid hemagglutinins produced during viral multiplication.

Although the spectrum of red cell species that are agglutinated and the required conditions differ for different viruses, the phenomenon is basically similar in all cases: a virion or a hemagglutinin attaches simultaneously to two RBCs and bridges them, and at sufficiently high viral concentrations multiple bridging yields large **aggregates.**

HEMAGGLUTINATION ASSAY. The formation of aggregates can be detected in a number of ways. In the simplest, the **pattern method** (Fig. 44–15), the suspension of RBCs and virus is left undisturbed in small wells in a plastic plate for several hours. Nonaggregated cells sediment to the round bottom of the well and then roll toward the center, where they form a small, sharply outlined, round pellet. Aggregates, however, sediment to the bottom but do not roll; they form a thin film, which has a characteristic serrated edge. This method is used for **endpoint assays.** Serial twofold dilutions of the virus sample are each mixed with a standard suspension of RBCs (usually 10^7/ml). The last dilution showing complete hemagglutination is taken as the endpoint. This

titer has an inherent imprecision at least as large as the dilution step used (usually twofold).

A more refined method is to determine the proportion of aggregated cells by observing their sedimentation in a photoelectric colorimeter, since aggregated RBCs sediment faster than nonaggregated ones and can be measured separately. The titer obtained either way is expressed in **hemagglutinating units.** The photometric assay is the more sensitive and permits the demonstration that a single influenza virus particle agglutinates two RBCs.

The presence of neuraminidases on the surface of orthomyxovirus and paramyxovirus virions affects the course of hemagglutination. At 37°C the viral neuraminidase ultimately dissociates the viruses from RBCs by splitting N-acetyl neuraminic acid from receptors; the virus then spontaneously elutes off the RBCs, which disaggregate. At 0°C, in contrast, the enzyme is much less active, and the virion–RBC union is stable. After the virus has eluted, cells cannot be agglutinated again by a new batch of virus, since they have lost the receptors; these cells are said to be **stabilized.** (The eluted virus, on the contrary, retains all its activities.)

However, cells stabilized by a given orthomyxovirus or paramyxovirus can sometimes be agglutinated by another virus of these families. Indeed, it is possible to arrange the viruses in a series (called a **receptor gradient**) such that any virus will exhaust the receptors for itself and the viruses preceding it in the gradient, but not for those that follow it. This result indicates that viruses differ in the precise specificity of their neuraminidases.

Heating the virus inactivates its neuraminidase with-

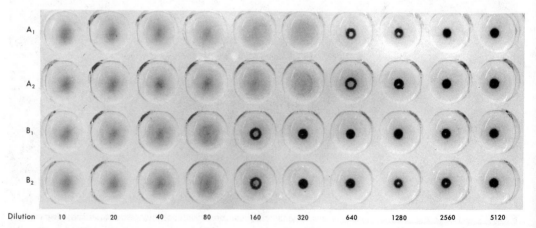

Figure 44–15. Results of a hemagglutination assay by the pattern method with influenza virus (an orthomyxovirus). Two samples, A and B, were diluted serially in steps: (1) 0.5 ml of each dilution was mixed with an equal volume of a red cell suspension, and (2) each mixture was placed in a cup drilled into a clear plastic plate and left for 30 minutes at room temperature. Each assay was made in duplicate. Sample A causes complete hemagglutination until dilution 320; sample B until dilution 80. In either case the subsequent dilution still shows partial hemagglutination. The hemagglutinating titer of A is 320; that of B, 80.

out destroying hemagglutinating activity. This **indicator** virus is useful for studying the union with receptors and mucoproteins without the complication of their enzymatic inactivation.

Assays Based on Antigenic Properties

Complement fixation (CF) or precipitation with antiserum can be used to measure amounts of virus. These methods have relatively low sensitivity and are used only for special purposes (see Chap. 50).

ASSAYS OF INFECTIVITY
Plaque Method

The plaque method is the fundamental assay method in virologic research, and it is also of great value in diagnosis: it combines simplicity, accuracy, and high reproducibility. First used with bacteriophages, this method was a key factor in the spectacular advances of research on phage and later also on animal viruses.

Bacteriophages are assayed in the following way. A phage-containing sample is mixed with a drop of a dense liquid culture of suitable bacteria and a few milliliters of melted soft agar at 44°C; the mixture is then poured over the surface of a plate (Petri dish) containing a layer of hard nutrient agar. The soft agar spreads in a thin layer and sets, and the bacteriophages diffuse through it until each meets and infects a bacterium. After 20 to 30 minutes the bacterium lyses, releasing several hundred progeny virions. These, in turn, infect neighboring bacteria, which again lyse and release new virus. The uninfected bacteria, in the meantime, grow to form a dense, opaque lawn. After a day's incubation the lysed areas stand out as transparent **plaques** against the dense background (Fig. 44–16*A*). The soft agar permits diffusion of phage to nearby cells but prevents convection to other regions of the plate; hence, secondary centers of infection cannot form.

With **animal viruses** a similar method is possible, the bacteria being replaced by a monolayer of cells growing on a solid support (see Chap. 47), and the nutrient medium is replaced by a solution containing the viral sample. Within an hour or so most of the virions attach to cells. Soft nutrient agar or some other gelling mixture is

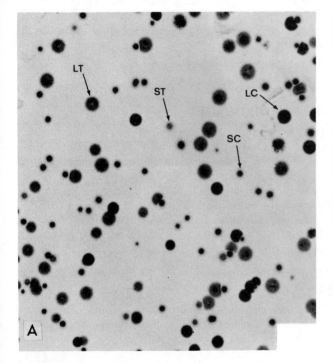
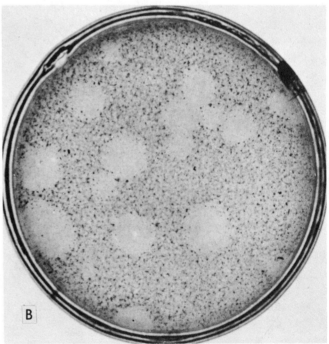

Figure 44–16. Plaque assay. **(A)** Phage. The progeny of cells infected by two phage types was diluted by a factor of 10^7; 0.1 ml of the diluted virus was assayed. The plate was counted 18 hours after plating. Four different plaque types, differing in plaque size and turbidity—large clear (*LC*), large turbid (*LT*), small clear (*SC*), and small turbid (*ST*)—can be distinguished, showing the great utility of plaque formation for genetic work with bacteriophages. Part of the plate is reproduced; a total of 407 plaques could be counted on the whole plate. The titer is 4.07×10^{10}/ml in the undiluted sample. The accuracy is ±10%. **(B)** Poliovirus (picornavirus). A sample of poliovirus type 1 was diluted by a factor of 2×10^5, and 0.1 ml was assayed on a monolayer culture of rhesus monkey kidney cells, with an agar overlay containing neutral red. The culture was incubated for 3 days at 37°C in an atmosphere containing 7% CO_2, which constitutes a buffer with the bicarbonate present in the overlay. Some of the plaques show partial confluence, but they can still be identified as separate plaques; 17 plaques can be counted on the photograph. The corresponding titer is 3.4×10^7/ml in the undiluted sample. The accuracy is ±50%.

poured over the cell layer. Plaques develop after 1 day to 3 weeks of incubation, depending on the virus (see Fig. 44–16B).

Plaques are detected in a variety of ways.

1. The virus often kills the infected cells, i.e., produces a **cytopathic effect;** the plaques are then detected by staining the cell layer with a dye that stains only the live cells (e.g., neutral red) or only the dead cells (trypan blue).

2. With certain viruses the cells in the plaques are not killed but acquire the ability to adsorb RBCs (see Maturation and Release of Animal Viruses—Enveloped Viruses, Chap. 48). The plaques are revealed by **hemadsorption,** i.e., by flooding the cell layer with a suspension of RBCs, then washing out those not attached to infected cells.

3. The infected cells may fuse with neighboring uninfected cells to form **polykaryocytes** (i.e., multinucleated cells), which are microscopically detectable (**syncytial plaques).**

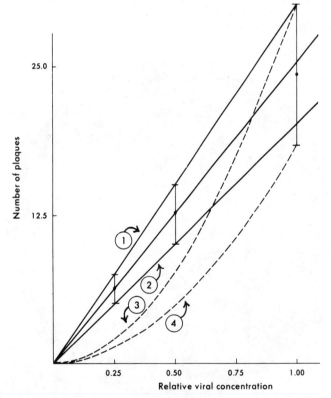

Figure 44–17. Dose–response curve of the plaque assay. The number of plaques produced by a sample of poliovirus type 1 at various concentrations was plotted versus the relative concentration of the virus; the accuracy of the assay (±2σ) is indicated for each point. The data are in agreement with a linear dose–response curve that falls between lines 1 and 2, and therefore with the notion that a single particle is sufficient to give rise to a plaque. Curves 3 and 4 give the range of data that would be obtained if at least two viral particles were required to initiate a plaque; the deviation is such that the hypothesis is ruled out (see Appendix).

4. Often the cells of the plaques contain large amounts of viral Ags, which can be detected by **immunofluorescence.**

The titer of the viral preparation is directly calculated from the number of plaques and the dilution of the sample, as shown in Figure 44–16B. As discussed in the appendix to this chapter, the accuracy of the assay depends on the number of plaques counted. An assay estimated from n plaques will be within $2/\sqrt{n}$ of the true value (e.g., with 100 plaques the range will be ±20%).

THE DOSE–RESPONSE CURVE OF THE PLAQUE ASSAY. The number of plaques in plates infected with different dilutions of the same viral sample is proportional to the concentration of the virus; i.e., the dose–response curve is linear (Fig. 44–17). A single virion is therefore sufficient to infect a cell. It follows that the viral population contained in a plaque is the progeny of a single virion, i.e., a clone, representing a genetically pure line. Plaques also provide useful genetic markers through their visible characteristics such as size, shape, and turbidity.

Pock Counting

When the chorionic epithelium of the chorioallantoic membrane of a chick embryo (see Fig. 48–1) is infected by vaccinia or herpes simplex virus, characteristic lesions (**pocks**) appear. They may be white or hemorrhagic; viral mutants may be distinguishable by the appearance of the pocks. This method, important initially, is now largely superseded by the plaque method.

Other Local Lesions

Tumor-producing viruses, such as the Rous sarcoma virus (see Chap. 65), can be assayed on monolayer cell cultures; they produce **proliferative foci,** each initiated by a single viral particle.

Many **plant viruses** can be titrated by counting the lesions produced on leaves rubbed with a mixture of virus and an abrasive material. The virus penetrates through ruptures of the cell walls caused by the abrasive, and the progeny spread to neighboring cells.

Endpoint Method

The endpoint method, used for assaying animal viruses before the advent of the plaque method, is still employed for certain diagnostic assays and for quantitating virulence or host resistance. The virus is serially diluted, and a constant volume of each dilution is inoculated into a number of similar **test units,** such as mice, chick embryos, or cell cultures. At each dilution the proportion of infected test units (**infectivity ratio**) is scored: for example, by (1) death or disease of an animal or embryo, (2) degeneration of a tissue culture, or (3) recognition of progeny virus *in vitro* (e.g., by hemagglutination).

The lower dilutions of the virus infect most of the test

units, and the highest dilutions infect none. A rough idea of the viral titer is given by the intermediate dilutions that produce signs of infection in only a fraction of the test units. The transition is not sharp, however, and only by combining the data from several dilutions is it possible to calculate the precise endpoint at which 50% of the test units are infected. At this dilution each sample contains on the average one ID_{50}, i.e., one **infectious dose for 50%** of the test units. One ID_{50} can be shown mathematically to correspond to 0.7 plaque-forming units (see Appendix).

The interpolation to obtain the ID_{50} can be carried out in a variety of ways. The method of Reed and Muench, though not mathematically derived, yields results in fair agreement with more rigorous methods. In this method (see Appendix) the dilution containing one ID_{50} is obtained by interpolation between the two dilutions that straddle the 50% value of the infectivity ratio. The interpolation assumes that in the proximity of the ID_{50} the infectivity ratio varies linearly with the log dilution. Usually the accuracy of the method is low, since the number of test units used at each dilution is small. When, for instance, six test units are employed at each tenfold dilution, as is common in diagnostic titrations, the titration is useful only to ascertain large differences in viral titer (50-fold or more) between two samples, which is adequate for many routine diagnostic procedures.

Viral titers obtained by the endpoint method are expressed in various equivalents of the ID_{50}: LD_{50} (lethal dose) if the criterion is death; PD_{50} (paralysis dose) if the criterion is paralysis; TC_{50} (tissue culture dose) if the criterion is degeneration of a culture.

COMPARISON OF DIFFERENT TYPES OF ASSAYS

The focal assay methods (plaques, foci, and pocks) are most satisfactory for their high efficiency combined with simplicity, reproducibility, and economy. For example, to match the precision obtained by counting 100 plaques on a single culture, on would require more than 100 test units per decimal dilution in an endpoint titration. The precision of any type of assay is adversely affected by a variability in the response of the cells or organisms used in the assay; the variabilities can be very large in the pock assay and even larger in endpoint assays using animals.

The various methods of assay have different sensitivities and measure different properties. Assays based on infectivity are as much as a millionfold more sensitive than those based on chemical and physical properties. Chemical and physical techniques, moreover, titrate not only infectious but also noninfectious virions (empty capsids, particles with a damaged nucleic acid). These methods can therefore be useful for studies requiring measurement of the total number of viral particles. Hemagglutination or immunologic methods can also ti-

TABLE 44–4. Ratio of Viral Particles to Infectious Units

Virus	Ratio
ANIMAL VIRUSES	
Picornaviruses	
Poliovirus	30–1000
Foot-and-mouth disease virus	33–1600
Papovaviruses	
Polyoma virus	38–50
SV40	100–200
Papilloma virus	$\sim 10^4$
Reoviruses	10
Alphaviruses	
Semliki Forest virus	1
Orthomyxoviruses	
Influenza virus	7–10
Herpesviruses	
Herpes simplex virus	10
Poxviruses	1–100
Adenoviruses	10–20
BACTERIAL VIRUSES	
Coliphage T4	1
Coliphage T7	1.5–4
PLANT VIRUSES	
Tobacco mosaic virus	$5 \times 10^4 - 10^6$

trate soluble components, obtained from breakdown of the virions or produced during intracellular viral synthesis.

The **ratio of the number of viral particles** (determined by electron microscopy) **to the number of infectious units** measures the **efficiency of infection,** which varies widely among different viruses, and even for the same virus assayed in different hosts. As is shown in Table 44–4, for most viruses the ratio is larger than unity. This result is due in part to the presence of noninfectious particles and in part to the failure of potentially infectious particles to reproduce. However, even with the highest ratio of particles to infectivity, infection is initiated by a single virion, since the dose–response curve remains linear. The ratio of total viral particles to hemagglutinating units is very high: about $10^{6.3}$ for influenza virus and 10^5 for polyoma virus.

Appendix

QUANTITATIVE ASPECTS OF INFECTION
Distribution of Viral Particles per Cell: Poisson Distribution

In a cell suspension mixed with a viral sample, individual cells are infected by different numbers of viral particles, and it is often important to know the distribution, i.e., the proportions of cells infected by zero, one, two, etc., viral particles.

These proportions depend on the **average number of viral particles per cell,** known as the **multiplicity of infection** (*m*). The relevant viral particles are those that initiate infection of a cell; inactive particles or particles that, for whatever reason, never enter a cell are neglected. Hence, *m* is related to the total number of viral particles (*N*) and of cells (*C*) by the relation $m = aN/C$, where *a* is the proportion of viral particles that initiates infection.

The proportion *P*(*k*) of cells infected by *k* viral particles is given by the *Poisson distribution*, assuming that the cells are all identical in their ability to be infected. In fact, cells vary in size, surface properties, and so forth, but usually the deviations are small enough to be negligible, at least as a first approximation.

According to the Poisson distribution:

$$P(k) = \frac{e^{-m}m^k}{k!} \tag{1}$$

The value of *m* can be derived from the known values of *N* and *C* if *a* can be determined; otherwise *m* can be calculated from the experimentally determinable proportion of uninfected cells, *P*(0). By making *k* = 0 in equation 1,

$$P(0) = e^{-m}, \text{ and} \tag{2}$$

$$m = -\ln P(0) \tag{3}$$

where ln stands for the natural logarithm.

The use of equations 1, 2, and 3 will now be illustrated with reference to two practical problems.

PROBLEM 1. 10^7 cells are exposed to virus. At the end of the adsorption period there are 10^5 infected cells. What is the multiplicity of infection?

$$P(0) = 0.99, m = -\ln(0.99) = 0.01$$

This problem emphasizes the point that the multiplicity of infection can assume any value from 0 to ∞. Values smaller than unity indicate that a small fraction of the cells is infected, mostly by single viral particles.

PROBLEM 2. What is the multiplicity of infection required for infecting 95% of the cells of a population?

$$P(0) = 5\% = 0.05, m = -\ln(0.05) = 3$$

The point of this problem is that even at very high multiplicities a certain proportion of the cell remains uninfected. The multiplicity of infection required to reduce the proportion of uninfected cells to a certain value can be calculated from equation 3.

Classes of Cells in an Infected Population

It is usually important to determine the proportion of only three classes of cells: **uninfected cells** (*k* = 0); **cells** with a **single infection** (*k* = 1); and **cells with a multiple infection** (*k* > 1). The proportions are:

Uninfected cells: $P(0) = e^{-m}$
Cells with single infection: $P(1) = me^{-m}$
Cells with multiple infection: $P(>1) = 1 - e^{-m}(m + 1)$*

PROBLEM 3. How do we determine the various classes of infected cells if the multiplicity of infection is 10?

$$P(0) = e^{-10} = 4.5 \times 10^{-5}$$

$$P(1) = 10 \times 4.5 \times 10^{-5} = 4.5 \times 10^{-4}$$

$$P(>1) = 1 - (4.5 \times 10^{-5})(10 + 1) = 1 - (4.95 \times 10^{-4}) = 99.95\%$$

With a population of 10^7 cells there are $4.5 \times 10^{-5} \times 10^7 = 450$ uninfected cells and 4500 cells with single infection; all the others have multiple infection.

PROBLEM 4. How do we determine the composition of the population of infected cells if the multiplicity of infection is 10^{-3}, or 0.001?

$$P(0) = e^{0.001} = 0.9990 = 9.99 \times 10^{-1} = 99.9\%$$

$$P(1) = 0.001 \times e^{0.001} = 10^{-3} \times 9.99 \times 10^{-1}$$
$$= 9.99 \times 10^{-4} = 0.0999\%$$

$$P(>1) = 1 - 0.9990(0.001 + 1) = 0.000001 = 10^{-6}$$

With a population of 10^7 cells there are $9.99 \times 10^{-4} \times 10^7 = 9900$ cells with single infection and $10^{-6} \times 10^7 = 10$ cells with multiple infection; most of the cells are uninfected.

MEASUREMENT OF THE INFECTIOUS TITER OF A VIRAL SAMPLE

To measure infectious titer, a viral sample containing an unknown number (*N*) of infectious viral particles is mixed with a known number (*C*) of cells. *N* is then calculated from the proportion of cells that remains uninfected according to equation 3: $m = -\ln P(0)$; since, as defined above, $m = a(N/C)$, $N = mC/a = -C \ln P(0)/a$, or

$$aN = -C \ln P(0) \tag{4}$$

Usually the factor *a* is not determinable, and therefore the number (*N*) of infectious viral particles present in the sample to be assayed cannot be calculated. In its place one obtains the product *aN*, the number of **infectious units.**

This is the basis for all measurements of the infectious viral titer. Its **application** is different in the plaque method and in the endpoint method.

---

* This value is obtained by subtracting from unity (the sum of all probabilities for any value of *k*) the probabilities *P*(0) and *P*(1).

Plaque Method

In the plaque method the number of plaques equals the number of infectious units. The actual number of cells employed in the assay is irrelevant, provided that it is in large excess over the number of infectious viral particles, so that m is very small; uncertainties connected with the counting of the cells are therefore eliminated.

THE DOSE–RESPONSE CURVE OF THE PLAQUE ASSAY.

As stated above, the number of plaques that develop on a series of cell cultures infected with different dilutions of the same viral sample is proportional to the concentration of the virus. We shall now show that this linearity proves that a single infectious viral particle is sufficient to infect a cell (**single-hit kinetics).**

Let us assume that more than one particle, say two particles, is required. There would then be two types of uninfected cells: those with no infectious viral particles and those with just one such particle. According to the Poisson distribution the proportions of cells in these two classes are e^{-m} and me^{-m}, respectively. Thus, under the foregoing assumption, $P(0) = e^{-m}(1 + m)$, which, for very small values of m, approximates to $P(0) = 1 - 1/2m^2$. Therefore, $P(i) = 1/2m^2$, and the dose–response curve would be parabolic rather than linear (see Fig. 44–17). If more than two particles were required to infect a cell, the curvature of the dose–response curve would be even more pronounced.

Endpoint Method

In the endpoint method the virus to be assayed is added to a number of test units (e.g., cultures or animals), each consisting of a large number of cells. A test unit is now equivalent to a single cell of the plaque assay. Therefore, m is the multiplicity of infection of a test unit, rather than of a cell.

The virus titer can be calculated from the proportion of noninfected units, $P(0)$, at the endpoint dilution, according to equation 3: $m = -\ln P(0)$. If at the endpoint $m = 1$ (i.e., there is one infectious unit per test unit), then on the average $P(0) = 0.37$.

Another approach, especially useful in quantitating virulence or host resistance, is the **method of Reed and Muench,** which is applicable to an assay involving a series of progressive dilutions of a virus. A constant volume of each dilution is inoculated in each animal of a group. An empirical pooling of the results obtained at all dilutions gives the dose at which 50% of the animals are infected (ID_{50}) or killed (LD_{50}).

In the example of Table 44–5, none of the dilutions gives a 50% endpoint; this lies between the third and the fourth dilution. The LD_{50} is calculated from the cumulated values, assuming that the proportion of the animals affected varies linearly with $\log_{10}$ dilution. The interpolated value is given by

$$h \frac{\text{\% animals affected at dilution next above 50\%} - 50\%}{\begin{array}{c}\text{\% animals affected at dilution next above 50\%} - \\ \text{\% animals affected at dilution below 50\%}\end{array}}$$

In this formula h is the log of a dilution step. The interpolated value is then added arithmetically (i.e., with the proper sign) to the log of the total dilution at the step just above 50% affected animals. In the example, interpolated

$$\text{value} = h \frac{71 - 50}{71 - 13} = h \frac{21}{58} = 0.36h \text{ (approximated to } 0.4h).$$

If $h = 1/10$, $\log h = -1$; total dilution at the third step is $(1/10)^3 = 10^{-3}$, and log dilution $= -3$. Interpolated value then is $-1 \times 0.4 = -0.4$. The log $LD^{50} = -3 + (-0.4) = -3.4$. The LD^{50} titer is expressed as $= 10^{-3.4}$; i.e., the virus sample contains $10^{3.4}$ LD^{50} doses. If, instead, $h = 1/2$, $\log h = -0.3$, total dilution at the third step $= (1/2)^3 = 1/8$, and log dilution $= -0.9$. Interpolated value $= -0.3 \times 0.4 = -0.12$; log $LD^{50} = -0.9 + (-0.12) = -1.02$, and LD^{50} titer $= 10^{-1.2}$.

TABLE 44–5. Example of Endpoint Titration

Dilution Step	Mortality Ratio	Died	Survived	Total Dead*	Total Survived*	Mortality Ratio	Mortality %
1	6/6	6	0	17	0	17/17	100
2	6/6	6	0	11	0	11/11	100
3	4/6	4	2	5	2	5/7	71
4	1/6	1	5	1	7	1/8	13
5	0/6	0	6	0	13	0/13	0

* Cumulated values for the total number of animals that died or survived are obtained by adding in the directions indicated by the arrows.
   (Modified from Lennette EH: General principles underlying laboratory diagnosis of virus and rickettsia infections. In Lennette EH, Schmidt NH [eds]: Diagnostic Procedures of Virus and Rickettsia Disease, p 45. New York, American Public Health Association, 1964)

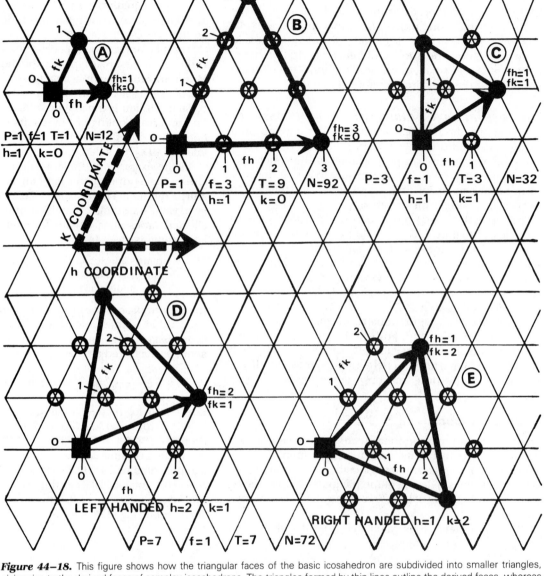

Figure 44–18. This figure shows how the triangular faces of the basic icosahedron are subdivided into smaller triangles, giving rise to the derived faces of complex icosahedrons. The triangles formed by thin lines outline the derived faces, whereas thick lines outline the faces of the basic icosahedron. The pentons (*closed circles*) are located at the corners of the basic faces, the hexons (*open circles*) at the corners of the derived faces. *(A)* The face of the basic icosahedron (T = 1) in which the derived and basic faces are identical. *(B)* The basic face is subdivided into nine derived faces: T = 9. The derived faces are all enclosed in a single basic face, using the same edges. *(C)* The basic face is subdivided into three derived faces: T = 3. The edges of basic and derived faces do not coincide: the basic face in fact contains six derived half-faces (see also Fig. 44–4). *(D and E)* T = 7. As in *C,* the edges do not coincide; moreover, the basic face can be subdivided into seven derived faces in two ways, generating a **left-handed** or a **right-handed** icosahedron. The relationship between derived and basic faces is in all cases given by the equation T = (fh)² + (fh)(fk) + (fk)² (see text), where fh and fk are the coordinates along the triangulation lines for a given value of T, measured from the full square. The parameter *P* (from T = Pf²) determines the relationship of the derived to the basic edges, which overlap for P = 1 *(A and B)*. Such capsids are **symmetric,** as are capsids for which h = k *(C)*; with other values of *P* capsids are **asymmetric** *(D, E)*.

The multiplicity corresponding to one LD_{50} (50% survival) is calculated from the relation $e^{-LD50} = 0.50$. Therefore, $LD_{50} = -\ln(0.50) = 0.70$. One LD_{50} corresponds to 0.70 infectious units.

PRECISION OF VARIOUS ASSAY PROCEDURES
Plaque Method

The statistical precision is measured by the **standard deviation** (σ) of the Poisson distribution, which is equal to the square root of the number of plaques counted. If the number of plaques counted is not too small, 95% of all observations made should fall within two standard deviations from the mean in either direction (i.e., $\pm 2\sigma$). Thus, 4σ is the expected range of variability of the assay. If n replicate assays are made, $\sigma = \sqrt{\bar{x}}/n$, where $\bar{x}$ is the mean value of plaque numbers in the replicate assays. The standard deviation relative to the mean (**coefficient of variation**) serves as a relative measure of precision: $\sigma/\sqrt{\bar{x}}$. This is $\sqrt{\bar{x}}/\bar{x} = 1/\sqrt{\bar{x}}$ for a single assay, and $1/\sqrt{n\bar{x}}$ for n replicate assays. The smaller the coefficient of variation, the higher the precision, which therefore increases as the square root of the number of plaques.

Example: If a total of 100 plaques are counted, the standard deviation is 10. If the same assay is repeated many times, its results will fall between 80 and 120 plaques in 95% of the cases; the coefficient of variation is 1/10. If 400 plaques are counted, the coefficient of variation is 1/20.

Reed and Muench Method

An approximate value, empirically derived, of the standard deviation of the titer determined by this method is $\sigma = \sqrt{0.79hR/U}$, where h is the log of the dilution factor employed at each step of the serial dilution of the virus, U is the number of test units used at each dilution, and R is the interquartile range, namely, the difference between the log of the dilution at which $P(i)$ is 0.25 and 0.75, respectively. In this calculation σ is expressed in logarithmic units. For the data of Table 44–5, with six assay units (animals) at each dilution, $h = 1.0$ and $R = 1.0$ (both in $\log_{10}$ units); $\sigma = \sqrt{0.79/6} = 0.36$ (in $\log_{10}$ units). The range of variation of the LD_{50} is therefore ± 0.72 in $\log_{10}$ units, and the highest expected value (within the 95% confidence limits) is 28 times (antilog of 1.44) the lowest value.

NUMBER OF CAPSOMERS IN ICOSAHEDRAL CAPSIDS

The number of capsomers that can exist in an icosahedral capsid is $10T + 2$. In fact, of the $60T$ subunits, 60 are in 12 pentons, $60(T - 1)$ in $10(T - 1)$ hexons, giving a total of $12 + 10(T - 1) = 10T + 2$. For describing all possible

TABLE 44–6. Value of Capsid Parameters and Numbers of Capsomers Found in Icosahedral Viruses

p*	f*	T*	No. of Capsomers	No. of Hexons
1	1	1	12	0
	3	9	92	80
	4	16	162	150
	5	25	252	240
3	1	3	32	20
	7	147	1472	1460
7	1	7	72	60

* For explanation of p, f, and T, see text.

arrangements of capsomers it is useful to represent the surface of the icosahedrons in a sheet covered with a grid of triangles, establishing two coordinates, h and k (Fig. 44–18). Each triangle is equivalent to one of the triangles inscribed in each face of the basic icosahedrons, according to the triangulation number. It is possible to define the relationship of the inscribed triangle to the face by outlining the face of the icosahedrons along the grid. In *A* there is only one triangle per face; that is, we deal with the basic icosahedron, $T = 1$. In *B* the side of the face reaches the third intersection, so that nine triangles are inscribed in the face; hence, $T = 9$. In these cases the sides of the face follow the grid, and the icosahedron is said to be **symmetric** with respect to the coordinates. In other cases (*C*, *D*, *E*) the sides of the face do not follow the grid: the icosahedron is **asymmetric** and can occur in either a left-handed (*D*) or right-handed (*E*) form.

With this system of coordinates, $T = Pf^2$, where f can be any integer, and P is $h^2 + hk + k^2$, where h and k are any two integers without common factors. The product Pf^2 measures the surface of the icosahedral face in units equal to the surface of the triangles of the grid. Identically, $T = (fh)^2 + (fh)(fk) + (fk)^2$, so that fh and fk can be used as coordinates, as done in Figure 44–18. When either h or k equals zero, the icosahedron is symmetric, with $T = n^2$, n being the number of intervals between capsomers along one side of the icosahedral face. For instance, it is easy to see that for the capsid of Figure 44–7, $T = 25$.

Only some of the permissible numbers of capsomers are found in icosahedral viruses; some are listed in Table 44–6.

Selected Reading

Abad-Zapatero C, Abdel-Meguid SS, Johnson JE et al: Structure of southern bean mosaic virus at 2.8 Å resolution. Nature 286:33, 1980

Baroudy BM, Venkatesan S, Moss B: Incompletely base-paired flip-flop terminal loops link the two DNA strands of the vaccinia virus genome into one uninterrupted polynucleotide chain. Cell 28:315, 1982

Burnett RM: The structure of the adenovirus capsid. J Mol Biol 185:125, 1985

Carp RI, Merz PA, Kascsak RI et al: Nature of the scrapie agent: Current status. J Gen Virol 66:1357, 1985

Caspar DLD: Design principles in virus particle construction. In Horsfall F, Tamm I (eds): Viral and Rickettsial Infections in Man, p 51. Philadelphia, JB Lippincott, 1965

Francki RIB: Plant virus satellites. Annu Rev Microbiol 39:151, 1985

Hogle JM, Chow M, Filman DJ: Three-dimensional structure of poliovirus at 2.9 resolution. Science 229:1358, 1985

Kirkegaard K, Baltimore D: The mechanism of RNA recombination in poliovirus. Cell 47:433, 1986

Klug A: Architectural design of spherical viruses. Nature 303:378, 1983

Matthews REF: Viral taxonomy for the nonvirologist. Annu Rev Microbiol 39:451, 1985

Newcomb WW, Boring JW, Brown JC: Ion etching of human adenovirus 2: Structure of the core. J Virol 51:52, 1984

Riesner D, Gross HJ: Viroids. Annu Rev Biochem 54:531, 1985

Robinson IK, Harrison SC: Structure of the expanded state of tomato bushy stunt virus. Nature 297:563, 1982

Stanley J: The molecular biology of geminiviruses. Adv Virus Res 30:139, 1985

Summers J, Mason WS: Replication of the genome of a hepatitis B–like virus by reverse transcription of an RNA intermediate. Cell 29:403, 1982

Wang K-S, Choo Q-L, Weiner AJ et al: Structure, sequence and expression of the hepatitis delta (δ) viral genome. Nature 323:508, 1986

45

Multiplication and Genetics of Bacteriophages

Model Systems

In spite of marked differences in structure and in genetic complexity, all viruses are similar in many basic aspects of multiplication. For many decades animal and plant viruses could be studied only in the intact host, and so the interaction of viruses with cells was first worked out with bacteriophages, especially the **"T-even" phages of Escherichia coli** (T2, T4, and T6). Though they were thought to be the simplest possible organisms, they turned out, in fact, to be among the most complex of all viruses, but their complexity was instrumental to many discoveries.

With respect to their effects of the host cells, bacteriophages are divided into two classes: **virulent phages,** which multiply without integration and often kill the host bacteria, and **temperate phages,** which integrate their genome in the host DNA, giving rise to the phenomenon of **lysogeny.** We will consider first the virulent phages, using as a model the T-even coliphages.

Multiplication

STRUCTURE

The virions of even-numbered T phages are made up of a head and a tail (Fig. 45–1). The **head** has the shape of two halves of an icosahedron connected by a short hexagonal prism, and it contains the DNA in association with polyamines, several internal proteins, and small peptides. The pentons and hexons of the head (see Chap. 44) are

795

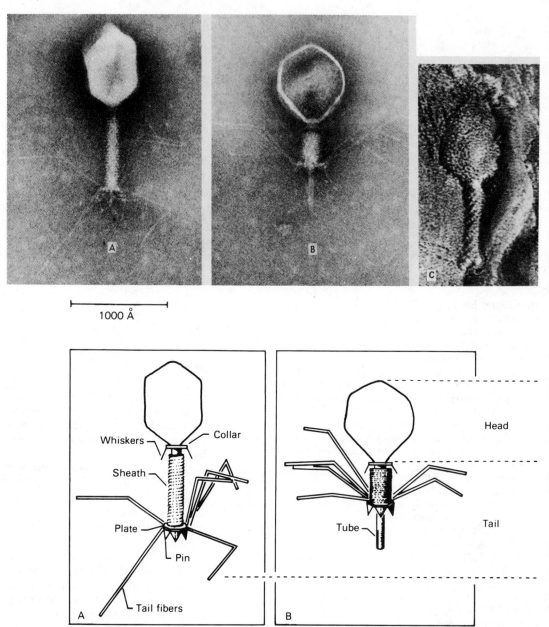

1000 Å

Figure 45–1. Electron micrographs of bacteriophage T2. *(A)* Phage before injection, with a full head and an extended sheath. *(B)* Phage after injection, with an empty head and a contracted sheath. *(C)* Helical structure of the sheath. *A* and *B*, negative staining. *C*, obtained by freeze-etching: the phage was embedded in ice, which was then fractured; the fracture was covered with a thin layer of evaporated metal, which was then photographed. *(A* and *B*, courtesy of E. Boy de la Tour; *C*, courtesy of M. E. Bayer.)

made up of different monomers. In other phages, such as *Salmonella* phages P1 and P2 and coliphage λ, the head is strictly icosahedral (see Fig. 44–3*F*). The T-even phage **tail** consists of a central helical **tube** (through which the viral DNA passes during cell infection), surrounded by a helical sheath capable of contraction. The **sheath** is con-

nected to the head through a thin disc or **collar** and to a **base plate** at the tip end. The plate is the organ of attachment to the wall of the host cell. It is hexagonal and of complex structure; it has a **pin** at every corner and is connected to six long, thin **tail fibers.** Each part of the virion is made up of several kinds of protein molecules.

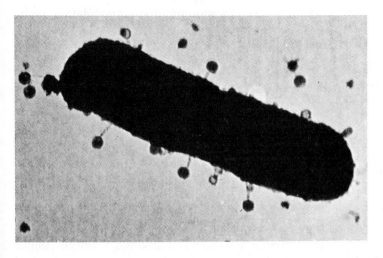

Figure 45–2. Electron micrograph of particles of phage T5 adsorbed to an *Escherichia coli* cell. The virions attach by the tips of their tails. Note also that the heads of some particles are clear (electron-transparent), having injected their DNA into the cells; others are dark (electron-opaque) and still contain their DNA. (Anderson TF: Cold Spring Harbor Symp Quant Biol 18:197, 1953)

About twenty are needed for the construction of a T4 head (see Fig. 45–14). Most other bacteriophages have tails, which vary greatly in dimensions and structure. Some small icosahedral phages, such as ϕX174, have no tail.

INFECTION OF HOST CELLS

The first step in infection is a highly specific interaction of the phage's **adsorption** organelle, such as the tail, with **receptors** on the surface of the host cell; then the DNA is **released** from the capsid and enters the cell.

Adsorption

All virions have a specialized structure for adsorption. In the T-even coliphages it is the base plate with its appendages. Electron microscopy shows that the tips of the **fibers** attach first and reversibly to the host cell receptors and are followed by the **tail pins,** which attach irreversibly. With all the tailed phages the adsorbed vi-

rion acquires a characteristic position with the tail perpendicular to the cell wall (Fig. 45–2).

The host cell receptors are proteins or lipopolysaccharide sugars located on the outer membrane where it is in contact with the inner membrane. Isolated receptors can bind to the phage tail, blocking adsorption of the phage to bacteria. This interaction of receptors with tail fibers is highly specific: mutations causing small changes in the receptors make the cells **resistant** to the phage. This principle is applied to *Salmonella* typing with the use of phages that adsorb to various forms of the O Ag. In T-even phages, resistance can be overcome by phage **host-range mutations** affecting the tail fibers. These coordinated changes illustrate the connection between the evolution of viruses and that of the host cells.

Separation of Nucleic Acid From Coat

In one of the most significant experiments of modern biology, Hershey and Chase demonstrated in 1952 that at infection the viral nucleic acid separates from the capsids (Fig. 45–3). They labeled the protein of T2 with ^{35}S or

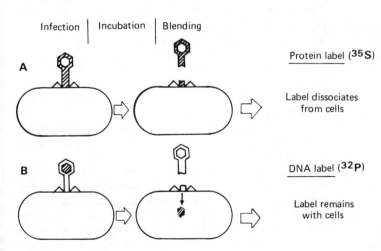

Figure 45–3. The Hershey and Chase experiment, showing the separation of viral DNA and protein at infection. *(A)* The phage protein was labeled by propagation in a medium containing ^{35}SO$_4^{2-}$. *(B)* Phage DNA was labeled by propagation in a medium containing ^{32}PO$_4^{2-}$. Phage was adsorbed to host bacteria, and after 10 minutes at 37°C, the culture was blended. Most of the ^{32}P remained associated with the cells, whereas most of the ^{35}S came off. Labeled components are shaded.

the DNA with ^{32}P, allowed the virus to infect bacteria, and by violent agitation in a blender, sheared the tails of the adsorbed virions. The experiment yielded two results that, at the time, seemed astonishing: (1) 80% of the ^{35}S label came off, whereas essentially all the ^{32}P label remained with the cells, and, since it was DNase-resistant, it was *within* the cells. (2) The blended bacteria produced progeny phage. These results strongly suggested that **phage DNA carries the genetic information of the phage into the cell.** This result provided the first evidence that the crucial event in viral infection is the penetration of the viral genome into the cell, and that the protein coat has only the function of guiding it there.

Mechanism of Penetration of the Nucleic Acid

The T-even phages have a highly specialized mechanism for releasing their DNA. After the tip of the tail has become anchored to the cell surface, the **contraction of the tail sheath** pulls the collar and the phage head toward the plate (see Fig. 45–1), pushing the tube through the cell wall locally digested by an enzyme contained in the tail. Because of this action, as well as its shape, the virion has been likened to a hypodermic syringe, and the release of the nucleic acid is called **injection.**

Contraction of the tail is the result of a **chain of conformational changes** initiated by the attachment of fibers and pins to the cell. The hexagonal base plate becomes starlike and separates from the tube, then the sheath shortens and thickens. Contraction is an irreversible reciprocal shift of the monomers, driven by the release of potential energy in the bonds between them. Many other tailed phages (such as T5 or λ) lack a contractile sheath and an injection mechanism. They simply release their DNA upon irreversible binding to the bacterial receptors. The released DNA, together with some proteins, penetrates through pores in the membranes, with which it remains associated. There it is exposed to nucleases but is protected by associated proteins and by DNA modifications (see DNA Modifications, below) or by other mechanisms.

TRANSFECTION. Bacteria can be infected by purified phage DNA after pretreatment with Ca^{2+} or conversion to spheroplasts; this property is important in DNA cloning (see Chap. 46). The efficiency of this transfection, however, is very low, because the DNA is likely to be degraded by exonucleases. The efficiency is higher (about 10^{-4}) for DNAs that are resistant to the enzymes because they either rapidly cyclize in the cells (e.g., λ DNA) or have a protein covalently bound at the ends (*Bacillus subtilis* phage φ29).

Effect of Phage Attachment on Cellular Metabolism

The attachment of the T-even and other phages *per se*, without expression of viral genes (e.g., in the presence of chloramphenicol to prevent new protein synthesis),

causes a **disorganization of the cell plasma membrane.** It causes massive flows of ions in either direction, depolarizing the membrane; even larger molecules, such as nucleotides, leak to the medium. These alterations cause profound **metabolic disturbances,** including an almost immediate cessation of cellular protein synthesis. The effects are only transient, however, and are rapidly **reversed** by the incorporation of several phage-specified proteins in the membrane. These proteins also make the cell "immune" to superinfection by phage of the same type. DNA-less phages (**ghosts**), lacking the needed genes, do not reverse the changes, and cause cell lysis.

MULTIPLICATION CYCLE

The process of viral multiplication, after penetration of the parental nucleic acid, involves many sequential steps, which end in the release of newly synthesized **progeny virions.** Analysis of this **multiplication cycle** requires synchrony of cell infection, which is achieved, as in the classic work of Delbrück, by allowing virus adsorption for only a brief time (**one-step conditions**). The remaining virus is then made ineffective either by diluting the culture or by adding phage-specific antiserum. If the **multiplicity of infection**—that is, the average number of viral particles that infect a cell—is high (e.g. >3), essentially all cells are infected; if it is low (e.g. <1), a large proportion of cells are not infected (see Appendix to Chap. 44). The cells that are infected and release progeny virus (**infectious centers**) can be enumerated because they produce plaques in the regular assay used for the virus (see Assay of Infectivity, Chap. 44).

One-Step Multiplication Curve

The multiplication curve, such as that of Figure 45–4, describes the production of progeny phage as a function of the time after infection. If the cells are disrupted immediately after the DNA is injected, they do not produce plaques. This temporary disappearance of infectivity, called **eclipse,** is due to the inability of the naked viral DNA to infect bacteria under ordinary conditions. After the eclipse period, infectious phage starts appearing in the cells, where it accumulates until it is released by the **lysis (burst)** of the cells. In a bacterial culture, lysis is detected by a drop in turbidity. The time interval between infection and the beginning of release is the **latent period,** which varies with the type of phage and the culture conditions. The average number of infectious units of virus per cell at the end of replication represents the **viral yield.**

With the T-even phages, lysis is delayed by more than an hour if an infected culture is heavily reinoculated before the time of normal lysis (**lysis inhibition**). The resulting increase in viral yield is useful for the purification of virions. **Rapid-lysis (r) mutants,** which are defective in a membrane protein, do not delay lysis, and their

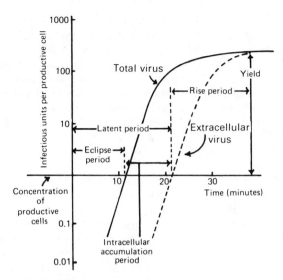

Figure 45—4. Diagram of the multiplication curve of bacteriophage T2. Bacteria and phage were mixed, and adsorption was allowed for 2 minutes; antiphage serum was then added to neutralize unadsorbed phage. The bacteria were recovered by centrifugation and were resuspended in a large volume of medium at 37°C in order to minimize readsorption of progeny phage to the bacteria. A sample was immediately plated to determine the concentration of productive cells (i.e., those able to produce phage). Other samples were taken from time to time and divided into two aliquots: one was shaken with chloroform to disrupt the bacteria and was then assayed **(total virus)**; the other was freed of bacteria by centrifugation, and the supernatant was assayed **(extracellular virus)**. The titers are compared with the concentration of productive cells as 1.0.

difference in plaque morphology from r⁺ (wild type; Fig. 45—5) is a valuable marker for genetic studies.

SYNTHESIS OF VIRAL MACROMOLECULES

A fundamental observation with T-even phages is that infection of bacteria causes a **profound rearrangement of all macromolecular syntheses.** Within a few minutes the synthesis of all DNA, RNA, and protein directed by the **cellular** genome ceases. The effect is unrelated to the transient inhibition produced by membrane damage during adsorption; it requires the expression of viral genes. Soon the cellular syntheses are entirely replaced by viral syntheses. This shift represents **the basis of viral parasitism:** the substitution of viral genes for cellular genes in directing the synthesizing machinery of the cell. With other phages the degree to which cellular functions are replaced by viral functions varies greatly, being minimal for some small filamentous phages the replication of which does not impede the multiplication of the host cells.

In cells infected by T-even and other large phages, the metabolic shift is determined by many new, viral proteins and enzymes that are synthesized after infection. Some of them turn off cellular syntheses, others carry out new viral syntheses.

Cessation of Synthesis of Host Macromolecules

Host macromolecular syntheses are stopped by three kinds of **turn-off proteins:** (1) Some phage proteins affect the host transcriptase, making it unable to recognize host promoters and consequently **shutting off host RNA syntheses.** (2) Some cause the **bacterial nucleoid to unfold;** the host DNA attaches to the cellular membrane where it is degraded. (3) Some cause **inhibition of host protein synthesis:** T-even phages cause the cleavage of a host tRNA, while T7 induces a translational repressor.

REGULATION OF TRANSCRIPTION OF PHAGE GENES

To achieve a smooth transition between cellular and viral syntheses, expression of genes is strictly regulated. An

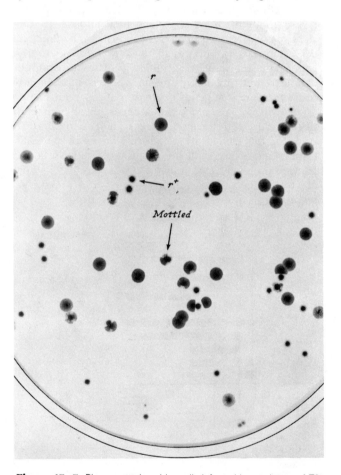

Figure 45—5. Plaques produced by cells infected by a mixture of T2r and T2r⁺ phage. Plaques of r type are large and without a halo; those of r⁺ type (wild type) are small and surrounded by a halo. The halo is produced by infected cells, with lysis inhibition caused by r⁺ phage. Cells infected by both r and r⁺ phage produce mottled plaques with a sectored halo (dark sectors, r phage; clear sectors, r⁺ phage). (Molecular Biology of Bacterial Viruses by Gunther S. Stent. W. H. Freeman and Company. Copyright © 1963)

important aspect of regulation is the **orderly temporal sequence** of expression of the genes. The regular succession of phage functions is determined mainly at the transcription level. Transcription of phage DNA generates viral mRNA, which, like bacterial mRNAs, are usually polycistronic.

The basic regulatory mechanism is the **successive appearance of new transcriptases** that recognize different sets of promoters or terminators. Some of the new transcriptases are specified entirely by viral genes, others are generated by changing the host transcriptase either by enzymatic modification or by association of viral proteins. For instance, coliphage N4 injects a transcriptase present in the virions; coliphages T3 and T7 cause the synthesis of new transcriptases after infection; T-even phages change the initiation specificity of the host transcriptase; and λ phage changes its termination specificity. **Changes of the phage DNA** also participate in this regulation: nicks and gaps may appear at some stage, as with T-even phages, or the DNA may enter the cells stepwise, as with phage T5, so that only a group of genes can be transcribed initially. The transcription changes occurring at any one stage are brought about by products or phage genes expressed at a previous stage.

We will now consider the **succession of transcription modes.** With the large phages, such as coliphage T4 or *B. subtilis* phage SPO1, several classes of genes are transcribed before replication of the phage DNA begins. **Immediate early and delayed genes** (Fig. 45–6), which are transcribed by the unaltered host RNA polymerase before replication of the phage DNA begins, encode

products that shut off cellular macromolecule syntheses and participate in the replication of the phage DNA. **Quasi-late** or **middle genes** also make products required for DNA replication and recombination but, in contrast to early genes, continue to be transcribed throughout infection. Their transcription begins at special promoters and requires other phage-specified proteins that interact with the host RNA polymerase. **Late genes** are transcribed by the host transcriptase in association with other phage-specified proteins after DNA replication has begun. Their products are capsid proteins and enzymes for lysing the cells.

With phage T4, late genes are transcribed from one DNA strand, called the "right" strand, whereas all the others are transcribed from the "left" strand, accentuating the differences between the two classes. Some genes are transcribed at different times and belong to more than one class. Coliphage N4 uses the injected transcriptases for early transcription after the DNA strands are separated by DNA binding proteins; for middle transcription it uses a new viral transcriptase made as a result of early transcription; for late transcription it uses the host transcriptase.

ANTITERMINATION. In the large phages, certain transcriptions units (Fig. 45–7) are subject first to immediate transcription, restricted to the promoter-proximal part by the host terminator *rho* factor. Later, delayed early transcription extends to the promotor-distal part, after proteins specified by immediate early genes prevent termination. Antitermination is especially important in the regulation of λ transcription (see Chap. 46).

POSTTRANSCRIPTIONAL REGULATION

Although most regulation occurs at transcription, there are important examples of posttranscriptional regulation. The **stability of the messengers** is highly variable. Thus the messenger for the T4 helix-destabilizing protein, gene product 32, is stabilized by the interaction of its 5′ leader sequence with transacting factors present in the infected cells. Another regulation mechanism is **intron splicing.** Phage transcripts, unlike those of eukaryotic viruses, usually do not have introns. However, the gene for thymidylate synthase (TS) of phage T4 has a 1-Kb intron, with a sequence similar to those of eukaryotic class I introns, such as that of **Tetrahymena rRNA.** Like other class I introns, the sequence is removed from the transcript by self-splicing, carried out by the RNA itself. The intron has regulatory function, for early in infection only the first exon of the gene is translated, generating an enzyme involved in binding of tetrahydrofolate to dUMP; later, after the intron is spliced out, TS is made. Introns also exist in other T4 genes.

Further regulation of gene expression occurs at

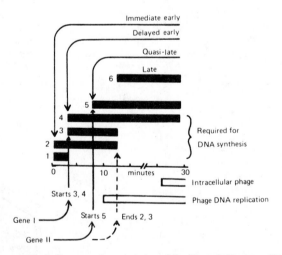

Figure 45–6. Program of transcription of *Bacillus subtilis* phage SPO1. Black bars (1,2,3 . . . 6) indicate the periods during which various classes of genes are transcribed. Phage genes I and II affect the beginning of synthesis of certain classes and the end of others, as indicated. Time is given in minutes from infection. (Modified from Gage P, Geiduschek EP: J Mol Biol 57:279, 1971. Copyright by Academic Press, Inc. [London], Ltd.)

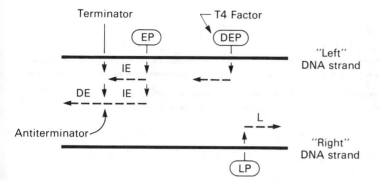

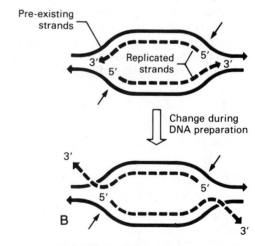

Figure 45–7. Transcription of different sets of genes on T4 DNA. Dashed arrows indicate newly synthesized RNA. *EP,* early promoters; *DEP,* delayed early promoters; *LP,* late promoters; *IE,* immediate early RNA; *DE,* delayed early RNA; *L,* late RNA. Delayed early messengers are transcribed either by interfering with termination of immediate early transcription (antitermination) or by initiating at new promoters. Early and late messengers are transcribed on different strands.

translation. For instance, the gene 32 protein inhibits its own production by binding to the messenger near the ribosome attachment site; that is, it is self-regulated. Many phages specify new tRNAs; they are essential to only some bacterial strains, which may be closer to those in which the phages have evolved.

VIRAL DNA REPLICATION

Many phages, such as T-even or T7 phages, have linear DNAs (see Chap. 44). These DNAs replicate in two phases: in the first one the amount of DNA increases; in the others, mature molecules are generated. In the **first phase** DNA replication **begins at a fixed internal origin** and proceeds **bidirectionally;** electron microscopy shows the origin of replication as a growing loop like that of Figure 45–8. The very long DNAs of T-even phages have several origins.

After several rounds of replication the mode changes to a **second phase,** which is characterized by giant molecules, called **concatemers,** generated by breakage and reunion, i.e., **recombination** (Fig. 45–9). The recombination intermediates characterized by single-strand nicks and gaps are the replication forks that from then on carry out most of the replication. The long concatemers generated by this mechanism have many branching points, and in electron micrographs appear as complex entanglements of filaments. With T-even phages, recombination continues to occur at a high frequency after concatemers are formed, leading to the dispersion of the parental DNA into many progeny molecules, each of which contains a small parental segment covalently linked to newly synthesized DNA.

Recombination is an essential step in the multiplication of T4 and other phages with linear DNA: mutants in recombination genes stop replication in the middle of infection. Recombination is important because it allows complete replication of their genomes. In their bidirectional replication from an internal origin, both DNA strands remain incompletely replicated at opposite ends

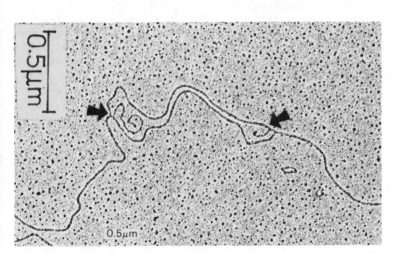

Figure 45–8. Evidence for bidirectional replication of T4 DNA. The electron micrograph of partially replicated DNA *(A)* shows a symmetric **growing loop,** with a "whisker" of single-stranded DNA *(arrows).* The sensitivity to specific nucleases shows that a whisker represents the 3' end of each growing strand. In all likelihood the whisker is formed as shown in *B,* because at each end of the loop the 3'-ended strand grows more rapidly than the 5' end (which is synthesized backward), and during the preparation of the DNA the two parental strands snap back to the point where replication is complete. (Modified from Delius et al: Proc Natl Acad Sci USA 68:3049, 1971)

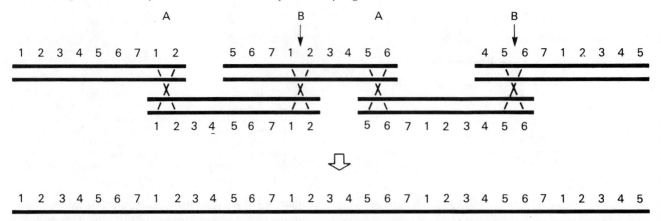

Figure 45–9. Concatemer formation by recombination. Crossovers of type B (*arrows*), between different parental molecules, cause genetic recombination, but those of type A, between identical molecules, do not. Numbers (arbitrary) indicate genes.

of a molecule if the synthesis of the last Okazaki segment (which grows backward) does not begin at the last nucleotide (Fig. 45–10). Joining the ends in concatemers permits their complete replication. At the end of replication the concatemers are cut in different ways to generate **mature molecules** with repetitious ends, which, in the case of T7 are completed by new synthesis (Fig. 45–11).

Biochemistry of Replication

After release from the virions, phage DNA, together with phage-specified proteins, becomes associated with the **cell plasma membrane,** where replication begins. Precursors derive from the medium and, for T-even phages, also from host DNA breakdown. For elaborating these precursors and synthesizing them into phage DNA, large phages (such as the T-even) specify many enzymes (Fig. 45–12), whereas the smallest phages depend almost entirely on enzymes of the host. With all phages a specific protein complex (**primosome**) is required during the first phase for **initiating phage DNA replication** at spe-

cific initiation sequences. As with bacterial DNA, phage primosomes cause the synthesis of short primer RNA segments, which are then elongated by DNA polymerase. With T-even phages, nicked molecules, which are intermediates in DNA recombination, act as primers in the second phase of replication.

B. subtilis phage φ29 DNA has a special method for initiating replication. The viral protein p3 is **covalently linked to both 5′ ends,** and it interacts with dATP to form a covalent complex, p3dAMP, the 3-OH group of which provides the replication primer. Synthesis then proceeds directly to the end of each strand. The linear, 18-Kb-long helical DNA can be replicated *in vitro* through the use of only p3 and a viral DNA polymerase.

The elongation of DNA chains is carried out by a complex of enzymes (at least 12 with T4)—some viral, some cellular—which includes DNA polymerase and accessory proteins, DNA unfolding protein, RNA polymerase, endonucleases and topoisomerases, a viral equivalent of *rec A* protein (see Recombination, Chap. 8) for the sec-

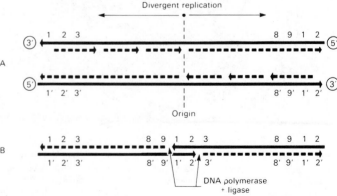

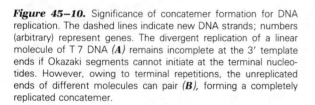

Figure 45–10. Significance of concatemer formation for DNA replication. The dashed lines indicate new DNA strands; numbers (arbitrary) represent genes. The divergent replication of a linear molecule of T7 DNA (**A**) remains incomplete at the 3′ template ends if Okazaki segments cannot initiate at the terminal nucleotides. However, owing to terminal repetitions, the unreplicated ends of different molecules can pair (**B**), forming a completely replicated concatemer.

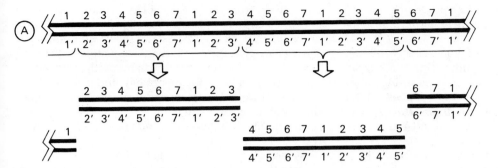

T4-type permuted molecules with repetitious ends

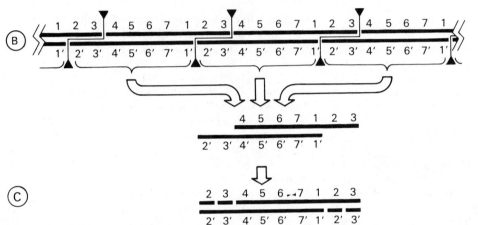

T7-type molecules with repetitious ends

Figure 45–11. Production of mature viral DNA molecules from concatemers. *(A)* Mechanisms generating permuted molecules with repetitious ends, as with phage T4. Constant lengths are cut off the concatemer, irrespective of sequences. *(B, C)* Mechanisms generating nonpermuted molecules with cohesive or repetitious ends. *(B)* Nucleases make staggered cuts on the two strands, recognizing specific sequences, and generate molecules with cohesive ends similar to those of mature phage λ DNA (see Chap. 46). *(C)* If the short strand at each end is continued by DNA polymerase as a complement of the longer strand, T7-type molecules with repetitious ends are generated. Black arrowheads indicate endonucleolytic nicking; numbers indicate sequences, primed numbers complementary sequences; dashed segments are replicated after cutting.

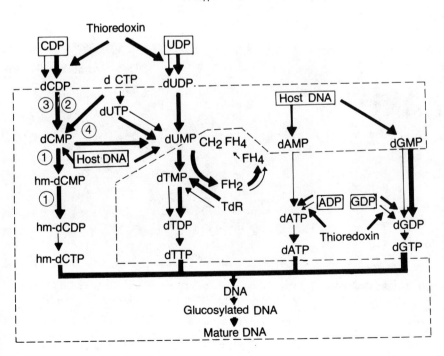

Figure 45–12. Enzymatic reactions involved in the synthesis of T4 DNA. Heavy arrows indicate enzymes specified by phage genes (whether or not there is a similar cellular enzyme with the same function). Thin arrows indicate cellular enzymes. The dashed line surrounds the machinery exclusive to T4 DNA reproduction. It includes enzymes for utilizing host DNA as a source of precursors, for replacing cytidine with hydroxymethylcytosine, and for synthesizing mature DNA. Boxed compounds are the normal source of precursors for DNA replication. *Circled numbers:* see text.

ond phase of phage T4, and enzymes producing nucleoside triphosphates. This arrangement favors speed oï synthesis.

Phages with special bases in their DNAs (see Chap. 44) specify enzymes not only for synthesizing the special nucleotide (see Fig. 45–12) but also for preventing incorporation of the usual one. Thus, T-even phages, which have **5-hydroxymethylcytosine** in their DNA, specify enzymes such as those indicated as 1, 3, and 4 in Fig. 45–12, that dephosphorylate dCTP, dCDP, and dCMP. This is an essential step because cytosine-containing phage DNA is unsuitable as a template for late transcription and is broken down by the nucleases of these phages that degrade the host DNA.

MATURATION AND RELEASE

Maturation and release are the last two of the series of events caused by the expression of viral genes in the infected cells. In **maturation** the various components become assembled to form complete or **mature** infectious virions; in **release** the virions leave the infected cells.

Assembly of the Capsid

The assembly of T-even bacteriophage is interesting as a model for the formation of biological structures containing many different component proteins and for their stabilization. The assembly was elucidated by using **conditionally lethal mutations** of phage genes, which under nonpermissive conditions each block the morphogenetic process at a specific step. Upon lysis the cells yield partly

and often erroneously assembled structures recognizable by electron microscopy (Fig. 45–13). In addition, certain pairs of defective lysates give rise to **complementation *in vitro*;** i.e., the accumulated incomplete structures can assemble spontaneously, when mixed, to form infectious virus. Such complementation studies have shown that the T4 capsid is assembled through three **independent subassembly lines,** which produce the phage head, the fiberless tails, and the tail fibers, respectively (Fig. 45–14), using mostly proteins belonging to the late class. Assembly of the head tail is initiated on the inner layer of the cell's plasma membrane, in connection with cellular proteins. The three structures, when completed, spontaneously assemble into capsids.

METHOD. In contrast to the simple icosahedral and helical capsids discussed in Chapter 44, the T4 head is not generated by self-assembly of the main capsid protein. By itself, this protein aggregates randomly into "lumps" or long cylinders (see Fig. 45–13). In fact, the head is assembled through a series of **sequential steps,** in which each protein molecule (except the first) undergoes a conformational change as it is assembled, revealing the binding site that is recognized by the next molecule.

The assembly of the head capsid is preceded by the formation of a **core** by self-assembly of a **scaffolding protein** and other proteins. Capsid proteins, especially the major capsid protein p23, assemble around the core, yielding first the rounded **procapsid I** (see Fig. 45–14). Formation of the cornered and expanded **procapsid II** occurs after the molecules of the main capsid protein p23 are shortened at their amino terminus by a protease,

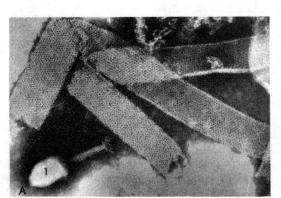
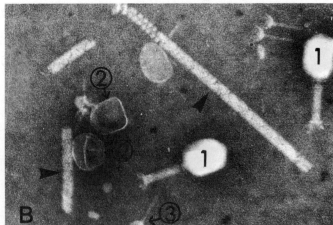

Figure 45–13. Electron micrographs of **polyheads** *(A)* and **polysheaths** *(B, arrow)* present in lysates produced by mutants of phage T4. In **B** one also sees "empty" head membranes *(2)* and tubes attached to base plates *(3)*. Both micrographs also contain some normal virions *(1)* because the cells were simultaneously infected with wild-type phage. The polyheads contain hexagonal capsomers that are no longer recognizable in regular phage, owing to further assembly steps; the polysheath has the diameter of a contracted regular sheath. *(A,* courtesy of E. Boy de la Tour; *B,* Boy de la Tour E: J Ultrastruct Res 11:545, 1964)

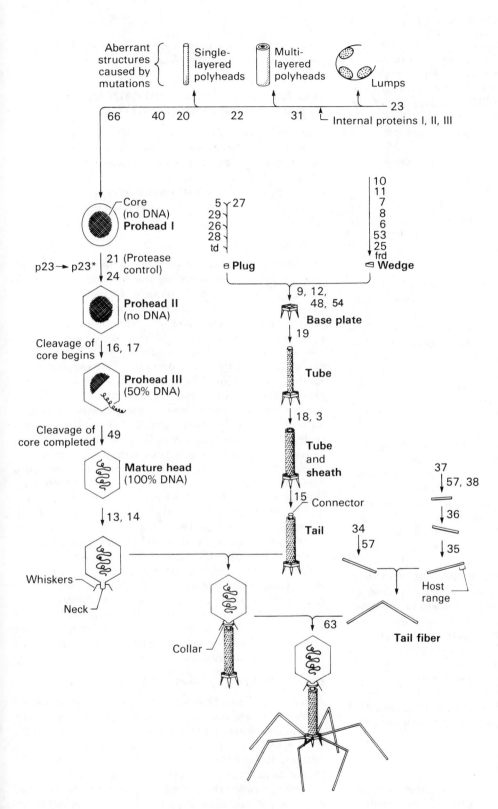

Figure 45–14. Assembly of T4 virions. Assembly occurs in three major subassemblies: head, tail, and tail fibers. Numbers indicate the T4 genes participating in a given step. *p23*, protein specified by gene 23; *p23**, product of cleavage of p23. The aberrant structures in head assembly accumulate when a mutation prevents the function of the next gene in the assembly line. "Lumps" are disorganized masses of p23 at the plasma membrane. (Data from Matthews CK, Kutter EN, Mosig J, Berget PB: Bacteriophage T4. Washington, American Society of Microbiology, 1983)

present in the core, to stabilize the structure. The core proteins are split by the protease into small fragments, some of which remain in the head (**internal peptides**). In *Salmonella* phage P22 the scaffolding protein is released intact from the maturing head and is reutilized for assembly of new proheads.

These mechanisms allow the orderly assembly of numerous components, synthesized at the same time in the same cell, to produce a capsid of a size adequate for holding the viral genome and to provide methods for capturing and holding the DNA (see below). Such mechanisms must be the result of a long evolution, during which the ability of the main components to form an icosahedral capsid by self-assembly was lost in order to allow the addition of other structures.

ASSOCIATION OF DNA AND CAPSID. Prohead I does not contain DNA. Cleavage of p23 causes extensive rearrangements, which expand the head and change its shape. These rearrangements also reveal chemical groups the binding of which to DNA probably provides the energy for "sucking" concatemeric DNA into the empty head, producing a "full" head. This process can be produced *in vitro* through the use of a mutant phage that produces heads but not DNA. DNA folding is facilitated by a **packaging enzyme** (the fragment cleaved off the p23 protein), polyamines, and basic peptides.

There are several DNA-packaging mechanisms. After the T4 head is filled with concatemeric DNA, the excess is cut off by an **endonuclease that works only when the head is complete.** Because this enzyme does not recognize DNA sequences, a "**headful**" of DNA is packaged; its length is precisely determined by the size of the capsid. With phages λ and T7 the nuclease recognizes special sequences, the positions of which precisely determine the length of the packaged DNA. Phages T1 and P22 are assembled by an intermediate mechanism in which packaging of a concatemer is initiated by cleavage at a specific **pac site** and is then continued by the headful mechanism. The encapsidated DNA need not be that of the phage: with some phages random fragments of cellular DNA can be encapsidated, giving rise to **generalized transduction** (see Chap. 46).

In the assembly of the hollow tail, which takes place separately, the precise length appears to be determined by the length of an internal tape protein. The assembled tail is then joined to the full head to produce complete (mature) virions.

Release

With T-even phages several gene products alter the plasma membrane, and then the **phage lysozyme** (from gene *e*) crosses the altered membrane and attacks the cell wall, causing lysis. With the very small phage φX174, lysis does not involve lysozyme but a host autolysin. Fila-

mentous phages are released by an entirely different mechanism, without lysis (see below).

DNA MODIFICATIONS: HOST-INDUCED RESTRICTION AND MODIFICATION

The mechanisms that allow the injected phage DNA to escape the action of membrane nucleases were unveiled by studying puzzling quasi-hereditary changes of the phage caused by the host. These studies led to the discovery of the **restriction endonucleases,** which now play such a central role in DNA cloning and sequencing (Fig. 45–15).

Methylation

Restriction and modification dependent on methylation were discovered by studying the behavior of phage λ infecting *E. coli* K12 cells lysogenic for phage P1 (designated K12 [P1]) instead of the nonlysogenic cells, which are the regular λ host. K12 (P1) cells are resistant to λ; rare infected cells, however, yield progeny phage, which can then grow regularly in K12 (P1) cells. It was soon recognized that the event **does not represent the selection of mutants,** for when the progeny phage is grown through a single cycle in cells not lysogenic for P1, the new progeny phage is again incapable of growing in K12 (P1). The explanation is that K12 (P1) cells contain a restriction endonuclease, specified by P1, which breaks down the unmethylated λ DNA entering the cells (see Fig. 45–15A). However, P1 also specifies the **modifying enzyme** that methylates cytosine in the DNA targets for the restriction endonuclease, protecting the DNA. This is a requirement for the survival of P1 itself and its host cell. When unmethylated λ DNA enters K12 (P1) cells, some molecules are methylated by the modifying enzyme before they are broken down. Made resistant, they multiply, generating DNA molecules that are immediately methylated. A single passage in nonlysogenic K12, which lacks the modifying enzyme, again yields unmethylated molecules, sensitive to the P1 restriction endonuclease. T3 and T7, although possessing an unmethylated DNA, can grow in K12 (P1) cells, because a viral enzyme methylates the DNA soon after its entry into the cells.

Glucosylation (see Fig. 45–15B)

E. coli B, the usual host for T-even phages, has a restriction endonuclease in the plasma membrane that breaks down unglucosylated phage DNA. In the T-even phages the DNA is glucosylated and therefore protected when entering the cells, and the newly formed DNA is rapidly glucosylated by phage enzymes (se Fig. 45–12). In bacteria lacking uridine diphosphate glucose (UDPG) the progeny viral DNA remains unglucosylated. The resulting virions, designated T*, are unable to grow; i.e., they are **restricted,** in any *E. coli* B strains, because their unglucosylated DNA is broken down. T* phage can, however,

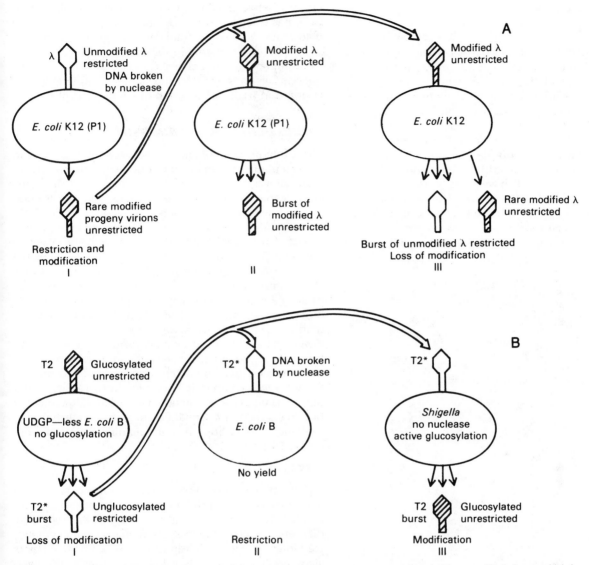

Figure 45–15. Two examples of host-induced restriction and modification. Shaded outlines indicate modified phage, which is unrestricted in the bacterial strains employed. *(A)* Restriction and modification in the same host. The regular λ phage is restricted and at the same time modified (by methylation) in *E. coli* K12 (P1) *(I)*; the modified phage then grows regularly in the restricting host *(II)*. After one growth cycle in *E. coli* K12 the modification is lost, except for rare virions that inherit a DNA strand from the parent *(III)*. *(B)* Restriction and modification occur in different hosts. The DNA present in wild-type T2 is glucosylated (i.e., modified). Unglucosylated phage T2* is produced after a growth cycle in a nonglucosylating host *(I)*. T2* is restricted in *E. coli* B *(II)*; it grows in *Shigella*, in which it is modified *(III)* to yield regular T2 again.

multiply in *Shigella*, which lacks the restriction enzymes. Moreover, since *Shigella* makes UDPG, the progeny DNA is glucosylated and is again unrestricted in *E. coli* B. In a parallel situation, a phage mutant that is unable to glucosylate (gt⁻) cannot grow in *E. coli*; it grows in *Shigella*, but it is not modified.

Significance

It is likely that restriction endonucleases, recognizing unmethylated targets, developed in bacterial evolution as a **defense against foreign DNAs including phages.** At the same time, modifying enzymes had to appear to protect the cell's own DNA. Phages, in turn, have developed defenses against the nucleases. It is likely that the replacement of base C with HMC in T-even phages is a defense against a restriction endonuclease, which cannot attack the modified HMC-containing DNA. This change, however, makes the phages susceptible to other nuclease systems of probably later development, against which glucosylation is the defense.

Phage Genetics

MUTATIONS

Genetics studies with phages have been instrumental in the elucidation of the nature of the gene, the molecular mechanism of mutation, and recombination. Because phages are haploid, many mutations prevent propagation, i.e., are **lethal.** Among the nonlethal mutations, **conditionally lethal mutants** that are temperature or suppressor sensitive can be isolated in most genes. Also useful are **plaque-type mutants,** such as the **rapid lysis (r) mutants** (see Fig. 45–5) and the **host-range (h) mutants** (Fig. 45–16), which have already been described (see Infection of Host Cells, above). The r_II mutants are also conditionally lethal because they multiply in *E. coli* B but not in *E. coli* K12(λ).

The study of wild-type **recombinants** in genetic crosses between two mutants, and of **complementation,** has established a fairly complete **phage map** (see below) and defined the limits of many genes. In complementation two mutants in different genes, each unable to multiply alone under restrictive conditions, multiply together when they infect the same cell, in which each supplies in trans the function missing in the other.

HOMOLOGOUS RECOMBINATION

The study of recombination is based on the proportion of recombinants (**recombination frequencies**) in the lysate of a culture infected by two mutant strains. This study, especially with the larger bacteriophages, is complicated because recombination takes place during DNA multiplication and involves many DNA molecules, which repeatedly recombine within the same cell. The observed recombination frequencies must therefore be subjected to a suitable mathematical analysis, which then yields the **distances between markers.** This is the basis for establishing the genetic map. The relationship of recombination frequencies and **physical distances** between markers is rather uniform for any given phage, although deviations are observed in some regions of the genome: for example, hot spots for recombination at the replication origins. The relationship varies for different phages. For instance, a map unit (corresponding to 1% recombination) is equivalent to about 100 nucleotide pairs in T4 but about 2000 in λ. The difference can be attributed to the much brisker breaking and rejoining activity of replicating T4 DNA.

A Physical Map

A physical map is derived through the use of restriction endonucleases for producing characteristic DNA fragments. The many available enzymes, which recognize different target sequences, yield many well-characterized fragments from a given viral DNA in a wide range of sizes, easily separable by gel electrophoresis. The overlaps of the fragments with larger pieces obtained by incomplete digestion reveal the **sequential order** of the fragments, thus allowing a physical mapping of the restriction sites.

Genes can be located on restriction maps by determining which fragments overlap a given marker. One method is **marker rescue by fragments:** transfection of a purified wild-type DNA fragment into a cell infected by a mutant phage can generate wild-type progeny by recombination if the fragment overlaps the mutation. Another method involves **transfection of a partial heteroduplex** containing a mutant complete strand and a wild-type fragment strand (Fig. 45–17). Wild-type progeny obtained either by DNA synthesis completing the fragment strand or by error correction in the heterozygous region localizes the gene as overlapping the mutation.

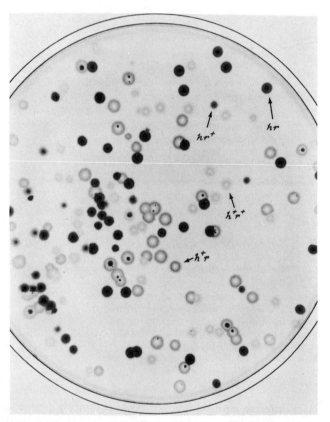

Figure 45–16. Plaques formed by a mixture of T2 phages carrying mutations at the h (host range) and the r locus, placed on a mixture of *E. coli* B and *E. coli* B/2 (i.e., resistant to T2h⁺ but sensitive to T2h). Phages with the h and those with h⁺ allele produce, respectively, clear plaques (dark areas in the photograph) and turbid plaques (gray areas in the photograph); phages with the r allele are larger than those with the r⁺ allele. Thus, all four possible combinations can be distinguished: T2h⁺r⁺ (wild-type), T2hr, T2h⁺r, and T2hr⁺. (From Molecular Biology of Bacterial Viruses by Gunther S. Stent. W. H. Freeman and Company. Copyright © 1963).

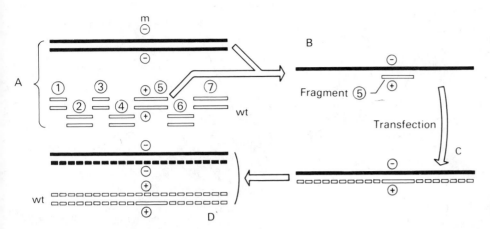

Figure 45–17. Marker rescue from synthetic partial heteroduplex. *(A)* Wild-type *(wt)* viral DNA is cut by restriction endonucleases, yielding characteristic fragments. Mutant DNA (mutation at −) and purified fragment 5 (which contains the corresponding wt allele +) are denatured and hybridized together. One of the products is the partial heteroduplex *(B)*, which is introduced into suitable cells by transfection. *(C)* The heteroduplex is completed by DNA synthesis (*dashed lines*) and after replication yields a wt molecule *(D)*. The mutant strand of the heteroduplex can also be converted to wt by error correction.

With the advent of DNA cloning and rapid sequencing technology, the genomes of many phages have been completely sequenced. Genes with known functions can be identified on such sequences by hybridization with DNA complementary to the messengers (cDNAs). This approach has led to a detailed knowledge of many genes not only with respect to their structural sequences but also to the regulatory sequences such as promoters, ribosome-binding sites, and termination signals.

Organization of the Genome

The arrangement of the genome of a phage has important implications for its function, as will be illustrated here with phage T4 and T7. The organization of the λ genome will be considered in Chapter 46.

Concerning the organization of the T4 genome, it should first be remarked that although the DNA in the virions is linear, the map (Fig. 45–18) is circular: if, starting at any marker, the map is completely covered by a series of crosses between pairs of markers at relatively close distance, the terminal marker is closely linked to the starting marker. The map is circular because the DNA molecules in the virions are **circularly permuted:** they are generated from a periodic concatemer by cutting off segments longer than the periodic unit. A segment can initiate at any gene and has long repetitive ends. Hence, any two genes that are adjacent to each other in the concatemers are also adjacent in most of the mature DNA molecules. In contrast, the map of phage T7 is linear (Fig. 45–19), because mature molecules are isolated by cutting concatemers at specific sequences.

The T4 map contains about 140 genes, and the functions of most are known. The map shows a high degree of organization: genes tend to be **clustered** according to their functions. Most of the genes for the proteins of the virions are together in one third of the genome, whereas the rest contains mostly genes for the various viral functions involved in DNA replication, transcription, and lysis. Genes specifying an organelle (head, tail, tail fibers) or a metabolic function (especially DNA replication) are of-

ten contiguous. A similar arrangement is found in the much simpler T7 genome. The significance of clustering is probably **functional:** contiguous genes can be efficiently regulated together, and if they are transcribed together on a polycistronic messenger, their products are generated in close proximity and timing. This pattern favors their assembly into multiprotein complexes, both in the virions and in multi-enzyme complexes in which substrates can flow rapidly from one enzyme to another.

Of the T4 genes, some are **essential,** their mutations blocking phage multiplication; others are not, their mutations only reducing the multiplication efficiency. Essential are almost all genes for the virion proteins but only half of those for metabolic functions. The essential genes include those specifying key enzymes for DNA replication or transcription, such as DNA polymerase, recombination enzymes, DNA-unfolding protein, subunits of the transcriptase, enzymes that generate dHMC or eliminate dC, and those that glucosylate the viral DNA (see Fig. 45–12). Of the **nonessential** genes, some perform functions that are not strictly necessary. Others duplicate cellular genes but work better because their products interact more efficiently with other viral proteins or with recognition signals on the viral DNA or RNA.

Among the three T-even phages (T2, T4, T6), most genes are highly conserved, implying that they are functionally important. Evidence for evolutionary divergence exists in the genes for the part of the tail fibers that recognizes the bacterial receptors. This evolution was probably promoted by the occurrence of phage-resistant bacterial mutants.

GENETIC REACTIVATION OF ULTRAVIOLET-INACTIVATED PHAGE

Phages have contributed much to our understanding of the biology of radiations, because effects on individual genes can be measured accurately. Thus in cells infected with ultraviolet-irradiated ("UV'd") phage, the **functional survival** of a phage gene can be determined directly

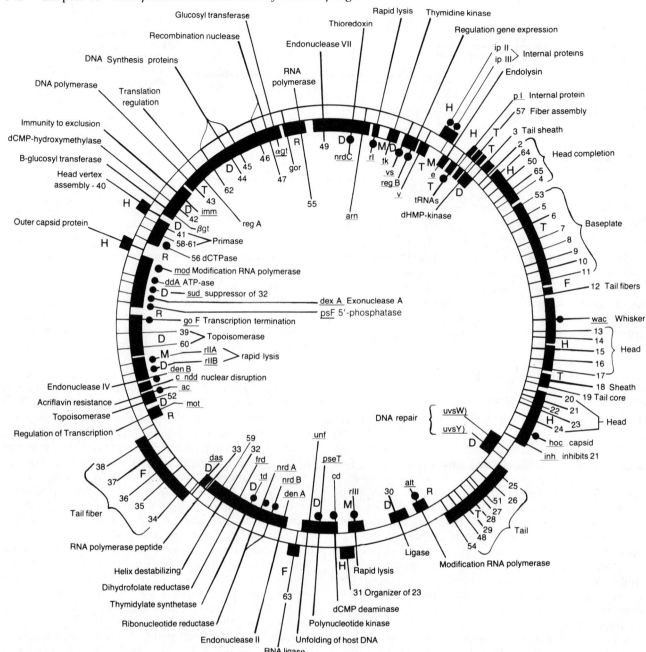

Figure 45–18. The circular genetic map of phage T4. Genes are indicated by numbers or acronyms. Blocks of genes with related functions are shown filled in black. Those on the inside of the circle specify functional proteins needed for DNA replication (*D*), mRNA synthesis (*R*), and translation (*T*) and proteins that participate in membrane functions (*M*). Genes on the outside specify structural proteins of the head (*H*), tail (*T*), or fibers (*F*). Genes identified by dots are dispensable. (Data from Matthews CK, Kutter EN, Mosig J, Berget PB: Bacteriophage T4. Washington, American Society of Microbiology, 1983)

from the amount of a gene product synthesized, or indirectly from its ability to complement a mutant gene infecting the same cells (Fig. 45–20). The functional survival depends on the size of the gene, its distance from the promoter (since UV damage interrupts transcription), and the efficiency of **damage repair.** Large phages, such as T4, employ several genes in repairing damage to their DNA. Small phages (e.g., φX174 or λ) rely in large part or completely on repair mechanisms of the host, which is then said to carry out **host-cell reactivation.**

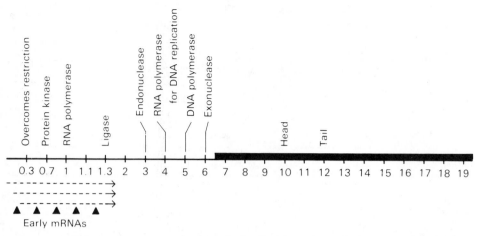

Figure 45—19. The linear genetic map of phage T7. The black bar indicates the late genes. Arrowheads are processing points of the early mRNAs that initiate on several closely spaced but distinct promoters.

In addition to the usual forms of repair of UV damage, T-even phages display strong reactivation based on recombination. One mechanism is **multiplicity reactivation.** When a cell is infected by irradiated phage, the probability of yielding infectious virus increases disproportionately to the multiplicity of infection (Fig. 45—21). The explanation is that different DNA molecules will have their UV lesions in different locations, and replicas of the undamaged segments can recombine to form concatemers containing the complete information of an intact molecule (Fig. 45—22). If recombination is prevented

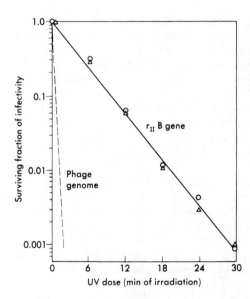

Figure 45—20. Kinetics of ultraviolet (*UV*) damage to a gene and to a genome. Functional survival of the $r_{II}B$ gene is compared with survival of the entire genome of T4 bacteriophage particles irradiated with UV light. Survival of the genome was measured from the fraction of K12(λ) cells yielding phage after single infection by irradiated $T4r_{II}B^+$ particles (*dashed line*). Survival of the $r_{II}B$ gene was measured by simultaneously infecting the same cells with unirradiated $r_{II}B$ mutant phage, which cannot multiply in this host unless complemented with an undamaged $r_{II}B^+$ allele. (Data from Krieg D: Virology 8:80, 1959)

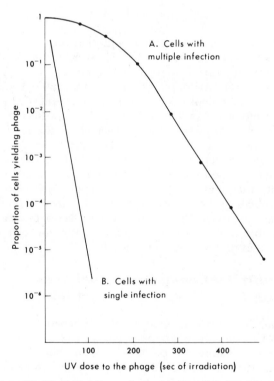

Figure 45—21. Multiplicity reactivation of UV-irradiated T2. In curve *A*, bacteria were each infected with an average of four T2 phages; the curve shows the fraction of the cells able to yield infectious phage for different UV doses given to the phage. Curve *B* shows the results obtained when the cells were infected at low multiplicity (i.e., mostly single infection). (Modified from Dulbecco R: J Bacteriol 63:199, 1952)

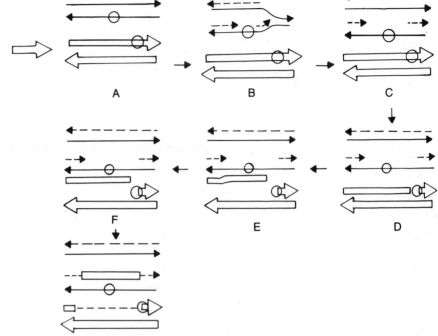

Figure 45–22. Reconstitution of an intact DNA strand *(G, black arrow)* from two UV-damaged strands *(A, open arrows)* by recombination. UV damages are indicated by crosses. *A* shows the homologous section of two DNA molecules. *(B)* The upper molecules replicate, but the new strand is interrupted at the UV lesion. *(C)* The gap is widened by the nuclease specified by genes 46 and 47. *(D)* The unreplicated damaged strand of the lower molecule is cut adjacent to the damage. *(E)* The cut lower strand pairs with the upper molecule at the gap. *(F)* The crossover is resolved by an endonuclease. *(G)* After repair synthesis, an undamaged strand *(arrow)* is formed. (Modified from Matthews CK, Kutter EN, Mosig J, Berget PB: Bacteriophage T4. Washington, American Society of Microbiology, 1983)

by mutations, multiplicity reactivation does not occur. This type of reactivation is much less evident with other phages in which recombination is less active.

A similar type of reactivation is **marker rescue** in a cell simultaneously infected by a lethally irradiated virion and by one or more undamaged virions. Recombination can incorporate a mutated gene from the irradiated genome into the undamaged DNA and hence into the progeny. Effective recombination must involve a partial replica of the UV'd phage containing the marker allele. Since this replica will initiate at a replication origin and terminate at the nearest unrepaired UV damage on each side, the probability of marker rescue decreases with the number of lesions in the irradiated DNA and with distance from the origin of replication.

Multiplication of Bacteriophages With Cyclic Single-Stranded DNA

The class of bacteriophages with cyclic single-stranded DNA includes two groups of phages with very different virions: **icosahedral** (ϕX174 and G4) and **filamentous** (f1 and M13). Surprisingly, the methods of infection and replication are similar.

These phages have only nine or ten genes, several of them expressing similar functions in the two groups. The genes encode structural proteins of the virions, proteins needed in DNA replication, and proteins for maturation.

INFECTION

Infection relies strongly on a **pilot protein,** which in ϕX174 is located in spikes at the 12 corners of the capsid, and in M13 at one end of the filamentous virion. This protein performs several important and seemingly unrelated functions: (1) it **causes the adsorption** of the virions to the cell receptors; (2) it **carries the viral DNA into the cells;** (3) it **initiates the replication** of the viral DNA, probably by linking it to the replicating machinery of the host at the cell plasma membrane; and (4) it is important for phage **morphogenesis.** The versatility of this protein is an example of the **genetic economy** of these phages. This economy finds another striking example in extensive gene overlaps in both ϕX174 and G4.

Most filamentous phages adsorb to the tip of pili specified by the F plasmid (see Plasmids, Chap. 7). As the DNA penetrates into the cell, the capsid protein becomes incorporated into the cell plasma membrane and is later reutilized during virus release (see below).

DNA REPLICATION

Replication of the phage DNA depends mostly on cellular enzymes. It takes place in three phases (Fig. 45–23).

1. Synthesis, by host enzymes, of a **complementary (minus) strand** on the infecting viral (plus) strand to form the **parental replicative form (RF).** This parental

RF, after being made superhelical by cellular gyrase, is transcribed into mRNAs with positive polarity, which are templates for the viral proteins.

2. **Replication of the parental RF by the rolling-circle model** (phase 1), generating ten to 20 **progeny RFs** per cell for ϕX174 and 100 to 200 for f1. This replication is initiated by a **multifunctional protein,** specified by a viral gene (protein A with ϕX74; see Fig. 45–23). As an endonuclease it nicks the positive strand (coming from the infecting virion) of the supercoiled parental RF at the origin of replication and becomes covalently bound, through a tyrosyl–dAMP phosphodiester bond, to the 5′ end it generated. The bound protein moves along the negative strand, separating the parental strands from each other ahead of replication while a new progeny positive strand is made by the host DNA polymerase. The two strands are kept separate by single-strand binding protein. As soon as replication is completed, the multifunctional protein cuts off the positive progeny strand, which becomes free. Then, acting as ligase, it causes cyclization of the released strand; the energy of the protein–DNA bond is utilized to seal the nick. The cyclic progeny strand can then be used to make a new RF by building a negative strand (as above) or for virion formation in phase 2.

3. In phase 2, **asymmetric synthesis of positive progeny strands** on progeny RFs occurs as in phase 1, except that a new viral protein (C with ϕX174) binds at the origin, causing the association of the growing progeny viral strand with a procapsid, forming a virion. The virions are then released by cell lysis. Some mutations will block both single-stranded synthesis and virion formation. Presumably they affect proteins that control the interaction of the procapsid with the nascent DNA strand.

Throughout replication the negative strand of the parental RF remains unnicked and acts as the template for all the positive strands that end up in progeny virions. Therefore, replication of these phages follows a **stamping-machine model.**

MORPHOGENESIS

Major differences exist between the two kinds of phage in the formation of mature virions and their release. With the **icosahedral ϕX174** the progeny positive strands become associated with virion proteins as they are synthesized.

In contrast, with **filamentous** phages the progeny viral strand, after becoming associated with a phage-specified DNA-binding protein, attaches to the plasma membrane at points of adhesion with the outer membrane. The inner membrane contains the main capsid protein and accessory proteins in transmembrane position, including both newly synthesized molecules and those initially imported by the infecting virions. As the viral DNA is extended through the membrane, it picks up protein monomers of either origin and releases the DNA-binding protein, which remains in the cytoplasm and is then reutilized for further single-strand synthesis. In this way virions cross the inner membrane without damaging it and leave the cells through gaps in the outer membrane. The **length of the virions depends on the length of the viral DNA,** a characteristic exploited for DNA cloning (see Vectors for DNA Cloning, Chap. 46).

The interaction between the capsid protein of filamentous phages and the cell membrane is **intimate and balanced.** Cell growth is retarded only a little, although about 1000 virions are excreted at each cell generation. However, phage mutations affecting virion proteins can kill the cells. This steady-state virus–cell interaction resembles that occurring with some animal viruses (see Chap. 51). Although there is no cell lysis, the slower growth of the infected cells causes the formation of **turbid plaques,** that is, with a lower bacterial density than in the surrounding lawn.

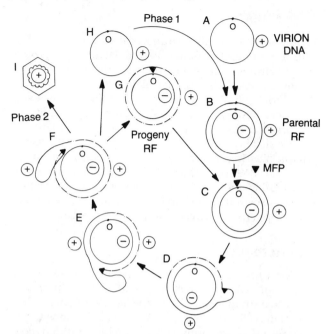

Figure 45–23. Replication of DNA of single-stranded phages. The virion DNA (the + strand; *A*) enters the cell, where it is converted to the ds parental RF *(B)*. The multifunctional protein *(MFP, black triangle)* cleaves the + strand at the origin and binds to it *(C)*. It causes the synthesis of a new + strand, displacing the old one *(D, E, F)*, which it finally ligates into a closed circle *(G)*; the protein remains bound to the replicated RF, which then commences a new cycle. The single + strand *(H)* is converted into a new RF in the first phase of replication; in the second phase it associates with a procapsid *(I)* and becomes incorporated in a progeny virion. (Data from Eisenberg S, Griffith J, Kornberg A: Proc Natl Acad Sci USA 74:3198–3202, 1977; Aoyama A, Hayashi M: Cell 47:99–106, 1986)

RNA Phage

The small RNA phages have an icosahedral capsid (T = 3) with the addition of one or two molecules of a protein called A protein, similar in function to the pilot protein of phage φX. RNA phages, like filamentous DNA phages, attach to F pili of male bacteria; i.e., they are male specific. Their RNAs show **extensive self-complementarity** and are therefore able to form complex secondary and tertiary structures. These phages are divided into several groups differing in serology but with considerable homology of RNA sequences: f2, MS2, and R17 are in one group, Qβ in another. The genomes of these phages have similar, exceptionally simple organization: they contain only four genes, of which two partially overlap.

RNA REPLICATION

The viral RNA acts as both genome and messenger. Its replication, which is similar to that of some animal viruses (see Chap. 48), involves special intermediates (Fig. 45–24). In cells infected with RNA-labeled virions the label is found in two forms: entirely double-stranded molecules, completely resistant to RNase, called **replicative form (RF)**; and molecules partially RNase resistant, called **replicative intermediate (RI)**, which have a double-stranded backbone with one or two single-stranded tails. The pattern of labeling after brief pulses of a radioactive precursor shows that the RF is produced by building a **complementary** negative strand on the infecting **viral** positive strand; the subsequent synthesis of a third, positive progeny strand on the double-stranded RF converts it into the RI, from which successive progeny strands are then released, as Figure 45–24 shows. The synthesis of the positive strands can be **semiconservative or conservative** in different RIs; only in the former is the label parental RNA accessible to RNase degradation.

RNA Replicase

The replicases of various phages are highly specific for phages of the same group; they do not replicate cellular RNAs. They recognize two CCC sequences placed in the proper steric arrangement by the secondary structure of the RNA, one of which is present at the 5′ end of all phage RNAs.

The replicase of phage Qβ is made up of **four subunits,** of which only one (subunit II) is phage specified; **the others are cellular proteins involved in protein synthesis.** Subunit I is the ribosomal protein S1; subunits III and IV correspond to two elongation factors of protein synthesis: EF-Tu and EF-Ts. The complex of subunits II, III, and IV can replicate the Qβ **negative** strand; replication of the **positive** (viral) strand requires subunit I and an additional host ribosomal protein. The phage-specified **subunit II is the true polymerase,** for it can carry out chain elongation alone. The interaction of the phage subunit with the protein synthesis factors perhaps indicates an evolutionary relationship between phage RNA and cellular messengers, as already suggested for some plant viruses (see Chap. 44).

The RNA replicase makes mistakes at a much higher frequency than DNA polymerase, probably because it lacks the editing function of the latter enzyme. As a result, **each viable phage differs at one or more bases** from the average population.

REGULATION OF TRANSLATION

In spite of the great simplicity of the genome, these viruses have a fine regulation of gene expression, perfectly attuned to the needs of multiplication. This regulation takes place at the level of translation. It takes advantage of changes of the **secondary structure of the RNA** and of its **interaction with proteins.** Thus the ribosome-binding region of the **A gene** is normally buried in the

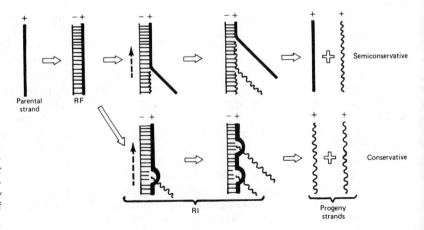

Figure 45–24. Intermediates in RNA replication. They can be distinguished because in the semiconservative type of replication the parental strand (*straight heavy line*) is exposed to RNase attack during replication, whereas in the conservative model it is not. *Wavy lines,* progeny strands; *dashed arrows,* direction of replication.

RNA folds; it may be accessible only once in the life of an RNA molecule (i.e., during synthesis), for as soon as the RNA folds up, it is permanently covered. The result is that very few A molecules are made. The **replicase gene** is translated early in infection, and the **coat protein** starts later, when new replicase molecules are no longer needed. Then the coat protein represses the translation of the gene of replicase by binding strongly to its ribosome-binding site. In this way the synthetic activity is ultimately concentrated on the synthesis of coat protein to encapsidate the RNA, and on a viral protein that triggers lysis to release the virions. Another approach to regulation is **gene overlap.** The coat protein gene overlaps with the **lysis gene,** which specifies a lysis protein made in minute amounts in infected cells. The lysis gene is out of phase and is read only occasionally by ribosomes that translate the coat gene.

Selected Reading

Alberts BM: The DNA enzymology of protein machines: Cold Spring Harbor Symp Quant Biol 49:1, 1984

Barrell BG, Air GM, Hutchinson CA III: Overlapping genes in bacteriophage ϕX174. Nature 264:34, 1976

Celis JE, Smith JD, Brenner J: Correlation between genetic and translational maps of gene 23 in bacteriophage T4. Nature 241:130, 1973

Eisenberg S, Griffith J, Kornberg A: ϕX174 cistron A protein is a multifunctional enzyme in DNA replication. Proc Natl Acad Sci USA 74:3198, 1977

Gage LP, Geiduschek EP: RNA synthesis during bacteriophage SPO1 development: Six classes of SPO1 RNA. J Mol Biol 57:279, 1971

Hsiao CL, Black LW: DNA packaging and the pathway of bacteriophage T4 head assembly. Proc Natl Acad Sci USA 74:3652, 1977

Kikuchi Y, King J: Genetic control of bacteriophage T4 baseplate morphogenesis. I. Sequential assembly of the major precursor *in vivo* and *in vitro*. J Mol Biol 99:645, 1975

Landers TA, Blumenthal T, Weber K: Function and structure in ribonucleic acid phage Qβ ribonucleic acid replicase. J Biol Chem 249:5801, 1974

Matthews CK, Kutter EM, Mosig G, Berget PB: Bacteriophage T4. Washington, American Society for Microbiology, 1983

Rashed I, Oberer E: Ff coliphages: Structural and functional relationship. Microbiol Rev 50:401, 1986

Sanger F, Air GM, Barrell BG et al: Nucleotide sequence of bacteriophage ϕX174 DNA. Nature 265:687, 1977

Schmidt FJ: RNA splicing in prokaryotes: Bacteriophage T4 leads the way. Cell 41:339, 1985

Zinder ND, Horiuchi K: Multiregulation element of filamentous bacteriophages. Microbiol Rev 49:101, 1985

46

Lysogeny and Transducing Bacteriophages

Lysogeny

Most of the bacteriophages described in the preceding chapter are **virulent;** i.e., they multiply vegetatively and kill the cells at the end of the growth cycle. The **temperate** phages, in contrast, besides multiplying vegetatively, can also produce the phenomenon of **lysogeny,** recognized in the early 1920s: the indefinite persistence of the phage DNA in their host cells, without phage production. Occasionally, however, the viral DNA in a **lysogenic cell** will initiate vegetative multiplication, generating mature virions. Lysogeny favors the persistence and spreading of a virus in a more subtle way than virulence: as Burnet has pointed out in connection with viral diseases in higher organisms, the best-adapted parasites are those that do not rapidly kill their hosts and thus deprive themselves of the opportunity to spread.

Temperate phages have provocative implications for many biological problems: they throw light on the origin of viruses and the evolution of bacteria, they provide an important mechanism for gene transfer between bacteria **(transduction),** and they supply a model for viral oncogenesis (see Chaps. 64 and 65), and for some forms of animal virus latency.

NATURE OF LYSOGENY

Lysogeny characterizes many bacterial strains freshly isolated from their natural environment. Such lysogenic cultures contain a low concentration of bacteriophage, which can be recognized because it lyses certain other related bacterial strains, known as sensitive or **indicator**

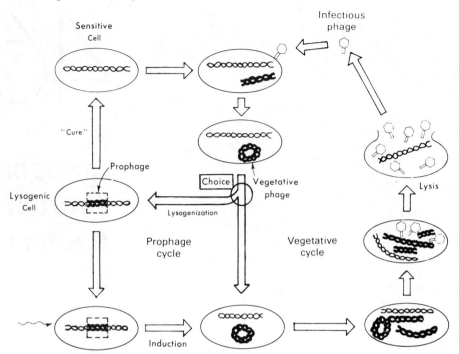

Figure 46–1. Development of a temperate bacteriophage.

strains. When a sensitive bacterial strain is infected by a temperate bacteriophage, one of two responses is seen (Fig. 46–1): some cells are lysed by phage multiplication, and others are lysogenized. Lysogenic strains thus produced are designated by the name of the sensitive strain followed by that of the lysogenizing phage in parenthesis, e.g., *Escherichia coli* K12(λ). Because temperate phages lyse only a fraction of the sensitive cells that they infect, they produce **turbid plaques.**

A bacterial strain can easily be recognized as lysogenic by streaking it on a solid medium across a strain sensitive to the phage released; a narrow zone of lysis is seen along the border of the lysogenic strain (Fig. 46–2). Since lysogeny cannot be recognized unless such a sensitive strain is available, many bacterial strains—perhaps most of those known—may be unrecognized as lysogens. Furthermore, many strains are lysogenic for several different phages.

The systems used most in experimental work on lysogeny are λ and related phages, active on *E. coli* K12; Mu, also active on *E. coli*; and P1 and P2, active on *Shigella dysenteriae* or on several strains of *E. coli*.

Relation to the Vegetative Growth Cycle

Lysogenic strains are not simply phage-contaminated bacterial cultures, since the ability to produce phage could not be eliminated by repeated cloning of the bacteria or by growth in the presence of phage-specific antiserum to prevent cell infection by virions present in the

medium. In 1925 Borden recognized that it was a hereditary property of the cells. Moreover, since disruption of the lysogenic cells does not yield infectious phage, the phage must be present in the cells in a noninfectious form. However, the ability of lysogenic cultures to produce virus without obvious lysis remained puzzling until Lwoff, in 1950, patiently observing the behavior of single cells in microdroplets, showed that phage is produced by **a small proportion of the cells;** these lyse and release phage in a burst (**induction**) just like cells infected by phage T4. The other cells of the culture do not give rise to a productive infection and are said to be **immune*** to the released phage. The phage adsorbs to the immune cells and injects its DNA, but **the DNA does not multiply** and does not cause cell lysis. **Immunity, therefore, is different from resistance,** which, as noted in the preceding chapter, prevents adsorption and injection (see Infection of Host Cells, Chap. 45).

These experiments made it clear that lysogeny involves a special, stably inherited, noninfectious form of the virus, called **prophage,** associated with immunity. The prophage occasionally shifts abruptly to the vegetative form and then reproduces just like a virulent phage. Lwoff further showed that the shift from the prophage cycle to the lytic cycle, normally a rare event, could be **induced** in all the cells of a culture by moderate ultraviolet irradiation (see Fig. 46–2).

---

* This term is totally unrelated to immunity as studied in immunology.

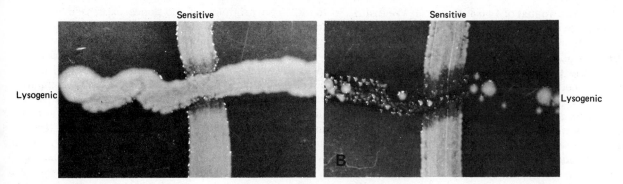

Figure 46–2. Cross-streaking of lysogenic and sensitive strains of *Escherichia coli* on nutrient agar. *(A)* Untreated. *(B)* Exposed to a small dose of ultraviolet (UV) light, after streaking, to induce the lysogenic cells. In *A* note the narrow bands of lysis of the sensitive strain (vertical streak) flanking the lysogenic strain (horizontal streak). In *B* note that the inducing treatment, by causing cell lysis, markedly reduces the colony density of the lysogenic streak, and the accompanying release of infectious phage causes pronounced lysis of the sensitive strain in the area of crossing.

THE VEGETATIVE CYCLE

The vegetative cycle of temperate phages is similar to that of virulent phages (see Chap. 45) but with some modifications. Virions of λ contain a double-stranded linear DNA, 48.5 Kb long, with a complementary single-stranded segment 12 nucleotides long at each 5′ end (Fig. 46–3). Under annealing conditions *in vitro*, these **"cohesive" ends** pair, generating a cyclic molecule with two staggered nicks. Infection with labeled phage reveals a similar cyclization *in vivo*, with ligase closing the two nicks. The evolution of the cohesive ends can be explained by the requirement for both a linear DNA in the virions, to allow encapsidation, and a cyclic form intracellularly, during replication and lysogenization (see The Prophage Cycle, below).

The Genetics of λ

As with other phages, the genes of λ are organized in three functional blocks independently regulated (Fig. 46–4): a left block specifying many functions needed for vegetative growth or lysogenization (left operon), a right block for DNA replication and capsid formation (right operon), and a central control block (immunity operon).

In Figure 46–4 the genome is represented as circular because within the cells the viral DNA is circular while the genes are expressed, i.e., during transcription. The **vegetative genetic map** (i.e., that based on recombination during vegetative growth) is linear, with the ends coinciding with those of the virion DNA (see Genetic Recombination, Chap. 45). This recombination is called **generalized** (to distinguish it from the specialized form, discussed below) and can be carried out either by the bacterial *rec BC* and *rec A* system (see Recombination, Chap. 8) or by a phage system (gene *red*, which encodes the recombination enzyme, and *gam*, which inhibits the host *rec BC* system; see Replication, below, for the role of *red* and *gam* genes).

Vegetative Transcription

The extraordinarily detailed study of λ transcription has led to a fairly complete understanding of the switching between vegetative and prophage cycles, which is an important model for the switching of genes in differentiation. Aspects important for the vegetative cycle will be reviewed now, and those specifically related to lysogenization will be reviewed later in this chapter.

The general pattern of vegetative λ transcription (see

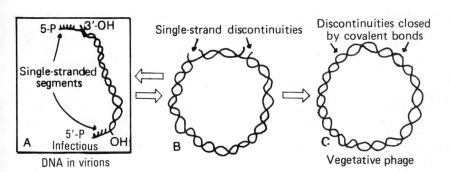

Figure 46–3. Different forms of phage λ DNA. *(A)* In the virions the DNA exists as a linear double-stranded molecule with complementary ends. *(B)* Under conditions of nucleic acid hybridization, the linear molecule can reversibly close into a ring by base pairing of the single-stranded ends. *(C)* Within the cell, the DNA forms completely covalently closed rings.

Fig. 46–4) is similar to that of T4 (see Chap. 45). We distinguish **immediate early** messengers (which appear in the presence of chloramphenicol), **delayed early,** and **late messengers**—all synthesized by the host transcriptase. As with T4, the transition from immediate to delayed early is produced by **interference with termination.** Thus, *in vitro*, in the presence of the bacterial termination factor rho, two short immediate early RNAs are formed. One is transcribed from the "left" DNA strand and extends leftward from promoter PL through gene N to the tL terminator; the other, transcribed from the "right" DNA strand, extends rightward from promoter PR through gene *cro* to the tR1 terminator, and some of this transcription continues further, through genes O and P

to tR2. The products of the genes expressed in these transcripts have important functions in viral development and lysogeny, which will be reviewed below.

The sequence of subsequent transcriptions is regulated as follows. After gene N is transcribed and translated, its product (indicated as pN), an antiterminator, allows both the leftward and the rightward transcriptions to proceed further. The mechanism of this antitermination is known in detail: pN binds to a characteristic *nut* (N-utilization) site downstream of each promoter, where it associates with cellular proteins (*nus*—for N-utilization substance—A, B, and E), forming a termination-resistant complex with the RNA polymerase.

The extended rightward transcription reaches as far

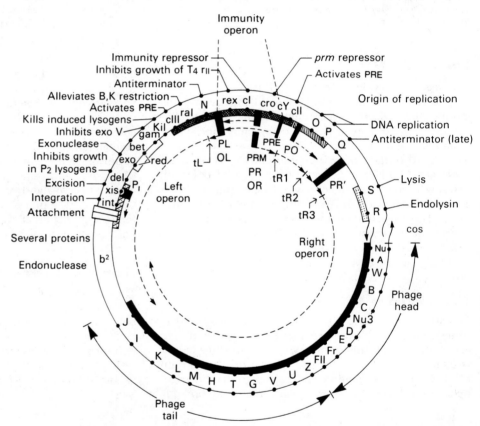

Figure 46–4. Genetic and functional organization of phage λ DNA. Capital letters indicate genes identified by nonsense mutations, which include most of those required for the vegetative cycle. The genes are arranged in functional groups, identified by the following bands (*left to right*): *dashed and dotted,* specialized recombination; *white,* generalized recombination; *crosshatched,* regulation; *dashed,* DNA replication; *dotted,* lysis; *black,* capsid. The DNA is represented in the cyclic configuration in which transcription occurs. In the virions the DNA is linear, with ends at *cos.* The map is linear; that is, markers close to *cos* but at opposite sides have the highest recombination frequencies. Transcription is indicated by dashed lines and proceeds in the directions indicated by the arrows. There are three main transcription segments designed as operons: leftward, rightward, and immunity operons. *PL, OL,* leftward promoter and operator; *PR, OR,* rightward promoter and operator; *PRE,* controller for repressor establishment; *PRM,* promoter for repressor maintenance; *PO,* promoter for replication-related transcription; *P₁,* promoter for *int* transcription; *tL, tR1, tR2,* terminators neutralized by the N gene product; *PR',* promoter for late transcription; *tR3,* terminator neutralized by the Q gene product.

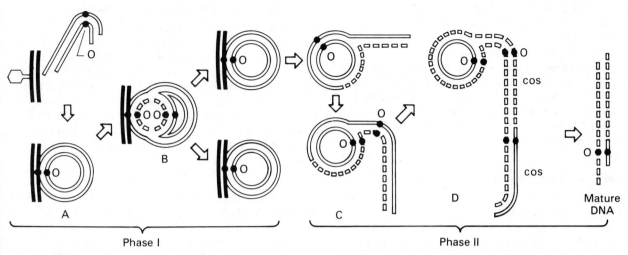

Figure 46–5. Replication of λ DNA. In phase I the DNA injected by the infecting virion first cyclizes *(A)*, then *(B)* it replicates symmetrically in association with the cell plasma membrane *(double line)*, initiating at a fixed origin *(O)*. In phase II the DNA, free of the membrane, replicates asymmetrically *(C)*, by the rolling circle model, generating linear concatemers. These are then cut at *cos* sites *(D)* to generate mature molecules with cohesive ends.

as gene Q, the product of which is another antiterminator. Together with protein *nus* A it binds to a *qut* (Q-utilization) site close to the promoter for late transcription (PR') just to the right of Q. The binding allows this transcription, which also proceeds rightward, to avoid terminator tR3 and thus to continue through the long series of genes for the vegetative proteins all the way to gene J and into the b₂ region.

Late transcription is strongly increased by DNA replication but also occurs in its absence.

Replication

The replication of λ DNA utilizes exclusively exogenous precursors, because the bacterial DNA is not destroyed. Replication occurs in two stages (Fig. 46–5). First the cyclic parental DNA associates with the cell membrane and replicates symmetrically, generating cyclic molecules. Initiation, at a unique site within gene O, requires the functions of viral genes O and P, as well as host functions. Replication proceeds in opposite directions and terminates where the two forks meet. It is initiated by the binding of the λO protein to the origin, followed by the λP protein and by several host proteins, giving rise to a *replication complex*.

In the second, *late* stage the progeny DNA leaves the membrane and replicates according to the rolling-circle model, initiating at variable locations on the cyclic DNA and generating long concatemers. They are required for packaging the DNA in the capsid at maturation. The control for the transition from early to late replication depends on phage genes under N dependence.

The function of gene *gam* is important in replication because it inhibits the host's *rec* BC exonuclease V,

which would otherwise degrade the concatemers. *Red⁻ gam⁻* phage, which does not form concatemers, can, however, replicate in a *rec* BC⁺ host that is also *rec* A⁺. The combined action of the corresponding proteins carries out homologous recombination between circular molecules, if they contain the eight-base *chi* sequence, generating circular dimers and higher oligomers. *Red⁺ gam⁺* phage, however, cannot grow in *E. coli* lysogenized by phage P2 (*spi* phenotype; that is, susceptible to P2 interference), whereas *red⁻ gam⁻* phage can; this property is exploited in the construction of vectors for DNA cloning (see Bacteriophages as Vectors for DNA Cloning, below).

In the formation of **mature molecules with cohesive ends,** a **terminase,** specified by phage genes *NU1* and *A*, binds to concatemers or oligomers at the sites corresponding to cohesive termini (*cos*; see Fig. 46–5) and produces staggered single-strand cuts 12 nucleotides apart. The terminase also functions in **packaging** a mature DNA molecule into a prohead. Packaging is polarized, and the same terminase molecule can sequentially package adjacent units of concatemer. Further stages in head assembly and capsid maturation generally follow the T-even model. Virions are released when the product of gene S stops cellular metabolism and weakens the cellular membrane, allowing the lysozyme produced by gene R to lyse the cell wall.

THE LYSOGENIC STATE

When a sensitive bacterium is infected by a temperate phage, the entering DNA has a **"choice"** between vegetative multiplication and lysogenization (see Fig. 46–1). The proportion of infected cells that are lysogenized varies from a small percentage to nearly all, depending on the system and the conditions.

The lysogenic state is determined by the activity of the **regulatory region** of the λ genome, which not only causes integration of the phage genome in the cellular DNA but also generates immunity. Immunity emerged as the central feature of lysogeny when it was shown, by Jacob and Wollman, to be produced by repression of phage genes, much like the repression of bacterial operons.

Immunity and Repression

Lysogenic cells contain the **immunity repressor** but no vegetative proteins or mRNAs; in induced cells the opposite is true. The repressor is specified by the cI gene in the immunity region. Mutations that alter the repressor (cI) prevent lysogenization but allow vegetative growth, thus producing clear plaques.* **Immunity to exogenous infection** is also the result of repression: it is not produced by cI⁻ phage, and when normal lysogenic cells are induced, it breaks down simultaneously with repression. In the presence of repression, infecting DNA cyclizes but is not replicated; it survives for many cell generations as an **abortive prophage.**

The **λ immunity repressor,** isolated by Ptashne, is an acidic protein with a monomer molecular weight of 26,000. In vitro, this compound, in oligomeric form, binds strongly to the DNA of the immunity region at two **operators** (OR, OL; see Fig. 46–4) that regulate transcription starting at the **rightward and leftward promoters** (PR, PL). This binding normally prevents the expression of most viral functions outside the immunity operon.

In **virulent mutants** (*vir*), both OR and OL are defective and fail to bind the repressor. Like the cI⁻ mutants that fail to make repressor, *vir* mutants do not lysogenize and form **clear plaques.** However, there is an important difference: immune cells, containing cI repressor, can be lysed by *vir* but not by cI⁻ phages, because the latter are sensitive to the repressor.

SPECIFICITY OF IMMUNITY. Immunity is highly specific: even closely related phages form cI repressors of different specificities, and each phage recognizes exclusively its own. No point mutation in a repressor gene is known to change its specificity into that of a different phage, even a closely related one. **Heteroimmune** recombinants, which have most genetic properties of one phage but the immunity of another, have played an important part in unravelling the mechanisms of lysogeny.

* Clear plaques are also produced by mutations in genes cII, cIII, and cY (*PRE*), which, as discussed below, participate in lysogenization but not in repressor formation.

Regulation of cI Repressor Formation

The problem of how lysogenization is produced, maintained, and reversed has attracted a large number of investigators. The basic mechanism is the antagonism between the immunity (*cI*) repressor, which causes immunity, and the *cro* repressor, which prevents immunity. Their complex balance involves two promoters for *cI* (for establishment and then for maintenance), both negative and positive feedback, and host and phage factors that influence the rate of synthesis of the two repressors.

CHOICE BETWEEN LYSOGENIZATION AND VEGETATIVE MULTIPLICATION. In the early period after infection (about 20 minutes) the host transcriptase initiates transcription at the PL and PR promoters (Fig. 46–6A). Gene *cro*, dependent on PR, immediately starts producing the *cro* repressor (*croR*); gene N, dependent on PL, simultaneously produces the pN antiterminator; *pN* in turn permits transcription of genes cII and cIII, the combined products of which transiently activate the **promoter for repressor establishment (PRE),** thus initiating transcription of the immunity operon and synthesis of the immunity repressor (*cIR*).

During this early period, *cIR* and *croR* both accumulate, and their actions on OR, the righthand operator, are the key to the choice between lysogenization and vegetative growth. OR is made up of three sites: OR1, OR2, and OR3, the interactions of which with the two repressors are outlined in Figure 46–7. OR1 adjoins the PR promoter, and OR3 adjoins PRM, the **promoter for CI repressor maintenance,** where the permanent transcription of the immunity operon initiates during the lysogenic state. *cIR* binds mainly to OR1 and OR2, with two effects: it blocks transcription of the right operon, and therefore of gene *cro*, at PR; and it promotes transcription of gene cI at PRM. *CroR* binds mainly to OR3, repressing transcription of gene cI at PRM; weaker effects on OR1 and OR2 repress transcription of gene *cro* itself at PR. The different effects result from the different binding affinities of the two repressors with the three sites, which in turn depend on the base sequences and the tertiary structure of the DNA. The overall result is an antagonistic action of the two repressors on PRM, *cIR* **stimulating its own synthesis** by positive feedback (Fig. 46–6B); lesser effects, noticeable only at high repressor concentrations, cause **autoregulation of both repressors** by negative feedback. The balance favors lysogenization over vegetative growth.

Once *cIR* and *croR* have reached sufficient concentrations, all transcriptions (and soon all syntheses of viral products) come to a halt. The role of *PRE* is now ended. At this stage the choice is determined by the concentrations of the two repressors. If *cIR* predominates (see Fig.

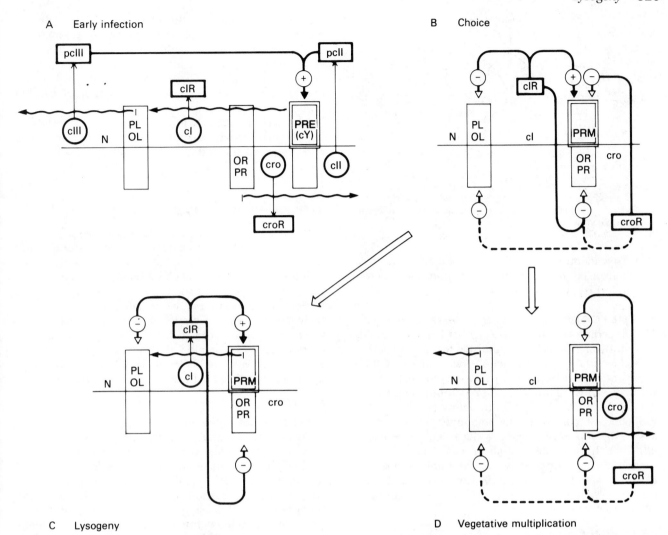

Figure 46–6. Regulation of repression in phage λ and determination of choice between vegetative replication and lysogeny. In the early period of infection *(A)* the left and right promoters (**PL, PR**) become active, allowing transcription (*wavy lines*) that, in the presence of pN, expresses **cII** and **cIII**. The products of these two genes (**pcII** and **pcIII**) activate the **controller for cI repressor establishment** (*PRE*), allowing transcription of the immunity operon (positive control, indicated by + and black arrowhead) and synthesis of immunity repressor, **cIR**. Cro repressor, **croR**, is also made. After about 20 minutes the various products have accumulated, and new synthesis temporarily ceases. *(B)* The choice is then determined by the competition between the negative control (−, *white arrowheads*) of the *cro* repressor (**croR**) and the positive control of the immunity repressor (**cIR**) on **PRM**. If **cIR** wins out *(C)*, it activates **PRM**, keeps it permanently activated by positive feedback control, and blocks **PL** and **PR**, resulting in the lysogenic state; if **croR** wins out *(D)*, **PRM** remains inactive, and transcription initiated at **PL** and **PR** causes vegetative multiplication. Active genes are circled. Heavy lines indicate the main actions of the gene products (*in rectangular boxes*); dashed lines indicate the weaker repression of the *cro* repressor on **PL** and **PR**, which forms a negative feedback control of vegetative multiplication. *OL, OR,* leftward and rightward operators.

46–6C), *PRM* is activated, *cIR* synthesis restarts, and the lysogenic state becomes established. If, on the contrary, *croR* predominates (see Fig. 46–6D), *PRM* is not activated, there is no *cIR* synthesis, and vegetative multiplication is established under the control of *croR* (see Plasmidial Prophages, below).

Once the choice is made, it is maintained by positive feedback. The choice is therefore determined during the first 20 minutes by the rates of synthesis of the two re-

pressors. Many factors influence these rates, especially the concentration of the cII product (an activator of *PRE*). Two *E. coli* genes, *hfl* (high-frequency lysogenization) A and B, specify a protease that breaks down the *cII* product, inhibiting lysogenization; their mutations promote lysogenization. Other *E. coli* mutations inhibit the synthesis of immunity repressor by decreasing the synthesis (or the action) of cyclic AMP (cAMP), which promotes lysogenization over the more expensive lytic multiplica-

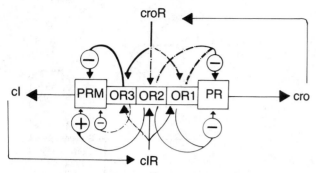

Figure 46–7. Interactions of cIR and croR with the three sites on **OR.** +, stimulation of transcription; −, repression; *solid lines* and *bold lines* main effects; *dashed lines* and *thin lines*, secondary effects taking place only at high concentrations.

tion. This action parallels the effect of cAMP in bacterial metabolism, i.e., mediating the adaptation to poorer food sources, in response to hard times.

SPECIAL FEATURES OF THE CONTROL OF λ IMMUNITY.
The preceding brief review shows that the control of the immunity operon has many unusual features, which coordinate and fine-tune the action and synthesis of the cI repressor: (1) *cIR* represses the operators of the rightward and leftward operons, but it **promotes transcription** of the immunity operon by acting on *PRM*. (2) The independent control of the immunity operon at two sites, *PRE* and *PRM*, separates the **initial synthesis** of *cIR*—which takes place in all infected cells—from the **permanent synthesis,** which occurs only in lysogenic cells. (3) A single operator, OR, controls two different operons, responding to the same repressor with opposite consequences.

Plasmidial Prophages

Plasmidial prophages include those that are not integrated but persist as plasmids, with a constant number of copies per cell. Examples are P1 and λDV, a λ derivative. The mechanism by which λ is maintained throws light on the relationship between plasmids and temperate phages. It contains the λ origin of DNA replication, two genes for replication proteins, the promoters pR and pL, and gene *cro* (see Fig. 46–4). The *cro* gene is crucial

for the maintenance of the plasmidial states. The *cro* repressor keeps the number of copies of the plasmid at a steady level by binding to PR and repressing, in a concentration-dependent fashion, the genes for DNA replication: if the number of copies increases, the higher production of repressor increases repression of PR, causing replication to slow down.

The derivation of λDV from λ shows the relatedness of temperate phages to plasmids. Temperate phages can be considered plasmids that have acquired blocks of genes for a virion's proteins, lysis, and lysogenization.

THE PROPHAGE CYCLE

When lysogenization occurs, the vegetative λ DNA becomes inserted into the cellular DNA as a **prophage** and replicates with it. Most prophages are integrated at **fixed locations** on the bacterial chromosome. In *E. coli*, phage λ and related phages usually settle in a unique site; P2 can occupy at least nine distinct sites, but two preferentially; and *μ*, which is a special case, can integrate anywhere. Some prophages (e.g., P1) exist separate from the chromosome as plasmids. P1, however, must occasionally interact with the bacterial chromosome, because it gives rise to specialized transduction (see below).

Insertion

Genetic studies show that prophage λ is **linearly inserted** in the bacterial chromosome (Fig. 46–8), but the order of the genes is permuted from that determined during lytic multiplication: the order is int-cI-U instead of U-int-cI. Campbell explained this permutation by suggesting that in lysogenization the **viral DNA in cyclic form is inserted linearly into the bacterial chromosome by a single reciprocal crossover,** which opens the ring at a point different from that where the ends of the mature DNA meet (Fig. 46–9). In fact, insertion involves recombination between a **phage attachment site (att P),** 240 bases long, and a **bacterial attachment site (att B),** only 25 bases long; the two sites have 15 bases in common. The exchange generates two recombinant **prophage attachment sites** flanking the prophage, left and right (*att L* and *att R*).

This is a special form of **site-specific recombination,**

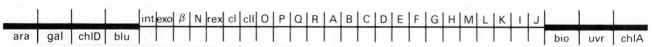

Figure 46–8. Evidence for linear insertion of the λ prophage in the bacterial chromosome. Prophage and bacterial genes were mapped by using deletions that entered the prophage from either side by taking advantage of the two *chl* (chlorate resistance) genes, A and D. To determine which prophage markers had also been deleted, the cells were induced and then superinfected with λ phage carrying distinguishable alleles of all the markers: the appearance (or nonappearance) of various prophage markers in the progeny phage indicated whether they were present in the partly deleted prophage. *Thin line,* phage DNA; *heavy lines,* bacterial DNA; *ara,* arabinose utilization; *gal,* galactose utilization; *blu,* stained blue by iodine; *bio,* biotin synthesis; *uvr,* ultraviolet light resistance. (Data from Adhya S et al: Proc Natl Acad Sci USA 61:956, 1968)

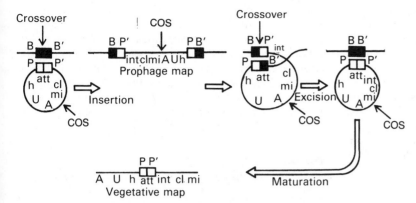

Figure 46–9. Campbell model for prophage integration explaining the permutation of the vegetative and prophage maps of λ DNA. Both the vegetative and the prophage maps can be derived from the same circle by opening it at different points: *cos* for vegetative multiplication and maturation and *att* for prophage insertion. The difference between the two maps is equivalent to shifting the block of markers (*int* to *mi*) from one end of the map to the other. For terminology, see Figure 46–4. *h,* host-range mutation; *mi,* minute plaque mutants; *heavy lines,* bacterial DNA; *thin lines,* phage DNA; *B* ■ *B′,* bacterial attachment site; *P* □ *P′,* phage attachment site; *B* ◨ *P′* and *P* ◧ *B′,* left and right prophage attachment sites, respectively, resulting from recombination between bacterial and phage sites.

similar to that carried out by some transposons (see Chap. 7), which requires little DNA homology. It starts with two single-strand cuts, staggered by seven base pairs within the homologous region. The cuts are carried out by the activity of a special **integrase,** specified by phage gene *int*. Recombination occurs in a complex containing the integrase, a host protein (integration host factor, IHF), and the two DNAs in **supercoiled** state: supercoiling favors the interaction of proteins with DNA.

Expression of *int* is regulated like that of *cI*, so the two main events of lysogenization—repression and integration—are coordinated. Thus, early in infection the cII-cIII products, which start *cI* repressor synthesis, also activate *int* transcription by acting at a **private promoter**, P_I (see Fig. 46–4); in the lysogenic state, *int* continues to be expressed at a low level, because P_I is insensitive to the cI repressor.

Excision

Excision of the prophage takes place when repression breaks down. It is the reversal of integration, i.e., a **reciprocal crossover between the attachment sites at the two ends** of the prophage, which yields a cyclic phage DNA molecule and an intact bacterial chromosome (see Fig. 46–9). Excision requires another viral function, that of gene *xis*, in addition to *int* and IHF (see Fig. 46–4). The *int* product is the basic recombination enzyme for both insertion and excision, and the *xis* product makes it conform to the different site configuration during excision (see Specificity of Attachment Sites, below).

Gene *xis*, in contrast to *int*, is transcribed from the PL promoter, under repressor control (see Fig. 46–4), and therefore is **not expressed in lysogenic cells.** The differential control of *int* and *xis* confers stability on the lysogenic state. If *xis* is expressed while repression persists, the prophage is detached but cannot multiply and is finally lost. IHF also performs a regulatory role because at high concentrations, such as those reached when the cells enter the resting phase, it inhibits excision, preventing phage multiplication under the unfavorable circumstances.

SPECIFICITY OF ATTACHMENT SITES. The differences in the sites involved in insertion and excision can be seen by considering the following equation of the prophage cycle:

$$POP' + BOB' \underset{int\text{-}xis}{\overset{int}{\rightleftharpoons}} BOP' + POB'$$

| Site: | Phage | Bacterial | Left prophage | Right prophage |

where P and P′ represent phage half-sites, B and B′ bacterial half-sites; O is the common central sequence, in which the crossover occurs. The sites existing after insertion (prophage sites) are recombinants between those of the phage and those of the bacterium. This difference explains the need for different enzymes in insertion and excision. Most important in determining the differences are the two parts of the prophage site, which is much longer than the bacterial site.

Induction of a Lysogenic Cell

The transition of prophage to vegetative phage represents a **breakdown of repression:** it can occur either spontaneously or, as already indicated, in response to an inducing stimulus. Then the disappearance of the repressor allows transcription to start at the PL and PR promoters. This transcription spreads to the whole genome (excluding the immunity region), as described above (see Vegetative Transcription), activating genes for prophage excision, DNA replication, recombination, virion proteins, and cell lysis. The prophage is excised as a covalently closed circle and begins to multiply as in the lytic cycle. Progeny virus is produced and leaves the cells as they burst.

Spontaneous induction may occur in rare cells as a result of the accidental activation of the induction machinery. Many prophages are induced by **ultraviolet (UV)**

light in doses too small to inactivate the phage. Prophages that are poorly inducible by UV light can be induced by thymine starvation, x-rays, alkylating agents, or some carcinogens. Some prophages cannot be induced at all; they do exhibit spontaneous induction but at a lower frequency than the inducible phages.

Induction of prophage λ has proved useful for the **identification of some carcinogenic chemicals,** which are strong inducers. Special lysogens are used, with cellular mutations for high permeability (since many carcinogens do not enter normal cells) and for elimination of excision repair (to enhance induction).

Mechanism of Induction

Induction is produced by conditions that remove the prophage from control by the repressor. Thus, when a lysogenic *Hfr* cell conjugates with a nonlysogenic F⁻ cell, induction occurs as soon as the prophage is introduced into the nonrepressive F⁻ cytoplasm (**zygotic induction).** A different mechanism is the infection of λ-lysogenic cells with a **virulent** λ mutant. Because the mutant is insensitive to the *cIR*, it produces in the cells all the gene products required for prophage excision and vegetative growth. The resident prophage is therefore induced despite the presence of its own repressor.

cIR inactivation is the most common mechanism of induction, generally as the consequence of changes initiated by UV light or other agents that produce, either directly or indirectly (i.e., during repair), **single-strand nicks or gaps** in DNA. The altered DNA causes activation of the cellular **rec A protease,** which cleaves the normal λ *cIR*. OR then synthesizes *croR*, which blocks *prm*.

This type of induction is part of a more general response of bacteria, whether or not lysogenic, to DNA damage. This "**SOS response**" (see Chap. 8), which tends to rescue the cell from genetic damage, includes activation of a new, error-prone DNA repair pathway and inhibition of bacterial division, with filamentous growth. The effect on phage allows it to abandon an irreparably damaged host.

EFFECT OF PROPHAGE ON HOST FUNCTIONS

Except for transducing phages (see below), which carry genes known to be derived from a recent bacterial host, most prophages exert no discernible effect on the bacterial phenotype other than immunity to superinfection. Certain prophages, however, change the cell's phenotype, either by expressing new functions (phage conversion) or by quantitatively modifying the expression of adjacent bacterial genes.

In **phage conversion** the new functions are viral, since they are abolished by phage mutations. Examples are changes of surface antigens in *Salmonella typhimu-*

rium and the formation of toxins by *Corynebacterium diphtheriae* and other bacteria. These effects are expressed by both vegetative phage and prophage, but other converting functions are expressed only by the prophage. For example, the resistance of *E. coli* K12(λ) to T-even phages with an r$_{II}$ mutation (see Conditionally Lethal Mutants, Chap. 45) is caused by the *rex* gene, which is located in the immunity operon and hence expressed only by prophage.

PHAGE Mu
Transposonlike Properties, Bacterial Termini

Phage Mu is a temperate phage of considerable interest because it is a transposon (see Chap. 8) in phage form. It has important applications in studies of bacterial genetics owing to its ability to integrate into, and inactivate, any genes. The name *Mu* derives, in fact, from this ability to **induce mutations.**

The mature genome of Mu is linear double-stranded DNA, 37 Kb long. It has the remarkable feature of possessing **heterogeneous ends of bacterial origin.** In Mu DNA we must therefore distinguish the constant central **viral part,** which is the **Mu genome,** and the short, variable bacterial ends. In different Mu DNA molecules the bacterial ends are different, and in a large population of molecules they encompass essentially all host sequences. The mechanism that generates these ends will become apparent below.

Invertible Sequence

Another special feature is that a sequence (**G segment),** about 3 Kb long within the viral DNA, can appear in **either orientation** in different molecules. It contains the COOH end of the gene for the tail fibers, the remainder of which is in the adjacent noninvertible region. A different sequence is therefore transcribed in each orientation. By inverting the G segment the phage can switch its receptor-binding specificity from one group to another in the bacterial lipopolysaccharide, and therefore from one host to another. The frequent inversions occur by a site-specific recombination between two identical inverted repeat sequences, 34 base pairs long, which bracket the invertible region. The inversion is analogous in both mechanism and significance to the phase shift in *Salmonella* (see Chap. 8) and to a similar mechanism for changing host range in phage P1. The invertase specified by the Mu gene *Gin* is 60% to 70% identical in amino acid sequence to the invertase of the other two systems and is interchangeable with them. It is also related to the resolvases of some transposons (see Chap. 8).

Lysogenization and Its Consequences

The regulatory system that controls the choice between lytic and lysogenic development of bacteriophage Mu includes a repressor gene C, comparable to λ cI, and a gene *ner*, comparable to λ *cro*. The biology of this bacteriophage is dominated by the activity of the viral DNA component as a **transposon** (see Chap. 8). The Mu genome lacks the terminal repeats that are characteristic of transposons but has repeats near the ends, which perform the same function.

The events unfolding in the infected cells have been clarified by studying *in vitro* the interaction of two plasmids, one containing the two ends of the Mu genome, and the other used to imitate the host genome. An extract of induced Mu-infected cells provided the needed enzymes and other proteins. As Fig. 46–10 shows, the two plasmids, held by proteins in a stable **transposome**, undergo staggered cuts, and two of the four ends join to form a **transposition intermediate (TI).** This can evolve in two ways. (1) **Non-replicative transposition** (see Fig. 46–10*A*) transfers the ends of the Mu genome, **without**

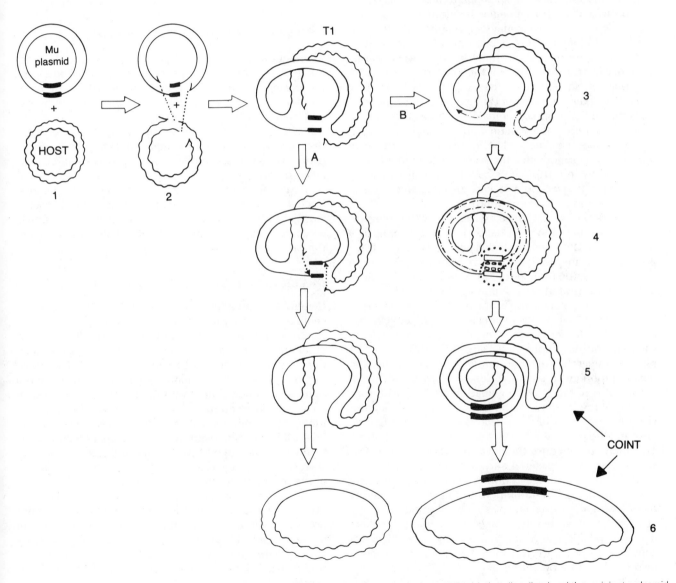

Figure 46–10. Transposition of the Mu genome *in vitro*. The donor is a plasmid (*thick lines*) containing Mu (*medium lines*) and the recipient a plasmid imitating the host genome (*thin lines; 1*). Cuts are produced at the two ends of Mu genome and in the host DNA (*2*); joining of the ends generates the transposition intermediate (*T1*). *(A)* Nonreplicative transposition by transfer of the genome without flanking sequences results in simple integration. *(B)* Replicative transposition. Elongation of the free ends of the host genome copies the Mu DNA (*3*), until the whole Mu genome with flanking plasmid sequences is replicated (*4*). An exchange at the two ends generates the cointegrate (*COINT; 5,6*). (Redrawn from Craigie R, Mizuuchi K: Cell 41:867–876, 1985)

the flanking plasmid sequences, to the host DNA, generating a simple insertion. (2) **Replicative transposition** (see Fig. 46–10*B*) extends the ends of the host genome to replicate the Mu-containing plasmid, **including the sequences flanking the Mu genome.** At the end of replication the free ends join, generating a **cointegrate,** which contains two copies of the Mu-containing plasmid integrated in the host genome. The choice between the two pathways is determined by the available enzymes, whether for DNA transfer or replication. Both simple insertion and replicative transposition require phage-specified protein A, the **transposase;** in addition, phage protein B increases the efficiency of transposition 100-fold.

When Mu infects a host bacterium, integration occurs by simple insertion of the genome, without the bacterial sequences, **at any place** in the bacterial DNA. Like transposons (see Chap. 8), the prophage is flanked by two 5-base-pair segments of duplicated host sequences. The ends of the prophage coincide with those of the Mu genome; therefore, the genetic maps of the phage and of the prophage are identical. The insertion of the prophage usually **inactivates** the bacterial gene in which it is inserted by interrupting its coding sequences, and by terminating transcription it can also inactivate distal genes in the same operon (**polarity**).

Induction does not cause excision, as with other prophages: instead, the prophage undergoes replicative transposition to a different site on the bacterial DNA. Replicative transposition goes on repeatedly, at each step doubling the number of Mu genomes, and generating many integrated copies of Mu DNA per cell.

A Mu DNA molecule leaves the host chromosome by a transposition that causes the detachment of a **cyclic hybrid molecule** containing a host segment adjacent to each end of the prophage. Because Mu DNA molecules may be integrated all over the host chromosome, the host component in such hybrids is highly variable. Encapsidation of Mu DNA contained in such hybrid rings occurs by the headful method, starting at a **packaging site** near one end of the phage genome and retaining only small parts of the host DNA from the cyclic hybrid. This method generates the linear molecules of Mu DNA with two variable bacterial ends, present in virions.

The hybrid rings may contain host markers or integrated episomes (**Mu-mediated mobilization of genes or episomes**). Conversely, phages or plasmids carrying Mu can be integrated into the chromosome by replicative transposition and are found flanked by two Mu genomes in identical orientation (**Mu-mediated integration of phage or episomes**).

SIGNIFICANCE OF LYSOGENY

Lysogeny indicates a close evolutionary relation between phages and transposing elements (see Chap. 8). All ly-sogeny depends on a site-specific recombination that is carried out by an enzyme with characteristics similar to those of the transposon resolvase. Moreover, transposable phage has all the characteristics of transposing elements.

Prophages give rise to **infectious heredity,** contributing new genetic characteristics to their host cells. Prophages that are not inducible and do not confer immunity cannot be distinguished from segments of cellular genetic material except by identifying their genes.

Phages as Transducing Agents

Transduction of bacterial genes from one cell to another by phages has been extensively used for mapping the bacterial chromosome (see Transduction, Chap. 7) and for studying gene regulation. Although now largely superseded in experimentation by DNA cloning and transfection, it still retains considerable interest as a natural process that interchanges bacterial and phage genes. The virologic aspects of the process will be considered here.

Two types can be distinguished: generalized transduction can transfer any bacterial genes, and restricted (specialized) transduction can transfer genes from only a very small region of the host chromosome adjacent to the prophage site.

GENERALIZED TRANSDUCTION

Generalized transduction is due to the encapsidation of cellular DNA in a phage coat by the headful mechanism (see Association of DNA and Capsid, Chap. 44). Apparently any marker of the donor bacterium can be transduced at a frequency of 10^{-5} to 10^{-8} per cell. The transducing DNA is not a replicon, and in the recipient cells a segment is incorporated into the host DNA by a double crossover, **in exchange for bacterial genes.** This homologous recombination is under the rec system of the host. Only closely linked markers can be **cotransduced** by the same phage particle because the piece of bacterial DNA carried by a phage corresponds to about 1% to 2% of the bacterial DNA.

Transduction is usually carried out with a high-titer phage preparation, which can be obtained from the donor strain either by lytic infection or by induction of lysogenic cells. Phage P1 is widely used in genetic studies of *Salmonella*, *E. coli*, and *Shigella*. Transduction occurs with different phages for many other bacterial genera.

Abortive Transduction

The introduced fragment of bacterial DNA (the **exogenote**) may persist without being integrated or replicated. Then it is transmitted **unilinearly,** i.e., from a cell to only one of its two daughters in which it expresses the functions of its genes. Such abortive transduction is easily recognized when the exogenote codes for an enzyme required for growth on a selective medium, for the restricted amount resulting from the unilinear inheritance yields **microcolonies** on minimal medium. The proportion of these to the large colonies generated by complete transduction reveals that **abortive transduction is several times more common;** hence, the probability of integration of the exogenote is rather small.

SPECIALIZED TRANSDUCTION

Phage λ can occasionally give rise to transduction in quite a different manner. It transfers only a **restricted group of genes** (the *gal* or *bio* regions) that are located near the prophage (see Fig. 46–11), and it is generated **only on induction of prophage,** but not (in contrast to generalized transduction) in lytic infection. The transducing genes are incorporated into the phage genome during abnormal excisions of the prophage.

The transducing λ virions have lost some λ DNA, to compensate in length for the incorporation of phage genes. As a result, most kinds of transducing particles are defective; i.e., they cannot multiply by themselves (e.g., λ*dgal,* λ*dbio,* where d stands for defective). However, they can replicate in mixed infection with regular λ as a **helper** to complement the missing functions. Some types of transducing particles (e.g., λ*gal,* λ*bio*) are infectious, because the missing phage genes are not essential for vegetative multiplication (Fig. 46–11).

Specialized transduction suggests an evolutionary relationship between bacteria and phages based on exchanges between their DNAs.

Bacteriophages as Vectors for DNA Cloning

BACTERIOPHAGE λ VECTORS

Phage λ is a suitable vector for DNA cloning because about one third of the genome (between genes J and N; see Fig. 46–4) is not needed for phage multiplication and can be replaced by foreign DNA. The total length of the hybrid DNA must be between 78% and 105% of that of the wild-type genome for efficient encapsidation. λ DNA contains multiple targets for restriction endonucleases, but variants with one or two targets, in the nonessential region, can be obtained by suitable selection or *in vitro* DNA recombination. Phage with a single target is suitable as **insertion vector:** its DNA is cut with the enzyme, and a fragment of foreign DNA is ligated in, reconstituting a

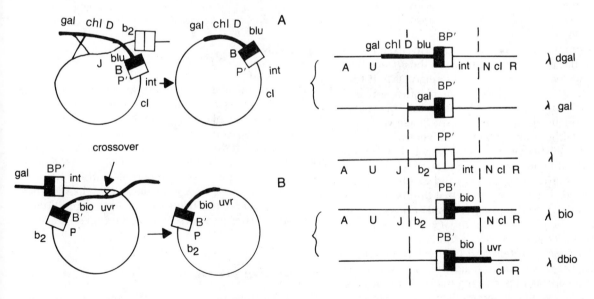

Figure 46–11. Production of transducing λ derivatives by crossovers outside the attachment sites. Crossovers on the left of the prophage *(A)* generate molecules containing *gal* and other bacterial genes (λ*dgal*) (where d stands for defective), which cannot replicate owing to loss of capsid genes. If the bacterium is deleted between *gal* and the prophage, *gal* genes can be incorporated in replacement of the nonessential b$_2$ region, and the phage is not defective (λ*gal*). Crossovers on the right *(B)* generate molecules containing *bio,* sometimes with other bacterial genes. Gene *bio* replaces recombination genes, and the phage can replicate (λ*bio*); if the replacement is longer (including N), the phage is defective (λ*dbio*). Phage λ*dgalbio,* which was useful for studying *int-xis*–promoted vegetative recombination, is obtained by recombination between λ*dgal* and λ*dbio.* The DNA between the two broken lines is not essential for replication. *Heavy lines,* bacterial DNA; *thin lines,* phage DNA.

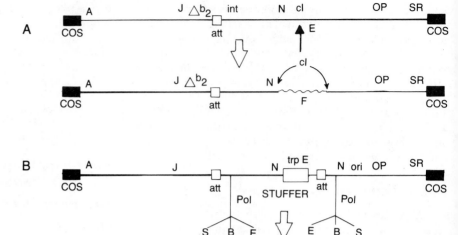

Figure 46-12. *(A)* Insertion vector λgt 10. This vector has a single site for restriction endonuclease EcoR1 *(E)* within the *cl* gene *(arrow).* The nonessential G$_2$ region has been partly deleted (Δb$_2$) to accommodate a longer insert. Insertion of a segment of foreign DNA *(wavy line)* inactivates the gene: the hybrid vector, *cl$^-$*, makes clear plaques, whereas the intact vector makes turbid plaques. *(B)* Replacement vector EMBL3. This vector is the result of many manipulations, during which the *E. coli* tryptophan E gene *(trp E)* was inserted in the immunity region, and the region around N and *att* was duplicated. Two polylinkers *(Pol)*, each carrying targets for three restriction endonucleases *(S,* Sal 1; *B,* Bam H1; *E,* EcoR1) were introduced near the two borders of the nonessential central region; their presence increases flexibility in the use of the vector. Using any of the three enzymes, the central "stuffer" segment is removed and is then replaced by the insertion of foreign DNA *(wavy line).* The resulting hybrid vectors are selected because, being red$^-$ gamma$^-$, they are Spi$^-$, and therefore able to grow on a P2 lysogen, whereas the intact, Spi$^+$, vector cannot. Lacking *int,* the hybrid vectors cannot lysogenize. For symbols, see λ map (Fig. 46–4).

complete genome with the addition. An example is λgt10, which has a single *EcoR1* target in the *cI* gene (Fig. 46–12*A*). Phage with an insertion of foreign DNA at that site becomes *cI$^-$* and produces clear plaques, a useful marker for selecting phages with insertion. This vector can accommodate up to 7 Kb of DNA. Phage with two targets is suitable as a **replacement vector** (see Fig. 46–12*B*). The DNA between the two targets is removed and replaced with a foreign fragment. Such a vector can accommodate between about 5 Kb and 22 Kb.

A favorable feature of λ vectors is that **the hybrid DNA can be packaged into the phage capsid *in vitro*,** greatly simplifying the cloning process. *In vitro* packaging employs two phage strains. One has a mutation in the gene for the major capsid protein and is therefore unable to make heads. The other makes heads but has mutations that make it incapable of packaging the DNA. In infected bacteria each accumulates incomplete phage particles. When extracts of the two kinds of infected bacteria are mixed together with hybrid DNA of a proper size, the two mutations complement each other: the DNA is packaged, and complete phage is made. Upon infecting sensitive cells, this phage injects the hybrid DNA, which multiplies and can be recovered in pure form.

COSMIDS

λ Vectors cannot accommodate DNA fragments larger than 23 Kb and so are unsuitable for cloning large genes. This difficulty is overcome by using cosmid vectors. These are small plasmids with the sequence *(cos)* for making cohesive ends and for packaging λ DNA (Fig. 46–13). They also have the origin of DNA replication of the plasmid, a drug-resistance gene to aid in selection of recombinants, and several different restriction targets. They are packaged in λ capsids *in vitro* like regular λ DNA. After injection of bacteria, hybrid DNA multiplies as a plasmid. These vectors can accommodate fragments up to 45 Kb.

PHAGE M13 VECTORS

The filamentous phage M13, with cyclic, single-stranded DNA (see Chap. 45), has been transformed into a vector by first inserting the β-galatosidase gene in a nonessential sequence (Fig. 46–14). Within this gene a **polylinker** (i.e., a series of targets for various restriction endonucleases) has been placed in a way that does not prevent expression of the gene.

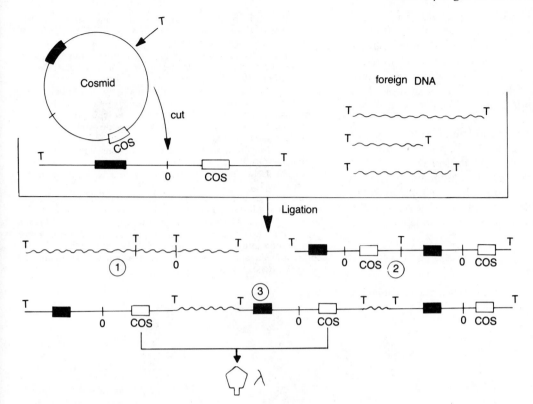

Figure 46–13. DNA cloning in a cosmid vector. The covalently closed vector contains a plasmid origin of replication (*0*), a gene for drug resistance (*black bar*), a target (*T*) for a restriction endonuclease, and the *cos* sequence. The vector and foreign DNA are cut with the restriction endonuclease and then ligated. Various products are formed: (*1*) a concatemer of foreign DNA fragments, (*2*) a concatemer of cosmids, and (*3*) a concatemer containing cosmids with foreign DNA insertions. Only the last ones are packaged in λ capsids because they possess *cos* sites at the proper distances. In an infected culture the vector-containing bacteria are readily selected because they produce drug-resistant colonies (Modified from Maniatis T, Fritsch EF, Sambrook T: Molecular Cloning. Cold Spring Harbor, NY, Cold Spring Harbor Laboratory, 1982)

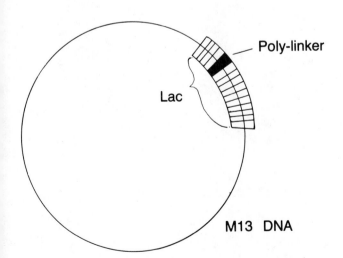

Figure 46–14. M13 cloning vector. A bacterial gene for β-galactosidase (*dashed*) is inserted in the nonessential region of the phage genome. The polylinker (*black*) within the gene by itself does not prevent β-galactosidase expression, which is abolished after foreign DNA is inserted at one of the targets. On plates containing a chromogenic β-galactoside, cells infected by the vector alone generate colored turbid plaques, while those with a foreign insertion make colorless plaques. (Modified from Maniatis T, Fritsch EF, Sambrook J: Molecular Cloning. Cold Spring Harbor, NY, Cold Spring Harbor Laboratory, 1982)

Through the use of one of the restriction sites of the polylinker, the foreign DNA is inserted into the double-stranded parental RF of the phage, which is then introduced into bacteria by transfection. The insertion destroys the function of the β-galactosidase gene. β-Galactosidase–negative turbid plaques produced by the transfected cells on indicator plates contain phage with the insert.

M13 vectors can accommodate widely different lengths of foreign DNA because during phage maturation the virions adjust their length to that of the DNA. The main use of this vector is for DNA sequencing: extraction of the progeny phage yields directly the single-stranded hybrid DNA that is needed for replication *in vitro*, in the presence of dideoxy nucleotides in the Sanger method.

Selected Reading

Buchari AI: Bacteriophage Mu as a transposition element. Annu Rev Genet 10:389, 1976

Craigie R, Mizuuchi K: Mechanism of transposition of bacteriophage Mu: Structure of a transposition intermediate. Cell 41:867, 1985

Friedman DI, Olson ER, Georgopulos C et al: Interaction of bacteriophage and host macromolecules in the growth of bacteriophage λ. Microbiol Rev 48:299, 1984

Friedman DI, Schauer AT, Olson ER et al: Proteins and nucleic acid sequences involved in regulation of gene expression by bacteriophage λ N transcription antitermination function. In Leive L (ed): Microbiology—1985, pp 271–176. Washington, American Society for Microbiology, 1985

Geider K: DNA cloning vectors utilizing functions of the filamentous phages of *Escherichia Coli*. J Gen Virol 67:2287, 1986

Glover DM: DNA Cloning: A Practical Approach. Washington, IRL Press, 1985

Ptashne M: A genetic switch; gene control of phage λ. Oxford, Cell Press and Blackwell Scientific Publications, 1986

Richet E, Abcarian P, Nash HA: The interaction of recombination proteins with supercoiled DNA: Defining the role of supercoiling in lambda integrative recombination. Cell 46:1011, 1986

Sadowski P: Site-specific recombinases: Changing partners and doing the twist. J Bacteriol 165:341, 1986

47

Animal Cells: Cultivation, Growth Regulation, Transformation

In animal cells growing in artificial media the effects of viruses can be detected by changes in the characteristics of the cells, and sometimes by cell death. The development of improved methods for cultivating the cells has been essential to the progress of animal virology. In particular, cell cultures provide quantitative techniques comparable to those used for bacteriophages, and with oncogenic viruses they provide methods for studying effects on the regulation of cell growth.

In this chapter we will consider the properties of cell cultures; the control of cell growth, including the roles of growth factors; and the genetic properties of cultured cells that are relevant for virology.

Characteristics of Cultures of Animal Cells

RELATION OF CELLS TO A SOLID SUPPORT. To prepare cell cultures containing separated animal cells, tissue fragments are first dissociated, usually with the aid of trypsin or collagenase. The cell suspension is then placed in a flat-bottomed **glass or plastic container** (a Petri dish, a flask, a bottle, or a test tube), together with a **liquid medium** (such as that devised by Eagle) containing required ions at isosmotic concentration, a number of amino acids and vitamins, and an animal serum in a proportion varying from a few percent to 50%. Bicarbonate is commonly used as a buffer, in equilibrium with

CO_2 (from 5% to 10%) in the air above the medium. After a variable lag the cells attach and spread on the bottom of the container and then start dividing mitotically, giving rise to a **primary culture.** Attachment to a rigid support is essential for the growth of normal cells (**anchorage dependence**) except those of the hemopoietic system.

Electron micrographs show that animal cells attach at a few points to the bottom of the vessel but elsewhere are separated by a layer of medium. The cells move actively, as shown by slow-motion pictures of living cell cultures under phase-contrast microscopy. The advancing part of a fibroblast is thin and rapidly moving (**ruffling**); the plasma membrane flows from the forward edge toward the nucleus, as seen from the motion of adhering particles. This flow is supported by the continuous arrival of membrane vesicles from the cytoplasm to the leading edge, where they fuse with the cell membrane, causing its expansion.

PRIMARY AND SECONDARY CULTURES. Primary cultures are maintained by changing the fluid two or three times a week. When the cultures become too crowded, the cells are detached from the vessel wall by either trypsin or the chelating agent EDTA, and portions are used to initiate new **secondary cultures (transfer).**

In both primary and secondary cultures the cells retain some of the characteristics of the tissue from which they were derived, and are mainly of two types: thin and elongated (**fibroblast like**), or polygonal and tending to form sheets (**epitheliumlike**). In addition, certain cells have a roundish outline and resemble epithelial cells but do not form sheets (**epithelioid cells**). The cells multiply to cover the bottom of the container with a continuous thin layer, often one cell thick (**monolayer**); if they are fibroblastic, they are **regularly oriented** parallel to each other. Primary cell cultures obtained from **cancerous tissues** usually differ from those of normal cells (see Cell Transformation, below).

CELL STRAINS AND CELL LINES. Cells from primary cultures can often be transferred serially a number of times. This process usually causes a selection of some cell type, which becomes predominant. The cells may then continue to multiply at a constant rate over many successive transfers, and the primary culture is said to have originated a **cell strain** (often called a **diploid cell strain**), the cells of which appear unaltered in morphologic and growth properties (Fig. 47–1). These cells must be transferred at a relatively high cell density to initiate a new culture, but eventually they undergo **culture senescence** and cannot be transferred any longer. For instance, with cultures of human cells the growth rate declines after about 50 duplications, and the life of the strain comes to an end.

During the multiplication of a cell strain some cells become **altered;** they acquire a different morphology, grow faster, and become able to start a culture from a small number of cells. The clone derived from one such cell is a **cell line;** in contrast to the cell strain in which it originated, it has unlimited life (**immortalization**). Cell lines derived from normal cells have a low **saturation density** under standard conditions (e.g., addition of 10%

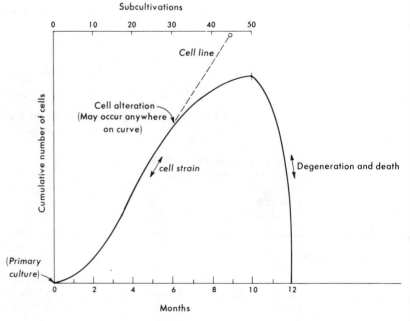

Figure 47–1. Multiplication of cultures of cells derived from normal tissues. The primary culture gives rise to a cell **strain,** the cells of which grow actively for many cell generations; then growth declines, and finally the culture stops growing and dies. During multiplication of the cell strain, altered cells may be produced, which continue to grow indefinitely and originate a cell **line.** The cumulative number of cells is calculated as if all cells derived from the original culture had been kept at every transfer. (Modified from Hayflick L: Analytic Cell Culture. National Cancer Institute Monograph, No. 7, 1962, p. 63)

serum and changes of medium two or three times weekly); they grow rapidly to form a monolayer and then slow down (**topoinhibition**).

MECHANISM OF CULTURE SENESCENCE. Senescence appears to depend directly on the **number of doublings** rather than on astronomical time. It does not depend on the special conditions of growth *in vitro*: **it also occurs *in vivo*,** as during serial transplantation from mouse to mouse of mouse mammary epithelium or of hemopoietic cells. Aging *in vitro* and *in vivo* are related: fibroblasts obtained from human donors of increasing ages or from patients with Werner's syndrome (premature aging), who have a shortened life span, can undergo fewer generations *in vitro*.

The mechanism of cellular senescence is obscure. A contributing factor may be the **accumulation of unrepaired damage** in cellular constituents. Accumulation of mutations in DNA may lower the growth ability of the cells and finally become lethal. Accidental errors in translation, causing changes in proteins that can in turn decrease the accuracy of information transfer (such as the aminoacyl-tRNA synthetases and DNA and RNA polymerases) may also cause progressive deterioration of cellular proteins, even independently of mutation. Indeed, in cultures of the mold *Neurospora* that are undergoing senescence, altered and partly inactive enzymes accumulate in the cells.

A second factor may be the **absence of efficient selection** against cumulative damage, because the culture of untransformed cells requires seeding at a relatively high cell density, and the cells also have their growth limited soon by **density-dependent growth inhibition.** In cell lines, in contrast, the cells initiate growth at low density, and selection against damaged cells is increased.

A third factor is the influence of **terminal differentiation** (see below), which limits life span *in vitro*. Thus, human keratinocytes on feeder layers of murine fibroblastlike 3T3 cells normally survive for about 50 cell generations (less if from old donors), then differentiate into squamous cells and die. If the cultures are grown in the presence of epidermal growth factor (EGF; see Growth Factors, below), their life span increases to about 150 generations, apparently because differentiation is delayed. Cellular changes preventing terminal differentiation may be responsible for lack of senescence in permanent cell lines.

LIQUID SUSPENSION CULTURES. Cell lines derived from cancers or from transformed cells (see below) sometimes produce cells with low adhesion to the container. These cells can be propagated in suspension by using a liquid medium poor in divalent ions and stirring constantly.

Such suspension cultures (e.g., derivatives of murine L cells) are very useful for virological studies.

STORAGE. Because cell strains tend to exhaust their growth potential on repeated cultivation, lines tend to change continually; it is useful to keep cells of early passages **in the frozen state.** Large batches of cells are mixed with glycerol or dimethylsulfoxide and subdivided in a number of ampules, which are then sealed and frozen. The additives allow the cells to survive the freezing. The frozen cells can be maintained for years in liquid nitrogen **with unchanged characteristics;** when the ampules are thawed, most of the cells are viable and can initiate new cultures.

SPECIAL PROPERTIES OF CELLS IN CULTURES

COMMUNICATION BETWEEN CELLS. Though the cells of a culture are separate in many respects, **gap** junctions form where the plasma membranes of two cells come in contact, providing some continuity. Channels in the junctions are revealed by a low electrical resistance between the cells and by the passage of fluorescent substances (of molecular weight up to 2000), injected into a cell, to adjacent cells. Through the channels, metabolic intermediates are exchanged between cells in sufficient quantities to allow cells with a metabolic defect to grow in mixed culture with normal cells (**metabolic cooperation**).

Gap junctions are visible by freeze-fracture electron microscopy (Fig. 47–2) as areas of closely packed particles, 8 nm to 9 nm in diameter, spanning the membrane where the plasma membranes of two cells touch each other. These particles each have a central channel that admits water and solutes.

STATE OF DIFFERENTIATION. Animal cells in culture retain, at least in part, the state of differentiation they had in the animal, but it may not be easily recognizable. However, specific products can sometimes be formed, e.g., collagen from fibroblasts, cytokeratins from epithelia, casein from mammary gland cells, and specific hormones from pituitary and other hormone-producing cells. A differentiation potential may also be expressed *in vitro*: thus, skin keratinocytes differentiate into squamous cells, and 3T3 cells (skin "fibroblasts") into fat cells.

CLONING OF ANIMAL CELLS

Colonies can be obtained from most cell strains or lines by transferring cells to new cultures at a very high dilution. For cell lines the proportion of cells that give rise to colonies (**efficiency of plating**) approaches 100%, but for primary cultures or cell strains it is very small. The efficiency of plating can be greatly increased if the cells are

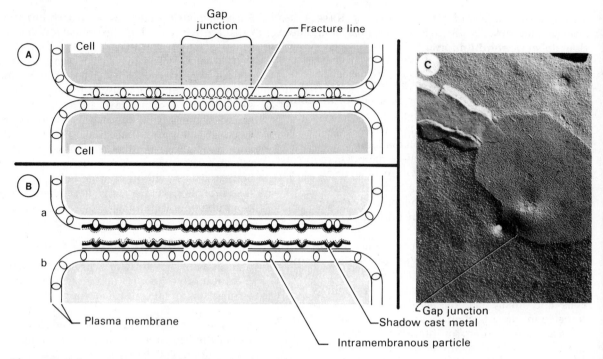

Figure 47–2. Intramembranous particles and gap junctions. A frozen cell preparation is fractured by hitting it with a knife. The fracture frequently goes through membranes, separating them into two layers. Where two cells are in contact *(A)* the fracture line *(broken line)* sometimes goes through a junction. The products of fracture *(B)* are coated with evaporated metal, and a replica of the surface is examined in the electron microscope. *(C)* Photograph of surface fracture *b* shows the gap junctions *(arrow)* and the intramembranous particles. (Courtesy of D. A. Goodenough)

mixed with a **feeder layer** of similar cells made incapable of multiplication by x-irradiation or mitomycin; these cells are still metabolically active and supply substances needed for growth. The efficiency of plating can also be increased by introducing individual cells into very small volumes of medium (as in sealed capillary tubes or in small drops of medium surrounded by paraffin oil),

which allow the cell products to reach an adequate concentration. In this way **clonal lines** are prepared.

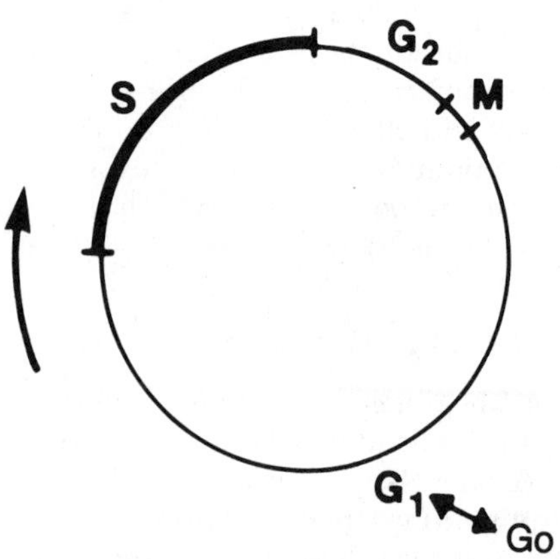

The Cell Growth Cycle

As with bacteria (see Chap. 3), the cells of a sparse culture in optimal medium multiply exponentially (i.e., with a fixed doubling time), although individual cells divide at random times. The cell growth cycle consists of four main phases (Fig. 47–3), each with a different biochemical and regulatory significance. DNA synthesis occupies only a fraction of the doubling time, the **synthetic (S) period,** which is separated from the **mitotic (M) period** by the **G2 period** (G for gap). After the mitotic phase and before the S period is the **G1 period,** which can vary enormously in length, depending on the cell type and the growth conditions.

The distribution of the cells of a culture in the various phases can be ascertained by **flow cytofluorometry,** as portrayed in Figure 47–4. From cells with a doubling time of 18 hours, typical lengths of the various periods are G1, 10 hours; S, 6 to 7 hours; G2, 1 hour; and M, about $\frac{1}{2}$ hour. Progress from one phase to another results from accumulation of specific substances within the cells, as

Figure 47–3. The cell growth cycle.

shown by the behavior of cell hybrids, obtained by the fusion of two cells. Thus, when the DNA of a cell in G1 is fused with a cell in S, it starts replicating, while it tends to condense into mitotic chromosomes when fused with a cell in mitosis.

SYNCHRONIZATION. The cell growth cycle is directly observable in synchronized cultures. The preferred method of synchronization is to start a culture with mitotic cells, which are weakly attached to the vessel and can be collected by shaking a randomly growing culture. However, after the first cycle, synchronization is rapidly lost because the G1 phases have different lengths in different cells.

GROWTH RESTRICTION IN G1. Cultures of untransformed cells stop growing after the depletion of serum or growth factors or, for certain cell types, of some amino acids or ions. The cultures then survive in a **quiescent state** known as **G0.** Growth resumes after addition of the depleted substance.

The growth of a quiescent culture can also be restored locally by removing a strip of cells (a **wound**) without replenishing the medium. Cells penetrating the wound from the edges initiate DNA synthesis within 12 hours and then divide. This phenomenon indicates that in such cultures growth stoppage also depends on local conditions (**topoinhibition**). A major source of topoinhibition is a boundary layer of the watery medium in contact with a continuous cell layer, through which medium factors can penetrate only by diffusion. Elimination of the boundary layer at the edges of a wound allows the factors to reach the cells much more efficiently by convection.

Cytofluorometry shows that **in quiescent untransformed cultures the cells are arrested in the G0 phase.** These cultures manifest a reduced uptake of glucose, phosphate, and other substances and a reduced synthesis of RNA and proteins; they display faster protein degradation and have most of the mRNAs free, rather than in polysomes.

The great variation in length of the G1 phase accounts for most of the variation in the total cycle time. Apparently, during the G1 phase the growth of untransformed cells must proceed through **restriction points** that are overcome by the availability of factors from the medium. A single factor may be sufficient for some cells, but several are needed for others. Serum contains many factors, but only one is usually limiting, causing the G1 lengths of different cells to follow a "single-event" distribution.

MECHANISM OF GROWTH CONTROL

We must distinguish between the **periodic doubling** of cell number and the **increase in cell mass.** Although

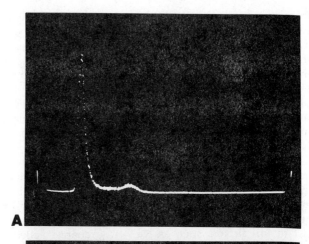

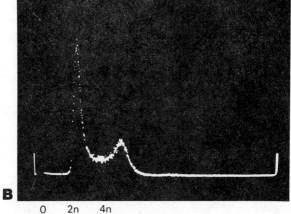

Figure 47–4. Flow cytofluorometry of fibroblastic cells. A single-cell suspension is exposed to an acridine dye, which, after intercalating in DNA, fluoresces green. The cells pass one at a time through a laser beam, and the excited fluorescence, which quantitates the amount of DNA, is measured. Each point in the graphs shows the number of cells that have the amount of DNA given in the abscissa. The tall peak at left measures the number of cells in G1 (with a diploid amount of DNA); the smaller peak at right measures the number of cells in G2 (with a tetraploid amount of DNA). Cells in S phase are between the two peaks. *(A)* Quiescent population, with most cells in G1 or G0. *(B)* Growing population, with a substantial proportion in S and G2. (Courtesy of R. E. Holley)

they go on at the same time in growing cultures, they are independently regulated. In early embryos, cells divide without increase in mass, and their size decreases at each division. Cultured cells can also be caused to initiate DNA replication without an increase in size by means of an alkaline shock, the rationale of which is discussed below. Studies with embryos show that the rapid periodic doubling involves only two phases, S and M.

The alternation of the two phases depends mainly on the alternative synthesis and destruction of a protein (**maturation-promoting factor,** MPF) that causes the cells to progress to the M phase. Influx or release of Ca^{2+}

from storage allows progress from M to S, apparently by causing MPF breakdown or inactivation. In somatic cells a protein, **cyclin,** perhaps similar to MPF, accumulates in the nucleus during S phase. DNA replication in S is controlled by the state of DNA or chromatin rather than by biosynthetic enzymes. Cycling is controlled by the cytoplasm: the enucleated cytoplasm of a fertilized oocyte undergoes periodic, cycle-connected changes, and plasmidial DNA injected into it replicates when the S phase is reached.

At later stages of embryonic development, and in adult animals, increase in cell mass occurs mainly during the G1 phase. In these cells multiple biochemical events take place after addition of a growth factor to quiescent cells (**pleiotypic response**). **Early events** consist in **ion fluxes,** such as Na^+-H^+ exchange activity, which increases the pH of the cytoplasm. This increase is required for growth: mutants lacking the ion exchange activity can grow only at alkaline pH. Ca^{2+} concentration increases by influx or by mobilization from membrane storage. The ionic changes activate energy-yielding and synthetic pathways. These early changes vary with cell type and growth factors, suggesting that different changes act as signals in different cells, perhaps depending on the specific blocks to be overcome in different cases.

The **late events** include many synthetic processes. The synthesis of polyamines increases; this is an essential step because its inhibition arrests cell growth. The polyamines may be needed for increasing transcription of DNA or for preparing it for replication. Later, the rate of protein synthesis increases by translation of mRNAs that had become dissociated from ribosomes in the period of quiescence; the synthesis includes cycle-specific proteins (e.g., receptors for other factors).

GROWTH FACTORS

Important for fibroblastic cells is a growth factor isolated by Ross from platelets (**platelet-derived growth factor, PDGF**). It is a small protein, made up of two chains, that is stored in the α granules of platelets and is released during blood clotting; hence, plasma has a much lower growth-promoting activity than serum. The **epidermal**

TABLE 47–1. Origins and Targets of Growth Factors

Growth Factor	Origin	Target(s)
Epidermal GF (EGF)	Submaxillary gland	Fibroblasts, epithelia
Tumor GF (TGFα) related to EGF	Cancer or embryonic	Fibroblasts, epithelia
TGFβ	Many cells	Many cell types, both stimulatory and inhibitory
Platelet-derived GF (PDGF)	Platelets	Fibroblasts, cells of mesodermal origin
Insulin	Pancreas	Fibroblasts
Insulinlike GF I	Liver	Fibroblasts, epithelia
Insulinlike GF II	Liver, placenta	Fibroblasts, epithelia
Interleukin-1 (IL-1)	Macrophages	Immune cells, astroglia; mediator of inflammation
Interleukin-2 (IL-2)	T-helper cells	T-helper cells, cytotoxic lymphocytes
Interleukin-3 (IL-3)	WEHI-3B leukemia	Hematopoietic stem cells; erythroid differentiation
Nerve GF (NGF)	Submaxillary gland	Sympathetic, sensory neurons
Endothelial GF or FGF (basic)	Bovine pituitary, brain, retina, adrenal, kidney	Endothelial cells, fibroblasts
Endothelial GF or FGF (acidic)	Bovine brain, retina	Endothelial cells, fibroblasts
Hemopoietin	Bladder, carcinoma line	Primitive multipotent hemopoietic cells
Erythropoietin	Liver	Erythroid precursor
Granulocyte-macrophage colony stimulating factor (GM-CSF)	Many tissues, especially lung	Hemopoietic stem cells, neutrophil activator
Granulocyte colony stimulating factor (G-CSF)	Id	Hemopoietic stem cells
Macrophage colony stimulating factor (M-CSF or CSF-1)	L cells	Macrophage progenitors; macrophage activator
B-cell stimulating factor 1 (BSF-1)	T cells	Resting B cell
Neurotransmitters		
Substance P	Neurons	Fibroblasts, vascular smooth muscle cells
Substance K	Neurons	Fibroblasts, vascular smooth muscle cells
Vasopressin	Neurons	Chondrocytes, bone marrow cells
Bombesin	Neurons	Bronchial epithelial cells
Transferrin	Liver	Lymphocytes
Thrombin	Plasma prothrombin	Fibroblasts
Phorbol esters*	Synthetic	Swiss 3T3 cells
Diglycerol analogs*	Synthetic	Swiss 3T3 cells
Ca^{2+} ionophore A23187*	Synthetic	T cells

* Drugs that simulate growth factor activity

growth factor (EGF), isolated by Cohen from the mouse submaxillary gland and also present in human urine, stimulates the growth of both epithelial and fibroblastic cells. Table 47–1 lists other growth factors, some of which also have other functions, such as proteolytic enzymes (thrombin), hormones (insulin), lectins (concanavalin A), ionophores, tumor promoters, and neurotransmitters. Cells produce factors required for their own growth, as shown by the enhancing effect of **conditioned medium** obtained from actively growing cultures on the growth of sparse cultures. **Tumor growth factors,** which cause normal cells to display characteristics of transformed cells, are produced by some normal and some transformed cells.

Growth factors overcome the blocks to replication that occur during the G0–G1 phases of the cell cycle. Best studied is the role of PDGF, which promotes the transition of fibroblastic cells from G0 to G1. Other growth factors, such as insulinlike growth factors, can then cooperate with PDGF in overcoming the subsequent G1 restriction points.

RECEPTORS FOR GROWTH FACTORS

As shown earlier for polypeptide hormones, growth factors act by binding to specific high-affinity receptors on the cell surface. These receptors are glycoproteins, with an **external,** a **transmembrane,** and a **cytoplasmic domain** (Fig. 47–5). Most receptors have a single polypeptide chain, but those for insulin and for insulinlike growth factor I have two chains, connected by disulfide bonds; the α-chain is external, while the β-chain has the transmembrane and the cytoplasmic domain. The binding of a factor to the external domain of a receptor has two effects. It changes the cytoplasmic domain, generating an internal signal that alters cellular characteristics, and it initiates a series of events that lead to disappearance of the receptor (**down regulation;** see below), a step in the regulation of the factor's activity.

CYTOPLASMIC SIGNALS

Two main mechanisms are known. In one, binding of the factor to the external domain activates a **protein kinase with specificity for tyrosine** in the cytoplasmic domain. Such receptors include those for EGF, PDGF, insulin, insulinlike growth factor I, and CSF-1. The responsible sequence of the cytoplasmic domain is similar in the various receptors. With ATP used as a phosphate donor, the kinase phosphorylates a number of different proteins along with itself. Which are significant for growth control is not known.

In the other mechanism, **phospholipase C splits phosphatidylinositol-4,5-bisphosphate (PIP2)** in the membrane (Fig. 47–6). This pathway, utilized by PDGF

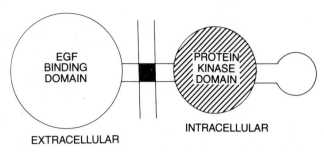

Figure 47–5. Arrangement of the EGF receptor showing the three domains: extracellular, transmembrane (*black*), and cytoplasmic, with two subdivisions, one of which is the protein kinase with tyrosine specificity. (Modified from Hunter T: Nature 311:414, 1984)

and many other receptors, is probably responsible for the early events in growth activation. Activation of the phospholipase may occur through **GTP-binding proteins** of the membranes, which, by hydrolyzing GTP to GDP, act as mediators between receptors and various kinds of regulatory proteins. For instance, adenyl cyclase is activated by such GTP-binding proteins in hormone-responsive cells.

The splitting of PIP2 generates two important activators of cellular functions: **inositol 1,4,5-triphosphate (IP3)** and **diacylglycerol (DG).** IP3 binds to receptors on the membranes of the endoplasmic reticulum, releasing bound Ca^{2+}; DG, in the presence of free Ca^{2+}, activates **protein kinase C,** a ubiquitous enzyme that phosphorylates serine and threonine (not tyrosine) in proteins. After binding DG in the presence of Ca^{2+}, the kinase sticks to the phospholipids of the membrane, where it phosphorylates various proteins. As shown below, these phosphorylations may have a regulatory role. A widely used growth and tumor protomer, TPA (tetradecanoyl phorbol acetate), acts like DG. The activation of protein kinase C increases the intracellular pH by about 0.15 units, probably by phosphorylating the Na^{+}-H^{+} transporter, which is activated during growth.

IP3 and DG have a variety of effects, not all related to growth control. Both have very short half-lives (minutes), because IP3 is rapidly dephosphorylated, and DG is phosphorylated to phosphatidic acid. The short life of these compounds is incompatible with a complete mitogenic role. They lead, however, to a prolonged effect, because IP3 is replaced by its longer-lasting 1,3,4 isomer, and the active form of protein kinase C persists. These two compounds and the tyrosine protein kinase probably initiate a cascade of reactions that generate the late events.

RECEPTOR TURNOVER

FORMATION OF RECEPTORS. As the polypeptide chains of the receptor glycoproteins are synthesized, they pene-

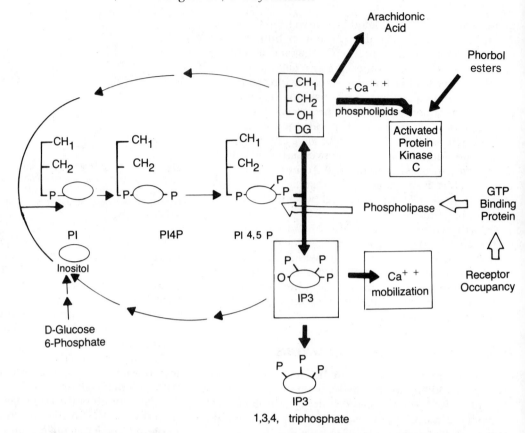

Figure 47–6. Inositol phospholipids in growth control. The thin lines indicate the turnover of inositol phospholipids. The boxes and heavy arrows indicate the compounds important in growth control; the open arrows indicate the activation pathway beginning at a receptor occupied by its ligand. *PI*, phosphatidylinositol; *PI4P*, phosphatidylinositol-4-phosphate; *PI4-5P*, phosphatidylinositol-4,5-diphosphate; *IP3*, inositol-1,4,5-triphosphate; *DG*, diacylglycerol. The significance of formation of arachidonic acid or inositol-1,3,4-triphosphate as well as inositol polyphosphates and cyclic phosphates (not shown) is unclear.

trate through the membrane of the rough endoplasmic reticulum (RER) by interaction of their **signal sequence** with a signal recognition ribonucleoprotein particle (SRP) and a membrane receptor (see Chap. 6). Within the tubules of the RER they remain connected to the RER membrane by an **anchor sequence** of hydrophobic amino acids. From the RER the proteins move in several steps, through the various sections of the Golgi stacks, where they undergo several modifications, such as addition of fatty acids and various kinds of sugars. Finally they reach the plasma membrane via transport vesicles.

INTERNALIZATION OF RECEPTORS. Receptors do not persist indefinitely at the cell surface because they are internalized (**endocytosis**) into the cells through special patches of membrane called **coated pits.** In electron micrographs of thin sections the pits, in the process of invagination, are seen to be coated at the cytoplasmic

side, by a layer of **clathrin,** bound to the membrane protein (Fig. 47–7).

The invagination of the pits generates small vesicles that fuse together, forming **endosomes.** An ATP-driven proton pump makes the lumen of the endosome acidic (pH 4.5–5.5). At this pH some ligands (e.g., Fe^{3+} bound to transferrin) dissociate from their receptors, cross the endosomal membrane, and are released into the cytoplasm; others (e.g., hormones) dissociate but remain in the endosome; in all cases the receptors remain membrane bound. Many viruses follow a similar pathway (see Chap. 48).

Agents that raise the pH of the endosomes block these effects. They include weak bases such as ammonium chloride, the antimalarial agent chloroquine, the antiinfluenzal agent amantadine, and some ionophores (e.g., monensin).

Each endosome progressively becomes subdivided

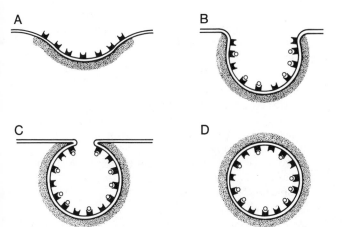

Figure 47–7. Endocytosis. A schematic representation from an electron micrograph. *(A)* Coated pit in a transverse section. The cell membrane *(double line)* is lined at the cytoplasmic side *(below)* by a layer of clathrin molecules. Receptors *(black)* protrude at the extracellular side. *(B)* As the ligand *(circles)* becomes bound to receptors, the pit deepens. *(C)* The pit closes into a vesicle still connected to the cell membrane. *(D)* The vesicle is free in the cytoplasm, as endosome, surrounded by the clathrin coating, with the ligand still attached to the receptors. See also Figure 48-2.

ferent cell needs: recycling reutilizes transport molecules that carry necessary metabolic precursors into cells, whereas down regulation prevents hormones or growth factors from having an excessive action. Down regulation may also play a role in determining the late events following exposure of cells to a growth factor. In fact, similar events may be produced, in the absence of factor, by antibodies to the receptors, which cause clustering and internalization but no cytoplasmic signals.

Cell Transformation

Oncogenic viruses (see Chaps. 64 and 65) can cause mutationlike changes in cultured cells that affect their growth and other properties. Such **transformation** (Fig. 47–8) can also occur spontaneously during the serial growth of cell lines. Radiation and certain chemicals may cause similar transformation in cultures, as well as cancer *in vivo*, by inducing mutations (**somatic mutations**). Ames has shown that most oncogenic chemicals (or their metabolic derivatives) are also mutagenic.

Various transformed cells have different sets of the following properties, which are absent in resting untransformed cells:

CULTURE BEHAVIOR

    Increased culture thickness
    Random cell orientation
    Increased saturation density (decreased topoinhibition)
    Decreased serum or growth factor requirement

into two compartments: one fuses with a lysosome, and the other rejoins the cell surface. Most of the released ligands reach the lysosomes and are destroyed. Some kinds of receptors are recycled to the surface, but others (such as EGF receptors) go to the lysosomes and are destroyed, giving rise to the phenomenon of receptor **down regulation.** These different pathways satisfy dif-

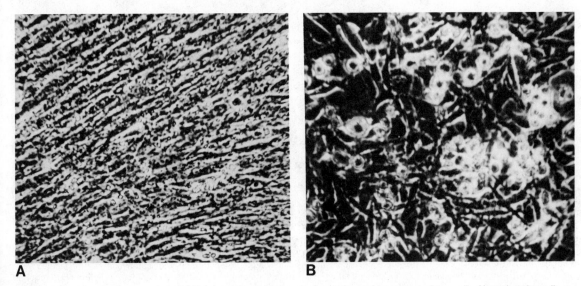

Figure 47–8. Viral transformation. *(A)* Uninfected crowded secondary culture of hamster embryo cells. Note that the cells are arranged in a thin (mostly single) layer with parallel orientation. *(B)* Similar culture transformed by polyoma virus (see Chap. 64). Note that cells lie on top of each other and are randomly oriented.

Increased efficiency of clone formation

Increased edge indentation and refractivity

Ability to form colonies on top of a layer of untransformed cells

Decreased anchorage dependence

Lack of G0 and arrest at various phases of the cell cycle, almost randomly, upon medium exhaustion

CELL SURFACE

Decreased fibronectin content (associated with disorganization of the attached cytoskeleton)

Shorter gangliosides

Reduced glycosyl transferase activity

Reduced adhesion to plastic

Increased receptor mobility (lectins)

Increased agglutination by lectins (Fig. 47–9)

Loss of receptors for hormones and toxins

Increased and unregulated transport activity (e.g., glucose, phosphate, nucleosides, K^+)

Increased glucose-binding protein

Presence of new antigens

METABOLIC CHARACTERISTICS

Increased protease production

Disaggregated microfilaments and reduction of actin-associated proteins

Increased aerobic glycolysis

Decreased intracellular concentration of cyclic AMP

Increased, abnormal collagen synthesis

Resurgent fetal functions

OTHER CHARACTERISTICS

Production of tumor by 10^6 or fewer cells inoculated

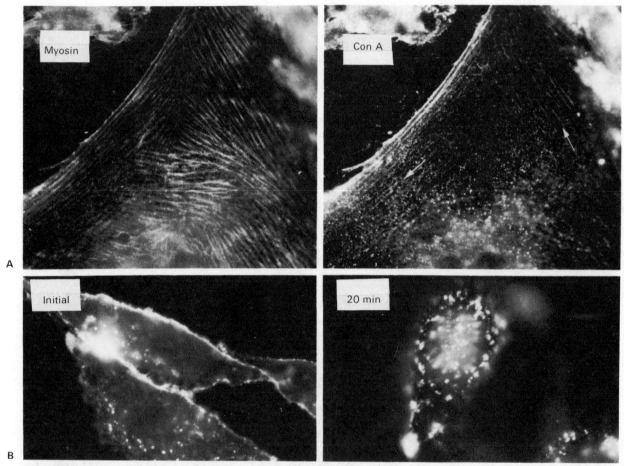

Figure 47–9. Surface and cytoskeletal alterations in transformed cells detected by the rearrangement of surface receptors induced by concanavalin A (conA, a plant lectin) and of myosin-containing cytoplasmic filaments. *(A)* At 20 minutes after exposure to conA, NRK (normal rat kidney) cells were fixed and treated with an anti-conA serum labeled with fluorescein (blue fluorescence, *right*), then treated with antimyosin serum labeled with rhodamine (red fluorescence, *left*). Through the use of appropriate light filters, the distributions of myosin (*left*) and of conA (*right*) were photographed in the same cell. The conA receptors, which were at first uniformly distributed over the cell surface, have formed very fine patches exactly aligned along the underlying myosin-containing stress fibers. *(B; right)* Large patches of conA receptors of Rous sarcoma virus–transformed NRK cells after 20 minutes of interaction with fluorescent conA. The initial uniform distribution is seen at left. (Ash JF, Singer SJ: Proc Natl Acad Sci USA 73:4575, 1976)

subcutaneously in immunologically accepting animals (syngeneic or athymic mice)

Chromosomal abnormalities

Absence of culture senescence

Some of the changes seen in transformed cells appear to derive from the persistent growth of transformed cells, since they are also found in growing untransformed cells. The genetic and epigenetic events controlling the various characteristics are not known; this is understandable given the limited methodology available for studying the complex genome in animal cells.

The spectrum of properties found in individual clones depends on the selection imposed during their isolation (e.g., whether by growth in agar, in low serum, or in dense cultures) and on the inducing agent (e.g., whether chemical or viral). Some kinds of transformed cells are malignant (i.e., they produce tumors in animals), others are not. The properties most closely associated with malignancy are loss of anchorage dependence, protease production, and reduction of fibronectin, but none is essential.

Genetic Studies With Cultured Cells: The Karyotype of Cultured Cells

The genetic characteristics of the cells are relevant for virological studies because many parameters of virus multiplication and its consequences depend on them. The analysis of the chromosomal constitution (**karyotype**) of tissue culture cells has acquired paramount importance in genetic studies since it became clear that karyotype anomalies of cultured cells are associated with certain human diseases. In addition, the karyotype gives an indication of the degree of abnormality that cells have attained during their cultivation *in vitro.*

Staining techniques allow not only the determination of the number of chromosomes in a cell but also their precise cytologic identification. Thus, characteristic **bands** are observed in mitotic chromosomes stained with the fluorescent dye quinacrine mustard and examined under ultraviolet light or stained after trypsin treatment.

In young cell strains, most cells tend to maintain the **diploid** ($2n$) chromosome number characteristic of the animal. The types of chromosomes are also usually normal, and the cells are said to be **euploid.** In contrast, the cells of older strains and cell lines (especially of transformed cells) deviate from the euploid pattern (**aneuploid** cells). The number of chromosomes may be different from diploid (**heteroploid**), either higher (usually between $3n$ and $4n$, i.e., **hypertriploid**) or lower (**hypodiploid**). In **quasidiploid** cells the number of chromosomes is $2n$, but their distribution is abnormal; for exam-

ple, a chromosome of one pair may be missing and replaced by an extra chromosome of another pair. In addition, **chromosomal aberrations** (e.g., **translocations** and **deletions**) often involve highly characteristic morphologic abnormalities in individual chromosomes, which are useful as **markers** for cell identification.

Although in some cell lines most cells are diploid, the majority of cell lines are constituted of heteroploid, especially hypertriploid, cells. **Individual lines are heterogeneous,** with cells containing different numbers of chromosomes. The most frequent (**modal**) number remains constant if the cells are grown under a constant set of conditions, but a change in conditions often results in selection of a type with a different modal number. The variation encountered in heteroploid cultures reflects frequent unequal segregation of chromosomes at mitosis.

SOMATIC MUTATIONS. Most mutations occurring in tissue culture cells, like those observed in prokaryotes, result in **structural changes in a protein.** The mutations are revealed indirectly by physical changes of the protein (e.g., isoelectric point, electrophoretic mobility, heat stability) or directly by amino acid changes. In aneuploid cell cultures a mutational phenotype can also be brought about by a **change in chromosome balance,** due to the loss or the gain of certain chromosomes by mitotic segregation, without structural protein changes. Variants of this type occur and revert at a relatively high frequency, which is not enhanced by mutagenic agents.

The study of mutability suggests that in some cells of permanent lines, diploid genes tend to become **functionally haploid,** as if one of the two homologues were lost or inactivated. Thus in quasidiploid cell lines, many recessive mutations in diploid (autosomal) genes are phenotypically expressed almost as frequently as are mutations in haploid (X-linked) genes, though they would be expected to require two homologous mutations and hence to be much less common. Moreover, in mutant cells resistant to α-amanitin (which acts on RNA polymerase II), essentially all the polymerase molecules are resistant to the drug, although it is unlikely that both the genes specifying the enzyme were mutated. The molecular basis of these findings is not known.

Selected Reading

Ash JF, Singer SJ: Concanavalin A–induced transmembrane linkage of concanavalin A surface receptors to intracellular myosin-containing filaments. Proc Natl Acad Sci USA 73:4575, 1976

Beguinot L, Lyall RM, Willingham MC, Pastan I: Down-regulation of the epidermal growth factor receptor in KB cells is due to receptor internalization and subsequent degradation in lysosomes. Proc Natl Acad Sci USA 81:2384, 1984

Bell RM: Protein kinase C activation by diacylglycerol second messengers. Cell 45:631, 1986

Carpenter G: Properties of the receptor for epidermal growth factor. Cell 37:357, 1984

James R, Bradshaw RA: Polypeptide growth factors. Annu Rev Biochem 53:259, 1984

Newport JW, Kirschner MW: Regulation of the cell cycle during early xenopus development. Cell 37:731, 1984

Nishizuka Y: Studies and perspectives of protein kinase C. Science 233:305, 1986

Rheinwald JG, Green H: Epidermal growth factor and the multiplication of cultured human epidermal keratinocytes. Nature 265:421, 1977

Ross R, Raines EW, Bowen-Pope DF: The biology of platelet-derived growth factor. Cell 46:155, 1986

Vara F, Schneider JA, Rozengurt E: Ionic responses rapidly elicited by activation of protein kinase C in quiescent Swiss 3T3 cells. Proc Natl Acad Sci USA 82:2384, 1985

Yarden Y, Escobedo JA, Kuang W-J et al: Structure of the receptor for platelet-derived growth factor helps define a family of closely related growth factor receptors. Nature 323:226, 1986

48

Multiplication and Genetics of Animal Viruses

Multiplication

The multiplication of many animal viruses follows the pattern of bacteriophage multiplication described in preceding chapters, but with important differences. For instance, as discussed in Chapter 44, some RNA genomes are segmented; some DNA genomes have unusual termini (such as inverted, repeated nucleotide sequences or covalent crosslinking of linear strands); some virions contain a transcriptase and other enzymes; and some viruses express their genetic information in a unique manner, by reverse flow from RNA to DNA. Moreover, animal viruses differ from bacteriophages in their interactions with the surface of the host cells (which do not have rigid walls) and in the mechanisms of release of their nucleic acid in the cell.

Animal viruses can be differentiated into virulent and moderate. Moderate viruses resemble temperate bacteriophages in their ability to establish stable relations with the host cells, but the differentiation is less sharp than with bacteriophages, and it is sometimes difficult to decide whether an animal virus is virulent or moderate.

The main characteristics of animal virus families are given in Table 48–1. Further details are found in later chapters.

HOST CELLS FOR VIRAL MULTIPLICATION

The first hosts for experimental or diagnostic work with animal viruses were adult animals, then chick embryos. Chick embryos have also contributed in an important way to the development of virology by conveniently pro-

845

TABLE 48–1. *Characteristics of Animal Virus Families*

Type	Nucleic Acid Strandedness	Symmetry of Nucleocapsid	Naked (N) or Enveloped (E)	Diameter of Virus (nm)	Family	Examples (Specific Viruses Mentioned in This Chapter)
RNA	Single-stranded	Icosahedral	N	21–30	Picornaviruses (see Chap. 55)	Poliovirus, Coxsackie virus, Mengo virus
			E	45	Togaviruses (see Chap. 60)	Semliki Forest virus, western equine encephalomyelitis virus, yellow fever virus, dengue virus
		Helical	E	80–120	Orthomyxoviruses (see Chap. 56)	Influenza virus, fowl plague virus
				125–300	Paramyxoviruses (see Chap. 57)	Sendai virus, measles virus, mumps virus, respiratory syncytial virus
				70–80x 130–240	Rhabdoviruses (see Chap. 59)	Rabies virus, vesicular stomatitis virus
				80–160	Coronaviruses (see Chap. 58)	Lymphocytic choriomeningitis virus, Lassa virus
		Unknown	E	110–130	Arenaviruses (see Chap. 60)	
				90–100	Bunyaviruses (see Chap. 60)	California encephalitis viruses
				100	Retroviruses (see Chap. 65)	Rous sarcoma virus, human T-lymphotropic virus, human immunodeficiency virus
	Double-stranded	Icosahedral	N	75–80	Reoviruses (see Chap. 62)	Reovirus, rotavirus
DNA	Double-stranded	Icosahedral	N	70–90	Adenoviruses (see Chap. 52)	Adenovirus
				43–53	Papovaviruses (see Chap. 64)	Polyoma virus, SV40, JC virus, BK virus
			E	180–200	Herpesviruses (see Chap. 53)	Herpes simplex virus, varicellazoster virus, cytomegalovirus, Epstein-Barr (EB) virus
		Complex	E*	200–250 250–350	Poxviruses (see Chap. 54)	Vaccinia virus, variola (smallpox) virus
				45	Hepadnaviruses (see Chap. 63)	Hepatitis B virus
	Single-stranded	Icosahedral	N	18–22	Parvoviruses (see Chap. 52)	Adeno-associated virus

* Lipid in outer coat, but no distinct envelope

viding a variety of cell types, susceptible to many viruses. Various cell types can be reached by inoculating the embryo by different routes (Fig. 48–1). These hosts have now been replaced almost completely by cultures of animal cells for detailed studies of viral replication.

Cell Strains and Cell Lines

Every type of animal cell culture discussed in Chapter 47 has found application in virology. The choice of species, tissue of origin, and type of culture (primary, cell strain, or cell line) depends on the virus and the experimental objectives. The systems used for the individual viral families will be given in the appropriate chapters.

HOST SUSCEPTIBILITY. Each animal virus can replicate only in a certain range of cells. Among **nonsusceptible cells** some have a block at an early step (e.g., they lack receptors for viral attachment or a factor required for expression of viral genes), so that the expression of all viral functions is prevented (**resistant cells**). Other cells lack a factor required for a later step, so that some, but not all, viral activities are expressed (**nonpermissive cells**). In either case a **heterokaryon,** formed by fusing a susceptible and a nonsusceptible cell, has the function and is usually susceptible.

PRODUCTIVE INFECTION
Role of Nucleic Acid—Transfection

That cells of higher organisms can be infected by naked viral nucleic acid, yielding normal virions, was first shown for tobacco mosaic virus RNA by Gierer and Schramm. The same was soon shown for the RNA or DNA of many animal viruses. In conjunction with the Hershey and Chase experiment with bacteriophage (see Separation of Nucleic Acid From Coat, Chap. 45), this result established the exclusive genetic role of the viral nucleic acid.

There are several important differences between infections by nucleic acid (transfection) and by virions.

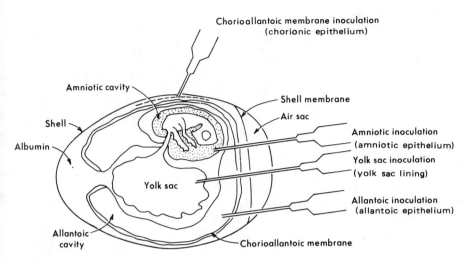

Chorioallantoic membrane inoculation
(chorionic epithelium)

Amniotic cavity

Shell membrane

Air sac

Shell

Albumin

Amniotic inoculation
(amniotic epithelium)

Yolk sac inoculation
(yolk sac lining)

Yolk sac

Allantoic inoculation
(allantoic epithelium)

Allantoic cavity

Chorioallantoic membrane

Figure 48–1. Chicken embryo (10–12 days old) and routes of inoculation to reach the various cell types (as indicated). For chorioallantoic membrane inoculation a hole is first drilled through the eggshell and shell membrane; the shell over the air sac is then perforated. Air enters between the shell membrane and the chorioallantoic membrane, creating an artificial air sac, where the sample is deposited, in contact with the chorionic epithelium. Yolk sac inoculation is usually carried out in younger (6-day-old) embryos, in which the yolk sac is larger.

1. **The efficiency of infection with nucleic acid is much lower,** by a factor of 10^{-6} to 10^{-8} in ordinary media, showing the important role of the viral coat in infectivity. The infectivity of nucleic acid is increased by several orders of magnitude in the presence of basic polymers (e.g., diethylaminoethyldextran) or by precipitation of the viral DNA onto cells with calcium phosphate. These additions appear to protect the nucleic acid against nucleases and to increase its uptake by the cells. Even under the most favorable conditions, however, the bare nucleic acid is no more than 1% as infectious as the corresponding virions. This limitation seems to arise from degradation of much of the nucleic acid within the cells. The efficiency is further increased by injecting the nucleic acid into the cells or by delivering it packaged in membranous vesicles (liposomes) that bind to the cell membrane and empty their contents into the cells.

2. **The host range is much wider with nucleic acids,** which can infect resistant cells. For instance, chicken cells, although resistant to poliovirus because they lack receptors for the virions, are susceptible to its RNA, but only a single cycle of viral multiplication takes place because the progeny are again virions and cannot spread to other cells.

3. **Infectious nucleic acid can be extracted even from heat-inactivated viruses** in which the protein of the capsid has been denatured; the nucleic acid can withstand much higher temperatures than the protein. The ability of nucleic acid infectivity to survive damage to the viral coat must be considered in the preparation of viral vaccines.

4. With some RNA viruses (e.g., poliovirus) **a DNA copy of the viral RNA is infectious.** This permits the preparation of viral genomes (such as those of vaccine strains) in large quantities by avoiding the high mutation rate in replication of RNA and its lability.

5. Finally, **the infectivity of nucleic acid is unaffected by virus-specific Abs,** which suggests that this form of a virus could be an effective infectious agent even in the presence of immunity. However, nucleases in body fluids probably greatly limit its role, because a single complete break in a molecule abolishes its infectivity. Indeed, naked viral nucleic acid plays a role in natural infection only as plant viroids (see Chap. 44), the tight secondary structure of which resists nucleases.

Of the animal viruses, papovaviruses, adenoviruses, some herpesviruses, togaviruses, and picornaviruses yield infectious nucleic acids. With retroviruses (see Chap. 65), infectious DNA can be extracted from infected cells or can be made by copying the viral RNA *in vitro*. Failure in other cases can be ascribed either to the difficulty of extracting a large DNA molecule intact or to **lack of virion enzymes** (e.g., a transcriptase) required for initiating the viral growth cycle.

Initial Steps of Viral Infection

Initially, as with bacteriophage infection, the viral nucleic acid must be made available for replication. Unlike bacteriophage, however, the entire animal virus nucleocapsid enters the cell, and the nucleic acid is then released. These early events can be investigated by studying the changes of viral infectivity or the fate of radioactively labeled viral components, or by electron microscopy. The following steps can be identified.

1. **Attachment or adsorption.** The virus becomes attached to the cells, and at this stage it can be **recovered in infectious form** without cell lysis by procedures that either destroy the receptors or weaken their bonds to the virions. Animal viruses have specialized attachment sites distributed over the surface of the virion: for instance, enveloped viruses such as orthomyxoviruses and paramyxoviruses attach through glycoprotein spikes (see The Envelope, Chap. 44), and adenoviruses attach through

the penton fibers (see Immunologic Characteristics, Chap. 50).

Adsorption occurs to **specific receptors,** which vary in number for different viruses from 5×10^2 to 5×10^5 per cell. Some receptors are glycoproteins (for myxoviruses or paramyxoviruses); others are phospholipids and glycolipids (for rhabdoviruses or some paramyxoviruses). They are usually macromolecules with specific physiological functions, such as complement receptors (for EBV), β-adrenergic receptor (for reovirus type 3), or Ia molecules of the major histocompatibility complex (for lactate dehydrogenase virus).

Whether or not receptors for a certain virus are present on a cell depends on the species and the tissue from which the cell derives and on its **physiologic state.** Cells lacking receptors for a certain virus are resistant to it, i.e., cannot be infected. Attachment is blocked by antibodies that bind to the viral or cellular sites involved. In epithelial cells the distribution of receptors may be polarized, i.e., confined to either the basolateral or the apical surface.

2. **Penetration** rapidly follows adsorption, and the virus can no longer be recovered from the intact cell. The most common mechanism of penetration is **receptor-mediated endocytosis,** the process by which many hormones and toxins enter cells: an area of cell membrane containing receptors with the attached virions—usually a clathrin-coated pit—invaginates to form a cytoplasmic vesicle. Virions can be recognized within the vesicles by electron microscopy (Fig. 48–2).

UNCOATING. The most common mechanism causing separation of the viral coat from the genome-containing core is an interaction of a coat component with the endosomal membrane. A key step is the **acidification** of the content of the endosome to a pH of about 5, owing to the activity of a proton pump present in the membrane. The low pH causes rearrangement of coat components, which then expose normally hidden hydrophobic sites. They bind to the lipid bilayer of the membrane, causing

extrusion of the viral core into the cytosol. For influenza virus (see Chap. 56) the acid-sensitive component is the HA_2 unit of the hemagglutinin; for adenoviruses it is the penton base. Ultimately the endosome fuses with a lysosome, where remnants of the viral coat as well as uncoated virions are destroyed. Paramyxoviruses are an exception: their fusion protein can carry out the fusion step at physiologic pH; hence, they penetrate and uncoat in a single step at the cell surface, rather than in endosomes.

Many weak bases, such as chloroquine or ammonium chloride, which accumulate in endosomes, prevent their acidification and block uncoating. Mutations in the proton pump have similar consequences. In both cases the cells become resistant to many viruses, as well as to hormones or toxins that use the same endocytic pathway. Amantadine, in contrast, affects only influenza type A and a few other viruses. Amantadine-resistant influenza mutants are altered in the hemagglutinin, which interacts with the endosomal membrane, and the connected matrix protein; these virions fuse with membranes in vitro at pH 7.0. This is a direct evidence for the role of membrane fusion in endosome for uncoating.

One-Step Multiplication Curves

As with bacteriophages, multiplication curves for animal viruses are obtained under one-step conditions (see Chap. 45) by means of cells from suspension cultures or from monolayer cultures dispersed by trypsin. For viruses the cell receptors of which can be easily destroyed (e.g., influenza viruses, polyomavirus) one-step conditions are possible even without dispersing the cell layers: the infected cultures are washed free of unadsorbed virus and then covered with a medium containing receptor-destroying enzyme, which prevents adsorption of released virus to the cells. For other viruses the same result is obtained by washing the monolayers with antiviral Ab after infection.

One-step multiplication curves of animal viruses (Fig. 48–3) show the same stages observed with bacterio-

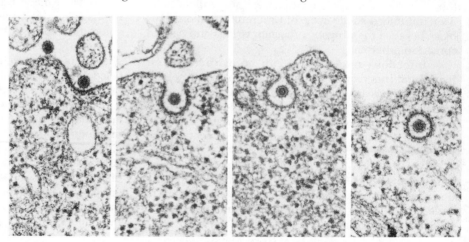

Figure 48–2. The first stages in infection of Semliki Forest virus, a togavirus. The electron micrographs show, from left to right, four stages in penetration. Of the two extracellular virions present in the first picture, one is attached to receptors in a coated pit; note the dark chathrin layer at the cytoplasmic site of the membrane. The virion-containing pit begins to deepen in the second picture and is almost closed in the third. In the fourth picture it has formed an endosome surrounded by chathrin and free in the cytoplasm. (Original magnification × 70,000; courtesy of J. Kartenbeck)

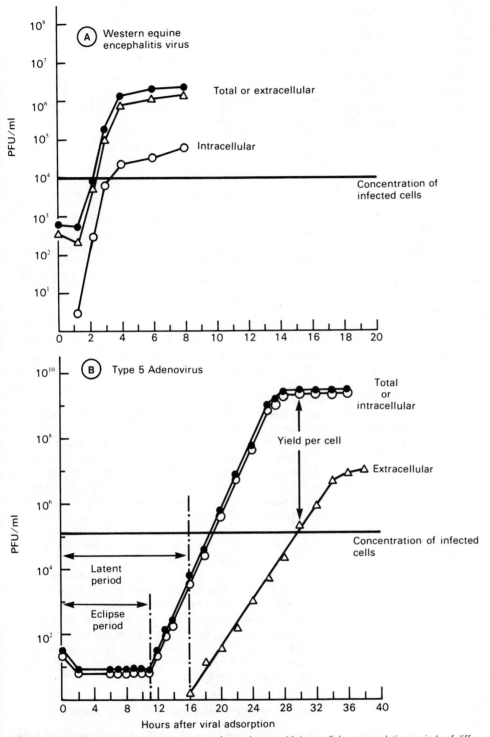

Figure 48–3. One-step multiplication curves of two viruses with intracellular accumulation periods of different lengths. Extracellular virus is measured in the medium surrounding the intact cells, intracellular virus after removal of the medium and disruption of the cells. *(A)* Western equine encephalitis virus multiplies in cultures of chick embryo cells with an extremely short accumulation period. *(B)* Type 5 adenovirus multiplies in cultures of KB cells with a long accumulation period. Intracellular (i.e., cell-associated) virus is measured by disrupting cells after they have been washed free of extracellular virus (i.e., virus already released into the medium). *PFU,* plaque-forming unit. *(A,* from data of Rubin H et al: J Exp Med 101:205, 1955; *B,* from data of H. S. Ginsberg and M. Dixon)

phages (see Chap. 45). The length of the **intracellular accumulation period** varies widely, however, with different viruses. It is very long with some, the progeny virions of which tend to remain within the cells, and is nonexistent with others, which mature and are released in the same act (by acquisition of an envelope at the cell surface). If the accumulation period is very short, the quantity of intracellular virus is at any time a small fraction of the total virus, as in Figure 48–3A.

Effect of Viral Infection on Host Macromolecular Synthesis

In these studies viral and cellular nucleic acids are separated and identified by their size, buoyant density, and configuration (e.g., cyclic), or their hybridization to the nucleic acid present in purified virions. Viral and cellular proteins can be distinguished immunologically or by their different rates of migration in acrylamide gel electrophoresis.

As with bacteriophages, **virulent viruses,** either DNA-containing (e.g., adenovirus, vaccinia virus, herpesvirus) or RNA-containing (e.g., poliovirus, Newcastle disease virus, reovirus), shut off cellular protein synthesis (Figs. 48–4 and 48–5) and disaggregate cellular polyribosomes, favoring a **shift to viral synthesis.** With most viruses the effect does not occur in the presence of inhibitors of protein synthesis (puromycin, cycloheximide), indicating that it is mediated by new virus-specified proteins. The replication and transcription of cellular DNA are

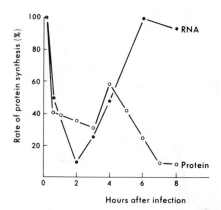

Figure 48–5. Inhibition of cellular RNA and protein synthesis in L cells infected with mengovirus (a picornavirus). The decline in incorporation of radioactive precursors begins immediately after infection. The resumption of synthesis at about 3 hours is due to synthesis of viral RNA and proteins. (Modified from Franklin RM, Baltimore D: Cold Spring Harbor Symp Quant Biol 27:175, 1962)

blocked by adenoviruses, herpesviruses, and poxviruses; chromosome breaks are often observed.

The **mechanisms of protein synthesis shut-off** vary even within the same viral family. Thus, among picornaviruses, poliovirus, using a viral protease, causes **cleavage of a 200-Kd cap-binding protein,** which is required for initiation of translation of capped cellular messengers. Viral messengers, being uncapped, are not affected. Viral mutants not carrying out the cleavage do not inhibit translation. In contrast, Mengo virus does not prevent initiation but causes an **elongation block of the initiation complexes** (ribosome, messenger, and Met-tRNA). With vesicular stomatitis virus the **leader sequence,** a transcript of a small part of the 3′ end of the genome, also blocks the initiation step, probably in conjunction with viral or cellular proteins. Herpesvirus induces degradation of cellular mRNAs; and an adenovirus gene (E1b) prevents the transport of cellular mRNAs to the cytoplasm during the late part of infection.

In contrast to virulent viruses, **moderate viruses** (e.g., polyomavirus) may **stimulate** the synthesis of host DNA, mRNA, and protein. This phenomenon is of considerable interest for viral carcinogenesis (see Viral Multiplication in Cell Culture, Chap. 64).

SYNTHESIS OF DNA-CONTAINING VIRUSES

There are **three classes of DNA-containing viruses,** based on genome structure: I, **double-stranded linear;** II, **double-stranded circular;** and III, **single-stranded linear.** All the linear DNAs possess some form of inverted repetitions, either at the termini of the genomes (e.g., adenoviruses) or in their substructure (e.g., herpesviruses). In addition, within these classes distinctive

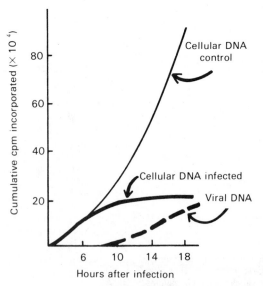

Figure 48–4. Inhibition of cellular DNA synthesis in L cells infected by equine abortion virus (a herpesvirus) in the presence of ³H-thymidine. Viral DNA was separated from cellular DNA because of its higher buoyant density in CsCl. (Modified from O'Callaghan DJ et al: Virology 36:104, 1968)

structural variations also occur. Biosynthesis follows patterns similar to those described for bacteriophages, but the structural differences in the viral genomes appear to dictate different modes of transcription, methods of posttranscriptional processing, and forms of DNA replication. The general reactions will be described here; more specific details will be found in the chapters that follow.

Transcription

In the synthesis of DNA-containing animal viruses, as in eukaryotic cells and unlike the process in prokaryotes, transcription and translation are not coupled. Except for poxviruses, transcription occurs in the nucleus and translation in the cytoplasm. Generally, the **primary transcripts,** generated by RNA polymerase II, are larger than the mRNAs found on polyribosomes, and in some cases as much as 30% of the transcribed RNA remains untranslated in the nucleus (e.g., adenovirus transcripts; see Chap. 52). The viral messengers, however, like those of animal cells, are monocistronic.

Transcription has a **temporal organization.** With most DNA-containing viruses only a fraction of the genome is transcribed into **early** messengers before replication has begun, and after DNA synthesis the remainder is transcribed into **late** messengers. The complex viruses have **immediate early** genes, which are expressed in the presence of inhibitors of protein synthesis, and **delayed early** ones, which require protein synthesis for expression. Interference with DNA synthesis by temperature-sensitive mutations or by inhibitors shows that the switch to late transcription requires prior DNA replication.

Regulation is carried out by proteins present in the virions, or specified by viral or cellular genes, interacting with regulatory sequences at the 5' end of the genes. Fusion of such sequences to a marker gene with easily measurable effects (e.g., the herpes thymidine kinase gene) show that the few hundred nucleotides preceding the coding sequences are essential for control. They have properties related to those of the **enhancers** of tumor viruses (see Chap. 64): they respond in *trans* to substances produced by other genes and act in *cis* on the associated genes, which they either stimulate or inhibit. For instance, with herpes simplex virus, regulatory events acting mainly on transcription cause the sequential appearance of different classes of mRNAs: **immediate early (α), delayed early (β),** and **late (γ^1 and γ^2)** (Fig. 48–6). In addition, late genes, especially those of the γ^2 class, are activated after viral DNA replication begins (see Multiplication, Chap. 53). These regulatory properties are generally similar to those of large bacteriophages (see Chap. 45).

Different classes of genes may be transcribed from **different DNA strands** and therefore in opposite direc-

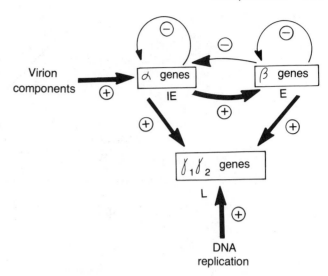

Figure 48–6. Regulation of transcription of the various classes of herpes simplex genes. +, *thick lines:* stimulation of transcription; −, *thin lines:* inhibition of transcription; *IE,* immediate early; *E,* early; *L,* late. α and β genes inhibit their own transcription through their products.

tions. Thus, with SV40, a papovavirus, unique regions on opposite strands code for early and late mRNAs (see Productive Infection, Chap. 64). In adenovirus (Fig. 48–7) **early transcription** occurs on both strands in five scattered regions of the genome. In contrast, synthesis of adenovirus **late messages** is mostly confined to the rightward-reading (r) strand: a unique large transcript is cleaved to generate five groups of messages (see Fig. 48–7) with identical 5' ends, each composed of a nontranslated cap and leader sequences, which are not contiguous to the message sequences in the genome. Each group has identical 3' ends. Similar is the arrangement of the two late mRNAs of both SV40 and polyomaviruses.

This complex method of producing mRNAs by **posttranscriptional processing** of primary transcripts serves to remove **intervening sequences** not destined to be translated. As with cellular mRNAs, their removal is essential for regulating the appearance of functional messages, and alternative splicings yield different messages and different proteins from the same segment of DNA. The complex regulation of transcription depends on proteins specified by both viral and cellular genes.

Like eukaryotic cell mRNAs, viral transcripts undergo other modifications: the addition of a **poly(A) chain** (100–200 adenine residues long) to the 3' end and a **methylated cap** at the 5' end. Except for poxviruses, these additions are made in the nucleus. As with cellular mRNA, the methylated capped 5' terminus appears essential for the stable attachment of viral mRNAs to the 40S ribosomal subunit and for effective translation.

The early transcription and processing of most DNA-containing viruses are carried out by host enzymes, us-

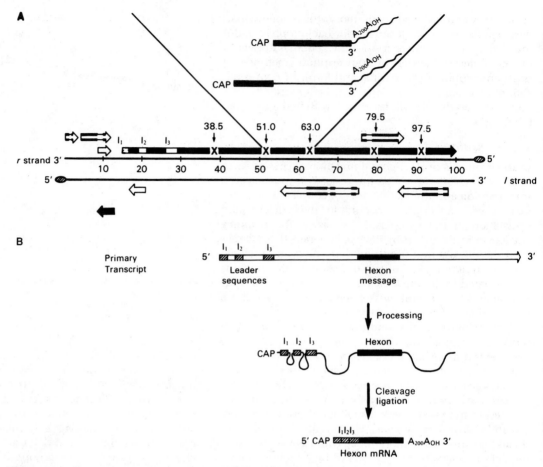

Figure 48–7. Transcription map of the type 2 adenovirus genome and a model for processing a late mRNA, the hexon message. *(A)* The encoded regions for the early and late mRNAs are indicated. *White arrows,* early transcripts (Protein IX RNA is expressed early and late from the 3' end of the E1B region, but the protein is made late and is a structural protein); *black arrows,* late transcripts. The thickened lines on the early transcripts indicate the regions that are included in one of the major mRNAs processed from transcripts of each region. The possible sites for cleavage and polyadenylation of the late transcript to produce the 3' termini of the messages are designated by Xs or small arrows. The cleavage and splice sites (see *B*) are each identified by a unique nucleotide sequence. The enlarged segment between positions 51.0 and 63.0 represents two late messages processed from large transcripts. They have different 5' ends and identical 3' ends; the region of the message translated into protein is designated by the heavy segment. *(B)* Primary transcript for late mRNAs on the r strand, and suggested model for processing this transcript to form the hexon mRNA. Only one mRNA can be derived from each transcript.

ing RNA polymerase II as transcriptase. Poxviruses, however, are profoundly different: they use enzymes present in the core of the virions, and their transcripts, without intervening sequences, are not spliced.

Synthesis of Viral Proteins

Viral proteins are synthesized on cytoplasmic polysomes in a temporal sequence corresponding to that of the viral mRNAs (Fig. 48–8): early proteins participate in DNA replication and transcription, the late ones are predominantly structural proteins of the virions. With most viruses these proteins are transported to the nucleus, where assembly takes place. Posttranscriptional control may participate in determining the temporal sequence;

for instance, with adenovirus a small viral RNA, VA1, enhances translation of late protein by stabilizing the initiation factor 2.

DNA Replication

DNA replication utilizes precursors derived from the medium, since cellular DNA is not degraded. The smaller DNA viruses rely on the host cell DNA polymerase, but the more complex adenoviruses, herpesviruses, and poxviruses use virus-encoded polymerases. Synthesis begins toward the middle of the eclipse period (see Fig. 48–3B), after the early viral proteins are made: it is blocked by mutations in some early viral genes or by inhibition of protein synthesis shortly after infection.

The mode of replication is **semiconservative,** but the nature of the **replicative intermediates** depends on the devices used for achieving complete replication—a problem already noted in Chapter 45 (see Fig. 45–10). Several methods of replication can be recognized (Fig. 48–9).

1. **Adenoviruses** (see Fig. 48–9A) show asymmetric replication, which initiates at the 3' end of one of the strands. The growing strand uses as primer cytidylic acid bound to the precursor of the terminal protein (see Chap. 44). That protein, together with the viral DNA polymerase and other proteins, becomes associated with a terminal repetition at the 3' end of the template strand. The growing strand **displaces the preexisting strand** of the same polarity and, with the template strand, builds a complete duplex molecule. The displaced single strand in turn replicates in a similar way after generating a panhandle structure by pairing the inverted terminal repetitions.

2. Several viruses use **circular intermediates. Herpesvirus** (see Fig. 48–9B) has a linear genome terminated by direct repeats of 300 to 400 base pairs, often in multiple copies. After the infecting viral DNA reaches the cell's nucleus, the ends undergo limited exonucleolytic digestion (see Fig. 48–9B, *top*) and then pair to form circles. In the **first phase** they replicate as cyclic molecules (see Fig. 48–9B, *middle*); in the **second phase** they form tandem **concatemers** in head-to-tail connection, probably by rolling circle replication (see Fig. 48–9B, *bottom*). During maturation, unit-length molecules are cut from the concatemers.

Papovaviruses (see Fig. 48–9C) have cyclic DNA in their virions. Replication is **bidirectional** and **symmetric,** via cyclic intermediates.

3. Replication of **parvovirus DNA** (see Fig. 48–9D), a single-stranded linear molecule, is directed by the unusual structure of its ends, which have **terminal palindromes** capable of forming hairpins. The replicative intermediates of the defective **adeno-associated virus DNA** include special concatemers, predominantly of double length, in which **a plus and a minus strand are covalently linked in the same strand.** They are probably produced in two self-priming steps (see Fig. 48–9D, *top* and *second from top*). Progeny molecules are generated by strand displacement (see Fig. 48–9D, *second from bottom* and *bottom*) and from double-stranded molecules, either monomeric or concatemeric.

4. **Poxvirus DNA** (see Fig. 48–9E) has, in addition to its large size, another striking feature: the two complementary strands are joined. The links are at the end of inverted terminal repetitions, so the two ends form two equal palindromes. The replicative intermediates, present in the cytoplasm, are special concatemers containing pairs of genomes connected either head-to-head or tail-to-tail. A model generating these structures is

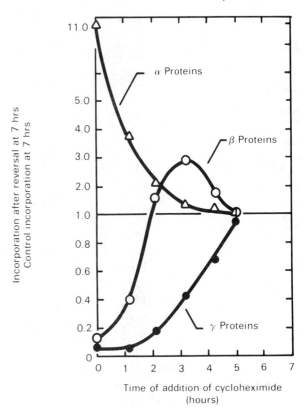

Figure 48–8. Sequential appearance of the three sets of type 1 herpes simplex virus proteins. These data show the rate of synthesis of representative α, β, and γ polypeptides following removal of cycloheximide 7 hours after infection. Cycloheximide was added to infected cultures at different times after infection (noted on the abscissa) and was removed from all cultures simultaneously. The relative rates of synthesis (plotted on the ordinate) were determined by measuring radioisotope incorporation into a specific polypeptide for 30 minutes after removal of cycloheximide as compared to the incorporation into the same viral polypeptide from infected cells to which inhibitor had not been added. (Modified from Honess RW, Roizman B: J Virol 14:8, 1974)

shown in Figure 48–9E, with head-to-head palindromes under the first part of the figure. Unit molecules are produced by staggered cuts and ligation.

5. **Hepatitis B** virus employs **reverse transcription** for multiplication (see Fig. 48–9F). The virions contain a partially double-stranded circular DNA with a complete negative strand (that is complementary to mRNA) in circular nicked form and an incomplete positive strand. Upon entering cells the positive strand is completed, generating a covalently closed, circular molecule, which is transcribed (see Fig. 48–9F, *top*). RNA transcripts are in turn reverse-transcribed into DNA by a viral enzyme in several steps, following very closely the model of retroviruses (see Chap. 65) including a jump of the nascent positive strand from one direct repeat (DR) to another (see Fig. 48–9F, *second and third from bottom*). The

A. Adenoviruses   B. Herpesvirus   C. Papovavirus   D. Parvovirus

E. Poxvirus   F. Hepatitis B Virus

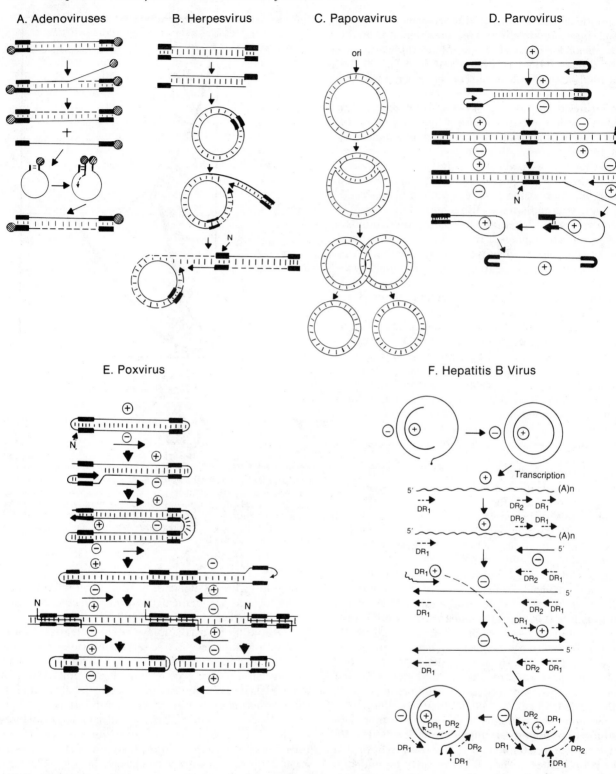

Figure 48–9. Models for the replication of viral DNAs. *(A) Dashed portions,* terminal protein. *(D)* +, −, strand polarity; *N,* endonuclease; *heavy lines,* palindromes; first and second from top are successive self-priming steps. *(E) Heavy arrows,* polarity of the helix; *N,* endonuclease. *(F) Wavy lines,* RNA; *thin lines,* DNA; *DR₁, DR₂,* direct repeats. **(D,** Senapathy P, Tratschin JD, Carter BJ: J Mol Biol 179:1, 1984; *E,* Moyer RW, Graves RL: Cell 27:391, 1981; *F,* Seeger C, Ganem D, Varmus HE: Science 232:477, 1986)

result is the uncompleted double-stranded molecule (see Fig. 48–9*F*, *bottom*).

With all viruses, as with bacteriophages, the newly synthesized viral DNA enters a pool from which it is subsequently removed to associate with virion structural proteins. Thus, if the infected cells are exposed to a short pulse of a radioactive DNA precursor at any time during the eclipse period, the label is distributed among virions finished at any subsequent time. In contrast to bacteriophage infection, viral DNA is made in excess, and much remains unused in the infected cells at the end of the multiplication cycle, often as a constituent of inclusion bodies.

Synthesis of RNA Viruses

The replication strategy of these genomes is dictated by the absence of multiple translation units within the same messenger, a characteristic of all animal cell messengers. To overcome this difficulty, three main strategies have developed: (1) With some viruses, the virion RNA, acting as messenger, is translated **monocistronically** into a **giant peptide,** which is then cleaved to generate distinct viral proteins. (2) In other viruses the virion RNA is **transcribed** to yield various **monocistronic mRNAs** by initiating transcription at different places. (3) Occasionally, the genome itself is a collection of **separate RNA** fragments that are transcribed into monocistronic mRNAs.

RNA-containing animal viruses can be placed in seven different classes, according to the nature of the viral RNA and its relation to the messenger, **which is taken to be of positive polarity** (Fig. 48–10).

In **classes I and II** the genomes have the same polarity as the messengers and are therefore defined as **positive-strand** viruses. In **class I** viruses (e.g., picornaviruses) the genome itself **acts as messenger,** specifying information for the synthesis of both structural and nonstructural proteins. The same RNA molecule must also initiate replication, because infection by a single viral particle occurs. Since RNA replication re-

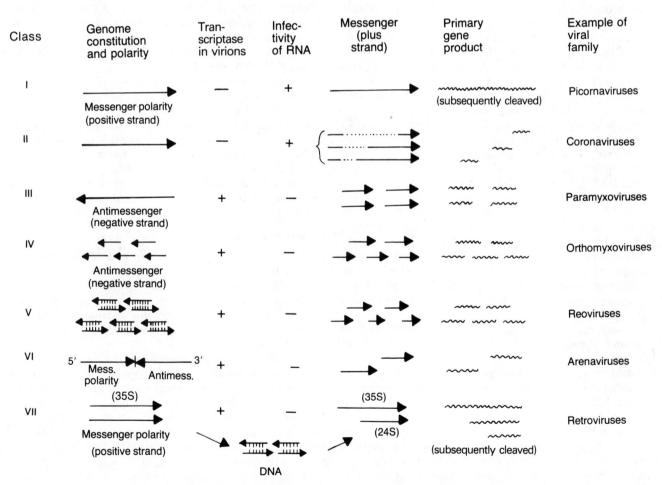

Figure 48–10. The various classes of RNA viruses and their primary modes of expression. The numbers of multiple genome pieces, messengers, and gene products are only diagrammatic representations and are not precise.

quires viral proteins (see below), the messenger function must be expressed first.

In **class II** viruses (e.g., coronaviruses) the genome generates first a negative-strand transcript, which is then transcribed into monocistronic mRNAs of different sizes. The way these are made is unique. Each begins with an identical short 5' leader that is joined to transcripts beginning at the start of the various genes and then continuing to the 3' end of the genome (**nested messengers**). These mRNAs are not produced by splicing a genomic-size transcript, because the virus, able to replicate in enucleated cells, does not require nuclear functions such as those required for splicing; instead, the leader probably remains attached to the polymerase and then acts as primer for the synthesis of the body of each messenger. Only one protein is made on each messenger, encoded in the 5' end of its body.

In **class III and IV viruses** the genomes have the polarity opposite that of the messenger and are defined as **negative-strand genomes.** In **class III** (e.g., paramyxoviruses) a **virion transcriptase** transcribes the genomes into separate monocistronic messengers initiating at a single promoter. The transcriptase stops and restarts at each juncture between different genes, generating the various messengers. **Class IV** viruses (orthomyxoviruses) have the additional feature that the genome is in several distinct, nonoverlapping pieces of single-stranded RNA; each segment gives rise to its own messenger. Most genomic segments contain a single gene, but two segments contain two overlapping genes: one is expressed by a full-length messenger, the other by a shorter messenger obtained by the former by splicing. The replication of these viruses has a nuclear phase, during which splicing occurs by means of the same signals and enzymes as eukaryotic transcripts.

In the synthesis of their messengers, orthomyxoviruses follow the peculiar strategy of using as primers capped 5'-end fragments obtained by endonucleolytic cleavage of host messengers. The use of cellular 5' ends might expose the viral messengers to a block of translation acting on cellular messengers in virus-infected cells (see Interferon, Chap. 49), but this effect is prevented by a viral protein.

Class V viruses (e.g., reoviruses) contain distinct, nonoverlapping segments of **double-stranded RNA** (ten in reoviruses); each is transcribed into an independent mRNA by a **virion transcriptase.** Most messengers are monocistronic, but one is bicistronic and expresses a second protein by initiating at an internal AUG in a different reading frame.

Class VI viruses (e.g., arenaviruses) have genomes that do not conform to any of the former classes. About half of the genome is of negative polarity and is transcribed into a messenger by a **virion transcriptase,** but the other half, of positive polarity, is transcribed twice: first a com-

plete transcript of the genome is made, then the messenger is transcribed from this transcript. These viruses are said to have an **ambisense genome,** because the genetic information is inscribed in opposite directions in its two parts. This is unusual for RNA but not for dsDNA, in which information is often inscribed in opposite directions in a strand: some segments are transcribed from that strand, others from its complement. In arenaviruses this is a device for independently regulating genome replication and virion maturation (see Chap. 60).

Rhabdoviruses (negative-strand genome) have a related organization, because they make two leaders, one by transcribing the viral strand (+ leader), the other its complement (− leader). But they are not messengers; they remain untranslated: the positive-strand leader is probably involved in host shutdown, whereas the negative-strand leader binds to a specific protein of unknown function.

Class VII viruses (retroviruses) are unique because their genomes are transcribed into DNA, not RNA. They contain two identical single-stranded RNAs of positive polarity, with a poly(A) tail at the 3'-OH terminus and a cap at the 5' end. In productive infection each is transcribed into DNA by a **reverse transcriptase** present in the virion; the functional mRNAs are then transcribed from this DNA (see Chap. 65).

Since RNA viruses of classes III to VII require a virion transcriptase for synthesizing a messenger, their purified viral RNAs are not infectious. Only those of viruses of classes I and II are infectious. Viruses of class VI behave aberrantly: the virion RNA is apparently of messenger, or positive, polarity but is not transcribed or translated.

With RNA virus there is no differentiation between early and late messengers in any of the preceding classes, with the possible exception of reoviruses (class V).

Viral Proteins

Viral proteins are synthesized in two different patterns that satisfy the monocistronic nature of the messengers.

1. When a virus has several messengers, each yields only one protein (two in exceptional cases; see above), and the number of viral proteins identifiable by acrylamide gel electrophoresis is equal or close to the number of messengers.

2. When, as with picornaviruses, the genome serves as a single messenger, a giant **polyprotein** is made, which is then cleaved (**processing**) to yield the viral proteins. The polyprotein is not normally recognized because it undergoes the first cleavage while being synthesized; inhibition of cleavage, by amino acid analogs incorporated into the precursor polyprotein or by high temperature, allows its detection. All viral proteins are generated in a series of successive cleavages (Fig. 48–11): the P1 region, at the amino terminus of the polyprotein, generates the

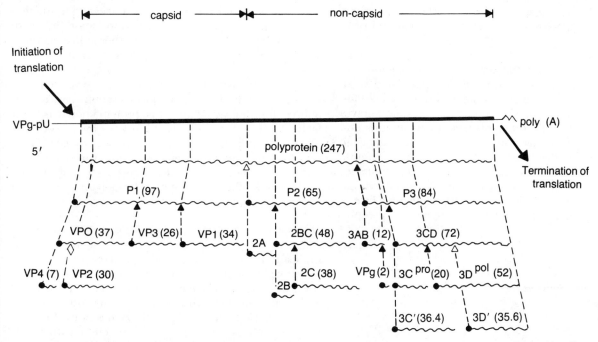

Figure 48–11. Posttranslational processing of the poliovirus polyprotein. *Solid line,* poliovirus genome; *wavy lines,* polypeptides. The polyprotein is rapidly cleaved into peptides P1, P2, and P3, which are then cleaved further. *Closed triangles,* cleavage at glutamine–glycine pairs by the virus-coded enzyme 3C; *open triangles,* cleavage at tyrosine–glycine pairs by viral enzyme 2A: *open diamonds,* cleavage at asparagine–serine pairs during capsid formation. 3C' and 3D' result from alternative cleavage. Numbers in parentheses indicate molecular weight in kilodaltons. (Modified from Emini EA, Schleif WA, Colanno RJ, Wimmer E: Virology 140:13, 1985)

structural proteins; the central P2 region generates proteins with unknown functions; and the P3 region at the carboxyl terminus generates noncapsid proteins, including the RNA polymerase and a cleavage enzyme. Cleavage is carried out by specific viral enzymes that are self-cleaved out of the polyprotein and recognize certain dipeptides, mainly glutamine-glycine, in the context of the secondary–tertiary structure of the protein.

REGULATION OF PRODUCTION. Regulation of class I viruses (picornaviruses and togaviruses) is governed by the posttranslation processing just described: proteins resulting from the first cleavage are available earlier in infection than those from later cleavages. With other viruses regulation is mainly transcriptional but is modulated by regulation of translation. This is evident when the synthesis of a gene product is shut off during the late period while the corresponding mRNA accumulates in the cytoplasm.

Replication of Single-Stranded RNA (Class I to V Viruses)

In all cases replication consists in building a **template strand** complementary to the viral strand and of the same length, which is then the template for **progeny viral strands.** These steps are carried out by a complex of enzymes of both viral and cellular origin, in association with the nucleocapsids of the infecting virions.

In many instances replication and transcription interfere with each other: with negative-strand viruses both template strands and transcripts are made from viral strands; and with positive-strand viruses a viral strand can be used as messenger or replication template. Initially in infection there is no interference: the messenger function is needed to provide proteins needed for replication. Later the supply of these proteins regulates the rate of replication. For instance, with vesicular stomatitis virus, a negative-strand virus, the amount of N protein regulates replication by binding to the progeny RNAs to form nucleocapsids. RNA replication can be abolished by preventing the binding of N-protein to the RNA, for instance by injecting into the cells a monoclonal antibody that combines with the free protein.

With the positive-strand poliovirus, replication occurs when the viral pVg protein becomes covalently linked at the 5' ends of the RNA, apparently initiating the formation of a replication complex.

Messenger and progeny strands are sometimes differentiated structurally. For instance, with influenza virus (an orthomyxovirus), the messenger strands differ in two ways from progeny strands: they have a capped leader derived from cellular messenger, and they lack 17 to 22 nucleotides at the 3' end. Moreover, replication requires ongoing protein synthesis to provide the required proteins, whereas transcription does not.

REPLICATIVE INTERMEDIATES. In RNA replication the newly made template strand remains associated with the viral strand on which it is made, forming a double-stranded structure the length of the viral genome, known as RF (**replicating form**). Synthesis of new strands occurs by conservative asymmetric synthesis; a single viral strand is made, displacing the preexisting viral strand, which then becomes associated with capsid proteins to generate a new nucleocapsid (Fig. 48–12). An RF with a nascent viral strand is known as an **RI** (**replicative intermediate**). RF molecules are fairly abundant during repli-

cation because after completion of a new strand the replicase appears to remain associated for some time with the template before reinitiating synthesis; RFs accumulate at the end of replication, when no more RIs are formed.

The mechanisms that form the double-stranded molecules are not well known. Poliovirus requires the association of the viral replicase with a protein known as "host factor," which can be replaced *in vitro* by oligo-U. The oligonucleotide acts as replication primer, suggesting that the host factor is a terminal uridyl transferase that adds a short chain of U's at the end of the poly(A). The chain of U's folding back along the poly(A) would form the replication primer.

SITE OF REPLICATION. The viral RNAs replicate in the cell's cytoplasm, except for orthomyxoviruses, which replicate in the nucleus. The **replicase,** present in infected cells, synthesizes new viral RNA strands of both polarities. Transcription occurs at the same site as replication. It is unclear whether replication and transcription are carried out by different enzymes or by the same enzyme variously modified by interaction with virion proteins, as is the case with RNA phages (see Chap. 45).

Replication of Double-Stranded RNA (Class VI Viruses)

Each segment of reovirus RNA is replicated independently. Replication is intimately tied to transcription of the genome by the **virions' transcriptase,** which generates mRNAs in the virion cores. A **replicase** uses the nascent messenger strand as template, making a negative strand, which then acts as template for a new positive strand. The two strands remain associated in a double-stranded molecule that ends up in a virion (Fig. 48–13). This replication is **asymmetric** and **conservative** because (1) the negative strand of the virion RNA

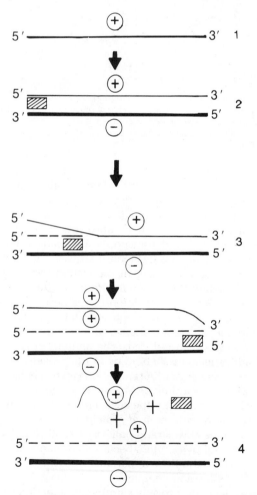

Figure 48–12. Replication of flavivirus RNA by strand displacement. The viral RNA (*1*) generates an RF (*2*). The replicase (*dashed*) builds a new + strand (*dashed*), displacing the RF + strand (thin line) (*3*). Finally, the preexisting + strand is released (*4*), while the RF and the replicase are ready to start a new cycle.

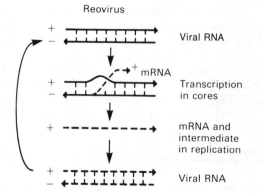

Figure 48–13. Transcription and replication of virion double-stranded RNA. In this conservative replication, information flows from **only one strand** (asymmetric), and both parental strands are conserved together.

serves as the initial template and (2) the parental RNA does not end up in the progeny (see Fig. 48–13).

Replication Through a DNA-Containing Replicative Intermediate (Class VII Viruses)

That the replication of retrovirus RNA occurs through a DNA intermediate was first shown by the blocking effect of inhibitors of DNA synthesis and transcription. To explain these observations Temin proposed that the viral replication proceeds through a double-stranded DNA RI, and that progeny viral RNA is obtained from it by regular transcription. Strong support for this theory was afforded by two discoveries: (1) a **reverse transcriptase,** present in virions, synthesizes DNA using the single-stranded viral RNA as template, and (2) viral DNA can be recognized in the infected cells, integrated into the cellular DNA as **provirus.** Transcription of the provirus by the cellular transcriptase yields the viral molecules that end up in virions. The complex process of reverse transcription is considered in detail in Chapter 65.

MATURATION AND RELEASE OF ANIMAL VIRUSES

Maturation proceeds differently for naked, enveloped, and complex viruses.

Naked Icosahedral Viruses

MATURATION. As with bacteriophages, maturation of naked viruses consists of two main processes: (1) assembly of the capsid and (2) its association with the nucleic acid. For **DNA viruses** the two steps are clearly separate, since DNA synthesis precedes the appearance of recognizable capsid components, sometimes by several hours. In contrast, with **naked icosahedral RNA viruses** the association of the capsid with the nucleic acid proceeds almost concurrently. The synthesis of viral RNA, measured either chemically or by infectious titer, is followed shortly by synthesis of mature virions; for poliovirus the time difference is 30 to 60 minutes. The fairly close temporal connection between synthesis and assembly may have evolved because of the inherent instability of the naked viral RNA in the cells.

ASSOCIATION OF THE CAPSID WITH THE NUCLEIC ACID. With icosahedral animal viruses, as with bacteriophages, preassembled capsomers are joined to form **empty capsids (procapsids),** which are the precursors of virions. In fact, in pulse-chase experiments with labeled amino acids added to infected cells, the label is incorporated first into nascent polypeptide chains, then capsomers, later procapsids, and finally complete virions. With poliovirus the capsomers are pentameric; with adenovirus they are both pentamers and trimeric hexons (see Chap. 44). With both viruses the assembly of capsomers to form

the procapsid is accompanied by extensive reorganization, which is revealed by changes of serologic specificity or isoelectric point.

With a number of viruses (e.g., picornaviruses, adenoviruses), polypeptides are processed while the nucleic acid associates with the procapsid. For example, in poliovirus maturation, the final step is the cleavage of the precursor polypeptide VP_0 into $VP_2 + VP_4$ (see Fig. 48–12). Presumably the viral RNA penetrates between the capsomers from the outside, triggering the cleavage reaction. VP_4 may be responsible for locking the RNA into the capsid, because its loss at uncoating (see Initial Steps of Viral Infection, above) or during heat inactivation is accompanied by separation of RNA from the capsid. In adenovirus morphogenesis, the viral DNA, linked to the 55 Kd terminal protein, enters the procapsid together with core proteins; subsequently proteins of both procapsid and core undergo cleavage. For viruses that form concatemers in DNA replication, specific sequences act as signals for DNA cleavage into monomers and for packing into the procapsid.

With reoviruses, the genome of which is segmented (class VI), the various progeny RNA pieces appear to assemble within an inner capsid in which they are held together, forming the virion core. Undefined final steps in morphogenesis lead to association of this core with the outer capsid (see Chap. 62).

After they are assembled, icosahedral virions may become concentrated in large numbers at the site of maturation, forming the intracellular crystals (Fig. 48–14) frequently observed in thin sections of infected cells.

RELEASE. Naked icosahedral virions are released from infected cells in different ways, which depend on both the virus and the cell type. Poliovirus, for instance, is **rapidly released,** with death and lysis of HeLa cells: the study of single infected cells, contained in small drops of medium under paraffin oil (Fig. 48–15), shows a total yield of about 100 plaque-forming units released over a period of $\frac{1}{2}$ hour. In contrast, virions of DNA viruses that mature in the nucleus tend to **accumulate** within the infected cells over a long period; they are released when the cells undergo autolysis, but in some cases they are extruded without lysis.

Enveloped Viruses

MATURATION. Viral proteins are first associated with the nucleic acid to form the nucleocapsid, which is then surrounded by the envelope.

In **nucleocapsid formation** the proteins are all synthesized on cytoplasmic polysomes and are rapidly assembled into capsid components (recognizable by immunofluorescence or electron microscopy). With most RNA viruses the nucleocapsids accumulate in the cytoplasm (Fig. 48–16), but with orthomyxoviruses (e.g., influ-

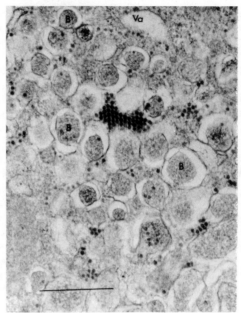
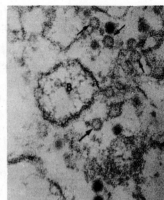

Figure 48–14. Electron micrograph of part of the cytoplasm of an HeLa cell infected by poliovirus (a picornavirus), showing a focus of viral reproduction. (*Left*) Many viral particles are present in the cytoplasmic matrix (some in small crystals) around or within membrane-bound bodies (*B*) and vacuoles (*Va*). (*Right*) Empty capsids (*arrows*). (Dales S et al: Virology 26:379, 1965)

enza and fowl plague virus) they are recognizable first in the nucleus (by 3 hours; Fig. 48–17) and later in the cytoplasm.

In **envelope assembly,** virus-specified envelope proteins go directly to the appropriate cell membrane (the plasma membrane, the endoplasmic reticulum, or the

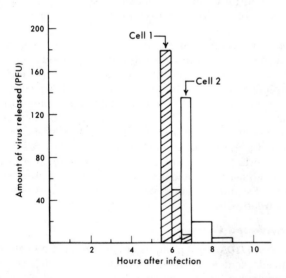

Figure 48–15. Kinetics of viral release from single monkey kidney cells infected by poliovirus. The cells were obtained by disrupting a monolayer of monkey kidney cells by trypsin; after being infected with poliovirus, each was introduced into a separate small drop of medium immersed in paraffin oil. Every half hour, the medium of each drop was removed, replaced with fresh medium, and assayed for infectivity by plaque assay. Note that with either cell the release was rapid (most virus came out in ½ hour), and note also the difference in the latent periods. (Data from Lwoff A et al: Virology 1:128, 1955)

Golgi apparatus), displacing host proteins. In contrast, **the lipids and carbohydrates are those produced by the host cell,** as shown by their composition and by their specific activities in virus-producing cells labeled before infection with a radioactive precursor. The viral envelope has the lipid constitution of the membrane where its assembly takes place (e.g., the plasma membrane for orthomyxoviruses and paramyxoviruses, the nuclear membrane for herpesviruses). A given virus will differ in its lipids and carbohydrates when grown in different cells, with consequent differences in physical, biologic, and antigenic properties (see also The Envelope, Chap. 44). The viral proteins, however, to a certain extent also select the lipids with which they aggregate; thus, two types of influenza virus (A and B) grown in the same cells may differ in the proportions of individual phospholipids.

The **formation of the envelope glycoproteins** is best understood for viruses that bud at the plasma membrane (e.g., orthomyxoviruses). The glycoproteins are synthesized on polysomes bound to the endoplasmic reticulum; immediately the hydrophobic N-terminal **signal sequence** penetrates the membrane and is cleaved off as it emerges at the other side (see Chap. 6). A hydrophobic **anchor sequence** holds the polypeptide in the membrane, usually as a transmembrane protein. From the endoplasmic reticulum the polypeptide moves via transport vesicles to the Golgi apparatus, where it attains its full **glycosylation** and other modifications, such as **fatty acid acylation** (palmitic or myristic acid). Some proteins are **proteolytically cleaved,** generating two S–S bonded peptides, as in the fusion protein of paramyxoviruses. These changes are important for the function of

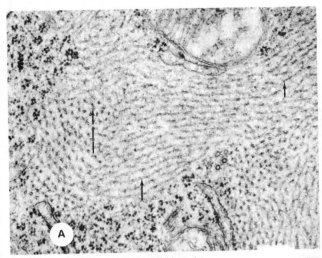

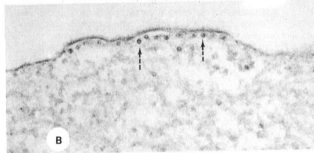

Figure 48—16. Maturation of an enveloped virus with a helical nucleocapsid (Sendai virus, a paramyxovirus) in infected chick embryo cells. *(A)* Accumulation of nucleocapsids in the cytoplasm, some cut transversely (*dashed arrow*), some longitudinally (*solid arrows*). *(B)* Transversely cut nucleocapsids under thickened areas of the plasma membrane, covered by spikes, preliminary to budding and virion formation. (Darlington RW et al: J Gen Virol 9:169, 1970)

the protein; thus, blocking N-linked glycosylation with tunicamycin or fatty acid acylation by mutation may prevent the appearance of the glycoprotein at the cell surface. After progressing through the various parts of the Golgi apparatus the glycoproteins, via other transport vesicles, reach the cell membrane, where they are exposed at the external surface of the cell.

The glycoproteins determine where virion maturation takes places: For instance the bunyavirus glycoproteins behave like intrinsic Golgi proteins, which reach the Golgi apparatus and are incapable of leaving it; as a result the virions mature and bud from the wall of Golgi vesicles into their lumen. From there they are transported to the surface by an unknown mechanism.

Matrix proteins that are present in viral envelopes are usually not glycosylated and stick to the cytoplasmic side of the plasma membrane through hydrophobic domains. Matrix proteins connect the cytoplasmic nucleocapsid with the cytoplasmic domains of the envelope glycoproteins and with the cell's cytoskeleton, and they gather the viral glycoprotein to form the virions (Fig. 48–18). The selection of viral glycoproteins is efficient but not exclusive: for instance, rhabdovirus virions contain 10% to 15% of nonviral glycoproteins. They may also contain glycoproteins specified by another virus infecting the same cell; such virions are known as **pseudotypes** (see Chap. 50).

FORMATION AND RELEASE OF VIRIONS. Envelopes are formed around the nucleocapsids by **budding of cellular membranes** (see Fig. 48–18). This budding is the result of an intimate adhesion of the nucleocapsid to the matrix (M) protein at the cytoplasmic side of the cell membrane where the viral glycoproteins are embedded;

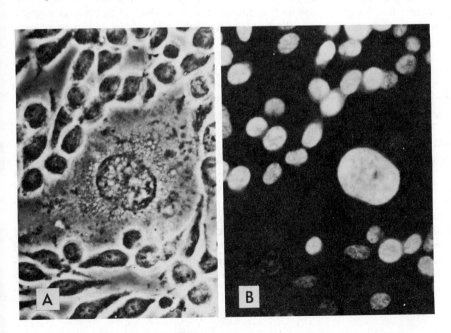

Figure 48—17. Localization of the nucleocapsid antigen of fowl plaque virus (an orthomyxovirus) in the nucleus 3 hours after infection of a culture of L cells. The cells were fixed and treated with fluorescent Ab to the viral Ag. *(A)* Phase contrast micrograph. *(B)* Micrograph of the same field in ultraviolet light, where only the Ag bound to the viral Ab is visible. The absence of fluorescence in the cytoplasm is especially evident in the giant cell. (Franklin R, Breitenfeld P: Virology 8:293, 1959)

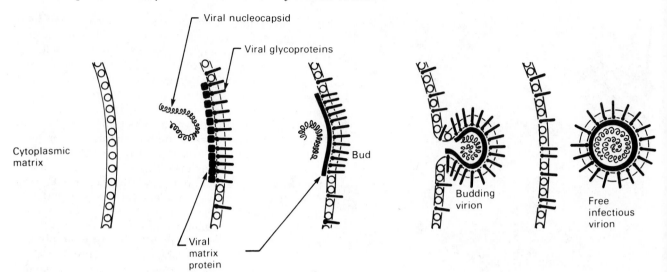

Figure 48–18. Budding of an enveloped virus (orthomyxovirus or paramyxovirus). *White circles,* host proteins of the plasma membrane (specified by cellular genes); *black spikes,* viral glycoproteins (the peplomers specified by viral genes), which become incorporated into the cell membrane, replacing host cell proteins, before budding of the viral particles begins. The viral **matrix (M) protein** attaches to the inner surface of the plasma membrane segment containing the viral glycoproteins and appears to serve as a recognition site for the nucleocapsid as well as a stabilizing structure.

the adhesion causes the membrane to curve into a protruding sphere surrounding the nucleocapsid. Interaction of matrix protein with actin-containing filaments seems to be important for budding.

The bud detaches from the membrane by a process that can be considered the reverse of penetration. If budding is from the surface membrane (e.g., paramyxoviruses), release occurs at the same time. If budding occurs in cytoplasmic vesicles (e.g., togaviruses), release requires subsequent fusion of the vesicle with the cell membrane. Either method of release is compatible with cell survival and can be very efficient, allowing a cell to release thousands of viral particles per hour for many hours. Herpesviruses bud out of the nuclear membrane into the cytoplasm and reach the outside through cytoplasmic channels and vesicles.

With some newly isolated influenza viruses (see Chap. 56) a deviation from the normal pattern of maturation leads to the formation of infectious cylindrical **filaments** with a diameter similar to that of the spherical particles. Their formation depends on genetic properties of the virus, type of host cell, and environment (e.g., in cell cultures it is greatly enhanced in the presence of vitamin A, alcohol, or surfactants).

A **polarized** viral budding is observed in cultures of epithelial cells in which the lipid and protein composition of the apical part of the plasma membrane differs from that of the basolateral part; the individuality of the two parts is maintained by the tight junctions between cells, which are barriers to diffusion within the plasma membrane. In MDCK cells (Madin-Darby canine kidney line), orthomyxoviruses and paramyxoviruses bud from the apical surface, whereas herpesviruses, rhabdoviruses, and retroviruses bud from the basolateral surface. The viral glycoproteins have distinguishing features that direct them to one or the other surface.

CELL SURFACE ALTERATIONS PRODUCED BY VIRAL MATURATION. With orthomyxoviruses and paramyxoviruses the viral glycoproteins incorporated in the membranes confer on the cell some properties of a giant virion. Thus, cells infected by these viruses may bind RBCs (**hemadsorption,** Fig. 48–19, the equivalent of hemagglutination) or viral antibodies, and paramyxovirus-infected cells may fuse with uninfected cells to form multinucleated syncytia, called **polykaryocytes** (Fig. 48–20), by fusion of their membranes. This fusion is equivalent to the fusion of the virion's envelope with the plasma membrane of the host cell at the onset of infection (see above, Uncoating). Polykaryocytes can also be formed by inactivated virions attached to the cell surface, provided that they have a functional fusion protein. This approach is used to fuse two different cell types, producing cell hybrids.

Complex Viruses

Maturation of the highly organized **poxviruses** takes place in cytoplasmic foci called "**factories.**" Membranes enclosing fibrillar material appear first; then viral DNA enters the particles when the membranes are almost complete, forming a dense, immature nucleoid (Fig. 48–21). As with other viruses, **peptide cleavage** appears to perform an important role. In contrast to simpler viruses, the poxvirus membrane contains **newly synthesized lipids** that differ in composition from cellular lip-

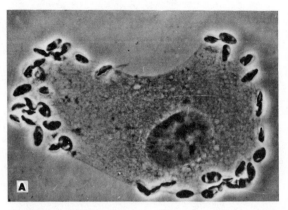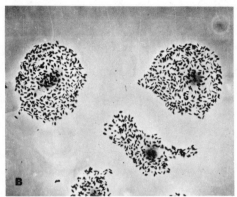

Figure 48–19. Hemadsorption of HeLa cells infected by Newcastle disease virus. Cells had been heavily irradiated with x-ray several days before infection; they stopped multiplying but increased in size and became giant cells, facilitating observations. The virus multiplies regularly in these cells. *(A)* Cell 5 hours after infection. The ability to adsorb chicken RBCs begins to appear at two opposite regions of the cell surface. At these regions new cell membrane appears to be laid down, allowing viral components to become incorporated together with the cellular components. *(B)* Cells at lower magnification, 9 hours after infection, showing that the entire cellular membrane has developed the capacity for hemadsorption. The RBCs are firmly attached to the cells and are not removed by repeated washing. (Marcus P: Cold Spring Harbor Symp Quant Biol 27:351, 1962)

ids. These viruses employ two pathways for releasing the progeny particles. Some become enveloped in Golgi-derived vesicles, which reach the cell surface, but the majority are released upon cell lysis.

The maturation of poxviruses after the precursors have been enclosed within the primitive membrane suggests that **poxviruses may be transitional forms toward a cellular organization.** Viral maturation, however, requires functions of the cellular nucleus, because it is blocked after the nucleus is removed or inactivated by UV light.

Assembly From Subunits in Precursor Pools

In a cell simultaneously infected by certain pairs of related viruses that differ in capsid Ags, such as poliovirus types 1 and 2, **phenotypic mixing** can occur because capsids made from building blocks of both viruses or either viruses may enclose a genome. Antiserum to either Ag may neutralize particles with mixed capsids (see Chap. 50). Hence, infection with a mixture of poliovirus of types 1 and 2 may yield six classes of virions (Fig. 48–22) with different combinations of genotype (RNA) and phenotype (protein). Similar mixing is seen with adenovirus, which yields capsids with fibers of different lengths and with random combinations of hexons, producing mixed antigenic types. Phenotypic mixing affecting envelope glycoproteins can occur even between unrelated viruses (such as rhabdoviruses and retroviruses), generating **pseudotypes.**

These observations show that the virions of animal viruses are assembled from building blocks more or less **randomly picked from pools.**

Genetics

Animal virus genetics has made impressive progress in recent years, owing to the extensive use of molecular methods. Yet it is not as well known as the genetics of bacteriophages, because the technical difficulties are

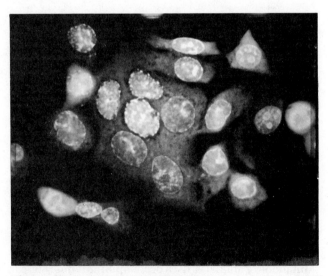

Figure 48–20. Formation of multinucleated syncytia (polykaryocytes) by Hep-2 cells infected by herpes simplex virus. Five cells have fused completely, and several others partly, into a central mass. Cells were stained with the fluorescent dye acridine orange and photographed in a dark field. (Roizman B: Cold Spring Harbor Symp Quant Biol 27:327, 1962)

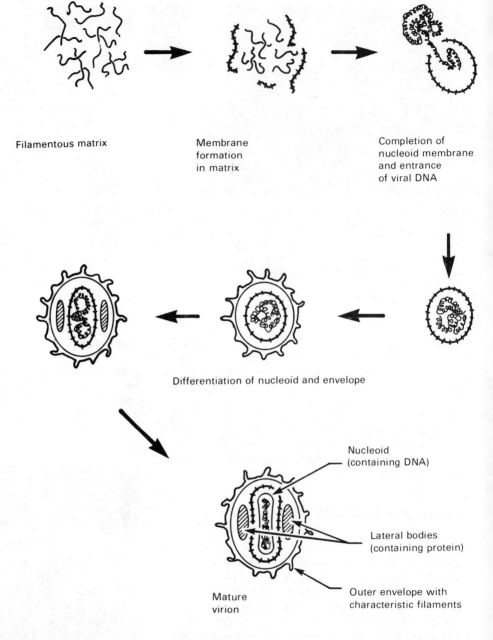

Filamentous matrix

Membrane
formation
in matrix

Completion of
nucleoid membrane
and entrance
of viral DNA

Differentiation of nucleoid and envelope

Nucleoid
(containing DNA)

Lateral bodies
(containing protein)

Outer envelope with
characteristic filaments

Mature
virion

Figure 48–21. Scheme of the development of vaccinia virions, reconstructed from electron micrographs (see Fig. 54–8). The entire process proceeds in "cytoplasmic factories."

greater, and with some viruses recombination is infrequent.

MUTATIONS

Mutations of animal viruses occur **spontaneously** or can be **induced** by various chemicals, including nitrous acid, 5-bromodeoxyuridine (BUDR), hydroxylamine, and nitrosoguanidine (fluorouridine is also useful for RNA viruses). Mutations can also be engineered after the viral DNA (or the complementary DNA from RNA viruses) is

cloned (see Chap. 8). With DNA viruses the spontaneous **mutation frequency** depends on the characteristics of the viral DNA polymerase, which can have either a mutator or an antimutator role (see Mutation, Chap. 8). The known **mutant phenotypes** are numerous and cover a larger range than bacteriophage mutations, because there are more ways for studying their properties (for instance, their various effects on animals).

The frequency of mutation, either spontaneous or induced, is higher with RNA than with DNA viruses because RNA polymerases and reverse transcriptases are

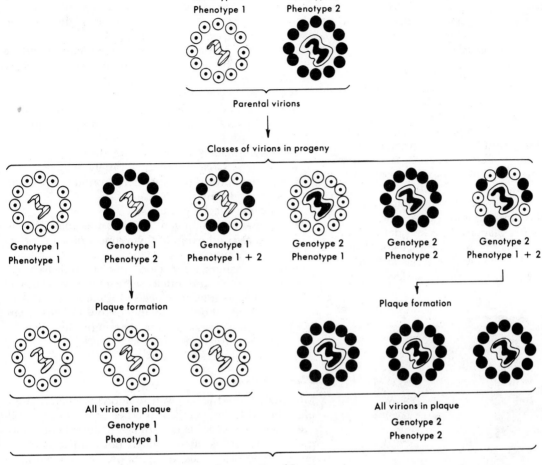

Genotype 1
Phenotype 1

Genotype 2
Phenotype 2

Parental virions

Classes of virions in progeny

Genotype 1
Phenotype 1

Genotype 1
Phenotype 2

Genotype 1
Phenotype 1 + 2

Genotype 2
Phenotype 1

Genotype 2
Phenotype 2

Genotype 2
Phenotype 1 + 2

Plaque formation

Plaque formation

All virions in plaque
Genotype 1
Phenotype 1

All virions in plaque
Genotype 2
Phenotype 2

Determination of Genotype

Genotype = the genetic information residing in the nucleic acid

Phenotype = the immunological characteristics residing in the capsid protein

Figure 48–22. Mechanism underlying phenotypic mixing of the antigenic specificity of poliovirus. Cells mixedly infected by types 1 and 2 produce virions of six genotype and phenotype combinations. Cloning of these by plaque formation yields unmixed virions, with phenotype determined by the genotype of the initiating virion, irrespective of the latter's phenotype.

much less accurate, by a factor of as much as 10^6. This high frequency causes **rapid drift** of the genome, as observed especially with othomyxoviruses and lentiviruses. As a result an RNA virus strain is always a heterogeneous collection of different genotypes, the composition of which depends on the selective conditions under which it is grown (see Viral Evolution, below).

Mutant Types

Only one class of **conditionally lethal mutations, temperature-sensitive (ts) mutations,** is useful in animal viruses. These mutations may affect the stability of the protein, its transport (by altering the membrane-binding domains), or its processing (such as cleavage or glycosylation). The ts mutations have been extremely valuable because they can be recovered in many (possibly all) genes. In spite of some defects, such as leakiness and a high reversion rate, they form the basis for most of our present knowledge of animal virus genetics. Some such strains of influenza virus are useful as vaccines because they are attenuated, i.e., less virulent.

Cold-sensitive mutants, which grow much better at 39°C than at 33°C, have occasionally been isolated. **Deletions** occur frequently in certain DNA genomes (such as parvoviruses); often the deleted sequences are located between direct repeats, 4 to 10 base pairs long. The mechanism seems to be slipped mispairing during replication. Frequent deletions in RNA genomes lead to formation of interfering particles and are discussed in Chapter 49.

Mutations affect many properties:

Host dependence (or host range). These mutants, occurring in many viruses, fail to multiply in certain nonpermissive cell types, which differ for the various viruses. Like the suppressor-sensitive mutants of phage, they can be propagated in permissive cells, are not leaky, and have a low reversion rate; however, they are limited to one or **a few genes** involved in overcoming the nonpermissiveness of the cells.

Plaque size or type (Fig. 48–23). These mutants are not as diverse as the corresponding phage mutants because animal virus plaques have less detail (they affect fewer and larger cells). Differences of plaque size may depend on differences either in features of the multiplication cycle or in the surface charges of the virions. Small charge differences affect plaque size because agar contains a sulfated polysaccharide that adsorbs the more highly charged virions, especially at certain pHs.

Cytopathic effect. Noncytopathic mutants produce plaques that are not lytic but are recognizable by other criteria (e.g., hemadsorption).

Pock type in poxviruses (see Chap. 54)

Surface properties, detected by physical methods or by appearance of extensive cell fusion (with herpesvirus)

Hemagglutination (in orthomyxoviruses)

Resistance to inactivation by a variety of agents

Resistance toward or dependence on inhibitory substances during multiplication

Pathogenic effect for animals

Functions of certain viral genes in the infected cells, such as production of thymidine kinase or induction of interferon

Physical changes, for instance, the length distribution of restriction endonuclease fragments with DNA, of oligonucleotides produced by RNAses with RNA, or the electrophoretic mobility of the proteins. Many mutations are **silent** and determine the extensive **polymorphism** observed in the base sequences of strains of the same virus.

Pleiotropism

Mutants selected for a given phenotypic alteration are often found to be changed in other properties as well. For instance, poliovirus mutants with altered chromatographic properties often (though not always) have decreased neurovirulence for monkeys. This pleiotropism reflects the effect of a single viral protein on several properties of the virus. Viral virulence is often affected because it depends on many viral functions. The connection between the properties is variable; for example, mutations that modify different charged groups of the viral capsid may have similar effects on chromatographic adsorption but different effects on the more specific adsorption to cells.

Pleiotropism has useful applications. Thus, by the application of characters that are detectable *in vitro* (such as temperature sensitivity of various functions or deficiency of cytopathic effect), it is possible to select **attenuated** (i.e., nonvirulent) strains for use in live virus vaccines. The more cumbersome animal testing is then reserved for final characterization. This approach has been used in the selection of live poliovirus vaccines.

Complementation

Complementation of ts mutants has been useful for determining the functional organization of the viral genome. When two ts mutants complement each other, the yield of a mixed infection, at the nonpermissive tem-

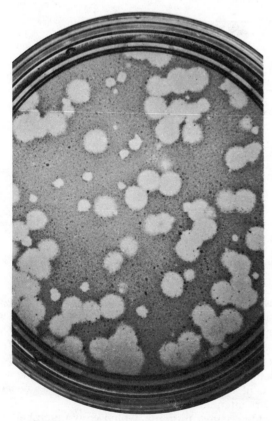

Figure 48–23. Two plaque-type mutants of fowl plague virus on a monolayer of chick embryo cells. The wild type produces large round plaques with fuzzy edges; a small-plaque mutant produces small plaques with irregularly indented outline and sharp edges. (Courtesy of H. R. Staiger)

perature, is greater than the sum of the separate yields at the same multiplicity of infection. Complementation is very efficient with the larger DNA viruses (adenoviruses, herpesviruses), for which the yield from mixed infection may approach 50% that of cells infected with wild-type virus. However, many animal viruses complement much less. Complementation is almost absent with picornaviruses, probably because their genome is translated into a larger polyprotein, and mutations that alter its tertiary structure prevent its cleavage into separate functional products. Probably for similar reasons, **asymmetric complementation** is observed with poliovirus: one mutant helps the other, but not vice versa.

In either DNA- or RNA-containing viruses, each complementation group usually corresponds to a different gene, as shown by different functional effects of different groups and by their effect on different proteins, recognizable by gel electrophoresis. Moreover, in viruses with a fragmented genome, in which each fragment is a gene, the number of the complementation groups is similar to that of the fragments.

GENETIC RECOMBINATION
DNA Viruses

In the large viruses with a linear DNA (adenoviruses, herpesviruses, poxviruses), recombination between pairs of ts mutants or between a ts and a plaque-type mutant occurs at frequencies comparable to those observed in some phages or bacteria. Generally, in recombination between mutants, the yield of mass cultures regularly contains the two reciprocal recombinant types, in comparable proportions. Recombination is also observed between viruses of different types within the same group (e.g., types 2 and 5 adenoviruses), but only at regions of high homology.

Little is known about the individual recombination events, except that they occur together with DNA replication, probably through the use of both viral and cellular enzymes. The proportion of recombinants between markers tested pairwise is additive. By a series of two- or three-factor crosses, the order of various mutations can be unambiguously established, in spite of the unusual structure or replication of these viral DNAs (see above). By this approach the herpesvirus map is 25 to 30 units long; hence, the frequency of recombination per unit length is much less than for phage T4, but of the same order as that of bacteriophage λ (see Chaps. 45 and 46). The maps are **linear**; i.e., distant markers are unlinked.

Maps have also been determined by molecular methods (Fig. 48–24), based on the fragments of the DNA generated by restriction endonucleases, the order of which is established from the overlaps of fragments produced by different enzymes. In **intertypic crosses,** differences in the fragments of the two parental DNAs reveal the crossover point in the DNA of a recombinant (see Fig. 48–24A). In **marker rescue** a fragment from wild-type virus is introduced into the cells by transfection together with viral DNA from a ts mutant; if the fragment overlaps the mutational site, wild-type virus can be generated by recombination (see Fig. 48–24B). With viruses having a cyclic DNA (e.g., polyomavirus), wild-type progeny virus can be obtained without recombination (see Fig. 48–24C): a strand of the wild-type fragment is annealed to the complementary complete strand of the mutated DNA, and the resulting hybrid is introduced into the cells. Extension of the fragment, by copying of the complementary strand, yields a wild-type strand if the fragment overlaps the mutation.

The maps obtained by molecular methods give the same gene order as those obtained by recombination, but the distances between genes do not agree well, suggesting that recombination occurs at different frequencies in different regions of the genome.

RNA Viruses—Reassortment

Burnet first recognized recombination between influenza virus strains in 1951. Some markers of this and other RNA viruses with **segmented genomes** (classes IV and VI) show high recombination frequencies, up to 50%. When the two parental viruses have corresponding segments that differ in size, these mutations can be assigned to different segments. In contrast, markers located to the same segment do not show recombination. Recombination among these viruses therefore results from random **reassortment** of segments. This is an important cause of variation: the major antigenic changes of influenza virus are primarily caused by reassortment between different species (see Evolution of Viral Antigens, Chap. 50).

RNA viruses with **continuous genomes** usually show little or no recombination; only picornaviruses and coronaviruses show measurable recombination, limited to some regions of the genome. This recombination probably arises from discontinuous replication by means of different templates, by a **copy choice** mechanism. An exceptionally high recombination frequency is found in the diploid retroviruses; recombination occurs in cells infected by **heterozygous virions,** in which the two RNA molecules carry different markers, probably by a copy choice mechanism.

GENE MAPS. For viruses **with a positive-strand continuous genome** that is translated into a single polypeptide chain (e.g., polioviruses), gene maps can be obtained **biochemically** (see Fig. 48–24D). A radioactive amino acid is added to the infected cell culture together with the antibiotic pactamycin, which inhibits initiation of protein synthesis. The label will be incorporated more by proteins corresponding to the distal (3' end) part of the RNA, which has the highest chance of being still untrans-

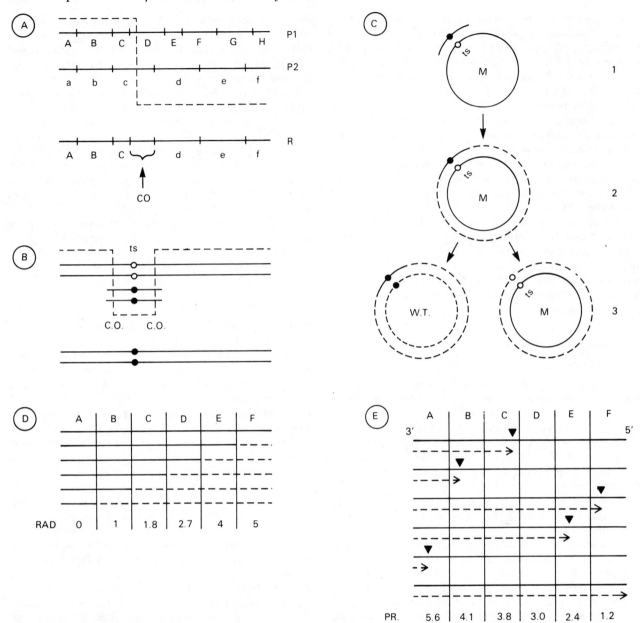

Figure 48–24. Molecular mapping. *(A)* In the intertypic cross of two viruses, **P1** and **P2,** the derivation of the DNA in the recombinant (R) can be ascertained from the restriction endonuclease fragments it contains; the position of the crossover point (CO) is delimited. *(B)* Mixed infection of cells with a viral DNA carrying a temperature-sensitive (ts) mutation and a wild-type (wt) fragment overlapping the mutation **(marker rescue)** produces a wt molecule by two crossovers (C.O.). *(C)* (1) A strand of a wt DNA fragment is annealed to a complete strand carrying a ts mutation (M); (2) after transfection (i.e., infection with pure DNA) the fragment is elongated; (3) replication yields a wt DNA molecule. *(D) Continuous lines,* a set of incomplete polyproteins at the time of addition of amino acid label + pactamycin; *dashed lines,* radioactive parts of the polyproteins when they are completed. The gradient of radioactivity (RAD) incorporated, after processing, establishes the order of genes (A to F). *(E)* Continuous lines, a set of viral genomes exposed to UV light; *arrowheads,* pyrimidine dimers; *dashed lines,* the transcribed segments; *numbers,* relative amounts of protein (PR.) synthesized for each gene (A to F). The gradient of synthesis establishes the order of genes.

lated when the label is added. The relative labeling of various proteins gives their location in the uncleaved polypeptide chain.

The gene order for several **negative-strand** viruses has also been determined by measuring the **effect of UV irradiation** of virions on the synthesis of the polypeptides specified by the various genes. The method is based on the blocking of the progress of transcription by the UV-induced pyrimidine dimers; therefore, a gene at the 5' end on the template strand has the highest sensitivity to the radiation because its transcription is blocked by any dimer along the whole genome, and the synthesis of the peptide it specifies undergoes the greatest reduction (Fig. 48–24E).

HETEROZYGOSITY. True heterozygosity is observed in retroviruses, which have two molecules of single-stranded RNA in the virion. **Multiploid heterozygosity** occurs in enveloped viruses that generate some particles with two nucleocapsids. This event is frequent in orthomyxoviruses and paramyxoviruses because two nucleocapsids can be readily accommodated in the floppy envelope; rhabdoviruses form occasional diploid particles of double length.

Reactivation of UV-Irradiated Viruses

CROSS-REACTIVATION; MULTIPLICITY REACTIVATION. With viruses that give rise to efficient recombination (large DNA viruses, influenza), markers from a UV-inactivated strain can be rescued by active virus simultaneously infecting the cells. The survival of a given marker, as a function of the UV dose, is much greater than the survival of the whole virus, as already seen with phages (see Genetic Reactivation, Chap. 45). Also, like bacteriophages, as multiplicity of infection with UV-inactivated virus is raised, the proportion of cells yielding infectious virus increases excessively. Both these reactivations are much more pronounced for RNA viruses with a segmented than with a continuous genome, in accord with the much higher frequency of recombination by reassortment of their genomic segments.

VIRAL EVOLUTION

The great ability to undergo variation is the background for the rapid evolution of viruses. The highest variability is expressed by RNA viruses, owing to the marked instability of RNA; further variability is contributed to some viruses by reassortment of genomic segments derived from different strains. Because of this tremendous variability, potentially no two RNA virions in the progeny of an infected cell should be identical. The extent of observed variability is, however, **controlled by selection** for effective interactions of virions with host cells and of viral proteins among themselves. Important in viral evo-

lution are viral antibodies and the type of host cells. Antibodies can explain the considerable evolution of influenza viruses in nature (see Chap. 50), and serial growth in different cell types causes considerable changes in a viral population.

The ability of viruses to evolve, however, seems to be subject to other types of control. This is especially seen in comparing different picornaviruses. Poliovirus exists in three serologic types, immunologically distinct but stable, whereas foot-and-mouth disease virus (FMDV) exists in seven main types with a larger number of subtypes, and new subtypes continuously emerge. The difference might be correlated with the ability of FMDV to infect a wide range of cloven-hoofed animals, whereas poliovirus infects only man. By shifting from one host to another, FMDV may have the opportunity of using more of its potential variability. Among picornaviruses, however, the rhinoviruses have a tremendous variety of strains, although they also infect only man. As discussed in Chapter 50, this variability may be based on the special selective conditions of viruses infecting mucosae. The limited evolution of poliovirus may be caused by internal restraints (e.g., in the processing step or in capsid assembly).

GENETIC CHANGES ASSOCIATED WITH CHANGES OF VIRULENCE. Many viruses cause severe diseases in animals or humans by attacking the cells of certain organs, such as the central nervous system or the liver. Such **virulent strains** can give rise to **attenuated strains,** which can multiply in the same host but fail to produce the disease (see Chap. 51). Some attenuated derivatives are used as live vaccines for immunizing animals or humans (see Chap. 50). They are usually obtained by growing a virulent strain serially through many generations in a different host, such as embryonated chicken eggs or cultures. For instance, attenuated poliovirus, lacking neurotropicity for humans and monkeys, is obtained by passaging the virus through monkey kidney cultures, and attenuated yellow fever virus and FMDV are obtained by passages through chick embryos. The passages probably select certain types of spontaneously occurring mutants. The approach is empiric, and the results vary from virus to virus; for viruses that can affect several hosts, attenuation in one host does not necessarily mean attenuation in another. Attenuation can also be obtained by selecting for variants with certain characteristics, such as cold-adapted for influenza or antibody-resistant for rhabdoviruses or bunyaviruses. In the reverse process, virulent strains can emerge spontaneously from attenuated ones and then remain stable.

Extensive genetic analyses have been carried out to try to identify the genes responsible for the changes of virulence. One approach is to compare the characteristics, and sometimes the base sequences, of closely related attenuated and virulent strains; the other is to determine the virulence of recombinants or reassortants between a virulent and an attenuated strain. These studies yielded different results in different systems. With some viruses many genetic changes contribute to determining virulence. For instance, the attenuated Sabin vaccine strains of poliovirus type 1 (see Chap. 55) differs from the original virulent strain in 55 bases and 21 amino acids, distributed all over the genome. Recombinants show that the 5' end of the genome is somewhat more important, but they afford no clear localization. With Sabin type 3 vaccine strain the situation is different: there are ten changes of bases and three of amino acids. Of these, a C → U change in the untranslated 5' end of the genome (N472) has predominant importance: its reversion to C, which occurs occasionally in vaccinated persons, restores the virulent phenotype. The revertant virus is strongly selected in humans but not in cultures. A similar precise localization of virulence-determining change restricted to a single amino acid was observed in the hemagglutinin of influenza virus and in the glycoprotein of rabies virus.

These differences in the changes involved in attenuation have important practical consequences. Spontaneous reversions to virulence occur easily when they can be brought about by a single change, but not when multiple changes are needed: whereas the type 3 Sabin vaccine strain is unstable, the type 1 vaccine is very stable.

USE OF ANIMAL VIRUSES AS VECTORS FOR IN VITRO DNA RECOMBINATION

Several animal viruses are useful vectors; some of them are oncogenic and will be considered in Chapter 65. Among the non-oncogenic ones, adenoviruses and herpesviruses are used. Here we will describe the use of vaccinia virus, which is suitable for the expression of recombinant genes in animal cells.

Construction of Recombinant Vaccinia Viruses

The principle is to introduce a foreign gene into a nonessential region of vaccinia virus DNA, such as the thymidine kinase gene (TK). For this purpose the selected gene is first introduced into the TK gene previously inserted into a plasmid vector. The TK gene is inactivated by the inserted gene, which becomes controlled by the TK gene promoter. The plasmid is then introduced by transfection into cells infected by wt vaccinia virus. Recombination between the resident and the transfected DNAs generates TK⁻ recombinant vaccinia DNA (**replication competent**), containing the inserted gene. During

growth in TK⁻ cells the recombinant virus is isolated by selection in medium containing 5-bromodeoxyuridine: for lack of the TK function, cells infected by the mutant do not incorporate the analog, and they escape its toxic effect. The cells express the foreign gene; if it specifies a membrane protein, the protein appears at the cell surface.

Selected Reading

Bishop DHL: Ambisense RNA genomes of arenaviruses and phleboviruses. Adv Virus Res 31:1, 1986

Boulan ER, Pendergast M: Polarized distribution of viral envelope proteins in the plasma membrane of infected epithelial cells. Cell 20:45, 1980

Evans DMA, Dunn G, Minor PD et al: Increased neurovirulence associated with a single nucleotide change in a noncoding region of the Sabin type 3 poliovaccine genome. Nature 314:548, 1985

Flint SJ: Regulation of adenovirus mRNA formation. Adv Virus Res 31:169, 1986

Futterer J, Winnaker EL: Adenovirus DNA replication. Current Topics Microbiol Immunol 111:41, 1984

Honess RW, Roizman B: Regulation of herpesvirus macromolecular synthesis. I. Cascade regulation of the synthesis of three groups of viral proteins. J Virol 14:8, 1974

Howard CR: The biology of hepadna viruses. J Gen Virol 67:1215, 1986

Kaariainen L, Ranki M: Inhibition of cell functions by RNA-virus infection. Annu Rev Microbiol 38:91, 1984

Kohn A: Membrane effects of cytopathogenic viruses. Prog Med Virol 31:109, 1985

Lodish HF, Porter M: Specific incorporation of host cell surface proteins into budding vesicular stomatitis virus particles. Cell 19:161, 1980

Mackett M, Smith GL: Vaccinia virus expression vectors. J Gen Virol 67:2067, 1986

Palese P, Young JF: Variation of influenza A, B, and C viruses. Science 215:1468, 1982

Scholtissek C, Koennecki I, Rott R: Host range recombinants of fowl plague (influenza A) virus. Virology 91:79, 1978

Seeger C, Ganem D, Varmus HE: Biochemical and genetic evidence for the hepatitis B virus replication strategy. Science 232:477, 1986

Senapathy P, Tratschin J-D, Carter BJ: Replication of adeno-associated virus DNA. J Mol Biol 178:179, 1984

Stanway G, Hughes PJ, Mountford RC et al: Comparison of the complete nucleotide sequences of the genomes of the neurovirulent poliovirus P3/Leon/37 and its attenuated Sabin vaccine derivative P3/Leon 12a₁b. Proc Natl Acad Sci USA 81:1539, 1984

Steinhauer DA, Holland JJ: Direct method for quantitation of extreme polymerase error frequencies at selected single base sites in viral RNA. J Virol 57:219, 1986

Stow NK, Subak-Sharpe JH, Wilkie NM: Physical mapping of herpes simplex virus type 1 mutations by marker rescue. J Virol 28:182, 1978

Wilson TMA: Nucleocapsid disassembly and early gene expression by positive-strand RNA viruses. J Gen Virol 66:1201, 1985

49

Interference With Viral Multiplication

Agents that interfere with viral multiplication are useful not only for therapy and prophylaxis but also for advancing our understanding of viral biology and of infection.

Control of Viral Diseases by Inhibition of Replication

Viral diseases result from a series of growth cycles that kill or alter cells (see Chap. 51). The maximal goal of antiviral treatment—to restore function to the infected cells—is usually unassailable because cellular macromolecules are damaged early in viral infections. Accordingly, the realistic goal is to stop viral replication and thus prevent spread to additional cells. But even this more limited goal presents considerable difficulties.

A major one is the problem of inhibiting the viruses without harming the cells. This selectivity is possible against bacteria because of their many metabolic, structural, and molecular differences from animal cells. Thus, sulfanilamide interferes with the function of *p*-aminobenzoic acid, which is a vitamin in bacterial but not in animal cells; penicillin interferes with the synthesis of the peptidoglycan, which is unique to bacteria; and streptomycin interacts with molecular features that are peculiar to bacterial ribosomes. The dependence of viral multiplication on cellular genes, in contrast, limits the points of differential attack.

Another limitation is that diseases become evident only after extensive viral multiplication and cellular alteration have occurred. Therefore, the most general approach to control is prophylaxis. Therapy is effective in localized viral diseases, such as herpetic keratoconjunctivitis (see Chap. 53), in which the killing of some uninfected cells can be tolerated if the damage is subsequently repaired. In addition, the special properties of herpesviruses permit the use of certain drugs for treating systemic herpes infections (see Agents Interfering With DNA Synthesis, below). With other viral diseases, therapy is limited to reducing their duration, the severity of symptoms, and the degree of viral shedding.

As with bacterial chemotherapy, a third important limitation of antiviral therapy is the emergence of **resistant mutants.** To avoid their selection, the principles valid for bacteria are equally applicable to viruses: adequate dosage, multidrug treatment, and avoidance of therapy unless clearly indicated. Fortunately, however, genetic resistance to two important antiviral agents— interferon and interferon inducers—does not seem to occur.

Viral Interference

When viruses of more than one type infect the same cell, each may multiply undisturbed by the presence of the others, except for possible recombination or phenotypic mixing. In certain combinations, however, the multiplication of one type of virus may be inhibited by the other. This inhibition is called **viral interference.**

The notion of interference developed first from observations with ring spot virus in tobacco plants. The initial lesions regress, but the virus persists, and if the plant is reinoculated with the same virus, no new lesions develop. Thus, the first infection interferes with the expression of the second infection. Subsequently it was found that in monkeys infection with a mild strain of yellow fever virus (a flavivirus) can prevent the usually lethal disease caused by a virulent strain or even by an antigenically unrelated flavivirus, showing that the protection is not due to Ab. Interference was later found with viruses in bacteria, thus opening the way for quantitative studies.

The study of interference with animal viruses took an important turn when Isaacs and Lindenmann, in 1957, discovered that influenza virus–infected cells produce a substance, which they called **interferon,** that accounts for many observed instances of viral interference.

DEMONSTRATION OF INTERFERENCE WITH ANIMAL VIRUSES

Interference was observed with many pairs of viruses in animals, but especially with influenza viruses in the allantoic epithelium of the chick embryo and recently with a variety of viruses in cell cultures. A typical experiment consists in inoculating the allantoic cavity with influenza A virus, as **interfering virus,** followed 24 hours later by influenza B virus, as **challenge virus:** the multiplication

of the second inoculum is partially or totally inhibited. The experiments can be simplified by using inactivated interfering virus; since it does not multiply, interference can be determined by measuring the yield of the challenge virus without the need to distinguish it from the interfering virus.

Interference depends on timing and on viral concentrations. Thus, if influenza A and B are inoculated **simultaneously** and at equal multiplicity in the allantoic cavity, they can multiply concurrently in the same cells, as shown by the production of phenotypically mixed progeny particles (see Assembly From Subunits in Precursor Pools, Chap. 48). Even viruses of different families can multiply in the same cells under proper circumstances.

We shall first consider in some detail the role of interferon in viral interference and shall then consider a heterogeneous group of other mechanisms.

INTERFERON

Interferon was discovered in the course of studying the effect of influenza virus inactivated by ultraviolet (UV) light on fragments of the chick chorioallantoic membrane maintained in an artificial medium. The supernatants, although devoid of viral particles, inhibited the multiplication of active influenza virus in fresh fragments. Subsequently, such "interferons" were shown to be produced by cells of many animal species infected by almost any animal virus, either DNA- or RNA-containing, and in tissue culture or in the animal.

Interferons (IFNs) are a family of small proteins first isolated from virus-infected or chemically activated fibroblasts and leukocytes (type I IFN); later, type II or immune IFN was isolated from T cells activated by mitogen or antigen. Type I IFNs are distinguished by serology into type α or β; type II is of one type, γ. IFN-α and IFN-β are stable at acidic pH (pH 2 in the cold), whereas IFN-γ is not. Cloning the genes showed the existence of a family of about twenty IFN-α genes, highly homologous to one another, including several inactive pseudogenes, and a single β gene, with 50% homology to α genes, all localized on human chromosome 9. These genes, which lack introns, encode proteins of 165 or 166 amino acids. Human IFN-α is not glycosylated, whereas IFN-β is. The single IFN-γ gene contains introns and has little homology to the other genes. It encodes a glycoprotein of 146 amino acids. At their 5' ends the genes contain sequences with the characteristics of enhancers that control their expression.

IFNs are produced in large quantities by animal or human cells: IFN-α by leukocytes infected with Sendai virus or lymphoblastoid cell lines carrying the Epstein-Barr (EB) virus genome (see Chap. 64), and IFN-β by fibroblastic strains or lines (see Chap. 47) exposed to poly(I):poly(C) (see below).

A much more convenient source became available after IFN genes were cloned from cDNAs in bacterial vectors, which then express the IFN proteins in bacteria. Produced IFNs have all the effects of IFNs made in animal cells, although they are not glycosylated. With appropriate vectors, production is also possible in yeast or in murine cells. In all cases IFNs are purified on columns of monoclonal antibodies attached to a solid support. These readily available and pure proteins made it possible to study the biological and antiviral activities of IFNs. Artificial recombinants between the various IFN genes obtained by DNA cloning express more IFNs with unusual properties.

IFN is usually **assayed** by determining its effect on the multiplication of a test virus, usually vesicular stomatitis virus (VSV, a rhabdovirus), which is very sensitive to IFN and infects cells of many vertebrate species. Serial IFN dilutions are added to the culture medium or to the agar overlay in a plaque assay, and the endpoint (a **unit**) is a 50% reduction in the viral yield or in the number of plaques. International units (IU) are expressed with reference to an international standard. A sensitive radioimmunoassay is also available, based on the use of monoclonal antibodies.

Effects

IFNs are among the most powerful drugs available: 10 to 20 molecules are sufficient to confer resistance on a cell. Each IFN has **antiviral action, inhibits cell proliferation, and modulates the immune response,** especially by activating natural killer (NK) cells; IFN-γ powerfully activates macrophages. Some of the activities are enhanced by combining IFN-α or β with IFN-γ. The **effects are generally species specific;** for instance, purified IFN of chick origin is less than 0.1% as effective in mouse cells as in chick cells. However, IFN produced in monkey kidney cells is effective in human as well as in monkey cells, and human IFNs are active in cells of several mammals, including nonprimates. IFN produced by an artificial recombinant gene obtained from two human IFN-αs has an even broader range: it is quite active in murine and feline cells.

The described effects are part of a general regulatory action of IFNs on cellular functions, which results in **activation or inactivation of expression of many genes.** Among activated genes not related to the antiviral action are those for major histocompatibility complex (MHC) Ags of classes I and II, β_2-microglobulin, tubulin, certain "tumor-associated antigens," and at least 12 unidentified proteins. Inactivated are growth-related genes, such as those stimulated in fibroblastic cells by platelet-derived growth factor. MHC Ag genes are strongly activated by IFN-γ but may be inhibited by IFN-α/β. All the induced proteins are also present in cells not exposed to IFN but in much smaller amounts. The genes are activated at the level of transcription by the interaction of an unknown protein with a regulatory DNA sequence common to all of them.

Of special relevance among activated genes is the Mx gene. Cells of Mx$^+$ mice exposed to IFN-α or -β acquire an antiviral state—limited to orthomyxoviruses—whereas Mx$^-$ mice do not. In Mx$^+$ mice a 75-kd protein is induced in the nucleus; homologous proteins are formed in other mammals, including man. The findings suggest that the mechanism of resistance varies with the virus type.

Production After Viral Infection

IFNs are produced by cells infected with complete virions, either infectious or inactivated. Very few viral particles (e.g., with reovirus, a single physical particle) are sufficient to induce a cell. Under one-step conditions of viral multiplication the **synthesis of IFNs** begins after viral maturation is initiated; if not interrupted by an early block in the synthesis of host macromolecules, it continues at the same rate for 20 to 50 hours, then stops (Fig. 49–1). The IFNs are released extracellularly. If the cells survive longer, as after infection by UV-inactivated virus, they cannot produce IFN again in response to reinfection until after a **refractory period** of at least two cell divisions.

Usually, good IFN inducers are viruses that multiply slowly and do not block the synthesis of host protein early or markedly damage the cells. For example, an attenuated mutant of poliovirus is a much better IFN inducer than the wild type, which multiplies better; and the paramyxovirus of Newcastle disease multiplies well in chick embryo cells but causes little IFN production,

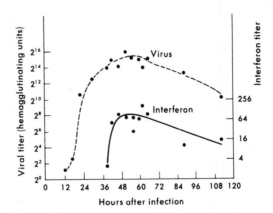

Figure 49–1. Time course of viral multiplication and interferon synthesis in the allantoic membrane of the chick embryo infected with influenza virus. Owing to the low multiplicity of infection, several cycles of viral growth were required before progeny virus could be detected; hence, the lag observed is much longer than the regular eclipse period of the virus. Note the considerable delay in the synthesis of IFN. (Modified from Smart KM, Kilbourne ED: J Exp Med 123:309, 1966)

while in human cells it causes a defective infection and induces abundant IFNs. However, many togaviruses induce large amounts of IFN, even though they multiply rapidly and have a pronounced cytopathic effect. Possible variables are effects on host macromolecule synthesis and amounts of inducer formed (see Chemical Induction, below).

Viral strains capable of high IFN production give rise to **autointerference** in endpoint assays: the dilutions containing the most virus may produce less virus because the IFN produced is sufficient to block further cycles of viral multiplication. Autointerference can also arise by a different mechanism (see Defective Interfering Particles, below).

Relation to Cells

Although animal cells of all types appear able to produce IFN-β, cells of the bone marrow and spleen and macrophages are the main producers of IFN-α. Thus, lethally x-irradiated mice grafted with rat bone marrow cells produce only rat-specific IFN. Moreover, antilymphocytic serum can inhibit IFN production in the animal. Bone

marrow cells constitutively produce small amounts of IFN, probably as regulator of cellular functions. Especially important is the regulatory role of IFN-γ. This IFN is produced by stimulated T-lymphocytes, and in vaccination against viral diseases it may activate macrophages, which then potentiate the action of Abs against cells (Ab-dependent cell cytotoxicity, see Chap. 50).

Chemical Induction

The nature of the stimulus to **interferon** production has been clarified by the Hilleman group's discovery that **double-stranded (ds)RNAs** such as reovirus RNA and certain synthetic polynucleotides can induce a large production of IFN in many animals and in tissue cultures. In human fibroblasts the effect of dsRNA is limited, however, to induction of IFN-β, whereas in the same cells viral infection induces both IFN-α and -β. The inducing activity resides in polyribonucleotides of a high molecular weight and resistant to enzymatic degradation, in which the 2' position of the ribose is unsubstituted. One of the best inducers is the double-stranded synthetic polymer consisting of one chain of polyriboinoisinic and one of polyribocytidylic acid (poly[I:C]). Other inducers are bacteria, rickettsiae, bacterial endotoxin, and phytohemagglutinin. Some inducers are active only in certain cell types. In cells, poly(I:C) causes the formation of transacting factors that interact with the 5' end of the IFN genes, allowing their transcription. Cells that are poor producers of the transactivators (such as the human HeLa cell line) produce little IFN upon induction.

ROLE OF dsRNA. It is likely that for most RNA viruses, dsRNA segments produced during replication (see Replication of Single-Stranded RNA, Chap. 48) mediate the induction of IFN. These viruses become much better inducers after mild UV irradiation, which inactivates viral genes required for initiation of progeny strand synthesis in the RIs, favoring accumulation of fully double-stranded RFs (Fig. 49–2). At high UV doses, however, the IFN-inducing activity decays in parallel to the activity of the transcriptase itself (and hence parallels the ability to form the RFs). Viruses containing dsRNA in the virions may induce without replication. For DNA viruses the inducer may be dsRNA resulting from symmetric transcription: double-stranded viral RNA extracted from cells infected with vaccinia (a DNA virus) induces IFN in tissue cultures.

CHARACTERISTICS OF PRODUCTION. In **virus-infected cells** the synthesis of IFN begins at about the time viral maturation initiates and then continues for many hours, unless the macromolecular syntheses of the host come to a halt. In cells exposed by poly(I:C), IFN production starts within about 2 hours; the rate of synthesis increases for several hours and then rapidly declines

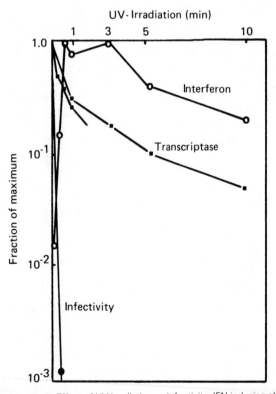

Figure 49–2. Effect of UV irradiation on infectivity, IFN-inducing ability, and transcriptase activity of Newcastle disease virus (a paramyxovirus). There is a marked enhancement of inducing ability after low UV doses, then it decays with a slope similar to that of transcriptase activity but much smaller than that of infectivity. (Modified from Clavell LA, Bratt MA: J Virol 8:500, 1971)

(shut-off). After shut-off, a new exposure of the cells to poly(I:C) does not restore IFN production for several hours (**hyporesponsiveness;** Fig. 49–3). Large concentrations of extracellular IFN inhibit the induction of IFN by either a virus or poly(I:C); in contrast, low concentrations enhance induction by an RNA virus (**priming).** The latter effect may be due to the demonstrable interference, by IFN, with the evolution of RFs into RIs.

Interferon is synthesized on membrane-bound polysomes and is then segregated into vesicles, which excrete it outside the cells. Until it is excreted, IFN does not act on the cell that produces it.

REGULATION OF SYNTHESIS. After induction by poly(I:C), IFN mRNA makes its appearance, and this event—as well as IFN production—is prevented by actinomycin D.

At the time of shut-off, functional interferon mRNA disappears; however, if the cells are exposed at that time to actinomycin D, the mRNA persists, shut-off does not occur, and IFN production is increased. This increase is even more pronounced if the cells are exposed for several hours to a reversible inhibitor of protein synthesis before actinomycin D (Table 49–1). Such a **superinduction** is probably caused by a **posttranslational effect** that increases the life of IFN mRNA in the cells.

Because IFN is produced by cellular genes, it is clear why **viruses that block cellular mRNA or protein synthesis are poor inducers of IFN production.** Moreover, it is understandable that IFN synthesis fails in tissue culture cells simultaneously infected by a good inducer and a poor inducer: the poor inducer evidently inhibits the required cellular functions. Interactions of this type presumably also occur in animals and may influence the pathogenesis of viral infections.

MECHANISM OF INTERFERON ACTION

IFNs cause antiviral resistance not directly but by **activating cellular genes encoding antiviral proteins.** Interaction of IFNs with the cell surface induces the cell response. Thus, IFN bound to polysaccharide particles (Sepharose) is as active as free interferon. IFN-α and -β interact with the same receptors, which differ from those for IFN-γ. The receptors contain gangliosides (glycosylated phospholipids); transformed cells (see Chap. 47), which are deficient in gangliosides, are less IFN sensitive than normal cells. In human cells a gene specifying the receptors for IFN-α and -β is present on chromosome 21, that for IFN-γ on chromosome 6. 21-Trisomic (Down syndrome) cells are especially sensitive to α and β IFNs.

Binding of IFN-β to its receptor causes a rapid and sharp increase of diacylglycerol in cells (see Chap. 47). This increase may be relevant for the gene activation

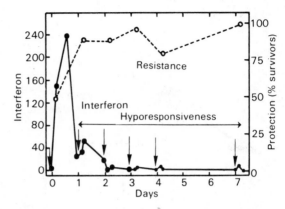

Figure 49–3. Refractory period following induction of interferon by double-stranded RNA injected into mice. After the first injection of RNA (*arrow at left*) there is a burst of interferon appearance in the serum, followed by the refractory period in which repeated injections (*other arrows*) do not cause further production. During this period, however, the mice are fully resistant to infection with encephalomyocarditis virus (a picornavirus), because the induced antiviral resistance persists. (Modified from Sharpe TJ et al: J Gen Virol 12:331, 1971)

caused by IFN. After binding IFN, the receptors are rapidly internalized through the endocytic pathway.

After the removal of extracellular IFN the inhibition of viral multiplication persists for a considerable period, the duration of which depends on the IFN concentration. The inhibition is overcome if cells are infected by virus at a high multiplicity of infection.

The **molecular mechanisms** of IFN-induced antiviral resistance are multiple and probably differ in different cell–virus systems. Effects on uncoating of the virus, on the stability or methylation of the viral RNA, and on transcription of the viral DNA have been reported. Retroviruses are affected at maturation, resulting in incorporation of nonviral proteins and altered processing of viral ones (see Chap. 65). However, *in vitro* studies with extracts of IFN-treated cells show that the **main target**

TABLE 49–1. Effect of Cycloheximide and Actinomycin D on Interferon Production*

Group	Cycloheximide (Hours of Treatment)	Actinomycin D at Hours 3–4	Interferon Yield
1	None	None	500
2	0–18	None	1,200
3	0–4	Yes	56,000
4	0–18	Yes	2,000

* Data show the effect that inhibition of RNA and protein synthesis has on interferon production in rabbit kidney cell cultures after poly(I:C) induction. The combination of the two inhibitors at suitable times and concentrations brings about dramatic enhancement of interferon production (compare groups 3 and 1).

(Data from Tan Yh et al: Virology 3:503, 1971)

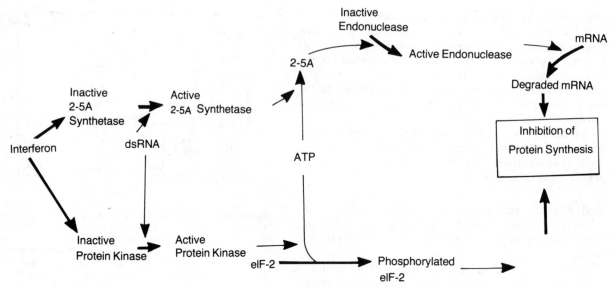

Figure 49—4. Effects of IFN and dsRNA on translation. *2-5A,* the adenine trinucleotide ''two-five A''; *eIF-2,* initiation factor.

of IFN action is translation, which is blocked by two mechanisms, involving a protein kinase and a nuclease (Fig. 49–4). In both the block requires the presence of minute amounts of **dsRNA,** which seems to signal to the cells the presence of a viral infection. As in the induction of interferon, the dsRNA may be that of a viral replicative intermediate, or it may result from symmetric transcription of the viral DNA; cellular dsRNA present in heterogeneous nuclear RNA is also adequate.

One of the **translation blocks** is caused by the activation of dsRNA-dependent **protein kinase,** which inactivates initiation factor eIF-2 by phosphorylating one of its subunits. The phorphorylation freezes the initiation complex formed by eIF-2, guanosine triphosphate (GTP), and Met-tRNAf with the small ribosomal subunit and mRNA. Because eIF-2 cannot be recycled, protein synthesis is inhibited or stopped. Some viruses can avoid this block: the VAI RNA of adenovirus prevents the activation of the kinase by dsRNA, reducing the effect of IFN.

The other translation block is due to **nucleolytic destruction of mRNA:** Kerr found that IFN induces the production of two **oligo A-synthetases** that, after activation by dsRNA, synthesize an **adenine oligonucleotide** containing three or more nucleotides of the form pppA2′p5′A2′p5′A with unusual 2′-5′ phosphodiester linkages—nicknamed "**two-five A.**" The oligonucleotide in turn activates an endoribonuclease, also induced by IFN, which cleaves mRNAs and ribosomal RNAs. Two-five A is important in antiviral resistance only in some virus–cell systems in which some analogs, which interfere with the RNase activity, inhibit the antiviral effect of IFN. In other systems, accumulation of two-five A in the cells has little effect on viral multiplication.

The blocks in translation may kill the infected cells,

but even so they halt the progress of infection. The two translation blocks occur in both infected and uninfected cells exposed to IFNs as part of the regulatory mechanism induced by this substance, but the effect is much more pronounced in virus-infected cells (containing dsRNA).

In mixed cultures of IFN-sensitive and IFN-resistant cells, antiviral resistance induced in the sensitive cells spreads to the resistant cells, presumably through channels of intercellular communication. Such a spread may favor the establishment of resistance throughout an organism.

Protective Role in Viral Infections

The protective role of endogenous IFN in viral infection of **cell cultures** is demonstrated by the establishment of **carrier cultures,** in which IFN produced in the cultures makes most of the cells resistant but cannot wipe out the infection; hence, only a small proportion are infected at any time (see Chap. 51).

A protective role of IFN **in animals** is suggested by many observations. (1) In mice recovering from influenza virus infection the titer of IFN is maximal at the time when the virus titer begins to decrease and before a rise in Abs can be detected. At this stage the IFN titer in the animals is sufficient to protect them against the lethal action of a togavirus. (2) Suckling mice, which are susceptible to coxsackievirus B1 (a picornavirus), produce little IFN in response to this virus, whereas adult mice, which are resistant, produce large amounts. Cortisone, which suppresses IFN production, makes adult animals susceptible. (3) Administration of a potent antiserum to IFN markedly increases the lethality of mouse hepatitis virus infection. (4) Mice naturally resistant to influenza virus or

VSV express a special protein the concentration of which is increased by IFN. This resistance-associated protein is maintained by the continued autocrine action of small quantities of IFN produced by the cells reacting with receptors of the same cells.

These studies suggest that IFN has a major protective role in at least some viral infections. Much depends on the **dynamics of the disease,** i.e., the relation between virus titer and IFN titer at various times. IFN is most effective when present before infection and when the dose of infecting virus is not too large (as at the beginning of most natural infections). The protection afforded may be especially useful because it develops more promptly than Ab production.

Clinically, effective **prophylaxis** was demonstrated against rhinovirus infection of human volunteers, with decreased incidence of infection and reduction of symptoms. Contacts of an infected patient can be protected by intranasal spray of large doses of IFN. Also reduced is cytomegalovirus reactivation in seropositive patients undergoing kidney transplant, with respect to both incidence of viremia and urinary shedding of the virus. In all cases the limiting factor is the extent of side-effects, which increase with dose in parallel with the beneficial effect.

POSSIBLE THERAPEUTIC USE. IFNs could theoretically be ideal antiviral agents, since they act on many different viruses and have high activity. However, their therapeutic value is limited by various factors: IFNs are effective only during relatively short periods and have no effect on viral synthesis that is already initiated in a cell. Moreover, at the high doses needed they have serious toxic effects on the host.

Attempts to use exogenous IFN for therapeutic purposes in human viral diseases have had some limited success. Thus, IFN-α had a prophylactic effect against influenza infection during epidemics, and local administration lessens the severity of respiratory diseases. In a large study, injection of large doses of recombinant IFN-α into genital warts (condyloma acuminatum) induced by papilloma virus (see Chap. 64) had a noticeable effect by causing their disappearance in one third of cases and reduced their surfaces in the other cases. Favorable effects have also been obtained after systemic treatment of warts of juvenile laryngeal papillomatosis, an aggressive disease also caused by a papilloma virus. A lessening of the pain of herpes zoster by IFN has been reported, as has a decreased spread of herpes simplex keratitis after local applications. However, the lesions produced by these viruses are not cured.

Effect on the Functions of Uninfected Cells

In vitro, IFNs inhibit cell replication and inhibit the activation of spleen lymphocytes by phytohemagglutinin. In human fibroblasts they increase the density of microfila-

ments at the cell membrane and the rigidity of the bilayer, while decreasing the mobility of surface receptors and endocytosis. *In vivo*, high doses inhibit liver regeneration, as well as the production of platelets and leukocytes, and enhance the expression of histocompatibility Ags on the lymphocyte surface.

IFN also profoundly affects the **immune response** in opposite ways: it reduces Ab production by stimulating T-suppressor cells, but it enhances the activity of cytolytic T cells; it also increases the cytotoxic activity of NK cells against virus-infected cells (see Chap. 50). These effects denote a **shift from humoral to cell-mediated immunity,** which has a defensive role in many viral infections. Some of these effects determine a pathogenetic role of IFN. Thus, administration of high doses to newborn mice induces a lethal liver degeneration and an autoimmune glomerulonephritis. Moreover, production of endogenous IFN contributes to the disease caused in mice by lymphocytic choriomeningitis virus (see Chap. 51), because it stimulates immune reactions. The combination of cell growth inhibition and enhancement of cell-mediated immunity accounts for the **antitumor** effect of IFN. Studies with highly purified IFN preparations show that all these effects are caused by the same molecule.

INTRINSIC INTERFERENCE (NOT MEDIATED BY INTERFERON)

An inability to detect IFN does not exclude its participation in an instance of viral interference, because the detection methods are relatively insensitive. However, if interference is established early in the infectious cycle, the participation of IFN can be considered unlikely because its production usually begins later.

Other mechanisms, grouped as intrinsic interference, have been studied with both bacteriophages and animal viruses.

Bacteriophage

Homologous or closely related phages (such as two mutants of the same strain, or T2 and T4) in the same cell must compete for the same precursors, cellular sites, and enzymes. The two strains can replicate more or less equally if they both infect the cell simultaneously and at low multiplicities. However, if they infect at different times or with different multiplicities, the phage with the advantage multiplies normally and interferes with (or even completely prevents) the multiplication of the other phage. In nonsimultaneous infection, interference appears to result from a change in the bacterial plasma membrane that prevents penetration of the DNA of the second phage.

With **unrelated** phages, one phage is excluded by a variety of mechanisms. Thus T-even bacteriophages probably exclude T1, T3, and λ by destroying the host cell DNA, the functions of which are needed for the multiplication of the excluded phages. Phage T4 excludes the RNA phage F2 both by inactivating a translation initiation factor that F2 requires and by rapidly degrading its RNA. If infection is not simultaneous, the phage that injects its DNA after another phage has taken over control of the cell machinery is always excluded.

Animal Viruses: Defective Interfering (DI) Particles

HOMOLOGOUS INTERFERENCE. As with bacteriophages, interference involving homologous animal viruses is most pronounced if one virus has an advantage, either in time or in multiplicity. This type of interference takes place with Newcastle disease virus (a paramyxovirus) at **adsorption,** through destruction of cellular receptors; with retroviruses at **penetration;** and with many viruses at **replication.**

Interference at replication is usually generated by **DI particles,** which accumulate after serial passages at a high multiplicity of infection. They are formed during infection with various kinds of RNA viruses, such as rhabdoviruses, togaviruses, orthomyxoviruses, and paramyxoviruses, coronaviruses, and of some DNA viruses (herpesviruses). With some viruses (e.g., VSV or Semliki Forest virus) the DI particles are smaller than regular particles and can therefore be obtained in pure form. They usually contain the normal virion proteins but have a shorter genome. DI particles are **replication defective:** they require as **helper** a regular virus coinfecting the same cells. In the early serial passages, DI particles rapidly increase in titer; then the yield of infectious virus, and finally the total particle yield, is progressively reduced (**autointerference**). In some cases these events lead to establishment of a **persistent infection** with a **carrier state** (see Chap. 51). Through autointerference the DI particles may limit the spread of viral infections in animals.

The genomes of DI particles are internally deleted but retain both ends, which are essential for the replication of RNA viruses. With DNA virus (e.g., herpesviruses) the origin of replication is always conserved and often repeated. These features show that to cause interference the DI genomes must replicate. They deprive the regular virus of its replicase by binding to it more effectively; moreover, they do not make a replicase of their own because they are always defective in the replicase gene.

The formation of DI genomes of RNA viruses is the consequence of the high variability of these genomes. With these viruses DI genomes are formed by a **copy choice** mechanism when the replicase, having replicated part of the template, skips to another part of the same or another template. With VSV and other negative-strand RNA viruses, the skipping generates defective genomes of four types: deletions, snapbacks, panhandles, and compounds (Fig. 49–5). In **deletions** the polymerase jumps to a site beyond, on the same template, skipping a segment. **Snapbacks** are formed when the

replicase, having transcribed part of the (+) strand, switches to using the just-made (−) strand as template; the resulting RNA, half of (−), half of (+) polarity, can produce a hairpin on annealing. A **panhandle** is formed by a similar mechanism, when the polymerase carrying a partial newly made (−) strand switches back to transcribing the extreme 5′ end of it; on annealing, the strand forms a panhandle. **Compound genomes** are made by a combination of deletions and snapbacks. Specific sequences may be involved in these irregularities. In fact, when a panhandle is formed in VSV the polymerase often jumps to a site 46 nucleotides from the 5′ end of the new (−) strand and then transcribes the remaining stretch; that site may be identified by its sequence. And the ends of deletions in Sendai virus DI particles have sequences related to transcription signals.

DI genomes may also have point mutations, not present in the regular viruses, and insertions, for instance of a cellular tRNA in the DI genomes of Sindbis virus.

The competition of DI genomes with competent genomes depends not only on the structure of the DI genome but also on that of the competent genome: different DI genomes may interfere to very different degrees with the same competent genome, and competent genomes may acquire mutations that make them resistant to the existing DI genomes. Subsequently, however, this resistance is overcome by new types of DI genome. During viral multiplication many types of DI genomes are continuously made; they are very heterogeneous. Both the DI genomes and the competent genome evolve continuously, increasing their ability to compete with each other.

HETEROLOGOUS INTERFERENCE. The mechanisms of heterologous interference vary in different systems, as shown by two examples. (1) Poliovirus arrests the multiplication of VSV and other RNA viruses, even when infecting later and at lower multiplicity. Apparently the mechanism is the poliovirus-induced alteration of the cap-binding protein (see Chap. 48): translation of the capped VSV or cellular messenger is prevented, but translation of uncapped poliovirus messengers is not. The interference may also involve other features of viral mRNAs because it does not occur with all RNA viruses. (2) Newcastle disease virus (NDV) RNA fails to replicate in cells previously infected by certain other RNA viruses, e.g., Sindbis virus (a togavirus). NDV RNA may form an inactive complex with the replicase induced by the interfering virus, because Sindbis mutants deficient in RNA replicase do not interfere.

SIGNIFICANCE OF VIRAL INTERFERENCE

Interference, both by IFN and by other mechanisms, is important in several aspects of viral infection. For in-

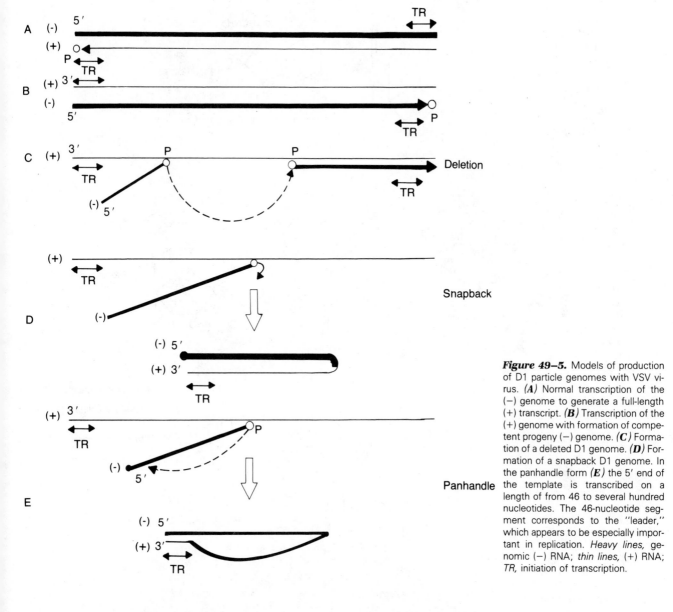

Figure 49–5. Models of production of D1 particle genomes with VSV virus. *(A)* Normal transcription of the (−) genome to generate a full-length (+) transcript. *(B)* Transcription of the (+) genome with formation of competent progeny (−) genome. *(C)* Formation of a deleted D1 genome. *(D)* Formation of a snapback D1 genome. In the panhandle form *(E)* the 5' end of the template is transcribed on a length of from 46 to several hundred nucleotides. The 46-nucleotide segment corresponds to the "leader," which appears to be especially important in replication. *Heavy lines,* genomic (−) RNA; *thin lines,* (+) RNA; *TR,* initiation of transcription.

stance, in human oral **vaccination** with attenuated poliomyelitis viruses (see Chap. 55) the three strains must be administered in a precise sequence or at specified concentration ratios to avoid interference of one strain with another. Similarly, the presence of various enteroviruses in the normal intestinal flora may hinder the establishment of infection by the vaccine strains. Viruses already present may also influence the response to a **naturally infecting virus.** For example, dengue virus infection in man is milder in the presence of an attenuated strain of yellow fever virus (both flaviviruses). IFN seems to play an important role in initiating recovery from some acute viral infections. The role of DI particles in animal infections is uncertain.

Chemical Inhibition of Viral Multiplication

SYNTHETIC AGENTS

The chemical structure of the more important synthetic agents is shown in Figure 49–6.

Selective Agents

Amantadine (adamantanamine), of peculiar structure, is active against influenza virus A and slightly against rubella and parainfluenza viruses. Being a base, it prevents the acidification of the endosomes and therefore the release of the viral genome to the cytoplasm (see

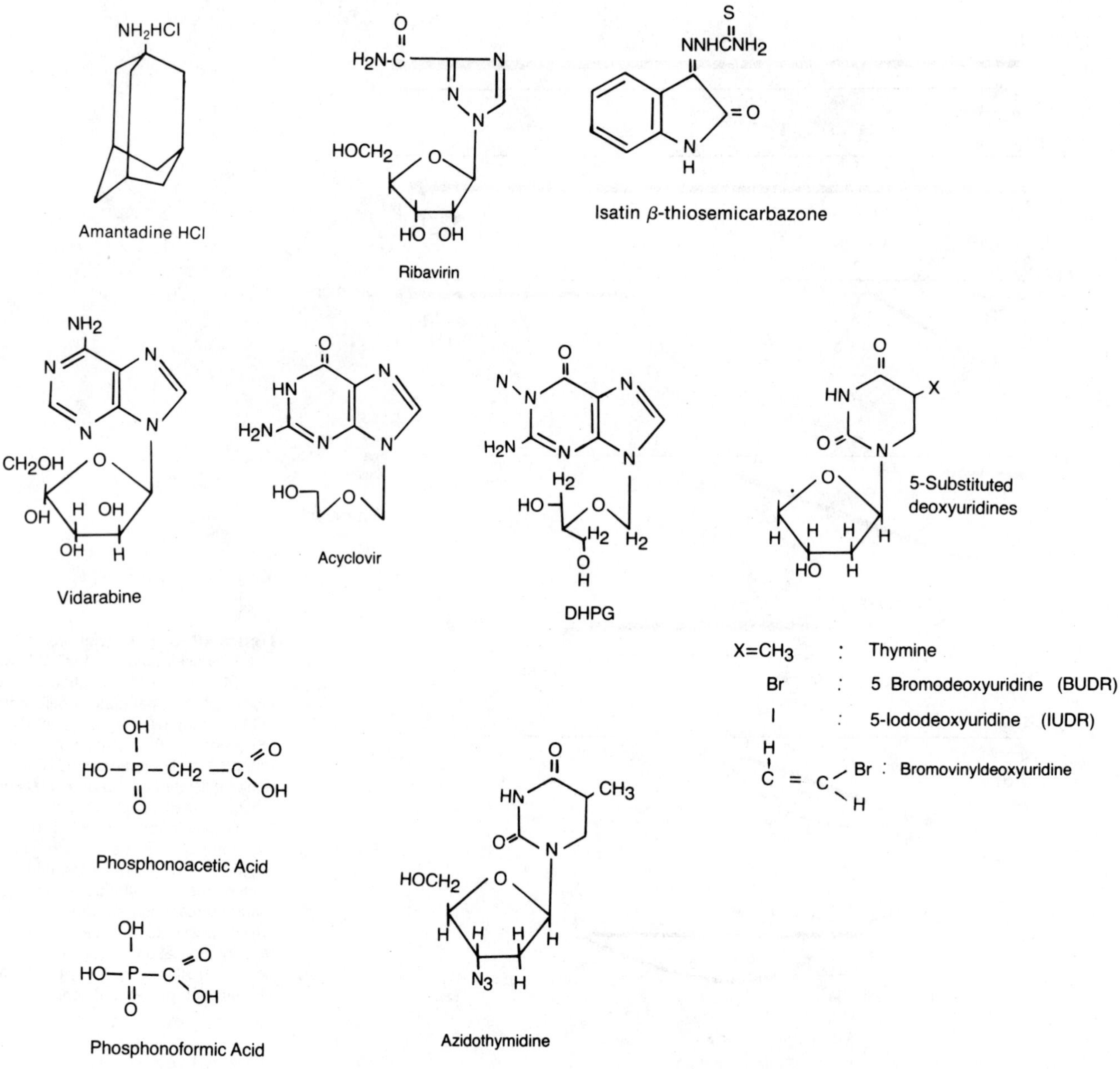

Figure 49–6. Chemical constitution of antiviral inhibitors.

Chap. 48). Drug-resistant mutants are changed in the hydrophobic part of the viral matrix protein, which is associated with the viral membrane and plays a crucial part in the release of the viral RNA from the endosome. Differences in the matrix protein between different viruses explain why the effect is limited to influenza A.

The compound, given orally, has prophylactic value against influenza A infections, attaining a 50% to 80% reduction of illness. Therapeutic effects are modest. The drug has limited side-effects, such as anxiety or insom-

nia, which rapidly dissipate on discontinuation of use. A methyl derivative, **rimantadine,** holds even better promise, because it is similarly effective but less toxic.

Ribavirin, a purine nucleoside analog, is phosphorylated in both virus-infected and uninfected cells. The phosphorylated derivative interferes with the synthesis of GMP, with resultant inhibition of both RNA and DNA synthesis and of mRNA capping. The toxic effect is stronger for virus-infected cells, which use more nucleic acid precursors than normal cells, owing to the synthesis of viral nucleic acids. *In vitro,* as well as in experimental animals, the drug has a broad antiviral spectrum that includes both DNA viruses (herpes simplex, vaccinia) and RNA viruses (influenza, parainfluenza, VSV).

In humans, ribavirin, especially by the IV route, is effective in the treatment of Lassa fever (see Arenaviruses, Chap. 62) if treatment is started within a week of onset of fever. Its administration by small-particle aerosol also appears to be somewhat effective in the treatment of influenza A and B within 24 hours of onset, and of respiratory syncytial virus infection in infants. Administered intravenously or orally, the drug causes hemolysis, which is rapidly reversible, but as an aerosol it has essentially no toxicity, probably because very little is absorbed.

Isatin-β-thiosemicarbazone and its N-methyl and N-ethyl derivatives inhibit the multiplication of several DNA and RNA viruses, especially poxviruses. They inhibit the synthesis of late poxvirus structural proteins, apparently by inactivating the late viral mRNAs. The result is the production of nearly spherical defective particles.

N-methylisatin-β-thiosemicarbazone (methisazone) had an impressive **prophylactic** success in preventing the spread of smallpox to contacts in an epidemic in Madras, India, in 1963. Among 1101 contacts vaccinated and treated with methisazone, three mild cases of smallpox occurred; in contrast, among 1126 vaccinated but not treated with the drug, 78 contracted smallpox, and 12 died. The much greater prophylactic effect of the drug can be attributed to its immediate effect on viral multiplication, contrasted with the delayed effect of the immune response to vaccination.

In contrast, the drug failed as a **therapeutic** agent in patients already suffering from smallpox. This failure is understandable, because the disease appears only after viral multiplication has reached a maximum.

Guanidine inhibits multiplication of some enteroviruses *in vitro* by interfering with the synthesis of viral single-stranded RNA without affecting cellular RNA synthesis. It does not show promise as a chemotherapeutic agent in animals, owing to the rapid emergence of **resistant viral mutants.** Viruses can also mutate to **dependence** on this drug.

Agents Interfering With DNA Synthesis

A considerable advance in antiviral chemotherapy has been the synthesis of analogs of purines and pyrimidines that inhibit the replication of certain viral DNAs much more than that of the cellular DNA. At the doses required for effective antiviral therapy they show little or moderate toxicity for the organism. Some of these compounds are the closest approximation to a selective antiviral therapy with limited cellular toxicity.

The most effective agents act against herpesviruses (see Chap. 53) and poxviruses (see Chap. 54), which, like

the T-even bacteriophages (see Chap. 45), have large genomes that specify many enzymes involved in DNA synthesis. The viral enzymes that differ markedly from the corresponding cellular enzymes are used to phosphorylate the drugs or are selectively inhibited by the drugs. Viruses with smaller genomes, which depend much more on cellular enzymes, cannot be selectively inhibited.

With herpesviruses, enzymes important for chemotherapy are the viral thymidine kinase and DNA polymerase, both different from the cellular enzymes in substrate specificity. Some drugs are converted to monophosphates by the viral enzyme and then to triphosphates by cellular enzymes. Other drugs are phosphorylated entirely by cellular enzymes. The triphosphates then block viral replication either by inhibiting the viral polymerase or by becoming incorporated into viral DNA. These substances have little effect on uninfected cells.

Vidarabine (ara-A) (9-β-D arabinofuranosyladenine) is phosphorylated entirely by cellular enzymes and is therefore active against all human herpesviruses, including cytomegalovirus and EB virus, which do not specify a thymidine kinase. The drug is also effective against vaccinia virus. A similar analogue of cytidine, **cytarabine (ara-C, arabinosyl cytosine),** has a similar action but is less selective.

Vidarabine, administered intravenously, has beneficial effects on the treatment of severe varicella or herpes zoster infections in immunosuppressed patients and of the often fatal herpesvirus infection in newborns. The drug is very useful in the therapy of herpesvirus encephalitis in man, reducing its mortality from 70% to 30%. The treatment must be initiated very early in the disease, which requires brain biopsy for early diagnosis. Vidarabine-resistant mutants occur and usually have an altered DNA polymerase. A drawback of vidarabine is its rapid deamination in the body to the hypoxanthine derivative, which is much less effective; a carbocyclic derivative (in which a methylene group replaces the oxygen atom of the carbohydrate ring), **cyclaradine,** is resistant to deamination and retains antiviral activity.

Acyclovir, an analogue of guanosine lacking part of the sugar ring, is phosphorylated exclusively by the viral kinase and therefore has little effect against cytomegalovirus and EB virus. Acyclovir triphosphate inhibits viral DNA polymerase and is incorporated into the viral DNA. Administered intravenously in man, acyclovir is even more effective than vidarabine in the treatment of herpes simplex encephalitis and varicella zoster virus infection in immunocompromised patients. It is equally effective in the treatment of herpesvirus infection in newborns. Oral acyclovir is promising for the prophylaxis of genital herpesvirus infections and of herpesvirus infection in patients undergoing bone marrow transplantation or intensive cancer chemotherapy, because it can be administered for long periods with little toxicity. Acyclovir-resistant viral mutants of herpes simplex virus are altered in the thymidine kinase or polymerase genes; no such mutants have been observed with varicella zoster virus.

Very promising is a drug closely related to acyclovir and with a similar mode of action, **DHPG.** *In vitro* it is more effective against cytomegalovirus and EB virus than acyclovir itself, and it is beneficial against serious cytomegalovirus infection in immunodeficient persons. It is also effective against some acyclovir-resistant mutants of human herpesviruses. Its most frequent complication is neutropenia.

Other Pyrimidine Nucleoside Analogues

Halogenated derivatives of deoxyuridine, such as 5-bromo-deoxyuridine (BUdR) and **idoxuridine** (5-iodo-2-deoxyuridine, IUdR), were among the first antiviral compounds to be synthesized; however, they are less selective and more toxic than the preceding compounds. These analogues are taken up by cells and phosphorylated by the viral and cellular thymidine kinase; the phosphorylated derivatives are incorporated into DNA instead of thymidine in both virus-infected and uninfected cells. The DNA continues to replicate but causes the synthesis of altered proteins. Indeed, in cells infected by herpesvirus in the presence of idoxuridine, viral maturation fails owing to defects of the capsid protein. If the drug is later removed, virions are formed; they contain DNA replicated in the presence of the drug, in which iodouracil replaces thymine.

In spite of its toxicity, idoxuridine is valuable for the topical treatment of surface lesions (e.g., keratitis) produced by herpes simplex or vaccinia virus. Some herpesvirus mutants are resistant.

5-Halogenovinyl pyrimidine analogues are also promising, especially **bromovinyldeoxyuridine,** which is most effective against herpesvirus type 1 and varicella zoster viruses, owing to the specificity of their thymidine kinases. Other drugs effective *in vitro* or in animals, especially against cytomegalovirus, are various fluorosubstituted arabinosyl-pyrimidine derivatives.

Phosphonoacetic acid and phosphonoformic acid, which inhibit the herpesvirus-specified DNA polymerase, markedly reduce the replication of this virus in cultures, as well as the severity of experimental infection in animals. Drug-resistant mutants are altered in the viral DNA polymerase.

Agents Interfering With Reverse Transcription

Reverse transcription (RT) is a replication strategy employed by retroviruses, hepadnaviruses, and some eukaryotic transposons. Interference with RT is important in the chemotherapy of retroviruses that are highly pathogenic for humans, such as HIV (see Human Immunodeficiency Virus, Chap. 65); because RT plays no role in the multiplication or function of animal cells, a high selectivity can be achieved.

Several antiviral drugs inhibit RT *in vitro* with little effect on cellular DNA replication: **suramin** and **ribavirin** are among those, but they are too toxic for use in humans. More selective are **dideoxynucleosides,** such as **3'-azidothymidine** and **dideoxycytosine.** In either case the nucleotide obtained after phosphorylation by host enzymes is incorporated into DNA, where, for absence of a 3'-OH, it blocks further chain elongation. These drugs have beneficial although partial effect in the treatment of acquired immune deficiency syndrome (AIDS; see Human Immunodeficiency Virus, Chap. 65). Prolonged treatment, however, is toxic for the bone marrow.

General Considerations

The drugs active against herpesvirus are important in the treatment of this infection because in addition to alleviating the symptoms, they reduce viral shedding and the spread of the virus. They are effective only against the acute manifestations; they do not affect latent infections, in which there is little replication of the viral genome and the virus-specified enzymes involved in the antiviral effect may not be expressed. By inhibiting viral multiplication, the drugs also decrease the production of antibodies to the virus, with possible adverse effect on subsequent infection. As in the case of other viral infections, these drugs are most effective if used prophylactically; they can be therapeutically effective only during the very early stages of disease, when viral spread to the susceptible cells is limited. Once all susceptible cells are infected, the disease is no longer modifiable.

ANTIBIOTICS

Antiviral activity against poxviruses and retroviruses is displayed by derivatives of **rifamycin** (e.g., rifampin) and by the related antibiotics tolypomycin and streptovaricin. In bacteria rifampin is known to inhibit initiation by RNA polymerase; and with retroviruses these antibiotics inhibit the activity of the reverse transcriptase and cause the formation of defective, RNA-deficient virions. With poxviruses rifampin acts by **interfering with virus maturation:** viral membranes begin to form at the periphery of the filamentous matrix (see Complex Viruses, Chap. 48) but remain incomplete. If rifampin is then removed, the membranes close and form virions (Fig. 49–7).

The mechanism of action of rifampin on poxvirus maturation is unknown. It may conceivably alter the structure of the uncleaved precursor peptides, inactivate the cleaving enzyme, or block transcription of a few viral genes important in maturation. The activities of the vari-

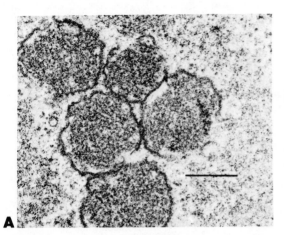
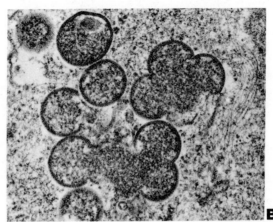

Figure 49–7. Effect of rifampin on the maturation of vaccinia virus in HeLa cells. *(A)* Electron micrograph from a thin section of infected cells treated for 8 hours with rifampin (100 μg/ml), showing the incomplete and disorganized viral membranes, each surrounding a matrix. Bar = 300 nm. *(B)* Thin section of similar cells 10 minutes after removal of rifampin, showing the rapid reorganization of the membranes to a morphology similar to that observed in normal maturation. (Courtesy of P. M. Grimley)

ous rifamycin derivatives toward retrovirus, poxvirus, or *Escherichia coli* transcriptase are uncorrelated, suggesting different modes of action. Poxvirus mutants resistant to rifampin and other antiviral rifamycin derivatives are readily isolated.

In vivo these compounds have some local effect; for instance, rifampin inhibits the development of vaccination lesions in man. They have little effect on systemic diseases in animals, perhaps because their high toxicity precludes the use of adequate doses.

Selected Reading

Balfour HH Jr: Acyclovir and other chemotherapy for herpes group viral infections. Annu Rev Med 35:279, 1984

Dolin R, Reichman RC, Madore HP et al: A controlled trial of amantadine and rimantadine in the prophylaxis of influenza A infection. N Engl J Med 307:580, 1982

Dolin R: Antiviral chemotherapy and chemoprophylaxis. Science 227:1296, 1985

Goeddel DV, Leung DW, Dull TJ et al: The structure of eight distinct cloned human leukocyte interferon cDNAs. Nature 290:20, 1981

Hall CB, McBride JT, Walsh EE et al: Aerosolized ribavirin treatment of infants with respiratory syncytial viral infection. N Engl J Med 308:1443, 1983

Hirsch MS, Schooley RT: Treatment of herpesvirus infections, parts 1 and 2. N Engl J Med 309:963, 1983

Lazzarini RA, Keene JD, Schubert M: The origins of defective interfering particles of the negative-strand RNA viruses. Cell 26:145, 1981

Lengyel P: Biochemistry of interferons and their actions. Annu Rev Biochem 51:251, 1982

McCormick JB et al: Lassa fever—effective therapy with ribavirin. N Engl J Med 314:20, 1986

O'Hara PJ, Nichol ST, Horodyski FM, Holland JJ: Vesicular stomatitis virus defective interfering particles can contain extensive genomic sequence rearrangements and base substitutions. Cell 36:915, 1984

Staeheli P, Haller O, Boll W et al: Mx protein: Constitutive expression in 3T3 cells transformed with cloned Mx cDNA confers selective resistance to influenza virus. Cell 44:147, 1986

Straus SE, Takiff HE, Seidlin M et al: Suppression of frequently recurring genital herpes. N Engl J Med 310:1545, 1984

Streissle G, Paessens A, Oediger H: New antiviral compounds. Adv Virus Res 30:83, 1985

Whitley RT et al: Vidarabine versus acyclovir therapy in herpes simplex encephalitis. N Engl J Med 314:144, 1986

Winship TR, Marcus PI: Interferon induction by viruses. VI. Reovirus: Virion genome dsRNA as the interferon inducer in aged chick embryo cells. J Interferon Res 1:4943, 1980

50

Viral Immunology

Induction of the Immune Response by Viruses

Viruses are usually strongly immunogenic and elicit two main types of response: a **humoral response,** caused by specific B cells with production of **antibodies** (Abs), and a **cellular response** caused by several varieties of T-lymphocyte clones, principally helper (T_h) and cytolytic (CTL) cells (see Chap. 15). B cells recognize free viral antigen (Ag), whereas T cells recognize viral Ags jointly with proteins of the major histocompatibility complex (MHC): CTLs with MHC-I and T_h with MHC-II proteins. Some specific cytolytic cells ($T_{h/c}$) recognize viral Ags together with MHC-II proteins. Participating in the organism's reactions are also "natural killer" (NK) cells, macrophages, various cells that are cytotoxic when activated by Abs (antibody-dependent cell cytotoxicity [ADCC]) and complement (complement-dependent cell cytotoxicity [CDCC]).

The repertoire of specificities of Abs and T cells relevant to an immune response is determined, as for other Ags, by rearrangements of the genes for immunoglobulins and for T-cell receptors (see Chaps. 16 and 17), as well as somatic mutations in the Ab genes. Abs and T cells formed in the same animal in response to a virus do not generally recognize the same antigenic groups (**epitopes**) of the virions. This is related to the different ways in which the antigen is presented to B or T cells. B cells see the free, unaltered proteins in their normal three-dimensional configuration on the viral surface; hence, Abs often recognize epitopes that depend upon the folded three-dimensional shape of the polypeptide chain. T cells usually see the Ag in denatured form or as fragments of the native antigen in conjunction with cellular MHC proteins. For instance, in the reaction to influenza hemagglutinin in mice, Abs almost regularly distinguish between different strains within the same subtype, whereas T cells show extensive cross-reactivities, sometimes even extending to different subtypes.

The characteristics of the immune reaction to the same virus may differ in different individuals, or in animals of non-inbred species, depending on their genetic constitutions; that is, depending on the available variable region genes for Abs or T-cell receptors and on the allele of the MHC genes expressed in different individuals.

Roles of the Immune Response

The humoral response and the cellular response have different consequences. Abs block the infectivity of virions (neutralization); those of the IgM or IgG class are especially relevant for defense against viral infections accompanied by viremia, whereas those of the IgA class are important in infections acquired through a mucosa (the nose, the intestine), because they can neutralize the virus at the entry portal. In contrast, the cellular response kills the virus-infected cells, which express at their surface viral proteins (such as the glycoproteins of enveloped viruses) and sometimes core proteins of these viruses (such as NP protein of influenza virus) or nonvirion proteins of nonenveloped viruses (such as the T Ag of papovaviruses).

Humoral Factors

Abs are elicited not only by surface components of intact virions and by internal components of disrupted virions, but also by viral products built into the surface of the infected cells or released by the cells (e.g., when they die). Although Abs provide the key to protection against many viral infections, they are sometimes pathogenic; e.g., deposits of Ab–Ag complexes in the kidneys of mice infected with lymphocytic choriomeningitis virus cause immune-complex disease. Abs are also useful in the laboratory for identifying, quantitating, and isolating virions (and also some of the unassembled components), for classifying viruses, and for serologic diagnosis of viral diseases. Especially useful for these purposes are **monoclonal Abs** obtained from **hybridomas** prepared with lymphocytes from mice immunized with viral material, or possibly from patients affected with viral diseases.

INTERACTIONS BETWEEN VIRIONS AND ANTIBODIES

Interactions of virions with Abs to different components of their coats have different consequences. Moreover, the many identical antigenic sites, regularly repeated on viral surfaces, interact with Abs in ways that would be impossible with isolated sites.

Reactions of viral Ags with their corresponding Abs are studied by both the usual immunologic tests and some special ones, such as hemagglutination inhibition and neutralization. Because neutralization is particularly characteristic of viruses and has widespread application, we shall consider it in detail.

NEUTRALIZATION

Viral neutralization consists of a decrease in the infectious titer of a viral preparation following its exposure to Abs. The loss of infectivity is brought about by interference by the bound Ab with any one of the steps leading to release of the viral genome into the host cells (see Chap. 48). Each one of these steps involves delicate molecular interactions between cellular and viral macromolecules in which the latter undergo characteristic conformational changes. The attachment of Abs to a virion macromolecule will perturb the step it carries out because the Ab binds with high affinity, preventing the physiologic conformational changes and often causing abnormal ones. In both cases viral replication is blocked. The **consequences** of the virion–Ab interaction therefore depend on many factors: (1) the structure of the virions; (2) the target of the Ab (e.g., Abs against the hemagglutinin but not against the neuraminidase neutralize influenza virus, and Abs against the hexon but not the penton neutralize adenovirus); (3) mutations affecting surface molecules that may alter susceptibility to certain Abs; (4) the type of Ab, especially its affinity for the components of virions; and (5) the number of Ab molecules attached to a virion. In addition, the interaction between viral and cellular macromolecules may be different in different cell types.

In neutralization we must distinguish readily reversible from stable virion–Ab complexes.

READILY REVERSIBLE VIRION–ANTIBODY COMPLEXES.
Readily reversible complexes are recognized by an experiment of the following kind. If influenza virus is mixed with Ab at 0°C and a sample of the mixture is added to an assay system (e.g., the allantoic cavity of chick embryos or cell cultures) ½ hour later **without dilution,** a decrease of the viral titer in comparison with untreated virus may be seen; but if the neutralization mixture is **diluted** by a large factor before assay, the original titer is restored (Fig. 50–1). Hence, there is a freely reversible equilibrium between dissociation and re-formation of the Ab–virion complexes: decreasing the concentration of the reactants diminishes the rate of complex formation but not the rate of dissociation.

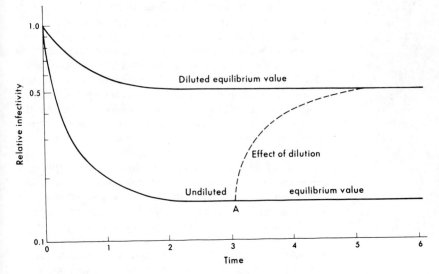

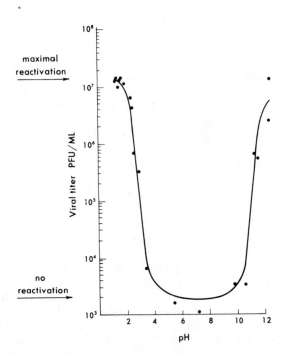

Figure 50–1. Time course of neutralization in a virus–Ab mixture with readily reversible Ab–Ag combinations. One mixture is undiluted; the other is diluted fivefold. Note the different equilibrium values reached. If at time *A* the undiluted mixture is diluted fivefold, the viral titer, corrected for dilution, increases, owing to dissociaton of virus–Ab complexes, and reaches the same equilibrium value as the originally diluted mixture.

Figure 50–2. Reactivability of neutralized Newcastle disease virus at different pHs, showing the dissociability of the virus–Ab complexes at acid and alkaline pHs. Virus and Abs were incubated together until a relative infectivity of about 10^{-4} was obtained (assayed after dilution). Aliquots of the mixture were then diluted 1 : 100 in cold buffer at various pH values, and after 30 seconds the pH was returned to 7 by dilution in a neutral buffer. The samples were then assayed. (Granoff A: Virology 25:38, 1965)

VIRION–ANTIBODY COMPLEXES STABLE ON DILUTION.

With time the virus–Ab complexes become more stable; if the assays are made **several hours after the virus has been mixed** with the Abs, neutralization persists after dilution (at neutral pH and physiologic ionic strength). Whereas reversible complexes form readily with little temperature dependence, the formation of irreversible complexes occurs very slowly at 0°C but rapidly at 37°C, suggesting the need for configurational changes.

Neither the virions nor the Abs are permanently changed in stable neutralization, for the unchanged components can be recovered. The neutralized virus can be reactivated by proteolytic cleavage of the bound Ab molecules into monovalent fragments and by other means, and intact Abs are recovered by dissociating the Ab–virus complexes at acid or alkaline pH (Fig. 50–2), by sonic vibration, or by extraction with a fluorocarbon.

PHYSICOCHEMICAL BASIS OF A STABLE ANTIBODY–VIRION ASSOCIATION.

The firm association of Abs with virions originates from the multimeric nature of the viral coat, which allows a single Ab molecule to establish specific bonds with two sites on a single virion: electron micrographs show that an Ab molecule can bridge two subunits of the virion's surface (Fig. 50–3). The stability of the complex is high, because whenever one of the bonds dissociates, the other holds, and the dissociated one has time to become reestablished.

Mechanism

Reversible neutralization is probably due to interference with attachment of virions to the cellular receptors, because many sites for adsorption on a virion have each been covered by an Ab molecule (or a monovalent frag-

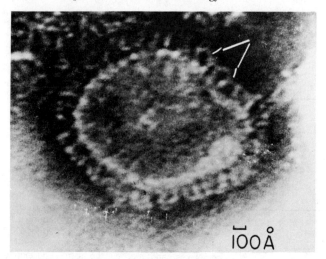

Figure 50–3. Electron micrograph of an influenza virion with Ab molecules attached to the spikes, some of them forming bridges between two spikes (*arrows*). (Lafferty KJ; Virology 21:91, 1963)

ment). In addition, aggregation by Abs may decrease the number of foci of infection.

Stable neutralization, in contrast, has a different mechanism: not only can it be shown that neutralized virions attach, but already attached virions can be neutralized. Moreover, **stable neutralization does not require saturation of the surface** of the virion with Ab molecules. Thus, phenotypically mixed virions with two types of surface monomers, produced by double infection (see Chap. 48; Fig. 50–4), can be neutralized by antisera specific for **either** monomer. In this type of neutralization the number of Ab molecules attached to a virion is much smaller than the number of protomers at the virion's surface. Fifty Ab molecules per virion are needed for 50% neutralization of influenza virus (1000 hemagglutinating units per virion) 3 or 4 molecules per virion for poliovirus (60 capsomers). Kinetic evidence shows that even a single Ab molecule can neutralize a virion (Fig. 50–5).

Stable neutralization is generally produced by Ab molecules that establish **contact with two antigenic sites** on different monomers of a virion, greatly increasing the stability of the complexes. That such double binding is obligatory for neutralization is shown by reactivation of poliovirus virions when the Ab is cleaved by papain and by their reneutralization if the Ab fragments are reconnected by an Ab to the neutralizing immunoglobulin.

The consequences of the double attachment are varied, as shown by some examples. (1) With poliovirus, neutralization often changes the isoelectric point (i.e., the balance of all + and − charges on the virion's surface) from pH 7 to 5.5 and also changes the accessibility of chemical groups on the virion's proteins to external

reagents. **The transition is all-or-none,** for there are no virions with intermediate isoelectric points. Apparently the binding of an Ab molecule to a capsomer **alters the capsomer's conformation;** the alteration then spreads to the whole capsid by a domino effect. (2) With bacteriophage M13, the DNA of which penetrates into the cells while the protomers of the capsid enter the plasma membrane (see Chap. 45), an Ab molecule blocks the latter process, presumably by holding two adjacent protomers together. Neutralization of some enveloped animal viruses may follow the M13 model. (3) With flavivirus the bound Ab **prevents the fusion** between the viral envelope and the membrane of the acidified endosome (see Chap. 48), blocking the release of the virion's core into the cytoplasm. The trapped virion is presumably handed over to a lysosome, where it is destroyed.

BOUND ANTIBODIES THAT DO NOT NEUTRALIZE. Since the kinetic data show that a single Ab can neutralize, while a higher number is actually bound when 50% of the virus is neutralized, the probability of neutralization by an attached Ab molecule is less than unity. One factor

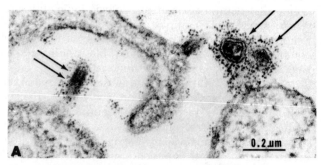

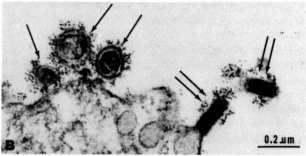

Figure 50–4. Immuno-electron microscopy of virions with a mixed envelope (pseudotypes) obtained by superinfecting a murine leukemia virus (MuLV)–producing cell with vesicular stomatitis virus (VSV). The virions are stained with ferritin-labeled anti-MuLV Abs: the ferritin molecules are recognizable as black spots. Single arrows point to uniformly labeled MuLV virions (spherical); double arrows to VSV (bullet-shaped) virions, some uniformly labeled (*A;* i.e., completely coated by MuLV-specific glycoproteins), others (*B*) with some glycoproteins VSV-specified and unlabeled and some MuLV-specified and labeled. (Chan JC et al: Virology 88:171, 1978)

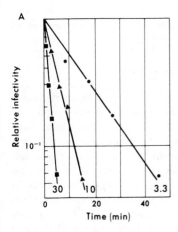

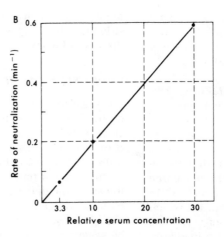

Figure 50–5. Kinetic curves of neutralization of poliovirus with stable Ab–virion complexes and Ab excess. Note the linearity of the curves in the semilog plot *A*, with different slopes corresponding to different relative concentrations of Abs (given by the numbers near each line). In *B* the slopes of the curves of *A* are plotted versus the concentration of the antiserum (in relative values), yielding a straight line. The linearity of the two types of curves implies that a single Ab molecule is sufficient to neutralize a virion. (Dulbecco R et al: Virology 2:162, 1956)

is heterogeneity of Ab molecules present in polyclonal sera; another is heterogeneity of the virions, even if clonal, owing to transient configurational changes. The virus–cell interaction is also important. Thus, in the endosomes, the lower pH favors partial dissociation of the Ag–Ab complexes, making some Abs incapable of interfering with the release of the viral genome. That the binding of Abs to the virions is not the sole factor in neutralization is dramatically demonstrated by effects of Abs on viruses (such as bunyaviruses) that can grow in both mammalian and insect cells: the same Abs may neutralize the virus in one but not the other cell type.

SENSITIZATION. The binding of Abs to virions without neutralizing them gives rise to the phenomenon of sensitization: the virions can be neutralized by Abs to the bound immunoglobulin. Sensitizing Abs are probably weakly bound and are stabilized when they are crosslinked by the second Ab. A related phenomenon is the appearance of a **persistent fraction** at high Ab/virion ratios (Fig. 50–6). The persistent fraction is often neutralized at least in part by addition of Abs to the bound immunoglobulin. The persistent fraction is larger when virions are neutralized by individual monoclonal Abs rather than by a polyclonal serum. A mixture of several monoclonal Abs to different epitopes of the same virion monomer usually decreases the persistent fraction to the level observed with polyclonal sera, showing **cooperation between Abs of different specificities.** Thus, the binding of Abs may induce a configurational change in the monomer that increases its affinity for another epitope on the same monomer.

A bound non-neutralizing Ab may, in some cases, increase rather than decrease the infectious titer of a virus. For instance, in flavivirus infection of macrophages, the Fc domain of Ab bound at low concentrations interacts with Fc receptors on the cells, increasing virion attachment. At higher Ab concentrations the effect disappears because neutralization takes place.

VIRION SITES FOR NEUTRALIZATION. Only epitopes on molecules involved in the release of the viral genome into the cells are targets for neutralization. In influenza virions only the hemagglutinins are targets, not the neuraminidase molecules; and in the large herpesvirus virions the main targets are the C and D glycoproteins. But in poliovirus all antigenic sites recognizable on the capsid are such targets, because the whole capsid is a unit

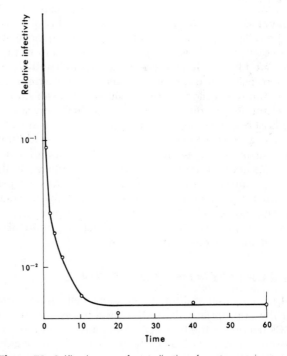

Figure 50–6. Kinetic curve of neutralization of western equine encephalitis virus (a togavirus), showing the rather abrupt change into a plateau as the time of incubation increases. This plateau is not justified by the A/V ratio employed, which would have allowed a far greater neutralization. The plateau corresponds to the persistent fraction. (Dulbecco R et al: Virology 2:162, 1956)

for releasing the nucleic acid. For adenovirus the main targets are the hexons, which are strongly interconnected and presumably work together for the release of DNA.

ANTIBODIES BOUND TO NON-NEUTRALIZING EPITOPES. Abs bound to non-neutralizing epitopes, together with those bound to neutralizing epitopes, are detected by nonbiological procedures such as complement fixation, immunoprecipitation, enzyme-linked sorption assay (ELISA), or radioimmunoassay (RAI). Some can also be detected by **neutralization in the presence of complement:** with enveloped virions the bound Ab activates the complement cascade (see Chap. 18), which then injects the C9 complexes into the virion envelope, causing its disruption. Complement can also inactivate virions by blanketing them. In primary infections of experimental animals, complement plays an important antiviral role initially, when Abs are of low affinity; thus, decomplementation by cobra venom factor (see Chap. 18) or genetic deficiency of component C5 increases the duration and severity of primary influenza.

PROTECTIVE ROLE OF NEUTRALIZING ANTIBODIES. The neutralizing power of a serum usually reflects the degree of protection in an infected animal. The correlation, however, is not always perfect. Discrepancies may be generated by differences in the neutralizability of a virus in the cells used for assay *in vitro* compared to those that the virus infects *in vivo*. For instance, the sera of mice protected from yellow fever did not neutralize the virus in Vero cells but did so in a mouse neuroblastoma cell line. Another reason for discrepancy is that an Ab that does not neutralize in cultures may act *in vivo* by activating host responses against the virus or the virus-infected cells (e.g., complement or macrophages). In addition, neutralizing Abs may fail to protect because rapid viral multiplication overcomes the neutralizing power. In the early period of immunization, low-affinity Abs act predominantly by activating complement and have low neutralizing power in cultures. The degree of protection is best estimated in cultures by carrying out **neutralization in the presence of complement.**

HEMAGGLUTINATION INHIBITION

With virions that agglutinate red blood cells (RBCs), adding the appropriate Abs to the virus before adding the RBCs decreases the hemagglutinating titer by hindering adsorption of the virions to the RBCs. In this **hemagglutination inhibition** (HI), unlike neutralization, Abs interfere with the adsorption of the virions, rather than with cell infection; and stable Ab–virion complexes do not appear to play a special role because univalent Ab fragments are effective. The number of Ab molecules per virion may have to be high enough to cover all the sites of the virion involved in adsorption.

EVOLUTION OF VIRAL ANTIGENS

The great selectivity of neutralization can be understood on the basis of the structure, genetics, and evolution of viruses. Animal viruses that have evolved in the ecology of mammalian organisms have been opposed by the neutralizing Abs, which are able to block viral infection. Viral evolution must tend to select for mutations that change the antigenic determinants involved in neutralization. In contrast, other antigenic sites would tend to remain unchanged, because mutations affecting them would not be selected for and could even be detrimental. A virus would thus evolve from an original type to a variety of types, different in neutralization (and sometimes in HI) tests, but all retaining some of the original mosaic of antigenic determinants recognizable by complement fixation.

These evolutionary arguments are consistent with the observation that the clearest differentiation of types within a family is present in viruses of rather complex architecture, in which the Ags involved in the interaction with the cell vary more than the proteins of other virions. Thus, enveloped viruses have a strain-specific envelope but a cross-reactive internal capsid; adenoviruses have type-specific fibers and family-specific (but also type-specific) capsomers (see Chap. 52). Moreover, the C Ag of polioviruses, which appears only after heating, cross-reacts in all three viral types (see Chap. 55). The heating reveals antigenic sites that are normally hidden and hence are not affected by selective pressure.

The extent of antigenic variation differs widely among viruses. It is most extensive with lentiviruses (see Chap. 65) and influenza virus, an orthomyxovirus (see Chap. 56). In influenza virus the hemagglutinins are the main sites of neutralization (see The Envelope, Chap. 44). Epidemiologic studies show that this variation occurs by the appearance every decade or so of strains in which the hemagglutinins are genetically unrelated to those of the previous years **(antigenic shift),** followed by the progressively smaller changes in the new strain in the following years **(antigenic drift;** see Chap. 56). Antigenic shift is probably due to the appearance of reassortants, in which the hemagglutinin gene has been replaced by another from a virus present in an animal reservoir (e.g., avian or equine); antigenic drift, in contrast, is due to the progressive accumulation of mutations that partly overcome the immunity prevalent in the host population. The important role of selection pressure in drift is shown by the similar evolution of two strains with the same hemagglutinin subtype (H1) in the periods 1950–1957 and 1977–

present. The same two areas of the hemagglutinin evolved in both cases, although by means of different amino acid substitutions.

HABITAT AND SELECTION. Drift is probably favored by the habitat of influenza viruses, namely, cells lining the respiratory tract: here they are exposed only to IgA Abs, which tend to form reversible complexes with virions and hence are less likely to neutralize. The virus can then multiply (although at a reduced rate) even in an immune host, producing a large population as a source of mutants; these, being less sensitive to the Abs, can then be selected. In contrast, viruses that cause viremia are more effectively neutralized by IgG; hence, mutants with a somewhat decreased binding of neutralizing Abs may still be eliminated. Thus, viruses such as mumps and measles, which are structurally similar to influenza viruses, have persisted as single immunologic types with only minimal antigenic variation. Structural constraints may also limit variability, especially in icosahedral viruses, as suggested by the large number of rhinovirus and aftovirus serotypes compared with the restricted number in poliovirus (see Genetics, Chap. 48).

Diagnostic Use of Immunology

Immunologic tests can be used with standard antisera to identify and characterize a virus isolated from a patient and, with standard Ags, to detect antiviral Abs in the patient's serum. These two applications of viral immunology involve a number of general problems that will be dealt with before considering the diagnostic methodology (described in the appendix to this chapter).

TYPES OF VIRUS-SPECIFIC ANTIBODIES

Different kinds of viral preparations elicit the formation of different Abs. (1) Immunization with virions that cannot multiply in the host (e.g., with **killed virions**) produces Abs predominantly directed toward **surface components** of the virions; these Abs have neutralizing and HI activities against the virions, as well as complement-fixation (CF) and precipitation activities against Ags of the viral coat. (2) In contrast, **viruses that multiply in the host** and produce a cytopathic effect in some cells—as in natural infection or in vaccination with "live" vaccines—lead to the formation of Abs against **all the viral Ags,** including Abs for surface Ags, CF or precipitating Abs for both surface and internal Ags, and Abs for nonvirion Ags. (3) Immunization with **internal components of the virions** produces CF and precipitating Abs active only toward the Ags of these components. (4) Immunization with *peptides* reproducing segments of virion proteins elicits Abs, the properties of which depend both on the protein and the specific sequences reproduced (see Immunologic Prevention of Viral Diseases, below).

SPECIFICITY OF TEST METHODS

The Abs that react in the different tests may overlap, though they may not be altogether identical. Neutralization is primarily caused by Ab molecules specific for the sites of the virion that are involved in the release of nucleic acid into the cells, while CF usually involves additional surface or internal Ags. Neutralization probably requires molecules with a higher affinity for virions than do HI and CF. Only certain classes of immunoglobulins can participate in CF. After viral infection the titers of Abs to different components rise and fall with quite different time courses, as will be discussed in the chapters on specific viruses.

Because of their high specificity, immunologic methods can differentiate not only between viruses of different families but also between closely related viruses of the same family or subfamily. By these means, **family Ags** may be identified; each family or subfamily may be subdivided into types (**species**) on the basis of **type-specific Ags;** some types can even be subdivided further (**intratypic differentiation**). The levels in this classification are obviously somewhat arbitrary. Usually, Abs detected by neutralization tend to be less cross-reactive and thus are useful to define the immunologic type, whereas those detected by CF tend to be more cross-reactive and are useful to define the family. By proper procedures, however, such as immunization with purified Ags, highly specific CF Abs can be prepared.

The resolving power of Abs is maximized by using **monoclonal Abs;** each is produced from a single clone of B cells and is therefore endowed with a single specificity. Monoclonal Abs to influenza or rabies virus can reveal antigenic differences that are not picked up by sera of immune animals, which usually recognize many specificities. Whereas all the methods for measuring viral antigens are needed for classifying a new isolate, the method of choice for diagnostic purposes is ELISA (see Chap. 12), for its high sensitivity, ready availability of reagents, and low cost.

Cell-Mediated Immunity

IMMUNITY BASED ON CYTOTOXIC T-LYMPHOCYTES (CTLs)

As will be discussed in Chapter 51, this cell-mediated immunity appears to be very important not only in localizing viral infections and in ultimate recovery but also in the pathogenesis of viral diseases.

CTLs are usually found in the blood or the spleen and sometimes in abundance in the lymph nodes draining local infection sites (e.g., in herpes simplex infection of mice and rabbits). CTLs are also present in exudates within affected organs; in mice they are found in the lung after infection with influenza virus or in the cerebro-spinal fluid after induction of meningitis by arenaviruses. CTLs kill virus-infected cells *in vitro* and probably *in vivo.*

In experimental animals primary CTLs reach maximal abundance about 6 days after a viral infection and then disappear as infection subsides. However, the organism subsequently contains, for a long time, virus-specific memory T cells, which can be recognized by culturing spleen cells together with virus-infected target cells: within a few days secondary CTLs appear in the culture, with much greater activity than in the initial response. A similar secondary response is probably produced in the body after a second infection.

Formation of CTLs is elicited by **cell-associated Ags** present at the cell surface, not only for enveloped viruses, the glycoproteins of which are incorporated into the plasma membrane (see Enveloped Viruses, Chap. 48), but also for other viruses when core or nonvirion proteins reach the cell surface. The specificity of the response depends on the types of viral proteins present at the cell surface. Thus, studies with reassortants between different influenza virus A types show that the hemagglutinin elicits both a type-specific and a cross-reactive immunity, and the matrix protein elicits cross-reactive immunity among several A types but not between A and B types. With vesicular stomatitis virus the response is directed mainly at the single-envelope glycoprotein. Larger viruses (herpesviruses, poxviruses) elicit both type- and group-specific responses because the viral glycoproteins contain determinants of both types.

Even noninfectious or inactivated viruses can elicit a cellular immune response, because their envelopes fuse with the cell plasma membrane in the initial stage of viral penetration. Moreover, the virions themselves may also be able to elicit the response after adsorbing to macrophages.

Both internal virion proteins and nonvirion proteins are often recognized by CTLs. An example is the nucleocapsid proteins of enveloped viruses, fragments of which reach the cell surface by an unknown route and are recognized very efficiently, giving rise mostly to cross-reactive CTLs. In animals infected by DNA-containing papovaviruses (see Chap. 64) the CTLs recognize the T Ag, a nonvirion Ag, exposed at the cell surface. Vaccinia recombinants expressing the protein of a foreign virus elicit a strong CTL response to it. Often, Abs to viral surface proteins do not block their interaction with CTLs, because the humoral and cellular responses recognize different epitopes: for instance, CTLs recognize Ags in association with MHC proteins rather than alone.

The spectrum of the initial and secondary cellular responses may differ. Thus, with influenza virus if the primary and the secondary infections are caused by the same viral type, the secondary response is type specific; but if the two types are different, it is cross-reactive. This mechanism can build a broad heterotypic cellular immunity, which tends to be highly cross-reactive.

ANTIBODY-DEPENDENT COMPLEMENT-INDEPENDENT CELL-MEDIATED CYTOTOXICITY

In the ADCC response the effector cells are **killer (K) cells,** which have monocyte or macrophage markers rather than T-cell markers and surface Igs. *In vitro* these cells kill virus-infected cells sensitized by IgG from immune donors, but not unsensitized targets. The cytotoxic cells are not themselves virus specific but acquire their specificity by reacting with the Fc region of the sensitizing Abs of suitable isotypes (see Chap. 14). The cytotoxic effect is inhibited by IgG F(ab')$_2$ fragments, which compete with the cell-bound IgG. This type of cytotoxic cell has been observed in humans and in animals infected by various enveloped viruses.

ADCC is very efficient *in vitro* against herpes simplex or varicella zoster–infected cells, preventing the usual spread of the virus from infected to neighboring uninfected cells; it may play a role in defense against human infections with these viruses.

NATURAL KILLER CELL CYTOTOXICITY

The so-called **natural killer (NK) cells,** which are found in the peripheral blood of most humans, are distinguishable from T- or B-lymphocytes, macrophages, and polymorphonuclear cells. Unlike K cells, they do not contain Fc receptors and are cytotoxic without requiring sensitizing Abs. They are not MHC restricted and attack a variety of isogeneic, allogeneic, or xenogeneic cell types, either infected by viruses or uninfected. NK cells are especially abundant in persons infected by many enveloped viruses or after vaccination with vaccinia virus. Their important role in the recovery from viral infection is suggested by an increased mortality of herpes simplex–infected mice after NK cells are depleted by means of the specific NK cells reagent anti-asialo GM1.

NK cells are not directly virus induced, because their presence is not related to a previous history of viral disease, but indirectly, by alpha **interferon** produced by virus-infected cells. In fact, interferon confers a viral specificity on NK cells by enhancing their cytotoxic action (as well as that of Ab-dependent K cells) on infected target cells while protecting uninfected cells from lysis. The NK action against virus-infected cells is blocked by monoclonal Abs specific for the viral proteins that they recognize as targets. There may be several classes of NK cells, recognizing different target molecules.

IMMUNOSUPPRESSION

The immune response is severely depressed in a number of viral infections by various mechanisms and with various consequences. Very important is immunodepression in humans infected by the lentivirus HIV (see Chap. 65), which infects and destroys T_h cells. As a result the patients become invaded by opportunistic parasites, including fungi, bacteria, and viruses. Measles virus blocks Ab synthesis by infecting lymphocytes. Immunodepression is observed in animals infected with oncogenic viruses (see Chaps. 64 and 65) containing either RNA (retroviruses) or DNA (Marek disease virus); it favors oncogenesis by helping the spread of the virus and reducing the rejection of transformed cells. This depression is manifested by an impaired responsiveness of lymphoid cells to T-cell mitogens (phytohemagglutinin or concanavalin A) and sometimes by a reduced response of B cells to immunization with other Ags. With herpesviruses, specific suppressor factors, produced by T suppressor cells, have been observed; this explains the earlier observation that thymectomy reduces the severity of the disease produced by a later infection. Cytomegalovirus induces suppression by infecting monocytes and inhibiting production of interleukin-1, which is essential for an immune response (see Chap. 15).

Immunologic Prevention of Viral Disease

Prevention is based on administration of vaccines, which generate humoral and cellular immunity against specific viruses. A vaccine may be made up of whole virions or of their components.

WHOLE VIRUS VACCINES

Whole virus vaccines contain nonpathogenic but immunogenic virions. Pathogenicity is eliminated either by chemical alterations that prevent expression and reproduction of the genome (**killed virus** vaccine) or by genetic changes that abolish pathogenicity but not the ability to reproduce (**attenuated live virus** vaccines). Both kinds of vaccine cause a polyclonal response, i.e., one directed at all or most of the epitopes of the surfaces of the virions; polyclonality is advantageous because neutralizing antibodies directed at different epitopes can collaborate (see Sensitization, above).

An example of killed vaccine is the Salk-type poliovirus vaccine, obtained by exposing the virus to formaldehyde. Attenuated vaccine strains are either iso-lated from a related host (e.g., vaccinia from cows to protect man against smallpox, Marek disease virus from turkeys to protect chickens) or selected for growth in a different cell type (e.g., poliovirus adapted to grow in monkey kidney cells to protect man against neurologic infection). Attenuated strains can also be obtained as mutants able to grow at low temperature (cold-adapted) or as recombinants or reassortants with defined genetic properties. A potential influenza live vaccine is based on a cold-adapted mutant, which can be extended to several serologic types by exchanging the RNA segment coding for the hemagglutinin (**cold-adapted reassortants**). A difficulty is the high reversion rate of the mutants. The genetic changes occurring during attenuation introduce some antigenic changes in the virus, but usually not sufficient to impair its immunizing activity.

Killed vaccines are administered by injection and elicit the formation of antibodies directed at surface epitopes of the virions, mostly IgG; they are less efficient in inducing an IgA response. The immunity they confer is of fairly short duration and must be maintained by repeated injections. They are unsuitable for viruses that are not easily neutralized (e.g., parainfluenza, respiratory syncytial virus) or are antigenically altered by the inactivating treatment (e.g., paramyxovirus F protein is damaged by formaldehyde). Abnormal responses, exacerbating rather than preventing subsequent disease, have been observed with formalin-killed vaccines to measles or respiratory syncytial virus. Attenuated live viruses, in contrast, can be administered orally or by inhalation; they initiate an inapparent infection that generates and maintains the immune response, both humoral and cellular, for many years. For viruses that enter the body at a mucosa site, they elicit production of IgA at that portal, a reaction that appears to be important for protection.

Drawbacks of attenuated live vaccines are their possible contamination with unknown infectious agents picked up from the organism or the cells in which they were prepared, genetic reversion to pathogenic forms (see Chap. 48), and sensitivity to interference (see Chap. 49) by other viruses present in the environment of the host. Another problem is the secondary spread of the vaccine strain, with possible enrichment of pathogenic revertants to which unvaccinated persons may be exposed.

COMPONENT VACCINES

Component vaccines have been made possible by the detailed knowledge of the viral genomes, of the structure of virions, and of how immunity works. Necessary for preparing component vaccines are (1) the identification of the components of the surfaces of the virions that elicit neutralizing Abs or other specific defenses; (2) the identification of neutralizing epitopes either by their alteration in **escape mutants** (i.e., mutants that escape neutralization by certain monoclonal Abs) or on theoretical grounds as special sequences of hydrophilic amino acids; and (3) the ability to produce virion proteins in large quantities by DNA cloning, or short peptides by artificial synthesis.

Component vaccines are of two types: subunit vaccines and peptide vaccines. **Subunit vaccines** employ whole viral proteins, which are injected either alone or in conjunction with adjuvants. An example is the hepatitis B vaccine, which was first made by means of molecules of the viral surface (HB_s) Ag present in the blood of chronic virus carriers. Through DNA cloning a similar vaccine can be made in yeast and in animal cells. For efficacy, the conformation of the protein in the vaccine must be similar to that in virions; for instance, the hepatitis B vaccine must contain dimers of the s Ag; monomers are not effective, perhaps because conformational changes alter the useful epitopes.

Peptide vaccines employ synthetically made peptides. The peptides are essentially haptens and elicit Ab formation only when they are conjugated to a protein, such as keyhole limpet hemocyanin. To boost the immunogenicity they are mixed with an adjuvant or are incorporated in membrane vesicles (liposomes). The conjugated peptides often elicit Abs of low affinity and not very cross-reactive with the intact protein; with some exceptions they are poor inducers of cellular immunity. Peptides derived from sequences that are known to bind neutralizing Abs sometimes do not elicit formation of such Abs but may **prime** the immune response: a subsequent exposure to complete virions will elicit a secondary response, much stronger than the primary response to the virions. Peptides can also cause a more intense cellular response in previously immunized animals.

ANTI-IDIOTYPIC ANTIBODIES (AB2) AS VACCINES. Abs (Ab2) raised against the variable region of the primary Ab (Ab1), which includes the binding sites, can replace Ag in inducing an immune response (Ab3) specific toward the Ag. Anti-idiotypic Abs (Ab2) capable of immunizing animals against polio or rabies viruses, among others, have in fact been prepared. An anti-idiotypic Ab can immunize by two different mechanisms. One is based on the fact that its binding site is the **internal image** of the Ag, because it is complementary to the complement of the Ag and can act like the Ag itself. A different mode of action is revealed by the ability of an Ab2 to immunize against poliovirus only mice of certain genetic constitutions, although all mice can be equally immunized by Ag. This Ab2 recognizes a special binding site of the primary Ab (Ab1) that is abundantly expressed in certain strains of mice. Ab2 activates the B cells displaying these Abs and acts by **idiotypic selection.** This type of anti-idiotypic Ab would not be suitable as vaccine in an outbred population because it is genetically restricted.

Anti-idiotypic Abs may also have an opposite effect: they may decrease the immune response to a virus, lowering the protection of the organism, perhaps through activation of specific T-suppressor cells.

VACCINES BASED ON VACCINIA VIRUS VECTORS. The surface proteins of many viruses, both DNA and RNA containing, have been introduced in vaccinia virus vectors (see Chap. 48). The proteins are regularly processed and are transported to the surface of the vector-infected cells in the proper orientation and configuration. Animals infected with such vectors have developed neutralizing Abs and T_cs specific for these proteins and have been protected from challenge with the corresponding virus. This is a promising approach for protecting animals and humans against viral disease.

LIMITATIONS OF VIRAL VACCINES

Vaccines are effective in protecting against diseases caused by viruses with genetically stable antigenicity, such as poliovirus. For viruses with a very large number of serologic subtypes, such as rhinoviruses or foot-and-mouth disease virus, vaccination is more problematic because a large number of vaccines would be required. Even greater difficulties are encountered with viruses that continuously vary, such as influenza viruses or the AIDS agents, HIVs. In the case of influenza, adequate protection can be obtained with killed vaccines made each year from the then-prevalent strain, because the emergence of variants is seasonal. If research identifies more invariant epitopes, then it might become possible to construct adequate peptide vaccines.

For practical use in humans, vaccines must satisfy stringent conditions of safety and efficacy. This caution delays the introduction of vaccines based on new principles, such as subunits, peptides, or anti-idiotypic vaccines. The use of vaccines based on vaccinia virus vectors entails infection of the organism with vaccinia virus, the consequences of which must be evaluated.

Appendix

MEASUREMENT OF NEUTRALIZING ANTIBODIES

The measurement of neutralizing antibodies rests on the points discussed in the body of this chapter. If the serum–virus mixtures are assayed **without dilution,** the relative concentration of Ab is derived from the proportion of neutralized virus, according to the **percentage law.** This method is simple to perform and measures both reversible and stable Ab–virion complexes; it is adequate and is widely used for diagnostic purposes, but is unsuitable for accurate measurement.

The percentage law, recognized by Andrews and Elford in 1933, states that under conditions of Ab excess, the proportion (percentage) of virus neutralized by a

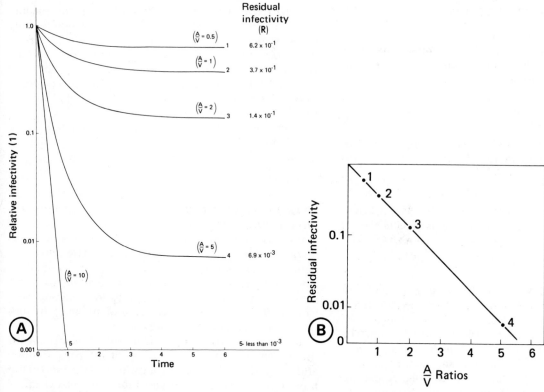

Figure 50–7. *(A)* Theoretical kinetic curves at different ratios of total Ab *(A)* total virus *(V)*–virion complexes. All the curves tend to plateau, the relative infectivity of which is a function of the ratio A/V (in arbitrary units). When the residual infectivity values are plotted semilogarithmically versus the A/V ratio, they generate a straight line *(B)*. This result affords additional evidence that neutralization of a virion requires only the binding of a single Ab molecule.

given antiserum is constant, irrespective of the viral titer. This law can be deduced from the mass law.

$$V + A \underset{k_2}{\overset{k_1}{\rightleftharpoons}} \overline{VA}; \frac{k_1}{k_2} = \frac{(\overline{VA})}{(V)(A)}; k(A) = \frac{(\overline{VA})}{(V)} \quad (1)$$

where V indicates the free virus, A the free Ab (assumed to have a much higher concentration than bound Ab), VA the Ab–virion complexes, and k their dissociation constant.

The formation of stable Ab–virion complexes is more precisely measured by means of *kinetic curves in Ab excess*. The curves obtained closely approach straight lines passing through the origin; the slopes are proportional to the concentration of the Ab and to its affinity for the virions and are independent of the virions' concentration (see Fig. 50–5). These curves follow the equation*

* This equation is equivalent to that used in the appendix to Chapter 44; *kt(A)* is the average number of neutralizing Ab molecules per virion after time *t*, since molecules of Ab (which is in large excess) continue to attach to the virions at a constant rate. Thus, *I* is the fraction of virions that have **no neutralizing molecule.** As discussed in the appendix to Chapter 8, equation 1 generates single-hit curves and is valid if a single Ab molecule is sufficient to produce neutralization; otherwise, the curve would have an initial shoulder (i.e., it would be a multiple-hit curve).

$$I = e^{-kt(A)} \quad (2)$$

and, taking the logarithm of both sides:

$$\ln I = -kt(A)$$

$$k(A) = \frac{\ln I}{t} \quad (3)$$

where I is relative infectivity, t the time after mixing the virus and the Ab (in minutes), and k the affinity; the other symbols are as in equation 1.

In Ag excess the residual relative infectivity, determined after dilution of the virus–serum mixture (Fig. 50–7), theoretically obeys the relations

$$Res = e^{-c(A/V)} \quad (4)$$

where *Res* is residual infectivity, c is a constant, A denotes the total amount of Ab, and V denotes the total amount of virus.†

† This equation is derived similarly to equation 1 above, except that the average number of neutralizing Ab molecules per virion is c(A/V). Again, this equation requires that a single Ab molecule be sufficient for neutralization; otherwise the curve would have an initial shoulder.

METHODS FOR ANTIGENIC ANALYSIS OF VIRUSES

We shall consider here only those immunologic methods that are peculiar to viruses: neutralization, HI, and immuno-electron microscopy.

Neutralization Tests

Neutralization tests are used mostly in typing viral isolates and in characterizing related viruses.

DETERMINING NEUTRALIZING ANTIBODY TITERS BY A 50% ENDPOINT METHOD. The titration is usually carried out with **constant virus and varying serum.**

METHOD 1: ENDPOINT TEST. To carry out a constant virus–varying serum titration, the serum is inactivated at 56°C for 30 minutes to destroy labile substances that have antiviral activity or that affect neutralization. The serum is then diluted serially, usually in two steps, and each dilution is added to a constant amount of virus (usually between 30 ID_{50} and 100 ID_{50}; see Appendix, Chap. 44). The amount of virus must be adequate to infect all the assay units in the subsequent titration and at the same time small enough to detect a low concentration of Abs. The mixtures are incubated for a selected time (at either 37°C or 4°C, depending on the virus employed); then a constant volume of each is assayed for infectivity by inoculation into 5 to 10 test units of a suitable assay system, such as mice, chick embryos, or tissue culture tubes. The neutralization titer of the serum is the dilution at which 50% of the units are protected (50% endpoint), calculated by the method of Reed and Muench (see Appendix, Chap. 44).

The accuracy of the assay can be calculated by the same methods as used for viral assays (see Appendix, Chap. 44). (Since the serum dilutions are closely spaced, the assay is more precise than the corresponding viral assays, which usually employ more widely spaced dilutions.) The constant virus–varying serum titration relies on the constancy of the virus employed; this requirement, however, is not critical because, according to the percentage law, the proportion of virus neutralized is (at least largely) independent of the titer of the virus.

This method is statistically more accurate than the **constant serum–varying virus** method because in virus–serum mixtures a small change in Ab titer usually produces a much larger change in the infectious titer of the virus. The reason is the exponential relation between residual infectivity and Ab concentration of equation 3 above.

METHOD 2: PLAQUE-REDUCTION TEST. In the plaque-reduction test an inoculum of about 100 plaque-forming units is incubated with serial dilutions of the serum; each mixture is then added to a monolayer culture, which is overlaid with agar and incubated. The endpoint is an 80% reduction in the number of plaques. The precision of the method depends on the number of plaques at the endpoint (see Appendix, Chap. 44).

These two methods are used either qualitatively, to demonstrate the presence of virus-specific Ab, or quantitatively, to compare Ab titers in different sera.

METHOD 3: DETERMINING THE RATE OF NEUTRALIZATION BY THE PLAQUE METHOD. Determining the rate of neutralization by the plaque method measures the slope (κ) of the kinetic curves described above. The values obtained are extremely reproducible; differences of about 20% are usually significant. Values obtained with the same serum provide a sensitive basis for distinguishing viral strains, including laboratory mutants (e.g., in work with vaccine strains of poliovirus).

In this test a virus sample of known titer is mixed with the antiserum; samples are taken at intervals, diluted, and assayed for plaques. The logarithm of the ratio of the titer of the sample to the original titer (the relative infectivity, I) is plotted against the time of sampling, yielding a straight line through or near the origin. The slope of that line is κ, which is characteristic for the serum and the virus; it is determined from the relation $\kappa = -\ln I/t(A)$, from equation 2 above, where I is the relative infectivity determined after t minutes of incubation of the neutralizing mixture and A is the concentration of the serum.

Example: At a serum dilution of 10^{-3} the relative infectivity is 3×10^{-2} after a 10-minute incubation. Since $\ln 3 \times 10^{-2} = -3.5$, $\kappa = 3.5/(10 \times 10^{-3}) = 350$.

Hemagglutination Inhibition

For the HI test a serial twofold dilution of heat-inactivated serum is prepared in saline solution, and from each dilution 0.25 ml is mixed with 0.25 ml of a viral suspension containing 4 hemagglutinating units (defined in Chap. 44, see Hemagglutination Assay). (If nonspecific HI substances are known to be present in the serum or the viral preparation, they must be removed in advance.) To each mixture is added 0.125 ml of a 1% RBC suspension. The tubes are shaken and then incubated at the temperature and for the time required for optimal hemagglutination with the virus used. The agglutination pattern is read after incubation, as discussed in Chapter 44. The **HI titer** is the reciprocal of the highest serum dilution that completely prevents hemagglutination.

Example:

	Initial Serum Dilution									HI Titer
	1:8	1:16	1:32	1:64	1:128	1:256	1:512	1:1024		
A	0	+	+	+	+	+	+	+	+	8
B	0	0	0	0	+	+	+	+	+	64

Immuno-electron Microscopy

Special techniques are especially useful for certain viruses (such as human rotaviruses; see Chap. 62) that cannot be grown in cell cultures or in convenient animal hosts and do not produce hemagglutination but have a high titer in the blood or excretions of infected persons. When the virus-containing sample is mixed with appropriate Abs, electron microscopic examination reveals virions of characteristic shape with an Ab halo.

Complications of Immunologic Tests

Interfering substances occasionally obscure the significance of immunologic tests. Although they concern the specialist carrying out the test, some knowledge of their nature is useful for evaluating test results.

NEUTRALIZATION TEST. Human and animal sera contain **nonspecific viral inhibitors,** especially active against influenza, mumps, herpes simplex, and togaviruses. They result from interactions with properdin and the alternate complement pathway. They are heat labile and can be eliminated by incubation at 56°C for 30 minutes.

HEMAGGLUTINATION-INHIBITION TEST. Most sera contain inhibitors of hemagglutination that are not Abs; they must be removed. The inhibitors for influenza viruses are inactivated by receptor-destroying enzyme (RDE; see Mechanisms of Hemagglutination, Chap. 44), trypsin, or periodate; those for togaviruses and flaviviruses are inactivated by extraction with acetone-chloroform.

COMPLEMENT-FIXATION TEST. Performance of the CF test is frequently hampered by the presence of anticomplementary substances in crude tissue suspensions used as Ag. This is especially true of the infected brain suspension used with togaviruses; it can be freed of the anticomplementary factors by thorough extraction with acetone in cold or by extraction with a fluorocarbon.

Selected Reading

Ada GL, Jones PD: The immune response to influenza infection. Curr Top Microbiol Immunol 128:1, 1986

Air GM, Laver G: The molecular basis of antigenic variation in influenza virus. Adv Virus Res 31:53, 1986

Al-Ahdal MN, Nakamura I, Flanagan TD: Cytotoxic T-lymphocyte reactivity with individual Sendai virus glycoproteins. J Virol 54:53, 1985

Arnon R: Peptides as immunogens: Prospects for synthetic vaccines. Curr Top Microbiol Immunol 130:1, 1986

Brown F: Synthetic viral vaccines. Annu Rev Microbiol 38:221, 1984

Chow M, Yabrov R, Bittle J et al: Synthetic peptides from four separate regions of the poliovirus type 1 capsid protein VP1 induce neutralizing antibodies. Proc Natl Acad Sci USA 82:910, 1985

Emini EA, Jameson BA, Wimmer E: Priming for and induction of anti-poliovirus neutralizing antibodies by synthetic peptides. Nature 304:699, 1983

Emini EA, Ostapchuk P, Wimmer E: Bivalent attachment of antibody onto poliovirus leads to conformational alteration and neutralization. J Virol 48:547, 1983

Ertl HCJ, Finberg RW: Sendai virus–specific T-cell clones: Induction of cytolytic T cells by an anti-idiotypic antibody directed against a helper T-cell clone. Proc Natl Acad Sci USA 81:2850, 1984

Gerhard W, Webster RG: Antigenic drift in influenza A viruses. I. Selection and characterization of antigenic variants of A/PR/8/34(HON1) influenza virus with monoclonal antibody. J Exp Med 148:383, 1978

Gollins SW, Porterfield JS: A new mechanism for the neutralization of enveloped viruses by antiviral antibody. Nature 321:244, 1986

Hurwitz JL, Hackett CJ, McAndrew EC, Gerhard W: Murine T_H response to influenza virus: Recognition of hemagglutinin, neuraminidase, matrix, and nucleoproteins. J Immunol 134:1994, 1985

Kennedy RC, Eichberg JW, Lanford RE, Dreesman GR: Anti-idiotypic antibody vaccine for type B viral hepatitis in chimpanzees. Science 232:220, 1986

Laver WG, Air GM (eds): Immune recognition of protein antigens. Current Communications in Molecular Biology. Cold Spring Harbor, NY, Cold Spring Harbor Laboratory, 1985

Morrison LA, Lukacher AE, Braciale VL et al: Differences in antigen presentation to MHC class I– and Class II–restricted influenza virus–specific cytolytic T lymphocyte clones. J Exp Med 163:903, 1986

Raymond FL, Caton AJ, Cox NJ et al: The antigenicity and evolution of influenza H1 haemagglutinin, from 1950–1957 and 1977–1983: Two pathways from one gene. Virology 148:275, 1986

Reagan KJ, Wunner WH, Wiktor TJ, Koprowski H: Anti-idiotypic antibodies induce neutralizing antibodies to rabies virus glycoprotein. J Virol 48:660, 1983

Schwartz RH: The value of synthetic peptides or vaccines for eliciting T-cell immunity. Curr Top Microbiol Immunol 130:79, 1986

Stitz L, Althage A, Hengartner H, Zinkernagel R: Natural killer cells vs cytotoxic T cells in the peripheral blood of virus-infected mice. J Immunol 134:598, 1985

Uytdehaag HF, Bunschoten H, Weijer K, Osterhaus A: From Jenner to Jerne: Towards ideotype vaccines. Immunol Rev 90:93, 1986

Watson RJ, Enguist LW: Genetically engineered herpes simplex virus vaccines. Prog Med Virol 31:84, 1985

51

Pathogenesis of Viral Infections

The consequences of a viral infection depend on a number of viral and host factors that affect pathogenesis, including the number of infecting viral particles and their path to susceptible cells, the speed of viral multiplication and spread, the effect of the virus on cell functions, the intracellular state of the viral genome, the host's secondary responses to cellular injury (edema, inflammation), and the host's defenses, both immunologic and nonspecific. Viral infection was long thought to produce only acute clinical disease, but other host responses are being increasingly recognized. These include asymptomatic infections, induction of various cancers, chronic progressive neurologic disorders, and possible endocrine diseases.

This chapter deals with the general features of viral pathogenesis, and, where possible, it describes the mechanisms involved. Subsequent chapters discuss the particular characteristics and special effects of various viruses that primarily infect man.

Cellular and Viral Factors in Pathogenesis

The effects of viral infection on cells depend on both the characteristics of the virus and the susceptibility of the cells.

VIRAL CHARACTERISTICS

Viral virulence, like bacterial virulence, is under polygenic control and cannot be assigned to any single viral property; it is, however, frequently associated with several characteristics that promote viral multiplication and cell damage. Thus, virulent viruses multiply well at the elevated temperatures that arise during illness (i.e., above 39°C), induce interferon poorly and resist its inhibitory action, block the biosynthesis of host macromolecules, and damage cell lysosomes or alter the cell membranes of the infected cells, producing damage in the infected animal or cytopathic effects in cell cultures. *Attenuated mutants*, including *conditionally lethal, temperature-sensitive (ts) mutants* (see Mutant Types, Chap. 48), produce less severe or no disease because they are altered in various of the above functions or manifest reduced attachment to specific receptors on particular target cells. However, viruses have genes that are nonessential for their replication but appear to be important for their virulence (e.g., the early region 3 of adenoviruses; see Chap. 52). Moreover, some viruses that are attenuated in their behavior in animals (e.g., poliovirus vaccine strains) cause the same cytopathic effects as wild-type virus in cultures, in which their multiplication is not restrained.

CELL SUSCEPTIBILITY

THE ROLE OF CELL RECEPTORS. The susceptibility of cells to viral infection is often determined by their early interactions with a virus: viral attachment or the release of its nucleic acid in the cells. With animal viruses, as was observed earlier with bacteriophages (see Chap. 45), resistance of the cells is often caused by failure of **viral adsorption;** hence, cells resistant to a virus may be susceptible to its extracted nucleic acid (see Productive Infection, Chap. 48). Indeed, differences in the adsorption of viruses to cells have been correlated with differences in organ susceptibility, and also with changes in host susceptibility with age (e.g., differences in types 1 and 3 reoviruses owing to their S1 genes; see Chap. 62).

Physiological and genetic factors affect the presence or activation of receptors for viral adsorption, as well as other cellular properties that influence susceptibility.

PHYSIOLOGICAL FACTORS. Cultivation may markedly alter the viral susceptibility of cells from that in the original organ. Hence, many viruses can be propagated in cells that are readily cultured, obviating the need for cells that are hard to culture, or for intact animals. For instance, polioviruses, which multiply in the nervous tissue but not in the kidney of a living monkey, multiply well in cultures derived from the kidneys, since receptors develop in the cultivated kidney cells.

Marked changes in susceptibility accompany the maturation of animals. Many viruses are much more virulent in newborn animals (e.g., coxsackieviruses, herpes simplex virus) and others in adults (e.g., polioviruses, lymphocytic choriomeningitis [LCM] virus). There are several mechanisms: with coxsackieviruses in mice the change in susceptibility is correlated with receptor activity, although it may also depend on changes in interferon,

endocrine function, and Ab production; with foot-and-mouth disease virus it involves the rate of viral multiplication; and with LCM virus it is due primarily to an immunologic mechanism (see below).

GENETIC FACTORS. Genetic differences in susceptibility have been demonstrated in mice (with togaviruses and influenza viruses) and in chickens (with oncogenic retroviruses). In crosses between resistant and susceptible animals the heterozygous first-generation (F_1) progeny are uniformly resistant or uniformly susceptible, depending on which allele is dominant. (Resistance is dominant with influenza and togaviruses, and susceptibility with retroviruses). Moreover, backcrosses of the F_1 person to the parent carrying the recessive allele yield 50% resistant animals, implying a difference in a single gene or a closely linked cluster. Some of these hereditary differences evidently involve the host cell–virus interactions, but others could reflect control of the immune response.

CELLULAR RESPONSES TO VIRAL INFECTIONS

Cells can respond to viral infection in four different ways: (1) no apparent change; (2) cytopathic effect and death; (3) hyperplasia, which may be followed by death (as in the pocks of poxviruses on the chorioallantoic membrane of the chick embryo; see Chap. 54); and (4) loss of growth control (topoinhibition or cell–cell contact inhibition), as in viral transformation of normal to cancer cells (see Chap. 64). The development of inclusion bodies and chromosomal aberrations may be special features of these cellular responses.

CYTOPATHIC EFFECTS. Virus-induced cell injury has been most extensively studied with cultured cells, since these are believed to reflect accurately the cell damage occurring *in vivo*, and their responses can be quantified. *In vitro* cell damage, termed the *cytopathic effect*, is recognized from various morphologic alterations, which are listed in Table 51–1; cell death usually follows.

The factors listed below appear to contribute to development of the various cytopathic effects.

EFFECTS ON SYNTHESIS OF CELLULAR MACROMOLECULES. Many virulent viruses cause an early depression of cellular syntheses. As noted in Chapter 48, DNA-containing viruses inhibit the synthesis of host cell DNA, but most do not affect host cell RNA and protein production until late in the multiplication cycle, whereas many RNA viruses inhibit host cell RNA and protein synthesis early in the multiplication cycle.

ALTERATION OF LYSOSOMES. Some viruses cause a reversible increase in lysosome permeability, without leakage of enzymes from the organelles. This change, the cause of which is unknown, is shown by an increased binding

TABLE 51–1. Cellular Response to Viral Infection

Virus	Cell Type*	Cellular Response	Inclusion Body
Adenoviruses	HeLa	Cell rounding and clumping	Nuclear
	Rat embryo	Transformed	Nuclear
Herpesviruses (herpes simplex)	HeLa	Polykaryocytes (some strains); cell rounding	Nuclear
Poxviruses (variola)	HeLa	Slow rounding; hyperplastic foci	Cytoplasmic
Picornaviruses (polioviruses)	Monkey kidney	Cell lysis	None
Orthomyxoviruses (influenza viruses)	Monkey kidney	Slow rounding	None
Paramyxoviruses (parainfluenza virus)	Monkey kidney	Fusion of cell membranes; syncytial formation	Cytoplasmic
Coronaviruses	Human diploid	Minimal; syncytia rarely	None
Togaviruses (eastern equine encephalitis virus)	Mouse L	Cell lysis	None
Rubella virus	Human amnion	Slow enlargement and rounding	Cytoplasmic
Reoviruses	Monkey kidney	Enlargement and vacuolation	Cytoplasmic
Rabiesvirus	Hamster kidney	Usually none	Cytoplasmic

* With many viruses several cell types can be used; in such instances, a commonly used type is listed.

of neutral red, the dye commonly used to stain the live cells in the plaque assay: the cells appear hyperstained and form "red plaques." Other viruses effect disruption of the organelles and discharge of their hydrolytic enzymes into the cytoplasm. The cells lose their ability to be stained with neutral red and form the usual "white plaques." This profound effect appears to be due to proteins synthesized late in the viral multiplication cycle, possibly capsid subunits.

ALTERATIONS OF THE CELL MEMBRANE. Many of the budding, enveloped viruses incorporate viral subunits, usually glycoproteins, into the infected cell membranes, as a prelude to the formation of the viral envelope (see Enveloped Viruses, Chap. 48). Even some viruses that do not bud from the cell surface, such as herpes simplex and vaccinia viruses, insert novel Ags into the plasma membrane. These changes may be recognized by reaction with virus-specific Abs, by **hemadsorption** (e.g., orthomyxoviruses and paramyxoviruses), or by absorption of increased quantities of plant lectins such as concanavalin A (e.g., poxviruses, paramyxoviruses). The inserted Ags make the cells targets for immunologic destruction by virus-specific Abs plus complement or by immune T-lymphocytes. In addition, effects on their membranes, as well as on the cytoskeleton, probably play a large role in altering the shape and function of cells. In a striking effect observed with paramyxoviruses, some herpesviruses, and the human immunodeficiency virus (HIV), the infected cells fuse with adjacent cells (i.e., establish a continuity between the plasma membranes, forming giant cells (**polykaryocytes).**

ABORTIVE INFECTION may also cause cytopathic effects although viral syntheses is incomplete: for example, in cultured HeLa cells influenza viruses synthesize Ags and damage the cells, though they do not form infectious virions. Incomplete viral replication (e.g., only early viral functions are expressed) may also activate cells such as

macrophages to elaborate cytokines (interleukin-1 [IL-1]; tumor necrosis factor [TNF]; and interferons, alpha and beta), all of which can produce inflammatory responses.

Viral toxic effects produce cell damage in animals and in cell cultures, owing to the accumulation of virions or viral structural proteins. In mice, for example, the intravenous injection of a concentrated preparation of influenza, mumps, or vaccinia virus causes hemorrhages and cellular necrosis in various organs, resulting in death within 24 hours; a large intracerebral inoculum of influenza virus produces necrosis of brain cells. Addition of adenovirus fiber protein to KB cells inhibits cellular DNA synthesis, and the penton base effects cell rounding and clumping. All these effects are produced without synthesis of viral components or with synthesis of only incomplete particles.

DEVELOPMENT OF INCLUSION BODIES. Intracellular masses may arise as accumulations, either of virions or of unassembled viral components, in the nucleus (e.g., adenovirus), in the cytoplasm (e.g., rabiesvirus Negri bodies), or in both (e.g., measles). These inclusion bodies appear to disrupt the structure and function of the cells and to contribute to their death. Other inclusion bodies do not contain detectable virions or their components but are "scars" left by earlier viral multiplication (e.g., the eosinophilic, intranuclear inclusion bodies that eventually appear in cells infected by herpes simplex virus; see Chap. 53).

INDUCTION OF CHROMOSOMAL ABERRATIONS. In primary cultures, chromosomal aberrations such as breaks or constrictions are commonly seen after infections with measles and rubella viruses; with several adenoviruses and herpes, parainfluenza, mumps, polyoma, and Rous sarcoma viruses; and with simian virus 40 (SV40). During natural infections, measles virus produces similar chromosomal abnormalities in peripheral leukocytes. The alterations often appear to be an early expression of the cytopathic effect in cells that will die later. Some of these aberrations have characteristic features; for example, herpes simplex virus induces breaks only at certain sites of two specific chromosomes, and chromatid breaks may continue to occur during the multiplication of cells surviving infection by herpes simplex or polyoma virus, suggesting a persistent or latent infection of the cell clones.

CELL TRANSFORMATION. Certain viruses that produce tumors or leukemia (see Chaps. 64 and 65) may have several effects on cultured cells: (1) stimulation of the synthesis of cellular DNA (e.g., polyoma virus); (2) surface alterations recognizable by the incorporation or uncovering of new antigenic specificities distinct from those of virion subunits and by increased agglutinability by plant lectins; (3) chromosomal aberrations and sister chromatid exchanges; (4) disruption of the cytoskeleton system; and (5) alterations of the growth properties of the cells, resulting in cell hyperplasia because their division is no longer subject to topoinhibition (i.e., inhibition of growth in a dense culture). Moreover, growth is less dependent on serum in the culture medium and does not require anchorage to the surface of a culture vessel—colonies of transformed cells grow in soft agar or methylcellulose. This conversion of a normal cultured cell to one resembling a malignant cell has been termed **transformation** (see Chap. 64). DNA-containing viruses (adenoviruses, herpes simplex, polyoma, SV40) can transform only nonpermissive cells, but at least a portion of the viral genome persists and continues to function. In contrast, cells transformed by RNA viruses (e.g., avian leukosis, murine leukemia) are permissive and usually continue to produce virions.

Patterns of Disease

In a host, viruses cause three basic patterns of infection: localized, disseminated, and inapparent.

LOCALIZED

In localized infections, viral multiplication and cell damage remain localized near the site of entry (e.g., the skin or parts of the respiratory or gastrointestinal tract). When the virus spreads from the first infected cells to neighboring cells by diffusion across intercellular spaces and by cell contact, the result is a single lesion or a group of lesions, as with warts. In a less strictly localized pattern, when virus is transported by excretions or secretions within connected cavities, infection causes diffuse involvement of an organ, as with influenza, the common cold, or viral gastroenteritis. Virus may in time spread to distant sites, but this dissemination is not essential for production of the characteristic illness.

DISSEMINATED

Disseminated infections develop through several sequential steps, as illustrated by Fenner's classic investigation of ectromelia (mousepox), summarized in Figure 51–1. Mousepox virus enters through an abrasion of the skin and multiplies locally; from there it spreads rapidly to regional lymph nodes, where it also multiplies. The virus then enters the lymphatics and the bloodstream, and this primary viremia causes the dissemination of the virus to other susceptible organs, especially the liver and spleen. Viral multiplication results in necrotic lesions in these organs and a more intense secondary viremia, which disseminates the virus to the target organ, the skin. There the virus undergoes extensive multiplication, producing papules that eventually ulcerate. With the appearance of the papular rash the asymptomatic incubation period terminates, and clinical disease begins.

The temporal relation among viral multiplication in the various organs, development of lesions, and formation of Abs should be noted (see Fig. 51–1A). It is particularly striking that overt disease begins only after virus becomes widely disseminated in the body and has attained maximum titers in the blood and the spleen.

This model of dissemination is applicable not only to exanthematous diseases such as smallpox and measles but also to nonexanthematous diseases such as poliomyelitis and mumps. Thus, the target organ for poliovirus is the central nervous system, and for mumps virus the salivary and other glands. In some instances, such as poliovirus infections (see Chap. 55), primary and secondary viremias are not distinguishable.

The dissemination of neurotropic viruses to the nervous system may occur by transmission along nerves as well as by viremia. In mice, for instance, such centripetal transmission of herpes simplex virus after foot pad inoculation can be followed by assaying segments of nerves at various times after infection. The virus may conceivably travel either by axonal transport or by multiplication in endoneural cells (Schwann's cells and fibroblasts), in which viral Ags can be localized by immunofluorescence.

For many years, before refined structural studies of virions became possible, animal viruses were classified primarily in terms of their viscerotropism, neurotropism, or dermotropism. The grouping of viruses on the basis of their target organs is presented in Table 51–2. However, the target organ for a given virus (where the susceptible cells are damaged) and the type of disease produced bear no relation to the taxonomic position of the virus, as defined in Chapters 44 (see The Viral Particles) and 48 (see Table 48–1). In fact, such unrelated viruses as influenza and adenoviruses may produce diseases that cannot be clinically differentiated, and such related viruses as parainfluenza, mumps, and measles may produce completely different clinical syndromes.

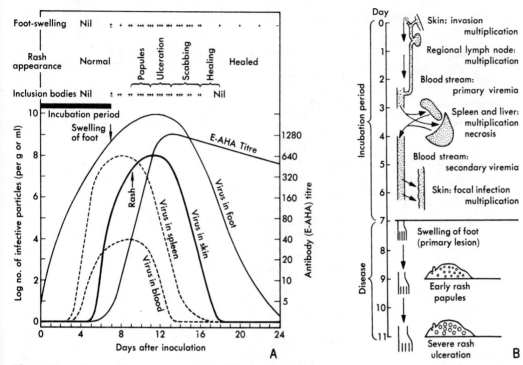

Figure 51–1. Sequential events in the pathogenesis of ectromelia (mousepox) in mice inoculated in the foot pad. *(A)* Relation among viral multiplication (in foot pad, spleen, blood, and skin), development of primary lesion and rash, and appearance of Abs (E-AHA). *(B)* Diagram of the dissemination of virus and the pathogenesis of the rash in mousepox. (Fenner F: Lancet 2:915, 1948)

INAPPARENT

Transient viral infections without overt disease (inapparent infections) are very common. Moreover, they have great epidemiologic importance, for they represent an often unrecognized source of dissemination of a virus, and they also confer immunity. For example, for every paralytic case of poliomyelitis in the United States before the days of widespread immunization, 100 to 200 inapparent infections could be detected serologically or by viral isolation.

Several factors are involved in the production of inapparent infections:

Moderate viruses or attenuated strains (as in live vaccines) usually cause inapparent infections.

When the host's defense mechanisms are effective, even viruses capable of causing acute disease may generate an inapparent infection. These defenses include the host's immunity, especially the ability to produce a prompt secondary response (Abs or cytotoxic T-lymphocytes), and the appearance of viral interference (see Chap. 49).

Failure of the virus to reach the target organ is also an expression of host defense, but of a more obscure

nature. Thus, as noted above, only about one of 200 nonimmune persons infected with poliovirus express symptoms of central nervous system (CNS) disease (see Chap. 55).

Effects of Viruses on Embryonic Development

The variation of susceptibility with age is especially striking for the embryonic period. Indeed, some viruses that produce mild disease in the adult produce extensive infection and severe malformations in the embryo. The role of viruses in the pathogenesis of congenital anomalies was not recognized until Gregg, in 1941, discovered that rubella virus may cause a variety of congenital anomalies if the mother is infected during the first 3 months of pregnancy (see Chap. 61). Of all the viral infections that may occur during the first trimester of pregnancy, rubella is the major cause of fetal death and congenital malformations. But a few other viruses also have teratogenic effects: **cytomegalovirus** induces a low incidence of microcephaly, motor disability, and chorioretinitis; **group B coxsackieviruses** are responsible for some congenital heart lesions; and **type 2 herpes simplex vi-**

TABLE 51–2. Grouping of Viruses by Pathogenic Characteristics in Man

Classification by Major Target Organs	Specific Virus(es)	Portal(s) of Entry	Other Affected Organs
Respiratory viruses	Influenza A, B, and C	Respiratory tract	
	Parainfluenza	Respiratory tract	
	Respiratory syncytial	Respiratory tract	
	Measles	Respiratory tract	Brain, skin, lung
	Mumps	Respiratory tract	CNS, testes, ovaries, pancreas
	Adenoviruses	Respiratory tract	
	Rhinoviruses	Respiratory tract	
	Coxsackieviruses (some)	Respiratory tract	CNS*
	Echoviruses (some)	Respiratory tract	CNS,* skin
	Reoviruses	Respiratory tract	?
	Lymphocytic choriomeningitis	Respiratory tract	CNS
	Coronavirus	Respiratory tract	
Enteric viruses	Polioviruses	Gastrointestinal tract	Muscles, CNS*
	Coxsackieviruses	Gastrointestinal tract	CNS,* skin
	Echoviruses	Gastrointestinal tract	CNS,* skin
	Rotaviruses (reovirus)	Gastrointestinal tract	
	Hepatitis A and B; non-A, non-B	Gastrointestinal tract, blood	Liver
Neurotropic viruses	Polioviruses	Gastrointestinal tract	Upper respiratory tract
	Coxsackieviruses	Gastrointestinal tract	Upper respiratory tract
	Echoviruses	Gastrointestinal tract	Upper respiratory tract
	Rabies	Skin and blood	
	Mumps	Respiratory tract	Testes, ovaries, pancreas
	Measles	Respiratory tract	Skin, lung
	Arboviruses	Blood	
	Herpes simplex virus	Respiratory tract, genitalia	Skin
	Virus B	Respiratory tract, blood	Respiratory tract
	Varicella zoster	Respiratory tract	Skin, cornea
	Lymphocytic choriomeningitis	Respiratory tract	Respiratory tract
	Kuru	Gastrointestinal tract	
	Creutzfeldt-Jakob	Unknown	
	BK and JC	Unknown	
Dermotropic viruses	Poxviruses	Respiratory tract	Respiratory tract, viscera, CNS
	Measles	Respiratory tract	Lung, brain
	Varicella zoster	Respiratory tract	CNS, cornea
	Coxsackieviruses	Gastrointestinal tract	Upper respiratory tract
	Echoviruses	Gastrointestinal tract	CNS, gastrointestinal tract
	Herpes simplex	Skin	Peripheral ganglia, cornea, genitalia
	Rubella	Respiratory tract	Respiratory tract
	Human wart (papilloma viruses)	Skin	
	Molluscum contagiosum	Skin	
Human T-cell tropic viruses	HTLV I and HTLV II	Blood	Spleen, lymph nodes
	Human immunodeficiency virus (HIV)	Blood	Organs containing lymphocytes, macrophages

* Major involvement in clinical disease
CNS, central nervous system

rus may cause microcephaly and other severe CNS malformations.

Passage of a virus across the placenta appears to be responsible for embryonic infection, and this probably occurs only when the mother is viremic. Multiplication of the virus in the placenta may favor transmission but is not strictly required, since the small coliphage ϕX174, which is unable to multiply in animals, is transmitted (though with very low efficiency).

Immunologic and Other Systemic Factors

CIRCULATING ANTIBODIES

PROTECTION. Abs in serum and extracellular fluids provide the main protection against primary viral infections; i.e., at the site of viral entry into the host. For those infections in which viremia is an essential link in the pathogenesis of the disease (i.e., measles, poliomyelitis, mumps, smallpox), the degree of protection is directly related to the level of neutralizing Abs in the blood when virus enters it. Furthermore, in experimental herpes simplex virus infections, the B-cell response limits the spread of virus to the CNS and reduces the establishment of latency in peripheral ganglia (see below). The mechanism by which Abs neutralize viruses has been considered in Chapter 50.

Protection of the respiratory and gastrointestinal tracts is associated with **IgA Abs** (see Chap. 14), which are secreted into the extracellular fluids. Hence, by inducing the secretion of IgA Abs, natural infections produce specific local as well as systemic immunity. Viral vaccines, particularly those containing live attenuated virus, also elicit the production of IgA Abs in the respiratory and gastrointestinal secretions. Although this feature theoretically affords a marked advantage to live viral vaccines, some vaccines produced with killed viruses and introduced parenterally, such as polioviruses and influenza viruses, have proved effective.

The protective role of Abs is also evident in the prophylactic effectiveness of **passive immunization.** Administration of immune serum or immune **γ-globulin** before infection or early in the incubation period can prevent or modify diseases with viremia and long incubation periods (greater than 12 days), such as measles, hepatitis A and B, poliomyelitis, and mumps. The striking protection of populations by some viral vaccines (Table 51–3) constitutes an additional demonstration of the prophylactic function of Abs. These specific vaccines will be discussed in the chapters that follow.

RECOVERY. Although humoral Abs generally develop during recovery from a viral disease, they appear to play a less prominent role in this process than in protection. Thus, intracellular virus may continue to increase, and pathologic lesions to evolve, even while Abs are being elaborated. Moreover, in most patients with agammaglobulinemia, recovery from viral diseases is usually normal, although some such affected children may have persistent and fatal echovirus infections. Furthermore, even patients with selective IgA deficiency do not develop more prolonged or more severe respiratory or enteric viral infections. These findings lend additional evidence that factors other than humoral Abs, such as natural killer cells, complement, and cellular immunity act to limit the course of and effect recovery from viral diseases.

The limited effect of humoral Abs on recovery is not surprising, since they are ineffective against intracellular viral precursors and virions. Furthermore, many viruses can spread directly to contiguous, uninfected cells, thus remaining inaccessible to Abs. However, Abs do serve an important function in restricting the dissemination of

TABLE 51–3. Viral Diseases in Which Immunization Has Been Effective

| | Vaccine | |
Disease	Attenuated Virus	Inactivated Virus
Smallpox	+	
Yellow fever	+	
Poliomyelitis	+	+
Measles	+	
Influenza	+*	+
Mumps	+	+
Rabies	+†	+
Adenovirus infection‡	+	+
Rubella	+	

* Experimental
† For veterinary use
‡ Caused by types 3, 4, 7, and 21

some viruses (e.g., polioviruses and togaviruses), the pathogenesis of which depends on a viremic stage.

PERSISTENCE OF ANTIBODIES. The time course and the persistence of Ab production and immunity vary with (1) the virus, (2) the nature of antigenic stimulus, and (3) the type of Ab. For example, (1) neutralizing Abs fall from their maximal level more rapidly, and to a lower titer, following influenza than following poliomyelitis infection; (2) immunity to measles persists for life following infection, but lasts only a few months following immunization with formalin-inactivated virus; (3) after infection, complement-fixing Abs generally appear earlier but decrease much sooner than neutralizing Abs.

Long-lasting immunity, with persistence of circulating Abs, follows infection with a number of viruses, especially those causing viremia. Thus, second attacks are extremely rare with measles, smallpox, yellow fever, or poliomyelitis, to mention only a few examples. In contrast, **second infections are common with most acute localized infections without viremia, particularly respiratory diseases** (probably because adequate quantities of neutralizing Abs do not persist in respiratory secretions, although sufficient circulating Abs are present). Adenovirus infections (see Chap. 52) are notable exceptions, perhaps because they frequently terminate in latent infections of lymphoid tissue in the respiratory and gastrointestinal tracts.

Latent infection with persistent synthesis of critical viral Ags offers the most reasonable explanation for the long-lasting immunity that follows many viral infections. **Repeated infections** by a prevalent virus or **secondary Ab response** in a disease with a long incubation period could also provide an explanation, but these possibilities seem much less plausible. Thus, neither of the latter mechanisms can account for the prolonged persistence of circulating Abs against smallpox or yellow fever in previously infected residents of the United States, where these diseases rarely, if ever, occur.

Panum's observations on a measles epidemic in the Faroe Islands offers a classic example of prolonged immunity in the absence of reexposure to the specific agent. Those persons who had been alive during the preceding epidemic, 67 years earlier, were immune, whereas the younger islanders were highly susceptible. Hence, not only did immunity persist in the absence of overt clinical reinfection, but the immune persons failed to infect their nonimmune contacts during all these years. This absence of transmission could be explained by incomplete viral multiplication, by the continued neutralization of the virus produced in the immune persons, or by persistence of memory cells rather than the existence of latent infection.

CELL-MEDIATED IMMUNITY

Dysgammaglobulinemias and drug-mediated immune suppression in humans have provided the strongest evidence that humoral Abs do not play the determinant role in recovery from many viral infections. Patients who lack immunoglobulins but develop cell-mediated immunity (CMI), which consists of cytolytic T-lymphocytes and Ab-dependent cell-mediated cytotoxicity (ADCC), ordinarily recover from viral diseases without difficulty, whereas patients with defective CMI but normal Abs recover poorly from certain viral infections. For example, in persons with defective CMI, smallpox immunization frequently leads to spreading of the virus, either with severe **generalized vaccinia** or extensive necrosis of the skin and muscle of the affected extremity (**vaccinia gangrenosa;** see Chap. 54). Moreover, these complications are unaffected by the administration of specific neutralizing Abs, but they are arrested by local injection of lymphoid cells from recently immunized donors, and development of a delayed hypersensitivity reaction to heat-inactivated vaccinia virus accompanies this recovery. Finally, in experimental animals, depression of CMI by antilymphocytic serum (which contains Abs to T cells) increases the severity or the duration of infection with a number of viruses, particularly those possessing envelopes (e.g., herpesviruses, poxviruses, and paramyxoviruses).

Cellular immunity also appears to play a critical role in **maintaining the latent viral infections:** activation of such infections has become common in patients with organ transplants or with malignancies whose CMI is suppressed by therapy. These latent infections include herpesviruses (varicella zoster, cytomegalovirus, and Epstein-Barr [EB] virus), adenoviruses, measles virus, hu-

man wart virus, and JC and BK viruses (papovaviruses similar to SV40). Herpesvirus infections are also often activated in patients with extensive burns (herpes simplex virus and cytomegalovirus) and in the aged (varicella zoster virus) owing to diminished CMI. Activation of these viruses is also a common and life-threatening event in patients with **acquired immune deficiency syndrome (AIDS)** owing to marked suppression of their T4-helper cells (see Chap. 65).

Pseudotolerance

Some viruses that infect the embryo or the newborn without damaging host cells give rise to apparent immunologic tolerance. Thus, chicks infected by avian leukosis virus produce virus throughout life without detectably producing neutralizing Abs. However, this phenomenon is not due to true tolerance, since Abs are formed, but they are complexed with the large amount of virus produced. Similarly, humans infected *in utero* with rubella virus or cytomegalovirus, and fetal mice infected with influenza virus, produce virus-specific Abs for long periods after birth. And although mice with **persistent LCM** or **murine leukemia virus** infection give birth to offspring who are viremic and lack detectable virus-specific circulating Abs, the infants synthesize Abs that complex with virus (see below). Such persistently infected mice, however, are deficient in cytotoxic T-cell production. Moreover, injection of specific cytotoxic T cells can reduce or even eliminate the persistent infection.

The virus produced in large amounts throughout the life of such **pseudotolerant** animals, usually with viremia, is **disseminated vertically** to their offspring through the ovum, placenta, or milk and **horizontally** to contacts through excretions and secretions. In such animals infection is asymptomatic for most of their life, but late in life a chronic disease may develop.

DISEASE BASED ON VIRUS-INDUCED IMMUNOLOGIC RESPONSE

The immune response, despite its protective and ameliorative effects, can also contribute to the production of disease, particularly with viruses that **antigenically alter the cell's surface membranes.** For instance, a severe, **hemorrhagic dengue,** often associated with a shock syndrome, occurs in those who have had prior infection with a different serotype, and children **immunized with inactivated measles** or **respiratory syncytial virus** develop unusually severe disease if subsequently infected by the same virus. These examples of **enhanced viral injury** could be due to one or a mixture of the following immunologic reactions with virus-infected cells: increased secondary response of cytotoxic T cells (see Chap. 50); specific Ab-dependent, cell-mediated lysis; Ab-mediated, complement(classic or alternate pathway)-dependent lysis; or enhanced binding of unneutralized virus-Ab complexes to cell surface Fc receptors, thus increasing the number of cells infected (i.e. *immune enhancement*). In another mechanism, circulating virus-specific **Ag–Ab complexes** may lodge in organs, such as the brain or kidney, inducing inflammation and disease.

The central role of the immune response in the development of some viral diseases is dramatically demonstrated in mice infected with **LCM** virus,* an arenavirus (see Chap. 60). In adult mice severe, often fatal disease follows about a week after intracerebral inoculation, but if the immune response has been suppressed (by neonatal thymectomy, chemicals, x-irradiation, or antilymphocytic serum), disease fails to develop although viral multiplication and spread are unrestrained. Moreover, after infection *in utero* or at birth, specific CMI is not detectable; the mice appear normal for 9 to 12 months in spite of widespread viral multiplication that produces persistent viremia and viruria, with viral Ags in most organs. Tissue injury can be initiated in such mice by transfer of spleen cells from a syngeneic immune donor but not by immune spleen cells treated with anti-θ serum (from animals immunized with Ag from T-lymphocytes) or by large amounts of immune serum.

In adult mice, viral replication and spread are relatively restricted in both neural and extraneural tissues, but the cell-mediated antiviral immune response is quick to develop and to elicit lethal disease by attacking the membranes of a critical number of involved cells. In contrast, in the fetus, neonate, or immunosuppressed adult mouse, with limited immunologic capabilities, infection proceeds unimpeded to eventual involvement of all tissues. The constant high level of virus that develops may conceivably depress the clonal expansion of virus-specific T-lymphocytes, but Abs are produced, only to be complexed with excess circulating viral Ags and complement. Filtration of these aggregates by the renal glomeruli initiates an inflammatory response, culminating in glomerulonephritis. In addition, necrotic lesions appear in the liver, brain, spleen, and other organs, apparently resulting from the reaction between virus-sensitized killer T-lymphocytes and viral Ags present on the surface of many cells. After intracerebral infection of an adult animal, the brain damage is generated by a similar T-cell–dependent immunologic mechanism. In contrast to the devastating effects of natural LCM infection, the immunization of mice with inactivated LCM produces humoral Abs that, upon subsequent infection, restrict viral spread and prevent disease.

These observations lead to the conclusion that in the absence of effective cellular immunity, LCM virus multiplies harmlessly for a long time in mice, producing an inapparent infection similar to the persistent infection that it causes in cell cultures (see below). Thus, every aspect of the disease, in both acute and chronic infection, can be shown to be immunologically mediated, and in this single animal model, LCM dramatically demonstrates both the benefits and the disadvantages of the immunologic response. **Anti-idiotypic Abs,** those directed against the Ab variable region (the antigen-combining site), usually develop during the immune response (see Chap. 14). Such Abs mimic viral Ag and, like viruses, may bind to receptors on the cell surface. This interaction of anti-idiotypic Abs and viral cell receptors could theoretically produce cell injury, although the precise role of these Abs has not yet been elucidated in the pathogenesis of viral diseases. Induction of this type of complication following a viral infection seems possible when it is realized that the viral receptors have not evolved for the benefit of viruses, but rather to accommodate substances required physiologically by the cell; for example, the human immunodeficiency (AIDS) virus (HIV) attaches to the T4-lymphocyte receptor, type 3 reovirus utilizes the mammalian β-adrenergic receptor, and EB virus combines with the complement C3d receptor on human B-lymphocytes.

NONSPECIFIC SYSTEMIC FACTORS

Nonspecific factors that influence resistance to viral infection include various **hormones, temperature, inhibitors** other than Abs, **natural killer (NK) cells,** and **phagocytes.** Nutrition may also affect the course of viral infections; e.g., measles has devastating consequences in malnourished children of West Africa. However, malnutrition influences so many aspects of the host defenses that specific analysis of cause and effect is difficult.

Infected cells may form and release an especially important factor, **interferon,** which inhibits viral multiplication by preventing the synthesis of viral proteins, and thus interferes with the infection of other cells by many viruses. Interferon also activates NK cells. Accordingly, interferon not only prevents the infection of cells but also limits viral spread and assists in recovery. This agent has been discussed in Chapter 49.

Phagocytosis does not appear to be as important a defense mechanism in viral as in bacterial infections. On the contrary, some viruses impair the antibacterial activity of **polymorphonuclear leukocytes** by producing leukopenia (e.g., measles virus) or by reducing phagocytic function (e.g., influenza virus). **Macrophages,** however, do appear to be important in viral infections; they rapidly take up certain viruses, and there is a correlation between host and macrophage susceptibility to viral infections (see Genetic Factors, above). Virus-infected macrophages can act as a source of infection for other cells, but with viruses that are unable to multiply in them,

---

* This virus can also infect humans, but it usually produces a mild respiratory infection, only occasionally followed by severe meningitis.

macrophages appear to play their usual role as scavengers.

Hormones have a potential effect on viral infections, as can be illustrated by several examples. Pregnancy increases the severity of several viral diseases: paralytic poliomyelitis is more frequent and more extensive; smallpox has a more severe course, and abortion is common; the complications of influenza, particularly pneumonia, are increased. Cortisone enhances the susceptibility of many animals to viral infection and commonly potentiates the severity of the disease; in humans it causes enlargement and perforation of herpetic corneal ulcers and induces extensive visceral spread of varicella virus that often terminates in severe pneumonia. These deleterious effects appear to result from the suppressive effects of cortisone on inflammatory reactions, CMI, and interferon production rather than from its action on the Ab response.

Temperature increase in the host may reduce viral replication by suppressing a temperature-sensitive step, by accelerating the inactivation of many heat-labile viruses (enveloped viruses), and by increasing interferon production. Conversely, in mice held at 4°C, rather than 25°C, after infection with coxsackievirus B1, viral multiplication is excessive in many organs, little interferon is produced, and the mortality is strikingly increased. A rise in body temperature may therefore contribute to recovery from viral disease.

Latent Viral Infections

In **latent infections,** overt disease is not produced, but the virus is not eradicated. This equilibrium between host and parasite is achieved in various ways by different viruses and hosts. The virus exists in latent infections either as an infectious and continuously replicating agent, termed a **persistent viral infection,** or in a truly latent **noninfectious occult form,** possibly as an integrated genome or an episomal agent.

Numerous experimental cell culture and animal models exemplify these two types of latent infections and permit understanding of both types of latent infections in humans. It is noteworthy that in humans, persistent viral infections may lead to chronic diseases, which appear some years after the initial viral infections. These persistent infections have been termed **slow viral infections** (see below) and are best exemplified by **subacute sclerosing panencephalitis** caused by a persistent, inapparent measles virus infection (see Chap. 57). In contrast, occult viral infections may lead to reactivation of the viral genome, perhaps akin to lysogeny in bacteria, resulting in productive viral replication and induction of acute disease, such as **fever blisters** caused by activated **herpes simplex virus** (see Chap. 53) or **shingles** similarly initiated by **herpes zoster virus** (see Chap. 53).

LATENT PERSISTENT INFECTIONS

Enveloped viruses such as **paramyxoviruses** (measles, parainfluenza, and mumps viruses), some herpesviruses (e.g., EB virus), **retroviruses,** and **arenaviruses** appear particularly suited to initiate persistent infections. Infection appears to persist because the virus does not disrupt the essential **housekeeping functions** of the cells (e.g., DNA, RNA, and protein synthesis), although they may affect **luxury functions.** For example, **LCM virus of mice** (see above) may turn off growth hormone production in the anterior lobe of the pituitary gland without altering the infected cells' vital processes, thus leading to retarded growth of the infected mice. Some persistently infected cells, as in measles subacute sclerosing panencephalitis (see below), may be assisted by the remarkable capacity of humoral Abs to **redistribute ("cap") viral Ags on the plasma membrane** (Fig. 51–2). This phenomenon promotes shedding of viral Ags from the cell surface, leaving the cell surface free of viral glycoproteins and the infected cell protected from either cell-mediated (CTL) or Ab-dependent cell-mediated (ADCC) immunologic destruction.

Defective viral particles, the genomes of which are partially deleted, produce effective interference with homotypic, nondefective virus, and they are therefore termed **defective interfering** (or DI) particles (see Chap. 49). DI particles appear to play a central role in steady-state infections in cell cultures and possibly in the establishment and maintenance of *in vivo* persistent infections.

LATENT OCCULT VIRAL INFECTIONS IN ANIMAL HOSTS

There is an increasing recognition that some viruses, both DNA- and RNA-containing viruses, may become undetectable following a primary infection only to reappear and produce acute disease. The mechanism by which this latency is established and the virus then reactivated must be accomplished in different ways, as the following examples illustrate.

1. **Herpes simplex virus** has a special pattern of **latency** and **recurrence.** This virus usually infects humans between 6 and 18 months of age, and the virus persists but cannot be found except during recurrent acute episodes, such as herpes labialis (fever blisters; see Chap. 53). The form in which the latent occult virus persists between recurrent episodes is uncertain. Virus cannot be isolated from tissue homogenates, but by cocultivating cells of sensory ganglia with susceptible cells,

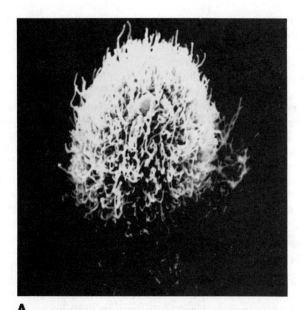

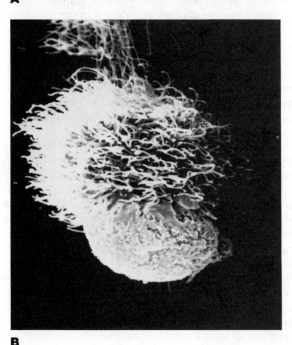

Figure 51–2. Distribution of measles virus Ags on the surface of infected HeLa cells before and after reaction with virus-specific Abs. *(A)* Scanning electron microscopy demonstrates the abundant fine microvilli randomly distributed when infected cells were not reacted with Abs. (In contrast, uninfected cells display shorter, thicker, and less abundant villi). *(B)* Marked redistribution ("capping") of viral Ags seen after infected cells were mixed with virus-specific Abs at 37°C. Serum without measles virus Abs or serum with Abs directed against Ags of other viruses did not cap the measles virus Ags. (Original magnification ×4000; Lampert PW et al: J Virol 15:1248, 1975)

virus has been detected in the human trigeminal (type 1 virus) and thoracic, lumbar, and sacral dorsal root ganglia (type 2 virus), as well as in sensory ganglia of experimentally infected mice, rabbits, and monkeys. DNA:DNA hybridization studies have detected the viral genome in normal brains as well as in peripheral ganglia. These data suggest that the DNA exists in a linear, unintegrated form, perhaps as episomes or in intact virions. It may be that, as in virus-carrier cultures, infection is confined to only a small proportion (about 0.01%–0.1%) of the ganglion cells by Abs, cellular immunity, viral interference (by interferon or DI particles), or metabolic factors. Because Abs are present, most of the extracellular virus is neutralized and goes undetected. Acute episodes, in which there is a burst of viral replication, probably depend on a transient change in the local level of immunity or changes in the susceptibility of the uninfected cells induced by a variety of physical and physiologic factors such as fever, intense sunlight, fatigue, or menstruation.

Experimentally, the role of cell susceptibility is shown by thymidine kinase–minus mutants, which cannot replicate in growth-arrested cells and do not establish latent infections of the trigeminal or cervical sensory ganglia following productive ocular infections. The role of shifts in the immune system is also illustrated by experimental infection of rabbits with herpes simplex virus. Herpes encephalitis can be reactivated 6 months after an acute encephalitis episode by inducing anaphylaxis with any Ag. Similarly, herpes keratitis can be provoked, after an acute corneal ulcer is healed, if the rabbit is made sensitive to horse serum and a corneal Arthus reaction is induced. **Nonspecific excitants** such as ultraviolet light, histamine or epinephrine injection, corticosteroids, or surgical manipulation of sensory ganglia and nerves can also **activate** experimental herpes simplex virus infection.

The other herpesviruses that infect humans also commonly produce latent infections: varicella zoster virus in sensory ganglia, cytomegalovirus in macrophages and lymphocytes, and EB virus in B-lymphocytes (see Chap. 53).

2. **Adenovirus infections** in humans are self-limited, but the virus frequently establishes a latent, persistent infection of tonsils and adenoids (see Pathogenesis, Chap. 52). Though these tissues fail to yield infectious virus when homogenized and tested in sensitive cell cultures, cultured fragments of about 85% of these "normal" tonsils and adenoids, after a variable time, show characteristic adenovirus-induced cytopathic changes and yield infectious virus. Viral DNA can be detected in tonsils and adenoids, as well as in peripheral lymphocytes.

Failure to recover infectious virus initially may be attributed to the paucity of virions, to their association with either Ab or receptor material, or to the absence of mature virions. The latent infection is probably not the result of lysogeny, since DNA in peripheral lymphocytes appears to be in a linear episomal form. The host's cytotoxic T cells probably fail to eradicate persistently infected cells because the carboxy-terminus of a 19,000 dalton glycoprotein (gp19kd), encoded in early region 3 (see Chap. 52), combines with one or more of the Class I major histocompatibility complex (MHC) Ags in the endoplasmic reticulum and prevents their transport to the infected cells' surfaces.

3. The **Shope rabbit papilloma virus** (see Chap. 64) illustrates latency due to the **replication of viral nucleic acid without viral maturation.** This virus produces warts equally well in the skin of domestic or of wild cottontail rabbits, but infectious virus and viral Ags can usually be detected only in the tumors of the wild animals,* in the keratinized cells of the outer epidermal layer but not in the growing basal layer. However, the basal layer of warts from either wild or domestic rabbits yields episomal, infectious, viral DNA when extracted with phenol.

In man the most dramatic example of **incomplete viral production** is the persistence and continued replication of **measles virus nucleocapsids** in lesions of **subacute sclerosing panencephalitis (SSPE),** which may develop years after acute measles infection (see Slow Viral Infections, below).

4. **Swine influenza virus,** an orthomyxovirus related to influenza A virus, illustrates a complex ecologic situation in which the virus is **latent in two intermediate hosts** and **requires assistance from a bacterium,** *Hemophilus influenzae suis,* to induce the acute respiratory disease in pigs (Fig. 51–3).

Shope showed that virus in the lung of a sick pig becomes associated, in occult form, with ova of the lungworm (a common parasite of most pigs), which is coughed up with pulmonary secretions, swallowed, and eventually passed in the pig's feces. The contaminated feces are then eaten by earthworms, in which the lungworm ova develop into larvae in which the virus can remain occult for at least 2 years. To complete the cycle the earthworm is eaten by a pig, and the lungworm larvae migrate to the pig's lungs, where they develop into mature lungworms. The virus remains noninfectious through this long odyssey, but when the parasitized pig is jolted by cold or by infection with *H. influenzae suis,* the occult virus is somehow induced to replicate; it may initiate an acute disease and induce viral spread. The nature of the viral occult form in the lungworm and earthworm and the exact role of the bacterium are unknown.

EPIDEMIOLOGIC SIGNIFICANCE OF LATENT INFECTIONS

As these examples indicate, latent viral infections affect the incidence and the pathogenesis of **acute viral diseases** in several ways. (1) In **herpes simplex** infection, **recurrent acute disease** is induced in the infected person when the balance that maintains the latent infection is intermittently disturbed (see Herpes Simplex Viruses, Pathogenesis, Chap. 53). (2) **Swine influenza** mimics the way in which a virus widely seeded among humans may initiate, in response to **environmental changes,** an **explosive epidemic by viral reactivation** in many areas at the same time, as noted in pandemics of influenza. Indeed, this intriguing animal model of latency may explain the manner in which influenza A virus "goes underground" only to **emerge,** often with **new antigenic characteristics,** many years later to produce widespread epidemics (see Epidemiology, Chap. 56). (3) A **reactivated latent (occult) virus may spread and initiate an epidemic** among susceptible contacts. Thus, a latent varicella virus, persisting in peripheral nerve ganglia after chickenpox, can be activated and produce the different clinical picture of herpes zoster (shingles), and the patient may then serve as a focus for initiating an epidemic of chickenpox (see Varicella–Herpes Zoster Virus, Epidemiology, Chap. 53). (4) Viral latency can also be seen in the **development of certain chronic diseases** dependent on an immunologic response, as for LCM, noted above, for SSPE, and possibly for some other so-called **slow viral infections.** (5) Some latent viral states **produce uncontrolled proliferation of cells,** i.e., tumors, as discussed in Chapters 64 and 65.

Slow Viral Infections

The term *slow virus* has become associated with those viruses that require prolonged periods of infection (often years) before disease appears. The term, however, is

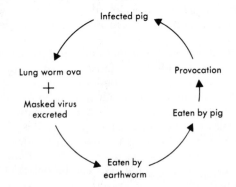

Figure 51–3. Natural history of swine influenza infection.

* Since the assay of this virus is extremely insensitive, it is not known whether failure to recover the virus signifies paucity or absence.

TABLE 51–4. *Examples of Slow Viral Infections*

Disease	Host	Organ Primarily Affected	Virus
Kuru	Man	Brain	Unknown
Creutzfeldt-Jakob disease	Man	Brain	Unknown
SSPE	Man	Brain	Paramyxovirus (measles)
Progressive rubella panencephalitis	Man	Brain	Togavirus (rubella)
Progressive multifocal leukoencephalopathy	Man	Brain	Papovavirus (SV40, BK, and JC)
Scrapie	Sheep	Brain	Unknown—? viroid; ? prion
Mink encephalopathy	Mink	Brain	Unknown—? viroid
Visna	Sheep	Brain	Retrovirus
Maedi	Sheep	Lung	Retrovirus
Progressive pneumonia	Sheep	Lung	Retrovirus
LCM	Mouse	Kidney, brain, liver	Arenavirus
Canine demyelinating encephalomyelitis	Dog	Brain, spinal cord	Paramyxovirus (distemper)
Disseminated demyelinating encephalomyelitis	Mouse, rat	Brain, spinal cord	Coronavirus (mouse hepatitis virus)
Aleutian mink disease	Mink	Reticuloendothelial system	Parvovirus
Hard pad disease	Dog	Brain	Paramyxovirus (distemper)

somewhat misleading, for although the virus is patient and the disease process develops over a protracted period, viral multiplication may not be unusually slow. Moreover, diseases of this group may be caused not only by unusual or "unconventional" viruses but also by others that ordinarily cause acute diseases. Table 51–4 lists some chronic degenerative diseases, particularly of the CNS, that belong to this group. Five that occur in humans are discussed: SSPE, progressive encephalitis, kuru, Creutzfeldt-Jakob disease, and progressive multifocal leukoencephalopathy. Claims have been made that other chronic diseases may have similar origins, but this has not been proved (e.g., multiple sclerosis, systemic lupus erythematosus, diabetes mellitus). Viral diseases that have a long incubation period but an acute course (e.g., type B hepatitis, AIDS, and rabies) are not considered to be slow viral infections and are not discussed here.

SSPE is the best substantiated example showing that even some common human viruses (i.e., measles virus) may occasionally give rise to chronic degenerative diseases. This progressive degenerative neurologic disease of children and adolescents (causing mental and motor deterioration, myoclonic jerks, and electroencephalographic dysrhythmias) was unexpectedly discovered to be caused by measles virus. With this finding it became clear that a single virus could induce both an acute contagious disease and a chronic illness. The following data implicate measles virus in this severe chronic disease: (1) all patients have had measles several years (up to 13) prior to onset of SSPE. (2) All have unusually high titers of measles Abs, even in the spinal fluid, and the Ab levels (IgM as well as IgG) often increase as the disease progresses. (3) Affected brain cells have nuclear and cytoplasmic inclusions similar to those seen in measles infections (see Fig. 57–10); the inclusions consist of filamentous tubular structures indistinguishable from the nucleocapsids seen in cells infected with measles virus (see Fig. 57–12). (4) Immunofluorescence study of the brain lesions reveals Ags that react with Abs to measles virus but not to distemper virus (a close relative of measles virus). (5) A virus very similar to measles virus has been isolated from brains of ferrets and newborn mice inoculated with brain material and by co-cultivation of affected brain cells with cells that readily support measles virus multiplication (e.g., African green monkey kidney cells, HeLa cells); though virus has not been directly isolated from homogenates of brain cells, when the affected cells are cultured *in vitro*, they show typical inclusion bodies as well as viral Ags and viral nucleocapsids. The RNA of the SSPE virus contains all the nucleotide sequences of measles virus RNA, but about 10% consists of additional sequences, which may have been derived by recombination with the RNA of another virus.

The finding of measles Abs in the spinal fluid of patients with multiple sclerosis raised the possibility that this chronic neurologic disorder is also a complication of prior measles. How the persistently infected cells escape immunologic eradication in the presence of apparently undisturbed T-cell levels and function, normal amounts of all components of complement, and large quantities of measles-specific Abs still requires explanation. Examination of brain biopsies during early clinical stages of SSPE showed general decrease in expression and syntheses of the viral genome. During the final stages of the disease, replication of the viral RNA is decreased, but nucleocapsid (RNA genomes and NP protein) levels are increased. Moreover, matrix protein, which is required for budding and virion assembly, is markedly decreased or absent. Thus, the block in viral replication and failure to express viral glycoproteins on surfaces of infected cells account for the slow development of pathologic changes, the accumulation of cell-associated viral components, the inability to isolate infectious virus, and the failure of elimination of infected cells in the face of a normal immune response. Thus, the surfaces of infected cells do not show budding viral particles or even surface viral glycoproteins, which are present intracellularly, and the viral matrix (M) protein, which is required for virion assembly, is present in decreased amounts or is not detectable. Patients do not have anti-M Abs, although Abs to all other viral Ags are made. Indeed, humoral Abs could affect these findings, since Abs produce "capping" and shedding of viral Ags (see above), and it has been demonstrated that Abs suppress synthesis of M protein in persistently infected cultures.

Progressive rubella panencephalitis, similar to but more rapidly progressive than SSPE, develops in a rare child who previously had congenital or early childhood rubella. **Rubella virus** (see Chap. 61), rather than measles virus, is recovered by culturing the affected brain *in vitro* with or without cocultivation with cells susceptible to rubella virus multiplication. Owing to the rare occurrence of this disease, little is known of the characteristics of the infecting virus.

Progressive multifocal leukoencephalopathy is a rare **subacute demyelinating disease.** Two different species of **papovaviruses** (see Chap. 64) have been isolated from the brains of victims and are also seen in the intranuclear inclusion bodies of affected oligodendrocytes. All the viruses isolated are of the **SV40-polyoma subgroup;** two viruses are almost identical to SV40, but all the others, termed **JC virus,** are closely related and distinctly different from SV40 immunologically, chemically, and biologically. JC virus multiplies only in human cells from very few organs (primary fetal glial cells are most sensitive for viral isolation). JC virus replicates very slowly, so it is truly a "slow virus." This disease generally develops in patients with **immunologic defects due to disorders of the reticuloendothelial system** (such as Hodgkin's disease and leukemias) or to immunosuppressive therapy. Most JC virus infections occur during childhood, and about 75% of adults have circulating Abs. Thus, the emergent viruses appear to be **opportunists** liberated from a latent infection in an immunologically compromised host.

Kuru, another slow viral disease of man, was first observed in 1957 in the Fore tribe of cannibals living in Stone Age conditions in New Guinea (*kuru* = shivering or trembling in the Fore language). It is transmitted by consumption of the brains of deceased relatives, a tribal ceremonial ritual for children and young women. This degenerative disease of the cerebellum, manifested by ataxia, disturbed balance, clumsy gait, and tremor, progresses inexorably to death in less than a year after onset. A striking decrease in kuru was seen after the tribal chiefs prohibited this custom of cannibalism.

The pathologic findings do not include the customary inflammatory evidence of an infectious process but do resemble the findings in scrapie, a disease of sheep proved to be transmissible and caused by an unusual agent (i.e., difficult to inactivate and without detectable nucleic acid). This resemblance suggested a viral etiology for kuru, and Gajdusek and Gibbs, using brain material from kuru patients, transmitted the disease serially to chimpanzees. (Subsequently, it was also transmitted to New and Old World monkeys and even to mink and ferrets.) The degenerative process, which had the same clinical and pathologic characteristics as kuru in humans (subacute spongiform encephalopathy), appeared 18 to 30 months after the initial inoculation of chimpanzees and after 1 year in subsequent passages.

Creutzfeldt-Jakob disease, a fatal presenile dementia of midadult life that is not geographically restricted and hence not so exotic, like kuru shows a **spongiform encephalopathy** and appears to be a **chronic viral disease.** A similar disease has been serially transmitted from the brains of patients to chimpanzees, several species of monkeys, guinea pigs, mice, hamsters, ferrets, goats, and cats. Its epidemiology is not clear, but the disease has been accidently transmitted in humans by a corneal transplant from a person who subsequently developed the fatal disease, by growth hormone prepared from human pituitary glands, and by electroencephalographic electrodes sterilized only with 70% ethanol and formaldehyde vapor after the electrodes had been used on a patient with the disease.

THE VIRUSES

Owing in part to long incubation periods and cumbersome assays, the etiologic agents of kuru and Creutzfeldt-Jakob disease, presumably viruses, have not been well characterized. The properties described, however, have been so difficult to study that it has not been possible to place these agents in a category with any of the well-known viruses of man and other animals.

The unconventional viruses that are of necessity present in brain extracts are highly resistant to inactivation by the usual chemical and physical sterilizing agents: formaldehyde, β-propiolactone, proteases, nucleases (RNases and DNases), ultraviolet irradiation at 254 nm, and heat at 80°C (they are incompletely inactivated at 100°C). Moreover, electron microscopic examinations of infected brain tissues (with as much as $10^{12}LD_{50}/g$) and virus concentrated in CsCl and sucrose gradients (10^7–10^8 LD_{50}/ml) did not reveal viral particles. Neither infectious nucleic acids nor viral Ags have been detected.

Neither immunosuppression (e.g., from x-ray or cyclophosphamide) nor immunopotentiation (e.g., with adjuvants) affects the pathogenesis of kuru or Creutzfeldt-Jakob disease in experimental animals, and B- and T-cell functions appear intact in the natural disease and in experimental infections. However, Abs directed against infectious extracts have not been detected in patients or infected animals. The characteristics of the agents of kuru and Creutzfeldt-Jakob disease are similar to those of scrapie and transmissible mink encephalopathy viruses. These indeed appear to be unique viruses, if they *are* viruses. Further characterization may show that the so-called slow or unconventional viruses are in fact a new type of infectious agent. Amyloid fibrils, associated with infectivity, have been purified from brains infected with unconventional viruses and termed **prions** or SAF (scrapie-associated fibrils). These fibrils are claimed to be free of nucleic acid. The amyloid present in the fibrils, which are found in abundance in the affected brains, differ only in quantity from amyloid molecules present in normal cells. It is possible that within such protein particles, a small nucleic acid molecule, such as a **viroid,** could be buried. A viroid consists of an infectious molecule of covalently closed circular single-stranded RNA (110,000–127,000 daltons) without associated protein (see Distinctive Properties, Chap. 44). Viroids depend entirely on host cell macromolecules for their replication. These agents have been described only as pathogens in plants. However, the single-stranded RNA of the **hepatitis delta virus,** which depends on the hepatitis B virus for its infectivity (see Chap. 63), has a high degree of nucleotide hormology with the potato spindle tuber viroid. Although the delta virus has not yet been proved to be a viroid, the history of earlier studies on the distribution of other novel microbes suggests that viroids will also be found in organisms other than plants, probably in animals.

The examples of slow viral infections of man are still few, and the evidence of causation is sparse. Nevertheless, suspicion of the role of viruses in chronic degenerative diseases is now high, and some conventional viruses (e.g., togaviruses, picornaviruses, paramyxoviruses) are being implicated in diseases such as multiple sclerosis and diabetes mellitus.

Selected Reading

Allison AC: Lysosomes in virus-infected cells. *Perspect Virol* 5:29, 1967

Blanden RV: Mechanisms of recovery from a generalized viral infection. II. Passive transfer of recovery mechanisms with immune lymphoid cells. J Exp Med 133:1074, 1971

Fulginiti VA, Kempe CH, Hathaway WE et al: Progressive vaccinia in immunologically deficient individuals. In Bergsiyia D, Good RA (eds): Birth Defects: Immunologic Deficiency Diseases in Man, p 129. New York, National Foundation, 1968

Gajdusek DC: Unconventional viruses and the origin and disappearance of kuru. Science 197:943, 1977

Galloway DA, Fenoglio C, Shevchuk M, McDougall JK: Detection of herpes simplex RNA in human sensory ganglia. Virology 95:265, 1979

Haase AT, Gantz D, Eble B et al: Natural history of restricted synthesis and expression of measles virus genes in subacute sclerosing panencephalitis. Proc Natl Acad Sci USA 82:3020, 1985

Klein RJ: Initiation and maintenance of latent herpes simplex virus infections: The paradox of perpetual immmobility and continuous movement. Rev Infect Dis 7:21, 1985

Notkins SL, Oldstone MBA (eds): Concepts in Viral Pathogenesis, I (1984) and II (1986). New York, Springer-Verlag

Ter Meulen V, Stephenson JR, Kreth HW: Subacute sclerosing panencephalitis. In Fraenkel-Conrat H, Wagner RR (eds): Comprehensive Virology, Vol 18, p 105. New York, Plenum Press, 1983

Walker DL, Padgett BL: Progressive multifocal leukoencephalopathy. In Fraenkel-Conrat H, Wagner RR (eds): Comprehensive Virology, Vol 18, p 161. New York, Plenum Press, 1983

52

Adenoviruses

Acute viral respiratory diseases continuously impose huge clinical and economic burdens. Thus, great efforts to isolate other major causative agents followed the isolation of influenza virus in 1933. The search was unsuccessful, however, until in 1953 two groups of investigators discovered **adenoviruses,** the first of several families now known to be etiologic agents of these acute infections. Rowe and colleagues, using cultures of human adenoids as a potentially favorable host for the elusive "common cold" virus, noted cytopathic changes in uninoculated cultures after prolonged incubation, as well as in cells inoculated with respiratory secretions. The pathologic alterations were shown to be due to the emergence of previously unidentified viruses from latent infections of adenoid tissues—hence the name *adenoviruses.* Hilleman and Werner, studying an epidemic of influenzalike disease in army recruits, isolated several similar cytopathic agents from respiratory secretions added to cultures of human upper respiratory tissues.

Adenoviruses cause acute respiratory and ocular infections. Although they are not the etiologic agents of the common cold, they are responsible for a small percentage of acute viral respiratory infections. It is evident, however, that certain specific types are etiologic agents of a broader range of infections such as hemorrhagic cystitis and infantile gastroenteritis.

General Characteristics

Several characteristics of adenoviruses (family **Adenoviridae**) are of particular interest: (1) Adenoviruses are simple DNA-containing viruses (i.e., composed of only DNA and protein) that multiply in the cell nucleus. (2) They induce **latent persistent** infections in tonsils, adenoids, and other lymphoid tissues of man, and they are readily activated. (3) Several adenoviruses are **onco-**

915

CHARACTERISTICS OF ADENOVIRUSES

Icosahedral symmetry
Diameter of 60–90 nm
Capsid contains 252 polygonal capsomers, 12 fibers, and four minor proteins.
Double-stranded DNA genome
Resistance to lipid solvents (absence of lipids)
Related by family cross-reacting soluble Ags (except for the chicken adenoviruses)
Multiplication in cell nuclei

genic for a number of newborn rodents (they were the first viruses of humans shown to have this property). (4) They serve as "helpers" for a group of small, defective DNA-containing viruses, the **adeno-associated viruses** (discussed at the end of this chapter), which cannot replicate in their absence. (Conversely, some adenoviruses cannot multiply efficiently in primary monkey cells unless the genetically unrelated simian virus 40 (SV40) is present as a helper [see Abortive Infections, Chap. 48].)

Adenoviruses are widespread in nature. The 93 accepted members of the adenovirus family have similar chemical and physical characteristics and a family cross-reactive Ag (see "Characteristics of Adenoviruses), but they are distinguished by Abs to their individual type-specific Ags: 41 are from humans and the rest from various other animals. Comparative studies of the viruses from humans permit their classification into several groups (Table 52–1).

Properties

STRUCTURE. Electron microscopy shows the virions to be 60 nm to 90 nm in diameter. In sections the viral particles have a dense central **core** and an outer coat, the capsid (Fig. 52–1). Negative staining reveals **icosahedral particles** with capsids composed of 252 **capsomers** (Fig. 52–2): 240 **hexons** make up the faces and edges of the equilateral triangles, and 12 **pentons** constitute the vertices. The hexons are truncated triangular or polygonal prisms with a central hole (Figs. 52–3 and 52–4). The pentons are more complex, consisting of a **polygonal base** with an attached **fiber,** the length of which varies with the viral type (Figs. 52–4 and 52–5). Four additional minor capsid proteins (IIIa, VI, VIII, and IX) are associated with the hexons or pentons in stoichiometric amounts (Fig. 52–6). These proteins confer stability on the capsid, form links with the core proteins, and function in virion assembly.

PHYSICAL AND CHEMICAL CHARACTERISTICS. Each virion contains one **linear, double-stranded DNA molecule** associated with **proteins** to form the **core.** The DNAs of different viral types vary in molecular weight and base composition (see Table 52–1): viruses within each subgroup share 70% to 95% of their nucleotide sequences (as shown by DNA–DNA, and DNA–mRNA hybridization), and the DNAs of viruses of different subgroups have only 5% to 20% homology.

The viral DNA has two novel features: (1) the terminal

TABLE 52-1. *Physical, Chemical, Oncogenic, and Hemagglutinating Characteristics of Human Adenoviruses*

Subgroup (Subgenus)	Type	Oncogenic* Potential	Viral DNA Percentage of Virion	Mol. Wt.	G + C (%)	Agglutination of RBCs Rhesus	Rat
A	12, 18, 31	High	11.6–12.5	20×10^6 (30 Kbp†)	47–49	0	Partial‡
B	3, 7, 11, 14, 16, 21, 34,§ 35	Weak	12.5–13.7	$23–25 \times 10^6$ (35–38 Kbp)	57–61	+	0
C	1, 2, 5, 6	None	12.5–13.7	23×10^6 (35 Kbp)	57–59	0	Partial
D	8–10, 13, 15, 17, 19, 20, 22–30, 32, 33, 36–39	None	12.5–13.7	$23–25 \times 10^6$ (35–38 Kbp)	57–60	+ or 0‖	+
E	4	None	12.5	23×10^6 (35 Kbp)	57	0	Partial
F–G#	40, 41						

* Highly oncogenic adenoviruses induce tumors in newborn hamsters within 2 months after inoculation; weakly oncogenic viruses induce tumors in fewer animals in 4 to 18 months. Even those viruses that are nononcogenic transform nonpermissive rodent cells *in vitro*, and the transformed cells produce tumors in syngeneic newborn animals and in nude mice.

† Kilobase pairs

‡ Complete hemagglutination occurs when heterologous Ab to a virus of the same subgroup is added to the reaction mixture, producing groups of fibers or aggregation of pentons into regular groups of 12.

§ Type 34 has hemagglutination characteristics of a subgroup D virus.

‖ Some types (9, 13, and 15) agglutinate rhesus RBCs but to a lower titer than rat RBCs.

These types have not yet been completely characterized. Hybridization shows a high degree of DNA homology, suggesting that they should be placed in the same subgenus, but their restriction endonuclease patterns are distinctly different.

RBCs, red blood cells

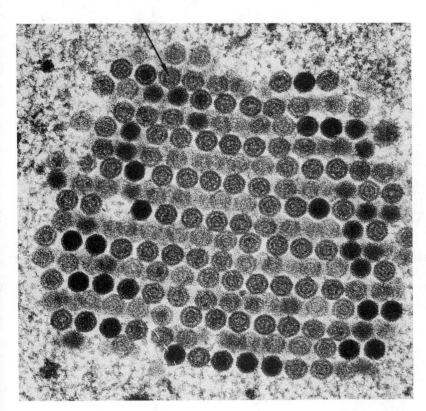

Figure 52–1. Thin section of a crystalline mass of adenovirus particles in a cell infected with type 4. Two types of particles can be seen: dense particles with no discernible internal structure, and less dense particles showing the central body of the viral particles, the core (*arrow*), and the capsid. The polygonal shape of adenoviruses is apparent in many particles. Differences in appearance of particles are probably due to the relation of the center of the virion to the plane of section. (Original magnification greater than ×110,000; courtesy of C. Morgan and H. M. Rose, Columbia University)

nucleotide sequences of each strand are **inverted repetitions** so that if the DNA is denatured, both strands form single-stranded circles through "panhandles" produced between the complementary ends, and (2) a small protein of about 55,000 daltons is covalently linked through the terminal deoxycytosine at the 5′ end of each strand (Fig. 52–7). The functions of these unique terminal structures of the viral genome are important in DNA replication.

The virion contains at least ten species of proteins associated with the capsid and the DNA–protein core (see Fig. 52–6). The capsid proteins have relatively strong noncovalent bonds between protomers in a capsomer, and weaker bonds between capsomers (see Chap. 44); hence, the capsid can be artificially disrupted into intact capsomers (see Figs. 52–3 and 52–4). Further dissociation of the hexons into their constituent polypeptide chains, in contrast, requires rigorous denaturing conditions (e.g., 6M guanidine hydrochloride and a sulfhydryl reagent to block formation of disulfide bonds). The penton base is the least stable of the capsomers. Noncovalent bonds associate the glycosylated fiber with the penton base.

The virion's core includes the covalently bonded **5′-terminal protein** and **two basic proteins** associated with the DNA to form a chromatinlike structure (see

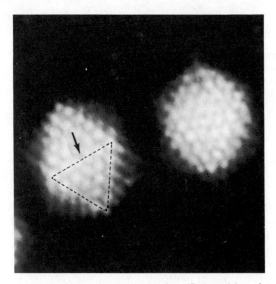

Figure 52–2. Electron micrograph of purified particles of type 5 adenovirus embedded in sodium phosphotungstate. The icosahedral symmetry (see Chap. 44) of the virion and subunit structure of the capsid are apparent. The arrow points to a virion's axis of twofold rotational symmetry. Capsomers at the apices of triangle are centers of the fivefold symmetry. The capsid parameters are P = 1, f = 5; hence, the capsid consists of 252 capsomers (see Number of Capsomers in Icosahedral Capsids, Appendix to Chap. 44). (Original magnification ×440,000, reduced)

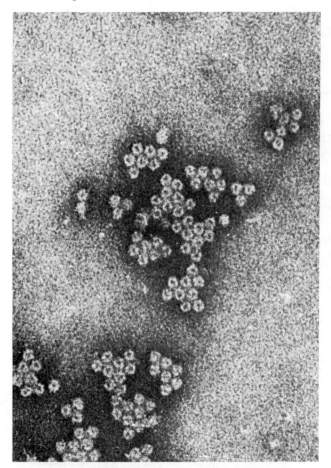

Figure 52–3. Electron micrograph of purified type 5 hexons embedded in sodium silicotungstate. The polygonal shape of the capsomer with the central hole is apparent. Groups of nine hexons are seen in different orientations so that both tops (those with large holes) and bottoms (small holes) are observed. The subunit structure can also be seen in many hexons. (Original magnification ×375,000; courtesy of M. V. Nermut, National Institute for Medical Research, London)

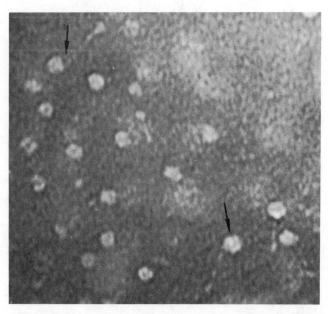

Figure 52–4. Electron micrograph of the capsid components of purified type 5 adenovirus particles disrupted at pH 10.5. Note the polygonal, hollow capsomers (i.e., the hexons, which are 7–8.5 nm in diameter with a central hole about 2.5 nm across) and the fibers (1–2.5 nm wide and 20 nm long), attached to polygonal bases (i.e., the pentons [*arrow*]). By actual count there are 12 pentons per virion. (Original magnification ×480,000, reduced)

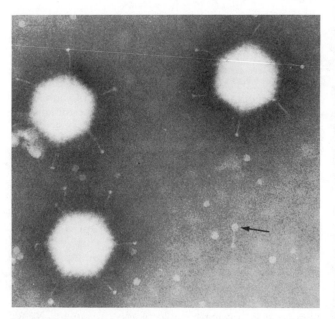

Figure 52–5. Electron micrograph of purified type 5 adenovirus particles embedded in sodium silicotungstate. Micrographs obtained in areas where the silicotungstate was thin revealed the fiber components of the penton projecting from corners of the virion. Free pentons (*arrows*) and hexons are also present. (Original magnification ×350,000; Valentine RC, Pereira HG: J Mol Biol 13:13, 1965)

Chap. 47). One of these (designated *protein VII;* see Fig. 52–6) is, like histones, rich in arginine (about 23 mol/dl).

STABILITY. Adenoviruses are relatively stable in homogenates of infected cells; they retain undiminished infectivity for several weeks at 4°C and for months at −25°C. Purified virions, however, are relatively unstable under all conditions of storage, owing primarily to the spontaneous release of pentons. Adenoviruses are resistant to lipid solvents.

HEMAGGLUTINATION. Human adenoviruses differ in their ability to agglutinate rhesus monkey or rat red blood cells (RBCs). Hemagglutination occurs when the tips of fibers on virions or on aggregated pentons (commonly arranged as dodecagons) bind to the RBC surface

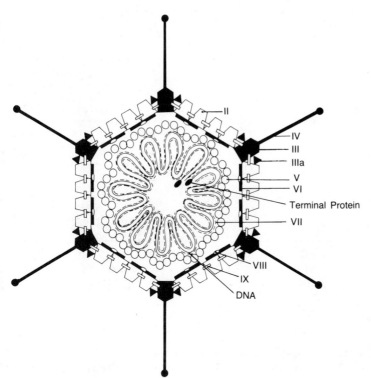

Figure 52–6. Model of an adenovirus particle, showing the apparent architectural interrelationships of the structural proteins (roman numerals) and the nucleoprotein core in the virion. The hexon (II), penton base (III), and fiber (IV) and the hexon-associated proteins (IIIa, VI, VIII, and IX) make up the capsid. Proteins V and VII are core proteins associated with the viral DNA; the TP (terminal protein) is covalently linked to the 5' end of the DNA.

and cause crosslinking. The nature of the fiber receptor on susceptible RBCs is not known. The combination of adenoviruses with cell receptors is stable, and spontaneous elution of the hemagglutinin (as seen with influenza viruses) does not occur.

There is a remarkable agreement among members of subgroups according to their hemagglutinin properties, viral oncogenicity, and DNA characteristics (see Table 52–1).

IMMUNOLOGIC CHARACTERISTICS. The major immunologic reactivities of adenoviruses are expressed by the hexon and penton proteins (Table 52–2). The **hexons** contain **family-reactive determinants,** which cross-react with a similar Ag in all except the avian adenoviruses. The hexons also possess a **type-specific reactive site,** which is the prevalent Ag exposed when hexons are assembled in virions (identified by neutralization titrations). Complement fixation (CF) and enzyme-linked immunosorbent assay (ELISA) titrations measure the family Ag on free hexons, but they are on the inner surface of the hexon in assembled virions.

The **pentons** provide minor Ags of the virions and a **family-reactive soluble Ag** found in infected cells. The **purified fibers** contain a **major type-specific Ag** as well as a **minor subgroup Ag.** Although the fiber is the organ of attachment to the host cell, Abs to the fiber or to the

intact penton only weakly reduce viral infectivity, probably by aggregating virions.

Neutralizing, hemagglutinin-inhibiting, and CF Abs appear about 7 days after the onset of illness and attain maximal titers after 2 to 3 weeks. Antibodies appear in

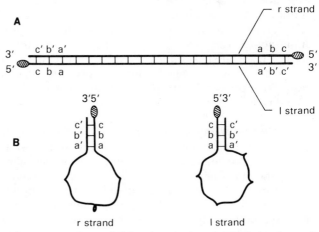

Figure 52–7. Diagram of the adenovirus genome, indicating the terminal inverted repetitions of nucleotide sequences and the protein covalently linked to a deoxycytosine at the 5' terminus of each strand. *(A)* The intact native linear viral DNA molecule. *(B)* The configuration assumed by each strand after denaturation owing to hybridization of the complementary 3' and 5' ends of the strands to each other, forming a "panhandle."

TABLE 52–2. *Characteristics of Major Type 5 Adenovirus Proteins* *

| Property | Hexon Protein | Penton Proteins | | | Internal Proteins‖ |
		Complete†	Base†	Fiber	
Immunologic reactivity	Type-specific and family cross-reactive	Family cross-reactive	Family cross-reactive	Type specific	?
Biologic activity	None known	Cytopathic; attachment of virions to cells	Cytopathic	Blocks biosynthesis of macromolecules; inhibits viral multiplication	Probably aid in assembly of viral DNA, TP for DNA replication
Hemagglutination	0	Partial	0	Partial	0
Molecular weight of native protein	315,000‡	419,000	236,000§	183,000§	
Polypeptide chains	105,000		80,000	61,000	55,000 (TP) 48,000 (V) 19,000 (VII)

* Proteins of capsid (≅58% of virion) consist of seven species; internal proteins (≅30% of virion) consist of three species.

† A DNA endonuclease is closely associated with but physically separable from the penton base; its function during infection is unknown.

‡ Molecular weights of hexons and fibers vary with type (e.g., type 2 hexon is 360,000 daltons).

§ Estimated from sedimentation coefficient

‖ See Figure 52-6.

nasal secretions at the same time or within a week after the detection of serum Abs. The CF Abs begin to decline 2 to 3 months after infection but are usually still present 6 to 12 months after infection. Neutralizing and hemagglutinin-inhibiting Abs persist longer, decreasing in titer only twofold to threefold in 8 to 10 years. Minor rises in heterotypic neutralizing Abs may follow adenovirus infections, especially when Abs to several types are already present at the time of infection.

The same type of adenovirus rarely produces a second attack of disease. Such persistent type-specific immunity is unusual among viral respiratory diseases, resistance of relatively short duration being the rule (see Immunologic Characteristics in Chap. 56 and Immunologic Characteristics under Parainfluenza Viruses in Chap. 57). This prolonged immunity probably results from the common latent, persistent infections of lymphoid cells.

TOXIN PROPERTIES OF THE PENTON. In addition to their immunologic reactivities, the penton and its individual components possess striking biologic activities. Thus, the intact penton causes rounding and clumping of cultured cells and detaches them from their support. Therefore, the penton is also termed **toxin,** or **cell-detaching factor.** Hydrolysis of the penton's base by trypsin, leaving the fiber intact, destroys the cytopathic effect. It is perhaps this same property of the penton that permits the virion to penetrate into the cellular matrix (see Viral Multiplication). The purified fiber, which is present in infected cells as a soluble protein as well as in pentons, has a different toxic action: in cultured cells it

blocks biosynthesis of DNA, RNA, and protein, stops cell division, and inhibits the capacity of cells to support the multiplication of related or unrelated viruses (see Table 52–2).

HOST RANGE. Adenoviruses from humans inoculated intranasally into cotton rats produce pulmonary disease that pathologically resembles that in man. Most adenoviruses of man, however, do not produce recognizable disease in common laboratory animals, but inapparent infections follow intravenous inoculation in rabbits or intranasal instillation in hamsters, piglets, guinea pigs, and dogs. In rabbits, type 5 virus persists for at least 6 months in the spleen, and it emerges when explants are cultured *in vitro* (similar to latent infection of human tonsils and adenoids; see Pathogenesis, below). Chick embryos are susceptible only to chicken adenoviruses. The members of subgroups A and B (see Table 52–1) produce tumors when inoculated in large amounts into newborn hamsters, rats, and mice (see Chap. 64). Rodent cells are nonpermissive for viral replication, but all adenoviruses can transform (immortalize) these cells. Only the E1A and E1B gene products are required to induce complete transformation of rodent cells (see Chap. 64).

A variety of **cultured mammalian cells** support the multiplication of adenoviruses to a high titer and evince characteristic cytopathic changes, including pathognomonic nuclear alterations (see Effect on Host Cells, below). Epithelium-like human cell lines (such as KB cells) and primary cultures of human embryonic kidney are most satisfactory for human adenoviruses; primary cultures of various other types of human and animal cells also support viral multiplication but give much lower yields. Human lymphocytes (T and B cells) also support viral replication; only low yields of virus are produced, and persistent infections can be maintained indefinitely in T cells.

MULTIPLICATION. The essential features of multiplication (Fig. 52–8) are similar for all adenovirus types. **Adsorption** to susceptible cultured cells is relatively slow, reaching a maximum after several hours. The viral particle then promptly penetrates the cell, primarily by a process analogous to phagocytosis; then, through the action of the penton base, when the pH of the phagocytic vacuole is reduced below pH 6 (Fig. 52–9), the endocytic vacuole's membrane is ruptured, permitting the virions to find their way into the cytoplasmic matrix for uncoating.

Uncoating of the viral DNA begins immediately after the virions have penetrated into the cytoplasm. It is detected biochemically when the nucleic acid becomes susceptible to DNase and by electron microscopy when the virion appears spherical rather than polygonal (see Fig. 52–9*B*). Initially, pentons and the immediate surrounding hexons are displaced, and this reduces the stability of the capsid. The other hexons and associated proteins then separate, and the naked viral core either enters the nucleus through nuclear pores or releases the viral DNA into a nuclear pocket (see Fig. 52–9*C*). The DNA thus gains access to the nucleus, where viral replication takes place (Fig. 52–10). Viral uncoating requires 1 to 2 hours.

Prior to and independent of viral DNA replication, **immediate early and early messenger RNAs** are transcribed from five separate regions of the genome (Fig. 52–11), corresponding to approximately 14% of the rightward(r)-reading strand and 27% of the leftward(l)-reading strand (designating the direction in which each strand is transcribed); these regions are identified by hybridization with restriction fragments of viral DNA and by electron microscopy of DNA–mRNA hybrids. Transcription from the early regions is not initiated simultaneously, but it is coordinately and sequentially regulated: E1A (see Fig. 52–11) is being transcribed within 1 hour after infection (termed **immediate early genes**), and its 13S mRNA gene product (a 289 amino acid protein) enhances transcription from the other early genes; E1B, E3, and E4 begin transcription about 2 hours after infection; and E2A and E2B are transcribed shortly thereafter. As early as 2 to 3 hours after infection, early messengers are present on polyribosmes and are translated into several early proteins, which are detected by SDS-polyacrylamide gel electrophoresis. Three of these proteins are required for replication of viral DNA: the E2A single-strand–specific DNA-binding protein (mol. wt. 60,000–72,000 daltons, depending on viral type); an E2B

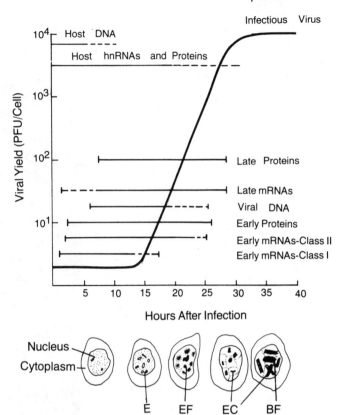

Figure 52–8. Diagram of the sequential events in the biosynthesis of type 5 adenovirus, its effect on synthesis of host macromolecules, and the concomitant development of nuclear alterations. *E,* eosinophilic masses; *EF,* eosinophilic masses with basophilic Feulgen-positive borders; *EC,* eosinophilic crystals; *BF,* basophilic Feulgen-positive masses; *PFU,* plaque-forming units. Types 1, 2, 5, and 6 have similar multiplication and nuclear changes.

DNA polymerase (about 140,000 daltons); and the DNA-terminal protein (55,000 daltons), which is required for initiation of DNA replication and is encoded in region E2B and synthesized as an 88,000-dalton precursor protein.

The activities of several enzymes involved in DNA synthesis may also increase prior to DNA replication, but these enzymes are not unique to virus-infected cells, and it is uncertain whether they are products of the viral or the host cell genome. Inhibition of the synthesis of early mRNA (e.g., by actinomycin C) or of early proteins (by cycloheximide or by amino acid analogues) prevents viral DNA synthesis.

Replication of viral DNA is semiconservative and is initiated at either end of the molecule with **the terminal deoxycytidine,** which is covalently linked to precursor terminal protein, serving as a primer. As elongation occurs, there is an asymmetric displacement of the other strand (see Fig. 52–11). Replication begins in the nucleus 6 to 8 hours after infection, attains its maximum rate by

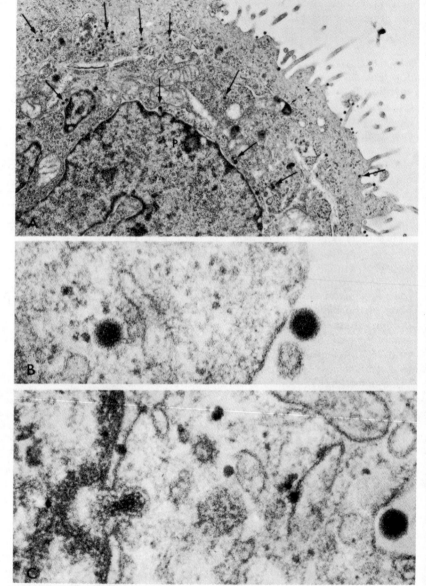

Figure 52–9. Adsorption, penetration, and uncoating of adenovirus in HeLa cells. *(A)* Numerous particles are adsorbed to the cell surface; others are present as free virions in the cytoplasm *(arrows)*. Some particles in phagocytic vacuoles are also noted. A nuclear pocket *(P)* is also present. (Original magnification ×15,000) *(B)* Higher magnification of a polygonal virion adsorbed to the plasma membrane and a virion that has assumed a spherical form in the cytoplasm, probably after penetration from a phagocytic vacuole. (Original magnification ×150,000) *(C)* Partially uncoated viral particle releasing core material into a nuclear pocket. For comparison, an unaltered virion is shown on the cell surface prior to engulfment. (Original magnification ×150,000; Morgan C et al: J Virol 4:777, 1969)

18 to 20 hours, and practically ceases by 22 to 24 hours after infection.

Transcription of late mRNAs begins in abundance adequate to produce viral structural proteins shortly after the initiation of DNA replication, although a small number of transcripts encompassing the L1 and L2 regions (see Fig. 52–11) can be detected during the early phase of infection. Hybridization to separate DNA strands shows that late mRNAs are predominantly encoded in the *r* strand. Only one late mRNA appears to

arise from the *l* strand (see Fig. 52–11). The mRNAs are generated by **processing of long primary transcripts and by splicing of noncontiguous leader sequences to sequences containing the message for a single protein** (see Chap. 48). Thus, at least 13 late messages are derived from primary transcripts stretching between the **major late promoter** (at 16.4 map units) and the end of the genome (100 map units). Processing probably regulates the relative proportions of late messengers, some of which are present in considerable abundance (e.g., those for the hexon and the 100K proteins). It follows that late proteins, which include the capsid proteins, are primarily products of the *r* strand; their formation depends on prior replication of the viral DNA. Although early mRNAs continue to be transcribed late, only about 30% of them are expressed (e.g., translation of the DNA-binding protein mRNA is meager during the period of late mRNA and protein synthesis).

Viral DNA and mRNAs are synthesized in the nucleus, and virions are assembled in the nucleus, but viral proteins, like host proteins, are synthesized on polyribosomes in the cytoplasm. **Translation of late viral mRNAs** is greatly facilitated by **VA I RNA** which is a small RNA transcribed from the *r* strand by the host RNA polymerase III (see Fig. 52–11). After their release from polyribosomes, the polypeptide chains are immediately transported into the nucleus, where they assemble into the multimeric viral capsid proteins (capsomers). **Assembly** of mature particles takes several steps that begin with formation of the procapsid about 2 to 4 hours after initiation of capsid protein production; this period is probably required to attain component pools of adequate size and terminates with entry of the viral DNA and final processing of the precursor structural proteins (pVI, pVII, and pVIII). The **eclipse period** lasts 13 to 17 hours.

EFFECTS ON HOST CELLS. Adenovirus infection has a profound effect on the physiology of host cells. Production of host DNA stops abruptly 8 to 10 hours after infection, and host biosynthesis of protein and RNA ceases 6 to 10 hours later (see Fig. 52–8). Accordingly, the division of infected cells also halts.

The hallmark of infection with adenoviruses is the development of characteristic **nuclear lesions** (see Fig. 52–8; Fig. 52–12), caused by the accumulation of unassembled viral components. In fact, the process of adenovirus assembly is quite inefficient; **only about 10% to 15% of the new viral DNA and proteins is incorporated into virions.** Some cellular changes may be produced by the E1B 55K protein and the E4 11K protein, which appears to collaborate to inhibit translation of host proteins, as well as the accumulation of fibers, which also blocks the synthesis of host macromolecules and of DNA endonuclease. The basophilic inclusion bodies (see Figs. 52–8 and 52–12) are composed of the excess viral DNA and structural proteins; the large basophilic crystals present in cells infected with type 3, 4, or 7 are made up of viral particles arranged in a crystalline lattice (see Figs. 52–1 and 52–12). In cells infected with subgroup C adenoviruses, prominent bar-shaped eosinophilic crystals are formed, mostly by the arginine-rich internal viral proteins.

Despite the extensive alterations, the infected cells remain intact, and the nuclei do not release the newly synthesized virions. Less than 1% of the total virus is in

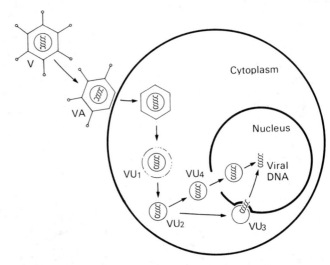

Figure 52–10. Diagram of uncoating of the adenovirus particle. *V,* intact virion; *VA,* attachment of the virion to the cell, followed by penetration of the virion into the cell; *VU₁*, the pentons are detached, leaving the virion somewhat spherical and the viral DNA susceptible to DNase; *VU₂*, the capsid disintegrates, leaving a viral core that migrates to the nucleus; *VU₃*, viral DNA is freed from the core into the nuclear pocket, and free DNA enters the nucleus; or, *VU₄*, the core enters the nucleus through a membrane pore, and DNA is then dissociated from proteins.

the culture fluid when the maximal viral titer is attained (as measured after cell disruption). The infected cells also remain metabolically active.

Pathogenesis

Progress in the study of pathogenesis has been impeded by the lack of satisfactory animal models. Accordingly, knowledge of human adenovirus infections is derived primarily from clinical observations and from experiments on volunteers. The recognized diseases (Table 52–3) predominantly involve the **respiratory tract,** the **eye,** and the **gastrointestinal tract.** The association of particular types with specific disease syndromes is striking. For example, **types 8, 19, and 37** are essentially the only adenoviruses associated with **epidemic keratoconjunctivitis,** the very fastidious adenoviruses **types 40 and 41** are the etiologic agents of **epidemic infantile gastroenteritis,** and type 11 adenovirus is an etiologic agent of **acute hemorrhage cystitis** in children (see Table 52–3). Adenoviruses usually cause either self-limited illnesses or inapparent infections, which are followed by complete recovery and persistent type-specific immunity.

Type 3 or 7 adenovirus has been isolated from a number of **fatal cases of nonbacterial pneumonia in infants,** and **type 7** from rare cases of **fatal pneumonia in military personnel.** The pulmonary lesions observed

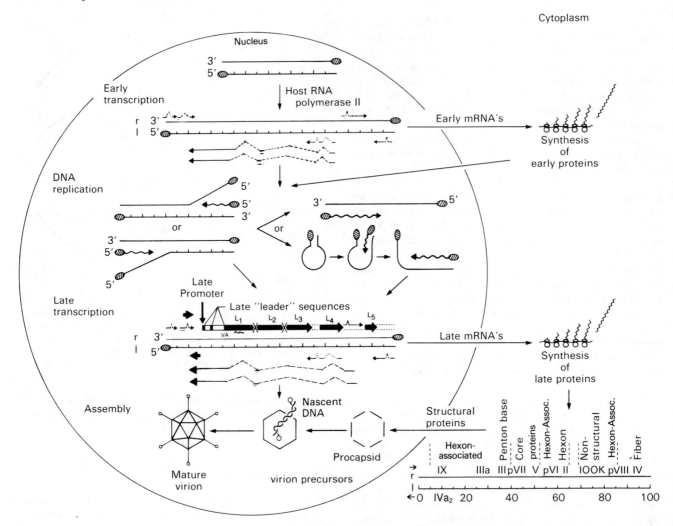

Figure 52–11. Diagram of the biosynthetic events in the multiplication of type 2 adenovirus (used as a model, since its transcription has been studied in greatest detail). Early mRNAs are transcribed from five separate regions of the genome; like late messages, they are processed from larger transcripts, and they have leader sequences transcribed from noncontiguous regions (the intervening absent sequences are indicated by a connecting caret [∧]). The semiconservative, asymmetric DNA replication is shown. A mechanism for replication of the displaced single strands, using the inverted terminal repetition to form a circlelike intermediate, is also suggested. The 80K 5' precursor terminal protein with a covalently linked deoxycytidine acts as a primer in initiation of DNA replication. Late mRNAs, except that for protein IVa$_2$, have a single promoter at 16.4 map units on the r (rightward) strand. Note that each late "megatranscript" contains only one set of leader sequences, and therefore only a single mRNA can be derived from each transcript. Also indicated are the regions of the genome in which the late viral proteins are encoded, and their known functions. The left terminus of the viral DNA initiates entry of the viral genome into preformed empty capsids.

are those of nonbacterial bronchopneumonia, but in addition there are numerous bronchiolar epithelial cells containing central basophilic masses in the nuclei, closely resembling the **inclusion bodies** produced by the same adenovirus types in cell cultures (see Fig. 52–12). The acute, mononuclear pulmonary infiltration produced in cotton rats, which is pathologically similar to that in humans, results from early viral gene functions in virus-infected bronchial and bronchiolar epithelial cells calling forth an inflammatory response of monocyte/ macrophages and lymphocytes, including specific cytotoxic T cells.

Virus introduced by feeding, or swallowed in respiratory secretions, multiplies in cells of the gastrointestinal tract and is excreted in the feces (where it is still infectious, owing to its stability), but, except for **types 40 and 41,** it usually does not produce gastrointestinal disease. However, some other adenoviruses, most often type 1, 2, 5, or 6, have occasionally been isolated from cases of acute infectious diarrhea, severe mesenteric adenitis, and intussusception, though an etiologic relationship between virus and illness has not been clearly demonstrated. Viremia is not observed in human infections, and virus is not commonly transmitted to distant organs. However, in cases of immune deficiency, viruses have been isolated from peripheral blood cells, and cases of meningitis, hepatitis, and nephritis have been described.

Most persons are infected with one or more adenoviruses before the age of 15. As a corollary, 50% to 80% of tonsils and adenoids removed surgically yield an adenovirus when explants are cultured *in vitro*. The most frequent types are 1, 2, and 5, the types responsible for most infections in young children. Adenoviruses have also been isolated from cultured fragments of mesenteric lymph nodes, and viral DNA has been detected in rare (10^{-4} to 10^{-5}) peripheral lymphocytes. It thus appears that following an initial infection, the virus frequently becomes latent in the lymphoid tissues, where it may persist for long periods. Although recurrent illness has not been shown to arise from these latent infections under usual circumstances, activation of latent adenoviruses does occur in patients with immunosuppression, as in those with the acquired immune deficiency syndrome (AIDS) (see Chap. 65).

It appears likely that latent persistent infections are

TABLE 52-3. Clinical Syndromes Caused by Specific Types of Adenoviruses

Disease Syndrome	Adenovirus Type	
	Most Common	Less Common
Acute respiratory disease of recruits	4, 7	3, 11, 14, 21
Pharnygoconjunctival fever; pharyngitis	3	5, 7, 21
Conjunctivitis	3, 7	2, 5, 6, 9, 10, 11
Epidemic keratoconjunctivitis	8, 19	37
Nonbacterial pneumonia of infants*	7	
Acute infantile gastroenteritis	40, 41	
Acute hemorrhagic cystitis*	11	

* Least common of the diseases produced

readily established because the infected cells are not lysed, and viral particles or viral genomes remain protected within their nuclei. In nature, the occult virus is confined to relatively few cells. Culturing tissues *in vitro*, however, alters the cellular environment in ways (including dilution of Abs) that permit the virus to multiply

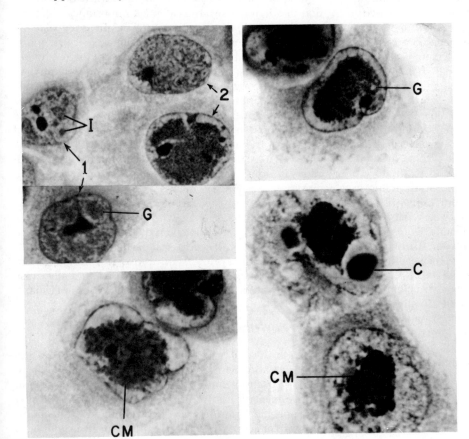

Figure 52-12. Sequential development of nuclear alterations in HeLa cells infected with type 7 adenovirus (types 3 and 4 produce similar effects). The earliest changes may be the formation of small eosinophilic inclusions (Feulgen-negative) *(I, 1)* and clusters of granules *(G)*. Clusters of granules gradually become larger *(2)* and more prominent (Feulgen-positive) and form a large central mass *(CM)*. In later stages the nucleus is enlarged, and crystalline masses (Feulgen-positive) are apparent *(C)*. (Original magnification ×1050; Boyer GS et al: J Exp Med 110:327, 1959)

more rapidly, to spread to uninfected cells, and to produce detectable cytopathic changes.

As noted above, some adenoviruses produce tumors in experimental animals after inoculation of large amounts. Ardent search, however, has not uncovered evidence that these viruses cause cancer in humans.

Laboratory Diagnosis

Adenovirus infection can be diagnosed serologically and by isolation of the offending virus from respiratory and ocular secretions, urine, and feces. For isolation, infected material is inoculated into cultures of continuous lines of human cells (e.g., HeLa or KB) or into primary human embryo kidney cells. If virus is present, cytopathic changes (rounding and clumping of cells) develop after 2 to 14 days, the time depending on the quantity of virus in the infected materials. Types 40 and 41, the fastidious **enteroadenoviruses,** cannot be isolated in the commonly used primary cell cultures or most continuous cell lines owing to their poor replication; therefore, electron microscopic examination of stool extracts has primarily been used for their identification and immunologic typing.

The virus is identified as an adenovirus by indirect immunofluorescence or CF titration with a hyperimmune rabbit serum or a convalescent human serum. This procedure detects the cross-reactive hexon and penton family Ags. The specific type of adenovirus can be ascertained most conveniently through hemagglutination-inhibition titrations; the required number of titrations can be reduced considerably by first determining the hemagglutination subgroup (see Table 52–2). To establish a virus as a new serotype, neutralization titration is the method of choice. A rapid presumptive diagnosis of adenovirus infection, but not of the specific viral type, can be made by examination of cells in respiratory or ocular secretions or urine by means of immunofluorescence or ELISA with rabbit serum containing Abs to the family Ag commonly employed. However, since each adenovirus type has a unique nucleotide sequence, and hence unique distribution of targets for restriction endonucleases, the specific type can be precisely identified by the restriction fragment patterns of its DNA.

The **serologic diagnosis** of an adenovirus infection is accomplished most conveniently by **CF titration,** which detects cross-reactive family Ags. Unfortunately, this assay identifies fewer than 50% of new infections, because many people have a constant high level of Abs from prior infections. A more precise diagnosis requires neutralization titrations with acute- and convalescent-phase sera. **Hemagglutination-inhibition** assay* for Abs is practi-

* Types 10 and 19 cross-react to such an extent that they cannot be distinguished by this procedure.

cally as sensitive as neutralization, is simpler and less expensive, and is almost as accurate if nonspecific inhibitors are removed from the serum. However, owing to the type-specificity of the reaction, all the common adenovirus types must be used in the test if an adenovirus has not been isolated from the patient.

Epidemiology

Man provides the only known reservoir for strains of adenoviruses that infect humans. Person-to-person spread in respiratory and ocular secretions is the most common mode of viral transmission, though dissemination in swimming pools has also been implicated in epidemics of **pharyngoconjunctival fever** and **conjunctivitis.** The spread of **epidemic keratoconjunctivitis** caused by types 8, 19, and 37 adenoviruses appears to be associated with conjunctival trauma produced by dust and dirt in shipyards and factories, or with improperly sterilized optical instruments. Adenoviruses are commonly present in the feces of infected persons, even those producing respiratory and ocular infections, but only types 40 and 41, the agents of infantile gastroenteritis, appear to be transmitted by the fecal–oral route.

Despite the large number and the worldwide distribution of adenoviruses, their clinical importance is largely restricted to epidemics of **acute respiratory disease (ARD),** an influenzalike illness in military recruits, and to limited outbreaks among children (except for keratoconjunctivitis caused by types 8, 19, and 37). Infections are observed throughout the year, but the greatest incidence and largest epidemics occur in late fall and winter. Types 7, 4, and 3 (in order of decreasing importance) are the viruses most frequently responsible for epidemics of acute respiratory and ocular diseases (see Table 52–3); types 11, 14, 21, 40, and 41 have been increasingly implicated in epidemics. Peculiarly, type 4 adenovirus commonly causes ARD in military recruits but rarely produces infections in civilians. This epidemiologic behavior of type 4 is without parallel; its explanation is unknown.

A relatively high proportion of adults have Abs to one or more types of adenoviruses (particularly types 1–3, 5, and 7), indicating previous infections. However, epidemiologic studies indicate that adenoviruses annually cause at most 4% to 5% of viral respiratory illnesses in civilians.

Prevention and Control

Isolation of sick persons has little or no effect on the spread of adenoviruses, since many healthy persons are carriers. Immunization, however, offers an effective preventive measure, as would be expected from the lasting type-specific immunity produced by natural infections. A highly effective live virus vaccine is used primarily to protect military recruits; a formalinized virus vaccine was experimentally successful in recruits, but its irregular antigenicity caused its abandonment. Successful immunization suppressed ARD caused by type 4 in recruits in the United States, but type 7 replaced it. Following continued immunization with types 4 and 7, other types have appeared (e.g., type 21, which had previously been responsible for epidemics of ARD in European defense forces).

Vaccines for military use should contain types 3, 4, 7, and 21 depending on the types prevalent. In closed populations, such as those in chronic-disease hospitals or homes for orphans, a vaccine containing types 1–7, 40, and 41 may be useful for infants and young children.

Parvoviruses

Small icosahedral viruses, 18 nm to 28 nm in diameter, were first discovered in association with adenoviruses and found to replicate in association with adenoviruses. These **adeno-associated viruses (AAVs)** led to the recognition of several other viruses of lower animals (latent rat viruses, minute mouse virus, and porcine virus) and another virus infecting humans (**human parvovirus**) that have physical and chemical properties similar to AAV. These viruses are grouped in the family *Parvoviridae* (its vernacular term is **parvovirus** (L. *parvus*, small)) and further divided into the subgroups (genera) composed of defective viruses, such as AAV (officially termed *Dependovirus*) and autonomous viruses (*Parvovirus*); a third genus of parvoviruses (*Densovirus*) infects only arthropods. **Defective parvovirus** depends totally on the multiplication of the unrelated adenoviruses or herpes simplex viruses (types 1 and 2); hence, it has been given the genus name *Dependovirus*. The viral genome consists of a linear molecule of single-stranded DNA with a molecular weight of only 1.5×10^6. The virions, however, can contain either a positive or a negative DNA strand that, when extracted from the viral particles, forms double-stranded molecules unless a reagent that blocks hydrogen bond formation (e.g., formalin) is present. The quantity of genetic information contained in this small DNA molecule is very limited and is utilized largely for specifying the three viral capsid proteins. The precise functions that the helper supplies are unknown, but studies with adenovirus mutants and microinjection of adenovirus' early mRNAs indicate that AAV utilizes early adenovirus proteins for each step in AAV replication. Thus, E1A provides a function to initiate AAV transcription, E4 is utilized for DNA replication, and adenovirus VA I is utilized for AAV translation. It is striking that the multiplication of adenovirus is itself inhibited when it offers assistance to the defective AAV (and AAV also reduces adenovirus oncogenicity in hamsters). Although

production of infectious AAV in cells coinfected with an adenovirus resembles complementation by two genetically related defective mutants (see Chap. 48), cross-hybridization of DNAs extracted from AAVs and several types of adenoviruses failed to detect homologous regions.

Five distinct immunologic types of AAVs have been identified as contaminants of human and simian adenoviruses, and AAV Abs are frequently found in humans and monkeys. About 70% to 80% of humans acquire Abs to AAV types 1, 2, and 3 within the first decade of life, and approximately 85% of adults maintain detectable Abs. AAVs types 1–3 can occasionally be isolated from fecal, ocular, and respiratory specimens during acute adenovirus infections, but not during other illnesses. Type 5 AAV, however, was isolated from a penile, flat, condylomatous lesion, and its seroepidemiology differs from that of the other types: the highest Ab titers are found in those 15 to 20 years old, and only about 60% of adults possess Abs.

In cell cultures, AAV DNA integrates into the host DNA and replicates with it, only to be excised and induced to replicate when the latently infected cells are coinfected with an adenovirus. Thus, AAVs may have a similar virus–host cell relationship in man as in cell cultures. They have been suspected of playing a role in the pathogenesis of "slow" viral infections (see Chap. 51), but so far this role is unconfirmed, and they appear to be only silent, unobtrusive partners of adenovirus infection.

AUTONOMOUS PARVOVIRUSES

One virus isolated from human sera during screening for hepatitis B virus Ag (see Chap. 63) has been shown to be a human pathogen, termed **human parvovirus,** and a number of species from lower animals (latent rat viruses, feline panleukemia virus, minute mouse virus, porcine virus, and many others) have physical and chemical characteristics similar to AAV except that they replicate without assistance of a helper virus. It is striking that although they are not defective, the **autonomous parvoviruses require actively dividing cells for productive infection.**

Since the initial detections of human parvovirus (termed B19) were not associated with specific illnesses, intense interest was not aroused until this virus was identified with aplastic crisis in two children with sickle cell disease. The association of human parvovirus with such aplastic crises has been strengthened by isolation from other cases, and viral isolations have been extended to adults with polyarthralgia syndrome and with aplastic crisis in sickle cell disease, as well as with several other hereditary hemolytic anemias such as hereditary spherocytosis, β-thalassemia, and pyruvate kinase activity. The pathogenic effect of human parvovirus in humans broadened when viral isolation, as well as clinical, epidemiologic, and immunologic evidence, indicated that it was the long-searched-for etiologic agent of erythema infectiosum ("fifth" disease), an acute, febrile, self-limited childhood disease.* Fifth disease and transient aplastic crisis share similar epidemiologic features in that they both spread within families and to close contacts, and they appear to confer lasting immunity. Children 5 to 10 years of age are at greatest risk for both infections.

Human volunteer experiments in adults free of Abs have further confirmed the etiologic role of human parvovirus as well as its pathogenic potentials. One week after inoculation, the volunteers developed a viremia accompanied by mild illness consisting of fever, malaise, myalgia, pruritus, and excretion of virus in respiratory secretions. A week later, reticulocytopenia, reduced platelets, neutropenia and lymphopenia, and a slight drop in hemoglobin developed. Seventeen to 18 days after inoculation, rash and arthralgia—typical adult erythema infectiosum—appeared.

The human parvovirus has all the chemical and physical characteristics of well-characterized parvoviruses. Its DNA does not have homology with AAV, but it does hybridize with the DNAs of other autonomous parvoviruses, implying that human parvovirus is a member of the genus *Parvovirus*. Productive replication of human parvovirus has been demonstrated in nuclei of human progenitor erythroid cells in bone marrow cultures supplemented with erythropoietin. Replication of viral DNA is similar to that of other parvoviruses, and its multiplication profoundly inhibits cell growth. These data indicate that the human parvovirus (B19) replicates autonomously and requires actively dividing cells, like other parvoviruses of this genus. It is not certain, however, that

an appropriate helper virus might not enhance its replication.

Selected Reading

BOOKS AND REVIEW ARTICLES

Berns KI (ed): The Parvoviruses. New York, Plenum Press, 1984

Challberg MD, Kelley TJ: Eukaryotic DNA replication: Viral and plasmid model systems. Annu Rev Biochem 51:901, 1982

Ginsberg HS (ed): The Adenoviruses. New York, Plenum, 1984

Moran E, Mathews MB: Multiple functional domains in the adenovirus E1A gene (minireview). Cell 48:117, 1987

Young N, Mortimer P: Viruses and bone marrow failure. Blood 63:729, 1984

SPECIFIC ARTICLES

Anderson MJ, Higgins PG, Davis LR et al: Experimental parvoviral infection in humans. J Infect Dis 152:257, 1985

Berget SM, Moore C, Sharp PA: Spliced segments at the 5′ terminus of adenovirus 2 late mRNA. Proc Natl Acad Sci USA 74:171, 1977

Berk AJ, Sharp PA: Structure of the adenovirus 2 early mRNAs. Cell 14:695, 1978

Cassant YE, Cant B, Field AM, Widdows D: Parvovirus-like particles in human sera. Lancet 1:72, 1975

Catmore SF, Tattersall P: Characterization and molecular cloning of a human parvovirus genome. Science 226:1161, 1984

Chow LT, Gelinas RE, Broker TR, Roberts RJ: An amazing sequence arrangement at the 5′ ends of adenovirus 2 messenger RNA. Cell 12:1, 1977

Evans R, Fraser N, Ziff E et al: The initiation sites of RNA-transcription of AD2 DNA. Cell 12:733, 1977

Hilleman MR, Werner JR: Recovery of a new agent from patients with acute respiratory illness. Proc Soc Exp Biol Med 85:183, 1954

Horne RW, Brenner S, Waterson AP, Wildy P: The icosahedral form of an adenovirus. J Mol Biol I:84, 1959

Konarska MM, Grabowski PJ, Padgett RA, Sharp PA: Characterization of a branch site in lariat RNAs produced by splicing of mRNA precursors. Nature 313:552, 1985

Rowe WP, Huebner RJ, Gilmore LK et al: Isolation of a cytopathogenic agent from human adenoids undergoing spontaneous degeneration in tissue culture. Proc Soc Exp Biol Med 84:570, 1953

Trentin JJ, Yabe Y, Taylor G: The quest for human cancer viruses. Science 137:835, 1962

---

* Termed *fifth disease* because it was the fifth childhood rash disease recognized after scarlet fever, rubeola (measles), rubella (German measles), and epidemic pseudoscarlatina

53

Herpesviruses

General Characteristics

The herpesviruses, a family (Herpesviridae*) of structurally similar viruses, are named (Gr. *herpein*, to creep) for those members responsible for two common diseases of man: **herpes simplex** (fever blister) and **herpes zoster** (chickenpox [varicella] and shingles) (Gr. *zoster*, girdle). The skin lesions of the herpetic diseases illustrate the affinity of most herpesviruses for cells of ectodermal origin. Like the poxviruses, another group of DNA viruses, herpesviruses exhibit focal cytopathogenicity, producing vesicles or pocks in patients and in egg membranes. Another prominent characteristic is the production of **latent** and **recurrent** infections; although the mechanism is not clear, it is noteworthy that herpesviruses, like adenoviruses (which also initiate latent infections), are DNA viruses and replicate in the cell nucleus.

The unusual epidemiologic features of the common herpes infections long puzzled physicians until techniques became available for identifying and characterizing the responsible viruses. Thus, the multiple recurrence of fever blisters in certain persons was bewildering until about 1950, when Burnet in Australia and Buddingh in the United States showed that herpes simplex virus often becomes latent after initiating a primary infection, usually in children, and is then repeatedly activated by subsequent provocations (see Latent Infections, Chap. 51). A similar mechanism was suspected in **chickenpox** (varicella); i.e., that it **recurs as herpes zoster** (shingles), since an outbreak of chickenpox was often observed to follow the sporadic appearance of zoster in an adult. However, because the initial and subsequent syndromes are so different, the relation was not certain until Weller,

---

* There are three subfamilies: Alphaherpesvirinae (includes the herpes simplex types 1 and 2 viruses and the varicella zoster virus), Betaherpesvirinae (cytomegalovirus), and Gammaherpesvirinae (Epstein-Barr virus).

in 1954, isolated in tissue cultures the same virus from patients with the two diseases. The virus closely resembles that of herpes simplex.

Besides the herpes simplex and varicella zoster viruses, the major herpesviruses that infect man are cytomegalovirus (inclusion or salivary gland virus of man), and EB (Epstein-Barr) virus. These viruses are widely separated in evolution despite their structural similarities (see Characteristics of Members of the Herpesvirus Family). They differ strikingly in their DNA composition, although some similarities exist in the manner in which the general structures of the viral genomes have long and short unique sequences separated by repeated sequences (Fig. 53–1). Herpes simplex viruses are immunologically related to each other but show no relatedness to other family members; and the other three human herpesviruses antigenically cross-react only slightly.

Herpesviruses have also been found in every other eukaryotic species examined, from fungi to monkeys. Ex-

CHARACTERISTICS OF MEMBERS OF THE HERPESVIRUS FAMILY

Size: 180–200 nm
Symmetry of capsid: Icosahedral
Capsomers: 162; 9.5 × 12.5 nm
Lipid envelope: Present
Sensitivity to ether and chloroform: Inactivates infectivity
Nucleic acid: Double-stranded DNA*
Site of biosynthesis of viral DNA: Nucleus
Site of assembly of viral particles: Nucleus
Inclusion bodies: Intranuclear, eosinophilic†
Common family antigen: None

* Molecular weights (daltons): herpes simplex viruses approximately 96×10^6, varicella zoster virus $80–86 \times 10^6$, cytomegalovirus 145×10^6 (231 kilobase pairs), EB virus 114×10^6. Guanine-cytosine content (mol/dl): cytomegalovirus 58.8%, herpes simplex type 1 67%, herpes simplex type 2 69%, varicella zoster 46%, and EB virus 59%. DNA–DNA hybridizations indicate that 40% to 46% of the base sequences are homologous in types 1 and 2 herpes simplex viruses.

† Cytomegalovirus-infected cells may also contain basophilic cytoplasmic inclusion bodies.

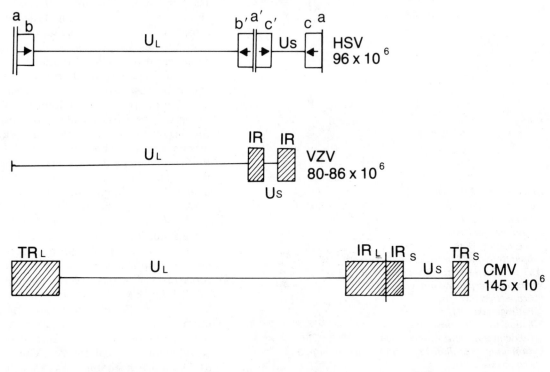

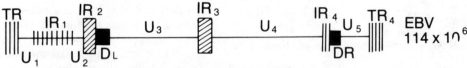

Figure 53–1. Diagrams of the physical structures of genomes of several viruses of the family Herpesviridae. The genomes are composed of unique (*U*) sequences with short (*S*) or a long (*L*) region, numbered where there are several (*EBV*). Terminal repeats (*TR*) bound the genome, and inverted repeats (*IR*) bound the unique regions. The rectangles contain reiterated sequences of more than 1000 base pairs. (Modified from maps presented by B. Roizman, L. D. Gelb, R. LaFemina, and G. Hayward, and Wathen and Stinski)

amples include **B virus of monkeys** (which may infect man accidentally), **pseudorabies virus** of pigs, **virus III** of rabbits, **cytomegaloviruses of animals** (inclusion virus of guinea pigs, inclusion virus of mice, and the agent of inclusion body rhinitis in pigs), oncogenic viruses (see Chap. 64) that produce **lymphoproliferative malignancies** in chickens (**Marek's disease virus**) and monkeys (**herpesvirus saimirii**), and several viruses that may be associated with renal carcinoma in frogs. These animal viruses appear to have only minor immunologic relatedness to human herpesviruses except for the marked cross-reactivity between herpes simplex virus and B virus. In this chapter only the viruses that infect man will be discussed.

Herpesvirus particles have a diameter from 180 nm (herpes simplex and varicella zoster viruses) to 200 nm (cytomegalovirus). Within a population of virions, many particles do not possess envelopes, and some are empty capsids (Fig. 53–2*B* and *D*). The virion components (Figs. 53–2 and 53–3) are arranged in (1) a DNA-containing **toroidal core** about 75 nm in diameter, (2) an **icosahedral**

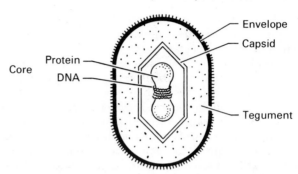

Figure 53–3. Diagram of a virion of herpes simplex virus. The DNA–protein core consists of DNA wrapped around an associated protein as on the spindle of a spool. The envelope contains a number of glycoproteins, the capsid is composed of at least four unique proteins, and the so-called tegument consists of about eight distinct polypeptides.

capsid 95 nm to 105 nm in diameter, (3) a surrounding **granular zone** (**tegument**) composed of globular proteins, and (4) an encompassing **envelope** possessing periodic short projections. The capsid is composed of 162 elongated hexagonal prisms (**capsomers**), each with a small, central hole.

The chemical composition of purified enveloped viral particles is consonant with their morphology. Herpes simplex virions contain 25 to 30 virus-specified proteins (70% of the virion); a large, linear, double-stranded DNA molecule (7% of the virion); envelope lipid (22% of the virion), which is chiefly host-specific phospholipid derived from the nuclear membrane; and small amounts of polyamines (spermine within the nucleocapsid and spermidine within the envelope). Other herpesviruses examined are similar.

Like other enveloped viruses, herpesviruses are relatively unstable at room temperature and are readily inactivated by lipid solvents.

Herpes Simplex Viruses

PROPERTIES

IMMUNOLOGIC CHARACTERISTICS. Types 1 and 2 herpes simplex viruses are the main immunologic variants that can be distinguished by neutralization titrations, although they cross-react strongly, and by their distinct clinical patterns. Some additional minor antigenic variations have been observed but do not warrant classification. Infected cells contain, along with virions, soluble Ags that elicit a delayed-type skin reaction in addition to the usual immunologic reactions. Infected cells are also antigenically altered by the insertion of four to five viral structural glycoproteins into their plasma membrane; the glycoprotein D (gp D) is particularly prominent in eliciting neutralizing Abs. These Ags make the infected

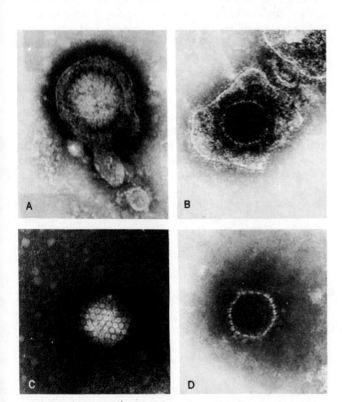

Figure 53–2. The four morphologic types of herpes simplex virus particles embedded in phosphotungstate. (**A**) Enveloped full particle showing the thick envelope surrounding the nucleocapsid. (**B**) Enveloped empty particle; the capsid does not contain viral DNA and therefore can be penetrated by the phosphotungstate. (**C**) Naked full particle; the structure of the capsomers is plainly visible. (**D**) Naked empty particle. (Original magnification ×200,000; Watson DH et al: Virology 19:250, 1963)

cells susceptible to damage and lysis by reaction with virus-specific Abs plus complement, or with specifically activated T-lymphocytes.

Specific Abs can be assayed by neutralization, enzyme-linked immunosorbent assay (ELISA) or complement fixation (CF) tests; they reach maximum titers about 14 days after infection. During the early stages after a primary infection, neutralizing Abs can be detected only in the presence of complement. Thereafter, complement is not required for neutralization, but its presence raises Ab titers fourfold to eightfold. Neutralizing Abs are primarily directed to the envelope glycoproteins; ELISA and CF Abs react with all the virion proteins.

Abs may drop to undetectable levels after the first infection, only to reappear with recurrent episodes. By adulthood, titers are generally high and persist indefinitely. Accordingly, an increase usually cannot be detected in recurrent adult disease, although infectious virus can be isolated readily from the lesion. Fetuses acquire maternal Abs via placental transfer, and they persist until about 4 months after birth; this persistence probably explains the common occurrence of primary infection in babies from 6 to 18 months of age.

Cell-mediated immunity also develops after primary infection and may be a major immunologic factor in maintaining a latent state. It appears that impairment of cellular immunity, as measured by diminished production of macrophage migration-inhibitory factor and diminished activity of sensitized T-lymphocytes, is correlated with episodic recurrences. Moreover, in immunosuppressed patients the virus is commonly activated and disseminated, leading to acute disease.

HOST RANGE. Humans are the natural host for herpes simplex viruses, but a relatively wide range of animals are also susceptible, including mice, guinea pigs, hamsters, and rabbits. The effects of infection depend on the route of inoculation. For example, inoculation of the cornea in the rabbit results in keratoconjunctivitis or keratitis, whereas intracerebral inoculation produces fatal encephalitis. The chick embryo has been a convenient host: the production of pocks on the chorioallantoic membrane affords a reproducible method for detection and assay, similar to that employed with poxviruses.

Many **cultured cell types** support multiplication of herpes simplex virus, undergo extensive cytopathic changes, and develop intranuclear inclusion bodies; chromosomal breaks and aberrations are also observed. The response of the cells varies with the strain of virus employed: some strains cause marked clumping of cells, and some produce typical plaques with suitable cells.

MULTIPLICATION. The **glycoproteins of the viral envelope** provide the normal **attachment** of the virions to susceptible cells. Following attachment, the viral envelope **glycoprotein B (gp B)** induces its **fusion** with the cellular plasma membrane, permitting the nucleocapsid to enter directly into the cytoplasm (see Chap. 48). Intact virions may also enter via endocytosis, from which they are released into the cytoplasm by similar viral envelope–membrane fusion. In the cytoplasm the capsid migrates to a nuclear pore, where the viral DNA is released into the nucleus and initiates viral multiplication. The **eclipse period** is 5 to 6 hours in monolayer cell cultures, and virus increases exponentially until approximately 17 hours after infection (Fig. 53–4); each cell has then made 10^4 to 10^5 physical particles, of which about 100 are infectious. Virions are **released** by slow leakage from infected cells.

As with other DNA-containing viruses (see Chap. 48), the **biochemical events** are **sequentially regulated,** presenting a cascadelike effect. Thus, after the viral DNA enters the nucleoplasm, even in the absence of protein synthesis, the host cell RNA polymerase II transcribes noncontiguous, restricted regions of the viral genome to produce five **immediate early (α) mRNAs** (Fig. 53–5). If translation is blocked, only these α mRNAs accumulate in the cytoplasm, and the larger, unprocessed transcripts remain in the nucleus. If protein synthesis is permitted, α **proteins** are made, leading to transcription of other regions of the genome and production of **delayed early (β) mRNAs.** The β **proteins** block further synthesis of α proteins and lead to transcription of a third set of RNAs and their processing into **late γ mRNAs.** Thus, the synthesis and translation of the mRNAs are **coordinately regulated:** formation of the α proteins is necessary for synthesis of the β proteins, and both of these nonstructural and minor structural proteins are necessary for synthesis of the **late major structural γ proteins.** It is noteworthy that synthesis of all the γ proteins is not dependent on viral DNA replication: $\gamma 1$ proteins such as gp B and the major capsid protein VP5 are made in the absence of viral DNA synthesis, although they are synthesized in relatively low abundance; but $\gamma 2$ proteins

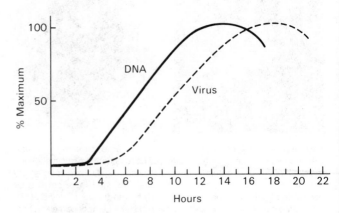

Figure 53–4. Temporal relationship between viral DNA replication and the production of infectious virus.

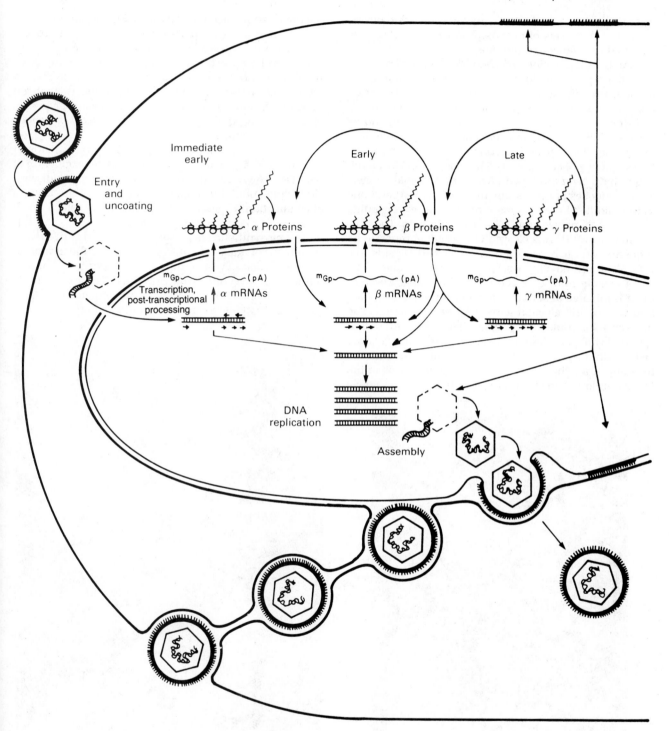

Figure 53–5. Sequence of events in the multiplication of herpes simplex virus from entry of the virus into the cell by fusion of the virion envelope with the membrane of the endocytic vacuole to assembly of virions and their exit from the cell through the endoplasmic reticulum. Also illustrated are transcription and coordinated sequential processing of mRNAs and synthesis of sets of proteins (α, β, γ) required for DNA replication and virion structures. (Modified from a diagram kindly supplied by B. Roizman, University of Chicago)

(e.g., glycoprotein C) strictly require amplification of viral DNA. The three sets of mRNAs produce an aggregate of about 50 virus-encoded proteins.

Viral DNA replication is carried out by both viral α and β proteins, which include a DNA polymerase and DNA-binding protein, and host cellular enzymes. The reactions are not yet precisely understood, but they appear to involve complex replicative intermediates, including "head-to-tail" concatemeric circular and linear–circular forms (see Chap. 48) generated by the reiterated nucleotide sequences (see Fig. 53–1). Three origins of DNA replication have been described: two in the terminal *c* reiterated sequences of the S segment (see Fig. 53–1) and one in the middle of the L segment near the genes encoding the DNA polymerase and DNA-binding protein. The concatemeric viral DNA is cleaved at a terminal reiterated *a* sequence, and it is packaged in preformed capsids (see Figs. 53–1 and 53–6). These particles are noninfectious and unstable until they acquire an envelope. Envelopment is initiated at sites on the inner nuclear membrane into which viral glycoproteins have been inserted. The nuclear membrane reduplicates (Fig. 53–7) to permit egress of viral particles into the cytoplasm, where it associates with the endoplasmic reticulum, and the viral particle appears either to complete envelopment or to become enveloped anew. Mature, infectious virus is slowly liberated from infected cells through the endoplasmic reticulum, but occasionally it also escapes by a process akin to reverse phagocytosis. Unlike the process with other enveloped viruses, envelopment and release of viral particles does not occur by budding from the plasma membrane. Rather, the plasma membrane is changed morphologically and contains virus-specific glycoproteins; this consequently makes the membrane a target for immunologic attack.

Only about 25% of the viral DNA and protein made in cell cultures is assembled into virions. The production of host DNA, RNA, and protein declines, concomitant with viral replication, and finally ceases within 3 to 5 hours after infection. Ultimately the productively infected cell dies.

The biosynthetic steps can be correlated with the development of nuclear inclusion bodies and the formation of viral particles. A basophilic, Feulgen-positive, granular mass of newly synthesized viral DNA develops centrally in the nucleus. The assembly of incomplete viral particles (see Fig. 53–6) begins within this material.

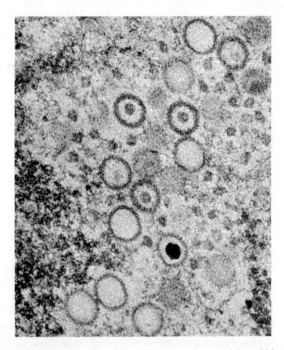

Figure 53–6. Formation of herpes simplex virus particles within the cell nucleus. Some capsids are in the process of assembling, while others are complete. Cores of varying density are forming within the capsids. Indistinct particles probably represent virus sectioned at one margin, with loss of density and overlapping structure. (Original magnification ×90,000; Nii S et al: J Virol 2:517, 1968)

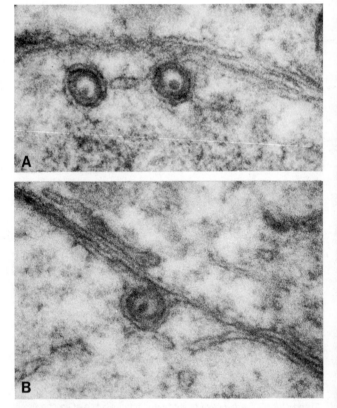

Figure 53–7. (*A* and *B*) Thin sections of mature particles of herpes simplex virus. The particles show the inner core and two or three membranes. In *B* the nuclear membrane partly surrounds a viral particle (apparently a step in the simultaneous assembly and egress of complete virions from the nucleus). (Original magnification ×87,000; Morgan C et al: J Exp Med 110:643, 1959)

The movement of viral particles from the nucleus into the cytoplasm is accompanied by the transport of soluble Ags into the cytoplasm; concomitantly the originally basophilic intranuclear inclusion body is converted into an eosinophilic, Feulgen-negative mass. Thus, the eosinophilic inclusion body that is usually observed in infected cells does not contain viral particles or specific viral Ags (detectable by immunofluorescence) but actually is the burnt-out remnant of a viral factory.

PATHOGENESIS

The most striking characteristic of herpes simplex virus infection is its propensity for persisting in a **quiescent** or **latent state** in humans, with recurrence of activity at irregular intervals. The initial infection occurs through a break in the mucous membranes (e.g., eye, mouth, throat, genitals) or skin, where local multiplication ensues. From this focus virus spreads to regional lymph nodes, where it multiplies further. On occasion virus disseminates into the blood and to distant organs. Viremia can occasionally be detected by isolation of virus from the cells of the blood buffy coat.

The initial infection ordinarily occurs in children 6 to 18 months of age; serologic surveys have demonstrated that it is most often inapparent. But 10% to 15% of those infected do develop a **primary disease,** usually **herpetic gingivostomatitis,** which is characterized by multiple vesicles in the oral mucous membranes and the mucocutaneous border. Similar lesions are less commonly seen in other regions, including the nostrils, the esophagus, the external genitalia or urethra, the cornea, and sites of trauma. More serious but rare complications include neonatal generalized infections, meningoencephalitis,* diffuse skin involvement in children with chronic eczema (Kaposi's varicelliform eruption, eczema herpeticum), and hepatitis.

During the initial infection, virus is taken up by adjacent nerve endings, and it migrates rapidly in axons of nerves to the ganglia. When the initial infection recedes, the virus persists, despite the presence of a high Ab titer, producing a latent infection in a sensory ganglion adjacent to the major site of the primary disease. The genome of the occult virus appears not to be integrated and probably persists in an episomal state; moreover, only α mRNAs are found. The balance may be readily upset, including viral replication in the nerve ganglion, thus provoking the second, **recurrent form** of herpes simplex disease. Because neutralizing Abs and cellular immunity are present, the new virus cannot disseminate, but it does migrate centrifugally from the ganglion along nerve axons to reach contiguous cells; recurrent herpes

simplex therefore usually remains localized. In a given person the clinical features are much the same with each episode. For example, if **gingivostomatitis** was the **primary disease,** the **recurrent form** is usually **herpes labialis** (fever blisters) in the same region of the lip; and if the primary disease was **herpetic keratitis,** the recurrent disease is also keratitis (which may lead to corneal scarring and is one of the major infectious causes of blindness).

Types 1 and 2 herpes simplex viruses differ significantly in their pathogenic potential. **Type 1 virus** is primarily associated with **oral** and **ocular lesions** and is transmitted in oral and respiratory secretions, whereas **type 2** is isolated primarily from **genital** and **anal lesions** and is passed through sexual contact. Changes in sexual mores, however, have somewhat altered this common pattern: occasionally, type 2 virus is isolated from oral lesions and type 1 virus from genital lesions. Mothers with **genital herpes** (a painful, persistent, recurrent infection) are the primary source of **neonatal infections** with type 2 virus, which are often severe and even fatal. It is also striking that in the United States more than 80% of women with cervical carcinoma have Abs to type 2 virus (see Chap. 64). However, a prospective study showed that this is not the result of a causal relation but probably only a reflection of lower socioeconomic status and, possibly, of a more promiscuous sexual activity of many who become victims of cervical carcinoma.

LATENCY. In experimental models in mice, labial strains of type 1 are characteristically found latent in neurons of cervical ganglia, and type 2 genital strains are found in sacral ganglia. Infectious virus is not detectable as such in ganglia, but it emerges when ganglion fragments are cultured *in vitro.* In humans the virus has similarly been detected in cultures of trigeminal ganglia (type 1) or sacral ganglia (type 2). Moreover, neurectomy of the facial branch of the trigeminal nerve (as therapy for persistent trigeminal neuralgia) characteristically activates latent herpes simplex virus, producing fever blisters. In experimental latent infections of mice and rabbits, trigeminal or sciatic nerve section likewise activates quiescent virus.

Viral multiplication and recurrent disease may also be induced in humans by naturally occurring factors such as heat, cold, or sunlight (ultraviolet light), and by immunologically unrelated hypersensitivity reactions, pituitary and adrenal hormones, and emotional disturbances. A few of these, such as epinephrine and hypersensitivity reactions, have evoked recurrences in experimental animals (see Latent Infections, Chap. 51).

LABORATORY DIAGNOSIS

The increasing occurrence of life-threatening herpesvirus infections in children with inherited T-cell defi-

---

* Encephalitis occurs more frequently in adults, either as a primary infection or as a flare-up of a latent infection.

ciencies and in patients who are immunosuppressed because of infection (e.g., with acquired immune deficiency syndrome [AIDS] virus), transplantation, or cancer therapy has given great importance to rapid, accurate, and economic laboratory procedures for an etiologic diagnosis. The development of effective chemotherapeutic agents is making rapid diagnosis even more imperative. The following methods are available: (1) The quickest and most economical diagnostic test consists of demonstrating characteristic multinuclear giant cells containing intranuclear eosinophilic **inclusion bodies** in scrapings from the base of vesicles. This procedure cannot, however, distinguish a herpes simplex infection from one produced by varicella zoster virus or cytomegalovirus. (2) **Electron microscopic examination** of biopsied tissues reveals cells that contain viral particles in various stages of maturation. (3) **Specific Ags** may be detected in cells from the lesions by ELISA or by immunofluorescent techniques. (4) **Virus** can be **isolated** by inoculating material from lesions (especially vesicular fluid or scrapings) into susceptible tissue culture cells or newborn mice. (5) **A rise in Ab titer** is detected by neutralization, CF, indirect hemagglutination, or ELISA through the use of serum obtained early in the primary disease and again 14 to 21 days after onset (paired sera). Following primary infections there is often also a small rise in neutralizing Abs for varicella zoster virus. Patients with recurrent disease have a high initial titer of circulating Abs and often do not show a significant increase.

EPIDEMIOLOGY, CONTROL, AND TREATMENT

Close person-to-person contact is the most common mechanism of viral transmission. Man is the only known natural host and source of virus. Secretions from lesions about the mouth (herpes labialis and stomatitis) and genitalia are the most frequent sources. Virus is also transmissible on eating and drinking utensils and other fomites for a brief period after contamination. Occasionally virus is found in the saliva of healthy persons, particularly children after the primary infection; the shedding may even continue for weeks or months.

Rare cases of primary infection have been reported in adults. Approximately 80% of adults have relatively high titers of neutralizing and CF Abs, as well as cellular immunity, and a substantial fraction of this population is subject to recurrent herpes.

Control is not feasible because of the large numbers of persons with inapparent infections and minor recurrent lesions from which virus is shed. However, it is important, whenever possible, to prevent contact between infants and persons who have herpetic lesions. Vaccines to prevent genital herpes are being prepared and experimentally studied. Such type 2 virus vaccines are being developed by means of specially constructed, attenuated virus; synthetic polypeptides consisting of a portion of the specific protective viral glycoprotein Ag; or an expression vector producing such a specific Ag.

Chemical therapy of herpesvirus infection provides the best example of developing chemotherapeutic agents that act specifically on viral rather than on host macromolecular synthesis, taking advantage of the unique characteristics of the biochemical reactants (see Chap. 49). Thus, **acylovir** [9-(2-hydroxyethoxymethyl) guanine] has been used successfully to treat the mucocutaneous lesions of oral and genital herpes simplex as well as encephalitis (successful treatment of encephalitis requires that acylovir therapy begin immediately upon suspicion of the diagnosis, before results of brain biopsy are known). It is noteworthy that although treatment of patients with recurrent oral or genital lesions significantly reduces the recurrences during therapy, the recurrent pattern resumes shortly after therapy is discontinued. Moreover, after prolonged therapy, resistant viral mutants, whose target DNA polymerase is markedly less affected by the drug, appear.

Vidarabine (adenine arabinoside; 9-β-arabinofuranosyladenine), also an inhibitor of herpesvirus-encoded, DNA polymerase, as well as virus-specific ribonucleotide reductase, has been employed locally for keratitis and herpes labialis and intravenously in cases of encephalitis and disseminated herpes simplex infections. Although vidarabine has been shown to be effective, acyclovir is more easily administered, has proved to be more effective in treatment of encephalitis, and is probably the present drug of choice. A number of other nucleoside analogues have been synthesized and studied: 5-iodo-2'-deoxyuridine (idoxuridine, IUdR) is useful for local treatment of herpetitic keratitis, but recurrences often follow cessation of therapy, and drug-resistant herpesviruses may emerge; and trifluorothymidine has proved to be even more successful than IUdR in the local treatment of herpes keratitis.

B Virus (Herpesvirus Simiae)

In its natural host, the monkey, B virus produces latent infections like those of herpes simplex virus in humans. However, in humans B virus can produce acute, ascending myelitis and encephalomyelitis. The increased handling of monkeys and the widespread use of monkey kidney cells in the commercial production of poliovirus vaccines augmented the transmission of this virus to humans: at least 24 cases have occurred in the past 30 years. Recognition of the danger is critical, since the disease in humans is usually fatal.

B virus closely resembles herpes simplex virus: the two are antigenically related but not identical. Antiserum from rabbits immunized with B virus neutralizes herpes simplex virus; however, Abs to herpes simplex virus neutralize B virus only slightly.

Varicella–Herpes Zoster Virus

The viruses isolated from patients with varicella (chickenpox) and from those with herpes zoster (shingles) are physically and immunologically indistinguishable (Fig. 53–8). Their identity has been further established by the production of typical varicella in children following inoculation of herpes zoster vesicle fluid.

PROPERTIES

Varicella zoster virus is relatively unstable even at −40°C to −70°C; the infectivity of virus from tissue cultures cannot be maintained reliably for longer than 2 months. Vesicle fluid from a patient, however, remains infectious for many months at −70°C, perhaps because of the high titers of virus and the high concentrations of protein.

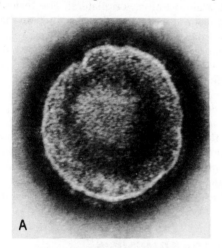

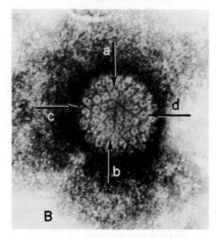

Figure 53–8. Morphology of varicella–herpes zoster virus particles embedded in sodium phosphotungstate. *(A)* Intact virion showing the envelope with surface projections and the centrally placed capsid. *(B)* Viral particle in which the envelope has ruptured, revealing the structure of the capsid more clearly. Arrows point to capsomers situated on axes of fivefold symmetry. (Original magnification ×200,000, reduced; Almeida JD et al: Virology 16:353, 1962)

IMMUNOLOGIC CHARACTERISTICS. The virions contain 30 to 33 polypeptides of which at least five are envelope-associated glycoproteins. A number of these Ags can be detected immunologically in vesicle fluids as well as in infected cells. In varicella, IgM Abs usually appear in the serum 2 to 3 days after onset of the exanthem; IgG Abs soon replace the IgM and continue to increase in titer for about 2 weeks. Titers of CF Abs decrease over a period of months, but neutralizing and immune adherence hemagglutinating Abs, as well as Abs to infected cell membrane Ags (detected by immunofluorescence), persist for many years after the primary infection. Epitopes inducing neutralizing Abs were identified on three of the glycoproteins; monoclonal Abs to two of the glycoproteins neutralized in the absence of complement, but one of the Ab sets required the addition of complement for viral neutralization. Cellular immunity, detected by peripheral blood and mucosal lymphocyte responsiveness to the viral membrane Ags, also persists and appears to play a protective role against reinfection, even in the absence of detectable circulating Abs. Most herpes zoster patients have a relatively high titer of viral IgG Abs at the onset of the disease, an indication that herpes zoster, like recurrent herpes simplex, occurs in previously infected, partially immune persons.

HOST RANGE. In contrast to herpes simplex virus, varicella virus does not cause reproducible disease in experimental animals or chick embryos, but it can be propagated in cultures of a variety of human and monkey cells. Little virus is found in the culture fluid, but stable virus can be obtained by sonic disruption of cells 24 to 36 hours after infection. Serial propagation is also accomplished by transfer of infected cells. Characteristic cytopathic effects and eosinophilic intranuclear inclusion bodies develop (see Fig. 53–9), and metaphase arrest and chromosomal aberrations have been observed.

MULTIPLICATION. Multiplication of varicella zoster virus is confined to the nucleus, and the developmental stages are similar to those of herpes simplex virus; the biochemical details have not been described. Viral DNA replication begins about 6 hours after infection, structural proteins can be detected 2 to 4 hours later, and a maximum quantity of virus is attained 24 to 36 hours after infection. Infectious virus after assembly does not emerge readily from infected cells in culture. Natural infections, however, are highly contagious, and the virus is present extracellularly in high titer in the vesicle fluid of lesions.

PATHOGENESIS

VARICELLA (CHICKENPOX). The primary disease produced in a host without immunity is usually a mild, self-limited illness of young children. The clinical picture strongly suggests that the virus is spread by respiratory secretions, enters the respiratory tract, multiplies locally and possibly in regional lymph nodes, produces viremia, and is disseminated by the blood to the skin and internal organs. The virus prefers ectodermal tissues, particularly in children.

After an incubation period of 14 to 16 days, fever occurs, followed within a day by a papular rash of the skin and mucous membranes. The papules rapidly become vesicular and are accompanied by itching. The lesions, which are painless (in contrast to herpes zoster), occur in successive crops, and all stages can be observed simultaneously.

In the infrequent adult cases the disease is more severe, often with a diffuse nodular pneumonia; the mortality may be as high as 20%. Varicella is also usually diffuse and intense in children receiving adrenocortical steroids and in persons with immune deficiencies.

The vesicles evolve from a ballooning and degeneration of the prickle cells of the skin, along with formation of giant cells with intranuclear eosinophilic inclusion bodies (Fig. 53–9). In disseminated fatal varicella, lesions containing similar giant cells appear in liver, lungs, and nervous tissue. Basically identical lesions may occur in dorsal root ganglia of patients with herpes zoster.

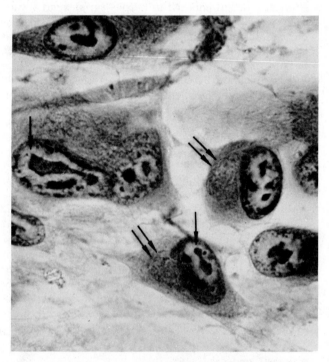

Figure 53–9. Typical eosinophilic inclusion bodies (*single arrows*) in the nuclei of human embryonic cells infected with varicella–herpes zoster virus. Poorly differentiated, pale eosinophilic bodies are also present in the paranuclear area of several cells (*double arrows*). (Original magnification ×1260; Weller TH et al: J Exp Med 108:843, 1958)

HERPES ZOSTER (SHINGLES). Herpes zoster (shingles) is the recurrent form of the disease, occurring predominantly in adults. It affects persons who were previously infected with the varicella zoster virus and who possess circulating Abs. The syndrome develops from an inflammatory involvement of sensory ganglia of spinal or cranial nerves, the virus having reaching the ganglia earlier during acute varicella by travelling along the nerves from the involved skin. The virus appears to remain latent in ganglionic nerve cells, and during activation it probably travels back along the nerve fibers to the skin.

Herpes zoster usually has a sudden onset of pain and tenderness along the distribution of the affected sensory nerve (frequently an intercostal nerve), accompanied by mild fever and malaise. A vesicular eruption, similar in pathology to varicella (except for its distribution), then occurs in crops along the distribution of the affected nerve; it is almost always unilateral. The vesicular eruption may last as long as 2 to 4 weeks; the pain may persist for additional weeks or months. Paralysis results if the inflammation spreads into the spinal cord or cranial nerves. Meningoencephalitis, which occurs rarely, is usually manifested as an acute illness with severe symptoms (headache, ataxia, coma, convulsions), but most patients recover completely.

Clinically, herpes zoster may be activated by trauma, by injection of certain drugs (arsenic, antimony), or by tuberculosis, cancer, or leukemia. Moreover, in persons with immunodeficiency states, particularly when these are induced in the therapy of lymphoproliferative diseases, the activated virus may disseminate and cause serious, often fatal, illness.

LABORATORY DIAGNOSIS

A clinical diagnosis of either varicella or herpes zoster seldom offers serious difficulties, but rarely the identification of chickenpox may require laboratory tests. This can be done most rapidly and easily by preparing a smear from the base of a vesicle and staining (by the Giemsa method) to detect typical varicella giant cells and cells with characteristic inclusion bodies. Immunofluorescence, ELISA, agar gel immunodiffusion, counterimmunoelectrophoresis, and electron microscopic examination of vesicular fluid provide rapid confirmation. For these rapid diagnostic techniques it is necessary to obtain clear viral fluid from early lesions—within the first 3 days for varicella and no more than 7 days with herpes zoster. In addition, virus may be isolated in cultured human or monkey cells and identified by serologic techniques. Antibody determinations on paired sera from patients may also be useful. Indirect immunofluorescence, immune adherence hemagglutination, and ELISA techniques are the most sensitive and rapid Ab assays. Antibody titrations are also useful to demonstrate susceptibility in seronegative adults or immunologically crippled children after exposure, as a basis for early prophylaxis with immune globulin.

EPIDEMIOLOGY AND CONTROL

Varicella virus is usually transmitted in respiratory secretions, producing a highly communicable disease with high clinical attack rate. Epidemics are common among children, especially in the winter and spring. Second attacks of chickenpox apparently do not occur. Herpes zoster, in contrast, is of low incidence, is not seasonal, is recurrent, and is predominantly confined to persons over 20 years of age. As has been pointed out, a case of herpes zoster may initiate an outbreak of chickenpox, and contact with chickenpox is said to provoke attacks of shingles in partially immune persons.

An attenuated viral vaccine has been developed and undergone intensive study in immunocompromised children, particularly those with leukemia receiving chemotherapy, as well in healthy, nonimmune young children. Mild rashes and fever follow immunization in as many as 35% to 40% of children undergoing therapy, and shingles may also subsequently appear. In leukemic children receiving maintenance chemotherapy, treatment is usually suspended from 1 week before to 1 week after immunization. Serum Abs appeared in approximately 90% of these children, the attack rate after exposure was reduced from about 90% to 20%, and all cases were extremely mild.

In view of the seriousness of varicella in adults, however, one might question the wisdom of attempts to prevent infection in healthy children unless the preventive procedure can offer as lasting protection as the natural disease. As in measles (see Measles, Prevention and Control, Chap. 57), chickenpox can be prevented or modified by administering high-Ab-titer IgG to contacts within 72 hours of exposure. Prophylaxis is of particular importance for susceptible adults and for children with impaired immunity. Adenine arabinoside (vidarabine) and acyclovir (see Chap. 49) have been used with apparent success to treat disseminated disease in the seriously ill (particularly in immunologically suppressed patients) as well as in some normal adults, but additional control studies are necessary.

Cytomegalovirus (Salivary Gland Virus) Group

Salivary gland virus disease of newborns is a severe, often fatal illness, usually affecting the salivary glands, brain, kidneys, liver, and lungs. M. G. Smith, in 1956, isolated the causative agent. The term *cytomegalovirus (CMV)* was applied to the group because of the large size of the infected cells and their huge intranuclear inclusion

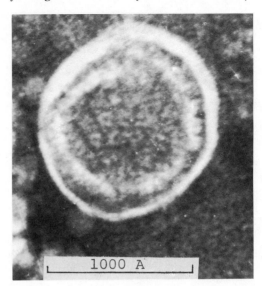

Figure 53–10. Enveloped full particle of human cytomegalovirus. (Original magnification ×405,000; Wright HT Jr et al: Virology 23:419, 1964)

bodies. Assignment to the herpesvirus family was based on the morphology of the viral particle (Fig. 53–10), the chemical composition of the virion (see Characteristics of Members of the Herpesvirus Family), and the characteristics of the intranuclear inclusion body present in infected cells (Figs. 53–11 and 53–12).

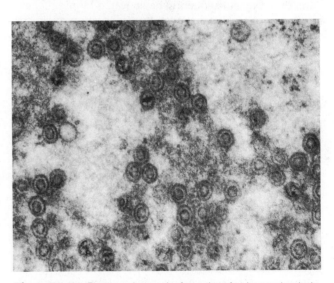

Figure 53–11. Electron micrograph of a portion of an intranuclear inclusion in a cell infected with human cytomegalovirus. The inclusion is made up of viral particles in various stages of development. Particles are composed of a central core about 40 nm in diameter, surrounded by a pale zone and, externally, by a thin membranous shell. Only a few particles have a dark central core, indicating the presence of nucleic acid. (Original magnification ×40,000; Becker P et al: Exp Mol Pathol 4:11, 1965)

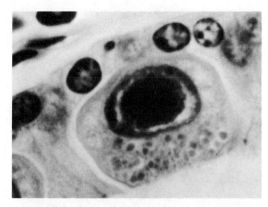

Figure 53–12. Epithelial duct cell from a human submaxillary gland, showing typical eosinophilic nuclear and basophilic cytoplasmic inclusions produced by infection with human cytomegalovirus. (Original magnification ×1500; Nelson JS, Wyatt JP: Medicine [Baltimore] 38:223, 1959)

Although primary disease is rare, infections are widespread: congenital and neonatal subclinical infections (acquired from the mother, before or at birth; see Pathogenesis) occur in 5% to 7% of live births. However, the incidence is much greater in those receiving blood transfusions, for example, in patients undergoing open heart surgery or organ transplants and receiving large quantities of blood. The virus commonly produces latent infections that may subsequently be activated by pregnancy, immunosuppression for organ transplantation or cancer chemotherapy, or viral infection (e.g., AIDS virus).

PROPERTIES

IMMUNOLOGIC CHARACTERISTICS. CMV-infected cells, like other herpesviruses, contain about 50 unique polypeptides of which 30 to 35 are virion structural proteins. The specific proteins that mediate the immune response, however, are only partially identified, but several have been shown to induce either humoral Ab or T-cell responses. Natural killer cell activity is also increased in acute CMV infections. Four membrane-associated glycoproteins have been characterized, of which three are disulfide linked and provide the antigenic epitopes for neutralizing Abs. As with herpes simplex virus, complement enhances the neutralizing capacity of Abs to some glycoprotein epitopes.

Human CMVs are not antigenically homogeneous, although their differences are not sufficient to warrant classification into distinct immunologic types. Moreover, DNA–DNA renaturation kinetics and restriction endonuclease maps indicate that the nucleotide sequences of different viral strains are largely homologous, although differences may be noted.

Humoral Abs develop relatively early during infection (IgM Abs are present at birth in the congenitally infected newborn) and persist at high levels during viral excretion. Cellular immunity, however, appears to play the major role in suppression of viral multiplication, leading to latent infection or, less commonly, to viral eradication.

HOST RANGE. Many species of animals are infected with their own specific CMVs, but no laboratory animal has proved susceptible to infection with the CMVs of humans. Virus has been isolated and propagated only in cultured human fibroblasts. *In vivo*, however, virus appears to multiply in a variety of cell types, including many of epithelial morphology. CMV also infects human lymphocytes and monocytes, but virus only undergoes an abortive replication cycle. In fact, in disseminated disease, virus has been detected in cells of essentially every organ.

MULTIPLICATION. Like herpes simplex viruses, viral replication is controlled by a coordinately regulated transcriptional program divided into three periods: **immediate-early,** which is independent of protein synthesis; **early,** in whose RNAs are encoded proteins required for DNA replication; and **late,** whose processed transcripts are translated into viral structural proteins. Synthesis of viral structural proteins depends on DNA synthesis. Viral replication is relatively slow as compared to herpes simplex viruses: viral DNA synthesis begins slowly after about 12 hours, but it is not maximally replicated until 24 to 36 hours after infection; virion-structural proteins are synthesized from 36 to 48 hours, and infectious virus is first detected 48 to 72 hours postinfection. Cytochemical and immunofluorescent techniques best reveal the synthesis of viral proteins and the development of the cytologic lesions that accompany viral multiplication, namely, focal lesions, followed by generalized cytopathic changes including rounding of cells and the appearance of large intranuclear eosinophilic inclusion bodies (see Fig. 53–12).

De novo biosynthesis of DNA and accumulation of early and late viral proteins are detected initially in the nucleus. Electron microscopic studies show that viral particles, like herpes simplex virions, are assembled in the nucleus (see Fig. 53–11), attain their envelope at the nuclear membrane, and migrate through reduplications of the nuclear membrane into the cytoplasmic endoplasmic reticulum. The maturation of viral particles appears to be inefficient: only rare, completely assembled virions can be detected among many incomplete particles (many of these are noninfectious dense bodies formed by enveloped viral proteins without DNA or assembled capsids). Hence, the yield of infectious virus in cell cultures is low, and as many as 10^6 particles are needed to initiate infection of a new culture. Most infectious virus remains cell associated, and the addition of intact infected cells to a culture therefore initiates viral propagation most efficiently.

Unlike herpes simplex viruses, CMV does not interrupt host macromolecular synthesis but rather stimulates host RNA and DNA synthesis in parallel with viral DNA replication. Accordingly, infected cells are not usually killed, and this explains why latent infections are frequently established.

PATHOGENESIS

CMVs are the most common cause of intrauterine infections. An increasing number of pregnant women excrete CMV as gestation proceeds, apparently owing to increasing levels of certain hormones (e.g., cortisol). Primary infection occurs in 19% to 20% of seronegative pregnant women, with subsequent infection of about 50% of the fetuses. In contrast, only 10% to 20% of pregnant women with latent infection transmit CMV to their fetuses. A mother with a primary or latent infection may transmit CMV to the fetus, either by transplacental transfer during pregnancy or by excreting virus into the genital tract at the time of birth. Protracted viral shedding may follow (although neutralizing Abs develop), and the infant carrier may serve as a source for dissemination (in different studies 15% to 60% of healthy children were shown to excrete virus during the first year of life). Although prolonged viral persistence is common following congenital infection, indefinite persistence is rare, and viral shedding is unusual in adults with Abs. Virus may also become latent in the newborn or during early childhood. Manifest illness infrequently occurs in newborns and infants up to 4 months of age, but if it appears, it usually has a relentless progression, with hepatic and renal insufficiency, pneumonia, neurologic symptoms, and eventual death.

Patients with neoplastic diseases and recipients of organ transplants, subjected to corticosteroids or other immunosuppressive drugs, or those with acquired immune deficiency diseases (e.g., AIDS) are particularly susceptible to viral activation or exogenous infection that results in localized or disseminated disease or inapparent infection. A syndrome resembling infectious mononucleosis (see below) may be observed in recipients of multiple transfusions of blood from latently infected donors. The syndrome has most frequently been reported in patients who have undergone open heart surgery, probably because of the large volumes of blood they receive. Reactivation of a latent infection or occurrence of primary disease, such as following multiple transfusions, is usually associated with an increase in suppressor-cytotoxic T cells (OKT8) and a decrease in helper cells (OKT4).

Like adenoviruses (see Chap. 52), CMVs can be isolated from explants of apparently normal adenoids and salivary glands cultured *in vitro* (see Pathogenesis, Chap. 52). Similar findings have been made with CMVs of mice, rats, hamsters, and guinea pigs.

The pathologic lesion is characterized by necrosis and pathognomonic cellular alterations. The affected cells are greatly increased in size; the nucleus is enlarged and contains a brightly stained eosinophilic inclusion body up to 15 μm in diameter (see Fig. 53–12), larger than that produced by any other virus infecting humans. In addition, the cytoplasm may be swollen and vacuolated and may show up to 20 minute basophilic and osmiophilic structures 2 μm to 4 μm in diameter; these contain DNA and polysaccharide and are therefore positive with Feulgen and periodic acid–Schiff stains.

LABORATORY DIAGNOSIS

Infection can be identified by viral isolation, immunologic assays, and exfoliative cytologic techniques:

Isolation of virus in cultures of human embryonic fibroblasts is the most sensitive method to detect infection in the newborn. Viral replication can be detected within 24 to 36 hours by means of **immunofluorescence, DNA–DNA hybridization** (or *in situ* DNA–RNA hybridization), or *ELISA* techniques. Thus, diagnosis can be made more rapidly, with high sensitivity and accuracy, and less expensively than with actual isolation and immunologic identification of the isolates.

Identification of characteristic cytomegalic cells with intranuclear and cytoplasmic inclusions (particularly in urinary sediment and bronchial and gastric washings) is an inexpensive diagnostic procedure. Detection of viral DNA or Ags by the techniques noted above can rapidly confirm the cytologic diagnosis.

Immunologic assays are valuable for diagnosis by demonstrating an increase in Ab titers. A variety of techniques are available: immunofluorescence, which can also distinguish a baby's IgM Abs from maternal IgG Abs; ELISA; indirect hemagglutination and latex particle agglutination, in which either tanned red blood cells or latex particles are coated with viral Ags; and CF. These techniques are rapid and inexpensive.

EPIDEMIOLOGY AND CONTROL

Infection with human CMV appears to be worldwide and common despite the relative rarity of clinical disease. About 5% to 10% of congenitally infected newborns display signs and symptoms of CMV disease, and from 10% to 18% of all stillborns show characteristic lesions at autopsy. In adults above 16 years of age, typical inclusions in salivary glands are rare, but in a sample taken in the United States, CF Abs were found in 53% of the population between 18 and 25 years old and in 81% of those over 35 years of age. Transplacental passage and infection at birth, during nursing, during blood transfusion, and during sexual intercourse are the most apparent mechanisms for transmitting virus, but person-to-person spread in urine and respiratory secretions seems likely. Latent virus has been detected in lymphocytes, a fact that highlights at least one means by which virus is transmitted while apparently noninfectious. Among pregnant women, 10% to 15% excrete virus during their third trimester, and at least 1% of newborns enter the world with viruria. Children and adults with immunologic deficiencies, naturally or iatrogenically acquired, are particularly susceptible to active disease. Vaccines consisting of attenuated strains and antiviral drugs (e.g., acylovir and interferon) are being studied, but effective measures for prevention and control will probably not be available until more is known of viral characteristics and transmission.

EB (Epstein-Barr) Virus and Infectious Mononucleosis

In a search for the cause of Burkitt lymphoma, Epstein and Barr, in 1964, observed herpeslike viral particles (termed *EB virus*; Fig. 53–13) in a small proportion (0.5%–10%) of the lymphoma cells repetitively cultured *in vitro*. The relation of EB virus to the malignancy is discussed in Chapter 64.

EB virus, however, has been shown to be the cause of infectious mononucleosis. The first indication of this relationship came 4 years after the discovery of EB virus, when G. and W. Henle discovered that lymphocytes from their technician, who had just recovered from infectious mononucleosis, could be serially cultured *in vitro*, unlike normal lymphocytes; and a small number of these cultured cells were found to contain EB virus. Further observations supported the conclusion that EB virus is the etiologic agent of infectious mononucleosis: (1) Transfusion of blood from such persons produces the disease in recipients devoid of Abs. (2) The virus persists in lymphocytes cultured from patients long after recovery from infectious mononucleosis. (3) Patients with infectious mononucleosis develop neutralizing and CF Abs, as well as Abs that react with EB virus–infected cells in an immunofluorescence assay. (4) The Abs persist for years, and their presence or absence is correlated with resistance or susceptibility to infectious mononucleosis. Finally, (5) EB virus has been isolated from pharyngeal secretions of patients with infectious mononucleosis.

PROPERTIES

Virions purified from cultured Burkitt lymphoma cells (Fig. 53–14) are structurally similar to those of other herpesviruses (see Fig. 53–2 and Characteristics of Members

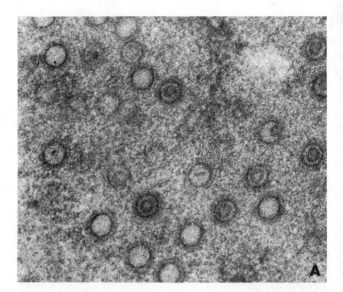
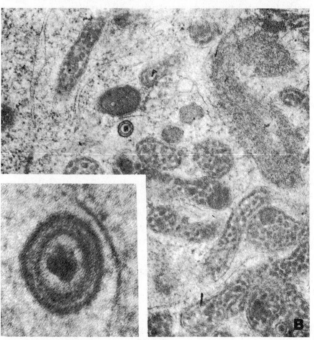

Figure 53–13. Structure of EB virus in cells cultured from Burkitt lymphoma. *(A)* Numerous developing immature particles in a thin section of a lymphoblast nucleus. (Original magnification ×76,500) *(B)* Mature viral particle with envelope, capsid, and nucleoid in the cytoplasm. (Original magnification ×42,000; *inset,* ×213,500; Epstein MA et al: J Exp Med 121:761, 1965)

of the Herpesvirus Family). The virion contains about the same number and size proteins as herpes simplex virus. The structure of the viral DNA isolated from infectious mononucleosis patients or from the transformed cell

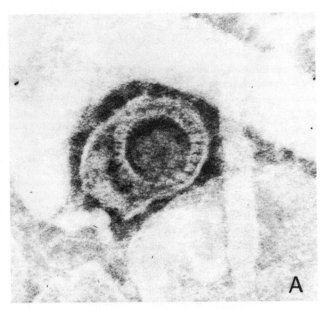 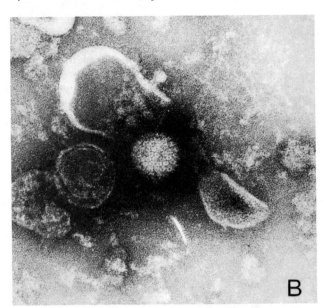

Figure 53–14. Structure of EB virus obtained from cultured Burkitt lymphoma cells. Electron micrographs are of purified, negatively stained virus. **(A)** Empty capsid enclosed in an envelope. (Original magnification ×200,000) **(B)** Viral particle with a disrupted envelope. A capsid (about 75 nm in diameter) similar to that of herpesviruses is clearly visible. (Original magnification ×120,000; Courtesy of K. Hummler)

lines is unique as compared with other herpesviruses (see Fig. 53–1). Indeed, EB virus DNA consists of five unique regions of DNA and seven regions of repeated DNA sequences, including the ends of the genome, which has six to 12 multiple tandem copies. It is also noteworthy that EB virus DNA shows considerable polymorphism among its isolates from patients. However, viral DNA from lymphoid cell lines derived from patients with infectious mononucleosis, though of the same size, differs in about 35% of the sequences when compared with EB virus DNA derived from Burkitt lymphomas. EB virus is immunologically unrelated to other herpesviruses.

The virus selectively infects human B-lymphocytes by means of a receptor related or identical to the receptor for the third component of complement, C3d. The hallmark of infection is **transformation** of the infected cell to a continuously dividing B-lymphocyte cell line—so-called **immortalized** cells. Infection primarily results in **latent infection** in which only limited, noncontiguous regions of the genome are transcribed, yielding at least three **nuclear Ags (EBNAs)** and a **membrane Ag** the precise functions of which are unknown. The most abundant transcripts detected during latent infections are two small, nonmessenger RNAs that appear to be transcribed by polymerase III. Following the immediate early events of infection, including production of a virus-encoded DNA polymerase and a DNase, the linear virion DNA is converted to a covalently closed circular mole-

cule via its large terminal repeated nucleotide sequences (see Fig. 53–1). The viral DNA replicates and primarily exists in this episomal form, although small numbers of integrated viral genomes have been detected in some cell lines and in tumor cells.

Latent infection can be converted to the **replicative** phase by several means. *In vitro* cultivation of lymphoid cells infected *in vivo* (e.g., lymphoid cells from patients with infectious mononucleosis) induces production of infectious virus in a small proportion of the cells. The replicative cycle can also be induced by a variety of chemical agents such as uridine analogues or the phorbol ester tumor promoter. The replicative cycle is marked by extensive transcription, increased DNA replication, and production of late proteins, which include capsid antigens and glycoproteins of which at least two (gp 350 and gp 220) are incorporated into the viral envelope and contain epitopes that induce neutralizing Abs. However, the induced cells produce relatively small amounts of infectious virus.

INFECTIOUS MONONUCLEOSIS
Pathogenesis

Primary infection ordinarily occurs via the oral route, and the virus initially replicates in the oropharyngeal epithelium and in the epithelium of salivary gland ducts. The intimate association of lymphoid and epithelial cells in the oropharynx permits ready infection of B-lymphocytes at this site and ensures entrance of EB virus–infected B cells into the circulation. In the largest proportion of the world population these events of primary infection occur during the first few years of life and usually produce only subclinical infection. In the developed countries, apparently owing to the improved hygienic conditions, primary infection is delayed until the age of 15 years or older, and this delayed infection results in the **clinical disease infectious mononucleosis** in up to 50% of the persons infected.

Infectious mononucleosis is an acute infectious disease, primarily affecting lymphoid tissue throughout the body. It is characterized by the appearance of enlarged and often tender lymph nodes, an enlarged spleen, and abnormal lymphocytes in the blood (from which the disease derives its name). In addition, fever and sore throat are common. Occasionally, other diverse manifestations are observed, including mild hepatitis, signs of meningitis or other central nervous system involvement, hematuria, proteinuria, thrombocytopenic purpura, and hemolytic anemia.

Following acute disease, EB virus persists for weeks to months in the oropharyngeal secretions of patients. In a small number of these patients, particularly in young adults (25–35 years), persisting illness and fatigue accompany the continuing viral replication. Whether EB virus causes the chronic illness or is an epiphenomenon is still unclear.

In addition to the EB virus–induced, polyclonal activation of B-lymphocytes, patients with infectious mononucleosis mount a specific Ab response to the viral infection. IgM and IgG Abs are directed against Ags produced during viral replication: early Ags, the viral capsid Ag, and the glycoprotein membrane Ags. The appearance of Abs to the EB virus nuclear Ags is a sign of the development of latent infection. Infection also induces a marked cell-mediated immune response, which is probably mainly responsible for the outcome of the acute EB virus infection. It is the marked proliferation of T-cell (T8) lymphoblasts that produces the characteristic atypical mononuclear cells that are prominent in the blood of patients with infectious mononucleosis. The expanded T-cell population consists to a large extent of EB virus–specific cytotoxic T cells. The increase in cytotoxic T cells results in a reversal of the T4/T8 ratio for 4 to 8 weeks. An increased activity of natural killer cells directed at a variety of Ags also appears early in infection.

Laboratory Diagnosis

Specific diagnosis depends on (1) detection of viral DNA, infectious virus, or viral Ags, (2) Ab response, and (3) observation of abnormal lymphocytes in the peripheral blood.

Intracellular viral DNA can readily be detected by DNA:DNA hybridization with *in vitro* labeled EB virus DNA probes. **Infectious virus** is isolated from peripheral blood, saliva, and lymphoid tissue with immortalization of human B-lymphocytes used as the assay (those from umbilical cord blood are most sensitive). **Viral Ags** are most easily identified by the **indirect immunofluorescence assay;** acute infection is diagnosed with Abs directed against either the capsid Ag in a cell line producing EB viruses or early Ag in nonproducer cell lines superinfected with EB virus. **ELISA** will probably also soon be available for diagnosis. **Serologic tests** can be used but are difficult to interpret owing to the long persistence of Abs following infection. Serologic diagnosis of acute infectious mononucleosis can best be accomplished by demonstrating IgM Abs to capsid Ag or development of Abs to EB virus nuclear Ags, since the nuclear Ags do not appear until late during primary infection.

These techniques for detection of virus or serologic response are specific and highly sensitive, but they are highly specialized and not yet suitable for the general hospital laboratory. A **practical laboratory diagnosis** can be made based on two unique findings:

- **Abnormal, large lymphocytes** with deeply basophilic, foamy cytoplasm and fenestrated nuclei appear, often accounting for 50% to 90% of the circulating lymphocytes. Initially there is a leukopenia, but by the second week of disease the count may rise to 10,000 to 80,000 cells/mm³.
- **Heterophil Abs** (i.e., agglutinins for sheep red blood cells) develop in 50% to 90% of patients during the course of the disease.

The immunogen eliciting the heterophil Abs is unknown, but it appears to be distinct from the EB virus. Thus, a small percentage of patients develop EB virus Abs but no heterophil Abs; heterophil Abs can be adsorbed from serum by bovine red blood cells without reducing the Ab titer to EB virus; and heterophil Abs are transient, but Abs to EB virus persist for years, perhaps for life.

Heterophil Abs also appear during serum sickness following injection of horse serum, and they may be present in serum from healthy persons. However, a differential adsorption test of a patient's serum distinguishes these Abs. Thus, heterophil Abs of infectious mononucleosis are adsorbed by bovine red blood cells but not by guinea pig kidney (which contains Forssman Ag); serum sickness agglutinins are adsorbed by both bovine red blood cells and guinea pig kidney; and normal serum heterophil agglutinins are adsorbed by guinea pig kidney but not usually by bovine red blood cells.

Epidemiology and Control

Infectious mononucleosis appears to be primarily a disease of relatively affluent teenagers and young adults (such as college students), in whom it causes proved disease in about 15% of the susceptible population. (About 75% of entering college students in the United States are free of detectable Abs). The peak incidence is at 15 to 20 years of age.

Successful infection appears to require extensive exposure, or unknown cooperating factors, for multiple cases in families are infrequent despite the presence of virus in pharyngeal secretions of infected persons. In cases of infectious mononucleosis the source of the infecting virus is rarely obvious, perhaps because persons with latent infections produce the virus in pharyngeal and oral secretions for prolonged periods after recovery. The common association of infectious mononucleosis with intensive kissing may reflect a requirement for a large inoculum. No adequate control procedures are available.

Human Herpesvirus 6 (HHV-6)

A previously unidentified member of the herpesvirus family was isolated from peripheral blood mononuclear cells of six patients with lymphoproliferative diseases in 1986. The virus has since been isolated from healthy adults who possessed HHV-6 Abs, as well as from patients with a variety of lymphoproliferative diseases, AIDS and AIDS-related complex (ARC) (see Chap. 65) in the United States, Great Britain, and parts of Africa. All of the isolates were immunologically related to each other but distinct from types 1 and 2 herpes simplex viruses, CMV, varicella-herpes zoster virus, and EB virus. HHV-6 is also immunologically unrelated to simian herpesvirus and Marek's disease virus. Like other herpesviruses the vi-

rion's capsid is icosahedral, composed of 162 capsomers, and enclosed in a lipid membrane envelope. The genome is a linear, double-stranded DNA molecule of about 150,000 base-pairs and a guanine + cytosine (G + C) content of about 40 percent. HHV-6 can infect and replicate in cultures of B-cells, T-cells, and monocyte/macrophages, but the natural host cells in humans is still unclear. Whether HHV-6 is the etiological agent of any disease or merely a latent virus that is occasionally activated is also uncertain.

Selected Reading

Gershon AA, Steinberg SP, LaRussa P, Ferrara A: The National Institutes of Allergy and Infectious Diseases Varicella Vaccine Collaborative Study Group: Live attenuated varicella vaccine: Efficacy for children with leukemia in remission. JAMA 252:355, 1984

Klein RJ: Initiation and maintenance of latent herpes simplex virus infections: The paradox of perpetual immobility and continuous movement. Rev Infect Dis 7:211, 1985

Pass RF: Epidemiology and transmission of cytomegolavirus. J Infect Dis 152:243, 1985

Rapp F: Persistence and transmission of cytomegalovirus. In Fraenkel-Conrat H, Wagner RR (eds): Comprehensive Virology, Vol 16, p 193. New York, Plenum, 1980

Rickinson AB, Yao QY, Wallace LE: The Epstein-Barr virus as a model of virus–host interactions. Br Med Bull 41:75, 1985

Roizman B (ed): Herpesviruses, Vols I and II. New York, Plenum, 1982

Wagner EK: Individual HSV transcripts: Characterization of specific genes. In Roizman B (ed): Herpesviruses, Vol 3. New York, Plenum, 1984

Wathen MW, Stinski MF: Temporal patterns of human cytomegalovirus transcription: Mapping the viral RNAs synthesized at immediate early, early, and late times after infection. J Virol 41:462, 1982

54

Poxviruses

The smallpox was always present, filling the churchyards with corpses, tormenting with constant fears all whom it had striken, leaving on those whose lives it spared the hideous traces of its power, turning the babe into a changeling at which the mother shuddered, and making the eyes and cheeks of the bethrothed maiden objects of horror to the lover.
—T. B. Macaulay: *The History of England From the Accession of James II,* Vol. IV

It now becomes too manifest to admit of controversy that the annihilation of the smallpox, the most dreadful scourge of the human species, must be the result of this practice (of vaccination).
—Edward Jenner: *The Origin of the Vaccine Inoculation,* 1801

Since the beginning of history, smallpox* has left its indelible mark on the medical, political, and cultural affairs of man. Records show severe epidemics from earliest times. Indeed, by the 18th century the disease had become endemic in the major cities of Europe. Terror of its presence was such that "no man dared to count his children as his own until they had had the disease."†

Because virulent smallpox strains appear to have no animal reservoir, and because vaccination is very effective, complete eradication of this scourge—long a dream of public health authorities—has now become a reality as the result of a vigorous World Health Organization (WHO) program of confinement and immunization initiated in 1966. Whereas in 1945 most of the world's inhabitants lived in endemic areas, October 1977 saw the last reported case of natural infection, detected in Somalia. Immunization has eliminated smallpox from the rest of the world (including India and Pakistan, where severe epidemics still occurred in 1973), and no documented case has been reported in the United States since 1949.

---

* A term initially employed to distinguish the disease from "large pox" (syphilis)

† The Comte de la Condamine, an 18th century French mathematician and scientist

In 1980 the WHO declared that smallpox had been globally eradicated. This remarkable feat has resulted in the saving of over $1 billion annually in global health expenditures, and in the United States it has brought a saving of about $150 million annually in the cost of vaccination and quarantine measures.

With the disappearance of the disease, and with the decline in enforced vaccination, susceptibility will slowly return, bringing a liability to massive epidemics if a source of infection should appear. Hence, it is still too early to be certain that this virus is buried in the graveyard of extinct organisms. There is no absolute certainty that a persistent, unrecognized focus of variola (smallpox) virus does not exist, that a member of another species of poxviruses (e.g., monkeypox or cowpox viruses) may not undergo genetic variation to virulence for humans, or that biological warfare—a horrifying possibility—would not reintroduce smallpox virus. To reduce the risk of escape of this virus from a laboratory (such as occurred in Birmingham, England in 1978, resulting in two cases), the WHO led the campaign to destroy stocks of smallpox virus throughout the world except in four designated laboratories. Thus, in the United States only a single reference stock is preserved, under stringent controls, at the Center for Disease Control in Atlanta.

It would clearly be unwise to ignore the smallpox virus entirely: continued knowledge and constant vigilance are still required. This chapter briefly presents the characteristics of poxviruses and how they replicate. Particular emphasis is placed on the properties of smallpox virus that permitted eradication of the disease it produces, and the methods employed in the eradication program.

General Characteristics

The smallpox (variola) virus is representative of the **poxviruses,** a group of agents that infect both humans and lower animals and produce characteristic vesicular skin lesions, often called **pocks.** Poxviruses (**family Poxviridae**) are the largest of animal viruses (see Characteristics of the Poxviruses): they can be seen with phase optics or in stained preparations with the light microscope. The viral particles (originally called **elementary bodies**) are somewhat rounded, brick-shaped, or ovoid and have a complex structure consisting of an internal central mass—the nucleoid—surrounded by two membrane layers (Figs. 54–1 through 54–3). The surface is covered with ridges that may be tubules or threads (see Fig. 54–2). Poxviruses contain DNA, protein, and lipid. They are relatively resistant to inactivation by common disinfectants and by heat, drying, and cold, characteristics that made their spread so easy in susceptible populations.

The **genus Orthopoxvirus** consists of viruses of certain mammals, including variola, vaccinia, monkeypox,

---

CHARACTERISTICS OF THE POXVIRUSES

Size: 250–390 nm × 200–260 nm

Morphology: Brick-shaped to ovoid (see Figs. 54–1, 54–9, 54–10)

Protein and lipid content: Present (vaccinia: 91.6% and 5%, respectively)

Stability: Relatively resistant to inactivation by chemicals (disinfectants) or by heat, cold, or drying; inactivated by chloroform; variably inactivated by ether

Nucleic acid: Double-stranded DNA*

Molecular weights (daltons) and base ratio: Vaccinia 150×10^6 (3.2% of the virion; 231 kilobase pairs); AT/GC = 1.67†

Fowlpox 200×10^6 (307 kilobase pairs); AT/GC = 1.84

Antigenicity: Common family and genus Ags

Multiplication‡: In cytoplasm of cells but requires host RNA polymerase II subunit from nucleus

Cytopathogenicity: Predilection for epidermal cells; eosinophilic inclusion bodies produced

* Complementary strands of vaccinia DNA are covalently crosslinked at or near the termini. Other poxviruses have not been examined for this structure.

† DNAs of cowpox, rabbitpox, and mousepox are similar.

‡ A DNA-dependent RNA polymerase in virion.

---

cowpox, ectromelia of mice, rabbitpox, camelpox and gerbilpox viruses. **Other genera** include viruses specific for birds (*Avipoxvirus*), ungulates (*Capipoxvirus*), and arthropods (*Entomopoxvirus*) and the tumor-producing (fibroma and myxoma) viruses of rabbits (*Leporipoxvirus*). Viruses of a sixth genus, which resemble other poxviruses in structure but not immunologically (hence termed *Parapoxviruses*), include **contagious pustular dermatitis (orf), paravaccinia (milker's nodules),** and

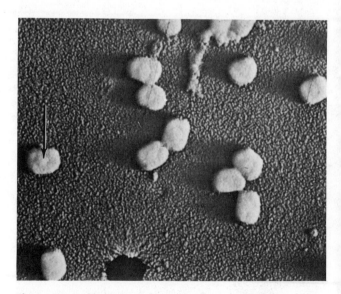

Figure 54–1. Morphology of vaccinia virus as revealed by electron microscopic examination of a shadowed preparation of purified viral particles. Note the central core surrounded by a depression (*arrow*). (Original magnification ×28,000; Sharp DG et al: Proc Soc Exp Biol Med 61:259, 1946)

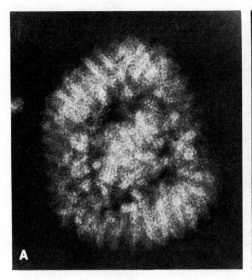

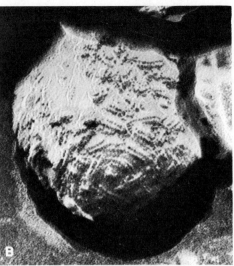

Figure 54–2. Fine structure of a mature vaccinia virion from a purified suspension of viral particles. *(A)* Virion negatively stained with phosphotungstate. The double tract of ridges and a suggestion of the subunit structure can be seen. The protrusion and sawtooth effect of the ridges are noticeable at the periphery. (Original magnification ×224,000) *(B)* Freeze-etched virion, showing subunits, length, and random orientation of the double ridge. (Original magnification ×224,000; Medzon EL, Bauer H: Virology 40:860, 1970)

bovine papular stomatitis viruses. Some poxviruses, such as the **molluscum contagiosum virus** and **Yaba monkey tumor virus,** cannot be classified immunologically in any of these genera.

All poxviruses studied are related immunologically by a common internal Ag extractable from viral particles. They can be divided into genera on the basis of their more specific Ags, nucleic acid homology, morphology, and natural hosts.

Genetic recombination may occur, but only between two viruses of the same immunologic group. The proportion of recombinants seems to be related to the degree of homology between the viral DNAs and parallels the degree of antigenic cross-reactivity.

Poxviruses vary widely in their ability to cause generalized infection, but they share a **predilection for epidermal cells,** in which they multiply in the cytoplasm and produce **eosinophilic inclusion bodies** (termed

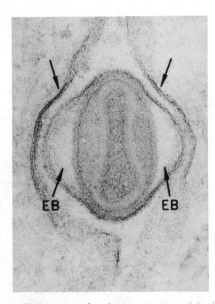

Figure 54–3. Thin section of an intact mature vaccinia virus particle showing the inner nucleic acid core and surrounding membranes. The elliptical body (*EB*) on each side of the nucleoid causes a prominent central bulging of the virion. The viral particle is lodged between two cells (*arrows*). (Original magnification ×120,000; Dales S: J Cell Biol 18:51, 1963)

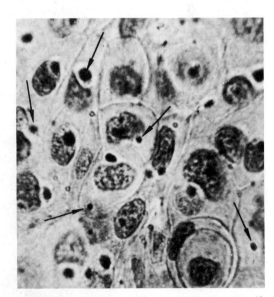

Figure 54–4. Eosinophilic cytoplasmic inclusion bodies (Guarnieri bodies) in corneal epithelial cells of a rabbit eye infected with vaccinia virus. (Original magnification ×900); Coriell LL et al: J Invest Dermatol 11:313, 1948)

Guarnieri bodies; Fig. 54–4). Fibroma and myxoma viruses have, in addition, a great affinity for subcutaneous connective tissues. Most poxviruses also multiply readily in epidermal cells of the chorioallantois of chick embryos, where they produce characteristic **nodular focal lesions,** termed *pocks* (Fig. 54–5). These lesions reflect a second characteristic of poxviruses: the **propensity to cause cellular hyperplasia** before cell necrosis. With myxoma, fibroma, and Yaba viruses the hyperplasia predominates, and tumors develop.

Variola (Smallpox) and Vaccinia

PROPERTIES

The virulence and contagiousness of smallpox virus have understandably limited its laboratory investigation. On the other hand, the closely related and much less dangerous vaccinia virus is one of the most thoroughly investigated animal viruses. Since the two viruses are very similar, they are discussed together.

Morphology

The morphology of vaccinia virions is revealed by various techniques of electron microscopy (see Figs. 54–1 through Fig. 54–3). Viral particles from smallpox crusts and vesicle fluids are morphologically indistinguishable from vaccinia particles. Thin sections (see Fig. 54–3) disclose a **central nucleoid** with a dumbbell-shaped dense coil composed of the viral DNA. The nucleoid is surrounded by **lipoprotein membranes,** and between the nucleoid and the outer viral coat is an **ellipsoidal body.**

In addition to the viral DNA, the viral cores contain several enzymes, primarily for transcription and modification of **immediate early mRNAs:** e.g., DNA-dependent RNA polymerase, polyadenylate polymerase, methyltransferase, and guanylyltransferase.

Chemical and Physical Characteristics

The chemical and physical characteristics of vaccinia virus, the first animal virus to be prepared in sufficient purity and quantity for detailed analysis, are summarized under Characteristics of the Poxviruses. The complexity of the virion is made apparent by the presence of more than 80 distinct species of polypeptides. Their precise localization in the core, lipoprotein membranes, and virion surface structures is only partially known. The majority of the polypeptides, however, are core components, either basic proteins needed for tight folding of the large DNA molecule or virion enzymes essential for uncoating and initiating viral multiplication.

Variola and vaccinia viruses are **relatively stable;** they resist drying and retain their infectivity for many months at 4°C and for years at −20°C to −70°C. Thus, exudates or crusts taken from patients with smallpox may yield infectious virus after almost a year at room temperature, and diagnostic specimens do not need refrigeration. The persistence of infectious variola virus on bedclothes caused a hazard not only for medical personnel but even for laundry workers. The relative resistance of the virus to dilute phenol and other common disinfectants complicated the decontamination of clothing, instruments, furniture, and so forth. However, variola and vaccinia viruses are inactivated by apolar lipophilic solvents (e.g., chloroform), by autoclaving, or by heating at 60°C for 10 minutes.

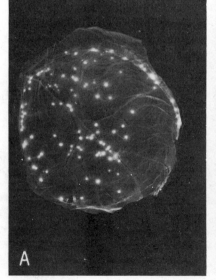 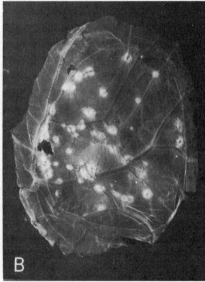

Figure 54–5. Pocks produced by variola virus (**A**) and vaccinia virus (**B**) 3 days after viral inoculation of the chorioallantoic membranes of chick embryos. Note the small gray-white pocks produced by variola virus and the large pocks made by vaccinia virus. (Downie AW, MacDonald A: Br Med Bull 9:191, 1953)

Antigenic Structure and Immunity

The antigenic structure of poxviruses has been examined largely with vaccinia virus, but smallpox virus is very similar. Viral strains from cases of severe smallpox (**variola major**) and those from cases of **variola minor (alastrim)** are immunologically indistinguishable. Moreover, it is striking that the antigens of smallpox viruses have not changed in their immunologic reactivity over the centuries that this virus has been a scourge throughout the world.

The Ags of poxviruses can be measured by all the usual immunologic techniques, including hemagglutination inhibition and neutralization of infectivity.

Stepwise dissection of purified virions with trypsin or chymotrypsin, 2-mercaptoethanol, and a nonionic detergent (e.g., Nonidet P40) permits localization of some of the Ags and polypeptides: (1) Two Ags responsible for neutralizing Abs are present in the tubules of the outer surface membrane; (2) Ags in the viral envelope evoke neutralizing Abs that protect against dissemination of virions throughout the body; (3) one large and three small Ags are identified in the core; and (4) one large Ag has been located between the core and the surface structures. The neutralizing Abs induced by the two surface Ags neutralize only viruses from the homologous subgroup. Neither of these sets of Ags is found on inactivated virus, a fact that explains the ineffectiveness of inactivated virus vaccines. A **family Ag,** which is a component of the core and one of the constituents of the NP fraction, can be extracted from virions with weak alkali; it cross-reacts, in complement fixation (CF) and precipitin assays, with a similar Ag from all poxviruses. Although it is not yet possible to identify the Ags with specific polypeptide chains, most of the polypeptides, have been topographically located in the virion.

Unlike other viruses, the **hemagglutinin** of variola and vaccinia viruses is not a component of the viral particle, and its Abs do not neutralize viral infectivity. It is a lipoprotein embedded in the membranes of infected cells and probably corresponds to a new surface Ag.

Antibody Response

Following infection or immunization, Abs to each of the viral Ags develop. The variations observed in their time of appearance and persistence depend on the nature and quantity of the Ag. Thus, neutralizing and hemagglutination-inhibiting Abs are first detected about the sixth day after onset of illness in the unvaccinated person, whereas CF Abs ordinarily appear 2 to 3 days later. Neutralizing and hemagglutination-inhibition Abs persist at least 20 years after infection, but CF Abs remain less than 2 years. In persons previously immunized, the various Abs generally appear 2 to 3 days sooner after onset of illness, reach higher titers, and persist longer.

Following natural infection, immunity to smallpox is long-lasting, if not persistent for life. In the rare reinfections that have been reported, the disease is usually atypical, very mild, and often without skin rash (variola sine eruptione). Immunity following vaccination, however, may last no longer than a year, and when smallpox was extant, immunization was recommended immediately following exposure regardless of when last vaccinated. If infection occurred in vaccinated persons, the clinical disease was also usually milder than in unimmunized neighbors.

The relative importance of **humoral** and **cellular immunity** remains largely unexplored, although cell-mediated immunity appears to be critical for recovery from infection. Thus, immunization with live vaccine has led to disease in persons with congenital defects of T-lymphocytes (see Chap. 50), as discussed under Complications of Vaccination, below.

Host Range

Variola virus has a much more limited host range than do vaccinia and other poxviruses. Monkeys are the only animals, other than man, known to be naturally infected; also, when variola virus is placed onto monkeys' scarified skin or inoculated intradermally, local lesions and fever follow. A few **animals** (chick embryos, rabbits, mice) and **cultured cells** (e.g., human embryonic kidney, monkey kidney, HeLa cells) are susceptible to experimental infection, and these have been valuable for diagnosis and research.

Multiplication

Although poxviruses contain DNA, **biosynthesis of the viral components and their assembly into viral particles take place entirely within the cytoplasm of the cell.** However, although most biosynthetic reactions can occur in enucleated cells, a large subunit of the nuclear host RNA polymerase II joins with a virus-encoded RNA polymerase subunit to transcribe a special set of mRNAs.

Virus attaches to uncharacterized host cell receptors, and it enters the cytoplasm primarily by the process of engulfment (see Chap. 48). After penetration, viral DNA is released by a **two-stage uncoating process** (see Chap. 48). The first stage is initiated almost immediately after engulfment by preexisting host cell enzymes, which break down the viral membrane part of the protein coat of the viral particle and the membrane of the endocytic vesicle to free the nucleoprotein core into the cytoplasm. The second stage results in breakdown of this core to liberate viral DNA. At the onset of this second stage, a DNA-dependent RNA polymerase present in the intact core transcribes about 25% of the viral genome. The resulting transcripts are processed within the core, and functional **immediate early mRNAs** emerge. They code for proteins required for the final uncoating events and for the enzymes necessary to produce the RNA for a second set of mRNAs, **delayed early.** Finally, after **viral DNA replication** begins, **late mRNAs** appear (derived from about 60% of the genome), while at least some early messengers continue to be made. Transcription continues until about 7 hours after infection. The kinetics of viral macromolecular biosynthesis are presented in Figure 54–6, and the sequential replication events are summarized diagrammatically in Figure 54–7.

Synthesis of **specific enzymes** and of a few **viral structural proteins** begins early in the biosynthetic process, before replication of viral DNA. The products include the second-stage uncoating proteins, three proteins associated with the nucleoprotein core, a protein essential for initiation of viral DNA replication, and enzymes related to DNA biosynthesis.

Viral DNA begins to be synthesized 1.5 to 2 hours after infection and attains its maximal concentration by the time newly made infectious virus is first detected (see Fig. 54–6). The **mode of DNA replication** is imposed by the unique covalent crosslinking of the two strands (see Synthesis of DNA-Containing Viruses, Chap. 48). Synthesis is initiated at either end of the genome. Large circular and forked replicating forms are found, indicating that an endonuclease cleaves the single-stranded crosslinks during replication. **Late viral proteins** are first detected about 4 hours after infection, and **infectious virus** is formed about 1 hour later by packaging viral DNA ran-

domly selected from the preformed pool (see Figs. 54–6, 54–7). **Posttranslational modifications** of several proteins (i.e., cleavage, glycosylation, and phosphorylation) are essential to virion maturation.

Concomitant with the biosynthesis of virus-directed mRNA and viral DNA, biosynthesis of host cell macromolecules is inhibited. Production of host proteins stops because initiation of polypeptide chain synthesis is blocked, and host cell polyribosomes are disrupted; host DNA ceases replicating; and the host mRNAs cannot leave the nucleus, although their synthesis continues unaltered for about 3 hours. How these controls of host cell biosynthesis are induced by the virus and whether they relate to cell injury are still unknown.

The morphologic counterparts of the foregoing biochemical events have been observed in thin sections of infected cells (Fig. 54–8). As viral DNA synthesis increases, regions of dense fibrous material appear in the cell cytoplasm. About 3 hours after infection, some of the early proteins form membranelike structures, which begin to enclose patches of viral components and proceed to form immature particles into which DNA enters. (Fig. 54–8A and B). After the envelope is completed, the nucleoid begins to take shape within the immature particle; an additional membrane encloses the condensing DNA; the lateral bodies differentiate; and, finally, the outer coat structures are laid down on the previously formed membrane, completing the assembly of mature virions (see Fig. 54–7).

Lysis of infected cells is not a prerequisite for liberation of newly formed virions. The viral particles seem to be released through cell villi. Radioautography and immunofluorescence reveal that viral materials may also be transmitted directly from cell to cell through villi.

SMALLPOX
Pathogenesis

Two basic forms of smallpox are recognized: **variola major,** which has a case fatality rate of approximately 25%, and **variola minor,** or alastrim, a less virulent form with a mortality rate below 1%. Although a variety of factors may influence the mortality rate in any epidemic, the epidemiologic evidence is convincing that severe and mild smallpox exist as distinct entities. Nevertheless, it is impossible to distinguish the viruses responsible for these two forms of the disease.

Virus multiplies first in the mucosa of the upper respiratory tract and then in the regional lymph nodes. A **transient viremia** then disseminates virus to internal organs (liver, spleen, lungs), where the virus propagates extensively. A **second viral invasion of the bloodstream** terminates the incubation period (about 12 days) and initiates the **toxemic phase,** characterized by prodromal macular rashes, fever, generalized aching, head-

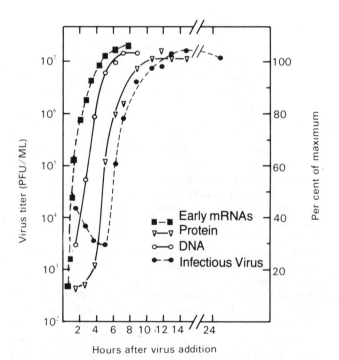

Figure 54–6. Biosynthetic events in the multiplication of vaccinia virus. (Modified from Salzman NP et al: Virology 19:542, 1963)

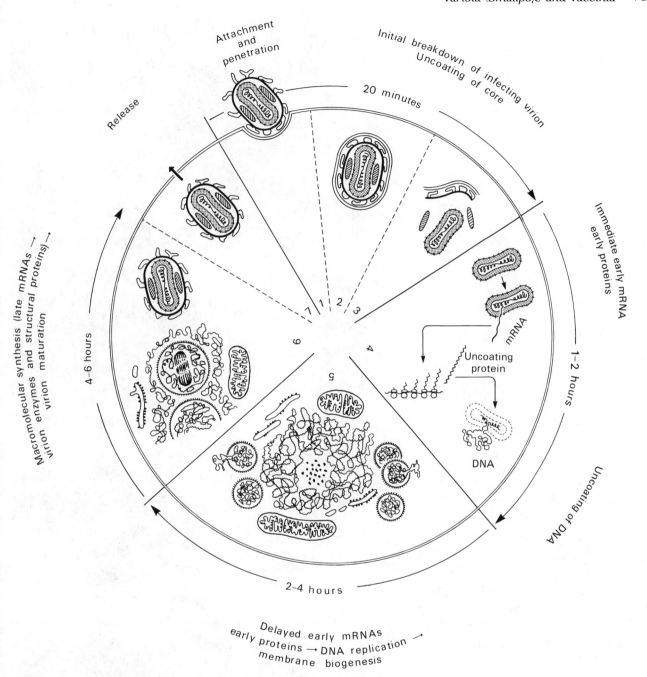

Figure 54–7. Diagram of the sequential events of vaccinia virus infection of a single cell.

ache, malaise, and prostration. Virus spreads to the skin and multiplies in the epidermal cells; the characteristic skin eruption follows in 3 to 4 days. Macular at onset, the rash progresses from papular to vesicular, finally becoming pustular in the second week of illness. In severe cases the rash may become hemorrhagic or confluent. The course of variola minor is similar but shorter, and the rash and other symptoms are less severe.

The **inclusion bodies,** or Guarnieri bodies, surrounded by a clear halo, characteristically develop in cells of the skin and mucous membranes infected with variola or vaccinia virus (see Fig. 54–4). Each inclusion body consists of an accumulation of viral particles and viral Ags. (Similar masses are observed in cells infected with other poxviruses).

A hypersensitivity response to the viral Ags may con-

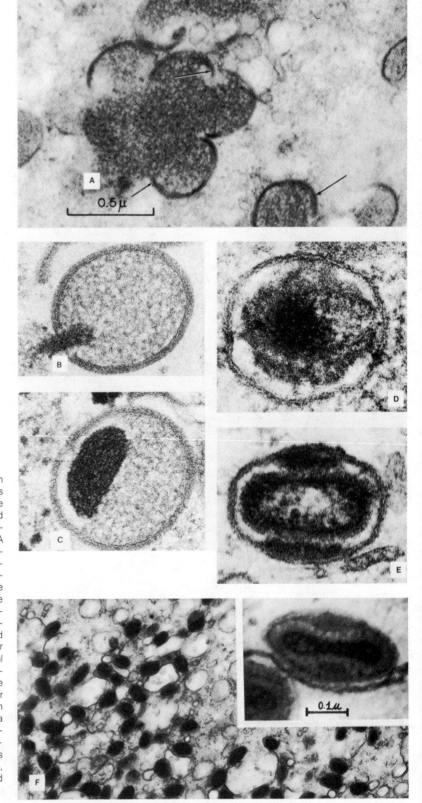

Figure 54–8. Developmental stages in the maturation and assembly of a vaccinia virus: electron micrographs of cells taken at intervals following infections. *(A)* Dense trilaminar viral membranes forming within and around clumps of dense fibrillar material in the cytoplasm. (Original magnification ×48,000) *(B)* Insertion of viral DNA and associated proteins into incomplete particles. (Original magnification ×150,000) *(C)* Condensation of nucleoprotein within the immature particle. (Original magnification ×150,000) *(D)* Maturation of a virion. The complete trilaminar lipoprotein envelope encloses the particle. Within is a dense nucleoid of fibrous nucleoprotein surrounded by a less dense homogeneous substance, thought to be material of the lateral bodies and core. (Original magnification ×170,000) *(E)* A further stage in a maturing virion. The core and two lateral bodies are clearly differentiated within the viral envelope. (Original magnification ×170,000) *(F)* A large group of mature vaccinia virions, smaller and denser than in their formative stages. (Original magnification ×24,000) The inset shows the internal structure of a single particle at higher magnification. The dense dumbbell-shaped core is surrounded by a zone of lower density. (Original magnification ×150,000) *(A* and *F,* Dales S, Siminovich L: J Biophys Biochem Cytol 10:475, 1961; *B* and *C,* Morgan C: Virology 73:43, 1976; *D* and *E,* Dales S, Mosbach EG: Virology 35:564, 1968)

tribute to the eruptive lesions of smallpox, for when the Ab response and hypersensitivity are inhibited in infected rabbits by x-irradiation or cytotoxic drugs, the characteristic pustules do not form, although viral multiplication is unrestricted. The toxinlike properties of the viral particles may also play a role in the cell necrosis. It is clear, however, that pustule formation does not result from secondary bacterial infection, since bacterial cultures of the pustule fluid are ordinarily sterile.

Laboratory Diagnosis

In the event of a recurrence of smallpox, the recognition of the disease will increasingly depend on laboratory procedures as physicians become less familiar with the clinical manifestations. These procedures either identify or isolate the virus, detect viral Ags, or measure a rise in titer of specific Abs. The recommended procedures and the specimens to be collected depend on the stage of the suspected disease (Table 54–1). The stability of the infectious virus and its Ags facilitates laboratory diagnosis because materials can be transported without danger of inactivation.

An early presumptive diagnosis can be made most rapidly by visualizing viral particles (elementary bodies) by electron microscopy, or even by light microscopy in a Giemsa-stained smear of scrapings from the bases of skin lesions. Virus is abundant in lesions during the active disease, but it is rarely detected during the incubation period and prodromal stage before the rash appears. A positive smear is decisive, but a negative result calls for further tests. Identification can be confirmed by viral isolation or by immunologic technique (see Table 54–1).

Epidemiology

Smallpox is confined to man and is **spread chiefly by person-to-person contact.** Although smallpox is considered to be highly contagious, spread is slow, and the probability of infection from a single exposure appears to be low.

Initially the virus is transmitted from the lesions of the upper respiratory tract in droplet secretions or by contamination of drinking or eating utensils; later, when the vesicles or pustules rupture and crusts are formed, the skin lesions also become a source of contagion. Dissemination by fomites is important because the virus is resistant to ordinary temperatures and drying. Airborne transmission of variola virus is unusual but can occur, as has been demonstrated epidemiologically and experimentally.

Although any person infected with variola virus is potentially contagious, the most dangerous disseminators are persons with unrecognized disease, e.g., the partially

TABLE 54–1. Diagnosis of Variola by Laboratory Tests

Method of Detection of Virus	Stage of Variola and Material Tested										Time Required for Test
	Pre-eruptive	Maculopapular and Papular			Vesicular		Pustular		Crusting		
	Blood	Blood	Skin Lesions	Saliva	Blood	Skin Lesions	Blood	Pustular Fluid	Blood	Crusts	
Microscopic examination (electron microscopy [most sensitive] or Giemsa-stained smears)			+			+		±		−	1 hour
Viral isolation (culture on chorioallantoic membrane of 12- to 14-day-old chick embryos or in tissue culture)	±	±	+	+	±	+		+		+	1–3 days
Antigen detection* (complement fixation, enzyme-linked immunosorbent assay [ELISA], agar-gel precipitation, immunofluorescence, or radioimmunoprecipitation)	±	±	+			+		+		+	3–24 hours
Detection of antibodies (hemagglutination inhibition, CF, ELISA, neutralization, or radioimmunoprecipitation)	−	±			+		+		+		3 h to 3 days

* Probably the most useful, economical, and efficient of diagnostic procedures. Positive results indicate a rise in Ab titer.

+, test usually positive; ±, test may or may not be positive; −, results usually negative; open spaces also indicate negative results.

(Modified from Downie AW, MacDonald A: Br Med Bull 9:191, 1963)

immune patient who has relatively few lesions. Such cases, easily overlooked or misdiagnosed, have been primarily responsible for introducing smallpox into countries free of the disease.

Prevention and Control

From the systematic beginnings by Jenner in England at the close of the 18th century, artificial immunization has become increasingly effective.* The worldwide eradication of smallpox by the WHO demonstrates the ultimate effectiveness of vaccination. This remarkable achievement was possible, however, primarily because of basic characteristics of the virus: the genetic stability of its Ags responsible for neutralizing Abs; the viremic stages of pathogenesis in which the virus is maximally exposed to Abs; and the lack of an animal reservoir. The eradication campaign was based on the principal of surveillance and containment, i.e., isolation of cases and early immunization of all their contacts. The alternative, eradication by immunizing the entire population of a country, was discarded because it proved impossible to reach all susceptible persons.

PREPARATION OF VACCINE. Since its original use for immunization against smallpox, cowpox virus has been propagated in many different laboratories under diverse conditions, and it is now believed, on the basis of its antigenic structure, to have been inadvertently replaced with an attenuated smallpox virus. The vaccinia virus used today is distinctly different from the cowpox virus encountered in nature.

Successful immunization requires the use of infectious (attenuated) virus, because of the marked lability of the protective Ag. The virus infects the skin at the site of inoculation and ordinarily does not produce viremia. The virus most commonly employed in the vaccine is a dermal strain of uncertain origin. It is prepared from scrapings of vaccinial lesions on the skin of calves or sheep, with 1% phenol added to kill contaminating bacteria and 40% glycerol added to increase the stability of the virus. WHO successfully used lyophilized vaccines to overcome the problem of inactivation of infectivity in hot climates.

---

* Variolation to protect against smallpox was practiced long before infectious agents and concepts of immunization were understood. The Chinese powdered old crusts and applied them to the nostrils; Brahmins in India preserved crusts and inoculated them into the skin of the unscarred; Persians ingested crusts from patients; and in Turkey, fluid from pocks was inoculated. It was this last practice that Lady Mary Wortly Montague, wife of the British ambassador to Turkey, introduced into England in 1718. Crusts and vesicle fluids were selected from patients during epidemics of mild disease (alastrim). The practice spread to the colonies, where it was more widely used than in the British Isles, but it never became popular because of the risks involved. Jenner introduced the use of attenuated (cowpox) virus in 1776, prompted by the clinical observation of milkmaids who acquired cowpox usually escaped smallpox, even when the disease was rampant in the community.

ADMINISTRATION OF VACCINE AND RESULTS. Classically, vaccine was administered intradermally by gently breaking the epidermis under a drop of vaccine; air jet has been particularly effective for immunization of large numbers, and this was the technique that the WHO employed in the eradication program. Puncture or scarification permits infectious virus to enter the skin, where it multiplies in the deeper layers of the epidermis. The extent of multiplication and spread of virus, and thus the type of reaction that ensues, depend on the state of immunity (and hypersensitivity) of the host. One of three **responses** is seen: (1) **primary** response; (2) **accelerated (vaccinoid)** response; and (3) **early immediate** response (Table 54–2).

Failure to elicit any dermal response is sometimes seen, but it is never the result of complete immunity; it simply indicates that the vaccination technique was faulty or the vaccine inadequate.

Eradication was possible because immunity developing 7 to 10 days after vaccination can protect those contacts of persons with smallpox who are vaccinated shortly after exposure (the incubation period is about 12 days). Protection lasts for 3 to 7 years, but mild smallpox may occur only 1 year after known successful vaccination.

COMPLICATIONS OF VACCINATION. Though vaccination is relatively safe, it gives rise to rare but occasionally fatal complications affecting the skin or central nervous system, especially with initial vaccinations (Table 54–3). Probably the most alarming complication is progressive spread of a primary vaccination response with extensive necrosis of skin and muscle (vaccinia gangrenosa) in those rare persons with thymic dysplasias, who cannot develop cellular immunity (about 1.5 cases per million primary vaccinees). It is essential that physicians and public health officers be aware of these complications and not attempt to vaccinate persons to treat unrelated diseases; e.g., physicians still unsuccessfully treat recurrent herpes simplex virus lesions by vaccination, occasionally resulting in severe complications including spread to unsuspecting contacts. Despite the eradication

---

TABLE 54–2. Immunologic Status Affecting Response to Vaccination

Response	Day of Appearance (Mean)	Interpretation
Primary	4	No immunity
Accelerated	3	Partial immunity; delayed hypersensitivity
Early or immediate	1	Delayed hypersensitivity; may or may not have immunity

TABLE 54–3. Incidence of Complications Associated With Smallpox Vaccination in the United States

Complication	Complications per 10^6 Primary Vaccinations (by Age, in Years, at Vaccination)					Complications per 10^6 Revaccinations (All Ages)
	<1	1–4	5–19	20+	*All Ages*	
Death (from all complications)	5	0.5	0.5	Unknown	1.0	0.1
Postvaccinial encephalitis	6	2	2.5	4	2.9	0.0
Vaccinia gangrenosa	1	0.5	1	7	0.9	0.7
Eczema vaccinatum	14	44	35	30	38	3
Generalized vaccinia	394	233	140	212	242	9
Accidental vaccinia infection	507	577	371	606	529	42

(Modified from Center for Disease Control Morbidity and Mortality Weekly Report 20:340, 1971)

of smallpox, it is still necessary to be aware of the reactions to and complications of vaccination because of the continued use of vaccination in the Armed Forces of the United States owing to the fear that smallpox virus might be used for biological warfare, and the proposed use of vaccinia virus as an expression vector for other immunization programs and gene therapy.

Other Poxviruses That Infect Humans

Several diseases other than variola and vaccinia are caused by poxviruses: monkeypox, cowpox, molluscum contagiosum, contagious dermatitis, milkers' nodules (paravaccinia), and tanapox.

MONKEYPOX

Human infection with monkeypox is clinically indistinguishable from smallpox. The disease is a rare zoonosis and was unrecognized in humans until smallpox was eradicated in the equatorial rain forest areas of west and central Africa. Most cases of human monkeypox have characteristic clinical and epidemiologic features. There is a 2-day prodrome followed by a typical smallpox rash, which evolves over 2 to 4 weeks; the lymphadenopathy is more prominent than in smallpox. The fatality rate is about 15%, and about 13% of cases are mild or very atypical, suggesting the possible occurrence of unrecognized cases. The interhuman transmission rate is much less than with smallpox, and cases resulting from tertiary transmission have not been observed. Thus, although there is concern that monkeypox virus might replace variola virus as a dangerous human pathogen, extensive genetic changes would be required in the monkeypox virus genome before it posed such a danger.

Seroepidemiologic surveys suggest that forest-dwelling monkeys, squirrels, and porcupines are involved in the natural cycle of viral transmission. The means by which humans are infected, however, have not been determined.

COWPOX

Cowpox is a self-limiting occupational disease of humans acquired from the udders and teats of infected cows. The vesicular inflammatory lesions are usually localized on the fingers, but the virus may accidentally be implanted on the face or other parts of the body.

Cowpox virus has properties similar to those of variola and vaccinia virus, but its antigenic structure differentiates it from the other agents in the subgroup. The host ranges of cowpox and vaccinia viruses are similar, but cowpox virus differs in several respects: (1) pocks appear more slowly on chorioallantoic membranes; (2) the virus has a tendency to invade mesodermal tissue, involving capillary endothelium and thus producing hemorrhagic ulcers in the pocks; (3) the inclusion bodies are larger and more eosinophilic than classic Guarnieri bodies; and (4) keratitis is produced slowly in rabbits, in comparison with the rapid development effected by vaccinia virus.

MOLLUSCUM CONTAGIOSUM

The molluscum contagiosum virus produces an uncommon skin disease affecting mainly children and young adults. The lesion is a chronic, proliferative process, restricted to the epithelium of the skin of the face, arms, legs, back, buttocks, and genitals. The virus has been shown to be sexually transmitted, producing inflamed or ulcerated lesions confused with those produced by herpes simplex virus. Electron microscopic observations reveal that the molluscum body (a large cytoplasmic inclusion body) is composed of virions indistinguishable from those of other poxviruses. Mature viral particles develop by a process resembling the formation of vaccinia virions. In addition to the relatively uncommon clinical infections, molluscum contagiosum virus has been transmitted experimentally to humans, and infections have been achieved in cultures of HeLa cells and primary human amnion and foreskin cells. Although virus could not be serially propagated in cultures, viral particles developed, as revealed by electron microscopic examination of thin sections, and cytopathic changes appeared.

The tendency to induce proliferative lesions is even more striking with molluscum contagiosum virus than with other poxviruses. This virus thus appears to provide a link between the common pathogenic viruses of man and tumor-inducing viruses. However, it should be noted that infected cells do not continue to synthesize DNA; it is the neighboring uninfected cells whose rate of cell division is stimulated. The mechanism of this stimulation is unknown.

MILKERS' NODULES (PARAVACCINIA)

Jenner recognized the existence of two diseases affecting the udder and teats of cows: classic cowpox and a second condition consisting predominantly of vesicular lesions. The latter disease is also transmitted to humans, producing painless smooth or warty "milkers' nodules" on the hands and arms. The lesions rarely become pustular. The infected cells contain eosinophilic cytoplasmic inclusion bodies and elementary bodies characteristic of poxvirus infection. Disease is associated with only mild constitutional symptoms and enlargement of regional lymph nodes.

Infection does not confer immunity to either cowpox or vaccinia viruses. Paravaccinia virus cannot be propagated on the chorioallantoic membrane of chick embryos or in laboratory animals usually susceptible to cowpox. The virus, which was isolated from a milkers' nodule of humans, has been serially cultured in fetal bovine kidney tissue cultures, as well as in diploid bovine conjunctival cells and human embryonic fibroblasts. In contrast to many poxviruses, it cannot be propagated serially in continuous human cell lines, such as HeLa cells. Its cytopathic effects resemble those produced by vaccinia virus,

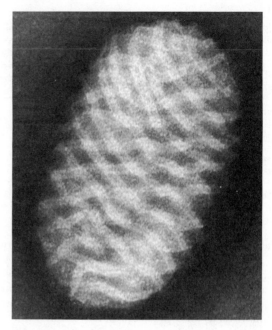

Figure 54–10. Mature contagious pustular dermatitis virus particle, negatively stained with phosphotungstic acid. The woven pattern of threads or tubules can clearly be seen. The apparent crisscrossing of the tubules results from the visualization of both the front and the back faces of the particle. (Original magnification ×600,000, reduced; Nagington J, Horne RW: Virology 16:248, 1962)

and infected cells prepared with Giemsa's stain show metachromatic cytoplasmic inclusion bodies.

Paravaccinia virus has stability characteristics similar to those of poxviruses. In thin sections the average viral particle measures 120 nm × 280 nm and has the typical morphology of a poxvirus. Electron microscopic observations of preparations stained with sodium phosphotungstate (Fig. 54–9) reveal ovoid virions whose size and surface structures are identical to those of contagious pustular dermatitis (Fig. 54–10) and bovine pustular stomatitis viruses.

CONTAGIOUS PUSTULAR DERMATITIS (ORF)

Although a natural affliction of sheep, mainly affecting lambs, contagious pustular dermatitis occurs rarely as an occupational disease of man. Sheep characteristically develop vesicles in the oral mucosa; these become encrusted and heal slowly after several weeks. In humans the infection usually causes a single lesion on a finger, beginning as a small, painless vesicle, which becomes pustular, encrusts, and finally heals. Transmission of infection from man to man has not been recorded.

The causative agent, contagious pustular dermatitis virus, can be isolated in various animal cell cultures or on the chick chorioallantoic membrane. It produces

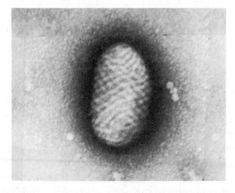

Figure 54–9. Electron micrograph of a viral particle isolated from a lesion of a milker's nodule. The negatively stained viral particle shows the characteristic morphology of a poxvirus. (Original magnification ×114,000; Friedman-Kien AE et al: Science 140:1335, 1963)

characteristic cytopathic changes but rarely gives rise to eosinophilic inclusion bodies. Electron microscopic study of the viral particles (see Fig. 54–10) reveals prominent tubule-like structures characteristic of poxviruses; the virion, in contrast to vaccinia and variola virions, is ovoid (160 nm × 260 nm) and is encircled in a regular pattern by the surface tubules.

TANAPOX VIRUS

A newly identified virus with characteristic poxvirus morphology has been isolated from two epidemics affecting several hundred tribesmen along the Tana River in Kenya. The disease is characterized by one or two pocklike lesions on the exposed upper part of the body and a febrile illness accompanied by severe aching and prostration. The lesion begins with a papule that develops into a raised vesicle and then umbilicates. Initially the pock resembles that of smallpox, but pustulation never follows. The virus has a host range limited to human and monkey cell cultures. It is serologically distinguishable from other orthopoxviruses, including the Yaba poxvirus of monkeys. The tanapox virus resembles a monkeypox virus that has affected monkeys in captivity in the United States, but in nature simian outbreaks have not been detected. Tanapox virus is probably a monkeypox virus that has been transmitted to man in Africa, where the natives use monkey meat and skins.

Selected Reading

BOOKS AND REVIEW ARTICLES

Behbalani AM: The smallpox story: Life and death of an old disease. Microbiol Rev 47:455, 1983

Dales S, Pogo BGT: Biology of poxviruses. Virol Monogr 18:1, 1981

Foege WH, Eddins DL: Mass vaccination programs in developing countries. Prog Med Virol 15:205, 1973

Fenner F: Portraits of viruses: The poxviruses. Intervirology 11:137, 1979

Mack TM: Smallpox in Europe, 1959–1971. J Infect Dis 125:161, 1972

Marsden JP: Variola minor: A personal analysis of 13,686 cases. Bull Hyg 23:735, 1948

Moss B, Winters E, Jones EV: Replication of vaccinia virus. In Cozzarelli N (ed): Proceedings of the 1983 UCLA Symposium on Mechanics of DNA Replication and Recombination, p 449. New York, Alan R. Liss, 1983

SPECIFIC ARTICLES

Arita I: Virological evidence for the success of the smallpox eradication programme. Nature 279:293, 1979

Arita I, Gramyko A: Surveillance of orthopoxvirus infections, and associated research, in the period after smallpox eradication. Bull WHO 6:367, 1982

Bladen RV: Mechanisms of recovery from a generalized viral infection: Mousepox. II. Passive transfer of recovery mechanisms with immune lymphoid cells. J Exp Med 133:1074, 1971

Councilman WT, MacGrath GB, Brinckerhoff WR: The pathological anatomy and histology of variola. J Med Res 11:12, 1904

Downie AW, Taylor-Robinson CH, Count AE et al: Tanapox: A new disease caused by a pox virus. Br Med J 1:363, 1971

Gerhelin P, Berns KI: Characterization and localization of the naturally occurring cross-links in vaccinia virus DNA. J Mol Biol 88:785, 1974

Immunization Practices Advisory Committee: Smallpox vaccine. Morbidity and Mortality Weekly report. 34:341, 1985

Kates J, Beeson J: Ribonucleic acid synthesis in vaccinia virus. I. The mechanism of synthesis and release of RNA in vaccinia cores. J Mol Biol 50:1, 1970

Morrison DK, Moyer RW: Detection of a subunit of cellular pol II within highly purified preparations of RNA polymerase isolated from rabbit poxvirus virions. Cell 44:587, 1986

55

Picornaviruses

History

Until the 1900s poliomyelitis (Gr. *poli,* gray, and *myelos,* spinal cord) was a disease primarily of infants (hence the name "infantile paralysis"), and this is still the pattern where sanitation is primitive. But with improved sanitation in many countries, in the 75 years prior to widespread immunization in 1960s, epidemics increased, the age distribution advanced, and the disease showed increasing severity as it appeared in young adults. This paradoxical response to improved sanitation was eventually explained by the findings that (1) practically everyone became infected, though the paralytic disease was rare, and (2) the consequences were usually negligible if infection was acquired early in life but might be serious when infection was postponed.

Clinically severe poliomyelitis was never very prevalent. In 1953 there were 1450 deaths and about 7000 cases with residual paralysis in the United States (versus about 500 deaths from measles, which was considered hardly more than a nuisance). However, the visibility of the crippled survivors caused even small epidemics to be terrifying. The problem was dramatized by the severe handicap of Franklin D. Roosevelt, who acquired poliomyelitis as an adult. The public's generous financial support of research (through the March of Dimes) led within 20 years to essentially complete control by immunization. Though the poliovirus was one of the most difficult to work with at the start of this program, it became a model for investigation of many other animal viruses.

In 1909 Landsteiner and Popper transmitted poliomyelitis to monkeys by intracerebral inoculation of a spinal cord filtrate from a patient, and the responsible agent was shown to be a virus.[*] However, progress depended

---

[*] Karl Landsteiner was also distinguished for his profound contributions to the understanding of immunologic specificity and for the discovery of human blood groups.

on the development of improved techniques for cultivating the virus. For example, as long as monkeys had to be used for experimentation, epidemiologic studies could demonstrate only that three antigenically distinct polioviruses exist. Adaptation of polioviruses to the cotton rat by Armstrong, in 1939, was a substantial step forward. The turning point came in 1945, however, when Enders, Weller, and Robbins showed that polioviruses can be isolated and readily propagated in cultures in nonneural human or monkey tissue. The incisive investigations that followed soon led to control of the disease.

Many related viruses were discovered as accidental by-products of the intensive pursuit of polioviruses. Thus, **coxsackieviruses*** were isolated in 1948 from the intestinal tract of children by intracerebral inoculation of newborn mice. The subsequent introduction of tissue culture techniques revealed the **echoviruses** (*e*nteric *c*ytopathic *h*uman *o*rphan viruses), a third group of viruses in the gastrointestinal tract of man. They were called orphans because initially they were not clearly associated with disease. A fourth group of related viruses, designated **rhinoviruses** (Gr. *rhino*, nose), was discovered in 1956 during studies of mild upper respiratory infections fitting the description of the common cold.

Classification and General Characteristics

Polioviruses, coxsackieviruses, and echoviruses are similar in epidemiologic pattern, in physical, chemical, and biologic characteristics, and in infecting the human gastrointestinal tract. They were originally given the name **enteroviruses,** but this term seemed inadequate when some coxsackieviruses and echoviruses were also found to produce acute respiratory infections. With the discovery of rhinoviruses, which have similar chemical and physical characteristics but produce primarily acute respiratory infection, **Picornaviridae** (vernacular, **picornaviruses**) was coined as the family designation (*pico*, implying small, and RNA, the nucleic acid component). However, because of differences in certain physical, chemical, and biological characteristics, human picornaviruses were classified into two genera: ***Enteroviruses*** (which occasionally cause respiratory rather than intestinal or neurologic disease) and ***Rhinoviruses*** (see Table 55–1 and "Characteristics of Picornaviruses"). To simplify classification and to avoid confusion caused by overlap of host range characteristics, newly isolated enteroviruses are no longer divided into coxsackieviruses and echoviruses. From type 68 upward only the species designation *enterovirus* is employed.

* Named after Coxsackie, NY, the town from which the initial isolates were obtained

TABLE 55–1. Classification of Picornaviruses Affecting Humans

Genus	Species	No. of Types
Enterovirus	Poliovirus	3
	Coxsackievirus	
	Coxsackievirus A	23*
	Coxsackievirus B	6
	Echovirus	32†
	Enterovirus	5‡
Rhinovirus	Rhinovirus	113

* Type 23 was shown to be identical to echovirus type 9; A23 has been dropped, and the number is unused.

† Type 10 has been reclassified as reovirus 1, and type 28 as rhinovirus 1; the numbers are now unused.

‡ Type 68–72

CHARACTERISTICS OF PICORNAVIRUSES*

Size: 22–30 nm
Morphology: Icosahedral
Capsomers: Probably 32
Nucleic acid: Single-stranded RNA
Reaction to lipid solvents: Resistant
Stability at room temperature: Relatively stable
pH stability: Enteroviruses: Stable at pH 3–9
              Rhinoviruses: Unstable below pH 6
Stability at 50°C: Enteroviruses: Relatively unstable
                   Rhinoviruses: Relatively stable
Density in CsCl: Enteroviruses: 1.33–1.34 g/cm^3
                 Rhinoviruses: 1.38–1.41 g/cm^3

* Viruses similar to human picornaviruses have been found in several species of lower animals: the agent of foot-and-mouth disease in cattle (a member of the genus *Aphthovirus* that is physically similar to the rhinoviruses), Teschen disease viruses of pigs, and Mengo and encephalomyocarditis viruses of mice (similar to enteroviruses) are members of the genus *Cardiovirus*.

The physical and chemical properties of picornaviruses are summarized under "Characteristics of Picornaviruses." They are small, contain RNA, and do not contain lipid. Polioviruses, described in detail in the following section, will serve as the prototype of the family.

Polioviruses
PROPERTIES

MORPHOLOGY. Electron micrographs of purified virus in thin sections of virus-infected cells reveal small particles with a dense core. Negative staining shows a capsid with a subunit arrangement consistent with icosahedral symmetry (Fig. 55–1). There appear to be 32 capsomers per virion, although clear capsomers are not discernible. Po-

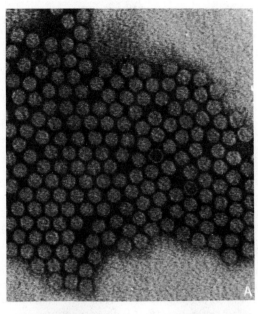

form a smaller peak ringed by promontories. Broad valleys surround the peaks at the fivefold axes, and shallow valleys separate the peaks at the threefold axes. VP4 is associated internally with the inner surface of the capsid and the viral RNA.

The virion RNA has the polarity of the viral mRNA (positive strand), it is infectious, and it can be translated *in vitro*. At its 3′ terminus is a poly(A) track of about 90 nucleotides, which is necessary for its infectivity. In addition, the virion RNA has two unusual features: (1) its 5′ end is not capped but terminates in pUp, and (2) a protein (**VPg**) of about 7000 daltons is covalently attached to its 5′ end. VPg is always covalently linked to the virion RNA; its presence is essential for initiation of RNA replication. However, the RNA remains infectious if VPg is

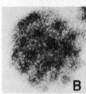

Figure 55–1. Electron micrograph of a purified preparation of poliovirus negatively stained. *(A)* Icosahedral symmetry of viral particles is evident. (Original magnification ×150,000) *(B)* Higher magnification of a viral particle printed in reverse contrast. Capsomers measure approximately 6 nm in diameter; their fine structure is not apparent. (Original magnification ×600,000) *(C)* Same particle as in *B,* marked to display two clear axes of fivefold symmetry (*white lines*). (Mayor HD: Virology 22:156, 1964)

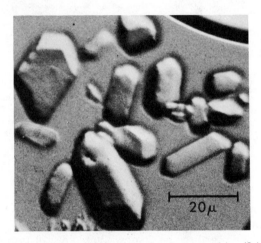

Figure 55–2. Crystals of purified type 1 poliovirus particles. (Schaffer FL, Schwerdt CE: Proc Natl Acad Sci USA 41:1020, 1955)

lioviruses and viruses of the other three picornavirus groups present only minor differences in size and structure.

PHYSICAL AND CHEMICAL CHARACTERISTICS. The characteristics of the polioviruses are given under "Characteristics of Polioviruses." Poliovirus was the first animal virus to be obtained in crystalline form (Fig. 55–2). A single molecule of single-stranded RNA constitutes about 30% of the virion; the remainder consists of four major (**VP1–4**) and one minor (**VPg**) species of proteins. Each surface subunit of the capsid, termed a **protomer,** is composed of three unique intimately associated polypeptide chains (VP1, VP2, and VP3; Fig. 55–3). At each fivefold axis of the capsid a pronounced tilt of the VP1 core forms a large ribbed peak, and at each threefold axis the cores of VP2 and VP3 alternate around the axis to

---

CHARACTERISTICS OF POLIOVIRUSES

Diameter of virion: 27–30 nm
Diameter of internal core: 16 nm
Diameter of capsomer: 6 nm
Molecular weight of RNA: 2.5×10^6 daltons (7.7 kilobases)
Base composition (G + C): 46 moles %*
Molecular weight of virion proteins†
  VP1: 35×10^3 daltons
  VP2: 28×10^3 daltons
  VP3: 24×10^3 daltons
  VP4: 6×10^3 daltons
  VPg: $\sim 7 \times 10^3$ daltons
Sedimentation coefficient of virion: 157–160 S_{20}
Particle mass of virion: 1.1×10^{-17} g
Molecular weight of virion: $8–9 \times 10^6$ daltons

---

* Composition is very similar for the three types.

† Virion proteins 1 through 4 are present in equal molar amounts.

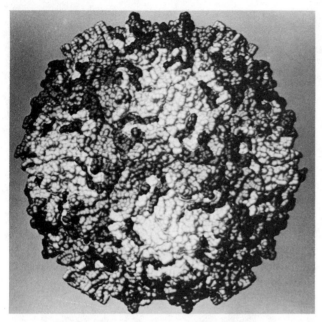

Figure 55–3. Folding of poliovirus major capsid proteins (VP1, VP2, and VP3) to form the outer surface of the virion (derived from computer analysis of x-ray crystallographic data). VP1 is light gray, VP2 is medium gray, and VP3 is dark gray. The three proteins form a protomer. VP4 is present in the inner surface of the capsid and is not visible. (Hogle JM, Filman DJ, Chow M: In Brown F, Chanock RM, Lerner RH [eds]: Vaccines 86: New Approach to Immunization, p 3. Cold Spring Harbor, NY, Cold Spring Harbor Laboratory, 1986)

removed by pronase because newly synthesized VPg is synthesized from the infecting genome.

There are three serotypes; their physical properties are identical, and their base compositions are very similar; the RNAs share 36% to 52% of their nucleotide sequences. Moreover, considerable nucleotide sequence homology exists between the RNAs of polioviruses, other enteroviruses, and rhinoviruses, as detected by cross-hybridization between RNA from virions and replicative forms of RNA from infected cells. This homology appears to be located in the viral RNA polymerase genes (at least between type 1 poliovirus and type 2 rhinovirus).

Polioviruses are more stable than many viruses (e.g., those with lipid envelopes). Hence, their transmission is facilitated because they can remain infectious for relatively long periods in water, milk, and other foods. However, polioviruses are readily inactivated by pasteurization and by many other chemical and physical agents. Magnesium chloride (1M) appears to stabilize their intercapsomeric bonds and hence markedly increases thermal stability.

IMMUNOLOGIC CHARACTERISTICS. The three distinct immunologic types of polioviruses can be recognized by neutralization, complement fixation (CF), gel-diffusion precipitation, and other immunoprecipitation reactions with type-specific sera.

There is no common poliovirus group Ag, but antigenic relations between types do exist. The cross-reactions are particularly prominent when heated virus is employed in CF titrations. The cross-reactivity, however, can be demonstrated only when sera are obtained from humans who have been infected with more than one type of poliovirus; i.e., after an initial infection the Ab response is strictly type-specific, but upon infection with a second type, Abs develop to two or all three of the viruses. Immunologic cross-reactivity between types 1 and 2 is also demonstrated in neutralization titrations by cross-absorption experiments and by the development of heterotypic Abs following natural infections or immunization. Slight cross-reactivity between types 2 and 3 can be detected by neutralization, but not between types 1 and 3. The immunologic kinship between types 1 and 2 Abs is epidemiologically substantiated: possession of type 2 Abs confers significant protection against the paralytic effects of subsequent type 1 infection.

Just as VP1, 2, and 3 polypeptides are closely associated on the surface of the virion (see Fig. 55–3), so each of these proteins can induce neutralizing Abs. VP1, however, is the **immuno-dominant Ag** for neutralizing Abs, and this surface protein contains at least four epitopes capable of inducing neutralizing Abs. VP2 and VP3 each contain a single epitope for neutralizing Abs.

Antigenic variants of types 1 and 2 viruses have been detected by precise plaque-reduction and CF studies with cross-absorbed sera. Through the use of monoclonal Abs, mutants resistant to neutralization, due to point mutations, can be isolated; when polyclonal sera are used, however, these antigenic differences do not affect the capacity of Abs induced by one strain to protect against infection by all other strains of the same type. Despite these minor intratypic differences, **polioviruses** actually **show marked antigenic stability,** both in nature and in laboratory manipulations.

Neutralizing Abs appear early in the course of poliovirus infection, and they have usually reached a high titer by the time the patient is first seen by a physician (Fig. 55–4). They attain a maximum titer 2 to 6 weeks after the onset of disease, decrease to about one fourth that level in 18 to 24 months, and then seem to persist indefinitely. Their presence confers clear protection against subsequent infection. CF Abs appear during the first 2 to 3 weeks after infection, reach maximum titers in about 2 months, and persist for an average of 2 years. Inapparent and nonparalytic infections result in Ab levels as high as those present after severe paralytic disease. Second attacks of paralytic poliomyelitis are rare and are invariably due to a different viral type from that producing the first illness.

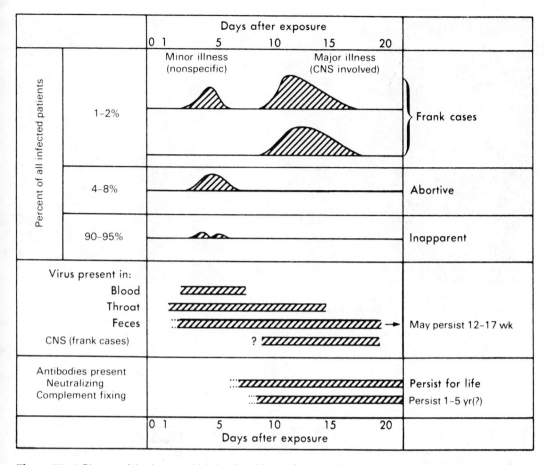

Figure 55–4. Diagram of the times at which the clinical forms of poliomyelitis appear, correlated with the times at which virus is present in various sites and with development and persistence of Abs. The high incidence of subclinical poliovirus infection is also noted. (Horstmann DM: Yale J Biol Med 36:5, 1963)

HOST RANGE. Humans are the only natural hosts for polioviruses. Abs are present in some monkeys and chimpanzees studied in captivity, but there is evidence that the infection is acquired only after capture.

Old World monkeys and chimpanzees are susceptible to infection (by the intracerebral, intraspinal, and oral routes) with fresh isolates as well as with laboratory strains. In contrast, nonprimates are relatively insusceptible. However, by serial passage, strains of poliovirus were adapted to cotton rats and mice. Strains of type 2 virus have also been adapted to suckling hamsters and the chick embryo.

An important development was the discovery that these viruses, hitherto considered purely neurotropic, can multiply and produce cytopathology in human extraneural tissues cultured *in vitro*. It then rapidly became evident that many tissues from primates can furnish cells susceptible to cytopathic changes (Fig. 55–5). Cultures of primate tissues are now widely used for isolation and identification of polioviruses and other picornaviruses, for production of vaccines, and for experimental studies.

MULTIPLICATION. To initiate infection, polioviruses attach rapidly to specific host cell receptors (composed of lipid and glycoproteins), which are much more prevalent in susceptible than in nonsusceptible tissues. Such **adsorption** to susceptible cells is independent of temperature but depends on the concentration of electrolytes. Infectious particles, but not empty particles, can adsorb, an indication that the conformation of the capsid is critical for attachment. Very soon after attachment the viral capsids are altered by loss of VP4, and about 50% of these particles also lose their RNA; these become noninfectious and elute from the cells. The remaining particles **penetrate** into the host cells, probably in endosomes, and rapidly **uncoat their RNA,** which becomes susceptible to RNase within 30 to 60 minutes after infection.

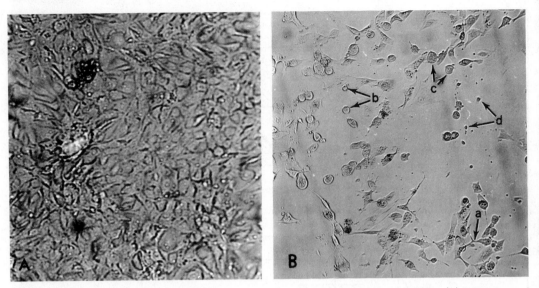

Figure 55–5. Cytopathic changes in monkey kidney cell cultures infected with type 1 poliovirus. *(A)* A monolayer of uninfected cells, unstained. (Original magnification ×200) *(B)* Advanced cytopathic changes in infected cultures, unstained. Polioviruses, like most enteroviruses that infect monkey kidney cells, produce marked cell retraction (*a*), rounding (*b*), and occasionally ballooning of cells (*c*), followed by rapid lysis, leaving a granular debris (*d*). (Original magnification ×200) (Ashkenazi A, Melnick JL: Am J Clin Pathol 38:209, 1962)

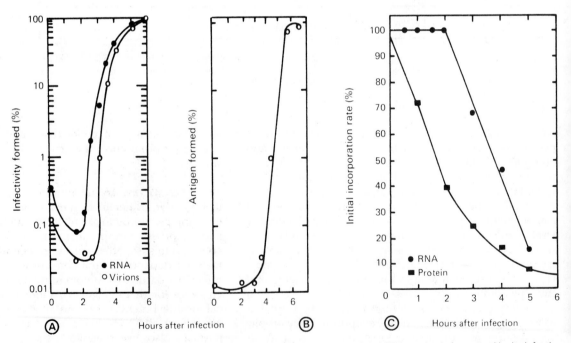

Figure 55–6. Biosynthetic events in poliovirus-infected cells. *(A)* Time course of viral RNA synthesis (measured by its infectivity) and of maturation of virions. *(B)* Biosynthesis of viral capsid proteins measured by incorporation of ^{14}C-labeled amino acids into Ab-precipitable material. *(C)* Rate of total RNA and protein synthesis in poliovirus-infected cells measured by the incorporation of ^{14}C-uridine or ^{14}C-L-valine into acid-precipitable material at the indicated times after infection. *(A,* Darnell JE Jr et al: Virology 13:271, 1961; *B,* Scharff MD, Levintow L: Virology 19:491, 1963; *C,* Zimmerman EF et al: Virology 19:400, 1963)

The **replication** of infectious virus follows the general pattern of viruses with positive-strand RNA, which initially serves as mRNA for the synthesis of viral proteins, including an RNA replicase. The RNA replicative intermediates then develop (see Synthesis of RNA Viruses, Chap. 48), serving first for synthesis of complementary negative strands and then for positive strands. The small **VPg** is covalently linked to the 5'-terminal oligonucleotide of all nascent RNAs (positive and negative strands); it is required for viral RNA synthesis, apparently serving as a primer for the formation of replication complexes. The VPg, however, is cleaved from about half of the plus strands, and these are destined to become uncapped messengers. Hence, VPg distinguishes virion RNAs from viral mRNAs of identical nucleotide sequences.

Replication of viral RNA is independent of biosynthesis of host cell DNA. The production of viral RNA commences within 15 minutes after viral uncoating is completed but all the early molecules, which are copied from the nascent complementary RNA templates, become messengers on very large cytoplasmic polyribosomes. Since internal initiation of protein synthesis on this message does not occur, this polygenic RNA of about 7000 nucleotides serves as a monocistronic message; it is **translated into a single long polypeptide,** termed a **polyprotein,** which is subsequently cleaved into the four individual viral capsid proteins plus VPg and the nonvirion proteins (see Chap. 48). Progeny RNA first appears in viral particles about 3 hours after infection (Fig. 55–6A); once **virion assembly** has started, production of capsid proteins (Fig. 55–6B) and RNA replication are closely coupled, and newly made viral RNA is incorporated into virions within 5 minutes after synthesis. The final step in morphogenesis (Fig. 55–7) appears to be the combination of viral RNA with a shell of viral proteins (VP0, VP1, VP3) termed the **procapsid** (see Chap. 48), during which one of the procapsid proteins (VP0) is cleaved to yield two of the final capsid structures (VP2 and VP4). Since complete viral replication occurs in cells enucleated with cytochalasin B, host cell nuclear functions are not required.

Final assembly of infectious particles is accomplished rapidly. Approximately 500 virions per cell are produced. Initially, virions are released through vacuoles, but after several hours they escape in a burst, accompanied by death and lysis of the host cell.

Synthesis of host cell proteins is inhibited very shortly after viral infection (Fig. 55–6C) owing to inactivation of initiation factors responsible for forming the host cap-binding protein complex. The cessation of host protein synthesis is accompanied by disruption of the host cell polyribosomes. Synthesis of normal host cell RNA ceases about 2 hours after infection, shortly after biosynthesis of viral RNA begins (see Fig. 55–6).

The **cytopathologic changes** accompanying these

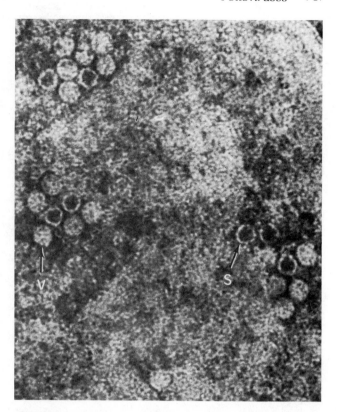

Figure 55–7. Development of poliovirus particles in pieces of the cytoplasmic matrix of artificially disrupted cells. Particles in various stages of assembly from empty shells (s) to complete virions (v) can be seen. (Original magnification ×200,000; Horne RW, Nagington J: J Mol Biol 1:33, 1959. Copyright by Academic Press, Inc. [London] Ltd.)

biosynthetic events are diagrammed in Figure 55–8. Intranuclear alterations, consisting of rearrangement of chromatin material with condensation at the nuclear membrane, are the first changes detected. One or more small intranuclear eosinophilic inclusion bodies of unknown nature form, and the nucleus becomes distorted and wrinkled and gradually shrinks. These events are probably related to the inhibition of synthesis of the host cell's protein and nuclear RNA (see Fig. 55–6C). The cytoplasm then develops a large eosinophilic mass, which is the site of replication and assembly of viral subunits (Figs. 55–8 and 55–9), and knobs appear on the cell membrane as the result of cytoplasmic bubbling associated with the release of virus. Finally the nucleus becomes pycnotic, the nuclear chromatin becomes fragmented, and the cell becomes rounded and dies.

GENETIC CHARACTERISTICS. The demonstration in 1953 that poliovirus contains only RNA stimulated great interest because it identified **RNA as genetic material.** The finding that polioviruses undergo mutations and re-

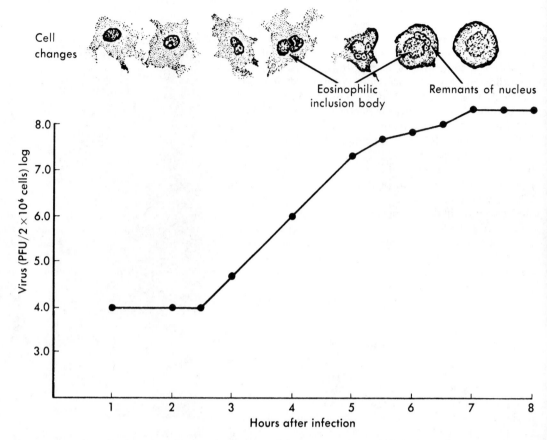

Figure 55–8. Diagram of the multiplication of poliovirus and the accompanying pathologic changes in infected cells. A perinuclear cytoplasmic eosinophilic mass (inclusion body) develops as viral multiplication reaches its maximum; the inclusion body impinges on the nucleus, which degenerates as the cell dies. *PFU*, plaque-forming unit. (Adapted from Reissig M et al: J Exp Med 104:289, 1956)

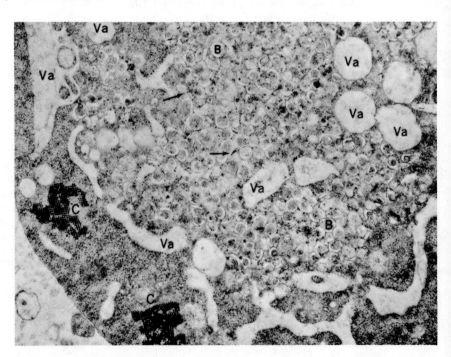

Figure 55–9. Cytoplasmic changes and assembly of virions in a poliovirus-infected cell. Large numbers of membrane-enclosed pieces of cytoplasm (*B*) accumulate in the central region of the cell, pushing the nucleus to one side (the nucleus is not shown in this photograph). Large cytoplasmic vacuoles (*Va*) also develop. A large number of virions (*arrows*) are present in the cytoplasmic matrix, both between and within the membrane-enclosed bodies (*B*). Two large crystals of virions are present (*C*). (Original magnification ×25,000; Dale S et al: Virology 26:379, 1965)

combination just as DNA viruses do provided a theoretical basis for developing attenuated mutants for use as a live virus vaccine. The number of mutant phenotypes observed (Table 55–2) is much larger than the number of viral genes, so that many phenotypes must arise from different mutations of the same gene.

Early studies revealed that recombination could occur between some of the mutants. With conditionally lethal, temperature-sensitive mutants several genes have been mapped: two genes for replication of viral RNA, one for synthesis of capsid proteins, and two for regulation of cell functions. Genetic maps have been obtained by the use of pactamycin to inhibit the initiation of protein synthesis; these maps locate the genes for virion proteins close to the 5' end of the RNA genome and in the order (5'→3') VP4→VP2→VP3→VP1. The nonstructural proteins are encoded toward the 3' end of the genome (see Chap. 48). Nucleotide sequence analysis of the entire genome and amino acid sequence determination of isolated gene products confirm the genetic map.

Genetic studies have also revealed that many mutations are **pleiotropic;** i.e., two phenotypic traits are changed by the same mutation, although the two phenotypes can also be changed separately. The *d* and *e* phenotypes (see Table 55–2), for example, can arise by a single mutation. Hence, mutations affecting neurotropism can be found among mutant phenotypes that are easily detectable *in vitro*, whereas their direct detection in primates would be much more limited and costly.

Several of the mutant phenotypes that are frequently associated with attenuation (see Table 55–2) affect the viral capsid, and others multiply preferentially at or below usual body temperatures. Thus, neurovirulence appears to depend on the ability of the virus to interact with certain cells and to replicate in febrile patients (rct/40 mutants). Furthermore, attenuated viruses induce the synthesis of more interferon than virulent viruses do, and are more readily inhibited by it (see Interferon, Chap. 49). However, the relatively common neurovirulent revertant of the type 3 Sabin vaccine strain does not conform to these patterns because it is due to a mutation changing the uridine at position 472 to cytidine in the small 5' noncoding region.

The ability to make infectious cDNA copies of the viral RNA genome will permit much more detailed genetic studies. In addition, intertypic and intratypic recombinants are being constructed to identify gene functions.

PATHOGENESIS

The major sequence of events in the multiplication and spread of polioviruses was revealed by studies in chimpanzees and man, as well as in cell cultures. In humans the progression of infection culminates in invasion of the target organs, the brain and spinal cord (Fig. 55–10).

Infection is initiated by the ingestion of virus and its **primary multiplication** in the oropharyngeal and intestinal mucosa. It is not known, however, whether virus multiplies in epithelial or lymphoid cells of the alimentary tract. The tonsils and Peyer's patches of the ileum are invaded early in the course of infection, and extensive viral multiplication ensues in these loci, so that as much as 10^7 to 10^8 infectious doses (i.e., 10^7 to 10^8 times the mean tissue culture infectious dose [see Chap. 44]) of virus per gram of tissue may accumulate. From the primary infectious sites of propagation the virus drains into deep cervical and mesenteric lymph nodes, but since its titer there is relatively low, these nodes may not be im-

TABLE 55–2. Characteristics of Some Poliovirus Mutants

Class of Mutants	Characteristic(s)	Marker Name
Factors that affect cell–virus interaction and therefore viral multiplication	Ability to multiply at 40°C	rct/40
	*Inability to multiply at 40°C	rct/40⁻
	*Ability to multiply at 23°C	rct/23⁺
	*Heat defectiveness (inability to multiply at 40°C, but usual multiplication at 36°C)	hd
	Plaque size	s
	*Resistance to heating in AlCl₃	a
	Resistance to heat inactivation of virion	t
	Inability to grow in MS cells	ms
Variants distinguished by presence or absence of inhibitory substance in media	*Sensitivity to agar inhibitor at acid pH	d
	Sensitivity to agar inhibitor at neutral pH	m
	Cystine inhibition of multiplication	cy⁺
	Cystine dependence	cyᵈ
	Tryptophan dependence	
	Adenine resistance	
	Guanidine resistance	gʳ
	Guanidine dependence	gᵈ
	Hydroxybenzylbenzimidazole (HBB) resistance	HBBʳ
	Resistance to normal bovine serum inhibitor	bo
	Resistance to normal horse serum inhibitor	ho
Mutants whose markers are physical characteristics of the virus	*Poor elution from Al(OH)₃ gel	Al(OH)₃
	*Greater adsorbability to DEAE-cellulose	e
Immunologic variants	Intratypic antigenic variants	

* Phenotypes associated with attenuated viruses

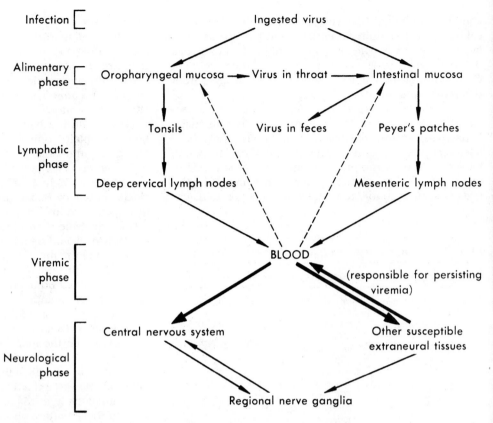

Figure 55–10. Pathogenesis of poliomyelitis. This model is based on a synthesis of data obtained in man and chimpanzees. (Adapted from Sabin AB: Science 123:1151, 1956; Bodian D: Science 122:105, 1955)

portant sites of viral replication for progressive infections. From the nodes the virus drains into the blood, resulting in a **transient viremia** that disseminates virus to other susceptible tissues, such as the brown fat (axillary, paravertebral, and suprasternal) and the viscera (probably in reticuloendothelial cells). In these extraneural sites the virus replicates, and it is continually fed back into the bloodstream to establish and maintain a **persistent viremic stage.** In most natural infections, even in nonimmune persons, only transient viremia occurs; the infection does not progress beyond the lymphatic stage, and clinical disease does not ensue.

Viral spread to the central nervous system (CNS) requires persistent viremia, which implies that direct invasion through capillary walls is the major pathway of penetration into the central nervous system. Therefore, the presence of specific Abs in the blood, even at the relatively low levels obtained by passive immunization, effectively halts viral spread and prevents invasion of the brain and spinal cord. However, transmission of virus along nerve fibers from peripheral ganglia may provide an additional route for entry into the CNS, because po-

lioviruses are found in these ganglia during the progression of infection, and virus can spread along nerve fibers in both peripheral nerves and the CNS.

Poliomyelitis generally conjures up the picture of a severe, crippling, and occasionally fatal paralytic disease. However, probably no more than 1% of infections culminate in that syndrome (see Fig. 55–4). A moderate number of infections induce transient viremia, resulting in a mild febrile disease, or so-called summer grippe.

The **course of classic paralytic disease** is initiated by a **minor disease,** which is associated with the viremia and is characterized by constitutional and respiratory or gastrointestinal signs and symptoms (see Fig. 55–4). There follows, after 1 to 3 days or often without any interval, the **major disease,** characterized by headache, fever, muscle stiffness, and paralysis associated with cell destruction in the CNS. Lesions causing **paralysis** occur most frequently in the anterior horn cells of the spinal cord (**spinal poliomyelitis**); similar lesions may occur in the medulla and brain stem (**bulbar poliomyelitis**) and in the motor cortex (**encephalitic poliomyelitis;** Fig. 55–11). Bulbar poliomyelitis is often fatal because of respira-

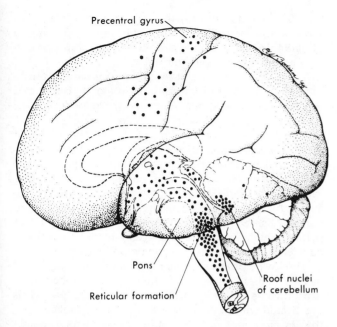

Figure 55–11. Lateral view of the human brain and the midsagittal surface of the brain stem. *Black dots,* usual distribution of lesions. Spinal lesions usually occur in the anterior horn cells; lesions in the cerebral cortex are largely restricted to the precentral gyrus; those of the cerebellum are largely found in the roof nuclei; lesions of the brain stem centers are widespread. (Bodian D: Papers and Discussions Presented at the First International Poliomyelitis Conference. Philadelphia, JB Lippincott, 1949)

Labels in figure: Precentral gyrus; Pons; Reticular formation; Roof nuclei of cerebellum

tory or cardiac failure; the other forms may result in survival with highly variable patterns of residual paralysis. Paralysis becomes maximal within a few days of onset and is often followed by extensive recovery, which may be aided by physiotherapy. The recovery represents, in part, compensatory hypertrophy of muscles that have not lost their innervation. In the aging this compensatory hypertrophy may be lost; and marked weakness, even paralysis, may return. In addition, although the virus-infected cells in the lesions are irreversibly damaged, neighboring uninfected neurons may also contribute to the paralysis through edema and by-products of necrosis, but paralysis from this cause is reversible. The temporal relation among clinical manifestations, distribution of virus, and the appearance of Abs is summarized in Figure 55–4.

Several host factors may alter the course of infection: fatigue, trauma, injections of drugs and vaccines, tonsillectomy, pregnancy, and age. These factors do not increase the incidence of infection but do affect the frequency and severity of paralysis. Trauma, including hypodermic injections, tends to localize the paralysis to the traumatized muscles. Tonsillectomy, recent or of long standing, markedly increases the incidence of bul-

bar poliomyelitis. The mechanisms of action of these localizing host factors are not certain. They may increase infection of peripheral nerve ganglia or transmission of virus along peripheral nerves associated with the affected area, or they may increase the permeability of blood vessels in corresponding areas of the CNS. The greater severity of paralysis in adults, and even more in pregnant women, may be related to endocrine factors: steroids, for example, greatly heighten the severity of infection in experimental animals.

LABORATORY DIAGNOSIS

Laboratory methods for the diagnosis of poliomyelitis are simple and efficient, because of the ready availability of excellent tissue culture methods and immunologic techniques. Virus is isolated most readily from feces or rectal swabs for about 5 weeks after onset, and from pharyngeal secretions for the first 3 to 5 days of disease. Multiplication of virus is detected by the development of characteristic cytopathic changes (see Fig. 55–5B) and by failure of the infected tissue cultures to become acid in 1 to 4 days after inoculation, revealed by incorporating phenol red in the medium (since this indicator shifts from red to yellow on acidification). The latter criterion arises from the inability of the dying infected cells to produce organic acids from glucose. Final identification of the virus is accomplished by neutralization tests by means of a standard serum for each of the three types. If an enterovirus other than poliovirus is also present, which is not uncommon, identification is more complex and requires multiple pools of antisera.

For serologic diagnosis, Ab levels are compared in sera obtained during the acute phase of the disease and 2 to 3 weeks after onset, by means of neutralization or, less often, CF titrations. Titration endpoints in neutralization are based on the inhibition of cytopathic effects or on continued acid production; the latter assay is especially convenient, since it can be carried out in disposable plastic trays and the endpoints can be determined rapidly without microscopic observations. CF tests are usually less dependable, because the different Ags from intact and incomplete virions are present in viral preparations, and Abs directed against each Ag appear at different times.

EPIDEMIOLOGY

Serologic surveys show that polioviruses are globally disseminated. In densely populated countries with poor hygienic conditions, practically 100% of the population over 5 years of age has Abs to all three types of poliovirus, epidemics do not occur, and paralytic disease is rare. In countries with improved sanitation, in contrast, the young are shielded from exposure, and prior to the effective use of vaccines, many who reached adulthood had escaped infection and were therefore without protective Abs. Because the incidence and severity of paralytic disease increase with age, if infection is delayed until susceptible persons are above age 10 to 15 years, more severe crippling disease occurs.

The widespread use of vaccines has strikingly altered the epidemiologic picture. In some countries (Sweden, Finland, Denmark, the Netherlands), paralytic poliomyelitis appears to have been eradicated. In the United States, epidemics have been eliminated except in pockets of lower socioeconomic groups, among whom immunization has not been widespread (although available free of charge); a recent study indicated that there were at least 20 million unimmunized children. Among those unprotected, small epidemics are again occurring in the very young (reviving the picture of "infantile paralysis") because, in contrast to the situation in countries with poor sanitation, polioviruses are not widely disseminated while babies are still protected by maternal Abs. However, the few cases of poliomyelitis that occur are also seen in older children and young adults.

TRANSMISSION. Poliomyelitis occurs primarily in the summer, like the common summer diarrheal diseases. This finding first suggested transmission by the fecal route. Indeed, a large amount of virus is excreted in the feces for an average period of 5 weeks after infection, even in the presence of a high titer of circulating Abs (see Fig. 55–4). A patient is maximally contagious, however, during the first week of illness, when pharyngeal excretion of virus also occurs. Multiple modes of infection probably account for the fact that infections can occur in any season of the year.

Person-to-person contact is the primary mode of spread, and transmission within families and schools appears to be the major mechanism of dispersion throughout a community. Presently, however, occurrence of the rare case in immunized populations does not produce secondary cases owing to the insufficient numbers of susceptible persons. Prior to widespread immunization, flies occasionally served as accidental vectors, but they were not an important mode of distribution. Water- and milk-borne epidemics caused by fecal contamination have also been reported. Dissemination of virus is rapid and extensive in nonimmune members of a family or in other contact groups, but the ratio of paralytic disease to inapparent infections is low, i.e., about 1:200 in temperate zones.

PREVENTION AND CONTROL

Until vaccine became available in 1954, the only approaches to the control of infection were passive immunization and nonspecific public health measures (isola-

tion of patients; closing of such gathering-places as schools and swimming pools; widespread spraying of insecticides); none of this proved successful in preventing or stopping an epidemic.

The present era of successful control can be attributed to three major discoveries: (1) Protection is required against the three distinct antigenic types of poliovirus. (2) Multiplication of poliovirus to a high titer in cultures of nonnervous tissues affords a practicable procedure for preparing large quantities of virus free of the nervous tissue that may induce demyelinating encephalomyelitis. (3) As the role of viremia in pathogenesis suggested, the infection can be interrupted before the CNS is infected. In addition, the protection of monkeys, mice, and man by passive immunization with immune serum or pooled γ-globulin proved that even low titers of Abs can be effective in preventing paralytic poliomyelitis.

The development of poliomyelitis vaccine proceeded by two different approaches: the preparation of an **inactivated virus vaccine,** based on evidence that poliovirus inactivated with formalin could immunize monkeys; and the development of a **live attenuated virus vaccine,** modeled on the successful control of smallpox and yellow fever by such vaccines.

INACTIVATED VIRUS VACCINE. Salk demonstrated that all three types of polioviruses could be inactivated in about 1 week by 1:4000 formalin, pH 7, at 37°C, with retention of adequate antigenicity. When purified virus is used, the inactivation follows pseudo–first-order kinetics. However, in crude viral preparations, aggregation of the viral particles results in a complex inactivation curve: the exponential rate of viral inactivation is not constant, and the inactivation curve tails off markedly. Failure to recognize this complication led to some serious initial difficulties in vaccine production, exemplified by an incident in which residual infectious virus in several lots of commercial vaccine induced 260 cases of poliomyelitis with 10 deaths. Fortunately, the errors were soon rectified, and a safe, highly effective vaccine was developed.* Extensive controlled studies showed an effective protection against paralytic poliomyelitis in 70% to 90% of those immunized, and subsequent use of vaccine in the general population confirmed its protective ability.

The inactivated vaccine has been supplanted by the live attenuated vaccine (see below) in the United States, but inactivated vaccine is still popular elsewhere. When

---

* In the presence of 1M MgCl₂, inactivation by formalin shows much less tailing off. Moreover, this procedure, which can be carried out at 50°C, inactivates adventitious viruses present in monkey cell cultures. These viruses, which include SV40 virus (see Chap. 64), are more resistant to formalin inactivation than poliovirus but are not stabilized by MgCl₂ against heat inactivation. Because 1M MgCl₂ also selectively reduced heat inactivation of infectious poliovirus, heating in its presence may similarly be used with infectious virus preparations to eliminate extraneous viruses such as SV40.

the inactivated vaccine is used in the United States (for example, for immunodeficient children), it is recommended that the vaccine containing all three poliovirus types be administered in three intramuscular or subcutaneous injections over a 3- to 6-month period and that a fourth injection be given after 6 to 12 months. In the early, extensive studies of this vaccine, Ab levels for all three types appeared to fall to approximately 20% of their maximum titer within 2 years, and thereafter to decline at a slower rate. The actual persistence of Abs was difficult to evaluate, however, because of the uncontrolled occurrence of reinfections. Booster injections of vaccine every 5 years are therefore recommended. More concentrated vaccines are being tested abroad, and it is believed that these preparations will not require more than two primary inoculations.

Immunization does not prevent reinfection of the alimentary tract unless serum Ab levels are very high (which is unusual except shortly after booster doses). However, infection of the oropharyngeal mucosa and tonsils is generally prevented, eliminating transmission by pharyngeal secretions. This effect may explain the decreased incidence of infection observed after the widespread use of inactivated virus vaccine.

LIVE ATTENUATED VIRUS VACCINE. Infection of the alimentary canal with attenuated live viruses offers several hypothetical advantages: (1) long-lasting immunity, similar to that following natural infections, (2) prevention of reinfection of the gastrointestinal tract and therefore elimination of this route for transmission of the virus, and (3) inexpensive mass immunization without the need for sterile equipment.

Three different sets of attenuated viruses were independently selected by Cox, Koprowski, and Sabin by multiple passage in a foreign host, most frequently tissue culture. The strains developed by Sabin were chosen by the U.S. Public Health Service for commercial production of vaccines. These strains lack neurovirulence for susceptible monkeys inoculated both intramuscularly and intracerebrally, but they occasionally cause paralysis following intraspinal inoculation. The type 1 and 2 strains are genetically stable, probably because they contain several mutations that decrease virulence (see Table 55–2), although a minor increase in neurovirulence may occur during passage in humans. Fortunately, however, the alimentary tract of humans does not offer a marked selective advantage to mutants with increased neurovirulence. In contrast, the type 3 vaccine strain reverts more frequently; it is estimated to produce approximately one case of paralytic poliomyelitis for every 3×10^6 vaccinated people, and the frequency is much greater in children with immunodeficiency diseases and in adult males. (Oligonucleotide mapping and the genetic markers in mutant strains used for immunization are of par-

ticular value in determining whether or not the vaccine was responsible for the rare postimmunization case of disease.)

In most persons, oral administration of a single type in a dose of 10^5 to 3.2×10^5 $TCID_{50}$ produces infection of the gastrointestinal canal, excretion of virus in high titer for 4 to 5 weeks, and development of Abs to a titer of approximately $1:128$ in 3 to 4 weeks. Serologic conversion occurs in over 95% of those without Abs to any of the three types at the time the vaccine is administered. During the period of relatively high Ab titers, natural reinfection of the alimentary tract is prevented, but the duration of this protection has not been clearly defined.

Since Abs and immunity persist following natural infections, a similar persistence was expected to follow immunization with infectious attenuated virus. In fact, however, Abs decrease at approximately the same rate as after immunization with inactivated viruses, i.e., a diminution in 2 years to about 20% of the maximum titer. Antibody levels are generally higher, however, following vaccination with live rather than with inactivated vaccines.

The three viruses are fed together, and interference, with multiplication of one or more types, which was initially feared, is minimized by adjusting the viral concentrations so that type 1 is present in the greatest quantity and type 2 in the lowest. For maximum Ab response, immunization with three doses of the trivalent vaccine during the first year of life, preferably from 3 to 18 months of age, is recommended; a booster is also advised for all children at the time of entrance to elementary school. Further vaccine administration is believed unnecessary unless one is exposed to a known case of poliomyelitis or anticipates travel to a region where poliomyelitis is endemic.

Preexisting infection of the alimentary canal with other enteroviruses may interfere with successful implantation of the poliovirus vaccine strains. Hence, community immunization programs are usually carried out in the winter or early spring, when enteroviruses are less prevalent.

CRITIQUE OF POLIOVIRUS VACCINES. Each class of the vaccines has advantages and disadvantages.

Inactivated virus vaccine, which is now of high potency and moderate purity, has the distinct **advantage** that it is safe and remarkably effective when properly employed. For example, the exclusive use of the inactivated vaccine in Finland and Sweden has apparently eliminated paralytic poliomyelitis in these countries. Indeed, there has not been a single case for more than 12 years; and in Finland, despite constant surveillance, no poliovirus has been isolated during this period. However, the inactivated vaccine has the following **disadvantages:** (1) logistic problems of administration by sterile injection to large numbers of people, especially children; (2) greater cost, both for administration and for several doses of vaccine; (3) requirement for booster immunizations every 5 years; and (4) failure to eliminate intestinal reinfection and fecal excretion. This last feature, however, could also be an advantage if immunity is not long-lasting, since natural infection could then occur at the usual rate, inducing immunity without producing paralytic disease.

The **live attenuated virus vaccine** has clear **advantages:** (1) it is easily administered; (2) it is relatively inexpensive; (3) it results in synthesis and excretion of IgA Abs into the gastrointestinal tract, thus producing alimentary tract resistance, decreasing spread within the population, and therefore conferring **"herd immunity"** as well as **individual immunity** (however, as noted above, it is unclear how long this persists); and (4) its effectiveness approaches 100%. The **disadvantages** of this vaccine as presently constituted are (1) reversion to increased virulence of the viruses employed, particularly type 3, and (2) dissemination of virus to unvaccinated contacts. The latter process might be advantageous by increasing the resistance of members of a group; it is, however, a potential hazard because the transmission is uncontrolled and may infect immune-deficient persons, and the viruses may be mutants of increased virulence.

Despite the safe immunization of millions with live virus vaccine in many countries, its acceptance for general use was slow in the United States, owing to the ear-lier accident with the inactivated virus vaccine and the fear of reversion of the attenuated strains to neurovirulence. The initial hesitancy has been overcome, however, and at present only the live virus vaccine is routinely used in the United States.

Whatever the advantages of either kind of vaccine may be, both have been used in the United States with remarkable effects (Fig. 55–12): In 1955, when the inactivated virus vaccine was approved for general use, 28,985 cases of poliomyelitis were reported in the United States; in the following year there were 15,140 cases; in 1964 there were only 122 cases; and in 1969 (after the shift to the live vaccine) a mere 20 cases of paralytic disease and no deaths were reported. From 1969 to 1981, 203 cases of paralytic poliomyelitis occurred, in four general categories: (1) 43 cases in three well-defined epidemics, affecting 22 unimmunized preschool children of Mexican–American parentage in South Texas in 1970, 11 unimmunized students in a Christian Science boarding school in Connecticut in 1972, and 10 cases in 1979 produced by a wild-type virus that spread from unimmunized persons in the Netherlands through Canada into four states; (2) 22 cases imported into the United States, most commonly from Mexico; (3) 41 endemic cases, unassociated with travel or vaccine; and (4) 100 vaccine-associated cases, occurring in persons who had either received the live virus vaccine or were in contact with recipients; of these, 14 cases were in persons with immunodeficiency diseases. **Indeed, the majority of**

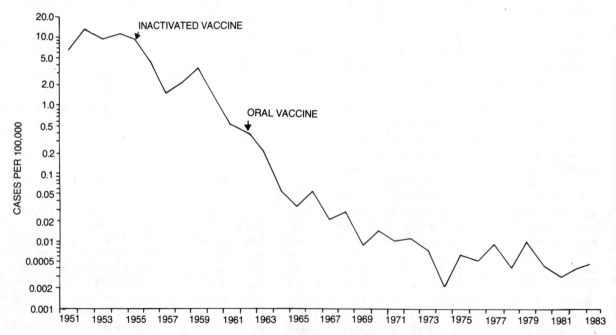

Figure 55–12. Number of cases of paralytic poliomyelitis after administration of killed virus vaccine (1955–1965) and live virus vaccine (1961–1983). Figures in parentheses give the total case rate per 100,000 population. (Data from United States Centers for Disease Control)

cases of paralytic disease in the United States now occur from vaccine administration, in either recipients or contacts. This disadvantage of the live virus vaccine could be revealed only as a consequence of its impressive effectiveness.

Because there is no reservoir for polioviruses other than humans, it is theoretically possible to eradicate the disease by global immunization. Owing to the practical problems of such a program, however, its fulfillment seems unlikely. Therefore, as sanitation improves and immunization decreases the prevalence of infection, as well as of disease, more and more people could reach adulthood, when disease is most dangerous, without ever encountering the virus, and therefore without protective Abs. Hence, the constant threat that virus will be introduced into a poliovirus-free, nonimmune population will probably make vaccination, at least of children, necessary indefinitely. It is depressing, however, that social and economic factors hamper the attainment of even this limited goal: as noted above, many of the economically disadvantaged are not vaccinated, and if the number of susceptible persons increases (for lack of early natural infection), the threat of devastating epidemics may once again arise.

Coxsackieviruses

Following the demonstration that yellow fever virus and other togaviruses (see Chap. 60) are more infectious and pathogenic for newborn than for adult mice, Dalldorf and Sickles attempted to utilize this unique host for studies of poliomyelitis. Instead they isolated a new virus from the feces of two children from Coxsackie, N.Y., in 1948. This new development offered the first major clue that many viruses other than polioviruses infect the intestinal tract of man.

Coxsackieviruses are distinguished from other enteroviruses by their much greater pathogenicity for the suckling than for the adult mouse. They are divided into two groups on the basis of the lesions observed in suckling mice: **group A viruses** produce a diffuse myositis with acute inflammation and necrosis of fibers of voluntary muscles; **group B viruses** evoke focal areas of degeneration in the brain, focal necrosis in skeletal muscle, and inflammatory changes in the dorsal fat pads, the pancreas, and occasionally the myocardium.

PROPERTIES

PHYSICAL AND CHEMICAL CHARACTERISTICS. Those few coxsackieviruses that have been appropriately examined are similar to polioviruses in physical properties and chemical composition (see "Characteristics of Polioviruses" and "Characteristics of Picornaviruses") but

differ significantly in RNA base composition. Hybridization analyses also show only about 5% nucleotide sequence homology. However, the replicase genes of the Coxsackie B3 virus and type 1 poliovirus show marked similarity.

IMMUNOLOGIC CHARACTERISTICS. Each of the 23 group A and six group B coxsackieviruses is identified by a type-specific Ag, measured by neutralization and *in vitro* assays (e.g., CF, enzyme-linked immunosorbent assay [ELISA]). In addition, all from group B and one from group A (A9) share a group Ag, which is detected by agar-gel diffusion. Cross-reactivities have also been observed between several group A viruses, but no common group A Ag has been found. A type-specific virion Ag of a few types (see Laboratory Diagnosis) causes agglutination of group O human red blood cells (RBCs) at 37°C (maximum titers are obtained with RBCs from newborns).

Type-specific Abs usually appear in the blood within a week after onset of infection in humans, and they attain maximum titer by the third week. Neutralizing Abs persist for at least several years, but CF Abs decrease rapidly after 2 to 3 months. Resistance to reinfection, according to epidemiologic data, appears to be long-lasting. Monoclonal Abs have detected at least five epitopes responsible for neutralizing Abs; their precise locations are not yet known, but purified VP2 can induce neutralizing Abs. In patients infected with group B or A9 viruses, the Ab directed against the so-called group-specific Ag appears earlier and persists longer than the type-specific Ab (suggesting a secondary response resulting from prior infection by a related virus).

HOST RANGE. Suckling mice inoculated by the intracerebral, intraperitoneal, or subcutaneous route are employed for propagation and isolation of coxsackieviruses. Mice 4 to 5 days old are still susceptible to infection by group A viruses, but group B viruses multiply best in mice 1 day old or less. Even adult mice can be rendered susceptible to group B viruses by cortisone administration, x-irradiation, continuous exposure to cold (4°C) during the period of infection, or severe malnutrition prior to and during infection. Denervation of the limb of an adult mouse increases susceptibility to group A viruses, with resulting myositis and muscle necrosis limited to the affected extremity.

The striking susceptibility of newborn mice may be partially explained by their failure to produce interferon when infected by coxsackieviruses. The increased susceptibility produced by cortisone may also be accounted for by inhibition of interferon synthesis (see Chap. 49).

Newborn mice infected with **group A viruses** develop a total flaccid paralysis, resulting from severe and extensive degeneration of skeletal muscles; there are no significant lesions elsewhere. Muscle necrosis may be so extensive that a marked liberation of myoglobulin results, causing renal lesions similar to those developing in the crush syndrome.

Group B viruses produce quite different manifestations in suckling mice, including tremors, spasticity, and spastic paralysis. Degeneration of skeletal muscle is focal and limited. The most prominent pathologic lesions are necrosis of brown fat pads, encephalomalacia, pancreatitis, myocarditis, and hepatitis. Adult as well as suckling mice develop pancreatitis, but in adult mice most of the other lesions do not appear or are so minimal that the mice survive. Necrosis of the myocardium, however, is often noted and is markedly increased by cortisone. Cortisone or pregnancy in adult mice transforms an inapparent infection into a fatal one.

Intracerebral inoculation of rhesus monkeys with A7 and A14 viruses produces widespread degeneration of ganglionic cells of the CNS, followed by flaccid paralysis similar to that caused by poliovirus. (Because of this behavior, A7 virus was initially mistaken for a new type of poliovirus.)

Tissue culture techniques have become increasingly valuable for study and isolation of coxsackieviruses and for obtaining attenuated strains by repeated passage of wild-type virus. The group B and A9 viruses multiply readily in various cell cultures, but most group A viruses do not (Table 55–3). The similar tissue culture host range of group B and A9 viruses parallels their antigenic relation and further suggests that these viruses are very closely related despite their dissimilar pathologic effects in suckling mice.

TABLE 55–3. Multiplication of Coxsackieviruses in Cell Cultures

Group and Type	Cell Culture		
	Monkey Kidney	HeLa	Human Amnion or Embryonic Kidney
GROUP A			
Types 1, 2, 4–6, 19, 22	−	−	−
Type 7	±*	±*	−
Type 9	+	±*	+
All others	±*	±†	±‡
GROUP B			
Types 1–6	+	+	+

* Not readily isolated in cell culture, but strains have been adapted to multiply in indicated cells.

† Types A13, 15, 18, and 21 multiply readily on first passage.

‡ Types A11, 13, 15, 18, 20, and 21 grow in human embryonic kidney cells.

(Adapted from Wenner HA, Lenahan MF: Yale J. Biol Med 34:421, 1961)

MULTIPLICATION. The multiplication cycle of coxsackieviruses is very similar to that of polioviruses. However, the assembled virions tend to remain within the cell rather than to be released rapidly into the culture medium. The cytopathic changes are also similar to those caused by other enteroviruses, but those produced by group A viruses develop much more slowly.

PATHOGENESIS

Most coxsackievirus infections in humans are mild; infections mimicking those of man have not been produced in laboratory animals. Hence, we have very little knowledge of the pathogenesis of human infections or the pathology of the lesions. The marked diversity of clinical syndromes, however, indicates that virus enters through either the mouth or the nose and follows a pathogenic course, from local multiplication through viremic spread, that is akin to that demonstrated in poliovirus infections (see Fig. 55–10). In biopsies obtained from a few patients with coxsackievirus A infections, focal necrosis and myositis were noted, but the lesions were not distinctive. In children who died of **myocarditis of the newborn,** a highly fatal disease caused by group B coxsackieviruses, the myocardium showed edema, diffuse focal necrosis, and acute inflammation; focal necrosis with inflammatory reaction also occurred in liver, adrenals, pancreas, and skeletal muscle, and occasionally there was diffuse meningoencephalitis. Group B coxsackieviruses also appear to cause mild interstitial focal myocarditis and occasionally valvulitis in infants and children.

The coxsackieviruses can produce a remarkable variety of illnesses (Table 55–4), and even the same virus may be responsible for quite different types of disease. Still, a number of group A viruses have not been definitely implicated as causative agents of any human disease. Some viruses in each group are associated with at least one distinctive syndrome, which can usually be diagnosed on clinical grounds alone. Thus, **herpangina*** is caused by certain group A viruses and **epidemic pleurodynia†** and myocarditis of the newborn by certain group B viruses. Other syndromes present no clinical features distinctive for coxsackieviruses: rarely, illness simulating paralytic poliomyelitis can be induced, particularly by A7

* Herpangina is an acute disease with sudden onset of fever, headache, sore throat, dysphagia, anorexia, and sometimes stiff neck. The diagnosis depends on recognition of the pathognomonic lesions in the throat: at the onset, small papules are present, but these soon become circular vesicles that ulcerate.

† Epidemic pleurodynia (epidemic myalgia; Bornholm disease) is an acute febrile disease with sudden onset of pain in the thorax (a "stitch in the side"), which is aggravated by deep breathing (simulating pleurisy) and by movement. The pain may be chiefly abdominal or associated with other muscle groups and may be accompanied by muscle tenderness.

Echoviruses

TABLE 55—4. *Clinical Syndromes Commonly Associated With Coxsackieviruses*

Clinical Syndrome	Coxsackieviruses	
	Group	Predominant Types
Aseptic meningitis	A	2, 4–7, 9, 10, 12, 16
	B	All
Paralytic disease	A	4, 7, 9,
	B	3–5
Herpangina	A	1–6, 8–10, 16, 21, 22
Fever, exanthema	A	2, 4, 9, 16
	B	4
Acute upper respiratory infection (cold)	A	2, 10, 21, 24
	B	2–5
Hand-foot-and-mouth disease	A	16 (4, 5, 9, and 10 [rarely])
Epidemic pleurodynia or mylagia	B	1–5
	A*	4, 6, 8, 9, 10
Myocarditis of the newborn	B	2–5
Interstitial myocarditis and valvulitis in infants and children	B	2–5
Pericarditis	B	1–5
Undifferentiated febrile illness	All	All

* Much less common than group B viruses

virus; a few group A and B viruses cause an acute upper respiratory illness; and pancreatitis, nephritis, and hepatitis have occasionally been associated with group A and B coxsackievirus infections.

Group B viruses may produce myocarditis of human newborns by intrauterine infection, as can certain group A viruses in mice. These findings suggest that coxsackieviruses may, like rubella virus, be responsible for some cases of congenital heart disease. Indeed, women with coxsackievirus infections during the first trimester of pregnancy have been shown to give birth to newborns with twice the normal incidence of congenital heart lesions.

LABORATORY DIAGNOSIS

The etiologic diagnosis of group A coxsackievirus infections depends on isolation of the causative agent from feces, throat secretions, or cerebrospinal fluid by inoculating suckling mice. However, for the initial isolation of group B and A9 viruses, inoculation of cell cultures is more suitable (see Table 55–3). In autopsies of patients with myocarditis and valvulitis, the Ag of group B viruses has been demonstrated by immunofluorescence.

A newly isolated virus is grouped as A or B on the basis of the lesions produced in suckling mice. Type identification is considerably more cumbersome, owing to the large number of types. One aid in identification is based on the fact that relatively few coxsackieviruses in-

duce hemagglutination of human group O RBCs at 37°C; these types (B1, B3, B5, A20, A21, and A24) are rapidly distinguished from other coxsackieviruses and can readily be identified by hemagglutination-inhibition titrations. With group A viruses, because of the large number of types, identification is initiated by neutralizing titrations by means of pools containing several type-specific sera, and final identification is accomplished with the individual type-specific sera.

While serologic diagnosis without viral isolation is not practicable because of the large number of possible viruses, **identification of an isolated virus as the cause of a particular illness requires serologic confirmation of infection** (by neutralization, immunofluorescence, CF, ELISA, or hemagglutination-inhibition titrations) because many enteroviruses appear to be present as harmless inhabitants of the intestinal tract rather than as etiologic agents of a current disease.

EPIDEMIOLOGY AND CONTROL

Coxsackieviruses are widely distributed throughout the world, as demonstrated by the occurrence of proved epidemics and by the results of serologic surveys. The type prevalent in any locality varies every few years, probably owing to the development of immunity in the population. For example, in 1947–1948, coxsackievirus B1 was predominant in epidemics observed in New York and New England, but by 1951 the B3 virus produced epidemics throughout the world, replacing the B1 virus.

Coxsackieviruses are highly infectious within a family or the closed population of an institution (about 75% of susceptible persons are infected). However, the mechanism of spread may vary with the strain of virus and the clinical syndrome. Most clinical infections and epidemics occur in summer and fall, and the viruses are frequently present in the feces, suggesting a fecal–oral spread. However, viruses may also be isolated from nasal and pharyngeal secretions and produce acute respiratory disease, suggesting spread by the respiratory route as well.

No effective control measures are yet available. Immunization is not practical because of the large number of viruses that induce human disease and the relative infrequency of epidemics caused by any single virus.

Echoviruses

The first echoviruses were accidentally discovered in human feces, unassociated with human disease, during epidemiologic studies of poliomyelitis. Viruses were termed **echoviruses** (an acronym for *enteric, cytopathic, human, orphan* viruses) if they were found in the gastrointestinal tract, produced cytopathic changes in cell cul-

TABLE 55–5. *Diseases Associated With Infection by Echoviruses*

Clinical Syndrome	Associated Echovirus Type(s)			
	Common		Uncommon	
	Epidemic	Endemic	Epidemic	Sporadic
Aseptic meningitis	4, 6, 9, 30		3, 7, 11, 16, 18, 19	1, 2, 5, 13–15, 17, 20–22, 25, 31–34
Neuronal injury				
Paralysis			4, 6, 30	1, 2, 9, 11, 16, 18
Encephalitis			3	2, 4, 6, 7, 9, 18, 19
Rash, fever	4, 9		16, 18	1–7, 14, 19
Acute upper respiratory infection		20?	19	4, 8, 9, 11, 22, 25
Enteritis	6		11, 14, 18	8, 12, 19, 20, 22–24, 32
Pleurodynia				1, 6, 9
Myocarditis				1, 6, 9, 19
Neonatal infections			11	4, 9, 17–20, 22, 31

tures, did not induce detectable pathologic lesions in suckling mice, and had the properties listed under "Characteristics of Picornaviruses." Most echoviruses, however, are no longer "orphans" in the world of human diseases but have been associated with one or more clinical syndromes ranging from minor acute respiratory diseases to afflictions of the CNS (Table 55–5).

Initially, 34 viruses were assigned echovirus serotype designations. However, once they were characterized, echoviruses 10 and 28 were reclassified (see Table 55–1).

PROPERTIES

Data on the characteristics of echoviruses are exceedingly fragmentary, and the viruses cannot be adequately compared.

PHYSICAL AND CHEMICAL CHARACTERISTICS. The morphology and general chemical characteristics are similar to those of polioviruses and coxsackieviruses. Infectious RNA has been extracted from a number of echoviruses, but it has not been studied in detail.

Echoviruses are generally stable, but there are marked variations, and some of these viruses are considerably less stable than polioviruses. Like polioviruses, heating at 50°C inactivates infectivity and alters the virion antigenic specificity; and as with polioviruses, 1M $MgCl_2$ stabilizes echoviruses to heat inactivation.

HEMAGGLUTINATION. Of the 32 echoviruses, 12 show **hemagglutinating activity** with human group O erythrocytes.* Maximum titers are obtained with RBCs from newborn humans (as with some coxsackieviruses), but the opti-

* Types 3, 6, 7, 11–13, 19–21, 24, 29, and 30.

mum temperature for the reaction varies with the virus.† The hemagglutinin is an integral part of the viral particle. Some types (3, 11, 12, 20, and 25) elute spontaneously from agglutinated RBCs at 37°C, but, unlike orthomyxoviruses and paramyxoviruses (see Chaps. 56 and 57), they do not remove the receptors from the cells, which are still agglutinable by the same or by other echoviruses.

IMMUNOLOGIC CHARACTERISTICS. The type designation of each echovirus depends on a specific Ag in the viral capsid, and neutralization titration is the most discriminating method for its identification. There is no group echovirus Ag, but heterotypic cross-reactions occur between a few pairs,‡ causing major difficulties in the identification of freshly isolated viruses and in the serologic diagnosis of infections.

Immunologic studies can also be carried out by CF, ELISA, and hemagglutination-inhibition titrations. The CF titrations have the advantage of simplicity but the disadvantage of increased cross-reactivity among echoviruses; it is also difficult to obtain satisfactory Ag for this assay from some isolates.

HOST RANGE. The original notion that echoviruses were not pathogenic for experimental animals has proved to be incorrect for at least 14 of the known viruses.§ Intra-

† Maximum titers are obtained at 4°C for types 3, 11, 13, and 19, and at 37°C for types 6, 24, 29, and 30. Titers for types 7, 12, 20, and 21 are independent of temperature.

‡ Types 1 and 8 show a major antigenic overlap by neutralization titrations, and type 12 cross-reacts to a lesser extent with type 29. Antibodies directed against type 23 neutralize type 22 virus, but the reciprocal reaction does not occur. Minor reciprocal cross-neutralization occurs between types 11 and 19 and between types 6 and 30.

§ Types 1–4, 6–9, 13, 14, 16–18, and 20.

spinal or intracerebral inoculation of virus into rhesus and cynomolgus monkeys initiates viremia, neuronal lesions, and meningitis, occasionally associated with detectable muscle weakness. Some strains of types 6 and 9 produce lesions in newborn mice similar to those induced by group B and A coxsackieviruses, respectively.

Cultures of kidney cells from rhesus or cynomolgus monkeys are most suitable for isolation and propagation of all echoviruses (Table 55–6). The final cytopathic changes produced by most echoviruses are similar to those induced by polioviruses and coxsackieviruses (see Fig. 55–5B).

MULTIPLICATION. Judging from the fragmentary data available, the multiplication of echoviruses resembles that of polioviruses.

Echoviruses replicate in the cytoplasm of infected cells. The virions appear to assemble and become oriented in columns supported by a fine filamentous lattice distinct from the endoplasmic reticulum (Fig. 55–13), a procedure similar to the assembly process of coxsackieviruses. Crystalline viral arrays may form. Viral particles are subsequently dispersed in the cytoplasm and released from the host cell through small rents in the plasma membrane or in cytoplasmic protrusions that are shed from the cell. Eventually, infected cells disrupt. Types 22 and 23 echoviruses, in contrast, appear to have a different mode of replication: they cause characteristic nuclear changes, and unlike all other echoviruses, they are not inhibited by 2(α-hydroxybenzyl)-benzimidazole or guanidine (see Chap. 49).

PATHOGENESIS

Echoviruses usually enter humans by the oral route; a few probably infect through the respiratory tract. The majority of infections probably remain limited to the primary cells infected in the alimentary or respiratory tract. It is obvious, however, from the clinical manifestations elicited (see Table 55–5), that virus occasionally disseminates beyond the initial organs infected, causing fever, rash, and symptoms of CNS infections. In fact, virus can be isolated from the blood in several of the syndromes

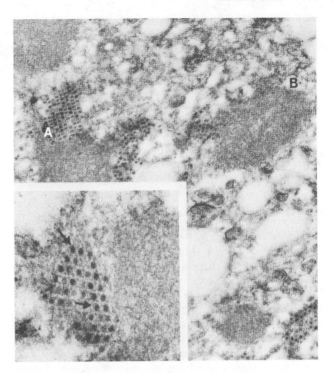

Figure 55–13. Assembly of type 9 echovirus particles in the cytoplasm of infected cells. Viral particles appear to differentiate into columns on a fine filamentous lattice at cytoplasmic template sites (*A*). Another crystal-like array of virions associated with finely granular masses is shown (*B*). (Original magnification ×50,800) (*Insert*) A mass at higher magnification. (Original magnification ×112,800) Transected fibrils lie between the particles (*arrows*). (Rifkind RA et al: J Exp Med 114:1, 1961)

listed, and from the cerebrospinal fluid in aseptic meningitis.

The pathologic effects of echovirus infection are still unknown, owing to the general mildness of the diseases. Cerebral edema and some focal destructive and infiltrative lesions have been noted in the CNS of the rare fatal cases examined, but the pathologic findings are not distinctive. Similar neurologic injury has been produced in monkeys and chimpanzees following intracerebral or intraspinal inoculation of the viruses.

LABORATORY DIAGNOSIS

Viral isolation in rhesus monkey kidney cells offers the most sensitive and reliable procedure for diagnosis of an echovirus infection. Feces and throat secretions are the most abundant sources of virus; infectious virus persists in feces longer than in any other body excretion or fluid. Use of kidney cell cultures from patas and rhesus monkeys is valuable for identification of the specific virus type isolated (see Table 55–6). The differential host sus-

TABLE 55–6. Susceptibility of Cell Cultures to Echoviruses

Culture	Virus
Rhesus and cynomolgus monkey kidneys	All
Patas monkey kidneys	Types 7, 12, 19, 22–25
Human amnion and kidneys	All
Continuous human cell lines	Poor until adapted

ceptibility noted and the limited number of viruses (12) possessing hemagglutinating activity afford convenient tools for preliminary grouping of an unknown echovirus and reduce the expense of the immunologic identification of a freshly isolated agent. Neutralization titrations provide the final criterion for identification because of their greater specificity.

Diagnosis solely by serologic analysis of the patient's paired sera is cumbersome* and expensive and is usually employed only during an epidemic caused by a single virus type.

EPIDEMIOLOGY AND CONTROL

The epidemiologic features of echovirus infections resemble those of other enteroviruses, especially coxsackieviruses. But for those echoviruses that cause respiratory infections (particularly for those, such as type 9, that produce extensive waves of infection), respiratory secretions may be a more significant route of viral transmission than feces. This route is also suggested by the rapid and pervasive spread of virus within the family unit.

Immunization does not appear practicable or warranted because of the large number of viruses and the relative infrequency of epidemics produced by a single agent.

New Enteroviruses

Newly identified picornaviruses that are not polioviruses but conform to the characteristics of enteroviruses are no longer separated into the species coxsackievirus and echovirus because of ambiguities presented by overlapping host range variations. Of the five such enteroviruses isolated (enteroviruses 68–72), two of these viruses, types 70 and 72, merit special attention. **Enterovirus 70,** which has the typical physical and chemical characteristics of other enteroviruses (see "Characteristics of Picornaviruses"), was isolated from many patients during epidemics of **acute hemorrhagic conjunctivitis** that swept through Africa, Asia, India, and Europe from 1969 to 1974. The disease is characterized by sudden swelling, congestion, watering, and pain in the eyes accompanied by subconjunctival hemorrhages. Symptoms subside rapidly, and recovery is usually complete within 1 to 2 weeks. In a rare patient the virus is neurovirulent and produces a poliomyelitis-like disease. The virus is readily isolated in diploid human embryonic lung fibroblasts and KB cells, but it can easily be adapted to propagation in primary monkey kidney cells. Enterovirus 70 multi-

plies best at 33°C but not at all at 38°C, usually a property of a rhinovirus rather than an enterovirus. This property correlates with its preferential infection of the conjunctivae.

Enterovirus 72 is the designation assigned to **hepatitis A virus,** which, after it could be propagated *in vitro,* was shown to have the physical and chemical characteristics of enteroviruses (discussed in detail in Chap. 63 to compare it with the other major viruses causing hepatitis).

Enterovirus 68 has been isolated from patients with acute respiratory infections. **Enterovirus 71,** which appears to be highly pathogenic, has been associated with epidemics of a variety of acute diseases, including aseptic meningitis, encephalitis, paralytic poliomyelitis-like disease, and hand-foot-and-mouth disease.

Rhinoviruses

Acute afebrile upper respiratory diseases, grouped clinically as the **common cold,** are the most frequent afflictions of man. Although the diseases are not serious, they cause much discomfort as well as the loss of more than 200 million man-days of work and school each year in the United States alone.

There have been many attempts to discover the etiology of this syndrome. Kruse, in 1914, showed that the common cold could be transmitted to man by a filterable agent, but subsequent studies in every conceivable animal failed to isolate the virus; only man seemed susceptible! From extensive human transmission experiments by Andrewes and his colleagues in England and by Dowling and Jackson in the United States, the notion emerged that the common cold was caused by a large number of viruses, rather than by a single agent, as had commonly been thought. (They also presented evidence that seems to explode the myth that cold, dampness, and thin clothes provoke the onset of a cold.) It is now known that viruses belonging to several different families can cause a common cold syndrome (see Epidemiology, Prevention, and Control, below).

Since the initial isolations of viruses from patients with common cold in 1956, at least 115 immunologically distinct but biologically related viruses have been isolated. Their chemical and physical characteristics led to their classification into the genus designated **Rhinovirus,** of the picornavirus family.

It is not clear why rhinoviruses were not isolated sooner, despite many efforts, since suitable cells were available, and the initial isolations were finally accomplished with methods employed unsuccessfully in earlier studies. The subsequent isolation of numerous types, however, was clearly facilitated by the important discovery that optimal propagation of rhinoviruses, in human

---

* Because of the virtual absence of shared Ags, it would require that each serum be tested with 32 different viruses.

embryo or monkey kidney cells, requires special conditions approximating those in the nasal cavities: an incubation temperature of 33°C and pH of 6.8 to 7.3. The viral multiplication and cytopathology are minimal—with some rhinoviruses, not even detectable—if the infected cell cultures are maintained under the more usual conditions of 37°C and pH 7.6.

PROPERTIES

STRUCTURAL PROPERTIES. Because of the relatively poor viral yield in cell cultures, only a few rhinoviruses have been investigated in any detail. The virion consists of a single molecule of RNA having a molecular weight like polioviruses (see "Characteristics of Polioviruses"). The capsid closely resembles that of other picornaviruses (see "Characteristics of Picornaviruses" and "Characteristics of Polioviruses"), as shown by x-ray crystallographic analysis (see Figs. 55–3 and 55–14), but the

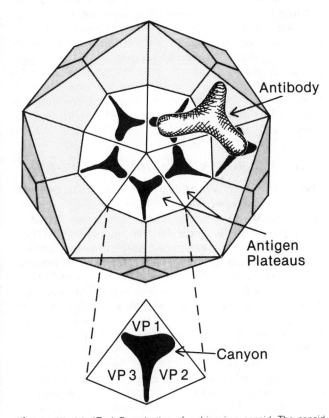

Figure 55–14. (*Top*) Organization of a rhinovirus capsid. The capsid consists of 12 pentamers, each at a fivefold axis (one is highlighted). Each pentamer comprises five wedge-shaped protomers. An Ab molecule is depicted bridging two protomers. (*Bottom*) Parts of the three unique polypeptide chains (VP1, VP2, VP3) are exposed at the protomer's surface (see Fig. 55–3), while the smallest polypeptide (VP4) is buried. The *canyon*, thought to bind host cell receptor near its base, is too narrow (about 20 Å) to accommodate the blunt-nosed binding site of the Ab. (Courtesy of R. R. Rueckert)

subunit structures seem to be more loosely bonded. There is also striking homology between the genomes of type 14 rhinovirus and type 1 poliovirus: from 65% homology of the regions encoding the replicase to 44% homology in the VP1 genes.

Rhinoviruses are sharply distinguished from other picornaviruses because they are **inactivated at low pH, maintain their infectivity at 50°C, and have higher buoyant density in CsCl** (see "Characteristics of Picornaviruses"). When rhinoviruses are held at pH 3 to 5 for 1 hour at 37°C, the virions are disrupted, yielding RNA, empty capsids, and free VP4; more than 99% of their infectivity is lost. The other picornaviruses are not affected by these conditions. Conversely, rhinoviruses are more stable than the other picornaviruses when heated at 50°C at neutral pH.

Not all rhinoviruses have yet been tested for heat stability, but the strains that multiply only in human cells (H strains) appear to be more stable than those that multiply also in monkey cells (M strains). Molar $MgCl_2$ partially stabilizes the M strains. The high buoyant density of rhinoviruses in CsCl is due to the permeability of their capsids to cesium ions (as many as 5000 cesium molecules may reversibly bind to an RNA molecule).

No hemagglutinating activity has been detected for rhinoviruses, but they have the novel ability to inhibit the spontaneous hemagglutination of trypsin-treated human RBCs.

IMMUNOLOGIC CHARACTERISTICS. Each of the distinct rhinoviruses identified possesses a type-specific Ag. There is not a common group Ag, but several consistent reciprocal cross-reactions (e.g., types 2 and 49, types 13 and 14) and more frequent unilateral heterologous neutralization reactions are noted with sera from immunized rabbits. Sequential immunization of rabbits with two or three different types further demonstrates immunologic relationships among rhinoviruses because acquired immunologic memory effects a secondary response to heterologous but related types. Thus several clusters of antigenically related rhinoviruses have been detected (e.g., types 13, 14, and 41; types 5, 17, and 42), a fact that may be utilized for the development of an effective vaccine.

Like polioviruses, the **capsid possesses four clusters of epitopes that induce neutralizing Abs,** with VP1 presenting the dominant antigenic sites (see Fig. 55–14). Natural human infections stimulate the production of type-specific neutralizing Abs (IgM, IgA, and IgG) that confer resistance to reinfection by virus of the same type (see Epidemiology, Prevention, and Control, below). Specific Abs appear in nasal secretions and serum 2 to 3 weeks after infection and continue to increase for 4 to 5 weeks after primary infection. The Ab response appears to be greater to the M than to the H strains.

HOST RANGE. Humans are the natural host for rhinoviruses. The chimpanzee is the only uniformly susceptible laboratory animal; after intranasal inoculation, virus multiplies in the nasal and pharyngeal mucosal cells, and type-specific Abs appear, but disease does not develop. Some types infect monkeys, but in these animals also, disease is not produced.

Cell and organ cultures are the only practical experimental hosts available. The **H viruses** multiply and produce cytopathic changes in human embryo kidney cells, in certain human diploid cell lines, and in a specially selected HeLa cell line, termed HeLa "R." The **M viruses** multiply and produce cytopathic changes in primary cultures of rhesus and monkey and human embryo kidney cells, human diploid cells, and continuous human cell lines (e.g., KB and HeLa cells). Organ cultures of human embryonic nasal and tracheal epithelium are particularly sensitive hosts for multiplication of rhinoviruses. A few recently isolated rhinoviruses multiplied only in these organ cultures, whereas others could be propagated in human cell cultures after preliminary isolation and several passages in organ cultures. Whether these rhinoviruses with limited host ranges to highly differentiated cells are new types or only uniquely fastidious strains of previously isolated types is unknown.

The **cytopathic changes** observed in cell cultures under optimal conditions qualitatively resemble those produced by other picornaviruses, but they are slower to develop and are usually incomplete. In infected organ cultures, ciliary activity diminishes, and superficial epithelial cells begin to shed 18 to 22 hours after infection. As in infections in humans, only the fully differentiated outer epithelial cells are injured; deeper cells appear unaffected.

MULTIPLICATION. The biochemical events in the replication of rhinoviruses do not differ significantly from those of other picornaviruses. For maximum replication, as for viral isolation, a temperature of 33°C is optimal. Higher temperatures restrict a temperature-sensitive step late in viral multiplication. A pH lower than usual (pH 7–7.2) also optimizes viral multiplication in many cell cultures.

PATHOGENESIS

Human infections appear to be confined to the respiratory tract and generally fit the **syndrome termed the common cold.** Virus infects and replicates in the ciliated epithelial cells lining the nose, and during the first 2 to 5 days of illness, viruses can be isolated from nasopharyngeal secretions but not from other secretions or body fluids. A small number of the infected epithelial cells are shed into the nasal secretions, but the nasal mucosa is not denuded. Symptoms appear to result from an inflammatory response triggered by the infection; the mechanisms of the response that effects increased mucus production is unknown. Rhinoviruses have also been associated with some exacerbations of chronic bronchitis and a few cases of bronchopneumonia in children and young adults (i.e., so-called primary atypical pneumonia; see Chap. 40). The absence of a satisfactory experimental animal has hindered detailed studies of pathogenesis.

LABORATORY DIAGNOSIS

Isolation of the etiologic agent from nasopharyngeal secretions is the only practical method of establishing the diagnosis. Organ cultures of human embryonic nasal or tracheal epithelium are the most sensitive hosts and are required for isolation of some rhinoviruses. Such cultures, however, are inconvenient for routine diagnostic purposes; therefore, monolayer cultures of primary human embryo kidney cells, human diploid cells, or HeLa "R" cells are generally used for primary isolations. The isolated virus can be typed by neutralization titrations with standard sera. Because of the existence of at least 115 distinct immunologic types, the number of titrations required is first narrowed by preliminary neutralization by means of pools containing several type-specific sera.

Routine serologic diagnosis is not practical, owing to the absence of a family cross-reacting Ag, the existence of so many distinctive types, and the small amounts of virus obtained in cell cultures.

EPIDEMIOLOGY, PREVENTION, AND CONTROL

The epidemiology of specific rhinovirus infections is that of the common cold. Seroepidemiologic surveys demonstrate that Abs to several prototype viruses are prevalent in many parts of the world and that rhinovirus infections are geographically widespread. Antibodies are found in relatively few infants and children, whereas the majority of adolescents and adults have high titers of Abs to one or more of the viruses studied. School children frequently introduce the virus into a family, where it spreads readily, particularly to those whose nasal secretions lack IgA Abs. The secondary attack rate may be as high as 70% in a family if the primary patient manifests symptoms of a common cold. Successful viral transmission appears to depend primarily on direct contact between infected and susceptible hosts. The high potential infectivity of rhinoviruses is further evident from a study of military recruits during their initial 4 weeks of training: 90% became infected with one or more different viruses, and 40% had two or more rhinovirus infections.

The incidence of isolation of rhinoviruses corresponds to the occurrence of minor respiratory infections, which is greatest in fall, winter, and early spring. Rhinoviruses play a significant role as causative agents of common colds, but clearly they are not solely responsible for production of these illnesses. For example, in one 2-year study of college students, rhinoviruses were isolated from 24% of patients with common colds, from 2% of those convalescing from a cold, and from 1.6% of healthy students; in a study of families with young children, 20% of upper respiratory infections were associated with rhinoviruses; and in a study of military recruits, rhinoviruses were isolated from 31.5% of those with common colds. These studies have also demonstrated that inapparent infections occur.

It is common knowledge that the same person may have repeated episodes of the common cold, even five or six times in a single year. One reason is the prevalence of a large number of immunologically unrelated viruses that cause this syndrome, including viruses other than rhinoviruses, e.g., A21 coxsackievirus and coronaviruses (see Chap. 58).

When volunteers were successively infected with four or five different rhinoviruses, the infection conferred specific immunity for at least 2 years to homologous but not to heterologous rhinoviruses. The degree of protection appears to depend on the Ab levels present at the time of reexposure, particularly the level of IgA Abs in nasal secretions. How long specific immunity persists is unknown.

It should theoretically be possible to prepare a vaccine that could induce immunity for any single virus or for all rhinoviruses. In fact, an inactivated type 13 vaccine has proved effective when administered intranasally to volunteers. However, many rhinovirus types are widespread (in contrast to the few predominant special types seen with other organisms), and several may be prevalent concurrently. A vaccine containing 113 different rhinoviruses appears to be impractical, but if the antigenically related clusters of rhinoviruses are sufficiently broad and encompass enough types, the development of an effective vaccine may yet be possible.

Selected Reading

POLIOVIRUSES
Books and Review Articles

Cooper PD: Genetics of picornaviruses. Compr Virol 9:133, 1977

Melnick JL: Portraits of viruses: The picornaviruses. Intervirology 20:61, 1983

Rueckert RR: On the structure and morphogenesis of picornaviruses. Compr Virol 6:131, 1976

Sangar DV: The replication of picornaviruses. J Gen Virol 45:1, 1979

Symposium: Biology of poliomyelitis. Ann NY Acad Sci 61:737, 1955

Specific Articles

Bodian D: Histopathologic basis of clinical findings in poliomyelitis. Am J Med 6:563, 1949

Enders JF, Weller TH, Robbins FC: Cultivation of the Lansing strain of poliomyelitis virus in cultures of various human embryonic tissues. Science 109:85, 1945

Hogle JM, Chow M, Filman DJ: Three-dimensional structure of poliovirus at 2.9 A resolution. Science 220:1358, 1985

Horstmann DM, McCallum RW, Mascola AD: Viremia in human poliomyelitis. J Exp Med 99:355, 1954

Horstmann DM: Control of poliomyelitis: A continuing paradox. J Infect Dis 146:540, 1982

Kim-Farley RJ, Schonberger LB, Nkowane BM et al: Poliomyelitis in the USA: Virtual elimination of disease caused by wild virus. Lancet 2:1315, 1984

Pollarsch MA, Kew OM, Semler BL et al: Protein processing map of poliovirus. J Virol 49:873, 1984

Racaniello VR, Baltimore D: Molecular cloning of poliovirus cDNA and determination of the complete nucleotide sequence of the viral genome. Proc Natl Acad Sci USA 78:4887, 1981

Rekosh D: Gene order of the poliovirus capsid proteins. J Virol 9:268, 1977

Sabin AB: Oral poliovirus vaccine: Recent results and recommendations for optimum use. R Soc Health J 2:51, 1962

Salk JE: A concept of the mechanism of immunity for preventing poliomyelitis. Ann NY Acad Sci 61:1023, 1955

Special Advisory Committee on Oral Poliovirus Vaccine: Report to the Surgeon General, USPHS. JAMA 190:49, 1964

Toyada H, Kohara M, Kataoka V et al: Complete nucleotide sequences of all three poliovirus genomes: Implication of genetic relationship, gene function and antigenic determinants. J Mol Biol 174:561, 1984

COXSACKIEVIRUSES
Books and Review Articles

Melnick JL, Wenner HAA, Phillips CA: The enteroviruses. In Lennette EH, Schmidt NJ (eds): Diagnostic Procedures for Viral and Rickettsial Disease, 5th ed. New York, American Public Health Association, 1980

Specific Articles

Burch GE, Sun S, Chu K et al: Interstitial and coxsackievirus B myocarditis in infants and children: A comparative histologic and immunofluorescent study of 50 autopsied hearts. JAMA 203:1, 1968

Dalldorf G, Sickles GM: An unidentified, filterable agent isolated from the feces of children with paralysis. Science 108:61, 1948

ECHOVIRUSES
Books and Review Articles

Moore M: Enteroviral disease in the United Sates, 1970–79. J Infect Dis 146:103, 1982

Wenner HA, Behbehani AM: Echoviruses. Virol Monogr 1:1, 1968

Specific Articles

Mirkovic RR, Kono R, Yin-Murphy M et al: Enterovirus type 70: The etiologic agent of pandemic acute hemorrhagic conjunctivitis. Bull WHO 49:341, 1973

RHINOVIRUSES
Books and Review Articles

Dingle JH: The curious case of the common cold. J Immunol 81:91, 1958

Gwaltney JM: Rhinovirus. In Evans AS (ed): Viral Infection of Humans: Epidemiology and Control, p 491. New York, Plenum, 1982

Specific Articles

Cooney MK, Fox JP, Kenney GE: Antigenic groupings of 90 rhinovirus serotypes. Infect Immun 37:642, 1982

Fox JP, Cooney MK, Hall CE: The Seattle virus watch. V. Epidemiologic observations of rhinovirus infections, 1965–1969, in families with young children. Am J Epidemiol 101:122, 1975

Pelon W, Mogabgab WJ, Phillips IA, Pierce WE: A cytopathogenic agent isolated from naval recruits with mild respiratory illness. Proc Soc Exp Biol Med 94:262, 1957

Price WH: The isolation of a new virus associated with respiratory clinical disease in humans. Proc Natl Acad Sci USA 42:892, 1956

Rossman MG, Arnold E, Erickson JW et al: Structure of a human common cold virus and functional relationship to other picornaviruses. Nature 317:145, 1985

56

Orthomyxoviruses

History and Classification

In 1918 to 1919 one of the most devastating plagues in history swept the world, killing approximately 20 million persons and afflicting a huge part of the human population. The underlying disease, influenza,* had been known to occur in large epidemics for several centuries. Indeed, the pandemics of 1743 and 1889–1890 were only slightly less disastrous than that of World War I.

The influenza bacillus (*Hemophilus influenzae;* see Chap. 31) was originally named as the primary cause of the disease by Pfeiffer in the great pandemic of 1889–1890. However, in 1933, Smith, Andrewes, and Laidlaw in England found that filtered, bacteria-free nasal washings from patients with influenza produced a characteristic febrile illness when inoculated intranasally into ferrets. The viral etiology was soon confirmed in other laboratories, and it eventually became clear that *H. influenzae* is only one of a number of bacterial pathogens (others include *Staphylococcus aureus* and *Streptococcus pneumoniae*) that may cause severe, often fatal secondary pneumonia in patients with influenza.

Further progress in the investigation of the virus and the disease was accelerated by the fortunate findings that influenza viruses can multiply to high titer in the chick embryo, a convenient and inexpensive laboratory animal, and that they cause **hemagglutination** of chicken red blood cells (RBCs; see Hemagglutination, Chap. 44). This reaction, discovered by chance in 1941 by Hirst and also by McClelland and Hare, proved to be of great practical and theoretical importance: It provided a simple method for detecting and quantitating influenza viruses; its specific inhibition by Abs to the virus pro-

---

* Derived from an Italian form of Latin *influentia* (influence), reflecting the widespread supposition that epidemics resulted from an astrologic or other occult influence such as an unhappy conjunction of the stars

vided a highly sensitive **hemagglutination-inhibition** test for measuring Abs; and its study revealed the mechanism of infection of host cells, since the receptor sites for the virus on the RBCs proved to be the same as those on the susceptible host cells. These **receptors** were shown to be mucoproteins possessing a **terminal *N*-acetyl-neuraminic acid (NANA) group.** As described earlier (see Hemagglutination, Chap. 44), absorption of virus leads to release of NANA by a viral enzyme, **neuraminidase;** the RBCs thereby become inagglutinable, and soluble mucoproteins present in respiratory secretions become nonreactive with fresh virus.

Of major interest in this family of viruses is the frequent emergence of novel antigenic variants as the source of pandemics, and the analysis of the mechanism responsible for this unusual genetic instability.

The successful investigations of influenza viruses, and the general availability of tissue cultures, led to the discovery of additional viruses (e.g., **parainfluenza viruses**) that agglutinate RBCs and react with similar mucoproteins. These were originally classified together with influenza viruses and termed *myxoviruses* (Gr., *myxo*, mucus), but later discovery of major physical and chemical differences among the viruses led to their separation into two families (Table 56–1): **Orthomyxoviridae*** and **Paramyxoviridae** (vernacular, orthomyxoviruses and paramyxoviruses), whose distinguishing characteristics are listed in Table 56–2. Orthomyxoviruses (influenza viruses) are described in this chapter, and paramyxoviruses are described in Chapter 57.

Influenza Viruses

After the isolation of the causative agent of influenza it soon became evident that a complex group of viruses was involved. The agents isolated from humans in England and the United States were found to be similar but not identical to the swine influenza virus isolated by Shope in 1931, and many viral strains isolated proved to be antigenic variants when compared with the initial isolates. In 1940 Francis and Magill, studying patients with influenza in the United States, independently isolated viruses that were immunologically distinct from the original strains. The agent isolated in 1933 was termed **influenza A virus,** and the second discovered was called **influenza B virus.** A third distinct antigenic type, **influenza C virus,** was subsequently isolated in 1949. Influenza C virus rarely produces clinical disease and has not been responsible for epidemics.

Since the discovery of influenza viruses **major new**

---

* **Orthomyxoviridae,** to contrast with **Paramyxoviridae,** is the designation assigned to this family by the International Committee on Viral Nomenclature.

TABLE 56–1. Classification of Orthomyxovirus and Paramyxovirus Families

Family	Genus (Type)	Species (Subtype)*
Orthomyxovirus	*Influenzavirus A*	
		H_1N_1 (A_1 human, $H_{sw}N_1$)†
		H_2N_2 (A_2)
		H_3N_2 (A_{HK}, A_3)
		$H_{eq}N_{eq}$ ($H_{eq2}N_{eq2}$)
		$H_{av}N_{av}$ ($H_{av8}N_{av8}$)
	Influenzavirus B	B‡ (human)
	Influenzavirus C	(human)
Paramyxovirus	*Paramyxovirus*	Parainfluenza 1–4
		Simian (SV5) parainfluenza
		Mumps
		Newcastle disease (NDV)
	Morbillivirus	Measles
		Rinderpest
		Canine distemper
	Pneumovirus	Respiratory syncytial

* Based on the immunologically distinct surface Ags, the hemagglutinin (H), and the neuraminidase (N), which undergo antigenic variation

† $H_{sw}N_1$, a virus isolated from swine in 1931 and humans in 1933 (previously designated H_0N_1), and the first major antigenic variant, H_1N_1, isolated in 1947, have very similar nucleotide sequences and are therefore classified as the same species. *sw*, swine; *eq*, equine; *av*, avian.

‡ Antigenic variations among strains are known, but the information is inadequate to enable division into subtypes.

---

antigenic variants (i.e., **species,** or **subtypes;** see Table 56–1) of influenza A and B viruses have continually emerged; the new variants are only remotely related to the earlier viruses or to each other. The frequent recurrence of the epidemic disease reflects the genetic variability of influenza viruses.

TABLE 56–2. Characteristics of Orthomyxoviruses and Paramyxoviruses

Characteristic	Orthomyxoviruses	Paramyxoviruses
Particle size	Small (80–120 nm)	Large (125–250 nm)
Diameter of internal helical core (nucleocapsid)	9 nm	18 nm
Localization of nucleocapsid	Nucleus	Cytoplasm
Segmented genome	+	–
Frequent genetic variation	+	–
Virion RNA polymerase	+	+
Separate hemagglutinin and neuraminidase	+	0
Filamentous forms	Common	Observed
Hemolysin	0*	+†
Prominent cytoplasmic inclusions	0	+
Syncytial formation	0	+

* At low pH they produce hemolysis.

† All species except pneumoviruses (respiratory syncytial virus)

Although bacterial types are narrow subgroups within the species, it should be noted that the original so-called **types** of influenza virus (see Table 56–1) are broad groups, now called **genera.**

PROPERTIES
Morphology

Influenza viruses are somewhat heterogeneous in size and shape, but are generally roughly spherical or ovoid (Fig. 56–1). Influenza A viruses have a mean diameter of 90 nm to 100 nm, whereas influenza B viruses are somewhat larger, approximately 100 nm in diameter. Filamentous forms of similar diameter occur in fresh isolates (Fig. 56–2).

Influenza virus particles (like paramyxoviruses) are distinguished by spikes or rods that cover the entire surface (see Fig. 56–1). These are evenly spaced and appear to be arranged in interlocking hexagons so that each rod has six neighbors. (Type C influenza virus particles display areas sparsely covered with spikes, revealing an underlying lattice of hexagons and pentagonal units.) Beneath the outer zone is a continuous membrane (Fig. 56–3). Disruption of the particle by lipid solvents uncovers an inner helical component, the nucleocapsid (see

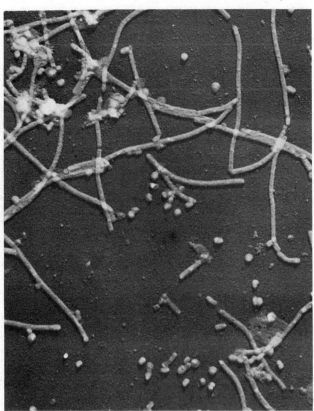

Figure 56–2. Electron micrograph of influenza H_2N_2 virus (third passage) showing filamentous viral particles as well as a few spherical ones. Chromium-shadowed preparation. (Original magnification ×10,400; Choppin PW et al: J Exp Med 12:945, 1960)

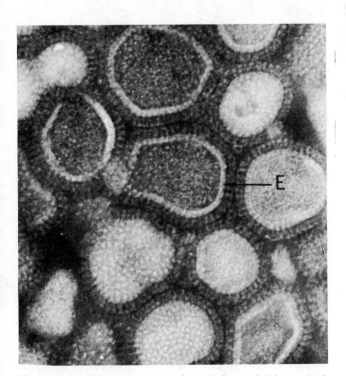

Figure 56–1. Electron micrograph of intact influenza A virions embedded in phosphotungstate. The virions are of variable shape and size and show evenly spaced, short surface projections covering the entire surface of the particles. *E*, envelope. (Original magnification ×300,000; Hoyle L et al: Virology 13:448, 1961)

Fig. 56–3). The purified nucleocapsid (Fig. 56–4) is composed of filaments of variable length (averaging 60 nm), each containing one of the segments of the viral RNA.

Upon complete disruption of the virion with sodium dodecyl sulfate (SDS) the **hemagglutinin** and the **neuraminidase** subunits can be separated by electrophoresis or rate zonal centrifugation. Each of these viral surface projections has a distinct structure (Fig. 56–5). The dispersed hemagglutinins, which are rod shaped, are univalent and therefore attach to RBCs but do not agglutinate them. When the SDS is removed, the hemagglutinins aggregate into clusters of radiating rods (Fig. 56–5C) that are multivalent and therefore produce hemagglutination. The neuraminidase subunits are mushroom-shaped and, after removal of SDS, aggregate into pinwheel-like structures (Fig. 56–5D); both the single and aggregated units have enzymatic activity. These arrangements originate from the mutual adherence of the terminal hydrophobic portions of the proteins, which are normally embedded in the lipid bilayer of the virion envelope.

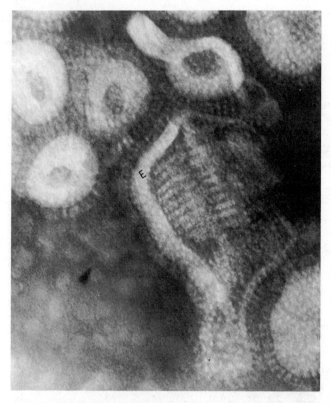

Figure 56–3. Partially disrupted influenza virus particle. The disrupted outer membrane or envelope (*E*), which is 6 nm to 10 nm thick, appears to have collapsed and become distorted, revealing the nucleocapsid folded in parallel repeating bands. (Original magnification ×300,000; Hoyle L et al: Virology 13:448, 1961)

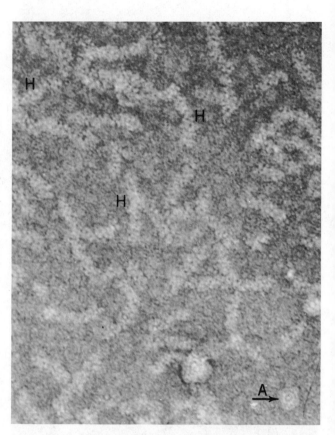

Figure 56–4. Preparation of highly concentrated nucleocapsid prepared by ether disintegration of purified influenza A virus particles and embedded in phosphotungstate. The helical structure of the nucleocapsid is apparent, particularly in regions marked *H*. The particle at *A* is interpreted as part of an elongated structure viewed along the particle axis. (Original magnification ×270,000; Hoyle L et al: Virology 13:448, 1961)

The **filamentous forms** of virus (see Fig. 56–2), often seen in freshly isolated strains, are very pleomorphic and frequently appear to be composed of spherical subunits; they may be as long as 1 μm to 2 μm and can be observed by dark-field microscopy. Evenly spaced spikes, similar to those of the more classic spherical particles, project from the surfaces. Filaments, which are apparently infectious, appear to assemble as a result of some defect in the development of particles and their emergence from the cell membrane. The capacity of an influenza virus strain to produce a predominance of filamentous forms is a stable genetic attribute of the strain.

Physical and Chemical Characteristics

The intact spherical particles contain approximately 0.8% to 1.1% RNA, 70% protein, 6% carbohydrate, and 20% to 24% lipids. A lower proportion of RNA is found in preparations containing numerous defective viral particles or filamentous forms.

Disruption of intact particles with lipid solvents, followed by removal of the hemagglutinin and neuramini-

dase by adsorption onto RBCs, reveals that the RNA is associated entirely with the **inner helical core** (the **S Ag**), which is 5% RNA by weight. In accord with electron micrographs of the nucleocapsid, gentle chemical extraction and physical separation of the nucleocapsid from other viral components yield nucleoproteins of three size classes. The **genome** extracted directly from the virion consists of **eight separate pieces of single-stranded RNA,** corresponding to segments of the nucleocapsid. (The influenza C genome, however, consists of only seven segments.) All the RNA pieces have almost identical 5′ ends consisting of a sequence of about 13 nucleotides ending with an Appp. In addition, the 3′ termini of all the genome RNAs have a high degree of conservation for the first 12 nucleotides (Fig. 56–6). Owing to the partial sequence complementarity between the 3′ and 5′ termini of each RNA, a panhandle holds each RNA in a circular form in virions and in infected

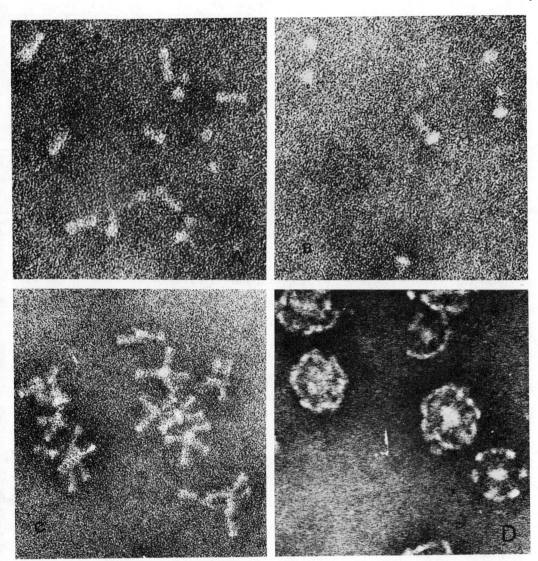

Figure 56–5. Morphology of the hemagglutinin and neuraminidase subunits of influenza A virus. *(A)* Single hemagglutinins appear as thick rods 14 nm × 4 nm in the presence of SDS. *(B)* Individual neuraminidase subunits dispersed in SDS are seen as oblong structures with a centrally located fiber possessing a terminal knob 40 nm in diameter. *(C)* Clusters of hemagglutinins formed by removal of SDS. *(D)* Neuraminidase subunits aggregated by the tips of their tails to form pinwheel-like clusters when SDS was removed. (Original magnification ×500,000; Laver WG, Valentine RC: Virology 38:105, 1969)

cells. It is striking that these conserved sequences at the 3′ and 5′ ends of the RNAs have extensive homology in all strains of types A, B, and C thus far examined. Since each RNA segment codes for a single viral protein, except segments 7 and 8, which encode two proteins each (Table 56–3), this physical structure is consistent with the marked genetic lability and very high recombination rate of influenza viruses (see Immunologic Characteristics and Genetic Characteristics, below).

Influenza virus RNAs are single-stranded molecules (total mol. wt. 5.9 to 6.3 × 10⁶ daltons, assuming one molecule of each RNA segment per virion). Influenza A, B, and C viruses are probably phylogenetically quite distant, for their genomes differ significantly in size and base compositions (the A + U/G + C ratio is about 1.25 for type A, 1.42 for type B, and 1.46 for type C).

Seven distinct **virion proteins** can be separated by polyacrylamide gel electrophoresis (see Table 56–3). Two

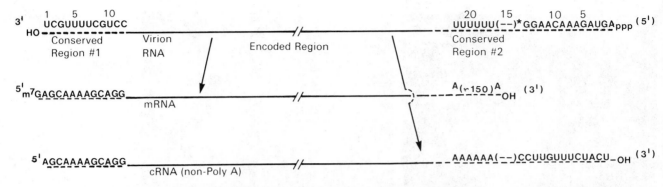

Figure 56–6. Diagram illustrating the nucleotide sequences of the two conserved regions of all orthomyxovirus genome RNAs and the two classes of transcribed cRNAs: polyadenylated incomplete transcripts (i.e., the mRNAs) and nonpolyadenylated complete transcripts, which are the templates for virion RNAs. The sequences 14–16 [(–)*] at the 5′ ends are variable. The mRNAs are copied by the virion transcriptase, whereas the complete cRNAs are transcribed by a polymerase modified by newly synthesized viral proteins. (Modified from Hay AJ, Skehel JJ: Br Med Bull 35:47, 1979)

other proteins, **nonstructural components NS$_1$ and NS$_2$,** are translated from two overlapping reading frames of RNA segment 8. The membrane **matrix (M$_1$) protein** (composed of identical small monomers) is the most abundant virion protein (see Table 56–3; Fig. 56–7); it is associated with the inner surface of the lipid bilayer and confers stability on the **viral envelope.** A second small polypeptide (**M$_2$**) is translated from a spliced RNA transcribed from segment 7, and it is inserted into the surface of infected cells but has not been detected in virions.

The **hemagglutinin** and **neuraminidase** are glycoproteins (containing glucosamine, fucose, galactose, and mannose). The rod-shaped hemagglutinin is synthesized as a single glycoprotein, but for virions to attain infectivity, its precursor must be proteolytically cleaved to two unique polypeptides (HA$_1$ and HA$_2$), which are held together by a single disulfide bond. The functional hemagglutinin consists of three noncovalently linked HA$_1$ and HA$_2$ polypeptides (see Fig. 56–7). The neuraminidase is a mushroom-shaped spike with a boxlike head composed

TABLE 56–3. Influenza A and B Virus Genome Segments and Encoded Proteins*

RNA Segment	Length (Nucleotides)	Encoded Polypeptide	Function
1	2341	PB$_2$	Host cell RNA cap "binding"; component RNA transcript
2	2341	PB$_1$	Initiation of transcription; component of transcriptase; possible endonuclease
3	2233	PA	Component transcriptase; elongation of mRNA
4	1778	HA	Surface glycoprotien; trimer; major antigenic component; CTL target Ag
5	1565	NP	Component of nucleoprotein complex, associated with each RNA segment; component of RNA transcriptase; expressed on cell surface; CTL target Ag
6†	1413	NA	Neuraminidase activity; glycoprotein on surface of viral envelope; tetramer
7	1027	M$_1$	Major component of virion; underlies lipid bilayer of viral envelope
		M$_2$	Nonstructural protein; CTL target Ag
8	890	NS$_1$	Nonstructural protein; function unknown
		NS$_2$	Nonstructural protein; function unknown
	Total: 13,588		

* A/PR/8/34 strain (H$_1$N$_1$) used as an example

† Influenza B virus encodes a second protein (NB), which is nonstructural and of unknown funciton.

(Modified from Lamb RA: In Palese P, Kingsbury DW [eds]: Genetics of Influenza Viruses, p 21. New York, Springer-Verlag, 1983)

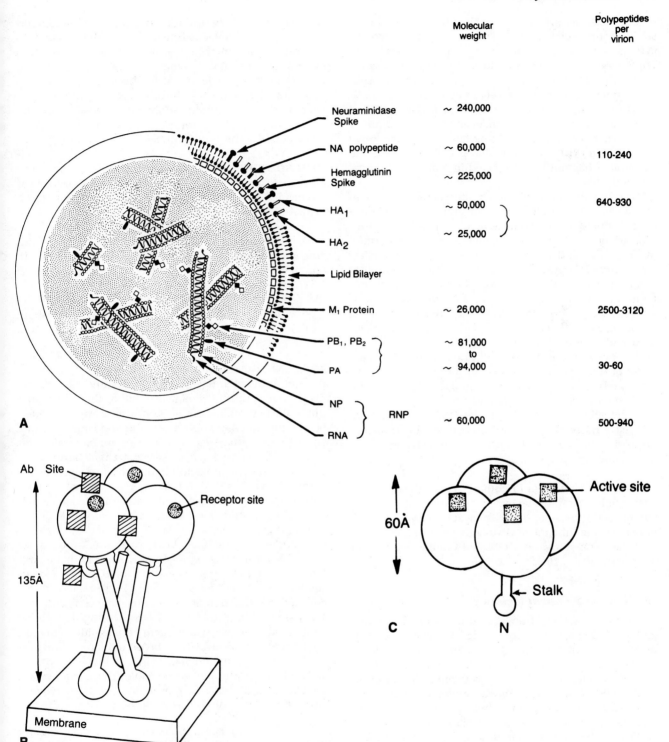

Figure 56–7. Schematic model of influenza virus particles. *(A)* The nucleocapsid is segmented and gives the appearance of a double helix owing to association of internal proteins (NP, PB₁, PB₂, and PA) with the single-stranded RNAs. Also shown is the estimated number of each polypeptide per virion. *(B)* The hemagglutinin spike is composed of three sets of HA₁ and HA₂ polypeptides. *(C)* The neuraminidase spike consists of four NA polypeptides. *(B,* modified from Wilson IA, Skehel JJ, Wiley DC: Nature 289:366, 1981; *C,* derived from Varghese JN, Laver WG, Colman PM: Nature 303:35, 1983)

of four identical glycosylated polypeptides joined by disulfide bonds (see Fig. 56–7). The **nucleocapsid protein (NP)** is a single phosphorylated polypeptide species. Three large internal polypeptides (PB$_1$, PB$_2$, PA), associated with RNA transcription and replication, are present in the nucleocapsid in relatively small numbers (see Fig. 56–7). Influenza B virus RNA segment 6 is transcribed into a bicistronic mRNA, which, in addition to neuraminidase, encodes a small, glycosylated, **nonstructural polypeptide (NB)** whose function is still unknown. The NB protein has not been detected in influenza A virus– infected cells.

Tryptic peptide maps show little difference between the nucleocapsid proteins from different strains of influenza A, but sharp differences between the hemagglutinins are noted. These striking differences are confirmed by nucleotide and amino acid sequences of many different strains. This result is consistent with evidence that within a given viral type (genus) the nucleocapsid proteins of different strains are antigenically similar, whereas the glycoprotein surface Ags are strain specific.

The lipid of the viral particle is two-thirds phospholipid and one-third unesterified cholesterol. The kinds and concentrations of the individual lipids resemble those of the plasma membrane of the host cells. Thus, when cells are labeled with ^{32}P before viral infection, the lipids incorporated into viral particles, except for phosphotidic acid, are seen to be derived from the host cell. At least a portion of the viral polysaccharide is also of host origin. In contrast, the RNA and proteins are specified by the viral genome.

STABILITY. The high lipid content makes these viruses susceptible to rapid inactivation by lipid solvents and surface-active reagents. As with most other viruses with lipid envelopes, the infectivity of influenza viruses is relatively labile on storage at $-15°C$ or $4°C$ but is retained for long periods at $-70°C$.

Immunologic Characteristics

VIRAL ANTIGENS. The **hemagglutinin,** which is the major surface glycoprotein Ag (see Figs. 56–5A and 56–7), is measured by direct hemagglutination, and its Abs are assayed by hemagglutination-inhibition, neutralization, complement fixation (CF), or enzyme-linked immunosorbent (ELISA) assays. The **neuraminidase,** which is the other surface glycoprotein of influenza A and B virions (Fig. 56–5B and 56–7), is assayed by enzyme activity. Antibodies specific for neuraminidase inhibit enzyme activity but do not neutralize infectivity. Influenza C viruses do not have neuraminidase activity.

The major structural **matrix protein of the viral envelop (M$_1$ protein)** is measured by CF, immunodiffusion, immunoprecipitation, and ELISA; its specific Abs cannot

neutralize infectivity or inhibit hemagglutinin and neuraminidase activities. The **internal** or **nucleocapsid (NP) Ag** corresponds morphologically to the internal helical component (the RNA-protein core; see Fig. 56–4) and is immunologically identical to the soluble Ag that is present in infected cells. Surprisingly, the NP protein is expressed on the surface membrane of infected cells and is a major target for cytotoxic T cells (CTLs). This Ag is assayed by CF titration or ELISA.

IMMUNOLOGIC GROUPING. On the basis of their nucleocapsid and M protein Ags the many influenza viruses are divided into three distinct **immunologic types (genera):** A, B, and C. The Ags of each type are unique and do not cross-react with those of the other two.

Within types A and B immunologic variants are distinguished by antigenic differences of the hemagglutinin (H) and neuraminidase (N). The antigenic variations of these two proteins, however, are genetically independent. Over the past few decades a major variant (i.e., **subtype**) of type A has emerged after varying intervals. The variant was either a new subtype (H$_1$N$_1$ → H$_2$N$_2$ → H$_3$N$_2$)* or a reemergence of an old one (H$_1$N$_1$ in 1977).

ANTIGENIC VARIATION. Influenza A virus undergoes two distinct forms of antigenic variation: **Antigenic drift** reflects minor antigenic changes in either the hemagglutinin or the neuraminidase, or both. **Major antigenic shift** occurs infrequently and reflects the appearance of viral strains with surface Ags that are immunologically only distantly related to those on earlier strains. The antigenic shift may involve either the hemagglutinin alone or the neuraminidase as well. Influenza A viruses have undergone three major antigenic shifts since 1933, detected by immunologic studies on sera from persons of different ages and on the viruses isolated. Such "seroarcheological" studies suggest that an H$_2$ virus was probably responsible for the large epidemic in 1890 and that a large epidemic in 1900 was caused by an H$_3$ virus. A virus similar to swine influenza virus (H$_{sw}$H$_1$)† presumably accounted for the human infections between 1918 and 1929, since sera from persons born during that period contain Abs to the swine agent; nucleotide sequence data show it to be an H$_1$N$_1$ subtype influenza A virus.

The first human influenza A virus (subtype H$_1$N$_1$)‡ was isolated in 1933; it was responsible for all influenza A infections until 1957; moreover, in sera from persons born during this period, regardless of their age when

---

*With the recognition that the hemagglutinin (H) and neuraminidase (N) glycoproteins vary independently and determine the antigenic characteristics of a viral strain, the subtypes are now named accordingly (see Table 56–1).

† Isolated by Shope in 1931 from pigs with a severe respiratory infection.

‡ The genus is termed type A; the subtype representing the first human influenza A virus to be isolated was originally called A$_0$.

tested, the highest influenza Ab titers are the H_1N_1 subtype prevalent at that time. In 1947 there emerged an H_1N_1 virus whose hemagglutinin's antigenicity had drifted to the extent that it was not efficiently neutralized by Abs to the 1933 H_1N_1 virus (see Table 56–1). The 1947 virus supplanted all prior strains, as indicated by isolations and by the appearance of Abs. In 1957 the H_2N_2 (Asian) influenza virus became prevalent. In 1968 another relatively large antigenic shift occurred, and the Hong Kong H_3N_2 virus emerged; the neuraminidase molecules are antigenically similar to those of the original H_2N_2 virus, but the hemagglutinin is chemically and immunologically unique. In 1976 swine influenza virus (H_1N_1) unexpectedly appeared at a U.S. Army post at Fort Dix, N.J., but it again disappeared after a brief encounter with about 200 soldiers. In the late fall of 1977 an H_1N_1 virus, another old acquaintance, emerged in the Soviet Union and Hong Kong, but this H_1N_1 was antigenically closer to the variants isolated in 1950 than to the original strains.

Influenza B viruses also undergo antigenic variations, but these are neither so extreme nor so frequent as those of A viruses, and some immunogenic cross-reactivity occurs among all the B variants. Hence, influenza B variants have not been classified into distinct subtypes. The originally isolated B virus was prevalent from 1936 to 1948, and the second variant appeared in 1954. Antigenic drift frequently occurred and eventually (in 1962) yielded an only distantly related antigenic variant.

The continual antigenic variation of influenza viruses is of considerable practical importance and theoretical interest. Each major shift has found a large proportion of the world population immunologically defenseless against the newly emerged virus. Furthermore, the neutralizing Abs induced by the vaccine current at the time did not react with the variant strain. The minor antigenic drifts that more frequently occur between pandemics, in contrast, may reduce the effectiveness of the vaccine but do not make it useless.

BASIS FOR ANTIGENIC VARIATIONS. The **minor antigenic variations** of antigenic drift result from mutations in the hemagglutinin and neuraminidase genes. The hemagglutinin mutations effecting antigenic drift are primarily confined to the four Ab combining sites in the H_1 polypeptide (see Fig. 56–7). The new variants always have mutations in two or more of the reactive epitopes. Therefore, the mutants emerge by selection of viruses that are less susceptible to neutralizing Abs prevailing in the population. In fact, experimental passage of viruses in the presence of small amounts of Ab in mice or chick embryos leads to similar selection of new variants.

A **major antigenic shift,** in contrast, cannot be explained by a simple mutation because the peptide maps of the hemagglutinins from different viral subtypes differ greatly, indicating extensive diversity in amino acid sequences. The change probably results from **recombination** (i.e., **gene reassortment**) between a human and an animal strain, both influenza A viruses. Such recombinants between different viral species have been produced experimentally in animals and have been selected by passage in immunized animals.

Each new major variant results from the adding of new major antigenic determinants while some of the previous ones are retained. Hence, **primary immunization** with H_2N_2 virus induces formation of neutralizing and hemagglutination-inhibiting Abs that react with H_2N_2 virus itself and with H_1N_1 subtype viruses, although the H_1N_1 virus does not elicit neutralizing or hemagglutination-inhibiting Abs able to react with the H_2N_2 virus. The complexity of the immunologic reactivities reflects the independent changes of the hemagglutinin and the neuraminidase, which are encoded in different genes (see Table 56–3). With a major antigenic change (a new subtype) the chemical changes of the hemagglutinin and neuraminidase, or of the hemagglutinin alone, are of such magnitude as to add antigenic reactivities that do not cross-react with the prior surface Ags. However, the antigenic specificities of the major internal NP and M proteins may not change even with major antigenic shifts.

On successive exposures to influenza viruses, whether by infection or by artificial immunization, the **Ab response is predominantly directed against the Ags of the viral strain with which one was initially infected.** Thus, if a child were infected first with an H_1N_1 virus in 1933 and then with an H_1N_1 virus in 1947, his Ab response in 1947 would be greatest to the 1933 H_1N_1 viral Ags, although he would also develop 1947 H_1N_1 Abs. With advancing age and an increased number of infections the Ab response to infection becomes broader, but the titer of Abs against the Ag of the original infecting virus remains the highest. This phenomenon, termed the **doctrine of original antigenic sin,** is reflected in the Ab levels of persons in different age groups (Fig. 56–8); it suggests that the initial encounter with influenza virus elicits a primary response and that with subsequent meetings a secondary response induces higher Ab titers owing to generation of an enlarged population of cross-reactive memory cells persisting since the primary antigenic response.

The prominent antigenic shift, resulting in the appearance of the major antigenic variants described, has led to speculation about whether an almost limitless number of major antigenic changes can occur. However, continued studies of "serologic archeology," which led to the concept of original antigenic sin, imply that the number of subtypes is limited, and the appearance and reappearance of viruses from H_1N_1 to H_3N_2 between 1889 and the present confirms the hypothesis that the repertoire of influenza A subtypes is limited (see Fig. 56–8).

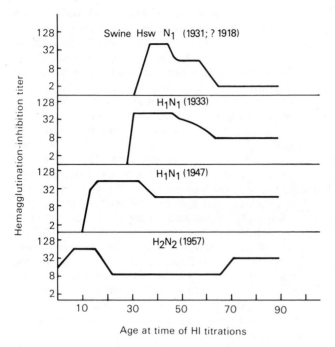

Figure 56–8. Age distribution, in the general population, of mean hemagglutination-inhibition Abs to subtypes of influenza A viruses. Sera were obtained in 1952 and 1958, and each was assayed with the viruses noted. The highest Ab titers for each virus tested were in those persons who were probably infected when that subtype first became prevalent (dates in parentheses). (Modified from Davenport FM et al: J Exp Med 98:641, 1953, with addition of data for H_2N_2 virus)

The observations, as well as the appearance first of the swine influenza H_1N_1 virus in 1976 and then of a similar H_1N_1 virus in 1977, strengthen the thesis that only a limited number of antigenic variations are possible. However, since the swine H_1N_1 did not flourish and spread and the 1933 H_1N_1 virus did not emerge after the H_3N_2 virus, it appears that the subtypes are not compelled to reappear in a set order, although the immune status of the population must serve as a major selective mechanism. It is striking that from 1977 to the present, for the first time since the influenza virus was isolated, two major subtypes, H_1N_1 and H_3N_2, have both persisted in the population. Moreover, this dual existence has resulted in the development of reassortment of RNA segments between the two subtypes as they spread in the population.

IMMUNITY. Either clinically evident or inapparent infection leads to immunity, and the immunity to viruses of the same antigenic structure appears to be long lasting. However, reinfections can be caused by variants with minor antigenic differences. **Immunity is induced by the hemagglutinin,** since it can be evoked by infection of purified hemagglutinin. Neuraminidase probably also

plays a role, however, for antineuraminidase Abs effectively reduce viral spread from infected cells and therefore diminish the impact of infection. Abs directed against the nucleocapsid Ag or other internal proteins, in contrast, do not confer immunity.

Since humoral immunity is highly type specific, and generally subtype specific, infection or artificial immunization with one influenza H_1N_1 virus affords immunity against infection with other H_1N_1 viruses but not against H_2N_2 viruses (nor, of course, against influenza B viruses). Circulating antihemagglutinin and antineuraminidase Abs are present for many years after infection, and disease is usually mild when due to reinfection by a subtype similar to one previously experienced.

CELL-MEDIATED IMMUNITY. In human and mouse infections virus-specific T-lymphocytes appear that are cytotoxic for infected cells, reacting with virus-specific glycoproteins (both the HA_1 and HA_2 hemagglutinin subunits) as well as with the broader-reacting M_2 and NP proteins. Thus, the immune cytotoxicity exhibits cross-reactivity between influenza viruses of the same genus (e.g., influenza A) as well as subtype specificity. The reaction requires that the virus-induced cytotoxic T cells and the infected cells share the host major class I histocompatibility complex. Cell-mediated immunity, and its persistence in man, plays an important role in recovery from influenza virus infections, as it does in many other viral infections (see Chaps. 50 and 51).

ARTIFICIAL IMMUNIZATION. Artificial immunization is limited not only by the marked antigenic variation of the viruses but also by the restriction of the infections to the respiratory mucous membranes, where secretory IgA Abs are required, and where Ab concentrations are only approximately 10% of those in the blood. Hence, minor antigenic modifications of the infecting virus permit it to escape neutralization more readily than it could if viremia were an essential part of the infectious process. The situation is analogous to the outgrowth of drug-resistant bacterial mutants when the drug concentration is borderline.

Genetic Characteristics

The remarkable genetic variability of influenza viruses involves not only antigenic subtypes but also other genetic markers. These include affinity for Ab, reactions with RBCs from animals of different species, virulence, reactions with soluble mucoprotein inhibitors, heat resistance, host range, and morphology. Only a few of these mutations have an obvious bearing on the behavior of influenza viruses in nature, but they illustrate the ease with which these agents vary and the potential types of selective pressures at work in nature.

Variation in the affinity of viruses for specific Ab (see

Chap. 50) is frequently noted. Thus, viruses isolated in the course of a single epidemic may vary in their susceptibility to neutralization by antiserum prepared with homologous virus (isolated during the same epidemic) or with heterologous strains. Strains isolated during the height of epidemics commonly react to high titer only with homologous Abs. Oligonucleotide mapping and nucleotide sequence analysis of such selected viruses reveal the potential frequency of mutations affecting the hemagglutinin epitopes responsible for neutralizing Abs and the number of antigenic variants that may circulate during an epidemic. The emergence of similar variants in nature may permit the persistence of virus in the population during interepidemic periods, but new subtypes appear to emerge from reassortment of RNA segments between two distinct viruses rather than sequential mutations.

Numerous mutants with increased virulence for a given host or organ system have been isolated. Conversely, **temperature-sensitive (ts) mutants** unable to multiply effectively at temperatures above 37°C and **cold-adapted mutants** (multiply best at 32°C) are less virulent and may prove valuable for live virus vaccines. The finding that such mutants revert to a wild-type phenotype at a relatively high frequency may, however, prove to be an insurmountable handicap to their use.

Genetic recombination, more properly termed **genetic reassortment,** has been extensively studied in influenza viruses because of its special epidemiologic and clinical implications for such a variable virus, the opportunity (which was initially unique) to investigate RNA as genetic material, and the numerous markers available.

The first evidence of recombination between animal viruses was obtained by Burnet in 1949, using influenza viruses: infections with mixtures of neurotropic and nonneurotropic strains of different antigenic identity yielded recombinants in which neuropathogenicity from one strain was combined with an antigenic character from the other. Subsequently, genetic recombination has been observed with many other naturally occurring strains carrying various markers and with conditionally lethal ts mutants. Extraordinarily high recombination frequencies between influenza viruses have been reported (up to 50%). The new genotypes, however, are not the consequences of true recombination (see Chap. 48) within an RNA molecule; rather, they emerge as the result of an independent assortment and segregation (i.e., reassortment) of separate segments of the viral genomes. The high frequency of reassortment recombination between influenza A viruses of different subtypes has made it possible to identify the viral protein encoded in a particular RNA segment by associating a given segment with a given polypeptide in recombinant viruses. This approach is possible because each RNA segment encodes only one or two proteins (Table 56–3) and because RNA and proteins

from different subtypes have unique electrophoretic mobilities. To complete the RNA segment assignments biochemical and biophysical analyses of the viral RNAs and proteins were required.

Reassortment is detected only within a genus, and not between influenza A and B viruses. When a mixed infection is initiated with high multiplicities of influenza A and B viruses, however, viral particles appear that have surface Ags of both parent viruses and are therefore neutralizable by Abs to either. This property results from **phenotypic mixing** (see Chap. 48) and is not passed on to the progeny.

Host Range

Strains of human influenza viruses are best propagated experimentally in the amniotic cavity of chick embryos (the most sensitive and the most convenient host) or in the respiratory tract of ferrets or mice. Many strains also multiply readily in cultures of monkey kidney, calf kidney, and chick embryo cells. Viruses can be readily adapted to propagation in the allantoic cavity of the chick embryo, as well as in the respiratory tracts of monkeys and many rodents.

Multiplication

ENTRY. Infection is initiated with the attachment of virions to susceptible host cells by reactions between the hemagglutinin spikes and specific N-acetylneuraminic acid–containing mucoprotein receptors.* The host receptors are similar to or identical with those on RBCs and with the soluble mucoprotein inhibitors in human and animal secretions. After attachment the viral particles, through the process of **endocytosis,** are engulfed into coated pits and vesicles, finally entering endosomes where they are exposed to about pH 5.0 (Fig. 56–9). This acidic pH activates the fusion function of the hemagglutinin, which permits the viral nucleocapsid to enter the cytoplasm. With this process infectivity is rapidly lost **(viral eclipse).**

REPLICATION. The initial steps in viral replication following entrance of the viral genome into the cell are still unclear. Unlike other RNA-containing viruses (e.g., picornaviruses), influenza viruses cannot replicate in enucleated cells. Moreover, ultraviolet irradiation, dactinomycin, or mitomycin C blocks viral multiplication if administered during the first 2 hours of infection but not thereafter (i.e., before synthesis of viral RNA is established). However, chemical inhibitors of DNA biosynthesis (e.g., arabinosylcytosine) do not reduce propagation

---

* Although the neuraminidase-containing spikes can also react with cell surface receptors, virions remain infectious after these spikes are removed by trypsin. Antibodies to neuraminidase cannot neutralize infectivity, although they block enzyme activity.

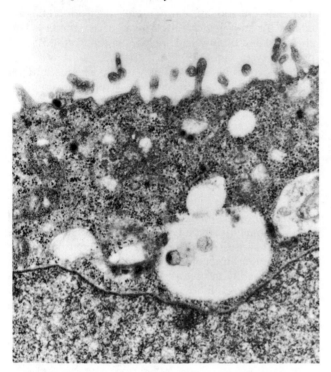

Figure 56–9. Attachment and phagocytic engulfment of influenza virus particles into clathrin-coated vesicles and endosomes. Some nucleocapsids have entered the cytoplasm as result of fusion of the viral envelope with the endosomal membrane. (Courtesy of A. Yoshimura and S. Ohnishi)

of infectious virus. Hence, **functioning but not replicating host DNA is essential for early events in multiplication of influenza viruses.** Amantadine, which inhibits RNA polymerase II, also blocks viral production. These phenomena ensue because the host continually supplies transcripts whose 5' ends are cannibalized to provide caps for the 5' termini of the viral mRNAs and to serve as primers for viral transcription.

Influenza viruses are **negative-strand (antimessenger) RNA viruses,** and therefore contain an **RNA-dependent RNA polymerase (RNA transcriptase)** within the virion to transcribe the virion RNA segments into mRNAs. The PB_1, PB_2, and PA virion proteins (see Table 56–3 and Fig. 56–7) in concert fulfill the RNA polymerase functions. Studies using temperature-sensitive mutants indicate that the PB_2 protein attaches to the cap structure of a nascent host mRNA, which is then cleaved by a viral endonuclease (apparently one of the viral P proteins). The cap structure then acts as a primer for transcription to produce the viral mRNA. PB_1, which is initially found at the first nucleotide added onto the primer, appears to catalyze the addition of each nucleotide. PB_2 dissociates from the capped primer, after the addition of the first 11 to 15 nucleotides, after which it associates with PB_1 and PA to move down the growing mRNA chain. Two classes of complementary RNAs (**cRNAs**) are made in infected cells: polyadenylated incomplete transcripts of the virion RNAs (terminated about 17 nucleotides from the conserved 5' ends of the

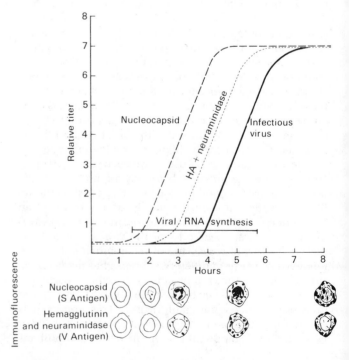

Figure 56–10. Multiplication of influenza A virus. Diagram of the biosynthesis of virions and viral subunits measured by titrations and immunofluorescence.

templates) that are associated with polysomes and serve as the mRNAs; and nonpolyadenylated complete transcripts, which are the templates for virion RNAs (see Fig. 56–6).

Primary virion transcription, detected with radiolabeled probes within the first hour of infection, can occur in the absence of protein synthesis and yields only mRNAs. Replication of the nonpolyadenylated cRNAs requires synthesis of viral proteins, apparently to modify the RNA polymerase, permitting production of complete transcripts. The complementary RNAs are predominant during the first 2 to 3 hours of infection, and virion RNAs predominate thereafter. However, the mechanism for regulating the synthesis of full-length transcripts (cRNAs) and virion RNAs, rather than mRNAs, is unknown. Both classes of complementary RNAs and the virion RNAs are made separately for each viral RNA segment through the usual intermediary replicative forms (see Chap. 48). Both the mRNAs and virion RNAs are synthesized in the nucleus.

The nucleocapsid protein (NP), which is about 90% of the protein associated with RNA-protein fragments, is associated with polymerase activity but probably only in a structural role. The NP (detected with fluorescein-labeled or ferritin-labeled Abs) is synthesized in the cytoplasm and is rapidly transported into the nucleus, where a significant proportion of the viral RNA is also found (Figs. 56–10 and 56–11). The newly assembled nucleocapsids subsequently move into the cytoplasm and migrate to the cell membrane. The hemagglutinin and neuraminidase proteins remain in the cytoplasm throughout replication (Fig. 56–10).

ASSEMBLY. About 4 hours after infection with influenza A virus the virion M_1 protein becomes associated with the inner surface of the cell plasma membrane, and discrete patches of the membrane thicken and incorporate hemagglutinin and neuraminidase molecules, which gradually replace the host proteins in these segments (Figs. 56–12 and 56–13). As segments of the helical nucleocapsid impinge on the altered membrane, it buds and forms viral particles, which are released as they are completed; virions cannot be detected within the cell.

Although the assembly of virions is an imperfect process, yielding virions of considerable morphologic heterogeneity and many noninfectious particles, it must have an effective control for packaging the appropriate set of nucleocapsid segments. Thus, **reassortants** derived from two subtypes containing distinguishable RNA segments never contain two copies of the same gene from different parents (e.g., a single virus does not contain the hemagglutinin genes from two parents).

Viral particles are released over many hours, without lysis of the infected cells, but eventually the cells die. The mechanism for releasing the budding virions is unclear.

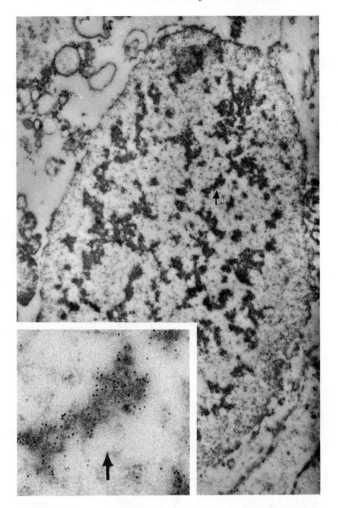

Figure 56–11. Nucleus of influenza virus–infected cell showing aggregates of dense material labeled with ferritin-conjugated specific Ab (*arrow*). The chromatin is sparse, and the nuclear membranes are disrupted. (Original magnification ×26,000) (*Inset*) Higher magnification of the portion of the nucleus marked by the arrow. Ferritin-conjugated Ab is present within the aggregates of dense material. The intervening nuclear matrix is nearly devoid of ferritin, i.e., nucleocapsid Ag. (Original magnification ×97,000; Morgan C et al: J Exp Med 114:833, 1961)

Neuraminidase may serve this function, since specific Abs to neuraminidase decrease viral release, though it cannot neutralize infectivity. However, univalent Fab fragments of this Ab do not reduce viral release, though they neutralize neuraminidase activity *in vitro*. The bivalent Ab may thus block viral release by binding virions to the membrane rather than by inhibiting specific enzyme activity.

The sequence of events with influenza B virus is similar, but the latent period (identical with the eclipse period for viruses that are assembled at the cell membrane) is 1 to 2 hours longer.

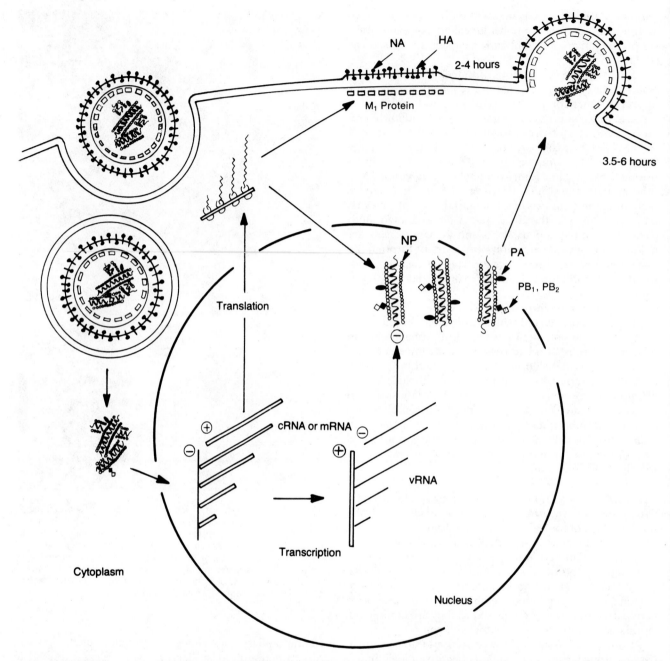

Figure 56–12. Schematic representation of the steps in the biosynthesis of influenza viruses, from adsorption, endocytosis, fusion of the viral envelope, and penetration of the nucleocapsid into the cytoplasm to insertion of newly made viral proteins into the cell's plasma membrane, assembly, and budding of the virion. The site of viral RNA transcription and replication is unknown but is probably the nucleus.

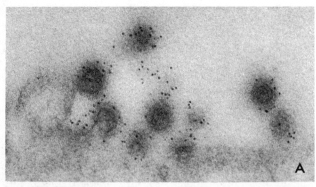

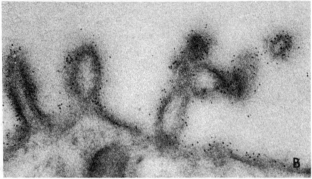

Figure 56–13. Development of influenza virus particles at the surface of an infected cell. Viral particles and components are labeled with ferritin-conjugated specific Ab. *(A)* In addition to fully formed viral particles, ferritin–Ab complexes have tagged one particle (*left of center*) presumed to be in the process of budding and two others (*below, right*) probably at early stages of differentiation. (Original magnification ×140,000) *(B)* Surface of an infected cell with several cytoplasmic protrusions with which ferritin–Ab complexes have combined as a result of the virus-specific antigenic change in the surface. No mature viral particles are evident. (Original magnification ×97,000; Morgan C et al: J Exp Med 114:825, 1961)

PATHOGENESIS

Influenza, an acute respiratory disease associated with constitutional symptoms, results from infection and destruction of cells lining the upper respiratory tract, trachea, and bronchi. Virus enters the nasopharynx and spreads to susceptible cells, whose membranes contain the specific mucoprotein receptors. The virus must first pass through respiratory secretions; and though these contain mucoproteins that can also combine with viral particles, infection is not blocked because the viral neuraminidase hydrolyzes the mucoproteins, rendering them ineffective as inhibitors.*

* The evolutionary selection of viruses containing neuraminidase is understandable. Were influenza virus devoid of its surface hydrolytic enzyme, the secretory mucoprotein would be as effective as Abs, and infection would be difficult to establish.

During acute illness the ciliated epithelial cells of the upper respiratory tract are primarily involved. Viral multiplication is followed by necrosis of infected cells and extensive desquamation of the respiratory epithelium, which is directly responsible for the respiratory signs and symptoms of the acute infection. Indeed, there is a direct correlation between the severity of disease and the quantity of virus produced and shed in nasopharyngeal secretions (peak titers range from 10^3 to 10^7 TCID$_{50}$/ml secretions). Those shedding less than 10^3 TCID$_{50}$/ml have only minor illness or are asymptomatic.

In nude mice or in mice treated with anti-θ serum, experimental infections are mild, implying that most of the cell damage is caused by virion-activated cytotoxic T-lymphocytes that recognize viral Ags on infected cells. Such activated T cells are also cytotoxic to cells infected with other influenza viruses of the same genus, probably because the related viral M_2 and NP proteins are the Ag signals.

Early in the course of the uncomplicated disease, constitutional symptoms—fever, chills, generalized aching (particularly muscular), headache, prostration, and anorexia—are more prominent than would be expected from a local infection of the respiratory tract. Viremia, however, is not an essential event in the pathogenesis of influenza infection, and although it has been detected on rare occasions, the constitutional symptoms are probably due to breakdown products of dying cells absorbed into the bloodstream. The liberation of endogenous pyrogen from polymorphonuclear leukocytes (PMNs), with which influenza viruses can react and enter, is probably not important in producing fever, since few such cells are found in the upper respiratory tract. However, the reaction of viral particles with PMNs *in vitro* inhibits the leukocytes from phagocytizing bacteria favoring their spread. Moreover, in experimentally infected mice, alveolar macrophages are greatly hampered in their capacity to clear bacteria from the lungs.

Normally, influenza is a self-limited disease lasting 3 to 7 days. About 10% of patients with clinical influenza have small areas of lobular pulmonary consolidation. **Secondary bacterial pneumonias** are the major cause of death. Although **fatal primary influenza virus pneumonia** without bacterial invasion is rare, it accounts for the unusual deaths from primary influenza. It occurs most frequently in persons with diminished respiratory function (e.g., those with mitral stenosis or chronic pulmonary disease, and women during the later stages of pregnancy). Viruses isolated from such fatal cases seem no more virulent in experimental animals than those causing minor illness.

Fatal nonbacterial pneumonia was more common in the 1918–1919 pandemic, and postmortem descriptions of the rare deaths in more recent epidemics are identical. The lungs appear unforgettably huge, distended with edema fluid and blood that pour out if the lung is cut. Microscopically, the tracheal and bronchial epithelium shows marked destruction and often denudation. The bronchioles and alveoli are distended with cell debris, blood, and edema fluid, but purulent exudate is absent. Fibrin-free, hyaline-like membranes often line the alveoli. Apparently, the pathogenesis of influenza pneumonia evolves in two stages: from bronchial and bronchiolar epithelial necrosis to hemorrhage and edema.

The highly fatal pneumonia during the pandemic of 1918–1919 was predominantly characterized by secondary bacterial complications. The most prominent invaders were *Staphylococcus aureus, Hemophilus influenzae,* and β-hemolytic streptococci. In recent epidemics, coagulase-positive *S. aureus* and pneumococci have been most frequent. In addition to the usual severe epithelial injury of influenza, the secondary bacterial pneumonias show **deeper invasion** of the walls of the bronchi and bronchioles by bacteria, destruction of alveolar walls, purulent exudate, abscess formation, and vascular thrombi.

The influence of influenza virus infection on bacterial invasion has been studied experimentally. Introduction of pneumococci, streptococci, or staphylococci into the lungs of healthy mice results in little if any inflammatory response, but extensive bacterial pneumonia develops in animals with pulmonary edema induced by influenza virus or irritant chemicals. This effect of influenza viruses is probably promoted by their capacity to inhibit phagocytosis of bacteria by alveolar macrophages as well as PMNs.

Extrapulmonary lesions have also been observed in fatal cases of influenza pneumonia, including central nervous system involvement such as the Guillain-Barré syndrome (ascending myelitis) or encephalitis; Reye syndrome (encephalopathy and fatty liver), which inexplicably has been particularly associated with influenza B epidemics; hemorrhage into the adrenals, pancreas, and ovaries; and renal tubular degeneration. Viruses have only rarely been isolated from such lesions, however, and the relation of viral infection to the lesions is obscure.

LABORATORY DIAGNOSIS

A presumptive diagnosis of influenza can often be made from clinical and epidemiologic considerations. Laboratory confirmation of a clinical diagnosis is generally too costly for individual or sporadic cases, but it is used to establish the presence of the agent in the community, to determine its specific type, and to carry out epidemiologic studies. Diagnosis may be established by viral isolation, demonstration of specific Ab increase, and im-

munofluorescent demonstration of specific Ags in epithelial cells present in nasal secretions or sputum.

Virus is usually **isolated** by inoculating nasal and throat washings or secretions into the amniotic sac of 11- to 13-day-old chick embryos or onto monolayers of monkey kidney cell cultures. The latter have the advantage of also supporting multiplication of many respiratory viruses other than influenza. Fresh isolates of influenza virus may fail to produce cytopathic changes in monkey kidney cells, and the presence of virus is best detected by the **hemadsorption** technique, employing guinea pig RBCs. With embryonated eggs, virus can be detected in the amniotic fluid, after 2 to 3 days' incubation, by **hemagglutination,** by means of guinea pig or human RBCs for influenza A and B viruses and chick RBCs for influenza C virus. The newly isolated virus from either chick embryos or cell cultures is usually typed by **hemagglutination inhibition** with standard antisera.

Immunologic methods are used most frequently for diagnosis of influenza infection. Because the majority of persons already have influenza virus Abs at the time of infection, it is essential to demonstrate an increase by comparing titers in serum specimens obtained during both the acute and the convalescent phases of the disease (paired sera). **Hemagglutination-inhibition (HI)** techniques are most often employed for this purpose, although they are handicapped by the troublesome presence in serum of **nonspecific** mucoprotein or protein **inhibitors.** These may be eliminated by treating the serum, after heat inactivation (56°C for 30 min), with either the receptor-destroying enzyme (RDE) from *Vibrio cholerae* (a neuraminidase), a mixture of trypsin and potassium periodate, or the adsorbent kaolin. **ELISA** and **solid-state radioimmunoassays** are at least as sensitive as the HI, but they are not used generally in hospital diagnostic laboratories.

The **complement-fixation (CF)** assay is equally sensitive, and it circumvents the difficulties presented by nonspecific serum inhibitors. With crude preparations, which contain the nucleocapsid antigen, CF has broad specificity and can identify only viral type, but if one utilizes the hemagglutinin separated from virions, the assay is just as strain-specific as hemagglutination inhibition. An increase in specific Abs can also be measured by **neutralization** titrations, but because of its greater expense and the time required, this procedure is employed only for special purposes.

Immunofluorescent techniques furnish a method for establishing the diagnosis of influenza while the patient is still acutely ill: fluorescein-conjugated Abs reveal the presence of virus-specific Ags in desquamated cells from the nasopharynx. This technique permits diagnosis of about 74% of the infections detected by viral isolation or by immunologic assays.

EPIDEMIOLOGY

Influenza occurs in recurrent epidemics that start abruptly, spread rapidly, and are frequently distributed worldwide. An influenza A epidemic generally appears every 2 to 4 years and an influenza B epidemic every 3 to 6 years, but the patterns have not been completely predictable. Although epidemics occur periodically in any given geographic locality, outbreaks occur somewhere every year. Epidemics of influenza A viruses are usually more widespread and more severe than those of influenza B. Influenza C virus has not caused epidemics, and it usually produces inapparent infections.

The incidence is highest in the age group of 5 to 9 years; above 35 it gradually declines with increasing age. The very young and the very old suffer the highest mortality, with about three-quarters of all influenza deaths occurring in those over 55 years of age. Indeed, even without virologic or serologic evidence an influenza epidemic is recognizable by the increased mortality due to pneumonia in the elderly. Other special groups showing elevated mortality include pregnant women and persons with chronic pulmonary disease or cardiac insufficiency. A striking exception to the usual age-related mortality rate, however, was noted in the severe 1918–1919 pandemic: The majority of the 20 million deaths occurred in young adults, probably because older persons had previous exposure to and hence some immunity against this unusually virulent influenza virus.

Epidemics are common from early fall to late spring. Outbreaks often develop in many places in a country at almost the same time and spread rapidly to neighboring communities and countries; with the common use of air travel, intercontinental spread has also become rapid. The rapid dissemination is not entirely due to the speed of modern transportation, however, for this characteristic was also noted when man could travel no faster than the speed of his horse. The pattern of epidemic spread may be related to the occurrence of sporadic cases and the probable seeding of the virus in the population several weeks prior to an explosive outbreak. Even during an epidemic, a **high ratio of infection to disease,** from 9:1 to 3:1, can be demonstrated serologically.

The pathway of widespread dissemination of the virus has now been exemplified by several well-studied episodes, such as the 1957 pandemic caused by a new variant, H_2N_2 (Asian) subtype, which apparently emerged from central China in February of 1957 (Fig. 56–14). The arrival of the virus in the United States was detected in naval personnel in Newport, RI, on June 2 and shortly thereafter in San Diego, Calif, without a traceable connection between the two episodes. The first civilian outbreak was observed in a conference in Davis, Calif, on June 20, followed by several similar small episodes else-where in California. From the conference the virus was carried directly by some of the more peripatetic members to a meeting of young people in Iowa, and from this location it was seeded throughout the country. This initial dissemination resulted in small, sporadic outbreaks until September, when epidemics occurred in almost all parts of the country. Similar spread along paths of travel occurred throughout the world.

In the summer of 1968, after an appropriate period of antigenic drift (11 years), another influenza A variant (H_3N_2) appeared in Hong Kong and produced a mild but widespread pandemic whose spread was strikingly similar to that of 1957. Although the 1968 Hong Kong virus had antigenic characteristics clearly different from the previously isolated H_2N_2 viruses, there was considerable immunologic relatedness, owing to the cross-reacting neuraminidase. The H_3N_2 viruses isolated from epidemics in 1969, 1970, and thereafter showed further antigenic drift.

When swine influenza $(H_{SW}N_1)$ virus (considered an H_1N_1 subtype) was isolated from a fatal illness and from approximately 200 nonfatal infections at Fort Dix, NJ, in the spring of 1976, it was postulated that this virus would be the next pandemic subtype. This prediction was based on the concept that the genetic variation of influenza A virus is limited (see Basis for Antigenic Variations, above) and that the emergence of subtypes is cyclic. However, the feared $H_{SW}N_1$ (H_1N_1) virus did not spread, and the previously prevalent H_3N_2 subtype (A Victoria) remained epidemiologically viable. The emergence of a different H_1N_1 virus in China and Russia in 1977 and its rapid spread to other continents heralds this subtype as a prevalent species and again suggests the limited variations of influenza viruses.

Many questions concerning the epidemiology of influenza remain unanswered. Not the least puzzling among the unknowns are the following: Why does the virus not spread rapidly at the time of the initial infections in a community? Where is the virus during interepidemic intervals? How does the virus become "masked" or "go underground" in the interval between its seeding and the occurrence of an epidemic? What provocative factors induce the epidemic?

After seeding, or during the interval between epidemics, virus may simply be transmitted slowly, producing inapparent infections or sporadic cases; remain latent in the persons previously infected; or reside, active or latent, in an animal reservoir. Influenza virus has rarely been isolated in nonepidemic periods, which speaks against the first possibility. The intriguing ecology of swine influenza virus, which is activated by cold weather in the presence of *H. influenzae suis* (see Latent Viral Infections, Chap. 51), offers one example of the second mechanism. Finally, human strains of influenza A virus

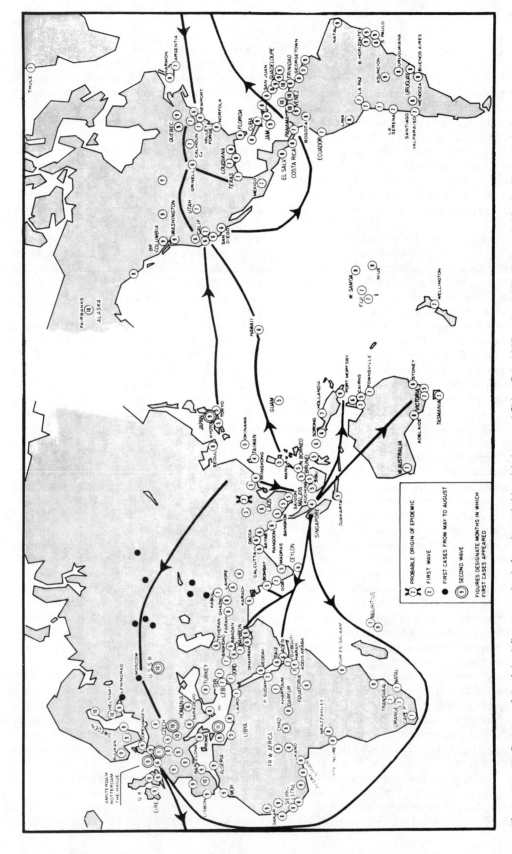

Figure 56–14. Progress of the Asian influenza pandemic from its probable origin in central China, Feb. 1957 to Jan. 1958. (Langmuir AD: Am Rev Resp Dis 83:1, 1961)

show immunologic and genetic relations to influenza viruses of horses, ducks, chickens, and pigs,* which supports the third mechanism and suggests that animals may serve as a source of new variants by reassortment with human strains.

The appearance of influenza viruses after a silent interval no doubt frequently depends on the development of a new antigenic variant that can escape an immunologic barrier existing in nature. However, "old" strains, having only minimal antigenic changes, also initiate epidemics, presumably because a sufficient number of previously uninfected persons enter the population, and the general Ab level falls below that necessary to prevent infections. The nature of the provoking factors that initiate an epidemic remains a mystery. It is also important to note that new variants, or even a different virus (e.g., type B), commonly emerge in a **heralding wave** of infections the spring before they produce fall and winter epidemics.

PREVENTION AND CONTROL

The high incidence of inapparent infections, the short incubation period, and the high infectivity preclude the successful use of isolation or quarantine procedures to control influenza. Quarantine of travelers entering a country can delay but not prevent the entrance of virus. In South Africa in 1957, for example, where ships were quarantined and the passengers and crew forbidden to land, infection did not enter through the ports, but the virus finally entered from the north, probably being carried by immigrant laborers traveling overland.

Artificial immunization can prevent influenza to a significant extent (reducing the incidence 60% to 80%), but not completely. Viruses propagated in chick embryos, partially purified, and inactivated by formalin or chemically disrupted, can provide a highly effective vaccine if the viruses utilized include a strain whose hemagglutinin and neuraminidase glycoproteins are closely related immunologically to the currently prevalent strain. This requirement is not always easy to satisfy. For example, although influenza vaccines containing an early H_1N_1 virus were highly effective in 1943 and 1945, the vaccine

employed in 1947 failed because it did not include the newly emerged H_1N_1 antigenic variant. Hence, influenza must be under constant global surveillance, including accurate antigenic characterization of isolated strains.† Vaccines currently employed contain a mixture of several strains of influenza A and B viruses in order to cover the known antigenic spectrum. New major antigenic variants are added as they appear.

Despite the proved value of the available inactivated viral vaccines, several factors have limited their use and possibly their effectiveness. (1) Pyrogenic reactions, accompanied by constitutional symptoms (not unlike the manifestations of mild influenza) and by local reactions, have been common, particularly in infants and young children; an incidence of 10% to 20% is not unusual in children less than 6 years of age, even when partially purified whole virus is used. Hence, the disrupted, purified component virus vaccine is recommended for children less than 12 years old. (2) Secretory IgA Abs in respiratory secretions are probably critical for successful protection, but subcutaneous injection of inactivated virus induces only low levels of such Abs in the respiratory tract. (3) Abs begin to decrease about 3 months after immunization, and immunity is often lost within 6 months.

Generally, a single subcutaneous injection of 0.25 ml to 0.5 ml containing 0.75 μg to 15 μg of each hemagglutinin subtype will confer immunity in 2 to 4 weeks. Persons immunized with a new subtype, especially children, show a primary immunologic response, whereas those who have had previous exposure to the Ags in the vaccine exhibit a secondary response. Therefore, if the vaccine contains a new major antigenic variant to which most individuals have no detectable Abs, such as H_2N_2 in 1957, a second injection is recommended a month after the first.

Influenza virus immunization is generally effective for all age groups. However, owing to the reactions to immunization and the limited nature of the disease in the general population, the vaccine is generally recommended for broadly defined high-risk groups and persons who provide essential general community services. Special groups recommended to be targeted for annual immunization are adults and children with chronic heart diseases, bronchopulmonary diseases, renal diseases, and metabolic disorders such as diabetes; residents of nursing homes and other chronic care facilities; persons more than 65 years of age; and medical personnel, policemen, and firemen.

New methods of preparation and administration of vaccines are being tested with encouraging results. (1) **Subunit vaccines,** consisting of hemagglutinin and neuraminidase components of disrupted virions, are be-

---

* The N_1 in human viruses extant during the late 1930s is immunologically related to the neuraminidase present in at least four of the avian influenza viruses as well as to that in the swine virus; the N_2 present in the H_2N_2 and H_3N_2 viruses is similar to the neuraminidase of a turkey influenza virus isolated in 1966; and the hemagglutinin of the H_3N_2 virus is immunologically similar to the hemagglutinin of an equine influenza virus ($H_{eq2}N_{eq2}$) as well as an avian hemagglutinin (H_{av7}). Indeed, every subtype of hemagglutinin (13 subtypes) and neuraminidase (nine subtypes) has been identified in avian influenza viruses. Moreover, viruses isolated from seals and whales, which have infected humans through laboratory contact, have been traced to be of avian origin. It therefore seems possible that new epidemic influenza viruses arise by reassortment with avian viruses.

† The World Health Organization has established centers throughout the world for this purpose.

ing used rather widely. This formulation permits administration of a greater antigenic mass, therefore effecting greater Ab responses, with fewer major toxic reactions. (2) **Attenuated infectious viruses** (selected by serial passage at low temperatures) have been widely used in the Soviet Union as well as in other countries, and those selected as cold-adapted mutants are being employed experimentally in the United States. The attenuated viruses have been shown to produce IgA Abs in respiratory secretions. With live vaccines, however, it is impossible to select and test rapidly a suitable derivative of the viral subtype that has recently emerged. (3) **Intranasal aerosol administration** of inactivated viral vaccine induces an adequate response of IgA Abs in nasal secretions as well as of specific IgA, IgM, and IgG Abs in serum, but this method has not yet been adequately evaluated. (4) **Recombinant DNA vaccine** in which the hemagglutinin gene is inserted into a heterologous viral vector (e.g., vaccinia virus) and expressed as the viral vector replicates.

A new approach to immunization has developed from the ability to "tailor-make" variants of influenza viruses by **genetic reassortment** of a new antigenic variant with an avirulent cold-adapted mutant, or with an established strain, in order to ensure propagation of the newly emerged subtypes to high titers. (The swine A influenza H_1N_1 vaccine virus used for nationwide immunization in 1976 was prepared by this method from the Fort Dix isolate.)

Widespread immunization has revealed an additional source of concern, at least with inactivated intact virus vaccine. Following immunization of more than 35 million persons with inactivated swine influenza (H_1N_1) virus in the fall of 1976, the Guillain-Barré syndrome occurred in 354 recipients, with 28 deaths. Most illnesses occurred 2 to 4 weeks after immunization. The incidence was about 1 in 100,000 persons who received the vaccine, almost six times greater than that in the nonimmunized population in the same period. Influenza virus vaccine produced after 1977 has not been associated with neurologic complication. Moreover, the etiology of the Guillain-Barré syndrome is not specifically related to influenza immunization. It has also been reported following other immunization procedures (e.g., rabies, smallpox), but the scale and the surveillance of the 1976 immunization program was never previously equaled so that an etiologic association could not be established with other immunogens. Such complications, in a mass program that retrospectively proved unnecessary, not only brought criticism on the use of influenza vaccine but unfortunately also discouraged public acceptance of other immunization programs.

CHEMOTHERAPY. The discovery that **amantadine (1-adamantanamine)** can inhibit an early step in the multiplication (uncoating) of some influenza viruses (see Chap. 49) reawakened hopes for the successful chemical control of viral diseases. Amantadine and rimantadine (an amantadine derivative) are about 70% effective in protecting against proven infections. Amantadine is also effective therapeutically in that virus is cleared more rapidly, and symptomatic improvement occurs about 1 day earlier if the drug is given within 24 to 48 hours after onset. Its clinical usefulness is limited, however, because its therapeutic value has been less striking than its prophylactic effect, its effectiveness is restricted to influenza A viruses (it does not affect influenza B), and it has neurologic toxic effects (particularly in the aged).

Ribavirin (1-β-D-ribofuranosyl-1,2,4-triazole-3-carboxamide, virazole), which inhibits synthesis of viral RNA by blocking guanine biosynthesis, has been more effective than amantadine in preventing experimental influenza A infection in cell cultures and animal models. Oral administration in clinical trials, however, has shown ribavirin to have only a small, inconsistent prophylactic or therapeutic effect.

Selected Reading

BOOKS AND REVIEW ARTICLES

Brachiale TJ, Brachiale VL: CTL recognition of transfected H-2 gene and viral gene products. In Notkins AL, Oldstone MBA (eds): Concepts in Viral Pathogenesis, Vol II, p 174. New York, Springer-Verlag, 1987

Burnet FM: Portraits of viruses: Influenza virus A. Intervirology 11:201, 1979

Lamb RA, Choppin PW: The gene structure and replication of influenza virus. Ann Rev Biochem 52:467, 1983

Mitchell DM, McMichael AJ, Lamb JR: The immunology of influenza. Br Med Bull 41:80, 1985

Murphy BR, Webster RG: Influenza viruses. In Fields BM (ed): Virology. New York, Raven Press, 1985

Palese P, Kingsbury DW (eds): Genetics of Influenza Viruses. New York, Springer-Verlag, 1983

Sweet C, Smith H: Pathogenicity of influenza virus. Microbiol Rev 44:303, 1980

Webster RG, Laver WG, Air GM, Schield GC: Molecular mechanisms of variation in influenza viruses. Nature 296:115, 1982

SPECIFIC ARTICLES

Broom J, Ulmanen I, Krug RM: Molecular model of a eucharyotic transcription complex: Functions and movements of influenza P proteins during capped RNA-primed transcription. Cell 34:609, 1983

Buonogurio DA, Nakada S, Parvin JD et al: Evolution of human influenza A viruses over 50 years: Rapid, uniform rate of change in NS gene. Science 232:980, 1986

Colman PM, Varghese JN, Laver WG: Structure of the catalytic and antigenic sites in influenza virus neuraminidase. Nature 303:41, 1983

Davenport FM, Minuse E, Hennessy AV, Francis T Jr: Interpretations of influenza antibody patterns of man. Bull WHO 41:453, 1969

Lamb RA, Zebedee SL, Richardson CR: Influenza virus M_2 protein is an integral membrane protein expressed on the infected-cell surface. Cell 40:627, 1985

Plotch SJ, Bouloy M, Krug RM: Transfer of 5′ terminal cap of globin mRNA to influenza viral complementary RNA during transcription in vitro. Proc Natl Acad Sci USA 76:1618, 1979

Practices Advisory Committee: Prevention and Control of Influenza. Morbidity and Mortality Weekly Report 34:261, 1985

Smith GL, Hay AJ: Replication of the influenza virus genome. Virology 118:96, 1982

Townsend ARM, McMichael AJ, Carter NP et al: Cytotoxic T cell recognition of the influenza nucleoprotein and hemagglutinin expressed in transfected mouse L cells. Cell 39:13, 1984

Wilson IA, Skehel JJ, Wiley DC: Structure of the hemagglutinin membrane glycoproteins of influenza virus at 3A resolution. Nature 289:366, 1981

Wiley DC,Wilson IA, Skehel JJ: Structural identification of the antibody-binding sites of Hong Kong influenza haemagglutinin and their involvement in antigenic variation. Nature 289:373, 1981

Yoshimura A, Ohnishi S: Uncoating of influenza virus in endosomes. J Virol 51:497, 1984

57

Paramyxoviruses

The paramyxoviruses (**Paramyxoviridae**) differ widely pathogenically. **Parainfluenza** and **respiratory syncytial viruses** produce **acute respiratory diseases, measles virus** causes a **generalized exanthematous disease,** and **mumps virus** initiates a **systemic disease** of which **parotitis** is a predominant feature. However, on the basis of chemical and several biological properties the paramyxoviruses are relatively homogeneous (Table 57–1). There are also sufficient differences in their characteristics to permit their classification into three genera: **Paramyxovirus, Morbillivirus,** and **Pneumovirus.** Respiratory syncytial virus, a pneumovirus that cannot hemagglutinate or cause hemolysis of red blood cells (RBCs), differs most sharply from the other paramyxoviruses.

General Properties

The characteristics that are similar for all paramyxoviruses are discussed in this section; the distinctive properties are described in the following sections on the individual viruses.

MORPHOLOGY

The virions are **roughly spherical enveloped particles** of heterogeneous sizes (see Table 57–1), larger than influenza viruses (see Table 56–2). Electron microscopic examination of negatively stained virions discloses that they appear similar to orthomyxoviruses. The intact viral particle has a well-defined **outer envelope,** about 10 nm thick, covered with short (8-nm to 12-nm) **spikes** that are more or less regularly arranged (Fig. 57–1). Disruption of the envelope reveals an inner **helical nucleocapsid** and serrations with a regular periodicity of about 5 nm (Figs. 57–2 through 57–4). The nucleocapsid is distinctly differ-

TABLE 57–1. *Characteristics of Human Paramyxoviruses*

Common Properties		Distinguishing Properties				
			Parainfluenza	Mumps	Measles	RSV
Average size	125–250 nm (range 100–800 nm)	Hemagglutinin*	+	+	+	−
Nucleocapsid diameter	18 nm (except RSV = 14 nm)	Hemadsorption†	+	+	+	−
Viral genome	5 × 10⁶ daltons (17–20 Kb); single negative-strand molecules	Hemolysin	+	+	+	−
Virion RNA polymerase	+	Neuraminidase	+	+	+	−
Reaction with lipid solvents	Disrupts	Antigenic types	4	1	1	1
Syncytial formation	+	Antigenic relationships	Mumps	Parainfluenza	−	−
Cytoplasmic inclusion bodies	+ (Measles virus nuclear)	Genus	Paramyxovirus	Paramyxovirus	Morbillivirus	Pneumovirus
Site of multiplication	Cytoplasm					

* Chicken and guinea pig RBCs

† Infected cells adsorb guinea pig RBCs.

+, present; −, absent

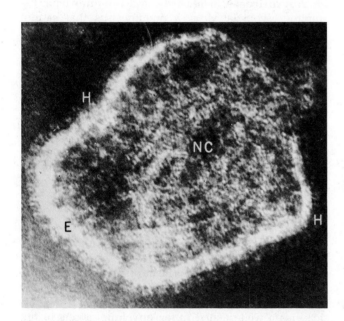

Figure 57–1. Electron micrograph of type 3 parainfluenza virus embedded in phosphotungstate. The envelope (*E*), peripheral short projecting spikes (*H*), and internal nucleocapsid (*NC*) are apparent. The helical nucleocapsid can also be seen escaping from a small break in the envelope. (Original magnification ×210,000; Courtesy of A. P. Waterson, St. Thomas's Hospital Medical School, London)

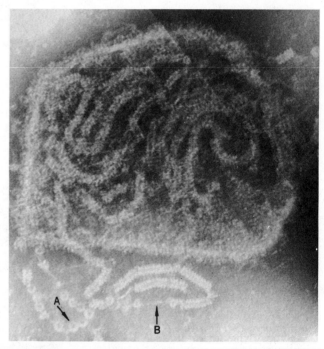

Figure 57–2. Partially disrupted mumps virus particle showing the envelope and the hollow helical strands forming the nucleocapsid. Several broken strands have been released, revealing periodic structures (*A*) that make up the helical nucleocapsid. Fine threads connecting separated pieces are visible (*B*). (Original magnification ×250,000; Horne RW, Waterson AP: J Mol Biol 2:75, 1960. Copyright by Academic Press, Inc. [London] Ltd.)

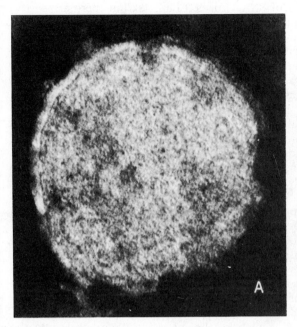
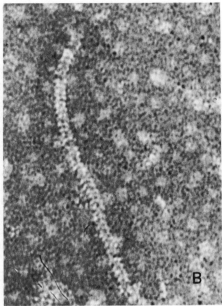

Figure 57–3. Fine structure of measles virus, revealed by negative staining with sodium phosphotungstate. *(A)* Particle showing the characteristic envelope and peripheral projections. The nucleocapsid is tightly packed and shows an appearance of concentric rings toward the periphery. (Original magnification ×280,000) *(B)* The portion of the helical nucleocapsid released from a disrupted virion. (Original magnification ×240,000; Horne RW, Waterson AP: J Mol Biol 2:75, 1960. Copyright by Academic Press, Inc. [London] Ltd.)

ent from that of influenza viruses (see Table 56–2): its diameter is approximately twice as great, its characteristic periodic serrations are more discrete, and it can be isolated from the virion as a single long helical structure. Filamentous virions are observed in thin sections of infected cells but not in negatively stained preparations, because they are apparently disrupted during fixation.

PHYSICAL AND CHEMICAL CHARACTERISTICS

The paramyxoviruses that have been purified and analyzed all have a similar protein, lipid, and RNA composition. The nucleocapsid consists of a single species of protein (NP) and **one large molecule of single-stranded RNA** of **negative polarity** (see Table 57–1). The viral envelope contains three proteins. Two glycoproteins form the surface projections (Fig. 57–5). One glycoprotein varies in viruses of the three genera: in parainfluenza and mumps virus it has both **hemagglutinin and neuraminidase activities** (termed **HN**); in measles virus it lacks neuraminidase activity (hence, termed **H protein**); and in respiratory syncytial virus it has neither hemagglutinin nor neuraminidase functions and is called the **G protein.** The other surface glycoprotein, which consists of two disulfide-linked subunits (F_1 and F_2), is responsible for the virion's **cell fusion** activity of all paramyxoviruses as well as the **hemolytic** function of

parainfluenza, mumps, and measles viruses (see Table 57–1). The third envelope protein (M), which is nonglycosylated, forms the **inner layer of the envelope,** maintaining its structure and integrity. The HN protein of parainfluenza and mumps virus is a dimer consisting of disulfide-linked, identical polypeptide chains.

Because the viral envelope has a high lipid content, organic solvents or surface-active agents rapidly inactivate the virions by dissolving their envelopes, thus liberating the envelope proteins and the nucleocapsids from the disrupted particles.

The virions are relatively unstable, losing 90% to 99% of their infectivity in 2 to 4 hours when suspended in a protein-free medium at room temperature or at 4°C.

MULTIPLICATION

The multiplication cycles do not appear to differ for each paramyxovirus, except for the great variations in the length of various phases. For example, the eclipse period is 3 to 5 hours for parainfluenza viruses, 16 to 18 hours for mumps virus, and 9 to 12 hours for measles virus. The basic biosynthetic events (predominantly derived from studies of parainfluenza and Newcastle disease viruses) are similar to those for other enveloped viruses that possess a negative single-stranded RNA and contain an RNA-dependent RNA polymerase within the virion (see Syn-

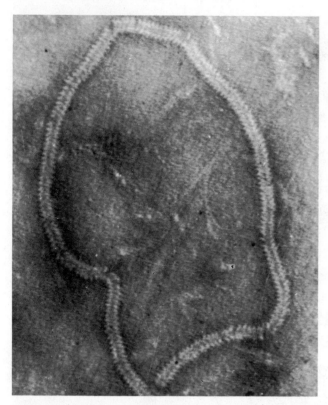

Figure 57-4. Strand of helical nucleocapsid of type 1 (Sendai) parainfluenza virus embedded in phosphotungstate. (Examination by tilting through large angles reveals the sense of the helix to be left-handed.) (Original magnification ×200,000; Horne RW, Waterson AP: J Mol Biol 2:75, 1960. Copyright by Academic Press, Inc. [London] Ltd.)

thesis of RNA Viruses, Chap. 48), but there are several unique features. In contrast to orthomyxoviruses, paramyxoviruses multiply without restraint in the presence of actinomycin D. The unsegmented virion RNAs of all paramyxoviruses consist of a linear series of linked genes. Because each gene produces a single mRNA, each contains conserved nucleotide sequences designating start and termination sites, the latter containing a poly(A) signal for its mRNA (Fig. 57–6). The genes are linked by a highly conserved **intergenic sequence,** GAA. The **P** and **L proteins** function for **RNA synthesis.** The **NP protein,** like its counterpart in orthomyxoviruses, does not have catalytic activity, but appears to provide the genomic RNA with the appropriate configuration for its **transcription and replication.** Since the genes in the viral genomes differ somewhat in each genus of the paramyxovirus family the genome maps also vary, but the basic structures are similar to that shown (see Fig. 57–6).

Virion infectivity, as well as hemolytic and cell fusion properties, requires **maturation of the F glycoprotein** by proteolytic cleavage of a larger precursor (F_0) by a cellular enzyme to produce two polypeptide chains, F_1 and F_2, which are linked by disulfide bonds into the functional dimer. With most paramyxoviruses the NP proteins of the nucleocapsid, as well as the HN (hemagglutinin–neuraminidase) protein, are detected only in the cytoplasm of infected cells, but the measles virus nucleocapsid is also present in the nucleus.

After viral RNA is synthesized in the cytoplasm, it is rapidly associated with the newly made nucleocapsid protein, but only a relatively small proportion of the nucleocapsids thus formed is assembled into virions. Occasionally, positive strands, owing to their excess, may be accidentally assembled into virions as well as nucleocap-

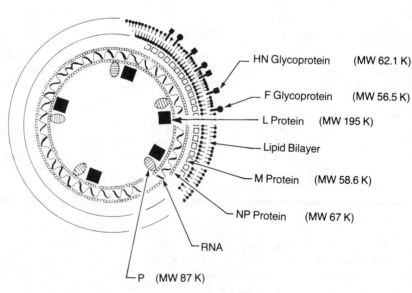

Figure 57-5. Diagram of a paramyxovirus. (Different forms are shown for the *F* and *HN* glycoproteins to indicate their chemical differences, although they are not distinguishable in electron micrographs.) The F and HN glycoproteins are anchored in the lipid bilayer, the F by its F_1 C terminus and the HN by its N terminus. The M protein forms the inner layer of the envelope and maintains its structure and integrity. The actual arrangements of the NP and L proteins in the nucleocapsid are unknown. *MW*, molecular weight; *K*, kilodaltons.

HN Glycoprotein   (MW 62.1 K)

F Glycoprotein   (MW 56.5 K)

L Protein   (MW 195 K)

Lipid Bilayer

M Protein   (MW 58.6 K)

NP Protein   (MW 67 K)

RNA

P   (MW 87 K)

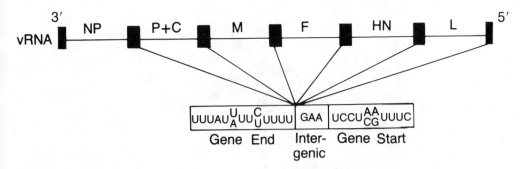

Figure 57–6. Diagram of the parainfluenza 3 virus RNA genome depicting the order of the genes (NP, P+C, M, F, HN, and L), the gene-end nucleotide sequences, the start sequences, and the intergenic sequences. The gene-end sequences contain the transcription termination sequences and the mRNA complementary poly(A) sequences. The 12 gene-end nucleotides are semiconserved, whereas the ten gene start nucleotides and the three intergenic nucleotides (GAA) are relatively well conserved for all five gene junctions. The nucleotide position of the translational start sites from the 5' end of the genes varies from 33 to 35 nucleotides for the M protein gene to 194 to 196 nucleotides for the F gene. (Data from Spriggs MK, Collins PL: Human parainfluenza virus type 3: Messenger RNAs, polypeptide coding assignments, intergenic sequences and genetic map. J Virol 59:646, 1986)

sids. The cytoplasmic inclusion bodies (Fig. 57–7) are predominantly accumulations of the excess nucleocapsids.

Electron microscopic examination of infected cells reveals the remarkable assembly and maturation of paramyxoviruses at the plasma membrane (Fig. 57–8). Strands of viral nucleocapsid can be seen to associate with the viral M protein lining the regions of thickened cell membranes containing virus-specific glycoproteins: these differentiated cell membranes are destined to become the viral envelopes. Intact viral particles are noted only at the cell membrane, where they are assembled

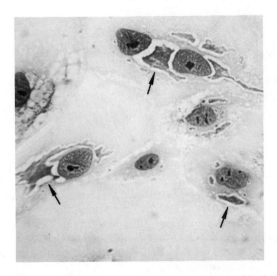

Figure 57–7. Eosinophilic cytoplasmic inclusions (*arrows*) in dog kidney cells infected with type 2 parainfluenza virus. Nuclei appear unaffected. (Original magnification ×450; Brandt CD: Virology 14:1, 1961)

and released from the cell by budding. The final assembly of the nucleocapsid and the specifically altered plasma membrane are especially prominent with these viruses (see Fig. 57–8).

Parainfluenza Viruses

Parainfluenza viruses were recognized in 1957 as important causes of acute respiratory infections of man and were initially termed *hemadsorption virus, croup-associated viruses,* and *influenza D.* At least four antigenic types infect man, and one infects monkeys.

The major characteristics of parainfluenza viruses infecting man are listed in Table 57–1.

PROPERTIES
Immunologic Characteristics

Each parainfluenza virus possesses three distinct Ags from which it derives its type specificity: The **HN (hemagglutinin–neuraminidase)** and the **F (fusion–hemolysin)** surface Ags, and an internal nucleocapsid Ag, the **NP protein** (see Fig. 57–5). Neutralizing Abs are directed against the HN glycoprotein, and at least four epitopes function in the neutralization and hemagglutinin-inhibition reactions. Distinct epitopes have also been identified with neuraminidase activity, indicating that neuraminidase and hemagglutinin functions are associated with unique regions of the HN glycoprotein. Parainfluenza viruses are immunologically unrelated to influenza viruses. Progressive major antigenic alterations have not been detected; only type 4 parainfluenza virus has subtypes, A and B.

Although there is not a single Ag common to all

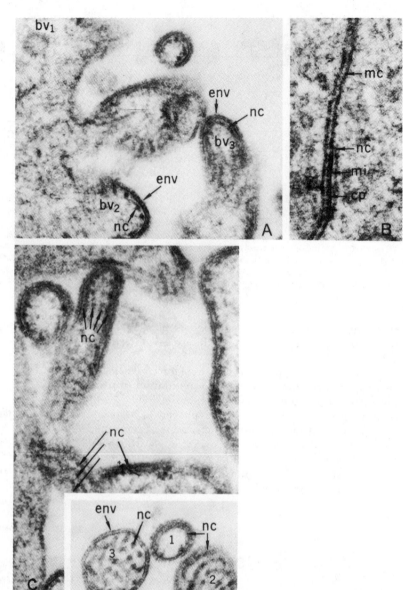

Figure 57–8. Parainfluenza virions forming at the cell membrane of a chick embryo cell and being released by budding. *(A)* Viral buds *(bv)* at various stages of development. The altered cell membrane forming the viral envelope *(env)* and the nucleocapsid *(nc)* beneath the envelope can be clearly distinguished. The nucleocapsid is cut transversely in two of the buds *(bv₁* and *bv₂)* and longitudinally in a third *(bv₃)*. (Original magnification ×105,000) *(B)* Differentiation of the viral envelope at the cell membrane. The cell membranes *(mc)* of two adjacent cells are shown. On contact with the nucleocapsid *(nc)* the cell membrane differentiates into the internal membrane of the envelope *(mi)* and the outer layer of short projections *(cp)*. (Original magnification ×105,000) *(C)* Arrangement of the nucleocapsid *(nc)* impinging on the altered cell membrane that is participating in the formation of the viral envelope. Notice the regularity of the arrangement of the nucleocapsid, seen in cross-sectional and longitudinal views. (Original magnification ×105,000) *(D)* Thin section of virions. Note the structure of the envelope covered with short projections *(env)* and the various arrangements of the nucleocapsids *(nc)*. In particle 1 the nucleocapsid is arranged parallel to the envelope. In particles 2 and 3 the nucleocapsid is arranged more irregularly. (Original magnification ×92,000; Berkaloff A: J Microsc 2:633, 1963)

parainfluenza viruses, there are immunologic relations among the parainfluenza viruses (at least types 1, 2, and 3) and with mumps viruses (see Table 57–1). These are noted by heterotypic Ab responses to infection in those who have had prior infections with one or more of the other viruses. The serologic response to the initial infection (the **primary response**) in humans, as well as in lower animal hosts, is strictly **type-specific.** Heterotypic Abs, particularly between types 1 and 3, subsequently appear in humans, probably as a result of repeated infections with different members of the group; each additional infection broadens the Ab response. The human heterotypic responses to infections are sufficiently frequent to permit the following conclusions: these agents constitute a group of viruses with cross-reactive Ags, the qualitative and quantitative characteristics of the heterotypic Ab response to infection depend on prior immunologic experience, and immunologic diagnosis of infection by a specific virus may be unreliable except following the initial infection.

Most adults have a relatively high titer of circulating Abs to all antigenic types but usually lack the critical neutralizing IgA Abs in nasal secretions. These appear following acute infections, but they decrease substantially within 1 to 6 months, although specific IgG serum Ab levels remain relatively high. Recurrent infections occur despite the presence of neutralizing Abs in the serum, although the severity of disease is reduced (perhaps owing to a secondary response of IgA Abs). The initial infection with a given type is the most severe and usually occurs in children; infections in adults are commonly afebrile and minor.

Reactions With Erythrocytes

The hemagglutinins and neuraminidases of parainfluenza viruses resemble those of influenza viruses in most biological characteristics (see Hemagglutination, Chap. 44). Maximum hemagglutination titers are obtained with chicken RBCs at 4°C (types 1 and 2) or with guinea pig RBCs at 25°C (types 1 and 3). The **hemolysin (F) glycoprotein** is inhibited by type-specific antiserum and is similar to the hemolysins of mumps and Newcastle disease viruses. For hemolytic activity to occur, intact mucoprotein receptors on RBCs are required, and therefore **anti-HN Abs** also inhibit hemolysis.

Host Range

Primary cultures of cells from monkey and embryonic human kidneys are the hosts of choice for primary isolations, neutralization titrations, and investigations of the biological properties of parainfluenza viruses. Organ cultures of human tracheal and nasal epithelium have similarly proved to be sensitive for primary isolations. Types 2 and 3 also multiply well in human continuous epithelium-like cell lines (e.g., HeLa cells). Type 1 virus has been adapted to HeLa and human diploid cells, but neither cell line is satisfactory for initial viral isolation.

In cell cultures cytopathic changes develop very slowly (particularly with type 4); infection is most quickly detected by hemadsorption of guinea pig RBCs. The cytopathic changes that eventually appear consist of stringiness or rounding of cells (types 1 and 4) or formation of large **syncytia** containing eosinophilic **cytoplasmic inclusion bodies** (types 2 and 3; see Fig. 57–7). Syncytia are produced by the viral surface F glycoprotein, which causes fusion and then dissolution of the fused membranes of infected cells (see Cytopathic Effects, Chap. 51). This remarkable capacity of parainfluenza viruses (even after ultraviolet or heat inactivation) to induce fusion of cells from many animal species has had great general utility for studying the genetics of eukaryotic cells as well as for virology.

Intranasal inoculation of very small amounts of virus into hamsters, guinea pigs, and cotton rats yields relatively high titers of virus in the lungs, but pulmonary lesions only develop in a particular species of cotton rats (*Sigmadon fulviventer*) **after type 3 infection.** The ani-

mals develop type-specific Abs and resist intranasal challenge with homologous virus for 1 to 3 months, but then susceptibility returns. This pattern mimics the relation of Abs and recurrent susceptibility in humans.

Type 3 virus is highly infectious for cattle. It appears to be harmless, however, except under conditions of stress, such as the herding of cattle together for transportation, when it may induce an acute febrile upper respiratory disease (hence the term *shipping fever*).

Parainfluenza viruses have been adapted to propagation in chick embryos.

PATHOGENESIS

Parainfluenza viruses cause a spectrum of illnesses, primarily in infants and young children, ranging from mid-upper-respiratory infections to croup or pneumonia (Table 57–2). In infants type 1 and 2 viruses are particularly prone to produce laryngotracheobronchitis (croup) and type 3 virus to cause bronchiolitis and pneumonia. Type 4, which consists of two subgroups (4A and 4B), is difficult to isolate, and apparently is a less common etiologic agent. The occasional infections of adults usually evoke a subclinical illness or a mild "cold." Even in children the majority of infections with parainfluenza viruses appear to be clinically inapparent. Conclusions concerning pathogenesis and development of lesions are derived from studies of infections in volunteers, observations of natural infections, and investigation of experimental infections in cotton rats, the best animal model. The virus enters by the respiratory route, and in most adults it multiplies and causes inflammation only in the upper segments of the tract. In infants and young children, however, the bronchi, bronchioles, and lungs are occasionally involved. **Viremia is neither an essential nor a common phase of infection.**

Parainfluenza viruses, like all other paramyxoviruses, can readily establish a persistent infection *in vitro* (see Chap. 51). Scattered findings suggest that similar chronic infections may follow acute diseases *in vivo*. Thus, a parainfluenza-like virus has been isolated by cocultivation of susceptible cells and brain tissue from a patient with multiple sclerosis, and structures resembling para-

TABLE 57–2. Clinical Syndromes Associated With Parainfluenza Viruses

Disease	Virus Type
Minor upper respiratory disease	1, 3, 4*
Bronchitis	1, 3
Bronchopneumonia	1, 3
Croup	1, 2

* Clinical disease uncommon

myxovirus nucleocapsids have been observed in electron micrographs of tissues from patients with various collagen diseases (e.g., systemic lupus erythematosus). However, no conclusive data exist indicating that a parainfluenza virus is the cause of any chronic disease, as measles virus has been shown to produce **subacute sclerosing panencephalitis** (see below and Chap. 51).

LABORATORY DIAGNOSIS

An etiologic diagnosis of parainfluenza virus infection requires laboratory procedures; the lack of distinctive clinical features precludes etiologic diagnoses on this basis. Measurement of a **rise in serum Abs** by enzyme-linked immunosorbent assay (ELISA), hemagglutination-inhibition, complement-fixation (CF), or neutralization titration permits diagnosis conveniently and economically. However, serologic techniques alone cannot reliably establish the specific type of virus that is responsible, because of the frequency and the degree of heterotypic Ab responses, as discussed earlier under Immunologic Characteristics.

The specific parainfluenza virus responsible for an infection can be identified by **viral isolation,** although the marked instability of the virions makes isolation difficult. For this purpose nasopharyngeal secretions containing antibiotics are added to primary tissue cultures of monkey or embryonic human kidney. Although cytopathic changes may not be detectable except with type 2 virus, or may develop very slowly, viral infection can be recognized rapidly and conveniently by **immunofluorescence** or by **adsorption of guinea pig RBCs** to infected cells. Hemadsorption to cells infected with types 1 and 3 viruses can usually be detected within 5 days after inoculation of the patient's secretions, but types 2 and 4 often require 10 days or more. The specific type can be identified by hemadsorption-inhibition techniques utilizing standard sera. Immunofluorescence can yield comparable diagnostic results in only 24 to 48 hours. It should be remembered that the simian parainfluenza virus SV5 is a common latent agent in monkey kidney cultures, and its emergence from this tissue must not be confused with its primary isolation from man.

EPIDEMIOLOGY

Parainfluenza viruses produce disease throughout the year, but the peak incidence is noted during the "respiratory disease season" (late fall and winter). Most infections are endemic; but sharp, small epidemics occasionally occur with types 1 and 2, and at present these epidemics usually occur simultaneously every other year. Parainfluenza virus infections are **primarily childhood diseases:** type 3 infections occur earliest and most

frequently, so that 50% of children in the United States are infected during the first year of life, and almost all are infected by 6 years of age; 80% of children are infected with types 1 and 2 by 10 years of age. Type 4 viruses induce few clinical illnesses but infections are common: By 10 years of age 70% to 80% of children have Abs.

Parainfluenza viruses are **disseminated in respiratory secretions.** Type 3 shows the most effective spread, and during outbreaks in closed populations (e.g., in institutions or hospitals) all children who are free of neutralizing Abs become infected. Under similar circumstances only about 50% of children are infected with type 1 or type 2 virus.

The epidemiologic patterns and the clinical manifestations of parainfluenza virus infections, in children and adults, emphasize the protective effect of neutralizing Abs as well as the lack of complete or long-lasting immunity (probably owing to an inadequate level of IgA Abs in the respiratory secretions). In contrast, young infants appear to be partially protected by passively acquired, maternal serum Abs. Febrile and severe illness is observed only with the initial infection. Reinfection may be produced by the same virus within as little as 9 to 12 months, but it results in a much milder disease.

PREVENTION AND CONTROL

Reducing the attack rate of respiratory diseases is an important social and economic goal. However, prevention of parainfluenza virus infections would probably reduce the incidence of acute respiratory illnesses by only about 15% in children less than 10 years old, and by much less in adults. Nevertheless, an effective vaccine, evoking an Ab response in the respiratory tract, would be of value for young children, especially in hospitals and institutions. Unfortunately, however, an effective vaccine is not available, although newer recombinant DNA techniques have raised hopes that one will be developed in the near future.

Mumps Virus

The unique clinical picture of mumps can be recognized in writings of Hippocrates from the fifth century B.C. The etiologic agent was not isolated and identified as a virus, however, until 1934, when Johnson and Goodpasture produced parotitis in monkeys by inoculating bacteria-free infectious material directly into Stensen's duct. No further major progress was made until the virus was propagated in the chick embryo and was found (in 1945) to agglutinate chicken RBCs, as do influenza viruses. The subsequently isolated parainfluenza viruses were found to have an even closer relation to mumps virus.

PROPERTIES

Immunologic Characteristics

Mumps virus, like parainfluenza viruses, contains the surface **hemagglutinin–neuraminidase (HN) glycoprotein** (also termed the **V [virion] antigen**), which induces protective Abs, **the hemolysis–cell fusion (F) glycoprotein Ag,** and the internal **RNA-protein nucleocapsid (NP)**, which is immunologically identical with the soluble Ag from cells (called the **S antigen**).

Antigenically, mumps virus exists as a single type; no immunologic variants have been detected. It cross-reacts significantly, however, with parainfluenza and Newcastle disease viruses. Therefore, a rise in heterotypic Abs to parainfluenza viruses is seen in the serum from mumps patients.

Antibodies against the nucleocapsid Ag appear within 7 days, and high titers are attained within 2 weeks after the onset of clinical illness. The HN Abs appear later (2–3 weeks after onset), attain maximum titers in 3 to 4 weeks, and persist longer than the nucleocapsid Abs. The HN Abs are measured by neutralization, hemagglutination-inhibition, ELISA, or CF assays with purified HN glycoprotein; they appear to reflect the degree of immunity. Nucleocapsid Abs, which are conveniently assayed by CF titrations, do not afford protection against subsequent infection. Humoral and cellular immunity develop after subclinical as well as clinical infections and usually persist for many years, although second infections have been reported.

Mumps infection induces delayed hypersensitivity that can be observed by a skin test with infectious or inactivated virus. A positive skin reaction correlates roughly with immunity, providing a useful epidemiologic tool, but false reactions (both positive and negative) occur.

Reactions With Erythrocytes

The viral particle **agglutinates RBCs** from several animal species (see Hemagglutination, Chap. 44). Mumps virus, however, has only weak neuraminidase activity against soluble mucoproteins, and therefore hemagglutination is highly susceptible to these inhibitors in serum or culture fluids. The hemagglutinin present on the surface of infected cells can also be detected in tissue culture by **hemadsorption.**

Mumps virus, like parainfluenza viruses, hemolyzes susceptible RBCs at 37°C by interacting with the same specific receptors as are involved in hemagglutination. Several viral particles per cell are required to produce hemolysis, and even under optimal conditions only about 50% of the hemoglobin is released. Calcium inhibits hemolysis. Viral hemagglutination, hemadsorption, and hemolysis are inhibited by Abs to the virion surface Ags (the HN and F glycoproteins).

Host Range

Humans are the only natural hosts for mumps virus, but the virus can infect monkeys and 6- and 8-day-old chick embryos (amniotic cavity or yolk sac); no pathologic lesions of the embryos are noted. After adaptation by serial passage in the allantoic sac of the chick embryo the virus can infect guinea pigs, suckling mice, hamsters, and white rats but has lost its virulence for man and monkey.

In culture, chick embryo and many types of mammalian cells (including monkey and human kidney cells) support multiplication of mumps virus. Infected cultures can be recognized by the appearance of viral particles (hemadsorption or agglutination of RBCs) and soluble Ag (CF), as well as by the slow development of cytopathic effects (cytolysis and development of giant cells with cytoplasmic inclusions; Fig. 57–9). Mumps virus can also replicate in human T-lymphocytes.

PATHOGENESIS

Mumps typically has an acute onset of parotitis (with painful swelling of one or both glands) 16 to 18 days after exposure. The virus is **transmitted in saliva and respiratory secretions** and its **portal of entry** in man is the **respiratory tract. Primary viral multiplication** also takes place in the respiratory tract epithelium and cervical lymph nodes; the salivary glands, the primary target organs, are infected via the bloodstream (Fig. 57–10). Thus, **viremia** begins several days before the development of mumps and before virus is present in the saliva.

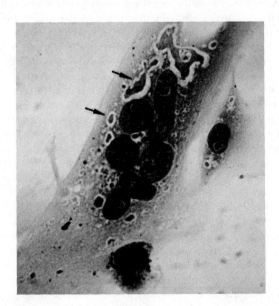

Figure 57–9. Eosinophilic cytoplasmic inclusions and giant cell formations in monkey kidney cells infected with mumps virus. Inclusions (*arrows*) develop in close proximity to the nuclei, which are unaffected. (Original magnification ×450; Brandt CD: Virology 14:1, 1961)

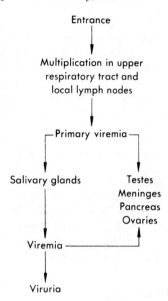

Entrance

↓

Multiplication in upper
respiratory tract and
local lymph nodes

↓

Primary viremia

Salivary glands   Testes
                           Meninges
                           Pancreas
                           Ovaries

Viremia

↓

Viruria

Figure 57–10. Schematic representation of the pathogenesis of mumps.

Virus is present in the blood and in saliva for 3 to 5 days after the onset of the disease, and since the kidney is frequently infected, **virus in the urine** is common for 10 days or more after the onset. The long incubation period reflects the time required for virus to establish a local infection, spread in the blood to the target organs, and multiply sufficiently to damage cells and induce inflammation. The occasional complications also suggest widespread dissemination of the virus.

The acute onset of fever and of salivary gland inflammation may be followed in 4 to 7 days by orchitis (in 20% to 30% of males past puberty),* by meningitis or meningoencephalitis (0.2% to 0.5% of cases, although cerebrospinal fluid pleocytosis occurs in over 50%), and occasionally by pancreatitis, oophoritis, myocarditis, or presternal edema. Even more rarely, nephritis or paralytic manifestations may appear. When infection occurs during the first trimester of the pregnancy, fetal wastage may also occur. The complications may develop at the same time as parotitis or even in the absence of salivary gland involvement.

The most complete pathologic descriptions of mumps virus lesions have been those of affected parotid glands and testes. The parotid lesions consist of interstitial inflammation of the gland and degeneration of the epithelium of the ducts. No characteristic inclusion bodies have been observed in patients' tissues, in contrast to tissue cultures (see Fig. 57–9). Testes show dif-

* Despite the commonly told tales, sterility rarely if ever results from mumps orchitis.

fuse degeneration, particularly of the epithelium of the seminiferous tubules, as well as edema, serofibrinous exudate, marked congestion, and punctate hemorrhages in the interstitial tissue. Meningoencephalitis or meningitis has been studied pathologically only in rare cases, and proof of etiology has often been lacking. The findings described are typical of postinfectious encephalitis, with perivascular demyelination.

LABORATORY DIAGNOSIS

Diagnosis can usually be made solely from clinical observations. However, to establish the diagnosis of mumps in atypical or subclinical infections (about one-third of infections) **viral isolation** and assays of **Ab response** are required. Virus can be isolated by inoculation of saliva, secretions from the parotid duct, or spinal fluid into the amniotic cavity of 8-day-old chick embryos or appropriate cell cultures; the latter appear to be more sensitive for primary isolation. Infection of test cells can be detected earliest by **immunofluorescence** or **hemadsorption** techniques. Since the virion is unstable at 4°C or at room temperature, specimens must be used immediately or stored at −70°C.

Immunologic diagnosis is made by demonstrating an increase in Abs after infection. **Complement fixation** with the **nucleocapsid (soluble) Ag** can detect a rise within the first 7 to 10 days after onset of illness. After 14 days serologic diagnosis is accomplished most readily with the **viral particles (HN Ag)** in **hemagglutination-inhibition, ELISA,** or **CF** titrations. The antigenic cross-reactions between the surface (HN) antigens of mumps and parainfluenza viruses complicate immunologic diagnosis, making it necessary to test all the Ags of related viruses; the highest Ab rise occurs in response to Ags of the infecting virus. When diagnosis is of critical importance, the **plaque neutralization** assay can detect Ab rises that may not be evident in other assays owing to the cross-reactive CF Abs and the nonspecific inhibitors of hemagglutination. If acute and convalescent sera are not available, serologic diagnosis may be made by testing for IgM Abs that appear early and do not persist.

Though the **skin test** may be useful in surveys for estimating immunity, it frequently leads to erroneous conclusions in individual cases and is not reliable for diagnosis. Indeed, because skin testing itself may induce a rise in Abs and confuse the interpretation of immunologic reactions, skin tests should not be used during the course of illness.

EPIDEMIOLOGY

Mumps is predominantly a **childhood disease** spread by droplets of saliva. Salivary secretions may contain infectious virus as early as 6 days before and as long as 9 days after the appearance of glandular swelling. Virus is also present in the saliva of patients with meningitis or orchitis, even in the absence of clinical involvement of the salivary glands. Although viruria develops, there is no evidence for transmission from this source.

Mumps is not nearly so contagious as the childhood exanthematous diseases (e.g., measles and chickenpox), and many children escape infection; hence, **disease in adults** is not uncommon (prior to artificial immunization about 50% of U.S. Army recruits were without Abs). **Subclinical infections,** detectable immunologically, are also much more frequent than in other common childhood diseases.

Mumps appears most often during the winter and early spring months, but it is endemic throughout the year. Large epidemics have been observed about every 3 to 5 years.

PREVENTION AND CONTROL

Because subclinical infections are common, control of infection by isolation is not effective. The disease can be prevented by immunization. **Infectious attenuated virus,** inoculated subcutaneously, induces development of Abs in about 90% of Ab-free subjects (both children and adults). Although vaccine induces infection, viremia and viruria are not detectable, clinical reactions do not occur, and virus does not spread to exposed contacts. The Ab response is not as great as that accompanying natural infections, but Ab levels and protection against clinical mumps persists for at least 12 years after immunization.

The live virus vaccine is of considerable value for susceptible adults in whom the disease is more severe and the complications more frequent. If widespread immunization of children is to be employed, the vaccine should induce persistent immunity, similar to that which follows the natural disease. It is not clear whether the infectious attenuated virus vaccine satisfies this requirement because sufficient data are not yet available.

Formalin-inactivated virus vaccine has been shown to induce a good Ab response and to be clinically effective. However, Abs decline 3 to 6 months after immunization, and neither the effectiveness nor the persistence of immunity appears to be as satisfactory as following the live virus vaccine.

Passive immunization with **γ-globulin from convalescent serum** has been employed to prevent infection after exposure, particularly in men, for whom orchitis is a relatively frequent and severely discomforting complication. Its effectiveness, however, has not been clearly demonstrated. Convalescent whole human serum was once used for similar purposes, but it is not recommended because of the considerable danger of contamination with hepatitis viruses (see Chap. 63) or the human immunodeficiency virus (HIV; see Chap. 65).

Measles Virus

Measles (**morbilli**)* is one of the most infectious diseases known, and it is almost universally acquired in childhood; fortunately, immunity is essentially permanent. It was first described as an independent clinical entity by Sydenham in the seventeenth century. Although measles was demonstrated as early as 1758 to be transmissible in volunteers, and was transferred to monkeys in 1911, it was not until 1954 that the virus, through Enders' persistent and careful search, was isolated reproducibly from patients and was shown to produce cytopathic changes in tissue cultures. This achievement led to a rapid advance in knowledge of the virus and to the development of an effective vaccine.†

PROPERTIES
Immunologic Characteristics

All measles strains studied belong to a **single antigenic type**.‡ Specific Abs are produced to each of the major viral Ags: the **hemagglutinin (H),** the **hemolysin–cell fusion (F),** and the **nucleocapsid (NP),** as well as the **matrix (M),** and the internal **P** and **L** proteins, all of which exist free in cell extracts as well as assembled in virions. Antibodies to the **virion surface glycoproteins** (hemagglutinin and hemolysis–cell fusion factor), in the presence of specific complement components (the alternate complement pathway), lyse infected cells, which contain these viral glycoproteins in their plasma membranes. These **cytotoxic Abs** probably play a role in certain aspects of the pathogenesis of the disease as well as in the elimination of infected cells during recovery. In the absence of complement, however, these same Abs cause the viral glycoproteins to accumulate ("cap") in a limited region of the infected cell surface, and finally to shed from the cell (see Chap. 51). It is likely that this phenomenon permits infected cells to escape immunologic destruction and to persist, possibly causing chronic infections such as **subacute sclerosing panencephalitis** (see Chap. 51).

Circulating Abs are detected 10 to 14 days after infection (i.e., when the rash appears or shortly thereafter) and reach maximal titer by the time the exanthem disappears. Antibody titers (neutralizing, CF, and hemagglutination-inhibiting) remain high following infection, and

---

* **Rubeola** is often employed as a synonym; unfortunately, this term has also been used as a synonym for rubella (German measles).

† This brief account illustrates only in part the unique role Enders played in leading the way to the recent control of two important diseases, poliomyelitis and measles.

‡ Measles virus, however, is related to the viruses of canine distemper and rinderpest (of cattle) in antigenic, physical, and biological properties. Considerable nucleotide sequence homology also exists between the genomes of measles and canine distemper viruses.

immunity persists for life (as shown by epidemiologic investigations; see Persistence of Antibodies, Chap. 51). In monkeys, reinfection can be produced 3 to 6 months after a primary infection, but clinical disease does not ensue. Abs directed against the hemagglutinin (H) and fusion (F) glycoproteins neutralize virus *in vitro;* passive immunity in experimental animals only requires the H Abs.

Like most orthomyxoviruses and paramyxoviruses, measles virus (or its separated hemagglutinin) agglutinates monkey RBCs. In contrast to orthomyxoviruses and other paramyxoviruses, measles virus does not elute spontaneously from agglutinated cells, the RBC receptors are not destroyed by *Vibrio cholerae* neuraminidase, and the virions do not contain neuraminidase molecules.

Cell-mediated immunity is also demonstrable by the time the rash appears. Human T-lymphocytes from normal as well as immune persons possess receptors for measles virus: the lymphocytes are agglutinated by purified virus, and they form rosettes upon reaction with infected cells. Following rosette formation, the virus-infected cells are killed. Although lymphocytes from both immune and susceptible persons are cytotoxic, the immune lymphocytes kill more effectively.

Host Range

Man is the natural host for measles virus, but this virus is highly contagious for both humans and monkeys. Monkeys in captivity commonly develop spontaneous measles, with humans probably serving as the source. Experimental measles infections have been produced in many animals other than primates; hamsters and mice have proved to be particularly useful.

Although unmodified measles virus from patients replicates poorly *in vitro*, multiplication has been achieved in a variety of mammalian as well as chick embryo cells. Both primary and continuous mammalian cell cultures are commonly employed.* Viruses adapted to propagation *in vitro* can also multiply in the amniotic sac or in the chorioallantoic membrane of chick embryos, and one strain has been adapted to propagation in brains of newborn mice.

The development of **large syncytial giant cells** is generally the major cytopathic effect produced by measles infection of cultured cells (Fig. 57–11). Eosinophilic inclusion bodies develop in both the nuclei and the cytoplasm of syncytial cells (see Fig. 57–11). The inclusions are composed of dense, highly ordered arrays of viral nucleocapsids (Figs. 57–12 and 57–13). Immunofluores-

---

* **Primary cultures:** human embryonic kidney, human amnion, monkey or dog kidney, chick embryo cells, bovine fetal tissue; **continuous cell lines of human origin:** HeLa, KB, Hep-2, amnion, heart, nasal mucosa, bone marrow, kidney. Primary cultures of human embryonic or monkey kidneys are most susceptible to unadapted viruses.

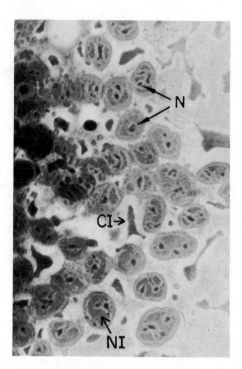

Figure 57–11. Inclusion bodies of cells infected with measles virus. A giant cell consisting of a large syncytium of cells is illustrated; each large round body is a nucleus. Large eosinophilic cytoplasmic inclusions are indicated by *CI* and numerous intranuclear eosinophilic inclusion bodies by *NI*. The nucleoli (*N*) are intact. (Original magnification ×750; Kallman F et al: J Biophys Biochem Cytol 6:379, 1959)

cence reveals specific viral Ags in both the nuclear and cytoplasmic inclusions.

PATHOGENESIS

Measles is a highly contagious, acute, febrile, exanthematous disease. The pathogenesis in man resembles the general pattern described for smallpox (see Chap. 54) and mumps (see Fig. 57–9), with **local multiplication** followed by **hematogenous dissemination.** Virus **transmitted in respiratory secretions** enters the upper respiratory tract, or perhaps the eye, and multiplies in the epithelium and regional lymphatic tissue. Virus may also disseminate to distant lymphoid tissue by a brief primary viremia. Viral multiplication in the upper respiratory tract and conjunctivae causes, after an incubation period of 10 to 12 days, the prodromal (i.e., pre-rash) symptoms of coryza, conjunctivitis, dry cough, sore throat, headache, low-grade fever, and Koplik spots (tiny red patches with central white specks on the buccal mucosa in which are noted characteristic giant cells containing viral nucleocapsids). Viremia occurs toward the end of the incubation period, permitting further wide-

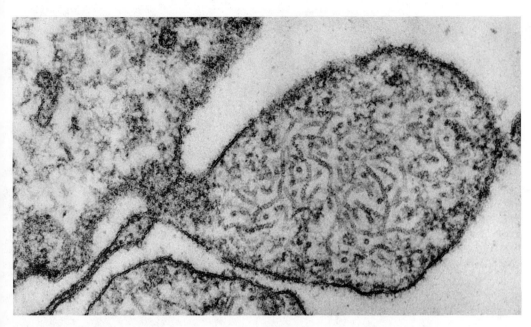

Figure 57–12. Measles virus particles budding from the surface membrane of an infected cell. Viral nucleocapsids are seen within the forming particles; the fuzzy structures on the surfaces of the virions probably correspond to the surface projections seen by negative staining (see Fig. 57–3). (Original magnification ×98,000; Nakai T et al: Virology 38:50, 1969)

spread dissemination of virus to the lymphoid tissue and skin. With the diffuse secondary multiplication of virus the prodromal symptoms are intensified and the typical red, maculopapular rash appears, first on the head and face and then on the body extremities.

Viral Ags and nucleocapsids are present in endothelial cells of the subcutaneous capillaries but usually infectious virus is not detectable in the affected superficial epidermal cells. The characteristic rash appears to result predominantly from interactions of immune T-lymphocytes with infected cells. It is striking that when children who are T-cell deficient owing to thymic dysplasia develop measles, they do not display a rash but manifest extensive giant-cell pneumonia.

Virus is excreted in the secretions of the respiratory tract and eye, and in urine, during the prodromal phase and for about 2 days after the appearance of the rash. **This early shedding of virus, before the disease can be recognized, promotes its rapid epidemic spread.** The blood, lymph nodes, spleen, kidney, skin, and lungs also contain detectable virus during this period. Measles virus can multiply in and has been isolated from human macrophages and lymphocytes, suggesting that these cells may play a role in its dissemination in the body and in the pathogenesis of the disease. The leukocytic involvement may also be responsible for the leukopenia observed during the prodromal stage as well as for depression of delayed-type hypersensitivity reactions (e.g.,

the tuberculin test). Measles virus can induce striking aberrations in the chromosomes of leukocytes during the acute disease. Although the chromosomal pulverization produced is probably lethal to the cell, a possible relation between some of the changes and the initiation of leukemia has been suggested.

The characteristic **viremia** in measles, in contrast to the more localized respiratory infections produced by influenza and parainfluenza viruses, probably contributes to the notably effective immunity conferred by the disease.

Complications

Bronchopneumonia and **otitis media,** with or without a bacterial component, are frequent complications of the disease. **Encephalomyelitis** is the most serious complication, appearing about 5 to 7 days after the rash. Its incidence in most epidemics is about 1 in 2000 cases (higher in children over 10 years); but in some outbreaks, particularly in the widespread infection of malnourished infants in Africa, the incidence has been much higher. However, cerebrospinal fluid pleocytosis may occur in as many as 30% of the cases. The mortality rate of encephalomyelitis is about 10%, and permanent mental and physical sequelae have been reported in 15% to 65% of survivors.

There is no evidence that measles encephalomyelitis, which occurs in certain epidemics, is due to viral strains

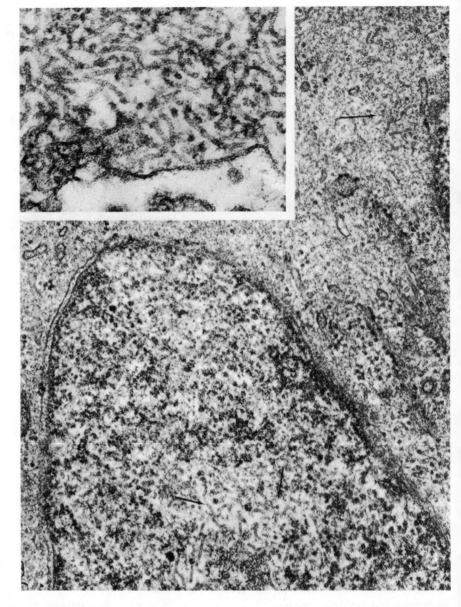

Figure 57–13. Electron micrographs of cell infected with measles virus, showing intranuclear and intracytoplasmic matrices containing viral nucleocapsids (*arrows;* original magnification ×60,000). (*Inset*) Higher magnification of an extensive accumulation of nucleocapsids. Where the tubules are favorably oriented, cross-striations of the nucleocapsids can be seen. (Original magnification ×140,000; Nakai T et al: Virology 38:50, 1969)

with increased virulence. Indeed, measles virus cannot be isolated from the brain, but lymphocyte infiltration and demyelination are prominent pathologic features, reminiscent of allergic encephalitis. These findings suggest that measles encephalomyelitis is a hypersensitivity response either to the measles virus or to virus-altered host tissue (i.e., an autoimmune phenomenon).

Giant cell pneumonia, a rare disease of debilitated children, or of those with immunodeficiency disease, was proved to be due to measles by isolation of virus.

Subacute sclerosing panencephalitis (SSPE), a progressive, fatal complication of measles, is an excellent example of a single virus inducing an acute disease and a chronic illness separated by a long interval during which there is restricted synthesis and expression of viral genes (see Slow Viral Infections, Chap. 51, for a complete description).

Pathology

The development of very large multinuclear **giant cells** (Warthin–Finkeldey syncytial cells) is the predominant and characteristic feature of the pathology of measles. These distinctive cells are found in nasal secretions during the prodromal stage of the disease, as well as in lymphoid tissue of the gastrointestinal tract, particularly the appendix. Giant cells are also often observed in sputum from patients with bronchopneumonia and may contain eosinophilic nuclear and cytoplasmic inclusions, similar to those seen in infected cell cultures; and such cells are characteristic of the rare **giant cell pneumonia.** These giant cells are presumably produced by cell fusions, like syncytial cell formation in infected cell cultures.

In **measles encephalomyelitis** the brain shows perivascular hemorrhage and lymphocytic infiltration early in the disease; areas of demyelination later appear in the brain and spinal cord.

Brains from patients with **subacute sclerosing panencephalitis** display a degeneration of the cortex and especially the underlying white matter. They contain characteristic intranuclear and intracytoplasmic inclusion bodies not unlike those noted in acute measles (see Figs. 57–11, 57–12, and 57–13), perivascular infiltration of plasma cells and lymphocytes, scattered degeneration of nerve cells, hypertrophy of astrocytes, microglial proliferation, and demyelination.

LABORATORY DIAGNOSIS

The epidemiologic and clinical features of measles are usually so characteristic that laboratory confirmation of the diagnosis is unnecessary except for investigative purposes. During the prodromal stage of the disease a rapid and simple presumptive diagnosis can be made by demonstrating specific viral immunofluorescence and characteristic giant cells in smears of the nasopharyngeal mucosa. Definitive diagnosis can be accomplished by isolation of virus from nasal or pharyngeal secretions, blood, or urine; viral isolations are best achieved in primary cultures of human embryonic or monkey kidneys. Serologic diagnosis can be made by comparing acute and convalescent sera using hemagglutination-inhibition, ELISA, or CF titrations, as described for other paramyxoviruses. Finding measles Abs in the cerebrospinal fluid is suggestive of injury to the blood–brain barrier, probably from an immunologic reaction, and is often a sign of severe neurologic disturbance such as acute encephalomyelitis or SSPE.

EPIDEMIOLOGY

Measles is a **highly contagious disease** in which virus is **spread in respiratory secretions.** It is predominantly a childhood affliction that occurs in epidemics during the winter and spring in rural areas. Since measles virus does not have a reservoir in nature other than humans, and since long-lasting immunity follows infection, persistence of the virus in a community depends upon endemic infections in a continuous supply of susceptible persons. It has been estimated that in urban areas 2500 to 5000 cases per year are required for continued transmission. Hence, it is clear why in the more highly developed countries epidemics tend to appear in 2- to 3-year cycles, as a sufficient number of nonimmune children arises in the population, and why the disease disappears from small, isolated communities. However, even in a highly immunized population exogenous introduction of virus can initiate a limited epidemic; for example, epidemics are now appearing in high schools and universities in which over 95% of the students were immunized as children.

In the United States the highest incidence is in children 5 to 7 years of age, and the disease is relatively mild. However, since 1973, after widespread immunization began, the age-specific incidence has steadily increased to older children and teenagers. Moreover, the disease is more severe in adults and in young children (but transplacental immunity usually protects newborns and babies up to the age of 6 months). In communities having primitive and crowded living conditions (e.g., in West Africa) most cases occur in infants less than 2 years old; the illnesses tend to be severe and often fatal (probably owing to malnutrition and a high rate of secondary infections), and epidemics occur yearly because the close contacts probably decrease the proportion of susceptibles required. If the virus is introduced into isolated, unimmunized communities, where the exposure is rare and measles has not struck in many years, the incidence is very high, and the illness is severe and frequently is fatal to very young children and to the elderly (e.g., the Faroe Islands; see Persistence of Antibodies, Chap. 51).

PREVENTION AND CONTROL

Public health measures alone, such as isolation, have not successfully prevented or even limited measles epidemics. Prior to the development of vaccines for active immunization, passive immunization with pooled γ-globulin[*] was used to furnish temporary protection. Because of the long incubation period, large doses, even when administered shortly after exposure, prevent the disease, and small doses reduce its severity. This procedure is still effectively employed for exposed susceptibles, particularly adults.

---

[*] Because the majority of adults in most countries have had measles, and because levels of circulating Abs remain high, pooled normal adult γ-globulin is effective in passive immunization.

After the successful cultivation of measles virus in tissue culture, vaccines were developed and effective control became possible. Following the methods that had proved so successful in the control of poliomyelitis both **attenuated live virus vaccine** and **formalin-inactivated virus vaccine were prepared.**

The initial "attenuated" virus induced mild measles with fever in about 80% of recipients, so that γ-globulin containing measles Abs was administered at a different site to reduce the reactions. Viruses of greater attenuation were eventually obtained, however, and they are now used without an accompanying injection of γ-globulin. Babies immunized prior to their first birthday often have a poor Ab response, and it is recommended that they be reimmunized when about 15 months old. In children older than 1 year, the live attenuated virus selected for general immunization induces an Ab response in almost 100% of those who previously lacked Abs, but the vaccine still produces reactions in 15% to 20% of children. The Ab titers are about 10% to 25% of the levels observed after the natural disease. Neutralizing Abs endure without significant decline for at least 2 years after immunization but decrease twofold to threefold by 5 years; CF Abs begin to decline in 6 to 8 months. Although effective immunity has been demonstrated at least 10 years after immunization, measles does occasionally occur in vaccinated children, particularly in those immunized during the first year of life. How long adequate protection persists after vaccination is still unclear, but the increasing number of measles outbreaks reported among adolescents and young adults who were previously immunized as young children suggests that the immunity may be less lasting than that following natural measles.

The vaccine does not cause acute neurologic complications and virus does not spread from vaccinees to susceptibles in the same family. Immunization with live virus vaccine has proved highly effective in large studies, and during epidemics it appears to prevent measles in more than 95% of children. In the United States, where widespread immunization has been employed, large epidemics have been eliminated and the incidence of measles has been reduced from about 450,000 reported cases per year prior to 1960 to 2543 in 1984 (Fig. 57–14).

The attenuated virus vaccine is distributed in a lyophilized form, usually mixed with other attenuated viruses. The most popular combination is measles virus mixed with mumps and rubella viruses. It is comforting that the multiple-virus formulation has neither increased the reaction rate to measles attenuated virus nor decreased the Ab response to any of the viral immunogens present.

A **formalin-inactivated** virus vaccine has been shown to elicit Abs in about 75% of the recipients after a course of three intramuscular injections. This vaccine has not received acceptance, however, because protection is only temporary, neutralizing Abs as well as CF Abs begin to decline rapidly within 3 to 6 months, and unanticipated severe disease has been reported in vaccinees who were subsequently infected naturally or reimmunized with live virus vaccine. (It should be noted, however, that this **"atypical" measles** is also observed in some recipients of live virus vaccine who subsequently develop natural measles.)

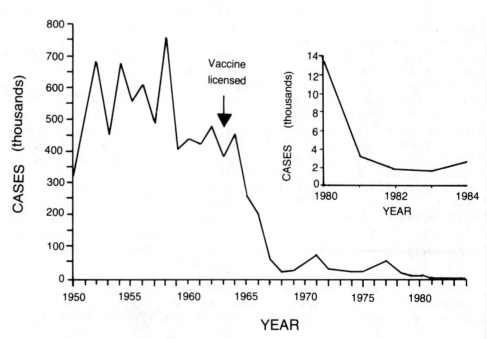

Figure 57–14. Reported cases of measles in the United States from 1950 to 1984. (Recreated from MMWR 34:308, 1985)

Respiratory Syncytial Virus

From a chimpanzee with coryzal illness, and from a laboratory worker who had been in contact with the animal, Morris and co-workers isolated a new virus in 1956. The following year Chanock isolated similar viruses from two infants with pneumonia and croup. Subsequent studies have indicated that **the virus is a major cause of lower respiratory tract disease during infancy and early childhood** throughout the world. Since it characteristically introduces formation of large syncytial masses in infected cell cultures, it was named **respiratory syncytial (RS) virus.**

PROPERTIES

The RS virus is related to parainfluenza, measles, and mumps viruses, but several distinctions led to its classification in a separate genus, *Pneumovirus* (see Table 57–1). In particular, hemagglutination, hemadsorption, hemolytic, and neuraminidase activities are not detectable despite the presence of regularly spaced clublike projections (peplomers) on the virion's surface (Fig. 57–15). Moreover, the virions and the nucleocapsids are extremely fragile, which makes preservation of infectivity difficult. In addition, filamentous virions are present in purified preparations (see Fig. 57–15) and in thin sections (Fig. 57–16); the filaments, unlike those of influenza viruses (see Fig. 56–2, Chap. 56), are often much narrower than the spherical virions, and they have the appearance of an elongated nucleocapsid rather than a folded helix covered with an envelope. Finally, the spherical virions are somewhat less variable in size and are slightly smaller (see Table 57–1) than the typical paramyxoviruses; the nucleocapsid has a slightly smaller diameter, and the helix has a regular periodicity slightly larger than for other paramyxoviruses.

The single-stranded RNA genome of RS virus is similar in size and organization to that of the other paramyxoviruses (see Fig. 57–6). However, the RS virus RNA encodes four additional proteins: two nonstructural proteins (NS_1 and NS_2); a third (SH), whose functions are unknown; and a second envelope membrane protein (22K).

Infectivity of RS virus is completely destroyed during storage at $-15°C$ to $-25°C$ for only several days. Viral suspensions can be preserved without complete inactivation by adding protein (5% to 10% normal serum or albumin), freezing rapidly, and maintaining at $-70°C$.

Immunologic Characteristics

Antigenic variants have been noted among the RS strains studied, but the immunologic cross-reactivity between variants is too great to permit division into distinct types. It is noteworthy that the antigenic differences do not appear to be progressive with successive epidemics.

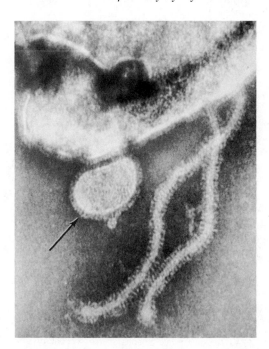

Figure 57–15. Intact respiratory syncytial virus particle (*arrow*) and two filaments negatively stained with phosphotungstate; note the regularly arranged clublike peripheral projections. (Original magnification ×110,000; Bloth B et al: Arch Gesamte Virusforsch 13:582, 1963)

Each variant has a specific surface Ag that can be detected by plaque neutralization assays in cell cultures with standard sera. Purified virions and extracts of infected cells contain the specific viral **surface Ags** and the other viral protein including the **major nucleocapsid (NP) Ag,** detectable by CF titration, that is common to all RS viruses but not to other paramyxoviruses.

Neutralizing Abs are directed primarily against the **fusion (F_1 and F_2) proteins.** Monoclonal Abs that react with the large **G surface glycoprotein** also neutralize virus and provide passive immunity to experimental animals.

Protection from reinfection is brief following RS virus infections, probably because the titer of IgA Abs in nasal secretions declines rapidly. Serum Abs persist, but even a level of neutralizing Abs as high as 1:256 does not provide adults with effective protection against reinfection. Babies during the first 6 months of life are most often infected and most seriously affected, despite the high level of serum IgG Abs derived from their mothers; and infants with neutralizing Abs may even develop bronchopneumonia on reinfection.

Host Range

RS virus has been observed to cause illness only in humans, chimpanzees, owl monkeys, and cotton rats. In addition, intranasal inoculation of virus into mice, fer-

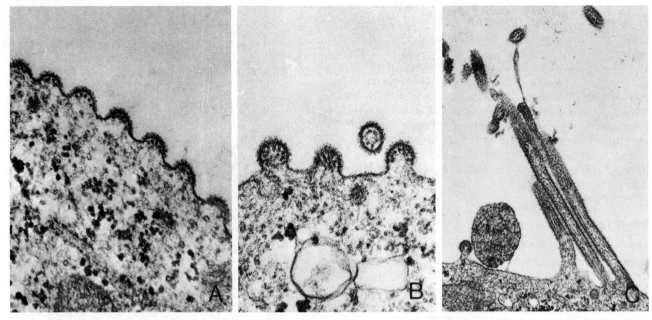

Figure 57–16. Electron micrographs of thin sections of a cell culture infected with respiratory syncytial virus. Different stages are seen in the morphogenesis of the viral particles at the plasma membrane. *(A)* Early stages of budding show thickening of the cell membrane with the appearance of fringelike projections. Submembranous accumulation of the nucleocapsid is also noted. (Original magnification ×75,000) *(B)* Later stages of viral budding and a single free virion are seen. The circular arrangement of the nucleocapsid in the spherical particles suggests an organized packing of this component. (Original magnification ×76,000) *(C)* Filamentous forms of viral particles are developing at the cell membrane. The linear arrangement of the nucleocapsid is visible within the filamentous particles. (Original magnification ×42,000; Norrby E et al: J Virol 6:237, 1970)

rets, monkeys, and many other mammals produces inapparent infections, from which virus can be recovered.

RS virus multiplies and produces cytopathic changes in continuous human epithelium-like cell lines, in human diploid cell strains, and in primary simian and bovine kidney cell cultures. About 10 hours after infection, virus-specific Ags, detected by immunofluorescence, appear in the cytoplasm of infected cells but not in their nuclei. As the quantity of Ag increases, it accumulates at the cell membrane, where virions assemble and bud from the altered cell membrane like other paramyxoviruses (see Fig. 57–16).

The formation of syncytia and giant cells, as in parainfluenza and measles virus infections, is the predominant and characteristic cytopathology (Fig. 57–17). Prominent eosinophilic cytoplasmic inclusions, consisting of densely packed material having a granular or threadlike appearance, are commonly found in infected cells, particularly in the syncytia (see Fig. 57–17). These inclusion bodies may be considered "scars" of the infection, for they do not contain RNA, viral particles, or accumulated virus-specific Ags.

PATHOGENESIS

The pathogenesis of RS virus infections has been largely surmised on the basis of clinical observations. The **initial infection** results from **viral multiplication in epithelial cells of the upper respiratory tract;** it most often ends at this stage in adults and older children. In about 50% of infected children less than 8 months old, **virus spreads into the lower respiratory tract**—the bronchi, the bronchioli, and even the pulmonary parenchyma—causing febrile upper respiratory disease, bronchitis, bronchiolitis, bronchopneumonia, and croup.

The dissemination of virus into the lower respiratory tract, with concomitant production of more serious disease, is probably due at least partially to the absence of IgA Abs in the respiratory secretions and to the slow development of Abs in the previously uninfected infant. With increasing age, and therefore repeated exposure and greater immunologic response to RS virus, infections are likely to be milder and confined to the upper respiratory tract and are most likely to be inapparent. In adults, because of the absence or limited quantity of virus-specific secretory (IgA) Abs in the respiratory tract, infections do occur despite the presence of circulating Abs; most frequently the disease is afebrile and clinically resembles the common cold.

Autopsy examination of infants dead of RS virus infection shows severe necrotizing lesions of the epithelium of the bronchi and bronchioles, and interstitial pneumonia consisting of mononuclear infiltration, patchy atelectasis, and emphysema. The exact mechanism of epithe-

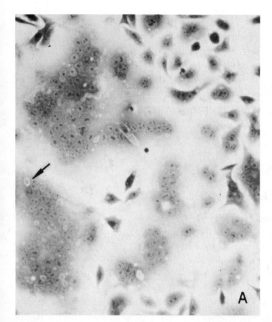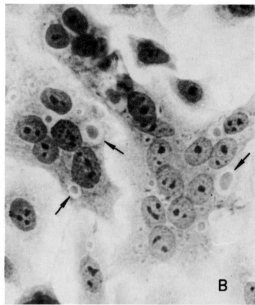

Figure 57–17. Syncytium formation and cytoplasmic inclusions (*arrows*) in Hep-2 cells infected with respiratory syncytial virus. Syncytia are characterized by the very large aggregates of intact nuclei and extensive cytoplasmic masses devoid of cell membranes. (*A,* original magnification ×125; *B,* original magnification ×540; Bennett CR Jr, Hamre D: J Infect Dis 110:8, 1962)

lial cell injury is unclear, but direct damage owing to viral replication rather than an immunologic response is probably the major cause. Cytoplasmic inclusion bodies are noted, but syncytial formation is not observed. These changes represent one end of the spectrum of disease produced by RS virus. In infants who die with bronchiolitis the lungs contain small amounts of virus and intracellular Ags that can be detected by immunofluorescence, whereas in infants with pneumonia large quantities of infectious virus and viral Ags are present.

LABORATORY DIAGNOSIS

Detection of RS viral Ags in exfoliated cells of the respiratory tract by **specific immunofluorescence** offers the most rapid and economic means for diagnosing acute infections. **A precise diagnosis of RS** virus infection, however, requires either **isolation of the virus** or demonstration of a **rise in Abs.** Serologic diagnosis is ordinarily the most reliable and easiest, using ELISA or CF (the most convenient and economical) or neutralization titrations. Very young infants, however, may not produce a detectable Ab response, in which case a laboratory diagnosis depends upon isolation of virus.

Because RS virus is highly labile, isolation is most efficient when nasal or pharyngeal secretions are inoculated directly from the patient into cultures of human continuous cell lines (Hep-2, HeLa, or KB). Characteristic giant cells develop within 2 to 14 days, but infection can be detected more rapidly by immunofluorescence. Virus can be isolated in about 70% of patients during the first week of illness. Newly isolated RS virus can be identified by CF, ELISA, or neutralization titrations with standard antisera.

EPIDEMIOLOGY

RS virus is a **major cause of respiratory disease in young children,** and the **most common cause of nosocomial infections** in pediatric wards. Infections have a worldwide distribution, and they occur in yearly epidemics of varying magnitude. Virus spreads rapidly through the susceptibles in a community, so that epidemics are sharply circumscribed and relatively brief. The outbreaks occur primarily in infants and children between late fall and early spring. Many adults may be infected during the episode, but they have mild disease or inapparent infections.

RS infections uniformly occur early in life. Indeed, RS virus is the only recognized virus that preferentially produces severe respiratory disease and has its maximum impact during the first 6 months of life. Severe pneumonia and bronchitis occur in infants between 6 weeks and 6 months after birth with the peak incidence in those 2 months old. Serious infections occur 30% more frequently in male babies and more commonly in white infants. Although infants have a poor Ab response to infection, approximately one-third of infants in the United States develop Abs in the first year of life, and 95% by 5 years of age. However, reinfections are common, and about 80% of previously infected children are reinfected in the second year of life.

PREVENTION AND CONTROL

Because RS virus ranks so high on the list of causes of respiratory disease in young children, preventive methods are highly desirable. Isolation or general public health measures are not adequate to control the spread of infection: it is difficult to recognize the disease early, and inapparent cases are frequent.

Experience with an alum-precipitated, formalin-inactivated vaccine was discouraging. Though the serum Ab response was good, the clinical response to subsequent RS virus infection was startling and paradoxic: both the **incidence and the severity** of disease **increased** strikingly, particularly in infants. These results resembled the severe reactions in children immunized with inactive measles virus and then naturally infected with measles virus. Animal models indicate that this frightening response was probably due to a cell-mediated hypersensitivity as well as to Ab–virus complexes producing an Arthus-type reaction. This dramatic failure of immunization was primarily the result of formalin damage to the neutralizing epitopes of the viral envelope F and G proteins.

Development of a live RS virus vaccine using selected attenuated viral variants, particularly temperature-sensitive mutants, was unsuccessful owing to the mutants' high reversion rates. Rapid progress is being made, however, in developing a vaccine consisting of a live viral vector, such as vaccinia virus or adenovirus, in which the F and G protein genes of RS virus are inserted to permit their expression. This approach has been successful in animals. Although the disease does not afford effective, lasting immunity, an effective viral vector vaccine administered early in infancy should prevent or reduce the serious effects of primary infection.

Newcastle Disease Virus

Newcastle disease virus (NDV) is primarily a respiratory tract pathogen of birds, particularly chickens, but it occasionally produces accidental infections in man. Human infections are almost exclusively confined to poultry workers and laboratory personnel. The disease is characteristically mild and limited to conjunctivitis without corneal involvement. Although predominantly of veterinary interest, this virus merits brief mention because of the prominent role it has played in the investigation of paramyxoviruses.

NDV possesses the characteristic properties of paramyxoviruses listed in Table 57–1. This virus particularly resembles parainfluenza and mumps viruses in morphology, chemistry, and reactions with RBCs. Moreover, many patients with mumps virus infection develop hemagglutination-inhibiting and CF Abs to NDV.

Selected Reading

PARAINFLUENZA VIRUSES
Books and Review Articles

Chanock RM, McIntosh K: Parainfluenza viruses. In Fields BN (ed): Virology. New York, Raven Press, 1985

Choppin PW, Compans RW: Reproduction of paramyxoviruses. Compr Virol 4:95, 1975

Specific Articles

Chanock RM: Association of a new type of cytopathogenic myxovirus with infantile croup. J Exp Med 104:555, 1956

Deshpande KL, Portner A: Monoclonal antibodies to the P protein of Sendai virus define its structure and role of transcription. Virology 140:125, 1985

Storey DG, Dimock K, Kang CY: Structural characterization of virion proteins and genomic RNA of human parainfluenza virus 3. J Virol 52:761, 1984

Yewdell J, Gerhard W: Delineation of four antigenic sites on a paramyxovirus glycoprotein via which monoclonal antibodies mediate distinct antiviral activities. J Immunol 128:2670, 1982

MUMPS VIRUS
Specific Articles

Julkunen I, Vaananen P, Penttinen K: Antibody responses to mumps virus proteins in natural mumps infection and after vaccination with live and inactivated mumps virus vaccines. J Med Virol 14:209, 1984

Levitt LP, Mahoney DH, Casey HL, Bond JO: Mumps in a general population: A seroepidemiologic study. Am J Dis Child 120:134, 1970

MEASLES VIRUS
Specific Articles

Fine PEM, Clarkson JA: Measles in England and Wales I: An analysis of factors underlying seasonal patterns. Int J Epidemiol 11:5, 1982

Frank JA Jr, Orenstein WA, Bart KJ et al: Major impediments to measles elimination. The modern epidemiology of an ancient disease. Am J Dis Child 139:881, 1985

Girandon P, Weld TF: Correlation between epitopes on hemagglutinin of measles virus and biological activities: Passive protection by monoclonal antibodies is related to their hemagglutination inhibiting activity. Virology 144:46, 1985

Norrby E: Measles. In Fields BN (ed): Virology. New York, Raven Press, 1985

Panum PL: Observation made during the epidemic of measles on the Faroe Islands in the year 1846. New York, American Publishing Association, 1940 (Reprint)

RESPIRATORY SYNCYTIAL VIRUS
Books and Review Articles

McIntosh K, Chanock RM: Respiratory syncytial virus. In Fields BN (ed): Virology. New York, Raven Press, 1985

Scott EJ, Taylor G: Respiratory syncytial virus. Brief review. Arch Virol 84:1, 1985

Specific Articles

Chanock RM, Roizman B, Myers R: Recovery from infants with respiratory illness of a virus related to chimpanzee coryza agent (CCA). I. Isolation properties and characterization. Am J Hyg 66:281, 1956

Collins PL, Dickens LE, Buckler-White A et al: Nucleotide sequences for the gene junctions of human respiratory syncytial virus reveal distinctive features of intergenic structure and gene order. Proc Natl Acad Sci USA 83:4594, 1986

Morris JA, Blount RE, Savage RE: Recovery of cytopathic agent from chimpanzees with coryza. Proc Soc Exp Biol Med 92:544, 1956

58

Coronaviruses

After the discovery that rhinoviruses are major etiologic agents of the common cold (see Chap. 55), more than 50% of illnesses still could not be associated with known causative agents. However, when Tyrrell and Bynoe in 1965 introduced the use of ciliated human embryonic tracheal and nasal organ cultures, they revealed a new group of viruses (and also improved the isolation of known agents). The unique properties of the new group included their distinctive club-shaped surface projections (Fig. 58–1), which give the appearance of a solar corona to the virion. Hence the family name **Coronaviridae** (L. *corona;* vernacular, *coronaviruses*, crown) was proposed to include the agents isolated initially as well as viruses propagated in human embryonic cell cultures by Hamre and Procknow from patients with acute respiratory diseases, and similar viruses from a variety of lower animals, presenting a total of 11 viral species.*

Properties

MORPHOLOGY

Electron microscopic examinations of negatively stained preparations reveal moderately pleomorphic spherical or elliptical virions. The surface is covered with distinctive, widely spaced, pedunculated projections (**peplomers**), 20 nm long, with narrow bases and club-shaped ends (see Fig. 58–1). Thin sections show virions with an outer membrane (envelope), an electron-lucent intermediate zone, and an inner nucleocapsid consisting of an electron-dense shell and a central zone containing

* Avian infectious bronchitis virus, calf neonatal diarrhea virus, murine hepatitis virus, porcine transmissible gastroenteritis virus, porcine hemagglutinating encephalitis virus, rat pneumotropic virus, rat sialodacryoadenitis virus, turkey bluecomb disease virus, bovine coronavirus, canine coronavirus, and feline infectious peritonitis virus

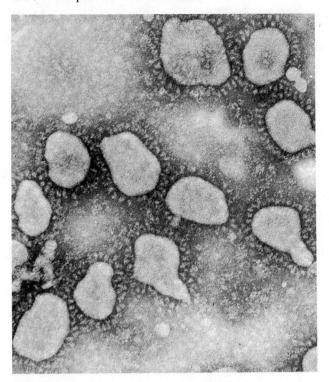

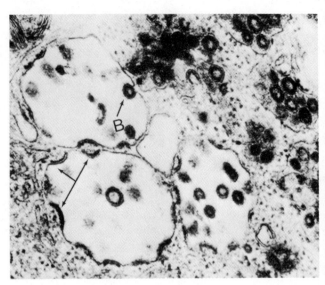

Figure 58–2. Development of a coronavirus in a human diploid cell. Thickened membranes (*arrows*) indicate sites of early morphogenesis. A particle budding into a vacuole (*B*) and several mature particles within vacuoles are also present. Mature particles show inner and outer shells with a translucent zone between them. (Original magnification ×50,000; Becker WB et al: J Virol 1:1019, 1967)

Figure 58–1. Coronaviruses. The negatively stained particles show the distinctive corona effect produced by the pedunculated surface projections, which are approximately 20 nm long and have a club-shaped end about 10 nm wide. The marked pleomorphism of the virions may be noted. (Original magnification ×144,000; Kapikian AZ: Diagnostic Procedures for Viral and Rickettsial Infections, 4th ed. New York, American Public Health Association, 1969)

amorphous material of variable density (Fig. 58–2). The nucleocapsid appears to be a loosely wound helix.

PHYSICAL AND CHEMICAL CHARACTERISTICS

The properties of all species studied are similar, but the most detailed characterization was done with the murine hepatitis virus owing to its ease of propagation and greater viral yield in cell cultures. Whenever comparable studies have been possible, the human coronaviruses proved to be comparable. The virion is enveloped in a lipid bilayer membrane (which projects two glycoproteins, E_1 and E_2) (Fig. 58–3). The most prominent projection, the **peplomer** or E_2 **spike,** consists of two polypeptide chains of equal sizes derived by proteolytic cleavage of a precursor protein. The E_2 protein and the hemagglutinin of influenza virus (see Chap. 56) are comparable. The E_1 **glycoprotein** spans the envelope; a small, glycosylated amino-terminal domain projects on the external surface, but the major portion of the protein (greater than 85%) is in the membrane and on the envelope's internal surface. Like the **matrix (M) protein** of orthomyxoviruses (see Chap. 56) and paramyxoviruses (see Chap. 57) this internal domain interacts with the nucleocapsid (see Fig. 58–3). The long, flexible, helical nucleocapsid consists of a single molecule of capped and polyadenylated infectious RNA (i.e., plus-stranded) associated with many molecules of a **basic phosphoprotein, the N protein** (see Fig. 59–2). The presence of lipid in the envelope makes the virion sensitive to lipid solvents. Deviations of as little as 0.5 units from the virion's optimal pH stability, which varies with viral strains, inactivate the virus, probably reflecting the lability of its envelope.

IMMUNOLOGIC CHARACTERISTICS

Coronaviruses contain three major antigens that are components of the virions: the peplomers (E_2), the matrix protein (E_1), and the nucleocapsid protein (N). Antibodies directed against these proteins divide human coronaviruses into two antigenic groups, of which the viruses 229E (isolated in cell culture) and OC43 (isolated in organ culture) are the prototypes. However, although 229E and OC43 viruses appear antigenically distinct by *in vitro* neutralization assays and other immunologic reactions carried out *in vitro,* infected children and adults develop Abs that react with both viruses following a single illness. Monoclonal Abs elicited by the three virion Ags indicate that the E_2 peplomer induces neutralizing

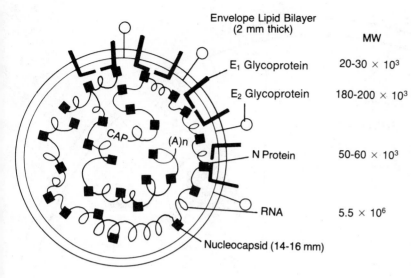

Figure 58–3. Model of coronaviruses schematically shows the helical nucleocapsid, consisting of a single-stranded RNA of positive polarity associated with N protein (only a few of the associated N [■] proteins are indicated); the association of the nucleocapsid with the cytoplasmic domains of the E₁ glycoproteins; and the surface projecting E₂ glycoprotein peplomer.

Abs, which are directed against three distinct epitopes. The E₁ membrane protein also induces Abs that neutralize, but this activity requires complement (see Chap. 51).

The peplomers of some coronaviruses effect hemagglutination with red blood cells (RBCs) from humans, mice, rats, and chickens. Unlike influenza and parainfluenza viruses, coronaviruses do not elute spontaneously from agglutinated RBCs, and treatment of susceptible RBCs with neuraminidase does not reduce hemagglutination, indicating that coronaviruses attach to different cellular receptors.

The viruses from humans appear antigenically unrelated to coronaviruses from other animals in neutralization tests, but complement fixation (**CF**) assays indicate a partial immunologic relatedness of some human types with mouse hepatitis virus.

HOST RANGE

Coronaviruses affecting man appear able to multiply in only a very limited range of host cells. Viruses isolated in organ cultures of ciliated human embryonic tracheal or nasal tissues (the OC type viruses) do not multiply well in monolayer cultures of human diploid or embryonic kidney cells, and vice versa; hence, both culture systems must be employed for viral isolations. The strains related to the 229E virus have the broadest host range in cell culture and can be propagated in primary or secondary human embryonic kidney cells, in human diploid fibroblast lines, and in heteroploid human embryonic lung cell lines. The highest yields of both types of coronaviruses are obtained in a human rhadomyosarcoma cell line, which is therefore probably the best for isolation of virus from clinical specimens. Two of the OC strains have been adapted to growth in the brains of suckling mice, but other laboratory animals have not proved to be susceptible to infection.

MULTIPLICATION

Coronaviruses infecting humans cannot be studied biochemically owing to poor replication and hence low yields. Their similarities of virion structure, including their genomes, to mouse hepatitis virus (MHV), however, suggest that MHV's method of multiplication also applies to human coronaviruses. Upon entry of virus into the cell via endocytosis, the viruses replicate entirely in the cytoplasm (Fig. 58–4). Shortly after entry a portion of the viral RNA genome, probably at its 5′ end, is translated into an "early" RNA-dependent RNA polymerase, which then transcribes the genome into a full-length complementary strand. This negative strand is transcribed into a set of seven viral mRNAs, transcribed by two different "late" RNA polymerases. These capped and polyadenylated mRNAs are uniquely arranged as a **nested set** of progressively decreasing size so that each smaller RNA contains all of the 3′ sequences except those of the gene translated from the next larger RNA (see Fig. 58–4). A second feature is that all the mRNAs, including the genomic RNA, have an identical 5′ leader sequence of about 72 nucleotides that is encoded only at the 5′ terminus of the genome RNA. This finding implies that all the viral mRNAs are formed by joining two noncontiguous RNAs. A study of the replicative intermediate RNAs, which are of genome length, indicates that the joining of the common 5′ leader to the body of each mRNA is not accomplished posttranscriptionally by splicing but occurs during transcription, an unusual biosynthetic process. The findings suggest that the leader RNA is synthesized independently and sequestered to prime transcription of

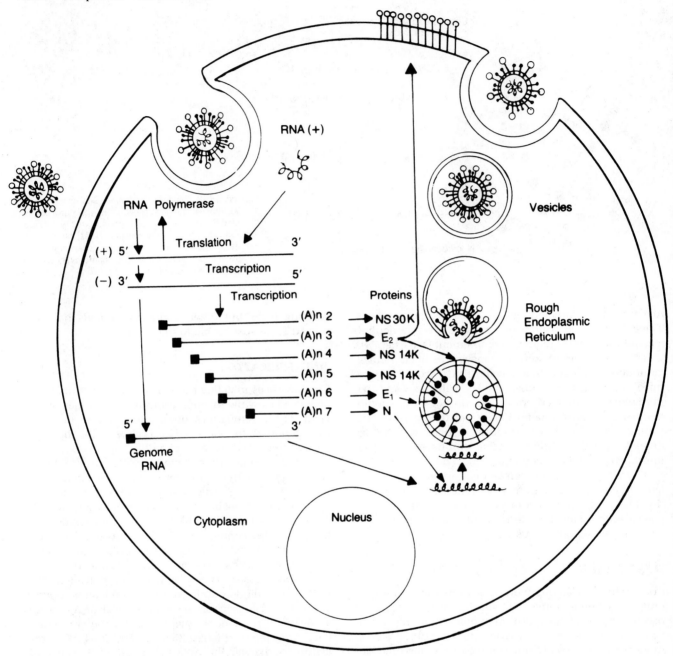

Figure 58–4. Schematic representation of the steps in replication of coronaviruses. ⌐, E₁ glycoprotein; ⌐, E₂ peplomer; ■, the 5′ common capsid, leader sequence on vested mRNAs; (A)n, 3′ poly(A) mRNA sequences; NS, nonstructural proteins. (Modified from Sturman LD, Holmes KV: The molecular biology of coronaviruses. Adv Virus Res 28:35, 1983)

each mRNA by binding to complementary intergenic initiation sites on the negative-strand RNA.

The translation of the structural proteins (E₁, E₂, and N) is associated with **assembly of virions** by budding into vesicles of the rough endoplasmic reticulum and the Golgi apparatus. The E₂ protein, which is cotransla-

tionally glycosylated, and the E₁ matrix protein, which is glycosylated in the Golgi apparatus, are inserted in the vesicle membranes and serve as the signals for association with the N-phosphoprotein–genome RNA complex, the **nucleocapsid** (see Fig. 58–4). Although the E₂ peplomers are also inserted into the plasma membrane, virions are not assembled at the cell surface. Rather, the virions are **released** by fusion of virion-filled vesicles with the plasma membrane, the cellular secretory process of exocytosis.

Viral multiplication is relatively slow compared with a number of other enveloped viruses such as orthomyxoviruses or togaviruses: the eclipse period lasts at least 6 hours, and maximum viral yield is not attained until about 24 hours after infection. Viral multiplication is optimal at 32°C to 33°C, as with rhinoviruses (see Chap. 55), and infectivity is rapidly lost at higher temperatures or with prolonged incubation.

Pathogenesis

Coronaviruses constitute another group of viruses responsible for common colds and pharyngitis. Patients from whom the viruses were recovered, and volunteers who were inoculated intranasally to establish the etiologic relation of coronaviruses to disease, exhibited signs and symptoms of acute upper respiratory infections: coryza, nasal congestion, sneezing, and sore throat were common; less frequent symptoms were headache, cough, muscular or general aches, chills, and fever. Pulmonary involvement has not been noted. In volunteers inoculated intranasally, viral multiplication occurred in superficial cells of the respiratory tract; viral excretion was detectable at the time symptoms were first noted, about 3 days after infection; and the mean duration of illness was 6 to 7 days. Although coronaviruses have many distinctive viral characteristics, the diseases they cause cannot be distinguished clinically from common colds produced by rhinoviruses or even from those occasionally initiated by influenza viruses.

Unfortunately, details of pathogenesis cannot be experimentally studied since an animal model for human coronaviruses does not exist. Other coronaviruses infect a variety of animals, however, producing hepatitis, transmissible gastroenteritis, encephalomyelitis, infectious peritonitis, and pneumonitis. Indeed, despite its being an enveloped virus whose infectivity is quite labile, especially at alkaline pH, it is transmitted by the fecal–oral route in many animals. Moreover, coronaviruses can be detected by electron microscopy in stools of infants with necrotizing enterocolitis, and two of these viruses have been isolated and passed in human fetal intestine organ cultures.

A number of coronaviruses infecting animals, particularly murine hepatitis virus, produce persistent infections. Moreover, some rodent coronaviruses infect the central nervous system, producing diverse pathology such as acute fatal encephalitis or slowly progressive, chronic demyelination, depending upon viral strain, as well as rodent age, strain, and route of inoculation. No such disease has been attributed to coronaviruses in humans, but some human viral strains can infect human and mouse brain cells, which suggests that neurotropism may have clinical implications in man.

Laboratory Diagnosis

Coronaviruses are so fastidious in their host requirements that isolation is not practicable for routine diagnosis. In principle, the diagnostic serologic procedures of CF, enzyme-linked immunosorbent assay (ELISA), neutralization, and hemagglutination-inhibition titrations can be used, but CF and ELISA titrations are the only practical procedures. Neutralization titrations are difficult and expensive, since they require human organ cultures and cell cultures; moreover, neutralizing Abs are present in 50% to 80% of the population, and although reinfection is common, an increase in titer is difficult to demonstrate. Hemagglutination has been obtained with only two viruses, both belonging to the same immunologic type of OC viruses.* For seroepidemiologic surveys, ELISA titrations are more informative than CF assays because CF Abs decline rapidly after infection. However, neutralization and hemagglutination-inhibition assays are more Ag-specific, although less sensitive than ELISA.

Epidemiology

Acute upper respiratory infections generally have their greatest incidence in children, particularly those between 4 and 10 years of age. It is therefore especially striking that coronaviruses are frequently associated with common colds in adults, and it is a member aged 15 years or older who most frequently introduces infection into a family. Virus is not commonly isolated from children, but neutralizing Abs have been detected in up to 50% of children 5 to 9 years old. Moreover, infection (diagnosed by an increase in Ab titer) is more common in older children and adults, although up to 70% of adults have Abs.

Available data indicate that coronavirus infections occur throughout all regions of the world studied. Infections occur predominantly during the winter and early spring and vary markedly from year to year. During a particular respiratory disease season only a single immunologic type appears to be the causative agent. In a seroepidemiologic study of adults covering a 4-year period in Washington, DC, coronavirus infections occurred in 10% to 24% of those with upper respiratory illnesses. A study

---

* Cultured human and monkey cells infected with OC43 viruses adsorb rat and mouse RBCs, so the hemadsorption-inhibition technique can therefore be used.

of Michigan families showed all age groups to be infected, from 0 to 4 years (29.2%) to over 40 years (22%),
with the highest incidence at 15 to 19 years. These findings contrast sharply to the situation with other respiratory viruses (e.g., respiratory syncytial virus), where there
is a marked decrease in disease incidence with increasing age. It is noteworthy that rhinovirus infections are
uncommon during the periods of prevalent coronavirus
infections. During epidemics all segments of the population are affected, but virus tends to spread preferentially
within families.

Coronavirus-like particles have been found in stools of
children and adults in many parts of the world. However,
the frequency of viral detection has been similar in the
sick and the healthy. The appearance of these viral particles in stools of newborns in hospital nurseries is poorly
understood; we understand neither the cause of illness
nor the way it is spread.

Prevention and Control

Additional data on duration of immunity following natural infection, on antigenic structure and immunogenic
potential of the virions, and on incidence of infections
are essential before the need for or the feasibility of a
vaccine is established. Indeed, the high frequency of reinfection accompanied by disease suggests that successful immunization may not be possible.

Selected Reading

BOOKS AND REVIEW ARTICLES

Siddell SG, Anderson R, Cavanagh D et al: Coronaviridae. Intervi-
    rology 20:181, 1983
Siddell SG, Wege H, Ter Meulen V: The biology of coronaviruses. J
    Gen Virol 64:761, 1983
Sturman LS, Holmes KV: The molecular biology of coronaviruses.
    Adv Virus Res 28:35, 1983

SPECIFIC ARTICLES

Baric RS, Stohlman SA, Razavi MK, Lai MMC: Characterization of
    leader-related small RNAs in coronavirus-infected cells: Further
    evidence for leader-primed mechanism of transcription. Virus
    Res 3:19, 1985
Hamre D, Procknow JJ: A new virus isolated from the human respi-
    ratory tract. Proc Soc Exp Biol Med 121:190, 1966
Hamre D, Kindig DA, Mann J: Growth and intracellular development
    of a new respiratory virus. J Virol 1:810, 1967
Tyrrell DAJ, Bynoe ML: Cultivation of a novel type of common-cold
    virus in organ cultures. Br Med J 1:1467, 1965

59

Rhabdoviruses

Were the basis for evolutionary development not so indelibly imprinted on scientific thought, a modern virologist might consider the emergence of the striking bulletlike morphology of rhabdoviruses (Gr. *rhabdos*, rod) a reflection of the violence of our times. This unique form, which was first described for vesicular stomatitis virus (VSV), a virus of cattle and horses, is also associated with rabies virus (Fig. 59–1) and at least 25 other viruses that infect a variety of mammals, fish, insects, and plants. Properties of the agents in this group are summarized under "Characteristics of Rhabdoviruses." Several rhabdoviruses replicate in arthropods as well as in mammals (e.g., VSV, Hart Park virus, Flanders virus, Kern Canyon virus) and hence were previously considered to be arboviruses. Rabies virus is the only member of the group known naturally to infect and produce disease in humans; it will be considered in detail. The Marburg virus,* a simian virus that only accidentally infects humans, has some similar features and will be discussed briefly.

Rabies Virus Group†

The terrifying change of a docile, friendly dog into a vicious, rabid (L. *rabidus*, mad) beast, often with convulsions, struck terror in those in its vicinity and was long considered the work of supernatural causes. The infectious nature of rabies was recognized in 1804, but it was Pasteur, in the 1880s, who suggested that the responsible etiologic agent was not a bacterium. He used his knowledge of the properties of infectious agents and his great intuition to demonstrate for the first time that the patho-

---

* The Marburg virus and the related Ebola viruses are officially classified in the family Filoviridae.

† Lyssavirus (Gr. *lyssa*, rage) is the official designation for this genus of the family Rhabdoviridae.

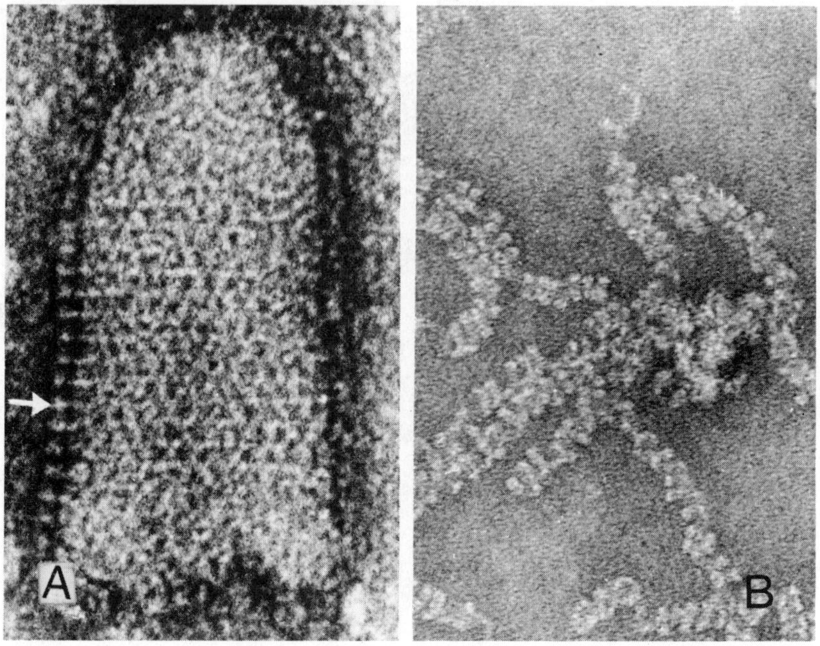

Figure 59–1. Morphologic characteristics of rabies virus. *(A)* Intact rabies virus particle embedded in phosphotungstate and viewed in negative contrast. On the left are well-resolved surface projections 6 nm to 7 nm long (*arrow*). (Original magnification ×400,000) *(B)* Helical nucleocapsid isolated from disrupted rabies virions. Note the tightly coiled and partially uncoiled regions of the single-stranded helix. (Original magnification ×212,000; *A*, Hummeler K et al: J Virol 1:152, 1967; *B*, Sokol F et al: Virology 38:651, 1969)

CHARACTERISTICS OF RHABDOVIRUSES

Morphology: Bullet-shaped; 130–240 nm × 70–80 nm
Nucleic acid: Single-stranded RNA of negative polarity; $3.5–4.6 \times 10^6$ daltons (11–14 Kb); noninfectious
Virion enzyme: RNA transcriptase
Nucleocapsid: Helical; 18 nm wide
Effect of lipid solvents: Disrupt virions; inactivate infectivity
Maturation: Budding at cytoplasmic membranes
Hosts: Wide variety of mammals, fish, invertebrates, and plants
Common antigens: None

genicity of a virus (before viruses had actually been identified) could be modified by serial passage in an animal other than its natural host. Fifty serial intracerebral passages in rabbits yielded a modified virus, **fixed virus** (as contrasted with the **wild-type** or **street virus**), which was used for immunization.*

Upon discovery of the filterable causative agent in 1903, Negri described the presence of prominent cytoplasmic inclusion bodies (**Negri bodies**) in the nerve cells of infected human beings and animals. Their characteristic appearance and easy recognition made possible the rapid pathologic diagnosis of infection.

Although rabies was one of the first diseases of man to be recognized as caused by a virus, the agent was stud-

ied very little until the late 1960s, when methods for propagating attenuated viruses in cell cultures overcame the dangers encountered in handling the virus and the difficulties involved in growing it to high titer.

PROPERTIES
Morphology

The virions (which average 180×75 nm) are cylindrical, resembling a bullet (see Fig. 59–1), with one rounded and one planar end, the latter probably arising by collapse of the region where the budding particle is sealed. Regularly spaced projections, each with a knoblike structure at the distal end, cover the surface of the virion. Shorter bullet-shaped and cylindrical particles, probably defective particles (see Chap. 48), are also occasionally observed in electron micrographs. The helical nucleocapsid is symmetrically wound within the envelope along the axis of the virion, often giving the appearance of a series of transverse striations (see Fig. 59–1A). The purified nucleoprotein is a ribbonlike helical strand, consisting of regular rodlike protein subunits attached to a thread of nucleic acid (see Fig. 59–1B).

Physical and Chemical Properties

The viral envelope consists of a lipid bilayer covered by external surface projections composed of a glycoprotein (**G protein**) and a **matrix nonglycosylated M protein (M_2 protein)** that reinforces the membrane internally (Fig. 59–2). The glycoprotein surface projections, which

---

* Since the fixed virus strain has residual pathogenicity for humans and other animals, it should be considered to be only partially attenuated.

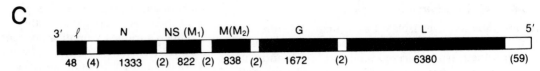

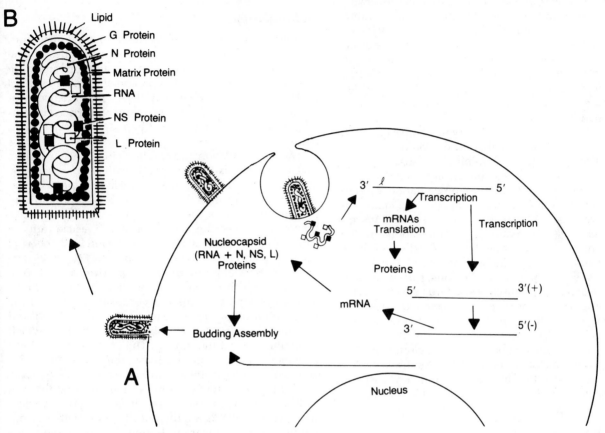

Figure 59–2. Model of rhabdovirus (vesicular stomatitis virus; VSV) virion, its genome, and the steps in viral multiplication. *(A)* The virion and its attachment, uncoating, transcription, translation, RNA replication, assembly, and budding from the infected cell. *(B)* Model of the virion. *(C)* Structure of the RNA genome of VSV, a typical rhabdovirus. The specific coding regions are indicated by the solid boxes; the open boxes indicate the intergenic sequences. The proteins encoded in the genome are noted above each gene, and the number of nucleotides in each gene and in the intergenic regions is noted below. ℓ designates the leader sequences transcribed and individually spliced on each mRNA transcribed. M_1 is the rabies protein comparable to NS, and M_2 is the rabies matrix protein comparable to M of VSV.

act as a hemagglutinin of goose **red blood cells (RBCs),** serve for virion attachment to host cells. The nucleocapsid consists of one molecule of **single-stranded RNA of negative polarity,** many identical copies of a **phosphorylated N protein,** and a few copies of the **RNA-dependent RNA transcriptase,** composed of a large **(L) protein** and a smaller **phosphorylated NS(M_1) protein.**

The rabies virus RNA genome has not been studied in detail. However, VSV, which is readily replicated in cell culture and easily purified, has been exquisitely investigated. Since the morphologic, physical, and chemical characteristics of VSV are so similar to those of rabies

virus, where comparable studies have been done, VSV will be considered the model for discussion of rabies virus structure and replication. Indeed, it is striking that the genome structure and the order of comparable genes of VSV (Fig. 59–2) are so similar to those of paramyxoviruses (see Chap. 57).

As with most enveloped viruses, infectivity deteriorates rapidly at room or refrigerator temperatures in the absence of protein from tissue or added normal serum or albumin. Inactivation is much slower in crude tissue extracts or in infected tissues stored in neutral glycerol. Infectivity is quite stable in frozen or lyophilized tissue extracts.

Immunologic Characteristics

All the rabies viruses isolated from man and other animals, throughout the world, appear to be of a **single immunologic type.** Selected modified (fixed) and wild-type (street) viruses, prepared by many different methods and propagated in different tissues, are also immunologically similar, although minor antigenic variants have been isolated. Several other viruses, immunologically related to rabies virus but distinguishable from it, appear to be limited geographically to regions of Africa and, in host range, primarily to lower animals and insects. However, some of these viruses have been isolated from human illnesses.*

The virion's surface structures, which consist of the G protein, are responsible for the production of neutralizing as well as hemagglutination-inhibiting Abs. Abs to the nucleocapsid proteins, in contrast, are recognized by complement fixation (CF), immunoprecipitation (e.g., enzyme-linked immunosorbent assay [ELISA]), and immunofluorescence. A third class of virus-specific Abs appears after either infection or immunization; in the presence of complement they lyse infected cells whose plasma membranes have incorporated viral Ags. **These cytolytic Abs may play a deleterious rather than a protective role in pathogenesis.** Virus-specific, cytotoxic T-lymphocytes have been demonstrated after infection and immunization, but their role in recovery or protection has not been demonstrated.

Owing to the long incubation period, circulating Abs may be present at the onset of illness. Neutralizing Abs also appear in high titer in the brain and cerebrospinal fluid of patients and can serve as a valuable indicator of infection.

Host Range

Rabies virus can infect all mammals so far tested. Among domestic animals, dogs, cats, and cattle are particularly susceptible. Skunks, bats, foxes, squirrels, raccoons, coyotes, mongooses, and badgers are the principal wildlife hosts. Birds are also susceptible, but less so than mammals.

To establish laboratory infections hamsters, mice, guinea pigs, and rabbits (in order of decreasing susceptibility) are employed. Intracerebral inoculations are more reliable than subcutaneous or intramuscular inoculations.

Rabies virus can be propagated in chick or duck embryos. Attenuated strains developed by multiple passage in embryonated eggs now serve as important sources for vaccines. Cultures of cells from many different animal species can also support viral multiplication. Hamster kidney, human diploid, and chick embryo cell cultures

maintained at 31°C to 33°C are most commonly used. Wild virus is propagated with greater difficulty than modified strains. Cytopathic changes are not usually observed in infected cultures, but intracytoplasmic Ag can be detected by immunofluorescence.

Multiplication

Despite the long incubation period in natural infections, and in experimental animals, the characteristics of viral multiplication in cell cultures are not unusual: the eclipse period is 6 to 8 hours, and the initial cycle of multiplication is completed in 19 to 24 hours. Since cytopathic changes are absent or minimal, carrier cultures or persistent infections (see Chap. 51) are established readily.

The family relationship of rabies virus to VSV suggests that the reactions in their multiplication are essentially identical. The virion attaches to specific receptors of susceptible cells through the viral surface glycoprotein projections and enters the cell in endocytic vesicles. Like influenza viruses, the acidic pH of the vesicle induces viral envelope–plasma membrane fusion and the viral nucleocapsid enters the cytoplasm (see Fig. 59–2). The **virion's RNA-dependent RNA polymerase (transcriptase),** which is composed of the L and NS (M_1) proteins associated with the nucleocapsid, transcribes the viral genome to produce five monocistronic, capped, and polyadenylated mRNAs and the short leader RNA, which is identical on all the mRNAs. The genome has a single promoter and the transcriptase therefore enters the genome at a single site and moves sequentially down it, so that production of each mRNA requires that the preceding 3' RNA be made first. It is not entirely clear whether the mRNAs are then produced by either terminating and restarting transcription at each intergenic sequence junction or processing a transcript of the entire genome. The rapid production of mRNAs *in vivo* and *in vitro*, the inability to demonstrate the processing of mRNAs from large transcripts, and the presence of conserved polyadenylation signals in the terminal 11 nucleotides of each gene suggests that the first mechanism is used to produce the mRNAs.

During viral replication cytoplasmic "factories" form prominent matrices of helical nucleocapsids. These masses of nucleocapsids appear as cytoplasmic inclusion bodies (i.e., Negri bodies) that can be identified by specific immunofluorescence. The virions then assemble by budding from cytoplasmic membranes (and from the basolateral surfaces of plasma membranes of cultured epithelial cells) (see Fig. 59–2).

PATHOGENESIS

A wound or abrasion of the skin, usually inflicted by a rabid animal, is the major portal of entry into man; the virus enters with the animal's saliva. (A dense population

---

* Duvenhaga virus, isolated from the brain of a man who had been bitten by a bat in South Africa; Lagos bat virus (Nigeria); and Mokola shrew virus (Nigeria)

of infected bats may also create an aerosol of infected secretions, by which virus appears to obtain entrance into the respiratory tract.) Virus multiplies in muscle and connective tissue but remains localized for periods that vary from days to months; it then **progresses along the axoplasm of peripheral nerves** to ganglia and eventually to the **central nervous system (CNS),** where it multiplies and produces severe and usually fatal encephalitis. Hematogenous spread of virus to the CNS has been claimed but not established. For transmission by a mammal, the virus must reach the salivary glands, but it apparently does so via efferent nerves rather than through blood and lymph vessels.

The **incubation period** is usually 3 to 8 weeks but can be as short as 6 days or as long as 1 year. It depends on the size of the viral inoculum, the severity of the wound, and the length of the neural path from the wound to the brain, that is, it is shorter following bites on the face and head. (These bites are also usually more extensive.) Illness is ushered in by a **prodromal period,** with irritability, abnormal sensations about the wound site, and hyperesthesia of the skin. **Clinical disease** becomes apparent with the development of the increased muscle tone and difficulty in swallowing, owing to painful and spasmodic contractions of the muscles of deglutition when fluid comes in contact with the fauces. Often the mere sight of liquids will induce such contractions; hence the common name *hydrophobia* (Gr., fear of water). The final stages of the disease result from the extensive damage in the CNS. A fatal outcome has been considered inevitable, but several patients with proved rabies have recovered after being given extensive care for sustaining vital functions. Epidemiologic data further suggest that recognizable rabies follows only 30% to 50% of proven exposures. For example, in an unintentional study about one-half of untreated persons developed clinical rabies and died following severe mutilation by a rabid wolf, which must certainly have effected a viral infection in all those attacked.

Pathologically, rabies is an encephalitis with neuronal degeneration of the spinal cord and brain. **Negri bodies** within affected neurons are characteristic and the only pathognomonic microscopic finding. These cytoplasmic inclusions are sharply defined, spherical or oval, eosinophilic, Feulgen-negative bodies, 2 μm to 10 μm in diameter, containing a central mass of basophilic granules (Fig. 59–3). Several may be found in a single cell. Immunofluorescence studies have demonstrated specific viral Ags in the Negri body, and electron micrographs show (Fig. 59–4) that it consists of a large matrix of viral nucleocapsids (eosinophilic material) and budding virions (the basophilic granules). Virions are also seen in intercellular spaces and in synaptic junctions.

Inclusion bodies are most abundant in Ammon's horn of the hippocampus but may also be found in large numbers in many other sites in the brain and in the posterior

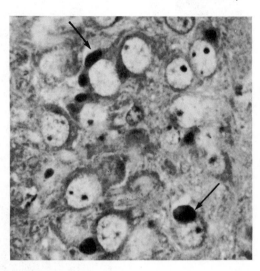

Figure 59–3. Negri bodies in the brain of a mouse infected with rabies virus. Numerous large dark cytoplasmic inclusion bodies (*arrows*) are present. The matrix of the inclusion body is stained intensely; the internal granules appear as light vacuoles. Stained by the dinitrofluorobenzene method for protein-bound groups. (Original magnification ×2000, reduced; courtesy of Dr. H. Koprowski, Wistar Institute, and Dr. R. Love, Jefferson Medical College of Thomas Jefferson University)

horn of the spinal cord. In the absence of identifiable Negri bodies a pathologic diagnosis of rabies cannot be made.

LABORATORY DIAGNOSIS

Definitive diagnosis of infections in humans, and in suspected animal vectors, depends on any one of the following findings: detection of viral Ags in specimens of brain, spinal cord, or skin by immunofluorescence (probably the method of choice, considering speed, accuracy, and cost); identification of Negri bodies in brain tissue; and isolation of virus from brain or saliva. Since the incubation period may be relatively short, the need for an immediate definitive diagnosis makes serologic techniques of little value early in the disease because circulating Abs appear slowly. Serum and cerebrospinal fluid (CSF) Abs eventually reach high levels, however, and if clinical doubts exist during later stages, Ab titrations (neutralization, CF, ELISA, immunofluorescence) can establish the diagnosis in an unimmunized patient.

Negri bodies are detected in impression smears prepared from the region of Ammon's horn. Seller's method, with a stain composed of a mixture of basic fuchsin and methylene blue, is commonly employed. Their distinctive stained appearance (**cherry red with deep blue granules**) differentiates them from other inclusion bodies, particularly those produced by distemper virus in dogs. Fluorescent Ab techniques provide reliable con-

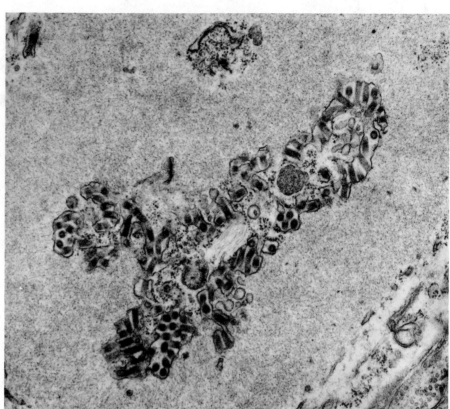

Figure 59–4. Electron micrograph of a Negri body containing several inner bodies composed of developing and mature virions. (Original magnification ×19,500; Matsumoto S: Adv Virus Res 16:257, 1970)

firmation of the specific nature of the inclusion body. The presence of Negri bodies is diagnostic, but **failure to detect them does not exclude rabies** and should be followed by attempts to isolate the virus.

Virus is preferably isolated by inoculating saliva, salivary gland tissue, or hippocampal brain tissue intracerebrally into infant mice. The mice develop paralysis after an incubation period of 6 to 12 days, depending upon the quantity of virus present. The illness is not pathognomonic of rabies, and the virus must be identified by immunologic techniques or by demonstrating Negri bodies in brain tissue from the inoculated animals.

EPIDEMIOLOGY

Although medical interest in rabies centers on infections of humans, epidemiologically this is a dead end to the infectious cycle, since humans contract rabies but do not normally transmit the disease. Dogs are generally the most dangerous source of infection for man, with cats next. In the United States, however, cattle are the most commonly infected domestic animals. The incidence of rabies in humans and dogs has decreased continuously in the United States since the institution of an effective immunization program and leash laws for dogs, and epi-

zootic canine rabies (dog-to-dog transmission) has become rare. But rabies still remains enzootic in wild animals, and therefore persists enzootic in dogs. Thus control measures remain essential. For example, human rabies dropped from 33 cases in 1946 to only 1 to 3 cases per year since 1960, and rabies in animals (detected annually in almost every state) has continued a slight but uneven decline (Fig. 59–5).

Wild mammals serve as a large and uncontrollable reservoir of **sylvan rabies,** which is an increasing threat to people and domestic animals throughout the world. The most frequent wildlife sources in North America are skunks, bats, raccoons, and foxes, in order of their potential danger. Moreover, an epizootic in foxes has reintroduced rabies into Western Europe, which once was relatively free of the disease. Worldwide, rabies in animals, including dogs, steadily increases. A worldwide total of about 1000 fatal human cases is reported annually to the World Health Organization (WHO), and the actual number must be several times greater.

Vampire and insectivorous **bats** are important reservoirs and could be one of the most important links in the ecology of rabies: experimentally, the virus can remain latent in these animals for long periods; and virus has been detected in the nasal mucosa, brown fat, and sali-

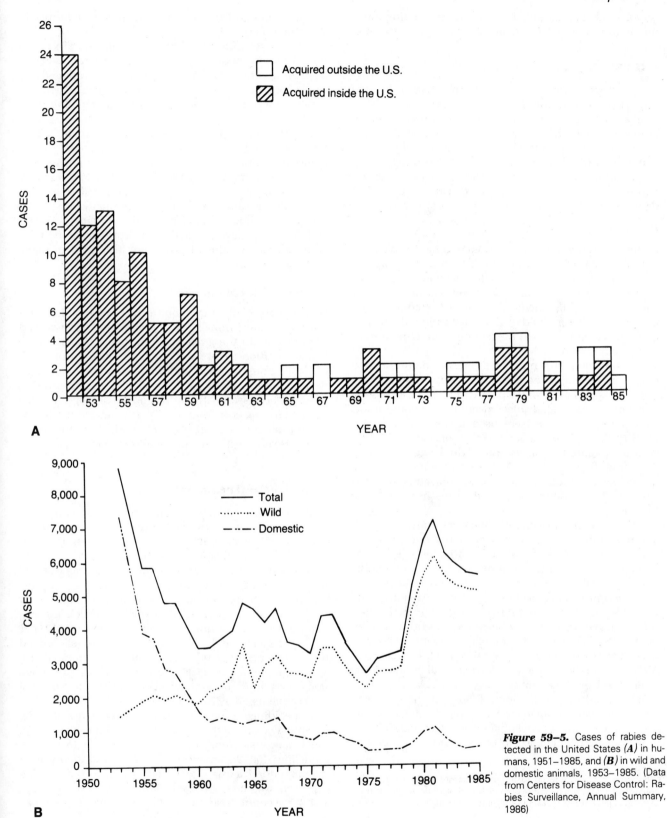

Figure 59–5. Cases of rabies detected in the United States *(A)* in humans, 1951–1985, and *(B)* in wild and domestic animals, 1953–1985. (Data from Centers for Disease Control: Rabies Surveillance, Annual Summary, 1986)

vary glands of apparently healthy bats, permitting transmission to man or other animals without a direct bite.

PREVENTION AND CONTROL

An effective program for rabies control must be directed toward preventing the disease in domestic animals, as well as in man. However, control measures directed against wildlife, which is now the main source of human cases, are impracticable. In fact, the primary rabies problem in the United States and many other countries is no longer human cases but the decision on whether to undertake immunization of humans, with its attendant dangers, after suspected exposure.

Vaccines

Pasteur's original vaccine was prepared by homogenization of partially dried* spinal cords from rabbits infected with modified (fixed) virus. Daily injections were given for 15 to 20 days with cords desiccated for progressively shorter periods. Frequent difficulties resulted, however, from the inexact method of viral inactivation, the lack of quantitative controls, and the complication of demyelinating allergic encephalitis.

Research led to a number of advancements in vaccines with development of **phenol-inactivated vaccines** (e.g., the Semple vaccine, which consisted of a 5% suspension of inactivated infected animal nervous tissue, usually rabbit), which were used in the United States until 1957. More recently, a vaccine consisting of rabies virus **propagated in embryonated duck eggs** and **inactivated by β-propiolactone** was prepared; this vaccine has a lower risk of allergic encephalomyelitis, but it is considerably less immunogenic than the nervous-tissue vaccines.

The low immunogenicity of the duck embryo vaccine and the continuing occurrence of allergic encephalomyelitis spurred efforts to replace it with a modified rabies virus propagated in cell cultures. Such a virus could be partially purified and concentrated in order to prepare highly immunogenic inactivated vaccines. An inactivated virus vaccine prepared from **virus grown in human diploid fibroblasts** is now being used in humans after being successfully tested in monkeys, rodents, dogs, and foxes. Five 1-ml injections (days 0, 3, 7, 14, and 28) elicit Ab levels superior to those following a full course of the phenolized or duck embryo vaccine. The new vaccine reliably produces high titers of Abs, and it has been shown to protect humans bitten by rabid animals; it also appears to be free of encephalitogenic factors. This vaccine is being widely used in Europe and was approved by the Food and Drug Administration in 1980 for use in the United States.

Alternatively, the **purified virion surface glycoprotein** produces neutralizing Abs and may eventually be used for immunization as a purified Ag or produced in a viral expression vector (e.g., vaccinia virus) in which a cDNA copy of the rabies virus G protein gene has been inserted.

Several types of **live attenuated virus vaccines** have been prepared from strains of virus adapted to chick embryos and to canine, feline, monkey, and murine cultured cells. Although considered unsuitable for humans, these vaccines have proved valuable for use in dogs, cats, and cattle. Live attenuated viruses after many passages in canine and feline cell lines have proved effective in dogs and cats, respectively. Inactivated viruses obtained from cultured cells of animal origin are also used in many parts of the world.

Public Health Measures

Primary control of rabies requires restriction of dogs and other domestic animals, as well as limitation of spread from wildlife to the greatest extent possible. The excellent WHO report (1973) recommends compulsory prophylactic immunization of dogs; registration of all dogs, destruction of stray dogs, and isolation and observation of suspect dogs; and attempted control of rabies in wildlife by trapping and other means. The danger of rabies is responsible for current severe restrictions on the transport of dogs across some national boundaries (e.g., Great Britain).

Prophylactic Treatment

Despite the low incidence of human rabies in many parts of the world, the question frequently arises as to the course to follow after an animal bite or scratch. The incidence of demyelinating encephalomyelitis, 1:500 to 1:8000, with a fatality rate of about 1:35,000 has resulted in the elimination of the use of a nervous tissue vaccine. The duck vaccine lacks nervous tissue and is presently recommended in parts of the world in which the cell culture vaccine is not affordable ($200 to $250 per course). Unfortunately, it has not completely eliminated the occurrence of encephalomyelitis (neuroparalytic reactions in about 1 in 25,000 immunized). Systemic reactions (fever, myalgia, etc.) also occur in about one third of the recipients after five to eight doses.

In deciding on the management of a person bitten by an animal suspected of being rabid a number of factors must be considered, but it is not possible to present guidelines for all situations. However, the following is recommended: if exposure to rabies appears definite or if a person was attacked by a nondomestic animal (e.g., skunk, raccoon), treatment with the human diploid cell

---

* Desiccation was employed to reduce infectivity, since Pasteur had noted earlier that dried cultures of chicken cholera bacteria lost their pathogenicity, but not their immunogenicity, for chickens.

vaccine and with human immunoglobulin* should be instituted promptly; vaccine should not be given to a person who has had only minimal contact with a questionable source of infection; and if the responsible animal can be captured alive, it should be observed for at least 10 days for the development of symptoms, since Negri bodies may not be detectable in the brain early in the disease, and the virus can appear in the saliva several days before the onset of symptoms. Suspected bats, however, should be killed and examined at once.

Prophylactic treatment is directed toward confining the virus to the site of entry. Local treatment of the wound consists of thorough cleansing (cauterization is no longer suggested) and infiltration with antiserum. Because of the long incubation period active immunization usually produces an adequate Ab level before the virus has reached its target organs in the CNS. **Combined inoculation with hyperimmune serum and vaccine** is the most effective regimen: serum Abs provide an immediate barrier to passage of virus, which lasts about 14 days, and meanwhile Abs are elicited by the vaccine. The use of hyperimmune serum, however, makes it mandatory to give the full course of vaccine injections in addition to two booster injections, since serum depresses Ab production. Antiserum alone should probably never be used.

Long-Term Prophylaxis

Veterinarians, laboratory workers, dog handlers, wildlife workers, and certain hobbyists (e.g., spelunkers) may be sufficiently exposed to rabies to justify prophylactic immunization. Members of this high-risk group should receive a course of vaccine followed in several months by a booster injection. Subsequent booster doses should be given every 2 to 3 years or following a suspected exposure.

Filoviridae—Marburg and Ebola Viruses

In 1967 in Marburg and Frankfurt, Germany, and in Yugoslavia, an acute febrile illness appeared in laboratory workers handling tissues and cell cultures from recently imported African green monkeys. The 31 cases that occurred, including cases of nosocomial infections in hospital personnel, resulted in seven fatalities. Similar episodes of hemorrhagic fever occurred in simultaneous epidemics in Zaire and the Sudan in 1976, resulting in over 500 cases and 430 deaths. From blood and organ suspensions from fatal cases, viruses, termed the Marburg and Ebola viruses, were isolated.

---

* A single injection of γ-globulin from hyperimmunized humans is recommended.

The viruses contain one molecule of linear, noninfectious RNA (presumably negative-stranded) and at least five major proteins. Virion infectivity is inactivated by lipid solvents. Electron microscopic examinations of negative-stained preparations reveal pleomorphic virions that are filamentous or somewhat rod-shaped, but with a variety of bizarre cylindrical and fishhook-like forms. The virions have a uniform diameter of 80 nm, but virions vary in length from 130 nm to as long as 14,000 nm, with the peak infectivity of Marburg virus at 790 nm and for Ebola virus at 970 nm. Like rhabdoviruses most particles have one rounded end; the other extremity is flat or occupied by a large bleb. Prominent cross-striations and an inner helical structure add to its similarities with rhabdoviruses. Marburg and Ebola viruses are not antigenically related. They are not considered to be rhabdoviruses, to which they are not immunologically related. They are now officially classified as members of a new family termed **Filoviridae.**

The illness produced by Marburg or Ebola virus is that of a severe hemorrhagic fever: a sudden onset with high fever, gastrointestinal upset, constitutional symptoms, and marked prostration, followed by uremia, rash, hemorrhages, and CNS involvement. Fatal cases show necrotic foci in many organs, including the brain; the liver and lymphatic tissues are most severely affected. Medical personnel should take great precautions when handling saliva, urine, or blood from patients.

Serologic surveys in Uganda and Kenya show that Marburg virus is present in monkeys and humans, producing **inapparent infections.** Hemorrhagic fever due to Marburg virus reappeared in South Africa in 1975 (three cases), in Kenya in 1980 (one case and the physicians who cared for the patient), and in Zimbabwe in 1982 (a single case).

Cases of Ebola virus hemorrhagic fever have also been observed since the initial episodes. In 1977 there was a single fatal case in Zaire, but in 1979 there were 34 cases resulting in 22 deaths at the same site in the Sudan as the original cases. The source of the virus has not been identified in any of the episodes, but serologic surveys show Abs in about 5% of the humans in the areas of Zaire where the cases occurred; 26% of the domesticated guinea pigs used as a food source also have Abs. However, there has not been any direct epidemiologic evidence that the guinea pigs were the source of virus infecting humans; rather it is suggested that both the humans and guinea pigs were infected from an unknown source.

The extensive use of primary monkey cell cultures, which may harbor Marburg or an Ebola virus, makes it imperative that physicians and virologists be aware of these simian viruses that on occasion cause disease in man.

Selected Reading

BOOKS AND REVIEW ARTICLES

Baer GM (ed): The Natural History of Rabies. New York, Academic Press, 1975.

Banerjee AK: Transcription and replication of rhabdoviruses. Microbiol Rev 51:66, 1987.

Dean DJ, Evans WM, McClure RC: Pathogenesis of rabies. Bull WHO 29:803, 1963.

Emerson SV: Rhabdoviruses. In Fields BM (ed): Virology, p. 1119. New York, Raven Press, 1985.

Expert Committee Report on Rabies: Sixth Report, WHO Technical Report Series No. 523, World Health Organization, Geneva, 1973.

Shope RE: Rabies. In Evans AS (ed): Viral Infections of Humans: Epidemiology and Control (2nd ed). New York, Plenum Medical Books, 1984.

Specific Articles

Appelbaum E, Greenberg M, Nelson J: Neurological complications following antirabies vaccination. JAMA 151:188, 1953.

Kabat EA, Wolf A, Bezer AE: The rapid production of acute disseminated encephalomyelitis in rhesus monkeys by injections of heterologous and homologous brain tissue with adjuvants. J Exp Med 85:117, 1947.

Kissling RE: Marburg virus. Ann NY Acad Sci 174:932, 1970.

Pasteur L: Methode pour prevenir la rage appres morsure. CR Acad Sci [D] (Paris) 101:765, 1885.

Tierkel ES, Sikes RK: Preexposure prophylaxis against rabies. JAMA 201:911, 1967.

U.S. Government: Recommendation of the Immunization Practices Advisory Committee (ACIP). Public Health Service, U.S. Department of Health and Human Services, Center for Disease Control, Atlanta, 1980

60

Togaviruses, Flaviviruses, Bunyaviruses, and Arenaviruses

The **arthropod-borne viruses (arboviruses)** multiply in both vertebrates and arthropods. In the cycle of transmission the former serve as reservoirs and the latter mostly as vectors, acquiring infection with a blood meal, but in some instances arthropods can also serve as reservoirs, maintaining the viruses by transovarian transmission. The virus is propagated in the arthropod's gut; and if it attains a high titer in its salivary glands, it can be transmitted when a fresh host is bitten. The viruses often cause disease in humans and other vertebrate hosts, but no ill effects are evident in the arthropods.

Most of the viruses described in this chapter were until recently classified, on epidemiologic grounds, as arboviruses. But increasing knowledge of their chemical and physical characteristics has revealed great heterogeneity among the arthropod-borne viruses. A number of these viruses with somewhat similar chemical and physical characteristics (Table 60–1), and of great medical significance to man, were previously grouped into a single family, **Togaviridae** (vernacular, **togaviruses;** *toga*, coat) comprising four genera. However, detailed characterization of a number of viruses clearly indicated that **flaviviruses,** previously classified as a genus in the family, were sufficiently distinct from other members that they should be designated as members of a separate family, **Flaviviridae** (see Table 60–1). Togaviridae comprise three genera: *Alphavirus* and *Rubivirus* (rubella virus; German measles virus), which are viruses infecting humans, and *Pestivirus*, a genus consisting of viruses that

TABLE 60–1. *Comparison of Viral Characteristics of Members of the Families Togaviridae and Flaviviridae*

Property	Togaviridae	Flaviviridae
Virion size	60–65 nm	45 nm
Envelope	+	+
Nucleocapsid	35–39 nm; cubic	30 nm; noncubic
RNA	Positive sense; 4.4×10^3 Kd (Sindbis virus, 11,274 nucleotides)	Positive sense; 3.8–4.2×10^3 Kd (yellow fever virus, 10,862 nucleotides)
Envelope proteins	gp E_1: 45–50 Kd gp E_2: 52–59 Kd gp E_3: 10 Kd*	gp E: 53 Kd M: 8.7 Kd
Nucleocapsid (C) protein	Nonglycosylated: 30 Kd	Nonglycosylated: 13.5 Kd
Nonstructural (NS) proteins	89, 82, and 16 Kd	About 7 species

* Present only in Semliki Forest virus

infect only animals (hog cholera virus and bovine diarrhea virus). The unique pathogenesis, epidemiology, and clinical problems of rubella, however, warrant its separate description (see Chap. 61). This chapter will also consider two other medically significant groups of viruses whose characteristics distinguish them sharply from togaviruses and flaviviruses. The family **Bunyaviridae** (previously called the Bunyamwera virus supergroup) includes the largest group of arthropod-borne viruses; it will undoubtedly be subdivided with further characterization. The family **Arenaviridae** (formerly included among the arboviruses) is also discussed in this chapter, although arthropod transmission is not observed.

The frequent association of an enveloped structure with transmission by arthropods may be more than coincidental: enveloped viruses lose infectivity readily (e.g., on drying, on exposure to bile) and must therefore be spread by either intimate contact (e.g., orthomyxoviruses, paramyxoviruses) or insect bite, whereas naked viruses, such as picornaviruses, tend to be more stable and can survive a more circuitous fecal–oral spread.

Arthropod-borne diseases, because of their vectors, depend strongly on climatic conditions: They are endemic in areas of tropical rain forests, and epidemics in temperate areas usually appear after heavy rainfall has caused an increase in the vector population. Apart from agents known to cause human diseases, a large number of additional arboviruses have been isolated from mosquitoes and ticks trapped in forests and from animals, especially monkeys, caged in the jungle as "sentinels" to permit insects to feed on them. These viruses are not known to cause prominent diseases of humans, but they are attracting a good deal of attention because of their threat as the world's expanding and increasingly mobile population impinges progressively on jungles. Over 350 arthropod-borne viruses have now been isolated (including some **rhabdoviruses** [discussed in Chap. 59] and **orbiviruses** [see Chap. 62]).

History

Yellow fever virus was the first arthropod-borne virus to be discovered, through the work of Major Walter Reed. He headed the United States Army Yellow Fever Commission, established in 1901 to try to overcome the disastrous effect of yellow fever on American troops in Cuba during the Spanish–American War. Reed and the members of the commission demonstrated transmission of this disease in bold experiments with human volunteers* built on the astute observations of Carlos Finlay, a Cuban physician, showing the association between yellow fever and mosquitoes. They also demonstrated the filterability of the agent. These studies established, for the first time, a virus as an agent of human disease, and an insect as the vector for a virus.

Their discoveries led to the eventual control of yellow fever, which for more than 200 years had intermittently been one of the world's major plagues and which, in fact, was a deciding factor in France's failure to complete the Panama Canal. This disease was by no means purely tropical; for example, an epidemic in the Mississippi Valley in 1878 caused 13,000 deaths, and substantial epidemics occurred in the nineteenth century as far north as Boston.

Immunologic Classification

The viruses isolated from arthropods may be divided into at least 34 distinct groups; many are still ungrouped. Table 60–2 lists the principal viruses that infect humans, the families and genera to which they have been assigned, and some of their clinical and epidemiologic characteristics.

* It should be noted that such experiments are not permitted today, and accordingly it is exceedingly difficult to establish whether a newly isolated virus is the cause of a disease or merely a fellow traveler with the undiscovered true etiologic agent.

TABLE 60–2. *Classification and Description of Arthropod-Borne Viruses and Clinically Related Viruses of Humans*

Family	Genus (Group)	Subgroup Complex	Viral Species	Vector	Clinical Disease(s) in Man	Geographic Distribution
Togaviridae*	*Alphavirus*	I	Eastern equine encephalitis (EEE)	Mosquito	Encephalitis	Eastern U.S., Canada, Brazil, Cuba, Panama, Philippines, Dominican Republic, Trinidad
		II	Venezuelan equine encephalitis (VEE)	Mosquito	Encephalitis	Brazil, Colombia, Ecuador, Trinidad, Venezuela, Mexico, Florida, Texas
		III	Western equine encephalitis (WEE)	Mosquito	Encephalitis	Western U.S., Canada, Mexico, Argentina, Brazil, British Guiana
			Sindbis	Mosquito	Subclinical or arthritis, rash	Egypt, India, South Africa, Australia, Sweden, Finland, Soviet Union
			(4 others) Semliki Forest	Mosquito	Fever or none	East Africa, West Africa
		IV	Chikungunya	Mosquito	Headache, fever, rash, joint and muscle pains	East Africa, South Africa, Southeast Asia
			Mayaro	Mosquito	Headache, fever, joint and muscle pains	Bolivia, Brazil, Colombia, Trinidad
		V–VII	Getah (each subgroup contains a single virus)	Mosquito	Subclinical or none known	
Flaviviridae	*Flavivirus*	I	St. Louis encephalitis	Mosquito	Encephalitis	U.S., Trinidad, Panama
			Japanese B encephalitis	Mosquito	Encephalitis	Japan, Guam, Eastern Asian mainland, Malaya, India
			Murray Valley encephalitis	Mosquito	Encephalitis	Australia, New Guinea
			Ilheus	Mosquito	Encephalitis	Brazil, Guatemala, Trinidad, Honduras
			West Nile	Mosquito	Headache, fever, myalgia, rash, lymphadenopathy	Egypt, Israel, India, Uganda, South Africa
			(8 other viruses)	Mosquito		
		II	Dengue (4 types)	Mosquito	Headache, fever, myalgia, prostration, rash (sometimes hemorrhagic)	Pacific islands, South and Southeast Asia, Northern Australia, New Guinea, Greece, Caribbean islands, Nigeria, Central and South America, Republic of China
		III	Yellow fever	Mosquito	Fever, prostration, hepatitis, nephritis	Central and South America, Africa, Trinidad
		IV	Tick-borne group (Russian spring–summer encephalitis group) 15 viruses	Tick	Encephalitis; meningo-encephalitis, hemorrhagic fever	Russian spring–summer encephalitis: U.S.S.R., Canada, U.S.; others: Japan, Siberia, Central Europe, Finland, India, Malaya, Great Britain (louping ill)

TABLE 60–2. *(Continued)*

Family	Genus (Group)	Subgroup Complex	Viral Species	Vector	Clinical Disease(s) in Man	Geographic Distribution
Bunyaviridae	*Bunyavirus* (Bunyamwera supergroup)	V–VII	(11 viruses) Rio Bravo (bat salivary gland) (16 others)	Mosquito Unrecognized Unrecognized	Encephalitis	California, Texas
		C group	Marituba and 10 others	Mosquito	Headache, fever	Brazil (Belem), Panama, Trinidad, Florida
		Bunyamwera group	Bunyamwera and 17 others	Mosquito	Headache, fever, myalgia, fever only, or none	Uganda, South Africa, India, Malaya, Colombia, Brazil, Trinidad, West Africa, Finland, U.S.
		California group	California encephalitis and 10 others	Mosquito	Encephalitis or none	U.S., Trinidad, Brazil, Canada, Czechoslovakia, Mozambique
		10 other subgroups (3 ungrouped members of genus)	46 viruses			
	Phlebovirus fever group	Phlebotomus	37 viruses	Phlebotomus	Sandfly fever; headache, fever, myalgia	Italy, Egypt
	Nairovirus	Crimean-Congo hemorrhagic fever group (4 others)	19 viruses	Tick	Fever, headache, gastrointestinal and renal symptoms, hemorrhages	Africa, Europe, Asia
	Unkuvirus	Uukuniemi group	Uukuniemi 7 others 8 unassigned viruses	Mosquito Tick		Finland
Arenaviridae	*Arenavirus*	Tacaribe	Tacaribe, Junin, Tamiami, Machupo, Pichinde, and 3 others Lymphocytic choriomeningitis Lassa		Headache, fever, myalgia, hemorrhagic signs	South and Central America
Ungrouped			Silverwater	Tick	None known	Canada
			Rift Valley fever	Mosquito	Headache, fever, myalgia, joint pains, hemorrhagic signs, rash	Africa
			Crimean hemorrhagic fever	Tick	Headache, fever, myalgia, hemorrhagic signs	Southern U.S.S.R.
			36 others	Mosquito	None known	
Others			48 viruses (14 groups of 2–8 viruses)	Mosquito Tick	None known in most cases	

* Rubivirus (rubella, or German measles, virus), also a togavirus, is discussed in Chapter 61.

Alphaviruses and flaviviruses are classified on the basis of hemagglutination-inhibition, neutralization, and complement fixation (CF) assays: members of a subgroup cross-react best with each other, but not with members of other families (Table 60–3). Bunyaviruses are classified into 10 subgroups by CF, which shows greater cross-reactivity among members of the family than does hemagglutination-inhibition, but many bunyaviruses are still unclassified. Species within a subgroup are identified by neutralization with standardized antisera; there is less cross-reaction with this test.

The immunologic cross-reactions seen within the ma-

TABLE 60–3. Results of Hemagglutination-Inhibition Titrations With Alphaviruses and Flavivirus

| Immune Serum | Genus | Viruses (Antigen) | | | | | | Semliki Forest | St. Louis Encephalitis |
		EEE	VEE	WEE	Sindbis	Chikungunya	Mayaro		
EEE	Alphavirus	**10,240**	80	160	20	40	20	20	<10
VEE	Alphavirus	160	**640**	80	20	80	80	40	<10
WEE	Alphavirus	80·	160	**10,240**	160	40	80	40	<10
Sindbis	Alphavirus	80	10	2560	**1280**	10	40	40	<10
Chikungunya	Alphavirus	20	20	40	<10	**1280***	80	80	<10
Mayaro	Alphavirus	40	40	320	40	640	**1280***	1280*	<10
Semliki Forest	Alphavirus	40	80	160	10	40	320	**2560**	<10
St. Louis encephalitis	Flavivirus	<10	<10	<10	<10	<10	<10	<10	**2560**

* Note cross-reactions among alphaviruses, but not between the alphaviruses and one flavivirus tested. Also note the cross-reactivity among some viruses forming two subgroups; EEE, VEE, WEE, Sindbis; and Chikungunya, Mayaro, Semliki Forest. When neutralization assays are employed instead of hemagglutination inhibition, EEE appears to be antigenically unique, and VEE shows less cross-reactivity with WEE and Sindbis viruses. At least seven subgroups of flaviviruses have also been identified.

(Modified from Casals J: Ann NY Acad Sci 19:219, 1957)

jor groups of arthropod-borne viruses suggest close phylogenetic relations. However, chemical analysis of the glycoprotein Ags and cross-hybridization of viral RNAs for characterizing genetic relatedness are just beginning to bring sharper taxonomic criteria into this field.

The immunologic cross-reactions among arthropod-borne viruses are of practical as well as theoretic interest. Thus, with the viruses that show cross-reactivity in hemagglutination-inhibition or CF tests, cross-reacting neutralizing Abs may be evident after repeated immunization, though not after primary immunization. Moreover, infection by one virus may confer a demonstrable increase in resistance to subsequent challenge with another. Epidemiologic evidence suggests that such cross-protection may be important in nature; vaccines are being developed to take advantage of these findings.

Togaviruses—Alphaviruses

The major alphaviruses pathogenic for man (see Table 62–2) produce severe encephalitis, particularly western and eastern equine encephalitis viruses (**WEE and EEE**, respectively).

PROPERTIES

Because of their wide distribution and the serious nature of illnesses caused by alphaviruses, particularly encephalitis, these viruses have been studied extensively. Most of them, however, are difficult and dangerous to work with, and the physical and chemical characterization is incomplete except for a few less pathogenic viruses that

can be readily propagated in cell cultures. Sindbis and Semliki Forest viruses, which are not usually pathogenic for humans, have been most extensively used for biochemical studies.

Morphology

The virions are roughly spherical; in thin sections they have an outer membrane (lipoprotein envelope) and a core of electron-dense material (ribonucleoprotein), and they tend to pack in crystalline arrays (Figs. 60–1 and 60–2). Negative staining shows an outer membrane covered with fine projections and a capsid, which appears to consist of 32 capsomers arranged in icosahedral symmetry (Fig. 60–3).

Physical and Chemical Characteristics

The purified virions that have been analyzed each contain one **positive-strand, infectious RNA molecule** (see Table 60–1), which amounts to 4% to 8% of the particle weight. The RNA, like most viral and eukaryotic cell mRNAs, has a polyadenylic acid-rich sequence at its 3′ terminus and a cap at its 5′ end. As with other enveloped viruses, the precise lipid composition reflects that of the host cells' plasma membranes.

Alphaviruses contain a basic nucleocapsid protein and either two or three envelope glycoproteins (Sindbis and Venezuelan equine encephalitis [VEE] viruses, two; Semliki Forest virus, three) that form the surface spikes that span the lipid bilayers to establish association with the capsid (Fig. 60–4).

The E_1 surface glycoprotein spike is the **hemagglutinin.** Virions agglutinate RBCs from newly hatched chicks or adult geese. Maximum hemagglutination (or **hemad-**

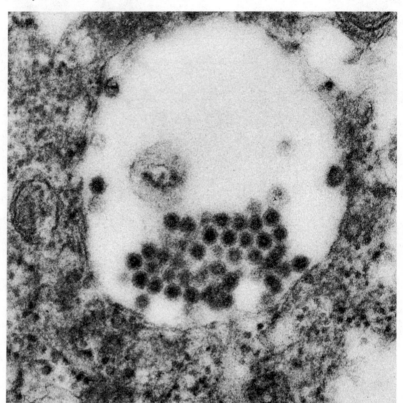

Figure 60–1. Thin section of a mature WEE virus within the cytoplasmic vacuole of an infected cell. The viral particle has a dark central nucleocapsid 30 nm in diameter and a peripheral membrane about 2 nm thick. Note the cubical shape of the virions aggregated in a crystalline-like array. (Original magnification ×100,000; Morgan C et al: J Exp Med 113:219, 1961)

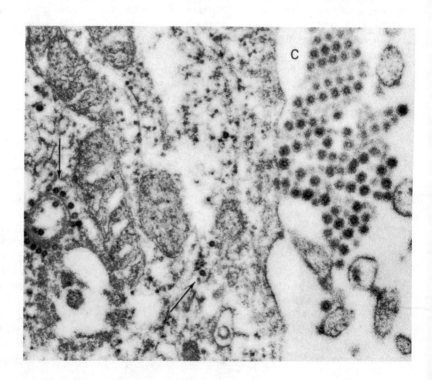

Figure 60–2. Extracellular crystal (*C*) composed of WEE virus particles. Dense precursor particles are scattered in the cytoplasm and are present on opposite sides of two concentric lamellae near the left border (*arrows*). Mature virions are seen only within vacuoles (see Fig. 60–1) or outside of cells. (Original magnification ×86,000; Morgan C et al: J Exp Med 113:219, 1961)

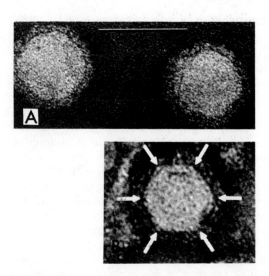

Figure 60–3. Morphology of a negatively stained alphavirus. *(A)* The spherical particles have a dense nucleocapsid and an envelope covered with fine projections. (Original magnification ×240,000) *(B)* In an occasional virion a nucleocapsid with a clear polygonal outline and the semblance of an ordered capsomeric structure is seen. Arrows point to the axes of fivefold symmetry of the icosahedron. (Original magnification ×360,000; Simpson RW, Houser RE: Virology 34:358, 1968)

sorption on infected cell cultures) is effected within narrow ranges of pH and temperature.* The E_1 protein also has **hemolytic activity.** The virions become firmly bound to the red blood cell (RBC) surface and do not elute spon-

* Maximum agglutination is attained at pH 6.4 and 37°C.

taneously. The surface glycoproteins also effect attachment to host cells.

Cell lipids inhibit hemagglutination; hence, detection of hemagglutinating activity in lysates of cells (particularly brain or spinal cord) requires preliminary extraction with lipid solvents. Moreover, treatment of virions with such solvents or with nonionic detergents inactivates infectivity and liberates the glycoproteins that induce production of species-specific neutralizing Abs.

The infectivity of most togaviruses decreases rapidly at 35°C to 37°C *in vitro;* infectivity and hemagglutinating activity have maximum stability at about pH 8.5.

Immunologic Characteristics

Alphaviruses also fall into immunologic subgroups whose members show cross-reactivity of the E_1 glycoprotein. The alphavirus cross-reactivity among subgroups, particularly subgroups I to IV (see Table 60–2), resides in the antigenic properties of the nucleocapsid protein. Monoclonal Abs to specific epitopes on the E_1 and E_2 glycoproteins neutralize virus and inhibit hemagglutination (see Table 62–3). Neutralizing Abs appear about 7 days after onset of disease and exist for many years, probably for life, which correlates with the persistence of solid immunity. Hemagglutination-inhibiting Abs appear at the same time and are easier to assay but less specific; CF Abs also rise early but are not detectable after 12 to 14 months.

Most togaviruses, in contrast to yellow fever and dengue flaviviruses (see below), maintain their immunoge-

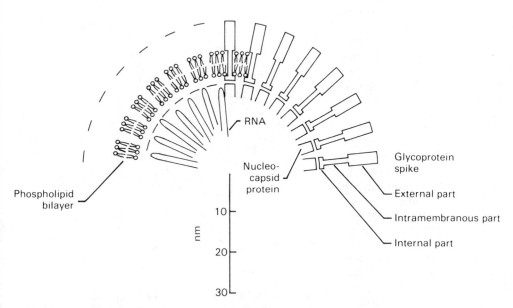

Figure 60–4. Diagram of the Semliki Forest virus, showing the glycoprotein spikes spanning the envelope lipid bilayer and associating with the protein of the nucleocapsid. (Modified from Simons K et al: In Capaldi RA [ed]: Membrane Techniques. New York, Marcel Dekker, 1977)

nicity and immunologic reactivity following destruction of infectivity by formalin, heat, or β-propriolactone.

Cross-reactive hemagglutination-inhibiting Abs develop after infection or artificial immunization; the degree of cross-reactivity increases up to about 1 month after the immunogenic stimulus. For example, an animal infected with EEE virus develops homologous Abs about 7 days after infection, and 3 to 6 weeks later develops relatively high titers of hemagglutination-inhibiting Abs against all alphaviruses. If the same animal is subsequently inoculated with EEE virus or another alphavirus, a rapid increase of hemagglutination-inhibiting Abs against all alphaviruses follows (a secondary group response); the Ab response is considerably greater than that following a single inoculation of either virus alone. Upon subsequent infection, or immunization, with a different but antigenically related virus the highest immunologic response is often to the first virus to which the subject was exposed—another example of the principle of original antigenic sin (see Influenza Viruses, Chap. 56). Proposed immunization procedures take advantage of this broad-ended secondary response.

Host Range

Alphaviruses multiply in a wide range of vertebrates and arthropods. Most of the viruses can also be propagated on a variety of primary and continuous cell cultures, including cultures of mosquito cells. They produce cytopathic effects (except in mosquito cells), and infected cells can also be detected by hemadsorption. A sensitive and reproducible plaque assay can be carried out with susceptible vertebrate cells. Because of their sensitivity and convenience, cell cultures are now the host of choice for experimental and diagnostic work.

The major vertebrate hosts for alphaviruses in nature are birds, rodents, and monkeys. Horses are readily and often fatally infected by the equine encephalitis viruses (whose initial isolation from horses, during epizootics, gave rise to their names). Monkeys are also useful hosts for studying the pathogenesis of infection.

Before its replacement by cell cultures the newborn mouse was the laboratory host of choice; it is highly susceptible to infection by all members of the family. Viruses multiply to high titer in brain, producing extensive pathogenic changes. Some of the viruses also multiply in muscle, lymphoid, or vascular endothelium cells. Resistance increases with age: most mice by age 3 to 6 months are quite resistant to infection by peripheral routes.

Wild birds and domestic fowl, particularly when newly hatched, can be infected artificially or by the bite of an infected mosquito. Embryonated chicken eggs are sensitive, convenient hosts for many studies. Mosquitoes (*Culex, Anopheles,* and *Mansonia*) are the arthropod hosts in nature for alphaviruses.

Multiplication

Togaviruses are positive-strand RNA viruses, which multiply in the cytoplasm. They show considerable variation in the lengths of their multiplication cycles, although the temporal differences are relatively minor within each subgroup. Thus, the duration of the cycle is relatively short for alphaviruses (e.g., WEE virus; Fig. 60–5); in contrast, flaviviruses multiply more slowly (e.g., the maximum yield of type 2 dengue virus is attained 20 to 30 hours after infection).

Virus is adsorbed rapidly by susceptible cells in culture and enters the cell in endocytic vesicles. Eclipse is evident within 1 hour. The uncoated parental genome serves as mRNA for the nonstructural proteins required for replicating RNA. The replication forms of viral RNA superficially resemble those in picornavirus-infected cells (see Chap. 48). However, in **alphavirus** infections two **RNA species** of positive polarity are synthesized: **49S virion RNA and 26S mRNA,** each of which is transcribed from a full-length copy (negative polarity) of the virion RNA (Fig. 60–6). The 26S mRNA is identical with the 3' OH terminal one-third of the 49S virion RNA and codes for the structural proteins, whereas the 49S RNA serves as messenger for translation of the nonstructural proteins (see Fig. 60–6). Extensive replication of 26S RNAs amplifies the messenger for structural proteins when they are most needed. As with picornaviruses, the 26S RNA acts as a **monocistronic mRNA** to produce a poly-

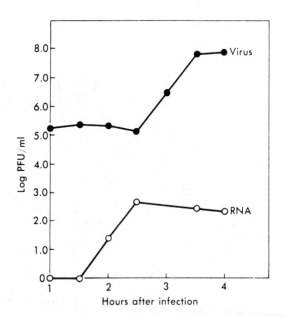

Figure 60–5. Temporal relation of the biosynthesis of infectious (viral) RNA and infectious WEE virus particles. *PFU,* plaque-forming units. (Wecker E, Richter A: Cold Spring Harbor Symp Quant Biol 27:137, 1962)

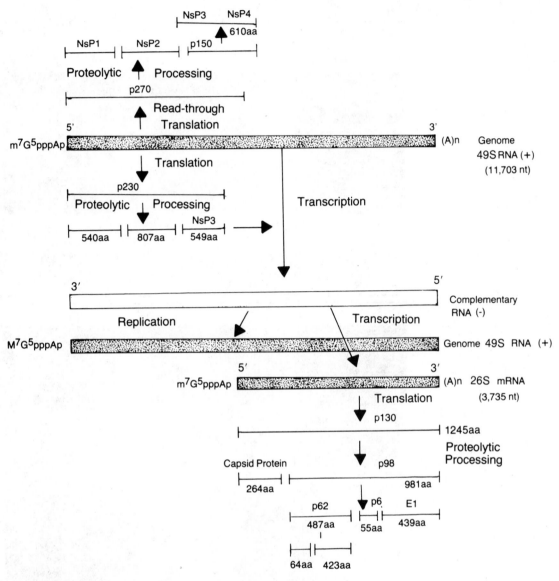

Figure 60–6. Replication of Sindbis virus, a model of alphavirus genome replication, transcription, and translation. The 49S genome (+) RNA is translated into polyprotein that is processed into the nonstructural proteins. The 26S mRNA, which is transcribed from the full-length negative-polarity RNA, is translated into polyprotein that is processed into viral structural proteins. (Recall that Sindbis virus envelope has two glycoproteins, E_1 and E_2, whereas Semliki Forest virus has an additional protein, E_3). *p*, indicates precursor protein; e.g., p 130 signifies a precursor protein of 130,000 daltons. (Modified from Strauss JH, Strauss EG, Hahn CS, Rice CM: In Rowlands DJ, Mayo M, Mahy BWJ [eds]: The Molecular Biology of the Positive Strand RNA Viruses, p 75. New York, Academic Press, 1987)

protein, which appears to have autoprotease activity, to process first the capsid protein and subsequently the other structural, virion proteins (see Fig. 60–6).

The envelope proteins are glycosylated and transported through the endoplasmic reticulum and Golgi apparatus to the plasma membrane, where they become transmembrane proteins. Nucleocapsids recognize the sites of insertion, and final **assembly of the virion** is accomplished by **budding at the cell surface.** The viral particle becomes infectious when it acquires its final coat (i.e., the envelope). Thus maturation of alphavirus particles (e.g., WEE and VEE) and release from the host cell are almost simultaneous (within 1 minute) (Figs. 60–7 and 60–8). Cells infected with Sindbis virus produce virions at the extraordinary rate of 10^4 per cell per hour for approximately 12 hours.

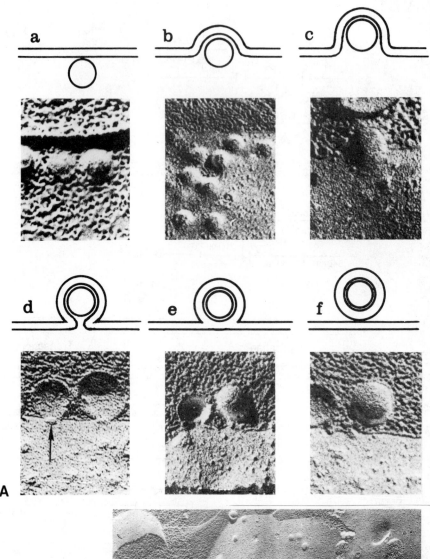

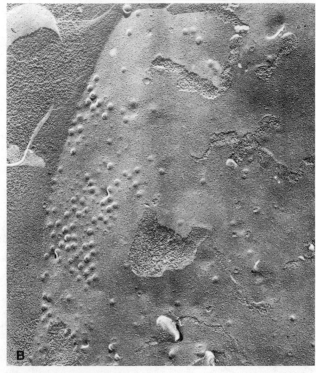

Figure 60–7. Morphogenesis of Sindbis virus (an alphavirus) at the plasma membrane of an infected cell as observed by freeze etching. *(A)* Schematic representation of viral maturation with corresponding electron micrographs. *(B)* Outer surface of the inner leaflet of a virus-infected cell, showing budding and mature virions. (Original magnification ×15,000; Brown DT et al: J Virol 10:524, 1972)

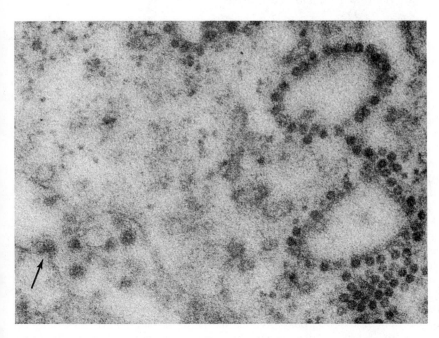

Figure 60-8. Characteristic formation of particles of WEE virus at the membrane of vacuoles in the cytoplasm of an infected cell. Extracellular virus is visible at lower left. One particle seems to be in the process of emerging from an adjacent cell membrane (*arrow*). (Original magnification ×96,000; Morgan C et al: J Exp Med 113:219, 1961)

PATHOGENESIS

When an infected mosquito bites a prospective host it injects virus from its salivary glands into the bloodstream or lymph of its victim. Successful infection depends on the presence of sufficient virus in the saliva of the mosquito and a paucity of neutralizing Abs in the host. Details of the pathogenesis of infections in humans are largely inferred from experimental studies in animals.

All alphavirus infections are similar in the initial stages. Virus is removed from the blood by, and multiplies in, skin and reticuloendothelial cells (mainly in the spleen and lymph nodes). Viremia follows, initiating the systemic phase of the clinical disease. Finally, virus invades various tissues—the central nervous system in the encephalitides; the skin, bone marrow, and blood vessels in the hemorrhagic fevers. The mechanisms by which encephalitis viruses invade the central nervous system are not yet understood: entrance may be effected directly through the blood–brain barrier, at nerve endings, or, less likely, by transmission along nerves.

Despite similarities in certain pathogenic characteristics, considerable diversity exists in the diseases produced by alphaviruses. Two types of **clinical syndromes** are seen (see Table 60–2): (1) EEE, WEE, and VEE, and Semliki Forest viruses produce a **systemic phase** of disease (chills, fever, aches) resulting from the viremia, and an **encephalitic phase** may follow after a variable time; (2) infections by Sindbis, Chikungunya, Mayaro, and Getah viruses are confined to the systemic phase, and the symptoms are primarily fever, arthritis,

and rash. Chikungunya virus also rarely produces hemorrhagic fever.

EEE virus may produce severe illnesses, with high mortality, and often with severe residual neurologic damage among survivors. WEE virus, in contrast, usually causes a less severe disease (most often appearing in infants and children), and most patients recover completely. WEE virus also frequently initiates abortive disease (fever and headache) or clinically inapparent infections. On rare occasions, WEE virus produces massive cerebral necrosis in newborns owing to transplacental transmission of the virus from infected mothers (like rubella virus) (see Chap. 61). VEE virus primarily infects horses; transmission to man usually results in a mild disease with variable systemic symptoms and only rarely causes severe encephalitis (e.g., in the summer of 1971 a devastating epizootic killed thousands of horses in Texas and Mexico, with mild disease occurring in over 100 humans as well).

Pathologically, severe alphavirus infections show gross involvement of viscera as well as of brain and spinal cord. The brain lesions caused by EEE virus are scattered in the white and gray matter, particularly in the brain stem and basal ganglia; the spinal cord shows milder changes. WEE infections, on the other hand, chiefly affect the brain, producing lymphocytic infiltration of the meninges and lesions of the parenchyma, predominantly in the gray matter. Lesions generally consist of necrosis of neurons, glial infiltration, and perivascular cuffing. Inflammatory reactions in walls of small blood vessels, and thrombi, may occur.

LABORATORY DIAGNOSIS

Togavirus infection is diagnosed by viral isolation or by serologic procedures. To isolate a virus from a patient, specimens are inoculated intraperitoneally and intracerebrally into newborn and suckling mice, or into susceptible cell cultures. The viremic phase of an alphavirus encephalitis is usually completed by the time a patient seeks medical assistance. Hence, isolation of virus from the blood and spinal fluid of patients during acute disease is unusual. With those viruses that produce fever, arthritis, and rash (e.g., Chikungunya virus), however, the responsible virus may be isolated from blood during the initial stages of illness. To obtain a virus from a fatal case of encephalitis, emulsions of brain and spinal cord are used.

A newly isolated virus is identified by hemagglutination-inhibition titrations with standard antisera, to determine its immunologic group, and by neutralization titrations, to establish its species.

Early serologic diagnosis can be made by detecting IgM Abs with the enzyme-linked immunosorbent assay (ELISA). Final serologic diagnosis is made with serum drawn during the acute illness and during convalescence. Antigens are obtained from infected cell cultures. Definitive diagnosis can be accomplished by showing a four-fold or greater increase in Ab titer by means of ELISA, hemagglutination-inhibition, CF, or neutralization assays. Neutralization titrations are the most specific, but *in vitro* assays are preferred because of their simplicity, speed, and economy. However, within an immunologic subgroup, rises in heterologous Ab may occur and obscure a precise etiologic diagnosis when *in vitro* assays are used. CF titrations are not adequate for epidemiologic surveys, moreover, because CF Abs do not persist as long as those measured by hemagglutination-inhibition or neutralization titrations.

EPIDEMIOLOGY

For most alphaviruses man is merely an incidental host. The mosquito is the common arthropod vector. The cycle of infection has been elucidated best for the equine encephalitis viruses, particularly **WEE** and **EEE,** and can be simply diagrammed as follows:

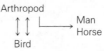

Despite the names of the diseases, the horse, like man, appears to be a dead end in the chain of infections (Fig. 60–9). In fact, horses are not significant reservoirs in nature for WEE and EEE viruses, probably because viremia does not usually reach sufficiently high levels to infect mosquitoes with regularity. It is noteworthy, however, that equine infections usually appear 2 to 3 weeks prior to the occurrence of disease in humans. Birds are the principal natural hosts of WEE and EEE viruses (see Fig. 60–9). Birds likewise appear to be the most likely hosts in

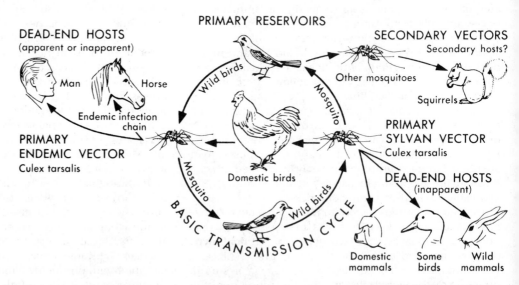

Figure 60–9. Epidemiologic pattern for WEE virus infections. The chains for rural St. Louis encephalitis are similar, except that horses are inapparent, rather than apparent, hosts. EEE infections also have a similar summer infection chain, but a few significant differences exist. (1) The identity of the vector infecting man is unknown. (2) Domestic birds do not appear to be a significant link in the chain. (3) It has a bird-to-bird secondary cycle in pheasants, whose role is unclear. (Hess AD, Holden P: Ann NY Acad Sci 70:294, 1958)

which viruses can persist in nonepidemic periods and during the seasons in which transmission by mosquitoes is not prominent (**overwintering**). Wild snakes and frogs, as well as some rodents, are probably secondary reservoirs for WEE. Hibernating mosquitoes are also a possible reservoir, for infectious virus can persist in them for at least 4 months.

WEE is generally found in the United States west of the Mississippi River, but increasingly the virus is also being isolated along the eastern seaboard. In contrast, EEE is confined to the eastern part of the United States and Canada. Both viruses are also found in the Caribbean, Central America, and South America.

The primary vector of WEE virus is the culicine mosquito, *Culex tarsalis* in central and western United States and *Culiseta melanura* in the northeast. The primary mosquito vector of EEE is not certain, but *Culiseta melanura* is susceptible to experimental infection and has been found infected in nature. Other mosquitoes also appear to be implicated in the epidemiologic cycles involving mammals.

VEE virus is distributed in the Everglades region of Florida (where it is endemic in rodents), in the southwestern United States, and in Central America, northern South America, the Amazon Valley, and southern Mexico. The natural cycle of infections involves mammals and mosquitoes; the natural reservoir is in small mammals rather than birds. **Aedes mansonia** and **psorophora** are the major vectors in epidemic spread of the virus. Horses are invariably infected when human disease occurs and appear to be the major source of virus for mosquitoes. An example, the severe outbreak of 1971, has been mentioned under Pathogenesis.

Chikungunya (African for "that which bends up") virus infections may be a notable exception to this general epidemiologic pattern: man is the only known vetebrate host, with *Anopheles* and *Aedes* mosquitoes the vectors.

PREVENTION AND CONTROL

Control measures are aimed at preventing transmission of the virus by eradicating, or at least reducing, the population of arthropod vectors and at increasing the host resistance by artificial immunization. The former procedure is the only effective means to prevent spread of the viruses, since humans and horses are dead ends, and this method has been relatively successful. Effective vaccines have been prepared against some of the viruses. Despite great effort, however, the viruses continue to exist and cases occur in the United States. In 1984 there were four human cases of EEE (two in Florida and two in Massachusetts) and two cases of WEE in South Dakota. Moreover, 103 EEE equine infections and three WEE equine infections were detected in the same year.

Formalinized chick embryo **EEE and WEE vaccines** produce effective Ab responses in horses. But these vaccines have not been utilized in humans except for protection of laboratory workers; their effectiveness in man has not been established. A live, attenuated **VEE virus vaccine** was successfully used to immunize horses in Texas in 1971; this procedure, along with strict quarantine of the equine population, halted the epidemic. An attenuated VEE virus vaccine has also been used experimentally in humans, but its effectiveness has not yet been demonstrated. The attenuated virus was also fomalin-inactivated and proved to be safe and highly immunogenic; its clinical effectiveness, however, is unproved.

Flaviviruses

The unique structural, morphologic, and replicative characteristics of **flaviviruses** led to their being separated into a family distinct from **Togaviridae** (see Table 60–1), although the viruses in both families have similar epidemiologic features (i.e., arthropod borne) and some produce similar clinical syndromes (see Table 60–2). Flaviviruses, however, do cause a greater variety of illnesses (encephalitis, hemorrhagic diseases, and severe systemic illnesses).

PROPERTIES

Despite the serious nature of many of the illnesses, the broad distribution of the viruses, and the recurrence of epidemics (particularly dengue fever), relatively few of the 60 members of the Flaviviridae family have been studied in detail. However, the marked similarity of those viruses investigated, although they are in different subgroups (see Table 60–2), permit generalities to be made.

Morphology

Flaviviruses are spherical and have a thin, unit membrane envelope, surface projections, and a dense core (i.e., nucleocapsid) whose symmetry is unclear. Thus, although their morphology is similar to that of togaviruses, flaviviruses are significantly smaller (see Table 60–1) and do not have distinct icosahedral symmetry of their nucleocapsids. In thin sections, however, flaviviruses frequently form crystalline-type arrays like togaviruses (see Figs. 60–1 and 60–2).

Physical and Chemical Characteristics

The flavivirus genome, like that of the togaviruses, is a single, linear **positive-strand RNA,** but there the similarity ends. The flavivirus genomes are significantly smaller (see Table 60–1); its 5' terminus is capped, but it does not have a 3' poly(A) tail. Moreover, the genome organization of flaviviruses is different in that the virion structural proteins are encoded in the 5'-terminal quarter, and the remainder encodes the nonstructural protein genes (Fig. 60–10). The virion contains only three structural proteins: a single envelope glycoprotein projection, the **E protein;** the envelope **membrane (M) protein;** and the **nucleocapsid C protein** (see Table 60–1). The number of nonstructural viral proteins is uncertain in flavivirus-infected cells; as many as 12 have been described, and at least three have been identified in yellow fever virus–infected cells (see Fig. 60–10). The nonstructural proteins detected appear to function in viral RNA replication, and at least one of the viral proteins must have protease activity.

The envelope E glycoprotein surface spikes are the viral **hemagglutinin** and effect **hemadsorption** to infected cells. Flaviviruses and togaviruses hemagglutinate similar species of RBCs, but the conditions of pH and temperature required for maximum hemagglutination (or hemadsorption) differ between the viruses of the two families.

Immunologic Characteristics

The **E glycoprotein,** which is on the surface of virions and infected cells, is the **major antigenic structure** of the virion possessing distinct but separate neutralization and hemagglutination-inhibition epitopes. The E protein has antigenic determinants that demonstrate virus-, subgroup-, and flavivirus-specific reactivities. The M and C proteins are also antigenic but do not play a critical role in either pathogenesis or viral classification. Of practical concern for prolonged immunity and artificial immunization is the finding that some flaviviruses isolated at different times (e.g., Murray Valley encephalitis viruses from 1956 and 1969) may be antigenically distinguishable.

Like togaviruses, most flaviviruses remain immunogenic after formalin inactivation. With yellow fever and dengue viruses, however, this treatment markedly impairs their capacity to elicit neutralizing Abs. Accordingly, preparation of successful vaccines required the development of attenuated viruses (see Prevention and Control, below). The existence of only a single known immunologic type of yellow fever virus accounts in part for the effectiveness of the vaccine.

The general immune response to flavivirus infection is similar to that of togaviruses (described previously). Indeed, the considerable cross-reactivity between members of the same subgroup, or even different subgroups, and the marked evidence of "original antigenic sin" response is critical for immunity and immunization procedures.

Host Range

Flaviviruses multiply in the same wide range of vertebrates, arthropods, and cell cultures as togaviruses. In addition to their prolonged replication in mosquitoes and ticks, some flaviviruses can survive in ticks for many months by **transovarian transmission** (e.g., Russian spring–summer encephalitis virus), and through periods of molting and metamorphosis, without apparent injury to the host; this survival during periods of poor transmission furnishes a possible mechanism of overwintering.

Multiplication

The initial stages of infection (i.e., attachment, entry, and uncoating) for flaviviruses are similar to those of togaviruses. Flaviviruses also replicate in the cytoplasm. Although replication of the viral genome is similar in both viral families, the production of the viral proteins is markedly different. Thus, the entire flavivirus genome is translated into a single polyprotein (like picornaviruses; see Chap. 55), which is processed by proteolytic cleavage into the virion structural proteins, from the sequences

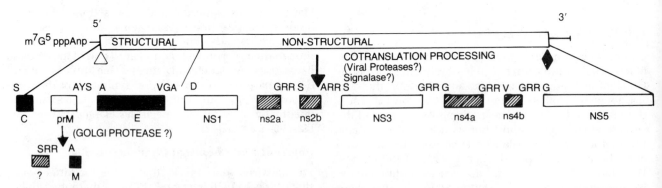

Figure 60–10. Structure of the 17D strain of yellow fever virus. The regions encoding the structural and nonstructural proteins are shown as an open box; the untranslated sequences at the 5′ and 3′ termini are shown as single lines. The cotranslational processing of the polyprotein encoded in the single open-reading frame is shown (open triangle indicates the initiation codon, AUG; and the solid diamond the termination codon, UGA); structural proteins, identified nonstructural proteins, and hypothesized (based on potential protease cleavage sites) nonstructural proteins are shown as solid, open, and hatched boxes, respectively. (Modified from Strauss JH, Strauss EG, Hahn CS, Rice CM: In Rowlands DJ, Mayo M, Mahy BWJ [eds]: The Molecular Biology of the Positive Strand RNA Viruses, p 75. New York, Academic Press, 1987)

encoded in the 5' quarter of the genomic plus-strand RNA, and the nonstructural proteins from the remainder (see Fig. 60–10). The processing of the polyprotein occurs rapidly and efficiently, essentially as the RNA is translated (**cotranslational processing**). The protease, which accomplishes the processing, is probably virally encoded but has not yet been identified.

Assembly of the virions characteristically occurs by budding into cytoplasmic vacuoles. Large numbers of virions accumulate in prominent vacuoles from which they are released through narrow canaliculi connecting the endoplasmic reticulum with the plasma membrane.

PATHOGENESIS

The initial insult—the vector bite and injection of virus, the spread of virus from site of local viral multiplication to lymph nodes, and spread of virus through lymphatics and blood into a variety of tissues, including the target organs—is not dissimilar from that of togaviruses (see preceding discussion).

Flaviviruses produce three types of clinical syndromes (see Table 60–2): **central nervous system disease,** manifested mainly as encephalitis (St. Louis, Japanese B, Murray Valley, Ilheus, and Russian spring–summer encephalitis viruses), with pathologic features similar to those produced by togaviruses; **severe systemic disease** involving viscera such as liver and kidneys (yellow fever virus); and **milder systemic disease** characterized by severe muscle pains and a rash that may be hemorrhagic (West Nile, dengue, and some of the tick-borne viruses). Despite the anxieties induced by the appearance of a flavivirus, most of these viruses, except for yellow fever and dengue, predominantly produce subclinical or mild infections that can be recognized only by laboratory diagnostic procedures.

The severity and extent of the **encephalitides** due to flaviviruses vary with the etiologic agent. For example, **St. Louis encephalitis** virus produces mild lesions, low mortality, and few residua compared with **Japanese B encephalitis** virus, which has a mortality rate of about 8% and causes neurologic residua in more than 30% and persistent mental disturbances in about 10% of clinically diagnosed infections.

The pathogenesis of **yellow fever** differs from that of other flavivirus infections: after primary multiplication in lymph nodes extensive secondary viral multiplication, with cell destruction, occurs in many viscera, including the liver, spleen, kidneys, bone marrow, and lymph nodes. The organs involved and the severity of the lesions vary with the infecting strain. Yellow fever may be a grave disease, with a mortality of about 10%.

The pathology of yellow fever is characterized by degenerative lesions of the liver, kidney, and heart, accompanied by hemorrhages and bile staining of tissues. The most distinctive lesions occur in the liver, where a pathognomonic midzonal, hyaline necrosis develops, with preservation of the basic liver architecture and without inflammatory reaction.

In uncomplicated **dengue fever** deaths are rare; hence, the pathologic lesions are not well known. Biopsies of the characteristic skin lesions reveal endothelial swelling, perivascular edema, and mononuclear infiltration in and about small vessels. In some epidemics, particularly in tropical Asia, hemorrhagic fever and shock syndrome may be prominent. **Hemorrhagic dengue** (characterized by high fever, hemorrhagic manifestations, shock, and a mortality as high as 15%) is most often seen in children sequentially infected with different immunologic types of virus during a limited period (about 2 years), suggesting a hypersensitivity or immune-complex type of disease. The pathologic findings and the marked depression of complement components (particularly C3) support this concept, suggesting that Ag–Ab complexes activate the complement system, with subsequent release of vasoactive peptides. However, primary cases have been reported, and their pathogenic mechanism must be explained.

LABORATORY DIAGNOSIS

Definitive diagnosis depends on viral isolation and serologic assays. Isolation of virus from blood is usually only successful in yellow fever, dengue, and tick-borne encephalitis; viral isolation is usually made during the first 2 to 4 days of the disease. For other flavivirus infections, viral isolation is most effectively made from brain tissue. Specific identification of the virus is best made using neutralization titrations, although hemagglutination-inhibition titrations with standard sera can also be employed to identify the immunologic group. Because of the marked cross-reactivity among flaviviruses, and particularly within the same subgroup, considerable care is required to identify the virus.

Serologic diagnosis can be made as described for togaviruses.

EPIDEMIOLOGY

The epidemiologic patterns of flavivirus infections are more varied than those of togaviruses. These patterns will be summarized for a few of the most important diseases.

St. Louis encephalitis[*] is the major flavivirus infection in the United States; despite its name, it occurs throughout the country. The most severe epidemic to occur since reporting was initiated took place in 1975,

---

[*] The first epidemic due to this virus was recognized in St. Louis, Mo, in 1933.

affecting the central part of the country; 1815 cases with 140 deaths were recorded. The epidemiologic pattern is similar to that described for WEE virus infections. Wild birds are the major reservoir of the virus, and *Culex taralis* and the *C. pipiens* complex are the most common mosquito vectors. Man is an accidental, dead-end host (see Fig. 60–9).

The epidemiology of **Murray Valley encephalitis, Japanese B encephalitis,** and **West Nile fever** is basically the same as that of St. Louis encephalitis except for the species of mosquito vectors and the avian reservoirs. Serologic surveys indicate that for each case of clinical disease produced by these viruses several hundred **inapparent infections** are also induced.

Yellow fever presents another complex ecologic situation.* Two distinct epidemiologic types exist, **urban** and **jungle yellow fever.** Each has a different cycle, but they may interact. In its simplest form the epidemiologic pattern of urban yellow fever simply involves man and the domestic mosquito, *Aedes aegypti:*

Aedes aegypti mosquito
└── Man ←─┘

Viremia in man begins 1 or 2 days before and persists for 2 to 4 days after the onset of clinical illness. Viremia is greatest during this period and mosquitoes taking a blood meal may be infected. A 10- to 12-day period of viral multiplication in the cells lining the mosquito's intestinal tract is then required (the **extrinsic incubation period**) until sufficient virus accumulates in the salivary glands to permit transmission to man.

Jungle yellow fever is transmitted by various jungle mosquitoes, primarily to monkeys. Man becomes an accidental host when he enters the animals' domain.

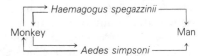

Infection of man may initiate a cycle of urban yellow fever.

Dengue fever resembles yellow fever epidemiologically. There is an urban cycle (man ⇌ *Aedes aegypti* mosquitoes), and probably a jungle cycle with the monkey as the mammalian host. *Aedes albopictus*, which has recently been introduced into the United States, can also serve as a vector. This disease is still prevalent in the Caribbean islands; more distant subtropical areas are also affected (see Table 60–2). A severe type 2 epidemic occurred in Cuba in 1981.

The **tick-borne** complex of viral infections introduces several unique features into the epidemiology of flavi-

---

* The monograph *Yellow Fever*, GK Strode (ed), New York, McGraw-Hill, 1951, reviews in exciting detail many of the important facts personally discovered by its authors.

virus infections: ticks may serve as reservoirs by **transovarian transmission** of virus; in addition to being transmitted by ticks (*Ixodes*), some of these viruses (e.g., **Russian spring–summer encephalitis virus**) may also be transmitted to man from the goat by milk instead of by an arthropod.

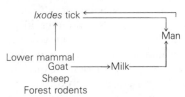

Omsk hemorrhagic fever virus is transmitted by *Dermacentor marginatus*, probably from muskrats, and **Powassan virus** (isolated in Canada and the United States) is transmitted by *Ixodes* ticks from small mammals, probably squirrels.

PREVENTION AND CONTROL

Yellow fever has played a special role in the development of concepts and methods for the control of insect-borne diseases. Reducing the population of the vector, *A. aegypti*, proved effective soon after Reed and his colleagues demonstrated the causative agent and the vector requirement. The use of modern insecticides has facilitated this control measure. It should be noted, however, that *A. aegypti* mosquitoes and other possible vectors are still present in many parts of the world, including the southeastern United States. Moreover, mosquito control measures cannot eliminate jungle yellow fever.

As noted earlier, the loss of immunogenicity of yellow fever virus upon inactivation made it necessary to seek a vaccine containing infectious virus. Theiler and his coworkers attenuated a mouse-adapted yellow fever virus by serial passage in tissue cultures, first of embryonic mouse tissues, then of embryonic chicks, and finally of embryonic chicks without brain or cord. For the most widely used vaccine, the attenuated virus (17D yellow fever virus) is propagated in embryonated chicken eggs. The 17D strain produces few reactions and has an excellent safety record. The duration of protection afforded by the 17D vaccine is not known, but Abs have been detected at least 6 years after immunization.

Eradication of yellow fever in the United States, and substantial reduction of its incidence in South America and other parts of the world, initially suggested that this disease would be eliminated throughout the world. However, the reservoir of jungle yellow fever was later discovered, and yellow fever has increased in incidence in parts of Central and South America and has been creeping northward. With this nidus present the danger of epidemics is real.

A **Japanese B encephalitis vaccine,** prepared by for-

TABLE 60—4. Properties of Bunyaviridae and Arenaviridae

Property	Bunyaviridae	Arenaviridae
Morphology	Spherical, enveloped, projecting spikes Diameter 80–110 nm Helical nucleocapsid	Spherical, pleomorphic; enveloped Diameter 110–130 nm average Beaded, circular nucleocapsid
Nucleic acid*	RNA, single-stranded; 3 (L, M, and S) segments: 2.1–3.1, 1.1–2.3, and 0.28–0.51 $\times$ 10^6 daltons (S segment of Phlebotomus viruses: 0.7 – 0.8 $\times$ 10^6 daltons)	RNA, single-stranded; two (L and S) segments, virus-specific 2–3.2 and 1.1 to 1.6 $\times$ 10^6 daltons (three species host RNA also in virions)
Virion proteins*	Two glycoproteins: (1) 75–120 and (2) 30–60 $\times$ 10^3 daltons; two nonglycosylated proteins: nucleocapsid (N) protein 19–60 $\times$ 10^3 daltons and RNA polymerase (L) protein 145–200 $\times$ 10^3 daltons	Two glycoproteins: (1) 42–72X and (2) 34–40 $\times$ 10^3 daltons; two nonglycosylated proteins: (N) 60–70 $\times$ and (L) 200 $\times$ 10^3 daltons
Effect of lipid solvents	Inactivate	Inactivate
Stability	Unstable below pH 7.0	Unstable
Hemagglutination	1-day chick or goose RBCs	None
Best animal host	Suckling mice; chickens	Various rodents

* Molecular weights vary with different viral species.

malin inactivation of virus propagated in chick embryos, has been employed with apparent success in children in Japan. However, a similar vaccine was ineffective in U.S. Army personnel stationed in Japan and the Far East. An effective **dengue vaccine** containing infectious, attenuated virus has not yet been developed, although efforts continue, particularly with temperature-sensitive mutants. In addition, the development of live virus expression vectors (e.g., a vaccinia virus vector) containing the cDNA encoding the dengue virus E glycoprotein is under active investigation and offers considerable promise. However, until we explicitly understand the role of viral Ag–Ab complexes in the pathogenesis of dengue hemorrhagic fever and shock syndrome such vaccines should be used with caution.

The marked antigenic cross-reactivity of flaviviruses may prove useful for immunization purposes. For example, in experimental animal studies, immunization with an infectious attenuated virus, such as yellow fever virus, and subsequent injection of one or more inactivated or live attenuated heterologous viruses, resulted in a broad immunologic response that protected against a variety of flaviviruses.

Bunyaviruses

On the basis of morphologic, chemical, and structural features, more than 200 of the so-called arboviruses have been grouped into a single family, Bunyaviridae (see Table 60–2), the largest family of RNA-containing viruses. Based on immunologic and genetic differences, this large family has been further divided into four genera: *Bunyavirus*, *Phlebovirus*, *Nairovirus*, and *Unkuvirus*. Phle-

boviruses, however, appear to have a unique genome and therefore a different replication strategy (discussed later), and these viruses will probably be classified in a separate family. The large *Bunyavirus** genus, which consists of 124 viruses, includes the California encephalitis, Bunyamwera, and C subgroups, which are the major ones affecting humans (additional members of the genus, the Bwamba, Capim, Guama, Koongol, Patois, Simbu, and Tete virus groups, have similar properties). Sandfly (or *Phlebotomus*) fever virus and Rift Valley fever virus (genus *Phlebovirus*), Crimean-Congo hemorrhagic fever virus (genus *Nairovirus*), and Hantaan virus (unassigned) are other members of the family associated with human epidemics.

PROPERTIES

The **structures** of all viruses studied show marked similarities to each other (Table 60–4) and clear distinctions from togaviruses and flaviviruses. The virions are spherical particles, clearly larger than togaviruses. Their envelopes are unit membranes covered with surface projections, which are indistinct for most bunyaviruses but arranged in a regular lattice on the phleboviruses and Uukuniemi virus. These spikes consist of two glycoproteins, G_1 and G_2, present in equimolar amounts; they have hemagglutinating activity and induce hemagglutination-inhibiting and neutralizing Abs. The envelope does not possess a matrix protein. The nucleocapsid, when released from the virion, appears to have helical symmetry and is present in three distinct segments

* Named for Bunyamwera, Uganda, where the type species virus was isolated.

(each consists of a common N protein and a unique RNA molecule), often seen in circular forms. However, the three species of RNA are linear. The circles are formed by pairing of complementary segments at the free 3′ and 5′ ends of the RNA molecules: in fact, free RNAs of the Uukuniemi virus are circular under nondenaturing conditions and can reform circles on annealing after denaturation. The viral RNAs are **negative strands,** their 3′ ends are not polyadenylated, their 5′ ends are not capped, and they are not infectious. The virions contain an RNA-dependent RNA polymerase, probably the transcriptase.

Immunologic Characteristics

Bunyaviridae, like togaviruses and flaviviruses, can be studied by hemagglutination-inhibition, CF, and neutralization titrations. In contrast to these viruses, however, the cross-reactivity of bunyaviruses, except for phleboviruses, is maximal in CF rather than in hemagglutination-inhibition titrations. For example, CF titrations with one or two standard sera can identify an agent as a group C virus, and specific viral identification can be accomplished by hemagglutination-inhibition and neutralization titrations. Thus CF titrations show all bunyaviruses to be antigenically related through the cross-reacting nucleocapsid protein, but neutralization and hemagglutination-inhibition titrations can subdivide members of the *Bunyavirus* genus into 13 subgroups (serogroups). Similarly, the viruses of each of the three other genera are immunologically related through the nucleocapsid N protein, and members of each genus are divided into serogroups (see Table 60–2). Viruses of one genus are immunologically unrelated to members of the other genera.

Host Range

Suckling and newly weaned mice are the laboratory animals of choice for isolation of the viruses by intracerebral inoculation. These viruses also multiply and produce cytopathic changes and plaques in a variety of cultured cells; among the most useful are continuous human (e.g., HeLa) lines and baby hamster kidney (**BHK21**) cell lines.

Multiplication

Only a few members of the Bunyaviridae family have been studied in detail, but the data obtained indicate that these viruses replicate like orthomyxoviruses (see Chap. 56), except for the phleboviruses (see later). After attachment to susceptible cells via the virion surface glycoproteins, the particles are engulfed and uncoated, and the nucleocapsids enter the cytoplasm. RNAs are immediately transcribed, and, like influenza viruses, the mRNAs attain their 5′ caps by cannibalizing host cellular mRNAs (see Chaps. 48 and 56). These viral mRNAs are translated, after which the genome RNA is transcribed to make a full-length positive-sense strand (Fig. 60–11).

The multiplication of a single phlebovirus, the Punta Toro virus, has been extensively investigated, but these studies imply that members of this genus have unusual genomes. The nucleotide sequence of the S RNA of Punta Toro virus indicates that the 5′ position of the RNA directly encodes the NS protein and is therefore positive-sense RNA. However, the 3′ region, from which the nucleocapsid N protein is derived, is negative-sense RNA,

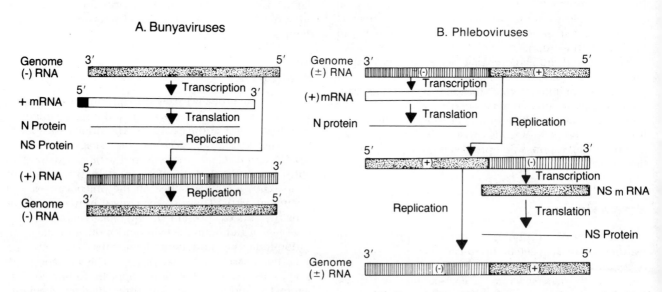

Figure 60–11. Replication strategy of the bunyaviruses (**A**) and phleboviruses (**B**). The models, which include transcription, translation, and replication of the segment of genome RNA, depend on the nucleotide sequences of the small (S) segment of the snowball hare bunyavirus (**A**) and the ambisense genome of the Punta Toro phlebovirus (**B**). (Bishop DHL et al: Nucleic Acids Res 10:3703, 1982; Ihara T et al: Virology 136:293, 1984)

like other bunyaviruses. Thus, the proteins are not encoded in overlapping reading frames as in other bunyaviruses, and therefore it must undergo unique replication as shown in Figure 60–11. The phleboviruses are said to have "ambisense" polarity. Whereas the Punta Toro virus S RNA is about twice the molecular weight of the bunyavirus S RNA, the L and M RNA segments are similar in size to those of other bunyaviruses, and it is assumed that their replication follows similar reactions.

Viruses of the Bunyaviridae family have an additional unusual feature: morphogenesis of the virions is accomplished by budding into the vacuoles of the Golgi apparatus (Fig. 60–12) rather than at the plasma membrane or into undifferentiated cytoplasmic vacuoles, like flaviviruses.

PATHOGENESIS AND EPIDEMIOLOGY

Bunyamwera virus, which is the prototype virus from which the family and genus names were derived, was first isolated from a mixed pool of *Aedes* mosquitoes trapped in Uganda. Eighteen immunologically related but distinct viruses have been recognized, including strains isolated in the United States (Florida, Virginia, Colorado, Illinois, and New Mexico). Disease attributed to the Bunyamwera group (see Table 60–2) is rare and usually mild. Like togaviruses and flaviviruses, the virus enters the body when the infected vector bites and partakes of a blood meal. Viremia occurs, and the resulting disease depends on the organs susceptible to a particular virus.

The **California serogroup encephalitis viruses,** which were initially isolated from mosquitoes in the San Joaquin Valley of California, are widely distributed. They produce prominent clinical illnesses, manifested by fever, headache, and mild or severe central nervous system involvement, particularly in children. Recovery is usually complete, although mild residua and even rare deaths have been recorded. The LaCrosse encephalitis virus is the most common arthropod-borne virus to cause human encephalitis in the United States. The snowshoe hare and Jamestown Canyon viruses are other members of this serogroup to cause encephalitis in North America. Clinical disease has been reported from 13 states in all regions of the United States as well as in the countries noted in Table 60–2. The natural reservoir of these viruses is unknown, but the agents have been found in the blood of rabbits, squirrels, and field mice in titers adequate to infect mosquitoes. Although California encephalitis viruses have been isolated from several *Aedes* and *Culicine* species, *Aedes triseriatus* appears to be the principal vector. Moreover, transovarian passage of the virus in this vector may furnish an important mechanism for its maintenance during the winter.

Among a large number of viruses isolated from experi-

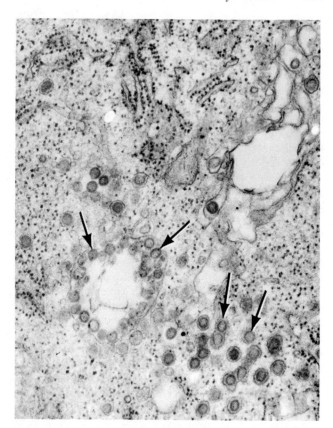

Figure 60–12. Development of Bunyamwera virus in the cytoplasm of a neuron in a mouse brain. Viral particles are present in the cytoplasm and budding into Golgi vacuoles and cisternae of the endoplasmic reticulum. Virions have a mean diameter of 90 nm to 100 nm, a nucleocapsid core of 60 nm to 70 nm in diameter, and an envelope of 15 nm to 20 nm thick. (Original magnification ×39,500; Murphy FA et al: J Virol 2:1315, 1968)

mental (sentinel) monkeys caged in the forested Belem area of Brazil seven different viruses were recognized as being immunologically related to each other but distinct from togaviruses and flaviviruses. Several other immunologically distinguishable but related viruses have been isolated in the Florida Everglades and Central America. These viruses, previously called **group C arboviruses,** but now recognized as a division of the *Bunyavirus* genus, produce mild disease in man, consisting of headache and fever; recovery is complete.

The natural reservoir of C viruses appears to be in monkeys and other forest mammals (e.g., opossums, rats, sloths). The specific mosquito vector has not been established, but culicine and sabethine mosquitoes are likely candidates.

Among the many other viruses of this family some species of the phlebovirus genus, the phlebotomus fever (or sandfly fever) viruses, and Rift Valley fever virus are known to produce disease in man. Most of the viruses were isolated from insects (particularly mosquitoes and ticks) and animals captured in the wild.

The **Congo-Crimean hemorrhagic fever virus,** a **Nairovirus** transmitted by *omma* ticks, initially was considered to cause serious illness that was often fatal. As it became more widely recognized, however, it was realized that the virus did not always cause severe disease but that it caused widespread zoonosis wherever its vector existed (from South Africa through the Middle East and Asia into China).

Arenaviruses

On the basis of morphologic, immunologic, and clinical characterizations the seemingly disparate Lassa virus, lymphocytic choriomeningitis (LCM) virus, and Tacaribe group of viruses, previously considered to be arboviruses, are now classified into a single family called **Arenaviridae** (vernacular, **arenaviruses;** L. *arena*, sand), a term derived from the unique electron microscopic appearance of the virions (Fig. 60–13).

Complement fixation reveals the immunologic relatedness of the arenaviruses, owing to the marked cross-reactivity of the nucleocapsid (N) protein; the Tacaribe viruses, however, are more closely related to each other than to Lassa or LCM virus. Neutralization titrations show the immunologic specificity of each arenavirus.

Although arenaviruses were initially grouped together because of their immunologic relations and similar morphology, they also have comparable epidemiologic, ecologic, and pathogenic patterns. Tacaribe group, LCM, and Lassa viruses do not require arthropods for spread; the natural hosts of all arenaviruses appear to be rodents, in which they often produce chronic infections.

PROPERTIES

The viral particles (see Table 60–4) are spherical or pleomorphic. As viewed in thin sections the virions consist of a dense, well-defined envelope with prominent, closely spaced projections and an unstructured interior containing a varying number of electron-dense granules, probably host ribosomes (see Fig. 60–13), which cause the unique pebbly appearance from which the viruses gained their name. Negative-contrast electron micrographs also show spherical or pleomorphic virions with an envelope having pronounced and regularly spaced club-shaped surface projections.

Within the virion are several species of ribonucleoproteins, which are both virus specific and host cell derived (see Table 60–4). The host cell ribonucleoproteins have characteristics of ribosomes, with 28S and 18S RNAs. The two viral RNA segments are single-stranded RNAs of "ambisense" polarity with the same characteristics as the S RNA of phleboviruses (see Fig. 60–11). The virions contain two glycoproteins associated with the envelope and two nonglycosylated proteins, the N protein (a component of the nucleocapsid) and a large (L) minor protein

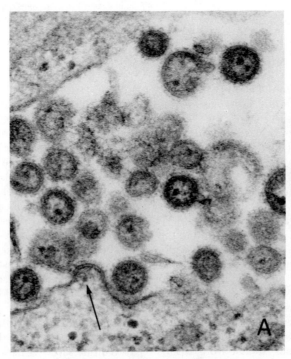
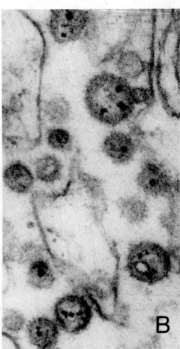

Figure 60–13. *(A)* Machupo virus (a Tacaribe group virus) particle budding *(arrow)* from the plasma membrane of an infected cell; the thickened membrane of the budding particle is prominent compared with the neighboring membrane. Many extracellular mature virions (mean diameter of 11 nm to 13 nm) are present: Their prominent surface projections and internal, ribosome-like particles are readily seen. (Original magnification ×114,000). *(B)* Lymphocytic choriomeningitis (LCM) virus particles in an infected culture of mouse macrophages. The morphology is strikingly similar to that of the Tacaribe group virus in *A.* (Original magnification ×82,000; Murphy FA et al: J Virol 4:535, 1969)

(probably the transcriptase; see Table 60–4). Epitopes on the G$_1$ glycoprotein are the major antigenic determinants for neutralizing Abs. The S viral RNA segment encodes the N protein in its negative-sense 3′ half and the glycoprotein (GPC)—the precursor to the G$_1$ and G$_2$ glycoproteins—in its positive-sense 5′ half. The intergenic region is GC rich, forms a hairpin structure, and appears to serve as a termination signal for both transcriptions.

The biochemical events of **viral multiplication** follow the patterns described for phleboviruses. The appearance of ribosomal RNAs in the virions is inhibited by dactinomycin (actinomycin D) (0.15 μg/ml), but neither synthesis of viral RNAs nor production of infectious virus is affected. Electron microscopic studies show that virions are formed by budding, chiefly from plasma membrane (see Fig. 60–13). At the sites of budding, the host cell membrane becomes thickened, more clearly bilamellar, and covered with projections. The ribosome-like particles are present within the budding particles before separation from the infected cell. (Their significance is unknown.)

PATHOGENESIS AND EPIDEMIOLOGY

Arenaviruses commonly produce chronic carrier states in their natural hosts, possibly because viral multiplication in animals, as in cell culture, is not associated with extensive cell damage; rather, cell death results from cytotoxic T cell attack as in LCM infections in mice (see Chap. 51). The virus may be isolated from the animals' urine, as well as from their blood and internal organs.

The **Tacaribe group of viruses** (Tacaribe, Machupo, Junin, Tamiami, and five others) has been isolated principally from bats and cricetid rodents in the Western Hemisphere. Junin and Machupo viruses have been frequently isolated from cases of Argentinian and Bolivian hemorrhagic fevers, respectively, and appear to be the etiologic agents of these severe illnesses. Thus, the Tacaribe group viruses, similar to LCM virus of mice, appear to be **spread to humans in excretions of the naturally infected rodents.** Except for Lassa virus, there is no evidence of viral spread from patient to patient.

LCM virus rarely infects humans. When it does, it is usually under conditions in which the indigenously infected mouse population is very dense or from contact with infected hamsters. The disease is generally mild and is manifested most often as a lymphocytic form of meningitis or an influenzalike illness, but occasionally as a meningoencephalitis. Leukopenia and thrombocytopenia frequently develop. Very rarely, LCM virus produces severe and even fatal illnesses associated with hemorrhagic manifestations.

Lassa virus, first isolated in 1969 from an American missionary working in Nigeria, has attracted considerable interest because it is **highly contagious** and produces a **serious febrile illness.** The disease is characterized by severe generalized myalgia, marked malaise, and sore throat accompanied by patchy or ulcerative pharyngeal lesions. Fatal cases also develop myocarditis, pneumonia with pleural effusion, encephalopathy, and hemorrhagic lesions. The virus persists in the blood for 1 to 2 weeks, and during this period it can be isolated from urine, pleural fluid, and throat washings. It is more stable than togaviruses and flaviviruses in body fluids, which probably permits its person-to-person contagion and accounts for the hazard it presents for laboratory isolation or study. Arthropods collected in Nigeria, the only known locale of natural infections, have not yielded virus, and insect cell cultures are insusceptible to viral propagation. The only cycle of Lassa virus transmission outside humans has been detected in the wild rodent *Mastomys natalensis*, which suggests that rodent control may limit viral transmission to man. Lassa virus produces an infection in mice similar to LCM virus infection, and chronic latent infections can be established.

General Remarks

Only a few of the known viruses that multiply in arthropods and vertebrates have been discussed in this chapter. The characteristics of only a few of the viruses have been studied in detail (e.g., Sindbis, yellow fever, dengue viruses), and the properties of most of these agents, and even their clinical and epidemiologic behavior, are known in only a fragmentary fashion. Some, such as the phlebotomus (sandfly) fever virus, transmitted by the bite of the female sandfly *Phlebotomus papatasii*, assumed importance to the U.S. Armed Forces during World War II, when the disease (which is not serious) appeared in military personnel in the Mediterranean area.

Many of the arthropod-borne viruses, including some that can cause serious disease, also produce a very much larger number of inapparent infections in endemic areas; hence, the native human population carries a high level of immunity but the insect population is still highly infectious because of the viral reservoir in lower animals. Such diseases could increase dramatically in quantitative significance when ecologic alterations cause development of a dense population of infected athropods next to a nonimmune human population or when a large, immunologically virginal human population (e.g., military personnel) moves into an endemic area.

Because of their close antigenic relation to human pathogens, those arthropod-borne viruses that have not been associated with human disease cannot be ignored by medical investigators, however esoteric they may seem. Several such viruses have been isolated in the United States or Canada—for example, the Rio Bravo virus (flavivirus group, U.S.), California encephalitis and

Trivittatus viruses (California group, U.S.), and Silverwater virus (Bunyaviridae ungrouped, Canada). Since a change in either the host reservoir, the vector, or the genetics of the viral population might permit these agents to infect man, they remain a potential hazard.

The comforting realization that as many as 200 arthropod-borne viruses of seemingly diverse immunologic groupings, or even without obvious relatives, may be segregated into one family, the Bunyaviridae, on the basis of physical and chemical characteristics, indicates that order is appearing in what previously seemed unmanageable. Thus, the ecologic–epidemiologic classification of otherwise disparate viruses as "arboviruses" is being replaced by classification on a broader base into several new families. In addition, a few viruses initially isolated from arthropods have been placed into well-established families (reoviruses, rhabdoviruses, and picornaviruses), and the arenaviruses have been shown not to be associated with arthropod vectors.

Selected Reading

BOOKS AND REVIEW ARTICLES

Bishop HL, Shope RE: Bunyviidiae. Compr Virol 14:1, 1979

Lehmann-Grube F: Portraits of viruses: Arenaviruses. Intervirology 22:121, 1984

Matthews REF: Classification and nomenclature of viruses (Third Report of the ICTV). Togaviridae. Intervirology 17:1, 1982

Schlesinger RW (ed): The Togaviruses. New York, Academic Press, 1980

Schlesinger RW: Dengue Viruses. Vienna, Springer-Verlag, 1977

Schlesinger S, Schlesinger M (eds): The Togaviruses and Flaviviruses. New York, Plenum Press, 1986

Strauss JH, Strauss EG, Hahn CS, Rice CM: The genomes of alphaviruses and flaviviruses. In Rowlands DJ, Mayo M, Mahy BWJ (eds): The Molecular Biology of the Positive Strand RNA Viruses, p 75. New York, Academic Press, 1987

SPECIFIC ARTICLES

Hewlett MJ, Pettersson RE, Baltimore D: Circular forms of Unkuniemi virion RNA: An electron microscopic study. J Virol 21:1085, 1977

Ihara T, Akashi H, Bishop DHL: Novel coding strategy (ambisense genomic RNA) revealed by sequence analysis of Punta Toro phlebovirus S RNA. Virology 136:293, 1984

Iroegbu CV, Pringle CR: Genetic interactions among viruses of the Bunyamwera complex. J Virol 37:383, 1981

Pardigon N, Vialot P, Girard M, Buloy M: Panhandles and hairpin structures at the termini of Germiston virus (Bunyavirus). Virology 122:191, 1982

Reed W, Carroll J, Agramonte A, Lazear JW: The etiology of yellow fever: A preliminary note. Philadelphia Med J 6:790, 1900

Rice CM, Strauss JH: Nucleotide sequence of yellow fever virus: Implications for flavivirus gene expression and evolution. Science 29:726, 1985

61

Rubella Virus

Dr. George Maton in 1814 realized that a family epidemic of an acute febrile illness with rash, previously considered to be scarlatina (scarlet fever) or rubeola (measles), was a unique disease, which in 1866 was finally given the name *rubella*. This disease resembles measles but is milder and does not have the serious consequences often seen with measles in the very young. Because rubella seems to be such a harmless disease, it did not receive much attention earlier, although its probable viral etiology was demonstrated in experiments with human volunteers in 1938. However, interest in rubella was much increased when Gregg, an Australian ophthalmologist, noted in 1941 that women contracting rubella during the first trimester of pregnancy frequently gave birth to babies with congenital defects. Nevertheless, the cultivation of rubella virus was not achieved until 1962, when Parkman, Buescher, and Artenstein detected the virus through its interference with type 11 echovirus in primary grivet monkey kidney cultures, and Weller and Neva demonstrated unique cytopathic changes (Fig. 61–1) in infected primary human amnion cultures.

Rubella virus is classified as a **togavirus** (genus *Rubivirus*) on the basis of its physical and chemical characteristics (see Chap. 60). However, owing to the worldwide importance of German measles in humans and its unique clinical features and pathogenesis, a separate chapter is devoted to this virus.

Properties

MORPHOLOGY

The virion is roughly spherical and has an average diameter of about 60 nm, in both thin sections and negatively stained preparations; it consists of a roughly isometric core of 30 nm, covered by a loose envelope (Fig. 61–2).

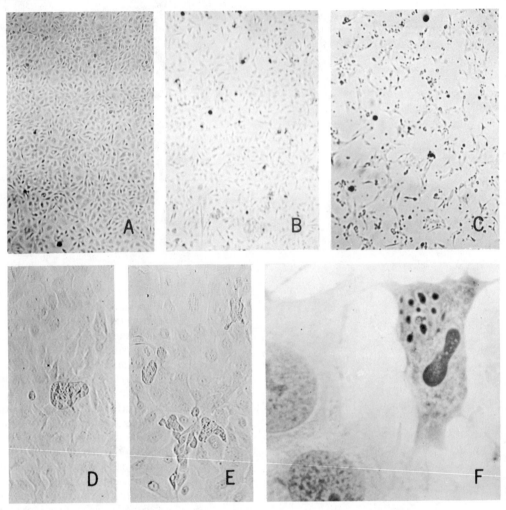

Figure 61–1. Cytopathic effect of rubella virus in human amnion cultures. *(A)* Appearance of normal amnion cell culture as viewed microscopically under low magnification. (Original magnification ×33) *(B)* Rubella-infected culture with estimated 20% destruction of cells on the 14th day after inoculation. (Original magnification ×33) *(C)* Rubella-infected culture with 80% cell destruction on the 28th day after inoculation. (Original magnification ×33) *(D)* Single affected cell with adjacent uninvolved cells on the tenth day after inoculation. (Original magnification ×132) *(E)* Scattered infected cells showing ameboid distortion on the tenth day after inoculation. (Original magnification ×132) *(F)* Infected cell with a large eosinophilic cytoplasmic inclusion and basophilic aggregation of nuclear chromatin, as well as portions of two normal cells. (H&E stain, original magnification ×3500; Neva FA et al: Bacteriol Rev 28:444, 1964)

Negative staining techniques reveal small spikes projecting 5 nm to 6 nm from the envelopes of most particles. Gentle disruption of the envelope with sodium deoxycholate uncovers an angular core; definite symmetry of the nucleocapsid is obscure, but ringlike subunit structures are discernible.

The morphology and growth characteristics of rubella virus resemble those of the alphatogaviruses (see Chap. 60).

CHEMICAL AND PHYSICAL PROPERTIES

The virion contains one molecule of single-stranded RNA with a molecular weight of 3.8×10^6 daltons (11 Kb), significantly smaller than the RNAs of other togaviruses. Two glycoproteins (E_1 and E_2) are present in the envelope, and an arginine-rich nucleocapsid (C) protein is associated with the RNA. Each nucleocapsid capsomer consists of two disulfide-linked C proteins. The virion

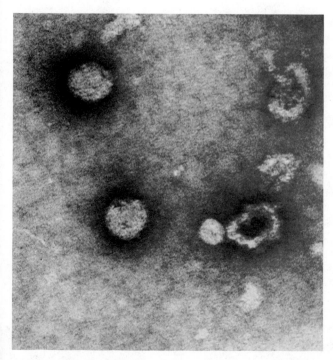

Figure 61–2. Morphology of rubella virus. Note the nucleocapsids within and dissociated from the envelopes. The nucleocapsid cores are somewhat angular and when separate from the envelopes show a subunit structure. (Horzinek MC: Arch Gesamte Virusforsch 33:306, 1971)

RNA is infectious, like that of other togaviruses, and therefore has a positive polarity; it has a 5'-terminal cap and a 3'-terminal poly(A) tract.

Like other enveloped viruses, rubella virus is rapidly inactivated by ether, chloroform, and sodium deoxycholate; it is relatively labile when stored at 4°C and relatively stable at −60° to −70°C.

The **hemagglutinin** and hemolytic activities reside in an integral component of the virion, the E_1 glycoprotein. The hemagglutinin, however, remains biologically active after gentle disruption of the viral particle. It is most effectively assayed with newborn chick, pigeon, goose, and human group O red blood cells (RBCs). As with the other togaviruses, the hemagglutinin does not elute spontaneously from the affected RBCs, and neuraminidase does not render the RBCs inagglutinable (see Mechanism of Hemagglutination, Chap. 44).

IMMUNOLOGIC PROPERTIES

Rubella virus is immunologically distinct from the other togaviruses; only a single antigenic type has been detected. Neutralizing and hemagglutination-inhibiting Abs, which are directed to the E_1 protein, develop during the incubation period of the disease and are commonly

present when the rash appears (see Pathogenesis, below); they attain maximal titer during early convalescence and persist (along with immunity) for many years, if not for life. It must be noted, however, that the hemagglutination-inhibiting Abs and the neutralizing Abs are responses to different epitopes of the E_1 protein, since they can vary independently following German measles or immunization. Complement-fixing Abs appear about 6 to 10 days after onset, begin to diminish after 4 to 6 months, and disappear after a few years.

MULTIPLICATION

Rubella virus can replicate in a variety of primary, continuous, and diploid cell cultures of monkey, rabbit, and human origin. When cells are initially infected, the eclipse period is 10 to 12 hours. The viral titer reaches a maximum 30 to 40 hours after infection and may remain high for weeks (indeed, carrier cultures are readily established; see Chap. 51).

As with other togaviruses, the infectious virion RNA initiates viral replication by serving as an mRNA for viral protein synthesis. Viral multiplication is confined to the cytoplasm, and its RNA synthesis proceeds through intermediate replicative forms. Similar to other togaviruses, a 24S RNA as well as 40S RNA is made. The 24S RNA encodes the structural proteins with the gene order NH_2-C-E_2-E_1-COOH (see Synthesis of RNA Viruses, Chap. 48, and Viral Multiplication, Chap. 60).

Morphogenesis of the virions occurs at cell membranes (particularly the plasma membrane), which differentiate by incorporating viral proteins. Nucleocapsids then bud through the thickened vacuolar and surface membranes to form mature viral particles (Fig. 61–3). Unlike other togaviruses, however, nucleocapsids do not accumulate in the cytoplasm. Because viral components, including the hemagglutinin, are incorporated into the cell surface membrane during budding, the infected cells can be detected by hemadsorption.

In many infected cell cultures (e.g., grivet monkey kidney) an increase in viral titer is associated with **increased resistance** to infection with some challenge viruses (e.g., picornaviruses, orthomyxoviruses, measles virus), which provides another procedure for detecting infected cells and isolating viruses. Propagation of rubella virus induces the interference, and it is not consistently associated with interferon production (see Viral Interference, Chap. 49).

Cytopathic changes are not detectable in most rubella-infected cell cultures, but in cultured primary human cells distinctive cellular alterations appear slowly over 2 to 3 weeks. Affected cells are enlarged or rounded, and they often have ameboid pseudopods; staining reveals a disappearance of the nuclear membrane, promi-

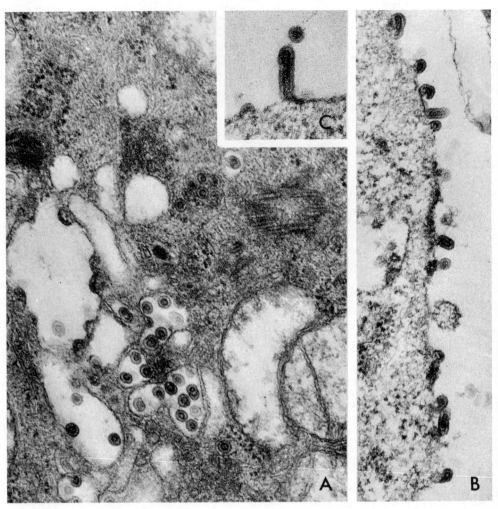

Figure 61–3. Development of rubella virus in the surface and cytoplasmic membranes of infected cell cultures. *(A)* Viral particles budding from cytoplasmic membranes into vacuoles and into the cytoplasm. Numerous mature virions are present with vacuoles. (Original magnification ×60,000) *(B)* Viral particles budding from the surface of an infected cell. (Original magnification ×60,000) *(C)* An elongated form in the budding process. (Original magnification ×84,000; Oshiro LS et al: J Gen Virol 5:205, 1969)

nent clumping of nuclear chromatin, and round or irregular eosinophilic cytoplasmic inclusion bodies (see Fig. 61–1). The cytopathic effects are associated with inhibition of the biosynthesis of host macromolecules and the inability of infected cells to divide. However, the infected cells do not lyse.

In cultures of human diploid cells that are chronically infected (**carrier cultures**) many chromosomal breaks are evident. Such breaks may have a bearing on the pathogenesis of congenital lesions in the infected fetus.

Pathogenesis

The rash appears 14 to 25 days (average 18 days) after infection with rubella virus. During this prolonged incubation period viremia occurs and viral dissemination is widespread throughout the body, including the placenta during pregnancy. Virus multiplies in many organs, but few signs are manifested except for a relatively common arthralgia and arthritis in women, accompanying infection of synovial membranes; leukopenia from viral replication in lymphocytes; occasional thrombocytopenia but uncommon purpuric manifestations; and rare encephalitis. (A chronic progressive disease simulating measles-induced subacute sclerosing panencephalitis infrequently occurs.) The virus can be isolated from nasopharyngeal secretions (and occasionally from feces and urine) as early as 7 days before and as late as 7 days after the appearance of the exanthem. Respiratory secretions are probably the major vehicle for transmitting the virus.

The disease is not unlike measles, except that it is milder, is of shorter duration, and has fewer complications. It is initiated by a 1- to 2-day prodromal period of fever, malaise, mild coryza, and prominent cervical and occipital lymphadenopathy. During the prodromal illness, and for 1 to 2 days after the rash appears, virus can be isolated from the blood. It can also be isolated from the skin lesions.

No characteristic pathologic lesions have been described in rubella, except for the **serious damage induced in infected fetuses.** This damage seems to involve tissues of all germ layers and results from a combination of rapid death of some cells and persistent viral infection in others. The continued infection, in turn, frequently induces chromosomal aberrations and, finally, reduced cell division. The infant infected during the first trimester may be stillborn; if it survives, it may have deafness, cataracts, cardiac abnormalities, microcephaly, motor deficits, or other congenital anomalies in

addition to thrombocytopenic purpura, hepatosplenomegaly, icterus, anemia, and low birth weight (the **rubella syndrome).** The greater susceptibility of the early embryo to damage is correlated with the greater placental transmission of virus at that stage: when infection occurs during the first 8 weeks of pregnancy, the virus can be isolated as often from an aborted fetus as from the placenta, whereas in later infections viral isolations are less frequent from the fetus.

PERSISTENCE

When a woman has clinical rubella during the first trimester of pregnancy, the chance that the baby will have a structural abnormality is approximately 30%. Deformed infants born 6 to 8.5 months after intrauterine infection, and even those clinically normal, may still excrete virus in their nasopharyngeal secretions, although high titers of neutralizing IgM and IgG Abs and cell-mediated immunity are present (Fig. 61-4). Viral shedding persists until the clones of infected cells that are still able to divide eventually disappear. Indeed, one infant continued to shed virus in the presence of circulating Abs 2 years after birth, and in another the virus was isolated from cataract tissue at 3 years of age.

The Ab response in congenital rubella, like that noted in congenital cytomegalovirus infections (see Chap. 53) and congenital syphilis (see Chap. 37), indicates that in-

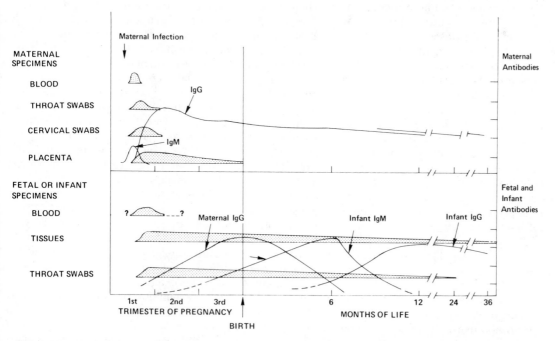

Figure 61–4. Virologic events (*shaded areas*) and antibody response in maternal–fetal rubella infection. (Modified from Meyer HM et al: Am J Clin Pathol 57:803, 1972)

trauterine rubella infections **do not induce immuno-logic tolerance** to rubella virus Ags. However, immunity following congenital rubella shows differences from that following postnatal or childhood infections: some congenitally infected infants fail to develop atypical Ab responses, others lose detectable Abs by 5 years of age, and others show depressed or absent cell-mediated immunity.

Laboratory Diagnosis

Rubella may be clinically confused with measles as well as with infections produced by a number of echoviruses and coxsackieviruses (see Chap. 55). The diagnosis may be confirmed by inoculating infected materials (usually nasopharyngeal secretions) into susceptible cell cultures. The **interference assay,** in primary grivet monkey kidney cultures, is the quickest and most sensitive procedure for initial viral isolation. Infection may also be detected by the development of cytopathic changes in susceptible cell cultures, by immunofluorescence, and by hemadsorption. Serologic diagnosis can be efficiently accomplished by hemagglutination-inhibition titrations, but care must be used to remove lipoprotein nonspecific inhibitors of hemagglutination (e.g., by adsorption of serum with dextran sulfate-CaCl$_2$). The hemagglutination-inhibition titration serves as a standard, since it correlates well with neutralization titrations. Solid-phase immunoenzyme assays (enzyme-linked immunosorbent assays [ELISAs]) are also reliable, and they are now most frequently used for diagnostic purposes because of the ease of performance and rapidity of completion. Complement fixation titrations are now used less often because Abs appear later and decrease earlier than Abs measured with the other techniques.

Evaluation of the immune status is of particular importance for women who are exposed to German measles during the first trimester of pregnancy (even a past history of rubella or previous immunization is not an absolute guarantee of immunity), women of childbearing age who wish to determine whether they should be immunized, and neonates born to a mother who was exposed to rubella during pregnancy or who have suggestive signs of the rubella syndrome.

Epidemiology

Rubella is a highly contagious disease, spread by nasal secretions. Unlike measles or chickenpox, however, **rubella infection is often inapparent,** thus fostering viral dissemination and rendering isolation of patients virtually useless. The ratio of inapparent infections to clinical cases is low (approximately 1 : 1) in children but as high

as 9 : 1 in young adults. Patients are most infectious during the prodromal period, owing to the large amount of virus present in the nasopharynx, but communicability may persist as long as 7 days after the appearance of the rash. Transmission usually occurs by direct contact with infected persons, mostly children 5 to 14 years of age. However, **the apparently normal infant excreting virus acquired *in utero* is perhaps the most dangerous carrier:** his infection is unrecognized, and he comes in close contact with nurses, physicians, hospital visitors (including future mothers early in pregnancy), and, later, other children at home.

In urban areas of Europe and the Americas, during the winter and spring months, minor outbreaks are noted every 1 or 2 years. Major epidemics recur every 6 to 9 years, and superepidemics erupt at intervals of up to 30 years. This epidemic pattern succeeds in immunizing 85% of the population up to 15 years of age (the age span of susceptibles is significantly more than that in measles). Infection is almost always followed by long-lasting protection against clinical disease, although reinfections do occur. Most inapparent infections occur in those whose immunity has partially waned; the reinfection induces a secondary immune response (IgG Abs), which probably prevents or reduces the extent of viremia.

Prevention and Control

The extensive epidemic in the United States during 1964 resulted in congenital disabilities in approximately 20,000 infants, causing enormous anguish and an economic loss of well over 1 billion dollars. To avoid these dire consequences, prevention of maternal infection is of utmost importance. Isolation procedures are rarely practical, and passive immunization is of questionable value. However, effective live **attenuated viral vaccines** have been developed and are presently being used effectively to prevent the recurrence of such a devastating experience. The vaccine (RA27/3 strain) currently used in the United States is one isolated in human fetal kidney cells and attentuated by passage in fetal kidney fibroblasts and WI-38 diploid cells at 30°C. The vaccine requires a single injection and is immunogenic in at least 95% of the recipients, but Abs appear later than those following natural infection, and at levels as much as tenfold lower. Nevertheless, immunization effectively protects the recipients from clinical rubella following exposure for at least 15 years, even after extensive exposure during epidemics. Accordingly, vaccination has markedly reduced the incidence of the congenital rubella syndrome (Fig. 61–5), but congenital rubella continues to occur because 10% to 20% of the childbearing-aged population continue to be susceptible. As the presently immune young children increasingly enter the childbearing period, con-

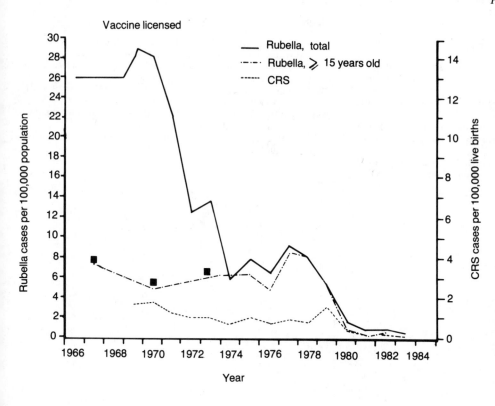

Figure 61–5. Incidence rate of reported rubella cases and congenital rubella cases, United States, 1966–1985. *CRS*, congenital rubella syndrome. (Modified from MMWR 33: 551, 1986)

genital rubella will decrease further, but this process will take 10 to 30 years. Hence, efforts must increase to immunize the susceptibles who are of age to have children.

Though the vaccines employed are highly protective some drawbacks exist. (1) In 2 to 3 weeks after immunization, small amounts of infectious virus appear in the nasopharynx. Viremia is unusual, however, and transmission to susceptible contacts has not been observed. (2) At the time of nasopharyngeal viral shedding, mild arthralgias and occasional arthritis occur in 1% to 2% of children and in 25% to 40% of adult women; adults also occasionally experience mild rash, fever, and lymphadenopathy. (3) The Ab levels attained confer solid immunity, but the long-lasting immunity that follows natural infection may not occur (unfortunately, the most attenuated viruses used in vaccines also are the least immunogenic). (4) A tenfold higher reinfection rate is observed in vaccinees than in those who have had natural infections. (5) An effective herd immunity is not produced, even when as many as 85% of 1- to 12-year-olds are immunized. (6) Despite the marked reduction in incidence of clinical disease, infection is frequently not prevented, even with exposure only 2 to 3 months after immunization. However, the inapparent infection could serve to induce a life-long immunity similar to that following the natural disease.

It should be emphasized that immunization has a unique goal: to protect an unborn fetus rather than the recipient of the vaccine. This goal has been approached by two almost opposing plans: immunization of teenage girls, who are the prospective mothers, or immunization of children 1 to 12 years of age, who are the major viral transmitters, thereby indirectly protecting pregnant women. In the United States the latter alternative has been chosen; that is, routine immunization of all children. In addition, immunization is recommended for all women of childbearing age who are without protective Abs. (Birth control must be rigidly practiced for 2 to 3 months following immunization.)

The immunization program pursued in the United States has elicited great concern, since the vaccine may not confer long-lasting immunity and therefore the women may become susceptible during their childbearing years. In Great Britain immunization is given to all girls between 10 and 14 years old and to women of childbearing age who do not have detectable hemagglutination-inhibiting Abs. It is not yet clear which approach is more successful in attaining the goal of preventing fetal damage.

If preventive measures fail, many physicians recommend therapeutic abortion when rubella occurs during the first trimester of pregnancy.

Selected Reading

BOOKS AND REVIEW ARTICLES

Horstman DM: Rubella. In Evans AS (ed): Viral Infections of Humans: Epidemiology and Control, 2nd ed, p 519. New York, Plenum, 1984

Rawls WE: Congenital rubella: The significance of virus persistence. Prog Med Virol 10:238, 1968

Krugman S, Hinman AR, Burke JP (eds): International symposium on the prevention of congenital rubella infection. Rev Infect Dis 7:1, 1985

Preblud SR, Serula MK, Frank JA Jr et al: Rubella vaccination in the United States: A ten year review. Epidemiol Rev 2:171, 1980

SPECIFIC ARTICLES

Davis WJ, Larson HE, Simsarian JP et al: A study of rubella immunity and resistance to infection. JAMA 215:600, 1971

Gregg NM: Congenital cataract following German measles in the mother. Trans Ophthalmol Soc NZ 3:35, 1941

Oker-Bloom C: The gene order for virus structural proteins is NH_2-C-E_2-E_1-COOH. J Virol 51:354, 1984

Sedwick WD, Sokol F: Nucleic acid of rubella virus and its replication in hamster kidney cells. J Virol 5:478, 1970

Vaheri A, Hovi T: Structural proteins and subunits of rubella virus. J Virol 9:10, 1972

62

Reoviruses and Epidemic Acute Gastroenteritis Viruses

Classification and General Characteristics

The term *reovirus* (respiratory enteric orphan virus) refers to a group of RNA viruses that infect both the respiratory and the intestinal tracts, usually without producing disease. Though originally considered members of the echovirus group (and classified as type 10 echovirus), reoviruses are larger and differ in producing characteristic cytoplasmic inclusion bodies. Moreover, these inclusion bodies, which contain specific viral Ags, stain green-yellow with acridine orange, like cellular DNA, rather than red, like the usual single-stranded RNA. This striking observation led to the discovery that **reovirus RNA is double stranded** with a secondary structure similar to that of DNA. This finding was the first indication that such an unusual nucleic acid exists in nature. Viruses with similar chemical and physical properties have since been found to be widely disseminated in vertebrates, invertebrates, and plants. These viruses (more than 150) have been grouped into the family **Reoviridae** (vernacular, **reoviruses**).

All these viruses have segmented, double-stranded RNA genomes. They are similar in morphology (Table 62–1), but differences in structure, antigenicity, stability, and preferred hosts are the bases for dividing Reoviridae into several genera: *Orthoreovirus* (**reovirus**) includes species that infect humans, birds, dogs, and monkeys; *Orbivirus* (Latin *orbis*, ring) comprises members that multi-

TABLE 62–1. Characteristics of Reoviridae That Infect Man

Characteristic	Reoviruses	Rotaviruses	Orbiviruses*
Morphology	Icosahedral; double capsid; no envelope	Icosahedral; double capsid; no envelope	Icosahedral; double capsid—outer is skinlike
Size (diameter)	75 nm; inner capsid 50 nm	70 nm; inner capsid 50 nm	70 nm; inner capsid 50 nm
Nucleic acid	RNA; double-stranded; 10 segments, mol. wt. $0.7–2.7 \times 10^6$, total 15×10^6 daltons (46 Kb)	RNA; double-stranded; 11 segments, mol. wt. $0.23–2.04 \times 10^6$, total 10×10^6 daltons (31 Kb)	RNA; double-stranded; 10 segments, mol. wt. $0.3–2.7 \times 10^6$, total 12×10^6 daltons (37 Kb)
Effect of lipid solvents	Infectivity stable	Infectivity stable	Infectivity stable
Virion polypeptides	8	10	8

* Blue-tongue virus, the best-characterized orbivirus, was used for this comparative analysis. The size range for the genus is 60 nm to 80 nm.

ply in insects, including Colorado tick fever virus, which infects humans; *Rotavirus* (Latin *rota*, wheel) includes some major etiologic agents of infectious infantile diarrhea in humans and several other animals; *Cypovirus* includes the **cytoplasmic polyhedrosis viruses,** which consist of viruses that infect Lepidoptera and Diptera; *Phytoreovirus* contains viruses that infect many different types of plants (e.g., rice dwarf virus and clover wound tumor virus); and *Fijivirus* also contains viruses that infect plants as well as insects (e.g., maize rough dwarf virus). Only the viruses infecting humans will be discussed.

MORPHOLOGY

The virions of all Reoviridae have similar sizes, icosahedral symmetry, and not one but two icosahedral capsids. Fine-structure electron microscopy (Fig. 62–1) reveals that the outer capsid is probably constructed of 32 large capsomers (18 nm in diameter) and that neighboring capsomers share subunits (see Fig. 62–1), which is apparently a unique feature of this family. The inner capsid has 12 prominent projections at its vertices and an undetermined number of intervening capsomers. Each projection is composed of five molecules of $\lambda 2$ proteins into which the $\sigma 1$ dimer is anchored (Fig. 62–2). Rotaviruses are slightly smaller than reoviruses (see Table 62–1) but have similar double capsids.

Orbiviruses (e.g., blue-tongue virus of sheep, the type species) show another morphologic variation: the capsomer arrangement of the outer capsid is usually obscure, but exposure of the virions to CsCl below pH 8 removes a thin outer layer, revealing a capsid of 32 large, ring-shaped capsomers (hence, its Latin derivation, *orbis*). Colorado tick fever virus has not been adequately studied.

Reoviridae of different genera do not display any immunologic relatedness.

CHEMICAL AND PHYSICAL CHARACTERISTICS

The virions of Reoviridae are composed of protein and about 15% RNA. The double-stranded nature of the RNA is shown by many properties: complementary base ratios (G = C = 20 mol/dl); sharp thermal denaturation (T_M 90°C to 95°C); pronounced hyperchromicity on denaturation; resistance to a concentration of ribonuclease A that completely degrades single-stranded RNA; and characteristic density in $CsSO_4$. Electron micrography reveals stiff filaments, like those of DNA, and x-ray diffraction patterns are consistent with double-stranded molecules.

The **genomes** of Reoviridae consist of **ten or 11 distinct segments,** which are distributed in **three size classes** (Fig. 62–3). That these are distinct components of the virion rather than products of artificial fragmentation is shown by the following characteristics: the fragment sizes are reproducible within a genus; the different pieces do not cross-hybridize; each fragment contains two free 3'-OH termini and two 5'-terminal diphosphates; and electron micrographs of gently disrupted virions demonstrate molecules of viral nucleic acid of the expected lengths.

Orthoreovirus virions (other genera have not been examined) also contain about 3.7×10^6 daltons of a heterogeneous collection of small, single-stranded oligonucleotides, produced by aborted transcription but whose function is unknown.

The **orthoreovirus** and **orbivirus virions** contain eight species of polypeptides, and those of rotaviruses contain ten polypeptides; their molecular weights are distributed in three size classes. Since the structural proteins (Table 62–2) can be separated only after denaturation of the virion, it is impossible to identify directly their specific functions (i.e., hemagglutination, RNA polymerase, nucleoside phosphohydrolase, group antigenicity, and type-specific antigenicity). However, association of each polypeptide with a virion structure (or a nonstructural protein), the identification of the RNA segment

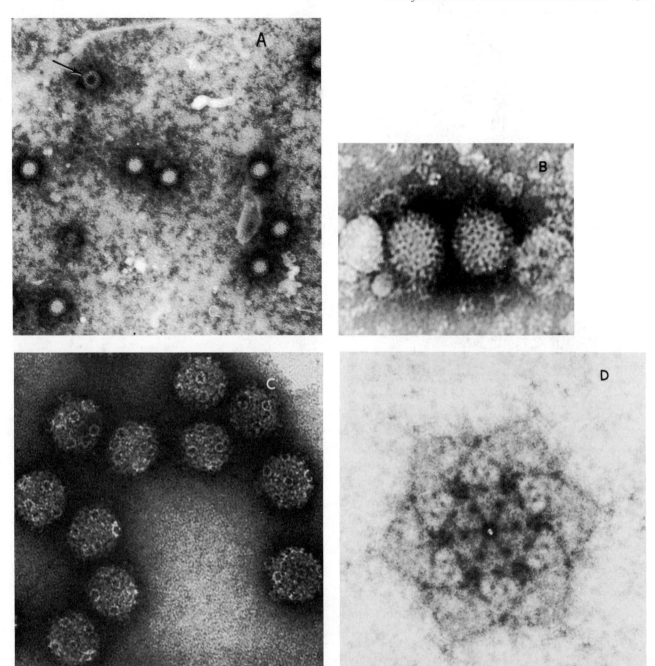

Figure 62–1. Electron micrographs of negatively stained orthoreovirus virions, cores, and capsomers. The virion is 75 nm to 80 nm in diameter. Cubic symmetry, the structure of the capsid, and the absence of an envelope are illustrated by low *(A)* and high *(B)* magnification. Note the empty particle in *A* in which the inner coat that covers the core is apparent *(arrow).* (*A,* original magnification ×75,000; *B,* original magnification ×375,000) *(C)* Cores prepared from purified virions by chymotrypsin degradation of the outer capsid followed by equilibrium centrifugation in a CsCl density gradient. Note the hollow spikes located at the 12 vertices of the icosahedral core. (Original magnification ×280,000) *(D)* Cluster of capsid subunits in which the central capsomer was enhanced by an n = 6 rotation. Rotational enhancement of image detail makes evident the structure of the central capsomer, which is made of six wedge-shaped subunits that exhibit sharing with neighboring capsomers. Note also that each wedge-shaped subunit is also composed of subunits (i.e., polypeptide chains). (Original magnification ×1,200,000; *A, B,* Gomatos PJ et al: Virology 17:441, 1962; *C,* White CK, Zweerink HJ: Virology 70:171, 1976; *D,* Palmer EL, Martin ML: Virology 76:109, 1977)

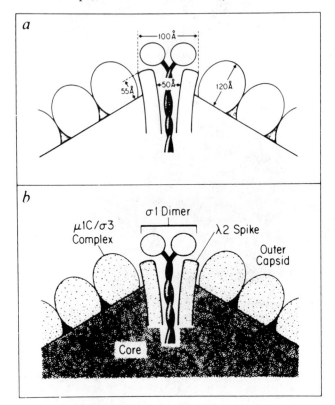

Figure 62–2. Schematic representation of the morphology of the outer capsid of orthoreovirus type 3. *(a)* Dimensions of the virion. *(b)* Orientation of the σ1 protein in the virus. The α-helical region is shown to extend throughout the λ2 channel into the viral core. The globular structure sits on top of the λ2 channel and interacts with host cell receptors. (Bassel-Duby R et al: Nature 315:421, 1985)

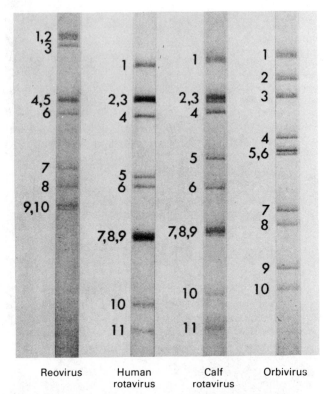

Figure 62–3. Electrophoresis of the virion RNA of orthoreovirus type 3, human rotavirus, calf rotavirus, and an orbivirus on 7.5% polyacrylamide gels (migration was from top to bottom). RNA segments for each virus are distributed in three size classes (L,M,S). (Modified from Schnagl RD, Holmes IH: J Virol 19:267, 1976)

(i.e., the gene) in which each polypeptide is encoded, and the correlation of some polypeptides with function have been possible using genetic and biochemical techniques (see Table 62–2). The outer capsid has a complex structure (see Fig. 62–2) that provides stability to the virion.

The σ1 outer capsid protein is a dimer consisting of the two carboxy-terminal globular receptor-interacting domains and the α-helical coil structure formed from the amino-terminal portions of the polypeptides (see Fig. 62–2). The σ1 protein is also responsible for hemagglutination by all three immunologic types (types 1 and 2 agglutinate human red blood cells (RBCs); type 3 agglutinates bovine RBCs). Orthoreoviruses agglutinate and elute from RBCs, but unlike orthomyxoviruses, they do not destroy the receptor sites on the RBCs, although the reovirus receptors are hydrolyzed by neuraminidase. The RBC receptor is probably a glycoprotein, since either trypsin or periodate inactivates, it and *N*-acetyl-D-glucosamine blocks hemagglutination by binding to the viral capsid.

Orthoreoviruses

PROPERTIES

Immunologic Characteristics

The σ1 outer capsid protein induces specific neutralizing and hemagglutination-inhibiting Abs that distinguish **three immunologic types** of reoviruses. The three types of reoviruses are antigenically related, however, by three or four cross-reacting Ags that can be measured by complement fixation (CF) and immunoprecipitin tests. For example, heterotypic reovirus Abs appear in the serum of about 25% of persons who have primary infections with type 1 reovirus. Type-specific Abs to reoviruses appear 2 to 4 weeks after infection.

Host Range

Reoviruses appear to be ubiquitous in nature: specific viral inhibitors (presumably Abs) have been found in the serum of all mammals tested except the whale; and humans and many other species (including cattle, mice, and monkeys) are naturally susceptible to reoviruses.

TABLE 62–2. Correlation Between Classes of Orthoreovirus* Genomic Segments and Polypeptides in Virions and Infected Cells

Genome				Polypeptides				
Size Class	Segment	Mol. Wt. ($\times 10^{-6}$)	Time of Expression	Size Class	Component†	Mol. Wt. ($\times 10^{-3}$)	Origin‡	Function§
L	1(L$_1$)	2.7	Early‖	λ	λ3	135	Core	RNA synthesis
	2(L$_2$)	2.6	Late		λ2	148	Core	
	3(L$_3$)	2.5	Late		λ1	155	Core	
M	4(M$_1$)	1.8	Late	μ	μ2	70	Core	
					μ1	80	Core	
	5(M$_2$)	1.7	Late		μ1c	72	Outer capsid	
	6(M$_3$)	1.6	Early‖		μNs	75	Nonstructural	
S	7(S$_1$)	1.1	Late	σ	σ1	49	Outer capsid	Cell association, hemagglutination induction neutralizing Abs
					σ1x**	?	?	
	8(S$_2$)	0.85	Late		σ2	38	Core	RNA synthesis
	9(S$_3$)	0.76	Early‖		σNs	36	Nonstructural	RNA synthesis
	10(S$_4$)	0.71	Early‖		σ3	34	Outer capsid	

* Type 3 (Dearing strain) is given as an example. Sizes of the RNA segments and polypeptides are different for each type.

† Identification of a polypeptide with a double-stranded RNA segment was accomplished by *in vitro* translation of specific mRNAs and by intertypic genetic recombination, which takes advantage of the different sizes of RNA segments in different viral types.

‡ Determined by controlled disruption of purified virions and SDS-polyacrylamide gel electrophoresis of infected cell cytoplasmic extracts

§ Identified by genetic studies with temperature-sensitive mutants

‖ Predominant messages transcribed during early stages of infection; mRNAs made in the presence of cycloheximide added at time of infection

Processed from μ1

** Translated from second open-reading frame in S$_1$ RNA; function unknown

Newborn mice are particularly vulnerable to experimental infection, which is often fatal; when infected with type 3 reovirus they occasionally develop a chronic illness similar to runt disease (see Chap. 20).

Cell cultures, including primary cultures of epithelial cells from many animals and various continuous human cell lines, are used to isolate and study reoviruses. The infection causes gross cytopathic changes and permits **hemadsorption** of human **group O RBCs.** Distinctive eosinophilic **inclusion bodies** (Fig. 62–4) are seen in the cytoplasm of infected cells.

Multiplication

The eclipse period is long (6 to 9 hours, depending on viral type and size of inoculum), compared with that of other RNA viruses with icosahedral symmetry (Fig. 62–5; see Chap. 48). Virus then increases exponentially, reaching a maximum titer (from 250 to 2500 plaque-forming units per cell) by approximately 15 hours after infection. Infected cells are not rapidly lysed following viral replication, and release of infectious virus is incomplete.

Owing to the unique structure of the capsid and the novel nucleic acid, replication of orthoreoviruses presents some unusual features. The virus is capable of utilizing the β-adrenergic receptor on the host cell for attachment and cell entry. After **cell penetration,** by receptor-mediated endocytosis, the virions become associated with lysosomes, whose proteolytic enzymes hydrolyze about half of the outer capsid (all of polypeptides σ1 and σ3 and an 8000-dalton piece of polypeptide μ1c), forming a **subviral particle** that is smaller than the virion but larger than the viral core (inner capsid and RNAs). Thus, the core is only partially uncoated and the double-stranded RNA genome segments are not released free into the cytoplasm.

TRANSCRIPTION. The virion RNAs do not function as messengers; but, like DNA, they are first transcribed. However, transcription is **conservative, only the negative (−) strands serve as templates,** and the transcripts are processed into single-stranded mRNAs. This transcription ensues entirely within the subviral particles, which leave the lysosomes after the uncoating process. Initially (beginning 2 to 4 hours after infection), four segments (1, 6, 9, and 10 seen in Fig. 62–3 and Table 62–2) of the viral genome are predominantly transcribed, although all genome segments are copied. An RNA polymerase (transcriptase) contained within the core of the

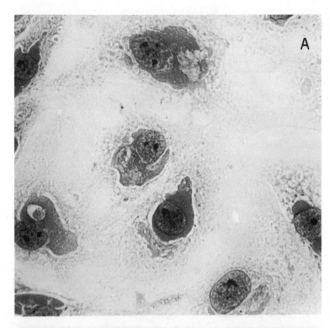

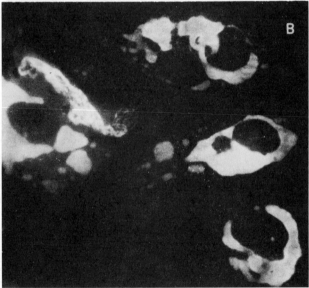

Figure 62—4. Large eosinophilic cytoplasmic inclusion bodies in monkey kidney cells infected with type 1 orthoreovirus. *(A)* H&E stained and viewed with a light microscope. (Original magnification ×1000) *(B)* Stained within fluorescein-conjugated Ab and viewed with ultraviolet optics. (Original magnification ×1500) (Rhim JS et al: Virology 17:342, 1962)

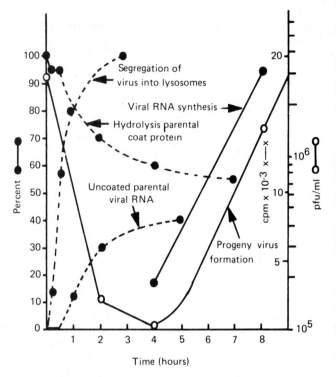

Figure 62—5. Sequential events in the uncoating and replication of orthoreovirus. *cpm*, counts per minute; *pfu*, plaque-forming units. (Silverstein SC, Dales S: J Cell Biol 36:197, 1968)

By 6 hours after infection the ten segments of the viral genome are transcribed at comparable rates. The sizes of the mRNAs correspond to those of the virion RNAs (see Fig. 62–3, Table 62–2), and each hybridizes specifically to one strand of the segment of the viral genome of corresponding size. Most of the newly synthesized single-stranded RNA molecules leave the subviral particles, rapidly become associated with polyribosomes, and appear to function as monocistronic mRNAs. These mRNAs are capped, but unexpectedly they are not polyadenylated at their 3′ ends, though the virion contains an oligoadenylate synthetase activity and is relatively rich in poly(A) oligonucleotides.

RNA REPLICATION. Unlike double-stranded DNA molecules (see Chap. 48), orthoreovirus double-stranded RNA is **replicated conservatively.** The negative strand of each segment is copied in great excess into plus single strands (i.e., with the same polarity as the mRNA), and these then serve as templates for synthesis of the minus strands. Free minus strands are not detected because they remain associated with their templates to form the various double-stranded RNA segments.

Replication of the viral RNA requires continuous protein synthesis, apparently to supply the virus-encoded replicase and transcriptase functions. Newly replicated

virion is responsible for this early transcription, which is accomplished without synthesis of new proteins or replication of the viral genome. Four additional enzymatic activities within the virion (nucleotide phosphohydrolase, guanyltransferase, and two methyltransferases) are responsible for synthesizing the caps at the 5′ termini of the mRNAs.

RNA molecules of all ten size classes are found in infected cells, further strengthening the evidence that the viral genome is indeed segmented. The segmented structure of the genome explains the remarkably high recombination frequency (i.e., 3% to 50%) detected with temperature-sensitive mutants (due to reassortment, as with influenza viruses; see Chap. 56).

TRANSLATION. About 75% of the newly synthesized plus strands become associated with cytoplasmic polyribosomes, which serve as the sites for synthesis of viral proteins. All eight virion structural proteins can be detected in infected cells as early as 3 hours after infection, but only seven of these are primary gene products: μ1c (see Table 62–2) is derived from μ1 by cleavage. In addition, two nonstructural viral polypeptides, μNs and σNs, whose functions are unknown, are also synthesized.

ASSEMBLY. Infectious virions begin to appear 6 to 7 hours after infection (Fig. 62–5), but how the ten genomic segments (which may be likened to chromosomes) are segregated in the appropriate number remains unexplained. Excess viral Ags accumulate and viral particles assemble in close association with the spindle tubules (Figs. 62–6 and 62–7). However, the mitotic spindle is not essential for viral multiplication, since viral synthesis proceeds unhindered in nondividing cells arrested in metaphase by colchicine, which disaggregates the spindle. Unassembled, newly synthesized double-stranded RNAs and the excess viral Ags accumulate in large masses (see Fig. 62–4), forming the characteristic cytoplasmic inclusion bodies that give green-yellow fluorescence with acridine orange staining.

Orthoreovirus infection inhibits biosynthesis of host cell DNA and proteins within 6 hours, and cell division ceases. In such cells the mitotic index increases more than threefold, but the mitotic sequence is not completed and abnormal mitotic figures form, perhaps because of the viral association with mitotic spindles.

PATHOGENESIS

Orthoreoviruses have frequently been isolated from the feces and respiratory secretions of healthy persons, as well as from patients with a variety of clinical illnesses, particularly minor upper respiratory and gastrointestinal disease. The relation of these viruses to disease is not clear, and human transmission experiments have not

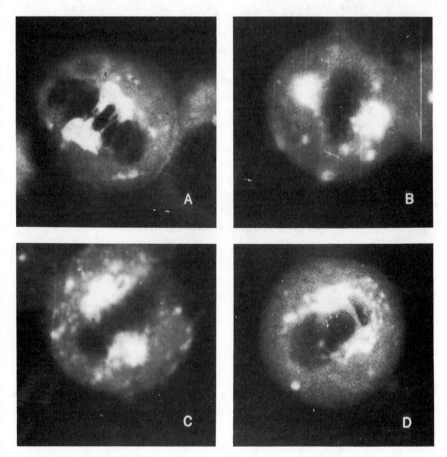

Figure 62–6. Orthoreovirus-infected cells stained with fluorescein-conjugated Ab. Viral Ag is closely associated with the mitotic spindle of virus-infected cells. Cells were examined by dark-field microscopy with ultraviolet illumination. (Original magnification ×750; Spendlove RS et al: J Immunol 90:554, 1963)

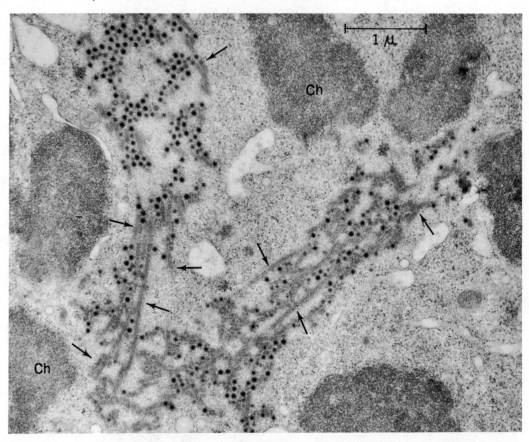

Figure 62-7. Electron micrograph of a cell infected with type 3 reovirus. The section was made through the spindle and chromosomes (*Ch*) of an infected cell in mitosis, showing aggregates of viral particles closely associated with the tubules of the spindle, indicated by arrows). (Original magnification ×15,000; Dales S: Proc Natl Acad Sci USA 50:268, 1963)

been decisive: afebrile respiratory illnesses only occurred in one-third of the volunteers, the symptoms were irregular, and the illnesses were very mild.

In the few deaths that have been attributed to type 3 orthoreoviruses, the pathologic lesions noted (encephalitis, hepatitis, and pneumonia) were similar to lesions found in experimental animals.

LABORATORY DIAGNOSIS

Reoviruses may be isolated from throat washings or fecal specimens by means of cell cultures (e.g., human embryonic or monkey kidney), and they are usually identified as belonging to the reovirus genus by CF or **ELISA** tests. The specific immunologic type can then be identified by hemagglutination-inhibition or neutralization assays.

To permit recognition of Abs in a patient's serum by hemagglutination-inhibition titrations the serum should be pretreated with trypsin or periodate, or adsorbed with kaolin, to remove nonspecific mucoprotein inhibitors.

Since orthoreoviruses are also frequently isolated from healthy persons, an increase in serum Ab titer must be demonstrated before an illness can be assumed to be caused by a reovirus.

EPIDEMIOLOGY AND CONTROL

Though orthoreovirus infections do not seem to be of great clinical importance, studies should be continued to monitor their pathogenetic potential. Both the respiratory and the gastrointestinal tracts may well be sources of their spread. Unrecognized infections are common, for approximately 10% of children by 5 years of age and 65% of young adults in the United States have reovirus Abs in their sera. Antibodies are also frequently found in various wild and domestic animals, but it is not known whether the animals serve as reservoirs for human infections.

Since the meager data assign a limited pathogenicity to these viruses, specific immunization procedures are not warranted.

Rotaviruses

Acute **nonbacterial gastrointestinal infections** (epidemic gastroenteritis and infantile diarrhea) are second only to acute respiratory infections as the cause of illness in families with young children. Hence, the discoveries of viruses that are major causes of these infections encourage the hope that these common illnesses will be better understood and controlled. **Rotaviruses** (initially termed *human reovirus-like agent*) have been identified as a major cause of **sporadic acute enteritis** in infants and young children. In addition, two immunologically distinct viruses that resemble caliciviruses have been shown to be etiologic agents of **epidemic acute gastroenteritis** (discussed separately below).

These new viruses were discovered by direct electron microscopic observation of fecal extracts, duodenal fluid, and duodenal mucosa; none was detected by isolation in a cell culture or animal. A major diagnostic advance, **immune electron microscopy,** was of special utility: sera from convalescent patients were used as a source of specific Abs to agglutinate the virions and make them more easily recognizable and to identify the virus as one that had actually produced an acute infection with an attendant Ab response (Figs. 62–8 and 62–9).

PROPERTIES

The **physical and chemical characteristics** of rotaviruses are similar to those of orthoreoviruses (see above) except that the viral genome consists of 11 double-stranded RNA segments (see Fig. 62–3). The electrophoretic patterns of the 11 segments vary with strains isolated at different times and different locations. These so-called electropherotypes are useful for molecular epidemiologic studies. The physical characteristics of the virion RNAs and the proteins they encode are summarized in Table 62–3. The functions of the individual nonstructural proteins are still unclear, particularly those responsible for transcription and RNA replication.

Rotaviruses isolated from humans belong to **four immunologic serotypes** (1 to 4) based upon neutralization titrations. The outer capsid protein VP7 is the major Ag inducing neutralizing Abs; VP4, which is responsible for hemagglutination, is a minor neutralization Ag. Marked cross-reactivity of human rotaviruses with each other, and with many animal rotaviruses, can be detected by CF, ELISA, and immunofluorescence assays owing to VP6, a major core Ag that makes up about 80% of the virion's protein mass. On the basis of immunologic cross-reactivities (e.g., by CF, ELISA, immunofluorescence, im-

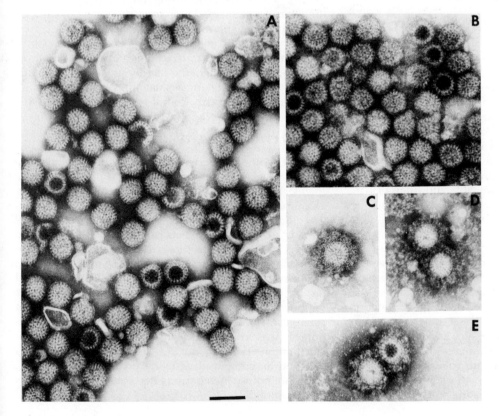

Figure 62–8. Identification of a rotavirus from man by immune electron microscopy. *(A)* Viral particles in stool filtrate. Note the capsomer structure and the appearance of a double capsid in the empty particles. *(B)* Filtrate incubated with acute-phase serum. *(C* through *E)* Viral particles in the same stool preparation incubated with convalescent serum from the same patient. (Kapikian AZ et al: Science 185:1049, 1974. Copyright 1974 by the American Association for the Advancement of Science)

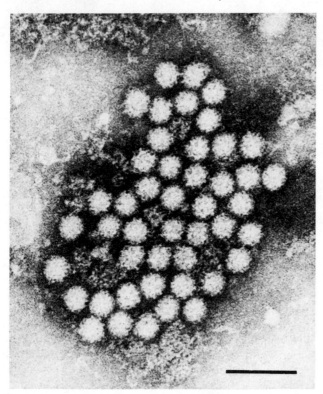

Figure 62–9. Electron micrograph of an aggregate of acute nonbacterial gastroenteritis virus (Norwalk agent) particles in stool from an acutely ill patient. (Original magnification ×200,000; Kapikian AZ et al: J Virol 10:1075, 1972)

mune hemagglutination) all rotaviruses are divided into two serogroups (I and II). A few viruses having the physical characteristics of rotaviruses do not share either group Ag and are called **pararotaviruses.** Serotypes 1 and 2 include only human rotaviruses, but serotypes 3 and 4 include a number of animal rotaviruses. Some animal rotaviruses, however, are distinct and form serotypes 5 to 7. It is noteworthy that the antigenic characteristics of the serotypes are genetically stable and do not correlate with variations of RNA electrophoretic patterns.

Human rotaviruses are fastidious viruses that do not replicate well in cell cultures except after serial passage in the presence of trypsin or when host range mutants are selected by passage in a susceptible animal host (e.g., type 1 multiplies in piglets), or by selecting reassortants after cocultivation with a related animal rotavirus. Thus, although human rotaviruses can now be propagated in cell cultures after adaptation, most data concerning physical and chemical characteristics and multiplication of rotaviruses derive from experiments using animal viruses, particularly SA11, simian rotavirus, which is closely related to human serotype 3 viruses.

Unadapted human rotaviruses induce an abortive in-fection in cell cultures, and infectious virus is usually not produced or is made in small numbers. However, extensive studies of the simian SA11 virus indicate that replication of rotaviruses follows the same steps in attachment, entry, uncoating, biosynthesis, and assembly as followed by orthoreoviruses (see above). One step in rotavirus morphogenesis, however, is more striking than what is seen with orthoreoviruses: precursor viral particles bud into the cisternae of the endoplasmic reticulum, thus becoming enveloped; but the enveloped stage is transient, and the envelope is stripped to form mature particles. The ability of trypsinization to increase the infectivity of many strains may be due to an enzymatic amplification of the latter step of virion maturation.

PATHOGENESIS

Severe diarrhea and fever, occasionally accompanied by vomiting, is a common syndrome in children less than 2 years old, particularly infants. About half of the most severe illnesses of babies seen in hospitals are caused by the human rotavirus; during the fall and winter the incidence is particularly high. Biopsies of the duodenal mucosa show it to be a principal site of viral multiplication and pathologic lesions, which may account for the symptoms observed. (Whether other parts of the gastrointestinal tract are also affected is uncertain.) Viral excretion in feces is maximal during the first 4 days of illness, but it has been detected as long as 21 days after the onset of diarrhea. In experimental infections of newborn, gnotobiotic calves and piglets, viral replication and pathologic lesions occur in mucosal and submucosal cells of the villous epithelium of the duodenum and spread caudally throughout the entire small intestine, but the large bowel and other organs do not appear to be involved.

LABORATORY DIAGNOSIS

Identification of rotavirus infection requires a laboratory diagnosis because so many agents can produce similar manifestations of gastroenteritis. **Electron microscopic examination** of a negatively stained stool specimen is the quickest, most sensitive, and most reliable method (see Fig. 62–8); it also detects protorotaviruses, which do not share Ags with rotaviruses. However, many laboratories have neither the equipment nor the expertise to use electron microscopy, and therefore the **ELISA** technique has become the mainstay in most laboratories. RNA dot hybridization is a reliable and rapid method to detect rotaviruses in stool specimens and rectal swabs. Isolation of virus from stools can be accomplished; but the isolation rate is only about 75%, and considerable time is required as compared with the preceding techniques. Immunofluorescence permits detection of infected cells more rapidly.

TABLE 62–3. Rotavirus Genomic RNAs and Encoded Proteins*

Genome		Polypeptide			
RNA Segment	Mol. Wt. $(\times 10^{-6})$	Designation	Mol. Wt. $(\times 10^{-3})$	Location in Virion	Function
1	2.05	VP1	125	Core	
2	1.68	VP2†	94	Core	
		VP2‡	88		
		VP4‡	84		
3	1.60	NSVP1(?)	Not identified		
4	1.60	VP3†	88	Outer capsid	Hemagglutinin
		VP5‡	60		Minor neutralization
		VP8‡	28		
5	0.98	NSVP2	53		
6	0.81	VP6	41	Core	
7	0.5	NSVP3	34		
8	0.5	NSVP4	35		
9	0.5	VP7	32	Outer capsid	Major neutralization Ag (? glycoprotein; maturation)
10	0.3	NSVP5	20		
11	0.2	VP9	26	Outer capsid	

* Data obtained from the best-studied rotavirus, simian SA11

† Precursor protein proteolytically cleaved

‡ Designates polypeptide as a cleavage product

Ab response is a common and economic means to diagnose rotavirus infections. Owing to the acquisition of Abs at an early age, the illness must induce a fourfold or greater increase in Abs to make a positive diagnosis. There are many serologic techniques to diagnose rotavirus infections; CF, ELISA, immunofluorescence, and viral neutralization titrations (in primary African green or cynomolgus monkey kidney cell cultures) are the most commonly employed.

EPIDEMIOLOGY AND CONTROL

Acute gastroenteritis caused by a rotavirus is a worldwide, sporadic disease, found primarily in young children 6 to 24 months of age. It is a leading cause of childhood deaths in developing countries. Rotaviruses are the third most common cause of gastroenteritis. Their prevalence is demonstrated serologically: over 90% of children in the Washington, DC, area were found to have CF Abs by age 3 years. Nosocomial infections are common in newborns, although clinical illness is rare. The basis for this unexpected finding is unknown. Although the virus is probably transmitted by the fecal–oral route, infection is most common during the cooler part of the year, unlike bacterial diarrheas and dysenteries. The virus is spread successfully because it is present in large amounts in feces (e.g., 10^{11} viral particles per gram of feces), and it is very stable on ordinary surfaces at room temperature.

Outbreaks of rotavirus infections do occur in adults, but subclinical infections are the rule. Indeed, in a small study at least one parent in the family had an inapparent infection at the time illness began in the baby, suggesting that the child's source of virus might literally have been the hand that fed it.

Prevention of this major disease in young children is an important goal whose attainment seems possible but requires additional immunologic and epidemiologic data. The major issues that require resolution before immunoprophylaxis can be generally successful are the following: (1) Does homotypic immunity prevent reinfection and disease? (2) How effective is heterotypic immunity, and how many viral serotypes or type-specific Ags that induce neutralizing Abs must be included in the vaccine? (3) If immunity is homotypic, must the vaccine contain the genes (RNA 9 and RNA 4) for the major and minor neutralizing Ags, respectively? The findings that rotaviruses are genetically stable and that immunologic variants do not continuously arise—as with influenza viruses (see Chap. 56)—despite their similar segmented genomes and ease of genetic reassortment, imply that immunoprophylaxis through vaccination should be successful. Several of the following approaches to develop a rotavirus vaccine are being explored, any or all of which might be effective: **Live attenuated viral vaccine,** which could consist of attenuated human viruses or an animal rotavirus serologically related to human serotypes (e.g., rhesus rotavirus similar to human type 3). **Cloned ro-**

tavirus genes encoding the neutralizing antigens and inserted into either an animal virus such as adenovirus or vaccinia virus or a bacterial vector that transiently colonizes the small intestine. **Synthetic peptide vaccine** can be readily made, since the amino acid sequences of the major and minor neutralizing Ags are known. **Reassortant viral vaccine,** taking advantage of the genes encoding the neutralizing Ags from human rotaviruses and the ability to propagate animal rotaviruses to high titers.

A recent field trial of the rhesus rotavirus vaccine in 247 infants 1 to 10 months old showed that this vaccine protected 68% of infants against type 3 rotavirus infections during a 1-year period. This study also suggested that immunity is homotypic.

Colorado Tick Fever Virus (Orbivirus)

Colorado tick fever is the only tick-borne viral disease recognized in the United States, though Powassan virus, a tick-borne flavivirus (see Chap. 60), had been isolated in Canada. The virions morphologically are classified as orbiviruses (see Table 62–1) having an outer indistinct capsid and an inner capsid. Unlike other orbiviruses, however, the genome of the Colorado tick fever virus consists of 12 segments whose electrophoretic pattern differs from those of other orbiviruses. Its genome is larger than that of any other member of the Reoviridae family. The virus multiplies readily in hamsters, suckling and adult mice, and some continuous human cell lines. Virions replicate, in large numbers, free in the cytoplasm and unassociated with cell membranes or mitotic spindles.

Colorado tick fever virus consists of two serotypes and neither is immunologically related to reoviruses and rotaviruses. The virus is partially inactivated by ether, probably owing to its skinlike outer coat; but it is not inactivated by sodium deoxycholate (in contrast to viruses with classic envelopes, such as togaviruses, which are also transmitted by insects).

Colorado tick fever is an acute, febrile, nonexanthematous infection characterized by acute onset of fever, chills, headache, and severe pains in the muscles of the back and legs. The course of the disease usually consists of two febrile periods of 2 to 3 days separated by a short, afebrile remission. Recovery appears to be complete but infectious virus often persists in RBCs as long as 4 months. Although the disease is uncommon, this viral persistence provides a problem in selecting blood donors in the locale where Colorado tick fever virus infections occur. Infection induces long-lasting, probably lifelong, immunity.

The disease occurs in the western United States, where its major vector, the tick *Dermacentor andersoni,* is found. The virus has also been isolated from the tick *D. variabilis,* collected on Long Island, NY, but no human infections have been reported from this locality. The golden ground squirrel appears to be the major animal reservoir; the virus has also been isolated from chipmunks, other squirrels, and a deer mouse. Infection of man is only incidental and is a dead end in the chain of transmission.

Prevention is directed primarily toward avoiding ticks, either by not entering infested areas or by wearing suitable clothing and using arthropod repellents.

Other Epidemic Acute Gastroenteritis Viruses

NORWALK VIRUS GROUP
Properties

Epidemiologic studies in families and human volunteer experiments suggested that two immunologically distinct viruses cause acute nonbacterial gastroenteritis, one of the most common illnesses in the United States, and second only to acute respiratory illnesses in families. The value of **immune electron microscopy** to detect and characterize rotaviruses (see Fig. 62–8) soon led to the detection of the second group of viruses; the agent initially isolated was termed *Norwalk virus** (see Fig. 62–9). Although these viruses are unrelated to viruses of the family Reoviridae, they will be described in this chapter, since their taxonomic niche is uncertain, and their pathogenesis and epidemiology are so similar to rotavirus infections (which, however, are generally more severe).

The Norwalk virus is the prototype of a group of related viruses that are extremely fastidious and have not been successfully isolated in cell cultures or animals. Electron microscopy has been the primary technique used to characterize these viruses. The virions are nonenveloped, 23-nm to 34-nm, spherical particles with suggestions of surface indentations (see Fig. 62–9). On the basis of morphology, buoyant density in CsCl, resistance to acid and heat inactivation, and failure to lose infectivity when extracted with ether, the viruses were originally considered to be parvovirus-like (see Chap. 52). However, the virions are slightly larger than parvoviruses, the nature of their nucleic acid is unknown because of the inability to obtain adequate quantities of purified virions from fecal specimens, and they contain a single protein of about 39,000 daltons. This latter characteristic distinguishes the Norwalk viruses from parvoviruses, which contain three structural proteins ranging from 60,000 daltons to 85,000 daltons. Thus, the Norwalk and related viruses are not parvoviruses but are similar to **cali-**

---

* The first viruses were identified during an epidemic in Norwalk, Ohio, and were termed the *Norwalk agents.*

civiruses (see below), which also contain only a single structural protein of about 65,000 daltons.

Pathogenesis and Epidemiology

The disease occurs in outbreaks and is characterized by a combination of nausea, vomiting, diarrhea, low-grade fever, and abdominal pain. The illness is self-limited, usually lasting 1 to 2 days; it is commonly found in families or even in community-wide outbreaks. In contrast to the sporadic form of acute gastroenteritis caused in infants by rotaviruses, acute epidemic gastroenteritis mainly affects **school-aged children and adults** and often spreads to family contacts. Both forms of viral gastroenteritis occur most frequently from September to March.

Virions appear in stools with the onset of disease and are shed in greatest number during the first 24 hours of illness, and for not more than 72 hours after onset. Virus has not been detected during the relatively short incubation period (about 48 hours). Antibodies develop following infection, but their persistence and effect on resistance to subsequent infection are still unknown. Only 50% of persons 40 to 60 years of age have detectable Abs to Norwalk virus, whereas 90% of the same persons have rotavirus Abs. **Three distinct immunologic types** have been identified by immune electron microscopy. However, the frequent occurrence of disease in older children and adults may be due to the existence of many different immunologic types of viruses (like rhinoviruses) rather than to failure of Abs to persist or to produce resistance to infection.

Diagnosis of Norwalk virus group infection can be made by radioimmunoassay as well as by immune electron microscopy. The former technique is the more useful, since it is more economical and requires less equipment and expertise.

CALICIVIRIDAE

The virions possess a characteristic six-pointed starlike shape whose surfaces have cup-shaped (chalice) indentations, a morphology that suggested the family name. Most caliciviruses infect animals other than humans (swine, horses, and even sea lions), but one member of the family causes gastroenteritis in children. Unfortunately, the caliciviruses infecting humans cannot be propagated in cell cultures or in animals, but the caliciviruses of lower animals replicate readily *in vitro*. The classical caliciviruses are about 31 nm to 35 nm in diameter and have genomes consisting of a linear single-stranded RNA, and the virion contains a single, major structural protein.

The epidemiologic and clinical features of calicivirus infections are similar to those of rotaviruses, but the occurrence of family and nosocomial infections is considerably less. Epidemics have been studied in Scandinavia, Canada, Japan, and England, but infections have not been reported in the United States. Like rotaviruses, Abs are acquired between 6 and 24 months of age, and over 90% of adults show immunologic evidence of having been infected.

Selected Reading

BOOKS AND REVIEW ARTICLES

Cukor G, Blacklow NR: Human viral gastroenteritis. Microbiol Rev 48:157, 1984

Estes MK, Graham DY, Dimitrov DN: The molecular epidemiology of rotavirus gastroenteritis. Prog Med Virol 29:1, 1984

Joklik, WK (ed). The Reoviridae. New York, Plenum, 1983

Kapikian AZ, Chanock RM: Rotaviruses. In Fields BN et al (eds): Virology. New York, Raven Press, 1985

Kapikian AZ, Hashino Y, Flores J et al: Alternative approaches to the development of a rotavirus vaccine. In XIth Nobel Conference: Development of Vaccines and Drugs Against Diarrheal Diseases, Stockholm, 1985

SPECIFIC ARTICLES

Bassel-Duby R, Jayasuriya A, Chatterjee D et al: Sequence of reovirus hemagglutinin predicts a coiled-coil structure. Nature 315:421, 1985

Fields BN, Green MI: Genetic and molecular mechanisms of viral pathogenesis: Implications for prevention and treatment. Nature 300:12, 1982

Gomatos PJ, Tamm I: The secondary structure of reovirus RNA. Proc Natl Acad Sci USA 49:707, 1963

McCrae MA, Joklik WK: The nature of the polypeptide encoded by each of the 10 double-stranded segments of reovirus type 3. Virology 89:578, 1978

Mustoe TA, Ramig RF, Sharpe AH, Fields BN: Genetics of reovirus: Identification of ds RNA segments encoding the polypeptides of the μ and σ size classes. Virology 89:594, 1978

Smith RE, Zweerink HJ, Joklik WK: Polypeptide components of virions, top component and cores of reovirus type 3. Virology 39:791, 1969

63

Hepatitis Viruses

The infectious nature of hepatitis was long unrecognized because the disease tends to occur sporadically and because jaundice, a prominent clinical sign, has many diverse causes. Since the time of Virchow the disease was believed to result from obstruction of the common bile duct by a plug of mucus, and it was known as **acute catarrhal jaundice.** In 1942 Voeght first transmitted hepatitis by feeding a patient's duodenal contents to volunteers. Subsequently, it was found that the etiologic agents are filterable and that the disease may be transmitted in two ways: by the intestinal–oral route (**infectious hepatitis**) or by the injection of infected blood or its products (**serum hepatitis**). However, the differences in transmission are not absolute, since the virus of so-called infectious hepatitis can also produce disease when inoculated parenterally, and experimentally, the virus of serum hepatitis has been transmitted orally. The viruses causing these two types of hepatitis showed other differences, particularly the absence of cross-immunity in human transmission experiments. Accordingly, new names were assigned: **hepatitis A virus (HAV)** and **hepatitis B virus (HBV)** for infectious and serum hepatitis viruses, respectively. Epidemiologic and serologic data indicated that there are at least three additional hepatitis viruses.

Evidence for the existence of more than one hepatitis virus evolved from the serendipitous discovery of the so-called **Australia antigen** (also called **hepatitis-associated Ag [HAA]** or **SH Ag**), which appears only in patients with hepatitis B (serum hepatitis) and is identified as the HBV surface Ag (HB$_s$Ag). This Ag was first detected by Blumberg in the serum of an Australian aborigine. In a search for new serum alloantigens he happened to employ test serum from two hemophiliacs who had received multiple blood transfusions. The sera from these subjects, which contained Abs to the so-called Australia

Ag, were then found to react with serum from a variety of patients who had received multiple transfusions or who resided in institutions (e.g., for mental defectives or for lepers) in which the inmates had a high incidence of hepatitis. The detection of Australia Ag was then recognized as signaling the presence of active or inactive serum hepatitis. The discovery of this novel Ag has permitted further characterization of hepatitis B virus and has allowed diagnostic differentiation of the clinical disease.

Of these two viruses only HAV has been propagated in cell cultures, but both can produce infection in chimpanzees and monkeys, and their distinct morphologies can be identified by electron microscopy. Moreover, the identification of hepatitis A and B viruses has led to the recognition that there are at least two other hepatitis viruses, which are unrelated to HAV or HBV. These viruses, termed **non-A, non-B hepatitis viruses,** are at present the major etiologic agents of hepatitis following transfusions in the United States. The continued high incidence of hepatitis (e.g., in the United States approximately 53,000 cases were reported in 1978) and its great morbidity have stimulated increasing interest in these viruses.

Although the hepatitis viruses are taxonomically distinct, their clinical and epidemiologic associations merit their discussion in a single chapter. Similarly, the **delta virus,** which is a defective virus whose replication and transmission requires the help of HBV and which in return makes the HBV disease more severe, will also be included. The properties of these viruses will be described separately, but the similarities of the diseases they produce indicate that their pathogenesis, epidemiology, and control be discussed and compared together.

Properties of Hepatitis A Virus

A 27-nm viral particle (Fig. 63–1) present in the stools of patients with hepatitis A is clearly the etiologic agent of the disease: the particles (recognizable by electron microscopy) are found in the stools of patients with clinical hepatitis A during the peak of the disease and its associated biochemical changes; these particles are not found in patients with serologically identified hepatitis B or non-A, non-B hepatitis; hepatitis A patients develop Abs that react with the viral particles (recognized by neutralization, immune adherence, and complement fixation [CF]); and the particles have been detected, by immune

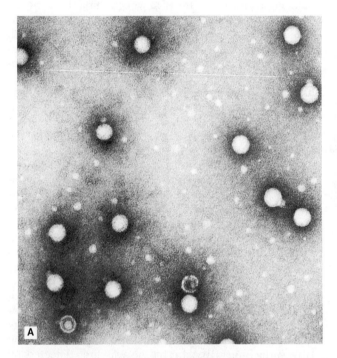
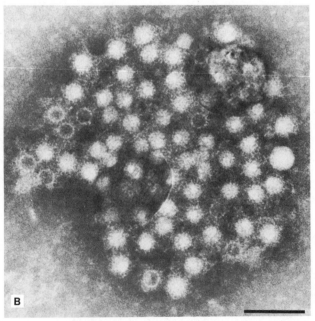

Figure 63–1. Electron micrographs of hepatitis A virus (HAV) particles negatively stained with phosphotungstic acid. *(A)* Virions purified from human stools. Note the fuzzy margins of the virions and the lattice of Ab molecules connecting the virions. (Original magnification ×150,000) *(B)* Immune electron microscopy of HAV virions aggregated by serum from a late-convalescent patient with naturally acquired hepatitis. (Original magnification ×230,000; *A,* courtesy of Dr. John Gerin, Oak Ridge National Laboratory; *B,* Kapikian AZ et al: In Pollard M [ed]: Perspectives in Virology, Vol 9, p 9. San Francisco, Academic Press, 1975)

electron microscopy, in the serum, liver, and feces of marmosets and chimpanzees to whom the disease was transmitted with feces or blood from patients with hepatitis A.

In **morphology** the virions are similar to other picornaviruses (see Chap. 55), with an average diameter of 27 nm, icosahedral symmetry, and no envelope (see Fig. 63–1; see "Properties of Hepatitis A Virus [HAV]"). The **physical and chemical characteristics** of purified hepatitis A virions are like those of enteroviruses: a single-stranded RNA genome, of positive polarity with a 5'-terminal protein (VPg) and a 3' poly(A) tail. The capsid consists of four structural proteins and is even more stable to acid and heat than other enteroviruses (see "Properties of Hepatitis A Virus [HAV]"). The chemical and physical characteristics have led to its formal classification as **enterovirus type 72.** As with most viruses, including HBV, infectivity is inactivated by ultraviolet irradiation, formalin (1:400 dilution) for 3 days at 37°C, and heat for 5 minutes at 100°C (these properties are important for vaccine development). The virions are relatively resistant to common disinfectants, however, and therefore special cleansing procedures must be used to prevent hospital spread.

Human transmission studies and extensive epidemiologic data suggest that the virus exists as a **single immunologic type** and that long-lasting immunity follows infection. Antibodies appear shortly after the onset of clinical disease (CF Abs being detectable earliest); Ab levels rise slowly and persist for years (Fig. 63–2).

Initially, only marmoset-adapted HAV could be propagated in explant cultures of marmoset livers and in a fetal monkey kidney cell line. Presently, however, **viral multiplication** can be carried out in African green monkey and fetal rhesus monkey cells, Vero cells, human diploid lung cells, and a human liver hepatoma cell line. Although viral titers as high as 10^8 TCID$_{50}$ per milliliter are attained in cell culture, cytopathic effects do not occur. Despite the ability to propagate virus *in vitro*, biochem-

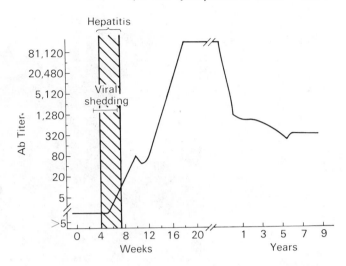

Figure 63–2. Sequential relationship of viral shedding to clinical hepatitis, and the development of virus-specific Abs during HAV infection. (Modified from Krugman S, Friedman H, Lattimer C: N Engl J Med 292:1141, 1975

ical studies of viral synthesis have been difficult to carry out. Nevertheless, it is possible to isolate HAV directly from patients' feces in cell cultures, and the replication of virus *in vitro* has made the production of a vaccine possible (see later).

Although direct biochemical studies of viral replication have not been done, the entire genome has been sequenced from cloned cDNAs. These studies showed that the genome is organized like other picornaviruses, that it can encode a polyprotein with the viral structural proteins at the amino-terminal portion and the RNA polymerase in the remainder.

Properties of Hepatitis B Virus
MORPHOLOGY

Serum from patients with clinical hepatitis B commonly contains three distinct structures (Fig. 63–3) that possess the hepatitis B surface antigen (HB$_s$Ag; see Antigenic Structure, later). The **Dane particle** (named for its first observer) is the least common form, but it alone has the structure attributed to viruses and appears to be infectious. This particle is a complex sphere, 42 nm in diameter with an electron-dense core 28 nm in diameter (Fig. 63–3) surrounded by an envelope. Negative stain can penetrate the Dane particles, revealing the 7-nm outer layer or envelope. Occasional particles lack the core and have a translucent center. The core structures can be isolated by reacting Dane particles with sodium dodecyl sulfate. **Spherical particles** with an average diameter of about 22 nm (range, 16 nm to 25 nm) are most numerous.

PROPERTIES OF HEPATITIS A VIRUS (HAV)

Size: 27–32 nm
Morphology: Icosahedral; naked
Genome: Single-stranded RNA; 2.25–2.28 × 10⁶ mol. wt. Positive polarity
Structural proteins:
   VP1—30–33 Kd
   VP2—24–27 Kd
   VP3—21–23 Kd
   VP4— 7–14 Kd
   VPg—
Stability
   Ether: Stable
   Acid: Stable, pH 3.0
   Heat: Stable (60°C/60 min)

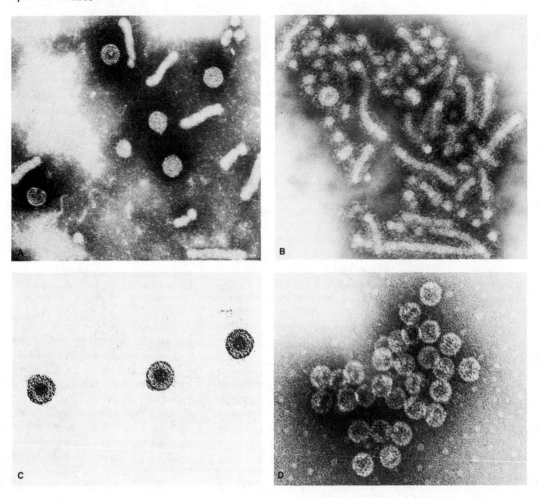

Figure 63–3. Electron micrographs of negatively stained forms of hepatitis B virus (HBV). *(A)* Dane particles, filaments, and 22-nm HB$_s$Ag particles present in the serum of a patient with active infection. (Original magnification ×150,000) *(B)* Immune electron microscopy of Dane particles, filaments, and 22-nm HB$_s$Ag particles aggregated by serum from a late-convalescent patient. (Original magnification ×150,000) *(C)* Purified Dane particles stained with uranyl acetate to show the DNA core. (Original magnification ×200,000). *(D)* Cores of HBV isolated from the liver of a patient with active hepatitis. (Original magnification ×200,000) *(A–C,* courtesy of Dr. John Gerin, Oak Ridge National Laboratory; *D,* Kaplan PM et al: J Virol 17:885, 1976)

These particles are unlike any known virus. Their surfaces appear to have a subunit structure similar to that of Dane particles, but no uniform symmetry is discernible. **Filamentous forms,** about 22 nm in diameter and ranging in length from 50 nm to greater than 230 nm, are also plentiful and have a similar surface structure. When the filaments are mixed with a nonionic detergent, they form spheres that are morphologically and antigenically similar to the 22-nm particles, suggesting that the filaments are aggregates of the spherical particles.

The ease with which the preceding forms can be observed is a reflection of their amazing abundance in patients' sera. In one serum sample, for example, 3×10^{13} 22-nm particles per milliliter were counted, with 1/15 as many filaments and 1/1500 as many Dane particles. A serum may be infectious for humans in a 10^{-7} dilution.

PHYSICAL AND CHEMICAL CHARACTERISTICS

The abundance of viral structures in blood (see Fig. 63–3; Fig. 63–4) has made physical and chemical analyses possible despite the inability to propagate the virus in cell cultures (Table 63–1).

Virions (Dane particles) and isolated 28-nm cores (nucleocapsids) contain the **viral genome, a circular, partially double-stranded DNA molecule,** which consists of a long (L) strand of constant length with a free 3′ terminus and a 5′ terminus that is covalently linked to a

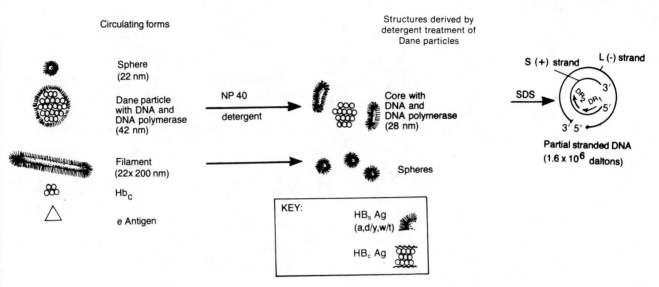

Figure 63–4. Schematic diagram of forms of HBV and the DNA structure. (Modified from Robinson WS, Lutwick LI: N Engl J Med 295:1232, 1976)

TABLE 63–1. *Physical and Chemical Characteristics of Hepatitis B Viral Forms*

Characteristic	22-nm Spheres	Filamentous Forms	Dane Particles (42-nm Spheres)	Core Particles
Buoyant density (CsCl)	1.20 g/ml³	1.20 g/ml³	1.25 g/ml³	1.36 g/ml³
Sedimentation coefficient	39–54S		58.5S	110S
Protein	+		+	+
Glycoproteins	3		3	0
Lipid	+		+	0
Nucleic acid	0		+	0
			Circular, interrupted double-stranded DNA	Circular, interrupted double-stranded DNA

small protein and a short (S) strand that varies from 15% to 60% of the circle length (see Fig. 63–4; Fig. 63–5). The positions of the 5′ termini of the L(−) and S(+) strands are fixed, whereas the 3′ end of the S(+) strand is variable. The 5′ ends of both strands are base-paired, which assures the circular form of the double-stranded DNA. In addition, at both sides of the cohesive 5′ ends there is an 11-base-pair direct repeat (5′TTCACCTCTGC); similar direct repeats (DR1 and DR2) are found in all the hepadnaviruses,* which suggests that they play an important role. This DNA is smaller than that of any known animal virus containing double-stranded DNA. The nucleocap-

* Viruses with the same morphologic, chemical, and physical characteristics as HBV have also been found in woodchucks, ground squirrels, and Peking ducks. Indeed, hepatitis and hepatocarcinoma are associated with the infection of woodchucks. Accordingly, these viruses have been taxonomically grouped into the family **Hepadnaviridae.**

sid consists of the core Ag (HB$_c$Ag), a DNA polymerase, and a protein kinase. The DNA polymerase of the virion is dependent on the four deoxynucleoside triphosphates and Mg^{2+}; it completes the single-stranded regions without any added DNA or RNA primer, producing covalently closed, double-stranded circular DNA. The polymerase also serves as a reverse transcriptase (see below).

The viral envelope contains three glycoproteins, termed the *major, middle,* and *large proteins* (see Fig. 63–4). The **hepatitis B surface Ag (HB$_s$Ag),** which is the predominant component of the 22-nm particles found in the blood of patients with active disease and carriers, is a disulfide-bonded dimer of two molecules of the major protein. In the middle protein a 55 amino acid sequence, which is the region distinct from the major protein, probably contains the receptor for polymerized human serum albumin that appears to mediate the attachment

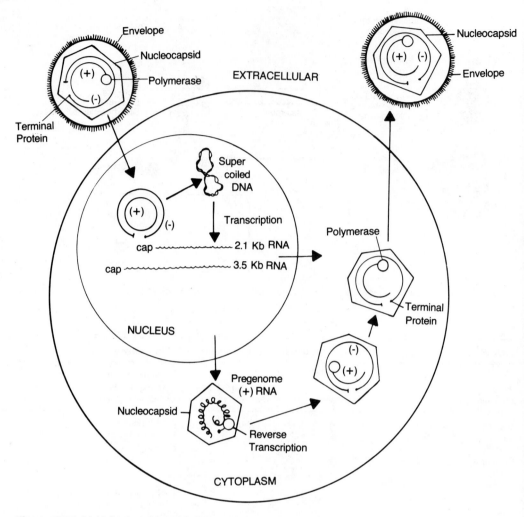

Figure 63–5. Multiplication of hepatitis B virus in hepatocytes.

of the virus to hepatocytes. The large protein consists of the middle protein plus about 128 amino acids added to its N terminus; this exposed additional sequence appears also to be important for attachment to hepatocytes.

A virion contains 300 to 400 molecules of major proteins and 40 to 80 of the middle and large proteins; filaments have the same protein composition as virions. However, the spherical 22-nm particles are different: in chronic carriers in which active viral replication ensues, they contain the same relative numbers of major and middle proteins but 20 times fewer large proteins; in the absence of viral replication they contain mostly the major protein, less than 1% of middle protein, and no large protein.

The **nucleocapsid** contains only a single protein, the **core protein,** which possesses **protein kinase activity**

capable of phosphorylating itself. The core protein is expressed as the **HB$_c$Ag,** and when the capsid is disrupted *in vivo,* proteolytic cleavage uncovers the **HB$_e$Ag** determinant. The core protein also interacts with the HBV genome through its arginine-rich C-terminal region.

ANTIGENIC STRUCTURE

The 42-nm enveloped virion containing DNA has two distinct major Ags, the **surface Ag (HB$_s$Ag)** and the **core Ag (HB$_c$Ag).** The HB$_s$Ag is the only Ag on the two other hepatitis B particles circulating in the blood, that is, the 22-nm spheres and the filamentous particles (see Fig. 65–4).

The HB$_s$Ag contains several antigenic determinants: a **group-specific determinant, a,** which is present in all HB$_s$Ag-containing material, and two sets of generally mutually exclusive type-specific determinants, **d** or **y** and **w** or **r**, which represent sets of alleles of two independent genetic loci. In addition, four variants of the **w** allelic determinant have been observed. Thus, a number of phenotypic combinations or subtypes are possible (Table 63–2). A few sera containing surface antigenic reactivity of mixed subtype (**adyw, adyr, awr, adwr,** and **adywr**) have also been reported; whether these arise from mixed HBV infection or unusual phenotypic mixing is unclear.

The subtypes of HB$_s$Ag are not associated with different biological activities of the viruses, and no clinical differences have been observed in the infections caused by the various subtypes. These subtypes are valuable as markers for studies of the epidemiologic behavior of the virus.

Chemical reduction and alkylation of 22-nm particles and purified HB$_s$Ag markedly reduces its antigenicity, which emphasizes the critical importance of its disulfide-linked dimeric structure. Deglycosylation also greatly diminishes this reactivity of the HB$_s$Ag.

The **HB$_c$Ag** is of a **single antigenic type** and is found only in the core of the 42-nm Dane particle and in free core particles present in the nuclei of hepatocytes from infected livers. Hence, to detect the HB$_c$Ag in plasma one must disrupt the enveloped 42-nm particles with lipid solvents to expose the core Ag, whereas the HB$_s$Ag can be readily detected in serum during acute hepatitis B and in chronic carriers. Some HB$_s$Ag-positive sera contain an additional specific Ag, designated **e (HB$_e$Ag),** which is considerably smaller than either the HB$_s$Ag or the HB$_c$Ag particle (about 12S); it is also distinct from the viral DNA polymerase. The HB$_e$AG is specific for hepatitis B virus infection. Two subdeterminants (HB$_e$Ag/1 and HB$_e$Ag/2) have been detected. The HB$_e$Ag, in part bound to immunoglobulins, appears during the incubation period of acute hepatitis B, just after the appearance of HB$_s$Ag and prior to clinically apparent liver injury. Antibodies to HB$_e$Ag occur frequently in HB$_s$Ag-containing serum and even in serum having anti-HB$_s$Abs. The function of the e Ag is unknown, but epidemiologic evidence indicates that the presence of this viral gene product in serum is associated with active viral replication and liver pathology. Patients with HB$_e$Ag are those most likely to have active disease and to be efficient transmitters of infection.

IMMUNITY

Antibodies directed against the surface and core Ags appear at different times and show different patterns of disappearance (Fig. 63–6). Antibodies to HB$_c$Ag increase rapidly during the early phase of clinical disease; their appearance is usually associated with reduced viral replication and beginning resolution of disease. However, these Abs are also consistently present in chronic carriers of HB$_s$Ag, and they may be a sensitive indicator of continued viral replication. The presence of anti-HB$_e$Abs does not uniformly indicate a good prognosis, and serum from such patients may even be infectious.

Cell-mediated immunity to HB$_s$Ag appears near the end of the acute phase of hepatitis, and its increase is correlated with the disappearance of the circulating Ag. In contrast, Abs to HB$_s$Ag do not appear until months after termination of the clinical illness (Fig. 63–6). It is also noteworthy that in chronic HB$_s$Ag carriers specific cell-mediated immunity is generally decreased and circulating anti-HB$_s$Abs are not demonstrable, but electron microscopic examination of serum detects HB$_s$Ag–Ab complexes.

An increase in Abs to HB$_s$Ag is clearly correlated with immunity. Thus, human γ-globulin containing these Abs is of value in preventing hepatitis B; and immunization in humans with purified HB$_s$Ag induces formation of Abs to HB$_s$Ag, accompanied by immunity to challenge. In addition, immunization of chimpanzees with purified HB$_s$Ag results in resistance to challenge with HBV-infected serum (see Prevention and Control).

MULTIPLICATION

Without a susceptible cell in which HBV can replicate, data on the steps in viral multiplication were derived entirely from identification of viral structures detected in hepatocytes from patients with acute and chronic HBV hepatitis and from ducks and ground squirrels infected with the hepatocytes. These studies led to a unique model of biosynthesis of a DNA virus (see Fig. 63–5). Following entry and uncoating of the virion into susceptible cells, the viral DNA reaches the nucleus and utilizing the virion DNA polymerase forms complete double-stranded circles that attain a supercoiled configuration. Host cell DNA-dependent RNA polymerase then transcribes the DNA minus-strand to make multiple complete RNA cop-

TABLE 63–2. Phenotypic Combinations or Subtypes of HB$_s$ Antigens Observed in Patients

| Group Determinant | Subtype Determinant | |
	d/y	w/r
a	y	w$_1$
a	y	w$_2$
a	y	w$_3$
a	y	w$_4$
a	y	r
a	d	r
a	d	w$_2$
a	d	w$_4$

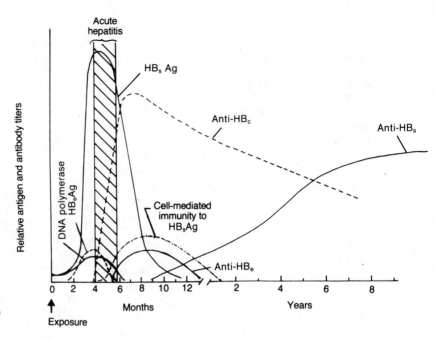

Figure 63–6. Diagram of the time course of circulating HBV Ags and the immune response. Note that HB$_c$Ag is not found free in the plasma.

ies termed the **pregenome RNA**, as well as a smaller capped RNA (see Chaps. 48 and 65). The RNAs are transported into the cytoplasm where the core protein is made and rapidly encapsidates the pregenome RNA as well as the newly synthesized viral polymerase and the DNA terminal protein. There follows a unique reaction for DNA viruses, reverse transcription of the pregenome RNA, with the DNA-linked terminal protein probably serving as a primer to initiate synthesis of the DNA minus-strand. As viral DNA is synthesized, the pregenome RNA is degraded, except for a small fragment of about 20 base pairs derived from the 5′ end that appears to act as a primer for synthesis of the DNA plus-strand from the newly made minus-strand template. The progeny particles usually contain only partially double-stranded viral DNA. They obtain HB$_s$Ag-containing envelopes, probably by budding from the cell's plasma membrane, and become infectious virions.

Thus, hepadnaviruses employ a strategy similar to that of retroviruses for genome replication. However, hepadnaviruses employ the strategy of initiating and terminating the synthetic cycle with DNA rather than RNA genomes. Hepadnaviruses differ from retroviruses in one other characteristic: whereas the retrovirus RNA is always transcribed from an integrated DNA molecule, hepadnavirus can transcribe the pregenome RNA from free as well as integrated viral DNA. It is striking to note that there is significant homology in nucleotide sequence (particularly in the **pol** gene) between the genomes of HBV and several retroviruses.

Properties of Non-A, Non-B Hepatitis Viruses

The sensitive immunologic and electron microscopic methods used to detect the viruses and Ags of hepatitis A and B viruses have made it possible to identify at least two other viruses. One of these has been transmitted to chimpanzees, and the virus has been identified by immune electron microscopy. The virions are nonenveloped icosahedrons about 27 nm in diameter, which resemble caliciviruses in morphologic and physical characteristics. A second virus, which can also infect chimpanzees, is larger; inactivated by lipid solvents; and has a positive-sense single-stranded RNA genome. This latter non-A, non-B hepatitis virus resembles a togavirus or a flavivirus (see Chap. 60). The non-A, non-B hepatitis viruses do not crossreact immunologically with Ags of hepatitis A or B viruses.

Properties of Delta Hepatitis (D) Virus

In 1977 a new Ag termed delta Ag was noted in nuclei of hepatocytes in patients with chronic hepatitis B, but neither the HB$_c$Ag nor other HBV Ags were detected in the cells containing the delta Ag (δ Ag). Indeed, the delta Ag is found only in patients with chronic and often severe HBV hepatitis; it is not noted in patients with non-A, non-B, or HAV hepatitis. The delta virus genome is a 1.75 Kb single-stranded, circular RNA that does not have any homology with the HBV genome. However, the nucleotide sequence of the delta virus RNA shows extensive homology with a common viroid (see Chap. 51). The genome of extracellular delta virus found in blood is associated with δ Ag and encoated by the HB$_s$Ag to form particles of 35 nm to 37 nm.

Studies in chimpanzees and woodchucks, which are susceptible to infection with δ virus as well as HBV, indicate that the δ virus is defective, and its replication requires coinfection with HBV or the woodchuck virus (WHV) to act as a helper virus. Moreover, δ virus replication appears to depress replication of HBV, just as coinfection of cells with the defective adeno-associated virus (AAV) and an adenovirus results in multiplication of AAV and a decreased yield of its helper adenovirus (see Chap. 52). The HB$_s$Ag or WHV Ag covers the δ virus particle and probably serves to protect the δ virus RNA genome as well as to permit the particles' attachment to and entry of the host hepatocytes.

Pathogenesis

The response of humans to infection with hepatitis viruses ranges from inapparent infection and nonicteric hepatitis to severe jaundice, liver degeneration, and death; the disease is often debilitating and convalescence is prolonged. Though clinical differences in type A and type B hepatitis have been described, the acute disease may be clinically indistinguishable, so that the two infections are often differentiated (Table 63–3) mainly by the routes of infection, the length of the incubation periods, and the laboratory identification of specific viruses, Ags, and Abs.

Hepatitis A virus (HAV) usually enters by the oral route and multiplies in the gastrointestinal tract (probably in the epithelium, although, as in poliovirus infection, mesenteric lymph nodes may also be involved). Viremia eventually occurs, and virus spreads to cells of the liver, kidney, and spleen. Virus can be detected in the feces and duodenal contents and in the blood and urine during the preicteric and the initial portion of the icteric phases (Fig. 63–7). When quantitative immune electron microscopy is used, HAV is first detected during the **preicteric period** and attains its highest concentration in the feces prior to the appearance of jaundice (see Fig. 63–7). Indeed, the onset of jaundice usually heralds the approaching termination of viral shedding. More sensitive human transmission studies, however, indicate that virus may be shed in the feces for slightly longer periods. When virus is present in the feces it is also found in liver cells and in the bile. Antibodies to HAV appear as the viral titer decreases and liver damage becomes apparent (see Fig. 63–7). This timing suggests that liver damage may be effected, at least in part, by immunologic mechanisms (although HAV–Ab complexes have not been de-

TABLE 63–3. Differentiating Characteristics of Hepatitis Types A and B

Property	Type A	Type B
Usual transmission	Fecal–oral	Parenteral inoculation*
Characteristic incubation period†	15–40 days	60–160 days
Type of onset	Acute	Insidious
Fever >38°C	Common	Uncommon
Seasonal incidence	Autumn and winter	Year-round
Age incidence	Most common in children and young adults	All ages; most common in adults
Size of virus	27 nm	42 nm
Virus in feces	Incubation period and acute phase	Not demonstrated
Virus in blood	End of incubation period and briefly during acute phase	Incubation period and acute phase; may persist for years
Appearance of HB$_s$Ag	Absent	14–50 days after infection
Detection of HB$_s$Ag		Blood (less often in feces, urine, semen, and bile)
Duration of HB$_s$Ag		60 days to years
Prophylactic value of γ-globulin	Good	Good if titer of anti-HB$_s$Ag is high

* Parenteral injection is probably not the predominant mode of transmission in developing countries where the means of spread is unknown.

† Considerable overlapping in the duration of incubation periods for types A and B has been noted in volunteers as well as in patients during epidemics, that is, as long as 85 days for type A hepatitis and as short as 20 days for type B hepatitis.

tected in either chimpanzee or man, and the appearance of specific cytotoxic T cells has not been studied).

Hepatitis B virus (HBV) enters predominantly by the parenteral route, but its primary site of replication is unknown. However, HB$_c$Ag is present in the nuclei of hepatocytes as early as 2 weeks after experimental infection in chimpanzees, who develop a disease closely akin to that in man. During the latter half of the incubation period (see Fig. 63–6), 5 to 8 weeks after infection, the blood becomes infectious (a danger if used for transfusion), and it contains detectable HB$_s$Ag and viral DNA polymerase. The HB$_s$Ag has also been identified in bile, urine, semen, feces, and nasopharyngeal secretions. It is striking that the HB$_s$Ag and DNA polymerase usually begin to decline in the blood before acute symptoms disappear and are not detectable by the time liver functions return to normal.

Whether immune reactions play a role in the pathogenesis of hepatitis B is still unclear but, as noted earlier, anti-HB$_c$Abs appear at the onset of disease; HB$_s$Ags are present in large quantity weeks before anti-HB$_s$Abs appear; and cell-mediated immunity to HB$_s$Ag becomes detectable during the active disease, and its increasing de-

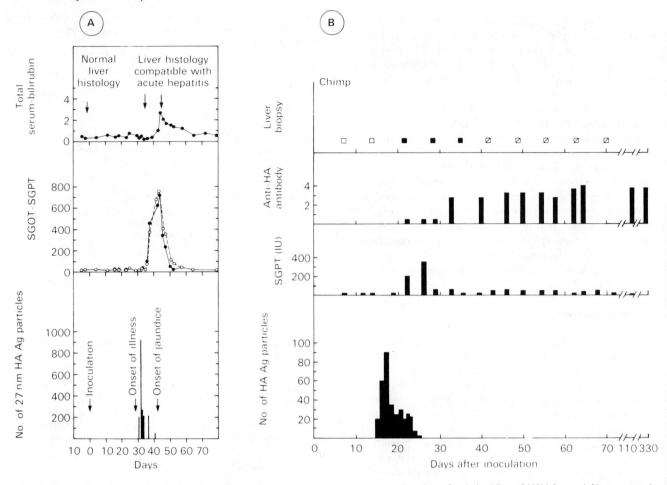

Figure 63–7. Temporal relationship of clinical illness, liver pathology, serum enzyme alterations, fecal shedding of HAV Ag, and Ab response in experimental HAV infection *(A)* in man and *(B)* in the chimpanzee. *SGOT* and *SGPT,* serum glutamic–oxaloacetic and pyruvic transaminases. Liver histology: □, normal; ■, acute hepatitis; ▨, resolving hepatitis. (Dienstag JL et al: Lancet 1:765, 1975; Dienstag JL et al: J Infect Dis 132:532, 1975)

velopment correlates with the fall in HB$_s$Ag titer (see Fig. 63–6).

Both HAV and HBV infections primarily affect the liver. When jaundice occurs, it is usually preceded by anorexia, malaise, nausea, diarrhea, abdominal discomfort, fever, and chilliness. This preicteric phase may last from 2 days to 3 weeks. The icteric stage of hepatitis A usually has an abrupt onset with a sharp rise in temperature, whereas that of hepatitis B characteristically appears more insidiously and with less fever. Nevertheless, **hepatitis B is ordinarily a more severe disease,** the fatality rate sometimes being as high as 50%, whereas in hepatitis A fatalities rarely exceed 1% (although convalescence is often prolonged). These differences, however, may not reflect only the characteristics of the viruses, for persons receiving blood or plasma transfusions are usually ill at the time of inoculation.

Liver biopsies obtained during the course of the illness have revealed early cloudy swelling and fatty metamorphosis at the time clinical symptoms begin and diffuse parenchymal destruction by the time jaundice has developed. No inclusion bodies are seen in affected cells; intracellular HB$_s$Ag, however, can be detected by immunofluorescence early in the course of type B hepatitis, and occasionally 20-nm to 30-nm virus-like particles (probably the nucleocapsids or cores) are seen in liver biopsies. The degeneration of cells is not localized to any one part of the liver lobule, in contrast to the findings in yellow fever (see Chap. 60) or chemical hepatitis. With recovery, hepatic cells regenerate; scar tissue (cirrhosis) develops only after extensive or long-standing destruction of cells, which is primarily associated with hepatitis B. In fatal infections, the liver parenchyma is often almost completely destroyed (**acute yellow atrophy).**

In 10% to 20% of adult patients and about 35% of children HB$_s$Ag persists in the blood for extended periods, but less than half of these become **chronic Ag carriers.** More than half of the chronic carriers continue to manifest biochemical and pathologic evidence of chronic liver disease. Although the mechanism of persistent infection with antigenemia is unexplained, defects in cell-mediated immunity (e.g., that directed at HB$_s$Ag) or other forms of immunodeficiency seem likely. The delta virus produces its most deleterious effects when it infects chronic HB$_s$Ag carriers. Simultaneous infection with HBV and δ virus does not produce a disease different from that induced by HBV alone.

It has been proposed that HBV infection is causally related to hepatocarcinoma based on the evidence that there is a close correlation between the geographic distribution of hepatitis B and the incidence of hepatocarcinoma, HB$_s$Ag is detected in patients with hepatocarcinoma with an unusually high frequency, and integrated and free viral DNA is found in many, but not all, hepatocellular carcinomas. The striking association between the woodchuck hepatitis virus infections and hepatocarcinomas in these animals adds support to the hypothesis that HBV is an oncogenic virus.

Laboratory Diagnosis

Immunologic techniques provide the most sensitive and economical approach for detecting viral Ags and Abs. Immune electron microscopy can be used to identify HAV in feces and HBV in blood or liver biopsy tissue. If a liver biopsy is obtained, both viruses can be identified by immunofluorescent techniques. The HAV Ags or Abs can be easily assayed by CF, immune adherence, enzyme-linked immunosorbent assay (ELISA), or radioimmunoassay (RIA). The CF Abs are detectable first. The ELISA and solid-phase RIA are the most sensitive of these techniques, but the immune adherence titration (which requires purified HAV Ag or standardized serum, guinea pig complement, and human group O red blood cells [RBCs] is simpler, less costly, and faster, as well as being quite sensitive and specific. Since Abs are usually present at the onset of illness (see Fig. 63–7), serologic diagnosis requires detection of HAV-specific IgM Abs. The Abs in serum from clinical cases also neutralize HAV in cell culture, as well as in chimpanzees and marmosets, but this procedure is too expensive and time-consuming.

A number of tests have been devised to detect and measure HBV Ags, particularly the HB$_s$Ag. The most sensitive techniques now available are RIAs and ELISAs with either a micro-solid-phase method or a double-Ab immunoprecipitation procedure. The passive hemagglutination assay (using RBCs coated with either HB$_s$Ag or anti-HB$_s$Abs) is also an accurate and very sensitive method for quantitating either Ag or Ab. Agar gel diffusion and countercurrent immunoelectrophoresis are of considerable value for identifying the subtype Ags and the e Ag. Since HB$_c$Ag does not circulate in the blood, its measurement is not useful for clinical diagnosis. Detection of Abs to HB$_c$Ag is valuable, however, since their presence appears to reflect viral replication. Similarly, HB$_e$Ag has been associated with viral infectivity and therefore signifies specific HBV infection.

Epidemiology

Predominantly, the **type A hepatitis virus** (of the **short-incubation disease** previously called *infectious hepatitis*) is spread by ingestion (particularly in epidemics), and **type B hepatitis virus** (of the **long-incubation disease** formerly termed *serum hepatitis*) is disseminated by parenteral inoculation. However, the viruses of both diseases can be rarely transmitted by both the oral and the parenteral route. The diseases produced by **non-A, non-B hepatitis viruses** may have a relatively short incubation period, but their major spread is also by parenteral inoculation. However, an epidemic form of non-A, non-B hepatitis, probably spread by the fecal–oral route, has been observed in several areas of Southeast Asia and North Africa. Epidemic non-A, non-B hepatitis, which predominantly affects adults, has not been detected in the United States or Western Europe, but it is not known whether the etiologic agent(s) exists in these regions.

HEPATITIS A

Hepatitis A mimics poliomyelitis in many of its epidemiologic features. When environmental factors favor widespread intestinal–oral transmission, the disease is **endemic,** and infection (usually mild or inapparent) occurs in the very young. Under these conditions the disease in adults is uncommon and epidemics are rare. On the other hand, under good sanitary conditions, spread of the virus is restricted, and adulthood is frequently attained without immunity. In such nonimmune populations, especially in military groups, **epidemics** are likely, and the source of virus can usually be traced to **contamination of water or food** by infected humans.

The danger of HAV dissemination from an infected person is greatest during the latter part of the incubation period, when viral shedding in the feces is greatest but is unrecognized because jaundice is not yet present (see Fig. 63–7). Long-term intestinal carriers of the virus have not been detected. Because **subclinical infections,** particularly in children, often predominate, secondary person-to-person spread and contamination of food and drink are common. Such transmission is particularly favored by the unusual stability of hepatitis A virus and its notable resistance to disinfectants, such as chlorine at ordinary concentrations in water. Not only contaminated water but also **shellfish** that live in it (and concentrate the virus) may be sources of infection: for example, raw oysters and clams obtained from polluted waters have been the origin of numerous epidemics throughout the world. Hepatitis A virus is not a common cause of transfusion hepatitis because viremia is usually brief and chronic viremia occurs rarely, if ever.

Subhuman primates, particularly chimpanzees, are the only known natural nonhuman hosts. Hepatitis has developed among handlers 3 to 6 weeks after infected animals arrived in the United States from Africa. Apparently, the young animals were infected by man after capture and subsequently excreted HAV in their feces, and hence infected their handlers. (Some animals showed clinical manifestations of disease.)

HEPATITIS B

Hepatitis B is readily distinguishable from hepatitis A not only by morphologic and immunologic properties but also on epidemiologic evidence, such as the long incubation period, parenteral transmission, increasing incidence with age, and nonepidemicity (see Table 63–3).

Despite sensitive immunologic techniques to detect viral carriers by screening the blood of donors for HB$_s$Ag, blood and its products continue to be a potential source of hepatitis in the United States. However, only a portion of these cases are caused by undetected hepatitis B virus. Indeed, about 90% of the cases now transmitted by **transfusion*** in the United States are caused by **non-A, non-B hepatitis viruses.** The unrecognizable chronic carriers of hepatitis B or a non-A, non-B virus are the pernicious sources of infection, spreading virus via transfusions of infected blood, plasma, or convalescent serum; via contaminated fibrinogen; and via inadequately sterilized syringes, needles, or instruments (medical and dental) containing traces of contaminated blood. The last source, which includes common stylets for blood counts and syringes for drawing blood, has been essentially eliminated in many parts of the world by the use of disposable instruments. However, needles used in tattooing and communal equipment used by drug addicts are still a common means of viral dissemination. Injection of as little as 10^{-6} ml to 10^{-7} ml of contaminated blood may transmit infection, as predicted by the electron microscopic finding of as many as 10^7 Dane particles per milliliter of blood.

The large amount of virus and its Ags in blood and the demonstration of HB$_s$Ag (and the probable presence of

---

* Overt hepatitis follows about 1% of blood transfusions in the United States. On the assumption that even more inapparent infections are produced, it has been estimated that 2% to 3% of the adult population carries a hepatitis virus.

virus) in other body fluids as well also explain why type B hepatitis is an **occupational disease** of health personnel—dentists, physicians, nurses, and ward personnel who are frequently exposed to the unrecognized chronic carriers; laboratory workers who handle blood; and technicians who process human plasma and blood products.

Health personnel who work in hemodialysis units and in cancer therapy wards, where the chronic carrier rates among patients are high, appear to be particularly vulnerable. It is striking that infected professionals serving in renal dialysis units, for example, develop acute hepatitis, whereas the patients, who have various forms of immunodeficiencies, do not manifest clinical disease. The mechanism by which virus is transmitted from carriers to these healthy workers is not entirely clear. Many infected workers do not recall any accidental parenteral injections, although possible viral entrance through skin abrasions cannot be ignored. It should be recalled that HB$_s$Ag is detectable in the saliva, urine, and feces of chronic carriers, as well as in blood and its products, so that entrance of the virus through membranes of the eye or mouth must be considered a plausible route of infection.

Additional epidemiologic observations provide further evidence that transmission of HBV by means other than parenteral injection is also likely when chronic infection exists. It is now clear that HBV has disseminated and persists throughout the world, even in remote and insular localities where medical care is primitive and blood and its products are not commonly used for therapeutic or prophylactic purposes. Indeed, there is evidence suggesting that all biological fluids from HBV-infected persons are infectious and potentially able to transmit the virus. Hence, nonparenteral transmission of virus must occur. Furthermore, family clusters of type B hepatitis are being observed with increasing frequency; these cases are grouped around an index case with whom family members have had close person-to-person contact but no known exchange of blood. As noted previously, experimental oral transmission has been demonstrated, and sexual transmission is also probable. Neonates may be infected during gestation by placental transmission (cord blood often contains HB$_s$Ag), at the time of delivery, or in the postnatal period.

Although hepatitis B is usually sporadic, epidemics may occur when many samples of serum or plasma are pooled. For example, in the early 1940s more than 28,000 cases of serum hepatitis in American military personnel resulted from the use of yellow fever vaccine containing contaminated human serum to stabilize the live virus.

NON-A, NON-B HEPATITIS

Sensitive immunologic techniques used to screen blood donors for HBV Ags and to establish the diagnosis of viral hepatitis have sharply reduced the incidence of hepatitis B infections, but they have also revealed another agent (or agents) as a cause of posttransfusion hepatitis. **Non-A, non-B hepatitis** is now the major form of posttransfusion hepatitis in the United States. The incubation period is usually 6 to 8 weeks; however, periods as short as 10 days and as long as 11 weeks have been recorded (which further implies that more than one virus is responsible for non-A, non-B hepatitis). Indeed, in large outbreaks that were epidemiologically similar to those produced by HAV, virions morphologically akin to a picornavirus were detected in feces by means of immune electron microscopic techniques.

Prevention and Control

No specific therapy is available for any of the viral hepatitides, although some antiviral drugs (e.g., acyclovir and adenine arabinoside) have been tried experimentally. In all proved or suspected cases of viral hepatitis great care should be taken in the disposal of feces and of all syringes, needles, plastic tubing, and other equipment used for blood sampling and parenteral therapy. Whenever possible, disposable equipment (including needles and plastic syringes and even thermometers) should be used in hospital and office practice. A syringe, once used, should not be reused with a fresh needle, even merely to obtain a blood specimen. Nondisposable equipment and supplies (e.g., dishes and bed clothing) should be autoclaved at 15 lb pressure (121°C), boiled in water for at least 20 minutes, or heated to 180°C for 1 hour in a sterilizing oven.

Subjects giving a history of jaundice or with detectable HB$_s$Ag in their blood should not be used as blood donors. Blood HB$_s$Ag has been reported in about 0.3% of blood donors in New York and 0.2% to 1.2% of different groups of blood donors in Tokyo; the carrier rate among commercial donors, particularly drug addicts, is 3 to 10 times higher than that among volunteers. However, the incidence of hepatitis non-A, non-B Ags in the population is unknown. Because minute amounts of contaminated plasma can initiate infection, the practice of pooling plasmas should be avoided: then plasma from an infected individual, used unwittingly, will infect only one person.

The protection of individuals exposed to patients, carriers, or contaminated blood requires additional consideration. Since hepatitis A patients usually shed virus only briefly after jaundice appears (see Fig. 63–2), and viremia is transient, these patients in hospitals and at home constitute a hazard for their contacts for only a short period. In contrast, hepatitis B (and probably non-A, non-B hepatitis) patients are potential sources of virus for transmission over a prolonged period, whether they are suffering from acute icteric hepatitis or are chronic carriers without clinical liver disease. Accordingly, all close contacts of carriers or possible carriers of HBV must take every precaution to prevent exposure to blood (and to objects potentially contaminated with blood—e.g., toothbrushes, razors) and to body excreta. These precautions are of greatest significance for personnel working in hemodialysis units, intensive care units, and custodial mental institutions; for dentists; for technicians in clinical laboratories and blood processing facilities; and for close family contacts (particularly spouses).

Type A hepatitis may be prevented by **passive immunization.** Pooled human γ-globulin* reduces the incidence of icteric disease (but not of infection) when given early in the incubation period. Initially, inconsistent results were obtained in preventing hepatitis B with pooled γ-globulin. However, the advent of assays for anti-HB$_s$Abs has made it apparent that immune γ-globulin containing a high titer of anti-HB$_s$Abs is partially effective; that is, in different recipients it prevents disease, decreases the severity of hepatitis, or markedly prolongs the incubation period. Therefore, γ-globulin containing anti-HB$_s$Abs is recommended for prophylaxis in exposed persons; however, for those who are at a high risk of acquiring HBV infection owing to their occupation, newly developed vaccines are more effective. For the newborn of a mother positive for HB$_s$Ag and HB$_c$Ag, a regimen combining one dose of HB$_s$Ab-positive γ-globulin at birth with an HB$_s$Ag vaccine soon after birth is 85% to 90% effective in preventing infection.

The ability to propagate virus in cell cultures is leading to the development of an attenuated virus HAV vaccine. Trials in marmosets, chimpanzees, and humans are in progress. The potential is also great for the production of a subunit Ag vaccine in *Escherichia coli* through the use of a plasmid vector or in animal cells by means of an animal virus vector, such as vaccinia virus or adenovirus (see Chap. 50). For hepatitis B the relatively large amounts of HB$_s$Ag in the serum of chronic carriers make it possible to purify the Ags that are essential for inducing neutralizing Abs, and allow the use of this material for immunization after inactivation of any infectious virus present. This vaccine has been licensed and is now successfully used. A purified HB$_s$Ag prepared in yeast by a recombinant DNA-vector technique has also proved to be effective experimentally and is now available for general use. An experimental vaccine with infectious vacci-

---

* Infection with hepatitis A virus is so widespread that the serum of many adults contains anti-HAV Abs, and a relatively high titer is present in concentrated γ-globulin pools. HAV and HBV have been eliminated from these pools, along with the fibrinogen, in the usual cold ethanol fractionation of plasma. The recommended dose of γ-globulin is 0.02 ml/kg of body weight, administered by intramuscular injection as soon after exposure as possible.

nia virus as a vector has been shown to produce immunity in chimpanzees, and one with an adenovirus vector in vaccines is under study.

Selected Reading

Dienstag JL, Alter HJ: Non-A, non-B hepatitis: Evolving epidemiologic and clinical perspective. Semin Liver Dis 6:67, 1986

Feinstone SM: Hepatitis A. Prog Liver Dis 8:299, 1986

Hilleman MR: Newer directions in vaccine development and utilization. J Infect Dis 151:407, 1985

Immunization Practices Advisory Committee: Recommendations for protection against viral hepatitis. Morbidity and Mortality Weekly Report, CDC 34:313, 1985

Miller RH, Robinson WS: Common evolutionary origin of hepatitis B virus and retroviruses. Proc Natl Acad Sci USA 83:2531, 1986

Purcell RH, Rizzetto M, Gerin JL: Hepatitis delta virus infection of the liver. Semin Liver Dis 4:340, 1984

Rizzetto M, Verone G, Gerin JL, Purcell RH: Hepatitis delta virus disease. Prog Liver Dis 8:417, 1986

Seeger C, Ganem D, Varmus HE: Biochemical and genetic evidence for the hepatitis B virus replication strategy. Science 232:477, 1986

Ticehurst JR: Hepatitis A virus: Clones, cultures, and vaccines. Semin Liver Dis 6:46, 1986

Tiollais P, Pourcel L, Dejian A: The hepatitis B virus. Nature 317:489, 1985

Zuckerman AJ: The history of viral hepatitis from antiquity to present. In Deinhardt F, Deinhardt J (eds): Viral Hepatitis: Laboratory and Clinical Science, p 3. New York, Marcel Dekker, 1983

64

Oncogenic Viruses I: DNA-Containing Viruses

Unity of Oncogenic Viruses

The first tumor-producing (oncogenic) virus was discovered in 1908 by Ellerman and Bang, who demonstrated that seemingly spontaneous leukemias of chickens could be transmitted to other chickens by cell-free filtrates. Later (1911) Rous found that a chicken sarcoma, a solid tumor, can be similarly transmitted. The viruses responsible turned out to be retroviruses (see Chap. 65). These virus-induced tumors were then considered by many as a biological curiosity, either not true cancers or perhaps a peculiarity of the avian species. These notions, however, were shaken when DNA-containing viruses were shown to produce a cutaneous fibroma and a papilloma of wild rabbits (by Shope, in 1932), and the renal adenocarcinoma of the frog (Lucke, 1934).

The later discovery of virus-induced tumors in mice provided a particularly suitable system for experimental work. In 1936 Bittner demonstrated that a spontaneously occurring mouse adenocarcinoma is caused by a virus transmitted from the mother to the progeny through the milk, and in 1951 Gross discovered the first of many retrovirus-induced murine leukemias. These studies revealed that the viral etiology of a cancer can easily go unrecognized for several reasons: cancer can be caused as a rare effect by ubiquitous viruses, which may easily be considered as innocuous bystanders; with some oncogenic viruses the viral particles are heterogeneous, and most infect cells without inducing cancer; the disease may not develop until long after infection; and the cancers do not seem contagious, because the method of transmission of the virus is not apparent (e.g., through the embryo or the milk).

Further impetus to investigations of tumor viruses arose from the later discovery of a new group of DNA-containing viruses that cause cancer in mice and other rodents: polyoma virus and simian virus 40 (SV40) (as a passenger virus in cultures of rhesus monkey kidney cells). Finally, the **human** adenoviruses, papilloma viruses, and herpesviruses were also shown to have oncogenic activity in rodents. Moreover, by this time the study of bacterial lysogeny had clearly shown that the genetic material of viruses can become permanently integrated with that of the host. These realizations led to an explosive development of interest in viral carcinogenesis.

Soon the oncogenic effect of several viruses was demonstrated also in tissue cultures, in the form of **cell transformation** (see Chap. 47). Studies in this model system led shortly to a shattering conclusion: **a virus that has induced cancer is often no longer recognizable in the culture by its infectivity,** or by antigenicity. Traces could, however, be found in the form of viral DNA, RNA, and new Ags, in ways reminiscent of lysogeny. It thus became clear that time-tested techniques and approaches for the identification of viral agents of disease may not be adequate in the search for viral agents of human cancer.

The discovery of many new oncogenic viruses in the 1960s revealed a puzzling distribution. Most classes of DNA-containing viruses were found to produce tumors in animals, whereas only one family of RNA-containing viruses, the group now called **retroviruses,** did so (Table 64–1). The replication of retroviruses also displayed a sensitivity, peculiar for RNA viruses, to agents that interfere with DNA replication or transcription. This property was explained when Temin and Baltimore independently discovered that the oncogenic retroviruses, unlike other RNA viruses, replicate through a DNA-containing intermediate, made by a **reverse transcriptase** (RNA-dependent DNA polymerase). This discovery brought unity into the field of oncogenic viruses, suggesting that **oncogenesis is an attribute of viral DNA.** This unification has become stronger more recently with the demonstration that all oncogenic viruses cause cancer and transformation through **oncogenes** they carry or activate.

These developments, and the problems they raise, will be analyzed in this and the next chapter by examining the characteristics of cell transformation induced by several viruses. Many of the findings in animals will be analyzed in detail as the basis for results more recently obtained in humans.

TABLE 64–1. Distribution of Oncogenic Viruses Among Animal Virus Families

Nucleic Acid in Virions	Viral Group (or Family)	Oncogenic Viruses
RNA	Picornaviruses	None
	Togaviruses	None
	Orthomyxoviruses	None
	Paramyxoviruses	None
	Rhabdoviruses	None
	Coronaviruses	None
	Arenaviruses	None
	Retroviruses*	Oncoviruses: leukosis viruses, sarcoma viruses
	Reoviruses	None
DNA	Adenoviruses	Many types
	Papovaviruses	Polyoma virus, SV40, SV40-like human viruses, papilloma viruses
	Herpesviruses	Virus of neurolymphomatosis of chickens (Marek disease), Lucke's virus of frog renal adenocarcinoma, herpes simplex virus (cell transformation),† Epstein-Barr virus (Burkitt lymphoma, nasopharyngeal carcinoma), cytomegalovirus,† primate herpesviruses
	Hepadnaviruses	Hepatitis B virus
	Poxviruses	Fibroma virus
	Parvoviruses	None

* See Chapter 65.

† Transformation *in vitro* after ultraviolet irradiation

Oncogenes

ONCOGENES AND PROTO-ONCOGENES

The study of oncogenic viruses has allowed the identification of a set of genes, also expressed in seemingly spontaneous animal and human cancers, which initiate the cancer process. Many of them play an important role, not only in cancer but also in normal cell growth and differentiation. The illegitimate expression of these genes is responsible for the processes of transformation and neoplasia. This fundamental discovery was made studying the transforming activity of an oncogenic retrovirus, the Rous sarcoma virus (RSV; see Chap. 65). Genetic studies by Martin and Vogt first identified in this virus the *src* gene, responsible for transformation; then M. Bishop and collaborators, probing the genome of normal chicken cells with probes made from the *src* gene, identified a very similar gene, the **cellular *src*** gene (or *c-src*). The normal gene is known as *src* **proto-oncogene,** and the related gene present in the virus as *src* **oncogene** or *v-src*. *v-src* is incorporated in the RSV genome as a consequence of the recombination of a nontransforming retrovirus with *c-src*. The *c-src* is highly conserved in animal species, suggesting that it performs some important function.

THE v-src ONCOGENE. The possible function of *v-src* was clarified after Erikson identified its protein product by translating *in vitro* RSV RNA: it is a phosphoprotein of 60 Kd, known as **pp60**$^{v\text{-}src}$**.** He then showed it to be a **protein kinase.** Hunter discovered that it has the unusual property of **phosphorylating tyrosine** in proteins, whereas most other kinases phosphorylate serine or threonine. This finding suggests that the function of *c-src* is somehow related to cell growth regulation, because tyrosine phosphorylation is carried out by many growth factor receptors (see Chap. 47).

v-src VERSUS c-src. The protein expressed in normal cells by the *src* proto-oncogene is similar but not identical to that expressed by *v-src,* and does not cause transformation. This difference might be attributed to two circumstances: one is that the *v-src* gene differs from the *c-src* gene in its 3′ end and lacks a phosphorylation site (tyr-527) apparently crucial for normal control; the other is that the viral gene is more strongly transcribed. Transfection experiments with a cloned *c-src* gene show that the alteration is more important than the overexpression. Apparently the altered gene escapes its normal regulatory restraints, becoming a transforming gene.

OTHER ONCOGENES. After *v-src* many other oncogenes were discovered in oncogenic viruses; and DNA extracted from human cancers was also shown to contain oncogenes able to transform NIH 3T3 cells. Some of these cancer-related oncogenes are similar to those previously recognized in viruses. More than 30 oncogenes of various origins are now known and are listed in Table 64–2.

ONCOGENES OF DNA VIRUSES. Whereas the oncogenes present in oncogenic retroviruses are altered cellular proto-oncogenes that confer no advantage on the virus except that of being selected by the experimenter, the oncogenes present in oncogenic DNA viruses lack sequence homology with known cellular proto-oncogenes and do perform essential functions for the virus. These viruses multiply in resting cells, which lack the enzymes needed for the replication of the viral DNA. The viral oncogenes cause the production of the enzymes by activating the machinery for cellular DNA replication. In all likelihood the growth stimulation is responsible for transformation. Whether or not the oncogenes of DNA

TABLE 64–2. Oncogenes

Oncogene	Location	Function
ONCOGENES PRESENT IN DNA VIRUSES		
E1A	Nucleus, cytoplasm	Regulates transcription
E1B		
PV-ST	Cytoplasm	
PV-MT	Plasma membrane	Binds and stimulates pp60$^{c\text{-}src}$ and pp62$^{c\text{-}yes}$
PV-LT	Nucleus	Initiates DNA synthesis and regulates transcription
SV40-ST	Cytoplasm	
SV40-LT	Nucleus, plasma membrane	Initiates DNA synthesis, regulates transcription and binds p53
ONCOGENES PRESENT IN RETROVIRUSES (see Chap. 65)		
abl	Plasma membrane?	Tyrosine protein kinase
erb A	Cytoplasm	Thyroid hormone receptor
erb B	Plasma and other membranes	EGF receptor Tyrosine protein kinase
ets	Nucleus	
fes	Plasma membrane	Tyrosine protein kinase
fgr	id	id
fms	id	CSF-1 receptor (tyrosine protein kinase)
fos	Nucleus	
fps (see *fes*)		
kit	Membranes	Tyrosine protein kinase
mil/raf	Cytoplasm	Serine/threonine protein kinase
mos	id	Serine protein kinase
myb	Nucleus	
myc	Nucleus	
ras	Plasma membrane	GTP-binding protein
raf (see *mil*)		
rel	Cytoplasm	
ros	Cytoplasm	Tyrosine protein kinase
sis	Cytoplasm and secreted	PDGF subunit
src	Plasma membrane	Tyrosine protein kinase
ski	Nucleus	
yes		Tyrosine protein kinase
ONCOGENES NOT PRESENT IN VIRUSES		
bcl—human follicular lymphoma		
bcr—human chronic myelogenic leukemia		
int-1, 2, 3, and *4*—breast cancer in rodent		
met—chemically transformed human cell line		
neu—rat neuroglioblastoma (similar to *erb B*)		
p53—active in transformed cells		
ret—human lymphoma DNA		
rho—similar to *ras*		

viruses derive from cellular proto-oncogenes, they have evolved independently for the sake of the virus.

MODE OF ACTION OF ONCOGENES. Most of the known oncogenes encode **proteins important in cell growth control** (see Chap. 47): some are related to growth factor subunits (platelet-derived growth factor [PDGF] by *v-sis*), others to growth factor receptors (an amputated epithelial growth factor [EGF] receptor by *v-erb B*). The truncation of the external domain of these receptors presumably keeps the cytoplasmic domain active all the time, in the absence of activation from the outside. Many oncogene products are protein kinases with tyrosine specificity (the *src* family), two (oncogenes *mos* and *raf/mil*) are protein kinases with threonine-serine specificity, others (the *ras* family) are plasma membrane guanosine triphosphate (GTP)–binding proteins implicated in signal transduction. Several oncogenes encode nuclear proteins (*myc*, *myb*, *fos*, E1A, LT) some of which (E1A, LT) are known to regulate gene transcription.

The normal counterparts of oncogenes, the proto-oncogenes, appear therefore to specify proteins that are parts of regulatory pathways that initiate at the cell surface and terminate at the genes, activating cell growth. The oncogenes with nuclear products, which have no known relationship to proteins regulating growth, may represent the proximal end, close to the genes, of these pathways. The important differences in base sequences of proto-oncogenes performing the same function (e.g., tyrosine protein kinase) suggest that there are multiple similar but distinct regulatory pathways that are active in different cell types or that respond to different signals. In normal cells these pathways function only occasionally, in response to well-defined stimuli; the continuous activity of a pathway when a proto-oncogene becomes an oncogene would cause the cell to grow without restraint and would alter the activity of its genes, causing it to be transformed.

This model of transformation is supported by the following observations. (1) In normal cells some cellular proto-oncogenes (e.g., *c-fos*) are expressed only in response to a growth stimulus, in a transient way; (2) normally, each cellular oncogene is strongly expressed only in some cell type (e.g., *c-src* in brain cells, *c-fos* in differentiating macrophages) and at different stages of development (*c-fos* in expressed in placenta); (3) cells transformed by the oncogene *v-sis* encoding a PDGF subunit revert to normality when the medium contains antibodies to the PDGF. The latter result suggests that the continued action of PDGF produced by the cells on the cells' own PDGF receptors maintains the state of transformation.

ACTIVATION OF CELLULAR ONCOGENES IN VIRUSES AND CANCERS. The principal method by which a proto-oncogene is converted into an oncogene with unregulated function is by structural alterations of its coding or control sequences. The coding sequences are altered in the majority of cases. The changes may be single-base mutations, causing the replacements of critical amino acids, frame shift mutations, deletions, or insertions. In retroviruses, fusion of parts of a proto-oncogene with a viral gene may also contribute to the activity of the oncogene. As a result of the alterations, the oncogene may have unregulated transcription (e.g., *v-myc*) or translation (e.g., *v-fos*), or its protein may have lost targets for regulatory modifications (e.g., *v-src*). Proto-oncogenes may become deregulated by interaction with other cellular constituents; an example is the deregulation of *c-src* by complexing with polyoma virus MT protein (see Association of T protein With Other Oncogene Proteins, below).

An oncogene may be generated without viral intervention when a proto-oncogene is altered by physical or chemical carcinogenic agents or by translocation. Important in all cases is a high expression by an active enhancer, either viral or cellular.

Enhancers

Enhancers are DNA sequences activating transcription, which are present in both DNA viruses and retroviruses as well as in cellular genes (e.g., for immunoglobulins, insulin, chymotrypsin). Although the enhancers of different genes share common properties such as repeats, they vary greatly in sequences. Best known is the SV40 enhancer, which is made up of two 72-base-pair repeats; it increases transcription of viral or of some heterologous genes 10 or more times, in comparison with enhancer-free genomes. An enhancer is usually close to the promoter it controls; it is remarkable, however, that they continue to act on the promoter if displaced to positions several thousand base pairs removed in either direction, although with decreasing efficiency at great distances, and they can be turned back-to-front without losing activity. An enhancer acts only on some promoters: for instance, the SV40 enhancer acts strongly on the β-globulin promoter but weakly on the α-globulin promoter.

Enhancers are specifically **activated** by *trans*-acting factors, which may be of viral or cellular origin, and therefore confer cell or tissue specificity on the expression of genes they control. For instance, the SV40 enhancer does not increase transcription by the herpesvirus promoter in human cells unless the LT protein, an SV40 regulator, is present. Embryonal cells (e.g., undifferentiated embryonal carcinoma cells) produce transacting factors that **inhibit** some viral enhancers. Viral mutants capable of replicating in these cells have altered enhancers (see "Papovaviruses: Polyoma and Related Viruses," below).

Enhancers appear to operate by facilitating access of the transcriptional machinery to DNA. They are in fact recognized in SV40 minichromosomes as segments devoid of nucleosomes (nucleosome gaps), which are highly sensitive to attack by many nucleases. This property may be associated with the presence of Z-DNA sequences, which cannot fold to form nucleosomes and bind special proteins.

Cooperation of Oncogenes

Various oncogenes have two main effects on cultures of embryonic rat cells: **immortalization** and **transformation.** Immortalized cells do not undergo *in vitro* senescence, have reduced requirements for growth factors, may be unable to undergo terminal differentiation, and may be morphologically transformed. However, they do not grow in suspension in agar and do not produce tumors in syngeneic animals or in immunodeprived nude mice. Transformed cells are capable of growing in agar and forming tumors but may undergo senescence. For complete transformation and induction of tumor formation both immortalization and transformation are needed in this cell system. Typical immortalizing oncogenes are *v-myc* and *v-fos* among retroviral genes and *E1A* and *Py-LT* among those of DNA viruses; they encode nuclear proteins that may act directly on cellular genes. Among transforming oncogenes are the retroviral *v-ras* and the DNA virus *E1B* and *Py-MT*; they specify membrane proteins that, through intracellular mediators, may alter the regulation of genes.

Studies with other cells show that the distinction between the two classes of oncogenes is not absolute: the effects depend on many variables, such as the species and the type of cell used and the strength of expression of the oncogene. It is likely that the effects of an oncogene are influenced by the balance of expressed cellular genes. But even with these limitations, it is clear that there are different classes of oncogenes, although perhaps not as rigidly defined, and oncogenes of different classes can cooperate to produce a more pronounced oncogenic effect than either alone. This concept is corroborated by observations with oncogenic viruses, to be detailed later, and in the following chapter, which show that neoplasia is a multistep process and that different oncogenes can carry out different steps. Permanent cell lines, in which the effects of oncogenes are much more pronounced than in short-term cultures, have probably undergone one or more of these steps.

Oncogenic DNA Viruses

PAPOVAVIRUSES: POLYOMA AND RELATED VIRUSES

Prominent among DNA-containing viruses for understanding the mechanism of carcinogenesis are papovaviruses. The first virus, isolated by Stewart and Eddy, was found to produce various kinds of neoplasia when injected into newborn mice; it was therefore named **polyoma virus** (PyV), that is, agent of many tumors. The virus is widespread in mouse populations, both wild and in the laboratory; it is normally transmitted to animals after birth, through excretions and secretions. The structurally similar **SV40** was discovered by Sweet and Hilleman as an agent that multiplies silently in rhesus monkey kidney cultures (used for propagating poliovirus) but was found to produce cytopathic changes in similar cultures from African green monkeys *(Cercopithecus aethiops)*. It was later shown to produce sarcomas after injection into newborn hamsters.

Subsequently, **human papovaviruses** were isolated, first from the brain of a patient with progressive multifocal leukoencephalopathy (PML); next, others from patients with Wiskott–Aldrich syndrome (defects in cellular and humoral immunity, and reticulum cell sarcomas, due to an X-linked recessive allele); and then, frequently, from the urine of immunosuppressed individuals. These SV40-like viruses are designated by the initials of the persons from whom they were isolated (e.g., JC virus, from a PML patient; BK virus, from urine). These viruses produce tumors in hamsters and transform hamster cells *in vitro*. Since 70% of humans have Abs to the SV40-like viruses, they may be the human equivalent of the widespread SV40 of rhesus cultures and polyomavirus of mice.

Properties

The virions of PyV, SV40, and SV40-like human viruses are small, naked icosahedrons with a diameter of 45 nm and with 72 capsomers (see Chap. 44). They contain a minichromosome made up of a **cyclic double-stranded** DNA, about 5 Kb long, associated with octamers of cellular histones (H2a, H2b, H3, H4) to form nucleosomes similar to those present in cellular chromatin. Removal of the proteins upon extraction causes a deficit in intrinsic helical turns, which is compensated by twisting of the double helix (**supercoiling**). The SV40 genome is very similar in sequences to those of the SV40-like viruses. It also has significant, although lower, homology to the PyV genome, suggesting a common origin in evolution.

All papovaviruses are very resistant to inactivation by heat or formalin; hence, SV40 (from rhesus kidney cultures) survived in some early batches of formalin-killed poliovirus vaccine.

Multiplication in Cell Cultures

These viruses can produce either a **productive** or a **nonproductive** infection. The outcome depends on the species of the cells and their physiological state, because viruses with such small genomes depend heavily on cellular functions. Thus, cells of certain **permissive** species (Table 64–3) are killed by infection and yield virus, whereas those of **nonpermissive** species are **transformed** without virus production. In **semipermissive** cultures some cells are transformed while others are killed and yield virus (probably depending on the state of

TABLE 64–3. Some Permissive and Nonpermissive Cells Used With Polyoma Virus and SV40

Cell	Virus	Type of Culture
Permissive	Polyoma virus	Secondary cultures of mouse embryo cells
		Primary cultures of mouse kidney cells
		3T3 and 3T6 cell lines (mouse subcutaneous tissue)
	SV40	Primary cultures of African green monkey kidney cells
		BSC-1 CV-1 } cell lines (African green Vero } monkey kidney)
Nonpermissive or semipermissive	Polyoma virus	Secondary cultures of hamster embryo cells
		Secondary cultures of rat embryo cells
		BHK cell line (baby hamster kidney)
	SV40	Secondary cultures of hamster, rat, or mouse embryo cells
		3T3 cell line (mouse subcutaneous tissue)

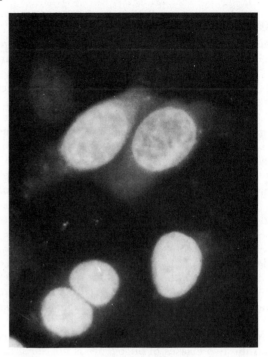

Figure 64–1. Fluorescence photomicrograph of cultured mouse kidney cells productively infected by polyoma virus. The accumulation of capsid Ag in the nuclei is revealed by its combination with fluorescein-conjugated Abs, which emit green fluorescence under ultraviolet light.

the cells). Permissive cells can be transformed by virus when viral multiplication is prevented by viral mutations or by damage in the viral DNA.

PRODUCTIVE INFECTION. As with most DNA viruses, viral DNA replication and capsid assembly occur in the cell nucleus (capsid Ag is detected there by immunofluorescence [Fig. 64–1] and virions by electron microscopy); each nucleus can produce up to 10^8 viral particles. As with other naked viruses, release depends upon **disintegration of the cells.**

Transcription of the supercoiled DNA is carried out by the host polymerase II. In the **early transcription** (Fig. 64–2) genes for DNA replication are transcribed from the "early" DNA strand; in the **late transcription,** which starts after DNA replication has begun, genes for virion proteins are transcribed from the opposite, "late" DNA strand, at a much higher rate than the persisting early strand transcription. Early transcription is **autoregulated** because it is inhibited by the large T Ag (see Viral Proteins, below).

Both early and late transcription initiate in the **control region,** which includes the origin of DNA replication (see Fig. 64–2), between the early and the late regions of the genome, and proceed in divergent directions. The control region regulates all phases of transcription as well as DNA replication. In SV40 (Fig. 64–3) it contains a series of repeats with different functional significance. Three 21-base-pair repeats, each containing

two GC-containing hexamers, act as **promoters** for early transcription. At the downstream end of the repeats is a **TATA box;** at the upstream end two 72-base-pair repeats constitute the **enhancer.** Each control sequence (the 21-base-pair repeats, the TATA box, the enhancer) binds activation factors specified by cellular genes, the presence of which makes the cells permissive for the virus. Especially important is the enhancer: although SV40 does not multiply in lymphoid cells, a construct of SV40 DNA associated with the enhancer from an immunoglobulin gene will. The three regulatory elements operate in concert and are somewhat redundant: deletion of several hexamers of the 21-base-pair repeats reduces only slightly the efficiency of viral multiplication. Artificially changing the distances between the elements has worse effects, suggesting that regulation depends on interactions among the proteins.

The regulatory elements control both early and late transcription. Early transcription is dependent on all three types of elements. It begins at several different sites, which change as infection proceeds (see Fig. 64–3). Late transcription depends on two of them: the 21-base-pair repeats and the enhancer; it also has heterogeneous starting points. The switch from early to late transcription is brought about by the binding of the large T Ag (see

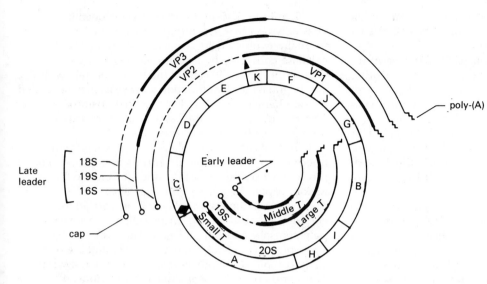

Figure 64–2. Polyoma virus mRNAs and proteins. Heavy lines indicate the translated parts of the mRNAs; wavy lines are untranslated parts; dashed lines (introns) are parts removed by splicing. The middle T is known only for polyoma virus. The two black triangles indicate shifts of the reading frame.

later) to specific sites in the control region and also by the replicating state of viral DNA.

In PyV the general organization is the same, but the different regulatory elements partially overlap with each other and the binding sites for T Ag. The PyV enhancer is made up of two domains, one homologous to the SV40 enhancer, the other to the enhancer of the E1A region of adenovirus (see below), showing the evolutionary relatedness of DNA oncogenic viruses. The function of PyV enhancer is blocked by E1A-encoded peptides, explaining its inactivity in cells (such as murine embryonal carcinoma cells) that express an E1A-like function. The activity is restored by viral mutations that modify the enhancer, changing the host range of the virus.

VIRAL PROTEINS (see Fig. 64–2). During the early infection with PyV, three **early proteins** are synthesized, collectively known as T (tumor) antigens. They are detected by immunofluorescence or immunoprecipitation of infected cell extracts with the serum of an animal bearing a large virus-induced tumor. They are the nuclear **large T (LT)** Ag, the cytoplasmic as well as nuclear **small T (ST)** Ag, and the membrane-bound **middle T (MT)** Ag. Both LT and MT have the properties of oncogenes. These proteins are specified by three different early mRNAs with a common leader sequence and different splices: parts of the PyV LT and MT mRNAs derive from the same DNA segment, but in different phases. In contrast, during SV40 infection only two T Ags are made: LT and ST. A function

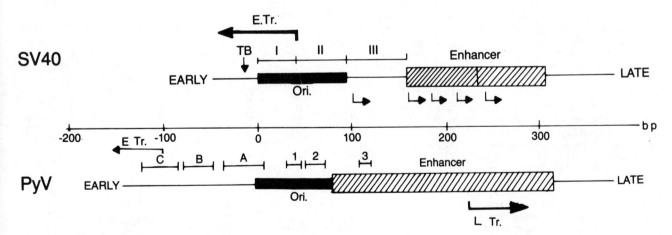

Figure 64–3. Organization of the control regions of SV40 and PyV. The early region of the genome is on the left, the late region on the right. *TB,* TATA box; *E.Tr,* beginning of early transcription; *L.Tr,* beginning of late transcription (at multiple sites in SV40); *Ori.,* origin of replication; *I, II, III, 1, 2, 3, A, B, C,* binding sites for LT. Distances are in base pairs from the origin. (Data from Frisque RJ, Bream GL, Cannella MT: J Virol 51:458, 1984 for SV40; Cowie A, Kamen R: J Virol 52:750, 1984 for PyV)

equivalent to that of PyV MT is carried out by a fraction of the SV40 LT, which, like MT, is present in the cell plasma membrane.

In both viruses LT performs **several different functions** on viral multiplication and transformation. During multiplication, by binding to different sites in the control region of the viral DNA, it causes the initiation of viral DNA replication, blocks early transcription, and promotes late transcription. In transformation it acts like an immortalizing oncogene. In addition, the C terminus of SV40 LT has a function absent in PyV LT, the **helper function** for adenovirus (see Viruses With Hybrid DNA, below).

Of the four **late proteins,** three are in the virions: the main capsid protein (virion protein 1, VP1) and two minor proteins, VP2 and VP3 (the sequence of VP3 being contained in that of VP2). The three capsid proteins are synthesized on three different late mRNAs with a common untranslated leader and different splices (see Fig. 64–2). The VP2 and VP3 peptides end at a common terminator about halfway through the late region; VP1 is read on a different frame. The fourth protein (**agnoprotein,** i.e., of unknown function), small and very basic, is encoded in the mRNA leader; it probably participates in the assembly of virions. Thus, like small bacteriophages (see Chap. 45), the small genome of these papovaviruses expresses several distinct proteins from the same DNA segment in both its early and late region.

Viral **DNA replication** begins after an unusually long lag of 10 to 12 hours. During this time **cellular genes essential for viral replication are activated.** In crowded quiescent cultures infection stimulates the **synthesis of cellular DNA,** mRNAs, and histones to a level comparable to that of growing cultures. It also stimulates formation of **enzymes involved in DNA synthesis:** thymidine kinase, deoxycytidylate deaminase, and DNA polymerase α. The induced thymidine kinase is that normally expressed in growing cells, showing that the cells are converted by the virus to a growing state. This conversion, probably caused by the MT protein with PyV and by the equivalent function with SV40, may be related to the changes the virus induces in transformation; its obvious advantage for the virus would then explain why these viruses have transforming genes.

DNA replication takes place in supercoiled replicative intermediates (Fig. 64–4); it initiates at a palindrome at the viral origin (see Fig. 64–3) after LT binds to the origin region, especially sites I and II in SV40, and then proceeds bidirectionally. Replication is carried out by a complex of host enzymes, including a primase, DNA polymerase α and β, topoisomerases I and II, RNAse H. Some of the viral DNA molecules generated are recycled back to replication; others become associated with histones and are then encapsidated into virions.

MUTATIONS AFFECTING PRODUCTIVE INFECTION. The analysis of mutants (**temperature sensitive [ts], host range, plaque size, and deletions**) identifies **four regions** in the PyV or SV40 genome. Two regions are expressed **early:** (1) Mutations in region A affect LT: they make it heat labile, prevent viral DNA replication, and cause overproduction of early mRNAs by removing the negative regulation of LT. (2) PyV hr-t mutations (for the host range-transformation), which are not temperature sensitive, affect ST and MT Ag and restrict viral multiplication to special cell types. Two genes are expressed **late:** mutations in region B/C affect VP1, producing either heat-sensitive virions or small plaques; mutations in region D affect VP2 and VP3, preventing penetration.

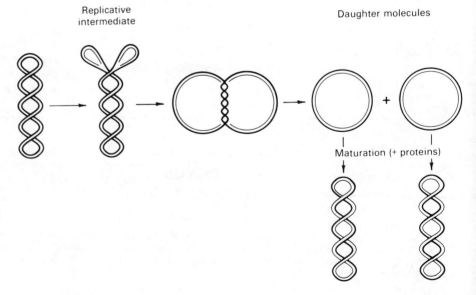

Figure 64–4. Replication and maturation of polyoma virus DNA. The replicative intermediate is partly supercoiled, partly relaxed, and therefore has intermediate buoyant density in CsCl-ethidium bromide gradients. When replication is almost complete, it yields two daughter molecules, each with a gap in the new strand at the replication terminus. These molecules are then sealed and, in conjunction with cellular histones, are converted to chromatin containing covalently closed DNA supercoils. Supercoiling is caused by unwinding of the helix by topoisomerase after it binds the histones.

Replicative intermediate

Daughter molecules

Maturation (+ proteins)

Cell Transformation

After nonpermissive rodent cells are exposed to the virus, transformed clones are usually identified by their distinct morphology (Fig. 64–5), ability to form foci overgrowing a monolayer of untransformed cells, or ability to grow in suspension in agarose or methylcellulose. The various procedures select for different subsets of transformed cells, with somewhat different properties. The number of stable transformed clones generated by a viral sample is much less (10^{-3} to 10^{-5}, depending on the cell type) than the number of plaques on permissive cells. Yet transformation of a cell is caused by a single virion, because its frequency is proportional to the viral titer (see Dose Response Curve of the Plaque Assay in the appendix to Chap. 44).

Isolation of transformed clones in soft agar allows a distinction between cells undergoing **stable transformation,** which form rare large colonies, and those undergoing **abortive transformation,** which form small but much more frequent colonies. In abortive transformation the cells return to normality after four to six generations and stop growing in suspension; however, they continue to grow if transferred to a dish with liquid medium. Abortive transformation is due to failure of integration (see later).

INTEGRATION OF THE VIRAL DNA INTO THE CELLULAR DNA. Cells permanently transformed by PyV or SV40 contain one or a few viral genomes per cell, as shown by the kinetics of hybridization of their DNA with labeled viral DNA. During fractionation the viral DNA sequences are always found associated with the cellular DNA, even when completely denatured to single strands (by sedimentation in an alkaline sucrose gradient). Hence, the viral DNA is integrated, that is, covalently bound to the cellular DNA as the prophage of lysogenic cells (see Chap. 46). The integrated viral genomes are often duplicated in tandem (i.e., head-to-tail) and often have rearrangements or deletions. A fraction of the early region at its 5′ end is always present, because the function of the MT Ag (in PyV) or the N-end of the LT Ag (in SV40) is required for the expression of the transformed state. Integration occurs by a nonhomologous recombination between the cyclic viral DNA and the cellular DNA and needs the activity of the LT Ag: ts A mutants do not integrate at nonpermissive temperature, causing abortive transformation.

To locate the **viral and the cellular integration sites,** fragments containing viral DNA generated by restriction endonucleases from the DNA of transformed cells or from the virus are compared with each other. Evidently, only the hybrid linker fragments (containing both cellular and viral DNA), which derive from the two ends of the integrated genome, differ from those obtained from the free viral DNA, showing in which fragment the viral DNA has been opened at integration. The lengths of the hybrid fragments depend mostly on the integration site in the cellular DNA; hence, these sites can be compared in different clones of transformed cells.

The results show that **neither the viral nor the cellular sites of integration are constant** for the same integrated genome in cell clones that derive from independent transformation events; hence, it is unlikely that integration causes transformation by inserting the viral genome in a specific cellular gene.

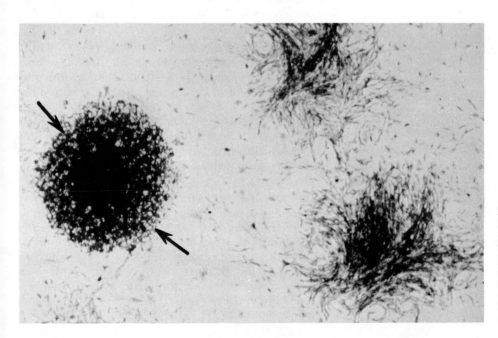

Figure 64–5. Colonies of the BHK line (hamster kidney) infected by polyoma virus. One colony is transformed (*arrows*) and is recognizable by its considerable thickness and the random orientation of its cells. The untransformed colonies are thin and contain cells that tend to orient parallel to one another. (Courtesy of M. Stoker)

TRANSCRIPTION OF THE INTEGRATED GENOME. Only the early region of the integrated viral DNA or the part of it that is essential for maintaining transformation is transcribed in nonpermissive cells. The restriction of transcription is caused by the structure of the chromatin rather than by the specificity of the host transcriptase. Thus, with transcription *in vitro* by *Escherichia coli* transcriptase, chromatin extracted from SV40-transformed cells yields the same RNA as is synthesized *in vivo*.

ROLES OF VIRAL PROTEINS IN TRANSFORMATION. All T Ags are normally expressed in cells transformed by PyV or SV40. The function of the various proteins is dissected by studying mutants and by transfecting nonpermissive cells with vectors that express selected parts of the early regions.

The best understanding is obtained with **polyoma virus,** which specifies three early proteins. With cells of **permanent rat lines** neither LT nor ST alone causes transformation or appreciable changes, whereas MT causes transformation and abolishes requirement for growth factors. With **primary rat embryo cultures** MT causes transformation if strongly expressed; LT only immortalizes the cells. The effect of MT is graded: in cells containing a vector with a promoter controlled by dexamethasone, which can be stimulated to different degrees, the effect varies from morphologic transformation to focus formation, anchorage-independent growth, or tumorigenesis, depending on the degree of MT expression. Mutations, such as hr-t, that alter MT, abolish transformation. The ts A mutations, which affect LT, prevent the onset of transformation at the nonpermissive temperature; once transformation has taken place at the permissive temperature, it may or may not revert at the higher temperature, depending on the location of the mutation. The ST Ag has an accessory function in transformation by both PyV and SV40, especially in primary cultures; in some types of cell it confers a more extreme transformed phenotype. It acts especially on actin components of the cytoskeleton. The cooperation of the three proteins, as in infection with complete PyV, causes the most pronounced transformation of primary cultures.

With **SV40,** LT performs the functions of both PyV LT and MT; the majority of the molecules go to the nucleus and cause immortalization, whereas a small proportion, after fatty acid acylation, go to the plasma membrane as transmembrane proteins, performing functions similar to those of MT. In fact, mutants blocked in nuclear transport still transform cells of permanent lines (an MT function), but not of primary cultures because they lack the immortalization function (an LT function). The transforming functions reside at the 5' end of the LT gene: mutations affecting the other half of the gene do not interfere with transformation, although they may interfere with viral multiplication in permissive cells.

Replication of the viral DNA is not needed for transformation, for many mutations dissociate the two functions. Moreover, SV40 genomes in which the origin of replication is deleted efficiently transform permissive human cells because they do not kill them for lack of late proteins.

ASSOCIATION OF T PROTEINS WITH OTHER ONCOGENE PROTEINS. In infected cells the PyV MT is associated with the phosphoprotein specified by the proto-oncogene *c-src* ($pp60^{c\text{-}src}$, see above) and *c-yes* ($pp62^{c\text{-}yes}$); the complex is precipitated from cell extracts by antibodies to either protein. The precipitate has strong protein kinase activity with tyrosine specificity, which belongs to the $pp60^{c\text{-}src}$ and $pp62^{c\text{-}yes}$, and is strongly enhanced by the association with MT; MT itself is phosphorylated at tyrosine by this activity.

Formation of this complex is very important for transformation, for in MT mutants the ability to transform and to activate the protein kinase is similarly affected. Association with MT enhances the kinase activity of the oncogene proteins. In $pp60^{c\text{-}src}$ this is accompanied by a change of the site of phosphorylation from tyr-527 to tyr-416, as in the *v-src* present in Rous sarcoma virus. Transformation by PyV and by RSV, two unrelated viruses, appears therefore to share a common mechanism, the activation, by different mechanisms, of a cellular oncogene product. The SV40 LT is associated with another cellular phosphoprotein, p-53, which is strongly expressed in embryonic and neoplastic cells. The SV40 LT-p-53 complex also has protein kinase activity, but with specificity for serine and threonine. It is likely that the association is important for transformation.

COMPLEXITY OF TRANSFORMATION. Transformation requires a complex of factors. It involves the expression of two or three oncogenes or their equivalent, the formation of complexes between the proteins encoded by these genes and other cellular proteins. It is affected by the strength of the expression of the oncogenes and by the nature and species of the cells in which they are expressed. All these requirements evidently have the role of minimizing the danger of transformation for cells.

REVERSION OF TRANSFORMATION. Reversion, whereby the cells again acquire normal characteristics, can occur by three mechanisms: (1) **Alterations of the integrated viral genome,** especially deletions resulting from recombination. (2) **Excision and loss** of the integrated genome: in the presence of LT function an integrated viral genome containing the origin of replication can repeatedly undergo local replication. Recombination within the replicated segment may cause excision of a complete viral genome, leading to viral replication in permissive or semipermissive cells (**induction**). This event may lead to death of the cell. In nonpermissive cells, excision of the integrated genome may give rise to revertants if the sequences required for transformation are completely excised. (3) **Changes of cellular genes.** Reversion may be caused by changes of cellular genes that control the expression of the integrated viral genome. Either an "antioncogene" becomes activated or a gene producing a needed transacting factor becomes inactivated.

Changes of cellular genes play an important role in transformation in other ways. They are responsible for the increase in malignancy (**progression**) during prolonged growth of the transformed cells either in culture or in the animal.

IMMUNOLOGIC CONSEQUENCES OF TRANSFORMATION. PyV- or SV40-transformed cells display new antigenic determinants (**transplantation antigens**) that make them foreign in an isogeneic host, and therefore liable to attack by cytotoxic T and other immune cells (see Chap. 50). New determinants are contributed by the PyV MT or SV40 LT present at the cell surface.

SV40 Genome in Transgenic Mice

The microinjection of plasmids containing SV40 DNA associated with a suitable promoter–enhancer combination into the male pronucleus of a fertilized mouse oocyte gives rise to a transgenic mouse with SV40 sequences in its genome. Such animals usually develop tumors localized in cells in which the viral control region can be expressed. If the SV40 genome is connected to its own control region, **intracranial choroid plexus tumors** usually develop, because the virus has tropisms for these cells (see below). If the genome is connected to the control region of an insulin gene, insulinomas are produced. Cells containing and expressing the viral genomes (usually as LT) may remain normal, but if they are kept in culture for a long time they may become transformed. Apparently the expression of the viral genome induces changes in cellular genes that then cause the transformed phenotype.

Role of SV40 and SV40-like Viruses in Human Pathology

SV40, although able to grow in human cells, does not transform them: the cultures grow for many generations until they undergo a **crisis** and die. The SV40-infected cells, however, can be transformed by infecting them with a murine sarcoma virus (see Chap. 65), implying collaboration of oncogenes. The virus is not oncogenic for humans: this was shown in the 1950s when large numbers of people were accidentally inoculated by SV40

present, unrecognized, in early batches of poliovirus vaccine. Epidemiologic studies have since shown no oncogenic effect.

SV40 has a tropism for the brain. A persistent infection is sometimes responsible for the chronic human brain disease **progressive multifocal leukoencephalopathy (PML).** All affected cells have nuclear LT, but few produce virus; they contain nonintegrated viral DNA and express only early functions. The cells are stimulated to multiply, and display many chromosomal abnormalities. These are probably produced by the ability of LT to induce local and generalized DNA replication and nonhomologous recombination.

JCV and BKV are very similar to SV40 in general genome organization. The main differences are in the control regions, especially the enhancers, which determine the type of human cells in which they grow. BKV is restricted to the kidney and multiplies in primary cultures of human embryonic kidney cells. Many adults have a latent kidney infection with BKV, which can be activated by immunodepression. Like SV40, JCV has tropism for the brain and can give rise to PML. The virus is restricted to glial cells, and multiplies in primary cultures of human fetal brain rich in spongioblasts, or in a line of human fetal glia cells (astroglia) immortalized by infection with origin-defected SV40. Transgenic mice that express the T Ag of JCV in the brain have impaired myelin formation with destruction of oligodendrocytes, as in PML.

Both JCV and BKV are oncogenic in some animal hosts. JCV induces a variety of tumors in hamsters and in primates, mostly of neural type. BKV, with the exception of some mutants, is not oncogenic in hamsters, but it collaborates with oncogene Ha-*ras* in transforming human embryonic kidney cells.

An oncogenic simian papovavirus called **B-lymphotropic papovavirus** isolated from a B-lymphoblastoid line derived from an African green monkey is related to SV40 and BKV. It transforms hamster embryo cells *in vitro*. Antibodies to this virus are frequent among humans and primates, suggesting a widespread infection with it or some antigenically related virus.

Viruses With Hybrid DNA

SV40 DNA can integrate in viral DNAs, with which it has very little homology, as it does in cellular DNA. Recombinants with adenovirus DNA enclosed in adenovirus capsids (**adeno-SV40 hybrids**) have been powerful tools for dissecting the function of the SV40 genome in transformation. They were observed in adenovirus grown in monkey cells, in which occult SV40 helps adenovirus multiplication. The recombination occurs in the adenovirus E_3 region, which is nonessential for its multiplication (see Chap. 52). The SV40 **helper function,** which resides in the last 113 amino acids at the C-terminal portion of LT, is expressed in the hybrids and provides an initiation factor required for synthesis of adenovirus late proteins. All hybrids may have various defects in other SV40 functions. Those expressing early SV40 proteins transform cells, which are indistinguishable from cells transformed by SV40 alone.

PAPOVAVIRUS: PAPILLOMA VIRUSES

The first papilloma virus was discovered in rabbits by Shope, who produced warts in the skin of either wild or domestic rabbits *(Oryctolagus cuniculus)* by inoculating extracts of warts of wild cottontail rabbits *(Sylvilagus floridanus)*. The papilloma virions are structurally similar to polyoma virus virions, but somewhat larger (55 nm); they also contain a cyclic double-stranded DNA (about 8 Kb in length). Papilloma viruses are, however, unrelated to polyoma viruses in DNA sequences. Papilloma viruses infect many animal species, producing **benign warts,** called **papillomas,** and probably malignant tumors (e.g., cervical carcinoma in humans). About 50 types are known for the human virus, at least six for the bovine viruses. The types are defined on the basis not of serology, as for other viruses, but of DNA homology: different types have less than 50% homology. The human types form 12 groups on the basis of residual DNA homology (Table 64–4). The genomes of the various types have the same general organization but may differ considerably in length, DNA sequences, and diseases they produce.

Multiplication and Pathogenesis

In most species papilloma viruses induce papillomas in the skin and some mucous membranes in individuals of the same or related species, but cattle virus can also produce mesenchymal tumors in horses and hamsters. Bioassay, based on wart formation in the skin, shows that the virus infects with extremely low efficiency. The ratio of physical particles to infectious units ranges between 10^5 and 10^8. These viruses do not propagate in tissue cultures; the main sources of virus are skin papillomas. Nonproductive infection, however, may occur *in vitro:* DNA of human papilloma type 5 (HPV5) transfected into a line of mouse cells (C127) causes them to grow in agar and form tumors in nude mice; and other HPVs transform human epithelial cells grafted to nude mice. Bovine papilloma virus (BPV) has an especially broad host range: it replicates in both epithelial and fibroblastic cells, causes tumors in hamsters, and transforms the C127 and other murine cells as well as epithelial cells of bovine origin. For these properties it is especially useful in experimental work. Human viruses can produce a latent infection in cervical and laryngeal epithelium.

GENE ORGANIZATION AND TRANSCRIPTION (Fig. 64–6).

All papilloma viruses have the same organization. The genome contains ten open reading frames, eight (E_1 to E_8) in the **early region,** which encompasses 70% of the genome, and two (L_1 and L_2) in the **late region.** Transcription takes place on only one strand. In productive infection, as in cottontail warts, the whole genome is transcribed; in unproductive infection, as in domestic rabbit warts, only the early region is transcribed. Beginning and ending of transcription are separated by a noncoding area of approximately 1000 base pairs, which contains sequences that regulate DNA transcription and replications. A trans-activator of transcription acting on one such sequence is encoded by gene E_2. Transcripts are spliced in different ways, generating several messengers.

TABLE 64–4. Human Papilloma Virus Homology Groups

I	II	III	IV	V A	V B	V C	VI	VII	VIII	IX	X	XI	XII
1	2	6	4	5	9	24	7	16	18	30	34	35	41
	3	11		8	15			31	32				
	10	13		12	17			33	40				
	26	27		14	37			34	42				
	27	27		19	38								
	28	32		20									
	29			21									
				22									
				23									
				25									
				36									

Underlined groups, associated with carcinomas

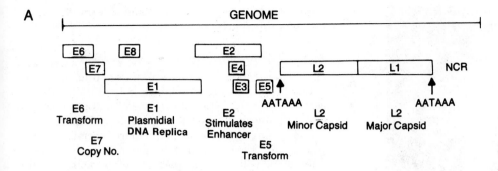

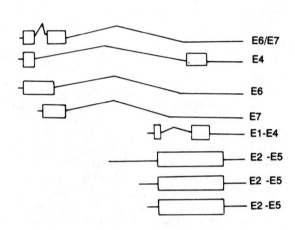

Figure 64–6. (A) The genome of bovine papilloma virus, showing the open reading frames (*boxed*) with their functions (below, two polyadenylation sites [AATAAA]). *NCR,* noncoding region with the origin of DNA replication (as cyclic plasmid), enhancer, and promoter. *(B)* Transcripts of the early region found in transformed cells. Coding sequences are boxed. Slanted lines, spliced-out sequences. (Chen EY, Howley PM, Levinson AD, Seeburg PH: Nature 299:529, 1982; Yang Y, Okayama H, Howley PM: Proc Natl Acad Sci USA 82:1030, 1985)

DNA REPLICATION. The viral DNA is present in the nucleus of papilloma cells or transformed culture cells as cyclic, highly methylated molecules that replicate autonomously but in synchrony with the cellular DNA. The progeny molecules segregate equally to the daughter cells, which thus maintain a **constant copy number** per cell (**plasmidial state),** usually 100 to 200 but as much as 10,000 for BPV in terminally differentiated keratinocytes. Autonomous replication and maintenance of copy number depend on the function of viral genes. Replication requires the activity of the E_1 gene, which has some homology with the SV40 sequences for LT Ag; copy number depends on gene E_7. In the absence of the E_1 function (e.g., in cancer cells; see below) the viral DNA cannot replicate autonomously and persists in the cells only if it becomes integrated.

Oncogenic Activity—Papillomas

Skin papillomas begin as a proliferation of the dermal connective tissue, followed by proliferation and hyperkeratinization of the epidermis. In warts of wild cottontail rabbits the nuclei of the keratohyaline and keratinized layer contain viral capsid Ag (recognizable by immunofluorescence) and viral particles (recognizable by electron microscopy and infectivity). The proliferating

connective tissue and basal epidermis, in contrast, contain neither Ag nor virions (Fig. 64–7), but they do contain viral DNA, which is probably responsible for the stimulus to proliferate.

Papillomas, including human warts, often **regress spontaneously.** If a rabbit has several separate papillomas, they all regress simultaneously, suggesting an **immunologic mechanism.** In contrast, the papilloma-derived carcinomas in rabbits usually do not regress and can be serially transplanted. Presumably they are less immunogenic, or their high growth potential overcomes the allograft reaction (see Chap. 17).

CARCINOMAS. It is likely that papilloma virus infection does not itself cause the cells to become cancerous, but this happens as the result of **additional events.** In fact, papillomas of cottontail rabbits do not regularly evolve to malignant cancers, and then only after a period of 1 to 2 years. The progression is much more frequent in domestic rabbits, showing the role of genetic factors; it is also favored by exposure to carcinogenic polycyclic hydrocarbons. Papillomas produced with bovine papilloma virus type 4 in the alimentary canal frequently evolve into carcinomas in cattle that eat bracken. This fern contains carcinogens that cooperate with the virus, inducing pro-

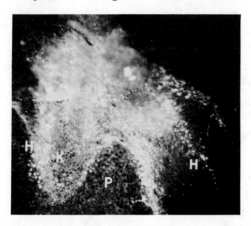

Figure 64–7. Fluorescence photomicrograph of a frozen section of wild rabbit papilloma stained with fluorescent antiviral Abs. Capsid Ag is present in nuclei and therefore appears as small, discrete, bright areas; it is restricted to the keratohyaline (*H*) and keratinized (*K*) layers of the epidermis. There is no capsid Ag in the cells of the proliferating basal layer (*P*). (Noyes WF, Mellors RC: J Exp Med 104:555, 1957)

gression. The rabbit cancers retain the viral genome in the form of plasmids, whereas the bovine ones have only **integrated** viral genomes; they often lack the viral genome altogether, showing that it is required for **initiating** the cancer but not for progressing to the malignant state.

Role of Papilloma Viruses in Human Tumors

The tumorigenic activity of papilloma viruses is demonstrated experimentally by the transformation of cells in culture or in grafts and by the evolution of both rabbit and bovine papillomas to carcinomas.

Several kinds of human tumors are associated with the various types of human papilloma viruses (HPV; see Table 64–3). They include various forms of warts, premalignant lesions, and malignant cancers of various origins, which have viral DNA sequences in their cells. Viral DNA is also frequently detected in anogenital tumors, such as the common genital wart (**condylomata acuminata**) of the cervix, vulva, and anus. Those with irregular mitoses may evolve into **squamous carcinomas.** Regularly associated with HPV DNA is **epidermodysplasia verruciformis,** a rare, lifelong disease characterized by disseminated flat warts and macular lesions, which may develop into cancers after several years. A third HPV-associated disease is the **juvenile-onset laryngeal papillomatosis;** the papillomas are benign but resist treatment, recur stubbornly, and tend to spread through the respiratory tract. Certain types of HPV are typically associated with carcinomas (see Table 64–4), especially types 16 and 18; their presence in cervical dysplasias carries a high risk of progression to cancer. Malignant cancers tend to contain integrated HPV genomes, whereas premalignant lesions

always contain genomes in plasmidial form; the significance of this difference is unknown.

ETIOLOGIC CONSIDERATIONS. The regular association of certain HPV types with several kinds of human tumors, although not proving an etiologic role of the virus, suggests it strongly, especially in view of the recognized transforming and tumor-inducing ability of the virus. For the squamous carcinomas of the uterine cervix this concept is supported by its high frequency in women having intercourse with multiple partners, who themselves also have multiple partners. Such promiscuity appears to favor the spread of genital viruses such as HPV, which is present in human semen.

MECHANISM OF TRANSFORMATION. The mere presence of viral DNA integrated in cells does not entail a neoplastic transformation, for HPV16 DNA is commonly found in the normal epithelium surrounding a cervical carcinoma. The finding suggests that among a population of DNA-carrying cells, some become neoplastic, owing to the interplay of additional events. As to the viral role in transformation, studies with mutant or deleted papilloma virus genomes of animals, especially bovine, as well as transfection of cells with cloned DNA fragments, have identified two genomic regions that are essential for transformation of cultured cells or tumor induction in animals. They are the E_6–E_7 and the E_5 regions of the early part of the genome. E_6 encodes a peptide present both in the nucleus and in membranes, whereas E_5 encodes a small hydrophobic peptide, probably membrane-bound. Each region alone can transform mouse cells, but together they act synergistically and produce a more complete transformation, a situation analogous to that encountered with polyoma viruses. In transformed or tumor cells the two regions are transcribed by two separate mRNAs from which the E_1 region is spliced out. The absence of this gene makes integration the only means for persistence of the viral genome in the cancer cells. In human cervical carcinomas, which contain only integrated viral DNA, the integration is such as to allow expression limited to the E_6–E_7 region. The function of these transforming genes is necessary and sufficient for initiating cell transformation or the formation of benign warts in lower animals, but insufficient for producing recognizable changes in human cells. These viral functions are insufficient for the progression of the cells to the malignant state in any species.

HUMAN ADENOVIRUSES

Human adenoviruses cause a productive infection of human cells and kill the cells (see Chap. 52). Many of these viruses, however, transform nonpermissive hamster or rat fibroblasts, in which infection is nonproductive, and cause tumors when injected into newborn hamsters. Tumors are induced at high frequency and rapidly by viruses of serologic group A (**highly oncogenic**); those of group B are **weakly oncogenic;** the others are **nononcogenic.** Viruses of all groups transform hamster cells *in vitro.* Permissive human cells can be transformed by subgenomic viral DNA fragments, which lack genes necessary for DNA replication and cell killing.

The virus-transformed cells contain integrated fragments of the viral DNA, usually multiple and in nonequimolar amounts, corresponding altogether to a fraction of the genome, sometimes to its entirety. Cells transformed by viruses of any group contain at least **four tumor (T) Ags:** two specified by the E1A region of the genome and two by the E1B regions. They are revealed by Abs present in tumor-carrying animals.

MECHANISM OF TRANSFORMATION. The four genes that specify the tumor Ags are located in the early region at the extreme left segment of the viral DNA (see Chap. 52); DNA fragments containing that segment of the genome can transform cells. These and other early genes are transcribed in nonpermissive transformed cells; late genes either are absent in the proviral DNA or are not transcribed, ensuring cell survival. The cooperation of the four genes has results comparable to those of the polyoma virus early genes. Like PyV LT, E1A has an immortalizing function; like PyV MT+ST, E1B contributes a complete transforming function. E1A, like other immortalizing oncogenes, can cooperate with a *ras* oncogene in transforming primary cells.

The E1A region specifies a transactivator of transcription of viral genes; it also has profound effects on the cellular genome. It initiates cellular DNA replication, often in a disorderly way, causing irregularities in chromosome numbers and chromosomal aberrations, and has contrasting effects on transcription of cellular genes. It enhances the activity of cellular regulatory factors that activate growth-stimulatory genes; it inhibits the function of some viral enhancers, such as those of PyV and SV40. The E1A region of highly oncogenic adenoviruses inhibits transcription of the gene for the heavy chain of the class I major histocompatibility (MHC) antigen in both rodent and human cells, with important consequences for the tumorigenicity of the cells they transform (see below). With the latter effect the E1A region mimics the function of certain regulatory cellular genes expressed in early embryonic cells, which also prevent expression of class I MHC genes. Nononcogenic adenoviruses (such as Ad 5) do not inhibit transcription of MHC-I genes; on the contrary, the introduction of the E1A region of Ad 5 into cells transformed by Ad 12 restores MHC-I transcription.

Cells morphologically transformed (an incomplete transformation) by nononcogenic adenoviruses, upon continuous cultivation, acquire the ability to grow in agar and to produce tumors in syngeneic animals. This evolution to full oncogenicity is comparable to the **progression** of malignant cancers; it may be caused by the chromosomal rearrangements induced by the virus. A similar mechanism may explain how some rodent tumors induced by highly oncogenic adenoviruses retain the tumorigenic property upon loss of the viral genome.

ROLE OF MHC EXPRESSION. **Highly oncogenic** adenoviruses produce tumors that grow indefinitely in immunologically competent syngeneic animals, showing no sign of rejection. Resistance to rejection is apparently due to lack of expression of class I MHC Ags on the tumor cells, which prevents the MHC-restricted activity of cytotoxic T (CTL) lymphocytes (see Chap. 50). Lack of expression is due to the modulation of transcription of cellular genes by the products of the EIa gene, which activates certain promoters while inhibiting others. Introducing an MHC gene by transfection restores MHC expression and abolishes tumorigenicity. Cells transformed *in vitro* by highly oncogenic adenoviruses behave similarly when transplanted into immunocompetent animals. In contrast, cells transformed *in vitro* by nononcogenic adenoviruses express the MHC Ags and form tumors only in immunocompromised animals, such as nude mice, that lack a CTL response. Suppression of class I MHC genes is therefore important for tumor formation in animals but not for transformation *in vitro.*

ONCOGENIC HERPESVIRUSES

Members of all three subclasses (α, β, and γ) of the herpesvirus (HSV) family have a demonstrated or suspected oncogenic activity. They are herpes simplex types 1 and 2 in the α subclass; cytomegalovirus in the β subclass; and Epstein-Barr, herpesvirus saimiri, and the Marek disease virus of chickens in the γ subclass.

All these viruses are able either to immortalize or to transform cells *in vitro.* Epstein-Barr virus, herpesvirus saimiri, and Marek disease virus produce malignant tumors in animals. Moreover, the human viruses are implicated in some human malignancies by epidemiologic observations.

Alphaherpesviruses

UV-irradiated human herpesvirus of either type 1 or type 2 transforms hamster embryo cell cultures *in vitro.* The transformed cells produce tumors when injected into weanling hamsters. Some fragments of viral DNA immortalize the cells, which then become tumorigenic upon serial passages. With intact virus, transformation cannot be seen because the cells are killed. The rationale for UV treatment is that in some virions the radiation, with its random effects, inactivates cell-killing genes but not transforming genes. Using transfection of cloned viral DNA fragments, the transforming region has been located at map units 0.31 to 0.42 for HSV-1 and 0.58 to 0.62 for HSV-2 (see Chap. 53). A characteristic of these transformants is that the infecting viral DNA fragment is unstable and can be lost. Lack of viral DNA sequences, although the cells remain transformed, suggests involvement of cellular genes in transformation.

Human herpesvirus type 2 has been implicated in **squamous cervical and vulvar cancer** in women. However, although the cancer cells often contain herpesvirus proteins, recognizable serologically, and herpesvirus DNA, a prospective epidemiologic study did not confirm an etiologic herpes 2 role. Given the frequent occurrence of herpes 2 infection in promiscuous women, the virus is likely to be an occasional passenger in the cancer cells.

Betaherpesviruses

Like HSV-1 or -2, UV-irradiated cytomegalovirus (HCMV), as well as some cloned fragments of the viral DNA, transform hamster or rat embryo cells in cultures, making them tumorigenic. The fragments assign the transforming sequences to the immediate early region of the genome. However, there is no clear indication that HCMV is oncogenic in humans or animals.

Gammaherpesviruses

Epstein-Barr virus (EBV) was discovered in electron microscopic sections of the **Burkitt lymphoma,** a neoplasm of B-lymphocytes that affects the bones of the jaws and abdominal viscera. The lymphoma cells have a characteristic cytologic appearance and display at their surface immunoglobulins (Igs), all of the same kind in a given tumor; that is, the tumors are **monoclonal.** Subsequently, the virus was recognized in other human cancers, such as the **nasopharyngeal carcinoma (NPC),** some cases of **primary intracerebral lymphoma** and of **lymphoepithelioma-like carcinomas of the thymus,** as well as in **polyclonal lymphoproliperative disorders in immunodeficient persons.** The virus induces a lymphoma in New World monkeys such as marmoset monkeys and cotton-top tamarins. EBV is also the agent of **infectious mononucleosis (IM),** an extensive but self-limiting lymphoid proliferation (see Chap. 53).

STATE IN TUMOR CELLS. Cell cultures derived from BLs usually do not produce EBV virus, but some **producer** lines do, in small amounts. In both kinds of cultures EBV is present in all or most cells as a **latent infection.** The cells contain viral DNA, of which one or two copies are randomly **integrated** in the host DNA; the others (50 to 100 per cell) are present extrachromosomally, as nuclear **plasmids** (as papilloma virus DNA in papillomas). Of the large EBV genome only a fraction is transcribed, generating three mRNAs, which correspond to two regions: one specifying a nuclear Ag, the other a membrane antigen.

The **nuclear Ag** (called EBNA, from EB virus nuclear Ag) is a soluble complement-fixing agent recognized by antibodies in the patient's serum. It contains five proteins. Of these, one is free in the nucleus; another, containing repeats of the dipeptide glycine-alanine, binds to metaphase chromosomes, probably to a periodic structure, such as chromatin. In this way it may regulate the host genome. The **surface Ag,** present in the cell plasma membrane, contains two proteins; it is recognized by immunofluorescence by means of an antiserum to a protein made in bacteria from a cloned EBV DNA fragment. This Ag elicits a cell-mediated immune response against the infected cells. One of the surface Ags confers tumorigenicity on cells to which it is transfected. It therefore appears to be a **transforming gene,** possibly equivalent to PyV MT.

Except for producer lines, no other viral gene is expressed in BL cells; EBV DNA is replicated as a plasmid by cellular enzymes. As with papilloma virus, the replication is **synchronous** with that of the host DNA and maintains a **constant copy number** per cell. Maintenance appears to depend on the action of the EBNA-1 protein on the origin of replication of the viral DNA. EBNA-1 may therefore be equivalent to the PyV LT.

INDUCTION. Viral multiplication can be induced in latently infected cell lines by tumor promoters (perhaps through activation of protein kinase C; see Chap. 47) or butyrate, or, more significantly, by introducing into the cells certain cloned fragments of viral DNA. The expression of two viral genes (EB1 and EB2) generates a *trans*-activating factor, the absence of which determines latency. The first new gene products appearing after induction, before replication of the viral DNA, are several polypeptides of the **early Ag.** In some cell lines no other genes are activated, giving rise to an **abortive infection.** In more permissive lines the early Ag is followed by the **viral capsid Ag** and a new DNA polymerase, which makes **linear viral DNA molecules,** equal to those present in virions; this enzyme, in contrast to the cellular enzyme, is **inhibited by phosphonoacetic acid or acyclovir** (see Chap. 49). These cells release progeny virions. In producer cell lines spontaneous induction frequently takes place in rare cells.

INFECTIVITY OF RELEASED VIRUS. Virus released through induction of BL cells is infectious for human cells carrying **receptors** for the C3d–CR2 component of complement, which are also receptors for the virus. They are present on resting human B-lymphocytes and epithelial cells of oral and nasopharyngeal squamous epithelia, and the prickle cell layer of the tongue. Infected human cord blood lymphocytes are induced to differentiate into Ig-secreting blast cells, capable of indefinite multiplication; they give rise to permanent **lymphoblastoid cell lines,** which are immortalized but not transformed. Cells lacking receptors can be infected by circumventing their need, either by transfection with purified viral DNA or by exposure to the DNA enclosed in the envelope of another virus. Resistant cells can also be made sensitive by the injection of the receptor gene; receptors then appear on the surface. These approaches permit the infection of a variety of cell types.

The ability of the virus to immortalize B-lymphocytes shows that it performs in human cells one of the functions needed for transformation. In New World monkeys it displays a complete oncogenic potential by inducing lymphomas.

VIRAL TRANSMISSION AND CONSEQUENCES OF INFECTION IN HUMANS. The virus is transmitted horizontally. In underdeveloped countries, because of poor hygiene and overcrowding, essentially all children are infected by the age of 3 years. In developed countries infection occurs later, and about 20% of the people escape infection altogether. Primary infection takes place through the throat. The virus productively infects epithelial cells around the oropharynx, which are recognized as being EBNA-positive; they give rise to abundant viral shedding. A small number of B-lymphocytes are also infected, but latently, and are immortalized. These lymphocytes express different Igs at their surfaces (**polyclonal reaction**). Because these cells also express the viral surface Ag, they are killed by the cytotoxic T-cell response of the organism; the infection remains clinically silent. Primary infection in adolescents or young adults through kissing, in contrast, frequently generates infectious mononucleosis (IM). Again, this polyclonal B-cell proliferation is brought under control by a strong T-cell reaction. Most circulating lymphocytes present during the acute phase of the disease are cytotoxic T cells specific for the viral surface Ag. In both subclinical infection and IM the infected person is finally seroconverted, produces Abs to a variety of EBV Ags, and becomes solidly immune to a new infection. Virus production persists for life in the buccal cavity and is the main source of viral transmission. The persistence of the infected epithelial cells may be attributed to their failure to express or to present adequately the viral surface Ag, thus avoiding the cellular immune response of the host.

CONSEQUENCES OF INFECTION IN IMMUNODEFICIENT PERSONS. Immunodeficient persons include organ transplant patients made immunodeficient for safeguarding the transplant and persons with genetic or acquired defects of the immune system. In these persons, infected B cells persist, giving rise to a massive polyclonal B-cell proliferation, which itself can be lethal. In some

cases the disease evolves to a monoclonal lymphoma owing to the occurrence of an additional, rare event of unknown nature. Immunodeficiency may also favor the development of a BL (see later).

BURKITT LYMPHOMA. BL is a cancer that has the greatest incidence in certain areas of the world, especially central Africa and New Guinea (**endemic BL**), where it affects children from 2 to 16 years of age; in other places it is very rare (**sporadic BL**). Cells derived from endemic BL regularly contain many copies of the viral genome, but those derived from sporadic BL usually lack them. The discrepancy suggests that the virus performs a function, probably immortalization, that can also be supplied in other ways. An important factor in the development of BL is the activation of the proto-oncogene *c-myc* (located on chromosome 8) by characteristic chromosome translocations, which are regularly present in BLs. The translocations bring the *c-myc* gene close to one of the immunoglobulin loci. Most frequently the translocation involves the heavy-chain Ig locus (chromosome 14), more rarely the locus for the κ light chain (chromosome 2) or for the λ light chain (chromosome 22). The Ig produced by a particular tumor is usually specified by the gene involved in the translocation: BLs with an 8–2 translocation produce a κ-chain Ig; those with the 8–22 translocation produce a λ-chain Ig. This suggests that the *c-myc* is activated only if translocated near an active Ig gene. There is great variability in the localization of the break point in respect to both the *c-myc* and the Ig genes, but the 5' end of *c-myc* is always altered; this alteration may be the cause of *c-myc* activation. The translocation and *c-myc* activation abrogate the immune response against the surface Ag, probably by reducing its expression; the mechanism is unknown.

The endemic forms of BL occur in areas with high incidence of ***Plasmodium falciparum* malaria.** The suppression of T-cell activity and stimulation of B-cell proliferation caused by the parasite probably favor the development of the tumor. Malaria immunosuppression may also contribute to the early age of primary EBV infection in endemic areas.

BL is therefore produced by three functions. The virus performs the immortalizing function in endemic areas, where infection in children is widespread. The activation of *c-myc* contributes the transforming function; and a favoring function is caused by malaria, probably by allowing the formation of a large population of immortalized B cells susceptible to transformation. In nonendemic areas some other unknown, less frequent event provides the immortalizing function. It is interesting that in BL cells the activated *myc* gene acts as a transforming oncogene as it does in avian cells infected by the MC29 virus (see Chap. 65); in contrast, in rodent primary cells *myc* acts as an immortalizing oncogene. These differences point to the importance of the species of the cells, and therefore the state of the rest of the genome, in determining the effect of an oncogene.

NASOPHARYNGEAL CARCINOMA (NPC).

NPC is one of the most frequent cancers in males in certain ethnic groups in southern China, where a high consumption of Cantonese-style salted fish during childhood appears to provide a necessary cofactor. The tumors contain proliferating epithelial cells as well as lymphocytes: EBV DNA is present in the epithelial cells in multiple (100 to 150) copies as plasmids. As in the abortive infection of B-lymphocytes, only the early Ag is produced. The patients have Abs of G and A isotypes to this Ag. The Abs are useful for early diagnosis because their appearance precedes by 1 to 2 years the onset of the tumor and because they are easily screened; during this time the mucosa displays characteristic hyperplasia and atypia. The titers of the Abs are related to tumor burden, so they are a good indicator of the course of disease.

HERPESVIRUS SAIMIRI.

Herpesvirus saimiri naturally infects squirrel monkeys without producing any clinical symptoms. Virus can be isolated from normal animals and propagated in cultures of owl monkey kidney cells. In New World monkeys, especially marmosets, the virus is highly oncogenic, rapidly producing T-cell lymphomas and acute leukemias. *In vitro* the virus immortalizes owl monkey T cells, making them independent of the interleukin-2 growth factor (see Chap. 47). Immortalized cells as well as tumor cells contain large numbers of viral DNA molecules in stable plasmidial form; it is not known whether the cells also have integrated DNA. This virus is therefore similar to EBV except that it affects T cells rather than B cells. A small proportion of the genome, extremely variable among strains, is responsible for oncogenesis; these sequences are not needed for viral multiplication in owl cells.

MAREK DISEASE VIRUS.

Marek disease virus (MDV), a chicken herpesvirus, causes both a **productive** infection in the epithelium of feather follicles and an **abortive** infection, with neoplastic transformation, in lymphoid T cells; the tumor cells infiltrate many visceral organs and the peripheral nerves. Most lymphoma cells contain little or no infectious virus, but their inoculation into healthy chickens transmits the disease. The involvement of T cells in the neoplasia, and the formation of suppressor cells, leads to severe **immunosuppression,** which favors development of the disease by decreasing the immunologic defenses.

A successful live vaccine against MDV infection of chickens has been developed, using a virus adapted to the turkey that is altered in the presumptive transforming region of the genome. The vaccine has markedly decreased the incidence of lymphoma.

HEPATITIS B VIRUS

Infection with **hepatitis B virus (HBV;** see Chap. 63) is intimately associated with **primary hepatocellular carcinoma (PHC)** in humans, which is the leading cause of death from cancer worldwide, and in some animals, such as the woodchuck, the ground squirrel, and Peking ducks. The virus has wide distribution: more than 10% of individuals are infected worldwide. It multiplies only in cultures of human hepatocellular carcinoma cells and does not transform any type of cells *in vitro.* The virions contain a cyclic, partially double-stranded molecule, which in the cells is replicated by reverse transcription through an RNA intermediate (see Chaps. 48 and 65).

In the hepatocellular carcinomas of man and the woodchuck and in lines derived from them, the HBV genome is found **integrated.** The opening of the DNA circle for integration appears to occur at various places, but the sequences for the surface (s) Ag are usually uninterrupted, suggesting an important role in cancer induction. Often multiple copies (five to seven) are integrated, scattered over the cellular genome. In some cases short direct repeats (11 base pairs to 12 base pairs) flank the genome, as is the case with transposons and retroviruses, to which the virus is related by the use of reverse transcription for DNA replication (see Chap. 8). In cell lines derived from human hepatocellular carcinomas the integrated viral genome and the host flanking sequences are often heavily rearranged, but they may be less so in the cancer cells themselves. The cancer cells may express the surface (s) Ag (earlier termed *Australian Ag*), but not core (c) Ags. The gene for this Ag is in highly methylated form in the cancer cells; in culture, 5-azacytidine, which prevents methylation of the newly made DNA, elicits the production of c Ag. Some cancers do not express any viral antigen.

Experimental evidence for an etiologic role of HBV in PHC is based on the experimental induction in the woodchuck. In humans such a role is supported by a striking correlation between the incidence of PHC and that of chronic HBV infection. Both are common in many parts of Africa and Asia but rare in North America and Europe. In the south coast provinces of China, in which PHC constitutes 50% of all cancer deaths in males and 25% in females, 86% of the patients are serologically positive for s Ag. An important factor for cancer development seems to be infection at young age, frequently from the mother; the infected children end up as virus carriers with chronic hepatitis and develop PHC 30 to 40 years later. A prospective epidemiologic study in Taiwan showed that the risk of PHC is 200 or 300 times higher in **chronic carriers** than in noncarriers. Alcoholic liver cirrhosis does not provide a background for this cancer. In the carriers the HBV DNA is not integrated in the liver cells, whereas it is in the cancers.

The mechanism of cancer induction by HBV is unclear. The virus does not seem to contain any oncogene, nor does the integration activate neighboring cellular proto-oncogenes, as happens with retroviruses (see Chap. 65), because it occurs at random sites. The tumors are monoclonal in respect to the mode of integration, suggesting the need of other events for cancer formation. Rearrangement of cellular DNA induced by the virus may contribute the additional event through alteration of cellular genes. In all likelihood several factors concur in generating the cancer, including environmental factors, such as mycotoxins. The prevalence of the cancer in males may be related to the presence of hormone-responsive control elements in the viral genome.

DNA TUMOR VIRUSES AS CLONING VECTORS

Many viral genomes of DNA tumor viruses have been converted into cloning vectors (see Gene Manipulation, Chap. 8). **SV40 DNA** was the first to be used and is present in several currently used vectors. They contain the basic SV40 replicon, that is, its origin of replication and the LT gene, the rest being foreign DNA. In cells coinfected with a ts A virus as helper maintained at 41°C the hybrid DNA replicates and is encapsidated by the capsid proteins of the helper. The SV40 replicon is also incorporated in plasmids (such as pBR322; see Chap. 8), together with selective markers, converting them into **shuttle vectors,** which can replicate in either animal cells (using the SV40 replicon) or in bacteria (using the plasmidial replicon). The LT gene can be dispensed with if the vector is grown in **cos cells** in which LT is generated by the expression of an integrated SV40 genome.

    Bovine papilloma virus (BPV) DNA is useful as a vector, owing to its persistence in cells, because extrachromosomal plasmids allow easy purification. Sixtynine percent of the genome is required for replication and maintenance. It can accept at least 16 Kb of foreign DNA; with larger inserts it tends to integrate into the host DNA. Fused to pBR322 it constitutes a useful shuttle vector. Foreign genes introduced at the BVP–pBR322 junction are properly regulated in animal cells.

    Also useful as cloning vectors are the EB virus, herpes simplex virus, and adenovirus.

Selected Reading

Baker CC, Howley PM: Differential promoter utilization by the bovine papillomavirus in transformed cells and productively infected wart tissues. EMBO J G: 1027, 1987

Bishop JM: Viral oncogenes. Cell 42:23, 1985

Brinster RL, Chen HY, Messing A et al: Transgenic mice harboring SV40 T-antigen genes develop characteristic brain tumors. Cell 37:367, 1984

Das GC, Niyogi SK, Salzman NP: SV40 promoters and their regulation. Nucleic Acids Res Mol Biol 32:218, 1985

Fluck MM, Staneloni RJ, Benjamin T: Hr-t and ts-a: Two early gene functions of polyoma virus. Virology 77:610, 1977

Greenfield C, Fowler MJF: Hepatitis B virus and primary liver cell carcinoma. Mol Biol Med 3:301, 1986

Hanahan D: Heritable formation of pancreatic β-cell tumours in transgenic mice expressing recombinant insulin/simian virus 40 oncogenes. Nature 315:115, 1985

Hunter T, Cooper JA: Protein tyrosine kinases. Ann Rev Biochem 54:897, 1985

Kato S, Hirai K: Marek's disease virus. Adv Virus Res 30:225, 1985

Khoury G, Gruss P: Enhancer elements. Cell 33:313, 1983

Kingston RE, Baldwin AS, Sharp PA: Transcription control by oncogenes. Cell 41:3, 1985

Klein G, Giovanella BC, Lindhal T et al: Direct evidence for the presence of Epstein-Barr virus DNA and nuclear antigen in malignant epithelial cells from patients with poorly differentiated carcinoma of the nasopharynx. Proc Natl Acad Sci USA 71:4737, 1974

Kovesdi I, Reichel R, Nevins JR: Identification of a cellular transcription factor involved in E1A *trans*-activation. Cell 45:219, 1986

Lewis AM, Cook JL: The interface between adenovirus-transformed cells and cellular immune response in the challenged host. Curr Topics Microbiol Immunol 110:1, 1984

Li JJ, Peden KWC, Dixon RAF, Kelly T: Functional organization of the Simian Virus 40 origin of DNA replication. Mol Cell Biol 6:1117, 1986

Lupton S, Levine AJ: Mapping genetic elements of Epstein-Barr virus that facilitate extrachromosomal persistence of Epstein-Barr virus–derived plasmids in human cells. Mol Cell Biol 5:2533, 1985

Manos MM, Gluzman Y: Simian Virus 40 large T-antigen point mutants that are defective in viral DNA replication but competent in oncogenic transformation. Mol Cell Biol 4:1125, 1984

McKnight S, Tjian R: Transcriptional selectivity of viral genes in mammalian cells. Cell 46:795, 1986

Mounts P, Shah KV: Respiratory papillomatosis: Etiological relation to genital tract papilloma viruses. Progr Med Virol 29:90, 1984

Palmiter RD, Brinster RL: Transgenic mice. Cell 41:343, 1985

Rassoulzadegan M, Cowie A, Carr A et al: The roles of individual polyoma virus early proteins in oncogenic transformation. Nature 300:713, 1982

Ratner L, Josephs SF, Wong-Staal F: Oncogenes: Their role in neoplastic transformation. Am Rev Microbiol 39:419, 1985

Sefton BM: The viral tyrosine protein kinases. Curr Topics Microbiol Immunol 123:39, 1986

Spector DH, Spector SA: The oncogenic potential of human cytomegalovirus. Progr Med Virol 29:45, 1984

Tiollais P, Pourcel C, Dejean A: The hepatitis B virus. Nature 317:489, 1985

Tosato G, Blaese RM: Epstein-Barr Virus infection and immunoregulation in man. Adv Immunol 37:99, 1985

van Beveren C, Verma IM: Homology among oncogenes. Curr Topics Microbiol Immunol 123:1, 1986

van der Ebs AJ, Bernards R: Transformation and oncogenicity by adenoviruses. In Doerfler W (ed): The Molecular Biology of Adenovirus 2. New York, Springer-Verlag, 1984

Wang D, Liebowitz D, Kieff E: An EBV membrane protein expressed in immortalized lymphocytes transforms established rodent cells. Cell 43:831, 1985

Yang Y-C, Okayama H, Howley PM: Bovine papillomavirus contains multiple transforming genes. Proc Natl Acad Sci USA 82:1030, 1985

Zuckerman AJ: Prevention of hepatocellular carcinoma by immunization against hepatitis B. Int Rev Exp Pathol 27:60, 1985

65

Oncogenic Viruses II: RNA-Containing Viruses (Retroviruses)

The family of **Retroviridae** (L. *retro*, backward; vernacular, **retroviruses**) is characterized by the presence of a reverse transcriptase in the virions. It includes several genera (Table 65–1), some of which are not oncogenic. The tumorigenic retroviruses are members of the three genera of **oncoviruses** (Gr. *oncos*, tumor). They induce sarcomas, leukemias, lymphomas, and mammary carcinomas. Retroviruses exist in the most diverse species, from fish to humans. They can be transmitted both horizontally and vertically; occasionally they incorporate and transmit sequences of the host DNA.

The virions are enveloped and ether-sensitive, about 100 nm in diameter; the capsid, probably icosahedral, encloses the single-stranded RNA genome.

Retroviruses have an unusual method of multiplication. Within the cells the viral RNA, released from the envelope, gives rise to a double-stranded DNA copy by **reverse transcription.** This copy moves to the nucleus and becomes **integrated** in the cellular DNA as **provirus.** The provirus is **transcribed** by the DNA-dependent RNA polymerase II, generating RNA copies, some of which are the genomes of progeny virions; others are processed to mRNAs.

Components of Virions

The viral RNA is a positive-sense, single-stranded molecule of about 9 Kb in oncovirus, 10 Kb in lentivirus, and

TABLE 65–1. Retroviridae

Genus	Subgenus	Species
Cisternavirus A Mice, hamster, guinea pig		
Oncovirus B Mammary carcinomas in mice		Mouse mammary tumor viruses: MMTV-S (Bittner's virus), MMTV-P (GR virus), MMTV-L
Oncovirus C	Human	Human lymphotropic viruses I and II (HTLV-I and II)
	Avian	Rous sarcoma virus (RSV) Rous-associated viruses (RAV) Other chicken sarcoma viruses Leukosis viruses (ALV) Reticuloendotheliosis viruses Pheasant viruses
	Mammalian	Murine sarcoma viruses (MSV) Murine leukosis virus G (Gross or AKR virus) Murine leukosis viruses (MLV)-F,M,R (Friend, Moloney, Rauscher viruses) Murine radiation leukemia virus Murine endogenous viruses Rat leukosis virus Feline leukosis viruses Feline sarcoma virus Feline endogenous virus (RD114) Hamster leukosis virus Porcine leukosis virus Bovine leukosis virus Primate sarcoma viruses (woolly monkey; gibbon ape) Primate sarcoma-associated virus Primate endogenous viruses: baboon endogenous virus (BaEV), stumptail monkey virus (MAC-1), owl monkey virus (OMC-1)
	Reptilian	Viper virus
Oncovirus D Primates		Mason-Pfizer monkey virus (MPMV) Langur virus Squirrel monkey virus
Lentivirus		Human immunodeficiency virus (HIV) Visna virus of sheep Caprine arthritis-encephalitis virus Equine infectious anemia
Spumavirus F		Foamy viruses of primates, felines, humans, and bovines

shorter in some defective viruses (see later). Like cellular mRNAs, it has a poly(A) tail at the 3′ end, a cap at the 5′ end. Electron micrographs of the RNA extracted from several type C viruses show that **each virion contains two RNA molecules** held together by a dimer linkage structure near the 5′ end. The RNA dimer (70S) separates upon denaturation into the two genetically identical molecules; hence, the virion is **diploid.** The virions also contain some cellular RNAs of low molecular weight; among them are tRNAs, which, as seen below, perform an essential function.

As shown in Fig. 65–1, the viral RNA contains three basic genes: *gag, pol,* and *env* in 5′ to 3′ direction. Human oncoviruses have an additional gene, and lentiviruses have five (see below). The two ends of the RNA have distinctive features, which, as will be seen below, are very important for the functions of the virus. The 5′ end contains, in 5′ to 3′ direction, the **cap; a terminal redundancy (R)** of from 10 to 80 nucleotides, depending on the virus; the **U5 sequence** (meaning unique 5′); and the **primer binding site** (PBS) of 16 to 18 nucleotides complementary to the 3′ end of a tRNA, which is bound to it. Avian viruses have tryptophan tRNA; murine and feline viruses have proline tRNA; the mouse mammary tumor virus and lentiviruses have lysine tRNA. The bound tRNA is the **primer** for reverse transcription. The AUG codon at beginning of the **gag** protein is several hundred nucleotides beyond the cap site. In this interval there are two important sequences: the **dimer linkage site (DLS),** where the two copies of the RNA present in virions are held together, and the **packaging signal** (ψ), which allows the packaging of the RNA in the virions.

The 3′ end contains, beyond the end of the *env* gene: the **+ strand primer region** (+P) of 12 bases rich in purines, which is important in reverse transcription; the **unique (U3) sequence,** which contains important signals for the transcription of the provirus; the **terminal redundancy (R),** identical to that at the 5′ end; and a **poly(A)** chain. The U3 sequence is quite long and variable in different viruses. It has 150 to 170 bases in type C avian oncoviruses, but over 1200 in mouse mammary tumor virus (type B), which has the only U3 sequence with an open reading frame capable of encoding a small protein.

The general organization of the genome, with its terminal repeats enclosing the genes, is similar to that of bacterial and eukaryotic transposons (see Chap. 8). Additional similarities will emerge later.

Multiplication (Fig. 65–2)

Most retroviruses are not cytopathic and do not appreciably alter the metabolism of the cells they infect. In cultures, infected cells continue to multiply while releasing progeny particles. The adsorption of virions (through

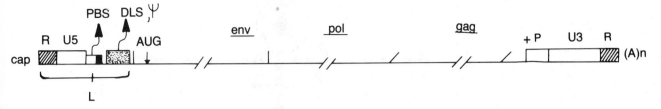

Figure 65–1. Features of a retroviral genome. *R*, terminal redundancy; *U5*, unique 5′ end region; *PBS*, primer binding site; *DLS*, dimer linkage site; ψ, packaging signal; *AUG*, initiation codon for *gag* protein synthesis; +*P*, plus-strand primer region; *U3*, unique 3′ end region; *L*, leader region; (*A*)*n*, poly(A). *gag, pol,* and *env* are the three genes.

their glycoproteins to specific cell receptors) and penetration take place as with other enveloped viruses (see Chap. 48).

The outstanding feature of oncovirus multiplication is the **DNA intermediate** in the replication of the viral RNA. Such an intermediate was predicted by Temin from the extraordinary sensitivity of oncornavirus multiplication to agents that inhibit DNA replication or transcription (BUdR, FUdR, or actinomycin D) and from the presence of sequences complementary to the viral RNA in the DNA of infected cells. The ability of this DNA to infect other cells, which then produce virus, later supplied direct evidence for a viral DNA.

Less than 1 hour after infection of growing chicken cells with an avian oncovirus, viral DNA synthesis begins in the cytoplasm. A continuous **minus strand** (complementary to the viral RNA) is made by the viral reverse transcriptase (Fig. 65–3), and even before it is completed, the synthesis of the **plus DNA** strand (complementary to the minus strand) begins. When the minus strand is completed, the part of the viral RNA still paired to it is degraded by RNase H.

Initially, the viral DNA is a double-stranded **linear** molecule containing gaps, with a continuous minus strand and a discontinuous plus strand. Between 6 and 9 hours after infection the gaps are filled, and the DNA moves to the nucleus and becomes **cyclic;** by 24 hours several DNA molecules have become integrated in the cellular DNA as **proviruses** at different random sites in each cell. The **linear, cyclic,** and **proviral forms** of the viral DNA contain a complete genome because they are **all infectious.** The viral DNA does not undergo independent replication either in linear or in cyclic form, because it is not a complete replicon. Progeny RNA is generated by regular transcription of the integrated provirus.

As a consequence of this method of replication the **double-stranded viral DNA is different from the virions' RNA,** having increased its length by 500 to 600 nucleotides. The differences are at the two ends, which have become equal (Fig. 65–4); they are known as **long terminal repeats (LTRs).** Each LTR consists, in the 5′ to 3′ direction, of a U5, R, and U3 region. Each LTR contains

a signal for cap addition, a TATA and a CAT site determining the beginning of transcription, as well as a site for addition of poly(A). The provirus utilizes only the initiation signals of the upstream (5′) LTR because the advancing transcription interferes with initiation at the downstream LTR. The 3′ LTR contributes the termination signals but can initiate transcription if the 5′ LTR is missing. Like the insertion sequences present at each end of bacterial transposons, each LTR has at the two ends short direct repeats of the cellular integration site (five to 13 base pairs in different proviruses).

A salient feature of LTRs is a **transcriptional enhancer** (see Chap. 64), consisting of a tandem repeat of an 85-base-pair (in a murine virus) sequence, which upon interaction with trans-acting factors of both viral and cellular origin, controls the rate of transcription in *cis.* Enhancers have cell-specific activity: the range is broad for some oncoviruses that are transcribed in many kinds of cells, narrow for others. In this way the LTRs contribute to determining the viral host range.

INTEGRATION

The LTRs are crucial in the integration of the viral DNA into the cellular DNA. Only covalently closed cyclic molecules, with the two LTRs connected end to end in a direct repeat, are integrated (Fig. 65–5). The integrase cuts the two strands separately at the U5–U3 junction; it makes two staggered cuts in the cellular DNA and inserts the viral DNA into it. After the gaps are repaired, the inserted viral DNA, or **provirus,** is four base pairs shorter than the cyclic DNA (they will be replaced at the next reverse transcription) and is flanked by the short repeats of cellular DNA, which are the hallmark of integrated transposons (see Chap. 8). Regular transcription, initiating at the 5′ LTR and ending at the 3′ LTR, generates the viral RNA present in virions. These proviruses are rarely excised by recombination between the LTRs.

The complex method of retroviral genome replication is similar to that of other eukaryotic transposons, such as the Ty elements of yeast and the *copia*-like elements of *Drosophila.* It also has some similarity to the mechanism

(Text continues on p 1128.)

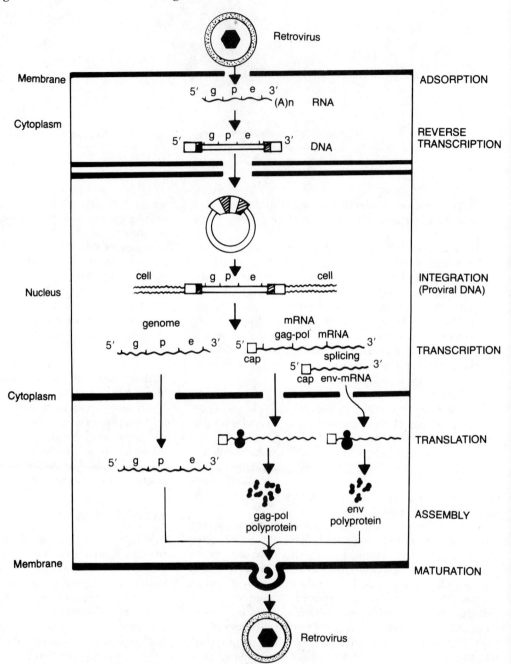

Figure 65–2. The retroviral life cycle, from entry of the infecting virions (*above*) to release of progeny virions (*below*). (Modified from Verma I: In Becker Y [ed]: Replication of viral and cellular genomes, p 275. Boston, Martinus Nijhoff, 1983)

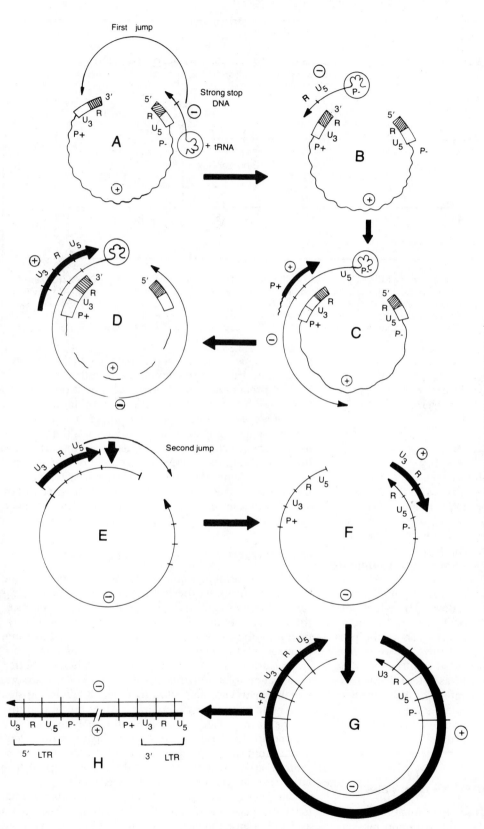

Figure 65–3. Model of reverse transcription of a retrovirus RNA. *(A)* Synthesis of the minus(−)-strand DNA initiates at the tRNA primer bound to the primer binding site (*P−*) close to the 5' end of the RNA and continues to the 5' end. This step yields the **strong stop DNA** attached to the tRNA primer. *(B)* The strong stop DNA (−) has "jumped" to the terminal redundancy (*R*) at the 3' end of the RNA. *(C)* The minus DNA strand grows toward the 5' end of the RNA. At the same time plus-strand synthesis begins at an RNA primer connected to the viral DNA minus strand at the plus primer binding region (*P+*) in proximity to its 5' end. The primer is isolated by the RNase H function of the reverse transcriptase from the viral RNA. *(D)* The plus DNA strand grows toward the tRNA primer and stops at its beginning. *(E)* The tRNA primer and the viral RNA are degraded by RNase H. *(F)* The plus DNA has "jumped" to the other (3') end of the minus DNA strand. *(G)* Both plus and minus strands are completed, generating a double-stranded DNA molecule bounded by two LTRs *(H)*. The "jumps" must be considered exchanges between the two ends, which are held in close proximity by proteins, including the reverse transcriptase. The exchanges may occur between ends of the same molecule or between those of the two molecules forming a dimer in the virions. (Modified from Verma I: In Becker Y [ed]: Replication of Viral and Cellular Genomes, p 275. Boston, Martinus Nijhoff, 1983)

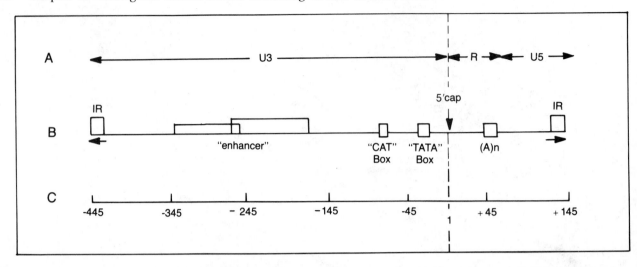

Figure 65–4. Organization of one of the LTRs flanking an Mo-MuLV provirus. *(A)* The main LTR regions (symbols are as in Fig. 65–1). *(B)* Map of the LTR. *IR,* inverted repeats of 11 base pairs in the integrated LTR. The unintegrated DNA contains two additional A-T pairs at each end. *"TATA" Box* is the polymerase II initiation site; *"CAT" Box* is a sequence associated with polymerase II activity; *(A)n* is the signal for poly(A) addition; *5' cap* is the site for cap addition *(arrow).* When the provirus is transcribed, the cap site (nucleotide #1) marks the beginning of the RNA. *(C)* Distances in base pairs. (Modified from Verma I: In Becker Y [ed]: Replication of Viral and Cellular Genomes, p 275. Boston, Martinus Nijhoff, 1983)

of integration of temperate bacteriophages, such as lambda (see Chap. 46). In fact, the site created by the joining of the two LTRs in the cyclic molecules is referred to as the **att** site, and the integrase is referred to as the **int** enzyme.

REVERSE TRANSCRIPTASE

The crucial protein reverse transcriptase, specified by gene *pol,* is a multifunctional enzyme with the following activities: (1) **RNA-dependent DNA polymerase** that builds a DNA strand complementary to the **template** plus RNA strand as an extension of the tRNA bound to the template acting as primer. The two strands remain together in a **hybrid** (RNA–DNA) **helix.** (2) **DNA-dependent DNA polymerase,** which builds a plus DNA strand complementary to the newly built strand, generating a double-stranded DNA helix. (3) **RNase H,** which degrades the RNA strand in RNA–DNA hybrids, leaving an oligonucleotide as primer for the synthesis of the plus DNA strand, and cuts off the primer tRNA. (4) **Integrase,** which integrates the double-stranded viral DNA into the cellular DNA. The polymerase, RNase H, and integrase functions are carried out by separate parts of the protein. Of the various functions only the integrase is virus-specific; the enzyme of one virus performs the other functions on the RNAs of all other viruses and on nonviral RNAs.

SYNTHESIS OF VIRAL PROTEINS (Fig. 65–6)

Synthesis of viral proteins begins at the same time as that of the viral DNA and takes place on two main messen-

gers. A 35S messenger, probably identical to the RNA that ends up in virions, is the template for synthesis of the *gag* protein precursor. The adjacent *pol* gene is out of frame with *gag* and is read 5% of the time by frame-shifting ribosomes, generating a *gag–pol* polyprotein. A second 24S messenger, spliced from the 35S RNA, is the template for the *env* precursor, which is also read on a different frame. The various precursors (*gag* polyprotein, *gag–pol* polyprotein, *env* polyprotein) are later cleaved into the final products (see Fig. 65–6). Processing is carried out by a viral protease recognizing cysteine, which is specified by a sequence between the *gag* and *pol* sequences.

MATURATION (see Fig. 65–2; Fig. 65–7)

The *env* polyprotein enters the tubes of the endoplasmic reticulum during synthesis and moves to the Golgi apparatus, where it is glycosylated. From the Golgi it moves to the plasma membrane. Most of the *gag* polyprotein remains in the cytosol, but a fraction follows the same pathway of the *env* polyprotein, is glycosylated, and reaches the outer side of the plasma membrane. About 8 hours after infection the *gag* and *gag–pol* precursors, together with viral RNA, start to assemble nucleocapsids under the cell plasma membrane while budding of the virions takes place (Fig. 65–8); the polyproteins are cleaved in the process. The nucleocapsids bind to *env* polyprotein, which is then cleaved into the transmembrane matrix protein p15E and the external gp 70. The latter remains bound to p15E by S–S bonds.

The packaging sequence ψ of the viral RNA is essential for nucleocapsid assembly. If it is deleted, no virions are assembled, but the virus can supply the proteins to an

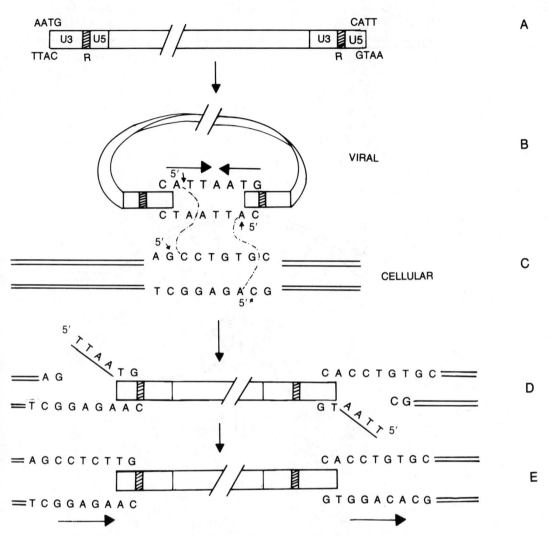

Figure 65–5. Integration of proviral DNA. *(A)* Linear form of proviral DNA. It closes covalently to form a circle (*small arrows*). *(B* and *C)* The integrase function of the polymerase makes two staggered cuts in the cellular DNA and two in the viral DNA (*large arrows*). The 3' ends of the cut viral DNA join the 5' ends of the cut cellular DNA. *(D)* Four bases of the proviral DNA are removed at each end (*underlined*). *(E)* The gaps are filled by copying the two single-stranded cellular sequences, generating two direct repeats (*arrows*). (Modified from Panganiban AT: Cell 42:5, 1985)

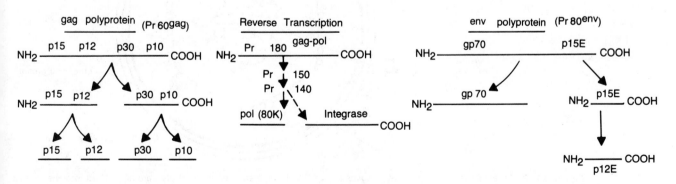

Figure 65–6. Processing of the polyproteins of a murine retrovirus. *Pr,* precursor protein.

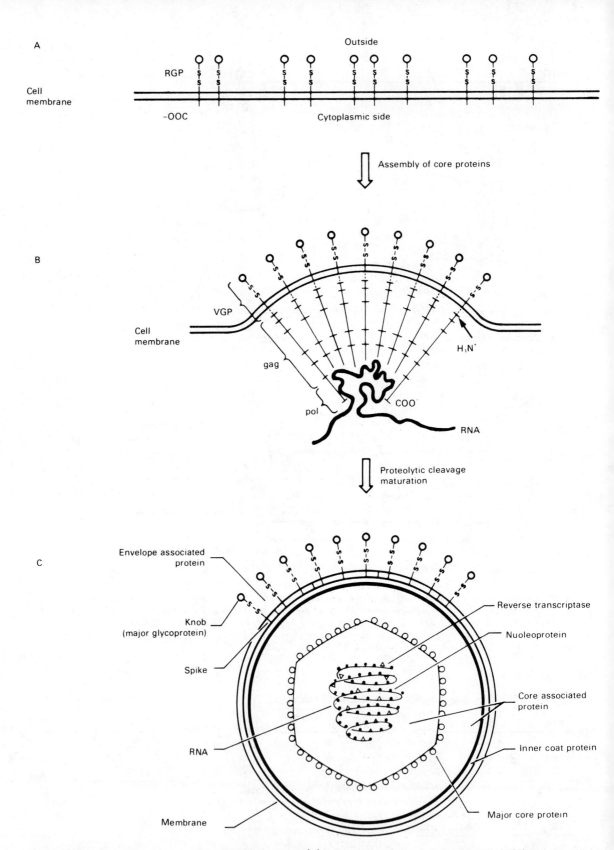

Figure 65–7. Assembly and maturation of a leukosis virus. *(A)* Incorporation of the viral glycoproteins (*VGP*) into the cellular membrane. *(B)* Assembly of the core polyprotein under the cellular membrane; interaction with VGP and viral RNA. *(C)* Mature virions. (Modified from Bolognesi DP et al: Science 199:183, 1978. Copyright 1978 by the American Association for the Advancement of Science)

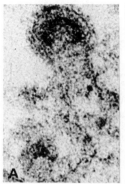
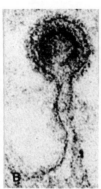
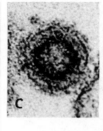
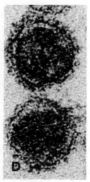

Figure 65–8. Thin sections of type C particles from cells producing a mouse leukosis virus. *(A* and *B)* Two phases of budding of the virions at the cell surface. *(C)* Detached immature virion, with an electron-lucent nucleoid. *(D)* Two mature particles with dense nucleoids. (Courtesy of L. Dmochowski)

intact genome, which will then be assembled. The packaging sequence is present in the 35S RNA but not in the *env* mRNA, from which it is removed with the intron; lacking the sequence, this messenger is not packaged. This explains why only genomic RNA is present in virions. Moving the packaging sequence to the 3' end of the genome by *in vitro* DNA recombination allows the packaging of *env* messengers.

PHENOTYPIC MIXING

In cells infected by more than one kind of oncovirus some progeny virions contain glycoproteins not specified by the enclosed genome. In this way defective genomes, incapable of specifying virions' proteins, can form virions in a cell that is also infected by a normal genome, which acts as **helper.** The glycoproteins may even derive from an **unrelated virus,** such as vesicular stomatitis virus (VSV). Such **pseudotypes** have a **host range determined by the envelope,** which may be broader than the host range of the genotype. Thus, a murine sarcoma virus genome in an envelope derived from a feline or primate virus can induce tumors in the usual host of the latter virus.

Genetics

Many markers are available for genetic studies in both avian and murine viruses: **temperature-sensitive (ts) mutations** affecting the reverse transcriptase or the cell-transforming ability; differences in the **host range** or **antigenicity** determined by the glycoproteins; differences in the **electrophoretic mobility** of individual proteins; **restriction endonuclease fingerprints** of the various forms of the viral DNA; and, for Rous sarcoma virus (RSV), morph mutants (see Fig. 65–11), which produce **transformed cells of fusiform,** rather than round, morphology.

Oncoviruses have a **high mutation frequency,** suggesting frequent errors by the reverse transcriptase. For example, an avian sarcoma virus unable to infect duck cells generates mutants that are able to do so, with a frequency of 10^{-4} to 10^{-5} per generation.

In genetic crosses with avian viruses **the frequency of recombination is very high,** 10% to 20% between *env* and *pol* and between *env* and *src.* Indeed, the progeny may have undergone two to five crossovers per molecule. Vogt has proposed that this high frequency, far exceeding that of any other animal virus (DNA or RNA), is due to the diploidy of the virions. It can be shown that in crosses between two strains with different markers **heterozygous virions** are produced during the first multiplication cycle. In the next cycle they generate recombinants, possibly because the synthesis of the minus DNA strand frequently switches from one RNA molecule to its partner (after the initial switch required for replication; see Fig. 65–3). Recombination has helped in **mapping** the viral genes, establishing their order as shown in Figure 65–1.

Viral Assay

IN VITRO. Virus can be identified and assayed by several characteristics. In fibroblastic cultures oncogene-carrying viruses transform cells, which then form colonies **(foci)** over the normal resting cells. **Syncytial plaques** are produced by the fusion of XC cells (rat cells transformed by RSV) plated together with cells infected by murine leukosis viruses. **Immunofluorescence plaques,** revealed by fluorescent Abs to a viral Ag, are produced by many viruses. Virions in sufficient concentrations are assayed by measuring the **reverse transcriptase activity.**

IN VIVO. Some assays use as endpoints the induction of leukemias or tumors; the production of spleen foci is used for Friend virus (Fig. 65–9), and an increase in spleen weight is used for Rauscher virus.

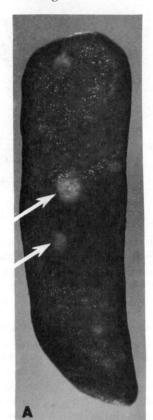

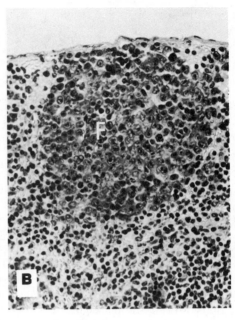

Figure 65–9. Foci in the spleen of C3H mice inoculated with Friend leukemia virus. *(A)* Macroscopic appearance of the foci *(arrows)* in whole spleen. *(B)* Microscopic appearance at low magnification of a section of spleen with one focus *(F)*. The focus contains large cells, characteristic of Friend's leukemia. (Axelrod AA, Steeves RA: Virology 24:513, 1964)

Immunologic Reactions of Virion Proteins

The virion proteins possess various kinds of antigenic sites that are useful for classifying the viruses. Abs elicited against the envelope glycoproteins react only with those of the same virus (**type-specific** Abs); Abs elicited against core proteins (**gs Ag**) also react with proteins of other viruses of the same viral species (**group-specific** Abs); some Abs react with viruses of other species as well (**interspecies** Abs). In the mammalian viruses two specificities can be distinguished in the same polypeptide chain of the major capsid protein: gs^1 is common to all viruses of a given species but does not cross-react with viruses of other species, while gs^3 is common to all mammalian (but not avian) oncoviruses, suggesting a **common origin** for all mammalian type C oncoviruses. The reverse transcriptase too is antigenic and contains type, group, and interspecies determinants.

Antibodies to various determinants may have different effects, for example, immunoprecipitation or neutralization. In the presence of complement, antibodies against envelope proteins are cytotoxic for infected or transformed cells carrying these proteins in their plasma membranes (**complement-dependent cytotoxicity;** see

Chap. 50). In the absence of other signs of infection such surface Ags have in the past been mistaken for genuine cellular Ags. Thus, GIX, originally recognized as a thymocyte differentiation Ag, was later shown to be a type-specific determinant of the main envelope glycoprotein (gp 70) of AKR virus. Antibodies against glycoproteins are useful for **preventing viremia** in cats and, consequently, preventing the horizontal spreading of infection. Heterologous Abs, which are active especially toward interspecies Ags, can prevent tumor formation by murine or feline viruses even if administered several days after the virus.

Antibodies against viral glycoproteins in chronically infected mice (especially of the NZB strain) are correlated with an **autoimmune disease.** The same mechanism may be involved in the pathogenesis of human **lupus erythematosus,** because in this disorder the kidneys contain Ags that cross-react with the group-specific Ags of mammalian type C viruses.

Oncoviruses

Oncoviruses are classified (Table 65–2) according to their appearance in electron micrographs of thin sections:

TABLE 65–2. Comparative Morphologic and Biochemical Properties of Infectious Type A, B, C, and D Oncoviruses

Characteristic	Type A	Type B	Type C Avian	Type C Mammalian	Type D
Prototypes	M432*	MMTV	RSV RAV	MuLV SSV BaEV	MPMV
Presence of intracytoplasmic A particles	−	+	−	−	+
Complete nucleoid at budding	+	+	−	−	+
Preferred cation for DNA polymerase activity	Mg^{2+}	Mg^{2+}	Mg^{2+}	Mn^{2+}	Mg^{2+}
Mature particle					
Nucleoid morphology	Centric	Eccentric	Centric	Centric	Eccentric
Envelope spikes	NA	Long, with knobs	Short	Short	Short
Hormone responsiveness of virus	No	Yes	No	No	No

* M432 is an endogenous virus from *Mus cervicolor* containing extensive sequence homology with type A intracisternal A particle (IAP) genes (4). There is no extracellular form of the IAP; budding taking place into endoplasmic reticulum.

NA, not applicable

(Chin IM, Callahan R, Tronick SR et al: Science 223:364, 1984)

mature **B particles** have an acentric core; **C particles** have a central core; **D particles** have a morphology intermediate between **B** and **C** particles. **A particles,** found only within cells, have a double shell with an electronlucent center.

CLASSIFICATION OF TYPE C ONCOVIRUSES

Avian type C viruses have seven subgroups (A to G); murine viruses have three: G (AKR virus), FMR (Friend, Moloney, and Rauscher viruses), and NZB xenotropic; feline viruses also have three (A, B, C). This classification is based on serology, interference, and host range. These properties depend mostly on the envelope glycoprotein.

Serology depends on antigenic differences of the glycoproteins. **Interference** is the resistance to further infection of cells already harboring an identical or related virus whose envelope glycoproteins block the cell receptors for the superinfecting virus. The block is at the adsorption–penetration step.

HOST RANGE. With **avian** viruses susceptibility of different breeds of chicken (and their cultured cells) is controlled by several dominant cellular genes that specify the cell surface receptors; susceptibility is dominant. The viruses are classified according to the genotype of the cells they infect. In contrast, with **murine** viruses, resistance of **mouse cells** takes place at a stage between penetration and integration. It is mainly controlled by the cellular Fv-1 gene, which exists in the *n* or *b* alleles (so named from prototype mouse strains). Virus strains that grow in Fv-1^{nn} cells (e.g., Swiss NIH mice) are called N-tropic; those that grow in Fv-1^{bb} cells (e.g., BALB/c mice) are B-tropic. Heterozygous strains of mice (Fv-1^{nb}) are resistant to both viruses; hence, in contrast to the avian case, resistance is dominant. The tropism of the virus is determined by a *gag* protein; restriction can be overcome by viral mutations generating NB-tropic viruses, or by treating cells with glucocorticoids. Another mouse gene, **FV-2^r**, prevents focus formation by the Friend virus; susceptibility is dominant.

CATEGORIES OF TYPE C ONCOVIRUSES OF LOWER ANIMALS
Oncoviruses Not Carrying Oncogenes

Exogenous oncoviruses, which are acquired by animals through infection, were discovered in mice and chickens because they induce various forms of leukemias after a **long latent period** but do not transform cells *in vitro*. Among the exogenous **murine leukosis viruses (MuLVs)** the Moloney MuLV induces T-cell lymphomas; the Rauscher and Friend MuLVs cause erythroblastosis, and then erythroleukemia, with characteristic foci in the spleen. **Avian leukosis viruses (ALVs)** and **feline leukosis viruses (FeLVs)** produce B-cell lymphomas. We will see below that these neoplasias do not result from the activity of viral genes, but from the activation of proto-oncogenes present in the cells. Some retroviruses of this class, however, can directly produce changes in the host: an example is the **osteopetrosis** induced by an avian retrovirus, a proliferative disease of the bone caused by abnormal growth and differentiation of osteoblasts (the bone-forming cells).

Endogenous oncoviruses, which are produced by proviruses present in the cells, were recognized through observations in inbred mouse strains. Some strains were selected for a high incidence of leukemia at a young age (e.g., AKR, C58), others developed the disease infrequently and at an older age (e.g., BALB/c, C57BL, C3H/He), and some (e.g., NIH Swiss) were essentially leukemia free. Gross found that filtered extracts of AKR leukemic cells could transmit leukemia to newborn low-leukemia (C3H) animals; a virus (called **AKR** or **Gross virus**) was identified as the agent.

Gross also showed that animals of a high-leukemia strain did not need postnatal infection in order to develop leukemia, because their fertilized ova, when implanted into the uterus of a female of a low-leukemia strain, developed into mice with a high incidence of leukemia—evidently **the virus is transmitted congenitally (vertically).** Another murine virus of this category, isolated by Kaplan from x-irradiated mice, produces a low incidence of thymic lymphomas (**radiation leukemia virus**).

Several groups of **avian leukosis viruses** are transmitted vertically. Most induce lymphatic leukemia, with B cells as targets; some do not induce neoplasia of any sort.

ORIGIN OF ENDOGENOUS VIRUSES. The demonstration that murine endogenous viruses are vertically transmitted shows that they are not ordinary infectious agents. In fact, in crosses between high- and low-leukemia mouse strains, transmission follows Mendelian genetics, as expected of integrated proviruses. In the AKR strain all mice have such a provirus, Akv, but individual mice may have several, all evidently copies of Akv. They are probably derived from infection of oocytes by virus generated after activation of the original Akv provirus (see below). This view is corroborated by the production, in the laboratory, of mice with Moloney MuLV proviruses by infecting oocytes with Mo MuLV virus. With viruses that produce pronounced viremia in their host, establishment of a new provirus in the germ line occurs frequently (once every 10 to 30 years of inbreeding). This mechanism also explains the presence in cats of the RD114 provirus, which is closely related to a provirus present in baboons.

Endogenous proviruses (as well as **provirus-related sequences**) are common in the DNA of many animal species, up to 100 or so proviruses per haploid genome. Because detection depends on suitable hybridization probes, many may still be undiscovered.

EXPRESSION OF ENDOGENOUS PROVIRUSES. A few proviruses are capable of generating virus; the majority are not, because they are defective or are not expressed. Expression depends on the state of the cellular genome. Thus, cellular genes determine whether chicken cells containing a RAV-0* provirus will make infectious RAV-0 or just its envelope proteins. Also important for expression is the stage of differentiation of the cells that affects the state of the chromatin at the site of integration: only proviruses located in active chromatin and with undermethylated enhancers are expressed. Expression of proviruses with highly methylated enhancers is promoted by 5-azacytidine, which inhibits methylase activity. Demethylation probably favors the interaction of the enhancer with activating factors, but it is not itself sufficient for expression. Spontaneous induction of proviruses frequently occurs in the genital tract (ovary, placenta, testes, prostate) or in the embryo.

A competent but inactive provirus can be **induced** to generate virus, using agents that also induce prophages (see Chap. 46), such as halogenated pyrimidines, chemical carcinogens, radiations, or inhibitors of protein synthesis. Induction may also occur after infection with other oncoviruses. Each procedure may induce some proviruses but not others in the same cell.

VARIOUS KINDS OF MURINE PROVIRUSES. Each animal generally contains different kinds of endogenous proviruses; the mouse has three kinds. Upon induction, **ecotropic** proviruses, probably of recent origin, generate virus able to infect mouse cells. **Xenotropic** proviruses generate virus that does not infect mouse cells, but cells of other species; the difference is in the *env* gene and the LTRs. **Amphotropic** proviruses—found in wild mice—generate virus that infects both murine and nonmurine cells. The origin and evolutionary state of the latter two classes of proviruses are not known.

CONSEQUENCES OF ENDOGENOUS PROVIRUSES. Endogenous proviruses can have important consequences for cells: (1) Generation of **leukemia** or **lymphoma,** as is the case for Akv. (2) Contributing genetic information to other viruses by **recombination** (see Recombinant Viruses later). (3) **Replication help** for defective viruses in the form of virion proteins or polymerase. (4) **Inactivation of host genes** inside which they are integrated. In the mouse a provirus inserted into a gene for coat color generates the **dilute** mutation. Excision of the provirus (by recombination between the LTRs) causes reversion of the mutation. (5) Insertion of the proviral glycoprotein into the cell membrane may confer **new antigenic specificity** on the cells, or **resistance to infection** by related retroviruses by blocking their receptors (interference). This is the mechanism of a mouse mutation (Fv-4) that renders cells

---

* *RAV*, Rous-associated virus. Such viruses are isolated from stocks of defective Rous sarcoma virus, in which they act as helper. Each one is identified by a number.

resistant to many ecotropic murine leukemia viruses. (6) Evolutionary spreading of the provirus through the host genome by reverse transcription like other eukaryotic transposons (see Transposons, Chap. 8).

BASES OF ONCOGENICITY. Neoplasia develops with a lag of 6 months or longer after the body of an animal is invaded by a replication-competent type C oncovirus generated by either **infection** with an exogenous virus or spontaneous **induction** of an endogenous provirus. The long time is required either for the integration of a new provirus at a specific site or for the production of special recombinants.

INSERTIONAL ACTIVATION OF ONCOGENE. The most general mechanism of oncogenicity is the insertional activation of the oncogene. It was discovered by Hayward and collaborators in the generation of bursal lymphomas in chickens by ALV. In the neoplastic cells a new provirus, absent in other cells, is localized in the proximity of the *c-myc* proto-oncogene, most frequently in the control area at the 5′ end of the gene, increasing its rate of transcription. The provirus is usually defective but always contains one LTR. These characteristics suggest that *c-myc* is activated by the enhancer function of the LTR, which replaces the normal controls; structural changes caused by the insertion or occurring independently also contribute to the activation. Another example is the activation of *c-erb B* by ALVs to induce erythroblastosis in chickens. In other neoplasias the provirus is localized at a number of constant sites in the tumor cells, activating new presumptive oncogenes, the role of which in tumor induction is in some cases supported by their involvement in translocations characteristic of some nonviral neoplasias.

Insertional oncogene activation generates **monoclonal neoplasias** in which all malignant cells (i.e., capable of producing tumors in isogeneic hosts) have the provirus at the same localization. This stage is often preceded by a stage of **polyclonal** proliferation of cells that are not malignant (they do not produce tumors in isogeneic hosts) and that contain proviruses integrated at various locations. The large number of infected cells produced at this stage increases the chance of provirus insertion near the oncogene, which generates the malignant cell. Such a cell overgrows all others, giving rise to the monoclonal neoplasia.

RECOMBINANT VIRUSES (See Fig. 65–9; Fig. 65–10). In murine leukoses two types of recombinant viruses are important intermediates in oncogenesis. They are formed when an ecotropic oncovirus, of either exogenous or endogenous origin, induces endogenous xenotropic proviral sequences and recombines with them. The recombinants are of two kinds: the mink cell focus-forming viruses and the spleen focus-forming viruses.

The genomes of **mink cell focus-forming viruses (MCFV)** are mostly ecotropic, with part of the *env* gene and of the U3 region of the LTR of xenotropic origin. They usually result from separate acts of recombination with different endogenous proviruses. The recombinants are **replication competent** and **dualtropic,** owing to the xenotropic component; in addition to infecting mouse cells, they produce **necrotic foci** on a line of mink lung cells. MCFVs were first observed during the spontaneous development of **thymic lymphomas in AKR mice,** in which the Akv ecotropic provirus is spontaneously induced in various organs after birth, causing viral spread through the organism. Soon MCFVs appear in the thymus, where lymphomas are formed later, at the age of about 6 months. MCFVs persist in the lymphoma cells. Similar recombinants were subsequently recognized in leukemias induced by exogenous MuLVs.

MCFVs in oncogenesis are classified by their properties. They have a **special host range** that enables them to efficiently infect certain cell types not efficiently infected by the parental ecotropic virus. For instance, some will infect only T-lymphocytes, others B-lymphocytes. This property depends on the enhancer in the U3 region: replacing the U3 region with that of another virus may change the host range.

MCFVs have a direct tumorigenic effect: inoculation of MCFV into newborn AKR mice accelerates the production of lymphomas, whereas inoculation of ecotropic

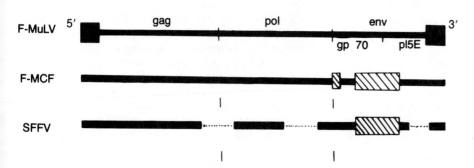

Figure 65–10. Main features of two recombinant viral genomes (FMCF and SFFV) derived from Friend MuLV, compared with the original genome. Xenotropic sequences are shown as hatched segments, ecotropic sequences as solid lines, and deletions as dotted lines. (Gonda MA, Kaminchick J, Oliff A et al: J Virol 51:306, 1984)

AKR virus does not. Clearly, the injected MCFV bypasses the need for *ex novo* formation from AKR. That MCFVs are **required** for oncogenicity is shown by abrogation of lymphoma formation by a mouse mutation that prevents the replication of MCFV but not of the ecotropic AKR virus. The mechanism of oncogenesis is oncogene activation by promoter insertion. In AKR lymphomas MCF proviruses are often integrated at several distinct **specific sites.** One is within (or in the proximity) of the *c-myc* oncogene; others are near presumptive oncogenes designated variously, for instance, *Mlvi, Pim*. Activation of the oncogene is caused by structural changes, increased transcription, or messenger stabilization. As in other cases of insertional activation, the onset of clonal neoplasia is preceded by a polyclonal cell proliferation of non-tumorigenic cells, which lasts until a provirus becomes localized near an oncogene; then this cell initiates the monoclonal tumor. The sequential activation of several presumptive or recognized oncogenes such as *Pim-1*, *Pim-2*, and *myc* in the same cell, appears to bring about the evolution of the lymphoma to its malignant state by synergistic action.

Spleen focus-forming viruses (SFFV) are probably formed by recombination between ecotropic and MCFV genomes in mice infected by the erythroleukemia-inducing Friend or Rauscher MuLVs. They have a structure similar to MCFVs, but with deletions in the *env* region, which is largely of MCFV origin, and are therefore defective. They replicate using the parental MuLV as helper; therefore, each SFFV can exist only in a complex with its helper. SFFV is required for oncogenicity: injected into an **adult** animal the complex produces rapid erythroleukemia, which is at first reversible but then progresses to malignancy through additional steps. In contrast, the replication-competent Friend or Rauscher viruses, which act as helper, do not produce erythroleukemia in adult mice but do produce it when they are inoculated into **newborns;** they must first generate the SFFV.

Owing to the *env* deletion, SFFVs make an abnormal, short glycoprotein, of 52 Kd to 55 Kd instead of 70 Kd, which is incorporated into the cell membrane but not in the virions; in the progeny, SFFV genomes have envelopes containing helper glycoproteins. The altered glycoprotein gene confers on SFFVs two crucial properties: tropism for erythroblasts and a growth-promoting activity for these cells. These changes are essential for tumorigenicity, which is abolished if the recombinant *env* gene is mutated.

The role of the SFFV is to generate the initial polyclonal nontumorigenic erythroid proliferation in which the clones of tumorigenic cells will later appear. For this purpose the SFFV must reach a high titer in the thymus. In fact, an intrathymic injection of helper-free SFFV has no effect; several injections are needed to induce a transient splenomegaly with polyclonal proliferation of growth-factor-independent erythroid cells. A malignant leukemia is only obtained by repeating the injections for many days. In the natural infection a sustained SFFV replication is maintained by the helper; in some of the SFFV-infected cells an additional event leading to malignancy will then occur. The nature of these additional events is unknown. In rats, however, SFFVs are not required: the Friend MuLV by itself causes erythroleukemia, without production of SFFV. (Rat cells do not have equivalent xenotropic proviruses.) The initial polyclonal proliferation is probably produced by the MuLV itself.

In infected animals, a large number of different MCFVs or SFFVs are formed. Only those with sequences especially suitable for performing the specific growth-promoting effect are important for carcinogenesis.

FELINE LEUKEMIA VIRUSES. Cats have two main types of **endogenous** viral genomes. One type is represented by the RD114 provirus, which is homologous to a baboon endogenous virus. The RD114 provirus is present in only some of the *Felidae* species, showing that it was acquired at some point during their evolution, probably by cross-species infection from baboons. Cats have some 20 proviruses of this kind, mostly defective; one or two are replication competent. They are expressed, producing *gag* proteins, in tumors and during embryonic life and are induced, producing infectious virus, in mixed cultures of feline cells with heterologous cells. Other endogenous genomes are related to the exogenous FeLVs and are defective.

The **exogenous** FeLVs belong to three serologically distinct groups: A, B, and C. Whereas viruses of group A occur alone, those of groups B and C occur in conjunction with A and may be generated by it. Oral or nasal infection with exogenous FeLV through saliva occurs frequently in cats; 2% of all cats become persistently infected. Transplacental transmission also occurs. In the cats the virus replicates in hematopoietic cells. The animals generate antibodies to FOCMA (feline oncornavirus associated membrane antigen, a product of the *gag* gene) and to the glycoproteins of the virions. The latter Abs are neutralizing. There is a persistent infection of the bone marrow revealed by appearance of the *gag* protein p27 in serum or by relapsing viremia.

The viruses produce leukemias of both lymphoid and myeloid type, probably by insertional activation of an oncogene; the *c-myc* gene is activated in about one-third of the cases. The viruses, especially those of group C, also produce anemia and **immunosuppression,** through the action of structural proteins of the virions—especially p15E—on immune and erythroid cells. For these multiple effects FeLVs are useful as a model for immunosuppression by human retroviruses (see below).

Immunologic Effect. The virions elicit the formation of neutralizing Abs, especially after removal of the carbohydrate side chain of the envelope glycoprotein. Some of the Abs are cross-reactive among most strains. Abs to the envelope Ags can protect cats against the development of lymphomas. Subunit vaccines reproducing parts of envelope glycoprotein prepared in yeast seem effective in protecting cats against FeLV infection.

Oncogene-Containing Oncoviruses

Oncogene-containing oncoviruses are called **acutely transforming viruses (ATVs)** because upon injection into a suitable host they produce tumors within a few months. They also transform fibroblastic cells *in vitro*, producing characteristic **foci** (Fig. 65–11) that are useful for assay. Both properties are due to the presence of an activated oncogene (see Oncogenes, Chap. 64) in the viral genome. Peyton Rous isolated the first strain of ATV, which is known as **Rous sarcoma virus (RSV),** from a chicken with a spontaneous sarcoma. Many other strains were subsequently isolated in various species.

ATVs are all **defective,** with the exception of two RSV strains (Prague C, Schmidt-Ruppin), and all contain one or more oncogenes in replacement for normal viral sequences (Fig. 65–12). The two nondefective RSV strains, which also contain an oncogene, were probably generated from a defective genome by recombination with other oncoviruses. The oncogenes were captured by rare illegitimate recombination with the normal proto-oncogenes of the cells, in which both viral genes and the proto-oncogene were altered. Deletions of the viral genome explain the defectiveness of ATVs; alteration of the proto-oncogene explains its activation (see Oncogenes, Chap. 64).

The deleted genomes of ATVs, being **replication defective,** require a **helper** for their multiplication; ATVs are then generated as **pseudotypes** with helper envelope. **Nonproducer** transformed cells, which do not contain helper, can be obtained by transforming cells at low multiplicity with the ATV–helper mixture—to obtain cells infected by ATV alone—or, in the murine system, using helper-free ATV. Such virus is obtained from cells harboring a Ψ-free helper, which helps the production of ATV but is not itself packaged into virions.

AVIAN SARCOMA VIRUSES (Table 65–3). The prototype is the Rous sarcoma virus, but the group contains many other viruses unrelated to it. RSV contains the oncogenic *v-src,* which is inserted in replacement of *env* sequences, and is transcribed by a special short mRNA in which it is connected directly to the leader sequence.

ROLE OF **v-src.** The *v-src* oncogene encodes a tysosine-specific protein kinase, the phosphoprotein $pp60^{v-src}$, which is endowed with much higher activity than the product of *c-src.* Transformation is caused by the activity of the kinase, for when cells transformed by ts mutants in the *src* gene are shifted to a nonpermissive temperature, they lose the transformed phenotype within an hour, as soon as the *v-src* protein is denatured. Deletions within the *v-src* gene give rise to **transformation-defective (Td)** strains. When injected into chickens, some of them

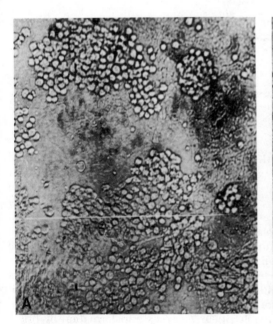 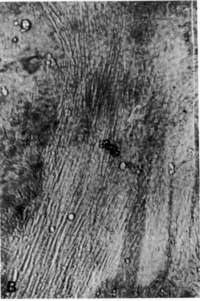

Figure 65–11. Transformation of cultures of the iris of the chick embryo by either wild-type Rous sarcoma virus (*A*) or its morph^f mutant (*B*). Cells transformed by the wild-type virus are round, whereas those transformed by morph^f virus are fusiform and form bundles. The untransformed cells form an epitheliumlike sheet and can be recognized because they contain various amounts of black pigment, whereas both kinds of transformed cells are almost colorless. (Courtesy of B. Ephrussi and H. Temin)

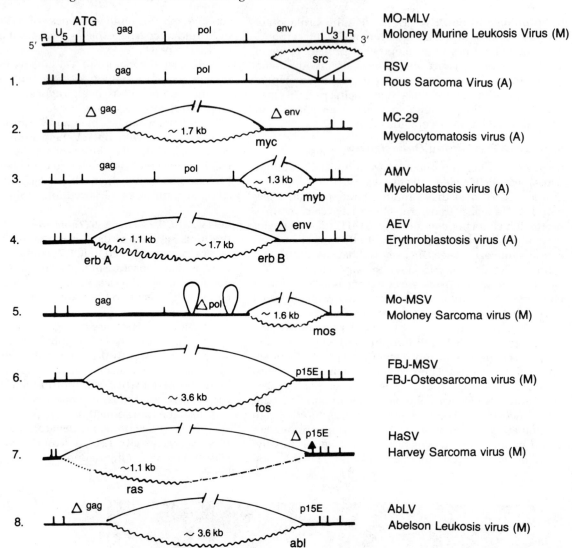

Figure 65–12. Organization of viral genomes containing oncogenes, compared with the Moloney murine leukemia virus (*Mo-MuLV, top*). Wavy lines indicate oncogenes, with attached denominations. Dotted lines at *7* indicate sequences derived from a rat endogenous retrovirus; thin lines indicate deleted MuLV sequences; heavy lines indicate retained sequences. A triangle preceding a gene indicates that the gene is truncated. AEV (*4*) has two oncogenes.

unexpectedly produce tumors, which, in contrast to those induced by regular RSV, arise after a lag period of many months, and far from the site of inoculation. Hanafusa isolated oncogenic virus from the unusual tumors and showed that it is derived by recombination of the Td RSV genome with the cellular *src* proto-oncogene. Rescue only takes place if the 3′ end of the *v-src* oncogene persists in the Td mutants; these sequences are essential for conferring a high tumorigenic activity on *v-src*. Complete replacement of *v-src* with the *c-src* proto-oncogene abolishes the transforming activity; a single amino acid replacement in *c-src* can restore it if the gene is strongly expressed. Strong expression of *v-src* and of other oncogenes as well, however, can be lethal for the cells, showing that transformation depends on a delicate balance of genes.

For transformation, pp60^{v-src} must be connected to the cell plasma membrane through a fatty acid (myristic acid) bound to its N-terminal glycine. Replacing glycine with another amino acid, which prevents myristylation, prevents transformation. Mutants in which the protein is myristylated but does not bind to the membrane also fail to transform.

Presumably pp60^{v-src} causes transformation by phos-

TABLE 65–3. *Avian Sarcoma Viruses*

Virus	Genome Size (Kb)	Oncogene	Oncogene Protein
Rous sarcoma virus (RSV)	Varies	v-src	pp60^{src}
Fujinami sarcoma virus (FSV)	4.5	v-fps	p140$^{gag\text{-}fps}$
PR6 II	4.0	v-fps	p105$^{gag\text{-}fps}$
Y73	4.8	v-yes	p90$^{gag\text{-}yes}$
UR-2	3.3	v-ros	p68$^{gag\text{-}ros}$
ASV-17	3.5	v-jun	p55$^{gag\text{-}jun}$
Myelocytomatosis virus MC-29	5.6	v-myc	p110$^{gag\text{-}myc}$
OK10	8.2	v-myc	p200$^{gag\text{-}pol\text{-}myc}$ p57$^{gag\text{-}myc}$
CM II	6.0	v-myc	p90$^{gag\text{-}myc}$
MH2	6.0	v-myc v-mil	p100$^{gag\text{-}mil}$
Reticular endoteliosis virus	5.5	v-rel	p56$^{env\text{-}rel}$
Avian erythroblastosis virus (AEV)	3.0	erb A erb B	p75$^{gag\text{-}erb\,A}$ p44$^{erb\,B}$
Avian myeloblastosis virus (AMB)	7.0	myb	p48^{myb}
E26	5.7	myb ets	p135$^{gag\text{-}myb\text{-}ets}$
Sloan-Kettering viruses	5.7–8.9	ski	p110$^{gag\text{-}ski\text{-}pol}$ p125$^{gag\text{-}ski}$
S13	8.5		gp 155

(Note: MC-29, OK10, CM II, and MH2 are bracketed together as a "family.")

phorylating cellular proteins. Several such proteins are known, but it is not clear whether any of them are directly involved in transformation. Gene activation by promoter insertion does not play any role in transformation, for the site of localization of the RSV provirus in the host genome is different in different tumors. The localization is important, however, in mammalian cells transformed *in vitro* by RSV. In these cells the strength of viral transcription and the degree of transformation depend on the state of the chromatin around the provirus, as detected by nuclease sensitivity, and the degree of methylation of the enhancer DNA.

Tumors induced by RSV in chickens tend to regress spontaneously because the cells are killed by the cell-mediated immune response of the organism to the helper glycoprotein present in the cell membrane.

Other avian acutely transforming viruses produce sarcomas and other tumors different from sarcomas: MC-29 produces myelocytomatosis, endotheliomas, and carcinomas; avian erythroblastosis virus (AEV) produces an erythroblastic leukemia; and avian myeloblastosis virus (AMV) causes a myeloblastic leukemia. These viruses carry a variety of oncogenes (see Table 65–3), which specify proteins of different groups: some are tyrosine-protein kinases, at least in structure if not in function (*src, fps, yes, ros, fms, kit,* and *erb B*), and are associated with the cell plasma membrane. One (*mil*) is a cytoplasmic serine/threonine-specific protein kinase. *Myc, fos,* and *myb* have nuclear localization; *erb A* and *rel* have

cytoplasmic localization. In most viruses the oncogene replaces part of the *gag* gene (see Fig. 65–12) and is expressed in the same messenger. The oncogene protein is then a **gag–onc fusion protein.** Whereas most ASVs have one oncogene, some have two: MH-2 (related to MC29) has *v-myc* and *v-mil*; avian erythroblastosis virus has *v-erb A* and *v-erb B*; E-26 (related to avian myeloblastosis virus) has *v-myb* and *v-ets*. In these cases the added oncogene confers on the virus either more extreme transforming power (as in AEV) or the ability of y to cause different tumors (as in E-26, which transforms cells of the erythroid lineage), showing the importance of cooperation between oncogenes. Cooperation can occur in various ways. In MH-2, which transforms macrophages, *v-myc* is the transforming gene, whereas *v-mil* causes cell immortalization by inducing the production of a growth factor needed by the macrophages themselves (**autocrine growth**). With the reticuloendotheliosis virus, the single oncogene *rel* cooperates in the tumors with *c-myc*, which is activated by the helper virus integrated within its regulatory sequences. This is one of the few cases in which the helper virus participates in causing cell transformation. Other significant helpers are those of avian myeloblastosis virus (called MAVs: myeloblastosis-associated viruses), which by themselves produce kidney and bone tumors.

The **murine sarcoma viruses (MuSVs;** Table 65–4) were all derived from Mo-MuLV during passages in mice or rats. They contain several types of oncogenes; their

TABLE 65–4. Murine Sarcoma Viruses

Virus	Genome Size (Kb)	Oncogene	Oncogene Protein
Harvey-MuSV	5.5	Ha-ras	p21
Kirsten-MuSV	4.5	Ki-ras	p21
BALB-MuSV	6.8	bas	p21
Mo-MuSV	5.8	mos	p37
Myeloproliferative sarcoma virus (MPSV)	7.0	mos	p37
Abelson leukemia virus	4.0	abl	p130$^{gag\text{-}abl}$
Rat SV	6.7	ras	p29
FBJ osteosarcoma virus ⎫ FBR osteosarcoma virus ⎭		fos	p55 p75$^{gag\text{-}fos}$
3611 MSV		raf	p75$^{gag\text{-}raf}$

TABLE 65–5. Feline Sarcoma Viruses

Virus	Oncogene	Oncogene Protein
Snyder-Theilen FeSV	fes/fps	p85$^{gag\text{-}fes}$
Gardner-Arnstein FeSV	fes/fps	p110$^{gag\text{-}fes}$
Hardy-Zuckerman-1	fes/fps	p95$^{gag\text{-}fes}$
Susan McDonough	fms	p160$^{gag\text{-}fms}$
Gardner-Rasheed	fgr	p70$^{gag\text{-}actin\text{-}fgr}$
Parodi-Irgens	sis	p75$^{gag\text{-}sis}$
Hardy-Zuckerman-2	abl	p95$^{gag\text{-}abl}$
Hardy-Zuckerman-4	kit	p80$^{gag\text{-}kit}$

proteins are expressed by themselves, except for that of the Abelson murine leukosis virus, which is expressed as a *gag-abl* fusion protein. Some of the oncogenes originate from the mouse genome, others from the rat genome. In the case of Harvey sarcoma virus, the oncogene is enclosed in sequences of a rat leukemia virus, which presumably captured it first.

Transformation by MuSV occurs in steps, possibly produced by cooperation among oncogenes. In fact, in Abelson MuLV-transformed cells that contain the *v-abl* oncogene, *c-myc* is often amplified and strongly expressed; transformation is decreased when there is lack of expression of p53, a presumptive oncogene protein, or of the EGF receptors, which mediates the effect of tumor growth factor α produced by the same cells. In contrast, in highly malignant cells the *v-abl* oncogene may be absent, suggesting that other genes maintain the malignant state.

In addition to transforming fibroblasts, some of the murine sarcoma viruses affect hemopoietic cells. The myeloproliferative sarcoma virus stimulates the growth of hematopoietic stem cells and of myeloid and erythroid precursors; the special host range is determined by the U3 sequence. Ha-MSV and Ki-MuSV stimulate the growth of erythroid cells; Ki-MuSV, in addition, transforms human keratinocytes immortalized by adeno-SV40 hybrid virus, again showing the importance of cooperation between oncogenes. The Abelson virus causes lymphoid and mast cell tumors.

FELINE SARCOMA VIRUSES (FeSV; Table 65-5). Defective, oncogene-carrying derivatives of FeLV cause sarcomas in FeLV-infected young cats. Virus obtained from the tumors produces fatal tumors in young cats; in older cats cell-mediated immunity causes tumor rejection. Ten different strains of feline sarcoma viruses have been identified. They carry a variety of oncogenes: *fms*, *fes*, *fgr*, *sis*, *abl*, and *kit*. In addition, T-cell lymphomas are produced by a defective FeLV derivative containing the *myc* gene. In all cases the oncogenes are expressed as *gag–onc* fusion proteins. A puzzling finding is that one third of the naturally occurring lymphoid tumors in cats contain neither infectious FeLV nor its genome (tracked through its U3 region), yet epidemiologic evidence shows that they are associated with exposure to FeLV. Perhaps the virus induces secondary changes that maintain the neoplastic state and is then lost.

ROLE OF ONCOVIRUSES IN CHEMICALLY AND PHYSICALLY INDUCED NEOPLASIA AND CELL TRANSFORMATIONS

Though mutagens and viruses have long appeared to provide different mechanisms for inducing cell transformation, they are now understood to act in a similar way: by activating oncogenes. The various agents can cooperate, because many viruses produce transformed foci in cell cultures in conjunction with carcinogens but not without them. Presumably, just as different viruses can cooperate by introducing or activating different oncogenes, so can oncogenes activated by carcinogens cooperate with the viral ones.

After the radiation leukemia virus was obtained from an x-ray-induced thymoma, viruses seemed the answer to physical or chemical carcinogenesis. A viral origin of tumors induced by these agents is not general, however, because many radiation-induced thymomas can be shown not to be virus mediated. Moreover, chemically induced AKR thymic lymphomas lack the integrated MCFs that are regularly present in tumors induced by virus. The unifying factor is probably represented by oncogenes.

Role of Type C Oncoviruses of Lower Animals in Human Neoplasia

Since the viral etiology of leukemias and related tumors in many animal species has been recognized, a possible role of these viruses in human leukemias has been suspected. The viruses of cats have especially been scrutinized, because feline leukemia and sarcoma viruses are shed in the saliva of infected cats and can infect human cells in culture. However, in epidemiologic studies disease in pets does not correlate with human infection.

PRIMATE AND HUMAN TYPE C ONCOVIRUSES
Primate Leukemia Viruses

Type C viruses are present in many primates, such as baboons, Old World monkeys, and great apes. **Endogenous** viruses have been recognized in some species: baboons have about 100 proviruses related to the **baboon endogenous virus (BaEV)**, of which only some can be induced to multiply and release infectious virus; colobus and other Old World monkeys have 50 to 70 related copies of other proviruses. **Exogenous** viruses belong to the **gibbon ape leukemia virus (GaLV)** group, which were isolated from various kinds of tumors or leukemias and induce the same neoplasias in young gibbon apes. To this group belongs the defective **simian sarcoma virus (SSV)**, the only known oncogene-carrying virus among the primate viruses: it carries the *sis* oncogene, which is expressed in a p28 protein corresponding to the B chain of the platelet-derived growth factor (PDGF). Binding of p28, expressed at the cell surface, to the PDGF receptors of the same or other cells is required for transformation, which is therefore based on self-stimulation of growth. In fact, *v-sis*–transformed fibroblasts behave *in vitro* like normal fibroblasts stimulated by PDGF. Additional steps are presumably required for attaining the malignant phenotype in the sarcomas.

Primate leukemia viruses do not show extensive homology with other type C viruses, but share with them some common antigenic determinants of the reverse transcriptase and the p30 *gag* protein. They share gp-70 determinants with D-type primate viruses. T-lymphotropic simian viruses are discussed later, together with human viruses.

Human Oncoviruses

Several types of **endogenous** proviruses have been identified by hybridizing probes from simian viruses to human DNA under conditions, allowing detection of moderate homology. Some are in multiple copies (50 to 100) in the human genome; others are as a single copy. Some have the length and organization of a complete oncoviral genome, but none can give rise to infectious virus, owing to termination codons and frame shifts; others are highly defective. Evidently there has been evolutionary restraint to their expression, which has caused their divergence. These proviruses are related to other mammalian C-type viruses, but some are recombinants with mouse mammary tumor virus (type B) or D-type viruses. The similarity of some of these proviruses to endogenous simian proviruses shows that they originated before the separation of man from other primates.

Human endogenous viruses, although not expressed in adult tissues, are expressed in placentas in which antigens of p30 *gag* are recognizable, and type C particles—probably not infectious—are frequently seen budding from cells of the trophoblastic syncytium.

Exogenous human type C oncoviruses are of a single family, which includes the **human T-lymphotropic viruses (HTLV-I and -II);** they are unrelated to human endogenous retroviruses. HTLVs are similar in organization to **bovine leukemia viruses** and some **simian T-lymphotropic viruses** and differ from other oncoviruses in several properties. (1) They have a very restricted host range, limited to helper T-lymphocytes and other cells expressing the OkT4—also known as Cd4—antigen; this Ag is the receptor for viral adsorption. (2) They induce the formation of multinucleated syncytia in certain indicator cell lines, a useful diagnostic tool. (3) Their *gag* gene is shorter and specifies only three proteins; it lacks the equivalent of the MuLV p12. (4) They have additional sequences that encode a *trans*-acting activator of the viral promoter.

HTLV-I and -II. HTLV-I is associated with a special form of leukemia, **adult T-cell leukemia (ATL),** also known as mycosis fungoides or Zésary cutaneous T-cell leukemia. The closely related HTLV-II has been associated with two cases of hairy cell leukemia (also of T cells). HTLV-I was discovered by Gallo by growing T cells from patients with ATL *in vitro* in the presence of interleukin-2 (IL-2; T-cell growth factor). The cells then release HTLV-I into the medium. Clonal cultures of helper T cells infected by the virus have abnormal properties. They are nonspecifically activated: they have IL-2 and transferrin receptors and provide the helper function to B cells in the absence of antigen, causing polyclonal production of antibodies (see Chap. 16); but some have lost helper activity or are alloreactive. These cells express on their surfaces altered major histocompatibility (HLA) antigens, together with HTLV-I *env* products, gp 61, and gp 45.

RELATION OF HTLV-I TO ATL. An important role of the virus seems likely: the virus immortalizes normal human T cells *in vitro;* and in leukemic individuals the leukemic cells, but not the normal cells, contain the HTLV-I provirus. The leukemias are **clonal,** having the provirus at the same site in all cells of the same individual, although the site varies in different individuals. Clonality shows that a leukemia arises from a single cell already harboring the provirus, excluding a secondary infection after the leukemia was established. It is likely, however, that additional changes are required for generating the leukemic clone.

HTLV-I does not have an oncogene and must therefore act by changing the expression of cellular gene. It does not act in *cis* on a cellular oncogene, because the provirus does not have unique localizations. It probably promotes proliferation of quiescent T cells by changing the expression of cellular genes in *trans* through the expression of the *tax* gene (also present in **bovine leukemia virus**) which specifies a *trans*-activator of transcription. The main effect is the activation of genes for the IL-2 receptor and for synthesis of IL-2, which allow the cells to multiply autonomously. The *tax* gene, located at the 3' end of *env* and extending into the U3 region, is highly conserved among the various isolates of the HTLV-I virus; it is expressed by a double-spliced mRNA, which is not produced by other oncoviruses (Fig. 65–13), and encodes a nuclear 40-Kd protein that acts on enhancerlike sequences present in the viral LTR, stimulating viral transcription. Gene *tax* may be comparable to the adenovirus E1A gene (see Chap. 64). The regular preservation of the gene in the leukemic cells harboring a defective provirus suggests that it plays an important role in leukemogenesis.

EPIDEMIOLOGY. Antibodies against viral *gag* and *env* antigens are present in ATL patients and in some unaffected persons in endemic areas in the southwestern United States, the Caribbean islands, parts of South America and south Italy, many parts of Africa, and the southern islands of Japan. The virus and the disease persist in migrant populations from these areas. Not all ATL cases, however, are HTLV-I positive. The virus is also implicated in a neurologic disease (tropical spastic paraparesis) that is prevalent in areas where HTLV-I is endemic.

OTHER ONCOVIRUSES
Oncovirus B

MOUSE MAMMARY TUMOR VIRUSES (MMTV). Most mice, both wild and inbred, have **endogenous MMTVs.** These proviruses are related to each other but vary in location, number, and degree of completeness. They were probably acquired by different and fairly recent infections of the germ line. More distantly related sequences are either precursors of these proviruses or products of their divergence. The proviruses can be expressed to various degrees, probably depending on their location in the mouse genome. Except for the GR mouse, these endogenous MMTVs seem to play little or no oncogenic role.

Exogenous viruses are important for oncogenesis. The prototypes are the **Bittner virus,** derived from the C3H mouse strain, and a related virus derived from the RIII strain. Both are **high-cancer strains,** in which mammary cancers appear in 90% of the animals by 1 year of age. In contrast, **low-cancer strains,** such as BALB/c, have a 20% to 50% incidence of mammary tumors by 2 years of age.

The Bittner virus was discovered as a result of questioning the seemingly obvious genetic basis of the high incidence of mammary cancers in C3H mice. In 1936 Bittner showed that newborns of a low-cancer strain nursed by females of a high-cancer strain acquire a high incidence and vice versa. This simple experiment revealed that the cancer is induced by a transmissible agent present in the milk (the **milk agent),** later recognized as a virus. The virus is generated in the lactating mammary gland by induction of an endogenous provirus, MTV-1, which in the absence of exogenous infection gives rise to a low frequency of mammary cancers by spontaneous induction later in life (18 to 24 months).

PROPERTIES. The virions are generally similar to those of the C type described earlier, but they differ in some details, such as the presence of spikes (Fig. 65–14) and the eccentricity of the cores (Fig. 65–15). One major difference is the organization of the LTRs, which contain an open reading frame of 1.1 Kb, coding for a 36-Kd protein. Other differences include the molecular weights of the peptides, and a Mg^{2+} preference of the reverse transcriptase (containing two subunits) compared to a Mn^{2+} preference for type C viruses.

Viral replication in lines of rat or mink cells is similar to that of type C viruses. However, the **viral yield** in cultures is markedly **increased by glucocorticoids** and, in some cells, by progesterone. A 120-base-pair sequence within the LTR is responsible for this effect. Either hormone binds to its receptor in the cytoplasm; the complex moves to the nucleus where it binds to the LTR enhancer, increasing both viral multiplication and oncogenicity. Hormonal activation of LTRs is responsible for the predominant localization of the effects of the virus to the mammary gland.

ASSAY. A slow and qualitative bioassay uses as endpoint the development of breast cancer in mice. Physical, biochemical, and serologic methods are also available.

Figure 65–13. Genome organization of HTLV-I. Underneath is the constitution of the double-spliced mRNA that expresses the *tax* gene. Solid lines, messenger sequences; dashed lines, spliced-out sequences.

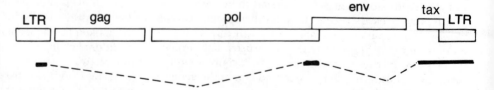

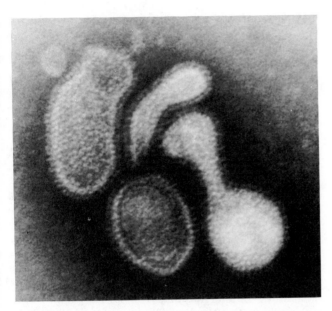

Figure 65–14. Electron micrograph of the purified mouse mammary tumor virus (MMTV) with negative staining. Note the envelope, covered by spikes, which surrounds an internal component. (Lyons MJ, Moore DH: JNCI 35:549, 1965)

PATHOGENESIS. Suckling animals infected through the milk with the C3H or the RIII virus develop **hyperplastic alveolar nodules (HANs)** and **adenocarcinomas.** The cancers induced by the RIII virus are dependent on ovarian hormones for growth, whereas those induced by the C3H viruses are independent.

The hyperplastic nodules, which are constituted of normal-looking, milk-producing mammary tissue (Fig. 65–16) containing large amounts of virus, are **preneoplastic lesions** (i.e., have a high tendency to evolve into cancer). Thus, pieces of infected mammary gland transplanted to gland-free mammary fat pads of isologous,

virgin, virus-free females undergo neoplastic transformation more frequently if they contain nodules. In the GR mouse, virus produced by spontaneous induction of the MTV-2 provirus under hormonal stimulation during pregnancy also proliferates in lactating glands, causing the formation of **plaques,** benign tumors that regress at the end of pregnancy (not to be confused with those used for virus assay in cultures; see Chap. 44). However, after several pregnancies they tend to generate pregnancy-independent carcinomas. In all cases, therefore, MMTVs induce hyperplastic lesions (nodules, plaques) whose progression to cancer requires other events.

The exogenous Bittner virus causes HANs and mammary cancers in the same way as the avian leukosis viruses: by activating cellular proto-oncogenes. In the cancers the MMTV proviruses are localized almost always near one of the oncogenes *int-1*, *int-2*, *int-3*, or *int-4*, which are normally silent, and cause their transcription. *Int-1* is normally expressed only in precursors of male germ cells and in the embryonic nervous system, but stimulates cell growth upon transfection into normal mammary cells.

HOST AND HORMONAL FACTORS IN CANCER INDUCTION. The importance of hormonal factors is evident in the pregnancy dependence of the plaques induced in GR mice by the MTV-2 virus. Moreover, with the Bittner virus the cancer incidence is low in virgin infected females but high in infected females that are force-bred (i.e., made to bear litters in quick succession without nursing them) or given estrogen. It is even more striking that when virus-infected males are castrated and are injected with estradiol and deoxycorticosterone over a long period, they frequently develop mammary cancer, whereas normal males have no mammary cancer at all. All these effects can be attributed to the hormonal activation of the LTRs, which allow extensive viral multiplication, and subsequent occasional provirus insertion near an *int* gene.

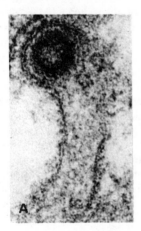
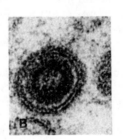
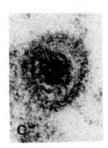

Figure 65–15. Electron micrographs of thin sections of a mammary tumor producing mouse mammary tumor virus. *(A)* Budding of the virions at the cell membrane. *(B)* Immature virion with an electron-lucent core. *(C)* Mature B-type particle with a dense, eccentric core. (Courtesy of L. Dmochowski)

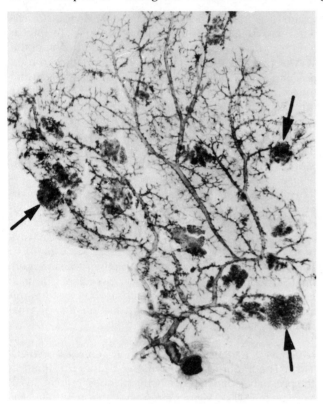

Figure 65–16. Hyperplastic alveolar nodules in the mammary gland of a multiparous C3H female mouse bearing a mammary tumor. The nodules (some indicated by *arrows*) are filled with milk. (Whole mount of gland, hematoxylin staining, original magnification ×6) (Nandi S et al: JNCI 24:883, 1960)

GENETIC FACTORS. The expression of an MMTV is strongly affected by the genetic constitution of the host, which determines the time of tumor appearance. For instance, resistance of the C57BL strain to the Bittner virus (of which they are normally free) is determined by several genes that affect viral multiplication. Moreover, the development of cancers in the presence of the virus is controlled by two additional genes. Various H2 alleles also affect the incidence of tumor formation.

RELEVANCE IN HUMAN BREAST CANCER. It is not known whether viruses similar to MMTVs are involved in the genesis of human breast cancer. Particles containing 70S RNA dimers and a reverse transcriptase have been isolated from neoplastic tissues, which sometimes contain Ags related to the viral core Ag of MMTV. Nucleic acid homology and serologic specificity show that the particles bear some relatedness to MMTV. Cell cultures from human breast cancers shed a protein immunologically related to the MMTV glycoprotein.

Oncovirus D

The retroviruses of the oncovirus D group differ from others in virion morphology, nucleic acid sequences, and antigenicity. The virions resemble those of B oncoviruses in the budding mechanism and in the preference of their reverse transcriptase for Mg^{2+}; they resemble type C virions in morphology and in the sizes of their peptides. Two **endogenous** type D viruses have been isolated from Old World monkeys, one from cells of a spectacled langur and the other from those of a squirrel monkey.

Among **exogenous** viruses, **Mason-Pfizer monkey virus (MPMV)** was isolated from a mammary carcinoma and normal tissues from rhesus monkeys. Its genome seems to have evolved from a recombinant between a murine B oncovirus and a primate C oncovirus related to the baboon endogenous virus (BaEV). The virus is propagated in rhesus or human cell lines and transforms rhesus foreskin cultures; as with MMTV, the yield is increased by dexamethasone. A syncytial plaque assay uses cells of a human glioma line transformed by RSV. In rhesus monkeys the virus is not oncogenic but induces **T-cell deficiency** resulting in a wasting disease with opportunistic infections, lymphoadenopathy, and thymic atrophy. Similar viruses have been isolated from cases of spontaneous immunodeficiency syndrome in rhesus monkeys kept in several regional primate centers in the United States (see simian HIV-related viruses, later).

Cisternavirus A

Two kinds of intracisternal A particles (IAPs) with a double shell and a clear core are observed by electron microscopy in the cisternae of the endoplasmic reticulum in rodent tissues: large ones are present in oocytes and in various kinds of tumors, especially plasmocytomas; small particles occur in the cells of early embryos. Both are noninfectious. Their genomes are present in about a thousand copies per cell in the DNA of all mouse species, in Syrian hamsters, and in rats. In the mouse they are highly heterogeneous, the largest being 7.3 Kb. The genomes, flanked by LTRs of 300 to 400 base pairs, contain the three oncovirus genes, and have considerable homology to parts of the oncovirus B and C genomes. The products are a *gag*-like protein, p73, the main component of the IAP inner shell, and a Mn^+-dependent reverse transcriptase; many stop codons prevent *env* expression. Variants of the *gag* protein are secreted by some cells as IgE-binding factors, which regulate IgE synthesis by B-lymphocytes. The viral genomes are, like transposons, mobile within the host genome, giving rise to **activation or inactivation of genes** by inserting near or within them. Insertional activation of the *c-mos* proto-oncogenes has been observed in a mouse myeloma and of the IL-3 gene (see Chap. 47) in a myelomonocytic leukemia. Insertional inactivation has been observed in an im-

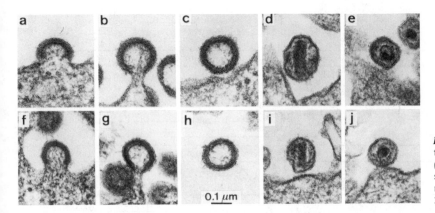

0.1 μm

Figure 65–17. Electron micrographs of thin secretions of cells in various stages of the release of HIV (***a*** to ***e***) or the Visna virus of sheep (***f*** to ***j***). Note the similar bar-shaped nucleoids in ***d*** and ***i***. (Original magnification ×100,000; Gonda M et al: Science 227:173, 1985)

munoglobulin gene. IAP genomes may represent a gene pool important for retroviral evolution.

Lentiviruses

Lentiviruses give rise to slowly developing diseases. One of them, the human immunodeficiency virus (HIV) is responsible for the human **acquired immunodeficiency syndrome (AIDS).** Other viruses cause slow diseases in animals: the **visna-maedi virus,** which causes an encephalitis (**visna**) or pneumonia (**maedi**) of sheep; the **caprine arthritis-encephalitis virus;** and the **equine infectious anemia virus.** A **feline lentivirus (FIV)** causes an immunodeficiency syndrome in cats. The diseases are characterized by a long incubation period and protracted course. The viruses cause an infection, mostly latent, of monocytes and macrophages, and from them spread to other cells.

Lentiviruses have the following distinctive characteristics: The virions have a bar-shaped rather than spherical nucleoid and contain proteins with an arrangement similar to other retroviruses, but of different sizes. The larger genome (approximately 10 Kb) contains genes not present in other retroviruses. It uses a tRNA^lys as primer for negative-strand synthesis, whereas most other infectious mammalian retroviruses use tRNA^pro. Genes *pol* and *env,* which overlap in oncoviruses, are separated in HIV by a region that includes sequences for other genes (see below). The genomes of lentiviruses have homology with each other but not with other retroviruses. The main targets of lentiviruses are mononuclear phagocytes (monocytes and tissue macrophages). Their precursor cells in the bone marrow undergo latent infection, which becomes productive when the cells reach the various tissues and mature to macrophages. Release of lymphokines may then give rise to inflammation and disease. A factor contributing to the protracted course of disease is the high mutability of the viral genome, with production of mutants capable of evading the immune response.

HUMAN IMMUNODEFICIENCY VIRUS*

Human immunodeficiency virus (HIV) occurs in many strains, some of which are given special names. HIV-1 is the collective denomination of strains isolated in Europe, America, or Central Africa; HIV-2 is a strain isolated from prostitutes in West Africa. Both cause the lethal AIDS disease, although HIV-2 tends to produce milder forms. The disease is characterized by severe **immunodepression,** with large reduction of the ratio of CD4+ to CD8+ cells, and **opportunistic infections** of various kinds: fungal (pneumonia from *Pneumocystis carinii,* oral or esophageal *candidiasis*), bacterial (salmonellosis, tuberculosis), and viral (cytomegalovirus, SV-40 like JC virus). The disease is also accompanied by secondary neoplasias, such as **Kaposi's sarcoma** and **B-cell lymphomas.** **Brain lesions** with dementia are frequently present and may be the only manifestation. The viruses can also cause less severe symptoms, of which the **lymphoadenopathy syndrome** is the most common, sometimes as a prelude to the immunodepression.

The virus was isolated by Montagnier from patients affected by the lymphoadenopathy syndrome by cultivating lectin-activated peripheral blood lymphocytes (PBLs) with IL-2. He observed expression of reverse transcriptase and production of viral particles, which, like those of other lentiviruses, have a **bar-shaped nucleoid.** Subsequently many other isolations of similar viruses followed. Like HTLV-I and -II, all strains have strong tropism for CD4+ (helper) lymphocytes.

GENETIC PROPERTIES (FIG. 65–18 A AND B). The genome of HIV (approximately 10 kb) contains nine genes, with important differences between HIV-1 and -2. Like other retroviruses both viruses contain the *gag, pol,* and *env* genes. The products of the *gag* and *pol* genes are processed by a viral protease, which is part of the *pol*

---

* The virus is also known as LAV (lymphoadenopathy virus), HTLV-III (for its tropism toward CD4+ cells), or ARV (AIDS-related virus).

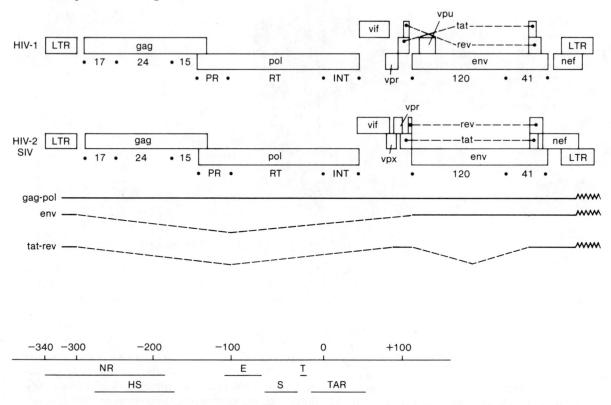

Figure 65–18. *(A)* The genomes of the HIV-1 and -2 proviruses. They differ in genes *vpu* and *vpx*, as well as in the frames of the various exons. In both viruses, genes *tat* and *rev* have two separate exons. 17, 24, 15: proteins p17, p24, p15 derived from processing of the *gag* polyprotein. PR, RT, INT: protease, reverse transcriptase, integrase, resulting from processing of the *pol* polyprotein. 120, 41; glycoproteins gp120 and gp41 derived from processing of the gp160 *env* polyprotein. Below the genomes are the main splicing patterns of the transcript, which lead to expression of *gag-pol, env,* and *tat-rev.* *(B)* The regulatory region of HIV-1. Numbers: base pairs upstream (−) or downstream (+) to the cap site (0). NR: negative regulatory region; HS: region homologous to IL-2 and IL-2 receptor genes; E: enhancer; S: SP1 binding region; T: TATA box; TAR: *tat*-responsiveness region.

polyprotein, whereas the 160-Kd product of the *env* gene is processed by a cellular protease into a gp-41 transmembrane glycoprotein and a gp-120 external protein. Both viruses have five other small genes: *tat, rev, nef, vif,* and *vpr*; in addition, HIV-1 has *vpu,* whereas HIV-2 has *vpx.* Mutations in genes *tat* and *rev* strongly inhibit viral multiplication, whereas those in *nef* enhance it. These genes specify proteins that act in *trans,* regulating the expression of other viral genes.

Gene *tat* specifies a **transactivator** that, in collaboration with a cellular protein, enhances expression of all viral genes by increasing the production of active messengers. In cooperation with cellular factors, it acts as **antiterminator,** preventing premature termination of transcription at the 59th base downstream from the cap

site, in the TAR region of the genome (see later discussion in Regulation of Provirus Transcription) where, as in other terminators, the RNA is capable of forming a hairpin loop.

The *rev* protein is required for the expression of the *gag, pol,* and *env* genes but not for *rev* and *tat.* Because all genes are transcribed in a single transcript, which is then spliced in various ways (Fig. 65–18A) the *rev* protein must affect a posttranscriptional step. In the *env* gene the protein, by binding at a site within the 3'-half of the gene, overcomes an inhibition of translation caused by the interaction of cellular regulatory factors with two other sites within the gene. The *rev* protein may also inhibit splicing of the *env* transcript, so that *tat* and *rev* messengers are produced at the expense of *env* messengers. The mode of action of *rev* on the *gag* and *pol* genes may be similar. The combination of the *tat* and *rev* proteins greatly increases viral replication by amplifying the effect resulting from transcriptional activation of the genome (see the following section, Regulation of Provirus Transcription).

The *nef* protein downregulates the transcription of the HIV genome by acting on its NR (negative regulatory) region. This protein has properties similar to those of the p21 product of the *ras* oncogene: it is myristoylated, binds GTP, is phosphorylated by protein kinase C, and has GTP-ase activity. Mutations in the gene increase the viral yield 3 to 4 times, suggesting that this gene may be involved in the regulation of the latent state. The *vif*, *vpu*, *vpr*, and *vpx* genes probably specify virion proteins that increase the efficiency of infection.

REGULATION OF PROVIRUS TRANSCRIPTION. (FIG. 65–18 B). Transcription of the HIV genome is stimulated or inhibited by the binding of suitable regulatory factors of either viral or cellular origin to the 5' LTR. Thus the inhibitory NR region responds to the *nef* protein and to a cellular protein, Ppt-1, expressed in nonactivated T cells, which also inhibits expression of the IL-2 receptor gene. Several regions (the SP1 binding sites, the enhancer, the TATA box) increase transcription in response to many cellular factors, such as NFk-B, which also acts on an immunoglobulin gene. These factors are produced in T lymphocytes activated by Ag or mitogens and act on cellular genes. In this way cell activation serves also to activate a resident latent HIV provirus. Transcription is also activated by the products of some viral genomes, such as HTLV-I and -II (gene *tax*), EBV, cytomegalovirus, herpes simplex virus type 1, and adenoviruses (gene E1A), which interact with the enhancer.

CELL INFECTION. The virus infects cells expressing at their surface the 58 Kd CD4 protein, which is the viral receptor. Among these cells are T helper lymphocytes, antigen-presenting cells, (such as macrophages, their monocyte precursors, and the dendritic cells of lymph nodes), astroglia, B-lymphocytes, especially if immortalized by EBV, colonic epithelia in culture. Any human cell transfected with the CD4 gene and expressing the protein at its surface can be infected. In contrast, mouse cells similarly transfected are not infectible, although they can produce virus if transfected with the cloned HIV provirus. Thus other molecules besides CD4 are also necessary for infection. Among animals, some primates and rabbits can be infected, offering possible models for studying the biology of the virus; it seems, however, that they do not develop the AIDS disease. Immunodeficient *scid* mice reconstituted with human hemopoietic cells are susceptible to HIV infection; they may be an important tool for research.

Important in infection are the two cleavage products of gp160, the *env* product, of which gp41 is anchored to the cell membrane, whereas gp120 is connected to gp41 by noncovalent bonds. Gp120 binds to the host CD4 protein, a step blocked by certain monoclonal Abs specific for CD4. Mutational studies show also a requirement for the extracellular N-terminus of gp41, which has a **fusogenic** property (see Chap 48, Initial Steps of Viral Infection). It is likely that the binding of gp120 to CD4 exposes the gp41 terminus, allowing its interaction with an undefined receptor at the cell surface; its penetration into the host cell membrane would cause its fusion to the viral membrane. By this mechanism the viral core would directly enter the cytoplasm of the host cell. By a similar mechanism the *env* protein present at the surface of the infected cells may cause their fusion to CD4+ uninfected cells, with formation of **syncythia** (Fig. 65–19). This phenomenon is pronounced with some cell lines, but is not of general occurrence. HIV virions have also been seen in endosomes, suggesting that the virus can also enter the cells through the endocytosis pathway (see Chap. 48, Initial Steps of Viral Infection). CD4 endocytosis may be caused by its phosphorylation, through the phosphokinase C pathway, following the attachment of HIV virions.

An important consequence of infection is the progressive disappearance of the CD4 protein from the cell surface (**CD4 downregulation**), by a posttranscriptional mechanism, with a profound impairment of the function of the cells. As with other retroviruses (see above, Classification of type C oncoviruses), the mechanism of downregulation is, at least in part, interference, because the *env* protein, by binding the CD4 protein intracellularly, prevents the expression of the latter at the cell surface. Indeed, intracellular complexes of CD4 with gp160 or gp120 can be precipitated from cell extracts by certain MoAbs to CD4. Moreover, introduction into the cells of a vaccinia virus vector that expresses only the *env* protein causes substantial downregulation of CD4. This may not be, however, the only mechanism, because a vaccinia vector expressing only the *nef* gene also causes CD4 downregulation.

The consequence of infection for cell survival may vary. T-helper lymphocytes infected in vitro may undergo a **latent infection,** with little production of viral proteins and persistence of the viral genome as an integrated provirus; but when these cells are activated by Ag or mitogen, they enter **productive infection,** with a burst of viral replication and release of infectious virus, followed by cell death. Cells of certain permanent human CD4+ cell lines (such as H9) are infected by HIV but are not killed; they are the source of the virus used for experimental work and diagnostic assays. Cells of the monocyte lineage tend to undergo a productive infection that can last for a long time, with accumulation of

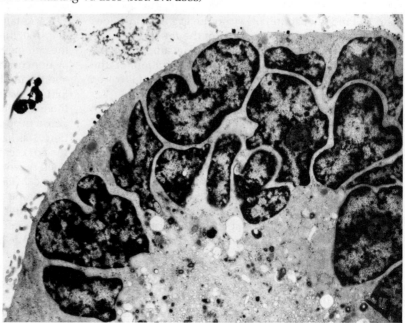

Figure 65–19. Electron micrograph of a giant multinucleated cell of a cultured T4+ lymphocyte from a culture infected with HIV (original magnification ×8000). (Klatzmann D et al: Science 225:59, 1984)

virions in intracellular vacuoles but poor extracellular release.

The death of productively infected cells is not due to the formation of syncytia, as formerly thought. A lethal factor may be the gp41 across the cell membrane, because amputation of its cytoplasmic domain can abolish cell killing, and some gp41 peptides, conjugated to a protein carrier, can slowly kill cells. Its role may be related to that of p15E in FLV infection (see previous discussion of Feline Leukemia Viruses). Another factor in cell death may be the accumulation of unintegrated viral DNA, a characteristic of lentiviruses.

HYPERVARIABILITY. A characteristic of HIV-1 and -2, as of other lentiviruses, is a very high genetic variability caused by a reverse transcriptase that causes mutations at a rate of a million-fold higher than that observed in the replication of DNA viruses. In fact, independently isolated viral strains differ from each other owing to mutations, deletions and insertions, and even in the same individual variant strains continue to appear all the time. In the *env* gene, the gp120 part has five hypervariable regions; the *gag* and *pol* genes are less variable, probably because constraints in viral assembly and enzymatic activity limit the range of acceptable mutations. A consequence of the variability is the emergence of strains with **tropism** for certain cell types. Thus, virus isolated from infected macrophages multiplies in macrophages much more readily than in T lymphocytes, and vice versa. Another consequence is the rapid emergence, often by a

single aminoacid change, of **Ab-resistant variants** during viral growth in the presence of antibodies.

IMMUNE RESPONSE. HIV-infected persons develop a humoral and a cell-mediated response to virion Ags, both internal (such as p24 or the reverse transcriptase) and external (such as gp41 and gp120).

HUMORAL RESPONSE. Seropositivity appears after HIV infection more slowly than in most other viral infections, leaving a fraction of potentially infectious individuals unrecognizable for some time by serological tests. Abs to p24 and to some gp41 epitopes are recognized first but decreased markedly as symptoms appear, whereas those to gp120 remain more constant; the neutralizing titers are relatively low. The epitopes recognized are type-specific, but each serum has a broad specificity for viral strains because it contains Abs to many different epitopes; within one individual the epitopes recognized vary with time.

CELL-MEDIATED RESPONSE. A response of T-helper lymphocytes can be recognized by growth stimulation of PBLs exposed in vitro to cells presenting viral Ags. In infected but symptom-free individuals the response is strong for p24 but weak for gp120. CTLs capable of lysing cells with HIV Ags on their surfaces are present in the peripheral blood and other body fluids. They may be restricted to either class I or class II HLA Ags. Infected macrophages present viral Ag in the context of class I Ag, but in CD4+ cells that bind gp120 to surface CD4 molecules, the complex undergoes endocytosis, and Ags are presented in association with HLA class II Ags. The peripheral blood also contains mononuclear cells with characteristics of Natural Killer cells, which are capable of lysing HIV-infected target cells; there are also lymphocytes that lyse these targets in the presence of specific Abs (ADCC).

The various forms of immune response are highest in infected symptomless individuals, but decline in strength as the disease progresses. The causes for the decline may be multiple: killing of T-helper and antigen-presenting cells by HIV infection; killing of T-helper cells by cell-mediated immunity against adsorbed or processed viral Ags; virus-induced CD4 down-regulation; reduced production of lymphokines, such as IL-2 or IFN-gamma, that are needed for the operation of some effector cells; production of suppressor factors by the infected cells; genetic variation affecting crucial viral epitopes.

PATHOGENESIS. Infection occurs by transfer of body fluids containing either free virus or infected cells. The main vectors are blood and semen, but virus is also present in tears, saliva, bronchial secretion, and milk. Entry of the virus or virus-infected cells into the body is followed by infection of antigen-presenting cells and CD4+ lymphocytes. A long latent phase follows, during which the HIV provirus is recognized in a small fraction of PBLs by DNA hybridization using viral probes, but immunocytology fails to reveal viral proteins. These appear in a small proportion of PBLs in the phase of productive infection, in CD4+ cells that are activated. Activation may be caused initially by alloantigens introduced with the infecting inoculum (blood cells, spermatozoa) and subsequently by antigens introduced by infecting agents. These activated cells transmit the infection to new susceptible cells. The infected persons remain as **asymptomatic carriers** for an undetermined period of time, some perhaps indefinitely. It seems that many, perhaps most of the infected persons will ultimately develop the disease; after a large proportion of CD4+ cells and antigen-presenting cells have disappeared or become nonfunctional, immunodepression and the AIDS disease develop, months or years following the onset of infection. Profound **perturbations of the immune system** become detectable at this stage by the study of PBLs: a decrease of CD4+ in comparison to CD8+ lymphocytes; reduced in vitro growth response to anamnestic Ags (such as tetanus toxoid, or CMV Ags), reduced response to T-cell mitogens, deficient synthesis of lyphokines important in antimicrobial defense (IL-2, IFN-gamma), reduced expression of HLA class II Ags, and decreased response to IFN-alpha connected to downregulation of

receptors, probably caused by accumulation in the serum of an unusual acid-labile IFN-alpha.

Frequently in HIV-1 infected persons, B cells, although not HIV-infected, undergo a **polyclonal activation** with release of large amounts of Abs of various isotypes into circulation. Stimulation may be provided by HIV virions or by abnormal production of lymphokines. Concurrent infections such as EBV and CMV may also contribute to the lymphoadenopathy. **Brain disease** is accompanied by the presence in the cerebrospinal fluid of virus-specific Abs as well as viral Ags, which are produced by HIV-infected macrophages and glial cells.

The origin of the **neoplasias** developing in some AIDS cases is uncertain. Changes similar to those of Kaposi's sarcoma (KS) were observed in transgenic mice expressing the HIV-1 *tat* gene. In these animals the gene is expressed in the epidermis, but the KS-like lesions are localized in the underlying subcutaneous tissue; they lack *tat* expression. The neoplastic changes may be induced by a factor produced by the *tat*-expressing epithelia. Opportunistic infections (EBV, CMV) may be involved in the origin of the lymphomas.

LABORATORY DIAGNOSIS. Infected peripheral blood cells produce viral proteins, demonstrable serologically, or an increase of reverse transcriptase, upon cocultivation with H9 or similar cells. Infection is also revealed by demonstration of viral DNA in PBLs by hybridization or by the polymerase chain reaction technique. ELISA assays are most widely used for the detection of serum Abs that bind to HIV proteins, both core (p24) or surface (gp 120, gp41), or to specific immunodominant and conserved peptides of these proteins. More sensitive is the western blot, based on the detection of electrophoretically separated viral proteins adsorbed on paper, using Abs from the patients. **Seroconversion** becomes detectable after a period of several weeks after infection, depending on the assay used.

EPIDEMIOLOGY. HIV infection has reached pandemic proportions. Virus is transmitted by infected persons, usually asymptomatic carriers who may be even more infectious than AIDS patients, in which viral multiplication is reduced by the disease of the helper and antigen-presenting cells. Transmission through the blood is observed especially among drug addicts who share syringes, in hemophiliacs who receive blood concentrates, and in individuals receiving transfusion after surgery, although the contribution of the latter class is now minimized by screening the donated blood for HIV Abs. Sexual transmission, originally observed among homosexuals, occurs also in heterosexual intercourse, in both directions. Through heterosexual contacts the disease, which was originally prevalent in men, has rapidly spread to women, closing the gap between the two sexes. The practice of rectal sex appears to be particularly responsible for heterosexual transmission. Infection is frequent among prostitutes, especially in central Africa, and in groups with pronounced sexual promiscuity. Transmission also occurs from an infected mother to her child, either transplacentally or perinatally (by contamination with mother's blood). In contrast, nonsexually related persons living together with infected persons, or providing health care to them, have a very low risk of infection, except through rare needle-stick accidents or exposure of wounds or skin abrasions to infected blood. These studies indicate that transmission through contacts not involving blood or sexual secretions is highly exceptional. Exposure to high titer virus in the laboratory may however lead to infection.

CONTROL. The best approach to control is **prevention.** Reduction of sexual promiscuity and adoption of prophylactic measures (such as the use of condoms) can reduce sexual transmission. Transmission through shared needles by drug addicts may be reduced by education. Transmission via blood or blood concentrate may be eliminated or at least markedly reduced by serologic screening of donated blood; the use of coagulation factors produced by recombinant DNA technology will eliminate this risk altogether. Transmission from mother to child can be reduced by recognizing infection and preventing or interrupting pregnancy in infected women. **Vaccination** attempts have been carried out, but the information available is still very limited. In humans a CTL response was obtained in Zaire in a group of healthy volunteers immunized with a vaccinia vector expressing the *env* protein, and later boosted with injection of *env* peptides. Chimpanzees inoculated with viral Ags have responded with Ab production and cell-mediated immune response, but the animals were not protected, because they became infected after challenge with the virus. The difficulties of vaccination are compounded by the latency of infection, viral transmission upon cell contact, and the great variability of the virus. In chimpanzees, **passive immunization** with high titer *env* Abs did not prevent infection.

Control by **chemotherapy** is of some use, because many **dideoxynucleosides** (among which is 3'-azidothymidine [AZT]; see Chap. 49) have selectivity, that is, they can block DNA synthesis through reverse transcription more effectively than regular DNA replication. These substances have other advantages: they are active orally, have moderate toxicity, and penetrate the blood-brain barrier. AZT has been shown to prolong survival of AIDS patients, but it is not suitable for long term treatment of asymptomatic carriers, owing to bone marrow suppression. **Interferon alpha** has shown some success in a fraction of cases against Kaposi sarcoma.

OTHER HIV STRAINS AND HIV-RELATED SIMIAN VIRUSES. A virus related to HIV (simian immunodeficiency virus, SIV) causes an AIDS-like disease in monkeys (SAIDS, simian AIDS). Various strains were isolated from captive rhesus monkeys (*Macaca mulatta*) in a primate research center in USA, as well as from monkeys caught in the wild; the isolates are more closely related to HIV-2 than to HIV-1. Abs to SIV are found in many monkey species, although they do not develop disease. The precise genealogical connections between human and monkey viruses are not clear.

Selected Reading

Chen ISY: Regulation of AIDS virus expression. Cell 47:1, 1986

Coffin JM: Genetic variation in AIDS viruses. Cell 46:1, 1986

Evans LH, Cloyd MW: Friend and Moloney murine leukemia viruses specifically recombine with different endogenous retroviral sequences to generate mink cell focus-forming viruses. Proc Natl Acad Sci USA 82:459, 1985

Felber BK, Paskalis H, Kleinman-Ewing C et al: The pX protein of HTLV-I is a transcriptional activator of its long terminal repeats. Science 229:675, 1985

Friend C, Pogo BG-T: The molecular pathology of Friend erythroleukemia virus strains. Biochim Biophys Acta 780:181, 1985

Gallo RC: The AIDS virus. Sci Am 256:46, 1987

Ghysdael J, Bruck C, Kettmann R, Burny A: Bovine leukemia virus. Curr Topics Microbiol Immunol 112:1, 1984

Gartner S, Markovits P, Markovitz DM et al: The role of mononuclear phagocytes in HTLV-III/LAV infection. Science 233:215, 1986

Gonda MA, Kaminchick J, Oliff A et al: Heteroduplex analysis of molecular clones of the pathogenic Friend virus complex: Friend murine leukemia virus, Friend mink cell focus-forming virus, and the polycythemia- and anemia-inducing strains of Friend spleen focus-forming virus. J Virol 51:306, 1984

Guyader M, Emerman M, Sonigo P et al: Genome organization and transactivation of the human immunodeficiency virus type 2. Nature 326:662, 1987

Hahn BH, Shaw GM, Taylor ME et al: Genetic variation in HTLV-III/LAV over time in patients with AIDS or at risk for AIDS. Science 232:1548, 1986

Haseltine WA, Sodrowski JD, Patarca R: Structure and function of the genome of HTLV. Curr Topics Microbiol Immunol 115:177, 1985

Hirsch V, Riedel N, Mullins JI: The genome organization of STLV-3 is similar to that of the AIDS virus except for a truncated transmembrane protein. Cell 49:307, 1987

Hull R, Covey SN: Genome organization and expression of reverse transcribing elements: Variations and a theme. J Gen Virol 67:1751, 1986

Ju G, Cullen R: The role of avian retroviral LTRs in the regulation of gene expression and viral replication. Adv Virus Res 30:180, 1985

Levy JA: Mysteries of HIV: Challenges for therapy and prevention. Nature (London) 333:519, 1988

Neel BG, Hayward WS, Robinson HL et al: Avian leukosis virus-induced tumors have common proviral integration sites and synthesize discrete new RNAs: Oncogenesis by promoter insertion. Cell 23:323, 1981

Panganiban AT: Retroviral DNA integration. Cell 42:5, 1985

Rabson AB, Martin MA: Molecular organization of the AIDS retrovirus. Cell 40:477, 1985

Robert-Guroff M, Markham PD, Popovic M, Gallo RC: Isolation, characterization, and biological effects of the first human retrovirus: The human T-lymphotropic retrovirus family. Curr Topics Microbiol Immunol 115:7, 1985

Rosen CA, Terwilliger E, Dayton A et al: Intragenic cis-acting *art* gene-responsive sequences of the human immunodeficiency virus. Proc Natl Acad Sci USA 85:2071, 1988

Ruscetti S, Wolff L: Spleen-focus forming virus: Relationship of an altered envelope gene to the development of a rapid erythro-leukemia. Curr Topics Microbiol Immunol 112:21, 1984

Siliciano RF, Lawton T, Knall C et al: Analysis of host-virus interactions in AIDS with anti-gp120 cell clones: effect of HIV sequence variation and a mechanism for CD4+ cell depletion. Cell 54:561, 1988

Sonigo P, Barker C, Hunter E, Wain-Hobson S: Nucleotide sequence of Mason-Pfizer monkey virus: An immunosuppressive D-type retrovirus. Cell 45:375, 1986

Stevenson M, Meier C, Mann AM et al: Envelope glycoprotein of HIV induces interference and cytolysis resistance in CD4+ cells: sistance in CD4+ cells: mechanism for persistence in AIDS. Cell

Verma IM: Retroviral vectors for gene transfer. In Microbiology—1985, pp 229–232. Washington, American Society for Microbiology, 1985

Vogel J, Hinrichs SH, Reynolds RK et al: The HIV gene *tat* induces dermal lesions resembling Kaposi's sarcoma in transgenic mice. Nature (London) 335:606, 1988

Vogt PK (ed): Leukemia virus. Curr Topics Microbiol Immunol 115, 1985

Weiss R, Teich N, Varmus H, Coffin J (eds): RNA Tumor Viruses. Cold Spring Harbor, NY, Cold Spring Harbor Laboratory, 1984

Whitlock CA, Witte ON: The complexity of virus–cell interactions in Abelson virus infection of lymphoid and other hematopoietic cells. Adv Immunol 37:74, 1985

Wong-Staal F, Gallo RC: Human T-lymphotropic retroviruses. Nature 317:395, 1985

Yamanoto N, Hinuma Y. Viral aetiology of adult T cell leukemia. J Gen Virol 66:1641, 1985

Index

Numbers in **boldface** indicate a figure; t following a page number indicates tabular material; n following a page number indicates a footnote.

ISBN 0-397-50689-9

90000